Study Guide for

Essentials for Nursing Practice

Eighth edition

Patricia A. Castaldi, DNP, RN, ANEF
Director
Practical Nursing & Allied Health Programs
Union County College
Plainfield, New Jersey

ELSEVIER

ELSEVIER
MOSBY

3251 Riverport Lane
St. Louis, Missouri 63043

STUDY GUIDE FOR
ESSENTIALS FOR NURSING PRACTICE, EIGHTH EDITION

ISBN: 978-0-323-18778-7

Notices

Knowledge and best practice in this field are constantly changing. As new research and experience broaden our understanding, changes in research methods, professional practices, or medical treatment may become necessary.

Practitioners and researchers must always rely on their own experience and knowledge in evaluating and using any information, methods, compounds, or experiments described herein. In using such information or methods they should be mindful of their own safety and the safety of others, including parties for whom they have a professional responsibility.

With respect to any drug or pharmaceutical products identified, readers are advised to check the most current information provided (i) on procedures featured or (ii) by the manufacturer of each product to be administered, to verify the recommended dose or formula, the method and duration of administration, and contraindications. It is the responsibility of practitioners, relying on their own experience and knowledge of their patients, to make diagnoses, to determine dosages and the best treatment for each individual patient, and to take all appropriate safety precautions.

To the fullest extent of the law, neither the Publisher nor the authors, contributors, or editors, assume any liability for any injury and/or damage to persons or property as a matter of products liability, negligence or otherwise, or from any use or operation of any methods, products, instructions, or ideas contained in the material herein.

Executive Content Strategist: Tamara Myers
Senior Content Development Specialist: Tina Kaemmerer
Book Production Team Leader: Deepthi Unni
Senior Project Manager: Divya Krish
Cover Designer: Gopalakrishnan Venkatram

Printed in the United States

Last digit is the print number: 9 8 7 6 5 4 3 2 1

To John and Dan for all of your love and support.
To the faculty, students, and all of my colleagues who have inspired me throughout the years.

Patricia A. Castaldi

Introduction and Preface

This guide is designed to correspond, chapter by chapter, to *Essentials for Nursing Practice* (eighth edition). Each chapter in this guide contains study aids to assist in learning and applying the theoretical concepts from the text.

The comprehensive chapter review sections allow you the opportunity to evaluate your own level of comprehension after reading the text. Use of the study group questions with fellow students may help in your overall understanding of the nursing content as well as provide a way to further evaluate your familiarity with that content. There are also short-answer, priority order, and multiple-response questions to promote your preparation for classroom examinations and the alternate-format items on the NCLEX® examination. You may find that there are questions that require you to apply information from other chapters or use other reference sources to answer them.

General study tips to use while reading, taking classroom notes, and preparing for and taking examinations are also included in this guide. Other students have found these ideas to be helpful in their nursing course experiences.

Answers for all of the questions and activities can be found at the end of the study guide.

STUDY CHARTS

While reading through the chapters in the text, you may create study charts to assist you to organize the material that is covered. The charts allow for a comparison of key concepts in the chapter. Suggestions for creating charts are provided in the chapters of this text. An example follows.

Routes of Injection

The learning activities presented in this study guide should assist in your review of the text material and your application of the nursing concepts to classroom and clinical experiences.

Route	**Angle of Insertion/Needle Size/Maximum Amount of Medication**
Intradermal	
Subcutaneous	
Intramuscular	

General Study Tips

While Reading

- Read before the scheduled class: Highlight key points or outline content in the text that will be covered in the classroom. Don't highlight everything! Clarify with your instructor(s) what the expected readings are for your class. Tables and boxes in the text can help to summarize critical information.
- Look up definitions: Find the meanings of words you do not recognize while you are going through the text. It helps to have a medical dictionary and a regular dictionary handy!
- Make notes: Write down a list of topics that you do not understand while you are reading so that you may clarify them with the instructor.
- Compare notes: Use notes taken from the book and in class to create a complete picture of the content.
- Use study/comparison charts: Put facts and ideas in an organized form so that you can refer to them easily at a later point, such as when studying for an examination.
- Use references: Go back to texts and notes used in other courses (such as anatomy and physiology) to help in understanding new material.

In the Classroom

- Make notes: Do not try to write everything down. Note the essential information from the class. Use the margins of notebook paper or type in your mobile device any questions that you may have as you go along so that you remember to ask them at some point. Before the end of the class, note any areas that you need to clarify with the instructor.
- Ask questions: Remember to take advantage of the expertise of the instructor. Do not go away from the class without trying to clear up areas of confusion!
- Digital recordings/audiotape: Make recordings of classroom discussions, *only with instructor permission*, if
  1. There is time to listen to them at some point (such as in the car).
  2. There are positive results from this process, with better understanding of the material and improved examination grades.

On Your Own

- Use available resources: Take advantage of all of the resources at the school, such as the library, computer laboratory, and skill laboratory. Make time to practice nursing techniques, watch DVDs or videos, and complete computer learning programs.
- Join/create a study group: Get together with other students in your class to review material. Study groups offer an opportunity to share information, challenge one another, and provide mutual support.
- Use time management techniques: Use available time as efficiently as possible. For example, the time that is spent waiting for an appointment or riding on public transportation may be used to read over materials or complete assignments.

Before an Examination

- Try to remain calm: Easy to recommend, but hard to do! Learn and use relaxation skills. Do not jump immediately into the examination. Relax and get focused first, and then start the test.
- Be prepared: Check with the instructor to be sure you have covered the content that will be on the examination. Bring the right materials: pencils, pens, erasers, computer passwords, and so on. Leave enough time to get to the examination area to avoid last-minute "rushing in."

During the Examination

- Read the questions carefully: Determine what the question is asking. Stay focused on the actual question without reading into the situations. If allowed to mark on the examination paper, underline key words or cross out unnecessary information to assist in getting to the heart of the question.
- Do not keep changing your answers: Most of the time, the first answer selected is correct. Do not change an answer unless you have remembered the correct response.
- Stay focused: Take brief moments during the examination, if necessary, to stop and use relaxation techniques to compose yourself.
- For multiple response ("Select all that apply"), approach each answer as being true or false in relation to the question.
- When doing math of pharmacology, think about the answer that you obtain to see if it makes sense. How often would you give 10 tablets or 10 mL IM? If the answer does not seem realistic, recalculate!

General Suggestions for Classroom-Based and Online Courses

- Review the syllabus in advance to identify the course requirements and expectations.
- Make a calendar to keep track of dates for examinations, quizzes, and assignments.
- Schedule time to study or complete assignments, especially if you are working.
- Connect with other students in the course electronically, by telephone, or in person.

- Take advantage of all of the available resources, such as online or on-campus tutorial programs.
- If your study habits are leading to positive results in the class, then don't make major changes. If, however, you are finding that you are not passing or just getting by in the course, you should talk with an instructor about how to change your approach to be more successful. Don't wait until it is too late to make a difference in your grade!
- Keep in contact with the instructor! Do not forget to ask questions.
- Maintain professional behavior with your instructors and classmates.

Contents

1 The Nursing Profession

CASE STUDY

1. Mr. R., 24 years old, decides that he would like to become a nurse researcher.
   a. What formal education does Mr. R. need to reach this career goal?
   b. To maintain or enhance this role, what other education may be needed?

CHAPTER REVIEW

Match the description/definition in Column A with the correct term in Column B.

	Column A	*Column B*
_____	1. Demonstrate self-care activities.	a. Communicator
_____	2. Act on behalf of the patient's interests.	b. Manager
_____	3. Provide emotional support.	c. Educator
_____	4. Coordinate members of the staff.	d. Advocate

Complete the following:

5. Identify the main purpose of the following nursing organizations:
   a. National League for Nursing (NLN)
   b. American Nurses Association (ANA)
   c. International Council of Nurses (ICN)

6. Identify four career paths that you can choose as a nurse.

7. Nurses and their professional organizations have lobbied on behalf of:

8. The three components of nursing care are:

9. Select all of the accurate statements regarding Nurse Practice Acts in the United States.
   a. Regulate the scope of practice _____
   b. Determine ethical guidelines _____
   c. Use standards from the ANA _____
   d. Vary greatly from state to state _____
   e. Originate from federal legislation _____

10. Identify four core roles for the advanced practice nurse (APRN).

11. Provide at least three examples of essential skills for nurses.

12. To become a nurse educator or advanced practice nurse, an individual needs what minimum level of formal education?

13. What is the difference between continuing and in-service education?

Match the description/definition in Column A with the correct person in Column B.

	Column A	Column B
_____	14. Founder of the American Red Cross	a. Lillian Wald
_____	15. Began the Henry Street Settlement	b. Dorothea Dix
_____	16. First professor of nursing at Columbia University	c. Harriet Tubman
_____	17. Superintendent of the female nurses in the Union army	d. Mary Adelaide Nutting
_____	18. Active in the Underground Railroad movement	e. Mary Mahoney
_____	19. Founder of the Nurses' Associated Alumnae of the US and Canada	f. Clara Barton
_____	20. First professionally educated African-American nurse	g. Isabel Hampton Robb

21. Identify at least three external influences on the practice of nursing today.

22. Provide examples of workplace hazards that are faced by nurses.

23. Nurses recognize that the use of genomics in health care allows providers to:

24. Select all of the examples of the QSEN competency for patient-centered care:
    a. Determining the patient's meal preferences _____
    b. Using a flow chart for the nursing care plan _____
    c. Identifying the cultural needs of the patient _____
    d. Documenting on the patient's electronic health record _____
    e. Resolving a staff conflict over vacation time _____
    f. Implementing a patient fall protocol _____

25. The ANA Standards of Professional Performance include which of the following areas? Select all that apply.
    a. Consultation _____
    b. Education _____
    c. Prescriptive authority _____
    d. Quality of practice _____
    e. Ethics _____
    f. Assessment _____
    g. Leadership _____

Select the best answer for each of the following questions:

26. The nurse is aware that a characteristic of today's health care system is:
    1. costs are decreasing.
    2. more services are hospital based.
    3. there are less underserved individuals.
    4. the population aged 65 and older is increasing.

27. An inaccurate statement regarding nursing and health care is:
    1. the majority of the public rank nurses highest among professionals for honesty.
    2. acting in a professional manner influences consumer perceptions of health care providers.
    3. public policy can be influenced by nursing involvement.
    4. there is less public access to health care information.

28. The nurse, in considering the difference between autonomy and accountability, recognizes that autonomy is:
    1. initiating nursing interventions that do not require medical orders.
    2. the legal responsibility for nursing interventions.
    3. incorporating values into practice.
    4. generating knowledge to support practice.

STUDY GROUP QUESTIONS

- How did the profession of nursing develop? Who were some of the founders of the profession?
- What are some of the major influences on nursing today?
- What is professionalism in relation to nursing? What are the characteristics of professional practice?
- How are the standards for nursing practice developed? What are the legal and ethical aspects of practice?
- What are the varied responsibilities and roles of nurses?
- How can individuals prepare to be nurses? What career opportunities are available?
- What professional nursing organizations exist and what are their goals/purposes?
- What are the current trends in nursing?

STUDY CHART

Create a study chart to compare the *different levels of nursing education* and the career roles that may be attained at each level.

2 Health and Wellness

CASE STUDIES

1. A personal friend has been experiencing severe stomach and intestinal distress for a few months. She is 35 years old and is employed as an advertisement salesperson for a local newspaper. During the past year, she has been pressured to create more income for her department. When you ask her if she has sought medical treatment, she responds, "I don't have the time to go to the doctor." In addition to her job responsibilities, she is a single parent of a grade school child who enjoys several after-school activities.
   a. What physical and lifestyle factors are present in this situation?
   b. What initial responses/interventions may be helpful for this individual?

2. Mr. G., 44 years old, has recently been diagnosed with diabetes mellitus. He requires a change in his diet and activity, and he will need to take insulin.
   a. Identify factors that could influence his coping with or managing of the disease.
   b. What illness behaviors could Mr. G. possibly demonstrate?
   c. What impact can this illness have on Mr. G.'s wife?
   d. How can the QSEN competency of safety be applied?

CHAPTER REVIEW

Match the description/definition in Column A with the correct term in Column B.

	Column A	Column B
_____	1. A person's definition and interpretation of symptoms and use of the health care system	a. Health belief model
_____	2. A belief that patients have the authority to be active participants in determining their health and well-being	b. Internal variables
_____	3. Longer than 6 months' duration	c. Body image
_____	4. A subjective concept of physical appearance	d. Holistic health
_____	5. Developmental stage, intellectual background, emotional and spiritual factors	e. Illness behavior
_____	6. Short term and severe	f. Acute illness
_____	7. Addresses the relationship between a person's beliefs and behaviors	g. Chronic illness

Complete the following:

8. Health is the absence of disease.
   True _____ False _____

9. Identify at least one health promotion concern for older adults.

10. Identify Maslow's hierarchy of needs on the pyramid:

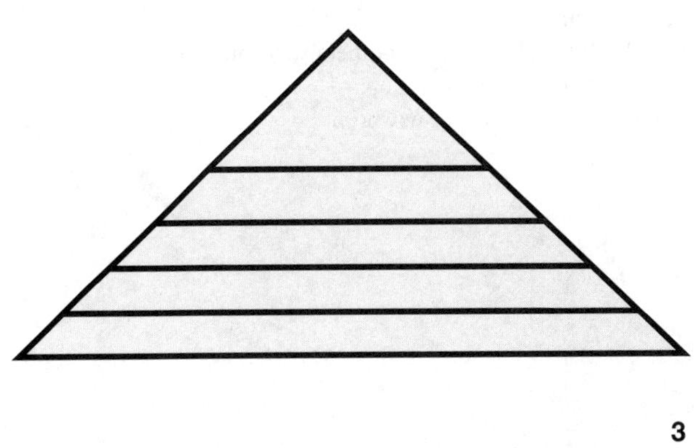

11. Identify whether the following are internal or external variables that influence health beliefs and practices.
    a. Financial status

    b. Family health behaviors

    c. Cognitive abilities

    d. Cultural values

12. What is an example of a positive health behavior?

13. What is an example of a negative health behavior?

14. What are two goals of *Healthy People 2020*?

15. Identify all of the external variables that may influence a person's illness behaviors. Select all that apply.
    a. Visibility of symptoms _____

    b. Disruption of normal routine _____

    c. Accessibility of the health care system _____

    d. Acuity of the illness _____

    e. Cultural background _____

    f. Economics _____

Select the best answer for each of the following questions:

16. At the tertiary level of prevention, a nurse would prepare an educational program for a group requiring:
    1. chemotherapy.
    2. cardiac rehabilitation.
    3. genetic screening.
    4. sex education.

17. At the secondary level of prevention, what is the intervention with which a nurse expects to assist or provide instruction?
    1. Immunization
    2. Referral to outpatient therapy for monitoring
    3. Performance of a biopsy
    4. Parent bathing a newborn

18. A nurse is working with a patient who is experiencing chronic joint pain. To assist the patient to manage or reduce the pain, the nurse decides to use a holistic health approach. With this in mind, the nurse specifically elects to include:
    1. aroma therapy.
    2. wound care.
    3. hygienic care measures.
    4. analgesic medications.

19. A nurse is completing an assessment for a patient who has gone to a medical clinic. Variables that influence the patient's health beliefs and practices are being determined. The nurse is aware that an internal variable for this patient is the:
    1. way in which the patient celebrates family occasions.
    2. manner in which the patient deals with stress on the job and at home.
    3. frequency of the family's visit to the health care agency.
    4. amount of insurance coverage that is provided by the patient's employer.

20. A nurse recognizes that primary prevention is a critical aspect in health care. The target group for a program on hand hygiene for this level of prevention is:
    1. fourth grade children at the elementary school.
    2. patients in a cardiac rehabilitation program at the medical center.
    3. parents of a child with a congenital heart defect.
    4. patients with diabetes at the outpatient clinic.

21. A nurse is leading a group of community members who are trying to quit smoking. In the precontemplation phase of health behavior change, the nurse anticipates that the group members will respond by:
    1. discussing previous attempts at quitting.
    2. recognizing the benefits of not smoking.
    3. expressing irritation when the topic of quitting is introduced.
    4. requesting phone numbers of support people who have participated in the group.

22. A young adult student has gone to the university's health center for a physical examination. The nurse conducting the initial interview is looking for possible lifestyle risk factors. The nurse is specifically alerted to the student's:
    1. mild hypertension.
    2. mountain climbing hobby.
    3. family history of diabetes.
    4. part-time job at the auto factory.

23. According to Maslow's hierarchy of needs, a patient's priority should be:
    1. physical safety.
    2. psychological safety.
    3. self-esteem.
    4. adequate nutrition.

24. To determine a patient's stage in the process of changing behaviors in reponse to being diagnosed with diabetes, a nurse can conclude that the patient is in the maintenance stage on the basis of what response?
    1. "I don't believe I need injections because I feel okay."
    2. "I may need to adjust my diet a little."
    3. "I take my insulin daily as ordered."
    4. "I have been trying to learn the diet plan."

25. A nurse recognizes an environmental risk for illness upon learning that the patient:
    1. works in a chemical plant.
    2. has a history of heart disease.
    3. admits to intermittent substance abuse.
    4. is older than 65 years of age.

STUDY GROUP QUESTIONS

- What are the different health models and how can they be applied to different patient situations? What are the advantages and disadvantages of each model?
- What are the different internal and external variables that are present in health practices and illness behavior? Give specific examples of the different variables and possible nursing interventions.
- What behaviors may be observed in a patient during illness? What impact may the patient's illness have on the family and significant others?
- How do the levels of prevention relate to the nursing care of patients in different health care settings?

STUDY CHART

Create a study chart to compare the *Levels of Prevention* that identifies patient and nursing activities associated with each level.

3 The Health Care Delivery System

CASE STUDIES

1. An 80-year-old female patient has just been diagnosed with an inoperable cancerous growth in the brain. After being told of the poor prognosis, she opts to refuse chemotherapy.
   a. Where could this individual be referred for terminal care?

2. You are working as a unit manager on a busy medical unit in a hospital.
   a. What are some considerations that are involved in the management of care?
   b. How will you use the QSEN competency of teamwork and collaboration in the management of the unit?

CHAPTER REVIEW

Match the description/definition in Column A with the correct term in Column B.

Column A

_____ 1. Nationwide health insurance program that provides benefits to individuals older than 65 years of age

_____ 2. Integration of best knowledge, clinical expertise, and patient values

_____ 3. Fixed amount of payment for services per enrollee

_____ 4. Short-term relief for persons providing care to ill, disabled

_____ 5. Income eligibility for coverage below the federal poverty level

_____ 6. Patient responses directly related to nursing care

_____ 7. Administrative control over primary health care services practice for a defined patient population

_____ 8. Worldwide in scope

_____ 9. A set of providers and services organized to deliver a coordinated continuum of care to the population of patients in a specific market

_____ 10. A program to recognize health care organizations that achieve excellence in nursing practice

Column B

a. Medicaid
b. Capitation
c. Globalization
d. Managed care
e. Magnet status
f. Medicare
g. Respite care
h. Integrated delivery networks (IDNs)
i. Nursing-sensitive outcomes
j. Evidence-based

Complete the following:

11. A(n) ________________________ is a system of family-centered care designed to allow patients to live with dignity while dealing with a terminal illness.

12. In an acute care setting, when does discharge planning begin?

13. Technology influences health care delivery by:

14. The main purpose of a utilization review is to:

5 Legal Principles in Nursing

CASE STUDIES

1. In preparation for surgery, you are to have the patient sign the consent form for the procedure. During discussions about postoperative care, the patient does not appear to fully understand what will be done during the surgery.
   a. What are your responsibilities in this situation?

2. You are reviewing the doctor's orders for the medications to be given to the patient. One of the medication orders is very difficult to read. The nurse in charge tells you that she is sure it is Lasix 40 mg PO.
   a. What should you do in this circumstance?
   b. What legal implications may be involved if the order is incorrect?

3. A child arrives in the emergency department in critical condition. His parents are divorced.
   a. What issues concerning consent for treatment may be involved in this child's case?

4. You have been observing a nursing colleague on your unit, and she appears to be taking narcotics from the medication cart. There have been occasions where her behavior has been erratic.
   a. What, if any, are your legal responsibilities regarding this colleague's behavior?

5. You are looking at a popular social media site and notice that a staff member has posted photos of a patient without permission.
   a. What should you do?
   b. What are the possible consequences of the staff nurse's posting?

CHAPTER REVIEW

Match the descriptions/definitions in Column A with the correct term in Column B.

	Column A	*Column B*
_____	1. Completed when anything unusual happens that could potentially cause harm to a patient, visitor, or employee	a. Tort
_____	2. Any willful attempt or threat to harm another person	b. Negligence
_____	3. A civil wrong or injury for which remedy is in the form of money damages	c. Living wills
_____	4. A crime of a serious nature that usually carries a penalty of imprisonment	d. Statutory law
_____	5. Limitation of liability for health care professionals offering assistance at the scene of an accident	e. Good Samaritan law
_____	6. Conduct that falls below the standard of care	f. Assault
_____	7. Any intentional touching of another person's body without consent	g. Common law
_____	8. A form of contemporary law created by elected legislative bodies	h. Battery
_____	9. Documents instructing physicians to withhold or withdraw life-sustaining procedures	i. Incident report
_____	10. A form of contemporary law created by judicial decisions in court when cases are decided	j. Felony

Complete the following:

11. The best way for a nurse to avoid being liable for negligence is to:

12. Two areas in which standards of care are defined are:

13. a. Informed consent requires that the patient:

    b. For informed consent, the nurse's role is to:

14. A 9-year-old boy arrives at the hospital after a fall from a tree. He will need emergency surgery. The 25-year-old brother who has brought him to the hospital may give legal consent.
    True _____ False _____

15. Professional negligence is termed:

16. Select all of the following correct statements regarding the Good Samaritan Law (1998):
    a. Health care providers are not liable for care provided during an emergency, even if they are not trained in the care they offer. _____
    b. In an emergency, nurses may treat minors without a parent's consent. ______
    c. Health care providers must follow through on care that is provided in an emergency, transferring the victim to EMTs or other emergency personnel. _____

17. A verbal or telephone order from a physician usually must be signed within ______ hours.

18. The two standards for determination of death are:

19. A "Do not resuscitate" (DNR) order may be given verbally by a physician.
    True _____ False _____

20. The elements of malpractice are:
    a. ____
    b. ____
    c. ____
    d. ____

21. The coroner is notified if the patient's death is:

22. Which of the following constitute a felony related to the Nurse Practice Act? Select all that apply.
    a. Giving the wrong medication to a patient _____
    b. Practicing without a license ______
    c. Misuse of controlled substances ______
    d. Not instituting safety protocols ______
    e. Sharing the patient's information with a co-worker ______

23. Advance directives act to:

24. Health care workers are required to report what incidents?

25. Provide an example of a preventable error.

26. A statute that encourages a health care provider to disclose patient care errors without admitting liability is called an:

27. Malpractice insurance carriers are required by law to report insurance settlements and verdicts to the:

28. Which of the following are examples of "never events"? Select all that apply.
    a. Patient falls _____
    b. Urinary tract infections ______
    c. Lost patient articles ______
    d. Omission of a drug dosage ______
    e. Intermittent catheterizations ______
    f. Pressure ulcers ______

29. Regulations specify that the use of physical or chemical restraint requires:

30. The Patient Self-Determination Act (1991) requires that health care institutions:

31. Place the following individuals in the order in which they will be approached for consent for organ donation:
    a. Guardian ______
    b. Adult son/daughter ______
    c. Spouse ______
    d. Parent ______
    e. Adult brother/sister ______
    f. Grandparent ______

6 Ethics

CASE STUDIES

1. You are the home care nurse for a 42-year-old male patient who has severe multiple sclerosis. He tells you on several occasions that he is tired of living this way, of not being able to do anything for himself. He says that he has read about individuals who have been "helped to die," and he asks if you can assist him in finding out more about this procedure.
   a. Apply the steps for processing an ethical dilemma to this situation.
   b. What is the role of the nurse in this situation?

2. The son of one of your patients asks you if he can look at his mother's medical record. He insists that he needs to know what is happening so that he and his sister can plan for the mother's care.
   a. What should you do in this circumstance?

CHAPTER REVIEW

Match the description/definition in Column A with the correct term in Column B.

	Column A	*Column B*
_____	1. Supporting the patient's right to informed consent	a. Ethics
_____	2. Considering the patient's best interest	b. Fidelity
_____	3. Avoiding deliberate harm	c. Justice
_____	4. Keeping promises	d. Morals
_____	5. Determining the order in which patients should be treated	e. Bioethics
_____	6. Consideration of standards of conduct	f. Autonomy
_____	7. Ethics within the field of health care	g. Beneficence
_____	8. Judgment about behavior	h. Nonmaleficence
_____	9. Personal beliefs about the worth of an idea	i. Values or object

Complete the following:

10. According to the Health Insurance Portability and Accountability Act of 1996 (HIPAA), access to a patient's medical record by a family member requires:

11. Identify an end-of-life issue that has ethical implications for nurses.

12. Identify the ethical theory for each of the following descriptions:
    a. Proposes that actions are right or wrong based on the essence of right and wrong in the principles of fidelity, truthfulness, and justice
    b. Discusses how ethical decisions affect women
    c. Proposes that the value of something is based on its usefulness

13. For the following areas, provide a specific example of how ethical concerns may be involved:
    a. Cost containment
    b. Cultural sensitivity

14. In applying the QSEN competency of informatics, explain how the digital transmission of patient information can be an ethical concern.

Select the best answer for each of the following questions:

15. A professional code of ethics includes:
    1. legal standards for practice.
    2. extensive details on moral principles.
    3. guidelines for approaching common ethical dilemmas.
    4. a collective statement of group expectations for behavior.

16. By administering medication to a patient on a unit in an extended care facility, a nurse is applying the ethical principle of:
    1. justice.
    2. fidelity.
    3. autonomy.
    4. beneficence.

17. A nurse has been working with a patient who had abdominal surgery. The patient is experiencing discomfort and has been calling for assistance often. The ethical principle of fidelity is demonstrated when the nurse:
    1. changes the dressing.
    2. provides a warm lotion back rub.
    3. informs the patient of the actions of the medications administered.
    4. returns to assist the patient with breathing exercises at the agreed-upon times.

18. A student nurse is assigned to work with parents who refuse to have essential medical treatment provided to their child. The medical center is pursuing a court order to force the family to accept the treatment plan that will assist the child. The nurse has strong feelings for the family's position, as well as the importance of the medical treatment. The first step for the nurse to take in attempting to resolve this ethical dilemma is to:
    1. examine personal values.
    2. evaluate the outcomes.
    3. gather all of the facts.
    4. verbalize the problem.

19. An example of advocacy in nursing practice is:
    1. documenting care provided to a patient.
    2. giving medication to a patient.
    3. assessing the patient's comfort level after surgery.
    4. contacting the physician to discuss the patient's response to the plan of care.

20. The last phase in the processing of an ethical dilemma is to:
    1. evaluate the action taken.
    2. consider treatment options.
    3. negotiate the options and outcomes.
    4. identify the problem.

21. Which one of the following situations represents an ethical rather than a legal consideration?
    1. Administering medications
    2. Providing care to someone without health insurance
    3. Sharing patient information with another health care worker
    4. Reporting a communicable disease to the public health officer

STUDY GROUP QUESTIONS

- What are ethics and what is the purpose of a code of ethics in a profession?
- What principles are promoted in a profession?
- How can a nurse be a patient advocate?
- What are the basic standards of ethics?
- What are values and how are they developed?
- How do values relate to ethics?
- How does a professional determine that an ethical dilemma exists?
- What are the steps for processing an ethical dilemma?
- What ethical dilemmas may arise in health care and nursing practice?

STUDY CHART

Create a study chart to identify and compare *Responsibility, Accountability, Confidentiality, Competence, Judgment, and Advocacy,* and provide examples of nursing behaviors for each.

7 Evidence-Based Practice

CASE STUDIES

1. You are working in a home care agency. One of your assigned patients is having difficulty with managing his daily insulin intake. You discover that he is having difficulty in getting an accurate blood glucose reading with his monitor. Because of the problem, the patient is self-administering too much or too little insulin. You remember that some of the other home care patients are also having some trouble with this particular glucose monitor.
   a. Use the PICO format to develop a possible question.
   b. What type of trigger is present in this scenario?

2. As a nurse for a surgical unit in a local medical center, you will be involved in identifying some quality improvement (QI) projects for your unit.
   a. What possible areas may be important for you, your fellow staff members, and the patients on your unit?

CHAPTER REVIEW

Match the description/definition in Column A with the correct term in Column B.

	Column A	*Column B*
_____	1. Characteristics, or traits, that vary among subjects	a. Pilot
_____	2. Prediction made about the relationship between study variables	b. Abstract
_____	3. To trial a new practice	c. Variable
_____	4. Brief summary of an article that quickly tells you if the article is research or clinically based	d. Hypothesis

Complete the following:

5. Evidence-based practice is:

6. Identify three valuable sources of non–research-based evidence.

7. A peer-reviewed article is:

8. A qualitative research study focuses on:

9. Provide an example of how a nurse integrates evidence into practice.

10. In the Quality Improvement model, what does PDSA stand for?
    P -
    D -
    S -
    A -

11. Provide an example of a patient outcome and measurement.

12. A randomized control trial (RCT) includes which of the following? Select all that apply.
    a. Subjects _____
    b. Experimental therapies _____
    c. A control group _____
    d. Subjective input from the researcher _____
    e. Analysis of the results _____

13. An evidence-based article includes which of the following? Select all that apply.
    a. An abstract _____
    b. The author's biography _____
    c. A literature review _____
    d. The study's design and methods _____
    e. The author's opinions about the subjects _____
    f. A conclusion relevant to the findings _____

14. Identify three of the competencies for evidence-based practice.

15. Sources for new scientific information are:

16. In a research study, the statistical analysis indicated a "p value" of 0.02. This is understood as being a good result. True _____ False _____

17. Two examples of comprehensive databases are:

18. Identify how evidence-based practice change can be communicated to others.

19. Root cause analysis is:

20. For the following study, identify each of the PICOT components:

    Over a 4-month period, the nursing staff on the unit is going to observe whether wound healing of pressure ulcers is improved if they are left open to air for 2 hours each day, rather than covered for 24 hours.

    P -
    I -
    C -
    O -
    T -

Select the best answer for each of the following questions:

21. A nurse recognizes which of the following as a sentinel event?
    1. An error is made and a medication dose is skipped.
    2. A wound infection is noted on a patient who has transferred from a nursing home.
    3. A patient dies within 48 hours of admission to the medical center.
    4. A hip replacement is performed on the wrong leg.

22. Which of the following is the best description of a case control study?
    1. A comparison of one group of subjects to another
    2. A focus on a subgroup with a known condition
    3. A prediction or explanation of phenomena
    4. A description of the responses to an independent variable

STUDY GROUP QUESTIONS

- What is evidence-based practice?
- How does a nurse become involved in the research process?
- What is PICO(T)?
- Where can reliable research-based data be found?
- What databases represent the scientific knowledge of health care?
- What types of evidence or studies are available for reference?
- How are evidence-based findings used in nursing practice?
- How are evidence-based changes communicated and evaluated?
- What is the relationship between evidence-based practice and quality improvement?

8 Critical Thinking

CASE STUDIES

1. You receive reports on your patient assignment for the day. You have six patients who require assessment and have orders for treatments and medications.
   a. How can you use critical thinking to approach this multiple patient assignment?

2. As a home care nurse, you have been assigned to visit a patient who requires dressing changes for a foot ulceration. When you arrive in the home, you see that the patient does not have any commercially packaged dressings or saline solution. You have used the last of your supplies and the drive to the office will take more than 1 hour. The dressing that the patient has on her foot is saturated with purulent drainage.
   a. What options are available to you in this situation?
   b. What further investigation about the patient and her living situation may be necessary?

3. A patient who has just been diagnosed with heart disease is being discharged to his home. He will be on a low-sodium and low-cholesterol diet.
   a. Using critical thinking skills, what areas will you focus on for this patient and his new diet?

CHAPTER REVIEW

Match the description/definition in Column A with the correct term in Column B.

	Column A	*Column B*
_____	1. Process of recalling an event to determine its meaning and purpose	a. Scientific method
_____	2. Series of clinical judgments that result in informal or formal diagnoses	b. Decision making
_____	3. End point of critical thinking that leads to problem resolution	c. Intuition
_____	4. Inner sensing that something is so	d. Diagnostic reasoning
_____	5. Process that moves from observable facts from an experience to a reasonable explanation of those facts	e. Reflection

Complete the following:

6. Identify one example of how critical thinking is used in each of the following steps of the nursing process:
   a. Assessment
   b. Nursing diagnosis
   c. Planning
   d. Implementation
   e. Evaluation

7. Identify the level of critical thinking demonstrated by each of the following:
   a. Trusting experts to have the right answers for every problem
   b. Analyzing and examining problems more independently
   c. Making choices without assistance and accepting accountability

8. Identify the elements of the critical thinking model.

9. Identify the attitude of critical thinking demonstrated for each of the following:
   a. Performing a skill safely and effectively
   b. Questioning an order that appears incorrect
   c. Performing a systematic and thorough pain assessment
   d. Developing a unique way to teach the patient how to change a dressing
   e. Admitting to the nurse manager that a medication was given in error

10. Provide an example of how the nurse can use each of the following critical thinking skills:
   a. Reflection
   b. Language
   c. Learning

11. What are two useful tools for developing critical thinking skills?

12. Which of the following statements are accurate regarding critical thinking attitudes? Select all that apply.
   a. Risk-taking is not desirable in patient care. _____
   b. Using disciplined thinking reduces creativity. _____
   c. Perseverance can indicate that one is always looking for available resources. _____
   d. Personal feelings should not be allowed to influence delivery of care. _____
   e. All sides of each situation should be considered. _____
   f. Intuition should be used as a primary tool in determining patient care. _____

Select the best answer for each of the following questions:

13. In employing critical thinking, the first step that the nurse should use is:
   1. evaluation.
   2. decision making.
   3. self-regulation.
   4. interpretation.

14. Having worked for a number of years in the acute care environment, a nurse achieved the ability to use a complex level of critical thinking. The nurse:
   1. acts solely on his or her own opinions.
   2. trusts the experts to have the answers to problems.
   3. implements creative and innovative options.
   4. applies rules and principles the same way in every situation.

15. Clinical care experiences have recently begun for a student nurse. When beginning to work with patients, the student nurse implements critical thinking in practice by:
   1. asking for assistance if uncertain.
   2. sharing personal ideas with peers.
   3. acting on independent judgments.
   4. relying on standardized, textbook approaches.

16. A nurse has an extremely large patient assignment this evening and begins to feel overwhelmed. Of the following, what is the nurse's priority activity?
   1. Sharing his or her feelings with colleagues
   2. Calling the supervisor and asking for assistance
   3. Reviewing the overall assignment to get his or her bearings
   4. Moving immediately to provide patient care, starting with the room closest to the nurse's station

17. Orientation for new nurses begins. The instructor assembled information on critical thinking and nursing approaches. The instructor recognizes that critical thinkers in nursing:
   1. make quick, single-solution decisions.
   2. act on intuition instead of experience.
   3. review data in a disciplined manner.
   4. alter interventions for every circumstance.

18. A nurse is caring for a patient who is experiencing a respiratory disorder. Intuition is a part of the critical thinking process for the nurse. While caring for the patient, the nurse demonstrates intuition by:
   1. reviewing care with the patient in advance.
   2. observing communication patterns.
   3. establishing a nursing diagnosis.
   4. sensing that the patient is not doing as well this morning as before.

19. Entering a room at 2:00 AM, a nurse notes that the patient is not in bed; the patient is sitting in the chair and states that she is having difficulty sleeping. Employing critical thinking, the nurse responds by:
   1. assisting the patient back into bed.
   2. asking more about the patient's sleep problem.
   3. positioning the patient and providing a warm blanket.
   4. obtaining an order for a hypnotic medication.

20. A nurse has a diverse patient assignment this evening. When reviewing the patients' conditions, the nurse determines that the first individual who should be seen is:
   1. the patient who is hypotensive.
   2. the patient receiving a visit from a family member.
   3. the patient being treated by the respiratory therapist.
   4. the patient waiting for the effects of an analgesic that was given 5 minutes ago.

21. In using the critical thinking skill of self-regulation, a nurse will:
   1. be orderly in data collection.
   2. look at all situations objectively.
   3. use scientific and experiential knowledge.
   4. reflect on his or her own experiences and improve performance.

22. During the process of reflection, what is the most appropriate question for a nurse to ask himself or herself?
    1. "What could I have done differently?"
    2. "What's going on right now?"
    3. "How can the patient's status change?"
    4. "What should I do to communicate this information?"

23. A nurse believes that substance abuse is a serious problem with negative consequences for patients and families. The nurse, however, provides excellent care to a patient who is admitted with this problem. The nurse is displaying the critical thinking attitude of:
    1. integrity.
    2. fairness.
    3. discipline.
    4. perseverance.

STUDY GROUP QUESTIONS

- How is critical thinking integrated into nursing practice?
- What attitudes are needed by a nurse to be a critical thinker?
- How are the competencies of critical thinking applied in clinical practice?
- Why is critical thinking important throughout the nursing process?

9 Nursing Process

CASE STUDIES

1. Mr. B., a 47-year-old male patient, goes to the annual community health fair. During a routine blood pressure screening, it is determined that his blood pressure is significantly above normally expected levels.
   a. What additional assessment data should be obtained from the patient and family?
   b. What limitations exist in this situation for completing an assessment?

2. Mr. B. returns for a follow-up visit at the medical center's adult health clinic. Mr. B. is diagnosed with hypertension and an antihypertensive medication is prescribed, but he appears unsure about how and when he should take the prescription. Mr. B. also identifies that his father died from a heart attack at 54 years old.
   a. Identify the relevant assessment data for this patient.
   b. Based upon this information, identify two nursing diagnoses.

3. During Mr. B.'s appointment at the adult health clinic, he was found to have high blood pressure, and antihypertensive medication was prescribed. Mr. B. did not have any previous knowledge of or experience with either hypertension or hypertensive medication. Mr. B. mentions again that his father died at age 54 years of a heart attack.
   a. Based on the nursing diagnoses that were developed, identify one long-term or short-term goal for each diagnosis and at least one expected outcome for each goal.

Nursing Diagnoses	Long-Term or Short-Term Goals	Expected Outcomes
1.		
2.		

   b. Identify two nursing interventions that may be appropriate in assisting the patient to achieve the expected outcomes and goals.

4. At his next visit to the adult health clinic, Mr. B. tells the nurse that he is taking the antihypertensive medication that was ordered by the physician "when he remembers." He says that he is trying to use the relaxation techniques that he was taught during his last visit, but he does not use them regularly.
   a. What nursing implementation methods should take priority at this time?
   b. What, if any, alterations must be made in the original plan of care?

5. Mr. B. returns to the adult health clinic for evaluation of his status. His blood pressure is lower than before but remains slightly above normal limits. He exercises once or twice a week and states that this is making him feel better. Mr. B. shows the nurse a calendar on which he has written down the times for taking his medication. Mr. B. relates that he has been trying very hard to use the relaxation techniques when he starts to feel anxious or overwhelmed. He identifies that he cannot control all of his "destiny," but he is trying to do things that may help him avoid what happened to his father.
   a. In accordance with previously identified outcomes, what nursing evaluation may be made on this patient's status?
   b. What areas, if any, may require reassessment?

6. A 4-year-old girl is newly diagnosed with diabetes mellitus. You are going to be working with the family to help them adjust to the treatment regimen.
   a. What assessment data is important to collect from the child and family?
   b. Identify a possible nursing diagnosis for the child or the family related to the new diagnosis.

CHAPTER REVIEW

Match the description/definition in Column A with the correct term in Column B.

	Column A	Column B
_____	1. Unintended effect of a medication, diagnostic test, or intervention	a. Subjective data
_____	2. Observations or measurements made by the nurse during assessment	b. ADLs
_____	3. Comparing data with another source to determine accuracy and relevancy	c. Adverse reaction
_____	4. Multidisciplinary, outcome-based care plan	d. Critical pathway
_____	5. Clinical judgment about patient responses to health problems or life processes	e. Nursing diagnosis
		f. Cue
_____	6. Information obtained through the senses	g. Objective data
_____	7. Activities performed in the course of a normal day	h. Scientific rationale
_____	8. Support for why a specific nursing action is chosen	i. Inference
_____	9. Interpretation of cues	j. Validation
_____	10. Information verbally provided by the patient	

Complete the following:

11. The three phases of an interview are:

12. Based on the following data clusters, identify possible nursing diagnoses for each of the following:
    a. Abdominal pain, three loose liquid stools per day, hyperactive bowel sounds

    b. Fatigue, weakness, tachycardia upon activity, exertional dyspnea

13. Identify at least one goal or expected outcome and one nursing intervention for the following nursing diagnoses:
    a. *Deficient Knowledge related to the need for postoperative care at home*
    Goal:

    Expected outcome:

    Nursing intervention:

    b. *Constipation related to lack of physical activity*
    Goal:

    Expected outcome:

    Nursing intervention:

    c. *Risk for injury*
    Goal:

    Expected outcome:

    Nursing intervention:

14. Identify whether the following are examples of cognitive, interpersonal, or psychomotor skills in patient care:
    a. Preparing and administering an injection
    b. Completing a health history
    c. Providing emotional support to a family member
    d. Changing a surgical dressing
    e. Recognizing the patient's need for nutritional instruction

15. Before implementing standing orders, the nurse should check:

16. The steps of the implementation phase of the nursing process are:

17. During interactions with a patient, a nurse gathers more data and identifies a new patient need. The nurse should:

18. A patient with diabetes mellitus goes to the outpatient center for care. There is a written plan for diet counseling, medication, and follow-up care. These specific procedures are termed a(n) _____________ for care.

19. An example of an indirect nursing intervention is:

20. Identify all of the following that typically may be delegated to unlicensed assistive personnel:
   a. Skin care _____
   b. Tracheostomy care _____
   c. Hygienic care _____
   d. Personal grooming _____
   e. Urinary catheterization _____
   f. Administration of IV medications _____
   g. Assistance with ambulation _____

21. Specify how the wording of the following patient outcome statements may be improved:
   a. Erythema will be less noticeable
   b. Pulse rate will be normal
   c. Patient's calorie intake will increase

22. Identify at least three (3) ways to create a good environment for an interview with a patient.

23. Indicate whether the following data are subjective or objective:
   a. "I feel tired."
   b. BP 124/64
   c. Pain level of 5 on a scale of 10
   d. Diaphoresis
   e. Wound edges dry and intact

24. What information can be found in a patient's medical record?

25. How would the following data be validated by the nurse?
   a. Patient states that he is fatigued.
   b. The pressure ulcer appears larger.

26. Provide examples of how the nurse can implement each of the following in the plan of care:
   a. Direct care
   b. Counseling
   c. Teaching
   d. Controlling adverse reactions

27. What are the steps in the evaluation process?

28. Provide an example of how the nurse can determine the patient's cultural needs or preferences.

29. For the nursing diagnosis *Feeding Self-care Deficit,* indicate two interventions that the nurse can implement to assist the patient.

Select the best answer for each of the following questions:

30. A new graduate is preparing to work with patients on a medical unit. The nursing process is applied as a:
   1. method for processing the care of many patients.
   2. tool for diagnosing and treating patients' health problems.
   3. guideline for determining the nurse's accountability in patient care.
   4. logical, problem-solving approach to providing patient care.

31. Upon admission, the nurse begins to assess the patient. The patient appears uncomfortable, stating that she has severe abdominal pain. The nurse should:
   1. inquire specifically about the discomfort.
   2. let the patient rest, returning later to complete the assessment.
   3. perform a complete physical examination immediately.
   4. ask the family about the patient's health history.

32. The following nursing diagnoses are proposed for patients on the medical unit. The diagnostic statement that contains all of the necessary components is:
   1. impaired gas exchange related to accumulation of lung secretions.
   2. imbalanced nutrition related to chemotherapy treatment.
   3. complicated grieving.
   4. pain related to abdominal surgery.

33. A nurse is working with patients who go to the community center for health screenings and educational sessions. An example of a wellness nursing diagnosis label that is appropriate for this group is:
   1. *Risk for Impaired Skin Integrity.*
   2. *Readiness for Enhanced Family Coping.*
   3. *Altered Parent-Infant Attachment.*
   4. *Fluid Volume Deficit.*

34. In reviewing the nursing diagnoses written by a new staff member, a supervisor identifies which of the following as a correctly written nursing diagnosis?
   1. *Altered Respiratory Function related to abnormal blood gases*
   2. *Urinary Infection related to long-term catheterization*
   3. *Deficient Knowledge related to need for cardiac monitoring*
   4. *Pain related to severe arthritis in finger joints*

35. A nurse is working with a patient who has the following symptoms: dyspnea, ankle edema, weight gain, abdominal distention, hypertension. The nursing diagnosis that is most appropriate for these signs and symptoms is:
   1. *Ineffective Tissue Perfusion.*
   2. *Disturbed Body Image.*
   3. *Impaired Gas Exchange.*
   4. *Excess Fluid Volume.*

36. A patient is to have abdominal surgery tomorrow. The nurse determines that an outcome for this patient that meets the necessary criteria is:
   1. patient will be repositioned every 2 hours.
   2. patient will express fears about surgery.
   3. patient will achieve normal elimination pattern before discharge.
   4. patient will perform active range-of-motion exercises every 2 hours while in bed.

37. There are a number of activities that are to be performed by a nurse during a clinical shift. In deciding to perform a nurse-initiated intervention, the nurse:
   1. administers oral medications.
   2. orders laboratory tests.
   3. changes a sterile dressing.
   4. teaches newborn hygienic care.

38. A nurse implements a preventive nursing action when:
   1. immunizing patients.
   2. assisting with hygienic care.
   3. inserting a urinary catheter.
   4. providing crisis intervention counseling.

39. A nurse has been working with a patient in the rehabilitative facility for 2 weeks. The nurse is in the process of evaluating the patient's progress. During the evaluation phase, the nurse recognizes that:
   1. nursing diagnoses always remain the same.
   2. time frames for patient outcomes may be adjusted.
   3. evaluative skills differ greatly from those for patient assessment.
   4. the number of nursing diagnoses and outcomes is most important.

40. An expected outcome for a patient is the following: "Pulse will remain below 120 beats per minute during exercise." If the patient's pulse rate exceeds 120 beats per minute one of every three exercise periods, the nurse appropriately evaluates the patient's goal attainment as:
   1. patient has achieved desired behavior.
   2. patient requires further evaluation of progress.
   3. patient's response indicates need for elimination of exercise.
   4. patient does not comply with therapeutic regimen.

41. The nurse is caring for a patient who has been medically stable. During the change-of-shift report, the nurse is informed that the patient is experiencing a slight arrhythmia. To avoid complications during the implementation of care, the nurse plans to first:
   1. evaluate the patient's vital signs.
   2. ask about the patient's previous diagnoses.
   3. contact the physician immediately.
   4. tell the nursing assistant to perform the usual care for the patient.

42. For a patient in the acute care facility, a nurse identifies several interventions. The statement that best communicates the specific nursing intervention to be performed is:
   1. assist with exercises.
   2. take the patient's vital signs.
   3. refer the patient to a therapist.
   4. provide 30 ml of water with the nasogastric tube feedings every 4 hours.

43. The nurse is working with a patient who has diabetes mellitus. The nursing diagnosis is "Deficient fluid volume related to osmotic diuresis." An appropriate patient outcome, based on this nursing diagnosis, is:
   1. patient will have an increased urinary output.
   2. patient will decrease the amount of fluid intake during a 24-hour period.
   3. patient will demonstrate a decrease in edema in the lower extremities.
   4. patient will have palpable peripheral pulses and good capillary refill.

44. A nurse is working with a patient who is experiencing abnormal breath sounds and thick secretions. The nurse identifies a nursing diagnosis of:
   1. *Deficient Fluid Volume.*
   2. *Ineffective Airway Clearance.*
   3. *Risk for Altered Mucous Membranes.*
   4. *Dysfunctional Ventilatory Weaning Response.*

45. In completing a health history, a nurse obtains from the patient psychosocial information that includes:
   1. the reason for seeking health care.
   2. past health problems.
   3. the primary language spoken.
   4. physical safety status.

46. A patient tells the nurse that she feels she may not be using the crutches correctly when ambulating. The best way for the nurse to validate this information is to:
   1. ask the family about the patient's ambulation.
   2. ask the physician how the patient was taught.
   3. discuss the problem with the other staff members.
   4. observe the patient using the crutches.

47. An example of the most appropriately written nursing diagnosis is:
    1. *Acute Pain related to surgery.*
    2. *Shortness of Breath related to immobility.*
    3. *Anxiety related to lack of knowledge about cardiac monitoring.*
    4. *Recurrent Infection related to improper catheterization procedure.*

48. In determining which of the following patients on the medical unit to visit first, a nurse selects the patient with which of the following diagnoses?
    1. *Imbalanced Nutrition: less than body requirements*
    2. *Ineffective Tissue Perfusion*
    3. *Deficient Knowledge regarding home care resources*
    4. *Impaired Physical Mobility*

49. An example of a physician-initiated intervention is:
    1. teaching a patient about the therapeutic diet.
    2. assessing a patient's skin.
    3. providing emotional support.
    4. preparing a patient for a diagnostic test.

STUDY GROUP QUESTIONS

- What is involved in patient assessment, and what priorities does a nurse have in completing an assessment?
- How does the patient assessment fit into the nursing process?
- Why does an error in the assessment phase influence the remaining implementation of the process, and how can a nurse avoid errors?
- What methods may be used to obtain patient data and what type of data is obtained with each method?
- What is involved in a patient interview?
- How can a nurse optimize the environment for a patient interview?
- How can a nurse use different communication strategies to obtain data during patient assessment?
- What is a nursing diagnosis?
- What are the components of a nursing diagnosis?
- How are actual and potential nursing diagnoses different?
- How are medical and nursing diagnoses different?
- What errors are possible in formulating nursing diagnoses, and how can they be avoided?
- Which nursing diagnoses become priorities in planning patient care?
- How are long-term and short-term goals different from each other?
- How are goals and expected outcomes different from each other?
- What are the guidelines for formulating goals and outcomes?
- In selecting nursing interventions, what are three essential nurse competencies?
- How are the three types of nursing interventions different from one another?
- What factors should be considered when selecting nursing interventions?
- What is the purpose of the care plan, and what types are available for use?
- How does a critical pathway differ from a "traditional" care plan?
- How does the consultation process begin, and who and what may be involved in the process?
- What is the focus of the implementation phase of the nursing process?
- What are standing orders and protocols, and how are they used in patient care situations?
- What are the five preparatory nursing activities that are completed before implementing the care plan?
- What are the nursing implementation methods?
- How is nursing implementation communicated to other members of the health care team?
- How is evaluation incorporated into the nursing process?
- How is evaluation used in patient situations and in nursing practice and health care delivery settings?
- What circumstances would lead to a modification of a care plan?

STUDY CHART

Create a study chart to compare the *Steps of the Nursing Process* that identifies the different activities involved in each step.

Create a *Concept Map* for one of the case studies in this chapter.

10 Informatics and Documentation

CASE STUDIES

1. Mrs. Q. has just been transferred to her room from the postanesthesia care unit (PACU) after right hip replacement surgery. She was accompanied by a nurse from the PACU. Vital signs were taken upon transfer and found to be within expected limits. A dressing is in place on the patient's right hip. Mrs. Q. does not appear to be having any difficulty at the moment.
   a. What information should be provided by the PACU nurse to the primary nurse on the surgical unit when Mrs. Q. is transferred to her room?
   b. What additional information may Mrs. Q.'s primary nurse want to obtain from the PACU nurse?

2. The primary nurse begins to plan and provide care for Mrs. Q. Upon entering the patient's room, Mrs. Q. is found to be grimacing and moaning in pain. She says that she is having intense pain in her right hip area. The dressing to her hip is dry and intact. Mrs. Q. says that she does not want to move because it really hurts. The primary nurse helps Mrs. Q. to get into a more comfortable position and begins to prepare the pain medication ordered by the physician. The primary nurse administers the pain medication, and, after approximately one-half hour, Mrs. Q. states that the pain has been reduced. Using SOAP or DAR methods, document the nursing interaction with Mrs. Q.

3. Mr. W. has just been diagnosed with type 1 diabetes mellitus and needs to learn how to self-administer his insulin injections.
   a. What information should be included in the patient record regarding the teaching provided to Mr. W. on the self-injection of insulin?

CHAPTER REVIEW

Match the description/definition in Column A with the correct term in Column B.

	Column A	*Column B*
_____	1. An oral or written exchange of information between health care providers	a. Record
_____	2. Information about patients provided only to appropriate personnel	b. POMR
_____	3. Permanent communication with the patient's health care management	c. Acuity recording
_____	4. Structured method of documentation with emphasis on the patient's problems	d. Report
_____	5. Documentation that requires staff to identify interventions and allows patients to be compared with one another	e. Confidentiality

Complete the following:

6. The following are guidelines for written documentation. Indicate the correct action to be taken by the nurse for each guideline.
   a. Never erase entries or use correction fluid, and never use pencil.
   b. Do not write retaliatory or critical comments about patients.
   c. Avoid using generalized, empty phrases.
   d. Do not cross out errors.
   e. Do not leave blank spaces.
   f. Do not speculate or guess.
   g. Do not record: "Physician made error."
   h. Never chart for someone else.
   i. Do not wait until the end of shift to record important information.

7. a. HIPAA (Health Insurance Portability and Accountability Act of 1996) has new regulations that require written consent for disclosure of all patient information.
   True _____ False _____
   b. Incident or occurrence reports should be documented in the patient's medical record in the nurse's notes section.
   True _____ False _____
   c. Poor written and verbal communication has been a top ten reason for sentinel events.
   True _____ False _____

8. Standards for health care agencies and documentation are set by the:

9. For each of the following, identify an example of how the patient record is used.
   a. Communication:
   b. Finance:
   c. Education:
   d. Research:
   e. Auditing/monitoring:

10. Provide an example of a malpractice issue related to charting:

11. Identify the five characteristics of quality documentation:

12. Subjective statements made by the patient are best documented by:

13. Demonstrate how a student nurse should sign a written patient record:

14. Identify what is wrong with the following notations and how they can be corrected:
    a. "Ate some breakfast."
    b. "Voided an adequate amount."
    c. "Provided wound care qd."

15. For telephone reports, identify what the SBAR acronym represents and give an example of each area:
    S:
    B:
    A:
    R:

16. Provide two items that should be included in a discharge summary:

17. Home care documentation is completed for quality control and as the basis for:

18. Completion of narrative notes only when there are abnormal patient findings is part of the concept of:

19. What are the purposes and advantages of nursing informatics?

20. Identify at least two ways in which electronic records are safeguarded for privacy and security:

21. Identify the four concepts included in informatics:

22. Which of the following are the correct nursing actions for a telephone order? Select all that apply.
    a. Identifying that Mr. J. is in Room 212 _____
    b. Asking the physician to repeat the medication order for Mr. J. three times _____
    c. Checking that 40 mg of the drug is what should be given _____
    d. Writing "TO" (telephone order) in the nurse's notes _____
    e. Asking another nurse to call the physician back to verify the order _____
    f. Having Mr. J.'s doctor cosign the order within 24 hours _____

23. What information is usually available to nurses on a clinical information system (CIS)?

24. A problem-oriented medical record includes: Select all that apply.
    a. Progress notes _____
    b. Narrative notes _____
    c. Initial care plan _____
    d. Problem list _____
    e. Incident reports _____
    f. Discharge summary _____

25. What information should student nurses leave off of written materials that are prepared for class?

26. Identify the errors in the following charting example:
    Patient says she feels ok. 140/82, 88, 14. Gained a little weight. Complained about her doctor. Says she didn't eat much breakfast today.

Select the best answer for each of the following questions:

27. A nurse is working in a facility that uses computerized documentation of patient information. To maintain patient confidentiality with the use of computerized documentation, the nurse should:
    1. delete any and all errors made in the record.
    2. give his or her password only to other nurses working with the patient.
    3. log off the file or computer when not using the terminal.
    4. remove sensitive patient information, such as communicable diseases, from the record.

28. The nurses on a medical unit in an acute care facility are meeting to select a documentation format to use. They recognize that less fragmentation of patient data will occur if they implement:
   1. source records.
   2. focus charting.
   3. charting by exception.
   4. critical pathways.

29. While caring for a patient on the surgical unit, a nurse notes that the patient's blood pressure has dropped significantly since the last measurement. The nurse shares this information immediately with the health care provider in a(n):
   1. flow sheet record.
   2. incident report.
   3. telephone report.
   4. change-of-shift report.

30. Documentation of patient care is reviewed during the orientation to the facility. The new graduate nurse understands that the method for written documentation that is acceptable is:
   1. using red ink to make entries on patients' charts.
   2. charting all of the patient care at the end of the shift.
   3. beginning each entry with the time of the treatment or observation.
   4. leaving space at the end of the notations to allow for additional documentation.

31. A nurse is caring for a patient who has had abdominal surgery. Accurate and complete documentation of the care provided by the nurse is evident by the following notation:
   1. "Vital signs taken."
   2. "Tylenol with codeine given for pain."
   3. "Provided adequate amount of fluid."
   4. "IV fluids increased to 100 mL per hour according to protocol."

32. A nurse is involved in patient care in an agency that uses military time for documentation. Which of the following represents 4:00 PM?
   1. 0400
   2. 0800
   3. 1400
   4. 1600

33. An example of the use of a clinical decision support system (CDSS) is:
   1. access to patient's lab reports.
   2. direct input to the medical orders by the health care provider.
   3. problem-oriented recording.
   4. an alert for incorrect drug dosages.

34. An appropriate action by a student nurse is demonstrated by:
   1. accessing records of other students' patients.
   2. writing the patient's name and room number on assignments.
   3. copying patient records for review and preparation of care plans.
   4. reading the patient's record in preparation for clinical care.

35. A nurse enters a patient's room and discovers a yellow pill on the bed under the patient's pillow. The patient receives Lasix 40 mg daily. Which of the following notations is appropriate to include on an incident or occurrence report?
   1. "Patient refused to take Lasix at 10 AM."
   2. "Yellow pill found on bed under pillow."
   3. "Lasix not administered by primary nurse."
   4. "Patient did not receive 10 AM diuretic."

36. The nursing information system (NIS) that follows a more traditional format is the:
   1. protocol design.
   2. critical pathway design.
   3. nursing process design.
   4. medical diagnosis design.

37. Which of the following statements made by a new staff nurse during a change-of-shift report requires correction?
   1. "The patient is uncooperative about doing his stoma care."
   2. "Oxygen is needed after ambulation. This is a change in priorities."
   3. "Ms. Q. is a 62-year-old with diabetes mellitus."
   4. "The abdominal surgical wound is healing slowly, with no drainage noted."

STUDY GROUP QUESTIONS

- What is the purpose of documentation and reporting?
- What are the legal guidelines for documentation?
- How do the guidelines influence nursing documentation and reporting?
- What methods are available for documentation of patient data?
- How do the different types of documentation (e.g., SOAP, DAR, and narrative) compare with one another?
- How does written documentation compare with computerized systems, and what are the advantages and disadvantages of each method?
- What types of forms are used for patient documentation?
- How does patient documentation change in different health care settings?
- What information is necessary when doing change-of-shift, telephone, transfer, and incident reports?
- What role do informatics play in heath care?
- How do nurses use information systems?
- What safety measures need to be taken by nurses when accessing electronic records?
- What type of patient information is accessible on electronic systems?

11 Communication

CASE STUDIES

1. For the following patient situations, identify the communication techniques that may be most effective in establishing a nurse-patient relationship:
   a. An older adult patient who has a moderate hearing impairment
   b. The Russian-speaking parents of a young child who has been taken into the emergency department after a bicycle accident
   c. A young adult patient who is blind and requires daily insulin injections
   d. A 60-year-old Hispanic woman who will be having her first internal pelvic examination
   e. A 45-year-old patient on a ventilator

2. You are working with a patient who appears to have literacy issues. There is a need to instruct the patient about the medical diagnosis.
   a. What strategies should you use to assist the patient to understand the diagnosis and treatment plan?

CHAPTER REVIEW

Match the description/definition in Column A with the correct term in Column B.

	Column A	*Column B*
_____	1. Person who initiates interpersonal communication	a. Therapeutic communication
_____	2. Information sent or expressed by the sender	b. Metacommunication
_____	3. Means of conveying messages	c. Sender
_____	4. Person to whom the message is sent	d. Intonation
_____	5. Indicates whether the meaning of the sender's message was received	e. Feedback
_____	6. Tone of the speaker's voice that may affect a message's meaning	f. Channels
_____	7. A message within a message that conveys a sender's attitude toward the self and toward the listener	g. Message
		h. Receiver
_____	8. Development of a working, functional relationship by the nurse with the patient, fulfilling the purposes of the nursing process	

Complete the following:

9. Determine what level of communication the following examples illustrate:
   a. Talking to oneself
   b. "He looks uncomfortable, and I want to show him that I'm concerned about his discomfort."
   c. The ability to speak to consumers on health-related topics

10. Provide an example of how compassion fatigue may develop.

11. Individuals maintain distances between themselves during interactions. Identify the zone (Intimate, Personal, Social, or Public) being used in each of the following examples:
   a. Speaking to a group of students in a classroom
   b. Conducting a small group therapy session
   c. Performing a physical examination
   d. Making patient rounds with a physician
   e. Changing a wound dressing
   f. Testifying at a hearing
   g. Completing a change-of-shift report

12. For an older adult with impaired communication, identify the appropriate communication techniques. Select all that apply.
    a. Maintaining a quiet environment that is free of background noise _____
    b. Shifting from subject to subject during the conversation _____
    c. Letting the person know if you are having difficulty understanding him or her _____
    d. Using explorative questions to facilitate conversation _____
    e. Using long sentences to explain subject matter _____

13. The following are examples of inappropriate communication by a nurse. Specify an effective strategy that should be used to correct the situation.
    a. Calling the patient "honey"
    b. Reporting to a nursing colleague about the "gallbladder in room 214"
    c. Talking about a patient to other nurses in the elevator
    d. Running into a patient's room to administer medications and then leaving immediately
    e. Informing a patient that the physician will be performing an abdominal hysterectomy and that she should expect a midline incision of approximately 10 cm

14. For the following examples, identify a question that the nurse could ask that would be more appropriate and obtain better information from the patient:
    a. "You're feeling okay today, right?"
    b. "You don't take any medication at home, do you?"
    c. "Are you having any lymphedema?"
    d. "The physician will be doing a paracentesis today. He said he explained it to you."

15. Identify the communication strategy that is being used for each of the following examples:
    a. Sitting with a patient who is crying
    b. Showing interest in the patient who is discussing concerns or sharing family information
    c. Saying "Go on" or "Tell me more"
    d. Asking the patient to verify the meaning of statements made
    e. Directing the attention of the patient to a particular idea in the discussion

16. For the nursing diagnosis *impaired verbal communication related to aphasia,* identify at least two nursing interventions to promote communication with the patient.

17. Nurses on a medical unit are discussing issues related to their work schedules. Identify the examples of positive responses:
    a. "There's nothing we can do about the staffing situation." _____
    b. "Don't talk to me like that!" _____
    c. "What do you think we can do to improve this situation?" _____
    d. "I want to hear what your concerns are." _____

18. A nurse takes into account cultural considerations when communicating with patients. Identify the appropriate action(s):
    a. Stroking the head of a Southeast Asian patient _____
    b. Assigning a female staff member to care for a female Amish patient _____
    c. Maintaining direct eye contact with a Native American patient _____
    d. Introducing oneself and using the patient's last name _____

19. For the acronym SOLER, identify the skills for attentive listening:
    S:
    O:
    L:
    E:
    R:

20. Identify the nursing actions/responses that occur during the Orientation Phase of the Helping Relationship. Select all that apply.
    a. Achieving a smooth transition for the patient to other caregivers as needed _____
    b. Providing information needed to understand and change behavior _____
    c. Reviewing available data, including the medical and nursing history _____
    d. Expecting the patient to test your competence and commitment _____
    e. Setting the tone for the relationship by adopting a warm, empathetic, caring manner _____
    f. Prioritizing patient problems and identifying patient goals _____

21. Rose is a new nurse on the cardiac unit. Her new colleagues, who have worked there for many years, do not help her and say things like, "Didn't you learn that in school?" This is an example of:

22. Identify three physiological alterations that could influence communication for the patient.

23. What is going on in the photo below that may interfere with communication between the nurse and the patient?

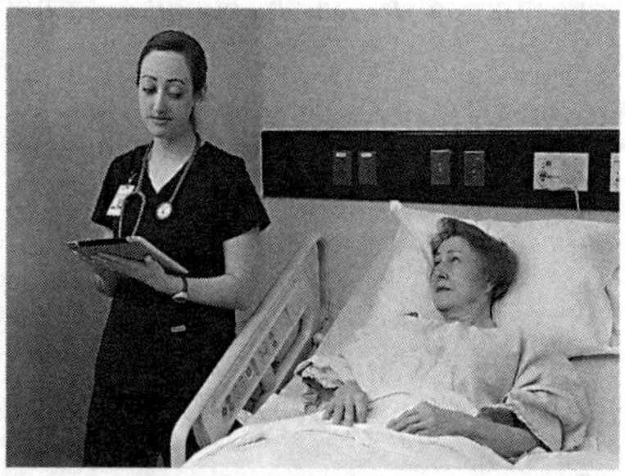

Select the best answer for each of the following questions:

24. A patient tells a nurse that he feels anxious and afraid. The nurse responds by saying, "I will stay here with you." The nurse is using the principle of effective communication known as:
    1. empathy.
    2. courtesy.
    3. availability.
    4. encouragement.

25. A patient states that he believes he may have cancer. The nurse tells him, "I wouldn't be concerned. I'm sure that the tests will be negative." The response by the nurse demonstrates the use of:
    1. assertiveness.
    2. false reassurance.
    3. professional opinion.
    4. hope and encouragement.

26. A nurse is assigned to a young adult male patient. Gender sensitivity is demonstrated when the nurse:
    1. uses sexual innuendo.
    2. engages in gender-oriented joking.
    3. stereotypes male and female roles.
    4. uses direct and indirect communication according to gender.

27. A patient regularly visits a medical clinic. A nurse establishes a helping relationship with the patient. During the working phase of a helping relationship, the nurse:
    1. encourages and helps the patient to set goals.
    2. reminisces about the relationship with the patient.
    3. anticipates health concerns or issues.
    4. identifies a location for the interaction.

28. A nurse is interviewing a patient who is in the outpatient area. The nurse uses paraphrasing communication with the statement:
    1. "This is your blood pressure medication. It will help to lower your blood pressure to the level where it should be."
    2. "Do you mean that the pain comes and goes when you walk?"
    3. "I would like to return to our discussion about your family."
    4. "If I understand you correctly, you are primarily concerned about your dizzy spells."

29. A patient tells a nurse that there are other people in the room who are watching her from under the bed. The nurse employs therapeutic communication when he or she:
    1. identifies that there are no people under the bed.
    2. tells the patient that he or she will help look for the other people.
    3. asks the patient why other people are watching her.
    4. reassures the patient that he or she will tell the people to go away.

30. While speaking with a female patient, a nurse notes that she is frowning. The nurse wants to find out about possible concerns by:
    1. asking why the patient is unhappy.
    2. telling the patient that everything is fine.
    3. identifying that the patient is frowning.
    4. asking if the patient is angry about the health care problem.

31. A patient's condition has deteriorated, and he has been transferred to the intensive care unit. The roommate asks the nurse what is wrong with the patient. The nurse should respond to the roommate by stating:
    1. "The patient's condition is no concern of yours."
    2. "Everything is fine. Don't worry. He'll be okay."
    3. "I recognize your interest in the patient, but I cannot share personal information with you without his permission."
    4. "Your roommate's condition worsened overnight, and he had to be moved to the intensive care unit for observation."

32. A patient is experiencing aphasia as a result of a CVA (cerebrovascular accident, or stroke). To promote communication, a nurse plans to:
    1. speak louder.
    2. use more questions.
    3. use visual clues, such as pictures and gestures.
    4. refer to a speech therapist to communicate with the patient.

33. A patient is talking endlessly about problems in the past with arthritic pain, but the nurse must get specific information for the admission assessment. The nurse's best response is:
    1. "You seem to have had difficulty managing the arthritis. What are you doing now for the pain?"
    2. "You can tell me more at another time. We need to move on to other information now."
    3. "You've given me a lot of information, but I have to ask you something else."
    4. "Are you taking medication for the arthritis?"

34. A nurse enters a room and finds the patient crying. The best action by the nurse is to:
    1. ask the patient why he or she is crying.
    2. tell the patient that things will get better.
    3. let the patient know that you will come back later.
    4. sit quietly with the patient.

35. A patient has a visual impairment. In communicating with this patient, a nurse should:
    1. use flash cards.
    2. use simple sentences.
    3. caution the patient before any physical contact.
    4. speak very loud and slow.

36. A nurse tells the patient's family that recovery may be "difficult." This may lead to an issue with:
    1. pacing.
    2. clarity.
    3. relevance.
    4. connotation.

37. A cultural group that may perceive continuous eye contact as intrusive or threatening is:
    1. Asian.
    2. Hispanic.
    3. African American.
    4. Northern European.

38. A nurse is working with a preschool-age child. An appropriate communication technique to use with an individual in this age-group is to:
    1. speak loudly and forcibly.
    2. communicate directly with the parents to determine the child's needs.
    3. sit or kneel down to be on the same level as the child.
    4. use medical terms when speaking with the parents so the child will not understand.

39. A patient's blood sample was dropped on its way to the lab. The patient asks the nurse why blood needs to be drawn again for the same test. The nurse's best response is:
    1. "One of the vials was dropped and broken by mistake. We will make sure that this sample gets to the lab safely."
    2. "We just have to do the test again."
    3. "Someone didn't do their job right the first time."
    4. "This kind of thing happens. It won't take long."

40. Which one of the following medications has the greatest potential to influence patient communication?
    1. Diuretics
    2. Antipsychotics
    3. Anticholinergics
    4. Antipyretics

41. A nurse is evaluating communication skills used during an interaction with a newly admitted patient. Of the statements made, the nurse responded therapeutically with:
    1. "Why aren't you able to keep taking the prescribed medications?"
    2. "We need to move quickly through the rest of the interview because it will be time for your therapy."
    3. "I can understand why you don't like that physician. I think you need to find another one."
    4. "I noticed that you didn't eat any of the lunch. Is there something that is bothering you?"

STUDY GROUP QUESTIONS

- What is therapeutic communication?
- What are the basic elements of communication?
- How do nurses and patients communicate verbally and nonverbally?
- What factors may influence communication?
- How may a patient's physical, psychosocial, and developmental status influence communication with the nurse?
- How is a helping relationship established with a patient?
- What are the principles/techniques of effective communication?
- How are the principles/techniques used by a nurse in a caring relationship?
- How is communication used within the steps of the nursing process?
- What are some of the barriers to effective communication, and how can they be overcome by the nurse?

STUDY CHART

Create a study chart to compare the *Components of Verbal and Nonverbal Communication* that identifies how each may influence the nurse-patient interaction (e.g., intonation).

12 Patient Education

CASE STUDIES

1. Your patient is a 47-year-old married woman who has gone to the medical clinic for evaluation. She has been diagnosed with hypertension and placed on an antihypertensive medication. She has no previous knowledge or experience with the diagnosis or the medication. There is a family history of coronary disease; her father died of a heart attack at 54 years old.
   a. What information about the patient may affect her motivation to learn?
   b. Formulate a teaching plan for the patient that includes goals and teaching strategies.

2. You are a nurse in a pediatrician's office. An 8-year-old boy has just been diagnosed with diabetes mellitus. His parents are very concerned about what this means for their son.
   a. What general information will the family need?
   b. How will you adapt your teaching for your 8-year-old patient?

3. There is a presentation tomorrow that you will give to a small group of patients.
   a. What do you need to take into consideration when preparing the setting for the teaching session?

CHAPTER REVIEW

Match the description/definition in Column A with the correct term in Column B.

	Column A	*Column B*
_____	1. Expression of feelings, attitudes, opinions, and values	a. Cognitive learning
_____	2. Mental state that allows for focus and comprehension of material	b. Motivation
_____	3. Acquiring skills	c. Attentional set
_____	4. Intellectual behaviors, including knowledge and understanding	d. Affective learning
_____	5. Desire to learn	e. Return demonstration
_____	6. Completion of a procedure to show competence	f. Psychomotor learning

Complete the following:

7. What are the six aspects of the ACCESS model and when would it be used?

8. A mild level of anxiety may motivate learning.
   True _____ False _____

9. From the following, select the appropriate topics for health education related to health maintenance and promotion and illness prevention. Select all that apply.
   a. First aid ______
   b. Occupational therapy ______
   c. Awareness of potential complications after a heart attack ______
   d. Hygiene ______
   e. Origin of symptoms ______
   f. Awareness of signs and symptoms of hypoglycemia ______
   g. Self-help devices ______
   h. Surgical intervention ______

10. Identify teaching activities for a(n):
    a. Infant
    b. Toddler
    c. Preschooler
    d. School-age child
    e. Older adult

11. A learner may find it difficult to concentrate in the presence of:

12. What characteristics does the patient need in order to learn psychomotor skills?

13. When selecting an environment for teaching, a nurse needs to consider:

14. Written materials used for teaching a patient with limited health literacy are usually presented at the ______ grade level.

15. Teaching sessions that are usually tolerated best last for _____ minutes. In planning the teaching session, essential information should be taught _____.

16. The patient becomes fatigued during the teaching session. You should:

17. For the nursing diagnosis *noncompliance with medication regimen related to insufficient knowledge of purpose and actions*, identify possible learning goals and outcomes and nursing interventions.

18. What is the preferred teaching style for the following types of learners?
    a. Visual
    b. Tactile
    c. Auditory

19. For the following, identify the domain of learning.
    a. Self-injection of insulin
    b. Coping with care of a family member
    c. Aware of potential complications after a heart attack
    d. Response of the family to a member's substance abuse
    e. Sterile dressing technique
    f. Aware of signs and symptoms of hypoglycemia

20. Identify an instructional technique that may be used in each of the following situations:
    a. A small group of patients in a cardiac rehabilitation group who need dietary information

    b. A patient with a leg cast who will be using crutches

    c. Students learning therapeutic communication skills to be used on a mental health unit

21. Explaining how a test will feel before the procedure is performed is an example of:

22. a. According to national reports, a total of ______% of adults in the United States have difficulty reading and understanding health information, including pamphlets and charts.
    b. What tools are available to assess your patients' literacy?

23. The nurse tells the patient that the injection will cause pain. What is a more effective way to communicate with the patient about the injection?

24. Identify what "teach-back" is and its purpose.

25. A focused assessment for patient education includes:

26. What should be included in the documentation of patient teaching?

Select the best answer for each of the following questions:

27. A nurse is preparing to teach a group of new parents about infant care. The nurse recognizes that learning can be enhanced with:
    1. previous unfamiliarity with the topic area.
    2. fear of health outcomes.
    3. moderate discomfort.
    4. mild anxiety level.

28. The patient who most likely has the greatest motivation to learn is the individual who is:
    1. waiting for the results of diagnostic tests.
    2. hypertensive, but has no symptoms.
    3. dealing with a family conflict.
    4. recovering from reconstructive surgery.

29. While preparing a teaching plan for a group of patients with diabetes, a nurse integrates the basic principle of education that:
    1. material should progress from complex to simpler ideas.
    2. prolonged teaching sessions improve concentration and attentiveness.
    3. learning is improved when more than one body sense is stimulated.
    4. previous knowledge of a topic area interferes with the acquisition of new information.

30. During a teaching session for a patient with heart disease, the nurse uses reinforcement to stimulate learning. An example of reinforcement for this patient is:
    1. allowing the patient to manage self-care needs.
    2. teaching about the disease process while delivering nursing care.
    3. outlining the exercise plan and providing explicit instructions.
    4. complimenting the patient on his or her ability to identify the action of prescribed medications.

31. After approximately 20 minutes have passed in the educational session, the nurse notices that the patient is slightly slumped in the chair and is no longer maintaining eye contact. The nurse should:
    1. reposition the patient in the chair.
    2. move the patient to a cooler, brighter room.
    3. reschedule the remainder of the teaching for another time.
    4. continue with the teaching session in order to cover the necessary content.

32. When preparing to teach the self-injection technique to a patient, the nurse begins with:
    1. having the patient demonstrate the procedure.
    2. discussing the procedure and the equipment used.
    3. providing written materials and having the patient practice the technique.
    4. demonstrating to the patient how to perform the procedure correctly.

33. After teaching a patient about a cerebrovascular accident (CVA/stroke), the nurse prepares to evaluate the patient's psychomotor domain of learning. This is accomplished by:
    1. observing the patient use a cane to ambulate.
    2. asking the patient about the basic etiology of a stroke.
    3. determining the patient's attitudes about the treatment regimen.
    4. having the patient complete a written schedule for daily activities at home.

34. When the teaching session has been completed, a nurse evaluates the patient's cognitive domain of learning to see if there are areas that require additional instruction. The nurse evaluates the patient's ability to:
    1. perform the range-of-motion exercises independently.
    2. identify the equipment necessary for surgical wound care.
    3. demonstrate the proper use of crutches to ambulate up and down stairs.
    4. discuss concerns about the difficulty in maintaining accurate records of the treatments.

35. Which patient appears to be demonstrating the greatest readiness to learn? The patient who says:
    1. "There's nothing wrong with me."
    2. "I think the doctor made a mistake."
    3. "I can manage on my own."
    4. "What do I need to know about this?"

36. A type of reinforcement that works well with children is:
    1. material.
    2. social.
    3. activity.
    4. negative.

37. A nurse recognizes that the most effective teaching strategy for a patient in the acceptance stage is to:
    1. share small bits of information.
    2. introduce only reality.
    3. provide simple explanations while doing care.
    4. focus on future skills and knowledge.

38. A patient is having difficulty communicating with other family members. Which one of the following would be the most effective teaching strategy for this patient?
    1. Demonstration
    2. Role-playing
    3. Telling
    4. Analogy

STUDY GROUP QUESTIONS

- What are the standards (e.g., The Joint Commission) for patient education?
- How does patient education promote, maintain, and restore health?
- What are the principles of teaching and learning?
- What factors may influence a patient's ability to learn?
- How does an individual's developmental status influence the selection of teaching methodologies?
- How does the teaching process compare with the communication and nursing processes?
- How does the nurse develop a teaching plan for a patient?
- What teaching approaches and instructional methods may be used by a nurse?
- How is patient education documented?

13 Managing Patient Care

CASE STUDY

1. As a nurse working on a busy surgical unit, this evening you have eight postoperative patients assigned to you.
   a. What types of activities could be delegated to an unlicensed nursing assistant?
   b. What determination do you need to make before safely delegating activities to the nursing assistant?
   c. What opportunities are available for doing more than one intervention at a time with the patient?

CHAPTER REVIEW

Complete the following:

1. Identify three responsibilities of a nurse manager.

2. A person who is reasonably independent and self-governing in decision making and practice is demonstrating:

3. The five rights of delegation are:

4. Provide the correct term for the following definitions:
   a. Duties and activities an individual is employed to perform:
   b. Official power to act:
   c. Being answerable for one's actions:

5. Case management is:

6. Provide at least one example of how staff members can be actively involved when decentralized decision making exists on a nursing unit:

7. For the QSEN competency of Teamwork and Collaboration, identify ways that team communication can be promoted.

8. A patient on the unit, who was admitted 2 days ago with ketoacidosis, has a blood glucose level of 425, which is far above the expected range. The patient was receiving a longer-acting insulin. There are concerns about the type of insulin and dietary management. Identify the way this information should be reported with the SBAR:
   S -
   B -
   A -
   R -

Select the best answer for each of the following questions:

9. A student nurse is working with a patient who has begun to have respiratory difficulty. It is the student nurse's initial responsibility to:
   1. call the pharmacy.
   2. alert the primary nurse.
   3. contact the attending physician.
   4. administer the prescribed medication.

10. The nurses on a medical unit are discussing plans to change the focus of the unit to the primary nursing care model. With this model, the assignment for nurse A is:
    1. Mrs. J., Mrs. R., and Mrs. T. for the length of their stays.
    2. to receive reports from the nursing assistant on the care of Mrs. J., Mrs. R., and Mrs. T.
    3. side 1 of the unit in cooperation with nurse B and the nursing assistant.
    4. medication administration for all of the patients on the unit while nurse B does the physical care with the nursing assistant.

11. A nurse in the long-term care facility is delegating care to the nursing assistant. It is appropriate for the nurse to delegate the care of the patient who requires:
    1. catheter care.
    2. an admission history.
    3. administration of oral medications.
    4. vital sign measurements after episodes of arrhythmias.

12. A student nurse is assigned to care for a patient in the hospital. While taking the patient's vital signs, the student cannot obtain the blood pressure reading after two attempts. The student should:
    1. keep trying to get the blood pressure measurement.
    2. use the closest measurement to the last reading.
    3. ask another nurse to obtain the blood pressure measurement.
    4. inform the instructor about the difficulty and request assistance.

13. A nurse is working with a patient who has just returned from surgery. The nurse has no experience working with the patient's postoperative surgical dressing. During an assessment, the nurse notices that the dressing has come loose and has fallen away from the surgical wound. The patient tells the nurse, "Oh, you can fix it." The nurse:
    1. asks the patient to help replace the dressing.
    2. replaces the loosened dressing as best as possible.
    3. asks the surgeon to replace the dressing.
    4. covers the wound with a sterile dry dressing until assistance is obtained.

14. A nurse has been assigned to work on a very busy medical unit in the hospital. It is important for the nurse to employ time management skills. The nurse implements a plan to:
    1. have all the patients' major needs met in the morning hours.
    2. anticipate possible interruptions by therapists and visitors.
    3. complete assessments and treatments for each patient at different times each day.
    4. leave each day unstructured to allow for changes in treatments and patient assignments.

15. The staff on a medical unit in an acute care facility is moving to a system where the nurse manager will lead a group of other RNs, LPNs, and aides. This is an example of:
    1. functional nursing.
    2. primary nursing.
    3. total patient care.
    4. team nursing.

16. A student nurse has a multiple patient assignment. In reviewing the report obtained from the primary nurse, the student should decide to see which patient first? The patient who is:
    1. experiencing nausea
    2. using a bedpan
    3. having a severe anxiety attack
    4. thirsty and wants another drink with breakfast

STUDY GROUP QUESTIONS

- To whom may a nurse delegate care responsibilities? What types of responsibilities may be delegated legally and safely?
- What is involved in decentralized decision making?
- How does the nurse manager function within the health care team?
- How do the different types of nursing care delivery models differ from one another?
- What is quality improvement (QI), and what does it mean to nurses?
- What is necessary for effective coordination and prioritization of care?

STUDY CHART

Create a study chart to compare and contrast the different *Nursing Care Delivery Models.*

14 Infection Prevention and Control

CASE STUDIES

1. An 86-year-old woman in an extended care facility has a urinary catheter attached to a drainage system.
   a. What precautions should be taken for this patient to prevent a urinary tract infection?

2. Yesterday a 45-year-old man had abdominal surgery. He has a large midline abdominal incision covered by a sterile dressing. He will require dressing changes twice daily.
   a. What precautions should be taken for this patient to prevent wound infection?

3. An 85-year-old man with MRSA requires isolation precautions. He is oriented to his surroundings and is concerned about whether his family will be able to visit him.
   a. What specific nursing care should be implemented for this patient?

CHAPTER REVIEW

Match the description/definition in Column A with the correct term in Column B.

	Column A	*Column B*
_____	1. Arises from microorganisms outside the patient	a. Exudate
_____	2. Cellular response to injury or infection	b. Aseptic technique
_____	3. Microorganisms that cause another infection because they are resistant to antibiotics	c. Health care–acquired infection
_____	4. Infection that developed that was not present at the time of patient admission	d. Sterilization
_____	5. Methods to reduce or eliminate disease-producing microorganisms	e. Colonization
_____	6. Microorganisms that do not cause disease but help to maintain health	f. Inflammation
_____	7. Process that eliminates all forms of microbial life	g. Flora
_____	8. Disease-producing microorganism	h. Pathogen
_____	9. Substance formed through the inflammatory process that may ooze from openings in the skin or mucous membranes	i. Endogenous infection
_____	10. Microorganism that grows but does not cause disease	j. Suprainfection
_____	11. Ability of microorganisms to produce disease	k. Exogenous infection
_____	12. Being more than normally vulnerable to a disease	l. Virulence
_____	13. Alteration of a patient's flora with a resulting overgrowth	m. Susceptibility

Complete the following:

14. Identify whether the following are performed using sterile technique in an acute care environment:
    a. Hand hygiene ______
    b. Postoperative dressing change ______
    c. Urinary catheter insertion ______
    d. Barrier precautions ______
    e. Intramuscular injection ______

15. An outcome for a patient with a 3-cm–diameter wound is:

16. Immunizations are available for which of the following? Select all that apply.
    a. Hepatitis A ______
    b. Diphtheria ______
    c. Rubella ______
    d. Tuberculosis ______
    e. AIDS ______
    f. Varicella ______

17. For the following, select all actions that require that equipment be discarded and/or the sterile field be redone.
    a. A mask is worn when opening the sterile tray. ______
    b. The sterile dressing package is torn. ______
    c. The tip of the sterile syringe touches the surface of a clean, disposable glove. ______
    d. A sterile basin is held out over the sterile field. _____
    e. A cup on the sterile field is touched with a sterile gloved hand. ______
    f. Sterile dressings are placed within the 1-inch edge of the sterile field. ______

18. Identify specific actions that a nurse can implement to interrupt the chain of infection.
    a. Control or eliminate the infectious agent:

    b. Control or eliminate the reservoir:

    c. Control the portals of exit:

    d. Control transmission:

    e. Control susceptibility of host:

19. What results would be expected for the following laboratory studies in the presence of an infection?
    a. WBC count
    b. Erythrocyte sedimentation rate
    c. Iron level
    d. Neutrophils
    e. Basophils

20. In relation to health care–acquired infections (HAI):
    a. How can they be reduced?

    b. Which patients are more susceptible to HAI?

21. A patient's gastrointestinal defenses against infection are altered by:

22. Select all the appropriate techniques for isolation precautions.
    a. Wash hands in the clean utility room after patient care. _____
    b. Provide for the patient's sensory needs during care. _____
    c. Prevent visitors from entering the patient's room. _____
    d. Keep face mask below the level of eyeglasses or goggles. _____
    e. Place disposable items in paper bags. _____
    f. Maintain each patient's personal protective equipment (PPE) within the patient's room. _____
    g. Keep PPE at the door to the room or in an anteroom area. ______

23. Handling of biohazardous waste includes:

24. Specify the order in which the following PPE should be applied before entering an isolation room:

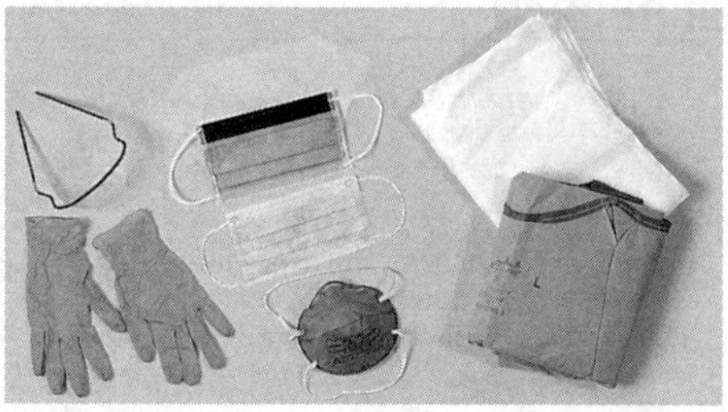

    a. Mask ______
    b. Gloves ______
    c. Gown ______

25. If a mask, gown, and gloves are worn into an isolation room, the first item(s) of PPE to be removed when exiting the room is/are the:

26. Select all of the following in which appropriate asepsis has occurred:
    a. Handling a sterile dressing with clean gloves ______
    b. Holding a sterile bowl above waist level using sterile gloves ______
    c. Keeping the hands above the elbows after a surgical scrub ______
    d. Turning away from and placing one's back to the sterile field ______
    e. Talking or coughing over the sterile field ______
    f. Discarding sterile packages that are wet ______
    g. Placing objects to the edge of the sterile field ______
    h. Discarding a small amount of solution before pouring the remainder into a sterile container on the field ______

27. For the nursing diagnosis *Impaired Skin Integrity related to 2-inch-diameter pressure ulcer on sacrum*, identify a patient outcome and nursing interventions.

28. Number the flaps on the sterile package in the figure according to which should be opened first, second, and last.

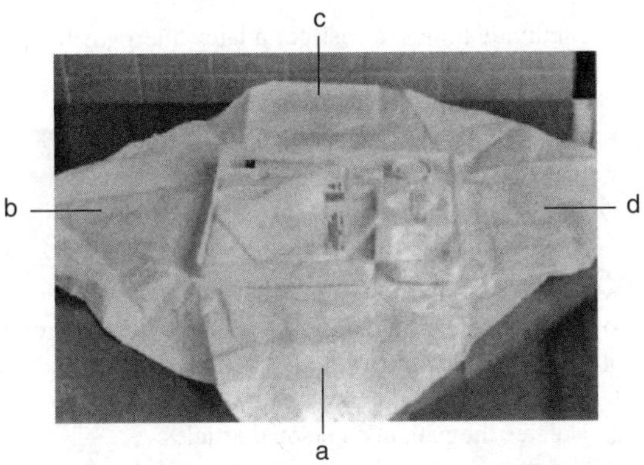

29. Proper disposal of contaminated sharps includes:

30. Provide an example of how the nurse needs to be aware of his or her own breaks in aseptic technique.

31. What equipment is needed to collect a urine specimen from the patient with an indwelling urinary catheter?

32. Select all of the following actions that are appropriate for hand hygiene.
   a. Cleaning under artifical nails ______
   b. Removing rings during washing ______
   c. Leaning against the sink ______
   d. Keeping the water temperature hot ______
   e. Washing the hands for at least 15 seconds ______
   f. Turning off the faucet with the elbows ______
   g. Keeping hands and forearms lower than the elbows during washing ______
   h. Drying from the forearms to the fingers ______

33. The patient sees the nurse using the hand sanitizer frequently and remarks, "I must be full of germs, since you're always cleaning your hands." How should the nurse respond?

34. Information on the current immunizations schedule can be found at the:

35. What are the three most common infections in long-term care?

36. Which of the following infectious organisms are transmitted through blood? Select all that apply.
   a. *Candida albicans* (fungi) _____
   b. HIV ______
   c. *Staphylococcus aureus* ______
   d. *Plasmodium falciparum* (protozoa) ______
   e. Streptococcus ______
   f. Hepatitis B ______

37. Place the following steps for specimen collection in an isolation room in the correct order. After changing the bed linens and changing the gloves, the nurse should:
   a. Perform hand hygiene ______
   b. Check the container label and send the specimen to the lab ______
   c. Place the specimen container on a clean paper towel in the bathroom ______
   d. Transfer the specimen to the containers ______
   e. Collect the specimen ______

38. When splashing or spraying of bodily fluids is anticipated, the nurse should use a:

39. Identify the breaks in isolation technique in each photo below:

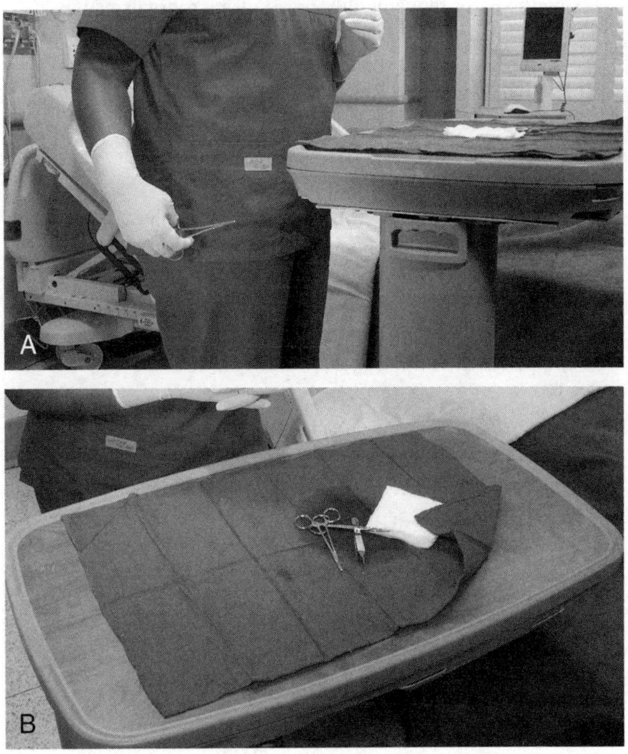

Select the best answer for each of the following questions:

40. At the community health fair, a nurse is asked by one of the residents about the influenza vaccine. The nurse responds to the resident that the influenza vaccine is recommended for individuals who are:
    1. Health care workers
    2. Traveling to other countries
    3. Younger than 6 years of age
    4. Between 40 and 65 years of age

41. A nurse is preparing a room for a patient with tuberculosis. The specific aspect for this tier of Standard Precautions that is different than tier 1 is that the care should include:
    1. a private room with negative air flow.
    2. hand hygiene after gloves are removed.
    3. eye protection if splashing is possible.
    4. disposal of sharps in a puncture-resistant container.

42. A nurse is preparing a teaching plan for patients about the hepatitis B virus. The nurse informs them that this virus may be transmitted by:
    1. mosquitoes.
    2. droplet nuclei.
    3. blood products.
    4. improperly handled food.

43. A nurse is working on a unit with a number of patients who have infectious diseases. One of the most important methods for reducing the spread of microorgaisms is:
    1. sterilization of equipment.
    2. the use of gloves and gowns.
    3. maintenance of isolation precautions.
    4. hand hygiene before and after patient care.

44. The assignment today for a nurse includes a patient with tuberculosis. In caring for a patient on droplet precautions, the nurse should routinely use:
    1. regular masks and eyewear.
    2. regular masks, gowns, and gloves.
    3. surgical hand hygiene and gloves.
    4. particulate filtration masks and gowns.

45. A nurse is caring for a patient who has a large abdominal wound that requires a sterile saline soak and dressing. While performing the care, the nurse drops the saline-soaked 4 × 4 gauze near the wound on the patient's abdomen. The nurse:
    1. discontinues the procedure.
    2. throws the gauze away and prepares a new 4 × 4 gauze.
    3. picks up the 4 × 4 with sterile forceps and places it on the wound.
    4. rinses the 4 × 4 with saline and places it on the wound using sterile gloves.

46. A nurse is checking the laboratory results of a male patient admitted to the medical unit. The nurse is alerted to the presence of an infectious process based on the finding of:
    1. iron: 80 g/100 mL.
    2. neutrophils: 65%.
    3. erythrocyte sedimentation rate (ESR): 13 mm per hour.
    4. white blood cells (WBC): 16,000/mm^3.

47. The individual most at risk for a latex allergy is the patient with a history of:
    1. hypertension.
    2. congenital heart disease.
    3. diabetes mellitus.
    4. cholecystitis.

48. A nurse is working with a patient who has a deep laceration to the right lower extremity. To reduce a possible reservoir of infection, the nurse:
    1. wears gloves and a mask at all times.
    2. isolates the patient's personal articles.
    3. has the patient cover the mouth and nose when coughing.
    4. changes the dressing to the extremity when it becomes soiled.

49. A nurse implements droplet precautions for the patient with:
    1. pulmonary tuberculosis.
    2. varicella.
    3. rubella.
    4. herpes.

50. A patient who has had a transplant will require what type of isolation?
    1. Contact
    2. Airborne
    3. Droplet
    4. Protective

51. For a patient with hepatitis A, the nurse is aware that the disease is transmitted through:
    1. feces.
    2. blood.
    3. skin.
    4. droplet nuclei.

52. A sign that is indicative of a systemic infection resulting from a wound is:
    1. redness.
    2. drainage.
    3. edema.
    4. fever.

53. There are small open wounds on the hands of the nurse. The nurse's most appropriate action is:
    1. asking to work at the nurse's station for the day.
    2. using clean, disposable gloves for patient care.
    3. applying antibacterial ointment before patient contact.
    4. providing patient care as usual and washing the hands more frequently.

54. A nurse is aware that older adults are more susceptible to infection as a result of:
    1. thickening of the dermal and epidermal skin layers.
    2. increased production of T lymphocytes.
    3. increased production of digestive juices.
    4. drying of the oral mucosa.

STUDY GROUP QUESTIONS

- What is the nature of the infectious process?
- What are the components of the chain of infection?
- What are the body's normal defenses against infection?
- What is a health care–associated infection, who are the patients at risk, and how can a nurse prevent this infection?
- How is the nursing process applied to infection control in the acute, extended care, and home care environments?
- What nursing measures may be implemented to prevent or control the spread of infection?
- What is included in Standard Precautions?
- What information may be taught to the patient and the patient's family for prevention or control of infectious processes?
- How does the nurse perform the procedures that are important for infection control?

15 Vital Signs

CASE STUDIES

1. You are volunteering at a community health fair. You have been asked to take blood pressure (BP) readings for the residents participating in the event.
   a. What blood pressure readings indicate that follow-up care should be recommended?
   b. What other information may be obtained from a patient while taking the blood pressure reading?

2. You are assigned to an orthopedic unit in the medical center. A patient was involved in an automobile accident and has bilateral casts on the upper arms.
   a. How will you obtain the patient's pulse rate and blood pressure?

3. You have just started your shift at the extended care facility. The nurse reporting off identifies that one of your assigned patients is febrile.
   a. What signs and symptoms do you expect to find with a patient who is febrile?
   b. What interventions are indicated for febrile patients?

4. The patient has been brought to the emergency room with signs of heat stroke.
   a. What interventions are anticipated for this patient?
   b. What teaching should be done to prevent the occurrence in the future?

5. A postoperative patient is being monitored with pulse oximetry. You are checking the reading, but the device does not appear to be working.
   a. What are the expected readings for oxygen saturation?
   b. What "troubleshooting" can you perform to determine if the pulse oximeter is working properly?
   c. How can you help postoperative patients to improve their saturation level?

CHAPTER REVIEW

Match the description/definition in Column A with the correct term in Column B.

	Column A	*Column B*
_____	1. Decrease of systolic and diastolic pressures below normal	a. Tachypnea
_____	2. Another word for fever	b. Bradypnea
_____	3. Rate and depth of respirations increase	c. Hypothermia
_____	4. Widening of blood vessels	d. Apnea
_____	5. Pulse rate less than 60 beats per minute for an adult	e. Bradycardia
_____	6. 140/90 mm Hg for two or more readings	f. Hypotension
_____	7. Rate of breathing abnormally rapid	g. Hyperventilation
_____	8. Decreased body temperature	h. Hypertension
_____	9. No respirations for several seconds	i. Vasodilation
_____	10. Rate of breathing abnormally slow	j. Febrile
_____	11. Normal breathing	k. Auscultatory gap
_____	12. Temporary disappearance of sounds between Korotkoff sounds	l. Eupnea

Complete the following:

13. Convert the following temperature readings:
    a. 97° F = _____° C
    b. 38.4° C = _____° F
    c. 102° F = _____° C
    d. 39.4° C = _____° F

14. What are the Fahrenheit and centigrade temperature readings that should alert the nurse to an alteration in the patient's temperature regulation?

15. Indicate on the model where the following pulses should be palpated:

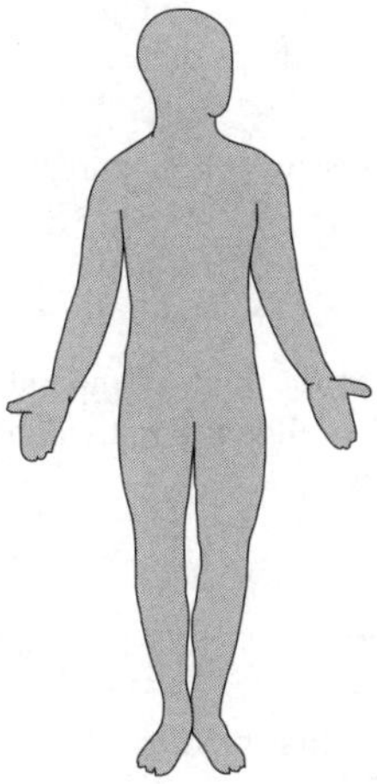

    a. Carotid
    b. Brachial
    c. Radial
    d. Apical
    e. Dorsalis pedis

16. Indicate on the aneroid scale where the following blood pressure reading would be noted:
    a. Korotkoff sounds first heard at 164 mm Hg and inaudible at 92 mm Hg

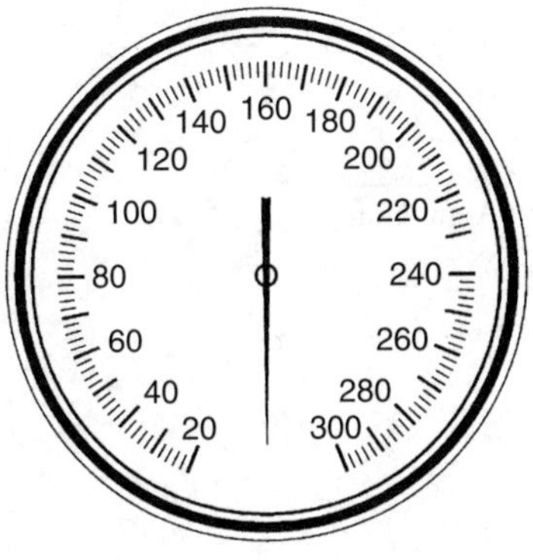

17. Vital sign measurements may not be delegated to unlicensed assistive personnel.
    True _____ False _____

18. Identify actions that will reduce body temperature in the following ways:
    a. Conduction:
    b. Convection:
    c. Evaporation:

19. A patient is on isolation precautions and temperature measurements are being used to monitor the status of the fever. The thermometer of choice in this situation is a(n):

20. A nurse identifies a pulse deficit. How was this assessed?

21. For a patient who has had a right mastectomy, the nurse should take the blood pressure:

22. Vital signs are usually recorded on the:

23. Decreasing hemoglobin levels will _______________ the respiratory rate.

24. To obtain arterial oxygen saturation for an adult patient, the pulse oximeter may be applied to:

25. The pulse pressure for a patient with a BP of 150/90 is:

26. Which of the following are correct for blood pressure measurement? Select all that apply.
    a. The cuff is 40% of the circumference of the limb being used. _____
    b. The bladder encircles 50% of the arm of an adult. _____
    c. The cuff is deflated at a rate of 2 to 3 mm Hg per second. _____
    d. The arm is kept below the level of the heart. _____
    e. The cuff is inflated to 30 mm Hg above the point where the pulse disappears. _____
    f. The systolic blood pressure is identified as the first onset of Korotkoff sounds. _____
    g. A difference of 30 mm Hg is expected between the left and right arm measurements. _____

27. A nurse is preparing to take the patient's oral temperature but discovers that he has just had a cup of coffee. The appropriate action is to:

28. Identify a situation when a patient's blood pressure may have to be palpated.

29. How are the following vital signs measured differently in children?
    a. Temperature:
    b. Blood pressure:

30. Which of the following are correct techniques for a tympanic temperature measurement? Select all that apply.
    a. Using the right ear if the patient has been lying on his/her left side in bed ______
    b. Pointing the probe midpoint between the eyebrows and sideburns for children younger than 3 years of age _____
    c. Pulling the ear pinna backward and down for an adult _____
    d. Moving the thermometer back and forth a little during the assessment _____
    e. Fitting the speculum tip loosely into the ear canal _____
    f. Waiting 2 to 3 minutes before repeating the measurement in the same ear _____

31. A patient's pulse is expected to be increased in the presence of which of the following factors? Select all that apply.
    a. Anxiety _____
    b. Hypothermia _____
    c. Unrelieved severe pain _____
    d. Asthma _____
    e. Hemorrhage _____
    f. Administration of beta blockers _____

32. What are the contraindications for the following temperature assessments?
    a. Axillary temperature
    b. Rectal temperature

33. End-tidal carbon dioxide ($ETCO_2$) values are used commonly for patients with:

34. For a blood pressure taken in the lower extremity:
    a. How should the patient be positioned?
    b. What artery is used for palpation?
    c. Is the reading expected to be higher or lower than the upper extremity?

35. Place the following steps for apical pulse measurement in the correct order:
    a. Count the rate for 1 minute. _____
    b. Replace the gown and position the patient for comfort. _____
    c. Locate anatomical landmarks. _____
    d. Place the diaphragm over the fifth intercostal space at the left midclavicular line. _____
    e. Warm the diaphragm in the hand for 5 to 10 seconds. _____
    f. Position the patient supine or sitting. _____

36. The danger of an increased temperature in young children is the potential for:

37. Provide three examples of antipyretic medications that may be ordered for a febrile patient.

38. How is orthostatic hypotension assessed?

39. Indicate the following for core temperature readings:
    a. Readings are invasive or noninvasive?
    b. Sites for core readings include:

40. What are the uses for the diaphragm and the bell of the stethoscope?

41. Indicate whether the body temperature is increased or decreased for the following individuals:
    a. Ovulating female
    b. Older adult

42. Indicate the correct techniques for pulse oximetry. Select all that apply.
    a. Recording the first reading after application of the probe _____
    b. Using the earlobe for a patient with tremors ______
    c. Applying the probe to the bridge of a toddler's nose _____
    d. Using fingers with acrylic nails, but no nail polish _____
    e. Expecting readings between 80% and 90% _____

43. How do the following influence respiration?
    a. Anxiety:
    b. Analgesic medications:
    c. Body position:

44. Which of the following can lead to hypotension? Select all that apply.
    a. Hemorrhage _____
    b. Stress _____
    c. Obesity _____
    d. Fluid deficit _____
    e. Cigarette smoking _____

Select the best answer for each of the following questions:

45. A nurse is working on a pediatric unit and assessing the vital signs of an infant admitted for gastroenteritis. The nurse expects that the vital signs are normally the following (BP is blood pressure in units of mm Hg, P is pulse rate in units of beats per minute, and R is respirations in units of breaths per minute):
    1. BP = 90/50, P = 122, R = 46
    2. BP = 90/60, P = 80, R = 20
    3. BP = 100/60, P = 140, R = 32
    4. BP = 110/50, P = 98, R = 40

46. While working in an extended care facility, a nurse expects the vital signs of an older adult patient to be:
    1. BP = 98/70, P = 60, R = 12
    2. BP = 120/60, P = 110, R = 30
    3. BP = 140/90, P = 74, R = 14
    4. BP = 150/100, P = 90, R = 25

47. A student nurse is taking vital signs for her assigned patients on the surgical unit. The student is aware that a patient's body temperature may be reduced after:
    1. exercise.
    2. emotional stress.
    3. periods of sleep.
    4. cigarette smoking.

48. While working in an emergency department, a nurse is carefully monitoring the vital signs of the patients who have been admitted. The nurse is alert to the potential for a decrease in a patient's pulse rate as a result of:
    1. hemorrhage.
    2. hypothyroidism.
    3. respiratory difficulty.
    4. epinephrine (adrenaline) administration.

49. A patient is being treated for hyperthermia. The nurse anticipates that the patient's response to this condition will be:
    1. generalized pallor.
    2. bradycardia.
    3. reduced thirst.
    4. diaphoresis.

50. Several friends have gone on a ski trip and have been exposed to very cold temperatures. One of the individuals appears to be slightly hypothermic. The best initial response by the nurse in the ski lodge is to give this individual:
    1. soup.
    2. coffee.
    3. brandy.
    4. warm cola.

51. When checking the temperature of a patient, a nurse notes that he is febrile. A nonsteroidal antipyretic medication is ordered. The nurse prepares to administer:
    1. digoxin.
    2. prednisone.
    3. theophylline.
    4. acetaminophen

52. A nurse has been assigned a number of different patients in the long-term care unit. When taking vital signs, the nurse is alert to the greater possibility of tachycardia for the patient with:
    1. anemia.
    2. hypothyroidism.
    3. a temperature of 95° F.
    4. a patient-controlled analgesic (PCA) pump with morphine drip.

53. While reviewing the vital signs taken by the aide this morning, a nurse notes that one of the patients is hypotensive. The nurse will be checking to see if the patient is experiencing:
    1. lightheadedness.
    2. a decreased heart rate.
    3. an increased urinary output.
    4. increased warmth to the skin.

54. Vital sign measurements have been completed on all assigned patients. The nurse will need to immediately report a finding of:
    1. pulse pressure of 40 mm Hg.
    2. apical pulses of 78, 80, 76 beats per minute.
    3. apical pulse of 82 beats per minute; radial pulse of 70 beats per minute.
    4. BP of 140/80 mm Hg left arm, 136/74 mm Hg right arm.

55. A nurse is preparing to take vital signs for the patients on the acute care unit. A tympanic temperature assessment is indicated for the patient:
    1. after rectal surgery.
    2. wearing a hearing aid.
    3. experiencing otitis media.
    4. after an exercise session.

56. Blood pressure monitoring is being conducted on a cardiac care unit. The nurse is determining whether an automatic blood pressure device is indicated for use. This device is selected for the patient with:
    1. an irregular heartbeat.
    2. Parkinson's disease.
    3. peripheral vascular disease.
    4. a systolic blood pressure greater than 140 mm/Hg.

57. A 34-year-old patient has gone to a physician's office for an annual physical examination. The nurse is completing the vital signs before the patient is seen by the physician. The nurse alerts the physician to a finding of:
    1. T: 37.6° C
    2. P: 120 beats per minute
    3. R: 18 breaths per minute
    4. BP: 116/78 mm Hg

58. A nurse is assigned to the well-child center that is affiliated with the acute care facility. A mother takes her 1½-year-old son to the center for his immunizations. The nurse assesses the child's pulse rate by checking the:
    1. radial artery.
    2. apical artery.
    3. popliteal artery.
    4. femoral artery.

59. A nurse determines that a patient's pulse rate is significantly lower than it has been during the past week. The nurse reassesses and finds that the pulse rate is still 46 beats per minute. The nurse should first:
    1. document the measurement.
    2. administer a stimulant medication.
    3. inform the charge nurse or physician.
    4. apply 100% oxygen at maximum flow rate.

60. The most important sign of heat stroke is:
    1. hot, dry skin.
    2. nausea.
    3. excessive thirst.
    4. muscle cramping.

61. The most accurate temperature measurement for an adult patient experiencing tachypnea and dyspnea is:
    1. oral.
    2. rectal.
    3. axillary.
    4. tympanic.

62. A nurse should insert a rectal thermometer into the adult patient:
    1. ¼ to ½ inch
    2. 1 to 1½ inches
    3. 1½ to 2 inches
    4. 2 to 2½ inches

63. A patient is determined to have an intermittent fever. This is supported by which of the following observations?
    1. A constant body temperature greater than 38° C (100.4° F)
    2. A fever that spikes and falls but does not return to normal
    3. Long periods of normal temperatures with febrile episodes
    4. Spikes in readings mixed with normal temperatures

64. Which of the following values indicates the correct pulse pressure for a patient with a blood pressure of 170/90?
    1. 80
    2. 170
    3. 260
    4. Value not known based on the information given

65. For a patient who is experiencing a febrile state, the nurse should:
    1. ambulate the patient frequently.
    2. restrict fluid intake.
    3. keep the patient warm.
    4. provide oxygen as ordered.

66. A nurse anticipates that bradycardia will be evident if a patient is:
    1. exercising.
    2. hypothermic.
    3. asthmatic.
    4. extremely anxious.

67. A nurse anticipates that a patient with hypertension will be receiving:
    1. diuretics.
    2. antipyretics.
    3. narcotic analgesics.
    4. anticholinergics.

68. To determine the arterial blood flow to a patient's feet, the nurse should assess the:
    1. radial artery.
    2. brachial artery.
    3. popliteal artery.
    4. dorsalis pedis artery.

69. A nurse anticipates an increase in blood pressure for the patient who is:
    1. sleeping.
    2. overweight.
    3. taking narcotics.
    4. hemorrhaging.

70. Prehypertension is classified as an average of repeated readings of:
    1. Systolic: 120 to 139 mm Hg; diastolic: 80 to 89 mm Hg
    2. Systolic: 140 to 159 mm Hg; diastolic: 90 to 99 mm Hg
    3. Systolic: 160 to 179 mm Hg; diastolic: 90 to 99 mm Hg
    4. Systolic: greater than 180 mm Hg; diastolic: greater than 100 mm Hg

STUDY GROUP QUESTIONS

- What are the guidelines for measurement of vital signs?
- When should vital signs be taken?
- How does the nurse determine what sites and equipment to use for measurement of vital signs?
- What body processes regulate temperature?
- What factors influence body temperature?
- How is the temperature measurement converted from centigrade to Fahrenheit and vice versa?
- What sites and equipment are used for temperature measurement?
- What nursing interventions are appropriate for increases and decreases in a patient's body temperature?
- What factors influence pulse rate?
- What sites may be used for pulse rate assessment?
- How should the stethoscope be used in pulse rate assessment?
- What changes may occur in the pulse rate and rhythm?
- What nursing interventions are appropriate for alterations in pulse rate?
- What is blood pressure?
- What factors may increase or decrease blood pressure?
- What are abnormal alterations in blood pressure?
- What equipment is used for blood pressure measurement?
- What nursing interventions are appropriate for increases and decreases in blood pressure?
- What body processes are involved in respiration?

- How are respirations assessed?
- What alterations may be noted in a patient's respirations?
- How does pulse oximetry function and what is its purpose?
- What are the procedures for assessment of temperature, pulse rate, respirations, blood pressure, and pulse oxygen saturation?
- What should be included in patient and family teaching for measurement and evaluation of vital signs?

STUDY CHART

Create a study chart to compare the *Vital Signs Across the Life Span* that identifies expected temperature, pulse rate, respiration, and blood pressure for each age group.

16 Health Assessment and Physical Examination

CASE STUDIES

1. You are assigned to assist with physical examinations in the outpatient clinic. On the schedule for today are three patients. One of the patients is a 72-year-old Hispanic woman, another is a 16-year-old girl, and the last is a 4-year-old boy.
   a. How can you assist each of these patients to feel more at ease before and during the physical examination?

2. A patient in the physician's office informs you that he is having trouble hearing when other people are speaking to him.
   a. What specific assessments will you perform on this patient?

3. You observe a lesion on the patient's abdomen that is draining fluid.
   a. What specific assessments should be made?
   b. How should you prepare to assess the lesion?

CHAPTER REVIEW

Match the description/definition in Column A with the correct term in Column B.

	Column A	*Column B*
_____	1. Black, tarry stools	a. Ptosis
_____	2. Fluid accumulation, swelling	b. Alopecia
_____	3. Loss of hair	c. Edema
_____	4. Drooping of eyelid over the pupil	d. Jaundice
_____	5. Tiny, pinpoint red spots on the skin	e. Bruit
_____	6. Curvature of the thoracic spine	f. Melena
_____	7. Yellow-orange discoloration	g. Kyphosis
_____	8. A hardened area	h. Petechiae
_____	9. Blowing, swishing sound in blood vessel	i. Erythema
_____	10. A red discoloration	j. Induration

Complete the following:

11. Identify the five skills used in physical assessment and briefly describe each.

12. Identify the following positions for physical examination.

a.

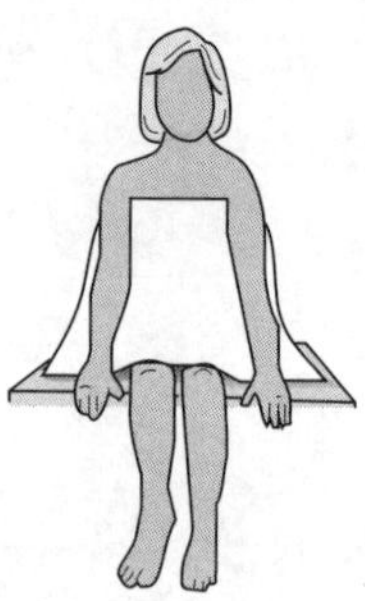

b.

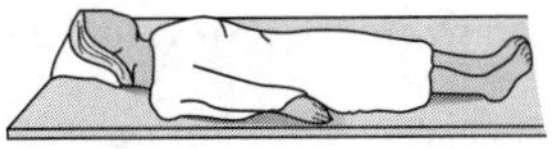

c.

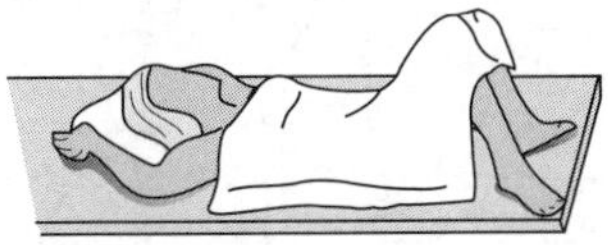

d.

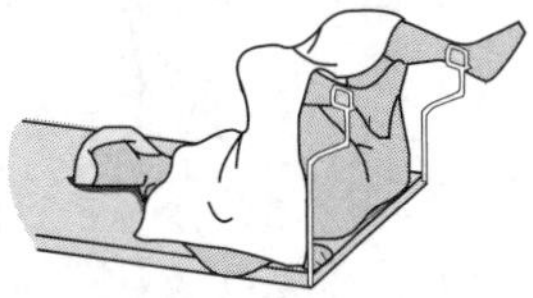

e.

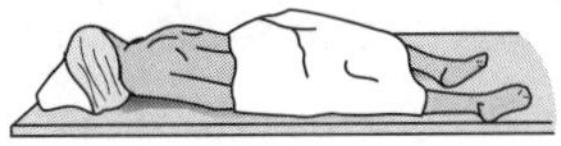

f.

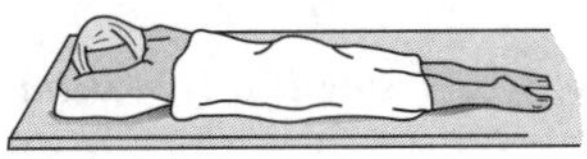

g.

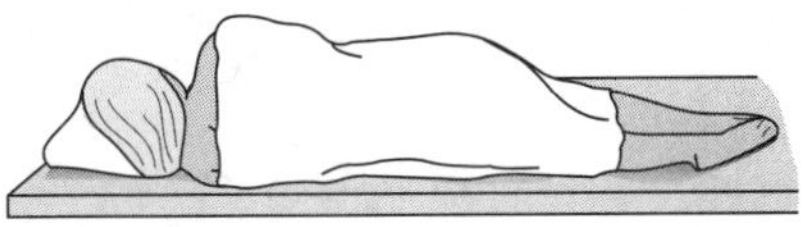

h.

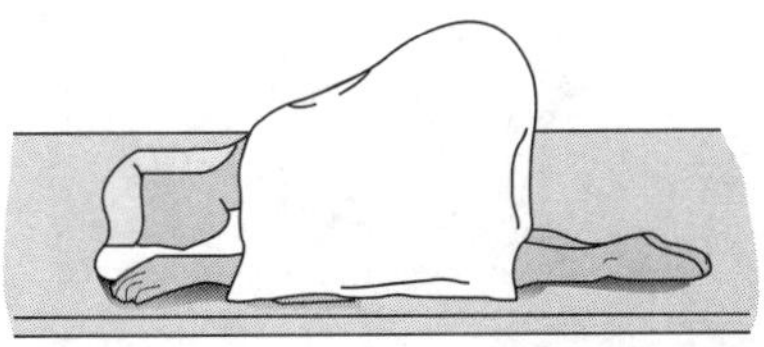

13. Identify which of the pulses is being palpated in each illustration.

a.

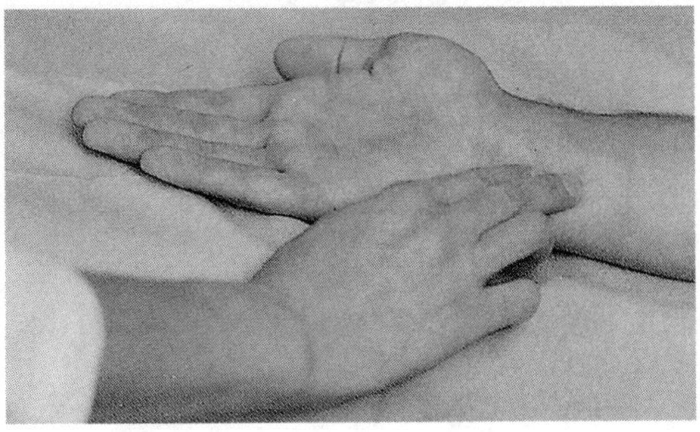

b.

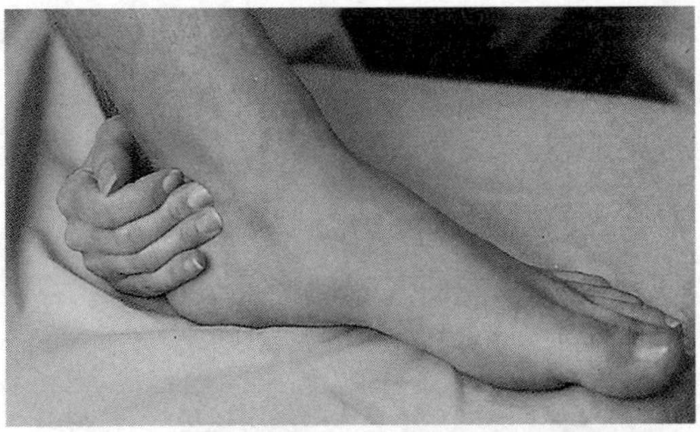

c.

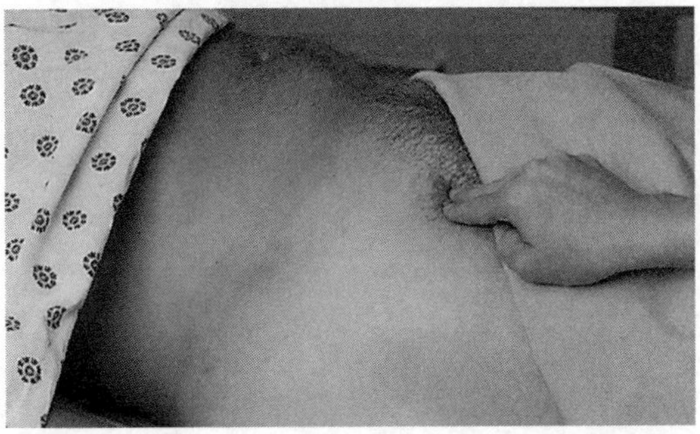

d.

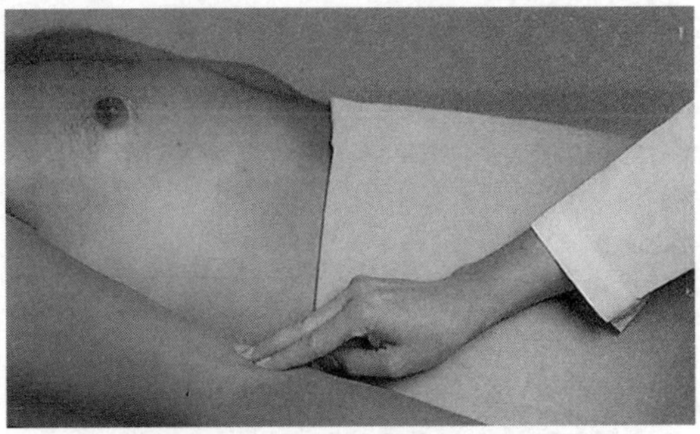

e.

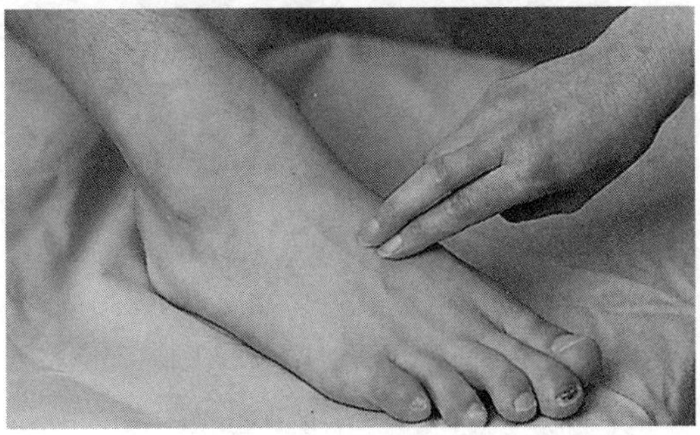

14. Correctly identify the primary skin lesion in each illustration.

a.

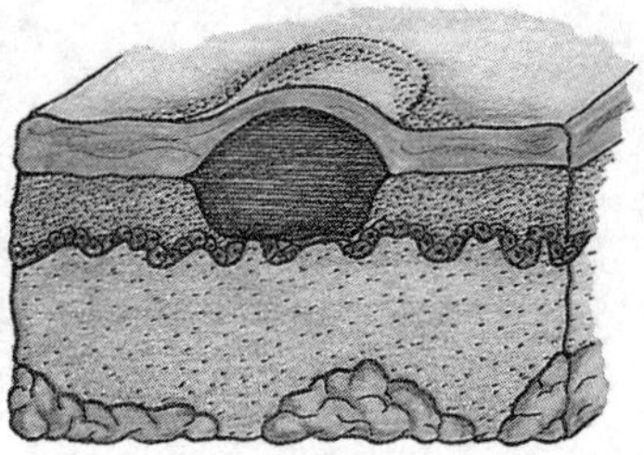

b.

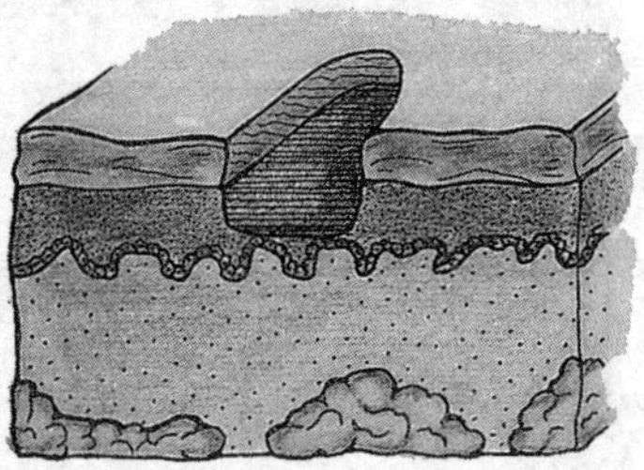

c.

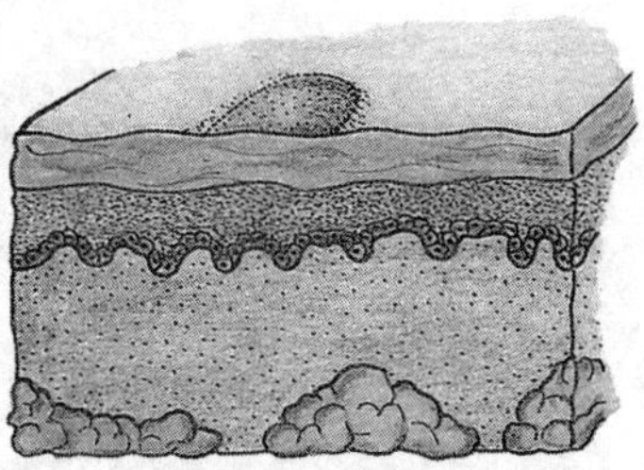

d.

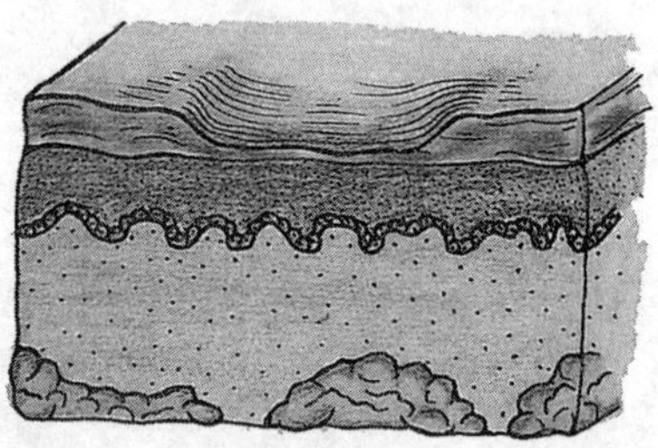

e.

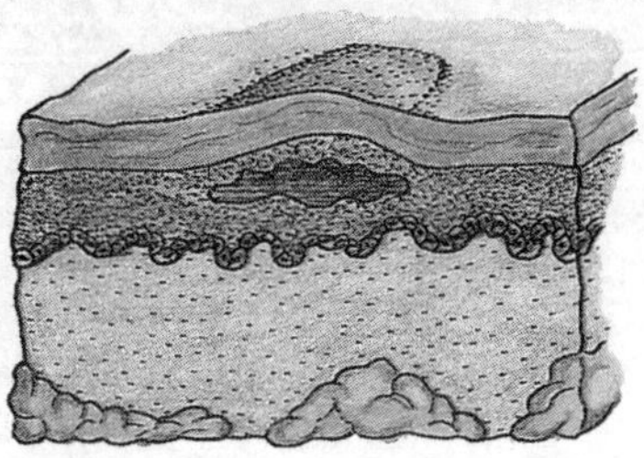

15. Identify on the illustration where the PMI is located.

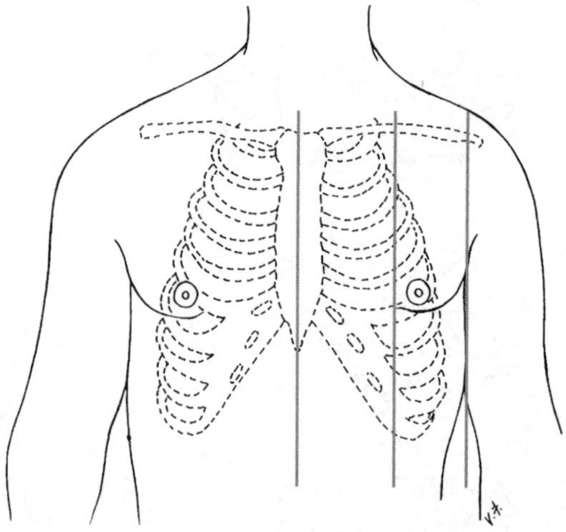

16. Identify a physical and a behavioral finding that may indicate abuse for the following:

	Physical	***Behavioral***
a. Child sexual abuse	______	______
b. Domestic abuse	______	______
c. Older adult abuse	______	______

17. Identify the abdominal structures that are assessed.

a.

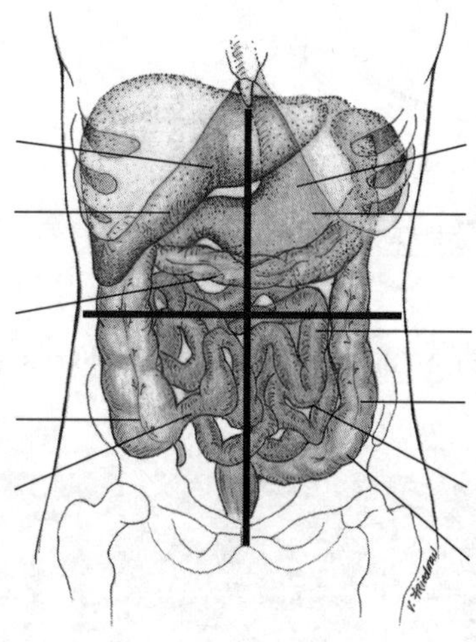

b.

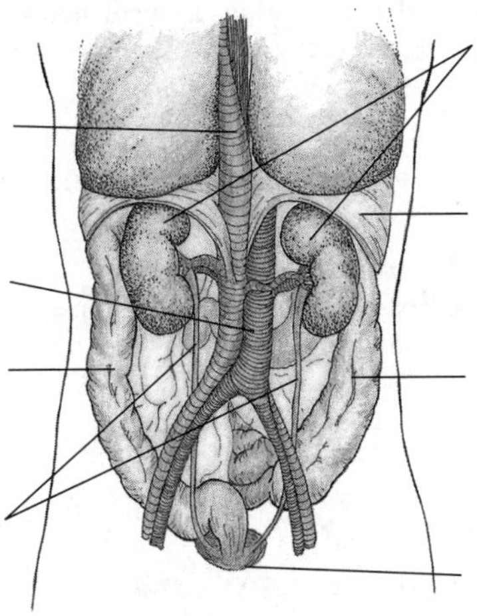

18. Mark each of the following physical assessment findings as either expected or unexpected. For unexpected findings, investigate what may be the possible etiology.

	Expected	*Unexpected*
a. Skin lifts easily and snaps back	______	______
b. Erythema noted over bony prominences	______	______
c. Hair evenly distributed over scalp and pubic area	______	______
d. Brown pigmentation of nails in longitudinal streaks (dark-skinned patient)	______	______
e. Pallor in face and nail beds	______	______
f. Clubbing of nails	______	______
g. PEERLA	______	______
h. Pupils cloudy	______	______
i. Yellow discoloration of sclera	______	______
j. Eardrum translucent, shiny, and pearly gray	______	______
k. Light brown or gray cerumen	______	______
l. Nasal septum midline	______	______
m. Nasal mucosa pale with clear, watery discharge	______	______
n. Sinuses tender to touch	______	______
o. Teeth chalky white, with black discoloration	______	______
p. Tongue medium red, moist, and slightly rough on top	______	______
q. Soft palate rises when patient says "ah"	______	______
r. Uvula reddened and edematous, tonsils with yellow exudate	______	______
s. Thyroid gland small, smooth, and free of nodules	______	______
t. Lungs resonant to percussion	______	______
u. Costal angle greater than 90 degrees between costal margins	______	______
v. Bulging of intercostal spaces	______	______
w. No carotid bruit present	______	______
x. Extra heart sound noted	______	______
y. Jugular vein distention at 45-degree angle	______	______
z. Dependent edema in ankles	______	______
aa. Female breasts smooth, symmetrical, without retraction	______	______
bb. Soft, well-differentiated, moveable lumps in the breasts noted	______	______
cc. Bowel sounds active and audible in all four quadrants	______	______
dd. Bulging flanks	______	______
ee. Flat or concave umbilicus	______	______
ff. Rebound tenderness found	______	______
gg. Perineal skin smooth and slightly darker than surrounding skin	______	______
hh. Bartholin glands palpable with discharge evident	______	______
ii. Glans penis smooth and pink on all surfaces	______	______
jj. Testes smooth and ovoid	______	______
kk. No crepitus found on range of motion	______	______
ll. Hips and shoulders aligned parallel	______	______
mm. Lordosis of spine noted	______	______
nn. Reflexes symmetrical	______	______
oo. Able to recall past events, unable to repeat series of five numbers	______	______
pp. Able to perform rapidly alternating movements	______	______

19. A patient has an area of discomfort. The nurse will examine this area:
    1. first.
    2. last.

20. When using the stethoscope, high-pitched sounds are heard best with a:
    1. diaphragm.
    2. bell.

21. To inspect an adult patient's ear canal, the nurse pulls the auricle:
    1. up and back.
    2. down and back.

22. The position to place the patient in for a genital examination is:

23. The position to place the patient in for an abdominal examination is:

24. Identify what a nurse is able to assess in a general survey of a patient:

25. A weight gain of 5 lb or 2.2 kg/day indicates:

26. What techniques are appropriate when assessing patients of different ages? Select all that apply.
    a. Speaking privately with adolescents about their concerns _____
    b. Using closed-ended questions to increase the speed of the examination _____
    c. Calling children and their parents by their first names _____
    d. Providing time for children to play _____
    e. Performing the examination for an older adult near bathroom facilities _____
    f. Proceeding rapidly through the examination of an older adult to finish it as quickly as possible _____

27. Patients older than 65 years should be instructed to have yearly eye examinations.
    True _____ False _____

28. A nurse is preparing to perform a skin assessment for an average adult patient. Select all of the following techniques that are correct:
    a. Using fluorescent lighting _____
    b. Keeping the room very warm _____
    c. Using disposable gloves to inspect lesions _____
    d. Looking for coloration changes by checking the tongue and nail beds _____

29. During a physical examination, a nurse notes that the patient appears to be very anxious. The nurse should:

30. One example of a test for colorectal cancer is:

31. Select the three best positions that a patient may be placed in for a cardiac assessment:
    a. Prone _____
    b. Supine _____
    c. Lithotomy _____
    d. Sitting _____
    e. Left lateral recumbent _____
    f. Dorsal recumbent _____
    g. Sims _____

32. Identify signs and symptoms that a patient may have if he or she has cardiopulmonary disease.

33. What are the risk factors associated with osteoporosis? Select all that apply.
    a. An active lifestyle _____
    b. Smoking _____
    c. African American background _____
    d. A history of falls _____
    e. A history of Cushing disease _____
    f. Exposure to sunlight _____
    g. A thin, light body frame _____

34. Identify at least two techniques that are used in assessment of the lymph nodes:

35. Continuous dilation of the pupils is found with the patient experiencing:

36. An expected response when testing the pupils for accommodation is:

37. What is used to weigh the following patients?
    a. Newborn infant
    b. Mobile adult

38. The primary nurse tells the student that the patient is experiencing tinnitus. The student expects that the patient will describe:

39. Three possible causes of hearing loss are:

40. To assess for a pulse deficit, the nurse should:

41. An irregular pulse is counted for ______ seconds.

42. Identify all of the risk factors for breast cancer. Select all that apply.
   a. Under 40 years old _____
   b. Recent use of oral contraceptives _____
   c. Late onset menarche _____
   d. Family history _____
   e. Childless _____

43. The nurse is preparing to do an assessment of the abdomen.
   a. The correct sequence for the abdominal exam is:
   b. Bowel sounds usually occur _____/minute.
   c. What finding is expected for the patient with ascites?
   d. Absent bowel sounds can result from:

44. When teaching the patient about the signs and symptoms of prostate cancer, the nurse should include what information?

45. How can the nurse test recent and past memory?

46. A patient is suspected of substance abuse. What physical findings would be found on the skin? Select all that apply.
   a. Loss of pigment _____
   b. Spider angiomas _____
   c. Hematomas _____
   d. Red, dry areas _____
   e. Burns on the fingers _____
   f. Irregularly shaped moles _____

Select the best answer for each of the following questions:

47. A nurse is assessing a patient's nail beds. An expected finding is indicated by:
   1. softening of the nail bed.
   2. a concave curve to the nail.
   3. brown, linear streaks in the nail bed.
   4. a 160-degree angle between the nail plate and nail.

48. A young adult woman arrives at the family planning center for a physical examination. For this patient with mature breasts, the nurse expects to find that the:
   1. breast tissue is softer.
   2. nipples project and areolae have receded.
   3. areolae are dark and have increased diameter.
   4. breasts are elongated and nipples are smaller and flatter.

49. A nurse has checked the medical record and found that a patient has anemia. The presence of anemia is accompanied by the nurse's finding of:
   1. pallor.
   2. erythema.
   3. jaundice.
   4. cyanosis.

50. A patient with asthma has gone to an urgent care center for treatment. On auscultation of the lungs, a nurse hears rhonchi. These sounds are described as:
   1. dry and grating.
   2. loud, low-pitched, and coarse.
   3. high-pitched, fine, and short.
   4. high-pitched and musical.

51. A patient is admitted to a medical center with a peripheral vascular problem. A nurse is performing the initial assessment of the patient. While assessing the lower extremities, the nurse is alert to venous insufficiency as indicated by:
   1. marked edema.
   2. thin, shiny skin.
   3. coolness to touch.
   4. dusky red coloration.

52. A nurse is performing a complete neurological assessment on a patient after a cerebrovascular accident (CVA/stroke). To assess cranial nerve III, the nurse:
   1. uses the Snellen chart.
   2. lightly touches the cornea with a wisp of cotton.
   3. whispers into one ear at a time.
   4. measures pupil reaction to light and accommodation.

53. Student nurses are practicing neurological assessment and determination of cranial nerve functioning. To assess cranial nerve X, the student nurse should ask the patient to:
   1. say "ah."
   2. shrug the shoulders.
   3. smile and frown.
   4. stick out the tongue.

54. While completing a physical examination, a nurse assesses and reports that a patient has petechiae. The nurse has found:
   1. light perspiration on the skin.
   2. moles with regular edges.
   3. thickness on the soles of the feet.
   4. pinpoint-size, flat, red spots.

55. A nurse reviews a chart and sees that a patient who has been admitted to the unit this morning has a hyperthyroid disorder. The nurse anticipates that an examination of the eyes will reveal:
   1. diplopia.
   2. strabismus.
   3. exophthalmos.
   4. nystagmus.

56. In preparation for an examination of the internal ear, a nurse anticipates that the color of the eardrum should appear:
   1. white.
   2. yellow.
   3. slightly red.
   4. pearly gray.

57. A patient with a history of smoking and alcohol abuse has gone to a clinic for a physical examination. Based on this history, the nurse is particularly alert during an examination of the oral cavity to the presence of:
    1. spongy gums.
    2. pink tissue.
    3. thick, white patches.
    4. loose teeth.

58. A patient in a physician's office has an increased antero-posterior diameter of the chest. The nurse should inquire specifically about the patient's history of:
    1. smoking.
    2. thoracic trauma.
    3. spinal surgery.
    4. exposure to tuberculosis.

59. When auscultating a patient's chest, a nurse hears what appears to be an S3 sound. This is an expected finding if the patient is:
    1. 10 years old.
    2. 35 years old.
    3. 56 years old.
    4. 82 years old.

60. A patient in a medical center has been prescribed bed rest for a prolonged period of time. There is a possibility that the patient may have developed phlebitis. The nurse assesses for the presence of this condition by:
    1. palpating the ankles for pitting edema.
    2. checking the popliteal pulses bilaterally.
    3. inspecting the thighs for clusters of ecchymosis.
    4. checking the appearance and circumference of the lower legs.

61. When teaching a 45-year-old patient in the gynecologist's office about breast cancer, a nurse includes information on recommendations for screening. The patient is informed that a woman her age should have:
    1. annual mammograms.
    2. biannual CT scans.
    3. physical examinations every 3 years.
    4. breast self-examinations every 3 months.

62. A patient has been experiencing some lightheadedness and loss of balance over the past few weeks. A nurse wants to check the patient's balance while waiting for the patient to have other laboratory tests. The nurse administers the:
    1. Allen test.
    2. Rinne test.
    3. Weber test.
    4. Romberg test.

63. Screenings are being conducted at the junior high school for scoliosis. A nurse is observing the students for the presence of:
    1. an S-shaped curvature of the spine.
    2. an exaggerated curvature of the thoracic spine.
    3. an exaggerated curvature of the lumbar spine.
    4. a bulging of the cervical vertebrae and disks.

64. While reviewing a medical record, a nurse notes that a patient has suspected pancreatitis. The nurse assesses the patient for:
    1. positive rebound tenderness.
    2. midline abdominal pulsations.
    3. hyperactive bowel sounds in all quadrants.
    4. bulging of the flanks with dependent distention.

65. An 80-year-old woman is being assessed by a nurse in an extended care facility. The nurse is assessing the genitalia of this patient and suspects that there may be a malignancy present. The nurse's suspicion is due to the finding of:
    1. scaly, nodular lesions.
    2. yellow exudates and redness.
    3. small ulcers with serous drainage.
    4. extreme pallor and edema.

66. A screening for osteoporosis is being conducted at an annual health fair. To determine the risk factors for osteoporosis, a nurse is assessing individuals for:
    1. multiparity.
    2. a heavier than recommended body frame.
    3. an African American background.
    4. a history of dieting and/or alcohol abuse.

67. A patient in a rehabilitation facility has experienced a cerebrovascular accident (CVA/stroke) that has left the patient with an expressive aphasia. The nurse anticipates that this patient will:
    1. be unable to speak or write.
    2. be unable to follow directions.
    3. respond inappropriately to questions.
    4. have difficulty interpreting words and phrases.

68. To assess a patient's visual fields, a nurse should:
    1. ask the patient to read text.
    2. turn the room light on and off.
    3. move a finger at arm's length toward the patient from an angle.
    4. shine a penlight into the patient's eye at an oblique angle.

69. A nurse exerts downward pressure on the thigh. This assessment is determining the muscle strength of the:
    1. triceps.
    2. trapezius.
    3. quadriceps.
    4. gastrocnemius.

70. Light palpation involves depressing the part being examined:
    1. ½ inch.
    2. 1 inch.
    3. 1½ inches.
    4. 2 inches.

71. A nurse teaches the male patient that he should notify a health care provider if he finds the following during a testicular self-examination:
    1. loose, deeper color scrotal skin with a coarse surface.
    2. cordlike structures on the top of the testicles.
    3. small, pea-sized lumps on the front of the testicle.
    4. smegma under the foreskin.

72. A nurse manager observes a new nurse on the unit performing a patient assessment. The new nurse's assessment should be interrupted if the manager observes the nurse:
    1. using the pads of the first three fingers to palpate the breast tissue.
    2. auscultating the abdomen continuously for 5 minutes.
    3. palpating both carotid arteries simultaneously.
    4. testing sensory function on random locations with the patient's eyes closed.

73. A nurse assesses a patient's skin and documents that vesicles are present. This observation is based on the nurse finding:
    1. flat, nonpalpable changes in skin color.
    2. palpable, solid elevations smaller than 1 cm.
    3. irregularly shaped, elevated areas that vary in size.
    4. circumscribed elevations of skin filled with serous fluid.

74. A nurse is assessing a patient's level of consciousness using the Glasgow Coma Scale. The following findings are documented: Eyes open to speech, responses are oriented, localized pain is noted. The score for this patient is:
    1. 15.
    2. 13.
    3. 11.
    4. 9.

75. To assess the temperature of the patient's skin, the nurse should use the:
    1. thumbs.
    2. fingertips.
    3. palm of the hand.
    4. dorsal surface of the hand.

76. The patient needs to sit upright to breathe easier. This is recorded by the nurse as:
    1. apnea.
    2. dyspnea.
    3. orthopnea.
    4. tachypnea.

STUDY GROUP QUESTIONS

- What are the purposes of the physical examination?
- How is physical assessment integrated into patient care?
- How does a nurse incorporate cultural sensitivity and awareness of ethnic physiological differences into the physical examination?
- What are the physical assessment skills, and what information is obtained through their use?
- How does a nurse prepare a patient and environment for a physical examination?
- What similarities and differences exist in the preparation and procedure for a physical examination of a child, adult, and older adult?
- What information is obtained through a general survey?
- What positions and equipment are used for completion of the physical examination?
- What is the usual sequence for performing the physical examination?
- What are the expected and unexpected findings of a complete physical examination?
- What self-screening procedures may be taught to patients?
- How does a nurse report and record the findings of a physical examination?

STUDY CHART

Create a study chart to compare the *Expected vs. Unexpected Findings in a Physical Examination,* working in sequential order of the exam from the integumentary system through the neurological system.

17 Administering Medications

CASE STUDIES

1. You are visiting a patient at home who has poor eyesight and occasional forgetfulness. The patient has four oral medications to take at different times of the day. He tells you that he doesn't think that he can remember to take them all and that he can't remember what information he was given by the prescriber.
   a. What strategies may be implemented to assist this patient in maintaining the medication regimen?

2. You are preparing to give medications to the patient in the long-term care facility, but the prescriber's handwriting is difficult to read.
   a. What should you do to prevent medication errors?

3. A patient in a long-term care facility is about to receive her medications, but you notice that she does not have an identification band.
   a. What is the appropriate next action?

4. You are going to administer an injection to a 6-year-old child on a pediatric acute care unit.
   a. What safety measures should you implement?

5. The patient has just received an immunization and appears to be having an anaphylactic reaction.
   a. What treatments are anticipated?

6. You are about to prepare a narcotic medication for administration to a patient. The record shows that 24 tablets should remain in the box but there are only 23 tablets left.
   a. What should you do?

7. You are caring for a patient who requires an antipyretic medication that is ordered for oral administration, but the patient has been experiencing severe nausea.
   a. What are your actions?

CHAPTER REVIEW

Match the description/definition in Column A with the correct term in Column B.

	Column A	*Column B*
_____	1. Placing medication under the tongue	a. Parenteral administration
_____	2. The effect of two medications combined is greater than each given separately	b. Inhalation
_____	3. Secondary effects of medication, such as nausea	c. Instillation
_____	4. Unpredictable effect of medications	d. Buccal
_____	5. Fluid administered and retained in a body cavity	e. Subcutaneous
_____	6. Injection into tissues below the dermis of the skin	f. Intraocular
_____	7. Severe allergic response characterized by bronchospasm and laryngeal edema	g. Idiosyncratic reaction
_____	8. Inserting medication into the eye	h. Polypharmacy
_____	9. Administering medications through the oral, nasal, or pulmonary passages	i. Sublingual
_____	10. Patient taking many medications	j. Synergistic effect
_____	11. Placing solid medication against the mucous membranes of the cheek	k. Side effects
_____	12. Injecting medication into body tissues	l. Anaphylactic reaction

Complete the following:

13. Provide an example of how a nurse's professional responsibility in administering medications is controlled or regulated.

14. a. Identify a strategy for a nurse to implement to avoid errors with medications that appear the same.

    b. Specify two acceptable patient identifiers.

15. Provide an example of how each of the following factors can influence the actions of medications.
    a. Dietary factors
    b. Physiological variables
    c. Environmental conditions

16. Identify the four routes for parenteral administration of medications.

17. For the following medication orders, identify the essential component that is missing. (Note: All have been correctly signed by the prescriber.)
    a. Apresoline IM stat
    b. Morphine sulfate 10 mg q3-4h
    c. Vancomycin 1 g IV
    d. Lasix 40 mg bid

18. Identify the six guidelines or "rights" that a nurse uses for administering medications.

    1. ____________________
    2. ____________________
    3. ____________________
    4. ____________________
    5. ____________________
    6. ____________________

19. Place the following steps in the correct sequence for removing medication from a vial for an IM injection.
    a. Select the correct needle and syringe. _____
    b. Dislodge air bubbles. _____
    c. Insert the needle through the rubber seal of the vial. _____
    d. Remove the syringe from the vial. _____
    e. Perform hand hygiene. _____
    f. Inject the air in the syringe into the air space in the vial. _____
    g. Remove the needle cap. _____
    h. Pull back on the plunger of the syringe and withdraw air equal to the volume of medication to be administered. _____
    i. Invert the vial and fill the syringe to the correct volume of medication. _____
    j. Remove the cap from the vial. _____

20. Identify the form of medication for the following.
    a. Solid dose form for oral use; medication in a powder, liquid, or oil form and encased by a gelatin shell:
    b. Solid dose form mixed with gelatin and shaped in form of pellet for insertion into body cavity:
    c. Clear liquid containing water and/or alcohol; designed for oral use; usually has a sweetener added:
    d. Finely divided drug particles dispersed in a liquid medium; when the liquid is left standing, particles settle to the bottom of the container:
    e. Semiliquid suspension used to cool, protect, or clean the skin:

21. An example of a commonly abused over-the-counter medication is:

22. Adherence to medication therapy:
    a. Noncompliance with or nonadherence to medication therapy may be related to:
    b. Identify at least one strategy to promote medication adherence.

23. MedWatch is a ______________________________.

24. For each of the following pairs, identify which of the two has the faster absorption or action in the body:

a.	IV _____	or	Oral _____
b.	IM _____	or	Subcutaneous _____
c.	Acidic oral medication _____	or	Alkaline oral medication _____
d.	Tablets _____	or	Solutions _____
e.	Large surface area _____	or	Smaller surface area _____
f.	Less lipid soluble _____	or	Highly lipid soluble _____
g.	Albumin binding _____	or	Nonalbumin binding _____

25. The time that it takes for a medication to reach its highest effective concentration is its:

26. Oral medication is contraindicated for a patient with:

27. What is a potential problem with this medication order? Lasix 40.0 mg

28. Identify the appropriate equivalents for the following:
    a. 1 mL = _____ gtt
    b. 60 mL = _____ ounces
    c. _____ L = 1 quart
    d. 3 g = _____ mg
    e. 0.25 L = _____ mL
    f. _____ mL = 1 teaspoon

29. Identify the five different types of medication orders and provide an example of each:
    1.
    2.
    3.
    4.
    5.

30. Verbal orders are usually required to be signed by the prescriber within what time frame?

31. A nurse calculates the medication order and determines that six tablets should be given to the patient for each dose. What should the nurse do first?

32. Describe the difference between an adverse and a side effect.

33. After a patient is given medications, the patient tells the nurse that the medicine looks different from the previous administrations of the medication. The nurse should:

34. Identify the correct techniques for medication administration. Select all that apply.
    a. Discard the patient's unopened unit-dose medication that was refused. _____
    b. Crush medication and mix it in a large amount of food to mask the taste. _____
    c. Note in the record if a patient refuses a medication. _____
    d. Record medications before administration. _____
    e. Give another nurse's medications to the patient. _____
    f. Administer non-time-critical medications within 1 to 2 hours of the scheduled time. _____
    g. Aspirate when giving immunizations. _____
    h. Document the patient's response in the record. _____

35. Identify the generic names for the following drugs:
    a. Levaquin
    b. Lasix
    c. Advil
    d. Haldol

36. A triple check to compare the medication label to the order should be done:
    1.
    2.
    3.

37. Identify a technique that may be used to facilitate administration of medications to children.
    a. Oral medications:
    b. Injections:

38. Identify a way that a nurse may minimize the discomfort of an injection.

39. How should a medication that is irritating to the tissues be injected?

40. Identify the correct angle for each of the following illustrations and the type of injection that is being administered.
    a. _________ b. _________ c. _________

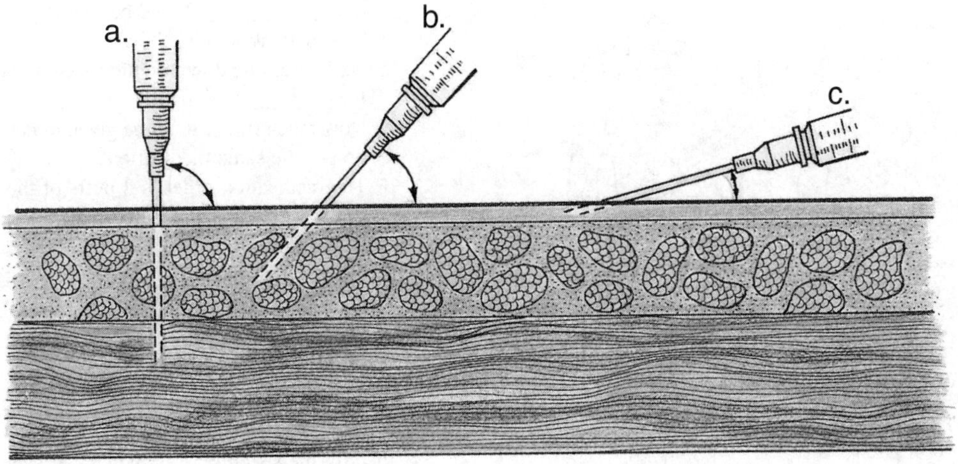

41. Identify three ways in which medication may be administered intravenously.
    a.
    b.
    c.

42. A wireless barcode scanner is usually used to identify:
    a.
    b.
    c.

43. Identify the meaning of the following abbreviations.
    a. ac: ____________________
    b. bid: ____________________
    c. prn: ____________________
    d. q4h: ____________________
    e. stat: ____________________

44. Check the orders and calculate the correct dosages for the following medication orders.
    a. Prescriber's order: Synthroid 0.15 mg PO daily
       In stock: Split tablets in a container labeled 75 mcg
       How many tablets should be given?
    b. Prescriber's order: Prilosec 40 mg PO bid
       In stock: Prilosec 20 mg tablets
       How much of the medication should be given?
    c. Prescriber's order: Lasix 20 mg IM stat
       In stock: Lasix 10 mg/mL
       How much medication should be given?
    d. Prescriber's order: hydrocortisone succinate 200 mg/day in two equal doses
       In stock: hydrocortisone succinate 50 mg/mL
       How much medication should be given for each dose?
       Mark the amount to be administered on the syringe.

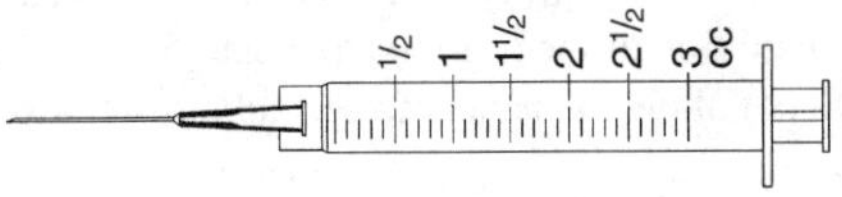

    e. Prescriber's order: regular insulin 24 units
       In stock: regular insulin U-100
       How much medication should be administered?
       Mark the amount to be administered on the syringe.

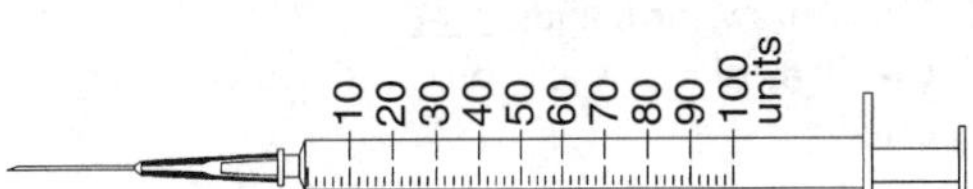

    f. Prescriber's order: cefazolin 500 mg q8h
       In stock: Keflex 250 mg tablets
       How many tablets should be given?
    g. The medication is mixed in 50 mL of fluid in a volume-controlled set and will be infused with a minidrip over 1 hour.
       The nurse sets the rate to infuse at: _______ drops/minute

45. Identify an area of patient assessment before administration of a parenteral injection.

46. Identify on the figure the sites recommended for subcutaneous injections.

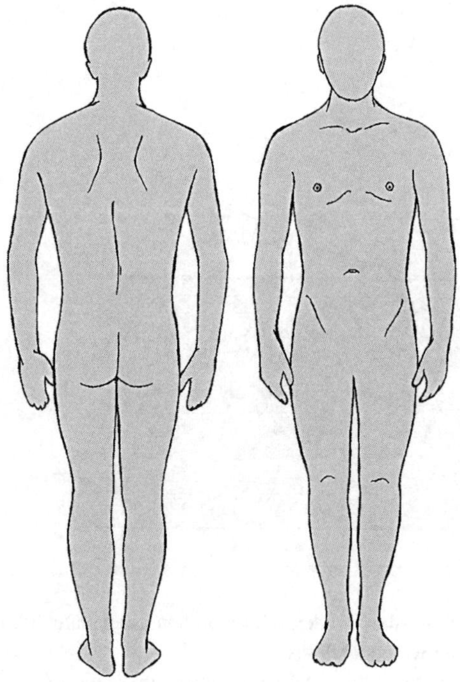

47. Select all of the following actions that are correct for the administration of medications to a patient with dysphagia.
    a. Do not allow the patient to self-administer, even if able. _____
    b. Position the patient upright. _____
    c. Turn the patient's head toward the weaker side to help the patient swallow. _____
    d. Use thinner liquids for the patient to take with the medications. _____
    e. Use a straw for liquids. _____
    f. Crush medication and mix with pureed food, if indicated. _____

48. For medication administration through an enteral/nasogastric tube:
    a. A priority assessment specifically for the patient receiving medication through a nasogastric tube is for the nurse to:
    b. The tube should be flushed with _________ mL of ___________________ in between each medication, and flushed after all medications are given with _________ mL.

49. Before administration of a topical, the nurse needs to:

50. Identify the following for the administration of ear drops:
    a. Position the patient:
    b. Pull ear pinna ________ for an adult patient.
    c. Irrigate with _____ mL of ________ temperature fluid.

51. For the use of a pressured metered-dose inhaler (pMDI):
    a. When the patient has difficulty coordinating the inhaler, a(n) __________ should be used.
    b. The patient should inhale for __________ seconds while pressing down on the canister and hold the breath for __________ seconds.
    c. How much time should be given in between administration of the same medication?
    d. The medication order is 2 puffs of the inhaler qid. The canister contains 160 puffs total.
    How many days will the canister last? _____________
    e. After the administration of a corticosteroid inhalation, the patient should:

52. The patient should be placed in ________________ position for the administration of a rectal suppository.

53. Identify the specific assessments that should be completed before administration of the following types of medications:
    a. Anticoagulant
    b. Antihypertensive
    c. Analgesic
    d. Cardiotonic

54. Eye drops should be administered directly onto the cornea.
    True _____ False _____

55. From the following, identify the guidelines that are appropriate for pediatric medication administration. Select all that apply.
    a. Identify the dosage based on the child's weight in pounds. _____
    b. Pediatric doses are usually given in micrograms and small syringes. _____
    c. IM doses are very small and usually do not exceed 1 mL in small children. _____
    d. Most medications are rounded to the nearest tenth. _____
    e. Mentally estimate a patient's dose before beginning the calculation, comparing the answer with the estimate before preparing the medication. _____
    f. Dosage ranges for 24-hour periods are similar to adult dosages. _____

56. Identify the correct sequence of actions for a saline flush.
   a. Pulling back gently on syringe plunger and checking for blood return _____
   b. Cleaning the lock's injection port with antiseptic swab _____
   c. Flushing the IV site with normal saline by pushing slowly on plunger _____
   d. Removing the saline-filled syringe _____
   e. Preparing two syringes filled with 2 to 3 mL of normal saline (0.9%) _____
   f. Inserting the syringe with normal saline 0.9% through injection port of IV lock _____

57. A nurse is responsible for administering an incorrect medication or dosage.
   True _____ False _____

58. For IV push or bolus medication administration:
   a. The medication should be infused at a rate of 2 mL over 2 minutes; this is how many milliliters (mL) every 30 seconds? ____________________.
   b. If the medication is incompatible with the IV fluid that is infusing, the nurse should:

59. Identify the site that may be used for an intradermal injection.

60. A tuberculin test has been administered.
   a. Results should be read in __________ hours.
   b. A positive test for an individual with no known risk factors is: ________________.

61. The patient is to receive a vaginal cream medication.
   a. The preferred position is: ____________________.
   b. The applicator is inserted: ________________ cm or ________________ in.

62. Provide examples of positive and negative synergistic effects.

63. An advantage of computerized physician order entry to medications is:

64. When do medication orders have to be rewritten by the prescriber?

65. What safety measures are used when withdrawing medication from an ampule?

66. The patient needs to have multiple subcutaneous injections. The basic rule for site rotation is to:

67. Place the steps for administration of an oral medication in the correct order.
   a. Label the medication. _____
   b. Compare the medication with the MAR. _____
   c. Identify the patient. _____
   d. Pour the liquid from the bottle into the cup. _____
   e. Perform hand hygiene. _____
   f. Compare the prepared medication with the MAR. _____
   g. Obtain the medication from the patient's drawer. _____

68. Identify the four (4) pharmacokinetic processes and an example of how each may be influenced.
   a.
   b.
   c.
   d.

Select the best answer for each of the following questions:

69. A nurse determines the location for an injection by identifying the greater trochanter of the femur, anterosuperior iliac spine, and iliac crest. The injection site being used by the nurse is the:
   1. rectus femoris muscle.
   2. ventrogluteal area.
   3. dorsogluteal area.
   4. vastus lateralis muscle.

70. Upon receiving the assignment for the evening, a nurse notices that two of the patients have the same name. The best way to identify two patients on a medical unit who have the same name is to:
   1. ask the patients their names.
   2. verify their names with the family members.
   3. check the patients' ID bands.
   4. ask another nurse about their identities.

71. A nurse is to administer a subcutaneous injection to an average-size adult. The nurse selects a:
   1. 27-gauge, ½-inch needle and 0.5-mL syringe.
   2. 25-gauge, ⅝-inch needle and 1-mL syringe.
   3. 22-gauge, 1-inch needle and 3-mL syringe.
   4. 20-gauge, 1-inch needle and 3-mL syringe.

72. A nurse has administered medications to all assigned patients on the medical unit. Upon assessing the response of the medications given, the nurse is alert to the possibility of a toxic reaction. This is indicated by the patient experiencing:
   1. itching.
   2. nausea.
   3. dizziness.
   4. respiratory depression.

73. The nursing staff is completing a review of the procedures used for the storage and administration of narcotics. A nurse implements the required procedure when:
    1. narcotics are kept together with the patient's other medications.
    2. small amounts of medication may be discarded without notation.
    3. the narcotic count is checked daily by the medication nurse.
    4. a separate administration record is kept in addition to the patient's medication administration record (MAR).

74. An order is written for a patient to receive potassium chloride (KCl) and vitamins intravenously. The nurse expects that this medication will be given via a(n):
    1. IV bolus administration.
    2. tandem administration.
    3. piggyback administration.
    4. large-volume administration.

75. While completing an admission assessment, a nurse discovers that a patient is allergic to shellfish. Later that morning when the nurse is preparing medications for this patient, the nurse will withhold medication that contains:
    1. iodine.
    2. alcohol.
    3. glucose.
    4. calcium carbonate.

76. A patient in a nurse practitioner's office is receiving penicillin for the first time. The nurse asks the patient to wait in the office after the administration of the medication. The nurse is observing for a possible anaphylactic response that would be demonstrated by:
    1. drowsiness.
    2. pharyngeal edema.
    3. an increased blood pressure reading.
    4. a decreased respiratory rate.

77. A drug that is to be given on a q4h schedule may be administered at:
    1. 10 AM and 10 PM.
    2. 10 AM, 2 PM, and 10 PM.
    3. 10 AM, 2 PM, 6 PM, and 10 PM.
    4. 10 AM, 2 PM, 6 PM, 10 PM, and 2 AM.

78. A specific assessment that a nurse should make before the administration of an anticoagulant is to check for:
    1. an allergy history.
    2. evidence of bruising.
    3. the patient's level of discomfort.
    4. increased blood pressure.

79. In the event of a mistake in the administration of medications, the first action that a nurse should take is to:
    1. complete an occurrence report.
    2. inform the patient of the problem.
    3. report the error to the nurse in charge or the physician.
    4. provide an appropriate antidote for the medication given.

80. The subcutaneous site that is most commonly used for low-molecular-weight heparin injections is the:
    1. abdomen.
    2. anterior thigh.
    3. scapular region.
    4. outer aspect of the upper arm.

81. A prescriber indicates to a nurse that a patient will be receiving an intermediate-acting insulin. The nurse anticipates that the patient will receive:
    1. insulin glargine (Lantus).
    2. insulin lispro (Humalog).
    3. isophane insulin suspension (NPH).
    4. protamine zinc insulin suspension (PZI).

82. A charge nurse is evaluating the injection technique of a new staff member. The correct technique for a Z-track injection is noted when the new staff member:
    1. uses the deltoid site.
    2. pulls the skin 1 to 1½ inches laterally.
    3. removes the needle immediately after the injection.
    4. releases the skin before the needle is removed.

83. For a subcutaneous injection to an average-size adult, which of the following techniques requires correction? The student nurse:
    1. selects a 25-gauge, ⅝-inch needle.
    2. injects the needle at a 45-degree angle.
    3. recaps the needle after injecting the medication.
    4. does not massage the injection site after administration.

84. A nurse is aware that a parenteral administration of a concentrated dose of medication in a small amount of fluid is a:
    1. bolus injection.
    2. piggyback infusion.
    3. volume control infusion.
    4. mini-infuser administration.

85. The patient who will most likely have a difficulty with the excretion of medication from the body is the individual who has:
    1. diabetes mellitus.
    2. renal failure.
    3. circulatory insufficiency.
    4. Parkinson's disease.

86. Which prescriber's order takes priority when preparing medications?
    1. PRN
    2. Now
    3. Stat
    4. Standing

87. The nurse anticipates that the medication that will be prescribed as an intraocular disk for the patient with glaucoma is:
    1. pilocarpine.
    2. azithromycin.
    3. iodoxamide.
    4. silver nitrate.

88. The medication that the patient is taking is ototoxic. Based on this information, the nurse knows to specifically assess the patient's:
    1. respiratory rate.
    2. urinary output.
    3. blood pressure.
    4. hearing.

89. The recommended maximum amount of IM medication that can be given safely at one time to an average-size older adult is:
    1. 0.5 mL.
    2. 1 mL.
    3. 2 mL.
    4. 3 mL.

STUDY GROUP QUESTIONS

- How are medications named and classified, and what forms of medications are available?
- What legislation and standards guide medication administration?
- How are medications absorbed, distributed, metabolized, and excreted from the body?
- What are the different types of medication actions?
- What are the different routes for medication administration, and what are the advantages, disadvantages, and contraindications for each route?
- What are the systems used for drug measurement, and how are amounts converted within and between the systems?
- How are dosages calculated for oral, parenteral, and pediatric medications?
- What are the roles of the health team members in the administration of medications?
- What are the six "rights" of medication administration?
- What patient assessment data are critical to obtain before administering medications?
- What equipment is used for the administration of medications via different routes?
- What are the sites or body landmarks for parenteral administration?
- What are the procedures for administration of medications?
- How can IV medication be administered?
- How is administration of medications adapted to patients of different ages and levels of health?
- What information is included in patient/family teaching for medication administration?
- How has technology influenced the administration of medications?

STUDY CHART

Create a study chart to compare *Parenteral Medication and Preparation* that identifies the equipment, needle gauge, amount of medication, site to be used, and angle of injection for subcutaneous, intramuscular, and intradermal injections.

18 Fluid, Electrolyte, and Acid-Base Balances

CASE STUDIES

1. The patient is diagnosed with heart failure and will be taking Digoxin and Lasix on a daily basis.
   a. What patient teaching is indicated in relation to possible fluid and electrolyte imbalances?

2. You are working with two patients today. One of the patients is unconscious and is experiencing a period of prolonged immobility. The other patient has a long history of alcoholism. You are alert to possible alterations in fluid and electrolyte imbalance.
   a. What specific signs and symptoms may these patients exhibit as a result of their present conditions?

3. An adult male patient has come to the outpatient clinic for an examination. During the initial interview, the patient tells you that he has smoked 2½ packs of cigarettes each day for the last 25 years.
   a. What physical signs do you anticipate finding because of the patient's history?
   b. What acid-base imbalance is this patient most likely to experience?

4. Following a motor vehicle accident, the patient had traumatic injuries and a significant hemorrhage. He will be receiving blood transfusions.
   a. What are the priority assessments that should be completed before administration of the blood?
   b. What safety measures should be implemented to reduce the possibility of complications?

CHAPTER REVIEW

Match the description/definition in Column A with the correct term in Column B.

	Column A	*Column B*
_____	1. Positively charged electrolytes	a. Anions
_____	2. Having the same osmotic pressure	b. Diffusion
_____	3. Movement of water across a semipermeable membrane	c. Filtration
_____	4. Movement of molecules from an area of higher concentration to an area of lower concentration	d. Active transport
		e. Cations
_____	5. Negatively charged electrolytes	f. Isotonic
_____	6. Movement of solutes out of a solution with greater hydrostatic pressure	g. Hypotonic
_____	7. Overall particle concentration	h. Osmosis
_____	8. Having a lower osmotic pressure	i. Osmolality
_____	9. Movement of molecules to an area of higher concentration	

Complete the following:

10. Identify the following terms:
    a. All fluids outside of the cell:
    b. Fluid between the cells and outside the blood vessels:
    c. All fluids within the cell:

11. Identify if the following electrolytes are cations or anions and whether they are primarily extracellular or intracellular:
    a. Sodium
    b. Potassium
    c. Calcium
    d. Magnesium
    e. Chloride
    f. Bicarbonate

12. Acid-base balance in the body is regulated by:

13. What age groups are most susceptible to fluid and acid-base imbalances?

14. Identify whether the following solutions are isotonic, hypertonic, or hypotonic:
    a. Dextrose 5% in water (D_5W)
    b. 0.45% sodium chloride (0.45% NS)
    c. 0.9% sodium chloride (0.9% NS)
    d. Lactated Ringer's (LR)
    e. Dextrose 5% in 0.45% sodium chloride (D_5½NS)

15. Identify three types of medications that may cause fluid, electrolyte, or acid-base imbalances.

16. Specify two possible nursing diagnoses for patients experiencing fluid, electrolyte, or acid-base imbalances.

17. Identify the sites for an IV infusion.

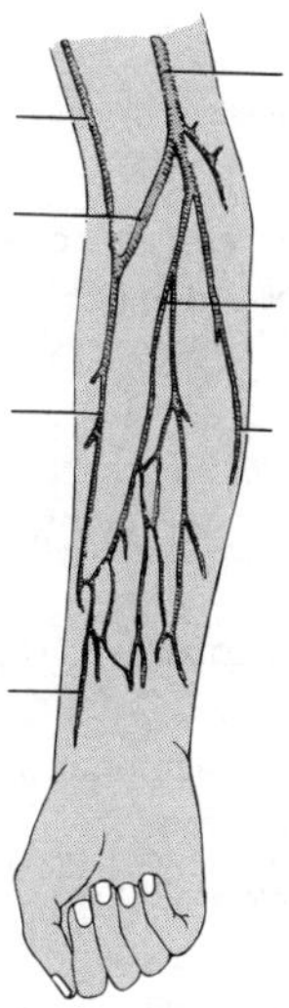

18. A patient who is NPO, with normal renal function, needs to have _____ added to the solution.

19. Identify the signs and symptoms that are associated with phlebitis at an IV site.

20. A patient with a peripherally inserted central catheter (PICC) line develops a fever and increased white blood cell (WBC) count. The nurse anticipates that the health care provider will order:

21. The patient had a rapid infusion of IV fluids and has developed crackles in the lungs, shortness of breath, and tachycardia. The nurse should:

22. Transfusion of a patient's own blood is termed:

23. Identify the electrolyte imbalance that is associated with each of the following test results:
    a. Serum sodium level—125 mEq/L
    b. Serum potassium level—5.8 mEq/L
    c. Serum ionized calcium level—3.7 mEq/L
    d. Serum magnesium level—1.2 mEq/L

24. Calculate the following IV infusion rates:
    a. IV 500 mL of D_5W to infuse in 5 hours; drop factor = 15 gtt/mL. How many gtt/min should infuse?
    b. IV 1000 mL of NS to infuse in 8 hours; drop factor = 10 gtt/mL. How many gtt/min should infuse?
    c. IV 200 mL of NS to infuse in 4 hours; drop factor = 60 gtt/mL. How many gtt/min should infuse?
    d. IV 2 L of D_5W to infuse in 18 hours. How many mL/hour should be set on the infusion pump?

25. Identify the following hormones that control fluid balance:
    a. Pituitary
    b. Adrenal

26. If a hypotonic solution is given intravenously to a patient, the fluid will move into the cells.
    True _____ False _____

27. Arterial pH is an indirect measurement of:

28. Oxygen moves into the lungs via the process of:

29. An average adult's daily intake of fluid is approximately _____ mL.

30. The nurse is going to perform a venipuncture to initiate IV therapy. Place the following steps in the correct order.
    a. Prepare the IV infusion tubing and solution. _____
    b. Re-apply the tourniquet. _____
    c. Perform hand hygiene. _____
    d. Cleanse the site. _______
    e. Select a large-enough vein. _____

31. The nurse is calculating the patient's intake and output for the last 8 hours. During this time, the patient consumed 1 cup of gelatin, ½ cup of juice, 1 cup of water, and 1 cup of tea. The IV infusion started with 750 mL in the bag, with 125 mL remaining at the end of the shift. The urinary output was 340 mL and there was 30 mL of drainage from the nasogastric tube.
Cup = 8 oz
What is the patient's intake and output?
I = _____ O = _____

32. Which of the following is/are most likely to lead to a fluid volume deficit? Select all that apply.
a. Vomiting _____
b. Heart failure _____
c. Corticosteroid administration _____
d. Fever _____
e. Increased sodium intake _____
f. Diuretic administration _____

33. A patient has a nursing diagnosis of *Deficient Fluid Volume related to excessive diaphoresis* from fever. Identify a related outcome and two nursing interventions for this patient.

34. When selecting a site to start an IV, the nurse should begin with the site that is: ______

35. The IV site is located in the right antecubital space. The nurse notes that the rate fluctuates when the patient flexes his right arm. The nurse should:

36. Identify the correct order of the following steps for the removal of an IV.
a. Turn off the roller clamp _____
b. Remove the IV catheter _____
c. Remove the dressing _____
d. Record the fluid infusion _____
e. Inspect the tip of the IV catheter _____
f. Perform hand hygiene and apply clean gloves _____
g. Place gauze over the site and apply light pressure _____

37. The nurse is preparing the IV fluid infusion. What should be checked when looking at the IV fluid?

38. In preparing to administer a blood transfusion, what are the critical assessments that need to be made?

39. It is suspected that the patient is experiencing hypokalemia. Identify all of the signs that support this assessment. Select all that apply.
a. Bilateral muscle weakness _____
b. Positive Chvostek's sign _____
c. Bradycardia _____
d. Diminished bowel sounds _____
e. Tetany _____
f. ECG abnormalities _____

40. Identify which of the following are correct when performing an IV site dressing. Select all that apply.
a. Apply tape over the IV insertion site. _____
b. Cleanse the site horizontally, vertically, and then in a outward circular pattern. ______
c. Use skin protectant where the tape will be. _____
d. Anchor the IV tubing. _____
e. Use clean technique for the procedure. _____
f. Use a catheter stabilization device. _____

Select the best answer for each of the following questions:

41. The IV site is swollen, pale, and cool to the touch. The nurse identifies this as:
1. phlebitis.
2. infiltration.
3. local infection.
4. allergic response.

42. A hypotonic IV solution is expected to be administered to a patient who is experiencing:
1. hypernatremia.
2. hypocalcemia.
3. hypervolemia.
4. hypokalemia.

43. The patient has hypernatremia with a fluid deficit. The nurse anticipates finding:
1. dry, sticky mucous membranes.
2. orthostatic hypotension.
3. abdominal cramping.
4. diarrhea.

44. The patient who is experiencing a gastrointestinal problem has had periods of prolonged vomiting. The nurse is observing the patient for signs of:
1. metabolic acidosis.
2. metabolic alkalosis.
3. respiratory acidosis.
4. respiratory alkalosis.

45. The nurse is working with a patient who has had emphysema for many years. The nurse believes that the patient has uncompensated respiratory acidosis. This belief is a result of an analysis of the patient's blood gas values that reveals:
    1. pH = 7.35, $PaCO_2$ = 40 mm Hg, HCO_3^- concentration = 22 mEq/L
    2. pH = 7.40, $PaCO_2$ = 45 mm Hg, HCO_3^- concentration = 28 mEq/L
    3. pH = 7.30, $PaCO_2$ = 50 mm Hg, HCO_3^- concentration = 24 mEq/L
    4. pH = 7.45, $PaCO_2$ = 55 mm Hg, HCO_3^- concentration = 18 mEq/L

46. The patient has been admitted to the medical center for stabilization of congestive heart failure. The physician has prescribed Lasix (a diuretic) for the patient. This patient should be observed for:
    1. diarrhea.
    2. edema.
    3. dysrhythmia.
    4. hyperactive reflexes.

47. The patient has a potassium level above the normal value. The nurse anticipates that treatment for this patient with hyperkalemia will include:
    1. fluid restrictions.
    2. foods high in potassium.
    3. administration of diuretics.
    4. IV infusion of calcium.

48. The patient has lost a large amount of body fluid. In assessment of this patient with hypovolemia (fluid volume deficit, FVD), the nurse expects to find:
    1. oliguria.
    2. hypertension.
    3. periorbital edema.
    4. neck vein distention.

49. The nurse is determining the care that is to be provided to the patients on the medical unit. There are a number of patients who have the potential for a fluid and electrolyte imbalance. A nurse-initiated (independent) intervention for these patients is:
    1. administration of IV fluids.
    2. monitoring of intake and output.
    3. performance of diagnostic tests.
    4. dietary replacement of necessary fluids/electrolytes.

50. For a patient who is experiencing a fluid volume excess, the nurse plans to determine the fluid status. The best way to determine the fluid balance for the patient is to:
    1. obtain diagnostic test results.
    2. monitor IV fluid intake.
    3. weigh the patient daily.
    4. assess vital signs.

51. The patient is admitted to the trauma unit after an accident while using power tools at home. The patient experienced significant blood loss and required a large infusion of citrated blood. The nurse assesses this patient for the development of:
    1. urinary retention.
    2. poor skin turgor.
    3. increased blood pressure reading.
    4. positive Chvostek's sign.

52. The patient is experiencing a severe anxiety reaction and the respiratory rate has increased significantly. Nursing intervention for this patient who may develop respiratory alkalosis is:
    1. placing the patient in a sitting position.
    2. providing the patient with nasal oxygen.
    3. having the patient breathe into a paper bag.
    4. having the patient cough and deep breathe.

53. A patient with normal renal function is to be maintained NPO. An IV of 1000 mL of D_5W is ordered to infuse over 8 hours. The nurse should:
    1. infuse the IV at a faster rate.
    2. add multivitamins to the solution.
    3. provide oral fluids as a supplement.
    4. question the prescriber about adding potassium to the IV.

54. A patient with an IV infusion may develop phlebitis. The nurse recognizes this condition by the presence at the IV infusion site of:
    1. pallor.
    2. swelling.
    3. redness.
    4. cyanosis.

55. The patient has had an IV line inserted. Upon observation of the IV site, the nurse notes that there is evidence of an infiltration. The nurse should first:
    1. slow the infusion.
    2. discontinue the infusion.
    3. change the IV bag and tubing.
    4. contact the prescriber immediately.

56. The nurse is reviewing the hospital policy for maintenance of IV infusions. The current guidelines for changing continuous IV tubing (non–blood administration sets) are every:
    1. 36 hours.
    2. 48 hours.
    3. 72 hours.
    4. 96 hours.

57. The patient has just started to receive the blood transfusion. The nurse is performing the patient assessment and notes the patient has chills and flank pain. The nurse stops the infusion and then:
    1. calls the physician.
    2. administers epinephrine.
    3. collects a urine specimen.
    4. sets up new tubing with an IV infusion of 0.9% saline.

58. A patient who has been admitted with a renal dysfunction is demonstrating signs and symptoms of a fluid volume excess (hypervolemia). Upon completing the patient assessment, the nurse anticipates finding:
    1. poor skin turgor.
    2. decreased blood pressure.
    3. neck vein distention.
    4. increased urine specific gravity.

59. The nurse is assisting the patient with a fluid volume deficit to select an optimum replacement fluid. The nurse suggests that the patient drink:
    1. tea.
    2. milk.
    3. coffee.
    4. fruit juice.

60. A patient with congestive heart failure and fluid retention is placed on a fluid restriction of 1000 mL/24 hours. On the basis of guidelines for patients with restrictions, for the time period from 7:00 AM to 3:30 PM the nurse plans to provide the patient:
    1. 250 mL.
    2. 400 mL.
    3. 500 mL.
    4. 750 mL.

61. The patient has come to the orthopedist's office for treatment of osteoporosis. The nurse is explaining to the patient some of the possible complications from this disorder that may affect fluid and electrolyte balance. The nurse informs the patient to report:
    1. low back pain.
    2. tingling in the fingers.
    3. muscle twitching.
    4. positive Trousseau's sign.

62. The patient has a history of alcoholism and is admitted to the medical center in a malnourished state. The nurse specifically checks the lab values for:
    1. hypercalcemia.
    2. hyponatremia.
    3. hyperkalemia.
    4. hypomagnesemia.

63. The patient who is most prone to respiratory acidosis is the individual who is experiencing:
    1. hyperthyroidism.
    2. an acute asthma episode.
    3. renal failure.
    4. an anxiety reaction.

64. Older adults have a greater risk of fluid imbalance as a result of:
    1. increased thirst response.
    2. decreased glomerular filtration.
    3. increased body fluid percentage.
    4. increased basal metabolic rate.

65. An example of a type of medication that can lead to metabolic acidosis is:
    1. aspirin.
    2. Lasix.
    3. potassium.
    4. Benadryl.

66. An appropriate technique when initiating an intravenous infusion is to:
    1. use hard, stiff veins.
    2. shave the arm hair with a razor.
    3. use the proximal site in the dominant arm.
    4. apply the tourniquet 4 to 6 inches above the selected site.

67. A unit of packed cells or whole blood usually transfuses over:
    1. ½ hour.
    2. 1 hour.
    3. 2 hours.
    4. 5 hours.

68. An individual with type O blood is able to receive:
    1. type A or type B.
    2. type AB.
    3. type O.
    4. all types.

69. A specific technique for initiating intravenous therapy for an older adult is to:
    1. select sites in the hands.
    2. use the largest possible IV cannula gauge.
    3. set the IV flow rate at 150 to 200 mL/hr.
    4. insert at a decreased angle of 10 to 15 degrees.

70. The patient lost 4 pounds since last week as a result of taking Lasix. This is approximately:
    1. ½ L of fluid.
    2. 1 L of fluid.
    3. 2 L of fluid.
    4. 4 L of fluid.

STUDY GROUP QUESTIONS

- How are body fluids distributed in the body?
- What is the composition of body fluids?
- How do fluids move throughout the body?
- How is the intake of body fluids regulated?
- What are the major electrolytes, and what is their function in the body?
- How is acid-base balance maintained?
- What are the major fluid, electrolyte, and acid-base imbalances and their causes?
- What signs and symptoms will the patient exhibit in the presence of a fluid, electrolyte, or acid-base imbalance?
- What diagnostic tests are used to determine the presence of imbalances?
- What information is critical to obtain in a patient assessment to determine the presence of a fluid, electrolyte, or acid-base imbalance?
- What health deviations increase a patient's susceptibility to an imbalance?
- What nursing interventions should be implemented for patients with various fluid, electrolyte, and acid-base imbalances?
- What information should be included in patient/family teaching for prevention of imbalances, or restoration of fluid, electrolyte, or acid-base balance?
- What are the nursing responsibilities associated with the initiation and maintenance of IV therapy?
- What are the responsibilities of the nurse with regard to blood transfusions?

STUDY CHARTS

Create study charts to compare

a. *Electrolyte Imbalances and Patient Responses,* including etiology, diagnostic test results, patient assessment, and nursing interventions for sodium, potassium, calcium, and magnesium imbalances
b. *Acid-Base Imbalances and Patient Responses,* including etiology, diagnostic test results, patient assessment, and nursing interventions for metabolic acidosis and alkalosis and for respiratory acidosis and alkalosis

19 Caring in Nursing Practice

CASE STUDIES

1. The daughter of a patient in an extended care facility has traveled from another state to visit. When she arrives with her husband and teenage son, she finds that her mother has deteriorated dramatically from the last time she spoke with her. The patient, in the terminal stages of liver disease, is now only minimally responsive with episodes of agitation and disorientation. The family, especially the daughter, is emotionally distraught.
   a. What can be done by the nurse to demonstrate caring for this patient's family?
   b. What can be done for the patient to demonstrate caring?

2. The nurse observes the student giving a bath to a bedridden patient. The door to the room is open and the patient is exposed. In addition, the student is not being very gentle with the patient.
   a. What caring behaviors are missing?
   b. How can the nurse help the student to recognize and incorporate caring behaviors?

CHAPTER REVIEW

Complete the following:

1. Match the theorists with the theoretical concepts:
   Patricia Benner and Judith Wrubel
   Jean Watson
   Madeleine Leininger
   Kristen Swanson
   a. Five processes and subdimensions _____
   b. Transpersonal caring _____
   c. Caring is primary _____
   d. Transcultural caring _____

2. For the following nursing behaviors, identify an example of a clinical intervention.
   a. Providing presence
   b. Touch
   c. Listening
   d. Knowing the patient

3. A patient is to have an IV line inserted. The nurse demonstrates caring behaviors by:

4. Describe how caring and spirituality are connected.

5. How can nurses care for each other?

Select the best answer for each of the following questions:

6. A nurse is discussing with her peers how much a patient matters to her. She states that she does not want the patient to suffer. The nurse is implementing the theory described by:
   1. Patricia Benner.
   2. Jean Watson.
   3. Kristen Swanson.
   4. Madeleine Leininger.

7. A patient was admitted to the hospital to have diagnostic tests to rule out a cancerous lesion in the lungs. The nurse is sitting with the patient in the room awaiting the results of the tests. The nurse is demonstrating the caring behavior of:
   1. knowing.
   2. comforting.
   3. providing presence.
   4. maintaining belief.

8. A nurse manager would like to promote more opportunities for the staff on the busy unit to demonstrate caring behaviors. The manager elects to implement:
   1. more time off for the staff.
   2. a strict schedule for patient treatments.
   3. staff selection of patient assignments.
   4. staff appointment to hospital committees.

9. A new graduate is looking at theories of caring. He selects Leininger's theory because it is most agreeable with his belief system. Leininger defines caring as a(n):
   1. new consciousness and moral idea.
   2. nurturing way of relating to a valued other.
   3. central, unifying domain necessary for health and survival.
   4. improvement in the human condition using a transcultural perspective.

10. A nurse is working with a patient who has been admitted to the oncology unit for treatment of a cancerous growth. This nurse is applying Swanson's theory of caring and demonstrating the concept of maintaining belief when:
    1. performing the patient's dressing changes.
    2. providing explanations about the medications.
    3. keeping the patient draped during the physical exam.
    4. discussing how the radiation therapy will assist in decreasing the tumor's size.

11. A new graduate is assigned to a surgical unit in which there are a large number of procedures to be performed during each shift. This nurse demonstrates a caring behavior in this situation by:
    1. avoiding situations that may be uncomfortable or difficult.
    2. attempting to do all the treatments independently and quickly.
    3. seeking assistance before performing new or difficult skills.
    4. telling patients that he or she is a new graduate and unfamiliar with all the procedures.

12. An example of the caring process of "enabling" is:
    1. performing a catheter insertion quickly and well.
    2. reassuring the patient that the lab results should be fine.
    3. providing pain medication before a procedure.
    4. assisting a patient during the birth of a child.

13. A subdimension of Swanson's process of caring—"doing for others as he/she would do for self"—involves:
    1. being there.
    2. performing skillfully.
    3. generating alternatives.
    4. offering realistic optimism.

14. In the Caring Assessment Tool (CAT), an example of mutual problem solving with a patient is when a nurse:
    1. discusses health issues with the patient and family.
    2. pays attention to the patient.
    3. provides privacy for the patient.
    4. includes the family members in the patient's care.

15. A nurse attempts to understand the specific cultural concerns of a patient and how they relate to his illness. What caring factor is applied?
    1. Attentive reassurance
    2. Encouragement
    3. Provision of basic human needs
    4. Appreciation of unique meanings

16. Additional teaching is required if a nurse observes that a nursing assistant working with an older adult patient:
    1. has the patient select the clothes to wear.
    2. addresses the patient as "Honey."
    3. carefully organizes the patient's personal items.
    4. combs and styles the patient's hair.

STUDY GROUP QUESTIONS

- What is "caring" in the nursing profession?
- What are the major theories of caring and the key concepts in each one?
- How is caring perceived by patients?
- What are caring behaviors?
- How can a nurse demonstrate caring to patients and families?

20 Cultural Awareness

CASE STUDY

1. For the following situations, identify how a nurse should approach the patient and significant others to recognize cultural concerns and health care needs:
   a. Large numbers of family members surround the patient on the acute care unit.
   b. Dietary practices of the patient prohibit the eating of meat or meat products.
   c. A traditional healer makes calls to the patient's home between the patient's visits to the physician.
   d. The patient and her family speak another language.

CHAPTER REVIEW

Complete the following:

1. Identify two possible nursing diagnoses that may be related to a patient's cultural needs.

2. Provide an example for how the nurse may develop each of the following.
   a. Cultural awareness
   b. Cultural skills

3. Identify an example of a question a nurse could use to elicit specific cultural information from a patient.

4. Identify a specific transcultural communication issue and an appropriate intervention.

5. Explain linguistic competence.

6. Identify four disadvantaged groups and their health care challenges.

7. What should be incorporated into "Teach-Back" to address cultural considerations?

8. Identify four important aspects for working with an interpreter.

9. What are the parts of the LEARN and RESPECT mnemonics?

L -	R -
E -	E -
A -	S -
R -	P -
N -	E -
	C -
	T -

Select the best answer for each of the following questions:

10. A nurse is meeting a patient for the first time for the admission interview. There are eight family members sitting around the patient's bed. After introductions, the most appropriate nursing action is to:
    1. ask the family members to leave immediately.
    2. proceed with the admission interview.
    3. come back at another time.
    4. ask the patient if he or she wants a family member present.

11. The community center where a nurse volunteers has a culturally diverse population. The nurse wants to promote communication with all the patients from different cultures. A beneficial technique for the nurse is to:
    1. explain nursing terms that are used.
    2. use direct and consistent eye contact and touch with all patients.
    3. call patients by their first names to establish rapport.
    4. expect and wait for responses to all questions that are asked.

12. A patient expresses to the nurse that traditional Western or American practices are used in the home for health promotion. The nurse expects that the patient will use:
    1. acupuncture.
    2. guided imagery.
    3. aromatic therapy.
    4. over-the-counter medications.

13. When working with an interpreter for a patient who speaks another language, the nurse should:
    1. direct questions to the interpreter.
    2. expect word-for-word translation.
    3. ensure that the interpreter speaks the patient's dialect.
    4. ask the interpreter to evaluate the patient's nonverbal behaviors.

14. The pregnant patient says that she goes to a woman who provides advice and comfort during and after childbirth. The nurse recognizes that the patient is referring to a(n):
    1. *Ayurvedic provider.*
    2. *Sabador.*
    3. *Imam.*
    4. *Doula.*

STUDY GROUP QUESTIONS

- What is culture?
- What are the major ethnocultural groups in the country/community, their health and illness beliefs and practices, and their traditional remedies?
- How can a nurse promote communication with individuals who are from other cultures and/or individuals who speak different languages?
- How can a nurse identify and respond to a patient's cultural needs?
- What information may be obtained from a cultural assessment?
- What nursing approaches may be successful in assisting multicultural patients in health care settings?
- What resources are available to assist a nurse in learning about and working with patients from other cultures?

21 Spiritual Health

CASE STUDY

1. A nurse is working in an acute care facility with a patient who practices Buddhism.
   a. What information should be obtained in relation to the patient's spiritual practices?
   b. What adaptations may have to be made by the nurse, the other members of the health care team, and the acute care facility to meet the patient's spiritual needs?

CHAPTER REVIEW

Match the description/definition in Column A with the correct term in Column B.

	Column A	*Column B*
_____	1. Does not believe in the existence of a supreme spiritual being or god	a. Faith
_____	2. Cultural or institutional religion	b. Hope
_____	3. Awareness of one's inner self and a sense of connection to a higher being	c. Connectedness
_____	4. Multidimensional concept that gives comfort while a person endures hardship and challenges	d. Atheist
_____	5. Awareness of that which cannot be seen or known in ordinary ways	e. Spirituality
_____	6. Belief that ultimate reality is unknown or unknowable	f. Self-transcendence
_____	7. Having close spiritual relationships with oneself, others, and a god or other spiritual being	g. Agnostic

Complete the following:

8. Identify general nursing interventions for promotion of spiritual health.

9. An example of a nursing intervention for a patient who has had a near-death experience is:

10. Identify two possible nursing diagnoses and patient outcomes relating to spirituality or spiritual health.

11. Identify what each letter in the FICA assessment tool acronym designates:
    F:
    I:
    C:
    A:

12. Formulate a question that may be asked to determine a patient's spiritual belief system.

13. There is an order for whole blood replacement for a patient. Before the blood administration, a nurse will check to see if the patient is a member of what religion(s)?

14. Provide at least two examples of rituals or practices associated with spirituality or religion.

15. Religious or spiritual practices may have an impact upon the provision of health care to a patient. For an individual who is of the Islamic faith, which of the following may have to be considered by a nurse and other health care providers? Select all that apply.
    a. Organ donation will be approved. _____
    b. Women prefer female providers/examiners. _____
    c. Euthanasia is practiced. _____
    d. Time will have to be set aside during the day for prayer. _____
    e. Faith healing may be used. _____
    f. Blood products and medicines may be refused. _____

16. Identify the four (4) dimensions of spiritual well-being.

17. Indicate which of the following statements about spirituality is/are correct. Select all that apply.
    a. Patients who identify a religious belief will all practice similar rituals. _____
    b. Promoting spirituality can help a patient cope with illness. _____
    c. Promoting a patient's spirituality may reduce the incidence of depression. _____
    d. The link between spirituality and physical health is well understood. _____
    e. Spirituality exists in all people regardless of their religious beliefs. _____

18. How does the nurse use *presence* to promote spiritual well-being?

19. The nurse wants to assist patients to achieve spiritual health. The nurse should:
    Select all that apply.
    a. Solve their spiritual problems. _____
    b. Employ his/her own personal religious practices with the patient. _____
    c. Explore meditation with the patient to assist in reducing stress. _____
    d. Integrate patient preferences into the plan of care. _____
    e. Provide an environment for expression of beliefs. _____
    f. Recognize that all patients experience spiritual problems. _____

Select the best answer for each of the following questions:

20. A patient is admitted to a medical center for surgery to repair a fractured hip. Upon reviewing the patient's admission history, a nurse finds that the patient attends religious services routinely. The nurse supports the patient's spiritual needs by stating:
    1. "Do you really go to services often?"
    2. "Don't worry. God will take care of you."
    3. "I'll call your minister and have him stop by to see you."
    4. "Is there any way that I may be able to help you with your spiritual needs?"

21. A patient who is of the Jewish faith is admitted to the long-term care facility. A nurse seeks to provide support of the usual health practices that are part of this religion. The nurse learns that one component of usual Jewish tradition states:
    1. No euthanasia should be used.
    2. A faith healer will be involved.
    3. Modern medical treatment should be refused.
    4. Physical exams should be performed only by individuals of the same sex.

22. While caring for a patient in the intensive care unit, the patient has a cardiac arrest. The patient is successfully resuscitated. After this near-death experience, the patient is progressing physically but appears withdrawn and concerned. The nurse assists the patient by stating:
    1. "The experience that you had is easy to explain and understand."
    2. "That was a very close call. It must be very frightening for you."
    3. "Other people have had similar experiences and worked through their feelings."
    4. "If you would like to talk about your experience, I will stay with you."

23. For a patient with a diagnosis of a chronic disease, a nurse wishes to encourage feelings of hope. The nurse recognizes that hope provides:
    1. a meaning and purpose for the patient.
    2. an organized approach to dealing with the disease process.
    3. a connection to the cultural background of the patient.
    4. a binding relationship with the divine being of the patient's religion.

24. A nurse is reviewing the plan of care for a 66-year-old home care patient who is experiencing the beginning stages of Alzheimer's disease. Several nursing diagnoses have been identified from the initial home visit and assessment. The nurse believes that the patient may need to be assessed for spiritual needs based on the diagnosis of:
    1. *Impaired Memory.*
    2. *Altered Health Maintenance.*
    3. *Ineffective Coping.*
    4. *Altered Thought Process.*

25. According to Erikson's stages of psychosocial development, with regard to spiritual beliefs it is expected that a 6-year-old child will:
    1. begin to ask about a god or supreme being.
    2. have spiritual well-being provided by the parents.
    3. interpret meanings literally.
    4. begin to learn the difference between right and wrong.

26. A nurse recognizes that a group whose members may reject modern medicine based on religious beliefs is:
    1. Hindu.
    2. Islamic.
    3. Catholic.
    4. Navajo.

27. According to Erikson's stages of psychosocial development, with regard to spiritual beliefs it is expected that a middle-age person will begin to:
    1. reflect on inconsistencies in religious stories.
    2. form independent beliefs and attitudes.
    3. review value systems during a crisis.
    4. sort fantasy from fact.

28. A young adult is diagnosed with a very aggressive form of cancer. He yells at the nurse, "Why did this happen to me?" The nurse's best response is:
    1. "Do you think that you did something wrong?"
    2. "You sound upset about your situation. Let's talk about it."
    3. "Tell me why you think this is unfair."
    4. "What makes you say that?"

STUDY GROUP QUESTIONS

- What is spirituality and how does it relate to an individual's health status?
- What are the concepts of spirituality/spiritual health?
- What spiritual or religious problems may arise during patient care?
- How can a nurse assess a patient's spirituality/spiritual health?
- What is the role of a nurse in promoting spiritual health?
- How can a nurse avoid imposing his or her own beliefs on a patient?
- What are the differences and similarities in spiritual practices and health beliefs between the major religious sects?
- How is hope related to spirituality?

22 Growth and Development

CASE STUDIES

1. A student nurse with an inpatient pediatric unit in a medical center has three patients: an infant, a 5-year-old child, and a 16-year-old adolescent.
   a. How should the nurse promote growth and developmental needs for these patients in the acute care environment?
   b. What would be included in a teaching plan for the new parents of the infant?

2. A patient in the extended care facility is an 86-year-old woman who is occasionally disoriented to time, place, and person.
   a. How should a nurse approach this patient to assist her in meeting her developmental needs?

3. A student nurse is working as a summer camp nurse with children 8 to 10 years old. It is the nurse's turn to select diversional activities for a group.
   a. What types of games or activities are appropriate for this age group?

4. A nurse is teaching the parents of adolescents the signs that may indicate a potential suicidal tendency in their children.
   a. What signs/behaviors will the nurse identify for these parents?

CHAPTER REVIEW

Match the description in Column A with the correct theorist in Column B.

	Column A	*Column B*
_____	1. Development of cognition	a. Freud
_____	2. Psychosexual focus	b. Erikson
_____	3. Based on human needs	c. Maslow
_____	4. Moral development	d. Piaget
_____	5. Psychosocial development	e. Kohlberg

Complete the following:

6. An example of a teratogen is:

7. The leading cause of death in the toddler and preschool age groups is:

8. Select the age group (infant, toddler, preschool age, school age, adolescent, young adult, middle-aged adult, or older adult) in which each of the following behaviors is evident or usually begins:
   a. Toilet training _____
   b. Tripling of birth weight _____
   c. Use of script handwriting _____
   d. Separation anxiety _____
   e. Moving away from the family _____
   f. Parallel play _____
   g. Search for personal identity _____
   h. Menopause _____
   i. Speaking in short sentences _____
   j. More graceful running and jumping _____
   k. Development of fears _____
   l. Presbycusis _____
   m. Loss of primary teeth _____
   n. Development of primary and secondary sexual characteristics _____
   o. Low risk of chronic illness _____
   p. Diminished skin turgor and appearance of wrinkles _____
   q. Socioeconomic stability _____
   r. Recognition of objects by their outward appearance _____

9. To promote awareness of time, place, and person in an extended care environment, a nurse implements:

10. Prescriptive use or administration of more medication than indicated clinically is termed:

11. Identify safety concerns in the home environment for the following age groups:
    a. Toddler
    b. Older adult

12. What are the expected physical assessment findings for a middle-aged adult? Select all that apply.
    a. Abnormal visual fields and ocular movements _____
    b. Palpable lateral thyroid nodes _____
    c. Pulse rate of 60 to 100 beats per minute _____
    d. Decreased strength of abdominal muscles _____
    e. Responsive sensory system _____
    f. Diminished motor responses _____

13. Identify a topic area that is age appropriate for a group of older adults in a senior housing development.

14. Indicate ways that the nurse can reduce stress for a hospitalized child.

15. What is a potential nursing diagnosis for an adolescent individual?

16. What are the characteristics of the adolescent age group? Select all that apply.
    a. Preference for same sex peers _____
    b. Risk-taking _____
    c. Search for personal identify _____
    d. Following the rules of new authority figures _____
    e. Adoption of the parents' moral standards _____
    f. Development of secondary sex characteristics _____

17. How is the "Sandwich Generation" a challenge for nurses?

18. Identify at least one health concern for toddlers and school-age children.

19. Indicate which of the following are true for older adult individuals. Select all that apply.
    a. Cognitive impairment is expected. _____
    b. Strong visual memory is retained. _____
    c. Delirium is potentially reversible. _____
    d. Depression is becoming more common in this population. _____
    e. Short-term memory is unaffected. _____
    f. Sense of touch remains strong. _____

Select the best answer for each of the following questions:

20. A nurse is assigned to prepare a teaching plan for a group of preschool-age children. For this age group, the nurse includes:
    1. appropriate use of medications.
    2. cooking safety including use of the stove.
    3. information on prevention of obesity and hypertension.
    4. guidelines for crossing the street or actions to take during a fire.

21. Children who are admitted to a hospital may be afraid about the hospitalization. To reduce the fear of school-age children in an acute care environment, a nurse:
    1. restrains them for all assessments and procedures.
    2. shows them the equipment that is to be used for procedures.
    3. provides in-depth information on how procedures are done.
    4. tells them that everything will be all right and the procedures will not hurt.

22. During a clinical rotation a student nurse is observing children in a day care center. The student is asked to assist with the activities for the preschool-age children. Children in this age group are usually able to:
    1. make detailed drawings.
    2. skip, throw, and catch balls.
    3. easily hold a pencil and print letters.
    4. use a vocabulary of more than 8000 words.

23. Parents of a toddler ask a nurse what their child should be able to do at the age of 2½ years old. The nurse identifies that the toddler will be able to:
    1. classify objects by size and color.
    2. speak in short sentences.
    3. solve difficult problems.
    4. recognize safety hazards.

24. Parents of a 1-year-old are asking about what can be expected of a child this age. A nurse informs the parents that a major milestone for a 1-year-old child is:
    1. tripling of the birth weight.
    2. sleeping 6 to 7 hours each day.
    3. walking with good balance.
    4. playing well with others.

25. A nurse is working with a group of young adults at the community center. There are many discussions about life and health issues. The nurse is aware that a health-related concern for young adults is that:
    1. attachment needs must be enhanced.
    2. "labeling" may alter their self-perceptions.
    3. adaptation to chronic disease is developing.
    4. fast-paced lifestyles may place them at risk for illnesses or disabilities.

26. A nurse is seeking to evaluate the effectiveness of information provided to the parents of an infant. The nurse determines that teaching has been successful when the parents:
    1. place small pillows in the infant's crib.
    2. position the infant on the stomach for sleeping.
    3. purchase a crib with slats that are less than 2 inches apart.
    4. prop up a bottle for the infant to suck on while falling asleep.

27. When presenting a program for a group of individuals in their middle-aged adult years, a nurse informs the members to expect the following physical change:
    1. A decrease in skin turgor
    2. An increased breast size
    3. Palpable lateral thyroid lobes
    4. A visual acuity that is greater than 20/50

28. Parents of a 3½-year-old boy are concerned when, after hospitalization, the boy begins to suck his thumb again. The boy had not sucked his thumb for over a year. A nurse informs the parents that:
    1. their health care provider must be informed about this behavior.
    2. the child was probably not ready to stop this behavior previously.
    3. the child is feeling neglected by his parents and they should spend more time with him.
    4. the behavior should be ignored as it is common for a child to regress when anxious.

29. An adolescent girl has gone to a family planning center for information about birth control. The patient asks a nurse what she should use to avoid getting pregnant. The nurse responds:
    1. "Are your parents aware of your sexual activity?"
    2. "You've been using some kind of protection before, right?"
    3. "What are your friends doing to protect themselves?"
    4. "What can you tell me about your past sexual experiences?"

30. A patient has gone to an outpatient obstetric clinic for a routine checkup. The patient asks a nurse what is happening with the baby now that she is in her third trimester. The nurse informs the patient that:
    1. the heartbeat can be heard.
    2. the fingers and toes are well developed.
    3. the organ systems are just beginning to develop.
    4. the brain is undergoing a tremendous growth spurt.

31. For a patient in a nursing center, the nurse suspects the potentially reversible cognitive impairment of:
    1. delirium.
    2. dementia.
    3. depression.
    4. disengagement.

STUDY GROUP QUESTIONS

- What are the principles of growth and development?
- How can growth and development be influenced internally and externally?
- What are the differences and similarities of the major developmental theorists?
- How can a nurse apply the different developmental theories to patient situations?
- What are the major physical, psychosocial, and cognitive changes that occur throughout the life span?
- What are the specific health needs for each developmental stage?
- How does the approach of a nurse differ for individuals in each developmental stage to meet their developmental needs?
- What are the different teaching/learning needs of each developmental stage?

STUDY CHART

Create a study chart to compare *Growth and Development Across the Life Span* that identifies the physical abilities, psychosocial/cognitive activities, and health promotion behaviors and strategies for each age group from infancy to older adulthood.

23 Self-Concept and Sexuality

CASE STUDIES

1. A 22-year-old man is admitted to a rehabilitation facility. He was seriously injured in an automobile accident and now is paraplegic. Although he is medically stable, it appears that he is having difficulty dealing with his physical limitations. The patient speaks frequently about his girlfriend and his involvement in athletics and other social activities.
   a. What self-concept and sexuality issues are involved in this situation?
   b. Formulate a plan of care for this patient.

2. A nurse suspects that a patient is the victim of sexual abuse.
   a. What behaviors may the patient be exhibiting that would lead to this assessment?
   b. What questions should the nurse ask to get more information from the patient about the possible abuse?

CHAPTER REVIEW

Match the description/definition in Column A with the correct term in Column B.

	Column A	*Column B*
_____	1. Set of conscious and unconscious feelings and beliefs about oneself	a. Sexuality
_____	2. Set of behaviors that have been approved by family, community, and culture as appropriate in particular situations	b. Self-concept
		c. Transgender
_____	3. Clear, persistent preference for persons of one sex	d. Self-esteem
_____	4. Emotional evaluation of self-worth	e. Sexual orientation
_____	5. Experiences and attitudes related to appearance and physical abilities	f. Role
_____	6. Sense of femaleness or maleness	g. Identity
_____	7. People whose gender identity or expression is different than their sex at birth	h. Body image
_____	8. Persistent individuality and sameness of a person over time and in various circumstances	

Complete the following:

9. Identify at least two examples of the following.
   a. Positive influences on self-concept

   b. Stressors to self-concept

10. Which of the following behaviors may indicate an altered self-concept? Select all that apply.
    a. Eye contact maintained _____
    b. Straight posture _____
    c. Hesitant speech _____
    d. Overly angry response _____
    e. Independence _____
    f. Passive attitude _____
    g. Able to make decisions _____
    h. Unkempt appearance _____

11. For the following patients, identify the potential concerns related to self-concept and sexuality.
    a. A woman who has had a mastectomy

    b. A woman who is undergoing chemotherapy for cancer and who has a young child at home

    c. A 7-year-old child who has been severely burned

    d. A middle-aged adult man who has had a heart attack

12. A way in which a nurse may promote self-concept in an acute care setting is by:

13. An example of an alteration in sexual health is:

14. Specify an area for patient education to promote sexual health.

15. For the nursing diagnosis *Situational Low Self-Esteem related to being unable to successfully pass a required college course*, identify a patient goal/outcome and nursing interventions.

16. The capacity for sexuality diminishes significantly in older adults.
    True _____ False _____

17. Cultural background does not directly influence self-concept.
    True _____ False _____

18. The best method of birth control to reinforce with patients is the least expensive selection.
    True _____ False _____

19. An example of an intervention that a nurse may implement to promote self-concept for an older adult is:

20. For tattoos and body piercings, identify the statements that are correct. Select all that apply.
    a. They are less common practices today _____
    b. There are more complications from piercings than tattoos _____
    c. Federal regulations are in place for these practices _____
    d. Sterile technique should be used for the procedures _____
    e. They are ways of expressing individuality _____

21. Provide an example of a role performance stressor.

22. The vaccine that is recommended for early adolescent males and females to reduce the risk for HPV-related cancers is:

23. What medical diagnoses can interfere with sexual functioning?

Select the best answer for each of the following questions:

24. A nurse recognizes that which of the following age groups is most vulnerable to identity stressors?
    1. Infancy
    2. Preschool
    3. Adolescence
    4. Middle-aged adulthood

25. An adolescent has gone to the nurse's office in a school to discuss some personal issues. The nurse wishes to determine the sexual health of this adolescent. The nurse begins by asking:
    1. "Do you use contraception?"
    2. "Have you already had sexual relations?"
    3. "Are your parents aware of your sexual activity?"
    4. "Do you have any concerns about sex or your body's development?"

26. During an interview and physical assessment of a female patient in the clinic, a nurse finds that the patient has multiple lacerations and bruises and that she has experienced headaches and difficulty sleeping. The nurse suspects:
    1. sexual dysfunction.
    2. emotional conflict.
    3. sexually transmitted infection.
    4. physical and/or sexual abuse.

27. A patient is admitted to a coronary care unit after an acute myocardial infarction. He tells the nurse, "I won't be able to do what I used to at the hardware store." The nurse recognizes that the patient is experiencing a problem with the self-concept component of:
    1. role.
    2. identity.
    3. self-esteem.
    4. body image.

28. An adolescent patient has just been diagnosed with scoliosis and will need to wear a corrective brace. She tells the nurse angrily, "I don't know why I have to have this stupid problem!" The nurse responds most appropriately by saying:
    1. "Tell me what you do when you get angry and upset."
    2. "Don't be angry. You'll be getting the best care available."
    3. "You'll heal quickly and the brace can come off pretty soon."
    4. "It's okay to be angry around your friends, but try not to be upset around your parents."

29. During an initial assessment at an outpatient clinic, a nurse wants to determine a patient's perception of identity. The nurse asks the patient:
    1. "What is your usual day like?"
    2. "How would you describe yourself?"
    3. "What activities do you enjoy doing at home?"
    4. "What changes would you make in your personal appearance?"

30. A patient has been in the rehabilitation facility for several weeks after a cerebral vascular accident (CVA/stroke). During the hospitalization, a nurse has identified that the patient has become progressively more depressed about his physical condition. Although the patient is able, he will not participate in personal grooming and now is refusing any visitors. At this point, the nurse intervenes by:
    1. telling the patient to think more positively about the future.
    2. helping the patient to get washed and dressed every day.
    3. leaving the patient to complete activities of daily living independently.
    4. contacting the physician to discuss a psychological consultation.

31. A nurse is working with a patient who has had a colostomy. The patient asks about resuming a sexual relationship with a partner. The nurse begins by determining:
    1. the patient's knowledge about sexual activity.
    2. how the patient has dealt with other life changes in the past.
    3. the partner's feelings about the colostomy.
    4. how comfortable the patient and the partner are in communicating with each other.

32. A nurse who is using Erikson's theory expects that a 5-year-old boy will begin to:
    1. accept body changes and maturation.
    2. incorporate feedback from peers into his personality.
    3. distinguish himself from the environment around him.
    4. identify with a specific gender group.

33. A patient asks a nurse about a prescription for tadalafil (Cialis). The nurse recognizes, however, that this drug is contraindicated for the patient who is taking:
    1. antibiotics.
    2. beta blockers.
    3. antihistamines.
    4. nonsteroidal antiinflammatory agents.

34. A nurse is aware that which of the following strategies is appropriate for teaching a patient for promotion of a positive sexual experience?
    1. Encouraging the use of only one position for intercourse
    2. Instructing couples to work harder at the beginning of intercourse
    3. Discussing side effects of medications that may alter responsiveness
    4. Emphasizing a shorter period of foreplay

35. Correction is required if a new nurse in the women's clinic is observed:
    1. closing the door during an examination.
    2. determining the patient's cultural beliefs.
    3. identifying physiological changes for the patient.
    4. discussing findings with the patient in the waiting room.

36. Which of the following is anticipated as a sexual change related to the aging process?
    1. Increased vaginal secretions
    2. Decreased time for ejaculation to be achieved
    3. Decreased time for maintenance of an erection
    4. Increased orgasmic contractions

37. During an initial assessment at an outpatient clinic, a nurse wants to determine a patient's level of self-esteem. The nurse asks the patient:
    1. "What is your usual day like?"
    2. "How do you feel about yourself?"
    3. "What hobbies do you enjoy doing at home?"
    4. "What changes would you make in your personal appearance?"

STUDY GROUP QUESTIONS

- What are the components of self-concept?
- What stressors may influence an individual's self-concept?
- How can a nurse promote an individual's self-concept in different health care settings?
- What is sexuality and how does it develop throughout the life span?
- How can sexual health be defined?
- What are some of the current issues related to sexuality and sexual health?
- How may sexual health be altered?
- What health-related factors may influence sexual function?
- How are self-concept and sexuality related?
- How can a nurse determine an individual's self-concept and sexual health?
- What adaptations may be made by a nurse in approaching different age groups for the assessment and promotion of self-concept and sexual health?
- How can a nurse apply critical thinking and nursing processes to the areas of self-concept and sexuality?
- What resources are available to assist individuals to promote optimum self-concept and sexual health?
- How can a nurse make the patient feel more at ease when completing an assessment of sexual health?

STUDY CHART

Create a study chart on *Stressors Affecting Self-Concept* that identifies how the components of self-concept may be influenced and nursing interventions that may be implemented to promote a patient's self-concept.

24 Family Context in Nursing

CASE STUDIES

1. A 65-year-old man has been admitted to the coronary care unit in a medical center. The patient experienced a myocardial infarction (heart attack) while working late in his store. His wife, who accompanied him to the medical center, not only has been the "homemaker" for the family for more than 25 years but also has assisted in the family business run by her husband. They have two children who live on their own. Their son lives with his male partner, whereas their younger daughter is married and has two children of her own. The patient and his wife speak readily about their daughter but avoid talking about their son.
   a. What factors related to family roles and function are involved in this situation?
   b. What stage of the family life cycle is this family in currently?
   c. What strategies may a nurse use to promote communication in this family?
   d. How may the role of the patient and his wife influence the health education plan?
   e. Identify a family-oriented nursing diagnosis for this situation.

2. The visiting nurse is working with a patient who has just been discharged from a rehabilitation facility after hip surgery.
   a. What should be included in the environmental assessment for this patient?
   b. What information about the patient's family should be assessed?

CHAPTER REVIEW

Match the family stage in Column A with the key principle identified for that stage in Column B.

	Column A (Family Stages)	*Column B (Key Principles)*
_____	1. Unattached young adult	a. Increasing flexibility of family's boundaries to include children's independence
_____	2. Newly married couple	b. Accepting parent-offspring separation
_____	3. Family with adolescents	c. Accepting shifting of generational roles
_____	4. Family with young adults	d. Committing to a new system
_____	5. Family in later life	e. Accepting a multitude of exits from and entries into the family system

Complete the following:

6. What is a family?

7. What genetic factors may have an influence upon a family?

8. Identify what is meant by the following:
   a. Family hardiness

   b. Family resiliency

   c. Family diversity

9. Identify the major concerns or challenges that may influence families today.

10. For families providing care for a family member:
    a. Identify possible indicators of caregiver stress.

    b. Identify a nursing diagnosis for a family coping with the difficult care of an older adult parent in the home.

11. Which of the following are correct statements regarding today's society? Select all that apply.
    a. Families are larger. ______
    b. Divorce rates have tripled since the 1950s. ______
    c. Fewer people are living alone. ______
    d. From the 1970s to the 1990s, the number of single-parent families has doubled. ______
    e. Less than one third of gay male couples live together. ______
    f. Father-only families have increased. ______
    g. The fastest growing age group is 65 years and older. ______

12. Identify an effect that inadequate functioning may have on a family.

13. What questions may be asked to determine the influence of culture on a family?

14. Provide examples of health promotion interventions for a family.

15. Identify factors that contribute to domestic violence.

16. How can the nurse care for a family that has experienced death?

17. What is a danger for a family with a rigid structure?

Select the best answer for each of the following questions:

18. A nurse is working with a family in which the parents, both previously divorced, have brought a total of three unrelated children together. This type of family structure is classified as:
    1. nuclear.
    2. extended.
    3. blended.
    4. multi-adult.

19. A community health nurse has been assigned to work with a patient who is being discharged from a psychiatric facility. The nurse recognizes when dealing with the family that:
    1. all family members do not need to understand and agree to the plan of care.
    2. health behaviors of the family do not influence the health of individual family members.
    3. a nurse needs to change the structure of the family to meet the needs of the patient.
    4. health promotion behaviors need to be tied to the developmental stage of the family.

20. Preparation for working with families includes understanding the life cycle stage that the patient is experiencing. A nurse is working with a family that is in the "launching children and moving on" stage. It is expected that a family in this stage may also need to deal with:
    1. a review of life events.
    2. determining career goals.
    3. the death of an older parent.
    4. development of intimate peer relationships.

21. A nurse is working with a family that has been taking care of a parent with Alzheimer's disease for several years in their home. A nursing diagnosis of *Risk for Caregiver Role Strain* is identified. The nurse initially plans for:
    1. respite care.
    2. more medication for the parent.
    3. placement in a long-term care facility.
    4. consultation with a family therapist.

22. After initial assessment of a family, a nurse determines that this is a healthy family. This assessment is based on the finding that:
    1. the family responds passively to stressors.
    2. change is viewed negatively and strongly resisted.
    3. the family structure is flexible enough to adapt to crises.
    4. minimum influence is exerted by the members upon their environment.

23. An older adult patient who had surgery is going to be discharged tomorrow. The patient has a visual deficit and will need dressing changes twice a day. To meet this specific need, the nurse first:
    1. refers the patient to an adult day care center.
    2. arranges for a private duty nurse to take care of the patient 24 hours a day.
    3. informs the patient that the dressing changes will have to be managed independently.
    4. investigates the availability of a family member or neighbor to perform the dressing changes.

24. A nurse is working in the community with an adult woman who is newly diagnosed with diabetes mellitus. The patient is married, has two school-age children, and works part time. The nurse is focused on assisting the patient to learn to manage the diabetes. At this point, the nurse is viewing the family as:
    1. patient.
    2. context.
    3. process.
    4. caregiver.

25. The concept of a family being able to transcend divorce and remarriage is termed:
    1. family resiliency.
    2. family diversity.
    3. family hardiness.
    4. family functioning.

26. To determine family form and membership, a nurse asks the patient:
    1. "How are financial decisions made?"
    2. "Who drives the children to school?"
    3. "Where do you go on vacation?"
    4. "Who do you consider your family?"

27. The nurse is asking the family how the tasks are divided in the household. This question is used to establish the family's:
    1. structure.
    2. function.
    3. status.
    4. form.

STUDY GROUP QUESTIONS

- What are the attributes of a family?
- What are the different family forms?
- What are the current issues/trends influencing families?
- How do the structure and function of a family influence family relationships?
- How does communication affect family relationships?
- How are the nursing approaches to the family as patient and the family as context similar/different?
- How may critical thinking and nursing processes be applied to family nursing?
- What specific assessments should a nurse make in relation to a family?
- How does a nurse plan for the educational needs of a patient within a family?
- What must a nurse consider to meet the health needs of patients within families?
- How are psychosocial/cultural factors involved in family processes and the nursing approach to families?
- What resources are available within the health care setting and community to assist and support family functioning?

STUDY CHART

Create a study chart for your own family and identify the relationships between the members and each person's role and function.

25 Stress and Coping

CASE STUDY

1. A young adult woman is preparing to be married in a few months. She has also received a recent job promotion that requires many additional hours to be spent at work. She is seen in a nurse practitioner's office for vague symptoms.
   a. What possible signs and symptoms may be demonstrated if this patient is experiencing a stress reaction?
   b. Identify a possible nursing diagnosis for this patient.
   c. Indicate an outcome for the nursing diagnosis.
   d. What relaxation techniques may be presented to this patient?

CHAPTER REVIEW

Complete the following:

1. Evaluating an event for its personal meaning is called:

2. Which of the following are correct statements about stress? Select all that apply.
   a. Increased self-confidence results in decreased tension. _____
   b. The emotional concern of others can increase negative effects. _____
   c. Shorter, less intense stressors increase the stress response. _____
   d. The same event can cause different stress levels in different people. _____
   e. The greater the perceived magnitude of the stressor, the greater the stress response. _____
   f. Stress is decreased if a person is unable to anticipate the occurrence of an event. _____

3. A priority nursing intervention for safety for a patient under extreme stress is to determine:

4. Depression in later adulthood is a common problem.
   True _____ False _____

5. An example of a positive benefit of exercise for stress reduction is:

6. For the following, select the type of stress-producing factor that is indicated: *Situational, Maturational, Sociocultural*
   a. Divorce _______________
   b. Poverty _______________
   c. Immigration status _______________
   d. Job change _______________
   e. Adolescent identity crisis _______________
   f. Hypertension _______________
   g. Children moving away from home _______________
   h. Homelessness _______________

7. Identify an indicator of stress for each of the following areas:
   a. Cognitive
   b. Cardiovascular
   c. Gastrointestinal
   d. Behavioral
   e. Neuroendocrine

8. Identify what stress management techniques can be taught to a patient.

9. The nurse is teaching the patient about reducing the sympathetic nervous system response to stress. A self-regulating approach is to do _____________ exercises.

10. Indicate an area that the nurse would discuss with the patient when using Pender's Health Promotion theory.

11. a. Compassion fatigue is most likely to be seen in a nurse who is working in a(n) ___________________ setting.
    b. What are the signs/symptoms of compassion fatigue?

12. In applying the QSEN competency of safety, what should the nurse assess in relation to stress and coping?

13. When does stress become a crisis?

14. The nurse is assessing a patient and is looking for outward indicators of stress. The following are objective signs associated with stress. Select all that apply.
    a. Twitching ______
    b. Hypotension ______
    c. Tachycardia ______
    d. Maintenance of eye contact ______
    e. Disheveled appearance ______
    f. Picking at the fingernails ______

15. Which of the following are components of cognitive therapy? Select all that apply.
    a. Empowerment ______
    b. Conflict resolution ______
    c. Change perspective ______
    d. Establishing support networks ______
    e. Interaction to express needs and desires ______
    f. Examine whether there is overestimation of the nature of the situation ______

Select the best answer for each of the following questions:

16. An individual who is coping by regressing will demonstrate which behavior?
    1. Becoming numb to the surroundings
    2. Refusing to discuss feelings
    3. Starting to act out in class
    4. Experiencing a loss of appetite

17. A patient has been hospitalized with a serious systemic infection. If the patient is in the resistance stage of the general adaptation syndrome and moving toward recovery, the nurse expects that the patient will demonstrate a:
    1. stabilization of hormone levels.
    2. greater degree of tissue damage.
    3. reduction in cardiac output.
    4. greater involvement of the sympathetic nervous system.

18. While working in a psychiatric emergency department, a nurse is alert to patients who are having severe difficulty in coping. A priority for the nurse is the safety of the patient and others; therefore the nurse asks patients:
    1. "How can we help you?"
    2. "Are you thinking of harming yourself?"
    3. "What physical symptoms are you having?"
    4. "What happened that is different in your life?"

19. As a result of a patient's health problem, the family is experiencing economic difficulty and demonstrating signs of crisis. As part of crisis intervention, a nurse:
    1. refers the patient for financial assistance.
    2. recommends inpatient psychiatric therapy.
    3. plans to teach the family about long-term health needs.
    4. has the patient avoid discussions about personal feelings and emotions.

20. A nurse working for the surgical unit notes that a patient has been exhibiting nervous behavior the evening before a surgical procedure. To assess the degree of stress that the patient is experiencing, the nurse asks:
    1. "Would you like me to call your family for you?"
    2. "How dangerous do you think the surgery will be?"
    3. "You seem anxious. Would you like to talk about the surgery?"
    4. "How would you like to speak with another patient who has had the procedure already?"

21. A nurse identifies that a patient is experiencing a stress reaction. To determine how the patient may cope with the event, the nurse should ask:
    1. "Are you taking any hypnotics?"
    2. "What do you think caused your stress?"
    3. "How long have you felt this way?"
    4. "Have you dealt with this reaction before?"

22. An 80-year-old patient was admitted to the hospital with a diagnosis of pneumonia. The patient is very lethargic and not communicating, and the patient's respirations are extremely labored. The nurse assesses that the patient is experiencing the general adaptation stage of:
    1. alarm.
    2. resistance.
    3. exhaustion.
    4. reflex response.

23. A patient has gone to the employee support center with complaints of fatigue and general uneasiness. The patient believes that the symptoms may be related to the increased amount of work that is expected in the job. The nurse initially recommends that the patient should attempt to reduce or control the stress by:
    1. leaving the job immediately.
    2. enrolling in a self-awareness course.
    3. seeking the assistance of a psychiatrist.
    4. employing relaxation techniques, such as deep breathing.

24. According to general adaptation syndrome (GAS), a nurse expects which of the following signs as part of an alarm reaction?
    1. Pupil dilation
    2. Decreased blood glucose levels
    3. Decreased heart rate
    4. Stabilized hormone levels

25. A nurse identifies that a patient is under stress. To determine the patient's perception of the stress, the nurse should ask:
    1. "Are you sure you are not taking drugs or alcohol?"
    2. "What does the situation mean to you?"
    3. "How did you handle this in the past?"
    4. "Why aren't you seeing a counselor?"

26. Which of the following patient observations does a nurse associate with the ego-defense mechanism of conversion?
    1. Assuming more job responsibilities
    2. Having difficulty sleeping
    3. Acting out inappropriately
    4. Refusing to talk about a problem

27. A patient has been having a hard time at home. He goes outside and begins to yell about the car and starts kicking the tires. This is an example of which of the following ego-defense mechanisms?
    1. Displacement
    2. Compensation
    3. Identification
    4. Denial

28. A nurse wants to assess whether a patient is using maladaptive coping strategies. The patient should be asked specifically about his or her:
    1. dietary intake.
    2. social activities.
    3. cigarette smoking.
    4. exercise plan.

STUDY GROUP QUESTIONS

- What is stress?
- What theories are associated with stress and the stress response?
- How does the general adaptation syndrome (GAS) work?
- How do nursing theorists explain stress and the stress response?
- What factors influence the response to stress?
- What assessment data may indicate the presence of a stress reaction?
- How does stress relate to illness?
- What are coping/defense mechanisms and how may they be used by individuals to deal with stress?
- What is the role of a nurse in reducing or eliminating stress for patients in health promotion, acute care, and restorative care settings?
- What is involved in crisis intervention?
- What are possible relaxation/stress reduction techniques?

26 Loss and Grief

CASE STUDIES

1. A woman's husband committed suicide and she is devastated by the event. In anticipation of potential difficulties, a nurse should be alert to the possibility of a complicated bereavement.
   a. What assessment data may indicate that the woman is experiencing a complicated period of bereavement?
   b. Identify a possible nursing diagnosis, goals/outcomes, and nursing interventions for an individual who is experiencing a complicated bereavement.

2. The family tells the nurse that the patient is interested in hospice care. The siblings have questions about what services are available. As the nurse, what do you tell them about hospice care?

CHAPTER REVIEW

Match the description/definition in Column A with the correct term in Column B.

	Column A	*Column B*
_____	1. A lifetime of normal developmental processes	a. Actual loss
_____	2. Loss that is uniquely experienced by a grieving person and often less obvious to others	b. Perceived loss
_____	3. The result of an unpredictable life event	c. Situational loss
_____	4. When a person can no longer touch, hear, see, or have valued people or objects	d. Maturational loss

Complete the following:

5. Grief resolution may be affected by:

6. Unexpected unemployment may be perceived as a loss. True _____ False _____

7. Provide an intervention that a nurse should implement for a family dealing with a patient's diagnosis of a terminal illness.

8. Which of the following interventions are appropriate for a terminally ill patient with constipation? Select all that apply.
   a. Maintenance of complete bed rest _____
   b. Increased intake of coffee _____
   c. Consumption of fresh vegetables _____
   d. Consumption of whole grain products _____
   e. Reducing fluid intake _____
   f. Obtaining an order for stool softeners _____

9. Identify at least two nursing measures that may be implemented to facilitate the mourning process.

10. Patients in the terminal stage of their lives may experience a sense of abandonment. What actions should a nurse implement to prevent or reduce this occurrence?

11. After a patient's death, there is federal and state legislation regarding policies and procedures for:

12. Formulate a question that a nurse could ask a patient regarding:
    a. The nature of a loss
    b. His/her cultural beliefs about loss
    c. How the family is coping with the loss

13. A patient has been in hospice care at home. A family member is taking care of the patient and is concerned about the patient's impending death, particularly what will happen to the patient. The nurse informs the family member that the signs of impending death include:

14. According to Worden, moving through the four tasks typically takes __________ (time frame).

15. What are the Rs in Rando's R Process Model?

16. In performing postmortem care, which are the correct actions? Select all that apply.
   a. Position the patient upright at 45 to 90 degrees. _____
   b. Ask the family members if they want to help with the care. _____
   c. Discard remaining personal items. _____
   d. Close the patient's eyes. _____
   e. Leave dentures in the patient's mouth. _____
   f. Remove all of the tubes and devices before an autopsy is performed. _____

17. Identify nursing interventions for the following symptoms that may be experienced by a patient who is dying.
   a. Fatigue:

   b. Decreased appetite

18. Provide an example of delayed grief.

19. When would an autopsy be performed?

20. Identify what should be included in the documentation after a patient's death.

21. What physical signs and symptoms can be associated with grief?

Select the best answer for each of the following questions:

22. A nurse is working with a patient who has been diagnosed with a terminal disease. The patient, who is moving into Kübler-Ross's denial stage of grieving, may respond:
   1. "I understand what the diagnosis means, and I know that I may die."
   2. "I would like to be able to make it to my son's wedding in June."
   3. "I think that the diagnostic tests are wrong, and they should be re-done."
   4. "I don't think that I can stand to have any more treatments. I just want to feel better."

23. While working with young children in a day care center, a nurse responds to instances that occur in their lives. Toddlers at the center generally experience loss and grief associated with:
   1. anticipation of loss.
   2. separation from parents.
   3. changes in physical abilities.
   4. development of their identities.

24. In a senior citizen center, a nurse is talking with a group of older adults. The recurrent theme associated with loss for this age group is a:
   1. confusion of fact and fantasy.
   2. perceived threat to their identity.
   3. change in status, role, and lifestyle.
   4. determination to reexamine life goals.

25. A nurse who has recently graduated from nursing school is employed by an oncology unit. There are a number of patients who will not improve and will need assistance with dying. The nurse prepares for this experience by:
   1. completing a detailed course on legal aspects of end of life issues.
   2. controlling his or her emotions about dying patients.
   3. experiencing the death of a close family member.
   4. identifying his or her own feelings about death and dying.

26. A patient has had a long illness and is now approaching the end stages of his life. To assist this patient to meet his need for self-worth and support during this time, the nurse:
   1. arranges for a grief counselor to visit.
   2. leaves the patient alone to deal with his life issues.
   3. asks the patient's family to take over his care.
   4. plans to visit the patient regularly throughout the day.

27. The spouse of a patient who has just died is having more frequent episodes of headaches and generalized joint pain. The initial nursing intervention for this individual is to:
   1. complete a thorough pain assessment.
   2. encourage more frequent use of analgesics.
   3. sit with the patient and encourage discussion of feelings.
   4. refer the patient immediately to a psychologist or grief counselor.

28. A patient is experiencing a very serious illness that may not be curable. The nurse promotes hope for this patient when:
   1. establishing firm goals.
   2. encouraging the development of supportive relationships.
   3. withholding information about the illness and its treatment.
   4. referring the patient for psychological counseling.

29. A patient in the long-term care facility is to receive palliative care measures only during the end stages of a terminal illness. The nurse anticipates that this will include:
   1. pain relief measures.
   2. emergency surgery.
   3. pulmonary resuscitation.
   4. transfer to intensive care if necessary.

30. A patient arrives for outpatient chemotherapy. During this visit the patient tells the nurse that she is experiencing periods of nausea. The nurse promotes patient comfort by providing:
    1. milk.
    2. coffee.
    3. ginger ale.
    4. orange juice.

31. The loss of a known environment is associated with:
    1. being hospitalized for several days.
    2. the death of a pet.
    3. amputation of the right leg.
    4. a recent burglary in the home.

32. Of the following, a situational loss occurs when a:
    1. parent requires physical assistance.
    2. family friend dies.
    3. child goes to college.
    4. job demotion and pay reduction occur.

33. An individual in Bowlby's second phase of mourning, yearning, and searching may be expected to:
    1. be unable to believe the loss.
    2. endlessly examine how the loss occurred.
    3. acquire new skills and build new relationships.
    4. experience emotional outbursts and sobbing.

34. A nurse recognizes exaggerated grief in the person who:
    1. has an active period of mourning that does not decrease and continues over time.
    2. postpones or holds back grieving and responds much later to the event.
    3. cannot function and is overwhelmed, with resulting substance abuse or phobias.
    4. is not aware that behaviors are interfering with daily activities, such as sleeping and eating.

35. The nurse is using Worden's four tasks of mourning to assess the family member's response to the death of a loved one. What is expected when the individual moves into Task III: *Adjust to the environment in which the deceased is missing*?
    1. Realizing that the loved one is gone
    2. Suppressing feelings over the loss
    3. Taking on roles of the loved one
    4. Forgetting the deceased and moving on

STUDY GROUP QUESTIONS

- What are loss and grief?
- What are the different types of loss and possible reactions to these losses?
- What are the differences and similarities between the theories of grief and loss?
- What is anticipatory grief?
- How may the grieving process be influenced by special circumstances?
- How are hope, spirituality, and self-concept related to loss and grieving?
- What behaviors are associated with loss and grieving?
- What resources are available for patient, family, and nurse that assist in the grieving process?
- What principles facilitate mourning?
- How may a nurse apply critical thinking and nursing processes to the patient/family experiencing loss and grieving?
- How are religious and cultural beliefs associated with loss, grief, death, and dying?
- How may a nurse intervene to assist a patient/family with loss and the grieving process?
- What is involved in care of the body after death?

27 Exercise and Activity

CASE STUDY

1. A nurse is assigned to work with an 80-year-old woman residing in a nursing home. There is conflicting information in the chart about her ability to move around independently. The nurse is concerned about meeting her needs for proper body mechanics as well as her safety.
   a. What important assessment information is needed to plan meeting the patient's needs?
   b. If the patient is unable to ambulate independently, what nursing interventions should be planned?

CHAPTER REVIEW

Match the description/definition in Column A with the correct term in Column B.

	Column A	*Column B*
_____	1. Awareness of the position of the body and its parts	a. Body mechanics
_____	2. Resistance that a moving body meets from the surface on which it moves	b. Prone
_____	3. Manner or style of walking	c. Range of motion
_____	4. Lying face up	d. Posture
_____	5. Lying face down	e. Dorsiflexion
_____	6. Movement of the foot where the toes point upward	f. Supine
_____	7. Maintenance of optimal body position	g. Friction
_____	8. Body alignment during walking, turning, lifting, or carrying	h. Gait
_____	9. Mobility of the joint	i. Proprioception

Complete the following:

10. Identify at least three components to assess to determine a patient's mobility.

11. Which of the following are correct principles of body mechanics? Select all that apply.
    a. Maintain a narrow base of support. _____
    b. Face the direction of movement. _____
    c. Maintain a higher center of gravity. _____
    d. Divide balanced activity between the arms and legs. _____
    e. Increase friction between the object and surface. _____
    f. Alternate periods of rest and activity. _____

12. The best way to determine a patient's level of pain is to observe for redness or swelling of the joints.
    True _____ False _____

13. For a patient who has been on prolonged bed rest:
    a. What should the nurse do to prepare the patient before ambulation?
    b. Transfers and position changes for this patient can lead to the development of:

14. Identify at least two pathological influences on alignment, exercise, or activity.

15. Range of motion can be determined by observing the patient's gait and ability to perform activities of daily living. True _____ False _____

16. An example of a physiological factor that may influence activity tolerance is:

17. Identify a nursing diagnosis associated with a change in a patient's ability to maintain physical activity.

18. For a patient who has severe arthritis and is unable to perform activities of daily living because of discomfort on movement, the priority is to:

19. A patient with a respiratory condition should be positioned in:

20. Complete the following about transferring patients.
    a. The general "rule of thumb" for transfers is:
    b. A nurse's priority during patient transfers is:

21. Identify the following patient positions:

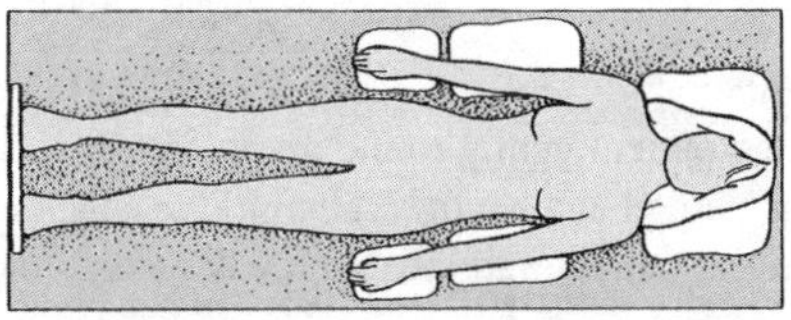

a. ______________________________

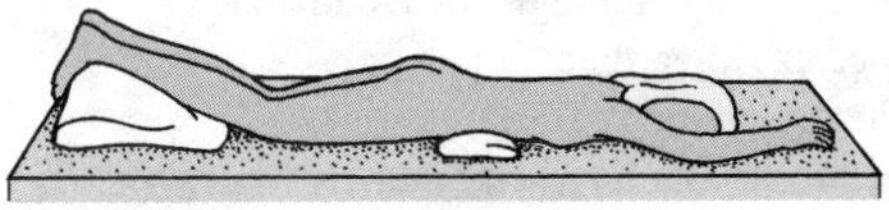

b. ______________________________

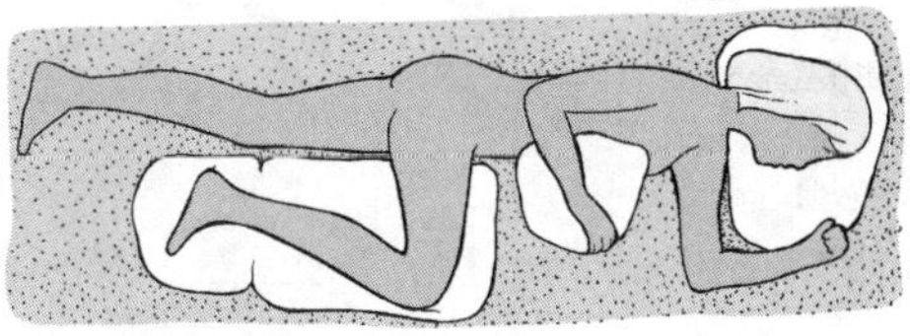

c. ______________________________

22. Which of the following are expected findings for assessment of a patient while standing? Select all that apply.
    a. Head is erect and midline. _____
    b. Body parts are asymmetrical. _____
    c. The spine has a lateral curve. _____
    d. The abdomen protrudes. _____
    e. The knees are in a straight line between the hips and ankles. _____
    f. The feet are pointed at an angle and close together. _____
    g. The arms hang comfortably at the sides. _____

23. Which of the following indicate correct care or technique for a patient who is using crutches? Select all that apply.
    a. The patient leans on the axillae to support his or her weight. _____
    b. Both crutches are transferred to one hand when preparing to sit. _____
    c. Crutches are placed 1 foot to the front and side of the feet. _____
    d. The patient has a non–weight-bearing left leg and is using a three-point gait. _____
    e. The unaffected leg is advanced first when the patient goes up the stairs. _____

24. Patients who are on prolonged bed rest need to be repositioned at least every _____ hours.

25. a. When transferring patients who are able to assist from the bed to a chair, the chair should be positioned:

    b. Identify the steps, in order, for the use of a mechanical lift.

26. Logrolling a patient in bed requires at least _____ caregivers to perform.

27. A nurse observes a patient and notes that there is limited range of motion in a few areas. This could be the result of:

28. The patient, who has some mobility in the upper arms and legs, needs to be moved up in bed. What should the nurse do to reduce friction when moving the patient?

29. Half of all back pain is associated with:

30. Improper positioning of patients in bed can lead to:

31. What position is contraindicated for a patient who is obese or has a respiratory condition?

32. A mechanical device that is used for specific repetitive joint exercise is a:

Select the best answer for each of the following questions:

33. A patient is able to bear weight on one foot. The crutch walking gait that the nurse teaches this patient is the:
    1. two-point gait.
    2. swing-through gait.
    3. three-point alternating gait.
    4. four-point alternating gait.

34. A nurse is working with a patient who is able only to minimally assist the nurse in moving from the bed to the chair. The nurse must help the patient stand. The correct technique for lifting the patient to stand and pivot to the chair is to:
    1. keep the legs straight.
    2. maintain a wide base with the feet.
    3. keep the stomach muscles loose.
    4. support the patient away from the body.

35. A nurse is assisting a patient who has been prescribed total bed rest to perform range-of-motion exercises. The nurse performs the exercises by:
    1. hyperextending the joints.
    2. working from proximal to distal joints.
    3. flexing the joints beyond where slight resistance is felt.
    4. providing support for joints distal to the joint being exercised.

36. A patient has experienced an injury to his lower extremity. The orthopedist has prescribed the use of crutches and a four-point gait. The nurse instructs the patient using this gait to:
    1. move the right foot forward first.
    2. move both crutches forward together.
    3. move the right foot and the left crutch together.
    4. move the right foot and the right crutch together.

37. The patient had a cerebrovascular accident (CVA/stroke) with resultant left hemiparesis. The nurse is instructing the patient on the use of a cane for support during ambulation. The nurse instructs the patient to:
    1. use the cane on the right side.
    2. use the cane on the left side.
    3. move the left foot forward first.
    4. move the right foot forward first.

38. A patient is admitted to the rehabilitation facility for physical therapy after an automobile accident. To conduct an assessment of the patient's body alignment, the nurse should begin by:
    1. observing the patient's gait.
    2. putting the patient at ease.
    3. determining the level of activity tolerance.
    4. evaluating the full extent of joint range of motion.

39. An average-size female patient who resides in the extended care facility requires assistance to ambulate down the hall. The nurse has noticed that the patient has some weakness on her right side. The nurse assists this patient to ambulate by:
    1. standing at her left side and holding the patient's arm.
    2. walking in front of her and having her hold on to her waist.
    3. standing behind her and encircling one arm around the patient's waist.
    4. standing at her right side and using a gait belt.

40. A patient has a cast on the right foot and is being discharged home. Crutches will be used for ambulation, and the patient has stairs to manage to enter the house and to get to the bedroom and bathroom. The nurse observes the patient using the correct technique in using the crutches on the stairs when the patient:
    1. advances the crutches first to ascend the stairs.
    2. uses one crutch for support while going up and down.
    3. uses the banister or wall for support when descending the stairs.
    4. advances the affected leg after moving the crutches when descending the stairs.

41. A patient is getting up to ambulate for the first time since a surgical procedure. While ambulating in the hallway, the patient complains of severe dizziness. The nurse should first:
    1. call for help.
    2. lower the patient gently to the floor.
    3. lean the patient against the wall until the episode passes.
    4. support the patient and move quickly back to the room.

42. One of the expected benefits of exercise is:
    1. decreased diaphragmatic excursion.
    2. decreased cardiac output.
    3. increased fatigue.
    4. decreased resting heart rate.

43. A nurse selects which of the following for maintaining dorsiflexion of a patient?
    1. Pillows
    2. Foot boots
    3. Bed boards
    4. Trochanter rolls

44. A nurse recognizes that the position that is contraindicated for a patient who is at risk for aspiration is:
    1. Fowler's.
    2. lateral.
    3. Sims'.
    4. supine.

45. A patient had total hip replacement surgery and requires careful postoperative positioning to maintain the legs in abduction. The nurse will obtain a:
    1. foot boot.
    2. trapeze bar.
    3. bed board.
    4. wedge pillow.

46. The patient is placed in bed in Fowler's position. To prevent external rotation of the hips, the nurse uses:
    1. foot boots.
    2. trochanter rolls.
    3. leg splints.
    4. side rails.

47. The first step in initiating an exercise program for a patient is to:
    1. select the equipment.
    2. design the fitness program.
    3. schedule time during the day.
    4. seek approval from the health care prescriber.

STUDY GROUP QUESTIONS

- What are body mechanics?
- How is body movement regulated by the musculoskeletal and nervous systems?
- What general changes occur in the body's appearance and function throughout growth and development?
- How can body mechanics be influenced by pathological conditions?
- What patient assessment data should be obtained regarding body mechanics?
- What is activity tolerance?
- How can proper body mechanics be promoted for patients in different health care settings?
- What safety measures should be implemented before patient transfers and ambulation?
- What are the proper procedures for range-of-motion exercises, transfers, positioning, and ambulation?
- How should a patient be instructed to use assistive devices, such as canes, walkers, and crutches?

STUDY CHART

Create a study chart to describe how to *Safely Use Assistive Devices for Ambulation* which identifies the nursing actions and patient instruction required to reduce possible hazards for the following devices: gait belt, cane, walker, crutches.

28 Safety

CASE STUDIES

1. You will be accompanying the visiting nurse to the home of a family with two young children who are ages 2 and 4 years.
   a. What general assessment information should be obtained regarding home safety during the visit?
   b. What specific safety observations should be made because there are two young children residing in the home?

2. A patient with diabetes mellitus is living at home and needs to take daily insulin injections.
   a. What are some of the precautions that this patient should take to avoid pathogen transmission and maintain safety?

3. You are currently working in a long-term care facility. There are a number of patients who are recognized as being at risk for falls. A restraint-free environment is desired.
   a. What specific interventions may be implemented to prevent falls and provide for patient safety without the use of restraints?

CHAPTER REVIEW

Complete the following:

1. Identify an example of a problem that may be encountered if a basic human need of a safe environment is not met.

2. Provide an example of a possible physical hazard that may be found in the home.

3. For older adults:
   a. Identify at least three (3) physiological changes that increase the risk of accidents for older adults.
   b. Indicate at least two (2) areas that should be included in teaching the older adult about:
      (1) Driving safety
      (2) Home environment safety

4. For each of the following, identify a nursing intervention that may be implemented to prevent injury and promote patient safety.
   a. Falls
   b. Patient-inherent accidents
   c. Procedure-related risks
   d. Equipment-related risks

5. The Centers for Medicare and Medicaid Services (CMS) have identified that payment will be denied for events that are not present on admission but occur during hospitalization. Which of the following are included in the listing of these "never events"? Select all that apply.
   a. Air embolism _____
   b. Blood transfusion _____
   c. Patient falls _____
   d. Wrong medication administered _____
   e. Surgical site infection _____
   f. Stage III pressure ulcer _____

6. Immunity that occurs as a result of injection of weakened or dead organisms and modified toxins is called:

7. For each of the following age groups, identify an example of a potential safety hazard.
   a. Infant, toddler, preschooler
   b. School-age child
   c. Adolescent
   d. Adult
   e. Older adult

8. During an assessment, a nurse determines that a patient with a high risk for injury is an individual experiencing:

9. For each of the following potential bioterrorist methods, identify a possible agent that may be used.
   a. Biological
   b. Chemical
   c. Radiological

10. There is a greater risk for poisoning as a result of finding multiple medications in the home of an older adult.
    True _____ False _____

11. An example of safety instruction for a school-age child would be:

12. The primary goal when using restraints (safety reminder devices) is to:

13. A restraint is indicated for a patient in the hospital. Which of the following are correct for the use of restraints? Select all that apply.
    a. Obtain renewals for restraint orders every 72 hours. _____
    b. Evaluate the patient at least every 2 hours. _____
    c. Pad the skin under the restraint. _____
    d. Remove the restraint at least every 2 hours. _____
    e. At least two fingers should fit under the secured restraint. _____
    f. Tie the restraint ends with a knot. _____
    g. Attach the restraint ties to the side rails. _____

14. Side rails may be used at any time to keep a patient in bed.
    True _____ False _____

15. An older adult patient who often forgets to take medication or does not remember if it was taken may benefit from a(n):

16. Identify an example of a medication safety strategy that is used in a health care agency.

17. For the following areas, identify a specific environmental adjustment that should be made to promote safety.
    a. Tactile deficit
    b. Visual deficit

18. Identify an example of an intervention that may be implemented as an alternative to patient restraint.

19. An example of a nursing diagnosis associated with patient safety concerns is:

20. Carbon monoxide poisoning can occur in the home.
    a. Identify the signs and symptoms associated with low concentrations.
    b. What safety measure is necessary to prevent exposure?

21. Explain the "Speak Up" campaign.

22. What resources/agencies are available for patient safety standards?

23. What are the leading causes of falls in the (a) home and (b) health care agency?

24. Information about chemical substances in the health care workplace can be found in:

25. The parents of an adolescent are concerned about possible substance abuse. What signs, symptoms, and behaviors are indicative of this problem?

26. For disaster management, hospitals are required to have what resources in place?

27. The application of physical restraints may be delegated to nursing assistive personnel.
    True _____ False _____

28. Identify the meaning of the following for fire management:

R -	P -
A -	A -
C -	S -
E -	S -

29. Match the type of fire extinguisher with the form of fire.
    Type A, Type B, Type C
    a. Grease fire __________
    b. Electrical fire __________
    c. Paper fire __________

30. The nurse notices that the plug for the infusion pump makes a spark when it is plugged into the wall socket. The nurse should:

31. Identify at least one (1) Patient Safety Goal identified by The Joint Commission for the following:
    a. Hospitals
    b. Home care

32. Place the steps for the Timed Get Up and Go Test in order:
    a. Stand still momentarily _____
    b. Sit down _____
    c. Walk 10 feet (3 meters) (in a line) _____
    d. Turn around _____
    e. Stand up from the armchair _____
    f. Walk back to chair _____
    g. Turn around _____

    What is an abnormal result for the test?

33. Indicate safety measures for the following:
    a. Use of home oxygen
    b. Food preparation

34. For the following patient scenario, identify the assessment findings that the nurse should focus on to prevent patient injuries.

    Upon entering the patient's home, the visiting nurse observed that the patient was wearing slippers with no back (slip-ons). The patient stated that she seemed always to leave her glasses somewhere. There were piles of newspapers and other items cluttering the floor around the living room chairs. The lighting in the stairway was less than 60 watts and there were throw rugs on the wood floors in the halls. When looking through the medicine cabinet with the patient, the nurse noted that some medications were expired. The patient admitted to falling once when getting up during the night to go to the bathroom.

Select the best answer for each of the following questions:

35. The nurse recognizes the importance of teaching the patient who is using oxygen at home that the leading cause of burns and fires is:
    1. smoking.
    2. the use of heating blankets.
    3. the misuse of the stove.
    4. damage to the oxygen tank.

36. An older adult patient is being discharged home. The patient will be taking furosemide (Lasix) on a daily basis. A specific consideration for this patient is:
    1. exposure to the sun.
    2. food consumption when taking the medication.
    3. the location of the bathroom.
    4. financial considerations for long-term care.

37. While walking through a hallway in the extended care facility, a nurse notices smoke coming from a wastebasket in a patient's room. Upon closer investigation, the nurse identifies that there is a fire that is starting to flare up. The nurse should first:
    1. extinguish the fire.
    2. remove the patient from the room.
    3. contain the fire by closing the door to the room.
    4. turn off all of the surrounding electrical equipment.

38. A patient is newly admitted to the hospital and appears to be disoriented. There is a concern for the patient's immediate safety. The nurse is considering the use of restraints to prevent an injury. The nurse recognizes that the use of restraints in a hospital requires:
    1. a physician's order.
    2. the patient's consent.
    3. a family member's consent.
    4. agreement among the nursing staff.

39. A nurse is completing admission histories for newly admitted patients to the unit. The nurse is aware that the patient with the greatest risk of injury:
    1. is 84 years of age.
    2. uses corrective lenses.
    3. has a history of falls.
    4. has arthritis in the lower extremities.

40. A child has ingested a poisonous substance. The parent is instructed by the nurse to:
    1. take the child to the hospital immediately.
    2. call the poison control center.
    3. take the child to the pediatrician.
    4. administer 30 mL of emetic.

41. A restraint that may be used to prevent an adult patient from pulling on and removing tubes or an IV is a(n):
    1. vest restraint.
    2. jacket restraint.
    3. extremity restraint.
    4. mummy restraint.

42. An older adult patient in the extended care facility has been wandering outside of the room during the late evening hours. The patient has a history of falls. The nurse intervenes initially by:
    1. placing an abdominal restraint on the patient during the night.
    2. keeping the light and the television on in the patient's room all night.
    3. reassigning the patient to a room close to the nursing station.
    4. having the family members check on the patient during the night.

43. A parent with three children has gone to the outpatient clinic. The children range in age from 2½ to 15 years old. A nurse is discussing safety issues with the parent. The nurse evaluates that further teaching is required if the parent states:
    1. "I have spoken to my teenager about safe sex practices."
    2. "I make sure that my child wears a helmet when he rides his bicycle."
    3. "My 8-year-old is taking swimming classes at the local community center."
    4. "Now my 2½-year-old can finally sit in the front seat of the car with me."

44. A bacteria that is spread through inadequate preparation or storage of food is:
    1. *Streptococcus.*
    2. *Candida.*
    3. *Listeria.*
    4. *Hepatitis B.*

STUDY GROUP QUESTIONS

- What are the basic human needs regarding safety?
- What are some physical hazards and how can they be reduced or eliminated?
- What developmental changes and abilities predispose individuals to accidents or injury?
- What additional risk factors may affect an individual's level of safety?
- What risks exist in a health care agency, and how can they be prevented?
- What safety measures and patient teaching should be implemented in different health care settings?
- What are the procedures for the correct use of side rails and restraints?
- How can a nurse avoid the use of patient restraints?
- What assessment information should be obtained regarding patient/family safety?
- How can a nurse assist patients and families in reducing or eliminating safety hazards?

29 Hygiene

CASE STUDIES

1. Your clinical experience is scheduled to be on a medical unit. It will be your responsibility to provide instruction to a patient who has just been diagnosed with diabetes mellitus.
   a. What specific information on hygienic care will be included for the patient's teaching session?

2. An older adult patient residing in an extended care facility requires assistance with hygienic care.
   a. What developmental changes are considered when assisting this patient to meet hygienic needs?

CHAPTER REVIEW

Match the description/definition in Column A with the correct term in Column B.

	Column A	*Column B*
_____	1. Inflammation of the skin characterized by abrupt onset with erythema, pruritus, pain, and scaly oozing lesions	a. Abrasion
_____	2. Thickened portion of the epidermis, usually flat and painless, on the undersurface of the foot or hand	b. Without teeth
_____	3. Inflammation of the tissue surrounding the nail	c. Plantar wart
_____	4. Scraping or rubbing away of the epidermis, resulting in localized bleeding	d. Xerosis
_____	5. Keratosis caused by friction and pressure from shoes, mainly on toes	e. Contact dermatitis
_____	6. Fungating lesion that appears on the sole of the foot	f. Corn
_____	7. Loss of hair	g. Gingivitis
_____	8. Edentulous	h. Paronychia
_____	9. Inflammation of the gums	i. Callus
_____	10. Abnormal drying of the skin	j. Alopecia

Complete the following:

11. Identify at least three (3) factors that contribute to a hygiene self-care deficit.

12. What modifications are done when providing hygienic care to a patient with dementia?

13. Which of the following techniques are appropriate for diabetic foot care? Select all that apply.
    a. Soaking the feet _____
    b. Rubbing the feet vigorously to dry them _____
    c. Walking barefoot to toughen the feet _____
    d. Applying lotion for dryness _____
    e. Wearing clean, white cotton socks _____
    f. Using a heating pad to warm the feet _____
    g. Applying a mild antiseptic to small cuts _____
    h. Avoiding elastic stockings _____

14. A nurse-initiated treatment for a skin rash is:

15. When cleansing a patient's eyes, the nurse should use:

16. The nurse recognizes that the skin goes through changes throughout the life span. Which of the following are accurate statements regarding the characteristics of the skin? Select all that apply.
    a. Neonatal skin is thinner. ______
    b. The sebaceous glands become active during the toddler years. ______
    c. Young adult skin should be elastic, firm, and smooth. ______
    d. The sweat glands are fully functional at puberty. ______
    e. Skin thickens progressively with aging. ______
    f. Lubrication from the skin glands diminishes over time. ______

17. For hygienic care, the nurse applies the ethical principle of autonomy, which means that the nurse should:

18. When is a standing shower contraindicated for a patient?

19. For the patient with a nursing diagnosis of *Activity Intolerance*, how can hygienic care be affected?

20. Identify ways that the nurse can promote healthy skin for the patient.

21. True/False:
    a. Cotton-tipped applicators should be used to remove earwax.
       True ______ False ______
    b. A 5- to 10-minute bath can add moisture to the skin of an older adult.
       True ______ False ______

22. The nurse wants to help the patient to have healthy teeth and gums. Which of the following recommendations should be made to the patient? Select all that apply.
    a. Change the toothbrush every 6 to 8 months. ______
    b. Use a soft-bristle toothbrush with a straight handle. ______
    c. Floss at least once each day. ______
    d. Brush the teeth at least once each day. ______
    e. Use a toothbrush cover to protect the bristles. ______

23. Evidence-based practice indicates that this product is more effective than soap in reducing the bacteria found in washbasins:

24. The patient's eyeglasses should be kept:

25. Ear irrigation is contraindicated in the presence of:

26. Asepsis is maintained during linen changes when the nurse:

27. Provide an example of how the nurse prepares a comfortable environment for the patient in the health care facility:

28. Identify physiological conditions that may place a patient at risk for impaired skin integrity.

29. How does the use of a commercial "bag bath" differ from a regular patient bed bath?

30. Identify a safety measure that is implemented when providing a tub bath for a patient.

31. How may patients' cultural background influence their hygienic care practices?

32. A nurse notes that a young adult patient has acne of the face and back. What care should be provided?

33. Identify at least three guidelines for patient bathing and skin care.

34. What patients may require special oral hygiene?

35. Place the steps of the bed bath in the correct order:
    a. Back ______
    b. Arms ______
    c. Face ______
    d. Abdomen ______
    e. Legs ______
    f. Perineal area ______
    g. Chest ______

36. Identify safety measures that should be implemented during oral care for an unconscious patient.

37. What is the procedure for irrigation of the ear?

38. Before providing nail care for a patient who is not diabetic, the nurse should:

39. During the bath, the nurse assesses the patient carefully. There are signs of vascular insufficiency in the lower extremities. This is determined based upon finding:

40. What special considerations are included for the hygienic care of the older adult?

41. For the patient who uses a hearing aid, which are the appropriate instructions for the nurse to provide to the patient? Select all that apply.
   a. Check for whistling sounds _____
   b. Wear the hearing aid continuously _____
   c. Store the hearing aid in a warm, heated place _____
   d. Use alcohol to clean the hearing aid _____
   e. Check the battery while the hearing aid is in the ear _____
   f. Remove the battery if the hearing aid is not going to be used for a day or two _____

Select the best answer for each of the following questions:

42. A nurse is caring for an older adult patient in an extended care facility. The patient wears dentures, and the nurse delegated their care to the nursing assistant. The nurse instructs the assistant that the patient's dentures should be:
   1. cleaned in hot water.
   2. left in place during the night.
   3. brushed with a soft toothbrush.
   4. wrapped in a soft towel when not worn.

43. A nurse determines, after completing an assessment, that an expected outcome for a patient with impaired skin integrity will be that the:
   1. skin remains dry.
   2. skin has increased erythema.
   3. skin tingles in areas of pressure.
   4. skin demonstrates increased diaphoresis.

44. A patient has been hospitalized following a traumatic injury. The nurse is now able to provide hair care for the patient. The nurse includes:
   1. using hot water to rinse the scalp.
   2. cutting away matted or tangled hair.
   3. using the fingernails to massage the patient's scalp.
   4. applying peroxide to dissolve blood in the hair and then rinsing with saline.

45. While completing a patient's bath, a nurse notices a red, raised skin rash on the patient's chest. The next step for the nurse to take is to:
   1. moisturize the skin with lotion.
   2. wash the area again with hot water and soap.
   3. discuss proper hygienic care with the patient.
   4. assess for any other areas of inflammation.

46. A nurse is planning patient assignment with a nursing assistant. In delegating the morning care for a patient, the nurse expects the assistant to:
   1. cut the patient's nails with scissors.
   2. use soap to wash the patient's eyes.
   3. wash the patient's legs with long strokes from the ankle to the knee.
   4. place the unconscious patient in high-Fowler's position to provide oral hygiene.

47. A patient is receiving chemotherapy and is experiencing stomatitis. To promote comfort for this patient, a nurse recommends that the patient use:
   1. a firm toothbrush.
   2. normal saline rinses.
   3. a commercial mouthwash.
   4. an alcohol and water mixture.

48. For a patient with dry skin, a nurse should:
   1. apply moisturizing lotion.
   2. use hot water for bathing.
   3. obtain a dehumidifier.
   4. wash the skin frequently.

49. Use of an electric razor is specifically indicated for a patient who is being treated with:
   1. diuretics.
   2. antibiotics.
   3. anticoagulants.
   4. narcotic analgesics.

50. When making an occupied bed, the first step for a nurse is to:
   1. cover the patient with a bath blanket.
   2. position the patient on the far side of the bed.
   3. explain the procedure to the patient.
   4. adjust the height of the bed to waist level.

51. The nurse is providing information to a group of parents. Which of the following statements provides accurate information about the teeth?
   1. Permanent teeth are in place at 13 years of age.
   2. Wisdom teeth erupt in the 35 and older age group.
   3. The first permanent teeth come in at around 3 years of age.
   4. Teething occurs after the child reaches 1½ to 2 years old.

52. The nurse manager is evaluating a new staff member's patient care. Which of the following interventions demonstrates correct technique?
    1. Placing the bedpan on the overbed table
    2. Returning extra linens from the patient's room to the linen cart
    3. Using side rails all the time to keep the patient safely in bed
    4. Moving the bed up to change the linen and reposition the patient

STUDY GROUP QUESTIONS

- What hygienic care measures are necessary for the integumentary system?
- What factors may influence a patient's hygienic care practices?
- How do growth and development influence hygienic care needs?
- What are the patient teaching needs for hygienic care across the life span?
- What assessments of the integumentary system are necessary to determine integumentary alterations and hygienic care needs?
- What are the correct procedures for providing hygienic care and a comfortable environment for patients?
- How does a patient's self-care ability influence the provision of hygienic care?
- How is physical assessment integrated into the provision of hygienic care?
- What actions should be taken if a patient refuses hygienic care?

30 Oxygenation

CASE STUDY

1. You are the nurse in an outpatient clinic in which a 32-year-old woman receives ongoing medical treatment. She tells you that she has had asthma since she was a young child. While speaking with the patient, you notice that she is exhibiting mild wheezing and a productive cough. She appears slightly pale.
   a. What additional assessment questions should be asked of this patient?
   b. Identify a possible nursing diagnosis for this patient.
   c. What nurse-initiated actions may be taken at this time?
   d. Identify general information that should be included in patient teaching for promoting oxygenation.

CHAPTER REVIEW

Match the description/definition in Column A with the correct term in Column B.

	Column A	*Column B*
_____	1. Collapse of alveoli, preventing exchange of oxygen	a. Hypoxia
_____	2. Tachypnea pattern of breathing associated with metabolic acidosis	b. Pneumothorax
_____	3. Need to sit upright to breathe easier	c. Atelectasis
_____	4. Collection of air in the pleural space	d. Kussmaul respiration
_____	5. Bloody sputum	e. Orthopnea
_____	6. Inadequate tissue oxygenation at the cellular level	f. Hemothorax
_____	7. Amount of blood in the ventricles at the end of diastole	g. Preload
_____	8. Collection of blood in the pleural space	h. Afterload
_____	9. Resistance of ejection of blood from the left ventricle	i. Hemoptysis
_____	10. Difficulty breathing, sensation of breathlessness	j. Dyspnea

Complete the following:

11. The average resting heart rate for an adult is _____ beats per minute.

12. Chest movement is affected by what conditions?

13. Identify whether the following signs and symptoms are associated with left ventricular or right ventricular heart failure:
    a. Distended neck veins _____
    b. Ankle edema _____
    c. Pulmonary congestion _____
    d. Increased arterial blood pressure _____

14. Which of the following may cause hyperventilation? Select all that apply.
    a. Anxiety _____
    b. Fever _____
    c. Severe atelectasis _____
    d. Head injury _____
    e. Excessive administration of oxygen _____

15. Provide an example of a physiological alteration or problem that may result in each of the following:
    a. Decreased oxygen-carrying capacity
    b. Decreased inspired oxygen concentration
    c. Hypovolemia
    d. Increased metabolic rate

16. A premature infant has a deficiency of ________ and is at risk for hyaline membrane disease.

17. An example of a controllable risk factor for cardiopulmonary disease is:

18. Which of the following pathophysiological changes in the heart and lungs occur with aging? Select all that apply.
    a. Thinning of the ventricular wall of the heart _____
    b. SA node becoming fibrotic from calcification _____
    c. Increased elastin in the arterial vessel walls _____
    d. Increased chest wall compliance and elastic recoil _____
    e. Decreased alveolar surface area _____
    f. Increased responsiveness of central and peripheral chemoreceptors _____
    g. Decreased number of cilia _____
    h. Increased respiratory drive _____

19. A patient awakes in a panic and feels as though she is suffocating. This is noted by the nurse as:

20. A musical, high-pitched lung sound that may be heard on inspiration or expiration is:

21. Identify the following two cardiac rhythms:
    a.

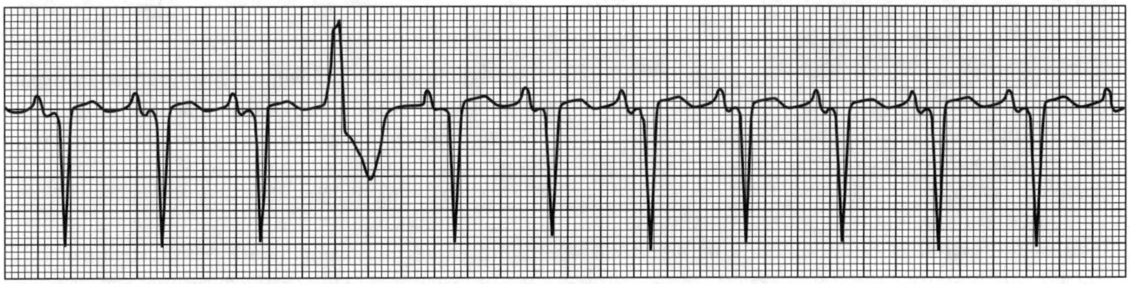

    b.

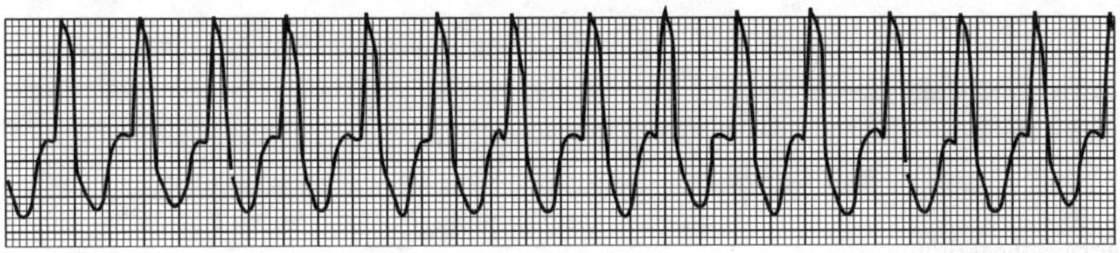

22. Briefly define the following abnormal chest wall movements:
    a. Retraction
    b. Paradoxical breathing

23. Which type of asepsis is used for tracheal suctioning?

24. Continuous bubbling in the chest tube water-seal chamber indicates:

25. Identify an example of a nursing intervention for promotion of each of the following:
    a. Dyspnea management
    b. Patent airway
    c. Lung expansion
    d. Mobilization of secretions

26. Identify the following types of oxygen delivery systems and the flow rate for each:
    a.

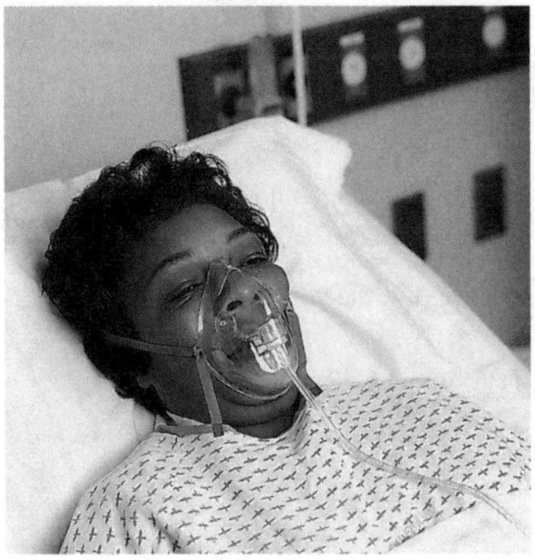

b. 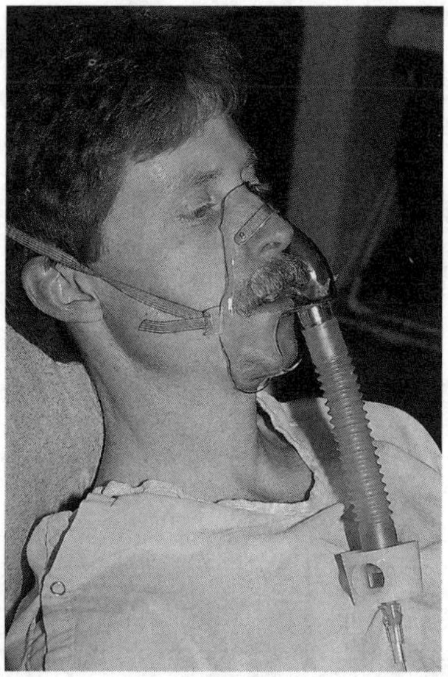

27. Identify the following for tuberculin (Mantoux) testing:
    a. A skin test is administered on a patient's:
    b. The test is read after _____ hours.
    c. A reddened, flat area is a(n) _________ reaction.
    d. The patient received a BCG vaccination, so the tuberculin skin test will most likely be:
    Positive ______ Negative ______

28. For chest percussion, vibration, and postural drainage:
    a. Chest percussion is contraindicated for a patient with:
    b. Vibration is used only during:
    c. The position for a 2-year-old for postural drainage is:

29. For continuous positive airway pressure (CPAP):
    a. CPAP is used for:
    b. The usual pressure setting is:
    c. A disadvantage of CPAP is:
    d. How is BiPAP different from CPAP?

30. For home oxygen therapy:
    a. It is indicated when the patient has an SaO_2 value of:
    b. What safety measures should be implemented when oxygen is used in the home?

31. The interventions in CPR are:
    C -
    A -
    B -

32. Defibrillation is recommended within _____ (time) for an out-of-hospital sudden cardiac arrest and within _____ (time) for an inpatient.

33. a. The prevalence of atrial fibrillation increases with age and is the leading contributing factor for stroke in the older adult.
    True _____ False _____
    b. Care of chest tubes can be delegated to a nursing assistant.
    True _____ False _____

34. The patient has oxygen via a nasal cannula. What specific nursing care should be provided for this patient?

35. For the nursing diagnosis *Ineffective Airway Clearance related to the presence of tracheobronchial secretions*, identify a patient outcome and a nursing intervention to assist the patient to meet the outcome.

36. Which of the following are appropriate interventions for patient suctioning? Select all that apply.
    a. Performing pharyngeal suctioning before tracheal suctioning _____
    b. Avoiding routine use of normal saline instillations when suctioning _____
    c. Applying suction for 30 seconds at a time _____
    d. Suctioning during the insertion and removal of the tube _____
    e. Allowing 1 to 2 minutes between suction passes _____
    f. Providing regular suctioning every 1 to 2 hours around the clock _____

37. Cardiac output is the result of the stroke volume × _____.

38. For a patient with hypoxia:
    a. What are the signs and symptoms?
    b. What treatment is anticipated?

39. Identify a possible nursing diagnosis for a patient with anemia.

40. Provide examples of dietary risks that may influence cardiopulmonary status and oxygenation.

41. The most effective positioning for a patient with cardiopulmonary disease is:

42. A method to encourage voluntary deep breathing for a postoperative patient is the use of an:

43. Identify at least two environmental or occupational hazards that may affect an individual's cardiopulmonary functioning:

44. Cardiac dysrhythmias may be caused by:

45. The nurse anticipates that atrial fibrillation will be treated with:

46. To reduce the incidence of ventilator associated pneumonia (VAP), the nurse will implement:

47. The nurse anticipates that treatment for hyperventilation will include:

48. Place the following steps for in-line suctioning in the correct sequence. The nurse has already positioned the patient and performed hand hygiene.
   a. Reassess pulmonary status. _____
   b. Insert the catheter until resistance is felt. _____
   c. Hyperoxygenate the patient. _____
   d. Withdraw the catheter, applying suction. _____
   e. Repeat the procedure, if indicated. _____
   f. Pick up the catheter enclosed in the plastic sheath. _____

49. Identify the areas on the chest tube system illustration below.

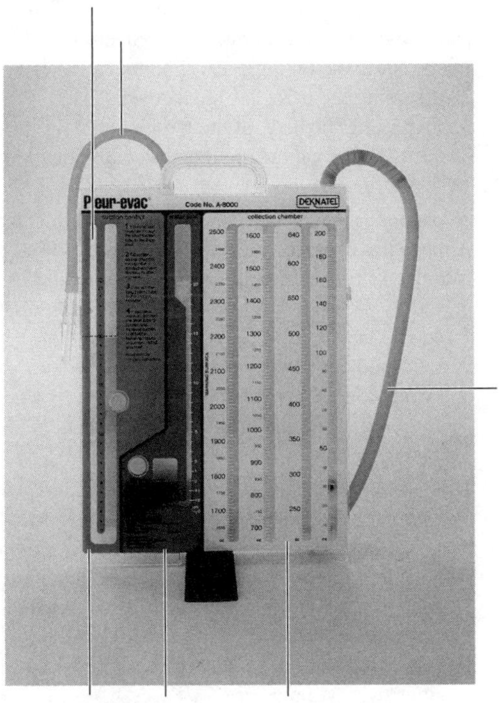

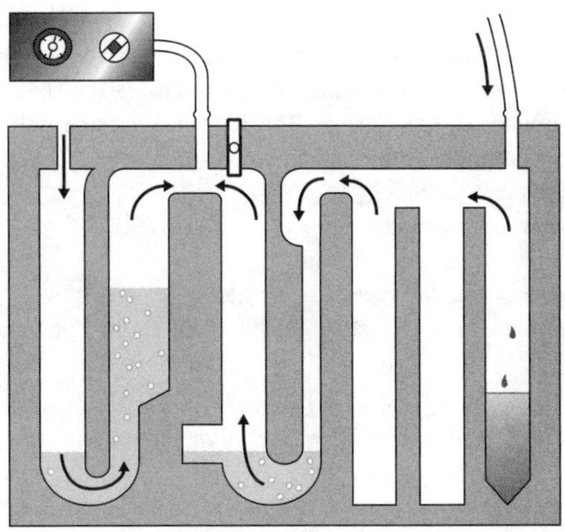

50. Identify the appropriate care for a patient with a closed chest tube drainage system in place. Select all that apply.
   a. Clamp the chest tube when the patient ambulates. _____
   b. Milk the tube for the patient who has just had thoracic surgery. _____
   c. Instruct the patient to inhale if the tube disconnects. _____
   d. Report more than 100 mL of sanguinous drainage after the patient is more than 8 hours postoperative. _____
   e. Keep the drainage unit upright. _____

51. Identify at least three (3) pathologies that reduce chest wall expansion.

52. Signs and symptoms of a myocardial infarction in women include:

53. What factors contribute to respiratory problems in infants and young children?

54. Which of the following are lifestyle factors that contribute to poor cardiopulmonary status? Select all that apply.
   a. Having a diet low in protein _____
   b. Participating in a daily exercise regimen _____
   c. Drinking significant amounts of alcohol _____
   d. Being a construction worker _____
   e. Having a high-stress job _____

55. An early sign that the patient's chronic cardiopulmonary disease is worsening is: ____________.

56. The patient becomes breathless and tired during the physical exam. The nurse should:

57. Nebulization is used in the administration of what types of medications?

58. A Yankauer suction catheter is used for ____________ ________ suction.

59. Positioning for the patient with right-sided atelectasis will be on the left or right side?

60. What medication is contraindicated for a patient with asthma?

61. Caution is used when administering oxygen to patients with chronic lung disease because:

62. Individuals have gone to the health fair to receive their free influenza vaccine. The nurse briefly discusses the medical backgrounds of the patients. The influenza vaccine will be withheld from the following individuals. Select all that apply.
    a. HIV-positive man _____
    b. Older adult woman _____
    c. Man with chronic arthritis _____
    d. Woman with a hypersensitivity to eggs _____
    e. Woman with a history of Guillain-Barré syndrome _____

Select the best answer for each of the following questions:

63. A patient has a chest tube in place to drain bloody secretions from the chest cavity. When caring for a patient with a chest tube, a nurse should:
    1. keep the drainage device above chest level.
    2. clamp the chest tube when the patient is ambulating.
    3. have the patient cough if the tubing becomes disconnected.
    4. leave trapped fluid in the tubing and estimate the amount.

64. A nurse is making a home visit to a patient who has emphysema (chronic obstructive pulmonary disease [COPD]). Specific instruction to control exhalation pressure for this patient with an increased residual volume of air should include:
    1. coughing.
    2. deep breathing.
    3. pursed-lip breathing.
    4. diaphragmatic breathing.

65. A patient has been admitted to a medical center with a respiratory condition and dyspnea. A number of medications are prescribed for the patient. For a patient with this difficulty, the nurse should question the order for:
    1. steroids.
    2. mucolytics.
    3. bronchodilators.
    4. narcotic analgesics.

66. After a patient assessment, the nurse suspects hypoxemia. This is based on the nurse finding that the patient is experiencing:
    1. restlessness.
    2. bradypnea.
    3. bradycardia.
    4. hypotension.

67. A patient has experienced some respiratory difficulty and is placed on oxygen via nasal cannula. A nurse assists the patient with this form of oxygen delivery by:
    1. changing the tubing every 4 hours.
    2. assessing the nares for breakdown.
    3. inspecting the back of the mouth q8h.
    4. securing the cannula to the nose with nonallergic tape.

68. A patient is being seen in an outpatient medical clinic. A nurse has reviewed the patient's chart and finds that there is a history of a cardiopulmonary abnormality. This is supported by the nurse's assessment of the patient having:
    1. scleral jaundice.
    2. reddened conjunctivae.
    3. symmetrical chest movement.
    4. clubbing of the fingertips.

69. A 65-year-old patient is seen in a physician's office for a routine annual checkup. As part of the physical examination, an ECG is performed. The ECG reveals a normal P wave, P-R interval, and QRS complex and a heart rate of 58 beats per minute. The nurse evaluates this finding as:
    1. sinus tachycardia.
    2. sinus bradycardia.
    3. sinus dysrhythmia.
    4. supraventricular bradycardia.

70. A patient is admitted to a medical center with a diagnosis of left ventricular congestive heart failure. A nurse is completing the physical assessment and is anticipating finding that the patient has:
    1. liver enlargement.
    2. peripheral edema.
    3. pulmonary congestion.
    4. jugular neck vein distention.

71. A patient has just returned to the unit after abdominal surgery. A nurse is planning care for this patient and is considering interventions to promote pulmonary function and prevent complications. The nurse:
    1. teaches the patient leg exercises to perform.
    2. asks the physician to order nebulizer treatments.
    3. demonstrates the use of a flow-oriented incentive spirometer.
    4. informs the patient that his secretions will need to be suctioned.

72. A nurse manager is evaluating the care that is provided by a new staff nurse during the orientation period. One of the patients requires nasotracheal suctioning, and the nurse manager determines that the appropriate technique is used when the new staff nurse:
    1. places the patient in the supine position.
    2. prepares for a clean or nonsterile procedure.
    3. suctions the oropharyngeal area first and then moves to the nasotracheal area.
    4. applies intermittent suction for 10 seconds while the suction catheter is being removed.

73. Chest tubes have been inserted into a patient after thoracic surgery. In working with this patient, a nurse should:
    1. coil and secure excess tubing next to the patient.
    2. clamp off the chest tubes except during respiratory assessments.
    3. milk or strip the tubing every 15 to 30 minutes to maintain drainage.
    4. remove the tubing from the connection to check for adequate suction.

74. A patient is being discharged home with an order for oxygen prn. In preparing to teach the patient and family, a priority for the nurse is to provide information on the:
    1. use of the oxygen delivery equipment.
    2. physiology of the respiratory system.
    3. use of PaO_2 levels to determine oxygen demand.
    4. length of time that the oxygen is to be used by the patient.

75. In discriminating types of chest pain that a patient may experience, a nurse recognizes that pain associated with inflammation of the pericardial sac is noted by the patient experiencing:
    1. knifelike pain to the upper chest.
    2. constant, substernal pain.
    3. pain with inspiration.
    4. pain aggravated by coughing.

76. A nurse is checking a patient who has a chest tube in place and finds that there is constant bubbling in the water-seal chamber. The nurse should:
    1. tighten loose connections.
    2. leave the chest tube clamped.
    3. raise the tubing above the level of the insertion site.
    4. prepare the patient for the removal of the tube.

77. The patient is admitted with a diagnosis of COPD. The appropriate oxygen delivery method for this patient is a:
    1. simple face mask with 5 to 8 L/min (50%) O_2.
    2. Venturi mask with 8 L/min (35% to 40%) O_2.
    3. nasal cannula with 1 to 2 L/min (28%) O_2.
    4. partial nonrebreather mask with 6 to 10 L/min (80%) O_2.

78. A nurse is completing a physical assessment of a patient with a history of a cardiopulmonary abnormality. A finding associated with hyperlipidemia is the patient having:
    1. cyanosis.
    2. xanthelasma.
    3. petechiae.
    4. ecchymosis.

79. During patient assessment, which of the following is an expected sign of hypoxemia?
    1. Pale conjunctivae
    2. Central cyanosis
    3. Dependent edema
    4. Splinter hemorrhages

STUDY GROUP QUESTIONS

- How do the anatomy and physiology of the cardiovascular and respiratory systems promote oxygenation?
- What physiological factors affect oxygenation?
- How do growth and development influence oxygenation?
- How do behavioral and environmental factors influence oxygenation?
- What are some common alterations in cardiovascular and pulmonary functioning?
- How are the critical thinking and nursing processes applied to patients having difficulty with oxygenation?
- What assessment information should be obtained to determine the patient's oxygenation status?
- What findings usually are seen in a patient who has inadequate oxygenation?
- How can the nurse promote oxygenation for patients in the health promotion, acute care, and restorative care settings?
- What specific measures and procedures should be implemented by the nurse to manage dyspnea, maintain a patent airway, mobilize secretions, and expand the lungs?
- What should be included in patient/family teaching for promotion and maintenance of oxygenation?
- What safety measures should be implemented for the use of oxygen in the home?

31 Sleep

CASE STUDIES

1. A middle-aged adult patient has gone to a physician's office to obtain a prescription for a "sleeping pill" because she has been having difficulty either falling or staying asleep. You are completing the initial nursing assessment and discover that the patient is recently divorced and trying to juggle extensive work and child care responsibilities.
   a. Identify a possible nursing diagnosis and outcome for this patient.
   b. Indicate nursing interventions and teaching areas for this patient.

2. A nurse has just been moved to the night shift in the hospital and starts to experience difficulty in getting to sleep when he gets home. He is finding it harder to focus at work.
   a. What can be done to assist the nurse in adapting to the change in his work schedule and sleep pattern?

CHAPTER REVIEW

Match the description/definition in Column A with the correct term in Column B.

	Column A	*Column B*
_____	1. Cessation of breathing for periods of time during sleep	a. Cataplexy
_____	2. A decrease in the amount, quality, and consistency of sleep	b. Sleep deprivation
_____	3. Awaking at night to urinate	c. Circadian rhythm
_____	4. Sudden muscle weakness during intense emotions	d. Parasomnia
_____	5. Difficulty falling or staying asleep	e. Sleep
_____	6. 24-hour day/night cycle	f. Sleep apnea
_____	7. Disorder that produces abnormal behavior or emotions	g. Insomnia
_____	8. Excessive sleepiness during the day	h. Nocturia
_____	9. A recurrent, altered state of consciousness that occurs for sustained periods.	i. Narcolepsy

Complete the following:

10. Provide examples of factors that may affect sleep.

11. Which of the following are appropriate nursing interventions to assist the older adult patient to achieve adequate sleep? Select all that apply.
   a. Altering the daily sleep and wake times ______
   b. Encouraging the patient to stay in bed even if not feeling sleepy ______
   c. Limiting the patient's caffeine intake in the late afternoon or evening ______
   d. Lowering the head of the bed as flat as possible ______
   e. Encouraging increased fluid intake 2 to 4 hours before sleep ______
   f. Avoiding use of sedatives and hypnotics, if possible ______
   g. Encouraging daytime naps of 1 to 2 hours ______
   h. Providing social activities and exercise ______

12. Identify a way in which a nurse can promote a restful environment in the acute care setting.

13. It is expected that during sleep the heart rate will decrease by 10 beats per minute from the daytime average rate.
True _____ False _____

14. Very few older adults experience sleep problems.
True _____ False _____

15. Normal sleep cycles usually last ______ (time) and are followed by ______ sleep.

16. Identify at least two nursing interventions that may be implemented related to a patient's sleep:
    a. Comfort measures
    b. Safety measures

17. A nurse tells a patient to include what information in a sleep diary?

18. What are the best types of bedtime snacks for promoting sleep?

19. A nurse recommends to the parents of a newborn that the best way to position the child for sleep is on his/her:

20. Identify at least one patient outcome related to sleep.

21. For sleep disturbances:
    a. What physical and behavioral problems may occur when individuals have an insufficient amount of sleep?
    b. What are the safety considerations for patients with narcolepsy, EDS, sleep deprivation, and/or nocturia?

22. Use of technology, such as cell phones, close to bedtime can lead to changes in sleep and excessive daytime sleepiness. True _____ False _____

23. What is the value of REM sleep?

24. Central sleep apnea is frequently seen in patients who have which pathological conditions?

25. Identify at least two questions to ask to assess a patient's sleep habits.

26. For a patient with chronic insomnia, the nurse should:

27. For the patient with obstructive sleep apnea, identify the recommendations for health promotion. Select all that apply.
    a. Weight loss ______
    b. Use of benzodiazepines ______
    c. Change of bedtime routine ______
    d. Use of analgesics ______
    e. Elevating the head of the bed ______

Select the best answer for each of the following questions:

28. Individuals experience changes in their sleep patterns as they progress through the life cycle. A nurse assesses that a patient is experiencing bedtime fears, restlessness during the night, and nightmares. These behaviors are associated with:
    1. infants.
    2. toddlers.
    3. preschoolers.
    4. school-age children.

29. A nurse is making rounds during the night to check on patients. When she enters one of the rooms at 3:00 AM, she finds that the patient is sitting up in a chair. The patient tells the nurse that she is not able to sleep. The nurse should first:
    1. obtain an order for a hypnotic.
    2. assist the patient back to bed.
    3. provide a glass of warm milk and a back rub.
    4. ask about activities that have previously helped her sleep.

30. A nurse is working on a pediatric unit at the local hospital. A 4-year-old boy is admitted to the unit. To assist this child to sleep, the nurse:
    1. reads to him.
    2. teaches him relaxation activities.
    3. allows him to watch TV until he is tired.
    4. has him get ready for bed very quickly, without advance notice.

31. A patient is found to be awakening frequently during the night. There are a number of medications prescribed for this patient. The nurse determines that the medication that may be creating this patient's particular sleep disturbance is the:
    1. narcotic.
    2. beta blocker.
    3. antidepressant.
    4. antihistamine.

32. A nurse suspects that a patient may be experiencing sleep deprivation. This suspicion is validated by the nurse's finding that the patient has:
    1. increased reflex response.
    2. blurred vision.
    3. cardiac arrhythmia.
    4. increased response time.

33. A nurse is working in a sleep clinic that is part of the local hospital. In preparing to work with patients with different sleep needs, the nurse understands that:
    1. bedtime rituals are most important for adolescents.
    2. regular use of sleeping medications is appropriate.
    3. warm milk before bedtime may help a patient sleep.
    4. individuals are most easily aroused from sleep during stages 3 and 4.

34. A nurse is visiting a patient in his home. While completing a patient history and home assessment, the nurse finds that there are many prescription medications kept in the bathroom cabinet. In determining possible areas that may influence the patient's sleep patterns, the nurse looks for a classification of medication that may suppress the patient's rapid eye movement (REM) sleep. The nurse looks in the cabinet for a:
    1. diuretic.
    2. stimulant.
    3. beta blocker.
    4. nasal decongestant.

35. A newborn is taken to a pediatrician's office for the first physical exam. The parents ask the nurse when they can expect the baby to sleep through the night. The nurse responds that, although there may be individual differences, infants usually develop a nighttime pattern of sleep by the age of:
    1. 6 weeks.
    2. 3 months.
    3. 6 months.
    4. 10 months.

36. A nurse is working with older adults in the senior center. A group is discussing problems with sleep. The nurse recognizes that older adults:
    1. take less time to fall asleep.
    2. are more difficult to arouse from sleep.
    3. have a significant decline in stage 4 sleep.
    4. require more sleep than middle-aged adults.

37. A patient with congestive heart failure is being discharged from the hospital to her home. The patient will be taking a diuretic daily. The nurse recognizes that, with this drug, the patient may experience:
    1. nocturia.
    2. nightmares.
    3. reduced REM sleep.
    4. increased daytime sleepiness.

38. During a home visit, a nurse discovers that the patient has been having difficulty sleeping. To assist the patient to achieve sufficient sleep, an appropriate question the nurse might ask is:
    1. "Do you keep your bedroom completely dark at night?"
    2. "Do you nap enough during the day?"
    3. "Why don't you eat something right before you go to bed?"
    4. "What kinds of things do you do right before bedtime?"

39. A patient has gone to the sleep clinic to determine what may be creating his sleeping problems. In addition, his partner is having sleep pattern interruptions. If this patient is experiencing sleep apnea, the nurse may expect the partner to identify that the patient:
    1. snores excessively.
    2. talks in his sleep.
    3. is very restless.
    4. walks in his sleep.

40. A nurse anticipates that the patient who is in non–rapid eye movement (NREM) stage 1 sleep is:
    1. easily aroused.
    2. completely relaxed.
    3. having vivid, full-color dreams.
    4. experiencing significantly reduced vital signs.

41. A nurse is working with a patient who has a history of respiratory disease. This patient is expected to demonstrate:
    1. longer time falling asleep.
    2. decreased NREM sleep.
    3. increased awakenings in the early morning.
    4. need for extra pillows for comfort.

42. To help promote sleep for a patient, a nurse recommends:
    1. exercise about 2 hours before bedtime.
    2. intake of a large meal about 3 hours before bedtime.
    3. drinking alcoholic beverages at bedtime.
    4. napping frequently during the afternoon.

43. An expected treatment for sleep apnea is:
    1. biofeedback.
    2. full body massage.
    3. administration of hypnotics.
    4. continuous positive airway pressure (CPAP).

44. As sleep aids, medications that are considered relatively safe to use are:
    1. nonbenzodiazepines.
    2. barbiturates.
    3. psychotropics.
    4. antihistamines.

45. An expected observation of a patient in REM sleep is:
    1. possible enuresis.
    2. sleepwalking.
    3. loss of skeletal muscle tone.
    4. easy arousal from external noise.

46. A parent asks the nurse what the appropriate amount of sleep is for her 11-year-old child. The nurse responds correctly by informing the parent that children in this age group should average:
    1. 14 hours per night.
    2. 12 hours per night.
    3. 10 hours per night.
    4. 7 hours per night.

47. Parents ask the nurse about having their child sleep in their bed with them. The nurse's best response is to:
    1. discourage the practice.
    2. identify that the child will probably sleep more soundly with them.
    3. recommend that lots of soft bedding be used to protect the child.
    4. indicate that there are risks associated with this practice.

STUDY GROUP QUESTIONS

- What is sleep?
- What are the physiological processes involved in sleep?
- How is sleep regulated by the body?
- What are the functions of sleep?
- What purpose do dreams serve?
- What are the normal requirements and patterns of sleep across the life span?
- What factors may influence sleep?
- What are some common sleep disorders and nursing interventions?
- What information should be included in a sleep history?
- How are the critical thinking and nursing processes applied with patients experiencing insufficient sleep or rest?
- What measures may be implemented by the nurse to promote sleep for patients/families?
- What information should be included in patient/family teaching for the promotion of rest and sleep?

STUDY CHART

Create a study chart to describe *Sleep Patterns Across the Life Span*, which identifies the sleep patterns and needs for infants, toddlers, preschoolers, school-age children, adolescents, adults, and older adults.

32 Pain Management

CASE STUDIES

1. A patient is going to be using a PCA pump with a morphine infusion after surgery.
   a. What assessments must be made before and while the patient uses the pump?
   b. What medications are usually prescribed for PCA?
   c. What information is needed in the teaching plan for this patient?

2. You are admitting a patient who is in labor. She tells you that this is her second child and that she had a "hard time having the first one because the pain was just horrible."
   a. What are the possible expectations of this patient?
   b. In applying the QSEN competency of patient-centered care, what nursing interventions do you include for this patient?

CHAPTER REVIEW

Match the description/definition in Column A with the correct term in Column B.

	Column A	*Column B*
_____	1. Local anesthesia, with minimal sedation, given between the vertebrae	a. Pain
_____	2. Unpleasant, subjective sensory and emotional experience	b. Analgesic
_____	3. Extends from the point of injury to another body area	c. Exacerbation
_____	4. Can cause the fight-or-flight response of the general adaptation syndrome	d. Radiating pain
_____	5. Rapid onset, lasts briefly	e. Acute pain
_____	6. Increase in the severity of symptoms	f. Chronic pain
_____	7. Classification of medication used for pain relief	g. Superficial pain
_____	8. Prolonged, varying in intensity	h. Epidural infusion

Complete the following:

9. Identify and briefly describe the four (4) physiological processes of pain.

10. The gate control theory of pain suggests that pain can be reduced through the use of:

11. Which of the following are physiological responses to acute pain as a result of sympathetic stimulation? Select all that apply.
    a. Decreased respiratory rate _____
    b. Increased heart rate _____
    c. Peripheral vasodilation _____
    d. Increased blood glucose level _____
    e. Diaphoresis _____
    f. Pupil constriction _____
    g. Decreased blood pressure _____

12. For a patient with chronic pain, identify the following:
    a. Associated symptoms
    b. An example of a lifestyle response to chronic pain

13. Identify two responses that an infant or child could have to pain.

14. The single most reliable indicator of pain is the:

15. Using the PQRSTU assessment guide, identify nursing interventions for the following.
    a. Quality
    b. Region
    c. Timing

16. Identify how a nurse may assess the level of pain for the following patients.
    a. Toddler

    b. Person for whom English is a second language

    c. Person with dementia

17. a. To determine the location of a patient's pain, a nurse should ask the patient to:
    b. The patient indicates that the discomfort is located in the right side of the abdomen. Provide an example of how the pain experience could be appropriately documented for this patient.

18. A pain rating of _____ on a scale of 0 to 10 is an emergency and requires immediate action.

19. For a patient who experiences discomfort upon ambulation or during a dressing change, a nurse should plan to:

20. An example of how a nurse may individualize a patient's treatment for pain is:

21. Which of the following are correct statements regarding transcutaneous electrical nerve stimulation (TENS)? Select all that apply.
    a. It is an invasive procedure. _____
    b. It requires a health care provider's order. _____
    c. Electrodes are applied directly onto skin. _____
    d. Controls are adjusted until the patient feels a buzzing sensation. _____
    e. It can be very expensive. _____

22. Which of the following medications are indicated for the treatment of mild to moderate pain? Select all that apply.
    a. Ibuprofen (Motrin) _____
    b. Morphine _____
    c. Codeine _____
    d. Fentanyl _____
    e. Acetaminophen (Tylenol) _____
    f. Propoxyphene (Darvon) _____

23. Identify two examples of nonpharmacological interventions that may be implemented to relieve pain.

24. An example of an adjuvant medication that may be used in conjunction with an analgesic to manage a patient's pain is:

25. The usual dosage of on-demand morphine in the PCA is:

26. Complete the following about analgesics.
    a. A priority nursing intervention specifically for the patient with an epidural analgesic infusion is:
    b. A priority nursing assessment for all patients before and while receiving analgesics is:

27. Identify an intervention that a nurse should implement to adapt or alter the environment to promote a patient's comfort:

28. A patient who may experience phantom pain is someone who has:

29. The term for patient-controlled oral analgesia is: ________________.

30. Whenever possible, the best way to evaluate the effectiveness of pain management is to: ________________.

31. The ABCDE approach to pain assessment and management is:
    A
    B
    C
    D
    E

32. Concomitant symptoms associated with pain include:

33. Identify whether the following statements are true or false.
   a. Nurses can allow their own misconceptions about or interpretations of the pain experience to affect their willingness to intervene for their patient.
      True _____ False _____
   b. The degree and quality of pain are related to the patient's definition of pain.
      True _____ False _____
   c. When patients are experiencing pain, they will not hesitate to inform you.
      True _____ False _____
   d. Fatigue decreases a patient's perception of pain.
      True _____ False _____
   e. A nurse should provide descriptive words for a patient to assist in assessing the quality of the pain.
      True _____ False _____
   f. Pain assessment can be delegated to assistive personnel.
      True _____ False _____
   g. Large doses of opioids for the terminally ill patient will hasten the onset of death.
      True _____ False _____
   h. Health care providers initially order higher doses than needed for patients with cancer pain.
      True _____ False _____
   i. The Joint Commission (TJC) has a standard that requires health care workers to assess all patients for pain.
      True _____ False _____
   j. Pain is a normal part of aging.
      True _____ False _____
   k. Nurses should anticipate that higher doses of oral opioids will be ordered after patients are converted from the IV form.
      True _____ False _____
   l. The least invasive pain management therapy should be tried first.
      True _____ False _____

Select the best answer for each of the following questions:

34. A patient is experiencing pain that is not being managed by analgesics given by the oral or intramuscular routes. Epidural analgesia is initiated. The nurse is alert for a complication of this treatment and observes the patient for:
   1. diarrhea.
   2. hypertension.
   3. urinary retention.
   4. an increased respiratory rate.

35. A patient had a laparoscopic procedure this morning and is requesting a pain medication. The nurse assesses the patient's vital signs and decides to withhold the medication based on the finding of:
   1. temperature = 99° F, rectally.
   2. pulse rate = 90 beats per minute, regular.
   3. respirations = 9 per minute, shallow.
   4. blood pressure = 130/80 mm Hg, consistent with prior reading.

36. A nurse is working with an older adult population in the extended care facility. Many of the patients experience discomfort associated with arthritis and have analgesics prescribed. In administering an analgesic medication to an older adult patient, the nurse should:
   1. give the medication when the pain increases in severity.
   2. combine opioids for a greater effect.
   3. use the IM route whenever possible.
   4. give the medication before activities or procedures.

37. One of the patients that a nurse is working with on an outpatient basis at the local clinic has rheumatoid arthritis. The patient has no known allergies to any medications, so the nurse anticipates that the physician will prescribe:
   1. amitriptyline.
   2. butorphanol.
   3. indomethacin.
   4. morphine.

38. An adolescent has been carried to the sidelines of the soccer field after experiencing a twisted ankle. The level of pain is identified as low to moderate. The nurse observes that the patient has:
   1. pupil constriction.
   2. diaphoresis.
   3. a decreased heart rate.
   4. a decreased respiratory rate.

39. A nurse on the pediatric unit is finding that it is sometimes difficult to determine the presence and severity of pain in very young patients. The nurse recognizes that toddlers may be experiencing pain when they have:
   1. an increased appetite.
   2. a relaxed posture.
   3. an increased degree of cooperation.
   4. disturbances in their sleep patterns.

40. A patient on the oncology unit is experiencing severe pain associated with his cancer. Although analgesics have been prescribed and administered, the patient is having "breakthrough pain." The nurse anticipates that his treatment will include:
   1. the use of a placebo.
   2. experimental medications.
   3. an increase in the opioid dose.
   4. administration of medications every hour.

41. A patient is experiencing pain that is being treated with a fentanyl transdermal patch. The nurse advises this patient to:
   1. avoid exposure to the sun.
   2. change the patch site every 2 hours.
   3. apply a heating pad over the site.
   4. expect immediate pain relief when the patch is applied.

42. A patient is experiencing severe pain and has been placed on a morphine drip. During the patient's assessment, the nurse finds that the patient's respiratory rate is 6 breaths per minute and shallow. The nurse anticipates that the patient will receive:
    1. naloxone.
    2. morphine.
    3. incentive spirometry.
    4. no additional treatment for this expected response.

43. An assessment tool that has the patient select words from a list that most accurately reflect his/her pain severity is the:
    1. Brief Pain Inventory (BPI).
    2. Visual Analog Scale (VAS).
    3. Verbal Descriptor Scale (VDS).
    4. Critical Care Pain Observation Tool (CCPOT).

44. A nurse is working for an oncology unit in the medical center. All of the patients experience pain that requires management. The nurse should visit first with the patient who is also exhibiting signs of:
    1. anxiety.
    2. fatigue.
    3. distraction.
    4. depression.

45. For a patient with a consistent level of discomfort, the most effective pain relief is achieved with administration of analgesics:
    1. PRN.
    2. every 3 to 4 hours.
    3. every 12 hours.
    4. around the clock.

46. A nurse anticipates that the patient with visceral pain will describe the pain as:
    1. sharp.
    2. cramping.
    3. burning.
    4. shooting.

47. Which of the following orders would the nurse question for the patient who has an epidural infusion for pain relief?
    1. Use of pulse oximetry
    2. Tubing changes every 24 hours
    3. An order for a sedative
    4. Use of fentanyl in the infusion

48. Because of the possible cardiovascular and neurological effects, which of the following analgesic orders for an older adult patient should be questioned?
    1. Acetaminophen
    2. Aspirin
    3. Ibuprofen
    4. Propoxyphene

STUDY GROUP QUESTIONS

- How may a nurse use a holistic approach to assist a patient in achieving comfort?
- What is pain?
- What are the physiological components of the pain experience?
- How may a patient respond, physiologically and behaviorally, to a pain experience?
- What factors influence the pain experience?
- How are acute and chronic pain different?
- How should a nurse assess a patient's pain?
- How may a patient characterize pain?
- What nonpharmacological measures may be used to relieve pain?
- What interventions may a nurse implement to promote comfort and relieve pain?
- What pharmacological measures are available for pain relief?
- How is a back rub/massage performed to achieve an optimum effect?
- What actions should a nurse take if comfort or pain relief measures are not effective?
- What information should be included in patient/family teaching for pain control or relief?

STUDY CHART

Create a study chart to describe the *Factors Influencing Pain and Comfort* that identifies how age, sex, culture, meaning of pain, and previous experience of a patient alter the pain experience.

33 Nutrition

CASE STUDIES

1. You are working with a patient who is being discharged from the acute care unit after a heart attack (myocardial infarction). The patient's primary care provider has prescribed medical nutrition therapy with a diet that is low in sodium and saturated fat. The patient comes from a family in which food plays an important role in traditional culture practices.
   a. What do you need to know about the patient and the family to assist in dietary planning?
   b. How can you assist this patient to meet the prescribed dietary requirements?

2. A pregnant woman is at the medical office for a prenatal checkup. What nutritional recommendations should be provided to this patient?

3. You are working in a home care agency and have a large older adult patient population. In planning care, what nutritional considerations should be taken into account for these patients?

4. As an occupational health nurse, you are concerned with positive health behaviors for the employees. You have noticed that some of the workers are overweight.
   a. Identify the nursing diagnosis and general goals based upon your observation.
   b. What should you include in a teaching plan to promote nutritional health for the employees?

CHAPTER REVIEW

Match the description/definition in Column A with the correct term in Column B.

	Column A	*Column B*
_____	1. Increase in blood glucose level	a. Anabolism
_____	2. Breakdown of food products into smaller particles	b. Hypoglycemia
_____	3. Production of more complex chemical substances through the synthesis of nutrients	c. Digestion
_____	4. All biochemical and physiological processes by which the body maintains itself	d. Anthropometry
_____	5. Organic substances in food that are present in small amounts and act as coenzymes in biochemical reactions	e. Catabolism
_____	6. Inorganic elements that act as catalysts in biochemical reactions	f. Nutrients
_____	7. Substances necessary for body functioning	g. Minerals
_____	8. Breakdown of complex body substances into simpler substances	h. Metabolism
_____	9. Decrease in blood glucose level	i. Hyperglycemia
_____	10. Measurement of size and makeup of body at specific sites	j. Vitamins

Complete the following:

11. Identify an example of a nutrition objective from *Healthy People 2020.*

12. For vitamins:
   a. Which vitamin is synthesized by the body?
   b. What are the fat-soluble vitamins?
   c. Identify an example of an antioxidant vitamin.

13. Identify whether the following represent carbohydrates, proteins, or fats.
    a. Starches ___________
    b. Meats ___________
    c. Linoleic acid ___________
    d. Fiber ___________
    e. 9 kcal/g of energy ___________
    f. Amino acids ___________
    g. Fruits ___________

14. For patients with alterations in bowel elimination, identify which type of fiber should be recommended:
    a. Prevention of diarrhea: ______________________
    b. Prevention of constipation: ______________________

15. What information can you provide to an individual at a health fair who is interested in general nutritional guidelines?

16. Provide an example of an alternative dietary pattern.

17. What are the roles of minerals in the body?

18. Describe the functions of water in the body.

19. For each area of nutritional assessment, identify specific elements to pursue with the patient.
    a. Food and nutrient intake
    b. Physical examination
    c. Anthropometric measurements

20. Which of the following are indicators of malnutrition? Select all that apply.
    a. Listlessness _____
    b. Straight arms and legs _____
    c. Some fat under the skin _____
    d. Paresthesia _____
    e. Loss of ankle reflexes _____
    f. Rapid heart rate _____
    g. No palpable masses _____
    h. Apathy _____
    i. Dry, scaly skin _____
    j. Reddish-pink mucous membranes _____
    k. Spongy gums with marginal redness _____
    l. Surface papillae present on the tongue _____
    m. Pale conjunctivae _____
    n. Corneal xerosis _____
    o. Firm, pink nails _____
    p. Calf tenderness and tingling _____

21. A nurse calculates a patient's body mass index (BMI) by dividing the weight in kilograms by the height in square meters. If the patient weighs 180 pounds and is 6 feet tall, what is the BMI?

22. A neurogenic cause of dysphagia is:

    A myogenic cause is:

23. A common sign or symptom of food-borne illnesses is:

24. A nurse on an acute care unit is concerned about the patient's appetite.
    a. What are the stressors in the environment that have an impact upon a patient's nutritional intake?
    b. Identify at least two interventions that should be implemented by the nurse to promote the patient's appetite.

25. Identify the interventions that a nurse should implement for the patient who is experiencing dysphagia.

26. An advantage of enteral nutrition over parenteral nutrition is that enteral nutrition:

27. Regarding enteral tube feedings:
    a. What are the contraindications to nasogastric tube placement?
    b. The most serious complication of tube feedings is:
    c. To avoid this complication, the nurse should:
    d. Displacement of a jejunostomy tube can lead to:
    e. The nasogastric tube becomes clogged. The nurse should:
    f. Intermittent nasogastric feeding tubes are clamped/closed to prevent:
    g. The method of choice for long-term enteral feeding for the patient who has not had upper GI surgery is:

28. On the food label pictured, what is/are the possible concerns?

Nutrition Facts

Serving Size: 1/2 cup (114 g)
Servings Per Container: 4

Amount per Serving	
Calories 260	
Calories from Fat 120	
	% Daily Value*
Total Fat 13 g	20%
Saturated Fat 5 g	25%
Trans Fat 0 g	
Cholesterol 30 mg	10%
Sodium 660 mg	28%
Total Carbohydrate 31 g	11%
Dietary Fiber 0 g	0%
Sugars 5 g	
Protein 5 g	

Vitamin A 4% • Vitamin C 1%
Calcium 15% • Iron 4%

*Percents (%) of a Daily Value are based on a 2,000 calorie diet. Your Daily Values may vary higher or lower depending on your calorie needs.

Nutrient	2,000 calories	2,500 calories
Total Fat	<65 g	<80 g
Saturated Fat	<20 g	<25 g
Cholesterol	<300 mg	<300 mg
Sodium	<2,400 mg	<2,400 mg
Total Carbohydrate	300 g	375 g
Dietary Fiber	25 g	30 g

1 g Fat = 9 calories
1 g Carbohydrate = 4 calories
1 g Protein = 4 calories

29. Identify foods that are choking hazards for toddlers.

30. What are the contributing factors to adolescent obesity and nutritional deficiencies?

31. The pH of the gastric aspirate for a patient who has been fasting is:

32. A parenteral nutrition formula that is hyperosmolar (greater than 10% dextrose) should be administered through a(n) ________________________ venous line.

33. A patient will be receiving parenteral nutrition (PN). Identify the following:
   a. The main reason for use of PN:
   b. A major nursing goal for the patient receiving PN:
   c. A nursing intervention to assist the patient in the prevention of metabolic complications related to PN therapy:
   d. Guidelines and precautions for lipid infusions:

34. Identify a dietary measure that should be implemented for a patient without teeth or with ill-fitting dentures.

35. A screening tool for older adults is the Mini Nutritional Assessment (MNA). Select all of the following correct statements about this tool.
   a. It is an 18-item tool. _____
   b. There are four sections to complete. _____
   c. The sections are divided into screening and assessment items. _____
   d. A score above 20 indicates a positive nutritional assessment. _____
   e. Anthropometric measures are required for the screening. _____

36. Indicate whether the following statements are true or false.
   a. Infants require more protein than adults.
      True _____ False _____
   b. Childhood obesity is five times higher than it was 30 years ago.
      True _____ False _____
   c. Unsaturated fatty acids have a minimal effect on blood cholesterol.
      True _____ False _____

37. What is the purpose of the ChooseMyPlate program?

38. What interventions should be implemented for a patient who is receiving enteral feedings? Select all that apply.
   a. Keep the head of the bed elevated to 30 to 45 degrees. _____
   b. Withhold the feeding if the residual is 50 to 100 mL. _____
   c. Tube placement is confirmed by monitoring the pH of aspirate. _____
   d. Gastric residual volume is measured daily. _____
   e. Continuous feedings are administered through an infusion pump. _____
   f. Tubing should be flushed with 200 mL of water before and after each feeding. _____

39. To decrease cholesterol levels, the best type of fatty acid intake is:

40. Complete a brief narrative documentation example that includes the following:
   10 Fr nasogastric tube, left side insertion, verification of placement, patient tolerance of procedure

41. The nurse is going to provide a continuous enteral feeding. Place the following steps in the correct order. Note: Certain steps have been completed, such as hand hygiene.
   a. Label the bag. _____
   b. Verify the order. _____
   c. Pour the feeding into the gravity bag. _____
   d. Bring the formula to room temperature. _____
   e. Check the expiration date on the formula. _____
   f. Connect the tubing to the gravity bag. _____
   g. Open the clamp and hang the bag on an IV pole. _____

42. What items are included in the Subjective Global Assessment (SGA)?

Select the best answer for each of the following questions:

43. A nurse is working with a patient who requires an increase in complete proteins in the diet. The nurse recommends:
   1. milk.
   2. cereals.
   3. legumes.
   4. vegetables.

44. A nurse is talking with a community resident who has gone to the health fair. The resident tells the nurse that he takes a lot of extra vitamins every day. Because of the greater potential for toxicity, the resident is advised not to exceed the dietary guidelines for:
   1. vitamin A.
   2. vitamin B_1.
   3. vitamin B_{12}.
   4. folic acid.

45. A nurse is working with a patient who is a lactovegetarian. The food that is selected as appropriate for this dietary pattern is:
   1. fish.
   2. milk.
   3. eggs.
   4. poultry.

46. A patient states that he does not eat fish anymore. An appropriate follow-up question by the nurse is which of the following?
   1. "Why don't you like fish?"
   2. "What caused you to lose interest in fish?"
   3. "Does fish make you feel ill in some way?"
   4. "Aren't you aware that fish is a valuable source of nutrients?"

47. A nurse is preparing to insert a nasogastric tube for enteral feedings. The nurse recognizes that this intervention is used when the patient:
   1. has a gag reflex.
   2. is not able to chew foods.
   3. is slow to eliminate food.
   4. is not able to ingest foods.

48. A nurse is preparing the enteral feeding for a patient who has a nasogastric tube in place. The most effective method that the nurse can use to check for placement of a nasogastric tube is to:
   1. perform a pH analysis of aspirated secretions.
   2. measure the visible tubing exiting from the nose.
   3. inject air into the tube and auscultate over the stomach.
   4. place the end of the tube into water and observe for bubbling.

49. A female patient who has gone to a family planning center is taking an oral contraceptive. This patient should increase vitamin B_6 and niacin intake. The nurse recommends that the patient consume more:
   1. tomatoes.
   2. whole grains.
   3. citrus fruits.
   4. green, leafy vegetables.

50. A patient tells the nurse that she is a vegan. Which of the following vitamin supplements is needed to promote health for this patient?
   1. Niacin
   2. Vitamin C
   3. Thiamine
   4. Vitamin B_{12}

51. A nurse is assigned to make home visits to a number of patients. Of the patients that the nurse visits, the patient with the greatest risk of a nutritional deficiency is the patient with:
   1. decreased metabolic requirements.
   2. an alteration in dietary schedule.
   3. a body weight that is 5% over the ideal weight.
   4. a weight loss of 3% within the past 6 months.

52. After surgery, a patient is having her dietary intake advanced. After a period of NPO, the patient is placed on a clear liquid diet. What food does the nurse request for the patient?
   1. Milk
   2. Soup
   3. Custard
   4. Popsicles

53. While completing an assessment during a home visit, a nurse discovers that the patient has a history of congestive heart failure and is taking digoxin 0.25 mg daily. Being aware that medications may influence the patient's dietary patterns, the nurse is alert to the patient experiencing:
   1. anorexia.
   2. gastric distress.
   3. an alteration in taste.
   4. an alteration in smell.

54. A patient on the unit has an enteral tube in place for feedings. When the nurse enters the room, the patient says that he is experiencing cramps and nausea. The nurse should:
    1. cool the formula.
    2. remove the tube.
    3. use a more concentrated formula.
    4. decrease the administration rate.

55. Which of the following statements made by the parent of an infant indicates the need for additional teaching?
    1. "I'll wait to give the baby regular cow's milk until he is a year old."
    2. "I'll start with cereal as the first solid food that I give to the baby after about 4 months."
    3. "I'll add a little honey to the baby's bottle to help him digest the formula."
    4. "When he can have them, I'll wait a few days in between giving the baby any new foods."

56. For the family that cans food at home, there is a need for specific instruction about ways to prevent:
    1. botulism.
    2. *E. coli.*
    3. salmonella.
    4. listeriosis.

57. The individual with the highest percentage of water in the body is a(n):
    1. infant.
    2. obese patient.
    3. lean patient.
    4. older adult.

58. A patient with a gastrostomy has an excessive residual volume of 200 mL. The nurse should:
    1. request an order for a chest x-ray.
    2. alter the type of feeding being given.
    3. request an order for an antidiarrheal agent.
    4. return the contents to the stomach.

59. A nurse is monitoring a patient's laboratory reports. Which of the following, if decreased, is indicative of anemia?
    1. BUN level
    2. Creatinine level
    3. Albumin level
    4. Hemoglobin level

60. A nurse is instructing the family of a patient who is on an National Dysphagia Diet Task Force (NDDTF) dysphagia puree diet to include:
    1. mashed potatoes.
    2. moistened breads.
    3. well-cooked noodles.
    4. soft fruits.

61. A nurse recognizes that a patient on a low cholesterol diet requires additional teaching if he indicates that he eats which of the following?
    1. oatmeal.
    2. pastries.
    3. dried fruits.
    4. green peppers.

62. A realistic weight loss goal for the patient who is overweight is:
    1. 1 pound per week.
    2. 3 pounds per week.
    3. 5 pounds per week.
    4. 7 pounds per week.

63. To prevent the presence of *E. coli* in food, a nurse specifically instructs a patient and family to:
    1. carefully can foods at home.
    2. boil shellfish completely.
    3. cook ground beef well.
    4. keep dairy products refrigerated.

64. A nurse is visiting a patient in the home and notes that additional teaching is required if the patient is observed:
    1. cooking poultry to 180° F.
    2. thawing frozen foods at room temperature.
    3. discarding all foods that may be spoiled.
    4. cleaning the inside of the refrigerator with bleach.

65. Tube feedings are ordered for a patient with a nasogastric tube. Unless the agency specifies otherwise, the nurse should:
    1. dilute the feedings with water.
    2. infuse the feedings over the course of 1 to 2 hours.
    3. begin with 150 to 250 mL at a time.
    4. increase feedings by 100 to 150 mL per feeding every 8 hours.

66. Which one of the following foods is avoided by the patient on a gluten-free diet?
    1. Cow's milk
    2. Oatmeal
    3. Canned fruit
    4. Coffee

67. The patient is receiving continuous enteral nutrition via a nasogastric tube and begins to vomit. The nurse should:
    1. slow down the feeding.
    2. remove the tube.
    3. aspirate remaining gastric content.
    4. place the patient in side-lying position.

68. During the insertion of a nasogastric tube, the unit nurse manager is observing the new nurse graduate. Correction is required when the new nurse:
    1. has the patient flex the head after the tube passes the nasopharynx.
    2. rotates the tube 180 degrees during the insertion.
    3. encourages the patient to swallow as the tube moves along.
    4. advances the tube during patient inspiration.

STUDY GROUP QUESTIONS

- What are the basic principles of nutrition?
- What body processes are involved in the intake, use, and elimination of foods?
- What are the six major nutrients, their purposes, and their food sources?
- What are the current recommendations for daily nutritional intake?
- How do nutritional needs change across the life span?
- How does culture/ethnicity influence dietary intake?
- What are some common alternative food patterns?
- How should a nurse assess a patient's nutritional status?
- What patients are at a greater risk for nutritional deficiencies?
- What nursing diagnoses may be appropriate for patients with nutritional alterations?
- How does a nurse assist patients to meet nutritional needs in the health promotion, acute care, and restorative care settings?
- What special diets may be prescribed for individuals?
- What are the nursing procedures for implementation of enteral and parenteral nutrition?
- What guidelines and precautions should be considered by a nurse in assisting a patient with enteral or parenteral nutrition?
- What general information should be included for patients/families for promotion or restoration of an adequate nutritional intake?

STUDY CHART

Create a study chart to describe the six nutrients that identifies the uses of each in the body and their food sources: carbohydrates, proteins, lipids, vitamins, minerals, and water.

34 Urinary Elimination

CASE STUDIES

1. A patient is going to the medical center for an intravenous pyelogram (IVP).
   a. What nursing assessments and patient teaching should be completed before this test is performed?
   b. What are the nurse's responsibilities for the patient after an IVP?

2. You will be working with unlicensed assistive personnel in an extended care setting.
   a. What urinary care may be safely delegated by a nurse?

3. On an acute care unit, a patient is to have her catheter removed. The primary nurse tells you that all that is necessary is to "cut it, wait for the balloon to deflate, and pull it out."
   a. How will you proceed with this catheter removal?

4. A clean-voided or midstream urine specimen is required from a male patient. He is able to perform activities of daily living, including hygienic care.
   a. How will you teach this patient to obtain the specimen?

5. A patient had surgery and an incontinent urinary diversion was created.
   a. What are the special needs of this patient and the interventions that you will implement?

CHAPTER REVIEW

Match the description/definition in Column A with the correct term in Column B.

	Column A	*Column B*
_____	1. Accumulation of urine in the bladder because of inability to empty bladder completely	a. Urgency
_____	2. Painful or difficult urination	b. Hematuria
_____	3. Difficulty in initiating urination	c. Oliguria
_____	4. Volume of urine remaining in the bladder after voiding	d. Retention
_____	5. Feeling the need to void immediately	e. Nocturia
_____	6. Voiding large amounts of urine	f. Frequency
_____	7. Urination, particularly excessive, at night	g. Dysuria
_____	8. Presence of blood in the urine	h. Residual urine
_____	9. Voiding very often	i. Hesitancy
_____	10. Diminished urinary output in relation to fluid intake	j. Polyuria

Complete the following:

11. An example of a noninvasive procedure that may be used to examine the urinary system is:

12. What are the indications for the use of intermittent and indwelling urinary catheterization?

13. What positions may be used for catheterization of a female patient?

14. a. The recommended daily fluid intake for dilution of urine, promotion of micturition, and flushing the urethra of microorganisms is:
    b. The minimum urinary output for an adult is _____ per hour.

15. Provide an example of how each of the following factors may influence urination:
    a. Sociocultural
    b. Fluid intake
    c. Pathological conditions
    d. Medications

16. Identify how the following pathological conditions can influence urination:
    a. Arthritis
    b. Diabetes mellitus
    c. Prostate enlargement

17. a. The type of urinary incontinence that results from increased intraabdominal pressure with leakage of a small amount of urine is called:
    b. The treatment for this type of incontinence includes:

18. Which of the following are the expected characteristics of a normal urine specimen? Select all that apply.
    a. pH 10 _____
    b. Protein 4 mg _____
    c. Presence of glucose _____
    d. Specific gravity 1.2 _____
    e. Amber color _____

19. What is a priority when managing a patient's condom catheter?

20. To maintain a patient's dignity and self-esteem when assisting with urinary elimination, the nurse makes sure to:

21. Manual compression of the bladder is called:

22. Which of the following statements are correct for urinary diversions? Select all that apply.
    a. A ureterostomy is a continent diversion. _____
    b. Continent diversions have pouches created to store urine. _____
    c. Patients with urinary diversions need special clothing and have activity restrictions. _____

23. For a patient on strict intake and output, identify how urinary output can be measured.

24. Identify a method that a nurse may implement to stimulate a patient to void:

25. To assist a patient to start and stop the urine stream, a nurse instructs the patient that a way to strengthen the pelvic floor muscles is by performing:

26. Identify the distance of catheter insertion:
    a. Female adult patient:
    b. Male adult patient:

27. Which of the following are appropriate techniques for indwelling catheter care? Select all that apply.
    a. Keep the drainage bag below the level of the bladder. _____
    b. Provide perineal care daily. _____
    c. Cleanse in a direction toward the urinary meatus. _____
    d. Attach the drainage bag to the side rail of the bed. _____
    e. Open the connection at the drainage bag to obtain a urine specimen. _____
    f. Avoid having any dependent loops of tubing. _____
    g. Drain all urine in the bag before patient ambulation or exercise. _____
    h. For the immobile patient, empty the drainage bag every 24 hours. _____

28. To prevent nocturia, a nurse instructs a patient to:

29. Identify how the mobility status of an older adult may influence urination.

30. Which of the following are expected signs or symptoms for a patient with acute onset urinary retention? Select all that apply.
    a. Tenderness over the symphysis pubis _____
    b. Hematuria _____
    c. Diaphoresis _____
    d. Oliguria _____
    e. Dysuria _____
    f. Incontinence _____

31. How can urinary infection be prevented or reduced for a patient with an indwelling catheter?

32. Which of the following statements are correct regarding a cystoscopy? Select all that apply.
    a. The procedure may be performed under general anesthesia. _____
    b. Fluids are restricted before and during the procedure. _____
    c. Antibiotics are often administered intravenously. _____
    d. An informed consent is not required. _____
    e. Bowel preparation is performed the evening before the test. _____
    f. The patient is NPO if the test is performed with local anesthesia. _____
    g. Bed rest is usually indicated immediately after the test. _____
    h. Bloody or cloudy urine may be observed after the test. _____
    i. Fluid intake is encouraged after the test is completed. _____

33. During a physical assessment, what techniques are used to:
    a. determine the presence of a kidney infection?
    b. assess the bladder?

34. Identify the following for a bladder scanner:
    a. Use:
    b. When to measure:

35. Identify the characteristic of the urine for a patient with:
    a. daily administration of furosemide (Lasix): _____
    b. liver disease: _____
    c. urinary tract infection: _____

36. Urinary specimens for analysis should be sent to the laboratory within _____ hours of collection.

37. Place the following steps for a clean-catch specimen in the correct order:
    a. Void in the toilet. _____
    b. Provide instruction to the patient. _____
    c. Void in a sterile urine cup. _____
    d. Cleanse the urinary meatus. _____
    e. Stop the urine stream. _____

38. The patient is going to have a computerized axial tomography (CT) scan to identify the possible presence of calculi. Identify the following:
    a. Preparation before the test:
    b. Care after the test:

39. The nurse observes that the patient has some problems with hygiene. To prevent a UTI, the nurse instructs the patient to:

40. Identify the correct urinary catheter (single, double, or triple-lumen) to use for each of the following interventions:
    a. Indwelling catheter with bladder irrigation:
    b. Intermittent catheterization:
    c. Indwelling catheter:

41. What are the responsibilities of the nurse after the removal of a urinary catheter?

42. Identify the following for a suprapubic catheter:
    a. Purpose of insertion:
    b. Nursing care:

43. The patient has an incontinent urinary diversion and requires care of the stoma. Place the nursing actions in the correct order:
    a. Apply the pouch and press firmly into place. _____
    b. Cleanse the skin around the stoma. _____
    c. Remove the protective backing from the adhesive surface on the pouch. _____
    d. Measure the stoma. _____
    e. Cut an opening in the pouch. _____

44. What types of medications are used to treat urgency urinary incontinence?

45. Which of the following foods can irritate the bladder and contribute to urgency? Select all that apply.
    a. Caffeinated beverages _____
    b. Breads _____
    c. Fish _____
    d. Spicy foods _____
    e. Cheese _____
    f. Citrus foods _____

46. Self-catheterization by the patient is done with clean technique.
    True _____ False _____

47. Timed voiding is based upon a fixed schedule and not on the patient's urge to void.
    True _____ False _____

48. The nurse is teaching the patient how to prevent UTIs. Identify the information that should be included in the instruction. Select all that apply.
    a. Cleanse the perineum from back to front. _____
    b. Void before and after sexual intercourse. _____
    c. Wear nylon underwear. _____
    d. Avoid bubble baths. _____
    e. Drink coffee or tea regularly. _____
    f. Try to empty the bladder completely with each voiding. _____

49. Identify at least four measures that the nurse should employ to reduce the chance of a catheter associated urinary tract infection (CAUTI).

50. What are three possible questions to ask the patient to determine if there are any urinary symptoms present?

51. In the photo, what intervention is needed to have appropriate urinary drainage?

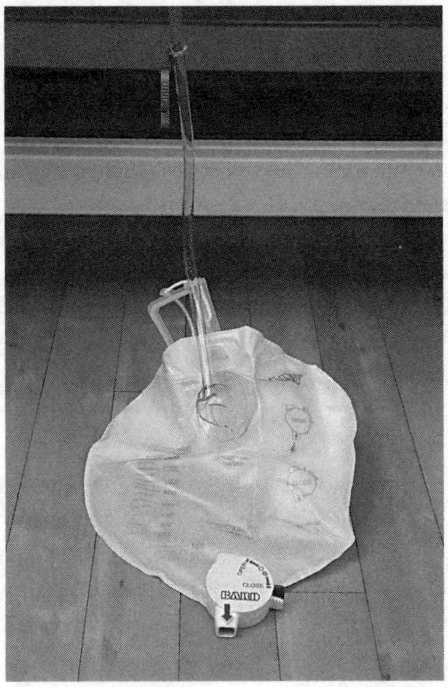

52. What lumen would be used to inflate the catheter balloon?

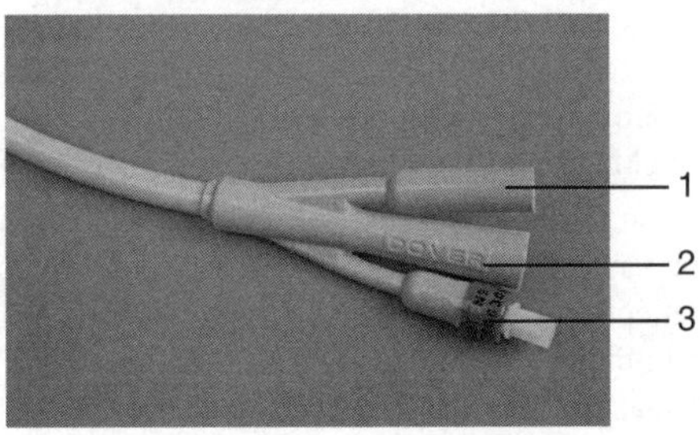

Select the best answer for each of the following questions:

53. The nurse recognizes that an intervention for a patient with stress incontinence is instruction regarding:
    1. use of a mobility aid.
    2. intermittent catheterization.
    3. pelvic muscle exercises.
    4. antimuscarinic medications.

54. The nurse is going to be catheterizing an average-size 9-year-old boy. The appropriate catheter size for this child is:
    1. 5 to 6 FR.
    2. 8 to 10 FR.
    3. 12 to 14 FR.
    4. 15 to 17 FR.

55. For the nursing diagnosis *Functional Urinary Incontinence,* the difficulty is related to the patient's:
    1. inability to completely empty the bladder.
    2. lack of sensation of a full bladder.
    3. difficulty in getting out of the chair and going to the toilet.
    4. pressure during coughing or sneezing.

56. For the patient who has had a continent urinary reservoir created, the nurse instructs the patient that there will be a need to:
    1. catheterize the pouch 4 to 6 times/day.
    2. eliminate urine through the intestine.
    3. use the Valsalva maneuver to empty the pouch through the urethra.
    4. restrict the intake of fluids.

57. The nurse is going to explain to new parents about toilet training. The parents are informed that early onset of a child's control of voluntary voiding does not occur until the age of:
    1. 6 months old.
    2. 12 months old.
    3. 18 months old.
    4. 4 years old.

58. A patient on the medical unit is scheduled to have a 24-hour urine collection to diagnose a urinary disorder. The nurse should:
    1. note the start time on the container.
    2. have the patient void while defecating.
    3. start with the first voiding sample from the patient.
    4. continue with the test if a specimen is flushed away.

59. One of a nurse's assigned patients is experiencing urgency urinary incontinence (UI). The nurse anticipates a medication that may be ordered for this difficulty is:
    1. propantheline.
    2. oxybutynin.
    3. bethanechol.
    4. phenylpropanolamine.

60. Several patients in a long-term care unit have indwelling urinary catheters in place. A nurse is delegating catheter care to the nursing assistant. The nurse includes instruction in:
    1. using lotion on the perineal area.
    2. disinfecting the first 2 to 3 inches of the catheter every 2 hours.
    3. ensuring that the drainage bag is secured to the side rail.
    4. cleansing about 4 inches along the length of the catheter, proximal to distal.

61. For a renal ultrasound, the patient is instructed to:
    1. not eat or drink for 8 hours before.
    2. have a full bladder.
    3. complete bowel cleansing.
    4. not do anything out of his/her routine, because there is no special preparation for this procedure.

62. Prevention of infection is a patient outcome that is identified for a patient with a urinary alteration and an indwelling catheter. The nurse assists the patient to attain this outcome by:
    1. emptying the drainage bag daily.
    2. draining all urine after the patient ambulates.
    3. performing perineal care q8h and prn.
    4. opening the drainage system only at the connector points to obtain specimens.

63. A patient being seen at a urologist's office suffers from urge incontinence. The nurse anticipates that treatment for this difficulty will include:
    1. biofeedback.
    2. catheterization.
    3. anti-muscarinic drug therapy.
    4. electrical stimulation.

64. A nurse notes that there is an order on a patient's record for a sterile urine specimen. The patient has an indwelling urinary catheter. The nurse will proceed to obtain this specimen by:
    1. withdrawing the urine from a urinometer.
    2. opening the drainage bag and removing urine.
    3. disconnecting the catheter from the drainage tubing.
    4. using a syringe to withdraw urine from the catheter port.

65. A patient had a laparoscopic procedure in the morning and is having difficulty voiding later that day. Before initiating invasive measures, the nurse intervenes by:
    1. administering a cholinergic agent.
    2. applying firm pressure over the perineal area.
    3. increasing the patient's daily fluid intake to 3000 mL.
    4. rinsing the perineal area with warm water.

66. To determine the possibility of a renal problem, a patient is scheduled to have an intravenous pyelogram (IVP). Immediately after the procedure, a nurse will need to evaluate the patient's response and be alert to:
    1. an infection in the urinary bladder.
    2. an allergic reaction to the contrast material.
    3. urinary suppression from injury to kidney tissues.
    4. incontinence from paralysis of the urinary sphincter.

67. A unit manager is evaluating the care that has been given to a patient by a new nursing staff member. The manager determines that the staff member has implemented an appropriate technique for clean-voided urine specimen collection if:
    1. fluids were restricted before the collection.
    2. sterile gloves were applied for the procedure.
    3. the specimen was collected after the initial stream of urine had passed.
    4. the specimen was placed in a clean container and then placed in the utility room.

68. A patient at the urology clinic is diagnosed with reflex incontinence. This problem was identified by the patient's statement of experiencing:
    1. a constant dribbling of urine.
    2. an urge to void and not enough time to reach the bathroom.
    3. an uncontrollable loss of urine when coughing or sneezing.
    4. no urge to void and being unaware of bladder fullness.

69. A female patient has an order for urinary catheterization. A nursing student will be evaluated by the instructor on the insertion technique. The student is identified as implementing appropriate technique if:
    1. the catheter is advanced 7 to 8 inches.
    2. a new cotton ball or swab is used for each wipe when cleansing the urethral meatus.
    3. the catheter is reinserted if it is accidentally placed in the vagina.
    4. both hands are kept sterile throughout the procedure.

70. A patient is diagnosed with prostate enlargement. The nurse is alert to a specific indication of this problem when finding that the patient has:
    1. chills.
    2. cloudy urine.
    3. polyuria.
    4. bladder distention.

71. Stress incontinence is associated with:
    1. irritation of the bladder.
    2. neurological trauma.
    3. alcohol or caffeine ingestion.
    4. coughing or sneezing.

72. For patients with diabetes mellitus, a nurse anticipates that the patients will experience:
    1. dribbling.
    2. hesitancy.
    3. polyuria.
    4. hematuria.

73. A nurse recognizes that one of the specific purposes of intermittent catheterization is for:
    1. prevention of obstruction.
    2. assessment of residual urine.
    3. urinary drainage during surgical procedures.
    4. recording of output for comatose patients.

74. A nurse notes that there is no urine in a drainage bag since it was emptied 1½ hours ago. The nurse should first:
    1. remove the catheter.
    2. provide additional fluids.
    3. check for kinks or bends in the tubing.
    4. apply external pressure on the patient's bladder.

75. The best way to remove urine from a patient's skin is for the nurse to use:
    1. alcohol.
    2. mild soap.
    3. an antibacterial agent.
    4. a hydrogen peroxide mix.

76. A nurse manager is observing a new nurse staff member provide care for a patient with a condom catheter. The manager determines that correction and additional instruction are required for the new employee if the staff nurse is observed:
    1. draping the patient and exposing only the genitalia.
    2. attaching the urinary drainage bag to the lower bed frame.
    3. using adhesive tape to secure the catheter to the patient's penis.
    4. clipping the hair at the base of the penile shaft.

77. A patient who is taking phenazopyridine needs to be instructed that a specific side effect of this medication is that:
    1. the urine will turn orange.
    2. there will be an increased urinary frequency.
    3. back pain will be moderately severe.
    4. occasional dizziness may be experienced.

78. A nurse anticipates that a treatment option for a patient with functional incontinence will include:
    1. catheterization.
    2. bladder training.
    3. electrical stimulation.
    4. hormone replacement.

STUDY GROUP QUESTIONS

- What is the normal anatomy and physiology of the urinary system?
- What factors may influence urination?
- What are some common urinary elimination problems, their causes, and patient signs and symptoms?
- How do growth and development influence urinary function and patterns?
- How can urinary drainage be surgically altered, and why would an alteration be necessary?
- What measures may be implemented to prevent infection in the urinary tract?
- How does a nurse assess a patient's urinary function/elimination?
- What noninvasive and invasive procedures may be used to determine urinary function?
- What diagnostic tests are used to determine the characteristics of urine?
- What are the expected characteristics of urine?
- What nursing interventions are appropriate for promoting urination in the health care and home care settings?
- What information should be included in teaching patients/families about promotion of urination and prevention of infection?

35 Bowel Elimination

CASE STUDIES

1. You have arranged with your instructor and the home care agency to visit a 76-year-old woman. In completing your initial assessment, the patient tells you that she has been having difficulty over the past 2 years in "moving her bowels." She takes you to the bathroom, where she shows you a collection of over-the-counter laxatives and enemas. The patient also tells you that, since the death of her husband, she does not do a lot of cooking, relying on sandwiches and prepared foods.
   a. Based on this information, identify a nursing diagnosis, patient goal(s)/outcomes, and nursing interventions related to bowel elimination.

2. A patient is scheduled to have a colonoscopy performed.
   a. Identify the patient teaching that is provided before the procedure.

CHAPTER REVIEW

Match the description/definition in Column A with the correct term in Column B.

	Column A	*Column B*
_____	1. Propulsion of food through the gastrointestinal (GI) tract	a. Stoma
_____	2. Agent used to empty the bowel	b. Hemorrhoids
_____	3. Artificial opening in the abdominal wall	c. Peristalsis
_____	4. Dilated rectal veins	d. Melena
_____	5. Blood in the stool	e. Cathartic

Complete the following:

6. Constipation in the older adult is usually the result of:

7. What types of patients should be cautioned against straining during defecation and why?

8. a. A common cause of diarrhea in health care facilities is:
   b. This common occurrence can be prevented by:
   c. If persistent diarrhea occurs, a patient is at risk for:

9. The most frequently reported GI complaints are:

10. Provide an example of the effect that fecal incontinence can have on an individual:

11. Which of the following factors will interfere with bowel elimination and decrease peristalsis? Select all that apply.
    a. Slower esophageal emptying _____
    b. Eating raw vegetables _____
    c. Immobilization _____
    d. Consumption of lean meats _____
    e. Anxiety _____
    f. Emotional depression _____
    g. Abdominal surgery _____
    h. Use of antibiotics _____
    i. Food allergies _____
    j. Parkinson's disease _____
    k. Use of narcotic analgesics _____
    l. Drinking fruit juices _____
    m. Tube feedings _____

12. Discuss how a patient's cultural background may influence care for elimination needs.

13. Identify a risk factor for colon cancer.

14. Identify two nursing interventions for a patient who is experiencing:
   a. Constipation
   b. Diarrhea

15. Provide an example of how each of the following factors influences bowel elimination:
   a. Positioning
   b. Pregnancy
   c. Diagnostic tests
   d. Diet
   e. Personal habits

16. How can a nurse promote comfort for a patient with hemorrhoids?

17. Identify at least three areas included in a GI assessment.

18. Enema administration:
   a. What is the correct position for an adult patient to receive an enema?
   b. The enema tube is inserted as follows:
      Adult: ________ inches or _______ cm
      Child: ________ inches or _______ cm
   c. The height of the bag for a regular adult enema should be _____ inches or _____ cm above the level of the anus.
   d. An enema that is used to treat patients with hyperkalemia is:
   e. A hypertonic enema works by:
   f. A commonly used over-the-counter hypertonic enema is:
   g. For a soapsuds enema, the only appropriate soap to use is:
   h. Provision of "enemas until clear" means:
   i. After administration of an enema, what assessments should be made?

19. The nurse anticipates that which of the osmotic laxatives could be prescribed for patients experiencing constipation: Select all that apply.
   a. Lactulose _____
   b. Loperamide _____
   c. Sorbitol _____
   d. Magnesium hydroxide _____
   e. Bisacodyl _____
   f. Polyethylene glycol _____

20. How is the QSEN competency for patient-centered care incorporated into the care of a patient with elimination needs?

21. A patient receiving tube feedings may experience diarrhea as a result of:

22. Identify what should be included in a focused assessment of a patient's bowel function.

23. What surgical procedures are anticipated for patients with:
   a. colorectal cancer?
   b. diverticulitis?

24. Which of the following are correct practices that should be included in the teaching plan for a patient with an ostomy? Select all that apply.
   a. Using creams around the peristomal skin _____
   b. Emptying the pouch when it is one-third to one-half full _____
   c. Washing the peristomal skin with a detergent soap _____
   d. Using sterile technique _____
   e. Anticipating a significant amount of bleeding _____
   f. Changing the entire pouching system daily _____
   g. Using the same manufacturer's flange and pouch _____
   h. Cutting the pouch opening approximately $^1/_{16}$ to $^1/_8$ inch larger than the stoma _____
   i. Applying a skin barrier around the stoma _____

25. Which of the following fecal characteristics are expected findings? Select all that apply.
   a. Yellow infant's stool _____
   b. A defecation frequency greater than three times per day for an adult _____
   c. White stool _____
   d. Tarry stool _____
   e. Soft, formed stool _____
   f. 150 mg/day average amount of stool _____

26. Before giving a patient a bedpan, the nurse should:

27. Select which of the following interventions may be delegated to assistive personnel.
   a. Digital removal of an impaction _____
   b. Enema administration _____
   c. Ostomy pouching _____
   d. Assisting the patient to use the bedpan _____

28. When determining placement of the nasogastric tube, the nurse expects that, if the tube is in the stomach, the gastric pH will be:

29. a. *Clostridium difficile* is transmitted by:
   b. Transmission of *C. difficile* can be prevented or reduced by:

30. Identify a positive outcome for a patient who has a colostomy.

31. Normal defecation in the acute or long-term care environment may be promoted by:

32. Nasogastric tube irrigation is usually done with ______ mL of ______ (solution). Suction applied to the NG tube is usually _______.

33. Place the following steps for nasogastric tube insertion in the correct order:
   a. Have the patient drink water and swallow. _____
   b. Perform hand hygiene. _____
   c. Auscultate for bowel sounds. _____
   d. Insert the tube past the nasopharynx. _____
   e. Prepare the equipment. _____
   f. Measure the distance to insert the tube. _____
   g. Ask the patient to talk. _____
   h. Identify the patient. _____
   i. Position the patient in high Fowler's. _____
   j. Lubricate the tube. _____

Select the best answer for each of the following questions:

34. For a patient with a nasogastric tube who has a painful, distended abdomen, the first most appropriate action by the nurse is to:
   1. remove the tube.
   2. irrigate the tube.
   3. pull the tube out farther.
   4. notify the supervisor.

35. A patient expresses a feeling of mild cramping during the administration of a saline enema. The nurse should first:
   1. discontinue the procedure.
   2. change the solution.
   3. lower the bag to slow the infusion.
   4. allow the solution to cool.

36. The patient begins to cough during the insertion of the nasogastric tube. The nurse should:
   1. remove the tube.
   2. lower the head of the bed.
   3. check the back of the throat.
   4. advance the tube further.

37. A nurse observes a nursing assistant carrying out bowel retraining with a patient in the extended care facility. The nurse identifies that the assistant implements an incorrect procedure when:
   1. allowing the patient adequate time in the bathroom.
   2. taking the patient to the bathroom at regular times throughout the day.
   3. pulling the curtain around the patient while on the commode.
   4. restricting fluids with breakfast and lunch meals.

38. For patients who have been prescribed extended bed rest, the prolonged immobility may result in reduced peristalsis and fecal impaction. A nurse is alert to one of the first signs of an impaction when the patient experiences:
   1. headaches.
   2. abdominal distention.
   3. overflow diarrhea.
   4. abdominal pain with guarding.

39. A patient has been admitted to an acute care unit with a diagnosis of biliary disease. When assessing the patient's feces, the nurse expects that they will be:
   1. bloody.
   2. pus filled.
   3. black and tarry.
   4. white or clay colored.

40. The nurse is documenting the appearance of the colostomy stoma. The term for a stoma that is above the abdominal skin level is:
   1. budded.
   2. flush.
   3. retracted.
   4. edematous.

41. A nurse is preparing to administer an enema to a 7-year-old child. When assembling the equipment, the nurse will prepare an enema of:
   1. 100 to 250 mL of fluid.
   2. 300 to 500 mL of fluid.
   3. 600 to 800 mL of fluid.
   4. 800 to 950 mL of fluid.

42. A nurse recognizes that the greatest challenge for skin care will be for a patient with a(n):
   1. ileostomy.
   2. sigmoid colostomy.
   3. descending ostomy.
   4. ileoanal pouch.

43. A nurse evaluates that a patient has normal bowel sounds by auscultating all four quadrants and finding:
   1. 4 sounds per minute.
   2. 15 sounds per minute.
   3. 40 sounds per minute.
   4. no bowel sounds after 1 minute.

44. A nurse instructs a patient who is taking an iron supplement that his stool may be:
    1. red and liquid.
    2. pale and frothy.
    3. mucus filled.
    4. black and tarry.

45. A nurse is caring for a patient with a Salem sump tube for gastric decompression. Which of the following actions by the nurse requires correction?
    1. Clamping off the blue lumen or air vent
    2. Using clean technique to insert the tube
    3. Anchoring the tube to the patient's gown
    4. Keeping the nares lubricated

46. A nurse recognizes that the intake of mineral oil to promote bowel elimination interferes with the absorption of:
    1. vitamin A.
    2. vitamin B_6.
    3. vitamin C.
    4. niacin.

47. Further follow-up is required if a patient informs the nurse that he regularly uses:
    1. Fleet enemas.
    2. tap water enemas.
    3. castile soap enemas.
    4. normal saline enemas.

48. During a digital removal of a fecal impaction, a nurse notes that the patient has bradycardia. The nurse should:
    1. provide oxygen.
    2. discontinue the procedure.
    3. turn the patient on the right side.
    4. instruct the patient to take rapid, deep breaths.

49. In the teaching plan for a patient who will be having a fecal occult blood test, which of the following foods should be noted for producing a false negative result?
    1. Fish
    2. Pasta
    3. Vitamin C
    4. Whole grain bread

50. The nurse is aware that a test for fecal ova and parasites requires:
    1. performing the test 3 times while the patient is NPO.
    2. keeping the sample at room temperature or warming.
    3. using a chemical fixative for the sample.
    4. saving the sample for 3 to 5 days.

STUDY GROUP QUESTIONS

- What is the normal anatomy and physiology of the gastrointestinal system?
- How is bowel elimination influenced by the process of growth and development?
- What are some common bowel elimination problems?
- How are continent and incontinent bowel diversions/ostomies different?
- What is included in the nursing assessment of a patient to determine bowel elimination status?
- What diagnostic tests may be used to determine the presence of bowel elimination disorders?
- How are the critical thinking and nursing processes applied to situations in which patients are experiencing alterations in bowel elimination?
- What nursing interventions may be implemented to promote bowel elimination and comfort for patients in the health promotion, acute care, and restorative care settings?
- What information should be included in the teaching plan for patients/families with regard to promotion and/or restoration of bowel elimination?

STUDY CHART

Create concept maps with nursing diagnoses, related assessment data, and nursing interventions for the following: constipation, diarrhea, and incontinence.

36 Immobility

CASE STUDIES

1. A patient has just gone to the rehabilitation facility. She has been immobilized with a spinal cord injury from an automobile accident. You are aware of the physical hazards of immobility, but her withdrawn behavior is your concern now.
   a. What can you do to prevent the possible psychological and emotional effects of the patient's period of immobility?

2. A patient will be getting out of bed for the first time after having surgery and receiving general anesthesia.
   a. What actions should be taken by the nurse to promote the patient's safety?

3. You are the nurse in a long-term care facility and your assignment includes several older adult patients who are immobile.
   a. What actions should be taken specifically for this older adult population?

CHAPTER REVIEW

Match the descriptions/definitions in Column A with the correct term in Column B.

	Column A	*Column B*
_____	1. Characterized by bone resorption	a. Renal calculi
_____	2. Temporary decrease in blood supply to an organ or tissue	b. Diuresis
_____	3. Capacity to maneuver around freely	c. Hypostatic pneumonia
_____	4. Permanent plantar flexion	d. Mobility
_____	5. Lung inflammation from stasis or pooling of secretions	e. Ischemia
_____	6. Increased urine excretion	f. Atelectasis
_____	7. Collapse of alveoli	g. Thrombus
_____	8. Bathing, dressing, eating	h. Activities of daily living
_____	9. Calcium stones in the kidney	i. Disuse osteoporosis
_____	10. Accumulation of platelets, fibrin, clotting factors, and cellular elements attached to the interior wall of an artery or vein	j. Footdrop

Complete the following:

11. The objectives or advantages of bed rest are:

12. Identify at least three pathological influences on mobility.

13. Which of the following pathophysiological changes occur with immobility? Select all that apply.
    a. Increased basal metabolic rate _____
    b. Decreased gastrointestinal motility _____
    c. Orthostatic hypotension _____
    d. Increased appetite _____
    e. Increased oxygen availability _____
    f. Hypercalcemia _____
    g. Increased lung expansion _____
    h. Decreased cardiac output _____
    i. Increased dependent edema _____
    j. Decreased stressors _____
    k. Increased urinary stasis _____
    l. Decreased passive behaviors _____

14. An example of a fluid and electrolyte imbalance that may occur with prolonged immobility is:

15. An example of a common behavioral change that may be observed in an immobilized patient is:

16. A nurse anticipates that a patient on prolonged bed rest will have a heart rate that is faster by _____%.

17. Virchow triad is related to ____________________, and the three associated problems are:

18. With an immobilized child, the nurse's focus is on:

19. An important concept when working with patients who are immobilized is to maintain the patient's autonomy. The nurse can accomplish this by:

20. Identify at least one major change that may occur in each of the following body systems as a result of immobility and a nursing intervention to prevent or treat the change.
    a. Cardiovascular system
    b. Respiratory system
    c. Integumentary
    d. Gastrointestinal
    e. Urinary
    f. Musculoskeletal

21. Using the algorithm for patient transfers, the appropriate intervention for a patient who is cooperative, has upper body strength, but cannot bear full weight should be: ____________

22. What areas are included in a focused assessment of patient mobility?

23. Identify for each of the following illustrations what range-of-joint-motion (ROJM) exercise is being performed:

    a.

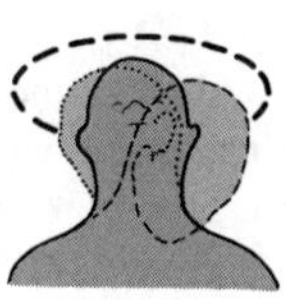

    b.

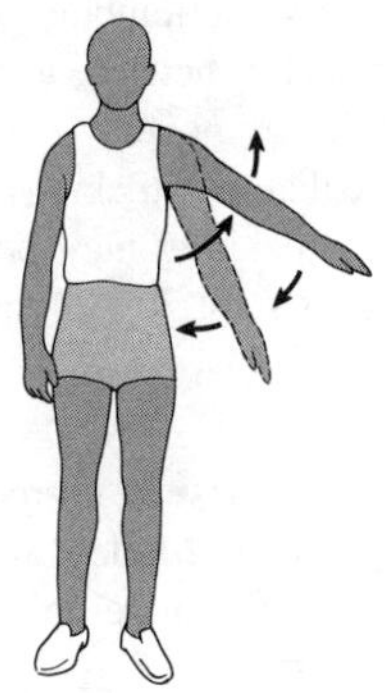

    c.

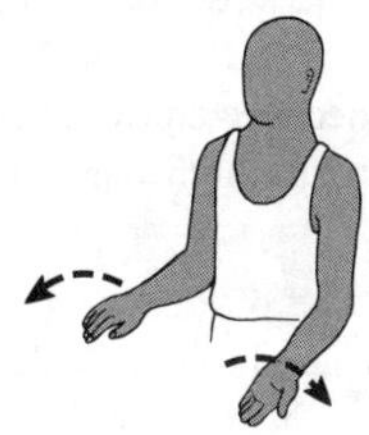

    d.

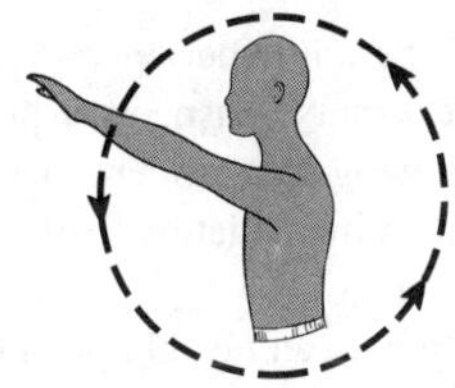

    e.

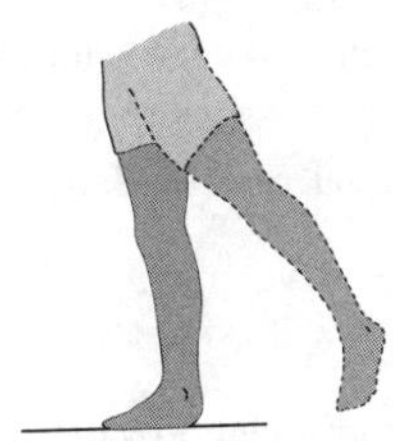

24. To evaluate muscle atrophy, a nurse should:

25. Where should a nurse check for edema in an immobilized patient?

26. For an immobilized patient, identify the usual frequency of assessment for the following:
    a. Respiratory status
    b. Anorexia
    c. Urinary elimination
    d. Intake and output
    e. Anthropometric measurements

27. Specific ROJM exercises to prevent thrombophlebitis include:

28. For a patient who will have antiembolic stockings:
    a. The contraindications for their use are:
    b. How often are they are removed?
    c. A nurse makes sure that the stockings are NOT:
    d. Application of the stockings may be delegated to an unlicensed nursing assistant.
    True _____ False _____

29. Which of the following actions are correct for the use of a sequential compression device? Select all that apply.
    a. The back of the patient's ankle and knee are aligned with markings on the sleeve. _____
    b. A hand width is left between the sleeve and the patient's skin. _____
    c. The sleeve and device are removed once daily. _____
    d. The unit is observed through one complete cycle after application. _____

30. a. A medication that is used to reduce the risk of thrombophlebitis is:
    b. It is usually given every _____ hours by the _____ route.

31. An immobilized patient is experiencing shortness of breath and chest pain. The nurse suspects a pulmonary emboli. Which of the following independent or nurse-initiated actions should be taken immediately? Select all that apply.
    a. Administering heparin _____
    b. Placing the patient in an upright position _____
    c. Drawing arterial blood gases _____
    d. Administering fluids _____
    e. Checking the patient's oxygen saturation _____

32. For a patient who is at risk for falls, which assessment should be used?

33. For a patient who had a cerebrovascular accident (CVA, or stroke) with right-sided hemiplegia, identify how the patient can be involved in joint exercise.

34. Identify at least two measures to prevent pressure ulcers.

35. Identify a nursing diagnosis for a patient who is immobilized.

Select the best answer for each of the following questions:

36. After a CVA (stroke) a patient is prescribed prolonged bed rest. During assessment, the nurse is especially alert to the presence of:
    1. an increased joint ROM.
    2. an increased hemoglobin level.
    3. an increased muscle mass.
    4. a unilateral increase in calf circumference.

37. An older adult patient had a fractured hip repaired 2 days ago. The patient is having more difficulty than expected in moving around, and the nurse is concerned about possible respiratory complications. In assessing the patient for possible atelectasis, the nurse expects to find:
    1. a decreased respiratory rate.
    2. wheezing on inspiration.
    3. asymmetrical breath sounds.
    4. rubbing sounds during inspiration and expiration.

38. For a patient who has been placed in a spica (full body) cast, the nurse remains alert to possible changes in the cardiovascular system as a result of immobility. The nurse may find that the patient has:
    1. hypertension.
    2. tachycardia.
    3. hypervolemia.
    4. an increased cardiac output.

39. A possible complication for a patient who has been prescribed prolonged bed rest is thrombus formation. For the nurse to assess the presence of this serious problem, the nurse should:
    1. attempt to elicit Chvostek sign.
    2. palpate the temperature of the feet.
    3. measure the patient's calf and thigh diameters.
    4. observe for hair loss and skin turgor in the lower legs.

40. A patient was prescribed extended bed rest after abdominal surgery. The patient now has an order to be out of bed. The nurse should first:
    1. assess respiratory function.
    2. obtain the patient's blood pressure measurement.
    3. ask if the patient feels light-headed.
    4. assist the patient to the edge of the bed.

41. A patient has been placed in skeletal traction and will be immobilized for an extended period of time. The nurse recognizes that there is a need to prevent respiratory complications and intervenes by:
    1. suctioning the airway every hour.
    2. changing the patient's position every 4 to 8 hours.
    3. using oxygen and nebulizer treatments regularly.
    4. encouraging deep breathing and coughing every hour.

42. Patients who are immobilized in health care facilities require that their psychosocial needs be met along with their physiological needs. A nurse recognizes a patient's psychosocial needs when telling the patient the following:
    1. "The staff will limit your visitors so that you will not be bothered."
    2. "We will help you get dressed so you look more like yourself."
    3. "We can discuss the routine to see if there are any changes that we can make with you."
    4. "A roommate can sometimes be a real bother and very distracting. We can move you to a private room."

43. A patient is transferred to a rehabilitation facility from the medical center after a CVA (stroke). The CVA resulted in severe right-sided paralysis, and the patient is very limited in mobility. To prevent the complication of external hip rotation for this patient, the nurse uses a:
    1. footboard.
    2. bed board.
    3. trapeze bar.
    4. trochanter roll.

44. A patient who has deep vein thrombosis is at risk for:
    1. atelectasis.
    2. pulmonary emboli.
    3. orthostatic hypotension.
    4. hypostatic pneumonia.

45. The equipment that is used on a bed to assist a patient to raise the torso is a:
    1. sandbag.
    2. bed board.
    3. trapeze bar.
    4. wedge pillow.

46. For exercise, which of the following is appropriate for an immobilized older adult?
    1. Gradual, extended warm-ups
    2. Rapid transitions and movements
    3. Sustained isometric exercises of at least a minute
    4. Slowing of exercise rate in the presence of angina or breathlessness

47. If all of the following are prescribed, the best nursing strategy for the prevention of renal calculi is:
    1. administration of diuretics.
    2. provision of a high-fiber diet.
    3. insertion of a urinary catheter.
    4. offering of 2 liters of fluid per day.

48. A nurse is instructing a patient on joint range of motion and performance of shoulder abduction. The nurse correctly instructs the patient to:
    1. raise the arm straight forward.
    2. move the arm in a full circle.
    3. move the arm until the thumb is turned inward and toward the back.
    4. raise the arm to the side to a position above the head.

49. To prevent plantar flexion, a nurse will obtain:
    1. trochanter rolls.
    2. foot boots.
    3. sandbags.
    4. hand splints.

50. A nurse is instructing a patient on ROJM and performance of forearm supination. The nurse correctly instructs the patient to:
    1. move the palm toward the inner aspect of the forearm.
    2. turn the lower arm and hand so the palm is up.
    3. straighten the elbow by lowering the hand.
    4. touch the thumb to each finger of the hand.

51. A patient has weakness to the upper and lower extremities and has been on bed rest for several days. Which of the following actions performed by the new staff nurse requires correction?
    1. Performing passive ROJM exercises
    2. Having the patient do as much of the bath as possible
    3. Massaging the lower extremities
    4. Assisting the patient to different positions every 1½ hours

52. A patient is being instructed to perform dorsiflexion of the foot. The nurse observes the patient's ability to:
    1. turn the foot and leg toward the other leg.
    2. move the foot so the toes point upward.
    3. turn the sole of the foot medially.
    4. straighten and spread the toes of the foot.

53. The nurse is applying a sequential compression device on the immobilized patient. Which of the following actions is appropriate?
    1. Make sure the red light is on so the unit will run.
    2. Remove the device after 2 to 3 days.
    3. Check for function after 10 or more complete cycles.
    4. Fit 2 fingers between the patient's leg and the device sleeve.

STUDY GROUP QUESTIONS

- What are the basic concepts of mobility?
- What is immobility?
- How is bed rest used therapeutically?
- What physiological changes may occur throughout the body as a result of immobility?
- What psychosocial and developmental changes may occur as a result of immobility?
- What assessments should be made by a nurse to determine the effect of immobility on the patient?
- What nursing interventions should be implemented to prevent or treat the effects of immobility?

37 Skin Integrity and Wound Care

CASE STUDY

1. You are a student nurse assigned to provide care to a patient in an extended care facility. While assisting the patient from the bed to the shower chair, you notice reddened areas on her sacral region and on both elbows and heels. The skin on these areas is intact, but the redness does not go away.
   a. Identify a nursing diagnosis, patient goal/outcomes, and nursing interventions related to this patient's assessment data.

CHAPTER REVIEW

Match the description/definition in Column A with the correct term in Column B.

	Column A	*Column B*
_____	1. Localized collection of blood under the tissues	a. Induration
_____	2. Separation of wound layers with protrusion of visceral organs	b. Approximate
_____	3. Wound edges come together	c. Abrasion
_____	4. Superficial loss of dermis	d. Laceration
_____	5. Pressure exerted against the skin when the patient is moved	e. Dehiscence
_____	6. Hardening of tissue resulting from edema or inflammation	f. Granulation tissue
_____	7. Removal of devitalized tissue	g. Hematoma
_____	8. Torn, jagged damage to dermis and epidermis	h. Evisceration
_____	9. Separation of skin and tissue layers	i. Debridement
_____	10. Red, moist tissue consisting of blood vessels and connective tissue	j. Shearing force

Complete the following:

11. Mark the areas on the body that are common sites for pressure ulcer development.

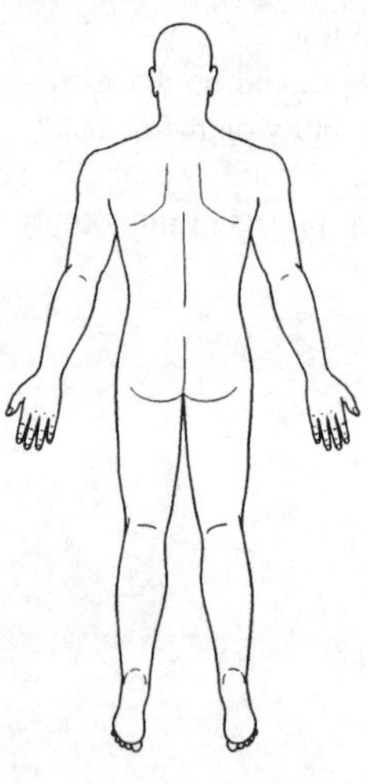

12. Identify the following stages of pressure ulcer development:

a.

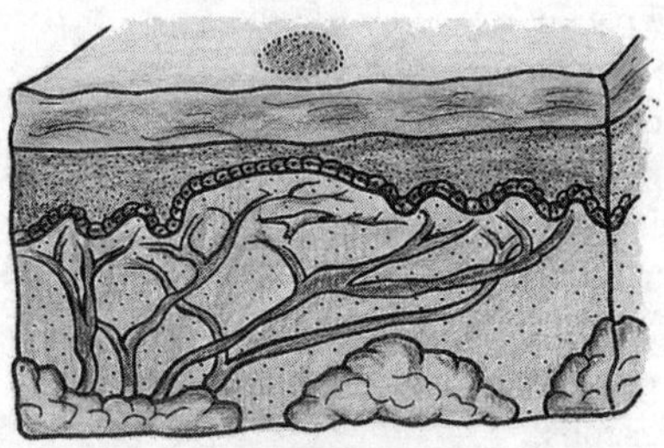

b.

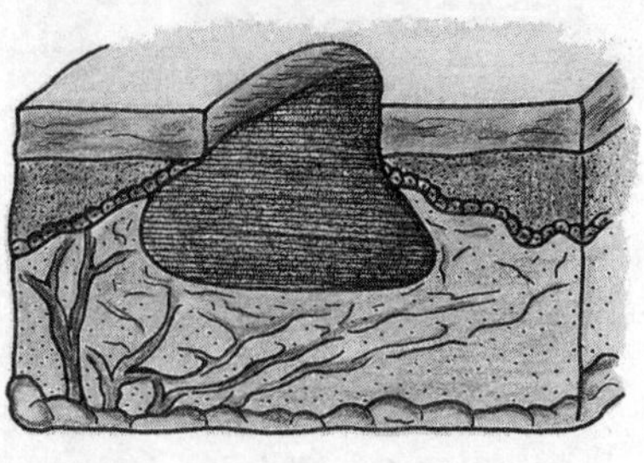

13. Provide an example of an external and internal contributing factor for pressure ulcer formation.

14. Patients in what age groups are at the highest risk for sensitivity to heat and cold applications?

15. The major change in an older adult's skin that contributes to pressure ulcer development is:

16. Identify the following related to wound healing.
    a. A clean surgical wound with little tissue loss heals by:

    b. A severe laceration or chronic wound heals by:

17. Identify if the following statements are true or false.
    a. Wounds that are kept moist for several days heal faster than those that are kept dry.
    True _____ False _____
    b. Specimens for wound cultures should be taken from wound areas with clean, healthy skin.
    True _____ False _____

18. Identify a complication of wound healing that is assessed by the nurse in the following examples.
    a. Separation of the layers of the skin with serosanguineous drainage noted
    b. Bluish swelling or mass at the site
    c. Fever, general malaise, and increased white blood cell (WBC) count
    d. Green, odorous local drainage
    e. Decreased blood pressure, increased pulse rate, increased respirations
    f. Visceral organs protruding through abdominal wall
    g. Wound edges swollen, painful, with redness extending from the edges outward

19. a. Assessment of a pressure ulcer includes:

    b. Identify the methods or indicators that are used for assessing darkly pigmented skin.

20. Identify an example of how each of the following factors influences wound healing.
    a. Age
    b. Obesity
    c. Diabetes
    d. Immunosuppression

21. Match each of the following types of wound drainage with its correct description.

Drainage	*Description*
a. Serous	1. Pale, more watery, with plasma and red blood cells
b. Sanguineous	2. Thick, yellow, green, or brown with organisms and white blood cells
c. Serosanguineous	3. Clear, watery plasma
d. Purulent	4. Fresh bleeding

22. Provide at least one nursing intervention that should be implemented to prevent pressure ulcer formation specifically related to:
    a. Pressure reduction
    b. Skin care

23. Arrange the steps for obtaining a wound culture in correct order.
    a. When tip is saturated, insert into appropriate sterile container. _____
    b. Complete lab slip providing clinical data, which includes wound site, time collected, and prior antibiotics. _____
    c. Moisten swab with normal saline. _____
    d. While applying pressure, rotate applicator within 1 to 2 cm^2 of clean wound tissue (try to draw out tissue fluid). _____
    e. Clean wound surface 1 cm^2 with an antiseptic solution. _____

24. A patient with a dirty penetrating wound is asked by the nurse whether a _______________ injection has been received within the last 10 years.

25. Identify how the nurse determines whether a wound is healing.

26. A patient who is sitting out of bed in a chair and requires assistance to move around should be limited to _____ hours sitting and should be repositioned every _____ hour(s).

27. A nurse can reduce friction or shear by:

28. Nursing care of an abrasion or laceration includes:

29. For use of a negative pressure wound therapy system:
    a. The purpose of the therapy is to:
    b. The tube is attached to:
    c. The dressing that is used for this system is:
    d. What should be done if the patient verbalizes an increase in discomfort with this treatment?

30. For wound irrigation, identify the following that are considered as safe guidelines.
    a. Syringe size
    b. Needle gauge
    c. psi
    d. The syringe should be held how far above the wound?
    e. During an irrigation, the nurse notes sanguineous return. The nurse should:
    f. It is noted that there is retained debris in the wound. The nurse should:

31. Identify what is pictured in the following illustrations:

a.

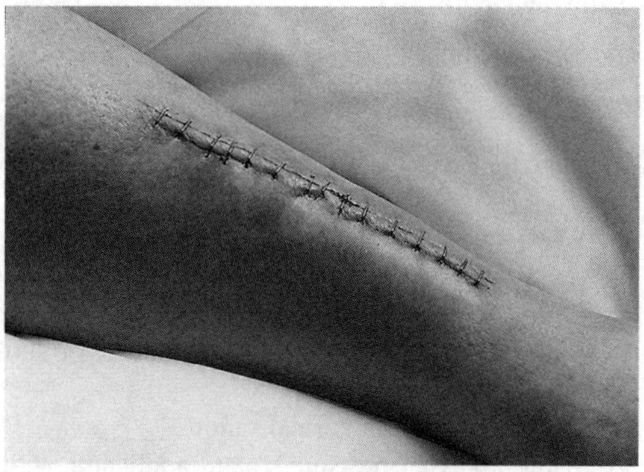

b.

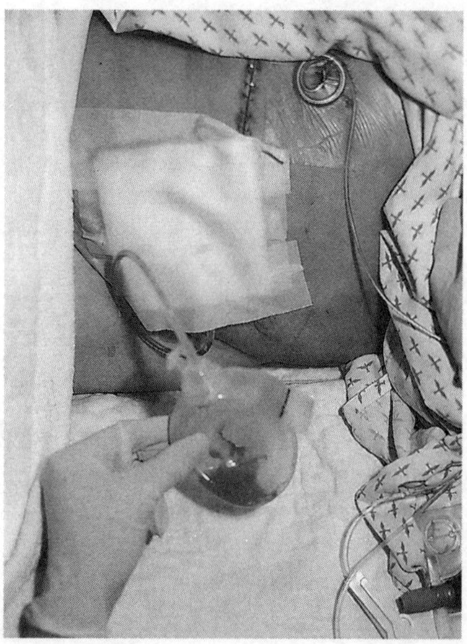

32. Which of the following are correct nursing interventions for elastic bandages? Select all that apply.
    a. Placing the body part to be bandaged in anatomical position _____
    b. Applying a bandage to an extremity from proximal to distal _____
    c. Positioning pins or knots toward the wound _____
    d. Overlapping turns by one half to two thirds the width of the bandage _____
    e. Assessing circulation once daily _____

33. Identify the steps in caring for a traumatic wound.

34. Specify whether the following effects are a result of heat (H) therapy, cold (C) therapy, or both.
    a. Vasoconstriction _____
    b. Decreased blood viscosity _____
    c. Increased tissue metabolism _____
    d. Decreased muscle tension _____
    e. Increased capillary permeability _____

35. a. Provide an instance in which the application of heat is contraindicated.
    b. Provide an instance in which the application of cold is contraindicated.

36. The usual duration of time for the application of heat or cold is:

37. Which of the following are correct for the application of heat or cold? Select all that apply.
    a. Providing a timer or clock so the patient may help time the application _____
    b. Allowing the patient to adjust the temperature setting _____
    c. Placing the patient in a position that prevents movement away from the temperature source _____
    d. Maintaining the temperature as hot or cold as the patient is able to tolerate _____
    e. Applying a heating pad or cold pack directly to the skin _____
    f. Adding hotter solution to a soak to maintain temperature while the patient remains immersed _____
    g. Keeping the rest of the patient draped or covered while receiving treatment _____

38. Using the Braden Scale, what is this patient's risk for pressure ulcer development?

		Score
Sensory	Very limited	______
Moisture	Occasionally	______
Activity	Chairfast	______
Mobility	Very limited	______
Nutrition	Probably inadequate	______
Friction/Shear	Potential problem	______
	Total Score	______
	Patient Risk	______

39. Which of the following are correct for application of a moist dressing? Select all that apply.
   a. Wringing out excess moisture from the dressing _____
   b. Pouring the solution directly onto the dressing in the wound _____
   c. Loosely packing sinus tracks or dead spaces in the wound _____
   d. Avoiding the use of secondary dressings _____
   e. Using Montgomery ties or straps perpendicular to the wound _____

40. a. Nonblanchable hyperemia is:
   b. This assessment signifies:
   c. When nonblanchable hyperemia is assessed, the stage is reversible if pressure is relieved.
   True _____ False _____

41. Which of the following are correct actions for a postoperative dressing? Select all that apply.
   a. Routinely changing the dressing soon after the procedure _____
   b. Reinforcing saturated dressings _____
   c. Providing the patient with an analgesic 30 minutes before the dressing change _____
   d. Expecting inflammation of the wound edges for at least a week after the surgery _____
   e. Noting the amount, color, consistency, and odor of wound drainage _____

42. A patient will need to continue to perform dressing changes when he is discharged to his home. Identify the necessary nursing assessments/evaluations before the patient's discharge.

43. Topical skin care for a patient should include: Select all that apply.
   a. Massaging reddened areas _____
   b. Examining the skin at least daily _____
   c. Using a mild cleansing agent _____
   d. Keeping the head of the bed at greater than a 30-degree angle _____
   e. Applying a moisture-barrier product _____
   f. Repositioning the patient in the chair every 3 hours _____

44. The usual wound care in the home environment is performed by the patient or family using sterile technique.
   True _____ False _____

45. Match the following wounds with the type of dressing that is most appropriate.

Wounds	***Dressings***
1. Occlusive, forming a gel with the wound surface, they protect the wound from contaminants _____	a. Gauze
2. Best for wounds with moderate drainage, deep wounds, undermining, and tunnels, moist or dry _____	b. Transparent film
3. Semipermeable to oxygen. Used as a primary dressing in wounds with minimal tissue loss that have very little wound drainage _____	c. Hydrocolloid

46. The correct way to remove old tape from the skin is to:

47. How can the nurse reduce discomfort during dressing changes?

48. Describe the correct application of a sling.

49. The desired temperature for a cold soak is _________.

Select the best answer for each of the following questions:

50. To avoid pressure ulcer development for an immobilized patient at home, a nurse recommends a surface to use on the bed. A surface type that is low-cost and easy to use in the home is a(n):
   1. foam overlay surface.
   2. air overlay surface.
   3. air fluidized surface.
   4. low air loss surface.

51. For a patient in the extended care facility who has a nursing diagnosis of *Impaired Physical Mobility*, a nurse will implement:
   1. massage of reddened skin areas.
   2. movement of the patient in the chair every 3 hours.
   3. maintenance of a position while in bed at 30 degrees or lower.
   4. placement of plastic absorptive pads directly beneath the patient.

52. A patient has experienced a traumatic injury that will require applications of heat. The nurse implements the treatment based on the principle that:
    1. long exposures help the patient develop tolerance to the procedure.
    2. the foot and the palm of the hand are the most sensitive to temperature.
    3. patient response is best to minor temperature adjustments.
    4. patients are more tolerant to temperature changes over a large body surface area.

53. A severely overweight patient has returned to the unit after having major abdominal surgery. When the nurse enters the room, it is evident that the patient has moved or coughed and the wound has eviscerated. The nurse should immediately:
    1. assess vital signs.
    2. contact the physician.
    3. apply light pressure on the exposed organs.
    4. place sterile towels soaked in saline over the area.

54. A patient with a knife protruding from his upper leg is taken into the emergency department. A nurse is waiting for the physician to arrive when a newly hired nurse comes to assist. The nurse delegates the new staff member to do all of the following as soon as possible except:
    1. assess vital signs.
    2. remove the knife to cleanse the wound.
    3. wrap a bandage around the knife and injured site.
    4. apply pressure to the surrounding area to stop bleeding.

55. A nurse is assessing a patient's wound and notices that it has very minimal tissue loss and drainage. There are a number of dressings that may be used according to the protocol on the unit. The nurse selects:
    1. gauze.
    2. alginate.
    3. negative pressure wound therapy.
    4. transparent film.

56. A nurse is completing an assessment of the patient's skin integrity and identifies that an area is a full-thickness wound with damage to the subcutaneous tissue. The nurse identifies this stage of ulcer formation as:
    1. Stage I.
    2. Stage II.
    3. Stage III.
    4. Stage IV.

57. A patient has a large wound to the sacral area that requires irrigation. The nurse explains to the patient that irrigation will be performed to:
    1. decrease scar formation.
    2. decrease wound drainage.
    3. remove debris from the wound.
    4. improve circulation in the wound.

58. A nurse is working with an older adult patient in an extended care facility. While turning the patient, the nurse notices that there is a reddened area on the patient's coccyx. The nurse implements skin care that includes:
    1. soaking the area with normal saline.
    2. cleaning the area with mild soap, drying, and applying a protective moisturizer.
    3. washing the area with an astringent and painting it with povidone-iodine solution.
    4. applying a dilute solution of hydrogen peroxide and water and using a heat lamp to dry the area.

59. A patient has a wound to the left lower extremity that has minimal exudates and collagen formation. The nurse identifies the healing phase of this wound as:
    1. primary intention.
    2. proliferative phase.
    3. secondary intention.
    4. inflammatory phase.

60. After neurosurgery, a nurse assesses the patient's bandage and finds that there is fresh bleeding coming from the operative site. The nurse describes this drainage to the surgeon as:
    1. serous.
    2. purulent.
    3. sanguineous.
    4. serosanguineous.

61. A patient has a surgical wound on the right upper aspect of the chest that requires cleansing. The nurse implements appropriate aseptic technique by:
    1. opening the cleansing solution with sterile gloves.
    2. moving from the outer region of the wound toward the center.
    3. cleaning the wound twice and discarding the swab.
    4. starting at the drainage site and moving outward with circular motions.

62. A nurse is working in a physician's office and is asked by one of the patients when heat or cold should be applied. In providing an example, the nurse identifies that cold therapy should be applied for the patient with:
    1. a newly fractured ankle.
    2. menstrual cramping.
    3. an infected wound.
    4. degenerative joint disease.

63. A patient will require the application of a binder to provide support to the abdomen. When applying the binder, the nurse uses the principle that:
    1. the binder should be kept loose for patient comfort.
    2. the patient should be sitting or standing when it is applied.
    3. the patient must maintain adequate ventilatory capacity.
    4. the binder replaces the need for underlying bandages or dressings.

64. A nurse is aware that malnutrition places a patient at a greater risk for tissue damage. The patient with the greatest risk is the individual who:
    1. experienced a 7% weight loss in 4 months.
    2. is between 45 and 60 years of age.
    3. has an albumin level of 5 mg/100 mL.
    4. has a transferrin level of 120 mg/dL.

65. The agent that is most effective and safest for cleaning a granular wound is:
    1. acetic acid.
    2. normal saline.
    3. povidone-iodine.
    4. hydrogen peroxide.

66. A nurse is working with a patient who has a stage III, clean ulcer with significant exudate. The nurse anticipates that which of the following dressings will be used?
    1. Composite film dressing
    2. Transparent dressing
    3. Calcium alginate dressing
    4. Gauze dressing

67. For a patient's optimal nutritional intake that will promote formation of new blood vessels and collagen synthesis, the nurse plans to teach the patient to include a sufficient intake of:
    1. fats.
    2. proteins.
    3. carbohydrates.
    4. fat-soluble vitamins.

68. The nurse notices that the skin surrounding a wound appears macerated. The nurse should:
    1. obtain a wound culture.
    2. monitor lab results.
    3. turn the patient more frequently.
    4. select a different dressing.

STUDY GROUP QUESTIONS

- What are pressure ulcers and what contributes to their development?
- Where are pressure ulcers most likely to develop?
- What are the stages of pressure ulcer development?
- What are the classifications of wounds?
- How do wounds heal?
- What are the possible complications of wound healing?
- How do pressure ulcers affect health care costs?
- What tools may be used to predict patients' risks for pressure ulcer development?
- What should be included in the nursing assessment of patients to determine their risk for pressure ulcer development?
- How are wounds managed in emergency and nonemergency health care settings?
- What types of drainage may be seen in wounds?
- How are wound cultures obtained?
- How can the nurse prevent pressure ulcer development?
- What nursing interventions may be implemented to treat pressure ulcers and wounds?
- What are the procedures for dressing changes and wound care?
- What criteria are used in the selection of dressings and sutures or staples?
- What are the principles involved in heat and cold therapy, including patient safety?
- What information should be included in patient/family teaching for prevention and treatment of pressure ulcers, wound care, and use of heat and cold therapy?

38 Sensory Alterations

CASE STUDIES

1. You are making a home visit to a patient with diabetes mellitus who is losing his eyesight (diabetic retinopathy).
   a. What interventions may be implemented with the patient to assist in maintaining adequate sensory stimulation?
   b. How can you promote a safe environment for him?

2. You have been assigned to care for a patient in the intensive care unit (ICU).
   a. What sensory alterations may this patient experience?
   b. How can you prevent the occurrence of these alterations or reduce their impact?

CHAPTER REVIEW

Complete the following:

1. Identify other terms for the following.
   a. Sight:
   b. Hearing:
   c. Taste:
   d. Smell:
   e. Touch:
   f. Position sense:

2. Identify one of the major diseases that can lead to visual impairment.

3. Provide the correct term for each of the following:
   a. A buildup of earwax in the external auditory canal
   b. Hearing loss associated with aging
   c. Opacity of the lens resulting in blurred vision
   d. Decreased salivary production or dry mouth
   e. Intermittent hearing loss, vertigo, tinnitus, and pressure in the ears

4. Identify how the following factors may influence sensory function:
   a. Age: older adulthood
   b. Medications
   c. Smoking
   d. Environment

5. How can a nurse evaluate a patient's vision and hearing during routine interactions or care?

6. For visual and hearing impairments in children:
   a. A common cause of blindness is:
   b. What information should be included when teaching parents about eyesight safety?
   c. Common causes of hearing impairment are:

7. Orientation to the environment for a patient with a sensory deficit should include:

8. Identify a way that a nurse can modify sensory stimulation in the health care environment.

9. A nurse may communicate with a hearing-impaired patient by:

10. For a patient with cataracts, the nurse anticipates which of the following signs and symptoms? Select all that apply.
   a. Cloudy vision _____
   b. Eye pain _____
   c. Glare _____
   d. Burning sensation _____
   e. Poor night vision _____
   f. Double vision _____

11. Indicate how a nurse may assist patients with the following deficits to adapt their home environments for safety:
   a. Hearing deficit
   b. Diminished sense of smell
   c. Diminished sense of touch

12. Identify a possible nursing diagnosis and goal/outcome for a patient with a sensory deficit.

13. In relation to screening for sensory deficits:
   a. Provide an example of a general screening that is conducted to determine visual and/or auditory deficits.
   b. The recommendation of frequency for hearing screenings is:

14. Which of the following are appropriate in promoting sensory stimulation in the home environment? Select all that apply.
   a. Reducing glare by using sheer curtains on windows ______
   b. Using pale colors on surfaces ______
   c. Serving bland foods with similar textures ______
   d. Using a pocket magnifier ______
   e. Introducing fragrant flowers ______
   f. Playing recorded music with high-frequency sound ______

15. A patient has gone to the local walk-in emergency center with flu-like symptoms. After seeing the physician, the patient shows the nurse the prescriptions the physician has written. The patient should be informed that ototoxicity may occur with the administration of which of the following medications? Select all that apply.
   a. Furosemide _____
   b. Vitamin C _____
   c. Acetaminophen _____
   d. Erythromycin _____
   e. Cough suppressant with codeine _____
   f. Aspirin _____

16. Identify at least one rationale for why a patient may not use his or her hearing aid.

17. A patient with a diminished tactile sense may be assisted with hygiene and grooming by:

18. What are the signs and symptoms associated with Ménière's disease?

19. The nurse is caring for a patient with a hearing aid. What is included in the care for this patient and the assistive device?

20. Behaviors that are specific for an adult with a visual impairment include: Select all that apply.
   a. Poor coordination ______
   b. Rocking ______
   c. Squinting ______
   d. No reaction to being touched ______
   e. Accidental falls ______
   f. Increase in appetite ______

21. Identify community resources where a patient with a sensory impairment may be referred.

22. The occupational health nurse wants to promote safety for the employees. What general safety measures may be implemented by the nurse in a work environment?

23. Provide an example of a patient who may experience sensory deprivation.

Select the best answer for each of the following questions:

24. An expected outcome for a patient with an auditory deficit should include:
   1. minimizing use of affected sense(s).
   2. preventing additional sensory losses.
   3. promoting the patient's acceptance of dependency.
   4. controlling the environment to reduce sensory stimuli.

25. A nurse is working with patients at the senior day care center and recognizes that changes in sensory status may influence the older adult's eating patterns. For patients who are experiencing changes in their dietary intake, the nurse will assess for:
   1. presbycusis.
   2. xerostomia.
   3. vestibular ataxia.
   4. peripheral neuropathy.

26. Parents arrive at the pediatric clinic with their 1½-year-old child. The parents ask the nurse if there are signs that may indicate that the child is not able to hear well. The nurse explains to the parents that they should be alert to the child:
   1. awakening to loud noises.
   2. responding reflexively to sounds.
   3. having delayed speech development.
   4. remaining calm when unfamiliar people approach.

27. A nurse is assessing a patient for a potential gustatory impairment. This may be indicated if the patient has a(n):
   1. weight loss.
   2. blank look or stare.
   3. increased sensitivity to odors.
   4. period of excessive clumsiness or dizziness.

28. Which of the following is a priority safety measure in the acute care environment for a patient with a sensory deficit?
   1. Encouraging the family to visit the patient
   2. Referring the patient to a support group
   3. Determining the patient's medical history
   4. Orienting the patient to the surroundings

29. A responsive patient had eye surgery, and patches have been temporarily placed on both eyes for protection. The evening meal has arrived, and the nurse will be assisting the patient. In this circumstance, the nurse should:
    1. feed the patient the entire meal.
    2. encourage family members to feed the patient.
    3. allow the patient to be totally independent and feed himself.
    4. orient the patient to the locations of the foods on the plate and provide the utensils.

30. After a cerebrovascular accident (CVA, or stroke), a patient is found to have receptive aphasia. The nurse may assist this patient with communication by:
    1. obtaining a referral for a speech therapist.
    2. using a system of simple gestures and repeated behaviors.
    3. providing the patient with a letter chart to use to answer questions.
    4. offering the patient a notepad and pen to write down questions and concerns.

31. A patient has been diagnosed with glaucoma. The nurse anticipates that the patient will report a history of:
    1. severe redness and itching of the eyes.
    2. cloudy and blurred vision.
    3. painless loss of peripheral vision.
    4. dark spaces blocking forward vision and distortion of lines.

32. A mother is taking her newborn for his first physical examination. She expresses concern because during her pregnancy she may have been exposed to an infectious disease, and the baby's hearing could be affected. The nurse inquires if the patient was exposed to:
    1. rubella.
    2. pneumonia.
    3. tuberculosis.
    4. a urinary tract infection.

33. For a patient with a hearing deficit, the best way for the nurse to communicate is to:
    1. approach the patient from the side.
    2. use visible facial expressions.
    3. shout or speak very loudly to the patient.
    4. repeat the entire conversation if it is not totally understood.

34. The school nurse recognizes that the most common type of visual disorder in children is:
    1. glaucoma.
    2. retinal detachment.
    3. nearsightedness.
    4. macular degeneration.

35. Because of the possibility of diminished independence for the patient with sensory losses, an important and specific ethical standard for the nurse to follow is the preservation of:
    1. autonomy.
    2. fidelity.
    3. justice.
    4. nonmaleficence.

STUDY GROUP QUESTIONS

- What are the human senses and their functions?
- What factors influence sensory function?
- What are some common sensory alterations?
- What types of patients are at risk for developing sensory alterations?
- How should a nurse assess a patient's sensory function?
- What behaviors or changes in lifestyle patterns or socialization may indicate a sensory alteration?
- How can a nurse promote sensory function and prevent injury and isolation in the health promotion and acute and restorative care settings?
- What screening processes are used to determine the presence of sensory alterations?
- How may the family/significant others be involved in the care of a patient with a sensory alteration?
- What information should be included in patient/family teaching for promotion of sensory function and prevention of injury?

39 Surgical Patient

CASE STUDIES

1. Your patient is scheduled to have extensive abdominal surgery with a large midline incision.
   a. How can you assist this patient to promote respiratory function postoperatively?

2. A patient is having outpatient surgery.
   a. How may preoperative teaching be conducted and what information should be included?
   b. The patient does not appear to have an understanding of the surgery or possible complications. What should you do?

3. While completing the preoperative checklist, you discover that a patient's temperature is 101° F.
   a. What action should be taken?

4. A patient insists that his good luck medallion must go with him everywhere, even to surgery.
   a. What should you do?
   b. What personal items or prosthetics should be accounted for before surgery?

5. A patient had laparoscopic surgery on his right knee and is going to be discharged to his home. His wife and young children have visited often during his hospital stay.
   a. What general information do you need to prepare the patient and the family for the discharge?

6. A patient has come into the ambulatory surgery center in the hospital for hernia repair. Upon admission to the PACU, the patient's oxygen saturation is 88% and he is not easy to arouse. There is no evidence of bleeding on the lower right abdominal dressing and no distention.
   a. What should you do for this patient in the PACU?
   b. After 3 hours, the patient has still not had any urinary output. What options are available?

CHAPTER REVIEW

Match the description/definition in Column A with the correct term in Column B.

	Column A	Column B
_____	1. Performed on the basis of the patient's choice; not essential for health	a. Palliative surgery
_____	2. Involves extensive reconstruction or alteration in body parts; poses risks to well-being	b. Transplant surgery
_____	3. Relieves or reduces intensity of disease symptoms; will not produce cure	c. Major surgery
_____	4. Must be done immediately to save life or preserve function of body part	d. Ablative surgery
_____	5. Surgical exploration that allows physician to confirm medical status; may involve removal of body tissue for analysis	e. Cosmetic surgery
_____	6. Performed to improve personal appearance	f. Emergency surgery
_____	7. Amputation or removal of diseased body part	g. Elective surgery
_____	8. Performed to replace malfunctioning organs or structures	h. Diagnostic surgery

Complete the following:

9. a. In relation to the operative experience, a patient who smokes cigarettes is at a greater risk for:
   b. Postoperative care for this patient requires more aggressive:

10. a. Identify a medical condition that may increase a patient's surgical risk.
    b. Malignant hyperthermia is associated with:
    c. The pregnant patient is at greater risk because of:

11. Identify an example of how changes in each of the following body systems place the older adult patient at risk during surgery.
    a. Cardiovascular
    b. Pulmonary
    c. Renal
    d. Neurological

12. Obesity places a patient at greater risk for surgery as a result of:

13. Identify a consideration for surgical patients who are taking the following medications:
    a. Insulin
    b. Antibiotics
    c. NSAIDs

14. Provide two examples of information that is usually included in preoperative teaching.

15. For preoperative screening, identify a routine screening test that may be ordered for a patient.

16. Identify the commonly used types of preoperative medications.

17. Identify two nursing diagnoses and related outcomes that may be formulated for a patient who will be having his or her first surgery.

18. The patient is going to receive general anesthesia for the surgical procedure. Specify the general NPO criteria for the following.
    a. No food or fluids _____ hours before surgery
    b. No meat or fried foods _____ hours before surgery

19. Identify the adverse effects associated with the following types of anesthesia.
    a. General anesthesia
    b. Regional anesthesia
    c. Local anesthesia
    d. Conscious sedation

20. Which of the following preoperative interventions are appropriate? Select all that apply.
    a. Completing bowel preparation before GI surgery _____
    b. Shaving the surgical site with a razor _____
    c. Providing antimicrobial soap for bathing _____
    d. Removing the patient's wig _____
    e. Leaving artificial fingernails intact _____
    f. Removing a hearing aid when the patient gets to the operating room (OR) _____

21. In the presurgical care unit (PSCU) and OR, how is verification done to determine:
    a. Right patient
    b. Right frame of mind of the patient
    c. Preparation for surgery

22. Identify whether the following tasks are responsibilities of the circulating nurse (C) or scrub nurse (S).
    a. Completion of preoperative assessments/verification _____
    b. Application of sterile drapes _____
    c. Establishment of the intraoperative plan of care _____
    d. Calculation of blood loss and urinary output _____
    e. Provision of sterile equipment for the surgeon _____
    f. Documentation of the procedure _____
    g. Maintenance of the sterile field _____

23. For the following, identify a nursing intervention for intraoperative patient care.
    a. Prevention of injury
    b. Maintenance of patient's body temperature
    c. Prevention of infection

24. Identify a specific nursing intervention to prevent the following postoperative complications.
    a. Pulmonary stasis
    b. Venous stasis
    c. Wound infection
    d. Gastrointestinal stasis

25. Which of the following assessment findings for a patient in the postanesthesia care unit (PACU) signify that the patient is qualified to be discharged from the unit? Select all that apply.
    a. Oxygen saturation 96% _____
    b. Rales on auscultation _____
    c. Pulse rate 110 beats per minute _____
    d. Bilateral peripheral pulses _____
    e. Abdominal distention _____
    f. Response to verbal stimuli _____
    g. Sluggish hand grasp and pupillary response _____
    h. Quarter-size sanguineous spot maintained on incisional dressing _____
    i. 30 mL per hour urinary output _____

26. A nurse is aware that a patient should void within _____ hours after surgery. For the patient who has not voided, what should the nurse do?

27. After general anesthesia, postoperative oral intake usually begins with an order for _____ (diet).

28. With regard to postoperative wound healing and care, which of the following statements are correct? Select all that apply.
   a. The surgical dressing is changed after the patient leaves the PACU. _____
   b. Any visible drainage on the surgical dressing should be marked. _____
   c. The patient who has an order for an oral analgesic should be medicated 20 minutes before an uncomfortable dressing change. _____
   d. Redness, warmth, and edema should be expected at the incision site. _____
   e. Wound drainage should be measured once a day. _____
   f. The patient should be draped during a dressing change to minimize exposure. _____

29. a. The patient in the illustration is demonstrating the use of a(n):

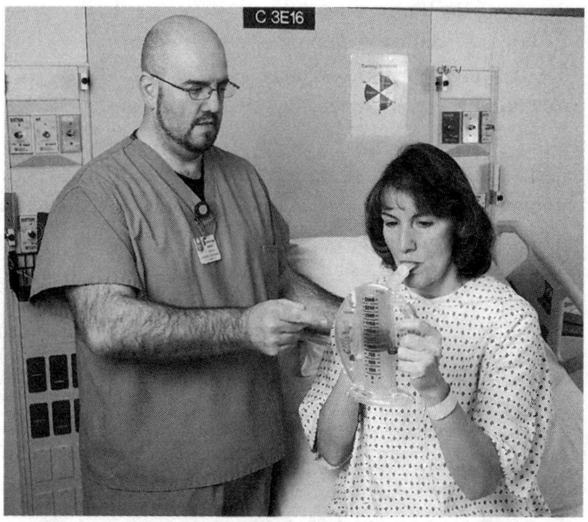

   b. This device is used to prevent:

30. For a patient who will be alert during a surgical procedure, what support should be provided by the nurse?

31. Identify examples of routine postoperative patient assessments and interventions.

32. What physical signs and symptoms are indicative of a latex allergy?

33. The American Society of Anesthesiologists recommends that postoperative analgesics be administered:

34. Indicate which of the following are appropriate interventions in the postanesthesia care unit (PACU). Select all that apply.
   a. Irrigating an existing N/G tube with normal saline _____
   b. Providing oral fluids _____
   c. Measuring I & O _____
   d. Yelling loudly to arouse the patient _____
   e. Checking for bleeding at the surgical site _____
   f. Administering analgesics _____

35. Research indicates that the use of preventive measures decreases the incidence of postoperative wound infection. Identify at least three (3) of those interventions.

36. What is included in the hand-off communication ANTICipate?

37. Identify two nursing diagnoses and a related outcome for each that may be formulated for a patient in the postoperative period.

Select the best answer for each of the following questions:

38. A nurse is starting the preparations for a patient who is having surgery tomorrow morning. The nurse prepares to have the consent form completed. The nurse recognizes that informed consent:
   1. is valid if the patient is disoriented.
   2. is signed by the patient after the administration of preoperative medications.
   3. indicates that the patient is aware of the procedure and its possible complications.
   4. requires that the nurse provide information about the surgery before the consent can be signed.

39. A patient is taken to PACU after surgery. A nurse is assessing the patient and is alert to the indication of a postoperative hemorrhage if the patient exhibits:
   1. restlessness.
   2. warm, dry skin.
   3. a slow, steady pulse rate.
   4. a decreased respiratory rate.

40. A nurse is checking the vital signs of a patient who had major surgery yesterday. The nurse discovers that the patient's temperature is slightly elevated. This finding is usually indicative of:
    1. a postoperative wound infection.
    2. an allergic response to latex.
    3. a response to the anesthesia.
    4. extensive neural damage.

41. A nurse is completing the preoperative checklist for a woman who will be having surgery. The nurse determines that the surgeon and anesthesiologist should be informed of which of the patient's laboratory results?
    1. Hemoglobin level: 10 g/dL
    2. Potassium level: 4.2 mEq/L
    3. Platelet count: 210,000/mm^3
    4. Prothrombin time: 11 seconds

42. A patient has received a spinal anesthetic during the surgical procedure. The nurse is alert to possible complications of the anesthetic and is assessing the patient for a:
    1. rash.
    2. headache.
    3. nephrotoxic response.
    4. hyperthermic response.

43. A patient is being evaluated for transfer from the PACU to the patient's unit. The nurse determines that the patient will be approved for transfer if the patient exhibits:
    1. increased wound drainage.
    2. pulse oximetry of 95%.
    3. respirations of 30 breaths per minute.
    4. nonpalpable peripheral pulses.

44. A patient is scheduled to have abdominal surgery later in the morning. At 9:00 AM, while completing the preoperative checklist, the nurse recognizes the need to contact the surgeon immediately. The nurse has identified that the patient:
    1. received an enema at 6:00 AM.
    2. admitted to recent substance abuse.
    3. ate a hamburger last evening at 6:00 PM.
    4. has bowel sounds in all four quadrants of the abdomen.

45. A patient is being positioned in the PACU after surgery. Unless contraindicated, the nurse should place the patient:
    1. prone.
    2. in high Fowler's.
    3. supine with arms across the chest.
    4. on the side with the face turned downward.

46. When a patient first arrives at PACU, the nurse will:
    1. provide oral fluids.
    2. allow the patient to sleep.
    3. provide a warm blanket.
    4. remove the urinary catheter.

47. A nurse is visiting a patient who had surgery 9 hours ago. The nurse asks if the patient has voided, and the patient responds negatively. At this time, the nurse:
    1. provides more oral fluids.
    2. inserts an IV and administers fluids.
    3. obtains an order for urinary catheterization.
    4. recognizes that this is a normal outcome.

48. During a patient assessment in the PACU, a nurse finds that the patient's operative site is swollen and appears tight. The nurse suspects:
    1. infection.
    2. hemorrhage.
    3. lymphedema.
    4. subcutaneous emphysema.

49. An immediate postoperative priority in providing nursing care for a patient is:
    1. airway patency.
    2. relief of pain.
    3. sufficient circulation to the extremities.
    4. prevention of wound infection.

50. A 54-year-old patient is scheduled to have a gastric resection. The nurse informs the surgeon preoperatively of the patient's history of:
    1. a tonsillectomy at age 10.
    2. employment as a telephone repair person.
    3. smoking two packs of cigarettes per day.
    4. taking acetaminophen for minor body aches.

51. A patient has been taking warfarin at home. The patient is going to be admitted for a surgical procedure, and the nurse anticipates that this prescribed medication will be:
    1. administered as usual.
    2. increased in dose immediately before the procedure.
    3. reduced in dose by half immediately before the procedure.
    4. discontinued at least 2 days before the procedure.

52. During the intraoperative phase, a nurse's responsibility is reflected in the statement:
    1. "I think that the patient requires more information about the procedure and its consequences."
    2. "There seems to be a missing sponge, so a recount must be done to see that all of the sponges were removed."
    3. "The patient has signed the request. I will prepare the medications and then get the record completed."
    4. "The patient appears reactive and stable. Dressing to wound is dry and intact. Analgesic administered per order."

53. A nurse is assisting a patient with postoperative exercises. The patient tells the nurse, "Blowing into this thing [incentive spirometer] is a waste of time." The nurse explains to the patient that the specific purpose of this therapy is to:
   1. stimulate the cough reflex.
   2. promote lung expansion.
   3. increase pulmonary circulation.
   4. directly remove excess secretions from the respiratory tract.

54. A patient is scheduled for surgery, and a nurse is completing the final areas of the preoperative checklist. After administering the preoperative medications, the nurse should:
   1. assist the patient to void.
   2. obtain the informed consent.
   3. prepare the skin at the surgical site.
   4. place the side rails up on the bed or stretcher.

55. At the ambulatory surgery center, a patient is having surgery using general anesthesia. The nurse will expect this patient to:
   1. ambulate immediately after being admitted to the recovery area.
   2. meet all of the identified criteria in order to be discharged home.
   3. remain in the phase I recovery area longer than a hospitalized patient.
   4. receive large amounts of oral fluids immediately entering the recovery area.

56. A nurse is preparing a patient for surgery and recognizes that the greatest risk of bleeding is for the patient with:
   1. diabetes mellitus.
   2. emphysema.
   3. thrombocytopenia.
   4. immunodeficiency syndrome.

57. A patient has a nasogastric tube in place after surgery and complains to the nurse of nausea. The nurse should first:
   1. remove the NG tube.
   2. provide oral fluids.
   3. move the patient side to side.
   4. irrigate the tube with normal saline.

58. Which of the following individuals is most at risk for postoperative wound infection?
   1. A pregnant patient
   2. A patient who smokes cigarettes
   3. A patient with poorly controlled diabetes
   4. A patient experiencing periods of sleep apnea

59. A patient's surgeon has previously discussed the procedure with the patient, but the patient has a few more questions. The best way for the nurse to approach this is to first:
   1. refer the patient back to the surgeon.
   2. determine what the patient has been told already.
   3. provide details of what the procedure will be like.
   4. get the consent form for the patient to read.

60. The nurse is alert for signs of a postoperative wound infection:
   1. within 24 hours of the surgery.
   2. 1 to 2 days after the surgery.
   3. 3 to 6 days after the surgery.
   4. 2 weeks after the surgery.

61. After surgery, the patient is suspected of having a pulmonary embolism. This is determined by the patient experiencing:
   1. restlessness, chills.
   2. dyspnea, sudden chest pain.
   3. hypotension, nausea.
   4. productive cough, crackles in the lungs.

STUDY GROUP QUESTIONS

- How are surgeries classified?
- What are some surgical risk factors, and why do they increase the patient's risk?
- How does the incision site influence a patient's recovery?
- How may previous surgical experiences influence the patient's expectations of surgery?
- What general information should be included in preoperative teaching?
- What is the purpose of the preoperative exercises that are explained and demonstrated to patients?
- What preoperative assessments should be made by a nurse?
- What are some common preoperative diagnostic tests that may be ordered for a patient?
- What nursing interventions are implemented in the preoperative care of patients?
- How does a nurse prepare and assist a patient in the acute care setting on the day of surgery?
- What are the roles of nurses in the operating room and in the recovery setting?
- What interventions are implemented to maintain patient safety and well-being in the operating room and postanesthesia care area?
- What nursing care is critical in the immediate postoperative stage?
- What are the similarities and differences between preanesthesia and postanesthesia care for patients in the acute care and ambulatory surgery settings?
- What general information should be included in postoperative teaching for patients/families in the acute care and ambulatory surgery settings?
- How may the family/significant other be involved in the patient's perioperative experience?

STUDY CHART

Create a study chart on Surgical Risk Factors that identifies how age, nutritional status, obesity, immunocompetence, fluid/electrolyte balance, and pregnancy may affect the patient's perioperative experience.

Answer Key

CHAPTER 1

Case Study

1. a. The preferred educational requirement for a nurse researcher is a doctoral degree, with at least a master's degree in nursing.
   b. To maintain this role, Mr. R. would need to continue his formal education in doctoral or postdoctoral study and/or participate in continuing education activities. In many states, continuing education hours are required to maintain nursing licensure as an LPN/LVN, RN, and APRN.

Chapter Review

1. c
2. d
3. a
4. b
5. a. The NLN advances excellence in nursing education to prepare nurses to meet the needs of a diverse population in a changing health care environment.
   b. The purpose of the ANA is to improve standards of health and the availability of health care, to foster high standards for nursing, and to promote the professional development and general and economic welfare of nurses.
   c. The ICN promotes national associations of nurses, improves standards of nursing practice, seeks a higher status for nurses, and provides an international power base for nurses.
6. Career paths that a nurse can choose are clinical practice, education, research, management, administration, and even entrepreneurship.
7. Nurses and their professional organizations have lobbied for creating smoke-free environments and stronger anti-tobacco laws, setting up anti-gang coalitions, establishing safer environments for walking and physical fitness in their communities, and advocating for breastfeeding.
8. The three components of nursing care are care, cure, and coordination.
9. Accurate statements about Nurse Practice Acts in the United States are a, c.
10. Four core roles for APRNs are clinical nurse specialist (CNS), nurse practitioner (NP), certified nurse midwife (CNM), and certified RN anesthetist (CRNA).
11. Essential skills for nurses include time management, therapeutic communication, patient education, and compassionate implementation of psychomotor skills.
12. To become a nurse educator or advanced practice nurse, a master's or doctoral degree is required.
13. Continuing education involves formal, organized educational programs offered by universities, hospitals, state nurses associations, professional nursing organizations, and educational and health care institutions. In-service education is instruction or training provided by a health care agency or institution designed to increase the knowledge, skills, and competencies of nurses and other health care professionals employed by the institution.
14. f
15. a
16. d
17. b
18. c
19. g
20. e
21. External influences on nursing include health care reform, demographic changes of the population, increasing numbers of medically underserved, workplace issues, the nursing shortage, and the threat of bioterrorism.
22. Workplace hazards that are faced by nurses include musculoskeletal injuries, such as back injury and repetitive motion disorders, and violence.
23. The use of genomics in health care allows providers to determine how genomic changes contribute to patient conditions and influence treatment decisions such as assessment and symptom management and titration of medications based on a patient's response.
24. The QSEN competencies for patient-centered care are a and c.
25. The ANA Standards of Professional Performance include b, d, e, and g.
26. 4
27. 4
28. 1

CHAPTER 2

Case Studies

1. a. This is an individual entering her middle adult years who is experiencing stress in her personal and professional life. She is being called upon by her employer and her child to meet their expectations, and she believes that this does not allow her the time to meet her health needs. The symptoms of gastrointestinal distress may be a response to the pressures in her life.
   b. Initially the nurse may spend time with this patient to discuss the patient's personal feelings and needs. The patient may benefit from instruction in stress reduction and relaxation techniques, along with a review of time management. The nurse may investigate with her if there are support people at work and in the neighborhood to assist her in keeping up with her busy schedule. This

individual also may be assisted in making an appointment for medical follow-up to determine her current health status.

2. a. There are several factors that could influence Mr. G.'s ability to manage his illness, including other health issues that he may have, how he perceives the illness, his prior lifestyle and social activities, family support, financial security, emotional stability, and his ability to comprehend the treatment regimen.
   b. Mr. G. could demonstrate illness behaviors, such as
      - losing motivation to participate in his care
      - becoming depressed, angry, anxious, or withdrawn
      - overly seeking or avoiding health care providers
      - assuming a dependent role
   c. Mr. G.'s wife could also exhibit emotional responses, including fear of her husband's ability to maintain his normal activities (work, socialization) and/or her ability to assist him with his care. She could also become overly protective of him or critical of his ability to manage his treatment. His wife could perceive that she will have to take on a larger role in keeping the household going.
   d. The QSEN competency of safety is applied in Mr. G.'s situation by making sure that he knows about the disease, his treatment requirements, and the indications when assistance should be sought. For example, Mr. G. needs to know what affect the combination of exercise and insulin will have on his physiology so that he does not experience a situation that could lead to a loss of consciousness and an injury.

Chapter Review

1. e
2. d
3. g
4. c
5. b
6. f
7. a
8. False
9. Health promotion for an older adult may include
   - Helping to maintain function and independence and improve quality of life.
   - Encouraging older adults to participate in group activities.
   - Monitoring older patients for acute and chronic diseases.
   - Encouraging physical activity.
10. The order, from lowest to highest need, is Physiological, Safety, Love and Belongingness, Self-Esteem, and Self-Actualization.
11. a. External variable
    b. External variable
    c. Internal variable
    d. External variable
12. Positive health behaviors include immunizations, adequate sleep, exercise, and good nutrition.
13. Negative health behaviors include smoking, substance abuse, poor diet, and refusal to take medication or follow a treatment regimen.
14. The goals of *Healthy People 2020* are to (1) attain high-quality, longer lives, (2) achieve health equality, (3) create social and physical environments that promote good health, and (4) promote quality of life across all life states.
15. Answers a, c, e, and f are external variables.
16. 2
17. 3
18. 1
19. 2
20. 1
21. 3
22. 2
23. 4
24. 3
25. 1

CHAPTER 3

Case Studies

1. a. This patient could benefit from the services of a hospice organization for either home care and/or inpatient care, depending on the program.
2. a. As a nurse on a busy medical unit it is important to be aware of the patients' needs and expectations to form effective partnerships to enhance the level of nursing care given. Managed care organizations expect patients who are hospitalized to be cared for and discharged within a projected time period. Therefore, as the nurse manager on the unit, you will have to use resources efficiently to help your patients successfully recover and return home. You will want to consider how to work efficiently with the staff to assess patients' needs, provide care, and prepare the patients for discharge.
   b. The QSEN competency of teamwork and collaboration can be applied by fostering open communication with the staff, demonstrating respect for them, and encouraging them to be part of the decision-making processes on the unit. For example, as the unit manager, you could ask the nursing staff for their input on strategies that will improve services, such as transport of patients to the radiology department.

Chapter Review

1. f
2. j
3. b
4. g
5. a
6. i
7. d
8. c
9. h
10. e
11. Hospice
12. Discharge planning should begin the moment the patient enters the health care agency; the planning assists in the transition of the patient's care from one environment to the other (such as from the hospital to the home). The patient's ongoing needs are anticipated and identified, and necessary services/resources are coordinated before the patient's discharge.
13. Developments in technology influence many aspects of health care delivery. New types of equipment for patient monitoring, computerization, and electronic communication and record-keeping systems create a need for health care providers to be up to date.
14. Utilization review is designed for review of admissions, diagnostic testing, and treatments provided by physicians or health care providers to patients. The purpose is to identify and eliminate overuse of diagnostic and treatment services.

15. a. Primary
    b. Tertiary
    c. Restorative
    d. Restorative
    e. Continuing
    f. Preventative
    g. Primary
    h. Preventative
    i. Secondary
    j. Continuing
    k. Secondary
    l. Restorative
16. The role of the case manager is to coordinate efforts of all the disciplines to achieve the most efficient and appropriate plan of care for the patient. The focus of case management is on discharge planning.
17. Vulnerable populations include children and women, older adults, the mentally ill, and the homeless.
18. Access to health care options are found in selections a, e, and g.
19. Patient referrals include
    - Involving the patient and family in the process, including selecting the necessary referral
    - Explaining the service to be provided, the reason for the referral, and what to expect from the referral's services
    - Making a referral as soon as possible
    - Informing the care provider receiving the referral of as much information about the patient as possible to avoid duplication of effort and exclusion of important information
    - Determining what the referral discipline (e.g., physical therapy, social work, diet and nutrition, radiology) recommends for the patient's care, and incorporating this into the treatment plan as soon as possible
20. The Patient Protection and Affordable Care Act of 2010 focuses on the major goals of increasing access to health care services for all, reducing health care costs, and improving health care quality. Provisions in the law include insurance industry reforms that increase insurance coverage and decrease costs, increased funding for community health centers, increased primary care services and providers, and improved coverage for children (HealthReform .gov, 2010).
21. Areas addressed in the Minimum Data Set for Resident Assessment include
    - Resident's background
    - Cognitive, communication/hearing, and vision patterns
    - Physical functioning and structural problems
    - Mood, behavior, and activity pursuit patterns
    - Psychosocial well-being
    - Bowel and bladder continence
    - Health conditions
    - Disease diagnoses
    - Oral/nutritional and dental status
    - Skin condition
    - Medication use
    - Special treatments and procedures
22. Cost is one of the biggest drawbacks to an assisted-living facility.
23. Two systems stimulated through health care reform are Accountable Care Organizations (ACO) and Patient-Centered Medical Homes (PCMH).
24. Nursing centers provide the services in selections a, b, and d.
25. Quality and safety are demonstrated by health care agencies through The Joint Commission, Six Sigma, and Value Stream Mapping.
26. Accurate statements about a critical access hospital include b and d.
27. The National Database of Nursing Quality Indicators include
    - Patient falls
    - Patient falls with injury
    - Pressure ulcers—community acquired, hospital acquired, unit acquired
    - Staff mix
    - Nursing hours per patient day
    - RN surveys on job satisfaction and practice environment scale
    - RN education and certification
    - Pediatric pain assessment cycle
28. Globalization and the nursing shortage are related because, in an effort to provide high-quality care, health care institutions may recruit nurses from around the world to work in the United States. The movement of nurses away from their home country can leave that country with its own shortage. The hiring of nurses from other nations also can require American hospitals to better understand and work with nurses from different cultures and with different needs.
29. The National Priorities Partnership focuses on
    - Patient and Family Engagement—providing patient-centered, effective care
    - Population Health—bringing increased focus on wellness and prevention
    - Patient Safety—focusing on eliminating errors whenever and wherever possible
    - Care Coordination—providing patient-centered, high-value care
    - Palliative Care—providing appropriate and compassionate care for patients experiencing advanced illnesses
    - Overuse—focusing on waste reduction to achieve effective, affordable care
    - Health Information Technology—providing safer, better coordinated care through use of electronic medical records and other sources of information technology
    - Disparities—reducing disparities through provision of culturally competent care
30. The purpose of a Professional Standards Review Organization (PSRO) is to review the quality, quantity, and cost of health care services provided through Medicare and Medicaid.
31. 3
32. 2
33. 1
34. 4
35. 2
36. 3
37. 4
38. 1
39. 2

CHAPTER 4

Case Studies

1. a. There are a variety of physiological, psychological, and sociocultural problems that the older adult may have, including the following:
   Physiological: Heart disease, hypertension, arthritis, stroke (cerebral vascular accident), diabetes, sensory impairments (failing eyesight and hearing), cognitive impairments (Alzheimer's disease), cancer, malnutrition

Psychological: Depression, anxiety, substance abuse, dependence, other altered coping abilities, loss
Sociocultural: Finances, housing, separation from family

b. The nurse should investigate what is already available for older adults. This information should be available at the local municipal building/center, library, and/or health department. If not already available, the nurse should look into the possibility of working with the local government, health department, and other members of the community to offer such services as the following: older adult day care; community activities (e.g., day trips and exercise groups) and transportation; health screenings; nutritional programs; in-person and telephone support groups; advice regarding security, financial, and housing concerns; and reduced or no-cost home maintenance assistance. Older adults should be encouraged, whenever possible, to become involved in activities that provide mutual satisfaction and stimulation, such as school programs where they can read to elementary school children or offer consultation to businesses in their area of expertise.

2. a. An assessment of the home environment should include
   - Overall appearance:
     - Condition of walls, floors, windows, doors, ceilings
     - Cleanliness, presence of vermin
   - Atmosphere: comfort, personal items
   - Utilities: water, heating/cooling, lighting
   - Neighborhood: safety, available resources (food, transportation, etc.)

   b. You will want to assess the patient's
   - Overall physical status, including a general survey, vital signs, glucose level, and ability to perform ADLs
   - Knowledge about diabetes and the care required, including therapeutic diet and medications
   - Ability to manage the health care regimen physically, emotionally, cognitively, and financially
   - Support systems: family, friends, local resources (clinics, pharmacies)

Chapter Review

1. The focus of community-based care is on health promotion, disease prevention, and restorative care.
2. Challenges for community-based nursing practice include increased sexually transmitted infections, pollution, new life-threatening diseases, lack of health care insurance, and underimmunization of infants.
3. The difference between public and community health nursing is that public health nursing focuses on the factors that influence health promotion and health maintenance needs of a population, while community health nursing focuses on the health care of individuals, families, and groups within the community.
4. Specific risks for vulnerable populations:
   a. Immigrant: Access to health care may be limited because of language barriers and lack of benefits, resources, and transportation. Some immigrant populations have specific health care risks such as hepatitis B, tuberculosis, and dental problems.
   b. Poor and homeless: People who live in poverty are more likely to live in dangerous environments, work in high-risk jobs, have less nutritious diets, and experience multiple stressors.
   Homeless patients are usually jobless, do not have the advantage of shelter, and must cope with finding a place to sleep at night and finding food. They may experience worsening chronic health problems because they do not get nutritious meals and have no place to store medications, if they can afford them. In addition, they lack a healthy balance of rest and activity.
   c. Mentally ill: Patients in the community are at a greater risk for abuse, assault, and injury. Many patients with pervasive mental illnesses are homeless or have poor housing and may lack the ability to maintain employment or to care for themselves.
   d. Older adult: There is a greater incidence of chronic disease and an increased need for health care services.
5. The role of the nurse in community-based practice is
   a. Case manager
   b. Educator/teacher
   c. Epidemiologist
6. The three components of a community are structure or locale, the people, and the social systems.
7. Interventions for a family with a member experiencing substance abuse include obtaining a drug use history; educating adults about safe drug storage and the risks for, drug-drug, drug-alcohol, and drug-food interactions; giving general information about drugs (e.g., drug name, purpose, side effects, dosage); instructing adults about pre-sorting techniques; counseling adults about substance abuse; promoting stress management to avoid the need for drugs or alcohol; and arranging for and monitoring detoxification if appropriate.
8. For a patient with Alzheimer's disease, interventions for the patient include maintaining high-level functioning, protection, and safety; encouraging human dignity; demonstrating to the primary family caregiver techniques to dress, feed, and toilet the patient; providing frequent encouragement and emotional support to the caregiver; acting as an advocate for the patient when dealing with respite care and support groups; protecting the patient's rights; providing support to maintain family members' physical and mental health; maintaining family stability; and recommending financial services if needed.
9. The potential safety hazards in the photo are: There is a wrinkled throw rug by her feet, along with an ottoman and other clutter that she could trip over. The folding table next to her is not steady enough to hold her weight, if she lost her balance. She uses a cane and may need the glasses (on the table) to see when she is ambulating. She appears to be wearing a medic alert necklace, which indicates that she may have other medical problems.
10. 3
11. 4
12. 1
13. 2

CHAPTER 5

Case Studies

1. a. A patient who does not appear to understand a procedure should not sign a consent form. The physician must be contacted to provide the information to the patient. The nurse's role in this situation is to witness the signing of the consent form only if the patient demonstrates an understanding of the procedure. Because the nurse will not be performing the procedure, it is not his or her responsibility to describe what will or will not be done during the surgery.
2. a. Any question of a written order should be clarified with the prescriber. You should not depend on the "guess" of another colleague, even if it is a supervisor.
   b. If the medication is administered according to the charge nurse's belief, and the order is not correct, then you are accountable for the result.
3. a. In an emergency situation, treatment may be provided to an individual without obtaining consent. If there is sufficient opportunity to obtain consent, the divorced parent who has legal custody of the child must be contacted.
4. a. You will have to investigate your state's statutes to determine what information is required to be reported for a colleague in a suspected substance abuse situation. In many states, the nurse is held accountable if he or she is knowledgeable about an impaired practitioner but does not report the situation to the Board of Nursing. In most instances, the situation is not acted on immediately; it is investigated further by the appropriate authorities.
5. a. Posting on social media sites, even when patients or colleagues are not specifically described, breaches a patient's trust and may be a form of lateral violence with respect to co-workers (ANA, 2011). This breach of confidentiality should be addressed with the staff member. It is important to know the employer's policies on the use of social media. The professional nurse has an obligation to report breaches of privacy and confidentiality.
   b. Inappropriate use of a patient's confidential information or image may be reported to the State Board of Nursing, and the nurse could face disciplinary charges (NCSBN, 2011).

Chapter Review

1. i	5. e	9. c
2. f	6. b	10. g
3. a	7. h	
4. j	8. d	

11. A nurse may avoid being liable by following the standards of care, providing competent care, communicating with other health care providers, documenting fully, and developing an empathetic rapport with patients.
12. Standards of care are defined in Nurse Practice Acts by boards of nursing, state and federal hospital licensing laws, professional and specialty organizations, and agency policies and procedures.
13. a. Informed consent requires that the patient
    - Understands the options and risks of the care provided
    - Has an opportunity to ask questions
    - Provides consent voluntarily
    - Is a competent adult

    b. The nurse is responsible for witnessing the patient's signature on the consent form and asking if he/she understands the procedure(s). If a patient denies understanding, or if it is suspected that he/she does not understand, then the physician or health care provider and nursing supervisor should be notified.
14. True
15. Professional negligence is termed malpractice.
16. The correct aspects of the Good Samaritan Law are choices b and c.
17. Verbal or telephone orders should be signed within 24 hours.
18. The two standards for determination of death are cardiopulmonary and whole brain.
19. False
20. The elements of malpractice are
    - The nurse owed a duty to the patient.
    - The nurse did not carry out the duty or breached the duty.
    - The patient was injured.
    - The patient's injury was caused by the nurse's failure to carry out that duty.
21. The coroner is notified if the patient's death is unforeseen or sudden or if the patient was not seen by a physician within 36 hours of death.
22. Felonies related to a Nurse Practice Act are b and c.
23. Advance directives act to instruct about withholding or withdrawing life-sustaining procedures in patients who are terminally ill.
24. Health care workers are required to report attempted suicide, rape, gunshot wounds, unsafe or impaired professional practice, child abuse, and certain communicable diseases.
25. Examples of preventable errors include patient falls, urinary tract infections, and pressure ulcers.
26. This is an apology statute.
27. Verdicts must be reported to the National Practitioner Data Bank (NPDB).
28. Examples of "never events" are a, b, and f.
29. Physical or chemical restraint requires a provider's order and careful oversight for appropriate use. They should only be used in emergency situations.
30. The Patient Self-Determination Act (1991) requires health care institutions to inquire whether a patient has created an advance directive, to give patients information on advance directives, and to document whether a patient states he or she has an advance directive.
31. The correct order for organ donation consent is: c, b, d, e, f, a.
32. HIPAA sets standards for the electronic exchange of private and sensitive health information.
33. Common sources of negligence are medication errors that result in injury to patients; IV therapy errors resulting in infiltration or phlebitis; burns to patients caused by equipment, bathing, or spills of hot liquids and foods; falls resulting in injury to patients; failure to use aseptic technique when required; errors in sponge, instrument, or needle counts in surgical cases, meaning an item was left in a patient; failure to give a report, or giving an incomplete report, to oncoming shift personnel; failure to adequately monitor a patient's condition; and failure to notify a health care provider of a significant change in a patient's status.

34. 2
35. 3
36. 4
37. 3
38. 1
39. 2
40. 1
41. 4
42. 1
43. 4

CHAPTER 6

Case Studies

1. a. **Step 1.** Is this an ethical dilemma?
Review of scientific data does not resolve the patient's situation, his question is perplexing, and your response and his action will have a profound relevance for human concern.
Step 2. Gather all the information relevant to the case.
The patient is a 42-year-old man with severe multiple sclerosis who is unable to perform the simplest activities of daily living. He appears to be aware of his situation and is seeking an alternative to his present lifestyle. You are his home care nurse and are aware of the patient's situation.
Step 3. Examine and determine one's own values on the issues.
Use of the values' clarification process may assist you in determining your beliefs about assisted suicide and the quality and sanctity of life.
Step 4. State the problem clearly.
The patient has an interest in being "helped to die," and he has involved you in a possible dilemma by asking you to assist him in getting more information about this method.
Step 5. Consider possible courses of action.
You may or may not be able to assist the patient in his actual pursuit of an assisted suicide because of your beliefs. In addition, the legal view on assisted suicide varies from state to state and will have to be investigated before any action is taken by you or the home care agency. A discussion with your supervisor and colleagues may assist in determining a course of action. (You should inform the patient that you will be sharing this information with other members of the health team.) If the patient is intent on finding out about, and possibly pursuing, an assisted suicide, his family members (if available) may become involved.
Step 6. Negotiate the outcome.
Communication with the patient may determine whether there are other alternatives to the patient's plan. Work with the patient to consider all of the possibilities, but respect the patient's wish, even if it is to pursue assisted suicide.
Step 7. Evaluate the action.
The actions taken by the nurse and other members of the home care agency should be documented. Recognize that satisfaction with the outcome by the patient and the nurse may not be possible. There are no right or wrong answers to ethical questions. Evaluation is based on the effectiveness of working through the problem to a reasonable solution.
b. The nurse in this situation should be the patient's advocate. The first step is to determine if the patient is truly intent on pursuing this alternative measure. If he really is interested, then the nurse may assist him in a number of ways. Information on assisted suicide may be obtained directly or indirectly for the patient. The nurse may not be able to become involved but can be supportive of the patient's decision to investigate the procedure. There are legal and ethical considerations that may inhibit the nurse from having any involvement, in which case the patient should be referred to others who may support him in his actions.
2. a. You cannot copy or forward medical records without a patient's consent. Health care workers are not allowed to share health care information with others without specific patient consent. This includes laboratory results, diagnosis, and prognosis. In addition, family members or friends of the patient are not permitted access to the patient's personal health information without the patient's consent.

Chapter Review

1. f
2. g
3. h
4. b
5. c
6. a
7. e
8. d
9. i
10. Access to a patient's medical record requires the patient's consent.
11. End-of-life issues include "do not resuscitate" (DNR) or "allow natural death" (AND) orders, assisted suicide/ euthanasia, living wills, and maintenance or removal of life-sustaining measures.
12. a. Deontology
b. Feminist ethics
c. Utilitarianism
13. a. Cost containment: not having enough staff or equipment with monetary cutbacks, having limitations on coverage and benefits, providing restricted hours and services
b. Cultural sensitivity: accepting a patient's refusal of treatment (e.g., Christian Scientist's beliefs), recognizing the need for special diets or concern for the body of the deceased
14. Digital transmission can be an ethical concern because there could be a question of where the information is being sent and who is able to access the information. Photos, lab results, and other sensitive data must be kept safe from public scrutiny.
15. 4
16. 4
17. 4
18. 3
19. 4
20. 1
21. 2

CHAPTER 7

Case Studies

1. a. Using the PICO format, you may develop a question based on the following:
P = Patient population of interest: home care patients, using this specific glucose monitor, who are having difficulty with the results and insulin management
I = Intervention of interest: determination of whether the problem is patient or equipment related
C = Comparison of interest: how the patients with other monitors are doing with their insulin management
O = Outcomes: Home care patients will have confidence in the use and results of their blood glucose monitors.

Their insulin management will be effective in controlling their glucose.

b. The trigger in this situation is problem focused.

2. a. Staff and patients on a surgical unit may be interested in the following areas for quality improvement:
   - Postoperative complications, such as the incidence of hemorrhage and infection
   - Patient response to pain management
   - Safety, including postoperative ambulation
   - Effectiveness of preoperative education
   - Ease of use and effectiveness of the preoperative checklist
   - Family involvement in care
   - Patient and family satisfaction with care

Chapter Review

1. c
2. d
3. a
4. b
5. Evidence-based practice is a problem-solving approach to clinical practice that combines the conscientious use of best evidence in combination with a clinician's expertise, patient preferences and values, and available health care resources in making decisions about patient care (Melnyk and Fineout-Overholt, 2011; Sackett et al., 2000). It incorporates quality research data into patient care.
6. Valuable non–research-based evidence may be found in
   - Performance improvement data
   - Risk management data
   - International and local clinical guidelines
   - Infection control data
   - Benchmarking
   - Retrospective or concurrent chart reviews
   - Clinicians' expertise
7. A peer-reviewed article is one submitted for publication and reviewed by a panel of experts familiar with the topic or subject matter of the article.
8. A qualitative research study focuses on trying to understand patients' experiences with health problems and the contexts of their experiences. It is descriptive rather than experimental.
9. The primary way that a nurse can integrate evidence into practice is by applying it into the plan of care for a patient. Evidence can also be incorporated into agency policies and procedures, teaching tools, clinical practice guidelines, and new assessment or documentation tools.
10. PDSA stands for: (P) Plan, (D) Do, (S) Study, and (A) Act.
11. Some examples of patient outcomes and measurements include the following:

Outcomes	*Measurements*
Patient will describe the signs and symptoms of hypoglycemia/hyperglycemia.	Communication with the patient
Patient's blood pressure will remain within therapeutic limits.	BP measurement every shift and as needed
Patient will be satisfied with outpatient surgery education.	Patient satisfaction survey

12. A randomized control trial (RCT) includes a, b, c, and e.
13. An evidence-based article includes a, c, d, and f.
14. Examples of competencies for evidence-based practice include
   - Demonstrate knowledge of basic scientific methods and processes
   - Describe EBP to include components of research evidence, clinical expertise, and patient/family values
   - Differentiate clinical opinion from research and evidence summaries
   - Describe reliable sources for locating evidence reports and clinical practice guidelines
   - Explain the role of evidence in determining best clinical practice
   - Describe how the strength and relevance of available evidence influences the choice of interventions in provision of patient-centered care
   - Discriminate between valid and invalid reasons for modifying evidence-based clinical practice based on clinical expertise or patient/family preferences
15. Sources for new scientific information are the standards and practice guidelines available from national agencies or organizations such as the Agency for Healthcare Research and Quality (AHRQ), the American Pain Society (APS), and the American Association of Critical-Care Nurses (AACN).
16. True
17. Examples of comprehensive databases include MEDLINE, CINAHL, and PubMed.
18. Evidence-based practice can be communicated to others through grand rounds, agency committees, professional organizations, abstracts, and posters and podium presentations at conferences.
19. Root cause analysis is a structured method used to analyze serious adverse events. A central tenet of RCA is to identify underlying problems that increase the likelihood of errors while avoiding the trap of focusing on mistakes by individuals.
20. The PICOT components for the example are

    P - Patient population of interest: patients with pressure ulcers

    I - Intervention of interest: wound healing when the ulcer is left open to air

    C - Comparison of interest: if there is a difference in healing for wounds with the typical dressings that are being used on the unit

    O - Outcome: pressure ulcers left open to air for 2 hours/day will heal faster than those that are covered all day

    T - Time: 4 months of observation
21. 4
22. 1

CHAPTER 8

Case Studies

1. a. In approaching a multiple patient assignment, you may benefit from doing the following:
   - Looking at the patients' backgrounds: diagnoses, baseline data, etc.
   - Determining the current status of each patient
   - Identifying the priority assessments and interventions
   - Making sure that what you need is available: equipment, medications, etc.
   - Organizing actions to maximize efficiency and patient safety and satisfaction
   - Writing specific notes for each patient, with the schedule for treatments and medications
   - Coordinating and communicating with patients and other staff members
   - Documenting actions as soon as possible
2. a. The nurse may choose to return to the office to obtain supplies and then make a later visit to this patient. This option is possible if the nurse has other patients to visit or if there is work to be done at the office. This option will, however, take time away from the nurse and extend visiting hours. The nurse may choose to purchase necessary items from a local pharmacy, but the nurse may not have the necessary funds or be able to be reimbursed for this purchase. It may be most appropriate for the nurse to investigate what alternative resources are available in the patient's home, such as clean cloths, boiled water, salt, and tongs (all to be used only with patient permission).
   b. The nurse should determine what resources the patient has in the home, including running water, waste disposal, and methods for heating and refrigeration. In addition, a financial screening may be needed if indicated for the determination of available funds and/or insurance coverage for supplies and equipment.
3. a. For this patient, there are a number of areas to focus on, including his
   - knowledge of the diagnosis and treatment
   - familiarity and comfort with the diet and food choices
   - support system—other family members, finances
   - need to do his own shopping and cooking
   - emotional response to the diagnosis

Chapter Review

1. e
2. d
3. b
4. c
5. a
6. Examples of critical thinking throughout the nursing process:
   a. Assessment: collecting and analyzing data
   b. Nursing diagnosis: identifying the appropriate patient problems
   c. Planning: establishing expected outcomes, prioritizing, collaborating, and delegating
   d. Implementation: performing nursing interventions safely
   e. Evaluation: determining achievement of outcomes, reassessing as indicated
7. The levels of critical thinking are
   a. Basic
   b. Complex
   c. Commitment
8. The elements of the critical thinking model are specific knowledge base, experience, competence, attitudes, and standards.
9. Examples of critical thinking attitudes:
   a. Confidence
   b. Thinking independently
   c. Discipline
   d. Creativity
   e. Integrity
10. a. Reflection allows the nurse to look back and learn from an experience and identify opportunities for improvement.
    b. Language must be used clearly and precisely to communicate effectively with patients, families, and other members of the health care team.
    c. Learning is a continuous process and necessary for nurses as the profession grows. With experience and learning, nurses get better at forming assumptions, presenting ideas, and making valid conclusions about patient care.
11. Two useful tools for developing critical thinking skills are reflective journaling and concept mapping.
12. Accurate statements regarding critical thinking attitudes are c, d, and e.

13. 4	17. 3	21. 4
14. 3	18. 4	22. 1
15. 1	19. 2	23. 2
16. 3	20. 1	

CHAPTER 9

Case Studies

1. a. The nurse should obtain additional data about the patient's medical history and current health status. The patient may be seeing a physician or other primary care provider and have medication prescribed for hypertension.
   b. A community health fair allows for general screening of large numbers of people, but it usually does not offer opportunity or space for privacy to complete health histories or physical assessments. Individuals demonstrating alterations from expected norms, such as this patient, are referred to clinics, personal physicians, or other health care delivery agencies, as appropriate.
2. a. The relevant assessment data obtained from the patient include
   - Being newly diagnosed with hypertension
   - Having a new prescription of an antihypertensive medication

- Demonstrating insecurity about the medication regimen
- Relating his father's death at age 54 from a heart attack

b. Nursing diagnoses for the patient may include
- *Knowledge Deficit* related to unfamiliarity with the diagnosis and treatment of hypertension
- *Knowledge Deficit* related to newly prescribed medication (as manifested by his verbalization of uncertainty as to how and when to take his medications)
- *Fear* related to possible repeat of father's medical history and early death

3. a. Sample diagnoses, goals, and outcomes for the patient:

Nursing Diagnoses	*Goals*	*Expected Outcome*
Knowledge Deficit related to newly prescribed medication (as manifested by his verbalization of uncertainty as to how and when to take his medications)	Patient will recognize the purpose of the hypertensive medication and prepare an administration schedule by the end of the clinic visit.	Patient will restate the use of the antihypertensive medication and scheduling of administration during the visit.
Fear related to possible repeat of father's medical history and early death (as manifested by verbalization of concern over similar family history)	Patient will demonstrate effective coping mechanisms within the next month. Patient will identify reduction or elimination of feelings of fear.	Patient will discuss his concerns about his father's medical history and early death during this visit. Patient will acknowledge his fear of repeating this history during his visits.
Knowledge Deficit related to unfamiliarity with diagnosis of hypertension	Patient will make specific lifestyle alterations and participate in the treatment regimen.	Patient will identify the etiology and therapeutic regimen for hypertension after the next two clinic visits.

b. Nursing interventions should include (1) teaching the patient about his medication and frequency of administration and (2) arranging uninterrupted time to sit with the patient and allow him to discuss his feelings and concerns regarding the diagnosis and family history. (Refer to the box below for interventions based on each diagnosis.)

Knowledge Deficit	*Fear*
• Assess patient's willingness and readiness to learn about his diagnosis and medication regimen. • Identify and present appropriate information about hypertension and the medication regimen counseling, as indicated. • Establish an environment and strategy for teaching patient that are conducive to learning. • Provide effective learning materials, including pamphlets, videos, photos, and charts, for example.	• Assess the degree of patient's fear. • Observe nonverbal and verbal responses. • Listen to patient's concerns and feelings. • Provide information on coping mechanisms to assist in reducing his level of fear. • Offer referral to a support program/counseling, as indicated.

4. a. For his hypertension to be controlled, the patient needs to take his medication on a regular basis. The nurse should focus on the implementation method of teaching. Counseling also may be involved, especially if the patient is experiencing other difficulties at work or home that are interfering with his ability to manage his therapeutic regimen. Emphasis may be placed on the patient taking his medication along with a daily routine, such as with meals or after bathing.

b. The nurse should look at the original goals, outcomes, and nursing interventions to determine what alterations may be necessary. The strategies for providing the information on the patient's diagnosis and medication may not have been appropriate. In addition, the patient's fear about his father's medical history may have been blocking his ability to focus and/or influencing his degree of motivation to participate in the therapeutic plan.

5. a. The patient appears to be achieving most of his goals. He states that he is exercising regularly and trying to use the relaxation techniques when he feels stressed. The patient also is expressing his method of coping with his father's medical history.

b. Areas for reassessment may include the patient's actual medication schedule (because his blood pressure is still slightly elevated) to determine that it is within the prescribed regimen. Determination also may be made to see if the patient may benefit from additional exercise (per review with the physician), and a review of his relaxation techniques may be conducted.

6. a. It is important for you to assess the following:
- Overall physical status of the child and how she has responded to the medical treatment
- Emotional response of the child and her parents
- Ability of the child and her parents to comply with the treatment regimen
- Home environment: socioeconomic considerations
- Child's preference for foods and activities

b. *Knowledge deficit* related to new diagnosis and lack of familiarity with treatment regimen

Chapter Review

1. c
2. g
3. j
4. d
5. e
6. f
7. b
8. h
9. i
10. a
11. The three phases of the interview are the orientation phase, working phase, and termination phase.
12. Possible nursing diagnoses are
    a. *Diarrhea*
    b. *Activity Intolerance*
13. a. *Knowledge Deficit related to the need for postoperative care at home*
    Goal: Perform, or obtain assistance in performing, postoperative care at home
    Expected outcome:
    - State the purpose and procedure for postoperative care
    - Demonstrate postoperative care before discharge
    Nursing intervention:
    - Provide appropriate materials for patient review of postoperative care before surgery
    - Review and demonstrate the postoperative care to patient after surgery
    - Observe the patient's independent performance of postoperative care before discharge
    b. Alteration in elimination: *Constipation related to lack of physical activity*
    Goal:
    - Reestablish normal pattern of elimination
    - Participate in specified daily physical activity, to tolerance
    Expected outcome:
    - Ambulate in hallway 3 times each day
    - Perform active range-of-motion exercises twice each day
    Nursing intervention:
    - Instruct and assist patient in performance of physical activity
    - Observe tolerance to physical activity
    - Assess elimination pattern daily
    - Promote additional measures to improve elimination, such as the intake of fluids and fiber
    c. *Risk for injury*
    Goal:
    - Patient will remain free of injury throughout hospital stay
    Expected outcome:
    - Change positions slowly
    - Sit on the edge of the bed before rising
    - Request assistance before ambulating if feeling dizzy
    Nursing intervention:
    - Instruct the patient to change positions slowly
    - Monitor the patient's blood pressure and other indications that could contribute to dizziness or instability
    - Assist the patient to ambulate
14. a. Psychomotor
    b. Interpersonal
    c. Interpersonal
    d. Psychomotor
    e. Cognitive
15. Before implementing standing orders, the nurse should determine the accuracy and appropriateness of the standing orders for the patient. In addition, the nurse should have the knowledge and competency necessary to carry out each order safely.
16. The steps of the implementation phase of the nursing process are as follows: reassess, review/revise the care plan, organize resources and care delivery, and anticipate and prevent complications.
17. If a new patient need is identified, the nurse should modify the care plan.
18. Specific procedures are termed a protocol for care.
19. Indirect nursing interventions include the following: delegation, environmental safety, infection control, documentation, and collaboration.
20. Activities a, c, d, and g can usually be delegated.
21. Examples of how patient outcomes may be improved are
    a. Erythema will be reduced in area by 2 inches within 2 days.
    b. Pulse rate will be within the patient's baseline of 60 to 70 beats per minute after medication administration.
    c. Patient will have a daily increase of 50 to 100 calories at each meal until ideal weight is achieved.
22. A good interview environment is
    - Free of distractions, unnecessary noise, and interruptions
    - Private and out of earshot of other patients, visitors, and staff
    - Scheduled when no other activities are planned to avoid interruptions
    - Well lit, warm, and with the patient in a comfortable position
23. The following data are subjective: a and c. Objective data are b, d, and e.
24. The medical record is a source for the patient's medical history, laboratory and diagnostic test results, current physical findings, and the health care provider's treatment plan. Data in the records offer a baseline and ongoing information about the patient's response to illness and progress to date.
25. a. The nurse can validate the patient's statement by observing him/her to see what the tolerance is to activity.
    b. The nurse can validate that the pressure ulcer is larger by measuring the ulcer daily and keeping track of the changes in its size.
26. a. Direct care: providing hygienic care, administering medications, performing dressing changes
    b. Counseling: allowing opportunities for the patient to discuss concerns, providing emotional support
    c. Teaching: giving information about the treatment for a disease, demonstrating how to perform care or prepare medications
    d. Controlling adverse reactions: evaluating the patient's response to a medication, checking for unexpected responses to treatments (i.e., redness by tape used on a dressing)
27. The evaluation process includes five elements: (1) identifying evaluative criteria and standards, (2) collecting data to determine if you met the criteria or standards, (3) interpreting

and summarizing findings, (4) documenting findings, and (5) terminating, continuing, or revising the care plan.
28. The nurse can ask the patient about particular preferences, as well as observe the patient's practices.
29. Interventions for the nursing diagnosis *Feeding Self-Care Deficit* can include assisting with the arrangement of food on the plate for easy access, obtaining utensils that are easier to hold, providing support of the patient's hand in using the utensils, sitting the patient up and feeding the patient slowly, and observing the patient's abilities and responses.

30. 4
31. 1
32. 1
33. 2
34. 3
35. 4
36. 4
37. 4
38. 1
39. 2
40. 2
41. 1
42. 4
43. 4
44. 2
45. 3
46. 4
47. 3
48. 2
49. 4

CHAPTER 10

Case Studies

1. a. A transfer report should include the following information:
   - Patient's name and age, name of primary physician, and medical diagnosis
   - Summary of medical progress to the time of transfer
   - Current physiological and psychological status
   - Current nursing diagnoses/plan of care
   - Critical assessments to be completed shortly after transfer
   - Any special equipment needed

   b. More specifically, the primary nurse may want to know about the surgical procedure, how it was tolerated by the patient, how the patient responded to the anesthesia, and observations made and treatments completed in the PACU.
2. Sample SOAP documentation for the patient:

   S: Patient states she is having intense pain in her right hip area and does not want to move because of the pain.

   O: Patient is grimacing and moaning in pain.

   A: There is an alteration in comfort related to new surgical incision to right hip.

   P: Reduce or eliminate discomfort by administering analgesic medication as ordered and assisting patient to more comfortable position.

   Sample DAR documentation for the patient:

   D: Patient is grimacing and moaning in pain. She states that she is having intense pain to right hip and does not want to move because it "really hurts." Dressing is dry and intact.

   A: Patient is assisted to more comfortable position, with leg supported. Analgesic administered per order.

   R: Patient expressed reduction in discomfort to tolerable level.
3. a. Documentation should include the information presented, method of instruction (e.g., discussion, demonstration, videotape, booklet), and patient response, including questions and evidence of understanding such as return demonstration or change in behavior. It would be important to note what material was presented to the patient regarding type I diabetes, including self-injection of insulin, dietary guidelines, and general care. The patient's response should be identified, such as his ability to prepare and administer the injections and specify foods to avoid in his daily diet.

Chapter Review

1. d
2. e
3. a
4. b
5. c
6. The proper guidelines for written documentation are
   a. Record all entries legibly and in black ink.
   b. Use only objective descriptions of the patient and use quotes for patient comments.
   c. Use complete, concise descriptions of patient interactions.
   d. Draw a single line through the error, write the word error above the line, initial or sign the error, and complete the correct notation.
   e. Use consecutive lines for charting and do not leave margins. Draw lines through unused space and sign your name at the end of the notation.
   f. Include only factual information in the notation.
   g. Identify that the physician was called to clarify an order for the patient.
   h. Have the other caregiver document the information, unless the individual calls with additional information. Document that the information was provided by another individual.
   i. Record pertinent information throughout the shift, signing each entry.
7. a. False
   b. False
   c. True
8. Standards are set by The Joint Commission (TJC) and National Committee for Quality Assurance (NCQA).
9. a. Communication: for continuity of care and accurate patient status
   b. Financial: for reimbursement, DRGs, insurance audits
   c. Educational: for teaching nursing and medical students
   d. Research: for statistical data and patient responses
   e. Auditing/Monitoring: for Joint Commission standards, incidence of patient falls, pain management
10. Malpractice issues related to documenting include the following: Failure to document, verbal orders, charting in advance of care, timing of events, incorrect data, and failure to report.
11. The five characteristics of quality documentation are factual, accurate, complete, current, and organized.

12. Subjective statements by the patient should be quoted and may be supported with objective findings.
13. Student nurses should sign their names, followed by either SN or NS and the school affiliation.
14. All of the notations are vague and should include more specific information. For example:
    a. Identification of the specific intake, such as "Consumed 8 ounces of hot cereal, 6 ounces of orange juice, and an 8-ounce cup of coffee for breakfast."
    b. Notation of an accurate output, such as "Voided 200 mL of clear, amber urine."
    c. Description of care, such as "10 AM Cleansed wound to left lower leg with normal saline and applied dry 4×4 dressing"; "qd" is removed, because it is not an acceptable abbreviation.
15. SBAR:
    S: Situation
    B: Background
    A: Assessment
    R: Recommendation
16. Discharge summaries should include the following: procedures that should be performed and the instructions given, medications prescribed and precautions, signs and symptoms of complications, names and phone numbers of health care providers, names of community resources, follow-up requirements, actual time of discharge, transportation used, and name of person accompanying the discharged patient.
17. Home care documentation is also completed for financial reimbursement.
18. The process of completing narrative notes only when abnormalities exist is part of "charting by exception."
19. Nursing informatics are the retrieval, storage, presentation, and sharing of data, information, and knowledge to provide quality, safe patient care. Nursing informatics facilitates the integration of data, information, and knowledge to support patients, nurses, and other providers in decision making in all roles and settings.
20. Electronic records are safeguarded through the use of passwords, firewalls, audit trails, and disaster recovery systems.
21. Four concepts included in informatics are data, information, knowledge, and wisdom.
22. The correct actions are a, c, d, and f.
23. Information available usually includes the multidisciplinary inpatient, outpatient, and emergency care provided, current health status and medical history, and medical orders and treatments, including medication administration and diagnostic test results.
24. Problem-oriented medical records include a, c, d, and f.
25. Written materials for class that are prepared based on clinical experiences should not have any patient identifiers on them, such as the patient's last name and room number, date of birth, medical record number, or other identifiable demographic information.
26. The errors in the charting example are: The word patient is not usually written in the narrative. The vital signs should be identified as BP, Pulse and Respiration and/or put in a flow sheet. The amount of weight gained should be indicated, as well as how much breakfast was eaten. Complaints about the physician should not be included in the record.
27. 3
28. 4
29. 3
30. 3
31. 4
32. 4
33. 4
34. 4
35. 2
36. 3
37. 1

CHAPTER 11

Case Studies

1. a. The following techniques may be effective for an older individual with a moderate hearing impairment:
       - Reducing background noise
       - Checking and cleaning a hearing aid
       - Speaking slowly and clearly
       - Using a low-pitched rather than high-pitched voice
       - Avoiding shouting at the patient
       - Using short, simple sentences
       - Facing the patient to allow for lip reading
       - Not covering the mouth while talking
       - Talking toward the unaffected ear
       - Using facial expressions and gestures
   b. The following techniques may be effective for individuals who do not speak English:
       - Speaking in a normal tone of voice
       - Establishing signals or methods of nonverbal communication
       - Obtaining an interpreter familiar with the language and culture
       - Allowing time for communication to take place
       - Developing a communication board, pictures, or cards for common requests
       - Having a dictionary available for reference
   c. The following techniques may be effective for an individual who is blind:
       - Announcing yourself when entering the room
       - Communicating verbally before touching the patient
       - Orienting the patient to the environment
       - Explaining the procedure in advance
       - Having the patient handle the equipment, as appropriate
       - Informing the patient when you are done and will be leaving the room
   d. The following techniques may be effective for an individual of another culture who is experiencing an invasive procedure for the first time:
       - Explaining the procedure in advance, using an interpreter if necessary
       - Recognizing possible discomfort with exposure and maintaining privacy
       - Staying with the patient to provide emotional support
   e. If the patient is not responsive:
       - Call the patient by name during interactions.
       - Communicate both verbally and by touch.
       - Speak to the patient as though he or she could hear.
       - Explain all procedures and sensations.
       - Provide orientation to person, place, and time as needed.

       If the patient is responsive:
       - Use a communication board
       - Provide a pen/pad

2. a. For an individual who is illiterate, you should implement the following:
    - Identify the patient's reading and comprehension level so that you do not communicate above or below his ability.
    - Organize what you want to say so that the most important points come first.
    - Break complex information into smaller and more understandable parts.
    - Use simple language, avoiding jargon, and define technical terms.
    - Use the active voice instead of passive (e.g., "You will receive the discharge instructions before you leave.").

Chapter Review

1. c	4. h	7. b
2. g	5. e	8. a
3. f	6. d	

9. a. Intrapersonal level
   b. Interpersonal level
   c. Public level
10. Compassion fatigue may develop in situations where nurses observe ongoing patient distress and pain, or participate in difficult relationships with fellow staff or physicians.
11. a. Public zone
    b. Social zone
    c. Intimate zone
    d. Social zone
    e. Intimate zone
    f. Public zone
    g. Personal zone
12. Appropriate communication techniques for the older adult with impaired communication include selections a, c, and d.
13. a. Courtesy should be used. The patient should be called by his or her name, such as Mrs. Jones or Mr. Brown.
    b. Courtesy should be used. The patient should be identified by name, not by room number or diagnosis.
    c. Confidentiality should be applied. The patient should not be discussed outside of the immediate patient area where anyone not involved in the patient's care may overhear the conversation.
    d. Availability should be applied. The nurse should spend time with the patient or identify to the patient when he or she will return to be with the patient.
    e. Avoidance of medical jargon should be considered. The nurse should explain to the patient, in understandable terms, what to expect of the procedure.
14. Examples of ways in which the nurse could enhance communication with the patient include
    a. "How do you feel today?"
    b. "Do you take any medications at home?" or "What types of medication do you take at home?"
    c. "Have you noticed any areas of swelling around your arms or legs?"
    d. "Do you have any questions about the procedure that will be done today?" or "Has the physician explained the procedure to you?"
15. The communication strategies being used are
    a. Using silence
    b. Attentive listening
    c. Encouraging conversation
    d. Clarifying
    e. Focusing
16. To assist the patient who has an aphasia, the nurse may
    - Use simple gestures and statements
    - Provide visual cues, such as pictures or flash cards
    - Listen and observe attentively
    - Allow time for responses, either verbal or nonverbal
    - Have call bells within easy reach
    - Encourage the patient to interact as much as possible
17. Positive responses include answers c and d.
18. Considering the patient's culture, actions b and d are appropriate.
19. The acronym SOLER is:
    S: Sit facing the patient
    O: Offer an open posture
    L: Lean toward the patient
    E: Establish and maintain intermittent eye contact
    R: Relax
20. Actions/responses during the Orientation Phase of the Helping Relationship include d, e, and f.
21. This is an example of lateral violence in the workplace.
22. Many altered health states limit communication, including facial trauma, cancer of the larynx or trachea, aphasia after a stroke, breathing problems, Alzheimer's disease, high anxiety, pain, and heavy sedation. Certain mental illnesses cause patients to have impaired communication like pressured speech, constant verbalization of the same words or phrases, or a slow speech pattern.
23. The nurse has an odd facial expression that can create a problem with communication, as well as not looking directly at the patient. Since the nurse is holding the chart, the patient could be concerned about what has been documented.

24. 3	30. 3	36. 4
25. 2	31. 3	37. 1
26. 4	32. 3	38. 3
27. 1	33. 1	39. 1
28. 4	34. 4	40. 2
29. 1	35. 3	41. 4

CHAPTER 12

Case Studies

1. a. The patient has no prior knowledge about her diagnosis or prescribed medication. She also has a family history of coronary disease, with her father dying of a heart attack at 54 years of age.
   b. Sample teaching plan for the patient:

Learning Need	*Resources*	*Objectives*	*Teaching Strategies*
Knowledge deficit related to newly diagnosed hypertension and antihypertensive medication therapy	Educational media: Video and audio programs on hypertension, written materials on the diagnosis and the medication, information from the physician and other health care providers (e.g., dietitian), nurse's knowledge of diagnosis and treatment regimen	Patient will be able to describe the diagnosis, etiology, treatment, and complications; describe the actions, side effects, and time of administration for the antihypertensive; identify when to contact the physician if complications or problems occur; independently monitor and record her blood pressure daily and as necessary; develop a meal plan for a week that incorporates the therapeutic diet	Provide patient with available educational media and written information on hypertension and antihypertensive medications; use illustrations to explain the functions of the heart and circulatory system and the effects of hypertension; demonstrate the technique for monitoring blood pressure, and have the patient and/or significant other return to demonstrate the procedure; involve significant others in the educational program

2. a. The family will need to know about the following:
   - Diagnosis, along with the prognosis, complications, and precautions
   - Treatment plan: insulin, diet, exercise
   - Health care support: when to contact the physician/nurse, follow-up office or clinic visits

   b. For the 8-year-old, you would include him in learning about the disease and how to manage it, including self-injection and how to recognize problems. Age-appropriate materials should be provided, including books, comics, and videos that will get his attention.
3. a. In preparing for the presentation, you should assess for distractions, noise, physical comfort (temperature, lighting, etc.), appropriate size and location, and the availability of necessary equipment (such as a computer).

Chapter Review

1. d
2. c
3. f
4. a
5. b
6. e
7. The six aspects of the ACCESS model are
   -**Assessment** of the cultural norms of the patient's lifestyle, health beliefs, and health practices
   -**Communication** with awareness of the many variations in verbal and nonverbal responses
   -**Cultural negotiation and compromise** that encourages awareness of various characteristics of the patient's culture and awareness of one's own biases
   -**Establishment** of respect for patient's cultural beliefs and values; establishment of a caring rapport as the basis of a therapeutic relationship
   -**Sensitivity** of how diverse cultures perceive their care needs and of the various patterns of communication (terms, concepts, tone, and style of communication)
   -**Safety** that enables patients to feel culturally secure and avoids disempowerment of their cultural identity
8. True
9. Examples of health maintenance and promotion topics include selections a, d, and f.
10. Specific teaching methods that may be implemented are
    a. Infant: Maintaining consistency in routines (bathing, feeding), holding the child firmly while smiling and speaking softly, and having the infant touch different textures
    b. Toddler: Using play to teach about procedures or activities, offering picture books, and using simple words to promote understanding
    c. Preschooler: Using role-playing, imitation, and play to make it fun to learn, encouraging questions and offering explanations, using simple explanations and demonstrations, and encouraging children to learn together through pictures and short stories
    d. School-age child: Teaching psychomotor skills needed to maintain health, and offering opportunities to discuss health problems and answering questions
    e. Older adult: Teaching when the patient is alert and rested, involving the adult in the discussion or activity, focusing on wellness and the person's strengths, using approaches that enhance reception of stimuli for patients with sensory alterations, and keeping teaching sessions short
11. The presence of pain, anxiety, and distractions may make it difficult for the learner to concentrate.
12. Patients need size, strength, coordination, and sensory acuity to learn psychomotor skills.
13. A nurse should consider the following factors when selecting an environment for teaching: privacy, room temperature, lighting, noise, ventilation, furniture, and space.

14. Written materials are generally at the fifth grade reading level or below.
15. Teaching sessions should last about 20 to 30 minutes, with critical information being taught first.
16. If the patient becomes fatigued during a teaching session, you should stop teaching and resume when the patient feels rested.
17. For the nursing diagnosis *Noncompliance with medication regimen related to insufficient knowledge of purpose and actions*, possible goals/outcomes and nursing interventions include
    Goal: Take medications as prescribed
    Outcome:
    - Verbalize purpose and actions of medication regimen
    Nursing interventions:
    - Provide information about prescribed medications, including purpose and actions; give patient written information about medications and their use; use visual aids as necessary to reinforce the material
    - Allow opportunity for patient to express concerns and ask questions
18. The preferred teaching styles are
    a. Visual: written materials (linguistic style) and pictures, models, and demonstrations (spatial)
    b. Tactile: writing, drawing pictures, and manipulating models of information
    c. Auditory listening, speaking, repeating the information to themselves or to others
19. The domains of learning are
    a. Psychomotor
    b. Affective
    c. Cognitive
    d. Affective
    e. Psychomotor
    f. Cognitive
20. Recommendations for instructional techniques are
    a. Lecture, group discussion
    b. Demonstration and return demonstration
    c. Demonstration and role-playing
21. Explaining in advance is preparatory instruction.
22. a. Almost 50% of adults in the United States have difficulty reading and understanding health information.
    b. Available literacy assessment tools: Single Item Literacy Screener (SILS) and The Newest Vital Sign
23. A better way to inform the patient about the injection is to identify the brief experience that will occur, such as a pinch. This reduces the anticipatory discomfort
24. "Teach-Back" is going through the process of asking the patient/family about components of the instruction to evaluate the level of understanding.
25. A focused assessment includes
    a. Learning needs
    b. Resources
    c. Ability to learn
26. Documentation of patient teaching should include
    Assessment data and related nursing diagnoses: Provide information and support for goals and outcomes.
    Interventions planned and used: Planned education provides continuity of care. Specifically describe subject matter so that other nurses can follow up and reinforce teaching (e.g., "verbalized side effects of digoxin").
    Evaluation of learning: Document evidence of learning (e.g., a return demonstration of coughing and deep breathing). This informs staff about the patient's progress and determines material that you still need to teach. Always use the Teach-Back method.
    Ability of patient and/or family to manage care: Identify needs for outpatient or home care follow-up after discharge. Appropriate referrals better meet the patient's needs.

27. 4	31. 3	35. 4
28. 4	32. 2	36. 1
29. 3	33. 1	37. 4
30. 4	34. 2	38. 2

CHAPTER 13

Case Study

1. a. After determining what needs to be done and prioritizing your interventions, you can delegate to the nursing assistant activities such as vital sign measurements, evening hygienic care, basic procedures (catheter care), and assistance with meals. The nursing assistant may also be asked to obtain necessary supplies and equipment for patient care. You also may have the assistant check on the general status of the patients and report any immediate problems.
   b. To safely delegate activities, you must determine the level of acuity of the patients and the knowledge and ability of the aide. If some of the patients are having abnormal vital signs, such as dysrhythmias, then it would not be appropriate to delegate pulse rate measurement to the nursing assistant.
   c. Some examples of opportunities for multiple tasks are
      - determining the patient's range of motion, communication patterns, and mental status when hygienic care is provided.
      - during treatments, discussing how the procedure may be done by the patient or family at home.
      - talking about the diet, food preparation, and/or shopping at mealtimes.

Chapter Review

1. The nurse manager responsibilities include:
   - Assist staff in establishing yearly goals for the unit and the systems needed to accomplish goals.
   - Monitor professional nursing standards of practice on the unit.
   - Develop an ongoing staff development plan, including one for new employees.
   - Recruit new employees (interview and hire).
   - Conduct routine staff evaluations.
   - Establish self as a role model for positive customer service (customers include patients, families, and other health care team members).
   - Serve as an advocate for the nursing staff to the administration of the institution.

- Submit staffing schedules for the unit.
- Conduct regular patient rounds and help to solve patient or family complaints.
- Establish and implement a quality improvement (QI) plan for the unit.
- Review and recommend new equipment needs for the unit.
- Conduct regular staff meetings.
- Conduct rounds with health care provider.
- Establish and support necessary staff and interdisciplinary committees.

2. A person who is reasonably independent in decision making is demonstrating autonomy.
3. The right task, right circumstances, right person, right direction/communication, and right supervision.
4. The correct terms are
   a. Responsibility
   b. Authority
   c. Accountability
5. Case management is the coordination and linking of health care services to patients and their families with the goal of promoting quality, cost-effective outcomes.
6. Staff members can be actively involved in a decentralized decision-making environment by:
   - establishing nursing practice or problem-solving committees.
   - encouraging collaboration between nurses and health care providers.
   - promoting interdisciplinary collaboration.
   - encouraging staff communication.
   - providing staff education.
7. Team communication can be promoted by respecting one another's ideas, sharing information, keeping one another informed, setting expectations of one another, always treating colleagues with respect, listening to the ideas of other staff members, and being honest and direct in what you say.
8. For the example the SBAR is:
   S - The patient's blood sugar is elevated well beyond expected limits.
   B - The patient was admitted 2 days ago with ketoacidosis and has been taking a longer-acting insulin.
   A - The insulin and dietary management are not managing the patient's blood sugar.
   R - A different type or dosage of insulin, along with a review of the dietary intake and other patient factors, is recommended.

9. 2	12. 4	15. 4
10. 1	13. 4	16. 3
11. 1	14. 2	

CHAPTER 14

Case Studies

1. a. The nurse should implement the following measures to prevent a urinary tract infection:
   - Provide personal hygiene, perineal care
   - Use aseptic technique when manipulating the catheter and drainage equipment
   - Keep the drainage bag unobstructed and below the level of the bladder
   - Provide ample fluids, within patient's limitations
2. a. To prevent a wound infection, the nurse should
   - Maintain sterile technique during dressing changes
   - Use medical asepsis in all interactions with the patient
   - Instruct the patient in hand washing/asepsis
   - Dispose of contaminated materials appropriately and promptly
   - Assist in keeping the patient and environment clean and dry
   - Limit the number of caregivers working with the patient
   - Provide optimum nutrition and fluids, within patient's limitations
   - Administer antibiotics, if prescribed
3. a. The nurse should include the patient and family/significant others in the preparation for instituting contact isolation precautions.
   The nurse should
   - Discuss the disease process and the need for isolation precautions
   - Explain and demonstrate isolation procedures
   - Teach the patient and family how to perform hand hygiene and apply PPE
   - Maintain a friendly, understanding manner; listen to the patient's concerns
   - Provide for the patient's sensory stimulation during isolation; encourage the family to bring the patient reading materials, puzzle books, etc.
   - Explain the patient's potential risk for depression or loneliness to family members
   - Encourage visitors to avoid negative expressions or actions concerning isolation; advise family members on ways to provide meaningful stimulation
   - Carefully observe the patient's response to isolation

Chapter Review

1. k	6. g	11. l
2. f	7. d	12. m
3. j	8. h	13. i
4. c	9. a	
5. b	10. e	

14. Sterile technique is required for options b, c, and e.
15. Examples of outcomes for this patient are the following: Wound will decrease in diameter by 1 cm in 2 days; wound will be free of signs of infection, including edema and drainage.
16. Immunizations are available for selections a, b, c, and f.
17. The nurse should discard the item or redo the sterile field in the case of b, c, and f.
18. Nursing interventions include
    a. Control or eliminate the infectious agent: clean, disinfect, and sterilize contaminated objects
    b. Control or eliminate the reservoir: remove sources of body fluids, drainage (dressings), or solutions that harbor microorganisms; discard disposable articles contaminated with infectious material

c. Control the portals of exit: avoid talking, sneezing, or coughing directly over a wound or sterile dressing field; teach patient to protect others; and handle all body fluids carefully (hand hygiene and use of gloves)
d. Control the transmission: disinfect equipment, provide a personal set of equipment for patients, do not shake linens or allow them to come in contact with the uniform, and perform hand hygiene
e. Susceptible host: hygienic care, adequate nutritional and fluid intake

19. a. White blood cell count: elevated in an acute infection, decreased in viral/overwhelming infections
b. Erythrocyte sedimentation rate: elevated with infectious processes
c. Iron level: decreased in chronic infections
d. Neutrophils: elevated with acute, suppurative infections; decreased with overwhelming bacterial infections
e. Basophils: remain normal during infections
20. a. Health care–acquired infections can be reduced with hand hygiene and the use of aseptic technique.
b. Patients more susceptible to HAI are those who have multiple illnesses, are older adults, are poorly nourished, have a lowered resistance to infection because of underlying medical conditions, have invasive treatment devices (such as catheters), or have been treated with multiple antibiotics for long periods of time.
21. A patient's gastrointestinal defenses are altered by the administration of antacids and histamine-2 blockers.
22. Appropriate techniques for isolation precautions include selections b, d, and f.
23. Handling of biohazardous waste includes "red" bagging for incineration or special handling.
24. The order for application of PPE is mask, gown, and then gloves.
25. The first items removed when leaving the isolation room are the gloves.
26. Appropriate asepsis is demonstrated in selections b, c, f, and h.
27. For the nursing diagnosis *Impaired skin integrity, related to 2-inch-diameter pressure ulcer on sacrum*, possible patient outcomes and nursing interventions include
Patient goal: Sacral ulcer will heal within 2 to 3 weeks
Outcomes:
- Sacral ulcer will reduce in size by 1 inch (within time frame).
- Skin will remain intact over remainder of body surfaces.
- Sacral ulcer will remain free of infection.

Nursing interventions:
- Provide wound care as prescribed using aseptic technique.
- Assess condition of ulcer.
- Provide skin care: Keep clean and dry, and apply moisturizers as needed.
- Turn and reposition patient every hour.
- Assess wound for presence of infection, and obtain culture if indicated.
- Provide for patient's nutritional and fluid needs.

28. c, d or b, then a
29. Disposal of contaminated sharps includes placing all needles (safety needles and needleless systems) into puncture-proof containers, which should be located at the site of use.
30. An example would be the nurse touching a nonsterile package with sterile gloves, recognizing the action as a break in technique, and then discarding the gloves and restarting the procedure.
31. To collect a urine specimen for a patient with an indwelling catheter, the nurse should obtain a sterile cup to collect 1 to 5 mL of urine, a needleless safety syringe to collect the specimen from the sampling port on the catheter, and an antiseptic wipe to clean the port (dependent upon the agency policy).
32. The correct actions for hand hygiene are b, e, and g.
33. Some patients perceive the simple procedures of proper hand hygiene as evidence of rejection. Help patients and families reduce some of these feelings by discussing the disease process, explaining the reason for the procedures, and maintaining a friendly, understanding manner.
34. The current immunization schedule can be found on the CDC website.
35. The three most common infections in long-term care are pneumonia, urinary tract infections, and pressure ulcers.
36. The organisms that are transmitted through blood are b, d, and f.
37. The correct steps for the procedure are c, e, d, a, b.
38. The nurse should use a face shield when splashing of bodily fluids is anticipated during care.
39. In the photo, the nurse has broken sterile technique by:
Photo A: The nurse is holding the sterile object below the level of the field on the table. It also appears that her gloved hand may be touching her scrubs.
Photo B: The sterile field is folded over, there is a wet spot and the dressing and instruments are sitting on the wet area.

40. 1	45. 2	50. 4
41. 1	46. 4	51. 1
42. 3	47. 2	52. 4
43. 4	48. 4	53. 2
44. 4	49. 3	54. 4

CHAPTER 15

Case Studies

1. a. Generally, an individual who has a blood pressure reading of above 120/80 mm Hg to 139/89 mm Hg on repeated assessments should be referred for medical follow-up. An average of two or more systolic readings higher than 140 mm Hg and diastolic readings higher than 90 mm Hg are usually indicative of hypertension.
b. Additional information should be noted, such as the arm used and the position (e.g., sitting, standing, lying down) of the patient during the measurement, previous blood pressure readings, known medical problems, and any medical care being received and medications being taken by the patient.
2. a. The patient's pulse rate and blood pressure reading may be obtained in the lower extremities. The pulses available include the femoral, popliteal, posterior tibial, and dorsalis pedis. The blood pressure is assessed by placing the thigh-sized cuff over the posterior aspect of the middle thigh region while the patient is in the prone position. The popliteal

artery is used for palpation and auscultation of the blood pressure. Measurement in the lower extremities may be 10 to 40 mm Hg higher in the systolic reading than that of the upper extremities.

3. a. A febrile patient may exhibit the following signs and symptoms:
      - Increased body temperature
      - Flushed, dry, warm skin
      - Chills
      - Feeling of malaise
      - Tachycardia
   b. Nursing interventions for febrile patients may include
      - Assessment of vital signs, especially temperature
      - Observation of patient response, including skin color and temperature, and chills
      - Promotion of patient comfort, responding to chills, thirst
      - Collection of appropriate specimens, such as blood cultures
      - Promotion of rest and reduction of activities that increase heat production
      - Promotion of heat loss by removing coverings and keeping the patient dry
      - Provision of care to meet increased metabolic demands, including oxygen, nutrition, and fluid requirements
      - Monitoring of ongoing status
4. a. You are anticipating that a patient who is brought to the emergency room with signs of heat stroke will have hypothermia blankets applied, receive intravenous (IV) fluids, and have irrigations of the stomach and lower bowel with cool solutions.
   b. To prevent future occurrences, the following information should be included in a teaching plan for the patient and family:
      - Avoid strenuous exercise in hot, humid weather.
      - Avoid exercising in areas with poor ventilation.
      - Drink fluids such as water and clear fruit juices before, during, and after exercise.
      - Wear light, loose-fitting, light-colored clothing.
      - Wear a protective covering over the head when outdoors.
      - Expose themselves to hot climates gradually.
5. a. The anticipated readings for oxygen saturation should be 95% to 100%, but at least above 90%.
   b. If the pulse oximeter does not appear to be working, there may be problems with light transmission or a rcduction of the patient's arterial pulsations. The site for measurement should be checked to determine that it is clean, warm, and dry; not directly near another light source; and receiving adequate circulation. The patient also may have to be reminded to limit excessive motion of the extremity that is being used for measurement.
   c. You can assist the alert patient to increase oxygen levels by taking deep breaths, especially if he/she has had general anesthesia. This will help to remove the residual from the lungs and improve oxygenation.

Chapter Review

1. f
2. j
3. g
4. i
5. e
6. h
7. a
8. c
9. d
10. b
11. l
12. k
13. a. $(97° F - 32) \times 5/9 = 36° C$
    b. $9/5 \times (38.4° C + 32) = 101.1° F$
    c. 38.9° C
    d. 102.9° F
14. The nurse is alerted to temperature alterations of above 100.4° F or below 96.8° F on an oral Fahrenheit thermometer, and measurements above 38° C or below 36° C on an oral centigrade scale. Rectal temperature readings may be 0.9° F or 0.5° C higher than oral measurements, with axillary readings ranging this same number of degrees lower than oral temperatures. Temperatures above 102.2° F for an adult and 104° F for a child can be harmful.
15. The pulses should be palpated as follows:

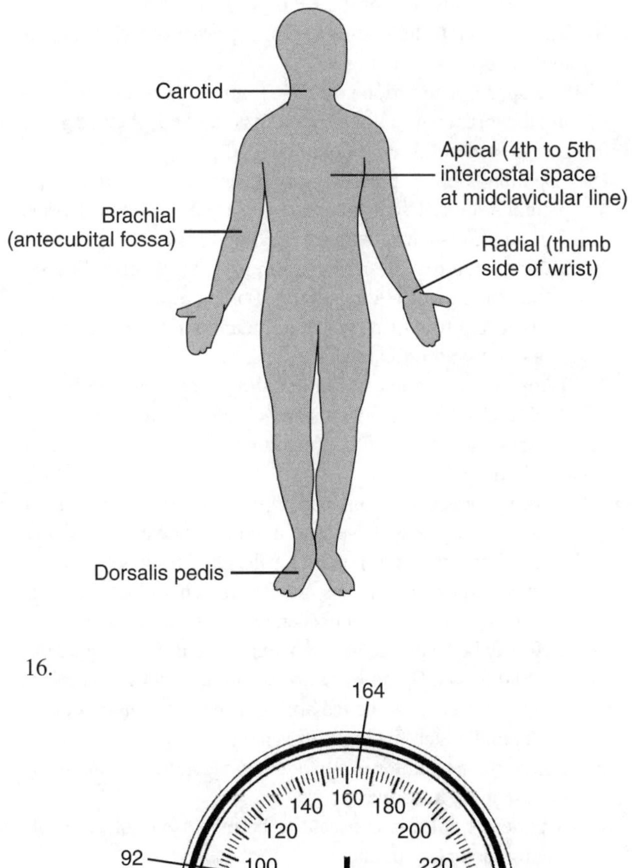

16.

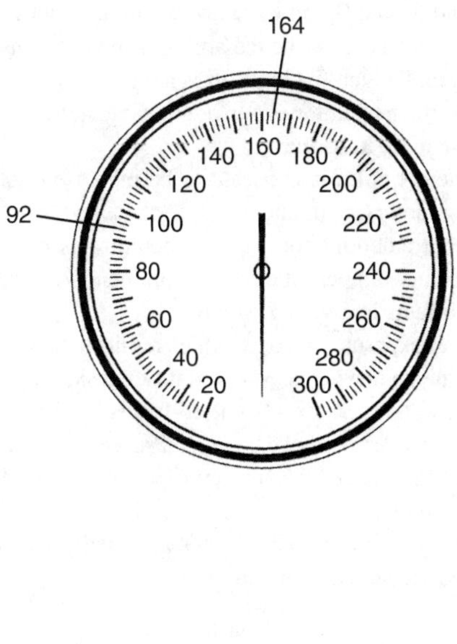

17. False
18. Interventions to reduce body temperature by
    a. Conduction: ice packs, tepid baths, heated blankets
    b. Convection: fans
    c. Evaporation: loss through the skin (diaphoresis) and respiration
19. The thermometer of choice for a patient in isolation is a disposable chemical dot thermometer.
20. A pulse deficit is assessed by two nurses who synchronize their measurement of the patient's apical and radial pulses. A deficit is found if there is a difference between the two readings.
21. For a patient who has had a right mastectomy, the left arm or lower extremities should be used for blood pressure measurement.
22. Vital signs are usually recorded on a graphic or flow sheet.
23. Decreasing hemoglobin levels will increase the respiratory rate.
24. A pulse oximeter may be applied to the earlobe, finger, or bridge of the nose.
25. The pulse pressure for the BP of 150/90 is 60.
26. The correct techniques for blood pressure measurement include options a, c, e, and f.
27. The appropriate action is to wait 15 minutes before measuring the temperature if the patient has smoked, chewed gum, or ingested hot or cold liquid or food.
28. A patient's blood pressure may have to be palpated if the patient's arterial sensations are too weak to create Korotkoff sounds, such as with severe blood loss.
29. a. Temperature: Sites for measurement vary depending on the child's age and condition. For example, it is contraindicated to take a tympanic membrane temperature on a child with otitis media.
    Tympanic membrane: Used in children age 2 and older
    Axilla: Used with newborns and children of any age
    Temporal artery: Used in premature infants, newborns, and children
    b. Blood pressure: An infant or child younger than 5 years of age lies supine with the arm supported at heart level. Older children sit. It is important for the child to be relaxed and calm. Allow at least 15 minutes for children to recover from recent activity or excitement before taking a reading. It may be helpful to have a parent present. You prepare the child for the BP cuff's unusual sensation during inflation. The cuff needs to be the appropriate width: infant cuff is 2½ to 3¼ inches; child cuff is 4¾ to 5½ inches.
30. The correct techniques for a tympanic temperature measurement are a, b, and f.
31. A patient's pulse is expected to be increased with the following factors: a, d, and e.
32. The contradictions for these temperature assessments are
    a. Axillary temperature: Not recommended to detect fever in infants and young children.
    Requires exposure of thorax, which results in temperature loss, especially in newborns. Not used if skin lesions are present.
    b. Rectal temperature: Not used for patients who have had diarrhea or who have had rectal surgery, rectal disorders, bleeding tendencies, or neutropenia. Not used routinely for infants.
33. End-tidal carbon dioxide values are used for patients who are on mechanical ventilation.
34. For a blood pressure reading in the lower extremity:
    a. The patient should be in the prone position, if tolerated. If such a position is impossible, flex the knee slightly for easier access to the artery.
    b. The popliteal artery is used for the palpation and auscultation.
    c. The systolic blood pressure is expected to be higher in the lower extremity.
35. The correct order of the steps for apical pulse measurement is f, c, e, d, a, b.
36. An increased temperature in young children can lead to dehydration and febrile seizures.
37. Commonly used antipyretic medications are acetaminophen, salicylates, indomethacin, ibuprofen, and ketorolac. Corticosteroids also may be used, but be alert to the masking of infection.
38. Orthostatic hypotension is assessed by obtaining pulse and blood pressure readings with the patient supine, sitting, and standing.
39. For core temperature readings:
    a. Readings are measured through invasive means.
    b. Sites include the pulmonary artery, esophagus, and bladder.
40. The diaphragm of the stethoscope is used to auscultate bowel, lung, and heart sounds (high-pitched sounds). The bell of the stethoscope is used to auscultate heart and vascular sounds (low-pitched sounds).
41. a. Increased temperature
    b. Decreased temperature
42. The correct techniques for pulse oximetry are b and d.
43. Respiration is influenced as follows:
    a. Anxiety - increases respiration rate and depth.
    b. Analgesics - depresses respiration rate and depth.
    c. Body position - Standing or sitting erect promotes full ventilatory movement and lung expansion; stooped or slumped position impairs ventilatory movement; lying flat prevents full chest expansion.
44. Hypotension can be seen with a and d.

45. 1	54. 3	63. 4
46. 3	55. 1	64. 1
47. 3	56. 4	65. 4
48. 2	57. 2	66. 2
49. 4	58. 2	67. 1
50. 1	59. 3	68. 4
51. 4	60. 1	69. 2
52. 1	61. 4	70. 1
53. 1	62. 2	

CHAPTER 16

Case Studies

1. a. For the 4-year-old boy, you are aware that the experience may be new and frightening. You can show the child the assessment procedures on a doll or model, while giving simple, understandable information, and he may handle equipment that will be used (as appropriate). The exam should be conducted in a comfortable environment, with time allowed for the child to play. The child may be

called by his first name, and he may be asked assessment questions that he will understand.

- For a 16-year-old girl, the nurse may begin the health assessment with the parent(s) in the room with the patient. There should be time, however, when the patient is by herself with the nurse to discuss concerns. The adolescent girl should be asked if she wants a parent present during the physical assessment, but the option is provided for the patient to not be accompanied. Procedures and findings should be explained to the parent(s) and the patient.
- The older Hispanic woman may have responses to the examination that are influenced by her culture. She will need to be informed and prepared for the breast and pelvic assessments, with consideration given to her privacy. This patient may desire another woman to be present during the examination or to conduct the physical. Care should be taken to determine that this patient understands the information and instruction provided by an examiner who may speak only English. An interpreter may be obtained if the patient is conversant in Spanish. The environment should be warm and comfortable. Ample time should be allowed for the patient to answer questions and assume necessary positions for the exam.

For each of the patients, opportunity should be provided to use the bathroom before, during, and after the examination.

2. a. For the patient who has expressed a difficulty in hearing, the nurse should do the following:
   - Have the patient remove any hearing aid if worn.
   - Note the patient's response to questions. Normally the patient responds without excess requests to have the questions repeated.
   - If you suspect a hearing loss, check the patient's response to the whispered voice. Test one ear at a time while the patient occludes the other ear with a finger. Ask the patient to gently move the finger up and down during the test. While standing 30 cm to 60 cm (1 to 2 feet) from the testing ear, cover your mouth so the patient is unable to read lips. After exhaling fully, whisper softly toward the unoccluded ear, reciting random numbers with equally accented syllables such as *nine-four-ten*. If necessary, gradually increase voice intensity until the patient correctly repeats the numbers. Then test the other ear for comparison.
3. a. The lesion and surrounding tissue on the abdomen should be assessed for location, size, shape, depth, and color. The drainage should be assessed for amount, color, consistency, and odor.
   b. After explaining the procedure, providing privacy, positioning the patient either dorsal recumbent or side-lying, and making sure there is adequate lighting, you should apply gloves and examine the area gently.

Chapter Review

1. f
2. c
3. b
4. a
5. h
6. g
7. d
8. j
9. e
10. i
11. The five skills used in physical assessment include
    - Inspection: Use of vision and hearing to detect characteristics of body parts and functions
    - Palpation: Use of the hands to touch body parts to determine temperature, texture, position, and movement
    - Percussion: Striking the body surface with the finger to produce a vibration and elicit sounds
    - Auscultation: Listening to sounds created in the body organs (use of stethoscope)
    - Olfaction: Use of smell to determine the presence of characteristic odors
12. The positions for the physical examination are
    a. Sitting
    b. Supine
    c. Dorsal recumbent
    d. Lithotomy
    e. Sims'
    f. Prone
    g. Lateral recumbent
    h. Knee-chest
13. The pulses being palpated are
    a. Ulnar
    b. Posterior tibial
    c. Femoral
    d. Brachial
    e. Dorsalis pedis
14. The skin lesions are
    a. Papule
    b. Ulcer
    c. Macule
    d. Atrophy
    e. Wheal
15. The PMI is located in the left anterior chest wall, at approximately the fourth to fifth intercostal space, at the midclavicular line.

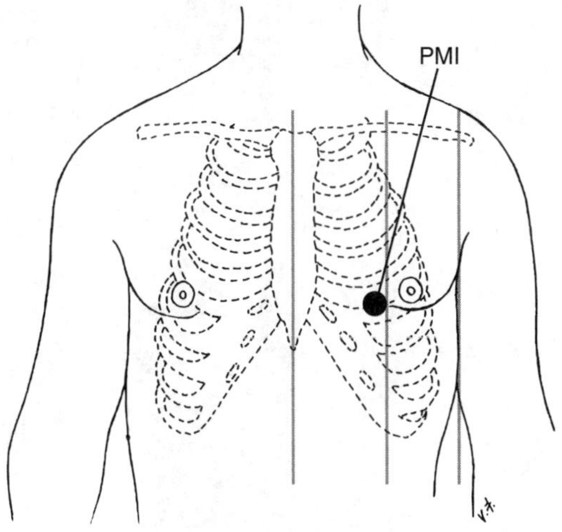

16. The following are findings that may indicate abuse:
    a. Child sexual abuse
    Physical findings:
    - Genital discharge, bleeding, pain, itching
    - Difficulty sitting or walking
    - Foreign bodies in genital tract or rectum

Behavioral findings:
- Problems eating or sleeping
- Fear of certain people or places
- Regressive or acting-out behavior
- Preoccupation with own genitals

b. Domestic abuse
Physical findings:
- Injuries and trauma inconsistent with reported cause
- Multiple injuries, burns, bites
- Old and new fractures

Behavioral findings:
- Eating or sleeping disorders
- Anxiety, panic attacks
- Low self-esteem
- Depression, sense of helplessness
- Attempted suicide

c. Older adult abuse
Physical findings:
- Injuries and trauma inconsistent with reported cause
- Bruises, hematomas, burns, fractures
- Prolonged interval between injury and treatment

Behavioral findings:
- Dependent on caregiver
- Physically and/or cognitively impaired
- Combative, belligerent

17. Abdominal assessment:

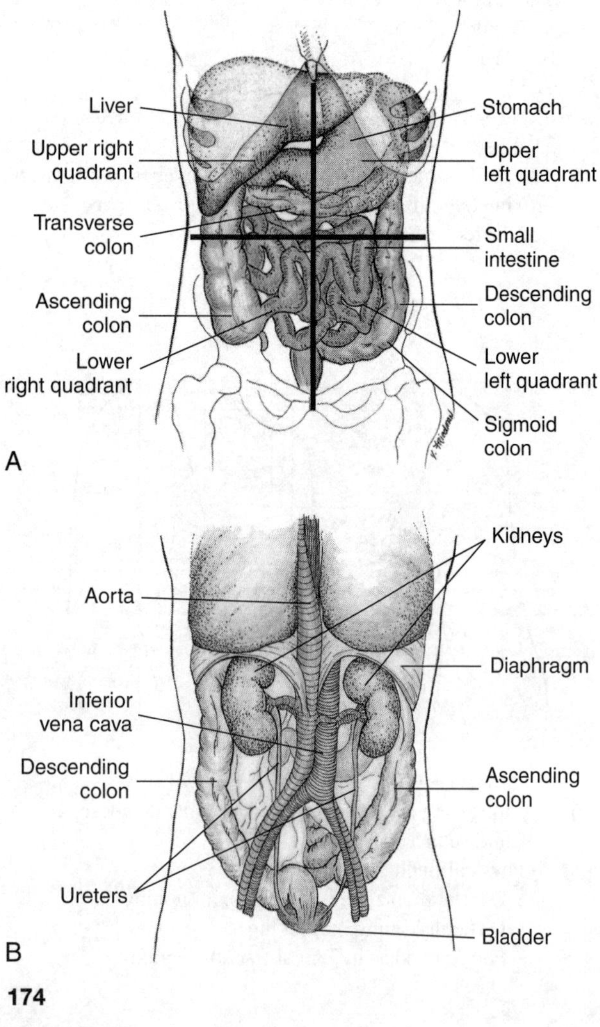

18. a. Expected
b. Unexpected
c. Expected
d. Expected
e. Unexpected
f. Unexpected
g. Expected
h. Unexpected
i. Unexpected
j. Expected
k. Expected
l. Expected
m. Unexpected
n. Unexpected
o. Unexpected
p. Expected
q. Expected
r. Unexpected
s. Expected
t. Expected
u. Expected
v. Unexpected
w. Expected
x. Unexpected
y. Unexpected
z. Unexpected
aa. Expected
bb. Unexpected
cc. Expected
dd. Unexpected
ee. Expected
ff. Unexpected
gg. Expected
hh. Unexpected
ii. Expected
jj. Expected
kk. Expected
ll. Expected
mm. Unexpected
nn. Expected
oo. Unexpected
pp. Expected

19. The nurse examines the area of discomfort last (b).
20. High-pitched sounds are best heard with the diaphragm of a stethoscope (a).
21. The nurse pulls the ear up and back (a).
22. The patient is placed in lithotomy position, if possible.
23. The patient is placed in the dorsal recumbent position.
24. In a general survey, the nurse assesses the patient's
    - Primary health problems
    - Behavior and appearance
    - Hygiene, skin condition, and body image; emotional state; recent changes in weight; and developmental status
25. A weight gain of 5 lb or 2.2 kg/day indicates fluid retention.
26. The correct examination techniques are answers a, d, and e.
27. True
28. The correct techniques are c and d.
29. For the anxious patient, the nurse should stop the examination, explain what is happening, ask the patient how he/she is doing, and postpone the procedure, if indicated.
30. Tests for colorectal cancer include fecal immunochemical test (FIT), fecal occult blood test (FOBT), colonoscopy, and barium enema.
31. Positions for cardiac assessment include answers b, d, and e.
32. Signs and symptoms of cardiopulmonary disease include chest pain or discomfort, palpitations, excess fatigue, cough, dyspnea, edema of the feet, cyanosis, fainting, or orthopnea.
33. The risk factors for osteoporosis are b, d, e, and g.
34. Techniques for assessment of lymph nodes include the use of a methodical approach to avoid overlooking any single node or chain. Examples:
    Neck: The patient relaxes with the neck flexed slightly forward. Inspect and palpate both sides of the neck for comparison. During palpation either face or stand to the side of the patient for easy access to all nodes. Using the pads of the middle three fingers of each hand, gently palpate in a rotary motion over the nodes.
    To palpate supraclavicular nodes, ask the patient to bend the head forward and relax the shoulders. Palpate these

nodes by hooking the index and third finger over the clavicle, lateral to the sternocleidomastoid muscle. Palpate the deep cervical nodes only with the fingers hooked around the sternocleidomastoid muscle.
Axilla: Palpate the axillary nodes with the fingertips gently rolling soft tissue. Normally lymph nodes are not palpable. Note the number, consistency, mobility, and size of palpable nodes.

35. Continuous dilation of the pupils is found with patients experiencing neurological pathologies, glaucoma, opioid withdrawal and trauma, or taking ophthalmic medication.
36. An expected response is that the pupils will converge and accommodate by constricting when looking at close objects. The pupil responses are equal.
37. a. Basket or platform scale
    b. A platform scale
38. Tinnitus is ringing in the ears.
39. Causes of hearing loss are working or living around loud noises, premature hearing loss from continued exposure to loud music through earbuds connected to electronic music devices or loud concerts, deterioration of the cochlea and thickening of the tympanic membrane in older adults, and ototoxicity resulting from high maintenance doses of antibiotics (e.g., aminoglycosides).
40. To assess for a pulse deficit, the nurse should auscultate the apical pulse first and then immediately assess the radial pulse (one-examiner technique). Assess the apical and radial rates at the same time when two examiners are present. When a patient has a pulse deficit, the radial pulse is slower than the apical.
41. An irregular pulse should be counted for at least 60 seconds (1 minute).
42. Risk factors for breast cancer are b, d, and e.
43. a. The sequence for the exam is inspection, auscultation, palpation, percussion.
    b. Bowel sounds usually occur 5 to 35 times/minute.
    c. A patient with ascites will have a distended abdomen, taut skin, and bulging flanks.
    d. Absent bowel sounds can occur as a result of lack of peristalsis, possibly because of a bowel obstruction, paralytic ileus (decreased or absent peristalsis), or peritonitis (inflammation of the peritoneum).
44. Signs and symptoms of prostate cancer include weak or interrupted urine flow, an inability to urinate, difficulty in starting or stopping the urine flow, polyuria, nocturia, hematuria, dysuria, or continuing pain in the lower back, pelvis, or upper thighs.
45. Recent memory can be tested by asking the patient to recall by repeating a series of numbers in the order they are presented or in reverse order. Patients normally recall five to eight digits forward or four to six digits backward. Another test for recent memory involves asking the patient to recall events occurring during the same day. To assess past memory, ask the patient to recall the maiden name of the patient's mother, a birthday, or a special date in history.
46. Findings on the skin of an individual who is suspected of substance abuse are b, d, and e.
47. 4
48. 2
49. 1
50. 2
51. 1
52. 4
53. 1
54. 4
55. 3
56. 4
57. 3
58. 1
59. 1
60. 4
61. 1
62. 4
63. 1
64. 1
65. 1
66. 4
67. 1
68. 3
69. 3
70. 1
71. 3
72. 3
73. 4
74. 2
75. 4
76. 3

CHAPTER 17

Case Studies

1. a. Your initial action is to review all of the medications prescribed for the patient and determine what he does remember about each one.

   A general teaching plan for medication administration should include
   - Adapt your approaches so that patients will understand instruction.
   - Provide information about the purpose of medications and their actions and effects.
   - Identify how to take a medication properly and what will happen if he or she fails to do so.
   - Demonstrate how to properly administer medications.
   - Teach ways to change medication schedules to fit into their lifestyles.
   - Teach family members or friends how to administer medications, if necessary.
   - Provide specially designed equipment such as syringes with enlarged calibrated scales for easier reading or Braille-labeled medication vials for patients with visual alterations.
   - Reinforce the basic guidelines for medication safety, including the proper use and storage of medications in the home.

   To assist this patient to maintain the medication regimen at home, you may create a large, colorful, easy-to-read schedule, chart, or calendar that the patient can use to check when medications have been taken. The patient's medications also may be arranged, by time of administration, in a commercially available or homemade container so that the patient also may be able to determine if the medications were taken as prescribed. (Some commercial devices "beep" when it is time for medications to be taken.)
2. a. If the prescriber's handwriting is illegible, it is unsafe to make assumptions about the medication order. To avoid errors, you should contact the prescriber as soon as possible and clarify the medication orders.
3. a. A patient without an identification band should not receive medications. To verify the identity of the patient, find another nurse or health care worker who is familiar with the patient. On verifying the name of the patient, obtain and provide the identification band for the patient. Asking the patient his or her name assists in verification but may be inaccurate if the patient is not aware or oriented to the surroundings.

4. a. When administering an injection to a child, you must be very careful to avoid injuring or severely agitating the child. An appropriate, well-developed muscle site should be selected. You also may need to have someone else assist in holding or distracting the child by talking. The injection should be given quickly and accurately. An anesthetic ointment may be applied to the site before the injection to decrease the amount of discomfort. Children should not be told that they are receiving a "shot" or that it will not hurt. A sleeping child should be awakened before being given an injection.
5. a. Expected treatment for an anaphylactic reaction includes notifying a patient's health care provider immediately; anticipating that antihistamines, epinephrine, and bronchodilators will be prescribed; and documenting medication allergies in the patient's medical record. Patients may require emergency treatment for airway constriction or obstruction, such as oxygen or intubation.
6. a. This discrepancy in the narcotic count should be reported immediately to the nurse in charge. Usually an attempt is made to determine if the missing dose can be accounted for by checking with all of the other staff members. If the missing medication cannot be tracked down, the discrepancy has to be documented on the computerized or written record. The agency's protocol for this situation then should be followed in relation to where and how the documentation is forwarded.
7. a. For the patient who requires an antipyretic but is experiencing nausea and vomiting, the nurse should contact the prescriber and have the medication order changed to a rectal suppository. For patients who have difficulty tolerating oral medications, the nurse should investigate alternative forms of the medication.

Chapter Review

1. i	5. c	9. b
2. j	6. e	10. h
3. k	7. l	11. d
4. g	8. f	12. a

13. Federal and state legislation, state Nurse Practice Acts, and agency policies and procedures control or regulate the nurse's administration of medications.
14. a. Strategies to prevent errors with look-alike medications include the following: ordering medications by the generic name, including the diagnosis on the prescription; repeating verbal orders to the prescriber; discussing the medications with the patient; reinforcing instructions with the patient; advising patients to check medication labels; and having the patient report any changes in the medication's appearance.
    b. Patient identifiers include name and patient identification number. Agencies may include other aids, such as the birth date or the bar code on the name band.
15. Factors influencing the actions of medications:
    a. Dietary factors: Drug and nutrient interactions can alter a drug's action or the effect of the nutrient; proper drug metabolism relies on good nutrition.
    b. Physiological variables: age, sex, weight, nutritional status, disease states
    c. Environmental conditions: stress, exposure to heat/cold, comfort of the setting
16. The routes for parenteral administration include intramuscular, intradermal, subcutaneous, and intravenous.
17. The components that are missing in the orders are
    a. Dosage
    b. Route
    c. Time for administration
    d. Route
18. The rights are
    1. Right drug
    2. Right dose
    3. Right patient
    4. Right route
    5. Right time
    6. Right documentation
19. The correct sequence for removing medication from a vial is e, a, g, h, j, c, f, i, b, d. Please note: air bubbles should first be dislodged while the needle is still in the vial.
20. The forms of medication are
    a. Capsule
    b. Suppository
    c. Elixir
    d. Aqueous suspension
    e. Lotion
21. Commonly abused over-the-counter medications include aspirin and cough and cold medicines.
22. a. Noncompliance or nonadherence may be related to a dislike of the side effects, the cost of the medication, or a busy lifestyle.
    b. Compliance with medication administration may be promoted by
    - Involving the patient in decisions about the schedule
    - Simplifying the schedule as much as possible
    - Clearly explaining about the medications
    - Providing aids to assist in remembering the schedule
    - Teaching patients about the medications and possible side effects
    - Encouraging patients to refill prescriptions before they run out
    - Checking the patient's medications to see that they are correct
23. MedWatch is a voluntary program for reporting when a medication causes serious harm.
24. Faster absorption or action is found with
    a. IV
    b. intramuscular
    c. acidic oral medication
    d. solutions
    e. large surface area
    f. highly lipid soluble medication
    g. nonalbumin-binding medication

25. This is the peak action of the drug.
26. Oral medications are contraindicated for the patient who has an NPO order, GI alterations, dysphagia, nausea, vomiting, gastric suction, NG tube, or received anesthesia.
27. The problem with this order is that the decimal point may be missed and the patient would receive 10 times the actual dose.
28. The equivalents are
    a. 15 gtt
    b. 2 ounces
    c. 1 L
    d. 3000 mg
    e. 250 mL
    f. 5 mL
29. The five types of medication orders are standing, prn, single (one-time), STAT, and now.
    Possible examples of the different orders:
    1. Standing: Lasix 40 mg PO daily
    2. prn: Morphine sulfate 10 mg IM q4h prn for pain
    3. Single: Versed, 6 mg IM on call to OR
    4. Give Apresoline, 10 mg IM STAT
    5. Give vancomycin 1 g IV piggyback now
30. Verbal orders are to be signed within 24 hours.
31. This number of tablets is not common, so the nurse should recheck the calculation to determine accuracy. Another nurse may be asked to verify the final calculation.
32. An adverse effect is an undesired, unintended, and often unpredictable response to a medication. A side effect is a predictable and often unavoidable adverse effect produced at a usual therapeutic dose.
33. If the patient identifies that the medication looks different, it is important for the nurse to check and make sure that the medication and the order are correct.
34. The correct responses regarding medication administration are c, f, and h.
35. The generic names are
    a. levofloxacin.
    b. furosemide.
    c. ibuprofen.
    d. haloperidol lactate.
36. When preparing medications, compare the label of the medication container with the medication administration order three times: (1) while removing the container from the drawer or shelf, (2) as you remove the amount of medication ordered from the container, and (3) at the bedside before administering the medication to the patient.
37. Techniques for administering medications to children include
    a. Oral medications: Give frozen juice bars, juice, or soft drinks after the medication is swallowed (as allowed).
    b. Injections: Wake the child before an injection, ask for assistance in holding the child, distract the child during the injection, give the medication quickly, avoid calling the injection a "shot," and inform the child that it may "pinch."
38. The discomfort of an injection may be minimized by
    - Using a sharp-beveled needle of the smallest possible size
    - Positioning the patient comfortably
    - Selecting the proper site
    - Diverting the patient's attention away from the procedure
    - Inserting the needle quickly and smoothly
    - Holding the syringe steady while injecting the solution
    - Injecting the medication slowly and steadily
    - Using the Z-track technique
    - Massaging the site, unless contraindicated
39. The Z-track technique should be used for medications that are irritating to the tissues.
40. a. Intramuscular: 90-degree angle
    b. Subcutaneous: 45-degree angle
    c. Intradermal: 5-degree to 15-degree angle
41. Medication may be administered IV via
    1. Mixtures with large volumes of IV fluids
    2. Injection (bolus) or intermittent access devices
    3. Piggyback through an existing IV line
42. A wireless barcode scanner is used to identify you (the nurse), the medication package, and the patient (armband).
43. a. ac = before meals
    b. bid = twice a day
    c. prn = as necessary
    d. q4h = every 4 hours
    e. STAT = immediately
44. Answers determined by dimensional analysis method.
    a. <u>150 mcg</u>
       75 mcg × 1 tablet = 2 tablets should be given
       Conversion of 0.150 mg to mcg: multiply 0.150 by 1000
    b. <u>40 mg</u>
       20 mg × 1 tablet = 2 tablets should be given
    c. <u>20 mg</u>
       10 g × 1 mL = 2 mL should be given
    d. 200 mg
       50 mg × 1 mL = 4 mL/day, but this is divided into two equal doses
       4 mL divided by 2 doses = 2 mL (marked on syringe)
    e. 100 units = 1 mL
       24 units/100 units = 0.24 mL
    f. <u>500 mg</u>
       250 mg × 1 tablet = 2 tablets should be given
    g. <u>50 mL</u> × <u>60 gtts</u>
       60 minutes 1 mL = 50 gtts/minute
       The hour time frame is converted to 60 minutes and the minidrip is 60 gtts (drops)/mL.
45. Patient assessments that should be completed before medication administration include:
    Parenteral injections: The size of the patient, condition of the injection site (integument and muscle condition), circulatory status
    For all patients, the type of medication and its effect on the patient are to be evaluated by the nurse.

46.

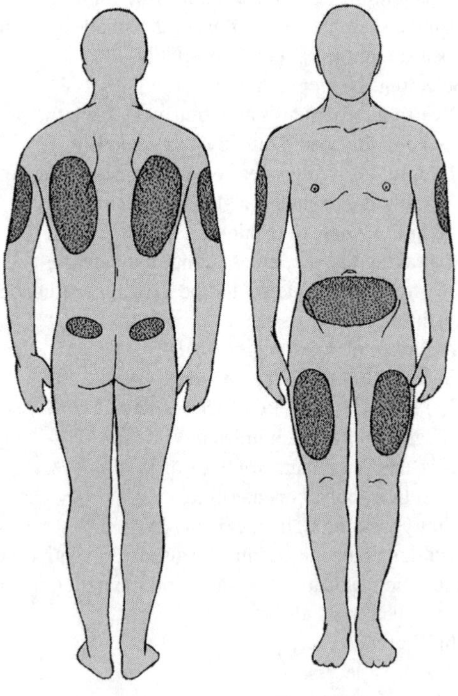

47. The correct techniques for administration of medications to patients with dysphagia are listed in answers b, c, and f.
48. a. Proper placement of the nasogastric tube is a priority assessment.
    b. The tube should be flushed with 15 to 30 mL of sterile water in between medications, with 30 to 60 mL of water given after all of the medications have been administered.
49. The nurse should apply clean gloves before administering topical medications. Sterile gloves may be indicated for medications applied to open wounds.
50. For administration of ear drops:
    a. Position the patient side-lying or sitting in a chair with the head tilted to the side.
    b. Pull the outer ear of an adult up and back.
    c. Irrigate with 50 mL of solution at room temperature.
51. For a pressured metered-dose inhaler:
    a. A spacer should be used.
    b. The patient should inhale for 3 to 5 seconds and hold breath for 10 seconds.
    c. 20 to 30 seconds should be given in between puffs of the same medication.
    d. This canister should last for 20 days (8 puffs/day, 160 total puffs in the canister).
    e. The patient should rinse out the mouth and/or brush the teeth after receiving a corticosteroid via the pMDI.
52. The patient should be placed in left Sims' position, if tolerated.
53. a. Anticoagulant: review of laboratory tests for clotting/bleeding times; assessment of the skin, mucous membranes, urine, and feces for signs of bleeding
    b. Antihypertensive: measurement of blood pressure
    c. Analgesic: completion of a pain assessment; measurement of vital signs, especially respirations and level of sedation
    d. Cardiotonic: assessment of apical pulse; measurement of vital signs; determination of the presence of cardiac-related signs and symptoms
54. False
55. For pediatric medications: b, c, e are correct.
56. The correct sequence is e, b, f, a, c, d.
57. True
58. a. The medication for an IV push/bolus should be given at a rate of 0.5 mL/30 seconds.
    b. If the medication is incompatible, the nurse should stop the IV fluids, clamp the IV line, flush with 10 mL of normal saline or sterile water, give the IV bolus over the appropriate amount of time, flush with another 10 mL of normal saline or sterile water at the same rate as the medication was administered, and then restart the IV fluids at the prescribed rate. This allows you to give IV push medication through the existing line without creating potential risks associated with IV incompatibilities. If IV infusion that is currently hanging is a medication (e.g., ranitidine), disconnect IV line and administer IV push medication to avoid giving a sudden bolus of the medication in the existing IV line to the patient. Verify institutional policy regarding the stopping of IV fluids or continuous IV medications. If unable to stop IV infusion, start a new IV site and administer medication using the IV push (IV lock) method.
59. Intradermal injections are given on the inner forearm and upper back.
60. a. Tuberculin tests are read within 48 to 72 hours.
    b. A positive test for an individual with no known risk factors is 15 mm or more of induration.
61. a. Dorsal recumbent position
    b. The applicator is inserted 5 to 7.5 cm (2 to 3 inches)
62. An example of a positive synergistic effect is: antihypertensives/vasodilators and diuretics. An example of a negative synergistic effect is CNS depressants and alcohol.
63. An advantage of computerized order entry by physicians is the ability to read the orders accurately and reduce errors from misinterpretation.
64. Orders must be rewritten by the prescriber when the patient goes for surgery, is transferred to another unit, or is discharged to home or another facility.
65. Care should be taken when breaking open the neck of the ampule and a filter needle should be used to withdraw the fluid. Medication cannot be saved in the ampule after it is opened.
66. For rotation of subcutaneous sites, the same general location should be used at the same time each day, but each injection should be at least 2.5 cm apart.
67. The correct sequence for administration of an oral medication is e, g, b, d, f, a, c.
68. The four pharmacokinetic processes are absorption, distribution, metabolism, and excretion.
    a. Absorption is influenced by the route of administration, ability of a medication to dissolve, blood flow to the site of administration, body surface area, and lipid solubility of a medication.
    b. Distribution is influenced by circulation, membrane permeability, and protein binding.

c. Metabolism is primarily influenced by the ability of the liver, along with the lungs, kidneys, blood, and intestines.
d. Excretion is influenced primarily by the function of the kidneys, along with the lungs, intestines, and skin.

69. 2	77. 4	84. 1
70. 3	78. 2	85. 2
71. 2	79. 3	86. 3
72. 4	80. 1	87. 1
73. 4	81. 3	88. 4
75. 1	82. 2	89. 3
76. 2	83. 3	

CHAPTER 18

Case Studies

1. a. A patient taking both digoxin and Lasix is more susceptible to fluid volume deficit (FVD) and hypokalemia. Digoxin strengthens the contraction of the heart muscle, improving the cardiac output and circulatory volume. Lasix is a potent diuretic that does not have a potassium-sparing effect. The patient should be instructed to be alert to the signs of decreased fluid and decreased potassium levels as follows:
   - Hypokalemia: weakness, fatigue, decreased muscle tone, intestinal distention, change in pulse rate or rhythm
   - FVD: poor skin turgor, thirst, sunken eyeballs, dryness, weakness, change in pulse rate or rhythm

   The patient also should be instructed in the technique for taking her own pulse rate and on the importance of dietary replacement of potassium (e.g., bananas, oranges, potatoes) or administration of prescribed supplements.
2. a. The patient on prolonged immobility is prone to hypercalcemia as a result of calcium being released from the bones into the bloodstream. The nurse is alert to changes in the cardiac rate and rhythm (e.g., tachycardia) and increases in the BUN and serum calcium levels. If the patient is conscious, there may be anorexia, nausea, vomiting, low back pain, and a reduction in the level of consciousness.

   Alcoholic patients are more susceptible to malnutrition and hypomagnesemia. The nurse is alert to muscle tremors, hyperactive reflexes, confusion, disorientation, dysrhythmias, positive Trousseau/Chvostek signs, and a serum magnesium level less than 1.5 mEq/L.
3. a. The nurse may anticipate that this patient will have signs and symptoms of diminished oxygenation, including dyspnea, wheezing, coughing, activity intolerance, restlessness, pallor/cyanosis, and possible lack of concentration.
   b. This patient most likely will experience respiratory acidosis.
4. a. The priorities before administration of the blood include
   - If the patient has IV access already in place, assess the site for signs of infection, infiltration, and patency. Determine the gauge of the IV cannula.
   - Assess the patient to determine if he or she knows the reason for the blood transfusion and whether the patient ever had a previous transfusion or transfusion reaction.
   - Ensure the patient or representative has signed the informed consent.
   - Check the blood products and the patient, and verify the compatibility of the blood and the patient. Some hospitals use bar code technology to identify patients and verify compatible blood before beginning transfusions.
   - Obtain the patient's baseline vital signs before a transfusion begins.

   b. The safety measures to be implemented to reduce complications are
   - Before a blood transfusion, two registered nurses or one registered nurse and a licensed practical nurse (see agency policy) must simultaneously check the label on the blood product against the patient's identification number, blood group, and complete name. ***If even a minor discrepancy exists, do not give the blood. Notify the blood bank immediately.***
   - Initiation of a transfusion begins slowly to allow for the early detection of a transfusion reaction.
   - Maintain the infusion rate, monitor for side effects, assess vital signs, and promptly record all findings.
   - It is important to stay with the patient during the first 15 minutes, the time when a reaction is most likely to occur. After that time period, continue to monitor the patient and obtain vital signs periodically during the transfusion as directed by agency policy. If a transfusion reaction is suspected, STOP the transfusion immediately. Disconnect the blood tubing, and connect the normal saline infusion to maintain an open IV line. Once the normal saline line is established, obtain vital signs and notify the health care provider. The unused blood product is returned to the blood bank.

Chapter Review

1. e	4. b	7. i
2. f	5. a	8. g
3. h	6. c	9. d

10. a. Extracellular fluid
    b. Interstitial fluid
    c. Intracellular fluid
11. a. Sodium: cation, extracellular—maintenance of water balance, nerve impulse transmission, regulation of acid-base balance, and participation in cellular chemical reactions
    b. Potassium: cation, intracellular—necessary for glycogen deposits in the liver and skeletal muscle, transmission and conduction of nerve impulses, cardiac rhythm, and skeletal and smooth muscle contraction
    c. Calcium: cation, intracellular—bone and teeth formation, blood clotting, hormone secretion, cell membrane integrity, cardiac conduction, transmission of nerve impulses, and muscle contraction
    d. Magnesium: cation, intracellular—enzyme activities, neurochemical activities, and cardiac and skeletal muscle excitability
    e. Chloride: anion, extracellular—follows sodium
    f. Bicarbonate: anion, both intracellular and extracellular—major chemical base buffer
12. The three types of acid-base regulators within the body are chemical, biological, and physiological.

13. Infants, young children, and older adults are most susceptible to fluid and acid-base disturbances.
14. a. Isotonic
    b. Hypotonic
    c. Isotonic
    d. Isotonic
    e. Hypertonic
15. The types of medications that may cause fluid, electrolyte, or acid-base disturbances include diuretics, steroids, potassium supplements, respiratory center depressants, antibiotics, and antacids.
16. Nursing diagnoses for imbalances include
    Ineffective Breathing Pattern
    Decreased Cardiac Output
    Deficient Fluid Volume
    Excess Fluid Volume
    Impaired Gas Exchange
    Impaired Skin Integrity
    Impaired Tissue Integrity
    Ineffective Tissue Perfusion
17.

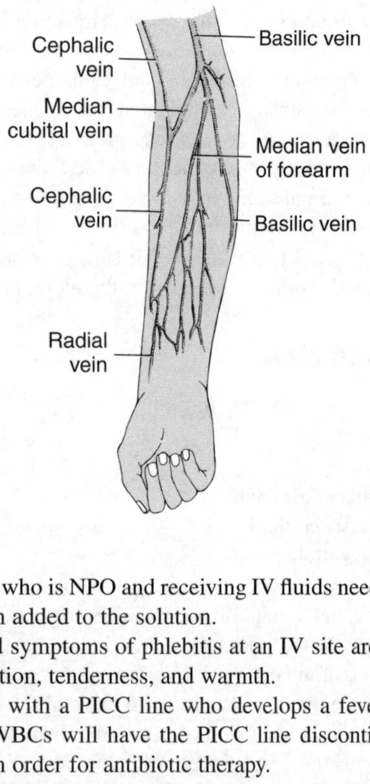

18. A patient who is NPO and receiving IV fluids needs to have potassium added to the solution.
19. Signs and symptoms of phlebitis at an IV site are redness, inflammation, tenderness, and warmth.
20. A patient with a PICC line who develops a fever and increased WBCs will have the PICC line discontinued and receive an order for antibiotic therapy.
21. Based on the patient's status, the nurse should slow the rate of IV infusion, notify the health care provider, raise the head of the bed, provide supplemental oxygen as ordered, and monitor the patient's vital signs.
22. Transfusion of a patient's own blood is an autologous transfusion.
23. a. Hyponatremia
    b. Hyperkalemia
    c. Hypocalcemia
    d. Hypomagnesemia
24. a. 500 mL in 5 hours (300 minutes) with 15 gtt/mL = 25 gtt/min
    b. 1000 mL in 8 hours (480 minutes) with 10 gtt/mL = 21 gtt/min
    c. 200 mL in 4 hours (240 minutes) with 60 gtt/mL = 50 gtt/mL
    d. 2000 mL in 18 hours = 111 mL/hr
25. a. Pituitary hormone—ADH (antidiuretic hormone)
    b. Adrenal hormone—aldosterone
26. True
27. Arterial pH is an indirect measurement of the hydrogen ion concentration.
28. Oxygen moves into the lungs by diffusion.
29. An average adult's daily intake of fluid is approximately 2200 to 2700 mL.
30. The correct order for the steps is c, a, e, b, d. Note that cleansing the area and re-application of the tourniquet may be interchanged.
31. Intake = 1465; Output = 370
32. Fluid volume deficit may be the result of a, d, and f.
33. The nurse anticipates that the patient who has insufficient fluid as a result of a fever will have orders for antipyretics and oral and/or IV fluids. The nurse will also provide comfort measures, such as keeping the patient dry if there is diaphoresis.
34. The IV should be started in the most distal site.
35. INS standards specify the use of an arm board or other joint stabilization device to protect the IV site by keeping the joint extended (INS, 2011). Use padding with arm boards because they may cause skin or nerve damage from pressure. It may be more comfortable for the patient to have an infusion started in a new location rather than relying on a site that causes problems.
36. The order for the steps when removing an IV are f, a, c, g, b, e, d.
37. When preparing the IV, the nurse should look at the fluid to note the type of fluid and amount, expiration date, integrity of the container, and clarity of the solution.
38. For patient safety, follow the agency's procedure to verify three things: the blood components delivered are the ones that were ordered; the blood delivered is compatible with the patient's blood type listed in the medical record; and the right patient receives the blood. An assessment of the patient before the administration is done to establish a baseline for comparison, in the event of a transfusion reaction.
39. For a patient experiencing hypokalemia, the correct signs are a, d, f.
40. In performing an IV site dressing, the nurse should do b, c, d, and f.

41. 2	51. 4	61. 1
42. 1	52. 3	62. 4
43. 1	53. 4	63. 2
44. 2	54. 3	64. 2
45. 3	55. 2	65. 1
46. 3	56. 4	66. 4
47. 3	57. 4	67. 3
48. 1	58. 3	68. 3
49. 2	59. 4	69. 4
50. 3	60. 3	70. 3

CHAPTER 19

Case Studies

1. One of the most important things that the nurse can do for the patient's daughter and her family is to sit with them and allow them to verbalize their feelings about the situation. Listening to the family and acknowledging their emotions lets them know that their feelings and concerns are important. It also demonstrates that the nurse is responsive to their needs and is involved in the holistic care of the patient. The nurse should explain how the patient's condition has progressed and the treatments that currently are being provided for comfort and support. The nurse may provide the daughter with the opportunity to assist with or observe the physical care being given to the patient. Providing information on available resources, such as hospice, is also important in demonstrating caring and concern for the well-being of the patient and her family.
2. a. The student giving the bath to the patient is missing the caring behaviors of comforting touch, maintaining dignity, and performing care appropriately.
   b. The nurse should enter the patient's room to provide privacy immediately. With the patient covered and safe, the nurse should speak with the student outside of the room about the observations. By being a role model and performing the bath in a caring manner, the nurse can demonstrate the appropriate method and reinforce the discussion with the student.

Chapter Review

1. The theories of caring are
   a. Swanson.
   b. Watson.
   c. Benner and Wrubel.
   d. Leininger.
2. Examples of clinical interventions for the following are
   a. Providing presence: staying with the patient while waiting for a procedure or test results
   b. Touch: holding the patient's hand, giving a massage, skillfully and gently performing a procedure
   c. Listening: opening the lines of communication, attentively listening to what the patient is saying, and responding appropriately
   d. Knowing the patient: centering on the patient and providing information that is relevant to the patient's circumstances
3. The nurse demonstrates caring behaviors during an IV insertion by explaining the procedure to the patient in advance and during the intervention, using skillful and gentle technique, and maintaining eye contact.
4. Caring and spirituality are connected in the way that the nurse identifies and provides for the patient's spiritual needs. Spirituality offers intrapersonal (connected with oneself), interpersonal (connected with others and the environment), and transpersonal (connected with the unseen, God, or a higher power) connectedness.
5. Nurses can care for each other by recognizing signs of compassion fatigue, providing mentorship, assisting in patient care activities, and allowing for discussion of concerns and feelings.

6. 1	10. 4	14. 1
7. 3	11. 3	15. 4
8. 3	12. 4	16. 2
9. 4	13. 2	

CHAPTER 20

Case Study

1. a. Involvement of the family is important in assisting the patient to achieve an optimal level of well-being, but there may have to be limits placed on the number of family members who may stay in the room, a reasonable time frame for visiting to allow the patient to rest and receive treatment, and the determination of where the family may gather to conduct discussions.
   b. The therapeutic diet may have to be adapted to avoid meat and meat products but still provide necessary nutrients (protein) or avoid unwanted ingredients (sodium). In an acute or restorative care setting, the dietitian should be involved in providing a menu that meets the patient's cultural preferences but is also tasteful, satisfying, and within therapeutic guidelines.
   c. A healer may provide emotional as well as health care support for the patient. The nurse should work with the health care team to integrate, as much as possible, the actions of the healer. Traditional remedies or treatments should be investigated, however, to determine if there may be any interaction with the prescribed medications or therapies.
   d. To promote communication with individuals and families who speak another language, the nurse should obtain an interpreter who is proficient in that language, use word signs or charts, refrain from speaking loudly, use appropriate titles and greetings, be attentive to nonverbal communication, and clarify uncertain areas.

Chapter Review

1. Nursing diagnoses related to cultural needs may include
   Impaired Verbal Communication
   Compromised Family Coping
   Ineffective Health Maintenance
   Impaired Social Interaction
   Noncompliance
2. a. Cultural awareness: Gain in-depth awareness of one's own background, stereotypes, biases, prejudices, and assumptions about other people.
   b. Cultural skills: Develop skills such as communication, cultural assessment, and culturally competent care.
3. A question may be, "Do you have any cultural practices or rituals that we should know about?" or "Do you use any traditional remedies?"
4. Examples of cultural patterns of communication that may influence the nurse-patient interaction:
   a. Differences in status and position, age, sex, and outsider versus insider perspectives that determine the content and process of communication
   b. Conflict seen as embarrassing or demeaning, with the use of indirect, face-saving communication

c. Awareness of a distinct linear hierarchy, with negotiation of conflict occurring between persons within the same level of position or authority
d. Nonverbal communication, including the amount of personal space that is comfortable, the degree of eye contact, the extent of touching, and how much private information is shared with others
e. Difference in language
Interventions: use of the mnemonics (e.g., LEARN), interpreters, understanding of cultural meanings related to communication

5. Linguistic competence is the capacity of an organization and its personnel to communicate effectively and convey information in a manner easily understood by diverse audiences. Those audiences include people of limited English proficiency, those who have low literacy skills or are not literate, individuals with disabilities, and those who are deaf or hard of hearing.
6. Disadvantaged groups are those who "have systematically experienced greater obstacles to health based on their racial or ethnic group; religion; socioeconomic status; gender; age; mental health; cognitive, sensory, or physical disability; sexual orientation or gender identity; geographic location; or other characteristics historically linked to discrimination or exclusion." The challenges faced include reduced access to health care, inequality in health services, and poor outcomes (e.g., higher infant mortality rates).
7. Cultural considerations are incorporated into "teach back" by specifically determining if the information was communicated effectively and understood by the patient, especially if he/she speaks a different language.
8. Working with an interpreter
   - Provide language assistance services free of charge to all patients who speak limited English or are deaf at all points of contact.
   - Notify patients, verbally and in writing, of their rights to receive language-assistance services.
   - Take steps to provide auxiliary aids and services, defined to include qualified interpreters, note takers, computer-aided transcription services, and written materials.
   - Ensure that interpreters are competent in medical terminology and understand issues of confidentiality and impartiality.
9. L - listen
E - explain
A - acknowledge
R - recommend
N - negotiate

R - rapport
E - empathy
S - support
P - partnership
E - explanations
C - cultural competence
T - trust
10. 4
11. 1
12. 4
13. 3
14. 4

CHAPTER 21

Case Study

1. a. The nurse should obtain information about the extent to which the patient practices Buddhism, including whether he or she is a vegetarian, fasts and refuses treatment on holy days, avoids alcohol, and hesitates to use medications. In addition, the patient's advance directives should be obtained because life support may be removed, if indicated.
b. Dependent upon the degree to which the patient practices his or her faith, adaptations may have to be made as follows:
   - Special dietary request for a vegetarian diet
   - Scheduling of treatments or tests, for example, on days that are not considered holy
   - Determination of medications that may be acceptable
   - Inquiry into the patient's ability to use medications or mouthwash with alcohol
   - Providing contact with a Buddhist priest

Chapter Review

1. d	4. b	6. g
2. a	5. f	7. c
3. e		

8. General nursing interventions for promotion of spiritual health include establishing presence, supporting a healing environment, using support systems, providing diet therapy, supporting practices and rituals, and allowing opportunities for prayer and/or meditation.
9. Nursing interventions for patients who had near-death experiences include the following: promoting open communication, providing a chance for the patient to explore the experience, supporting the patient's discussion with family/significant others.
10. Possible nursing diagnoses include
    - *Readiness for Enhanced Spiritual Well-Being*
    - *Spiritual Distress*
    - *Ineffective Coping*
    - *Anxiety*
    - *Hopelessness*
    - *Powerlessness*
    - *Risk for Spiritual Distress*

    Possible patient outcomes include
    Regain spiritual comfort, affirm a purpose in life, participate in religious practices, pray and meditate daily/prn, recognize/request need for spiritual support, communicate with family and/or significant others about spiritual health
11. The acronym stands for
F—Faith or belief
I—Importance of spirituality
C—Individual's spiritual **Community**
A—Interventions to **Address** spiritual needs
12. Examples of questions to determine a patient's spiritual belief system include
"What is most important in your life?"
"What gives your life meaning or purpose?"

13. The patient's religious background should be checked, because a Jehovah's Witness or Christian Scientist may refuse the blood.
14. Rituals or practices associated with spirituality and religion include participating in group or private worship or prayer, having baptism or communion, fasting, singing, meditating, scripture reading, making offerings or sacrifices, requiring burial or cremation, providing special care of the deceased, and/or having male children circumcised.
15. The correct responses are b, d, and e.
16. The four dimensions of spiritual well-being are
    - Personal dimension: refers to how you relate with yourself in finding meaning and purpose in life
    - Communal dimension: relates to the quality of your interpersonal relationships
    - Environmental dimension: describes how you interact in the world, including your sense of awe with the environment
    - Transcendental dimension: refers to the relationship between you and some higher power
17. The correct statements about spirituality are b, c, and e.
18. The nurse uses *presence* by spending quality time with patients, giving attention, answering questions, listening, having a positive and encouraging (but realistic) attitude, and offering closeness with a patient physically, psychologically, and spiritually.
19. The appropriate nursing actions to promote spiritual health are c, d, and e.

20. 4	23. 1	26. 4
21. 1	24. 3	27. 3
22. 4	25. 1	28. 2

CHAPTER 22

Case Studies

1. a. Promotion of growth and development for the hospitalized infant may include the following:
    - Having the parents/guardians provide most of the care to avoid interfering with the attachment process
    - Limiting the number of caregivers and following the parents' directions for care to promote trust
    - Limiting negative experiences and providing pleasurable sensations

    Promotion of growth and development for the hospitalized 5-year-old child may include the following:
    - Creating a comfortable environment for the child and parents
    - Providing consistent and appropriate care, if the parents are not available
    - Limiting the number of caregivers
    - Providing an environment of acceptance for regressive behavior and reassuring parents that the behavior is normal for children in this situation
    - Allowing children to examine equipment that may be used and participate in procedures, as appropriate
    - Providing comfort items, such as a tape with the parents' voice, pictures of family members, and favorite toys
    - Providing opportunities for play and social interaction with other children
    - Explaining routines in understandable language
    - Incorporating activities of daily living into the hospital routine

    Promotion of growth and development for the hospitalized 16-year-old may include the following:
    - Allowing for peers to visit or have telephone/Internet access
    - Addressing the adolescent rather than the parents during assessments
    - Providing the opportunity for the patient to make choices whenever possible
    - Supporting the amount of parental contact that the adolescent needs, whether intermittent visits or longer stays

   b. A teaching plan for the new parents of an infant should include information on
    - Safety in the environment
    - Feeding: breastfeeding or formula/bottles
    - Hygiene needs
    - Elimination patterns
    - Sleep patterns ("back to sleep")
    - Cord care: immediate neonatal stages
    - Immunization and medical follow-up schedule
    - Expectations for behavior
    - Support for each other
2. a. This patient may benefit from reality orientation, which includes the following:
    - Using time, date, place, and name in conversation
    - Reinforcing reality and providing meaningful things to do
    - Encouraging participation in activities
    - Ensuring that hearing aids or glasses, for example, are working or fitted correctly
    - Providing bowel and bladder training
    - Reinforcing positive behaviors
    - Being patient and allowing sufficient time for completion of activities
    - Speaking slowly and clearly, repeating as necessary
    - Providing clear, simple directions
    - Maintaining a caring and stimulating environment
3. a. Children in this age group usually are interested in games and sports. For indoor recreation, board games, electronic games, or word games may be suggested. Hobbies and crafts are also appropriate if they stimulate and maintain the children's interest. If the children will be outdoors, supervised games such as volleyball, softball/baseball, kickball, tennis, or relay races may be organized. Some sports may have to be modified to meet the physical abilities of the age group. Swimming, bicycling, rowing/canoeing, walking, and hiking are activities that do not have to involve competition but promote exercise.
4. a. Suicide is one of the main causes of death in adolescents and young adults. Parents should be aware of the following warning signs:
    - Diminished performance in school
    - Withdrawal from social activities with family and friends
    - Substance abuse
    - Changes in personality

- Disturbances in sleep, appetite, and usual activity levels
- Talking about death or suicide
- Giving away personal items

Chapter Review

1. d
2. a
3. c
4. e
5. b
6. Teratogens include communicable diseases, alcohol and drugs, smoking, and pollutants.
7. The leading cause of death in the toddler and preschool age group is accidents.
8. The behaviors are associated with the following age groups:
   a. Toddler
   b. Infant
   c. School age
   d. Infant
   e. Young adult
   f. Toddler
   g. Adolescent
   h. Middle adult
   i. Toddler
   j. School age
   k. Preschool age
   l. Older adult
   m. School age
   n. Adolescent
   o. Young adult
   p. Older adult
   q. Middle adult
   r. Preschool age
9. To promote awareness of time, place, and person, the nurse should implement reality orientation.
10. Prescription or use of more medications than indicated is called polypharmacy.
11. Safety concerns in the home environment include
    a. Toddler: access to poisons, such as cleaning supplies; electrical outlets; ability to exit the home; swimming pools; kitchen appliances; auto accidents; choking on small objects
    b. Older adult: poor lighting, slippery floors and unsecured rugs, excessive water temperature, stairs
12. The expected physical assessment findings for a middle-age adult are c, d, and e.
13. Age-appropriate topic areas for the older adult group are activity and exercise, communication with the health care provider, home and medication safety, nutrition, and skin care.
14. The nurse can reduce stress for a hospitalized child by reducing the number of different caretakers, having the parents remain with the child and bring in favorite toys/objects, limiting the amount of time that the child is restrained, providing simple explanations that the child will understand, and speaking in a soothing and comforting tone.
15. Examples of potential nursing diagnoses for adolescents include *Risk for Injury, Impaired Social Interaction,* and *Ineffective Coping.*
16. The characteristics for adolescents are b, c, and f.
17. Patients in the "Sandwich Generation" are responsible not only for themselves but for older parents and children. Multigenerational responsibilities can add stress to the patients' lives and create challenges in helping these individuals find time for their own health and medical care.
18. Concerns for toddlers and school-age children include safety, nutrition, sleep, and socialization/play.
19. The accurate statements for an older adult are b, c, d, and f.
20. 4
21. 2
22. 2
23. 2
24. 1
25. 4
26. 3
27. 1
28. 4
29. 4
30. 4
31. 1

CHAPTER 23

Case Studies

1. a. This young adult patient most likely will experience alterations in his self-concept, especially the perception of his body image and identity. Young adults may be very sensitive about their physical appearance and social status, and now the patient will have to cope with an alteration in his normal activities. In addition, the paraplegia will significantly influence his sexual functioning, an area in which he will have to adapt.
   b. Sample care plan:

Nursing Diagnosis	*Expected Outcome*	*Nursing Interventions*
Disturbed Body Image related to accidental injury and resultant lack of mobility and sensation to the lower extremities (as manifested by his verbalization of his prior social activities)	Patient will adapt to change in body image by • Discussing feelings about his injury and change in activity status • Participating in care as much as possible • Reflecting on personal strengths	Provide time for talking with the patient and discussing feelings; explore coping skills that the patient has used before, and encourage and support those skills; involve the patient in health care activities.
Ineffective Sexuality Pattern related to accidental injury and resultant lack of mobility and sensation to lower extremities	Patient will learn/use measures to attain sexual satisfaction within limitations by • Discussing feelings about sexual function and adaption • Participating in educational program on alternative measures to promote sexual response • Sharing response to measures used and suggesting possible alternatives	Provide time to talk with the patient and discuss feelings and concerns; provide information on sexual response and stimulation for patients with paraplegia; obtain a referral/consultation, if indicated, for additional support and information; have another young male paraplegic individual speak with the patient; provide for patient privacy.

2. a. The patient who you suspect may be a victim of sexual abuse may be found to have
    - Physical signs: bruises, lacerations, abrasions, burns, headaches, GI problems, eating disorders, abdominal or vaginal pain
    - Behavioral signs: sleep-pattern disturbances, nightmares, insomnia, depression, anxiety, fear, decreased self-esteem, substance abuse, frequent visits to health care providers

   b. Examples of questions that should be asked include
    - "Are you in a relationship in which someone is hurting you?"
    - "Have you ever been forced to have sex when you didn't want to?"
    - "Are you afraid of the situation that you are in?"

Chapter Review

1. b	4. d	7. c
2. f	5. h	8. g
3. e	6. a	

9. a. General positive influences on self-concept include words and actions of approval, interest, and acceptance; recognition and inclusion in decision making; trust; and support.
   b. Stressors that may influence self-concept include those that threaten body image, self-esteem, role, or identity, such as the effects of traumatic accidents, surgery, and acute or chronic diseases.
10. Behaviors that may indicate an altered self-concept include c, d, f, and h.
11. Potential concerns related to self-concept include
    a. Alteration in body image: Removal of breast can lead to questions of feminine image and sexual desirability.
    b. Alteration in body image and role: Loss of hair from chemotherapy, possible hospitalizations, and diminished strength may interfere with role as mother.
    c. Alteration in body image and identity: Physical changes in appearance and function (ability to play with others)
    d. Alteration in role and self-esteem: Possible inability to maintain current occupation, dependence on others
12. Ways in which the nurse may promote self-concept in an acute care setting include the following:
    - Arranging visits with someone who has experienced similar problems/changes
    - Listening, being sensitive to, and supporting the patient's needs
    - Being aware of nonverbal communication (e.g., reactions to the patient's mastectomy)
    - Including the patient, as much as possible, in decision making and self-care
13. Alterations in sexual health include infertility, sexual abuse, sexual dysfunction, and personal and emotional conflicts.
14. Patient teaching for the promotion of sexual health may include instruction about
    - Refraining from drinking alcohol 1 to 2 hours before sexual activity
    - Discussing behavior that provides the most sexual stimulation and satisfaction with the partner
    - Options available for contraception
    - Side effects of medications that alter sexual function and response
    - Use of usual positions and selection of times when patient feels rested (for individuals with cardiac dysfunction)
    - Safe sex practices
15. For the nursing diagnosis *Situational Low Self-Esteem related to being unable to pass a required college course*, examples are as follows:
    - Goal: increased self-esteem indicated in body image, behavior, and verbalization
    - Outcome: discusses positive aspects of self and future plans
    - Nursing interventions: spend time with the person to allow for discussion of feelings and concerns, establish sense of trust
16. False
17. False
18. False
19. Promotion of self-concept for an older adult may include
    - Clarifying what life changes mean
    - Being alert to preoccupation with physical complaints and encouraging verbalization of needs
    - Identifying positive and negative coping mechanisms and supporting effective strategies
    - Encouraging the use of storytelling
    - Communicating that the individual is worthwhile by actively listening to and accepting the person's feelings and concerns
    - Allowing additional time to complete tasks and reinforcing the person's efforts at independence
20. For tattoos and body piercings, the correct statements are b, d, and e.
21. Examples of role performance stressors include becoming parents, taking over the care of older parents, becoming a widow/widower.
22. The vaccine is Gardasil.
23. Cardiovascular disease, neurological disorders (stroke, Parkinson's), diabetes mellitus, respiratory disease, and arthritis are medical diagnoses that can interfere with sexual functioning.

24. 3	29. 2	34. 3
25. 4	30. 4	35. 4
26. 4	31. 4	36. 3
27. 1	32. 4	37. 2
28. 1	33. 2	

CHAPTER 24

Case Studies

1. a. The patient, who provides the major financial support to the family, has been hospitalized with a serious health problem. His wife has maintained a traditional role as "homemaker" while her husband has worked. The younger daughter has assumed a family life that appears to be more acceptable to her parents, whereas the older son is involved in an alternative family form. The younger daughter may be more involved in her parents' life because of her family pattern.

b. The family is apparently progressing from the "Family with young adults" to the "Family in later life" stage. There are elements of both stages within this situation.
c. The nurse may begin discussions with the father and mother initially, moving toward a total family meeting at a later date. Providing opportunities for family members to express their feelings about both the health care and the family situation may facilitate open communication about family structure and relationships. The family may need to be referred for ongoing counseling if there is a negative impact on the health/recovery of the patient.
d. The patient may have feelings about his business and family roles and his ability to resume them when he is discharged. His wife will need to be involved in the educational process to follow through with the plan of care. The patient's wife may need to assume a greater decision-making role with the patient to maintain the economic and emotional status of the family.
e. Possible family-oriented nursing diagnoses include
   - *Interrupted Family Processes*
   - *Ineffective Role Performance*
   - *Compromised Family Coping*

2. a. The visiting nurse should determine what the patient's home environment is like in regard to safety and accessibility. The nurse needs to know whether there is a ramp, stairs, or an elevator. If the patient will be using an assistive device, such as a walker or wheelchair, is there sufficient room for mobility within the home? How is the home arranged? Is it open or cluttered? Is there a shower or bath? Overall, does the patient have the necessary resources to manage post-hospital care?
   b. It is important to know whether there are family members living in the home or nearby. The patient may need assistance with household management, ADLs, or transportation to heath care agencies.

Chapter Review

1. b
2. d
3. a
4. e
5. c
6. A family is a set of interacting individuals related by blood, marriage, or adoption who usually live together and fulfill functions of socialization, division of labor, and economic provisions and cooperatively meet affective and emotional needs of the individuals within the family unit.
7. Family members may need to decide on whether or not to test for the presence of the disease and/or have children. Some families choose not to have children, whereas other families choose not to know genetic risks and have children; other families choose to know the risk and then determine whether to have children. With genetic risks for certain cancers, such as certain breast cancer, the family member may choose to have prophylactic mastectomies to reduce the risk for developing the disease.
8. a. Family hardiness is the intrafamilial system of support and structure that extends beyond the walls of the household. Through divorce, remarriages, or cohabitation new members are added to a family. In addition, an extended family also includes contact with former spouses or partners.
   b. Family resiliency is the ability of the family to cope with expected and unexpected stressors.
   c. Family diversity is the uniqueness of each family unit.
9. Current concerns or challenges that may influence the family today are: a changing family structure (which means fewer children, delayed childbirth, divorce, adolescent pregnancy, single parents, same-sex couples), changing economic status, homelessness, domestic violence, employment, and access to health care.
10. a. Caregivers may manifest the following signs and symptoms of caregiver strain:
    - Physical: fatigue, frequent illness/exacerbation of previous conditions
    - Psychological: changes in mood, anxiety, depression, anger

    b. A possible nursing diagnosis is *Caregiver Role Strain*.
11. The correct statements are b, d, f, and g.
12. Inadequate functioning can have many effects on the family, including stress, impaired cardiovascular and neuroendocrine functioning, and interference with decision making and problem solving.
13. Questions that may be asked to determine cultural influence on a family include
    a. "What types of foods do you eat?"
    b. "Who cares for sick family members?"
    c. "Have you or anyone in your family been hospitalized?"
    d. "Did family members remain at the hospital?"
    e. "Do you use some of your culture's health practices, such as acupuncture or meditation?"
    f. "What role do grandparents play in raising your children?"
14. Health promotion for a family can include healthy diets (e.g., low fat), exercise plans, safety instruction, immunizations, and regular health maintenance.
15. Factors contributing to domestic violence include stress, poverty, social isolation, psychopathology, learned family behavior, alcohol and drug abuse, pregnancy, sexual orientation, and mental illness.
16. The nurse can help the family by providing information, support, assurance, and presence (e.g., giving the family information about the dying process, helping to set up home care and obtain hospice, and offering grief support) and, if present at the time of death, being sensitive to the family's needs (e.g., by providing for privacy and allowing sufficient time for saying good-byes).
17. A family with a rigid structure is in danger of altered functioning. Rigid structures specifically dictate who accomplishes different tasks and also limits the number of persons outside the immediate family allowed to assume these tasks. For example, in a rigid family the mother is the only acceptable person to provide emotional support for the children and/or to perform all of the household chores. If something happens to the mother, the role is not easily managed by the father or other members of the family.
18. 3
19. 4
20. 3
21. 1
22. 3
23. 4
24. 2
25. 3
26. 4
27. 2

CHAPTER 25

Case Study

1. a. This patient may demonstrate the following:
   - Physical signs: increased heart rate, respirations, and blood pressure; headaches; fatigue; sleep disturbances; restlessness; gastrointestinal distress; weight gain or loss; backaches; amenorrhea; frequent or prolonged colds or flu
   - Psychological signs: forgetfulness, preoccupation, increased fantasizing, decreased creativity, slower reactions and thinking, confusion, decreased attention span
   - Emotional signs: crying tendencies, lack of interest, irritability, negative thinking, worrying
   - Behavioral signs: diminished activity or hyperactivity, withdrawal, suspiciousness, substance abuse, change in communication or interaction with others

   b. Possible nursing diagnoses for this patient include
   - *Anxiety*
   - *Ineffective Coping*

   c. Outcomes for these nursing diagnoses: The patient will
   - differentiate effective and ineffective coping patterns.
   - identify and express the need for help.
   - verbalize a decrease in stress.
   - work on time management.
   - recognize stressors and implement stress management techniques.
   - alter her lifestyle to reduce stress.
   - call upon her personal support system.

   d. A number of alternatives may be presented to this patient so that she may select those that are most beneficial to her. The nurse may use guided imagery, biofeedback, progressive muscle relaxation, hypnosis, music/art therapy, humor, assertiveness training, or journal/diary entry.

Chapter Review

1. Evaluating an event for its personal meaning is called primary appraisal.
2. The correct statements about stress are a, d, and e.
3. A priority nursing intervention for patient safety is to determine if the patient is suicidal or homicidal.
4. True
5. Positive benefits from exercise include increased muscle tone, decreased tension, increased relaxation, weight control, increased circulation, improved posture, and endorphin release.
6. a. Maturational
   b. Sociocultural
   c. Sociocultural
   d. Situational
   e. Maturational
   f. Situational
   g. Maturational
   h. Sociocultural
7. a. Cognitive: forgetfulness, denial, increased fantasy life, poor concentration, inattention to detail, orientation to the past, decreased creativity, slower thinking and reactions, learning difficulties, apathy, confusion, decreased attention span, calculation difficulties
   b. Cardiovascular: increased heart rate, increased blood pressure, tightness in chest
   c. Gastrointestinal: nausea, diarrhea, vomiting, weight gain or loss, change in appetite, bleeding
   d. Behavioral: change in activity level, withdrawal, suspiciousness, change in communication and interaction with others, substance abuse, excessive humor or silence, no exercise, hyperactivity
   e. Neuroendocrine: headaches/migraines, fatigue, insomnia/sleep disturbances, feeling of being uncoordinated, restlessness, tremors, profuse sweating, dry mouth
8. Stress management should include instruction about instituting positive workplace habits, avoiding excessive change, time management, relaxation techniques, exercise, and establishing support systems.
9. Kegel exercises
10. With Pender's Health Promotion theory, the nurse would discuss increasing physical activity, improving diet and nutrition, and using stress management strategies to become healthy and remain healthy.
11. a. Compassion fatigue is more likely to be seen in nurses working on oncology units or in hospice care.
    b. Signs and symptoms of compassion fatigue are feelings of hopelessness, being in a state of hypervigilance, anxiety, and emotional exhaustion.
12. Applying the QSEN competency of safety to stress and coping: the nurse is alert to overt signs of crisis, suicidal or homicidal thought processes, inattention, and physical and emotional fatigue/exhaustion.
13. Stress becomes a crisis when it overwhelms a person's usual coping mechanisms and demands mobilization of all available resources.
14. Objective signs of stress include a, c, e, and f.
15. Components of cognitive therapy are a, c, and f.

16. 3	21. 4	26. 2
17. 1	22. 3	27. 1
18. 2	23. 4	28. 3
19. 1	24. 1	
20. 3	25. 2	

CHAPTER 26

Case Studies

1. a. The patient may demonstrate the following behaviors indicative of complicated bereavement:
   - Overactivity without a sense of loss
   - Alteration in relationships with friends and family
   - Anger against particular people
   - Agitated depression: tension, guilt, feelings of worthlessness
   - Decreased participation in religious or cultural activities
   - Inability to discuss the loss without crying (a year or more after the loss)
   - False euphoria
   - Eliminating all signs of the deceased (e.g., pictures) or creating a "shrine"
   - Alterations in eating and sleeping patterns
   - Regressive behavior

b. Possible nursing diagnoses for the patient may be:
    - *Dysfunctional Grieving* related to sudden loss/suicide of husband
    - *Ineffective Coping* related to inability to deal with husband's loss/suicide

    Possible goals may be:
    - The patient will accept the reality of her husband's death.
    - The patient will renew activities of daily living and complete a normal grieving process.

    Nursing interventions may include:
    - Using therapeutic communication to promote the patient's verbalization of feelings concerning her husband's suicide
    - Demonstrating support of the patient by staying with her and using comfort measures, such as touch
    - Referring the patient to support groups, clergy, and/or counseling as appropriate for her needs
2. Hospice services center around the following:
    - Patient and family as the unit of care
    - Coordinated home care with access to inpatient and nursing home beds when needed
    - Symptom management
    - Physician-directed services
    - Provision of an interdisciplinary care team
    - Medical and nursing services available at all times
    - Bereavement follow-up after a patient's death
    - Use of trained volunteers for visitation and respite support

Chapter Review

1. d
2. b
3. c
4. a
5. Special circumstances that may influence grief resolution include suicide, sudden death, miscarriage, a child's death, and certain pathologies, such as AIDS.
6. True
7. Interventions that should be implemented for a family dealing with a patient's terminal illness include involving everyone in discussions, promoting open communication, answering questions, and providing caregiver support.
8. The correct interventions are c, d, and f.
9. Nursing measures that may be implemented to facilitate the mourning process include
    - Helping the patient accept that the loss is real
    - Supporting efforts to live without the deceased person or in the face of disability
    - Encouraging establishment of new relationships
    - Allowing time to grieve
    - Interpreting "normal" grief behavior
    - Providing continuing support
    - Being alert for signs of ineffective coping
10. The nurse may prevent a sense of abandonment by:
    - Answering patients' call lights promptly and assuring them that caregivers are available throughout the day and night
    - Being readily available to answer questions or interpret changes in the patient's condition; offering a calm, comforting presence
    - Avoiding placing patients in a private room
    - Reassuring family members that their presence is important
    - Allowing visitors to remain at all times with patients who are dying and relaxing other visiting restrictions
11. Federal and state legislation require that health care agencies formulate policies and procedures based on current laws to validate death, identify potential organ or tissue donors, request autopsy, and provide postmortem care.
12. a. Questions that may be asked about the nature of a loss:
    "How is the loss affecting your daily life?"
    "What past experiences have you had with loss?"
    "Tell me how you usually cope with disappointment or loss."

    b. Cultural beliefs about loss:
    "What do you believe about death?"
    "Who makes health care decisions in your family/culture?"
    "Tell me about your family's/culture's end-of-life and funeral practices."

    c. Coping strategies:
    "How are you managing with the care?"
    "What are you doing about your work and home responsibilities?"
    "Do you have plans for hospice care at home?"
    "Are you able to talk about your needs and feelings as a family?"
13. Signs of impending death include
    - Minimal intake of food or water
    - Increased sleeping and decreased consciousness
    - Disorientation and restlessness
    - Decreased urinary output and/or incontinence
    - Cool hands and feet
    - Noisy breathing
    - Irregular breathing patterns with long pauses

    At the time of death, you will note:
    - Absence of breathing and heartbeat
    - Bowel and bladder release
    - Unresponsiveness
    - Eyes fixed on a certain spot
    - Dilated pupils
14. Moving through Worden's four tasks can vary, but typically the process takes at least 1 year.
15. The Rs in Rando's R Process Model are recognizing the loss, reacting to the pain of separation, reminiscence, relinquishing old attachments, and readjusting to life after loss.
16. The correct actions for postmortem care are b, d, and e.
17. Nursing interventions include
    a. Fatigue: Help patient to identify valued or desired tasks; conserve energy for only those tasks. Assist with activities of daily living. Plan frequent rest periods in a quiet environment, and pace nursing care activities.

    b. Decreased appetite: Give patient whatever food or fluids patient enjoys. Offer frequent small meals and/or snacks rather than large meals. Do not force people to eat. Offer small portions of desired foods or home-cooked meals, per patient preference.

18. Delayed grief is seen when the survivor(s) attempts to return quickly to normal activities, pretending that everything is fine and then having a reaction at a later time.
19. An autopsy is performed in accordance with state legislation, usually in circumstances when death may have resulted from accident, homicide, or suicide.
20. Documentation should include information about the time and date of death, the name of the health care provider who pronounces the death, organ or tissue donation status, preparation of the body, medical devices left in or on the body, valuables or belongings left with the patient or given to the family, the time of discharge, and destination of the body.
21. Physical signs and symptoms associated with grieving include
    - Hollowness in the stomach
    - Tightness in the chest
    - Tightness in the throat
    - Oversensitivity to noise
    - Sense of depersonalization ("nothing seems real")
    - Feeling short of breath
    - Muscle weakness
    - Lack of energy
    - Dry mouth

22. 3
23. 2
24. 3
25. 4
26. 4
27. 3
28. 2
29. 1
30. 3
31. 1
32. 4
33. 4
34. 3
35. 3

CHAPTER 27

Case Study

1. a. The patient should be assessed for her ability to move independently, including her posture, muscle strength, range of motion, gait (if able), balance, activity tolerance, and cognitive status. If the patient is able to bear weight on both legs and maintain an erect position, the nurse must determine if she is capable of ambulating safely. Initial assessment of the patient's transfer out of bed should be accomplished with assistance in the event that the patient is unable to maintain a standing position.
   b. If the patient is not able to ambulate independently, she may be able to use an assistive device, such as a cane or walker. If possible, one or more nurses may use a gait belt to assist the patient in ambulating. Should the patient not be able to ambulate safely, even with assistance, a wheelchair may be necessary. To assist the patient in gaining muscle strength, a program of exercise may be implemented.

Chapter Review

1. i
2. g
3. h
4. f
5. b
6. e
7. d
9. c
10. Assessment of a patient's mobility includes range of joint motion, gait, exercise, balance, posture, and body alignment.
11. The correct principles of body mechanics are options b, d, and f.
12. False
13. a. Before ambulation, the patient should be placed in a sitting position with the legs dangled over the side of the bed.
    b. Care should be taken in making position changes slowly because orthostatic hypotension could occur.
14. Pathological influences on alignment, exercise, and activity include congenital defects; disorders of bones, joints, and muscles; central nervous system damage; and musculoskeletal trauma.
15. True
16. Examples of physiological factors that may influence activity tolerance are musculoskeletal abnormalities, diminished cardiovascular function, and diminished respiratory function.
17. Possible nursing diagnoses associated with a change in a patient's ability to maintain physical activity include
    - *Activity Intolerance*
    - *Disturbed Body Image*
    - *Risk for Injury*
    - *Impaired Physical Mobility*
    - *Impaired Skin Integrity*
    - *Acute* or *Chronic Pain*
18. The priority for this patient is pain relief.
19. The patient should be in Fowler's position—(head of the bed elevated 45 to 60 degrees) or semi-Fowler's position (head of bed elevated 30 degrees)
20. a. The general "rule of thumb" for transfers is to GET HELP to transfer a patient.
    b. Safety during transfers is the priority.
21. a. Supine
    b. Prone
    c. Lateral
22. Expected findings are answers a, e, and g.
23. The correct techniques are answers b, d, and e.
24. Patients should be repositioned at least every 2 hours.
25. a. The chair should be positioned on the patient's strong side at a 45-degree angle to the bed.
    b. More than one nurse is needed for this transfer. The correct sequence of steps for the use of a mechanical lift is the following:
       - Position the chair near the bed.
       - Raise the bed to working height with the mattress flat (as tolerated).
       - Roll the patient away from you (side rail is up on the far side).
       - Place the sling under the patient.
       - Roll the patient toward you.
       - Pull the sling through so that it is under the patient from the upper torso.
       - Check the position of the sling.
       - Move the lift under the bed and attach the sling to the lift.
       - Have the patient fold the arms over the chest.
       - Slowly lift the patient and maneuver the sling over the chair.

- Lower the patient into the chair and disconnect the lift.
- Position the patient for comfort and safety.

26. Logrolling requires at least three caregivers to perform.
27. Limited range of motion can be the result of inflammation, such as arthritis, fluid in the joint, altered nerve supply, or contractures.
28. The patient who is able to assist in positioning can be instructed to bend the knees and lift the hips and/or push up with the hands and arms. A draw sheet may also be used to move the patient up in bed.
29. Half of all back pain is associated with manual lifting tasks.
30. Improper positioning of patients in bed can lead to pressure ulcers and contractures.
31. A patient who is overweight or has a respiratory condition would not be placed in a prone position.
32. A mechanical device for repetitive motion is a continuous passive motion (CPM) machine.

33. 3	38. 2	43. 2
34. 2	39. 4	44. 4
35. 4	40. 4	45. 4
36. 1	41. 2	46. 2
37. 1	42. 4	47. 4

CHAPTER 28

Case Studies

1. a. You should assess some of the following areas regarding home safety:
   - Location of the home in the community
   - Security measures within the home
   - Environmental conditions: lighting, temperature, sanitation, stairways, floors/carpeting
   - Fire and electrical safety measures/hazards
   - Exposure to pollutants/pathogens

   b. With a toddler and a preschool child in the home, safety measures are extremely important. Accidents are one of the major problems for children, including falls and poisoning. If there are stairs in the home, gates should be in use or doors to the outside should be locked. For upper-level apartments or rooms, child-safety devices should be in place on the windows. Any household chemicals or medications should be out of reach and/or in a locked compartment. There also may be locks on other kitchen cabinets, drawers, and the refrigerator to prevent access. Electrical outlets should have covers, and plugs should be out of sight of the children. The family should have a fire safety plan, fire extinguishers, and smoke/fire alarms. Items that may be swallowed or broken should be out of reach. Additional safety measures may be in place in the kitchen and bathroom, such as faucet covers.
2. a. For the patient in the home who has diabetes mellitus and requires insulin injections, the following precautions should be taken:
   - Perform hand hygiene and maintain sterile asepsis for the injections.
   - Store the insulin properly.
   - Maintain an adequate supply of insulin and injection supplies.
   - Dispose of used needles and syringes appropriately; do not reuse the injection supplies (unless an insulin pen is used).
   - Have adequate light for preparation and administration of the injection.
   - Wear eyeglasses, if needed.
3. a. Guidelines that should be used to establish a safe, restraint-free environment include the following:
   - Involving patients and families in planning care; explaining all procedures and treatments to them
   - Encouraging family and friends to stay or using sitters
   - Using calm, simple statements and physical cues as needed
   - Using a knee band such as the Ambularm or an alarming seat belt to alert caregivers
   - Eliminating full side rails; using low beds with a floor mat at bedside
   - Assigning confused or disoriented patients to rooms near the nurses' station; observing these patients frequently and instituting regular patient checks
   - Providing appropriate visual and auditory stimuli
   - Providing ongoing pain assessment and nonpharmacological interventions
   - Using diversional activities appropriate for the patient
   - Instituting exercise and ambulation schedules as the patient's condition allows
   - Providing scheduled toileting, especially during peak fall times
   - Consulting with physical and occupational therapists to enhance strength, mobility, and exercise
   - Using protective devices such as hip pads, helmet, skid-proof slippers, and nonskid strips near bed
   - Providing prompt treatment and ongoing evaluation of medical problems

Chapter Review

1. Basic human needs in a safe environment and examples of what may affect them are
   - Oxygen: carbon monoxide, improper ventilation, pollutants
   - Degree of humidity: excessive dryness
   - Nutrition: improper storage/refrigeration, inadequate cleaning of cooking surfaces
   - Optimal temperature: excessive heat or cold
2. Inadequate lighting, clutter, lack of security, fire/electrical hazards, and temperature extremes are examples of physical hazards in the home.
3. a. Diminished vision, hearing, mobility, reflexes, and circulation are some of the reasons that older adults are predisposed to accidents.

   b. (1) Driving safety:
   Advise older adults to drive only short distances and in the daylight; avoid driving in inclement weather; use side and rear view mirrors carefully; look behind them toward their blind spot before changing lanes; and keep a window rolled down to hear sirens and horns.

(2) Home environment safety:
- Because of visual impairments in older adults, teach patients to keep living areas well lighted and free of clutter and to keep eyeglasses in good condition.
- Older adults have musculoskeletal changes that make movement difficult and increase the risk for falling. Teach patients to keep assistive devices in proper working order (canes, hand rails in tub and bathroom, and elevated seats) and to use nonskid strips in bathtubs.
- Advise older adults to avoid smoking in bed, to lower thermostats on water heaters, to avoid overloading electrical outlets, and to install and maintain smoke and carbon monoxide detectors in the house.

4. The following are examples of how the nurse may prevent health care agency risks:
   a. Falls: Complete a risk assessment, provide supervision, place the patient close to the nurses' station, orient the patient to the surroundings, use physical restraints if absolutely necessary.
   b. Patient-inherent accidents: Institute seizure precautions, remove foreign substances or hazardous items (sharps), provide supervision of the patient's activities.
   c. Procedure-related risks: Follow policies and procedures carefully, use appropriate technique for performing procedures.
   d. Equipment-related risks: Learn how to operate the equipment, have it checked regularly for proper functioning.
5. The "never events" are a, c, e, and f.
6. Active immunity is obtained through the injection of weakened or dead organisms and modified toxins.
7. Potential hazards include
   a. Infant, toddler, preschool: injuries, accidents, poisoning
   b. School-age child: sports, after-school activities, bicycle accidents, school bus injuries
   c. Adolescent: smoking, substance abuse, motor vehicle accidents, stress, sexual activity
   d. Adult: alcohol/substance abuse, motor vehicle accidents, stress-related activities
   e. Older adult: falls, medication misuse
8. Patients experiencing impaired mobility, diminished sensation and/or cognition, and decreased safety awareness are a high risk for injury.
9. Potential agents that may be used are
   a. Biological: anthrax, smallpox, typhoid, plague, botulism
   b. Chemical: cyanide, mustard gas, chlorine, nerve agents
   c. Radiological: nuclear device, "dirty bomb"
10. True
11. Teaching areas for a school-age child include crossing the street, stranger safety, bicycle safety, sport/activity safety, and personal hygiene.
12. The primary goal of restraints (safety reminder devices) is to prevent falls.
13. The correct actions for using restraints are b, c, d, and e.
14. False
15. An older adult having difficulty with medication administration in the home may benefit from the use of a medication organizer device or system.
16. In a health care agency, medication safety is promoted by properly identifying the patient, administering medicine correctly, maintaining accurate labeling and storage, and documenting promptly.
17. Environmental adjustments include
   a. Tactile deficit: Check/adjust the water heater temperature, clearly label the settings on the stove/oven, obtain easy-open medication containers.
   b. Visual deficit: Maintain adequate lighting, use stair treads and handrails, decrease clutter, use distinct colors, have large print on labels.
18. The following alternative measures may be implemented:
   - Orienting patients/families to the surroundings
   - Explaining routines and procedures
   - Encouraging family and friends to stay with the patient
   - Providing adequate stimulation, diversional activity
   - Using relaxation techniques
   - Instituting exercise and activity plans
   - Eliminating bothersome therapies as soon as possible
   - Maintaining toileting routines
   - Evaluating the effect of medications
   - Performing regular assessments of the patient's status
   - Using electronic bed and chair alarm devices
   - Placing the patient in a room near the nurses' station
19. Possible nursing diagnoses include the following:
   - *Risk for Imbalanced Body Temperature*
   - *Impaired Home Maintenance*
   - *Risk for Injury*
   - *Deficient Knowledge*
   - *Risk for Poisoning*
   - *Risk for Suffocation*
   - *Risk for Trauma*
20. a. Signs and symptoms of low concentration carbon monoxide poisoning are nausea, dizziness, headache, and fatigue. Higher concentrations are often fatal.
   b. There must be carbon monoxide detectors in the home.
21. The "Speak Up" campaign is designed to encourage patients to take a role in preventing health care errors by becoming active, involved, and informed participants in their health care (TJC, 2013b). For example, patients are encouraged to ask health care workers if they have washed their hands before providing care.
22. Resources/agencies that are available for patient safety include The Joint Commission, QSEN, CMS, OSHA, the Institute for Healthcare Improvement, the Agency for Healthcare Research and Quality, and the U.S. Department of Veterans Affairs.
23. (a) Most falls occur within the home, specifically in the bedroom, bathroom, and kitchen. Environmental factors such as broken stairs, icy sidewalks, inadequate lighting, throw rugs, and exposed electrical cords cause many accidents. Older adults typically fall while transferring from beds, chairs, and toilets; getting into or out of bathtubs; tripping over carpet edges or doorway thresholds; and slipping on wet surfaces or descending stairs.
   (b) Falls in the health care agency are usually the result of multiple factors:
   - *Intrinsic factors* are patient related and include physiological conditions such as vision disturbances,

urinary/stool frequency or incontinence, mental impairment, gait and balance disorders, polypharmacy, and older age.
   - *Extrinsic factors* are environmentally related and include room clutter, loose electrical cords, and spills.

24. Information about chemical substances in the workplace can be found on *Material Safety Data Sheets* (MSDS).
25. Signs, symptoms, and behaviors that are indicative of substance abuse are the presence of drug-oriented magazines, beer and liquor bottles, drug paraphernalia, blood spots on clothing, and the continual wearing of long-sleeved shirts in hot weather and dark glasses indoors. Psychosocial clues include failing grades, change in dress, increased absenteeism from school, isolation, increased aggressiveness, and changes in interpersonal relationships.
26. Hospitals are required to have an emergency management plan that addresses identifying possible emergency situations and their probable impact, maintaining an adequate amount of supplies, and having a formal response plan.
27. True
28. R – Rescue and remove all patients in immediate danger
    A – Activate the alarm. Always do this before trying to extinguish even a minor fire.
    C – Confine a fire by closing doors and windows and turning off oxygen and electrical equipment.
    E – Extinguish a fire using an appropriate extinguisher.
    Pull the pin. Hold the extinguisher with the nozzle pointing away from you, and release the locking mechanism.
    Aim low. Point the extinguisher at the base of the fire.
    Squeeze the lever slowly and evenly.
    Sweep the nozzle from side to side.
29. a. Type B
    b. Type C
    c. Type A
30. The nurse should report any equipment that does not appear to be working properly to the agency's maintenance, safety, or facilities department.
31. a. Hospitals
       - Identify patients correctly
       - Improve staff communication
       - Use medicines safely
       - Use alarms safely
       - Prevent infection
       - Identify patient safety risks (e.g., suicide)
       - Prevent mistakes in surgery
    b. Home care
       - Identifies patients correctly
       - Uses medicines safely
       - Prevents infection
       - Prevents patients from falling
       - Identifies patient safety risks (e.g., patients on oxygen, risk of fire)
32. The correct order for the steps of the Timed Get Up and Go Test is e, a, c, g, f, d, and b.
    An abnormal result is when a person takes more than 20 seconds to complete the test.
33. a. Use of home oxygen
       - Post "No Smoking" and "Oxygen in Use" signs.
       - Do not use oxygen around electrical equipment or flammable products.
       - Store oxygen tanks upright in carts or stands to prevent tipping or falling over.
       - Make sure that there is a sufficient supply on hand of oxygen and spare tubing.
    b. Food preparation
       - Proper refrigeration, storage, and preparation of food decrease risk of foodborne illnesses. Store perishable foods in refrigerators to maintain freshness.
       - Refrigerate foods at 40° F within 2 hours of cooking.
       - Thaw frozen foods in the refrigerator.
       - Wash hands for at least 15 seconds before preparing food.
       - Rinse fruits and vegetables thoroughly.
       - Avoid cross-contamination of one food with another during preparation, especially with poultry.
       - Use a separate cutting board for vegetables, meat, and poultry.
       - Cook foods adequately to kill any residual organisms.
       - Refrigerate leftovers promptly and label the date when leftovers are saved.
34. Based on the scenario, the following bold assessment findings require follow-up to prevent patient injuries:
    Upon entering the patient's home, the visiting nurse observed that the patient was wearing **slippers with no back**. The patient stated that she seemed to **always leave her glasses somewhere**. There were **piles of newspapers and other items cluttering the floor around the living room chairs**. The **lighting in the stairway was less than 60 watts** and there were **throw rugs on the wood floors** in the halls. When looking through the medicine cabinet with the patient, the nurse noted that some **medications were expired**. The patient **admitted to falling** once **when getting up during the night to go to the bathroom.**
    The patient should be wearing slippers that fit well and will not slide off and cause the patient to trip. The patient's glasses should be kept close by in a case or on a necklace, so that there is better vision. Clutter around chairs, poor lighting, and throw rugs can cause the patient to fall. Expired medications can be ineffective and dangerous to keep around. Nocturia is a concern, as is the admission of a prior fall.

35. 1
36. 3
37. 2
38. 1
39. 3
40. 2
41. 3
42. 3
43. 4
44. 3

CHAPTER 29

Case Studies

1. a. For the patient with diabetes mellitus, you should include the following instructions:
      - Carefully inspect the skin surfaces, particularly the extremities.
      - Perform daily foot care using lukewarm water, with no soaking; dry the feet well, especially between the toes.
      - Do not cut corns or calluses.
      - Apply bland powder if the feet perspire.
      - File the toenails straight across; no cutting.
      - Wear clean, dry socks daily.
      - Do not walk barefoot.

- Wear properly fitting, flexible shoes.
- Exercise regularly.
- Avoid application of hot water bottles or heating pads to the extremities.
- Clean minor cuts immediately and apply only mild antiseptics, if necessary.
- Avoid wearing elastic stockings, tight hose, or noncotton socks.
- Avoid crossing the legs.
- Avoid the use of commercial preparations for corn/callus removal, athlete's foot, or ingrown toenails.
- Consult a podiatrist as needed for foot problems.

2. a. The older adult patient may be experiencing changes in skin integrity. The skin is more fragile, so hot water and strong cleansing agents should be avoided. Older adults usually perspire less, so bathing need not be as frequent (unless personally desired). There may be an increased sensitivity or itching that may be relieved with the use of hydrocortisone cream, moisturizing soaps, lotions, or petrolatum. Humidity should be higher in the environment to alleviate skin dryness. The room temperature may have to be warmer. Care should be taken to avoid injury to the skin as wound healing is slower in this population. Range of motion should be assessed while assisting the patient. A shower or bath chair may be needed for the patient with reduced mobility.

Chapter Review

1. e	5. f	9. g
2. i	6. c	10. d
3. h	7. j	
4. a	8. b	

11. Factors that contribute to a hygiene self-care deficit are diminished mobility, chronic illness, pain, cognitive impairment, mental illness, and socioeconomic status.
12. For a patient with dementia, the nurse should use the towel bath technique. This is a person-centered in-bed approach in which a nurse uses a large towel, one or two regular-size towels, washcloths, a bath blanket, and no-rinse soap and water. This technique has been shown to produce a marked reduction in behavioral symptoms when comparing the in-bed approach to showering (Rader, 2006).
13. Appropriate techniques are answers d, e, g, and h.
14. A nurse-initiated treatment for a rash is a warm soak.
15. Plain water is used on the patient's eyes.
16. The accurate statements about the skin are a, c, d, and f.
17. The nurse should have the patient do as much of the hygienic care as possible, as well as participate in the decision making regarding his/her care.
18. A standing shower is contraindicated for a patient who is unable to safely stand, has a history of falls, and demonstrates fatigue, weakness, or unsteadiness.
19. A patient with the nursing diagnosis of *Activity Intolerance* would become easily fatigued and require rest periods and/or repositioning during the care.
20. Healthy skin can be promoted by inspecting the skin for changes in color or texture and reporting changes or abnormalities to the health care provider. Instruct patients to handle the skin gently, avoiding excessive or rough rubbing. Advise against use of hot water for bathing as well as too lengthy bathing sessions to prevent loss of oils and excessive drying of skin. Also encourage patients to consume a balanced diet including foods rich in antioxidants, vitamins, and minerals, and to consume adequate fluids. Stress safety concerns in the home such as failure to adjust the water temperature when bathing or showering or slipping on wet surfaces in the bathroom.
21. a. False
    b. True
22. The recommendations to make are b and c.
23. Chlorhexidene gluconate 4% is most useful.
24. Eyeglasses should be kept in a case on top of the bedside table or in a drawer of the bedside table when not in use.
25. Ear irrigation is contraindicated in the presence of a perforated tympanic membrane (eardrum).
26. Asepsis is maintained during linen changes by
    - Keeping soiled linen away from the uniform and off the floor
    - Placing soiled linen in the proper container
    - Avoiding fanning or shaking of linens
    - Discarding clean items that fall on the floor
27. The nurse prepares a comfortable environment for the patient by controlling the room temperature, providing for adequate ventilation and lighting, limiting noise, reducing odors, and keeping the room neat.
28. Conditions that may place the patient at risk include those that are associated with reduced sensation, vascular insufficiency, impaired cognition, incontinence, and/or decreased mobility (e.g., diabetes mellitus, cerebrovascular accident (CVA/stroke), spinal cord injury, and arterial insufficiency).
29. A commercial "bag bath" usually contains 8 to 10 premoistened towels. A single towel is used for each general body part cleansed. The towels may be microwaved for warmth.
30. When providing a tub bath for a patient, safety measures include
    - Assessing the patient's mobility
    - Placing rubber mat on tub or shower bottom and a disposable bath mat or towel on floor in front of tub or shower
    - Helping the patient to bathroom if necessary
    - Having the patient wear slippers to bathroom
    - Demonstrating how to use the call signal for assistance
    - Checking the temperature of the bathwater
    - Instructing the patient to use safety bars when getting in and out of tub or shower
    - Cautioning the patient against the use of bath oil in tub water
    - Instructing the patient not to remain in the tub longer than 10 to 15 minutes
    - Staying with the patient or checking on the patient every 5 minutes
    - Draining the tub of water before the patient attempts to get out of it
31. The patient's cultural background may influence hygienic care as follows:
    - Privacy may be a large concern, especially for women from cultures that value female modesty.
    - Exposure of the lower torso and the arms of Middle Eastern and East Asian women is not appropriate.

- Family members may want to participate in the care.
- Gender-congruent care may be needed or requested.
- In some cultures (e.g., Hindu, Orthodox Jewish, Muslim, Amish), touching between unrelated males and females is forbidden.
- The frequency of bathing may differ, as well as the products that are used.
- Many Asians (Chinese, Japanese, Koreans, and Hindus) consider the top parts of the body cleaner than the lower parts.
- Hindus and Muslims often use the left hand for cleaning, whereas the right hand is reserved for eating and praying.

32. Care for the patient's acne: Wash hair and skin each day with soap and warm water to remove oil. Use oil-free cosmetics because oily cosmetics or creams accumulate in pores and make acne worse. Eliminate foods from diet that aggravate condition. Use prescribed topical antibiotics for severe acne.
33. Guidelines for patient bathing and skin care include
    - Clean the skin at the time of soiling and at routine intervals. Individualize frequency of cleansing according to patient need and preference.
    - Avoid hot water and use a mild cleansing agent to minimize irritation.
    - Avoid the use of force and friction.
    - Minimize environmental factors that lead to skin drying.
    - Protect patients from injury by assessing and controlling the bathwater temperature.
    - Use assistive devices when indicated.
    - Use bathing as a time to interact with and assess a patient.
    - Assist patients through joint range-of-motion exercises to promote circulation and joint integrity.
    - For patients who fatigue easily, consider administering a partial instead of a complete bed bath.
34. Special oral hygiene will usually be required by patients who are unconscious or have artificial airways.
35. The correct order for the bath is c, b, g, d, e, f, a.
36. Safety measures for oral care of the unconscious patient include checking for the gag reflex, positioning and suctioning to prevent aspiration, checking for bleeding/anticoagulant therapy, and avoiding dislodging an E/T tube.
37. To irrigate the ear, have a patient sit or lie on the side with the affected ear up. Place a curved emesis basin under the affected ear. For adults and children over 3 years of age, gently pull the pinna up and back. In children 3 years of age or younger, the pinna should be pulled down and back. Using a bulb irrigating syringe, gently wash the ear canal with warm solution (37° C or 98.6° F), being careful to not occlude the canal, which results in pressure on the tympanic membrane. Direct the fluid slowly and gently toward the superior aspect of the ear canal, maintaining the flow in a steady stream. Periodically during the irrigation ask if the patient is experiencing pain, nausea, or vertigo. These symptoms indicate the solution is too hot or too cold or is being instilled with too much pressure. After the canal is clear, wipe off any moisture from the ear with cotton balls and inspect the canal for remaining earwax.
38. The hands and feet should be soaked for 10 minutes before nail care, unless the patient is diabetic.
39. Vascular insufficiency is indicated in the presence of decreased hair growth, absent or diminished pulses, foot infection, poor wound healing, thickened nails, shiny appearance of the skin, and blanching of the skin upon elevation.
40. For the older adult: The skin is more fragile, so hot water and strong cleansing agents should be avoided. Older adults usually perspire less, so bathing need not be as frequent (unless personally desired). There may be an increased sensitivity or itching that may be relieved with the use of hydrocortisone cream, moisturizing soaps, lotions, or petrolatum. Humidity should be higher in the environment to alleviate skin dryness. The room temperature may have to be warmer. Care should be taken to avoid injury to the skin because wound healing is slower in this population. Range of motion should be assessed while assisting the patient. A shower or bath chair may be needed for the patient with reduced mobility.
41. For the patient with a hearing aid, the correct instructions include a and f.

42. 3	46. 3	50. 3
43. 1	47. 2	51. 1
44. 4	48. 1	52. 4
45. 4	49. 3	

CHAPTER 30

Case Study

1. a. To gather further information from the patient about her current respiratory status, the nurse should ask the following questions:
    - "When do you experience shortness of breath/difficulty breathing?"
    - "What activities bring on the shortness of breath?"
    - "Does the shortness of breath interfere with your activities of daily living?"
    - "Do you find that it is hard to inhale or exhale?"
    - "Do you sleep with extra pillows at night?"
    - "Are you more tired than usual?"
    - "Do you smoke?"
    - "Are you exposed to smokers or other environmental hazards at home or at work?"
    - "When does the cough start?"
    - "Are there times when your breathing/coughing is better or worse?"
    - "What are you bringing up when you cough?"
    - "Have you been exposed to anyone with a respiratory infection?"
    - "Have you recently had an upper respiratory infection?"
    - "Have you had pain in your chest when you breathe?"
    - "Are you currently taking any medications?"

   b. Based on additional information from the patient, possible nursing diagnoses for this patient may be
    - *Activity Intolerance*
    - *Ineffective Airway Clearance*
    - *Impaired Gas Exchange*
    - *Risk for Infection*

   c. Nurse-initiated actions may include measurement of vital signs, auscultation of lung sounds, inspection of sputum, positioning for optimum respiratory function and comfort, and preparation of oxygen and suctioning equipment in case severe respiratory distress develops.

d. General teaching for health promotion should include the importance of
   - Receiving the pneumococcal and influenza vaccines (if she has not had them)
   - Limiting exposure to crowds and environmental pollutants
   - Avoiding smoking or secondhand smoke
   - Covering the mouth and nose if exposed to cold air
   - Determining and improving activity and exercise tolerance
   - Taking medications regularly
   - Performing breathing/coughing exercises

Chapter Review

1. c	5. i	9. h
2. d	6. a	10. j
3. e	7. g	
4. b	8. f	

11. The average resting heart rate for an adult is 60 to 80 beats per minute.
12. Conditions that may affect chest wall movement include pregnancy, obesity, musculoskeletal abnormalities, abnormal structural configuration, trauma, muscle diseases, and nervous system diseases.
13. a. Right ventricular heart failure
    b. Right ventricular heart failure
    c. Left ventricular heart failure
    d. Left ventricular heart failure
14. Hyperventilation may be caused by answers a, b, and d.
15. a. Decreased oxygen-carrying capacity: anemia, inhalation of toxic substances (carbon monoxide)
    b. Decreased inspired oxygen concentration: airway obstruction, higher altitudes
    c. Hypovolemia: fluid loss, dehydration, shock
    d. Increased metabolic rate: fever, pregnancy, hyperthyroidism
16. A premature infant may have a deficiency of surfactant.
17. Controllable risk factors include smoking, substance abuse, poor nutrition, lack of exercise, and stress.
18. Changes that occur in the cardiopulmonary system as a result of aging include answers b, e, and g.
19. This condition is noted by the nurse as paroxysmal nocturnal dyspnea (PND).
20. Wheezing is a high-pitched, musical lung sound that is heard on inspiration and/or expiration.
21. a. Ventricular fibrillation
    b. Ventricular tachycardia
22. a. Retraction is the visible sinking in of the soft tissues of the chest between and around firmer tissue and ribs, often seen in the intercostal spaces.
    b. Paradoxical breathing is asymmetrical or asynchronous breathing in which the chest contracts during inspiration and expands during expiration.
23. Surgical asepsis or sterile technique is used to suction the trachea.
24. Continuous bubbling in the chest tube water-seal chamber indicates an air leak.
25. Nursing interventions to achieve the following include
    a. Dyspnea management: administration of medications (e.g., bronchodilators), supervision of oxygen therapy, and instruction in breathing and coughing techniques and relaxation measures
    b. Patent airway: instruction in coughing techniques, suctioning, and airway placement
    c. Lung expansion: positioning, administering chest physiotherapy, instruction in the use of incentive spirometry, and management of chest tubes
    d. Mobilization of secretions: hydration of the patient, humidification/nebulization of oxygen therapy, and administration of chest physiotherapy
26. a. Simple face mask: 40% to 60% (5 to 8 L/min)
    b. Venturi mask: 24% to 60% (4 to 12 L/min)
27. For tuberculin (Mantoux) testing:
    a. Forearm
    b. 48 to 72 hours
    c. Negative reaction
    d. Positive
28. For chest percussion, vibration, and postural drainage:
    a. Bleeding disorders, osteoporosis, fractured ribs
    b. Exhalation
    c. Positioned on the nurse's/parent's lap
29. For CPAP:
    a. Sleep apnea, and improvement of ventilation for heart, neuromuscular, and pulmonary diseases
    b. 5 to 20 cm H_2O
    c. Hypercapnea, gastric distention, discomfort, risk for skin irritation, noise
    d. BiPAP (Bilevel positive airway pressure) works by providing assistance during inspiration and preventing airway closure during expiration. It provides two levels of pressure: inspiratory positive airway pressure (IPAP) and a lower expiratory positive airway pressure.
30. a. An indication for home oxygen therapy is an SaO_2 of 88% or less.
    b. Safety measures for home oxygen use include
       - Place "No smoking" signs on the patient's room door and over the bed. Inform the patient, visitors, roommates, and all personnel that smoking is not permitted in areas where oxygen is in use.
       - Determine that all electrical equipment in the room is functioning correctly and is properly grounded.
       - Know the fire procedures and the location of the closest fire extinguisher.
       - Check the oxygen level of portable tanks before transporting to ensure there is enough oxygen in the tank.
       - Have an alternative source of oxygen in case of a power failure.
31. The steps of CPR:
    C: Circulation
    A: Airway
    B: Breathing
32. Defibrillation is recommended within 5 minutes outside of a hospital/medical center and 3 minutes for an in-hospital victim.
33. a. True
    b. False
34. For the patient with a nasal cannula:
    - Verify setting on flowmeter and oxygen source for proper setup and prescribed flow rate.

- Monitor patient's response to changes in oxygen flow rate with pulse oximetry.
- Observe patient's external ears, bridge of nose, nares, and nasal mucous membranes for evidence of skin breakdown.
- Check cannula/mask every 8 hours.
- Keep humidification container filled at all times.

35. For the nursing diagnosis *Ineffective Airway Clearance related to the presence of tracheobronchial secretions*, possible patient outcomes and nursing interventions are the following:
    Patient outcomes:
    - Sputum clear within 24 to 36 hours
    - No adventitious lung sounds auscultated
    - Respiratory rate of 16 to 24 breaths per minute
    - Coughing and clearing airway within 24 hours

    Nursing interventions:
    - Instruct patient on coughing and deep breathing
    - Assist with position changes and ambulation
    - Provide 2000 to 2500 mL of fluid, if not contraindicated
    - Monitor vital signs
    - Suction prn
    - Provide chest physiotherapy, if indicated
36. The appropriate interventions for suctioning are b and e.
37. Cardiac output is the result of stroke volume × heart rate.
38. a. Signs and symptoms of hypoxia include tachycardia, peripheral vasoconstriction, dizziness, and mental confusion.
    b. Treatment may include cardiac and respiratory stimulant drugs, oxygen therapy, mechanical ventilation, and frequent analysis of blood gases.
39. Possible nursing diagnoses for a patient with anemia include *Activity Intolerance* and *Fatigue.*
40. Cardiopulmonary status may be influenced by the intake of a diet high in fat, cholesterol, salt, and calories, and low in iron and essential nutrients.
41. The most effective positioning for a patient is 45-degree semi-Fowler's.
42. An incentive spirometer will encourage the postoperative patient to breathe deeply.
43. Hazards include
    Environmental: air pollution, smog, and allergens (e.g., pollen)
    Occupational: exposure to asbestos, talcum powder, dust, and airborne fibers
44. Cardiac dysrhythmias may be caused by ischemia, valvular abnormality, anxiety, drug toxicity, caffeine, alcohol, or tobacco use, cardiothoracic surgery, or a complication of acid-base or electrolyte imbalance.
45. Atrial fibrillation is treated with synchronized cardioversion, rate control medication therapy, such as diltiazem or beta-blockers, interventions based on the underlying cause, and blood thinners such as warfarin (Coumadin).
46. To prevent the incidence of VAP, the nurse should
    - Monitor cuff pressure frequently to ensure there is an adequate seal to prevent aspiration of secretions.
    - Provide daily oral care with chlorhexidine.
    - Always drain ventilator circuit condensation away from the patient and into the appropriate receptacle. Drain the tubing hourly to prevent accumulation.
    - Keep the head of the patient's bed raised between 30 and 45 degrees unless other medical conditions do not allow this to occur.
47. Treatment for hyperventilation involves treating the underlying cause, improving tissue oxygenation, restoring ventilation, reducing respiratory rate, and achieving acid-base balance.
48. The sequence for in-line suctioning is c, f, b, d, a, e.
49. The areas on the chest tube drainage system are

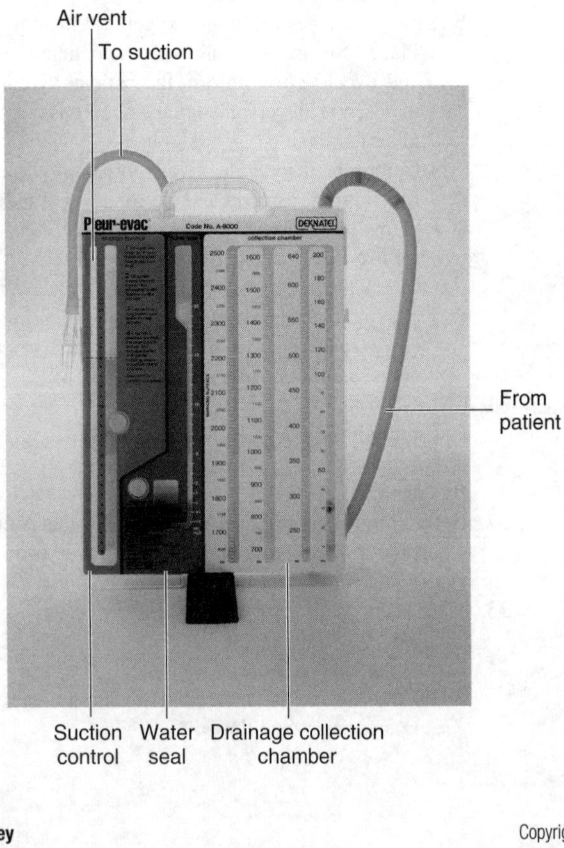

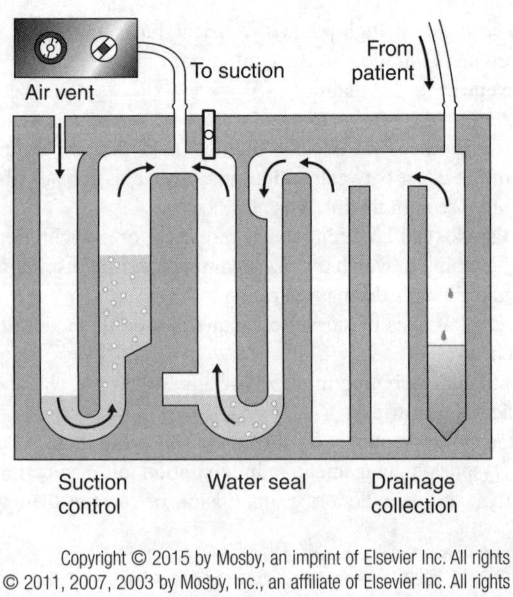

50. The correct responses for chest tube care are b, d, and e. Appropriate care for the patient with a chest tube includes
    - Assessment of respiratory status and system integrity:
        - Observation for air leaks, kinked tubes
    - Proper positioning of the patient with chest tubes to facilitate chest tube drainage and optimal functioning of the system
    - Careful ambulation and transfers
    - Identifying and reporting any changes in vital signs, level of comfort, SpO_2, or excessive bubbling in water-seal chamber
    - Immediately managing/reporting if there is a disconnection of the system, change in type and amount of drainage, bleeding, or sudden cessation of bubbling
    - Determining if milking/stripping is agency policy
51. Examples of pathologies that can reduce chest wall expansion are
    - Musculoskeletal abnormalities, such as pectus excavatum and kyphosis
    - Muscle diseases, such as muscular dystrophy
    - Nervous system diseases, such as myasthenia gravis, Guillain-Barré syndrome, and poliomyelitis
    - Disease or trauma involving the medulla oblongata and spinal cord
    - Trauma to the chest wall: multiple rib fractures, chest wall or upper abdominal incisions
52. The following signs and symptoms are indicative of cardiac pain in women: epigastric pain, complaints of indigestion, nausea or vomiting, or a choking feeling and dyspnea.
53. Factors contributing to respiratory problems in infants and children are prematurity (surfactant deficiency, respiratory syncytial virus [RSV] infection), frequent exposure to other children, exposure to secondhand smoke, nasal congestion from teething, and airway obstruction from foreign objects.
54. The lifestyle factors that contribute to poor cardiopulmonary outcomes are a, c, d, and e.
55. Fatigue is an early sign.
56. The nurse should complete the assessment in short sections to allow the patient to rest and recover. If the patient is breathless or fatigued, ask closed-ended questions, with yes or no answers. Focus the initial assessment on the patient's immediate problems.
57. Nebulization is used for the administration of bronchodilators and mucolytic agents.
58. A Yankauer suction catheter is used for oropharyngeal suctioning.
59. The patient should be positioned with the right side up, so he/she would be laying on the left side.
60. Bronchodilators and other ephedrine-containing products are contraindicated for patients with asthma.
61. Caution is used when administering oxygen to a patient with chronic lung disease because patients with COPD and hypercapnia (high carbon dioxide levels) have adapted to the higher carbon dioxide level. The carbon dioxide–sensitive chemoreceptors are no longer sensitive to increased carbon dioxide as a stimulus to breathe. Their stimulus to breathe is a decreased PaO_2.

    When you administer excessive oxygen to patients with COPD, this satisfies the body's oxygen requirement and negates the stimulus to breathe.
62. The patients who should receive the flu vaccination are d and e.

63. 3	69. 2	75. 3
64. 3	70. 3	76. 1
65. 4	71. 3	77. 3
66. 1	72. 4	78. 2
67. 2	73. 1	79. 2
68. 4	74. 1	

CHAPTER 31

Case Studies

1. a. A possible nursing diagnosis for this patient is *Disturbed Sleep Pattern related to current life situation: stress at home and work.* Goal includes
    - Patient will achieve an adequate amount of nightly sleep within 1 month.

    Outcomes include
    - Patient will identify and verbalize about current life stressors.
    - Patient will practice stress reduction/relaxation techniques as needed.

   b. The nurse may implement the following:
    - Sit with the patient and offer an opportunity for her to vent about her feelings and concerns.
    - Instruct the patient on stress reduction/relaxation techniques.
    - Advise about the value of exercise and activity before sleep.
    - Discuss manipulation of the environment to provide maximum comfort and minimum distraction.
    - Instruct the patient on the avoidance of heavy meals before bedtime and excessive caffeine or alcohol intake.
    - Have the patient maintain a log of sleep/rest patterns.
2. a. To assist the nurse to obtain sufficient sleep while adapting to the change in his work schedule, you should
    - complete an assessment of the nurse's sleep patterns and general health.
    - have the nurse complete a sleep diary to determine routines and previous success in getting to sleep.
    - suggest methods to promote a restful environment: reduce noise and light, adjust the temperature, have a comfortable bed/mattress and covering, turn off phones and other devices.
    - suggest methods to promote sleep: take a warm bath or shower, eat a nutritious snack, perform relaxation exercises, read for a little while.
    - for chronic insomnia, the nurse may need to be evaluated at a sleep center or request a change in schedule.

Chapter Review

1. f	4. a	7. d
2. b	5. g	8. i
3. h	6. c	9. e

10. Sleep may be affected by physical illness, medications/substances, lifestyle changes, sleep pattern alterations, emotional stress, environmental variations, exercise, fatigue, and food and caloric intake.
11. The correct responses are c, f, and h.
12. The nurse may promote a restful environment by checking that the:
    - patient's bed is clean and dry.
    - lights are lowered and not directed at patient's eyes.
    - temperature and ventilation in the room are at comfortable levels.
    - amount of noise is decreased.
    - number of distractions is decreased.
13. True
14. False
15. Sleep cycles usually last 90 to 110 minutes, followed by REM sleep.
16. a. Comfort measures for the patient:
        - Having loose-fitting nightwear
        - Having the patient void before bedtime
        - Giving a relaxing back rub
        - Removing minor irritants, such as changing wet dressings or diapers
        - Providing an extra blanket to prevent chilling
        - Applying dry or moist heat
        - Providing proper positioning
        - Administering pain medications 30 to 60 minutes before the patient goes to bed
    b. Safety measures for the patient:
        - Setting beds lower to the floor
        - Removing clutter and moving equipment from the path a patient uses
        - Assisting the patient to ambulate, if necessary
        - Making sure the call light is within the patient's reach
        - Positioning patients so that they will not fall out of the chair when sleeping; elevating the feet on an ottoman or small bench
17. A sleep diary usually includes information on waking and sleeping activities, such as exercise, work, mealtimes, alcohol and caffeine intake, the time and length of naps, evening and bedtime routines, the time the patient tries to fall asleep, time and number of awakenings, and the time of morning awakening.
18. The best type of bedtime snack is one containing protein and carbohydrates, such as cereal and milk or cheese and crackers, which contain L-tryptophan and help promote sleep.
19. Infants should be placed on their backs or sides for sleep.
20. Examples of possible outcomes:
    - Patient will fall asleep within ½ hour of planned time.
    - Patient will have less than two awakenings during the night.
    - Patient will identify factors that interrupt sleep patterns.
21. a. Physical and behavioral problems include fatigue, irritability, mood changes, blurred vision, decreased reflexes, slow response time, confusion, and alterations in motor performance, memory, and equilibrium. Sleep deprivation affects immune functioning, metabolism, nitrogen balance, protein catabolism, and quality of life. A loss of REM sleep often leads to confusion and suspicion.
    b. Safety considerations include instruction about the need for caution during activities, because attention is diminished and accidents are more prevalent.
22. True
23. REM sleep appears to be important for early brain development, cognition, and memory (Hobson, 2009). Researchers associate REM sleep with changes in cerebral blood flow, increased cortical activity, increased oxygen consumption, and epinephrine release. This association assists with memory storage and learning.
24. Central sleep apnea is associated with stroke, degeneration of the cervical spine, obesity, and encephalitis, and frequently is seen in patients with congestive heart failure.
25. Examples of questions to ask about sleep habits include
    - Tell me what you do just before going to bed.
    - Have you recently had any changes at work, school, or home?
    - How long does it take you to fall asleep?
    - How often during the week do you have trouble falling asleep or staying asleep?
26. For a patient with chronic insomnia, the nurse should refer the patient for medical follow-up and treatment and/or a sleep center for evaluation.
27. Recommendations for health promotion are a and e.

28. 3	35. 2	42. 1
29. 4	36. 3	43. 4
30. 1	37. 1	44. 1
31. 2	38. 4	45. 3
32. 2	39. 1	46. 3
33. 3	40. 1	47. 4
34. 2	41. 4	

CHAPTER 32

Case Studies

1. a. To successfully use a PCA pump, the patient must understand the purpose and use of the medication and pump, as well as be able to locate and push the button on the pump that controls the administration of the medication. The nurse should assess the IV site to ensure it is patent and without complications. The baseline blood pressure and respiratory rates should be recorded before the infusion begins. After the infusion starts, the vital signs are monitored as often as every 15 to 30 minutes for the first few hours until the patient gains relief at a constant dosage. If the patient's blood pressure or respirations decrease, the infusion rate is reduced according to the physician's or health care provider's order or agency policy. For severe respiratory depression, small doses of the opioid antagonist naloxone (Narcan) IV are administered, according to policy, to increase respiratory rate and depth.
    b. Usual medications for the PCA pump include opioids, such as morphine, hydromorphone, and fentanyl.
    c. Teaching for this patient should include
        - Use of the equipment
        - Purpose of PCA, action(s) of the medication, expected pain relief, precautions, and potential side effects of the medication (CNS depression)

- General precautions for an IV infusion
- Caution against family members/visitors operating the device for the patient

2. a. The patient may have an expectation that this labor and delivery experience will also be "horrible," which could predetermine her responses. She could be very fearful of repeating the severe pain and not getting any relief.
   b. Patient-centered care should include assessing the patient carefully, and providing the patient with explanations about her status and the procedures that are implemented. Demonstrating support and concern for her comfort is critical, so that she knows you will be her advocate and respond to her pain. Encouraging the presence of a family member or significant other can also assist in creating a supportive environment.

Chapter Review

1. h	4. g	7. b
2. a	5. e	8. f
3. d	6. c	

9. The four physiological processes of pain are transduction, transmission, perception, and modulation.
   Transduction: Transduction converts energy produced by these stimuli into electrical energy. The process begins in the periphery when a pain-producing stimulus sends an impulse across a sensory peripheral pain nerve fiber (nociceptor) initiating an action potential.
   Transmission: Pain-sensitizing substances surround the pain fibers in the extracellular fluid, spreading the pain message and causing an inflammatory response. Nerve impulses travel along afferent peripheral nerve fibers. Two types of peripheral nerve fibers conduct painful stimuli: the fast, myelinated A-delta fibers and the small, slow unmyelinated C fibers. The A fibers send sharp, localized, and distinct sensations that specify the source of the pain and detect its intensity. The small C fibers relay slower impulses that are poorly localized, visceral, and persistent.
   Perception: The pain impulse ascends to the brain and the central nervous system extracts information, such as location, duration, and quality of the pain impulse.
   Modulation: The brain releases inhibitory neurotransmitters such as endogenous opioids, serotonin, norepinephrine, and gamma aminobutyric acid (GABA). The neurotransmitters hinder the transmission of pain to help produce an analgesic effect.
10. The gate control theory suggests that heat, cold, transcutaneous electrical nerve stimulation (TENS), and pharmacological interventions will reduce pain.
11. The physiological responses to pain as a result of sympathetic stimulation include b, d, and e.
12. a. Associated symptoms of chronic pain include fatigue, insomnia, anorexia, weight loss, apathy, hopelessness, and anger.
    b. The influence of chronic pain on an individual's lifestyle can include the following: change of sleep patterns, inability to perform hygienic care, sexual dysfunction, alteration in home or work management, and interruption of social activities.
13. An infant may respond to pain by crying and by exhibiting changes in vital signs, facial expressions, or extremity movement. A child may respond to pain with crying, irritability, loss of appetite, quietness or restlessness, disturbed sleep patterns, or rigid body posture.
14. The single most reliable indicator of pain is the patient's self-report.
15. For the PQRSTU assessment:
    a. Quality: Suggest a change in medications if the quality of pain changes.
    b. Region: Position the patient so that body weight is shifted away from area of pain; apply heat/cold directly to the site.
    c. Timing: Administer medication so that the peak effect occurs when pain is most acute.
16. a. Toddler: Use of words that the child can understand ("boo-boo"), pictures ("Oucher" scale), and dolls to act out with, and pointing to areas of discomfort
    b. Person who speaks English as second language: Use of an interpreter, pictures (pain scale), and gestures, and pointing to areas of discomfort
    c. For the person with dementia, note their vocal response, facial movements, body movements, and inactivity.
17. a. In determining the location of the pain, the nurse should ask the patient to point to the area, or draw or trace the extent of the pain.
    b. Sample documentation: *Stating that pain is located on the R lower abdominal quadrant. Reports that the pain radiates upward slightly, with an intensity of 4 on a scale of 1-10.*
18. A pain rating of 7 or higher on a scale of 0 to 10 is an emergency.
19. The nurse should administer the pain medication about 30 minutes before painful activities.
20. Individualizing a patient's pain management may include
    - Using different types of pain relief measures
    - Providing pain relief measures before the pain becomes severe
    - Using measures that the patient believes are effective
    - Using the patient's ideas for pain relief and scheduling
    - Suggesting measures that are within the patient's capability
    - Choosing pain relief measures on the basis of the patient's responses
    - Encouraging the patient to try measures more than once to see if they may work
    - Keeping an open mind about nontraditional measures
    - Protecting the patient from more pain
    - Educating the patient about the pain
21. The correct statements regarding TENS are b, c, and e.
22. Medications used for mild to moderate pain include a and e.
23. Nonpharmacological interventions for pain relief include reduction/removal of painful stimuli, cutaneous stimulation, distraction, relaxation, guided imagery, anticipatory guidance, biofeedback, and hypnosis.
24. Adjuvant medications that may be used in conjunction with analgesics to manage pain are sedatives, anticonvulsants, steroids, antidepressants, antianxiety agents, and muscle relaxants.

25. The usual dosage of on-demand morphine for PCA is 1 mg every 10 minutes.
26. a. Priority nursing interventions for the patient with an epidural infusion include assessment of the site and patency of the tube along with maintenance of aseptic technique in site care.
    b. Priority assessment before and during administration of all analgesics is the patient's response to the medication, including respiratory status and degree of pain relief.
27. The nurse may adapt/alter the patient's environment to increase comfort by
    - Straightening wrinkled bed linen
    - Repositioning the patient
    - Loosening tight clothing or bandages (unless contraindicated)
    - Changing wet dressings or bed linens
    - Checking the temperature of hot/cold applications and bathwater
    - Lifting the patient up in bed, not pulling
    - Positioning the patient correctly on the bedpan
    - Avoiding exposure of the skin or mucous membranes to irritants (e.g., urine)
    - Preventing urinary retention by keeping the catheter patent
    - Preventing constipation by use of fluids, diet, and exercise
    - Reducing lighting that glares/shines directly on the patient
    - Checking the temperature of the room and the sensation of the patient
    - Reducing the level of noise and traffic
28. Phantom pain is seen in patients who have lost limbs or had strokes with paralysis.
29. Patient-controlled oral analgesia is Medication on Demand or MOD.
30. The best way to evaluate the effectiveness of pain management is to ask patients about their level of pain and/or observe their behavior.
31. The ABCDE approach is
    A: *A*sk about pain regularly. *A*ssess pain systematically.
    B: *B*elieve the patient and family in their report of pain and what relieves it.
    C: *C*hoose pain control options appropriate for the patient, family, and setting.
    D: *D*eliver interventions in a timely, logical, and coordinated fashion.
    E: *E*mpower patients and their families. ***E*nable** them to control their course to the greatest extent possible.
32. Concomitant symptoms associated with pain are nausea, headache, dizziness, urinary frequency, constipation, depression, restlessness, and anxiety.
33. a. True
    b. True
    c. False
    d. False
    e. True
    f. False
    g. False
    h. True
    i. True
    j. False
    k. True
    l. True

34. 3
35. 3
36. 4
37. 3
38. 2
39. 4
40. 3
41. 1
42. 1
43. 3
44. 4
45. 4
46. 2
47. 3
48. 4

CHAPTER 33

Case Studies

1. a. To assist this patient and the family with dietary planning, it is important to find out the following information:
      - Who prepares the food in the home?
      - Who buys the food, and where is the food purchased?
      - What foods are regularly eaten? Are there special foods for holidays or family occasions?
      - What are the patient's food preferences?

      In addition, the patient should keep a record of dietary intake (usually recorded for 3 to 7 days).
   b. Teaching about foods that are high in sodium and saturated fat is an important part of the plan for this patient. Reading labels and menus (if the patient eats out) will help in the selection of appropriate foods. The patient and family also may be informed about possible substitutions for foods, spices, and oils that are high in sodium and fat. Alternatives, such as polyunsaturated oils, lean meats, and egg substitutes, may be incorporated into meal preparation. A separate meal plan for the patient is usually not necessary because flavorings, such as lemon, can make foods attractive (as well as healthy) for the entire family. The most difficult times are often during holidays and special occasions, when food plays a central role in the family's activities. Low-salt and low-fat substitutions, wherever appropriate, should be used. Fresh or frozen fruits and vegetables, without sodium or fat-based sauces or additives, may be more flavorful than low-sodium canned foods. The patient also may be able to eat traditional foods, in moderation, on these occasions. Realistic expectations may work best for the patient rather than offering harsh, uncompromising restrictions.
2. Nutritional recommendations for a pregnant patient include
   - An increase of an additional 30 to 60 g protein daily
   - Calcium intake, especially critical in the third trimester
   - Supplemental iron
   - Folic acid intake increasing to 600 mcg daily during pregnancy
3. Nutritional considerations for an older adult patient include
   - Eating a balanced diet that contains a variety of foods; avoiding too much fat, cholesterol, sugar, and sodium or salt
   - Eating foods that have adequate amounts of starch and fiber, such as fruits and vegetables and whole-grain cereals and breads
   - Avoiding grapefruit and grapefruit juice
   - Drinking adequate fluids

- Consuming cream soups and meat-based vegetable soups as nutrient-dense sources of protein, with cheese, eggs, and peanut butter as useful high-protein alternatives
- Drinking milk for calcium and vitamin D; providing calcium supplements if lactose intolerance is present
- Taking vitamin and nutrient supplements, if necessary, for nutritional deficits

4. a. *Imbalanced Nutrition: More Than Body Requirements*
   General goals: safely achieve weight reduction, correct poor dietary patterns, achieve calorie or nutrient targets on a daily or weekly basis
   - Patient loses ½ to 1 lb per week.
   - Patient's daily fat intake is less than 30%.
   - Patient eliminates sugared beverages from diet.
   - Patient increases fruit and vegetable servings in diet to five servings per day.

   b. The teaching plan for these employees should include
   - Guidelines for nutrients and calories
   - Avoidance of foods high in fat, cholesterol, sugar, and sodium
   - Avoidance of "fast foods" and eating out too frequently
   - Label reading
   - Integration of exercise
   - Realistic weight loss goals
   - Avoidance of rapid weight loss plans or pills
   - Maintenance of the diet within the work environment and schedule

Chapter Review

1. i	5. j	9. b
2. c	6. g	10. d
3. a	7. f	
4. h	8. e	

11. The *Healthy People 2020* nutritional objectives are for individuals to decrease saturated fat intake in population 2 years and older; increase the variety of vegetable and fruit intake in the population 2 years and older; increase grain products intake and consumption of calcium in the population 2 years and older; reduce daily intake of sodium in the population 2 years and older.
12. a Vitamin K is synthesized by the body.
    b. Vitamins A, D, E, and K are fat soluble.
    c. Antioxidant vitamins are beta-carotene and vitamins A, C, and E.
13. a. Carbohydrates
    b. Proteins
    c. Fats
    d. Carbohydrates
    e. Fats
    f. Proteins
    g. Carbohydrates
14. Prevention of diarrhea: soluble fiber
    Prevention of constipation: insoluble fiber
15. Some general nutritional guidelines to share are
    - Eat a variety of foods; consume plenty of grains, fruits, and vegetables.
    - Balance the intake of food with the amount of physical activity.
    - Reduce the intake of sugar, sodium, fat/saturated fat, and cholesterol.
    - Moderate the intake of alcoholic beverages.
    - A copy of the ChooseMyPlate program may be provided and discussed with the patient.
16. Examples of alternative dietary patterns include vegetarians, ovolactovegetarians, and lactovegetarians. In addition, patients from diverse sociocultural backgrounds may have dietary patterns that are unique.
17. Minerals are inorganic elements that catalyze biochemical reactions. Macrominerals help to balance the pH of the body.
18. The roles of water in the body include transportation of nutrients and waste products; providing structure to large molecules (protein, glycogen); participation in metabolic reactions; serving as solvent, lubricant, and cushion; regulating body temperature; and maintaining blood volume.
19. a. Food and nutrient intake: 24-hour recall, percentage of meals consumed, food preferences, allergies, dislikes, and physical barriers to eating (oral discomfort, dysphagia)
    b. Physical examination: signs and symptoms of nutrient deficiencies, fat deposits, and poor muscle tone and skin turgor
    c. Anthropometric measurements: height, weight, and any changes in height or weight
20. Indicators of malnutrition include a, d, e, f, h, i, k, m, n, and p.
21. The nurse calculates this individual's BMI as 24.5, within the expected range of 18.5 to 24.9. The weight in pounds is rounded to 82 kg and the 6-foot height is 3.34 m^2.
22. Neurogenic causes of dysphagia include stroke, cerebral palsy, Guillain-Barré syndrome, multiple sclerosis, ALS, diabetic neuropathy, and Parkinson's disease.
    Myogenic causes include myasthenia gravis, aging, muscular dystrophy, polymyositis, and dermatomyositis.
23. A common sign of food-borne illnesses is diarrhea, often accompanied by cramping, nausea, and vomiting.
24. a. Stressors in the acute care environment include diagnostic testing (NPO, scheduling), pathologies, unit schedules, cafeteria food served, and medication administered.
    b. To promote a patient's appetite in the acute care setting, the nurse should
    - Enhance food presentation
    - Remove food covers from the patient's food tray
    - Clean the area and remove odors
    - Provide oral care
    - Provide for the best temperature and seasoning of the food
    - Include food preferences, as appropriate, within the diet
25. The patient with dysphagia should be
    - Provided with a rest period before eating
    - Positioned upright, with support as necessary, with the head flexed to a chin down position
    - Fed or taught to eat to the stronger side of the mouth
    - Given thicker fluids
    - Evaluated for the best level of diet
    - Fed slowly, provided smaller size bites, and allowed to chew thoroughly and swallow the bite before taking another
    - Allowed time to empty the mouth after each spoonful

26. Advantages of enteral nutrition include the following: decreased prevalence of hypoglycemia and electrolyte imbalances, increased use of nutrients, maintenance of structure and function of the GI tract, safer and less costly than parenteral nutrition.
27. a. Contraindications to N/G tubes are recent nasal surgery, basilar skull fractures, facial traumas, nosebleeds, and receiving anticoagulation.
    b. The most serious complication associated with tube feedings is aspiration.
    c. Aspiration can be avoided by positioning the patient upright (head of bed elevated at least 30 degrees).
    d. Displacement of the jejunostomy tube can lead to infusion of fluid into the peritoneal space, which can lead to serious complications.
    e. If the N/G tube becomes clogged, the nurse should
       - Verify that the tube is not misplaced or kinked.
       - Flush with warm water.
       - Flush the tube with water after checking the residual volume and periodically as ordered or per institutional protocol to avoid clogging.

       To prevent clogging:
       - Administer medications into the tube in liquid form whenever possible. If medications are appropriate to crush, ensure they are finely crushed and adequately diluted before administration.
       - Administer water before and after the administration of *each* medication.
       - Shake the formula in the feeding container periodically to reduce the settling of formula as sediment. Sediment at the bottom of the delivery container may clog the tube.
    f. Intermittent feeding tubes are clamped/closed to prevent air from entering the stomach.
    g. Gastrostomy tubes are preferred for enteral feeding longer than 3 weeks.
28. The label indicates that there are a fairly significant number of calories for only ½ cup. In addition, almost half of the calories are based on the fat content, with a significant percent being saturated fat. There is also more than ¼ of the recommended sodium, no fiber, and small amounts of vitamins and minerals.
29. Foods that could cause toddlers to choke are hot dogs, candy, nuts, grapes, raw vegetables, and popcorn.
30. Factors contributing to adolescent obesity and nutritional deficits include skipping meals or eating meals with wrong choices of calories, nutrients, and snacks.
31. The pH of gastric aspirate for a fasting patient is usually between 1 and 4.
32. A central venous line is used for a hyperosmolar solution.
33. a. PN is used because the patient is unable to ingest or digest enteral feedings.
    b. Nursing goals for PN are to prevent infection, maintain the PN system, prevent complications, and promote the patient's well-being.
    c. Nursing interventions to prevent complications of PN therapy include weighing the patient daily, monitoring I&O and caloric intake, testing urine or blood for glucose, obtaining blood samples for nutritional assessment, observing for fluid and electrolyte balance, and maintaining the correct infusion rate.
    d. The recommended infusion rate for lipids is 1 mL/min. Solutions should not be used if there is a separation of contents (oil/creamy layer on top) or if the solution is more than 12 hours old.
34. For patients without teeth or with ill-fitting dentures, a soft diet may be ordered. Patient preferences for foods should be taken into account, as well as consistencies, flavors, and colors.
35. The correct information for the Mini Nutritional Assessment (MNA) is found in a, c, d, and e.
36. a. True
    b. True
    c. True
37. ChooseMyPlate is directed at helping the obese and overweight population choose healthier foods and confront the obesity epidemic by providing a basic, visual guide for making food choices for a healthy lifestyle.
38. The correct interventions for the patient receiving enteral feedings are a, c, and e.
39. To decrease cholesterol, the best type of fatty acid intake is monounsaturated.
40. There will be slight variations to the documentation, depending on the record format, but the following should be indicated:
    10 Fr N/G tube inserted into left nare. Procedure tolerated without distress or complications. Placement verified via bedside X-ray.
41. The correct order to the enteral feeding is b, e, d, f, c, a, g.
42. The Subjective Global Assessment (SGA) includes a patient history, measurement of weight, and physical assessment.

43. 1	52. 4	61. 2
44. 1	53. 1	62. 1
45. 2	54. 4	63. 3
46. 2	55. 3	64. 2
47. 4	56. 1	65. 3
48. 1	57. 1	66. 2
49. 2	58. 4	67. 4
50. 2	59. 4	68. 4
51. 2	60. 1	

CHAPTER 34

Case Studies

1. a. Before the IVP, the patient should be assessed for
       - Allergies to shellfish, iodine, or contrast dyes.
       - Fluid status (avoid dehydration from bowel preparation because this may increase the potential toxicity of the contrast dye).
       - Medical conditions that increase risk (e.g., renal insufficiency).
       - Recent barium studies (tests within 2 to 3 days of the IVP will obscure findings).

       The patient should be instructed to
       - Take the cathartic the evening before the IVP.
       - Remain NPO after midnight.
       - Expect an IV infusion to be started for the injection of the dye.

- Expect a flushing sensation and a feeling of warmth, dizziness, or nausea when the dye is injected.
- Expect that a number of x-rays will be taken during the test and that voiding will be done near the end of the test.

b. After the IVP, the nurse will monitor I&O and report decreased or absent urination. The patient is informed that a normal diet may be resumed, fluid intake is encouraged, and any signs of an allergic reaction (e.g., itching or hives) should be reported.

2. a. The nurse may safely delegate the following urinary care measures: Assisting the patient with the use of the bedpan/urinal, monitoring I&O, maintaining aseptic technique, and promoting patient privacy and dignity. In some institutions, the established policy may allow for additional measures to be delegated, such as routine catheter care and specimen collection. Delegation to unlicensed assistive personnel requires that the nurse evaluate their ability to safely and accurately perform the specified measures.

3. a. The action proposed by the primary nurse is unsafe because it could result in serious damage to the patient's urethra. The correct procedure requires that you prepare a clean disposable towel, gloves, and a sterile syringe (same volume as the fluid in the catheter balloon). The patient is positioned in the same way as for catheter insertion, the syringe is attached to the balloon port, and the entire amount of fluid is aspirated. The catheter then is pulled out slowly and smoothly. If resistance is encountered, an additional attempt is made to remove fluid from the balloon. The catheter then is wrapped in a waterproof pad and disposed of in an appropriate container, along with the drainage tubing and bag (after emptying and measuring the remaining amount of urine). Perineal care then is provided to the patient, and the nurse will monitor the urinary output carefully.

4. a. The patient is provided with a sterile specimen cup, sterile disinfectant wipes, and clean gloves. He is instructed to apply the gloves and wipe the urinary meatus in a circular motion, moving up from the meatus to the glans penis. He also is cautioned against using the contaminated wipe repeatedly. After cleansing, the patient should discard the initial urination and begin collection in the sterile cup at the midstream portion of voiding. The cover of the specimen cup then is replaced, and the specimen is sent to the lab within 1 hour of the collection. If necessary to promote patient understanding, the use of more understandable terms, other than meatus and voiding, may be more effective.

5. a. With an incontinent urinary diversion, the urine drains continuously and the patient has no sensation or control over urinary output. This requires the application of a collection pouch at all times. The pouch will contain the urine and protect the skin from local irritation and skin breakdown as well as provide a barrier against odor. The pouch should be changed every 3 to 7 days, being cut to fit or a precut size. Each pouch may be connected to a bedside drainage bag for use at night. Consideration must be given to skin care to prevent breakdown. The patient may benefit from a referral to an ostomy support group.

Chapter Review

1. d	5. a	9. f
2. g	6. j	10. c
3. i	7. e	
4. h	8. b	

11. Noninvasive procedures for examination of urinary function include abdominal roentgenogram (radiograph of kidneys, ureters, and bladder [KUB]), intravenous pyelogram (IVP), renal scan, and computed tomography (CT).
12. Intermittent catheterization is used for immediate relief of bladder distention, long-term management of patients with incompetent bladders, sterile urine specimen collection, assessment of residual urine, and instillation of medication. Indwelling catheters are used for urinary outflow obstructions, patients having surgery of the urinary tract or surrounding structures, prevention of obstruction from blood clots, accurate monitoring of I&O and prevention of skin breakdown in critically ill or comatose patients, and provision of bladder irrigations.
13. A female patient may be placed in the lithotomy or Sims' position for catheterization.
14. a. The recommended daily fluid intake is 2000 to 2500 mL.
    b. The minimum urinary output for an adult is 30 mL per hour.
15. a. Sociocultural: Privacy needs for urination and schedule expectations (e.g., intermissions/recesses)
    b. Fluid intake: Increased intake will increase output (if fluid/electrolyte balance exists); alcohol, caffeine, and foods with high fluid content promote urination.
    c. Pathological conditions: Diabetes mellitus and multiple sclerosis cause neuropathies that alter bladder function, arthritis and joint diseases interfere with activity, renal disease influences amount and characteristics of urine, fevers reduce urinary output, and spinal cord injuries disrupt voluntary bladder emptying.
    d. Medications: Diuretics promote excretion of fluid and selected electrolytes, some drugs change the color of the urine, and some medications influence the ability of the bladder to relax and empty.
16. a. Arthritis can interfere with timely access to a toilet.
    b. Diabetes is associated with voiding frequently and the possibility of absent or weak bladder contractility.
    c. Prostate enlargement can result in hesitancy and interference with the ability to empty the bladder completely.
17. a. Stress incontinence
    b. Treatment for stress incontinence may include conditioning (Kegel) exercises, estrogen replacement, alpha-adrenergic agonists, intravaginal electrical stimulation, bladder neck suspension surgery, an artificial sphincter, or penile clamp.
18. Normal characteristics of urine are b and e.
19. The condom catheter should be changed every day, with the skin checked for signs of irritation and breakdown. Perineal care is provided with each catheter change. The tubing must be checked frequently to ensure that there are no kinks or other obstructions.

20. To maintain the patient's dignity when assisting with urinary elimination, the nurse should
    a. Provide comfort, privacy, time, access, and appropriate positioning.
    b. Provide gender-congruent care.
    c. Recognize cultural practices.
    d. Explain procedures.
21. Manual compression of the bladder is called Credé method.
22. Correct statements about urinary diversions are answers b and c.
23. For strict I&O measurement, the nurse should provide the patient with a urinal, bedpan, or urinary hat for the toilet.
24. To stimulate the patient to void, the nurse should run water near the patient, place the patient's hand in warm water, or stroke the inner thigh of a female patient.
25. To assist the patient to strengthen the pelvic floor muscles, the nurse teaches the patient Kegel exercises.
26. The length of catheter insertion is
    a. Female adult patient: 2 to 3 inches (5 to 7.5 cm)
    b. Male adult patient: 7 to 9 inches (17.5 to 22.5 cm)
27. Correct indwelling catheter care techniques are listed in options a, f, and g.
28. To prevent nocturia, the nurse instructs the patient to avoid drinking fluids at least 2 hours before bedtime. If the patient is taking a diuretic, the medication should be given early in the day.
29. An older adult may need to have an assistive device for ambulation to the bathroom, such as a walker. There may also be difficulty in removing clothes or getting on and off of the toilet.
30. For acute onset urinary retention, the correct items are a, c, d, and f.
31. Urinary tract infections may be prevented in patients with indwelling catheters by
    - Following good hand hygiene techniques
    - Not allowing the spigot on the drainage bag to touch a contaminated surface
    - Not opening the drainage system at connection points to obtain specimens or measure urine
    - Wiping the ends of the tube with antiseptic solution, if reconnection is necessary
    - Having a separate receptacle to measure urine for each patient
    - Not raising the drainage bag above the level of the bladder
    - Not allowing any dependent loops of tubing
    - Draining all urine from tubing into bag before the patient exercises or ambulates
    - Avoiding prolonged clamping or kinking of the tubing
    - Emptying the drainage bag at least every 8 hours
    - Removing the catheter as soon as possible upon health care provider order
    - Securing the catheter in place
    - Performing routine perineal hygiene every 8-hour shift and after defecation
32. With regard to a cystoscopy, answers a, c, e, g, h, and i are correct.
33. During a physical assessment:
    a. Presence of a kidney infection is determined by gently percussing the costovertebral angle (the angle formed by the spine and twelfth rib)
    b. The bladder is assessed by inspecting and observing a swelling or convex curvature of the lower abdomen. Upon gentle palpation of the lower abdomen, a full bladder is palpated as smooth and rounded. When a full bladder is palpated, patients will report a sensation of urinary urge tenderness or even pain. Percussion is an excellent technique to identify a full bladder. Gently tap the abdomen along the midline starting just above the umbilicus. The edge of the bladder is identified when the percussion note changes to a dull note.
34. a. The bladder scanner is used to determine the amount of residual urine.
    b. Measure post-void residual volumes 10 minutes after assisting the patient to void.
35. a. The urine for a patient taking Lasix will appear dilute.
    b. An individual with liver disease will have urine that is dark amber in color.
    c. With a urinary tract infection, the urine may be thick and cloudy with a foul odor.
36. Urinary specimens should be sent to the lab within 2 hours.
37. The correct order of steps is b, d, a, e, and c.
38. For the patient having a CT scan:
    a. Preparation before the test includes
        - Bowel cleansing (see agency or health care provider protocol)
        - Assessment for allergy to shellfish (iodine) or previous reaction to contrast media (if contrast is ordered)
        - Food and fluid restriction up to 4 hours prior to test (see agency or health care provider protocol)
        - Explain that they will be placed on a special bed that will move through a tunnel-like imaging chamber. They will need to lie still when instructed by the technician; some patients may feel claustrophobic.
    b. After the test:
        - Encourage fluids to promote dye excretion.
        - Assess for delayed hypersensitivity reaction to the contrast media.
39. To prevent a UTI, the nurse teaches the patient about hand hygiene and perineal care.
40. a. Triple lumen catheter
    b. Single lumen catheter
    c. Double lumen
41. After removal of a urinary catheter, the patient should have voiding monitored by using a voiding record or bladder diary. The bladder diary should record the time and amount of each voiding, including any incontinence. A bladder scan can be used to monitor bladder functioning by measuring post void residual (PVR). Careful monitoring should be done to observe for signs of a urinary tract infection.
42. For a suprapubic catheter:
    a. Suprapubic catheters are placed when there is blockage of the urethra (e.g., enlarged prostate, urethral stricture, after urological surgery) and in situations when a long-term urethral catheter causes irritation or discomfort or interferes with sexual functioning.
    b. Care of a suprapubic catheter involves daily cleansing of the insertion site and catheter. The same care for tubing and drainage bag as a urethral catheter applies

for a suprapubic catheter. The insertion site should be assessed for signs of inflammation and for the growth of over-granulation tissue. Site care applies principles of applying a dry dressing and institutional policy will indicate if aseptic or sterile technique is required.

43. The correct order for care of the stoma is b, d, e, c, a.
44. The medications used for urgency urinary incontinence are antimuscarinics, such as darifenacin, oxybutynin, and solifenacin.
45. Foods that can irritate the bladder include a, d, and f.
46. True
47. True
48. Urinary tract infections (UTIs) can be prevented by b, d, and f.
49. Measures to reduce the incidence of CAUTI are appropriate use, proper insertion and maintenance techniques, quality improvement programs, and ongoing surveillance for CAUTI and related causative factors.
50. Examples of possible questions are
    - Are you experiencing urgency, burning or painful urination, frequency, hesitancy, excessive urination, nocturia, dribbling, blood in the urine, straining to void, leaking urine on the way to the bathroom, leaking urine when you cough or sneeze?
    - Do you feel like you have completely emptied your bladder after you have urinated?
    - When did you last urinate?
    - Do you use a product to contain urine leakage? (adult brief, undergarment, pad)
    - How many containment products do you use during the day? At night?
51. The catheter tubing needs to be checked to make sure it is correctly anchored to the patient, as well as being hung above the floor on a part of the bed that does not move.
52. The lumen marked #3 is the one that would be used to inflate the balloon.

53. 3	62. 3	71. 4
54. 2	63. 1	72. 3
55. 3	64. 4	73. 2
56. 1	65. 4	74. 3
57. 3	66. 2	75. 2
58. 1	67. 3	76. 3
59. 2	68. 4	77. 1
60. 4	69. 2	78. 2
61. 2	70. 4	

CHAPTER 35

Case Studies

1. a. Nursing diagnosis: *Constipation related to overuse of laxatives/enemas and inadequate dietary fiber* (as manifested by patient's statement that she is having difficulty with bowel elimination)

   Goal: Patient will establish a regular defecation pattern within 1 to 2 months.

   Outcomes:
   - Patient will have a regular bowel movement within 3 days.
   - Patient's abdomen will be nondistended and nontender.
   - Patient will pass soft, formed stools at least every 2 to 3 days.

   Goal: Patient will maintain a diet that incorporates an adequate amount of fiber and fluids.

   Outcome:
   - Patient will identify and eat foods that are high in fiber and drink an adequate amount of fluid on a daily basis.

   Nursing interventions:
   - Providing instruction about foods high in fiber
   - Providing instruction on the importance of an adequate fluid intake
   - Allowing ample/regular time for defecation
   - Providing instruction on the adverse effects of reliance on laxatives/enemas
   - Investigating family and social contacts for stimulation of appetite
   - Identifying that daily bowel movements are not absolutely necessary

2. a. Before the colonoscopy, the patient should be instructed to
   - Drink clear liquids the day before.
   - Take some form of bowel cleanser (e.g., GoLYTELY).
   - Take enemas until clear, if ordered.

Chapter Review

1. c
2. e
3. a
4. b
5. d
6. Constipation in the older adult is usually the result of decreased fiber and fluid in the diet.
7. Patients should be cautioned against straining (Valsalva maneuver) on defecation if they have cardiovascular disease, glaucoma, increased intracranial pressure, or a new surgical wound.
8. a. *Clostridium difficile* is a common contributor to diarrhea in health care facilities.
   b. This occurrence may be prevented through proper hand hygiene and cautious use of antibiotics.
   c. As a result of diarrhea, the patient is at risk for fluid and electrolyte disturbances and anal irritation.
9. The most frequent complaints are related to functional bowel disorders.
10. Fecal incontinence can create skin breakdown, embarrassment, a change in body image, social isolation, depression, and diminished sexuality.
11. The following factors decrease peristalsis: a, c, d, f, g, j, and k.
12. Individuals from diverse cultural backgrounds may try to avoid exposure of the lower torso, refuse care from persons of the opposite gender, or not communicate issues related to bowel elimination.
13. Risk factors for colon cancer include
    - Age older than 50 years
    - Family history of colorectal cancer

- Ethnocultural background
- Personal history of inflammatory bowel disease
- High dietary intake of fats, with low fruit and vegetable intake

14. Examples of nursing interventions include
    a. Constipation: Increase intake of fiber (vegetables, fruits, whole grain cereals) and fluids, reduce caffeine intake, elevate the toilet seat, establish a routine, promote exercise, allow for privacy and time, provide chopped foods, rather than pureed (for poor dentition), provide mashed foods with fruit juices and hot tea (for difficulty swallowing).
    b. Diarrhea: Increase intake of low-fiber foods, replace fluids and electrolytes, reduce intake of milk/milk products and spicy foods, and provide perineal/perianal care.
15. a. Positioning: Squatting or sitting allows for intraabdominal pressure to be exerted and thigh muscles to be contracted to aid in defecation.
    b. Pregnancy: Constipation commonly occurs because of pressure of the fetus on the rectum.
    c. Diagnostic tests: Some tests require NPO or enemas in advance, and barium can harden and cause constipation if not eliminated after the test.
    d. Diet: Intake of fruits, vegetables, whole grain foods, and adequate fluid will promote bowel elimination.
    e. Personal habits: Failing to respond to the need to defecate and lack of privacy interfere with normal elimination patterns and lead to constipation. Hospitalized patients often share toilet facilities or use bedpans or bedside commodes. The resulting embarrassment causes them to ignore the urge to defecate.
16. The nurse may provide local application of heat, sitz baths, or topical medications (as prescribed) to promote comfort for the patient with hemorrhoids.
17. A GI assessment should include
    - Usual diet, fluid intake, and elimination patterns
    - Characteristics of the stool and recent changes, such as diarrhea
    - Health history: medications, illnesses, mobility, pain, surgery
    - Emotional status
    - Changes in appetite
    - Management of alterations: constipation, diarrhea, indigestion
18. a. The correct position for an adult patient is left Sims' position.
    b. 3 to 4 inches/7.5 to 10 cm for an adult and 2 to 3 inches/5 to 7.5 cm for a child.
    c. The height of the bag should be 12 inches or 30 cm.
    d. Kayexalate enema
    e. A hypertonic enema works by exerting osmotic pressure, pulling fluid from the interstitial spaces, and filling the colon with fluid. The distention in the colon promotes defecation.
    f. Fleet enema
    g. Castile soap
    h. "Enemas until clear" means that you repeat enemas until patient passes fluid that is clear of fecal matter. Check agency policy, but usually patients receive no more than three consecutive enemas, to avoid disruption of fluid and electrolyte balance. It is essential to observe contents of solution passed. Consider the results "clear" when no solid fecal material exists, but the solution is sometimes colored.
    i. The nurse assesses or delegates the assessment of the results of the enema, including the amount and color of the stool, and the patient's response.
19. The osmotic laxatives are a, c, and f.
20. The QSEN competency of patient-centered care is applied when the patient's needs and preferences are incorporated into the care.
21. The hyperosmolarity of enteral solutions draws fluid into the intestine and promotes defecation.
22. A focused assessment of a patient's bowel function should include
    - Chewing: Check the condition of teeth, gums, and mouth and ability to eat.
    - Mobility: Observe the gait, ability to assist with transfer, positioning, activity, and use of toilet facilities.
    - Anal sphincter function: Check for abdominal distention, impaction.
    - Abdominal muscle contractility: Observe muscle contraction (bearing down) while palpating lower abdomen.
23. a. Colorectal cancer: End colostomy
    b. Diverticulitis: Temporary end colostomy with pouch
24. The teaching plan for a patient with an ostomy should include b, g, h, and i.
25. The expected characteristics are a, e, and f.
26. Before giving a patient a bedpan, the nurse should position the patient with the head of the bed elevated at least 30 degrees, warm a metal bedpan, and provide privacy.
27. Skills b and d may be delegated to assistive personnel, if indicated in agency policy.
28. The gastric pH should be 5 or less.
29. a. *C. difficile* is transmitted by contact and factors that stimulate overgrowth (e.g., antibiotic use).
    b. Transmission of *C. difficile* can be reduced or prevented by employing hand hygiene with soap and water.
30. Examples of positive outcomes for a patient with a colostomy are
    - Skin surrounding the stoma will remain intact.
    - Patient will demonstrate proper peristomal skin care.
    - Patient will recognize and report complications.
31. Normal defecation can be promoted with a high-fiber diet, fluids, exercise/activity, and proper positioning and by allowing time and privacy.
32. Nasogastric tube irrigation is done with 30 mL of saline. Low intermittent suction should be applied.
33. The steps are completed as follows: b, c, e, h, i, b, f, j, d, a, and g. There are other interventions that are also done before and during these steps. These are some of the main actions related to the skill.

34. 2
35. 3
36. 3
37. 4
38. 3
39. 4
40. 1
41. 2
42. 1
43. 2
44. 4
45. 1
46. 1
47. 2
48. 2
49. 3
50. 3

CHAPTER 36

Case Studies

1. a. The patient may benefit the most from discussing her feelings, needs, and concerns with the nurse, and being involved, as much as possible, in the decision-making process for her plan of care. In addition, she may benefit from the following interventions:
   - Orienting her to the environment, routine/schedule, and staff members
   - Placing her with mobile patients who can interact with her
   - Encouraging frequent visits from family members and friends
   - Providing her with materials she enjoys, such as books and magazines
   - Providing stimulating diversional activity for her, such as music and games
   - Engaging in conversation with her during meals and implementation of nursing actions
   - Encouraging her to use any necessary assistive aids, such as glasses
   - Encouraging and assisting her (as necessary) to attend to daily grooming
   - Providing a stimulating physical environment, such as changing her view or decorating with personal objects
2. a. For the patient, there are safety considerations associated with the first time he will be getting out of bed. He could be prone to orthostatic hypotension, which is the drop in blood pressure from lying down or sitting to a standing position. When transferring from a supine position into a chair, move the patient gradually. First, obtain a baseline blood pressure and pulse with the patient in the supine position. Then raise the patient to a high-Fowler's position, and measure blood pressure and pulse again to detect decreases in blood pressure or elevations in pulse. Leave the patient in this position for 2 minutes to allow the body to adapt. Monitor the patient for dizziness or lightheadedness. The patient is now ready to sit at the side of the bed with the feet on the floor (dangling). If the patient experiences no dizziness, assist the patient to a chair. When transferring an immobile patient for the first time, make sure that assistance is available, if necessary.
3. a. Older adult patients are especially prone to the hazards of immobility. It is important to make sure that the following interventions are included in the patients' care:
   - Assess overall physiological and psychological status regularly
   - Skin: provide moisture, be gentle in moving and positioning
   - Respiratory: encourage deep breathing, coughing, moving
   - Musculoskeletal: incorporate range of motion into daily activities
   - Diet: make sure that sufficient fluids, vitamins and proteins are included
   - Elimination: assist in positioning, dietary intake of fluids and roughage
   - Cognitive/psychological: provide diversionary activities/stimulation, reality orientation, emotional support, explanations before care
   - Work with other members of the health care team to provide safe care and prevention of complications

Chapter Review

1. i
2. e
3. d
4. j
5. c
6. b
7. f
8. h
9. a
10. g
11. The objectives of bed rest are to decrease physical activity and oxygen needs, allow the ill/debilitated patient to rest, and prevent further injury.
12. Pathological influences on mobility include muscle and postural abnormalities, damage to the central nervous or musculoskeletal system.
13. The pathophysiological changes that occur with immobility include answers b, c, f, h, i, and k.
14. Fluid and electrolyte imbalances that occur with immobility include hypercalcemia and hypovolemia (initial phases).
15. An immobilized patient may react to the experience by exhibiting hostility, belligerence, inappropriate moods, altered sleeping patterns, withdrawal, confusion, anxiety, sadness, hopelessness, and depression.
16. The heart rate of an immobilized patient is generally 15% faster.
17. Virchow's triad refers to thrombus formation, and the three associated problems are (1) loss of integrity of the vessel wall, (2) abnormal blood flow, and (3) altered blood cells and clotting factors.
18. The nurse's focus for an immobilized child is on providing physical and psychosocial stimulation in order to keep pace with motor and intellectual development.
19. To maintain the patient's autonomy, the nurse encourages the patient to do as much as possible, demonstrate activities, and participate in goal setting and decision making.
20. The changes and interventions are
    - Cardiovascular system:
      - Orthostatic hypotension: Move the patient slowly from one position to another.
      - Increased cardiac workload: Place the patient in an upright position (if possible), provide regular exercise and adequate fluid intake.
      - Thrombus formation: Provide regular exercise, adequate fluid intake, and antiembolic stockings.
    - Respiratory system:
      - Hypostatic pneumonia and atelectasis: Encourage coughing and deep breathing, adequate fluid intake, and exercise; turning; upright positioning; and chest physiotherapy.
    - Integumentary:
      - Pressure ulcers: Assess the skin, use supportive devices, provide adequate nutrition and hydration, change position every 1 to 2 hours, and give meticulous skin care.

- Gastrointestinal:
  - Reduced appetite, inadequate/imbalanced nutrition, decreased peristalsis: Provide adequate nutrition (fruits, vegetables, fiber) and hydration, measure I&O, administer prescribed cathartics, promote activity or movement, and institute a bowel program.
- Urinary:
  - Urinary stasis resulting in greater risk for infection and calculi: Provide adequate hydration and promote activity and movement.
- Musculoskeletal:
  - Loss of strength and endurance, reduced muscle mass, decreased stability and balance, with possible contractures and disuse osteoporosis: Provide or encourage range-of-joint-motion exercises, turn every 1 to 2 hours, change position, and refer to physical therapy.

21. With the algorithm, a transfer aid should be selected for use.
22. Focused assessment of the patient's mobility includes range of joint motion (ROJM), pain, endurance, and activity.
23. a. Rotation of the neck
    b. Abduction of the arm
    c. Supination of the forearm
    d. Circumduction of the arm
    e. Hyperextension of the hip
24. To evaluate muscle atrophy, the nurse should perform anthropometric measurements—height, weight, and triceps skin folds.
25. The nurse checks for edema in the immobilized patient at the sacrum, hips, legs, and feet.
26. Assessment frequency (unless indicated by agency policy or changes in patient status):
    a. Respiratory status: every 2 hours
    b. Anorexia: at meals
    c. Urinary elimination: at the beginning or end of every shift
    d. Intake and output: every shift for daily measurement
    e. Anthropometic measurements: every 2 to 4 weeks
27. Specific exercises to prevent thrombus formation include ankle pumps, foot circles, knee flexion, and hip rotation.
28. For antiembolic stockings:
    a. Contraindications for use include dermatitis, open skin lesions, new skin grafts, and decreased circulation.
    b. The stockings are removed every shift.
    c. The stockings should not be partially rolled down or wrinkled, and the toes should not be uncovered.
    d. True
29. For a sequential compression device, options a and d are correct.
30. Newer Low Molecular Weight (LMW) heparins (anticoagulant) are usually given every 12 hours by the subcutaneous route.
31. For the immobilized patient with a suspected pulmonary emboli, actions b and e are correct.
32. The Morse Fall Scale should be used to assess the patient's probability of falling.
33. The patient can perform passive range of motion to the right side and active range of motion with the left side. Participation in ADLs, to the extent the patient is able, will also provide joint mobility.
34. The best ways to prevent pressure ulcers are to change the patient's position at least every 1 to 2 hours, assess the skin frequently, promote mobility, and provide moisture and hygienic care.
35. The following are examples of possible nursing diagnoses:
    - *Ineffective Airway Clearance*
    - *Risk for Constipation*
    - *Risk for Disuse Syndrome*
    - *Risk for Falls*
    - *Impaired Physical Mobility*
    - *Risk for Impaired Skin Integrity*
    - *Risk for Deficient Fluid Volume*
    - *Impaired Urinary Elimination*

36. 4	42. 3	48. 4
37. 3	43. 4	49. 2
38. 2	44. 2	50. 2
39. 3	45. 3	51. 3
40. 2	46. 1	52. 2
41. 4	47. 4	53. 4

CHAPTER 37

Case Study

1. a. Nursing diagnosis: *Risk for Impaired Skin Integrity related to prolonged pressure on bony prominences* (as manifested by reddened areas [reactive hyperemia] on sacrum, elbows, and heels)
   Goal: Integrity of skin and underlying tissues will be maintained.
   Outcomes:
   - Reactive hyperemia will subside and patient's normal skin coloration will return within 2 days.
   - Patient will assist, as possible, with turning and positioning every 1 to 2 hours.

   Nursing interventions:
   - Reposition or assist with repositioning every 1 to 2 hours.
   - Encourage the patient to shift weight when out of bed and in a chair.
   - Assess skin and underlying tissues with each position change.
   - Use supportive devices: padding for mattress and bony prominences.
   - Keep sacral area clean and dry.
   - Measure, document, and report reddened areas.

Chapter Review

1. g	5. j	9. e
2. h	6. a	10. f
3. b	7. i	
4. c	8. d	

11. Sites marked should include occipital bone (1), scapula (2), spine (3), elbow (4), iliac crest (5), sacrum (6), ischium (7), Achilles tendon (8), heel (9), and sole (10).

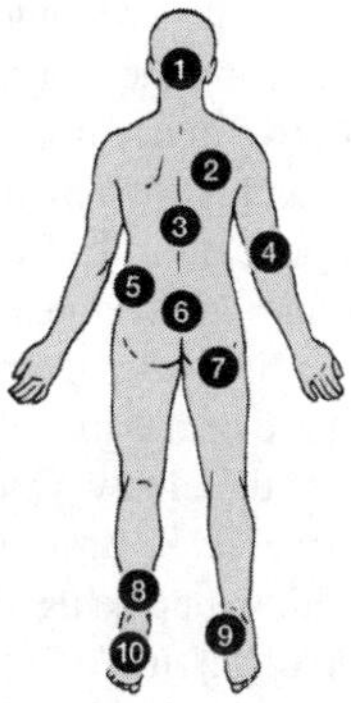

12. a. Stage I
    b. Stage III
13. External factors that contribute to pressure ulcers include shear, friction, and moisture on the skin.
    Internal factors include nutrition, infection, impaired peripheral circulation, obesity, and advanced age.
14. Infants, young children, and older adults are most susceptible to sensitivity to heat and cold therapy.
15. Dryness of the older adult's skin makes it less tolerant to pressure, friction, and shearing forces.
16. a. Primary intention
    b. Secondary intention
17. a. True
    b. True
18. a. Dehiscence
    b. Hematoma/bleeding
    c. Infection
    d. Infection
    e. Bleeding/shock
    f. Evisceration
    g. Infection
19. a. Assessment includes the location, extent of tissue damage, size (dimensions and depth of wound), tissue type (viable or nonviable) and percentage of wound tissue (e.g., viable versus nonviable), amount and color of wound exudate, and condition of surrounding skin.
    b. For darkly pigmented skin:
       - Look for changes in skin texture, temperature, and warmth.
       - Examine skin when pressure is applied and removed because the color can remain unchanged when pressure is applied.
       - Assess for color changes at the site of pressure that differ from patients with light skin color.
       - With a gloved finger, feel the area of potential skin damage as the skin in the injured area may feel cool to touch, indicating potential skin damage. Circumscribed area of intact skin is often warm to touch. As tissue changes color, intact skin feels cool to the touch.
       - If a patient previously had a pressure ulcer, that location maybe lighter in skin color.
       - Localized area of involved skin may be purple/blue or violet (eggplant) instead of red.
       - Edema may occur with induration and may appear shiny and taunt.
       - Patient may complain of discomfort at a site that is predisposed to pressure ulcer development.
20. a. Age: Infants and older adults may have decreased circulation, oxygen delivery, clotting, and inflammatory responses, with an increased risk of infection. Older adults have slower cell growth and differentiation, and scar tissue is less pliable.
    b. Obesity: Obese individuals have a decreased supply of blood vessels in fatty tissue (impaired delivery of nutrients to the site), and suturing of adipose tissue is more difficult.
    c. Diabetes: Individuals with this condition have small blood vessel disease (reduced oxygen delivery), and elevated glucose levels impair macrophage function.
    d. Immunosuppression: A reduced immune response leads to poor healing. Steroids also mask signs of inflammation/infection, and chemotherapeutic agents interfere with leukocyte production.
21. a. 3, serous
    b. 4, sanguineous
    c. 1, serosanguineous
    d. 2, purulent
22. a. Pressure reduction: Use of a supportive surface, regular and frequent turning and repositioning in the bed (q2h) and chair (q1h)
    b. Skin care: Keep skin clean and dry after incontinence, use skin barriers/protectants, turn or lift sheets to reduce friction and shear, maintain head of the bed at 30 degrees or lower, avoid vigorous massage of bony prominences or areas of redness
23. To obtain a wound culture, the steps are e, c, d, a, and b.
24. The patient who has a dirty, penetrating wound may require a tetanus toxoid injection.
25. The nurse determines wound healing by measuring the wound diameter and depth, assessing the wound tissue, checking the skin condition around the wound, and observing for exudate.
26. A patient who is out of bed in a chair should be limited to 2 hours sitting and repositioned at least every 1 hour.
27. The nurse reduces friction or shear by using a draw sheet, trapeze bar, and/or support when moving the patient and by providing skin care to maintain integrity.
28. Care of an abrasion or laceration includes control of any bleeding, rinsing of the wound under running water, gentle cleansing with mild soap, application of a prescribed or over-the-counter antiseptic, and protection with a bandage.
29. For a negative pressure wound therapy system:
    a. The purpose is to remove excess fluid, stimulate granulation tissue growth, and reduce wound bacteria.
    b. The tube is attached to suction to provide negative pressure.
    c. The dressing that is used is either black or white foam cut to fit the wound. The transparent dressing should cover

the wound, extend 3 to 5 cm beyond the wound edges, provide an occlusive seal, and be free of wrinkles.

   d. If there is an increase in discomfort and using black foam, switch to white foam. Notify the supervisor and/or provider.

30. For wound irrigation:
    a. Syringe size: 35 mL
    b. Needle size: 19 gauge
    c. psi: 8
    d. The syringe is held 1 inch (2.5 cm) above the wound.
    e. Reduce the irrigating pressure and notify the health care provider.
    f. Use more fluid or pressure.
31. a. Wound closed with staples
    b. Jackson-Pratt wound drainage system
32. The correct nursing interventions are statements a and d.
33. The steps in caring for a traumatic wound are
    - Stabilize the patient's cardiopulmonary function.
    - Promote hemostasis (stop any bleeding).
    - Cleanse the wound.
    - Protect the site from further injury.
34. a. Cold (C)
    b. Heat (H)
    c. Heat (H)
    d. Heat and cold (H and C)
    e. Heat (H)
35. a. Application of heat is contraindicated in the presence of active bleeding or acute inflammation, and for patients with cardiovascular disease.
    b. Application of cold is contraindicated in the presence of edema at the site, decreased circulation, and shivering.
36. Heat and cold are usually applied for about 20 to 30 minutes.
37. The correct interventions for application of heat and cold are a and g.
38. Total score = 13 points
    Patient risk = "at risk" status
39. The correct actions for a moist dressing are a, c, and e.
40. a. Nonblanchable hyperemia is redness that persists after palpation and indicates tissue damage.
    b. This signifies that deep tissue damage is present and is commonly the first stage of pressure ulcer development.
    c. True: Damage can be reversed with the removal of pressure.
41. For a postoperative dressing, the correct actions are b, c, and e.
42. Before the patient is discharged, the nurse will want to assess/evaluate the patient's
    - Wound and overall health status
    - Ability to perform the dressing independently
    - Concerns over the care and the appearance of the wound
    - Recognition of signs and symptoms that will require notification of the physician
    - Ability to obtain necessary supplies
43. Topical skin care should include b, c, and e.
44. False. It is usually clean technique.
45. 1. c; 2. a; 3. b
46. The correct way to remove old tape is to apply pressure against the skin away from the tape. It may be necessary to moisten the tape with normal saline, if it is very sticky.
47. Discomfort may be reduced during dressing changes by administering analgesics 30 minutes before, allowing "time-outs" during painful procedures, planning dressing changes when a patient is feeling best, soaking dried dressings before removal, avoiding aggressive packing, positioning and supporting the wound area, and using low adhesive or nonadhesive dressings.
48. A sling is correctly applied by having the patient sit or lie supine for a sling application. Instruct the patient to bend the affected arm, bringing the forearm straight across the chest. The open sling fits under the patient's arm and over the chest, with the base of the triangle under the wrist and the triangle's point at the elbow. One end of the sling fits around the back of the neck. Bring the other end up over the affected arm while supporting the extremity. Tie the two ends at the side of the neck so that the knot does not press against the cervical spine. You can fold the loose fold at the elbow evenly around the elbow and pin it. To prevent the formation of dependent edema, make sure the lower arm is always supported at a level above the elbow.
49. The desired temperature for a cold soak is 59° F or 15° C.

50. 1	57. 3	64. 1
51. 3	58. 2	65. 2
52. 3	59. 2	66. 3
53. 4	60. 3	67. 2
54. 2	61. 4	68. 4
55. 4	62. 1	
56. 3	63. 3	

CHAPTER 38

Case Studies

1. a. For this patient, you may implement the following interventions to maintain sensory stimulation:
    - Referring the patient to community agencies (e.g., Foundation for the Blind)
    - Recommending/assisting in obtaining books with larger print, audiotape books, and music
    - Recommending the introduction of brighter colors (e.g., red, orange, yellow) into the home environment (which also helps for him to better differentiate between surfaces and room objects)
    - Investigating family and social contacts
    - Allowing time for discussion of feelings, needs, and concerns

   b. To promote safety, you should
    - Assist in arranging the environment so that the patient knows where everything is and that clutter is out of the way
    - Instruct/assist in improvement of lighting in halls and stairways and use of color-coding (e.g., edges of stairs, medication bottles, and appliance dials)
    - Instruct about importance of follow-up visits to the ophthalmologist
2. a. A patient in an intensive care unit (ICU) may experience sensory overload from the intensity of sounds and activity and/or sensory deprivation from restricted visits of family and friends.

b. The nurse should try to organize care so that the patient is allowed opportunity for uninterrupted rest, whenever possible. Monitors at patient's bedside may have volume controls so that they can be turned down to a lower level. The nurse also should take time to sit with the patient, either quietly or for verbal stimulation. Visits from family members and friends should be encouraged but not to the point of patient fatigue. The environment may be arranged so that the patient has a different or more pleasant view, and personal items (e.g., photos) may be placed within the patient's field of vision. It may be a challenge for the nurse in this setting to adapt the patient's sensory input, so creativity, within realistic limits, is recommended.

Chapter Review

1. a. Visual
   b. Auditory
   c. Gustatory
   d. Olfactory
   e. Tactile
   f. Kinesthetic
2. Diseases that may lead to visual impairment include age-related macular degeneration, glaucoma, cataracts, and diabetic retinopathy.
3. a. Cerumen accumulation
   b. Presbycusis
   c. Cataract
   d. Xerostomia
   e. Ménière's disease
4. a. Age, older adulthood:
      - Decreased hearing acuity, speech intelligibility, and pitch discrimination
      - Increased dryness of cerumen, with obstruction of the auditory canal
      - Reduced visual fields; increased glare sensitivity; impaired night vision; reduced accommodation, depth perception, and color discrimination
      - Reduced sensitivity to odors and diminished taste discrimination
      - Difficulty with balance, spatial orientation, and coordination
      - Diminished sensitivity to pain, pressure, and temperature
   b. Medications: may cause ototoxicity or optic nerve irritation (chloramphenicol) or may reduce sensory perception (analgesics, sedatives, antidepressants)
   c. Smoking: may cause atrophy of taste buds and interference with olfactory function
   d. Environment: excessive stimuli, frequent activities, noise, TV, bright lights, pain, confinement
5. Assessment of vision and hearing:
   - Ask the patient to read.
   - Observe the performance of ADLs (activities of daily living).
   - Observe the patient's use of glasses, magnifiers, or hearing aids.
   - Observe patient's conversation/interaction with others.
6. a. Trauma is the leading cause of blindness in children, usually as the result of flying objects or penetrating wounds.
   b. Child eyesight safety includes avoiding toys with long, pointed handles or sharp edges; keeping the child from running with a pointed object; and keeping pointed objects and tools out of reach.
   c. Chronic middle ear infections and exposure to loud noise contribute to hearing loss in children.
7. Orientation to the environment should include
   - Keeping your name tag visible, addressing the patient by name, explaining the patient's location, and frequently identifying the time and date in conversations
   - Offering short and simple, repeated explanations and reassurance
   - Encouraging family and friends not to argue with or contradict a confused patient but to explain calmly their location, identity, and time of day
   - Walking the patient through a room to feel the walls and establish a sense of direction
   - Approaching a visually impaired patient from the front
   - Explaining the location of objects within the room, such as chairs or equipment
   - Keeping all objects in the same place and position and describing the location of key items
   - Placing necessary objects such as the call light, patient-controlled analgesia (PCA) button, glasses, water, or facial tissue in front of patients
   - Asking the patient how to arrange objects so ambulation is easier
   - Removing clutter and unnecessary equipment and keeping the path to the bathroom clear
8. Sensory stimulation may be modified in the acute care environment by
   - Increasing the patient's view outside and within the room
   - Arranging decorations, plants, photos, greeting cards, and the patient's personal items
   - Providing audio books and large-print reading material
   - Spending time with the patient; listening to and conversing with the patient
   - Playing pleasant music or turning on television shows that the patient enjoys
   - Providing attractive meals at the correct temperature
   - Providing a variety of textures and aromas to enhance the patient's appetite
9. The nurse may communicate with a hearing-impaired patient by
   - Making sure that a hearing aid, if needed, is in place and in working order
   - Approaching the patient from the front to get his or her attention
   - Facing the patient on the same level, with adequate lighting
   - Making sure that glasses, if needed, are worn and are clean
   - Speaking slowly and articulating clearly, using a normal tone of voice
   - Rephrasing, rather than repeating information that is not heard
   - Using visible expressions and gestures
   - Talking toward the patient's better ear
   - Using written information to reinforce spoken words
   - Not restricting the hands of deaf patients

- Avoiding eating, chewing, or smoking while speaking with the patient
- Avoiding speaking while walking away, in another room, or from behind the patient

10. Patients with cataracts exhibit a, c, e, and f.
11. a. Hearing deficit: Amplify low-pitch sounds, use lamps with sound activation, use assistive devices for telephones, and obtain closed captioning for the television.
    b. Diminished sense of smell: Use smoke and carbon monoxide detectors, take special care with disposal of matches and cigarettes, and check the expiration dates on foods.
    c. Diminished sense of touch: Lower the temperature of the water heater and use caution when checking the bath or shower water.
12. Nursing diagnoses for a patient with a sensory deficit include
    - *Disturbed Body Image*
    - *Fear*
    - *Hopelessness*
    - *Risk for Injury*
    - *Powerlessness*
    - *Self-Care Deficit, Bathing*
    - *Self-Care Deficit, Dressing*
    - *Risk for Situational Low Self-Esteem*
    - *Impaired Social Interaction*
    - *Social Isolation*

    Possible goals/outcomes include the following: The patient will manage self-care, ambulate safely, verbalize feelings, remain oriented to surroundings, communicate/interact with others, participate in planning care, identify community resources.
13. a. General screenings include examinations for congenital blindness and visual impairment in infants and young children, routine vision and hearing tests of school-age and adolescent children, regular medical eye/ear examinations every 2 to 4 years for individuals older than age 40 and every 1 to 2 years for those older than age 65.
    b. The specific recommendation for hearing screenings is for at least once every decade through age 50, and then once every 3 years.
14. The appropriate actions for promotion of sensory stimulation in the home are a, d, and e.
15. Drugs that may cause ototoxicity are a, d, and f.
16. A patient may not use his/her hearing aid because of its appearance, a denial of its need, fit, the difficulty in manipulating a small object, cost, or a lack of understanding of its use.
17. A patient with diminished tactile sense may be helped with the use of Velcro and zippers, and providing assistance with or encouragement for grooming (e.g., hairbrushing) of the affected side.
18. Ménière's disease is characterized by progressive low-frequency hearing loss, vertigo, tinnitus, and a full feeling or pressure in the affected ear.
19. Care for a hearing aid includes
    - Making sure your fingers are dry and clean before handling hearing aids
    - Inserting and removing the hearing aid over a soft surface
    - Placing the battery in hearing aid when it is turned off
    - Removing the hearing aid battery when not in use and storing it in a marked container in a safe place
    - Protecting hearing aids from water and excessive heat or cold
    - Using a soft dry cloth to wipe hearing aids and a soft brush to clean difficult to reach areas
20. Specific adult behaviors include a, c, and e.
21. Examples of available community resources are the American Foundation for the Blind, American Red Cross, Canine Companions, Lions Club, and public health/visiting nurse services.
22. The occupational health nurse reinforces the use of protective devices, such as eye goggles and earplugs, as well as participates in safety policy development and environmental and employee screening.
23. Patients who are more prone to sensory deprivation are those in medical isolation/private rooms, alone in the home, immobilized in hospitals or other facilities, separated from family and friends, and experiencing disabilities that restrict mobility and/or sensory function.

24. 2	28. 4	32. 1
25. 2	29. 4	33. 2
26. 3	30. 2	34. 3
27. 1	31. 3	35. 1

CHAPTER 39

Case Studies

1. a. Explain and demonstrate coughing and deep-breathing exercises with splinting of the abdominal incision. Assist in and encourage turning and positioning every 2 hours. Reinforce the use of the incentive spirometer. Explain and demonstrate range-of-motion exercises. Provide prescribed analgesia before activities, keeping in mind the action and dosage of the medication and its possible effect on the patient.
2. a. Preoperative teaching for the patient who is having ambulatory surgery may occur when the patient comes for preoperative tests and physical assessment. There also may be telephone contact with the patient on the evening before the surgery, as well as a 24-hour resource line for the patient to use for questions. Additional teaching may be conducted immediately before the procedure and before the patient's discharge. Information provided to the patient usually includes instructions specific to the surgery and anesthesia (e.g., dressings, activity and dietary restrictions), signs and symptoms of complications, and time frame for follow-up visits.
   b. If the patient does not appear to understand about the surgery or possible complications, then you should contact the surgeon, so that he or she can meet with the patient and review the procedure. It is not the nurse's responsibility or appropriate for the nurse to explain the procedure. The alert and oriented patient must have an understanding of the surgery that will be performed to sign the consent.

3. a. Any significant change in the patient's status should be reported to the surgeon and/or anesthesiologist immediately. Because of the effects of general anesthesia, temperature alterations are especially critical before surgical procedures. Surgery may be postponed until the patient's temperature has returned to normal.
4. a. The patient should be informed that, under usual circumstances, all loose items are removed before surgery. If the patient will be adversely affected by the removal of his "lucky" medallion, it may be pinned inside of the patient's gown or surgical cap, depending on the type of surgery. It is important, however, that the operating room personnel be informed that the patient has the medallion in place before the surgery. It may be the policy of the agency that the patient will have to sign a form stating that he has kept the medallion (or other jewelry) on his person in case of a loss.
   b. The other items that you will remove or account for before surgery are wigs, dentures, partial plates, caps/loose caps, and all removable prosthetics (eyes, limbs, etc.). If a patient has a brace or splint, check with the surgeon to determine whether it should remain with the patient, to be reapplied after surgery. Although patients must remove hearing aids, eyeglasses, and contact lenses, do not have them do this until just before the surgery.
5. a. Before the patient's discharge, it is important to know the following:
   - Degree of mobility that the patient should have and the prescription for exercise and rest
   - Pain relief measures
   - Wound care requirements
   - Patient and family expectations for recovery, including concerns about restrictions and length of time for convalescing
   - Schedule for medical follow-up
   - Recognition of the signs and symptoms indicating the need to seek medical follow-up
   - Nutritional needs
   - Other medical conditions that may have an impact upon the patient's recovery
   - Financial concerns
6. a. For the patient in the PACU, you will need to monitor his vital signs every 15 minutes or more frequently, especially the oxygen saturation. He will have to be aroused more often and reminded to breathe deeply. In addition, the abdomen and dressing will have to be assessed to make sure that there are no signs of internal hemorrhage.
   b. For this patient, you will want to palpate or use a scanner to see if his bladder is distended. If the patient is able, you can stand him up to urinate and provide oral fluid intake. Taking the patient to the bathroom, where there is privacy and the ability to run the water, may help to stimulate urination. In the event that the patient is unable to urinate after more than 8 hours, an order for catheterization may be required.

Chapter Review

1. g
2. c
3. a
4. f
5. h
6. e
7. d
8. b
9. a. The patient who smokes cigarettes is at a greater risk for bronchospasm or laryngospasm.
   b. Aggressive pulmonary hygiene should be instituted for this patient, including frequent turning, coughing and deep breathing, incentive spirometry, and chest physiotherapy.
10. a. The following medical conditions may increase a patient's surgical risk: bleeding disorders, diabetes mellitus, heart disease, upper respiratory tract infection, cancer, liver disease, fever, chronic respiratory disease, immunological disorders, and abuse of street drugs.
    b. Malignant hyperthermia is an inherited disorder that is associated with general anesthesia.
    c. Pregnant patients are at greater surgical risk because:
       - Cardiac output and respiratory tidal volume increase to keep up with the increase in metabolism and blood pressure decreases, making interpretation of vital signs and recognition of hypovolemic shock more difficult.
       - The high level of progesterone relaxes the lower esophageal sphincter (LES) and decreases gastrointestinal motility, which slows gastric emptying, resulting in an increased risk for aspiration of stomach contents.
       - Near term there is an increase in white blood cells beyond the normal range for that of non-pregnant women who have no infection.
       - There is an increased risk for deep vein thrombosis as a result of increased fibrinogen levels and decreased clotting time.
       - In addition, a pregnant patient and her family experience increased psychological stress because of fear of fetal loss or deformity.
11. a. Cardiovascular: Changes in structure and function reduce cardiac reserve and predispose the patient to postoperative hemorrhage, increased blood pressure, and clot formation.
    b. Pulmonary: Changes in structure and function reduce vital capacity, increase the volume of residual air left in the lungs, and reduce blood oxygenation.
    c. Renal: Changes in structure and function increase the possibility of shock with blood loss, limit the ability to metabolize drugs/toxic substances, increase the frequency of urination and the amount of residual urine, and reduce the sensation of the need to void.
    d. Neurological: Changes in function reduce the ability to respond to warning signs of complications and may lead to confusion after anesthesia.
12. Obesity places a patient at greater risk as a result of diminished ventilatory capacity and higher risk of aspiration. There may also be other issues relating to circulation, endocrine function, and musculoskeletal integrity.

13. a. Insulin: For a patient with diabetes, the need for insulin is reduced preoperatively because of NPO status. Dose requirements may increase postoperatively because of stress response and IV administration of glucose solutions.
    b. Antibiotics: Potentiation of anesthetics, possible respiratory depression from depressed neuromuscular transmission
    c. NSAIDs: Inhibited platelet aggregation and prolonged bleeding time
14. General information in preoperative teaching includes
    - Preoperative and postoperative routines
    - Expected sensations
    - Pain relief measures available (e.g., PCA)
    - Postoperative exercises
    - Activity and dietary restrictions
15. Routine preoperative screening tests include complete blood count, serum electrolyte analysis, coagulation studies, serum creatinine test, urinalysis, 12-lead electrocardiogram, and a chest x-ray.
16. Commonly used preoperative medications include
    - Sedatives: used for relaxation and decrease in nausea
    - Tranquilizers: used to decrease anxiety and relax skeletal muscles
    - Narcotic analgesics: used to sedate, decrease pain and anxiety, and reduce the amount of anesthesia needed
    - Anticholinergics: used to decrease mucous secretions in the oral and respiratory passages and prevent laryngospasm
17. Nursing diagnoses that may be formulated include
    - *Anxiety:* achieving emotional and physiological comfort and rest
    - *Deficient Knowledge:* understanding the physiological and psychological responses to surgery; understanding intraoperative and postoperative events
18. NPO criteria:
    a. 2 hours before
    b. 8 to 12 hours before
19. The uses and side effects of the types of anesthesia are
    a. General anesthesia: used for major procedures that require extensive tissue manipulation. Side effects include cardiovascular depression or irritability, respiratory depression, and liver and kidney damage.
    b. Regional anesthesia: used when operating on a specific body area. Side effects include a sudden decrease in blood pressure and respiratory paralysis.
    c. Local anesthesia: used for minor procedures, especially in ambulatory surgery, and after general anesthesia for postoperative pain relief. Side effects include local irritation and inflammation.
    d. Conscious sedation: used for procedures that do not require complete anesthesia. Respiration is maintained and the patient can respond to stimuli. Side effects include respiratory depression and decreased level of consciousness.
20. Appropriate preoperative interventions include a, c, d, and f.
21. Verification in the PSCU and OR includes
    a. Right patient: Ask patient to state name; inspect patient identification band for patient name and date of birth and compare with medical record.
    b. Right frame of mind: observe for signs of fear and anxiety, monitor vital signs for indications of excessive anxiety, and compare vital signs to baseline.
    c. Preparation for surgery: determine and mark the body area for the procedure, establish or verify IV, insert urinary catheter (if ordered), check that preoperative checklist and medications are done, and remove glasses and other prostheses.
22. a. Circulating nurse (C)
    b. Scrub nurse (S)
    c. Circulating nurse (C)
    d. Circulating nurse (C)
    e. Scrub nurse (S)
    f. Circulating nurse (C)
    g. Scrub nurse (S)
23. For intraoperative patient care:
    a. To prevent injury: sterile drapes, sponge and instrument counts, careful positioning, eye protection, grounding of electrical devices, availability of emergency equipment
    b. To maintain body temperature: warm room, warm irrigating solutions, warm blanket after surgery
    c. To prevent infection: standard precautions, sterile asepsis, skin scrubs
24. a. Pulmonary stasis: turning every 1 to 2 hours, coughing, deep breathing, incentive spirometry, chest physiotherapy
    b. Venous stasis: range-of-joint-motion (ROJM) exercises, turning, antiembolitic stockings, sequential compression device, adequate fluids
    c. Wound infection: sterile technique for dressing changes, standard precautions, adequate nutrition (proteins for wound healing)
    d. GI stasis: a gradual progression in dietary intake, promotion of ambulation and exercise, provision of an adequate fluid intake, administration of fiber supplements, stool softeners, enemas, and rectal suppositories as ordered, assisting with proper positioning, and stimulation of the patient's appetite; frequent oral hygiene and meals when the patient is rested and free from pain
25. The patient is qualified to be discharged based on options a, d, f, h, and i.
26. The patient should void within 8 hours of the procedure. For the patient who has not voided, the nurse should palpate the area above the symphysis pubis to determine the presence of bladder distention. A bladder scanner may be used to see if residual urine is present. The surgeon should be notified of the patient's inability to void.
27. The first oral intake is usually a clear liquid diet.
28. Appropriate care for an operative incision includes answers b, c, and f.
29. a. The patient in the illustration is demonstrating the use of an incentive spirometer.
    b. This device is used to prevent atelectasis and promote respiratory function.
30. For the patient who will remain alert during a surgical procedure, the nurse should explain the procedure, encourage questions, and warn the patient when unpleasant sensations will be experienced. Some settings provide music to mask unpleasant sounds and to promote relaxation.

31. Routine postoperative assessment includes
    - Monitoring vital signs and pulse oximetry
    - Respiratory assessment: monitoring respiratory rate, rhythm, and depth every 15 min × 4 or until stable, then every 30 min × 2, and then every hour × 4; comparing with baseline findings
    - Auscultating lung and heart sounds
    - Performing pain assessment with pain tool, including severity, location, description, measures used to relieve; assessing for any side effects of pain medication (altered mental status, depressed respirations, bradycardia, orthostatic hypotension, nausea or vomiting, urinary retention, constipation); observing patient's expressions, body position, ability to rest, or sleep
    - Wound assessment: observing surgical wound for redness, edema, warmth, drainage, and dehiscence; inspecting for amount of bleeding on dressing, in drainage systems, and underneath patient
    - Assessing level of consciousness and symptoms of restlessness or altered mental status
    - Observing skin, nail beds, and mucous membranes for color and hydration
    - Palpating peripheral pulses distal to surgical site, tight dressing, or cast if present
    - Inspecting any urine output; note color, consistency, and odor
    - GI assessment: inspecting for abdominal distention; auscultating for bowel sounds in all four quadrants at least every shift until discharge; palpating abdomen for firmness
    - Monitoring NG tube for patency and NG tube output for color and amount of drainage if present
    - Observing patient's ability and willingness to tolerate fluids and food
    - Monitoring laboratory values for signs of complications
32. A latex allergy is evident with the patient who has contact dermatitis with redness, inflammation, and blisters; has contact urticaria with pruritus, redness, and swelling; or has hay fever–like symptoms and anaphylaxis.
33. The recommendation is for systemic, around-the-clock analgesia.
34. The correct interventions are a, c, e, and f.
35. Interventions to decrease postoperative wound infection include the clipping of hair (vs. shaving), disinfection of the skin with an antiseptic agent such as chlorhexidene immediately before the incisional cut, administration of a prophylactic antibiotic, delay of dressing change until 48 hours after surgery, and adherence to principles of asepsis.
36. The hand-off communication is:
    A - **A**dministrative data, N - **N**ew clinical information must be updated, T - **T**asks to be performed by the covering provider must be clearly explained, I - **I**llness severity must be communicated, C - **C**ontingency plans for changes in clinical status must be outlined
37. Examples of postoperative nursing diagnoses are
    Ineffective Airway Clearance
    Anxiety
    Disturbed Body Image
    Ineffective Breathing Pattern
    Risk for Deficient Fluid Volume
    Risk for Infection
    Impaired Physical Mobility
    Nausea
    Acute Pain
    Delayed Surgical Recovery
    Examples of postoperative patient outcomes are stable vital signs, reduction in incisional pain, oxygen saturation above 92%, able to ambulate with assistance, and incision clean, dry, and infection free.

38. 3
39. 1
40. 3
41. 1
42. 2
43. 2
44. 2
45. 4
46. 3
47. 3
48. 2
49. 1
50. 3
51. 4
52. 2
53. 2
54. 4
55. 2
56. 3
57. 4
58. 3
59. 2
60. 3
61. 2

BRIEF CONTENTS

ESSENTIALS *for* NURSING PRACTICE

EIGHTH EDITION

Patricia A. Potter, PhD, RN, FAAN
Director of Research
Patient Care Services
Barnes-Jewish Hospital
St. Louis, Missouri

Anne Griffin Perry, EdD, RN, FAAN
Interim Dean and Professor
School of Nursing
Southern Illinois University—Edwardsville
Edwardsville, Illinois

Patricia A. Stockert, PhD, RN
President, College of Nursing
Saint Francis Medical Center College of Nursing
Peoria, Illinois

Amy Hall, RN, PhD, CNE
White Family Endowed Professor and Chair of Nursing
Dunigan Family Department of Nursing and Health Sciences
University of Evansville
Evansville, Indiana

ELSEVIER

ELSEVIER
MOSBY

3251 Riverport Lane
St. Louis, Missouri 63043

ESSENTIALS FOR NURSING PRACTICE ISBN: 978-0-323-11202-4

International Standard Book Number 978-0-323-11202-4

Executive Content Strategist: Tamara Myers
Senior Content Development Specialist: Tina Kaemmerer
Publishing Services Manager: Deborah L. Vogel
Senior Project Manager: Jodi M. Willard
Design Direction: Paula Catalano

Printed in Canada

Last digit is the print number: 9 8 7 6 5 4 3 2 1

CONTRIBUTORS

Michelle Aebersold, PhD, RN
Clinical Assistant Professor
School of Nursing
University of Michigan
Ann Arbor, Michigan

Brenda A. Battle, MBA, BSN, RN
Vice President for Care Delivery Innovations
Assistant Dean of Diversity and Inclusion
University of Chicago Pritzker School of Medicine
Chicago, Illinois

Linda Cason, MSN, RN-BC, NE-BC, CNRN
Manager
Employee Education and Development Department
Deaconess Hospital
Evansville, Indiana

Edith Claros, PhD, RN
Associate Professor of Nursing and Assistant Dean
School of Nursing
Massachusetts College of Pharmacy and Health Services
Boston, Massachusetts

Janice C. Colwell, RN, MS, CWOCN, FAAN
Advanced Practice Nurse
University of Chicago Medicine
Chicago, Illinois

Rhonda Comrie, PhD, RN
Associate Professor
School of Nursing
Southern Illinois University—Edwardsville
Edwardsville, Illinois

Christine Durbin, RN, JD, PhD
Assistant Professor
School of Nursing
Southern Illinois University—Edwardsville
Edwardsville, Illinois

Margaret Ecker, RN, MS
Nurse Consultant
Interim Director, Patient Care Services
Children's Hospital Los Angeles
Los Angeles, California

Jane Fellows, MSN, RN, CWOCN
Wound/Ostomy Clinical Nurse Specialist
Duke University Medical Center
Durham, North Carolina

Linda Felver, PhD, RN
Associate Professor
School of Nursing
Oregon Health & Sciences University
Portland, Oregon

Victoria N. Folse, PhD, APN, PMHCNS-BC, LCPC
Director and Associate Professor
Illinois Wesleyan University
Bloomington, Illinois

Lorri Graham, RN, MSN
Nursing Instructor
Saint Francis Medical Center College of Nursing
Peoria, Illinois

Janis Waite Hayden, RN, EdD
Professor
Saint Francis Medical Center College of Nursing
Peoria, Illinois

Tara Hulsey, RN, PhD, CNE, FAAN
Dean and Professor
Charleston Southern University
Charleston, South Carolina

Jerrilee LaMar, PhD, RN, CNE
Associate Professor of Nursing
University of Evansville
Evansville, Indiana

Kathryn A. Lever, RNC, MSN, WHNP-BC
Associate Professor of Nursing
University of Evansville
Evansville, Indiana

Suzanne Lugerner, RN, MS, LN, CNSC, CNS
Director, Clinical Nutrition
Department of Pharmacy Services
MedStar Washington Hospital Center
Washington, DC

Deborah L. Marshall, RN, MSN
Assistant Professor of Nursing
Dunigan Family Department of Nursing
University of Evansville
Evansville, Indiana

Judith A. McCutchan, RN, ASN, BSN, MSN, PhD
Professor/Dean, School of Health Sciences
Ivy Tech Community College
Evansville, Indiana

Carol McGinnis, DNP, RN, CNS, CNSC
Clinical Nurse Specialist
Sanford USD Medical Center
Sioux Falls, South Dakota

Jill Parsons, RN, PhD
Assistant Professor
MacMurray College
Jacksonville, Illinois

Kristine A. Rose, RN, MSN
Instructor
Saint Francis Medical Center College of Nursing
Peoria, Illinois

Matthew R. Sorenson, RN, PhD
Associate Professor
DePaul University
Chicago, Illinois

Donna L Thompson, MSN, CRNP, FNP-BC, CCCN
Continence Nurse Practitioner
Urology Health Specialists
Drexel Hill, Pennsylvania;
Continence Solutions
Media, Pennsylvania

Jelena Todic, MSW, LCSW
Manager, Education, Quality and Research
Barnes-Jewish Hospital;
Adjunct Professor
Brown School of Social Work
Washington University
St. Louis, Missouri

Ann Tritak, RN, EdD
Dean and Professor
School of Nursing
Saint Peters University
The Jesuit University of New Jersey
Jersey City, New Jersey

Pamela Becker Weilitz, DNP, APRN, ANP-BC
Adult Nurse Practitioner
VA St. Louis Health Care System
Maryville University
St. Louis, Missouri

Paige Wimberley, PhD, APN, CNS, CNE
Assistant Professor of Nursing
RN-BSN Coordinator
Arkansas State University
Jonesboro, Arkansas

Rita Wunderlich, PhD, RN, CNE
Associate Professor
Director, Upper Division Nursing Program
Goldfarb School of Nursing at Barnes Jewish College
St. Louis, Missouri

Valerie Yancey, RN, PhD
Associate Professor
Southern Illinois University—Edwardsville
Edwardsville, Illinois

REVIEWERS

Marianne Adam, MSN, CRNP
Assistant Professor
Moravian College
Bethlehem, Pennsylvania

Amy S. Adams, MSN, RN
Associate Professor
St. Elizabeth School of Nursing
Lafayette, Indiana

Cheryl Alberternst, RN, MSN
Nursing Faculty
Southeast Missouri State University
Cape Girardeau, Missouri

Suzanne L. Bailey, PMHCNS-BC, CNE
Associate Professor of Nursing
University of Evansville
Evansville, Indiana

Margaret E. Barnes, RN, MSN
Assistant Professor
Indiana Wesleyan University
Marion, Indiana

Anna Bruch, RN, MSN
Professor of Nursing
Illinois Valley Community College
Oglesby, Illinois

Pat Callard, MSN, RN, CNE
Assistant Professor of Nursing
College of Graduate Nursing
Western University of Health Sciences
Pomona, California

Kim Clevenger, EdDc, MSN, RN, BC
Associate Professor of Nursing
Morehead State University
Morehead, Kentucky

Michele C. Curry, MS, RN
Senior Lecturer
Indiana University East School of Nursing
Indiana University
Richmond, Indiana

Lauren Deichmann, MSN, FNP-BC
Family Nurse Practitioner
Barnes-Jewish Hospital Center for Preoperative Assessment and Planning
St. Louis, Missouri

Barbara Derwinski, MSN, RNC, WH, BC
Associate Professor
Bozeman College of Nursing
Montana State University
Billings, Montana

Holly J. Diesel, PhD, RN
Associate Professor
Goldfarb School of Nursing at Barnes Jewish College
St. Louis, Missouri

Dawna Egelhoff, MSN, RN
Assistant Professor
School of Nursing
Lewis & Clark Community College
Godfrey, Illinois

Amber Essman, MSN, APRN, FNP-BC, CNE
Assistant Professor
Chamberlain College of Nursing
Columbus, Ohio

Margie L. Francisco, EdD, MSN
Nursing Professor
Illinois Valley Community College
Oglesby, Illinois

Jacklyn Gentry, MSN, RN
Nursing Faculty
Brookline College
Phoenix, Arizona

Lorie Hacker, MSN, RN
Associate Professor
Ivy Tech Community College
Indianapolis, Indiana

Linda Hansen-Kyle, PhD, RN, CCM
Director, Nursing, San Diego Regional Center
Azusa Pacific University
San Diego, California

Pamela D. Korte, RN, MS
Professor of Nursing
Monroe Community College
Rochester, New York

Janis Longfield McMillan, RN, MSN, CNE
Nursing Faculty
Coconino Community College
Flagstaff, Arizona

Pamela S. Merida, MSN, RN
Assistant Professor, Nursing
St. Elizabeth School of Nursing
Lafayette, Indiana

Jeanie Mitchel, RN, MSN, MA
Nursing Professor
South Suburban College
South Holland, Illinois

Cindy Mulder, RNC, MS, MSN, WHNP-BC, FNP-BC
Instructor
The University of South Dakota
Vermillion, South Dakota

Elaine U. Polan, RNC, MS, PhD
Nursing Program Supervisor
Vocational Education & Extension Board Practical Nursing Program
Uniondale, New York

Anita K. Reed, MSN, RN
Department Chair Adult and Community Health Practice
St. Joseph's College
St. Elizabeth School of Nursing
Lafayette, Indiana

Rhonda J. Reed, MSN, RN, CRRN
Learning Resource Center Director
Technology Coordinator
Indiana State University
Terre Haute, Indiana

Kristine A. Rose, RN, MSN
Instructor
Saint Francis Medical Center College of Nursing
Peoria, Illinois

Carol Rueter, RN, PhD(c)
Bereavement Coordinator
Clinical Instructor
James A. Haley VA;
University of South Florida
Tampa, Florida

Susan Parnell Scholtz, PhD, RN
Associate Professor of Nursing
St. Luke's School of Nursing at Moravian College
Bethlehem, Pennsylvania

Gale Sewell, PhD(c), MSN, RN, CNE
Associate Professor
University of Northwestern
St. Paul, Minnesota

Cynthia M. Sheppard, RN, MSN, APN-BC
Assistant Professor of Nursing
Schoolcraft College
Livonia, Michigan

Emily G. Smith, MSN, RN, CRRN
Assistant Professor
School of Nursing
Endicott College
Beverly, Massachusetts

Ann D. Sprengel, EdD, MSN, RN
Professor
Department of Nursing
Southeast Missouri State University
Cape Girardeau, Missouri

Scott Carter Thigpen, RN, MSN, CCRN, CEN
Associate Professor of Nursing
South Georgia College
Douglas, Georgia

Kimberly Valich, MSN, RN
Department of Nursing Chairperson
Nursing Faculty
South Suburban College
South Holland, Illinois

Mary Walton, PhD, RN, ANP
Nursing Faculty
GateWay Community College
Maricopa Nursing
Phoenix, Arizona

Rachel West, MHA, MSN, RN
Nursing Faculty
Brookline College
Albuquerque, New Mexico

Kathleen S. Whalen, PhD, RN, CNE
Assistant Professor of Nursing
Loretto Heights School of Nursing
Regis University
Denver, Colorado

Angela Shirlean Williams-McCally, RN
Registered Nurse
Maury Regional Medical Center
Columbia, Tennessee

Jean Yockey, MSN, FNP-BC, CNE
Associate Professor
University of South Dakota
Vermillion, South Dakota

CONTRIBUTORS TO PREVIOUS EDITIONS

Jeanette Spain Adams, RN, PhD, CRNI, APRN

Elizabeth A. Ayello, RN, BSN, MS, PhD, CS, CETN

Marjorie Baier, RN, PhD

Sylvia Baird, RN, BSN, MM

Lois Bentler-Lampe, RN, MS

Peggy Breckenridge, MSN, FNP

Judith C. Brostron, RN, BA, JD, LLM

Victoria M. Brown, RN, BSN, MSN, PhD, HNC

Jeri Burger, RN, PhD

Gale Carli, MSN, MSHed, BSN, RN

Kelly Jo Cone, RN, BSN, MS, PhD

Roslyn Corcoran, RN, BSN

Eileen Costantinou, RN, MSN, BC

Ruth Curchoe, RN, MSN, CIC

Rick Daniels, RN, BSN, MSN, PhD

Carolyn Ruppel D'Avis, RN, BSN, MSN

Sharon J. Edwards, RN, BSN, MSN, PhD

Martha Keene Elkin, RN, MSN, IBCLC

Linda Fasciani, RN, BSN, MSN

Susan J. Fetzer, RN, BA, BSN, MSN, MBA, PhD

Leah Frederick, MS, RN, CIC

Cynthia S. Goodwin, RN, BSN, MSN

Lois C. Hamel, BS, MS

Maureen Huhmann, MS, RD

Judith Ann Kilpatrick, RN, MSN, DNSc

Carl A. Kirton, RN-C, BSN, MA, ACRN, ANP

Lori Klingman, RN, MSN

Kristine L'Ecuyer, RN, MSN, CCNS

Ruth Ludwick, RN, BSN, MSN, PhD, RN-C

Mary Kay Knight Macheca, RN, BSN, MSN(R), CS, CDE

Rita G. Mertig, RNC, MS, CNS

Mary Dee Miller, RN, BSN, MS, CIC

Elaine Neel, BSN, MSN

Geralyn A. Ochs, RN, AND, BSN, MSN

Marsha Evans Orr, RN, MS, CS, CNSN

Wendy R. Ostendorf, MS, EdD

Dula F. Pacquiao, EdD, RN, CTN

Nancy Panthofer, RN, BSN, MSN

Elizabeth S. Pratt, RN, MSN, ACNS-BC

Julia Balzer Riley, RN, MN, AHN-C, CET®

Janice J. Rumfelt, BSN, MSN, EdD, RNC

Marilyn Schallom, MSN, CCRN, CCNS

Sharon Souter, RN, BSN, MSN

Elizabeth Speakman, RN, EdD

Rachel E. Spector, BS, MS, PhD, CTN, FAAN

Susan Speraw, RN, PHD, CNP

Riva Touger-Decker, PhD, RD, FADA

Ellen Wathen, PhD, RN, BC

Joan Domigan Wentz, MSN, RN

Terry L. Wood, PhD, RN, CNE

Barbara Yoost, RN, BSN, MSN, CNS

I wish to dedicate this edition to the friends and professional colleagues who continue to inspire me.
I am so grateful to have chosen nursing as my profession.
Patricia A. Potter

To nursing faculty at Southern Illinois University—Edwardsville and Saint Louis University.
Your commitment to nursing and educational excellence inspires us all to be the guardians of the discipline.
To my grandchildren: Cora Elisabeth Bryan; Amalie Mary Bryan; Shepherd Charles Bryan, and Noelle Anne Bryan
Anne Griffin Perry

To nursing students everywhere—you have chosen a great profession!
To my family, Drake, Sara, and Kelsey, thanks for supporting me as I spent all those evenings and weekends writing. I love you all.
Patricia Stockert

To my very first mentor, Janice Boundy. Your belief in me and gentle guidance has inspired me to find qualities in myself that you already knew existed. You have been a great inspiration in my life, and I am always and forever grateful for your support, kindness and, most of all, friendship.

And to my family—thank you for your never-ending love and support.
I am so blessed to have you in my life.
Amy Hall

STUDENT PREFACE

Essentials for Nursing Practice was developed to provide you with all of the fundamental nursing concepts and skills in a visually appealing, easy-to-use format. We know how busy you are and how precious your time is. As you begin your nursing education, it is very important that you have a resource that includes all the information you need to prepare for lectures, classroom activities, clinical rotations, and exams—and nothing more. We have designed this text to meet all of those needs. This book has been designed to help you succeed in this course and prepare you for more advanced study. In addition to the readable writing style and abundance of full-color photographs and drawings, we've incorporated numerous features to help you study and learn. We've made it easy for you to pull out important content. **Check out the following special learning aids:**

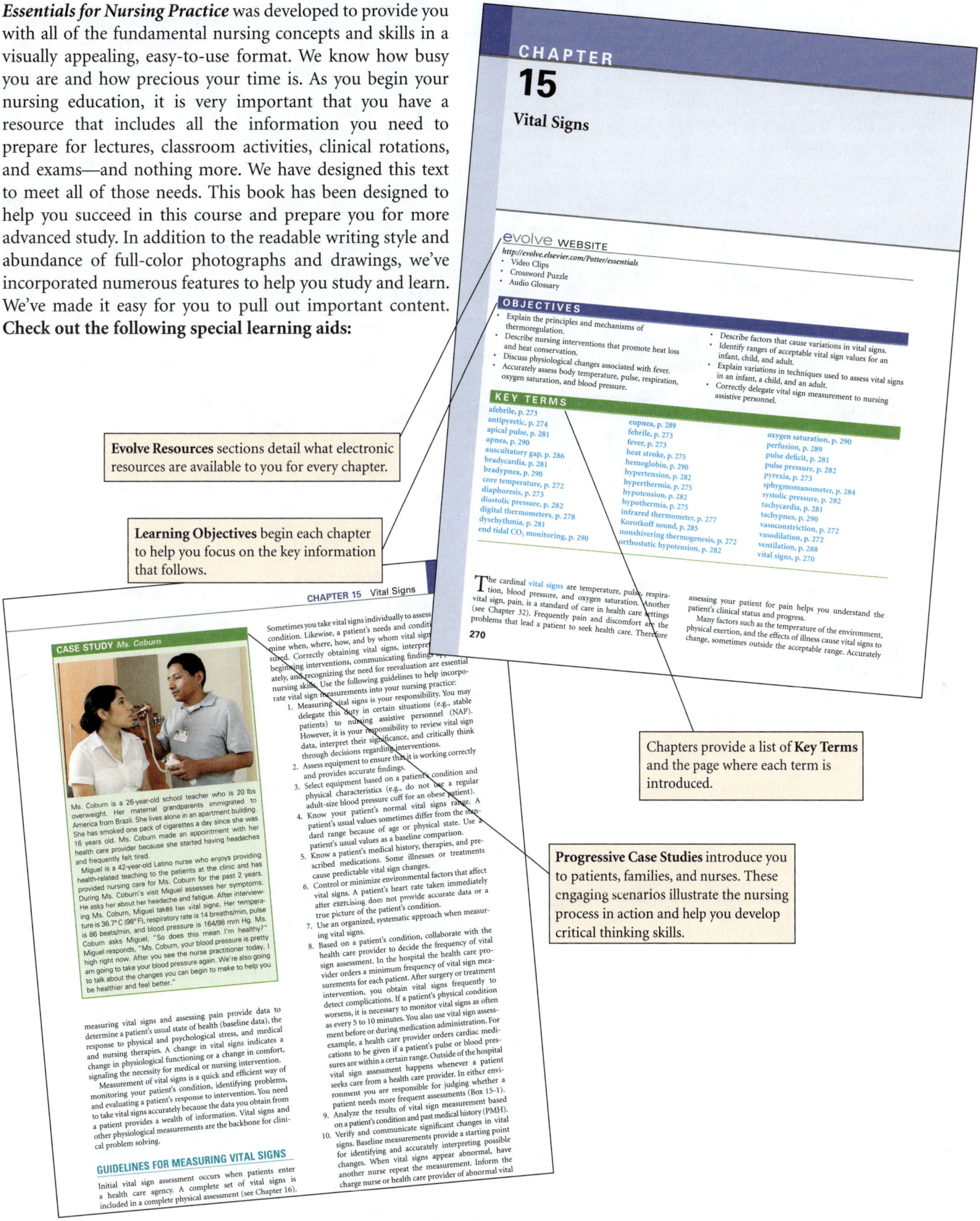
CHAPTER 15

Vital Signs

evolve WEBSITE

http://evolve.elsevier.com/Potter/essentials

- Video Clips
- Crossword Puzzle
- Audio Glossary

OBJECTIVES

- Explain the principles and mechanisms of thermoregulation.
- Describe nursing interventions that promote heat loss and heat conservation.
- Discuss physiological changes associated with fever.
- Accurately assess body temperature, pulse, respiration, oxygen saturation, and blood pressure.
- Describe factors that cause variations in vital signs.
- Identify ranges of acceptable vital sign values for an infant, child, and adult.
- Explain variations in techniques used to assess vital signs in an infant, a child, and an adult.
- Correctly delegate vital sign measurement to nursing assistive personnel.

KEY TERMS

afebrile, p. 273
antipyretic, p. 274
apical pulse, p. 281
apnea, p. 290
auscultatory gap, p. 286
bradycardia, p. 281
bradypnea, p. 290
core temperature, p. 272
diaphoresis, p. 273
diastolic pressure, p. 282
digital thermometers, p. 278
dysrhythmia, p. 281
end tidal CO_2 monitoring, p. 290
eupnea, p. 289
febrile, p. 273
fever, p. 273
heat stroke, p. 275
hemoglobin, p. 290
hypertension, p. 282
hyperthermia, p. 275
hypotension, p. 282
hypothermia, p. 275
infrared thermometer, p. 277
Korotkoff sound, p. 285
nonshivering thermogenesis, p. 272
orthostatic hypotension, p. 282
oxygen saturation, p. 290
perfusion, p. 289
pulse deficit, p. 281
pulse pressure, p. 282
pyrexia, p. 273
sphygmomanometer, p. 284
systolic pressure, p. 282
tachycardia, p. 281
tachypnea, p. 290
vasoconstriction, p. 272
vasodilation, p. 272
ventilation, p. 288
vital signs, p. 270

The cardinal vital signs are temperature, pulse, respiration, blood pressure, and oxygen saturation. Another vital sign, pain, is a standard of care in health care settings (see Chapter 32). Frequently pain and discomfort are the problems that lead a patient to seek health care. Therefore assessing your patient for pain helps you understand the patient's clinical status and progress.

Many factors such as the temperature of the environment, physical exertion, and the effects of illness cause vital signs to change, sometimes outside the acceptable range. Accurately

270

CHAPTER 15 Vital Signs

CASE STUDY *Ms. Coburn*

Ms. Coburn is a 26-year-old school teacher who is 20 lbs overweight. Her maternal grandparents immigrated to America from Brazil. She lives alone in an apartment building. She has smoked one pack of cigarettes a day since she was 16 years old. Ms. Coburn made an appointment with her health care provider because she started having headaches and frequently felt tired.

Miguel is a 42-year-old Latino nurse who enjoys providing health-related teaching to the patients at the clinic and has provided nursing care for Ms. Coburn for the past 2 years. During Ms. Coburn's visit Miguel assesses her symptoms. He asks her about her headache and fatigue. After interviewing Ms. Coburn, Miguel takes her vital signs. Her temperature is 36.7° C (98° F), respiratory rate is 14 breaths/min, pulse is 86 beats/min, and blood pressure is 164/98 mm Hg. Ms. Coburn asks Miguel, "So does this mean I'm healthy?" Miguel responds, "Ms. Coburn, your blood pressure is pretty high right now. After you see the nurse practitioner today, I am going to take your blood pressure again. We're also going to talk about the changes you can begin to make to help you be healthier and feel better."

measuring vital signs and assessing pain provide data to determine a patient's usual state of health (baseline data), the response to physical and psychological stress, and medical and nursing therapies. A change in vital signs indicates a change in physiological functioning or a change in comfort, signaling the necessity for medical or nursing intervention.

Measurement of vital signs is a quick and efficient way of monitoring your patient's condition, identifying problems, and evaluating a patient's response to intervention. You need to take vital signs accurately because the data you obtain from a patient provides a wealth of information. Vital signs and other physiological measurements are the backbone for clinical problem solving.

GUIDELINES FOR MEASURING VITAL SIGNS

Initial vital sign assessment occurs when patients enter a health care agency. A complete set of vital signs is included in a complete physical assessment (see Chapter 16).

Sometimes you take vital signs individually to assess condition. Likewise, a patient's needs and conditi[…] mine when, where, how, and by whom vital sign[…] sured. Correctly obtaining vital signs, interpre[…] beginning interventions, communicating findings […] ately, and recognizing the need for reevaluation are essential nursing skills. Use the following guidelines to help incorporate vital sign measurements into your nursing practice:

1. Measuring vital signs is your responsibility. You may delegate this duty in certain situations (e.g., stable patients) to nursing assistive personnel (NAP). However, it is your responsibility to review vital sign data, interpret their significance, and critically think through decisions regarding interventions.
2. Assess equipment to ensure that it is working correctly and provides accurate findings.
3. Select equipment based on a patient's condition and physical characteristics (e.g., do not use a regular adult-size blood pressure cuff for an obese patient).
4. Know your patient's normal vital signs range. A patient's usual values sometimes differ from the standard range because of age or physical state. Use a patient's usual values as a baseline comparison.
5. Know a patient's medical history, therapies, and prescribed medications. Some illnesses or treatments cause predictable vital sign changes.
6. Control or minimize environmental factors that affect vital signs. A patient's heart rate taken immediately after exercising does not provide accurate data or a true picture of the patient's condition.
7. Use an organized, systematic approach when measuring vital signs.
8. Based on a patient's condition, collaborate with the health care provider to decide the frequency of vital sign assessment. In the hospital the health care provider orders a minimum frequency of vital sign measurements for each patient. After surgery or treatment intervention, you obtain vital signs frequently to detect complications. If a patient's physical condition worsens, it is necessary to monitor vital signs as often as every 5 to 10 minutes. You also use vital sign assessment before or during medication administration. For example, a health care provider orders cardiac medications to be given if a patient's pulse or blood pressures are within a certain range. Outside of the hospital vital sign assessment happens whenever a patient seeks care from a health care provider. In either environment you are responsible for judging whether a patient needs more frequent assessments (Box 15-1).
9. Analyze the results of vital sign measurement based on a patient's condition and past medical history (PMH).
10. Verify and communicate significant changes in vital signs. Baseline measurements provide a starting point for identifying and accurately interpreting possible changes. When vital signs appear abnormal, have another nurse repeat the measurement. Inform the charge nurse or health care provider of abnormal vital

Evolve Resources sections detail what electronic resources are available to you for every chapter.

Learning Objectives begin each chapter to help you focus on the key information that follows.

Chapters provide a list of **Key Terms** and the page where each term is introduced.

Progressive Case Studies introduce you to patients, families, and nurses. These engaging scenarios illustrate the nursing process in action and help you develop critical thinking skills.

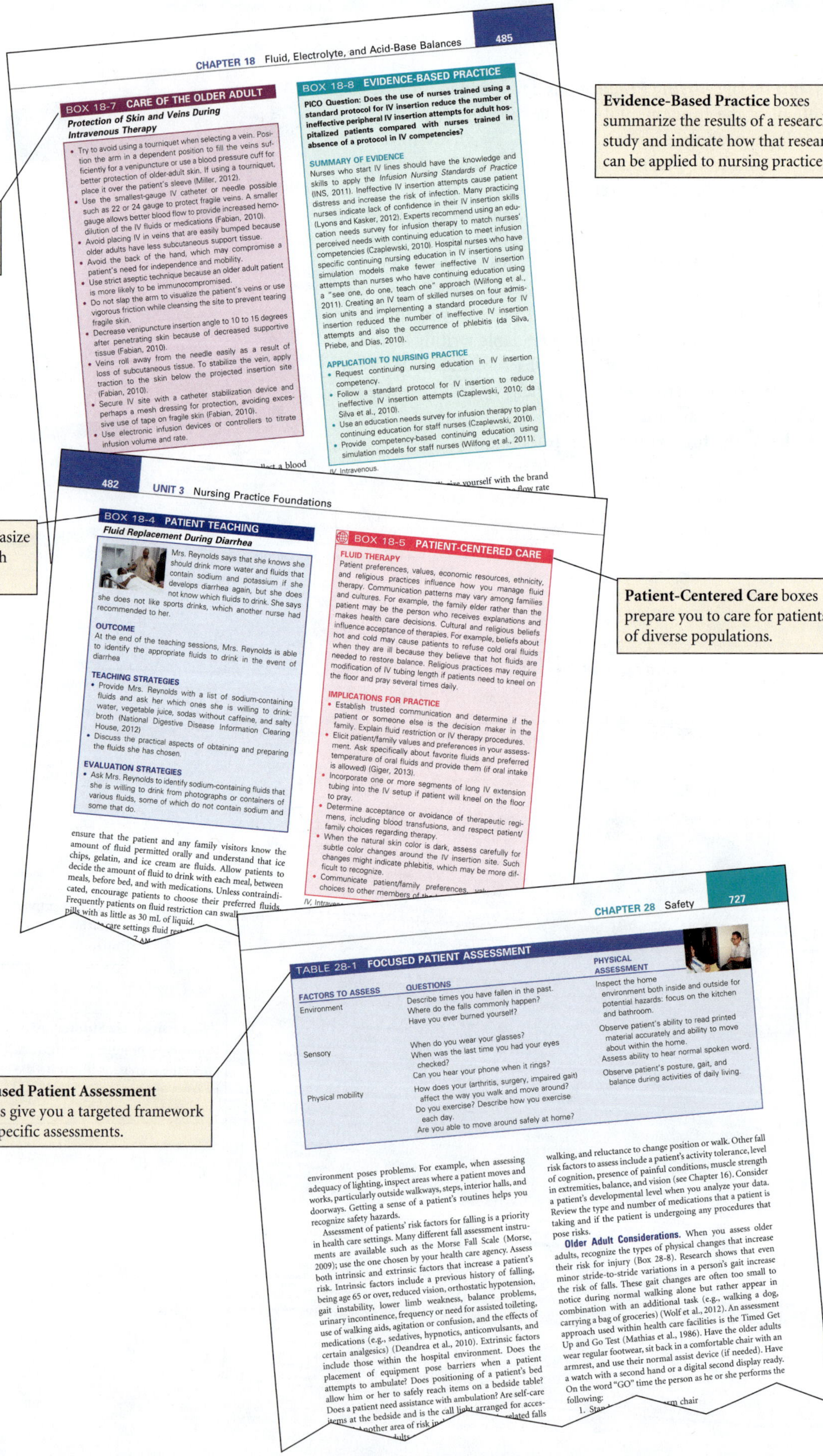

Evidence-Based Practice boxes summarize the results of a research study and indicate how that research can be applied to nursing practice.

Care of the Older Adult boxes highlight the care of this special population.

Patient Teaching boxes emphasize important information to teach patients.

Patient-Centered Care boxes prepare you to care for patients of diverse populations.

Focused Patient Assessment tables give you a targeted framework for specific assessments.

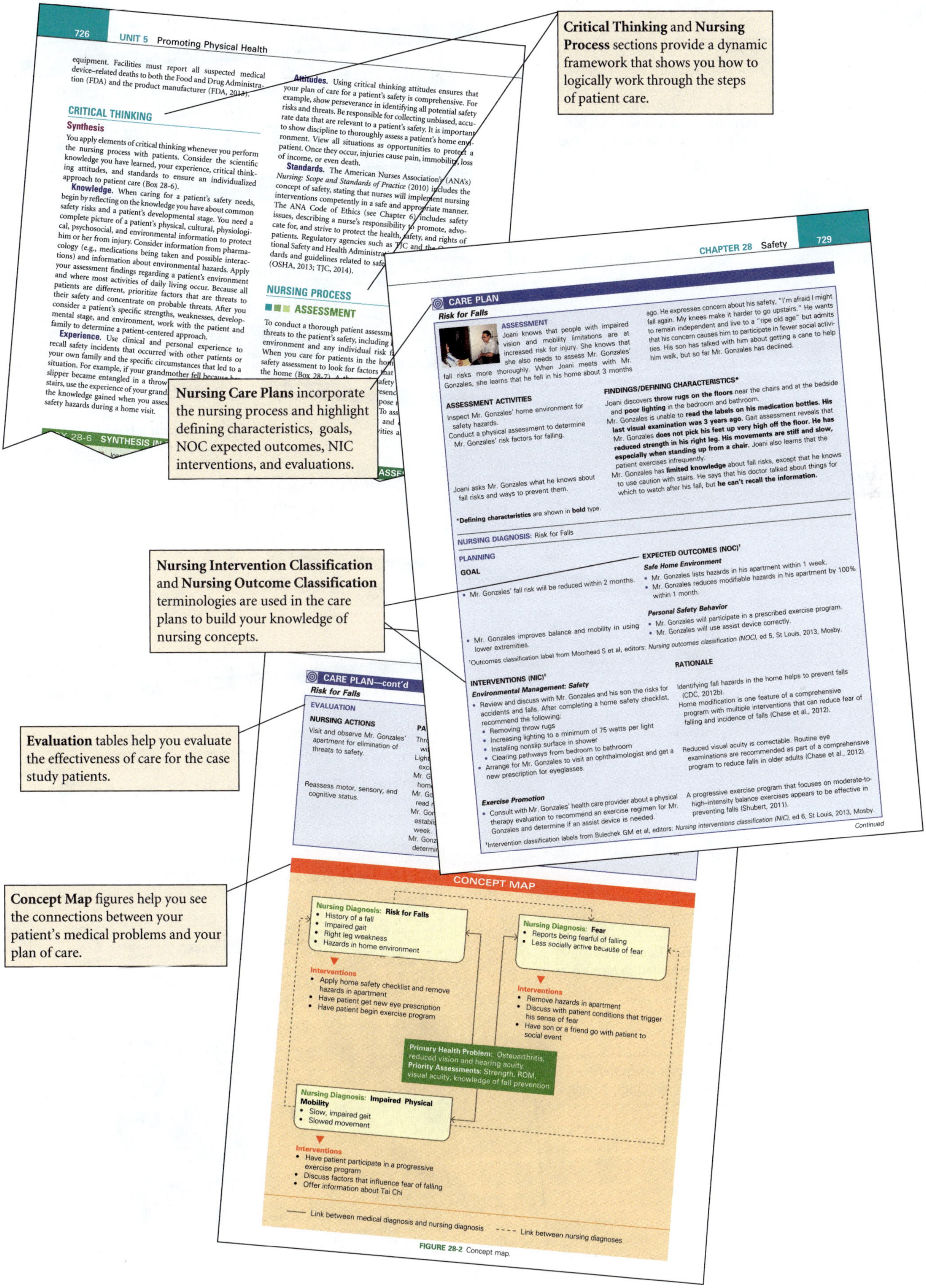

Critical Thinking and **Nursing Process** sections provide a dynamic framework that shows you how to logically work through the steps of patient care.

Nursing Care Plans incorporate the nursing process and highlight defining characteristics, goals, NOC expected outcomes, NIC interventions, and evaluations.

Nursing Intervention Classification and **Nursing Outcome Classification** terminologies are used in the care plans to build your knowledge of nursing concepts.

Evaluation tables help you evaluate the effectiveness of care for the case study patients.

Concept Map figures help you see the connections between your patient's medical problems and your plan of care.

Nursing Skills are presented in a clear, two-column format with steps and rationales so you learn why as well as how. Each skill begins with a **Safety Guidelines** section that will help you focus on safe and effective skill performance.

Video Icons indicate video clips associated with specific skills that are available on the Evolve Student Resources website.

Equipment lists show specific items needed for each skill.

Delegation Considerations guide you in delegating tasks to assistive personnel.

Clinical Decision Points alert you to important information to consider as you perform a skill.

Clear, close-up **photos** help you learn to perform important techniques.

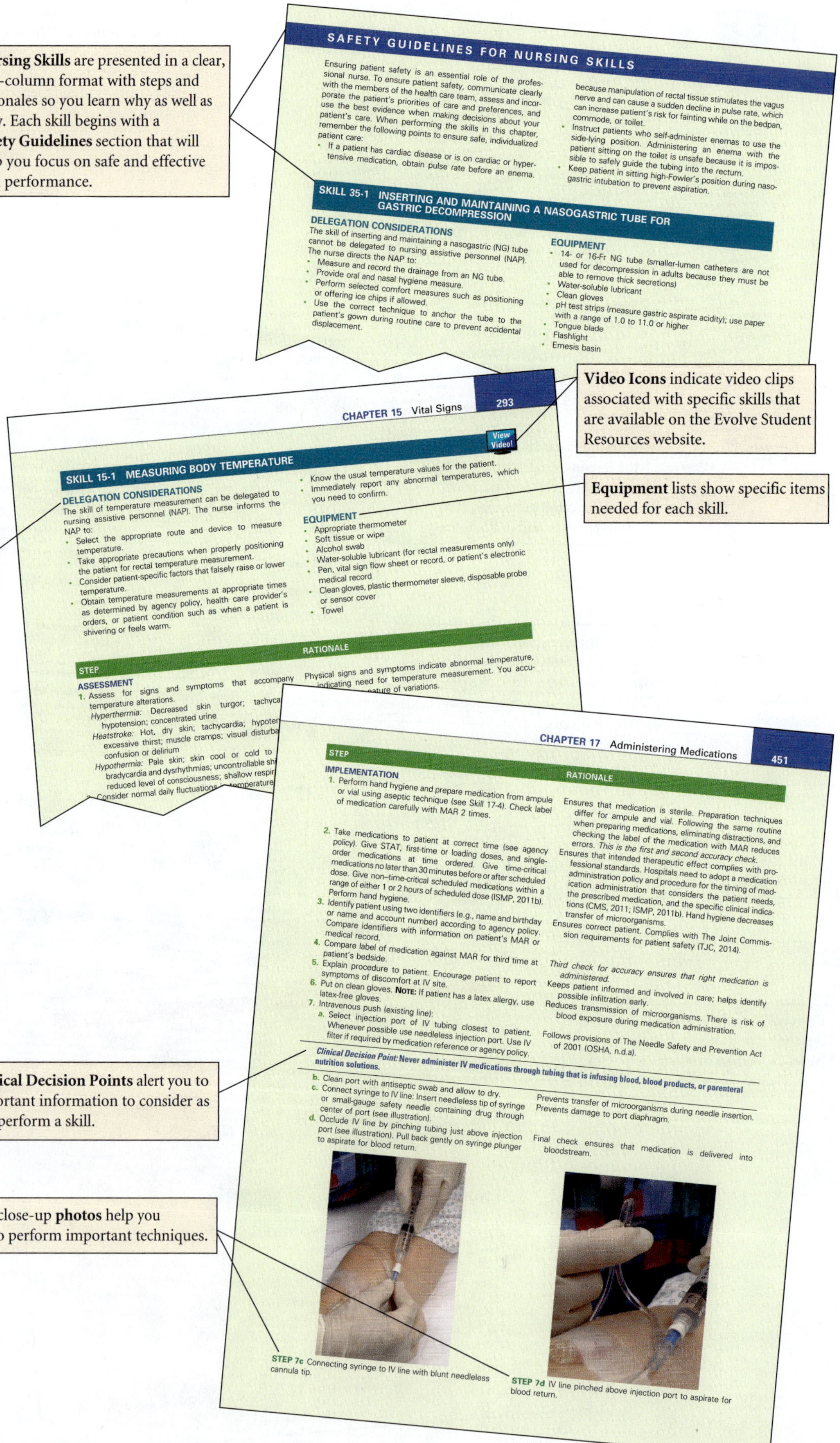

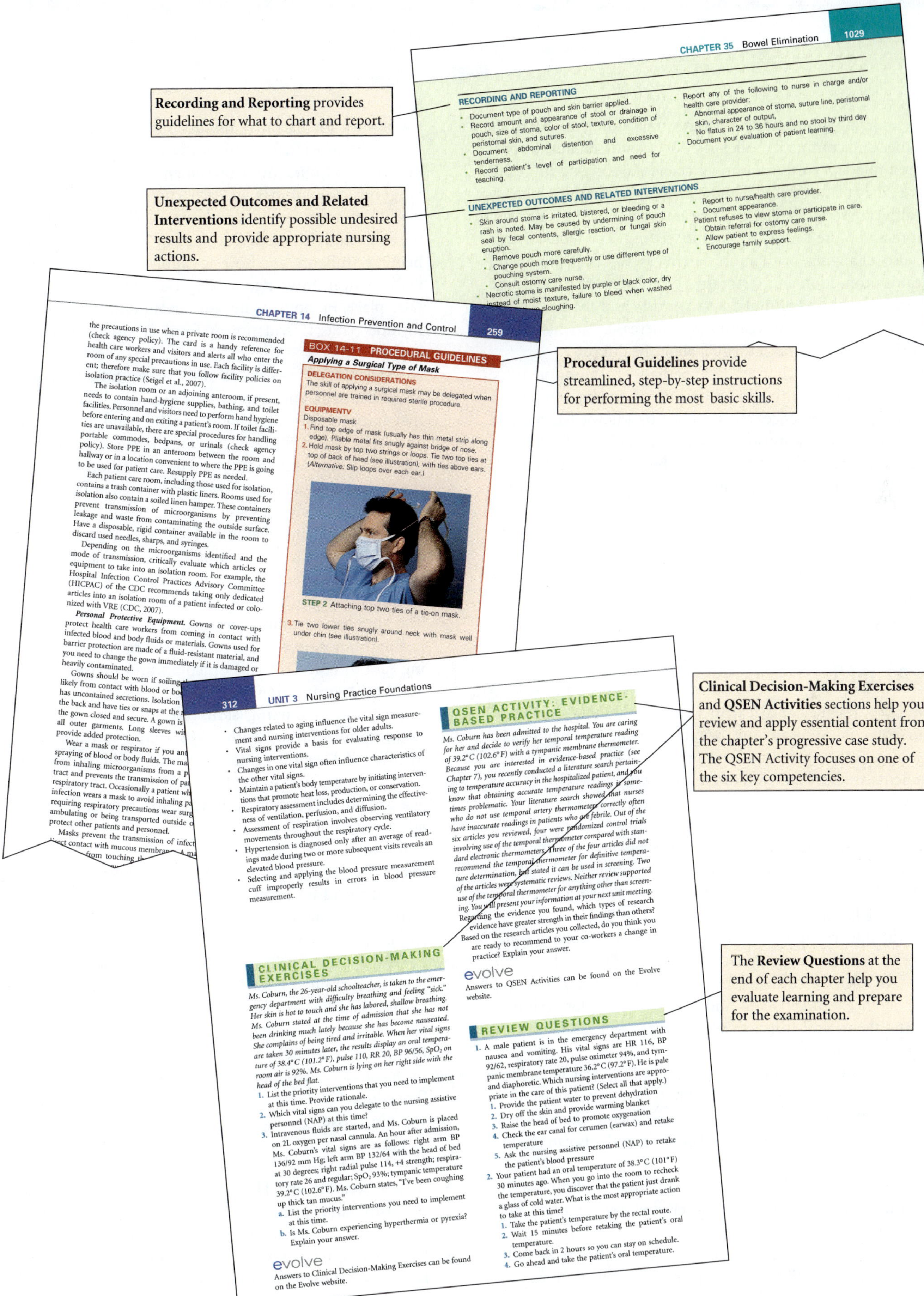

Recording and Reporting provides guidelines for what to chart and report.

Unexpected Outcomes and Related Interventions identify possible undesired results and provide appropriate nursing actions.

Procedural Guidelines provide streamlined, step-by-step instructions for performing the most basic skills.

Clinical Decision-Making Exercises and **QSEN Activities** sections help you review and apply essential content from the chapter's progressive case study. The QSEN Activity focuses on one of the six key competencies.

The **Review Questions** at the end of each chapter help you evaluate learning and prepare for the examination.

PREFACE TO THE INSTRUCTOR

The nursing profession is always responding to dynamic change and continual challenges. Today's nurses must be prepared to adapt to the continual changes occurring in health care. They play a vital role in the delivery of multidisciplinary health care services. The practice arena is changing—moving more and more to the community setting. The focus of care is also changing, with more emphasis is being placed on health promotion and restorative care. Even the patients are changing—more cultural diversity exists and the percentage of older adult patients continues to increase. Patients are far more involved in and informed about health care.

Despite these changes—or perhaps because of these changes—it is essential that the basics of nursing remain the foundation of practice. Nurses must be knowledgeable and professional. They must be both technically proficient and personally caring. And they must be able to synthesize a broad array of knowledge and experiences when providing care for their patients.

We continue to cover all of the fundamental nursing concepts, skills, and techniques that students must master before moving on to other areas of study. We address changes in practice that affect how and where nurses use the skills and knowledge they acquire.

FEATURES

We have designed this text to welcome the new student to nursing, communicate our own love for the profession, and promote learning and understanding. We know that today's students are busy and, too often, are overwhelmed by all that they must learn and do. They want their texts to focus on the most current, factual, and essential content and skills. We want to ensure that these students are ready to continue with their education and will, ultimately, be prepared for all of the challenges of practice. To this end, we have included the following key features:

- Students will appreciate the **clear, engaging writing style.** The narrative actually addresses the reader, making this textbook more of an active instructional tool than a passive reference. Students will find that even complex technical and theoretical concepts are presented in a language that is easy to understand.
- The **attractive, functional design** will appeal to today's visual learner. The clear, readable type and bold headings make the content easy to read and follow. Each special element is consistently color keyed so students can readily identify important information.
- Hundreds of **large, clear, full-color photographs and drawings** reinforce and clarify key concepts and techniques.
- The **five-step nursing process** serves as the organizing framework for all clinical chapters. This logical, consistent framework for narrative discussions is further enhanced by special boxes that highlight assessment, care plans, and evaluation of outcome achievement.
- **Ongoing case studies** in each chapter introduce "real-world" patients, families, and nurses. The chapter follows the case study through the steps of the nursing process, helping students see how to apply the process, along with critical thinking, to the care of patients. Cases take place in both acute and community settings and include patients and nurses from a variety of cultural backgrounds.
- **Nursing Care Plans** guide students on how to conduct an assessment and analyze the defining characteristics that indicate nursing diagnoses. The plans include NIC and NOC classifications to familiarize students with this important nomenclature. The evaluation sections of the plans show students how to evaluate and then determine the outcomes of care.
- **Concept Maps** included in each clinical chapter show you the associations among multiple nursing diagnoses for a patient with a selected medical diagnosis, as well and their relationship to nursing interventions.
- The implementation narrative consistently addresses health promotion, acute care, and restorative and continuing care to reflect a focus on **community-based nursing** and **health promotion.**
- **More than 35 nursing skills** are presented in a clear, two-column format with steps and rationales. Skills include delegation guidelines and clinical decision points that alert students to steps requiring special assessment or specific technique for safe and effective administration.
- **Procedural guidelines** provide streamlined step-by-step instructions for performing very basic skills.
- Care of the **older adult** and **patient teaching** are stressed throughout the narrative and are also highlighted in special boxes.
- **Learning aids** to help students identify, review, and apply important content in each chapter include Objectives, Key Terms, Key Points, Clinical Decision-Making Exercises, and Review Questions.
- **Printed lists** on the inside back cover provide information on locating specific assets in the book, including Skills, Procedure Guidelines, Nursing Care Plans, and Patient Teaching boxes.

New to This Edition

- A **new chapter on "The Nursing Profession"** addresses the history of nursing, forces that affect nursing today, and the various roles and responsibilities that nurses hold.
- Information related to the **Quality and Safety Education for Nurses (QSEN)** initiative is highlighted with activities

at the end of each chapter. These activities incorporate one of the six key competencies and relate back to the progressive chapter case study scenarios.

- **Evidence-Based Practice** boxes now include a PICO question, provide a summary of nursing research evidence related to that specific topic, and then explain its implications for nursing practice. These have been updated to reflect current research topics and trends.
- The latest **NANDA 2012-2014** diagnoses provide up-to-date content.
- **Review questions** have been heavily revised, with alternate format questions in each chapter.
- **New Procedural Guidelines** cover Blood Glucose Monitoring.
- A **new Skill** covers Patient-Controlled Analgesia.

LEARNING SUPPLEMENTS FOR STUDENTS

- The **Evolve Student Resources** are available online at http://evolve.elsevier.com/Potter/essentials and include the following valuable learning aids organized by chapter:
    - Chapter Review Questions from the book in an interactive format! Includes over 375 questions to prepare for examinations
    - Answers to and rationales for Chapter Review Questions
    - Answers to and rationales for Clinical Decision-Making Exercises
    - Answers to and rationales for QSEN Activities
    - Video clips to highlight common skills
    - Crossword Puzzle Activities
    - Animations
    - Case Study with questions
    - Printable versions of chapter Key Points
    - Audio glossary
    - Fluids & Electrolytes Tutorial
    - Nursing Skills Online reading assignments
    - Skills Performance Checklists for each skill in the text
    - Three practice quizzes to cover all Fundamentals content for further study
- A thorough **Study Guide** by Patricia A. Castaldi provides students with a wide variety of exercises and activities to enhance learning and comprehension. This study guide features case studies with related questions; chapter review sections with matching, fill-in-the-blank, and multiple-choice questions; study group questions; instructions for creating and using study charts; and printed answers for all questions.
- **Virtual Clinical Excursions** is an exciting workbook and CD-ROM experience that brings learning to life in a virtual hospital setting. The workbook guides students as they care for patients, providing ongoing challenges and learning opportunities. Each lesson in *Virtual Clinical Excursions* complements the textbook content and provides an environment for students to practice what they are learning. This CD/workbook is available separately or packaged at a special price with the textbook.

TEACHING SUPPLEMENTS FOR INSTRUCTORS

- The **Evolve Instructor Resources** (available online at http://evolve.elsevier.com/Potter/essentials) are a comprehensive collection of the most important tools instructors need, including the following:
    - **TEACH for Nurses** ties together every chapter resource you need for the most effective class presentations, with sections dedicated to objectives, teaching focus, nursing curriculum standards (including QSEN, BSN Essentials, and Concepts), instructor chapter resources, student chapter resources, answers to chapter questions, and an in-class case study discussion. Teaching Strategies include relationships between the textbook content and discussion items. Examples of student activities, online activities, and large group activities are provided for more "hands-on" learning.
    - The **Test Bank** contains a heavily revised set of more than 950 questions with text page references and answers coded for NCLEX Client Needs category, nursing process, and cognitive level. The ExamView software allows instructors to create new tests; edit, add, and delete test questions; sort questions by NCLEX category, cognitive level, nursing process step, and question type; and administer/grade online tests.
    - Completely revised **PowerPoint Presentations** includes over 1400 slides for use in lectures. New to this edition are the inclusion of art within the slides and progressive case studies that include discussion questions and answers.
    - The **Image Collection** contains hundreds of illustrations from the text for use in lectures.
- **Simulation Learning System** is an online toolkit that helps instructors and facilitators effectively incorporate medium- to high-fidelity simulation into their nursing curriculum. Detailed patient scenarios promote and enhance the clinical decision-making skills of students at all levels. The system provides detailed instructions for preparation and implementation of the simulation experience, debriefing questions that encourage critical thinking, and learning resources to reinforce student comprehension. Each scenario in *Simulation Learning System* complements the textbook content and helps bridge the gap between lectures and clinicals. This system provides the perfect environment for students to practice what they are learning in the text for a true-to-life, hands-on learning experience.

MULTIMEDIA SUPPLEMENTS FOR INSTRUCTORS AND STUDENTS

- **Nursing Skills Online 3.0** contains 18 modules rich with animations, videos, interactive activities, and exercises to help students prepare for their clinical lab experience. The instructionally designed lessons focus on topics that are difficult to master and pose a high risk to the patient if done incorrectly. Lesson quizzes allow students to check their learning curve and review as needed, and the module exams feed out to an instructor grade book. Modules cover Airway Management, Blood Therapy, Bowel Elimination/Ostomy, Chest Tubes, Enteral Nutrition, Infection Control, Injections, IV Fluid Administration, IV Fluid Therapy Management, IV Medication Administration, Non-parenteral Medication Administration, Safe Medication Administration, Safety, Specimen Collection, Urinary Catheterization, Vascular Access, Vital Signs, and Wound Care. Available alone or packaged with the text.

- **Mosby's Nursing Video Skills: Basic, Intermediate, Advanced, 4th edition,** provides 126 skills with overview information covering skill purpose, safety, and delegation guides; equipment lists; preparation procedures; procedure videos with printable step-by-step guidelines; appropriate follow-up care; documentation guidelines; and interactive review questions. Available online, as a student DVD set, or as a networkable DVD set for the institution.

ACKNOWLEDGMENTS

The eighth edition of *Essentials for Nursing Practice* is the result of a continued collaboration with Dr. Amy Hall and Dr. Patricia Stockert. Having professional colleagues to work with, trust, and challenge one another is a gift.

This textbook cannot be created without the support, guidance, and creative direction from our editorial team, designer, and production staff. Likewise, no book is successful without the hard work and dedication of its marketing team. We are also very fortunate regarding the manner in which staff from the electronic media division of Elsevier has produced products that complement the text and ensure its success.

Each of these divisions and the individuals within these groups contributed their time, talent, and energy to create a textbook that remains on the cutting edge with respect to the science and art of professional nursing. We wish to make special mention of some important individuals.

Tamara Myers, Executive Content Strategist, is a dedicated professional who continually challenges the author team to create a state-of-the-art revision and creates an environment for the editorial and production teams to develop a textbook that is creative and reflects contemporary nursing practice.

Tina Kaemmerer, Senior Content Development Specialist, is a dedicated professional whose organizational skills ensure that this project remains on target. She effectively tracks the manuscript through the publication process and is an invaluable resource for authors, contributors, and the production team.

Paula Catalano, our Book Designer, contributed to a clear, logical, and visually distinctive textbook design. She helped us achieve the goal of creating a text that is visually appealing yet easy for our readers to use. Paula is also credited for her creativity and vision for the design of the cover art and her direction in implementing the overall design of the text.

Many thanks and gratitude goes to members of the Production Team.

- Jodi Willard, Senior Project Manager, is a tireless and dedicated professional. As an accomplished project manager, she keeps us on deadline while ensuring consistency in formatting, presentation, and style. Her sense of humor and ability to always remain calm under pressure are invaluable attributes.
- Debbie Vogel, Publishing Services Manager, has contributed support throughout the editing and final pages.

Many thanks to Michael DeFilippo for his photographic excellence and to Barnes West Hospital, Creve Coeur, Missouri, for the generous use of their facility for our photo shoot.

A tip of the hat must always go to the sales and marketing team, headed by Pat Crowe and Katie Schlesinger, who provided us direction early on in the planning stage of *Essentials for Nursing Practice*. Their knowledge of market trends and needs helps us to make revisions of high quality.

Many thanks to our contributors, clinicians, and educators, who share their experiences and knowledge about nursing practice in helping to create informative, accurate, and current information. Their knowledge of their own clinical specialties ensures we have a state-of-the-art textbook. We are fortunate to be associated with excellent nurse authors who are able to convey standards of nursing excellence through the printed word.

A heartfelt thanks to our many reviewers for their expertise, candor, knowledge of the literature, and astute comments that assist us in developing a text with high standards that reflect professional nursing practice today.

After many years of collaboration, we find ourselves very fortunate and humble. *Essentials for Nursing Practice* and the other textbooks we have been able to develop have made important contributions to nursing practice. It remains a work of love.

Patricia A. Potter
Anne Griffin Perry
Patricia A. Stockert
Amy Hall

CONTENTS

UNIT 1 CONCEPTS IN NURSING

UNIT 2 PROCESSES IN NURSING CARE

CHAPTER

1

The Nursing Profession

evolve WEBSITE

http://evolve.elsevier.com/Potter/essentials

- Crossword Puzzle
- Audio Glossary

OBJECTIVES

- Discuss the characteristics of professionalism in nursing.
- Discuss the importance of education in professional nursing practice.
- Describe the purpose of professional standards of nursing practice.
- Describe the roles and career opportunities for nurses.
- Discuss the influence of social, political, and economic changes on nursing practices.

KEY TERMS

advanced practice registered nurse (APRN), p. 8
American Nurses Association (ANA), p. 2
caregiver, p. 7
certified nurse-midwife (CNM), p. 8
certified registered nurse anesthetist (CRNA), p. 8
clinical nurse specialist (CNS), p. 8
code of ethics, p. 6
continuing education, p. 5
genomics, p. 11
in-service education, p. 6
International Council of Nurses (ICN), p. 10
licensed practical nurse, p. 5
licensed vocational nurse, p. 5
National League for Nursing (NLN), p. 10
nurse administrator, p. 9
nurse educator, p. 9
nurse practitioner (NP), p. 8
nurse researcher, p. 9
nursing, p. 2
patient advocate, p. 7
professional organization, p. 9
Quality and Safety Education for Nurses (QSEN), p. 10
registered nurse (RN), p. 5

Nursing is an art and a science. As a professional nurse you learn to deliver care artfully with compassion, caring, and respect for each patient's dignity and personhood. As a science nursing practice is based on a body of knowledge that is continually changing with new discoveries and innovations. When you integrate the science and art of nursing into your practice, the quality of care you provide to your patients is at a level of excellence that benefits patients and their families. Your patients' health care needs are multidimensional. Thus your care reflects the needs and values of society and professional standards of care and performance, meets the needs of each patient, and integrates evidence-based findings to provide the highest level of care.

As a nurse you can choose a variety of career paths, including clinical practice, education, research, management, administration, and entrepreneurship. As a student it is important for you to understand the scope of nursing practice and how nursing influences the lives of your patients.

The patient is the center of your practice. The patient includes the individual, family, and/or community. Patients have a wide variety of health care needs, experiences, vulnerabilities, and expectations; but this is what makes nursing

CASE STUDY *Maria*

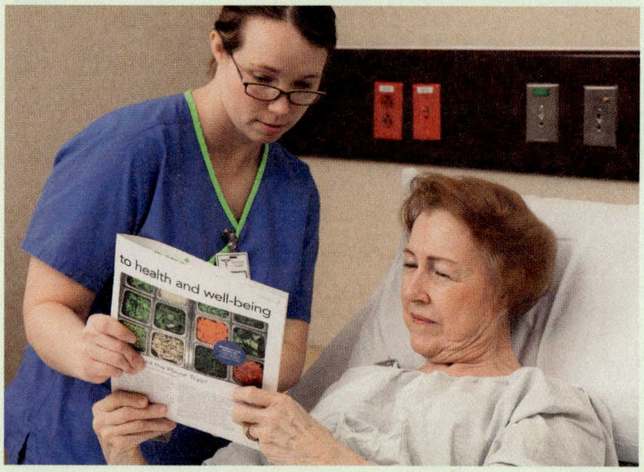

Maria is a nursing student in her final clinical nursing course. She is assigned to provide care for a 72-year-old patient, Mrs. Malone, on the rehabilitation unit. Mrs. Malone came to the unit following surgery for repair of a left hip fracture. She has improved strength, ability to walk and perform activities of daily living after participating in rehabilitation activities for the past 2 weeks, and is going home soon. Maria focused her nursing care plan on discharge teaching for Mrs. Malone. Mrs. Malone told Maria that she is excited about going home at the end of the week. This morning Maria is participating in the interdisciplinary team meeting to discuss Mrs. Malone's upcoming discharge.

both challenging and rewarding. Making a difference in your patients' lives is fulfilling. For example, you help a dying patient find relief from pain, help a young mother learn parenting skills, or find ways for older adults to remain independent in their homes. Nursing offers personal and professional rewards every day.

You need to provide nursing care according to standards of practice and follow a code of ethics (ANA, 2010b; 2010c). Professional practice includes knowledge from social and behavioral sciences, biological and physiological sciences, and nursing theories. In addition, nursing practice incorporates ethical and social values, professional autonomy, and a sense of commitment and community. The **American Nurses Association (ANA)** defines **nursing** as *the protection, promotion, and optimization of health and abilities; prevention of illness and injury; alleviation of suffering through the diagnosis and treatment of human response; and advocacy in the care of individuals, families, communities, and populations* (ANA, 2010b). The International Council of Nurses (ICN) (2010) has another definition: *Nursing encompasses autonomous and collaborative care of individuals of all ages, families, groups and communities, sick or well and in all settings. Nursing includes the promotion of health; prevention of illness; and the care of ill, disabled, and dying people. Advocacy, promotion of a safe environment, research, participation in shaping health policy and in patient and health systems management, and education are also key nursing roles.* Both of these definitions support the importance that nursing holds in providing safe, patient-centered health care to the global community.

Expert clinical nursing practice is a commitment to the application of knowledge, ethics, standards of practice, and clinical experience. Your ability to interpret clinical situations and make complex decisions is the foundation for your nursing care and the basis for the advancement of nursing practice and the development of nursing science (Benner, 1984; Benner, Tanner, and Chesla, 1997; Benner et al., 2010). Clinical expertise takes time and commitment. Critical thinking skills are essential to nursing (see Chapter 8). When providing nursing care, you need to make clinical judgments and decisions about your patients' health care needs based on knowledge, experience, and standards of care. Use critical thinking skills and reflections to help you gain and interpret scientific knowledge, integrate knowledge from clinical experiences, and become a lifelong learner (Benner et al., 2010). This includes integrating knowledge from basic science and nursing knowledge bases, applying knowledge from past and present experiences, applying critical thinking attitudes to a clinical situation, and implementing intellectual and professional standards (see Chapter 8). When you provide well–thought out care with compassion and caring, you provide each of your patients the best of the science and art of nursing care (see Chapter 7).

HISTORY OF NURSING

Nursing has responded and always will respond to the needs of its patients. Patients are most vulnerable when they are injured, sick, or dying. Since the beginning of the profession, nurses have studied and tested new and better ways to help them. Florence Nightingale studied and implemented methods to improve battlefield sanitation during the Crimean War in the 1850s, which ultimately reduced illness, infection, and mortality (Cohen, 1984). Think about the effect of Nightingale's actions so long ago. She set the stage for using evidence to direct nursing practice.

Nursing is a combination of knowledge from the physical sciences, humanities, and social sciences, along with clinical competencies needed for safe, quality patient-centered care (Gugliemi, 2010). Today nurses are active in determining the best practices for patient care related to problems such as skin care management, pain control, nutritional management, and care of older adults. Nurse researchers are leaders in expanding knowledge in nursing and other health care disciplines. Their work provides evidence for practice to ensure that we have the best available evidence to support our practices (see Chapter 7).

Nurses are also active in social policy and political arenas. With their professional organizations they lobby for health care legislation to meet the needs of patients. For example, they have lobbied for laws promoting smoke-free environments and stronger antitobacco laws, setting up anti-gang coalitions, establishing safer environments for walking and physical fitness in their communities, and advocating for breastfeeding (Mason et al., 2012).

Knowledge of the history of the nursing profession increases your ability to understand the social and intellectual origins of the discipline. Although it is not practical to describe all of the historical aspects of professional nursing, some of the more significant milestones are described in the following paragraphs.

Florence Nightingale

In *Notes on Nursing: What It Is and What It Is Not*, Florence Nightingale established the first nursing philosophy based on health maintenance and restoration (Nightingale, 1860). She saw the role of nursing as having "charge of somebody's health" based on the knowledge of "how to put the body in such a state to be free of disease or to recover from disease" (Nightingale, 1860). During the same year she developed the first organized training program for nurses, the Nightingale Training School for Nurses at St. Thomas' Hospital in London.

Nightingale was the first practicing nurse epidemiologist (Cohen, 1984). Her statistical analyses connected poor sanitation with cholera and dysentery. She volunteered during the Crimean War in 1853 and traveled the battlefield hospitals at night carrying her lamp; thus she was known as the "lady with the lamp." As a result of Nightingale's organization and improvement of the sanitation facilities at the battlefield hospitals, the mortality rate at the Barracks Hospital in Scutari, Turkey, was reduced from 42.7% to 2.2% in 6 months (Donahue, 2011).

The Civil War to the Beginning of the Twentieth Century

The Civil War (1860 to 1865) stimulated the growth of nursing in the United States. Clara Barton, founder of the American Red Cross, cared for soldiers on the battlefields, cleansing their wounds, meeting their basic needs, and comforting them in death. The U.S. Congress ratified the American Red Cross in 1882 after 10 years of lobbying by Barton. Dorothea Lynde Dix, Mary Ann Ball (Mother Bickerdyke), and Harriet Tubman also influenced nursing during the Civil War (Donahue, 2011). As superintendent of the female nurses of the Union Army, Dix organized hospitals, appointed nurses, and oversaw and regulated supplies to the troops. Mother Bickerdyke organized ambulance services and walked abandoned battlefields at night, looking for wounded soldiers. Harriet Tubman was active in the Underground Railroad movement and assisted in leading over 300 slaves to freedom (Donahue, 2011).

The first professionally educated African-American nurse was Mary Mahoney. She was concerned with relationships between cultures and races; and as a noted nursing leader she brought forth an awareness of cultural diversity and respect for the individual, regardless of background, race, color, or religion.

Isabel Hampton Robb helped found the Nurses' Associated Alumnae of the United States and Canada in 1896. This organization became the ANA in 1911. She authored many nursing textbooks, including *Nursing: Its Principles and Practice for Hospital and Private Use* (1894), *Nursing Ethics* (1900), and *Educational Standards for Nurses* (1907) and was one of the original founders of the *American Journal of Nursing* (Am J Nurs) (Donahue, 2011).

Nursing in hospitals expanded in the late nineteenth century. However, nursing in the community did not increase significantly until 1893, when Lillian Wald and Mary Brewster opened the Henry Street Settlement, which focused on the health needs of poor people who lived in tenements in New York City (Donahue, 2011). Nurses working in this settlement were some of the first to demonstrate autonomy in practice because they frequently encountered situations that required quick and innovative problem solving and critical thinking without the supervision or direction of a health care provider.

Twentieth Century

In the early twentieth century nursing evolved toward developing a scientific, research-based defined body of nursing knowledge and practice. Nurses began to assume expanded and advanced practice roles to meet the needs of society. Mary Adelaide Nutting was instrumental in the affiliation of nursing education with universities. She became the first professor of nursing at Columbia University Teachers College in 1906 (Donahue, 2011). In addition, the Goldmark Report concluded that nursing education needed increased financial support and suggested that university schools of nursing receive the money.

As nursing education developed, nursing practice also expanded, and the Army and Navy Nurse Corps were established. By the 1920s nursing specialization started to develop. Graduate nurse-midwifery programs began; in the last half of the century specialty-nursing organizations were created. Examples of these specialty organizations include the American Association of Critical Care Nurses; Association of Operating Room Nurses (AORN); Emergency Nurses Association (ENA); Infusion Nurses Society (INS); Oncology Nursing Society (ONS); and Wound, Ostomy, Continence Nurses Society (WOCN). In 1990 the ANA established the Center for Ethics and Human Rights (see Chapter 6). The Center provides a forum to address the complex ethical and human rights issues confronting nurses and designs activities and programs to increase ethical competence in nurses (ANA, 2010c).

Twenty-First Century

Today the nursing profession faces multiple challenges. Nurses and nurse educators are revising nursing practice and school curricula to meet the ever-changing needs of society, including bioterrorism, emerging infections, and disaster management. Advances in technology and informatics (see Chapter 10), the aging population, the high-acuity level of care of hospitalized patients, and early discharge from health care institutions require nurses in all settings to have a strong and current knowledge base from which to practice. In addition, nursing and the Robert Wood Johnson Foundation are taking a leadership role in developing standards and policies for end-of-life care through the *Last Acts Campaign* (see Chapter 26). The End-of-Life Nursing Education Consortium (ELNEC) offered collaboratively by the American Association of Colleges of Nursing (AACN) and the City of Hope Medical Center has brought end-of-life care and practices into nursing curricula and professional continuing-education programs for practicing nurses (Tilden and Thompson, 2009).

INFLUENCES ON NURSING

Multiple external forces affect nursing today, including health care reform, demographic changes of the population, increasing numbers of medically underserved, need for emergency preparedness, workplace issues, and the nursing shortage.

Health Care Reform and Costs

Health care reform affects not only how health care is paid for but how it is delivered. There will be greater emphasis on health promotion, disease prevention, and illness management in the future. More services will be in community-based care settings. As a result, more nurses will be needed to practice in community care centers, schools, and senior centers. This will require nurses to be more adept at assessing for resources, service gaps, and how the patient adapts to returning to the community. Nursing needs to respond to such changes by exploring new methods to provide care, changing nursing education, and revising practice standards (O'Neil, 2009).

Skyrocketing health care costs present challenges to the profession, consumer, and health care delivery system. As a nurse you are responsible for providing the patient with the best-quality care in an efficient and economically sound manner. The challenge is to use health care and patient resources wisely. Chapter 3 summarizes reasons for the rise in health care costs and its implications for nursing.

Demographic Changes

The U.S. Census Bureau (2008a) predicts that between 2010 and 2050 there will be a steady rise in the population. This change alone requires expanded health care resources. Add to the population change a steady increase in the population of people 65 years and older (U.S. Census Bureau, 2008b). To effectively meet all the health care needs of the expanding and aging population, changes need to occur as to how care is provided, especially in the area of public health, to address health care reform and meet the needs of the changing population. The population is still shifting from rural areas to urban centers, and more people are living with chronic and long-term illness (Presley, 2010). Not only are outpatient settings expanding, but more and more people want to receive outpatient and community-based care and remain in their homes or community (see Chapters 3 and 4).

Medically Underserved

The rising rates of unemployment, underemployment and low-paying jobs, mental illness, and homelessness and rising health care costs all contribute to increases in the medically underserved population. Caring for this population is a global issue; the social, political, and economic factors of a country affect both access to care and resources to provide and pay for these services (Mercer, 2011). In the United States some of the medically underserved population are individuals who are poor and on Medicaid. Others are part of the working poor (e.g., they cannot afford their own insurance, but they make too much money to qualify for Medicaid and as a result do not receive any health care). In addition, the number of underserved patients who require home-based palliative care services is increasing. This is a group of patients whose physical status does not improve and heath care needs increase. As a result, the cost for home-based care continues to rise, to the point that some patients opt out of all palliative services because of costs (Fernandes et al., 2010). Today nurses and schools of nursing are developing partnerships to improve health outcomes in underserved communities. Nurses work in these community-based settings providing health promotion and disease prevention to the homeless, mentally ill, and others who have limited access to health care or who lack health care insurance (McCann, 2010).

Need for Emergency Preparedness

The world is a changing place; the threats of terrorism are continuous. Many health care agencies, schools, and communities have educational programs to prepare for nuclear, chemical, or biological attack and other types of disasters. Nurses play an active role in emergency preparedness. The ICN works alongside national nursing associations to determine how to best educate and prepare nurses for future disasters (Robinson, 2010). For example, public health emergency simulation exercises allow nurses and students to work with community disaster-preparedness groups and hospitals to determine which specific nursing activities are needed (Morrison and Catanzaro, 2010). These activities sometimes range from participation in vaccine research, decontamination in the event of biological attack, and triage for mass casualty to crisis response units. Nurses have increased responsibilities in providing emergency preparedness education and preparing for disasters at the local, state, and federal levels (Zerwekh and Garneau, 2012).

Workplace Issues

Nurses are faced with multiple issues and hazards in the workplace. For example, they are at risk for ergonomic hazards that result in musculoskeletal injuries such as back injury and repetitive motion disorders (American Nurses Association, 2013). When looking for a new position, evaluate the workforce protection and safety plan that the hospital or health care organization has in place (Zerwekh and Garneau, 2012).

Another issue facing nurses is workplace violence. Workplace violence takes the form of bullying and acts of verbal or nonverbal aggression or harassment from co-workers and sometimes patients and families. Be sure to be familiar with the policies of your institution on workplace violence.

Nursing Shortage

There is an ongoing global nursing shortage, which results from insufficient qualified registered nurses (RNs) to fill vacant positions and the loss of qualified RNs to other professions (AACN, 2010; Flinkman et al., 2010). This shortage affects all aspects of nursing such as hospitals, long-term care facilities, administration, and nursing education (AACN, 2012); but it also represents challenges and opportunities for the profession. Many health care dollars are invested in strategies aimed at recruiting a well-educated, critically thinking, motivated, and dedicated nursing workforce (Benner et al., 2010). There is a direct link between RNs' care and positive patient outcomes, reduced complication rates, and a more rapid return of the patient to an optimal functional status (Aiken, 2010; Lucero et al., 2009).

With fewer nurses in the workplace, it is important for you to learn to use your patient contact time efficiently and professionally. Time management, therapeutic communication, patient education, and compassionate implementation of psychomotor skills are just a few of the essential skills you need. Most important, your patients leave the health care setting with a positive image of nursing and a feeling that they received quality care. Your patient should never feel rushed or that he or she was unimportant. If a certain aspect of patient care requires 15 minutes of contact, it takes the same amount of time to deliver the care in an organized manner as it would in a rushed, harried manner.

PROFESSIONALISM

Nursing is a profession. A person who acts professionally is conscientious in actions, knowledgeable in the subject, and responsible to self and others. This means that as a nurse you administer patient-centered care in a safe, conscientious, and knowledgeable manner. Professions possess the following characteristics:

- An extended education of members and a basic liberal education foundation
- A theoretical body of knowledge leading to defined skills, abilities, and norms
- Provision of a specific service
- Autonomy in decision making and practice
- A code of ethics for practice

Nursing shares each of these characteristics, offering an opportunity for the growth and enrichment of all of its members.

Licensed Practical Nurse/Licensed Vocational Nurse Education

A licensed practical or vocational nurse is educated in basic nursing techniques and direct patient care. The **licensed practical nurse (LPN)** or **licensed vocational nurse (LVN)** is a nurse who completes a practical nursing program and passes a licensure examination (NCLEX-PN®). The LPN/LVN practices under the supervision of an RN or other licensed person. The responsibilities and scope of practice are set by each state board of nursing. An LPN/LVN, or in Canada an RN assistant (RNA), generally receives 1 year of education and clinical preparation in a community college or other agency. Some RN programs allow an LPN to enter the program at an advanced level.

Registered Nurse Education

As a profession nursing requires that its members possess a significant amount of education. There are various educational routes for becoming a **registered nurse (RN)**. Currently in the United States an individual becomes an RN by completion of an associate degree, diploma, or baccalaureate degree program in nursing. The Canadian Nurses Association (2012) has identified the baccalaureate degree as the entry to practice standard for RNs in all provinces except Quebec. Nursing education provides the solid foundation for practice, and it responds to changes in health care created by scientific and technological advances.

Advanced Education

Some roles for RNs in nursing require advanced graduate degrees. The graduate degree provides the advanced clinician with strong skills in nursing science and theory, with an emphasis on the basic sciences and research-based clinical practice. A master's degree in nursing (e.g., Master of Arts in nursing [MA], Master of Nursing [MN], or Master of Science in nursing [MSN]) is for RNs with a Bachelor of Science in nursing (BSN) seeking roles as nurse educator, nurse administrator, or an advanced practice registered nurse (APRN) role. The degree provides the advanced clinician with strong skills in nursing science and theory with emphasis in the basic sciences and research-based clinical practice related to a specialty. Some roles within nursing require doctoral degrees. There are two doctorate degree options for nurses. The Doctor of Philosophy (PhD) has a focus on research, and the Doctor of Nursing Practice (DNP) has a focus on advanced clinical practice. The health care industry needs nurses prepared at the doctorate level with advanced academic and clinical preparation to educate nursing students and participate as members of the interdisciplinary health care team to provide evidence-based, competent, safe patient care (IOM, 2010). Nurses with doctorates advance the profession by promoting evidence-based practice, conducting and disseminating research, developing and testing theory, and influencing public policy and health care planning.

Continuing and In-Service Education

Continuing education programs are one way to promote and maintain current nursing skills, gain new knowledge about the latest research and practice developments, specialize in a specific practice area, and obtain new skills and techniques reflecting the changes in the health care delivery system (Hale et al., 2010). **Continuing education** involves formal, organized educational programs offered by universities, hospitals, state nurses associations, professional nursing organizations, and educational and health care institutions. An example is a program on caring for older adults with dementia offered by a university or a program on safe medication practices offered by a hospital. Often these programs provide the attendees with some type of continuing education credit.

In-service education programs are instruction or training provided by a health care agency or institution designed to increase the knowledge, skills, and competencies of nurses and other health care professionals employed by the institution. Often in-service programs are focused on new technologies or designed to fulfill required competencies of the organization. For example, a hospital offers an in-service program on safe principles for administering chemotherapy or a program on cultural sensitivity.

Theory

Professional nursing practice and knowledge have developed in part through nursing theories (global views that help to describe, predict, or prescribe activities for the practice of nursing). Theoretical models provide frameworks for how nurses practice. Typically a nursing school curriculum integrates a theoretical model. Examples of theories used in education and practice are Orem's self-care deficit theory, Benner's primacy of caring, and Roy's adaptation theory. Some nursing organizations adopt a nursing theory as the foundation for their standards of nursing care. The ongoing development of nursing theory or nursing science involves generating knowledge to advance and support nursing practice and health care (Alligood, 2010).

Service

Nursing is a service profession and a vital and indispensable part of the health care delivery system. Nurses in practice today maintain a consumer and service-based focus. Patients are more aware and knowledgeable about their health care problems, options, and rights. As a nurse you work with patients and families, individualizing care while incorporating their preferences and expectations. Show respect for patients by providing care on time, displaying a caring attitude, and considering patients' cultural and social differences. Collaborating with necessary health care providers ensures a smooth continuation of care from one setting to the next.

Autonomy and Accountability

Autonomy is essential to professional nursing and involves the initiation of independent nursing interventions without medical orders. It means that a person is reasonably independent and self-governing in decision making and practice. You reach autonomy through experience, advanced education, and the support of an organization that values the independent role of the nurse. With increased autonomy comes greater responsibility and accountability for the performance of nursing care activities. Accountability means that you are professionally and legally responsible for the type and quality of nursing care provided. To be autonomous and accountable carries the responsibility to keep current and competent in nursing and scientific knowledge and skills.

Code of Ethics

Nursing has a **code of ethics** that defines the principles that nurses use to provide patient-centered care (see Chapter 6). In addition, nurses incorporate their own values and ethics into practice. The ANA's *Code of Ethics for Nurses: Interpretation and Application* (2010c) provides a guide for carrying out nursing responsibilities to ensure high-quality nursing care and provide for the ethical obligations of the profession.

STANDARDS OF NURSING PRACTICE

Nursing is a helping, independent profession that provides services that contribute to the health of people. Three essential components of professional nursing are care, cure, and coordination. The *care* aspect is more than "to take care of"; it is also "caring about." Caring is relational and requires you as a nurse to understand a patient's needs so you can individualize nursing therapies (see Chapter 19). When you promote health and healing, you are practicing the *cure* aspect of professional nursing. To cure is to help patients understand their health problems and help them cope. The cure aspect involves the administration of treatments and the use of clinical nursing judgment in determining, on the basis of patient outcomes, whether the plan of care is effective. *Coordination* of care involves organizing and timing medical and other professional and technical services to meet the holistic needs of a patient. Often a patient requires many services simultaneously for care to be effective. A professional nurse also supervises, teaches, and directs all of those involved in nursing care.

As an independent profession, nursing has increasingly set its own standards for practice. These standards are guidelines for how nurses perform professionally and how they exercise the care, cure, and coordination aspects of nursing. Clinical, academic, and administrative nurse experts develop standards of nursing practice. As an example, the ANA has published *Nursing: Scope and Standards of Practice* (2010b). Within this document are Standards of Professional Performance and Standards of Practice for professional nurses. For detailed information on the ANA standards, go to http://www.nursingworld.org/scopeandstandardsofpractice.

In the practice setting it is important to have objective guidelines for providing and evaluating nursing care. Standards of nursing care are developed and established on the basis of strong scientific research and the work of clinical nurse experts. The purpose of a standard of care is to describe the common level of professional nursing care to judge the quality of nursing practice. An organization sometimes adopts a general set of standards for nursing care such as organizational protocols, policies, or procedures. For example, an organization has a written nasogastric tube protocol based on research findings. This protocol spells out the expected nursing care for patients with nasogastric tubes in that organization. Individual nursing units or work groups also establish standards of care to address the unique needs of patients for whom they care. For example, an oncology nursing unit develops standards of care for pain management and palliative care for patients with cancer. Standards of care are important if a legal dispute arises over whether a nurse practiced appropriately in a particular case (see Chapter 5). More important, they establish the guidelines for nursing excellence within an organization.

NURSING PRACTICE

You will have an opportunity to practice in a variety of settings, in many roles within those settings, and with caregivers in other related health professions. State and provincial Nurse Practice Acts (NPAs) establish specific legal regulations for practice, and professional organizations establish standards of practice as criteria for nursing care. The ANA is concerned with legal aspects of nursing practice, public recognition of the significance of nursing practice to health care, and implications for nursing practice regarding trends in health care. The ANA definition of nursing illustrates the consistent orientation of nurses to provide care to promote the well-being of their patients individually or in groups and communities (ANA, 2010a).

Nurse Practice Acts

In the United States each State Board of Nursing oversees its Nurse Practice Act (NPA) that regulates the scope of nursing practice for the state and protects public health, safety, and welfare. This protection includes shielding the public from unqualified and unsafe nurses. Although each state has its own NPA that defines the scope of nursing practice, most NPAs are similar. The definition of nursing practice published by the ANA is representative of the scope of nursing practice as defined in most states. In the last decade many states have revised their NPAs to reflect the growing autonomy of nursing and the expanded roles and scope of practice of advanced practice registered nurses.

Licensure and Certification

Licensure. In the United States RN candidates must pass the NCLEX-RN® examination administered by the individual State Boards of Nursing to obtain a nursing license. Regardless of educational preparation, the examination for RN licensure is exactly the same in every state in the United States. This provides a standardized minimum knowledge base for nurses. In all Canadian provinces except Quebec, new graduates must pass the Canadian Registered Nurse Examination (CRNE) to become an RN. Whether nurses are able to practice in a state or province other than their own depends on the agreement between the states or provinces involved.

Certification. Beyond the NCLEX-RN®, some nurses choose to work toward certification in a specific area of nursing practice. Minimum practice requirements are set based on the certification the nurse seeks. National nursing organizations such as the ANA have many types of certification to enhance your career such as certification in medical surgical or geriatric nursing. After passing the initial examination, you maintain your certification by ongoing continuing education and clinical or administrative practice.

RESPONSIBILITIES AND ROLES OF THE NURSE

As a nurse you are responsible for obtaining and maintaining specific knowledge and skills for a variety of professional roles and responsibilities. Nurses provide care and comfort for patients in all health care settings. Their concern for meeting the patients' needs remains the same whether care focuses on health promotion and illness prevention, disease and symptom management, family support, or end-of-life care.

Caregiver

As caregiver you help patients maintain and regain health, manage disease and symptoms, and attain a maximal level function and independence through the healing process. You provide healing through both physical and interpersonal skills. Healing involves more than achieving improved physical well-being. You need to meet all health care needs of a patient by providing measures that restore the patient's emotional, spiritual, and social well-being. As a caregiver you help the patient and family set goals and assist them with meeting these goals with minimal financial cost, time, and energy.

Advocate

As a patient advocate you protect your patient's human and legal rights and provide assistance in asserting these rights if the need arises. As an advocate you act on behalf of your patient, securing and standing up for your patient's health care rights (Hanks, 2010). For example, you provide additional information to help a patient decide whether or not to accept a treatment, or you find an interpreter to help family members communicate their concerns. You sometimes need to defend patients' rights in a general way by speaking out against policies or actions that put patients in danger or conflict with their rights.

Educator

As an educator you explain concepts and facts about health, describe the reason for routine care activities, demonstrate procedures such as self-care activities, reinforce learning or patient behavior, and evaluate patients' progress in learning. Sometimes patient teaching is unplanned and informal (see Chapter 12). For example, during a casual conversation you respond to questions about the reason for an intravenous infusion, a health issue such as smoking cessation, or necessary lifestyle changes. Other teaching activities are planned and more formal such as when you teach your patient to self-administer insulin injections. Always use teaching methods that match your patient's capabilities and needs and incorporate other resources such as the family in teaching plans (see Chapter 24).

Communicator

Your effectiveness as a communicator is central to the nurse-patient relationship. It allows you to know your patients, including their strengths and weaknesses and their needs. Communication is essential for all nursing roles and activities. You routinely communicate with patients and families, other nurses and health care professionals, resource persons, and the community. Without clear communication it is impossible to give comfort and emotional support, give care effectively, make decisions with patients and families, protect patients from threats to well-being, coordinate and manage patient care, assist patients in rehabilitation, or provide patient education. The quality of communication is a critical factor in meeting the needs of individuals, families, and communities (see Chapter 11).

Provider of Care

Most nurses provide direct patient care in an acute care setting. In the hospital some nurses choose to practice in a medical-surgical setting, whereas others concentrate on a specific area of specialty practice such as pediatrics, critical care, or emergency care. Most specialty care areas require some experience as a medical-surgical nurse and additional continuing or in-service education. Many intensive care unit and emergency department nurses are required to have certification in advanced cardiac life support and critical care, emergency nursing, or trauma nursing.

As health care returns to the home care setting, there are increased opportunities for you to provide direct care in a patient's home or community. Use the nursing process and critical thinking skills to provide care that is both restorative and curative. Educate your patients and families to promote health maintenance and self-care. In collaboration with other health care team members, focus your care on returning patients to their home at an optimal functional status.

Manager

Today's health care environment is fast paced and complex. Nurse managers need to establish an environment for collaborative patient-centered care to provide safe, quality care with positive patient outcomes. A manager coordinates the activities of members of the nursing staff in delivering nursing care and has personnel, policy, and budgetary responsibility for a specific nursing unit or agency. The manager uses appropriate leadership styles to create a nursing environment for the patients and staff that reflect the mission and values of the health care organization (see Chapter 13).

Career Development

Innovations in health care, expanding health care systems and practice settings, and the increasing needs of patients have been stimuli for the creation of new nursing roles. Today the majority of nurses practice in hospital settings, followed by community-based care, ambulatory care, and nursing homes/extended care settings.

Nursing provides an opportunity for you to commit to lifelong learning and career development to provide patients the state-of-the-art care they need. Career roles are specific employment positions or paths. Because of increasing educational opportunities for nurses, the growth of nursing as a profession, and a greater concern for job enrichment, the nursing profession offers expanded roles and different kinds of career opportunities. Your career path is limitless. You will probably switch career roles more than once. Take advantage of the different clinical practice and professional opportunities. These career opportunities include APRNs, nurse researchers, nurse risk managers, quality improvement nurses, consultants, and even business owners.

Advanced Practice Registered Nurse. The **advanced practice registered nurse (APRN)** is the most independently functioning nurse. An APRN has a master's degree in nursing; advanced education in pathophysiology, pharmacology, and physical assessment; and certification and expertise in a specialized area of practice (AACN, 2011). There are four core roles for an APRN: clinical nurse specialist (CNS), nurse practitioner (NP), certified nurse-midwife (CNM), and certified RN anesthetist (CRNA). The educational preparation for the four roles is in at least one of the following six populations: adult-gerontology, pediatrics, neonatology, women's health/gender related, family/individual across life span, and psychiatric mental health. APRNs function as clinicians, educators, case managers, consultants, and researchers within their area of practice to plan or improve the quality of nursing care for patients and their families.

Clinical Nurse Specialist. The **clinical nurse specialist (CNS)** is an APRN who is an expert clinician in a specialized area of practice (Box 1-1). The specialty may be identified by a population (e.g., geriatrics), setting (e.g., critical care), disease specialty (e.g., diabetes), type of care (e.g., rehabilitation), or type of problem (e.g., pain) (National CNS Competency Task Force, 2010). The CNS practices in all health care settings.

Nurse Practitioner. The **nurse practitioner (NP)** is an APRN who provides health care to a group of patients, usually in an outpatient, ambulatory care, or community-based setting. The major NP categories are acute care, adult, family, pediatric, women's, psychiatric mental health, and geriatric. The NP provides comprehensive care, directly managing the medical care of patients who are healthy or have chronic conditions and establishes a collaborative provider-patient relationship, working with a specific group of patients or with patients of all ages and health care needs.

Certified Nurse-Midwife. A **certified nurse-midwife (CNM)** is an APRN who is educated in midwifery and is certified by the American College of Nurse-Midwives. The practice of nurse-midwifery involves providing independent care for women during normal pregnancy, labor, and delivery and care for the newborn. It includes providing some gynecological services such as routine Papanicolaou (Pap) tests, family planning, and treatment for minor vaginal infections.

Certified Registered Nurse Anesthetist. A **certified registered nurse anesthetist (CRNA)** is an APRN with advanced

BOX 1-1 EVIDENCE-BASED PRACTICE

PICO Question: In chronically ill patients, does the education and support provided by a Clinical Nurse Specialist (CNS) compared to a non-CNS improve patient satisfaction?

SUMMARY OF EVIDENCE

A work analysis demonstrated that CNSs typically spend approximately 63% of their time in direct patient care or patient-related activities, including education and support (Norton et al., 2012). Clinical practice and education are two of the primary roles of a CNS (Mayo, Agocs-Scott, Khaghani, et al., 2010). In patients with chronic illnesses a review of the literature showed that CNS-provided education and care resulted in higher levels of patient satisfaction in a variety of patient groups (Moore and McQuestion, 2012). Breast cancer survivors were found to have a high level of satisfaction with the support provided by the CNS during the first year of treatment (Hardie and Leary, 2010).

APPLICATION TO NURSING PRACTICE

- Consider advancing your education to an advanced practice nursing role after you graduate from your basic nursing program.
- Participate in education programs conducted by a CNS for patients and staff (Policicchio et al., 2011).
- Schedule early follow-up appointments with the CNS for patients with chronic illness to assist with patient satisfaction (Moore and McQuestion, 2012).
- Partner with the CNS when able to provide support and education for patients (Moore and McQuestion, 2012).

education in a nurse anesthesia accredited program. Nurse anesthetists provide surgical anesthesia under the guidance and supervision of an anesthesiologist, who is a physician with advanced knowledge of surgical anesthesia.

Nurse Educator. A **nurse educator** works primarily in schools of nursing, staff development departments of health care agencies, and patient education departments. Nurse educators need experience in clinical practice to provide them with practical skills and theoretical knowledge. A faculty member in a school of nursing is responsible for teaching current nursing practice, trends, theory, and necessary skills in laboratories and clinical settings to educate students to become professional nurses. Nurse educators in schools of nursing usually have graduate degrees in nursing and additional education such as a doctorate or an advanced degree in nursing, education, or administration such as a Master's Degree in Business Administration (MBA). They usually have a specific clinical, administrative, or research specialty and advanced clinical experience.

Nurse educators in staff development departments of health care institutions provide educational programs for nurses within their institutions. These programs include orientation of new personnel, critical care nursing courses, assisting with clinical skill competency, safety training, and instruction about new equipment or procedures. These nursing educators often participate in the development of nursing policies and procedures.

The primary focus of the nurse educator in the patient education department of an agency is to teach patients who are ill or disabled and their families how to self-manage their illness or disability. These nurse educators are usually specialized and certified such as a certified diabetes educator (CDE) or an ostomy care nurse and see only a specific population of patients.

Nurse Administrator. A **nurse administrator** manages patient care and the delivery of specific nursing services within a health care agency. Nursing administration begins with positions such as the assistant nurse manager. Experience and additional education sometimes lead to a middle-management position such as nurse manager of a specific patient care area or house supervisor or an upper-management position such as assistant or associate director or director of nursing services.

Nurse manager positions usually require at least a baccalaureate degree in nursing, and director and nurse executive positions generally require a master's degree. Chief nurse executives and vice president positions in large health care organizations often require preparation at the doctoral level. Nurse administrators frequently have advanced degrees such as a Master's Degree in nursing administration, MBA or a Master's Degree in hospital administration (MHA), public health (MPH), or health service administration.

In today's health care organizations directors may have responsibility for more than nursing units. Often directors manage a particular service or product line such as medicine or cardiology. Management of a service line often includes directing supportive functions and the health care personnel within areas such as medicine clinics, diagnostic departments, or outpatient.

Vice presidents of nursing or chief nurse executives often have responsibilities for all clinical functions within a hospital. This may include all ancillary personnel who provide and support patient care services. The nurse administrator needs to be skilled in business and management and understand all aspects of nursing and patient care. Functions of administrators include budgeting, staffing, strategic planning of programs and services, employee evaluation, and employee development.

Nurse Researcher. The **nurse researcher** investigates problems to improve nursing care and further define and expand the scope of nursing practice (see Chapter 7). He or she often works in an academic setting, hospital, or independent professional or community service agency. The preferred educational requirement is a doctoral degree, with at least a Master's Degree in nursing.

PROFESSIONAL NURSING ORGANIZATIONS

A **professional organization** deals with issues of concern to those practicing in the profession. In North America two major professional nursing organizations are the

National League for Nursing (NLN) and the ANA. The NLN advances excellence in nursing education to prepare nurses to meet the needs of a diverse population in a changing health care environment.

The purposes of the ANA are to improve standards of health and the availability of health care, foster high standards for nursing, and promote the professional development and general and economic welfare of nurses. The ANA is part of the International Council of Nurses (ICN). The objectives of the ICN parallel those of the ANA: promoting national associations of nurses, improving standards of nursing practice, seeking a higher status for nurses, and providing an international power base for nurses. The ANA is active in political, professional, and financial issues affecting health care and the nursing profession. It is a strong lobbyist in professional practice issues.

Nursing students take part in organizations such as the National Student Nurses Association (NSNA) in the United States and the Canadian Student Nurses Association (CSNA) in Canada. These organizations consider issues of importance to nursing students such as career development and preparation for licensing. The NSNA often cooperates in activities and programs with the professional organizations.

Some professional organizations focus on specific areas such as critical care, nursing administration, nursing research, or nurse-midwifery. These organizations seek to improve the standards of practice, expand nursing roles, and foster the welfare of nurses within the specialty areas. In addition, professional organizations present educational programs and publish journals.

TRENDS IN NURSING

Nursing is a dynamic profession that grows and evolves as society and lifestyles change, as health care priorities and technologies change, and as nurses themselves change. The current philosophies and definitions of nursing have a holistic focus, which addresses the needs of the whole person in all dimensions, in health and illness, and in interaction with the family and community. In addition, there continues to be an increasing awareness for patient safety in all care settings.

Quality and Safety Education for Nurses

The Robert Wood Johnson Foundation sponsored the Quality and Safety Education for Nurses (QSEN) initiative to respond to reports about safety and quality patient care by the IOM (Barton et al., 2009). QSEN addresses the challenge to prepare nurses with the competencies needed to continuously improve the quality of care in their work environments (Table 1-1). The QSEN initiative encompasses the competencies of patient-centered care, teamwork and collaboration, evidence-based practice, quality improvement, safety, and informatics (Cronenwett et al., 2007). For each competency there are targeted knowledge, skills, and attitudes (KSAs). The KSAs are elements that are integrated in a

TABLE 1-1 QUALITY AND SAFETY EDUCATION FOR NURSES

COMPETENCY	DEFINITION WITH EXAMPLES
Patient-centered care	Recognize the patient or designee as the source of control and full partner in providing compassionate and coordinated care based on respect for patient's preferences, values, and needs. ***Examples:*** *Involve family and friends in care. Elicit patient values and preferences. Provide care with respect for diversity of the human experience.*
Teamwork and collaboration	Function effectively within nursing and interprofessional teams, fostering open communication, mutual respect, and shared decision making to achieve quality patient care. ***Examples:*** *Recognize the contributions of other health team members and patient's family members. Discuss effective strategies for communicating and resolving conflict. Participate in designing methods to support effective teamwork.*
Evidence-based practice	Integrate best current evidence with clinical expertise and patient/family preferences and values for delivery of optimal health care. ***Examples:*** *Demonstrate knowledge of basic scientific methods. Appreciate strengths and weaknesses of scientific bases for practice. Appreciate the importance of regularly reading relevant journals.*
Quality improvement	Use data to monitor the outcomes of care processes and use improvement methods to design and test changes to continuously improve the quality and safety of health care systems. ***Examples:*** *Use tools such as flow charts and diagrams to make process of care explicit. Appreciate how unwanted variation in outcomes affects care. Identify gaps between local and best practices.*
Safety	Minimize risk of harm to patients and providers through both system effectiveness and individual performance. ***Examples:*** *Examine human factors, basic safety design principles, and commonly used unsafe practices. Value own role in preventing errors.*
Informatics	Use information and technology to communicate, manage knowledge, mitigate error, and support decision-making. ***Examples:*** *Navigate an electronic health record. Protect confidentiality of protected health information in electronic health records.*

Adapted from Cronenwett L, et al: Quality and safety education for nurses, *Nurs Outlook* 57:122, 2007.

nursing prelicensure program (Jarzemsky et al., 2010). As you gain experience in clinical practice, you encounter situations in which your education helps you to make a difference in improving patient care.

Whether that difference in care is to provide evidence for implementing care at the bedside, identify a safety issue, or study patient data to identify trends in outcomes, each of these situations requires competence in patient-centered care, safety, or informatics. Although it is not within the scope of this textbook to present the QSEN initiative in its entirety, subsequent clinical chapters provide you an opportunity to address how to build competencies in one or more of these areas.

Genomics

Genetics is the study of inheritance, or the way traits are passed down from one generation to another. Genes carry the instructions for making proteins, which in turn direct the activities of cells and functions of the body that influence traits such as hair and eye color. **Genomics** is a newer term that describes the study of all the genes in a person and interactions of these genes with one another and with that person's environment (CDC, 2011). Using genomic information allows health care providers to determine how genomic changes contribute to patient conditions and influence treatment decisions such as assessment and symptom management and titration of medications based on a patient's response (Miaskowski and Aouizerat, 2012). For example, when a family member has colon cancer before the age of 50, it is likely that other family members are at risk for developing this cancer. Knowing this information is important for family members who will need a colonoscopy before the age of 50 and repeat colonoscopies more often than the patient who is not at risk. In this case nurses play an essential role in identifying a patient's risk factors through assessment and counseling patients about what this genomic finding means to them personally and to their family.

Public Perception of Nursing

Nursing is a pivotal health care profession. As frontline health care providers, nurses practice in all health care settings and constitute the largest number of health care professionals. They are essential to providing skilled, specialized, knowledgeable care; improving the health status of the public; and ensuring safe, effective quality care (ANA, 2010b). For the 11th year in a row, the Gallup survey found that 85% of the survey participants ranked nurses highest among professionals for honesty and ethics (Laidman, 2012).

Consumers of health care are more informed than ever, and with the Internet consumers have access to more health care and treatment information. This information affects the perception the public has of nursing. For example, the media frequently highlights incidents of preventable medical errors such as medication and surgical errors. Publications such as *To Err Is Human* (IOM, 2000) describe strategies for government, health care providers, industry, and consumers to reduce preventable medical errors. When you care for patients, realize how your approach to care influences public opinion. Always act in a competent professional manner.

Effect of Nursing on Politics and Health Policy

Political power or influence is known as the ability to influence or persuade an individual holding a government office to exert the power of that office to affect a desired outcome. Nurses' involvement in politics is receiving greater emphasis in nursing curricula, professional organizations, and health care settings. Professional nursing organizations at both the national and state level employ lobbyists to urge state legislatures and the U.S. Congress to improve the quality of health care (Mason et al., 2012).

You can influence policy decisions at all governmental levels. One way to get involved is by participating in local and national efforts (Mason et al., 2012). This involvement is critical in exerting nurses' influence early in the political process. The future is bright when nurses become serious students of social needs, activists in influencing policy to meet those needs, and generous contributors of time and money to nursing organizations and candidates who support efforts to improve access to and quality of health care (Mason et al., 2012).

KEY POINTS

- A profession possesses the characteristics of extended education, theory, service, autonomy, and a code of ethics.
- The essential components of professional nursing are care, cure, and coordination.
- Nursing standards of care offer evidence-based guidelines for nurses to provide and evaluate care.
- Nursing responds to the health care needs of society, which are influenced by economic, social, and cultural variables of a specific era.
- Changes in society such as increased technology, new demographic patterns, consumerism, health promotion, and the women's and human rights movements lead to changes in nursing.
- Nursing definitions reflect changes in the practice of nursing and help bring about changes by identifying the domain of nursing practice and guiding research, practice, and education.
- Professional nursing organizations deal with issues of concern to specialist groups within the nursing profession.

CLINICAL DECISION-MAKING EXERCISES

Maria is preparing a presentation for her professional nursing issues and trends course. Her presentation focuses on professionalism and the many opportunities for nurses today. She decides to discuss three career opportunities: the staff nurse, the advanced practice nurse, and the nurse administrator.

1. Which similarities and differences exist between staff nurses, advanced practice registered nurses, and nurse administrators that Maria should include in her presentation?
2. What are the characteristics of a professional nurse that Maria should discuss?
3. Reflect on the information in this chapter and think about your nursing career over the next 5 years. What are your goals for your professional nursing career? What strategies can you use to achieve your goals?

evolve
Answers to Clinical Decision-Making Exercises can be found on the Evolve website.

QSEN ACTIVITY: TEAMWORK AND COLLABORATION

Maria participates in the team meeting to help plan for Mrs. Malone's discharge.

To be an effective team member, which skills and competencies should Maria use to promote teamwork and collaboration during the planning process?

evolve
Answers to QSEN Activities can be found on the Evolve website.

REVIEW QUESTIONS

1. Match the advance practice nurse specialty with the statement about the role.

___1. Clinical nurse specialist	a. Provides independent care including pregnancy and gynecological services.
___2. Nurse anesthetist	b. Expert clinician in a specialized area of practice such as adult diabetes care.
___3. Nurse practitioner	c. Provides comprehensive care, usually in a primary care setting, directly managing the medical care of patients who are healthy or who have chronic conditions.
___4. Nurse-midwife	d. Provides care and services under the supervision of an anesthesiologist.

2. You are preparing a presentation for your nursing course on the topic of professional standards of care. Which statement(s) best describe(s) professional standards of care? (Select all that apply.)
   1. Describe a competent level of behavior in the professional role
   2. Protect the patient's confidentiality
   3. Are based on scientific research
   4. Ensure patient-centered care for all patients
   5. Define the principles of right and wrong to provide patient care
3. A nurse on the unit previously gave pain medication to the patient for incisional pain, which the patient rated as 7 out of 10 on the pain scale. The nurse now checks on the patient 30 minutes later and documents that the patient now rates the pain as a 1 out of 10 on the pain scale. Which standard of practice did the nurse perform?
   1. Diagnosis
   2. Evaluation
   3. Assessment
   4. Implementation
4. A patient on the surgical unit develops a surgical wound infection. The nurse irrigates the surgical wound and changes the dressing every 8 hours. Which standard of practice is performed?
   1. Planning
   2. Evaluation
   3. Assessment
   4. Implementation
5. The nurse spends time with the patient and family reviewing the dressing change procedure for the patient's wound. The patient's spouse demonstrates how to change the dressing. The nurse is acting in which professional role?
   1. Educator
   2. Advocate
   3. Caregiver
   4. Case manager
6. The nurse attends the interdisciplinary team meeting as director of the cardiac service line. The director presents information on the budget for the service line and the strategic directions for the next fiscal year. The nurse is acting in what professional role?
   1. Educator
   2. Nurse administrator
   3. Nurse manager
   4. Caregiver
7. A nurse conducted a literature review on effective methods for patient teaching. Based on the literature search, the nurse develops a unit-based protocol for using the Teach Back method when providing patient teaching. This is an example of which Quality and Safety in the Education of Nurses (QSEN) competency?
   1. Patient-centered care
   2. Safety
   3. Teamwork and collaboration
   4. Evidence-based practice

8. A nurse meets with the registered dietitian and physical therapist to develop a plan of care that focuses on improving nutrition and mobility for a patient. This is an example of which Quality and Safety in the Education of Nurses (QSEN) competency?
   1. Patient-centered care
   2. Safety
   3. Teamwork and collaboration
   4. Informatics
9. The nurses on an acute care medical floor notice an increase in the number of patient falls. The unit introduces a new patient rounding program. The nurse assigned to the project gathers data to monitor the effectiveness of the rounding program over a 6-month period. The nurse is practicing in which nursing role?
   1. Nurse manager
   2. Nurse administrator
   3. Nurse educator
   4. Nurse researcher
10. Nurses at a large medical center are participating in an education program led by staff educators to learn how to use an intravenous infusion pump to administer medications safely. This is which type of education?
   1. Continuing education
   2. Graduate education
   3. In-service education
   4. Professional registered nurse education

Rationales for Review Questions can be found on the Evolve website.

1. 1b, 2d, 3c, 4a; **2.** 1; **3.** 2; **4.** 4; **5.** 1; **6.** 2; **7.** 4; **8.** 3; **9.** 4; **10.** 3.

REFERENCES

Aiken LH: Economics of nursing, *Policy Politics Nurs* 9(93):73, 2010.

Alligood MR: *Nursing theory: utilization and application*, St Louis, 2010, Elsevier.

American Association of Colleges of Nursing: *Joint statement from the Tri-Council for Nursing on recent registered nurse supply and demand projections*, News Release, Washington, DC, 2010, The Association, http://www.aacn.nche.edu/Media/NewsReleases/2010/tricouncil.html. Accessed July 26, 2013.

American Association of Colleges of Nursing (AACN): *The essentials of master's education for advanced practice nursing*, Washington, DC, 2011, The Association.

American Association of Colleges of Nursing (AACN): *AACN nursing shortage fact sheet*, 2012, http://www.aacn.nche.edu/media-relations/NrsgShortageFS.pdf. Accessed July 26, 2013.

American Nurses Association (ANA): *Nursing's social policy statement: the essence of the profession*, Silver Spring, MD, 2010a, American Nurses Publishing.

American Nurses Association (ANA): *Nursing: scope and standards of practice*, ed 2, Silver Spring, MD, 2010b, The Association.

American Nurses Association (ANA): *Guide to the code of ethics for nurses: interpretation and application*, Silver Spring, MD, 2010c, The Association.

American Nurses Association (ANA): *Handle with care fact sheet*, 2013, http://www.nursingworld.org/MainMenuCategories/ANAMarketplace/Factsheets-and-Toolkits/FactSheet.html. Accessed August 27, 2013.

Barton AJ, et al: A national Delphi to determine developmental progression of quality and safety competencies in nursing education, *Nurs Outlook* 57(6):313, 2009.

Benner P: *From novice to expert: excellence and power in clinical nursing practice*, Menlo Park, CA, 1984, Addison-Wesley.

Benner P, Tanner CA, Chesla CA: The social fabric or nursing knowledge, *Am J Nurs* 97(7):16, 1997.

Benner P, et al: *Educating nurses: a call for radical transformation*, Stanford, CA, 2010, Carnegie Foundation for the Advancement of Teaching.

Canadian Nurses Association (CNA): *RN exam*, 2012, http://www.cna-aiic.ca/en/becoming-an-rn/rn-exam/. Accessed July 26, 2013.

Centers for Disease Control and Prevention (CDC): *Genomics and health frequently asked questions*, 2011, http://www.cdc.gov/genomics/public/faq.htm. Accessed July 25, 2013.

Cohen IB: Florence Nightingale, *Sci Am* 250(128):137, 1984.

Cronenwett L, et al: Quality and safety education for nurses, *Nurs Outlook* 57:122, 2007.

Donahue MP: *Nursing: the finest art—an illustrated history*, ed 3, St Louis, 2011, Mosby.

Fernandes R, et al: Home-based palliative care services for underserved populations, *J Palliative Med* 13(4):413, 2010.

Flinkman M, et al: Nurses' intention to leave the profession: integrative review, *J Adv Nurs* 66(7):1422, 2010.

Gugliemi M: Celebrating the freedom to leverage the power of nursing, *AORN* 91(5):533, 2010.

Hale MA, et al: Continuing education needs of nurses in a voluntary continuing nursing education state, *J Cont Educ Nurs* 41(3):107, 2010.

Hanks RG: Development and testing of an instrument to measure protective nursing advocacy, *Nurs Ethics* 17(2):255, 2010.

Hardie H, Leary A: Value to patients of a breast cancer clinical nurse specialist, *Nurs Stand* 24(34):42, 2010.

Institute of Medicine (IOM): *To err is human*, Washington, DC, 2000, The Institute.

Institute of Medicine (IOM): *The future of nursing: leading change, advancing health*, Washington, DC, 2010, National Academies Press.

International Council of Nurses (ICN): *ICN definition of nursing*, 2010, http://icn.ch/definition.htm. Accessed July 25, 2013.

Jarzemsky P, et al: Incorporating quality and safety education for nurses' competencies in simulation scenario design, *Nurse Educator* 35(2):90, 2010.

Laidman J: Nurses remain nations' most trusted professionals, *Medscape med news*, Dec 6, 2012, http://www.medscape.com?viewarticle/775758. Accessed July 24, 2013.

Lucero RJ, et al: Variations in nursing care quality across hospitals, *J Adv Nurs* 65(11):2299, 2009.

Mason DJ, et al: *Policy & politics in nursing and health care*, ed 6, Philadelphia, 2012, Saunders.

Mayo AM, Agocs-Scott LM, Khaghani F, et al: Clinical nurse specialist patterns, *Clin Nurse Specialist* 24(2):60, 2010.

McCann E: Building a community-academic partnership to improve health outcomes in an underserved community, *Public Health Nurs* 27(1):32, 2010.

Mercer MA: Global health needs and priorities in developing countries. In Cowen PS, Moorhead S, editors: *Current issues in nursing*, ed 8, St Louis, 2011, Mosby.

Miaskowski C, Aouizerat BE: Biomarkers: Symptoms, survivorship, and quality of life, *Semin Oncol Nurs* 28(2):129, 2012.

Moore J, McQuestion M: The clinical nurse specialist in chronic diseases, *Clin Nurse Specialist* 26(3):149, 2012.

Morrison AM, Catanzaro AM: High-fidelity simulation and emergency preparedness, *Public Health Nurs* 27(2):164, 2010.

National CNS Competency Task Force, Core Competencies, National Association of Clinical Nurse Specialists: *Core competencies*, Philadelphia, 2010, The Association.

Nightingale F: *Notes on nursing: what it is and what it is not*, London, 1860, Harrison and Sons.

Norton C, et al: An investigation into the activities of the clinical nurse specialist, *Nurs Stand* 26(30):42, 2012.

O'Neil E: Four factors that guarantee health care change, *J Prof Nurs* 25(6):317, 2009.

Policicchio J, Nelson B, Duffy S: Bringing evidence-based continuing education on asthma to nurses, *Clin Nurse Specialist* 25(3):125, 2011.

Presley S: Rural NPs embrace private practice, *Am J Nurs* 115(5):21, 2010.

Robinson JJA: Nursing and disaster preparedness, *Int Nurs Rev* 57(2):148, 2010.

Tilden VP, Thompson S: Policy issues in end-of-life care, *J Prof Nurs* 25(6):363, 2009.

US Census Bureau, Population Division: *Projections of the population and components of change for the United States: 2010 to 2050 (NP2008-T1)*, 2008a, http://www.census.gov/population/projections/data/national/2012.html. Accessed July 24, 2013.

US Census Bureau, Population Division: *Projections of the population by selected age-groups and sex for the United States: 2010 to 2050 (NP2008-T2)*, 2008b, http://www.census.gov/population/projections/data/national/2012.html. Accessed July 24, 2013.

Zerwekh J, Garneau AZ: *Nursing today: transition and trends*, ed 7, St Louis, 2012, Saunders.

CHAPTER

2

Health and Wellness

evolve WEBSITE

http://evolve.elsevier.com/Potter/essentials

- Crossword Puzzle
- Audio Glossary

OBJECTIVES

- Discuss the health belief, health promotion, basic human needs, and holistic health models of health and illness and their relationship to patients' attitudes toward health and health practices.
- Describe the variables influencing health beliefs and health practices.
- Describe health promotion and illness prevention activities.
- Explain the three levels of prevention.
- Discuss four types of risk factors and the process of risk-factor modification.
- Describe the variables influencing illness behavior.
- Explain the impact of illness on a patient and family.
- Discuss the nurse's role in health and illness.

KEY TERMS

active strategies of health promotion, p. 20
acute illness, p. 24
chronic illness, p. 24
health, p. 15
health belief model, p. 16
health beliefs, p. 16
health promotion, p. 20
health promotion model, p. 17
holistic health, p. 19
illness, p. 24
illness behavior, p. 24
illness prevention, p. 20
Maslow's hierarchy of needs, p. 17
passive strategies of health promotion, p. 20
primary prevention, p. 21
risk factor, p. 21
secondary prevention, p. 21
tertiary prevention, p. 21
wellness education, p. 20

In the past most individuals and societies viewed good health or wellness as the opposite or absence of disease. We now understand that some conditions of health lie between disease and good health. Therefore we view health from a broader perspective. As a nurse you use concepts of health, health promotion, wellness, and illness to help your patients achieve and maintain an optimal level of health. You use models of health and illness to understand and explain these concepts. In addition, you help patients make changes to their current health state to bring about improved health and wellness.

DEFINITION OF HEALTH

Defining health is difficult because each person has his or her own personal concept of health. The World Health Organization (WHO) defines health as a "state of complete physical, mental and social well-being, not merely the absence of disease or infirmity" (WHO, 1947). Individual views of health vary among different age-groups, genders, races, and cultures (Pender, Murdaugh, and Parsons, 2011). Pender (1996) explains that "all people free of disease are not equally healthy." **Health** is a state of being that people define in relation to their

CASE STUDY ***Charlie***

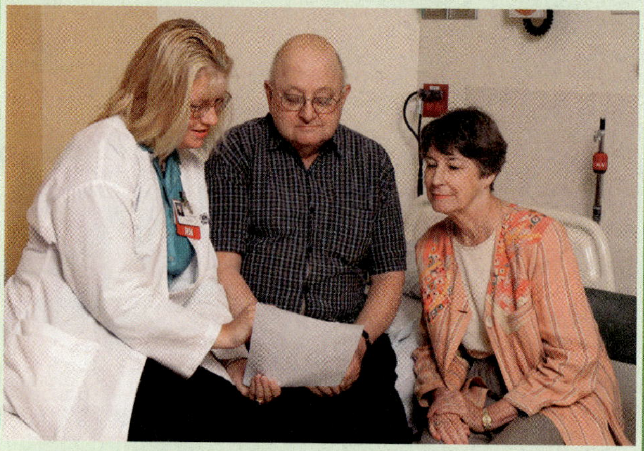

Charlie is a 56-year-old retired Navy officer who was recently diagnosed with high cholesterol and hypertension. Knowing that he has a family history of cardiac disease, Charlie has always tried to eat the right foods and exercise; but since retiring he has had difficulty adhering to a healthy diet and exercise regimen. He has been told by his doctor that he is 30 pounds overweight. Charlie has found it difficult to structure his time to exercise daily. His wife still works full time, and they often eat out during the week to accommodate her schedule.

Charlie comes to the clinic today for a routine follow-up after starting on medication to reduce his cholesterol. Liz, the cardiac nurse educator, is working with Charlie. This is their second visit. Charlie's laboratory values show some improvement in cholesterol levels, but his triglycerides are still high. His blood pressure is also still running on the high side of normal. Liz would like to work with Charlie on increasing his exercise and improving his eating habits to help him develop a healthier lifestyle and further reduce his risk for cardiovascular disease. She plans to assess his understanding of his personal cardiac risk factors and lifestyle choices and evaluate his readiness to change to manage his health.

own values, personality, and lifestyle. For many people, health is defined by the conditions of life rather than by pathological states (Pender et al., 2011). Nurses consider the total person and the person's environment to individualize nursing care and help patients identify and reach their health goals. Therefore health is a complex concept and means more than the absence of disease. People's thoughts about their health and how they take care of themselves influence individuals' definitions of health. For example, in addition to having good physical health, having a positive mental outlook, being cognitively alert, having a good memory, and being socially involved are all important (Laditka et al., 2009).

MODELS OF HEALTH AND ILLNESS

A model is a theoretical way of understanding a concept or an idea. Models offer ways to explain complex issues such as health and illness. Because health and illness are complex concepts, you need to use models to understand the relationships between health and illness and your patients' attitudes toward health and health practices. Health beliefs influence health practices. **Health beliefs** are a person's ideas, convictions, and attitudes about health and illness. They may be based on facts or misinformation, common sense or myths, or reality or false expectations. Because health beliefs influence health behavior, they can positively or negatively affect a patient's level of health. Nurses develop and use a variety of health models to understand patients' beliefs, attitudes, and values about health and illness to provide effective health care. These models allow you to understand and predict patients' health behavior, including how they use health services, participate in recommended therapy, and care for themselves.

Health Belief Model

Rosenstoch's (1974) and Becker and Maiman's (1975) **health belief model** (Figure 2-1) addresses the relationship between a person's beliefs and behaviors. It provides a way of understanding and predicting how patients will behave in relation to their health and how successful they will be in following health care therapies or regimens. Positive health behaviors are activities related to maintaining, attaining, or regaining good health and preventing illness. Common positive health behaviors include getting immunizations, maintaining proper sleep patterns, getting adequate exercise, and eating healthy foods. Implementation of positive health behaviors depends on an individual's awareness of how to live a healthy life and the person's ability and willingness to carry out such behaviors in a healthy lifestyle. Negative health behaviors include activities that are harmful to health such as smoking, abusing drugs or alcohol, following a poor diet, and refusing to take necessary medications.

The first component of the health belief model involves the individual's perception of susceptibility to an illness. For example, a patient needs to recognize the familial link for coronary artery disease. After recognizing this link, the patient perceives a personal risk for heart disease. The second component is the patient's perception of the seriousness of the illness. Demographic and sociopsychological variables, perceived threats of the illness, and cues to action (e.g., mass media campaigns and advice from family, friends, and medical professionals) all influence and modify this perception. The third component, the likelihood that the patient will take preventive action such as following a low-fat diet results from the patient's perception of the benefits of and barriers to taking action. Preventive actions include lifestyle changes, increased participation in recommended medical therapies, and a search for medical advice or treatment.

The health belief model helps you understand factors influencing patients' perceptions, beliefs, and behavior and plan care that will most effectively help patients maintain or restore health and prevent illness. Understand that each patient's views of health and wellness and individual belief systems influence the ability to make lasting changes in health

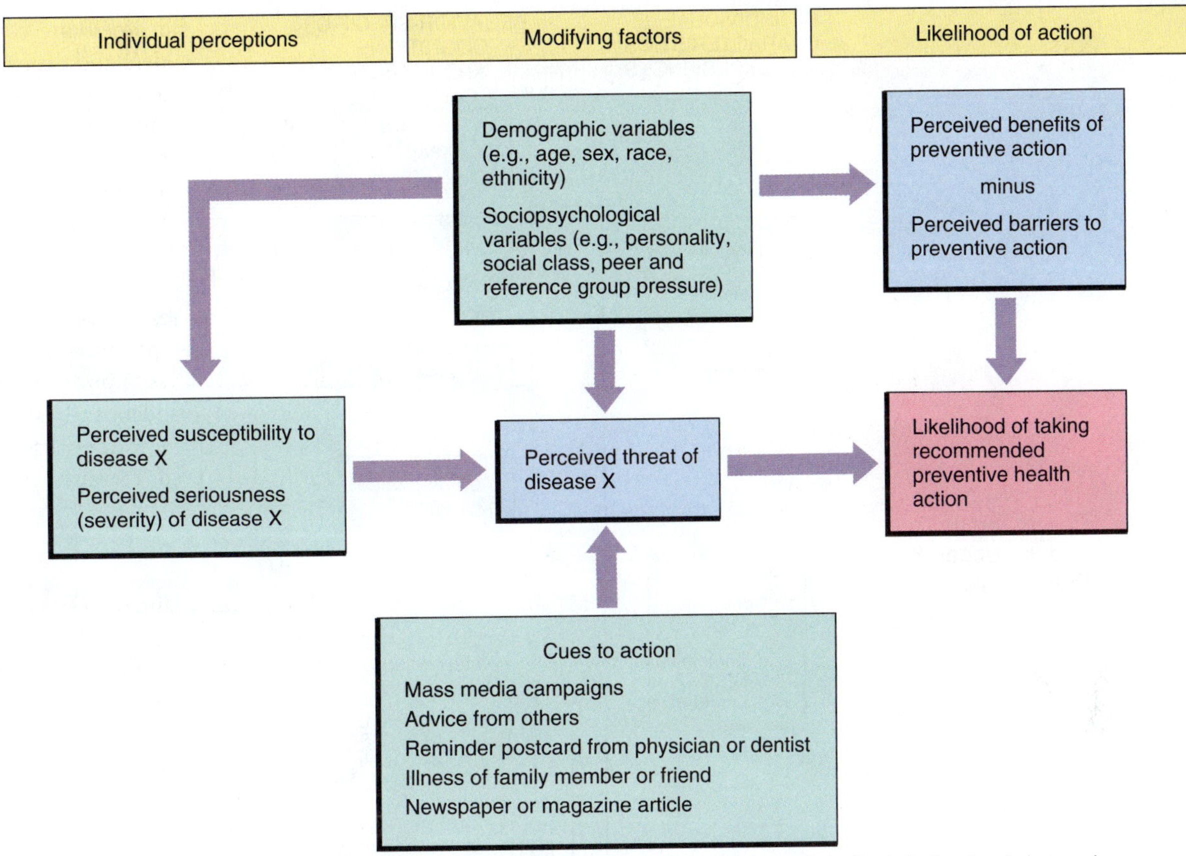

FIGURE 2-1 Health belief model. (Data from Becker MH, Maiman LA: Sociobehavioral determinants of compliance with health and medical care recommendations, *Med Care* 13(1):10, 1975.)

status. Do not make judgments when you encounter views and beliefs that differ from your own philosophies of health and wellness.

Health Promotion Model

The health promotion model proposed by Pender (1982, 1996; Pender et al., 2011) (Figure 2-2) defines health as a positive, dynamic state, not merely the absence of disease. The model was proposed as a framework for integrating the perspectives of nursing and behavioral science and the factors that influence health behaviors. Health promotion is behavior motivated by the desire to increase well-being and actualize human health potential; whereas health protection is behavior that is motivated by a desire to avoid illness, detect it early, or maintain function within the constraints of an illness (Pender et al., 2011). The **health promotion model** describes the multidimensional nature of people as they interact within their environment to pursue health (Pender et al., 2011). This model focuses on three areas:

1. Individual characteristics and experiences
2. Behavior-specific cognitions and affect
3. Behavioral outcomes

It also organizes cues into a pattern to explain the likelihood of a patient developing health promotion behaviors (Pender et al., 2011). The purpose of the model is to explain the reasons that individuals engage in health activities and is not for use with families or communities. You will use this model to help your patients carry out healthy behaviors in their daily lives.

Basic Human Needs Model

One way to understand an individual's motivation to achieve optimal health is to review Abraham **Maslow's hierarchy of needs** (1954). This model explains the basic needs of patients and families, their behaviors, and their readiness to take part in health promotion activities. Maslow's (1987) model describes human needs using a hierarchical pyramid divided into five levels (Figure 2-3). As people meet the needs of one level, they move up to the next level. According to Maslow, individuals have to meet lower-level needs before they are able to satisfy higher-level needs. Unsatisfied needs motivate human behavior.

The lowest level of needs on the hierarchy consists of very *basic physiological needs* such as oxygen, water, food, sleep, and sex. When these needs are not met, the affected person feels sick or irritated or complains of pain or discomfort. These feelings motivate the individual to satisfy the need (Maslow, 1970, 1987). The second level on the hierarchy of needs consists of *safety needs,* which include establishing stability and consistency. These psychological needs include the security of a home and a family. For example, a woman living in an abusive home is unable to move to the next level of love and belongingness because she is constantly concerned for her safety. The third level on the hierarchy is *love and*

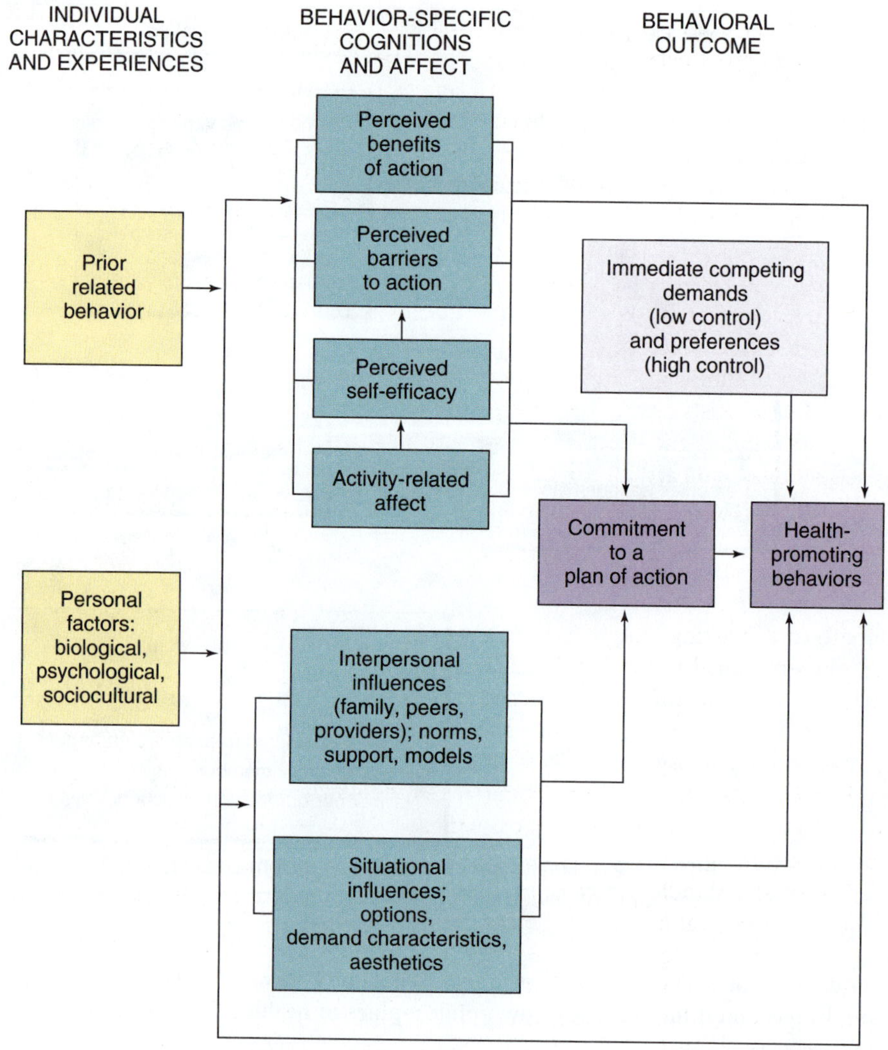

FIGURE 2-2 Health promotion model. (From Pender NJ, Murdaugh CL, Parsons MA: *Health promotion in nursing practice,* ed 5, Upper Saddle River, NJ, 2006, Prentice Hall.)

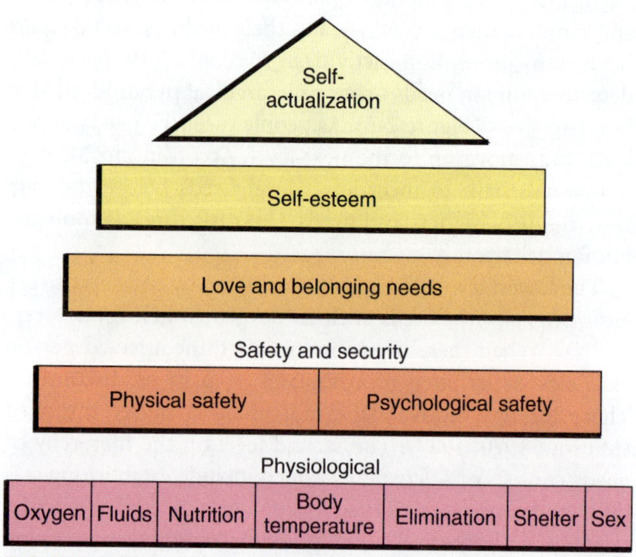

FIGURE 2-3 Maslow's hierarchy of needs. (From Maslow AH: *Motivation and personality,* ed 3, Upper Saddle River, NJ, 1987, Prentice Hall.)

belongingness, which is a desire to belong to groups. It consists of the need to feel love by others and to be accepted. The fourth level deals with the need for *self-esteem.* Self-esteem results from mastery of a task and also includes the recognition gained from others. The highest level of needs on the hierarchy is *self-actualization,* which is the desire to become everything that one is capable of becoming. Individuals at this level are concerned with maximizing their potential.

An understanding of Maslow's hierarchy of needs provides you with a framework to meet patient needs and prioritize care for your patients. Realize that, unless a patient's basic needs have been met, higher levels in the pyramid are not relevant and that patients of different generations approach life differently (Dols, Landrum, and Wieck, 2010). When using this model, you first ensure that basic needs of individuals are met. *For example, Charlie has a good relationship with his wife, but he is having trouble identifying ways to adjust his eating habits to reduce his cholesterol. Sally works with Charlie and his wife to develop a realistic meal plan.* The requirements to satisfy the needs of each level on the hierarchy vary from person to person. Needs are greater or lesser for different persons. Therefore a thorough and individualized assessment of needs is an important aspect of patient care. For example, in caring for patients with psychological issues such as depression or risk for suicide, safety and security needs are a priority. As a nurse you want to always provide patients with physical and psychological safety.

Wellness activities involving health promotion and illness prevention strategies help patients achieve and maintain optimal levels of health. Nurses identify actual and potential risk factors that predispose a person or group to illness. People have different attitudes and reactions to illness. Medical sociologists call the reaction to illness *illness behavior.* When you understand a patient's risks and how he or she reacts to illness, you are able to minimize the effects of illness and help patients and their families maintain or return to the highest level of functioning.

Holistic Health Model

Health care is taking a more holistic view of health by considering emotional and spiritual well-being and other dimensions of an individual as important aspects of physical wellness. **Holistic health** generally is a comprehensive view of a person as a biopsychosocial and spiritual being (Edelman and Mandle, 2010). The intent of the holistic health model is to empower patients to engage in their own recovery, thereby assuming some responsibility for health maintenance (Edelman and Mandle, 2010).

The holistic health model incorporates a variety of techniques based on recognition that personal health choices have a powerful impact on an individual's health. Some of the most widely used holistic interventions include aromatherapy, biofeedback, breathing exercises, massage therapy, meditation, music therapy, relaxation therapy, therapeutic touch, and guided imagery (see Chapter 32). Most holistic therapies are easy to learn and apply to almost any nursing setting and all stages of health and illness. For example, you use reminiscence to help relieve anxiety for an older patient dealing with memory loss or meditation with a patient dealing with the difficult side effects of chemotherapy. Surgical nurses use music therapy in the operating room to create a soothing environment. Relaxation therapy is useful in any setting to distract a patient during a painful procedure such as a dressing change. You help patients recognize the many options available and help them make choices to enhance health.

HEALTHY PEOPLE DOCUMENTS

Since the 1970s there has been a nationally focused initiative toward better health for the American people. *Healthy People* provides evidenced-based objectives to: (1) achieve increased quality and years of healthy life, and (2) eliminate health disparities (USDHHS, 2010). These objectives are updated every 10 years to meet a wide range of health needs, encourage collaboration in communities, help individuals make informed health decisions, and measure the impact of prevention activities. Currently there are four influential documents that outline specific national goals for improving the physical health of Americans: *Healthy People: The Surgeon General's Report on Health Promotion and Disease Prevention* (USDHHS, 1979); *Healthy People 2000: National Health Promotion and Disease Prevention Objectives* (USDHHS, 1990); *Healthy People 2010: Understanding and Improving Health* (USDHHS, 2000); and *Developing Healthy People 2020* (USDHHS, 2010).

Healthy People 2020 includes 600 objectives written in 42 topic areas to provide direction for health care efforts on an individual, community, and national level. New topic areas include adolescent health, health care–associated infections, and social determinates of health.

The document comprises four areas: (1) attain high-quality, longer lives, (2) achieve health equality, (3) create social and physical environments that promote good health, and (4) promote quality of life across all life states. The goal is to achieve or make improvements for each objective by the year 2020 (USDHHS, 2010).

VARIABLES INFLUENCING HEALTH BELIEFS AND HEALTH PRACTICES

Peoples' beliefs about their own health, their health practices, and the manner in which they care for themselves ultimately influence their health status. Health beliefs are a person's ideas and attitudes about health. These beliefs often directly influence health practices whether there is evidence to support them or not. Health practices are activities that individuals perform to care for themselves. They include activities of daily living such as bathing and brushing teeth and formal activities such as taking medications and visiting the health care provider for routine checkups. Today health care focuses on the role of patients and their responsibility for self-care. The ability to care for oneself is as important for healthy living as managing a complex medical regimen for a chronic illness. Many variables influence patients' health beliefs, health practices, and self-care. Internal and external variables influence how a person thinks and acts and how he or she will deal with an illness. Consider the impact of these variables and be able to incorporate appropriate interventions based on the person's unique characteristics. Internal variables include a person's developmental stage, intellectual background, and emotional and spiritual factors. External variables include family practices, socioeconomic factors, and cultural background.

Internal Variables

Developmental Stage. A person's concept of illness depends on his or her developmental stage (see Chapter 22). Knowledge of the stages of growth and development help you predict your patient's response to an actual illness or the threat of future illness. Your educational interventions need to be age appropriate to be effective. For example, use different techniques to teach healthy diet choices to a child and an adult.

Intellectual Background. A person's beliefs about health are shaped in part by knowledge (or misinformation) about body functions and illnesses, educational background, and past experiences. Cognitive abilities shape the *way* a person thinks, including the ability to understand factors involved in illness and apply knowledge of health and illness to personal health practices.

Emotional Factors. A person's degree of anxiety or stress influences health beliefs and practices. The manner in which a person handles stress throughout each phase of life influences the way that he or she reacts to illness. A person who generally is very calm often has little emotional response during illness, whereas a person normally unable to cope with stress either overreacts to illness or denies the presence of symptoms and does not take therapeutic action (see Chapter 25).

Spiritual Factors. Spirituality is reflected in how a person lives his or her life, including the values and beliefs exercised, the relationships established with family and friends, and the ability to find hope and meaning in life. Spiritual health often provides motivation during times of change in health status. Religious practices are one way people exercise spirituality. You need to understand patients' spiritual beliefs to involve them effectively in nursing care (see Chapter 21).

External Variables

Family Practices. The way that families use health care services generally influences their health practices. Perceptions of the seriousness of diseases and history of preventive care behaviors (or lack of them) influence how patients think about health. For example, a person raised in a family that believed in the importance of preventive care such as dental checkups twice a year is more likely to continue those health practices as an adult.

Socioeconomic Factors. Social and economic factors increase the risk for illness and influence the way in which a person defines and reacts to illness. Socioeconomic variables in part also determine how and where patients access medical care and receive treatment, how they pay for their health care, and the potential reimbursement to the health care agency or patient. Economic variables affect a patient's level of health by increasing the risk for disease and influencing how or at what point the patient enters the health care system. In addition, economic status also affects a person's participation in treatment to maintain or improve health. A person who has high utility bills, a large family, and a low income tends to give a higher priority to food and shelter than to costly drugs or treatment or expensive foods for special diets.

Cultural Background. Cultural background influences a person's beliefs, values, and customs. It influences the approach to the health care system, personal health practices, and the nurse-patient relationship. You need to recognize and understand cultural patterns of behavior and beliefs to effectively interact with each patient (see Chapter 20).

HEALTH PROMOTION, WELLNESS, AND ILLNESS PREVENTION

Health promotion activities are either passive or active. With **passive strategies of health promotion,** individuals gain from the activities of others without acting themselves. For example, the city puts fluoride in the municipal drinking water, or milk manufacturers fortify homogenized milk with vitamin D. These are passive health promotion strategies. With **active strategies of health promotion,** individuals adopt specific health programs. Weight reduction and smoking cessation programs require patients to be actively involved in measures to improve their present and future levels of wellness while decreasing the risk for disease.

You need to emphasize health promotion, wellness strategies, and illness prevention activities as important forms of health care because they help patients maintain and improve their health. **Health promotion** activities such as routine exercise and good nutrition help patients maintain or enhance their present levels of health and reduce their risks for developing certain diseases. **Wellness education** teaches people how to care for themselves in a healthy way and includes topics such as physical awareness, stress management, and self-responsibility (Box 2-1). **Illness prevention** activities such as immunization programs protect patients from actual or potential threats to health. The concepts of health promotion, wellness, and illness prevention are closely related and in practice overlap to some extent. All are focused on the future; the differences between them involve motivations and goals. Health promotion activities motivate people to act positively to reach more stable levels of health. Wellness strategies help patients achieve new understanding and control of their lives. Illness prevention activities motivate people to avoid declines in health or functional levels.

Illnesses, particularly chronic illnesses, often increase the cost of health care. Therefore health care has become increasingly focused on health promotion, wellness, and illness prevention. The rapid rise of health care costs has motivated people to seek ways of decreasing the incidence and minimizing the results of illness or disability. Improving self-management, preventive services, and curative services reduces health care needs and costs. You have an important role in educating patients about improving their ability to manage their health. You do this by helping them recognize their responsibility in the health-related choices they make and understand the effect their choices have on disease prevention. *In the case study of Charlie and the cardiac educator Liz, there is an obvious need for greater education for Charlie. Liz teaches him the importance of diet and exercise to manage his cholesterol and prevent long-term complications. She has Charlie plan a diet for a week to see if he can omit high cholesterol foods.* Health promotion, wellness activities, and illness prevention are all strategies aimed at decreasing the incidence of illness and minimizing the negative results of that illness or disability.

BOX 2-1 PATIENT TEACHING

Encouraging Exercise

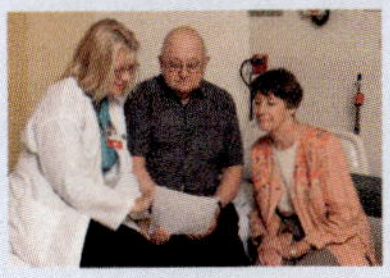

Because Charlie has been successful in exercising in the past, Liz decides to focus her teaching on the importance of routine exercise to improve his health and help reduce his risk of developing cardiac disease. She works with Charlie to establish a new routine for his daily exercise.

OUTCOME

By the end of the visit, Charlie will verbalize two reasons why it is helpful for him to stay physically active and one new strategy for adding exercise to his new daily routine.

TEACHING STRATEGIES

- Make sure that Charlie is aware of his risk for cardiac disease (Waldron et al., 2011).
- Make sure that Charlie understands how risk-reduction strategies such as exercise can help (Waldron et al., 2011).
- Help Charlie set achievable goals for change.
- Work with Charlie to establish realistic time lines for modification of exercise lifestyle habits.
- Reinforce the process of change with Charlie.
- Use active listening.
- Include Charlie's wife to support the lifestyle change.
- Identify community resources available to Charlie (e.g., walking track, fitness facilities).

EVALUATION STRATEGIES

- Have Charlie maintain an exercise log to track adherence; provide positive reinforcement and evaluate log at the next visit.
- Ask Charlie to discuss his success with lifestyle changes such as minutes spent in activity.
- Have Charlie identify community resources used in making change.

The Three Levels of Prevention

Nursing care directed at health promotion, wellness, and illness prevention can be understood in terms of health activities on primary, secondary, and tertiary levels.

Primary prevention is true prevention. It precedes disease or dysfunction and applies to patients considered physically and emotionally healthy. The purpose of primary prevention is to decrease the vulnerability of the individual or population to an illness or dysfunction (Edelman and Mandle, 2010). It includes passive and active strategies of health promotion. You provide it to an individual or to a general population, or you focus on individuals at risk for developing specific diseases. Primary prevention aimed at health promotion includes health education programs, immunizations, and physical and nutritional fitness activities. For Charlie, primary prevention means reducing his cholesterol through medications, diet, and exercise to prevent the development of cardiac disease.

Secondary prevention focuses on people who are experiencing health problems or illnesses and who are at risk for developing complications or worsening conditions. You direct activities at diagnosis and prompt intervention, thereby reducing severity and enabling the patient to return to a normal level of health as early as possible (Edelman and Mandle, 2010). A large portion of secondary-level nursing care is in homes, hospitals, or skilled nursing facilities. It includes screening techniques and treating early stages of disease to limit disability by delaying the consequences of advanced disease. Screening activities also become a key opportunity for health teaching as a primary prevention intervention (Edelman and Mandle, 2010). Secondary prevention for Charlie involves having him come to the clinic every 3 months to have his blood pressure checked until it is controlled.

Tertiary prevention occurs when a defect or disability is permanent, irreversible, and stabilized. It involves minimizing the effects of long-term disease or disability by interventions directed at preventing complications and deterioration (Edelman and Mandle, 2010). Activities are for rehabilitation rather than diagnosis and treatment. Care at this level helps patients achieve as high a level of functioning as possible, despite the limitations caused by illness or impairment. This level of care is called *preventive care* because it involves preventing further disability or reduced functioning.

Risk Factors

A **risk factor** is any situation, habit, environmental condition, physiological condition, or other variable that increases an individual's or a group's vulnerability to an illness or accident. The presence of risk factors does not mean that a disease will develop, but risk factors increase the chances that the individual will experience a particular disease. Risk factors play a major role in how you identify a patient's health status. They also influence health beliefs and practices if a person is aware of their presence. Risk factors are in the following interrelated categories: genetic and physiological, age, physical environment, and lifestyle.

Genetic and Physiological Factors. Physiological risk factors involve the physical functioning of the body. For example, physical conditions such as pregnancy or obesity place increased stress on physiological systems (e.g., the circulatory system), thus increasing susceptibility to illness. Heredity or genetic predisposition to specific illness is a major physical risk factor. In the case study Charlie has a family history of cardiac disease and therefore is at risk for developing the disease. Other examples of genetic risk factors include family histories of cancer, diabetes, and kidney disease.

Age. Age increases susceptibility to certain illnesses. The risks for birth defects and complications of pregnancy increase in women bearing children after age 35. Many kinds of cancer pose a greater risk for people over age 45 than for younger persons. The risk for heart disease increases with age for both genders. Box 2-2 discusses the importance of health promotion in older adults. Age risk factors are often closely associated with other risk factors such as family history and personal habits. You need to educate patients about the

BOX 2-2 CARE OF THE OLDER ADULT

Importance of Health Promotion

- Because individuals are living longer, health promotion activities are important to help maintain function and independence and improve quality of life.
- Focusing on self-care abilities and practices that foster health while aging is an important nursing intervention (Pender et al., 2011).
- Emphasize the need to engage in physical and social activity (Reed et al., 2011).
- Monitor older patients, especially those 75 years of age and older, for high blood pressure, obesity, and diabetes (Mokdad et al., 2004b).
- Physical activity extends years of active independent life, reduces disability, and improves the quality of life for older persons (Chodzko-Zajko, 2008).
- Promote self-care activities that maintain and improve functional status, including safe mobility and prevention of falls (Pender et al., 2011).
- Health care interventions often do not correspond with the patient's readiness to change. Use the stages of behavior change model (see Table 2-1) to identify older adults who are open to participating in health promotion activities.

importance of regularly scheduled checkups for their age-group. The Agency for Healthcare Research and Quality (n.d.), has developed guidelines for screening, counseling, and immunizations by age and gender. You can access scientific evidence, recommendations on clinical prevention services, chronic care, and information on how to implement recommended preventive services into practice at http://www.ahrq.gov/clinic/prevenix.htm.

Physical Environment. The physical environment in which a person works or lives increases the likelihood that certain illnesses will occur. A person's home environment often includes conditions that pose risks such as unclean, poorly heated or cooled, or overcrowded dwellings. These conditions often increase the likelihood that a person will contract and spread infections and other diseases. Also, some kinds of cancer and other diseases are more likely to develop when industrial workers are exposed to certain chemicals or when people live near toxic waste disposal sites. Screening for these environmentally based risk factors is directed at the short-term effects of the exposure and the potential for long-term effects (Edelman and Mandle, 2010).

Lifestyle. Lifestyle practices and behaviors have positive or negative effects on health. Practices with potential negative effects are risk factors. Examples of risk factors include overeating or poor nutrition, insufficient rest and sleep, and poor personal hygiene. Other habits that put a person at risk for illness include tobacco use, alcohol or drug abuse, and activities involving a threat of injury such as skydiving or mountain climbing. Some habits are risk factors for specific diseases. For example, excessive sunbathing increases the risk for skin cancer, and being overweight increases the risk for cardiovascular disease. Some examples of modifiable behavioral risk factors that are leading causes of mortality in the United States include tobacco use, poor diet, lack of physical exercise, alcohol consumption, and illicit drug use (Mokdad et al., 2004a; Mokdad and Remington, 2010). Although smoking remains the leading cause of mortality, poor diet and physical inactivity will soon be the leading cause of death. These data reflect the importance of a need for emphasis on preventive care and show the economic effect that lifestyle choices have on our health care system.

The effect of lifestyle behavior on the risk for developing disease has implications across the life span of a person. Understand that patients of all ages are vulnerable to the influences of unhealthy lifestyle patterns. You are able to influence the choices your patients make for preventing unhealthy behaviors and promoting healthy lifestyle patterns. Parents, family caregivers, school nurses, and teachers all influence the lifestyle practices of young children. Many adolescents encounter issues of seat belt use, gun possession, alcohol and drug use, and sexual promiscuity. Therefore you need to understand the relationship between growth and development and lifestyle behaviors and your patients' health status. Use evidence-based interventions when teaching your patients and the public about wellness-promoting lifestyle behaviors (Box 2-3).

BOX 2-3 EVIDENCE-BASED PRACTICE

PICO Question: In patients with diabetes, is diabetes self-management education (DSME) effective in controlling blood glucose levels?

SUMMARY OF EVIDENCE

Diabetes is a growing health concern, and nurses are in a strategic position to help patients manage their diabetes and achieve optimal blood glucose control. "Diabetes self-management education is the ongoing process of facilitating the knowledge, skill, and the ability necessary for diabetes self-care" (Funnell, p. S87, 2009). National standards were adopted in 2009 to support DSME. Interventions that are shown to be effective should focus on enhancing self-efficacy, problem solving, and social-environmental support (King et al., 2010). Among patients in a lower socioeconomic status, a problem-solving–based DSME was effective for the key clinical behavior (self-management) and outcomes (blood glucose control) (Hill-Briggs, 2011).

APPLICATION TO NURSING PRACTICE

- Determine the knowledge level and learning needs of each patient with diabetes.
- Help patients understand the importance of diabetes self-management in preventing long-term end organ disease.
- Assess the health literacy of your patients to determine the best way to educate.
- Use a health promotion theory such as the stages of behavior change whenever possible.
- Provide ongoing support to your patients and their family caregivers.
- Have patients monitor their glucose levels to determine the success of their diabetes self-management activities.

Risk Factor Identification. The goal of risk factor identification is to help patients understand the areas in their lives that they need to modify or even eliminate to promote wellness and prevent illness. You perform comprehensive health risk appraisals, using a variety of available health risk appraisal forms, to estimate a person's specific health threats based on the presence of various risk factors (Edelman and Mandle, 2010). You need to link findings from a health risk appraisal with educational programs and other community resources available to patients to provide a way for them to make necessary lifestyle changes and risk reduction. You will often find risk factors, often linked to the patient's age, documented in the patient's medical record. For example, when caring for adolescents, evaluate parenting practices, school performance, self-esteem, neighborhoods, and the community in general to identify at-risk youth (Riesch et al., 2012).

Risk Factor Modification and Changing Health Behaviors. Identifying risk factors is the first step in health promotion, wellness education, and illness prevention activities. Once you identify risk factors, implement appropriate and relevant health education programs that help a person to change a risky health behavior. This is called *risk factor modification.* Risk factor modification is a wellness strategy because it teaches patients to care for themselves in healthier ways. You need to emphasize wellness strategies because they have the ability to decrease the potential high costs of unmanaged health problems.

Aim your attempts to change a patient's behavior at stopping a health-damaging behavior (e.g., tobacco use or alcohol misuse) or adopting a healthy behavior (e.g., healthy diet or exercise) (Pender et al., 2011). Changing health behavior, especially behaviors that have become habits in people's lifestyle, is difficult. Many times adopting healthy behaviors and reducing risk factors require your patients to change. As a nurse you are challenged to motivate and facilitate health behavior change in working with individuals, families, and communities (Edelman and Mandle, 2010).

An understanding of the process of change helps you support difficult health behavior change in your patients. Current research shows that change involves movement through a series of five stages of behavior change (Table 2-1), ranging from precontemplation, when a person has no intention to change, to the maintenance stage, when a person maintains a changed behavior (Norcross and Prochaska, 2002). Most people acting on their own do not successfully get through all the stages on their first attempt (Norcross and Prochaska, 2002). As an individual attempts to change behavior, relapse and recycling through the stages occur frequently. When relapse occurs, the person returns to the contemplation or precontemplation stage before attempting change again. Relapse often feels like a failure, but the person needs to view it as a learning process. What he or she learns from relapse can be applied to the next attempt to change. You need to be able to identify your patient's stage of change to implement appropriate care (Box 2-4). Health promotion interventions have a greater effect if you time them appropriately to match a patient's specific stage of change. For example, you are not

TABLE 2-1 STAGES OF BEHAVIOR CHANGE

STAGE	DEFINITION
Precontemplation	Does not intend to make changes within the next 6 months. Patient is unaware of the problem or underestimates it. "There is nothing that I really need to change."
Contemplation	Considering a change within the next 6 months. Patient says that he or she is seriously considering a change. "I have a problem, and I really think I need to work on it."
Preparation	Has tried to make changes, but without success. Patient intends to take action in the next month. "I started to exercise regularly, but it didn't last long. I'll probably try again in a few weeks."
Action	Actively engaged in strategies to change behavior. This stage sometimes lasts up to 6 months. It requires commitment of time and energy. "I am really working hard to stop smoking."
Maintenance	Sustained change over time. This stage begins 6 months after action has started and continues indefinitely. It is important to avoid relapse. "I need to avoid people who smoke so I'm not tempted to start smoking again."

BOX 2-4 APPLICATION OF THE STAGES OF BEHAVIOR CHANGE MODEL

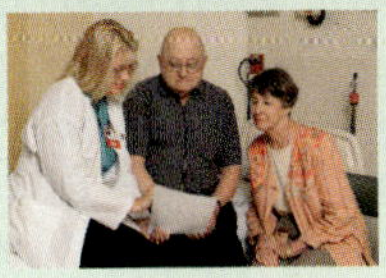

Liz wants to apply the stages of behavior change with Charlie. By using this model, Liz works with Charlie regarding what he is ready to do rather than simply telling him to be more active. To do this she first asks Charlie how he feels about exercise and what his plans are. When asked this, Charlie states, "I know that exercise would be good for me, and I should probably work on it." This tells Liz that Charlie is in the contemplation stage. She targets her teaching to helping Charlie see the benefits of exercise, how it could fit into his schedule, and what kinds of things he likes to do. She asks him to bring a list of benefits of exercise for him and three or four options for exercise to their next appointment. With this process she hopes to move Charlie into the preparation stage of behavior change for exercise at their next visit.

effective if you teach your patient who is in the contemplation stage and does not routinely eat fruits and vegetables to eat five fruits and vegetables a day. It is better to encourage your patient to think about the benefits of fruits and vegetables to encourage moving into the preparation stage.

The health care industry needs to do further work to design interventions and wellness strategies for people in all stages of behavior change. For example, patients are sometimes motivated to adopt needed health behaviors when health care professionals advise that a change in diet and an increase in exercise will prevent further problems. A patient can maintain changes over time only if you integrate the health behavior changes into the patient's overall lifestyle. In addition, understand that true change comes from the patient's desire to change. Maintenance of healthy lifestyles prevents hospitalizations and potentially lowers the cost of health care. Your advice and support may help patients adapt to a changed and healthier lifestyle.

ILLNESS

Illness is a state in which a person's physical, emotional, intellectual, social, developmental, or spiritual functioning is diminished or impaired compared with previous experience. Cancer is a disease process, but some patients with leukemia who are responding to treatment continue to function as usual. Some patients with breast cancer feel well physically but experience spiritual distress. Of interest, many patients find health within illness. An experience with illness sometimes motivates an individual to adopt more positive health behaviors.

Therefore illness is not synonymous with disease. Although you need to be familiar with different kinds of diseases and their treatments, be concerned more with illness, which includes not only the disease but also the effects on functioning and well-being in all dimensions.

Acute and Chronic Illness

Acute and chronic illnesses are two general classifications of illness used in this chapter. Both types affect functioning in many dimensions. An **acute illness** is usually short term and severe. The symptoms appear abruptly, are intense, and often subside after a relatively short period. A **chronic illness** usually lasts longer than 6 months. Patients fluctuate between maximal functioning and serious health relapses that are sometimes life threatening.

Because of successes in public health, medicine, and biomedical technology, acute and infectious diseases are no longer major causes of death, disease, and disability in the United States. Many health care analysts believe that the heaviest burden of illness today is caused by chronic diseases that are largely preventable. Beyond the prevention of these diseases, a major role for you as a nurse is to provide patient education that helps patients and their family caregivers manage their illnesses or disabilities to reduce the occurrence and improve the tolerance of symptoms (tertiary prevention). This education enhances wellness and improves quality of life for patients living with chronic illnesses or disabilities. Use a holistic approach when helping patients who have chronic illnesses better manage their care (Kralik, Price, and Telford, 2010). Include family caregivers when appropriate, because often they are the ones providing routine care and assistance. Self-management involves learning about responses to illnesses through daily life experiences and also as a result of trial and error. Taking responsibility for living well with illness strengthens patients. Therefore encourage patients to question the direction of their health care and make choices about it. The process of learning self-management skills is crucial to the transition of learning to live with a chronic illness. The management of chronic illnesses promotes health within illness and also addresses human comfort and quality of life. You as a nurse are able to reduce the impact of chronic illness on the individual and on society by providing quality, comprehensive, patient-centered care to patients living with chronic illness (Cumbie, Conley, and Burman, 2004).

VARIABLES INFLUENCING ILLNESS BEHAVIOR

People who are ill generally adopt **illness behaviors** (cognitive, affective, and behavioral reactions). These behaviors are influenced by sociocultural and social psychological factors. Illness behaviors affect how people monitor their bodies, define and interpret their symptoms, take remedial actions, and use the health care system (Mechanic, 1982). Personal history, social situations, social norms, and the opportunities and limits of community institutions all affect illness behaviors (Mechanic, 1995; Marks et al., 2005). Although people react to an illness in a variety of ways, patients often use illness behavior displayed in sickness to manage difficulties in life (Mechanic, 1995). If people perceive themselves to be ill, illness behaviors act as coping mechanisms. Illness behavior often results in patients being released from roles, social expectations, or responsibilities. For example, a young mother who is receiving chemotherapy for treatment of breast cancer is very tired and not expected to cook for her family every day. Instead the members of her church bring her family cooked meals, giving the mother more time to rest, heal, and be with her family. Remember, illness behavior is not deviant or needs to be fixed. Nurses must support their patients and understand the lived experience of their illness (Larsen, 2013).

Just as internal and external variables affect health behavior, they also affect illness behavior. The influences of these variables affect the likelihood of seeking health care and the participation in therapy, which ultimately affect health outcomes. Based on an understanding of these variables and behaviors, you individualize care to help patients cope with their illnesses at various stages. The goal of nursing is to promote optimal functioning in all dimensions throughout an illness.

Internal Variables

Internal variables influence the way patients behave when they are ill. These are a patient's perceptions of symptoms and the nature of the illness. If patients believe that the symptoms of their illnesses disrupt their normal routine, they are more likely to seek health care assistance than if they do not perceive the symptoms as disruptive. If they believe that the symptoms are serious or perhaps life threatening, they are also more likely to seek assistance. A person awakened by crushing chest pains in the middle of the night generally views this symptom as potentially serious and life threatening and will probably be motivated to seek assistance. However, sometimes such a perception also has the opposite effect. Some patients fear serious illness and react by denying it and not seeking medical assistance.

The nature of an illness, either acute or chronic, also affects a patient's illness behavior. Patients with acute illnesses are likely to seek health care and adhere readily to therapy. On the other hand, a patient with a chronic illness in which the symptoms are not curable but only partially relieved is sometimes not motivated to adhere to the therapy plan. Patients with chronic illnesses sometimes become less actively involved in their care, experience greater frustration, and adhere less readily to care. You generally spend more time than other health care professionals with patients who have chronic illnesses. You are in the unique position of being able to help patients overcome problems related to illness behavior.

External Variables

External variables influencing a patient's illness behavior include the visibility of symptoms, social group, cultural background, economic variables, accessibility of the health care system, and social support. The visibility of the symptoms of an illness affects body image and illness behavior. A patient with a visible symptom is more likely to seek assistance than a patient who does not have visible symptoms.

Patients' social groups help them recognize the threat of illness or support the denial of potential illness. Families, friends, and co-workers all influence patients' illness behavior. Patients often react positively to social support while practicing positive health behaviors. Cultural and ethnic background teaches a person how to be healthy, how to recognize illness, and how to be ill. The effects of disease and its interpretation vary according to cultural circumstances.

Economic variables influence the way a patient reacts to illness. Because of economic constraints, a patient will delay treatment and in many cases continue to carry out daily activities. This is especially common in patients who are underinsured. Patients' access to the health care system is closely related to economic factors. The health care system is a socioeconomic system that patients enter, interact within, and exit. For many patients entry into the system is complex or confusing, and some patients seek nonemergency medical care in an emergency department because they do not have access through insurance or do not know how to obtain health services otherwise. The physical proximity of patients to a health care agency often influences how soon they enter the system after deciding to seek care.

IMPACT OF ILLNESS ON PATIENT AND FAMILY

An illness of a family member affects the function of an entire family unit. A patient and family commonly experience behavioral and emotional changes and changes in body image, self-concept, family roles, and family dynamics.

Behavioral and Emotional Changes

Individual behavioral and emotional reactions depend on the nature of an illness, the patient's attitude toward it, the reaction of others to it, and the variables of illness behavior. Short-term, nonlife-threatening illnesses evoke few behavioral changes in the functioning of the patient or family. For example, a husband and father who has a cold lacks the energy and patience to spend time in family activities and is irritable and prefers not to interact with his family. This is a behavioral change, but it is subtle and does not last long. Some even consider such a change a normal response to illness.

Severe illness, particularly one that is life threatening, leads to more extensive emotional and behavioral changes such as anxiety, shock, denial, anger, and withdrawal. These are common responses to the stress of illness. You develop interventions to help patients and families cope with and adapt to this stress because the stressors usually cannot be changed.

Impact on Body Image

Body image is the subjective concept of physical appearance. Our perception of body image changes as we grow and develop (see Chapter 23). Some illnesses result in changes in physical appearance, and patients and families react differently to these changes. These reactions depend on the type of changes (e.g., the loss of a limb or an organ), the adaptive capacity of a family, the rate at which changes take place, and the support services available.

When a change in body image occurs such as results from a leg amputation, a patient generally adjusts by experiencing phases of the grief process (see Chapter 26). Initially the change or impending change shocks the patient. As the patient and family recognize the reality of the change, they become anxious and sometimes withdraw. As they acknowledge the change, they gradually move toward accepting their loss. At the end of the acknowledgment phase, they accept the loss. During rehabilitation the patient is ready to learn how to adapt to the change in body image.

Impact on Self-Concept

Self-concept is your mental self-image of all aspects of your personality. It depends in part on body image and roles but also includes other aspects of psychology and spirituality. Self-concept is important in relationships with other family members. A patient whose self-concept changes because of illness is sometimes no longer able to meet family expectations, leading to tension or conflict. As a result, family members change their interactions with the patient. In the course of providing care, you are able to observe changes in the patient's self-concept (or in the self-concepts of family members) and develop a care plan to help the patient adjust to the changes resulting from the illness (see Chapter 23).

Impact on Family Roles and Family Dynamics

People have many roles in life such as wage earner, decision maker, professional, and parent. When an illness occurs, the roles of the patient and family change (see Chapter 24). Such a change is either subtle and short term or drastic and long term. Patients and their families generally adjust more easily to subtle, short-term changes. However, long-term changes require an adjustment process similar to the grief process (see Chapter 26). The patient and family often require specific counseling and guidance to help them cope with the role changes.

Family dynamics is the process by which the family functions, makes decisions, gives support to individual members, and copes with everyday changes and challenges. Because of the effects of illness, family dynamics often change. Role functions stop or are delayed. Another family member sometimes needs to assume the patient's usual roles and responsibilities. This often creates tension or anxiety in the family. Role reversal is also common. If a parent of an adult becomes ill and is unable to carry out usual activities, the adult child often becomes the family caregiver and assumes many of the parent's responsibilities. Such a reversal leads to conflicting responsibilities for the adult child or direct conflict over decision making. You view the whole family and plan care to help them regain the maximal level of functioning and well-being (see Chapter 24).

KEY POINTS

- Health and wellness are not merely the absence of disease and illness. A person's state of health, wellness, or illness depends on the individual's values, attitudes, personality, and lifestyle.
- Unsatisfied needs motivate human beings. Basic human needs must be met before an individual is able to focus on higher-level needs.
- The health promotion model focuses on behaviors motivated by the desire to increase well-being and actualize human potential.
- Holistic health models of nursing promote optimal health by incorporating active participation of patients in improving their health state. Holistic nursing interventions complement standard medical therapy.
- Consider internal and external variables that influence patients' health beliefs and practices when planning nursing care.
- Health promotion activities maintain or enhance health. Wellness education teaches patients how to care for themselves. Illness prevention activities protect against health threats and thus maintain an optimal level of health.
- Nursing incorporates health promotion, wellness, and illness prevention activities rather than simply treating illness.
- The three levels of prevention are primary, secondary, and tertiary.
- Risk factors threaten health, influence health practices, and are important considerations in illness prevention activities. Risk factors involve genetic or physiological variables, age, physical environment, and lifestyle.
- Improvement in health often requires a change in health behaviors.
- Illness behavior influences how patients use the health care system.
- Illness has many effects on the patient and family, including changes in behavior and emotions, family roles and dynamics, body image, and self-concept.

CLINICAL DECISION-MAKING EXERCISES

Charlie and his wife have another appointment with Liz. In preparation for the visit, Liz reviews Charlie's medical record.

1. Based on what you know about Charlie throughout this chapter, identify risk factors that increase Charlie's susceptibility to problems with his elevated cholesterol and hypertension. Which questions would you ask Charlie to determine all of his risk factors?
2. Using the health belief model, identify two individual health perceptions that may be influencing Charlie.
3. As Liz begins the appointment, Charlie says, "I know I need to exercise and eat right. I just can't seem to figure out how to fit it into my day. When I was in the Navy I had a lot of structure to my life. Now it just seems like the day has no routine."
   a. Using the stages of the behavior change model, which stage best describes Charlie's desire to change?
   b. Which goals could Liz help Charlie set during this visit?

evolve

Answers to Clinical Decision-Making Exercises can be found on the Evolve website.

QSEN ACTIVITY: TEAMWORK AND COLLABORATION

Charlie has been attending classes at Preventive Cardiology for several weeks now. He finds the classes helpful but doesn't understand why so many different people are part of the education team. He has been seeing a nurse, registered dietitian, psychologist, and relaxation therapist. He thinks that it might be easier to just have one person do it all.

How would you explain to Charlie that each person has a critical role on the team?

evolve

Answers to QSEN Activities can be found on the Evolve website.

REVIEW QUESTIONS

1. You are caring for a patient who has just suffered a mild heart attack. You are developing his discharge education plan. Which statement by the patient indicates his readiness to change his behavior?
   1. "I don't think I really had a heart attack."
   2. "I already exercise 3 times a week."
   3. "I know my dad died early from heart disease."
   4. "I travel too much to eat healthy."
2. ____________ is behavior that is motivated by the desire to increase well-being and actualize human health potential, whereas ______________ is behavior that is motivated by a desire to avoid illness, detect it early, or maintain function within the constraints of an illness.
3. You are caring for a patient who was a victim of intimate partner violence. She tells you that she is very concerned about where she will stay once she leaves the hospital. According to Maslow's hierarchy of needs, with which level of needs are you most concerned?
   1. Physiological
   2. Self-actualization
   3. Love and belongingness
   4. Safety and security
4. Which of the following variables influence a patient's health beliefs and practices? (Select all that apply.)
   1. Developmental stage
   2. Emotional factors
   3. Family practices
   4. Genetic background
5. A 50-year-old woman decides to have an annual mammogram. Which level of prevention is this patient practicing?
   1. Primary prevention
   2. Secondary prevention
   3. Tertiary prevention
   4. Rehabilitation
6. A 55-year-old patient is being discharged from the hospital after a heart attack. He is being referred to a cardiac program where he will receive education on healthy eating, exercise, and stress reduction. This is an example of:
   1. Primary prevention
   2. Secondary prevention
   3. Tertiary prevention
   4. Rehabilitation
7. A __________ ______________ is any situation, habit, environmental condition, physiological condition, or other variable that increases the vulnerability of an individual to an illness.
8. A 30-year-old woman has just found out that her mother has been diagnosed with breast cancer. This is an example of which type of risk factor for the 30-year-old?
   1. Age
   2. Lifestyle
   3. Genetic
   4. Environment
9. A 45-year-old woman diagnosed with depression states, "I don't understand why everyone thinks I should seek counseling." This is an example of which state of behavior change?
   1. Precontemplation
   2. Contemplation
   3. Preparation
   4. Maintenance
10. Which of the following are examples of external variables influencing illness behavior? (Select all that apply.)
    1. Social group
    2. Cultural background
    3. Patient perception of the illness
    4. Accessibility of health care

evolve

Rationales for Review Questions can be found on the Evolve website.

1. 3; **2.** Health promotion/health protection; **3.** 4; **4.** 1, 2, 3; **5.** 2; **6.** 3; **7.** Risk factor; **8.** 3; **9.** 1; **10.** 1, 2, 4.

REFERENCES

Agency for Healthcare Research and Quality (AHRQ): *Preventive services*, n.d., http://www.ahrq.gov/clinic/prevenix.htm. Accessed February 10, 2013.

Becker MH, Maiman LA: Sociobehavioral determinants of compliance with health and medical care recommendations, *Med Care* 13(1):10, 1975.

Chodzko-Zajko W: *A national blueprint to get adults 50 and over up and moving, The Robert Wood Johnson Foundation*, 2008, http://pweb1.rwjf.org/reports/grr/048957.htm. Accessed July 16, 2013.

Cumbie SA, Conley VM, Burman ME: Advanced practice nursing models for comprehensive care with chronic illness: model for promoting process engagement, *Adv Nurs Sci* 27(1):70, 2004.

Dols J, Landrum P, Wieck KL: Leading and managing an intergenerational workforce, *Creative Nurs* 16(2):68, 2010.

Edelman CL, Mandle CL: *Health promotion throughout the life span*, ed 7, St Louis, 2010, Mosby.

Funnell MM: National standards for diabetes self-management education, *Diabetes Care* 32(1):S87, 2009. DOI: 10.2337/dc09-S087.

Hill-Briggs F, et al.: Effect of problem-solving-based diabetes self-management training on diabetes control in a low income patient sample, *J Gen Intern Med* 26(9):972, 2011.

King DK, et al: Self-efficacy, problem solving, and social-environment support are associated with diabetes self-management behaviors, *Diabetes Care* 33:751, 2010.

Kralik D, Price K, Telford, K: The meaning of self-care for people with chronic illness, *J Nurs Healthc Chronic Illness* 2(3):197, 2010. DOI: 10.1111/j.1752-9824.2010.01056.

Laditka SB, et al: Attitudes about aging well among a diverse group of older Americans: implications for promoting cognitive health, *The Gerontologist* 49(S1):S30, 2009. DOI:10.1093/geront/gnp084.

Larsen PD: *Illness behavior*, n.d., Jones and Bartlett Learning. http://www.jblearning.com/samples/076375126X/LARSEN_CH02_PTR.pdf. Accessed July 15, 2013.

Maslow AH: *Motivation and personality*, New York, 1954, Harper & Row.

Maslow AH: *Motivation and personality*, ed 2, New York, 1970, Harper & Row.

Maslow AH: *Motivation and personality*, ed 3, Upper Saddle River, NJ, 1987, Prentice Hall.

Marks DF, et al: *Health psychology: theory, research and practice*, ed 2, Thousand Oaks, CA, 2005, Sage.

Mechanic D: The epidemiology of illness behavior and its relationship to physical and psychological distress. In Mechanic D, editor: *Symptoms, illness behavior, and help seeking*, New York, 1982, Prodist.

Mechanic D: Sociological dimensions of illness behavior, *Soc Sci Med* 41(9):1207, 1995.

Mokdad AH, Remington P: Measuring health behaviors in populations, *Prev Chronic Dis* 7(4):A75, 2010.

Mokdad AH, et al: Actual causes of death in the United States, 2000, *JAMA* 291(10):1238, 2004a.

Mokdad AH, et al: Changes in health behaviors among older Americans, 1990-2000, *Public Health Rep* 119:356, 2004b.

Norcross JC, Prochaska JO: Using the stages of change, *Harv Ment Health Lett* 18(11):5, 2002.

Pender NJ: *Health promotion and nursing practice*, Norwalk, Conn, 1982, Appleton-Century-Crofts.

Pender NJ: *Health promotion in nursing practice*, ed 3, Stamford, Conn, 1996, Appleton & Lange.

Pender NJ, Murdaugh CL, Parsons MA: *Health promotion in nursing practice*, ed 6, Upper Saddle River, NJ, 2011, Prentice Hall.

Reed SB, et al: Social isolation and physical inactivity in older US adults: result from the third national health and examination survey, *Eur J Sports Sci* 11(5):347, 2011.

Riesch SK, et al: Health-risk behaviors among a sample of US preadolescents: types, frequencies and predictive factors, *Int J Nurs Stud* 50(8):1067, 2013.

Rosenstoch I: Historical origin of the health belief model, *Health Educ Monogr* 2:334, 1974.

US Department of Health and Human Services (USDHHS), Public Health Service: *Healthy people: the Surgeon General's report on health promotion and disease prevention*, Washington, DC, 1979, US Government Printing Office.

US Department of Health and Human Services (USDHHS), Public Health Service: *Healthy people 2000: national health promotion and disease prevention objectives*, Washington, DC, 1990, US Government Printing Office.

US Department of Health and Human Services (USDHHS), Public Health Service: *Healthy people 2010: understanding and improving health*, Washington, DC, 2000, US Government Printing Office.

US Department of Health and Human Services (USDHHS): *Developing healthy people 2020*, 2010, http://healthypeople.gov/2020/. Accessed November 11, 2013.

Waldron CA, et al: What are effective strategies to communicate cardiovascular risk information to patients? A systematic review, *Patient Educ Counseling* 82:169, 2011.

World Health Organization (WHO) Interim Commission: *Chronicle of WHO*, Geneva, 1947, The Organization.

CHAPTER

3

The Health Care Delivery System

evolve WEBSITE

http://evolve.elsevier.com/Potter/essentials

- Crossword Puzzle
- Audio Glossary

OBJECTIVES

- Describe the six levels of health care.
- Explain the relationship between levels of health care and levels of prevention.
- Discuss the types of settings in which professionals provide various levels of health care.
- Discuss the role of nurses in different health care delivery settings.
- Explain the advantages and disadvantages of managed health care.
- Compare the various methods for financing health care.
- Discuss the implications that issues challenging the health care system have for nursing.
- Discuss opportunities for nursing within the changing health care delivery system.

KEY TERMS

acute care, p. 31
adult day care centers, p. 39
assisted living, p. 38
capitation, p. 31
diagnosis-related groups (DRGs), p. 31
discharge planning, p. 34
evidence-based practice, p. 40
extended care facility, p. 37
globalization, p. 44
home care, p. 36
hospice, p. 39
integrated delivery networks (IDNs), p. 31
managed care, p. 31
Medicaid, p. 37
Medicare, p. 37
Minimum Data Set (MDS), p. 38
nursing-sensitive outcomes, p. 42
patient-centered care, p. 41
primary care, p. 33
professional standards review organizations (PSROs), p. 30
prospective payment system (PPS), p. 31
rehabilitation, p. 37
respite care, p. 39
restorative care, p. 31
skilled nursing facility, p. 37
utilization review (UR) committees, p. 30
vulnerable populations, p. 44

As you begin your career in nursing, you quickly realize that the U.S. health care system is very complex and constantly changing. Although health professionals offer a broad variety of services to the public, gaining access to services is difficult for those with limited health care insurance. The significant rise of patients without insurance has presented a challenge to health care and nursing because they are more likely to skip or delay treatment for acute and chronic illnesses (Kovner and Knickman, 2011). The continuing emergence of new technologies and medications contributes to ever-increasing costs of health care. Pressures to reduce costs come from declining reimbursement by third-party payers and from health care institutions being managed more as businesses than as service organizations. Challenges to health care leaders today are: reducing health care costs while maintaining high-quality care for patients,

CASE STUDY *Amy Sue Reilly*

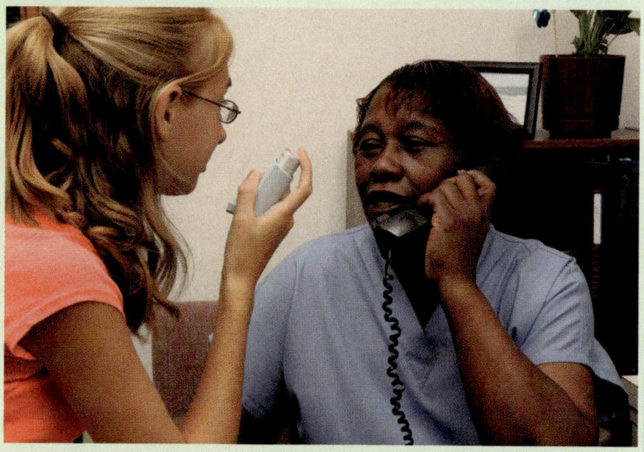

Amy Sue Reilly is a 15-year-old female of Irish descent. She is a freshman at a Catholic high school. Her parents are divorced. Her mother, Anne, is a cashier at a local grocery store; and her father, Joseph, is a lawyer. She has two brothers and lives at home with her mother. Although her parents are divorced, Amy Sue reports that her family is very close and that her parents work together to meet all their children's needs.

Amy Sue has had asthma since she was 5 years old. She has controlled it by taking oral medications and using her inhalers when needed. However, she recently has had some difficulty breathing, especially during gym class.

Corrine is a 45-year-old African-American nurse who recently accepted a job as a school nurse for the four Catholic schools in the area. Three of the schools are grade schools, and there is one high school. Corrine previously worked at a pediatrician's office. Amy Sue's difficulty managing her asthma is significant for Corrine because Corrine's daughter has asthma. In addition, because of her job in the pediatrician's office, Corrine has experience with caring for children with asthma and helping patients access the health care delivery system.

improving access and coverage for more people, and encouraging healthy behaviors (Knickman and Kovner, 2009). Many illnesses that required hospitalization 20 years ago are now treated in outpatient facilities or at home to reduce the costs resulting from lengthy hospitalization. As a result, hospitalized patients are sicker, and their treatment involves a higher level of technological care. Patients are discharged from hospitals sooner, often leaving families with the burden of providing care in the home setting. Nurses also face significant challenges of keeping individuals healthy within their homes and communities.

Nursing is a caring discipline. The profession's values are rooted in helping people to regain, maintain, or improve their health; prevent illness; and find comfort and dignity. The health care system of the new millennium is less service oriented and more business oriented because of cost-saving initiatives, which often causes tension between the caring aspect and business aspect of health care (Knickman and Kovner, 2009). The Institute of Medicine (2001) calls for a health care delivery system that is safe, effective, patient centered, timely, efficient, and equitable. The National Priorities Partnership is a group of 51 organizations from a variety of health care disciplines that joined together to work toward transforming health care (National Priorities Partnership, 2012). The group focuses on the following national priorities for health care transformation:

- Patient and Family Engagement—Providing patient-centered, effective care
- Population Health—Bringing increased focus to wellness and prevention
- Patient Safety—Focusing on eliminating errors whenever and wherever possible
- Care Coordination—Providing patient-centered, high-value care
- Palliative Care—Providing appropriate and compassionate care for patients experiencing advanced illnesses
- Overuse—Focusing on waste reduction to achieve effective, affordable care
- Health Information Technology—Providing safer, better coordinated care through use of electronic medical records and other sources of information technology
- Disparities—Reducing disparities through provision of culturally competent care

As a result of the transformations occurring in the health care system, the practice of nursing is changing. Nursing needs to lead the way in change by valuing and providing evidence-based, compassionate patient care and continuing in the role as patient advocate while meeting the challenges of new roles and new responsibilities (Singleton, 2010).

HEALTH CARE REGULATION AND COMPETITION

Through most of the twentieth century there were few incentives for controlling health care costs. There were few obstacles if patients needed to be in the hospital a few extra days for a wound to heal or for the family to prepare to take care of them at home. Insurers (third-party payers) paid for whatever a health care provider chose to order for a patient's care and treatment. However, as health care costs continue to rise out of control, regulatory and competitive approaches attempt to control health care spending. For example, **professional standards review organizations (PSROs)** review the quality, quantity, and cost of health care services provided through Medicare and Medicaid. Medicare-qualified hospitals are required to have physician-supervised **utilization review (UR) committees** to review admissions, diagnostic testing, and treatments provided by health care providers to patients. The purpose is to identify and eliminate overuse of diagnostic and treatment services. Many hospitals added nursing case managers to help meet the guidelines established by Medicare, Medicaid, and other payers.

One of the most significant factors that influenced health care payments, costs, and competition is the **prospective payment system (PPS).** Established by Congress in 1983, the PPS eliminated cost-based reimbursement. Hospitals serving Medicare patients were no longer paid for all costs incurred to deliver care to a patient. Instead inpatient hospital services for Medicare patients were combined into **diagnosis-related groups (DRGs).** Each group has a fixed reimbursement amount with adjustments for case severity, rural/-urban/regional costs, and teaching costs. Hospitals receive a set dollar amount for each patient based on the assigned DRG, regardless of the patient's length of stay or use of services in the hospital. Most health care providers (e.g., health care networks or managed care organizations) now receive capitated payments. **Capitation** is the payment mechanism in which providers receive a fixed amount per month per patient or enrollee of a health care plan (Kovner and Knickman, 2011). The purpose of capitation is to build a payment plan for select diagnoses or surgical procedures that includes the best standards of care and essential diagnostic and treatment procedures at the lowest cost. Bundled payment is a new form of payment. With bundled payments, a fixed amount is paid to the health care provider and the hospital for an episode of care or time period of care (Kovner and Knickman, 2011).

Payment methods influence the way health care professionals deliver care in all types of settings. The health care industry manages costs through efficiency and effectiveness so the organizations remain profitable. For example, when patients are hospitalized for lengthy periods, hospitals absorb the portion of costs not reimbursed. This simply adds more pressure to ensure that patients are managed effectively and discharged as soon as reasonably possible. Soon after implementing prospective payment, hospitals increased discharge planning activities and shortened hospital lengths of stay. Because patients are discharged home as soon as possible, home care agencies now provide complex technological care, including intravenous (IV) therapy, mechanical ventilation, and long-term parenteral nutrition.

The term **managed care** describes systems in which a payer has control over primary health care services delivery for a defined patient population. A provider or health care system receives a predetermined capitated payment for each patient enrolled in the program. In this case the managed care organization bears financial risk in addition to providing patient care. The focus of care of the organization shifts from individual illness care to concern for the health of its covered population. If people stay healthy, the cost of medical care declines. Systems of managed care focus on containing or reducing costs, increasing patient satisfaction, and improving the health or functional status of the individual (Sultz and Young, 2011). In theory, if people stay healthy, the cost of medical care declines. Managed care aims to increase access to care while decreasing costs. However, health care spending continues to rise. Increases are related to rising health care wages, increased costs of prescription drugs, higher insurance premiums, improved technology, and consumer demands.

Major health care reform came in 2010 with the signing into law of the Patient Protection and Affordable Care Act (Public Law No. 111-148). Health care reform of this magnitude has not occurred in the United States since the 1960s when Medicare and Medicaid were signed into law. The Patient Protection and Affordable Care Act focuses on the major goals of increasing access to health care services for all, reducing health care costs, and improving health care quality. Provisions in the law include insurance industry reforms that increase insurance coverage and decrease costs, increased funding for community health centers, increased primary care services and providers, and improved coverage for children (Adashi et al., 2010; National Conference of State Legislatures, 2010).

You do not have to be a health care financing expert in your role as a nurse. However, it is important for you to understand the basics of health care financing to recognize the effects on employers and patients. Table 3-1 summarizes the most common types of health care plans.

LEVELS OF HEALTH CARE

The health care industry is moving toward health care practices that emphasize managing health rather than illness because in the long term health promotion reduces health care costs. A wellness perspective focuses on the health of populations and their communities rather than just on finding a cure for an individual's disease. Larger health care systems have developed **integrated delivery networks (IDNs)** that include a set of providers and services organized to deliver a coordinated continuum of care to the population of patients in a specific market or geographic area (McDaniel, 2011). An integrated system reduces duplication of services, coordinates care across settings, and ensures that patients receive care in the most appropriate setting.

The health services pyramid (Figure 3-1) is a model of improving health care. The pyramid shows that the population-based health care services provide the basis for preventive services. Achievements in the lower tiers of the pyramid contribute to the improvement of health care delivered at the higher levels of the pyramid. An emphasis on wellness and health of populations and the environment enhances quality of life (Stanhope and Lancaster, 2012).

The health care system has six levels of care: preventive, primary, secondary, tertiary, restorative, and continuing care. Levels of care describe the scope of services and settings in which health care is offered to patients in all stages of health and illness. For example, the secondary level of care is the traditional **acute care** setting in which patients who have signs and symptoms of disease are diagnosed and treated. **Restorative care** includes settings and services in which patients who are recovering from illness or disability receive rehabilitation and supportive care. Levels of care are not the same as levels of prevention (see Chapter 2). Levels of prevention describe the focus of health-related activities: health promotion and disease prevention (primary prevention), curing disease (secondary prevention), and diminishing

TABLE 3-1 HEALTH CARE PLANS

TYPE	DEFINITION	CHARACTERISTICS
Managed care organization (MCO)	Provides comprehensive preventive and treatment services to a specific group of voluntarily enrolled people. Structures include a variety of models.	Focuses on health maintenance, primary care. All care is provided by a primary care physician. Referral is needed for access to specialist and hospitalization. May use capitated payments.
Preferred provider organization (PPO)	Type of managed care plan that limits an enrollee's choice to a list of "preferred" hospitals, physicians, and providers. An enrollee pays more out-of-pocket expenses for using a provider not on the list.	Contractual agreement exists between a set of providers and one or more purchasers (self-insured employers or insurance plans). Comprehensive health services at a discount to companies under contract. Focus on health maintenance.
Medicare	A federally administrated program by the Commonwealth Fund or the Centers for Medicare and Medicaid Services (CMS); a national health insurance program in the United States for people 65 years and older. Part A provides basic protection for medical, surgical, and psychiatric care costs based on diagnosis-related groups (DRGs). Also provides limited skilled nursing facility care, hospice, and home health care. Part B is a voluntary medical insurance; covers physician, certain other specified health professional services, and certain outpatient services. Part C is a managed care provision that provides a choice of three insurance plans. Part D is a voluntary prescription drug improvement (Sultz and Young, 2011).	Payment for plan is deducted from monthly individual Social Security check. Covers services of nurse practitioners. Does not pay full cost of certain services. Supplemental insurance is encouraged.
Medicaid	Federally funded, state-operated program that provides: (1) health insurance to low-income families, (2) health assistance to low-income people with long-term care (LTC) disabilities, and (3) supplemental coverage and LTC assistance to older adults and Medicare beneficiaries in nursing homes. Individual states determine eligibility and benefits.	Finances a large portion of care for poor children, their parents, pregnant women, disabled very-poor adults. Reimburses for nurse-midwifery and other advanced practice nurses (varies by state). Reimburses nursing home funding.
Private insurance	Traditional fee-for-service plan. Payment computed after patient receives services on basis of number of services used.	Policies typically expensive. Most policies have deductibles that patients have to meet before insurance pays.
Long-term care (LTC) insurance	Supplemental insurance for coverage of LTC services. Policies provide a set amount of dollars for an unlimited time or for as little as 2 years.	Very expensive. Often has a minimum waiting period for eligibility; payment for skilled nursing, intermediate, or custodial and home care.
State Children's Health Insurance Program (SCHIP)	Federally funded, state-operated program to provide health coverage for uninsured children. Individual states determine participation eligibility and benefits.	Covers children not poor enough for Medicaid.

complications (tertiary prevention). At any level of care nurses and other health care providers offer a variety of levels of prevention. For example, a nurse working in an acute care, tertiary setting monitors the recovery of a patient following open heart surgery while also providing health promotion information to the family concerning diet and exercise.

It is important for you to understand how the health care industry organizes and delivers different levels of care. Each level creates different requirements and opportunities for your role as a nurse. Box 3-1 highlights the types of services available to patients and families at each level of care. Changes unique to each level developed as a result of health care reform. For example, the health care industry now places greater emphasis on wellness; thus it directs more resources toward primary and preventive care. Nursing has the chance to provide leadership to communities and health care systems that are coordinating resources to better serve their populations. The ability to find strategies to better address patient

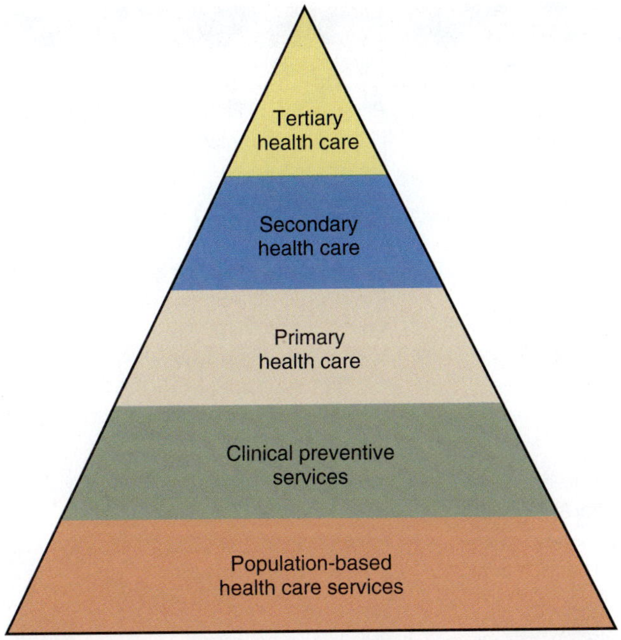

FIGURE 3-1 Health services pyramid. (US Public Health Service: *The core functions project,* Washington, DC, 1994/ update 2008, Office of Disease Prevention and Health Promotion. From Stanhope M, Lancaster J: *Public health nursing,* ed 8, St Louis, 2012, Mosby.)

BOX 3-1 EXAMPLES OF HEALTH CARE SERVICES

PREVENTIVE CARE
- Blood pressure and cancer screening
- Immunizations
- Poison control information
- Mental health counseling and crisis prevention
- Community legislation (seat belts, air bags, bike helmets)

PRIMARY CARE (HEALTH PROMOTION)
- Prenatal care
- Well-baby care
- Nutrition counseling
- Family planning
- Exercise classes

SECONDARY ACUTE CARE
- Emergency care
- Acute medical-surgical care
- Radiological procedures

TERTIARY CARE
- Intensive care
- Psychiatric facilities

RESTORATIVE CARE
- Cardiovascular and pulmonary rehabilitation
- Sports medicine
- Spinal cord injury programs
- Home care

CONTINUING CARE
- Assisted living
- Psychiatric and older-adult day care

needs at all levels of care is critical to the success of improving the health care delivery system.

Preventive and Primary Health Care Services

Health promotion is a major theme in the settings that deliver preventive and **primary care** such as schools, physicians' or health care providers' offices, occupational health clinics, and nursing centers (Table 3-2). Health promotion is a key to good-quality health care. Successful programs help patients acquire healthier lifestyles. The focus of health promotion is to keep people healthy through personal hygiene, good nutrition, clean living environments, regular exercise, rest, and the adoption of positive health attitudes. Health promotion programs lower the overall costs of health care by reducing the incidence of disease and minimizing complications, thus reducing the need to use more expensive health care resources. In contrast, preventive care is more disease oriented and focused on reducing and controlling risk factors for disease through activities such as immunization and occupational health programs.

Health care providers at the primary level of health care build interventions that lead to improved health outcomes for an entire population. The primary level of health care includes medical and health care services, health education, nutritional counseling, maternal/child health care, family planning, and control of diseases. Successful community-based primary health care programs take societal and environmental factors into consideration when addressing the health needs of communities (see Chapter 4).

Secondary and Tertiary Care

The diagnosis and treatment of illness are traditionally the reasons for the most commonly used services of the health care delivery system. With managed care these services are now often delivered at the primary care level. For example, more surgeons are performing simple surgeries in office surgical suites. However, if a patient develops a problem for which the surgeon or health care provider is not able to provide care, the patient needs a medical specialist. Care from a specialist sometimes requires hospitalization. Typically secondary care and tertiary care (also called *acute care*) are quite costly, particularly if patients wait to seek health care until after symptoms have developed.

Hospitals. Hospital emergency departments, urgent care centers, critical care units, and inpatient medical-surgical units are sites that provide secondary and tertiary levels of care. When you work in these settings, you are challenged to work closely with all members of the health care team. Your ability to think critically and identify patients' changing problems quickly and accurately is essential. Planning and coordination of care are necessary to deliver services in a competent and timely manner. You need to apply nursing research findings when selecting nursing interventions to improve patient outcomes. You constantly evaluate whether care is effective and how to improve it.

Quality, safe care is the focus of most acute care organizations. Patient satisfaction is a priority in a busy, stressful location such as an inpatient nursing unit. Patients expect you to treat them courteously and respectfully and involve them in daily care decisions. As a nurse you play a key role in bringing respect and dignity to each patient. It is necessary for nurses to be aware of patient needs and expectations early to form effective partnerships that ultimately enhance the level of nursing care given.

TABLE 3-2 PREVENTIVE AND PRIMARY CARE SERVICES

TYPE OF SERVICE	PURPOSE	AVAILABLE PROGRAMS/SERVICES
School health	Comprehensive programs integrate health promotion principles throughout a school curriculum. Services stress program management, interdisciplinary collaboration, and community health principles.	Positive life skills Nutritional planning Health screening Counseling Communicable disease prevention Crisis intervention
Occupational health	A comprehensive program is geared to health promotion and accident or illness prevention. Goal is to increase worker productivity, decrease absenteeism, and reduce use of expensive medical care.	Environmental surveillance Physical assessment Health screening Health education Communicable disease control Counseling
Physicians' offices	Provide primary health care and diagnose and treat acute and chronic illnesses. Beginning to focus more on health promotion practices. Advanced nurse practitioners often partner with a physician in managing patient population.	Routine physical examination Health screening Diagnostics Disease management
Nursing centers	Nurse-managed clinics provide nursing services with a focus on health promotion and health education, chronic disease assessment management, and support for self-care and caregivers.	Day care Health risk appraisal Wellness counseling Employment readiness Acute and chronic care management
Block and parish nursing	Nurses provide services to members of churches and neighborhoods (e.g., older patients or those unable to leave their home). Provides services that are not available in traditional health care system.	Running errands Transportation Respite care Homemaker aides Spiritual health
Community centers	Outpatient clinics that provide primary care to a specific patient population (e.g., well-baby, mental health, diabetes) that lives in a specific community. Sometimes affiliated with a hospital, medical school, church, or other community organization.	Physical assessment Health screening Disease management Health education Counseling

Managed care organizations expect patients who are hospitalized to be cared for and discharged within a projected time period. Therefore, if you work in a hospital, you need to use resources efficiently to help your patients successfully recover and return home. Many hospitals have redesigned nursing units to make more services available on nursing units, thus minimizing the need to transfer and transport patients across multiple diagnostic and treatment areas.

Hospitalized patients are acutely ill and need comprehensive and specialized tertiary health care. The services provided by hospitals vary considerably. Some small rural hospitals offer limited emergency and diagnostic services and general inpatient services. In comparison, large urban medical centers offer comprehensive, state-of-the-art diagnostic services, trauma and emergency care, surgical intervention, intensive care units (ICUs), inpatient services, and rehabilitation facilities. Larger hospitals hire professional staff from a variety of specialties such as social service, respiratory therapy, physical and occupational therapy, and speech therapy. The focus in hospitals is to provide the highest quality of care possible so patients are discharged early but safely to the home or another health care facility that will adequately manage any remaining health care needs.

Discharge Planning. Discharge planning is a centralized, coordinated, multidisciplinary process that ensures that a patient has a plan for continuing care after leaving a health care agency. *Discharge planning with coordination of services begins the moment a patient is admitted to a health care facility.* You play a large role in discharge planning if you work in a hospital. Discharge planning provides continuity of care within an acute care hospital. To achieve continuity of care, you use critical thinking skills and apply the nursing process (see Chapters 8 and 9). You anticipate and identify a patient's needs and work with all members of the multidisciplinary health care team to develop a plan of care that moves the patient from the hospital to another environment such as the patient's home or a nursing home.

Because patients leave hospitals as soon as their physical condition allows, they often have continuing health care needs when they go home or to another facility. For example, a patient still requires wound care after surgery or extensive ambulation training following a stroke. Patients and families worry about how they will care for the patient's needs and manage illness over the long term. As a nurse you help by anticipating and identifying patients' continuing needs before the actual time of discharge and coordinating health team members to achieve an appropriate discharge plan.

Some patients are more in need of discharge planning because of the risks they have. For example, some patients have limited financial resources or limited family support, others have long-term disabilities or chronic illness, and older adults there sometimes have cognitive and/or hearing impairments and poor health literacy (Bobay et al., 2010). Early discharge teaching is especially important to decrease older adults' readmission to a hospital (Bobay et al., 2010). However, any patient who is discharged from a health care facility with functional limitations or who needs to follow certain restrictions or therapies for recovery requires careful discharge planning. All health care providers who care for a patient with a specific health problem participate in discharge planning. The process is truly multidisciplinary and often includes family caregivers. For example, a patient with diabetes visiting a diabetes management center requires the collaboration of a nurse educator, dietitian, and health care provider to ensure that the patient returns home with the right information to manage the condition. A patient who had a stroke is not discharged from a hospital until caregivers have established plans with physical and occupational therapists to begin a program of rehabilitation.

Effective discharge planning often requires referring patients to various health care disciplines. In many agencies patients need a health care provider's order for a referral, especially when specific therapies are planned (e.g., physical therapy). Some tips on making the referral process successful include the following:

- Involve the patient and family in the referral process, including selecting the necessary referral. Explain the service to be provided, the reason for the referral, and what to expect from the services of the referral.
- Make a referral as soon as possible.
- Inform the care provider receiving the referral of as much information about the patient as possible. This avoids duplication of effort and exclusion of important information.
- Determine what the referral discipline (e.g., physical therapy, social work, diet and nutrition, radiology) recommends for the patient's care and incorporate this into the treatment plan as soon as possible.

Successful discharge planning involves the patient from the beginning, uses the strengths of the patient in planning, provides resources to meet the patient's limitations, and focuses on improving the patient's long-term outcomes. Discharge planning depends on comprehensive patient and family education (see Chapter 12). Patients need to know what to do when they get home, how to do it, and what to watch for when problems develop. The Joint Commission (2012a) requires the following when patients are discharged from health care facilities or transferred to other levels of care:

- A process that addresses the need for continuing care, treatment, and services after discharge or transfer
- The transfer or discharge of a patient to another level of care, treatment, and services; different professionals; or different settings is based on the patient's assessed needs and the capabilities of the hospital
- When patients are transferred or discharged, exchange with other service providers appropriate information related to the care, treatment, and services provided

Intensive Care. An ICU or critical care unit is a hospital unit in which critically ill, unstable patients receive close monitoring and intensive medical care. ICUs have advanced technologies such as computerized cardiac monitors and mechanical ventilators. Although many of these devices are on regular nursing units, the patients hospitalized within ICUs are monitored and maintained on multiple devices. Nursing and medical staff within an ICU are educated on critical care principles and techniques. An ICU is the most expensive delivery site for medical care because each nurse is usually assigned to care for only one or two patients at a time and because of all the treatments and procedures that the patients require.

Mental Health Facilities. Patients who have emotional and behavioral problems such as depression, violent behavior, and eating disorders often require special counseling and treatment in psychiatric facilities. Located in hospitals, independent outpatient clinics, or private mental health hospitals, psychiatric facilities offer inpatient and outpatient services, depending on the seriousness of the problem. Patients enter these facilities voluntarily or involuntarily. Hospitalization involves relatively short stays with the purpose of stabilizing patients before transfer to outpatient treatment centers. Patients with psychiatric problems receive a comprehensive multidisciplinary treatment plan that involves them and their families. Medicine, nursing, social work, and activity therapy collaborate to develop a plan of care that enables patients to return to functional states within the community. At the time of discharge from inpatient facilities, patients usually receive referrals for follow-up care at clinics or with counselors.

Rural Hospitals. Access to health care in rural areas has been a serious problem. Most rural hospitals have experienced a severe shortage of primary care providers. Many have been forced to close because of economic failure. In 1989 the Omnibus Budget Reconciliation Act directed the U.S. Department of Health and Human Services (USDHHS) to create a new health care entity, the rural primary care hospital (RPCH). The Balanced Budget Act of 1997 changed the designation for rural hospitals to Critical Access Hospital (CAH) if certain criteria were met (DHHS CMS, 2012). A CAH is located in a rural area and provides 24-hour emergency care, with no more than 25 inpatient beds for providing temporary care for 96 hours or less to patients needing stabilization before transfer to a larger hospital. Physicians, advanced practice nurses, or physician assistants staff a CAH. The CAH provides inpatient care to acutely ill or injured people before transferring them to better-equipped facilities. Basic radiological and laboratory services are also available.

With health care reform more big-city health care systems are branching out and establishing affiliations or mergers with rural hospitals. The rural hospitals provide a referral base to the larger tertiary care medical centers. Nurses who work in rural hospitals or clinics often function independently in the absence of a physician. Competence in physical assessment, clinical decision making, and emergency care is essential. Having a culture of evidence-based practice is important in rural hospitals; thus nurses practice using the best evidence to achieve optimal patient outcomes (Burns et al., 2009). Advanced practice nurses (e.g., nurse practitioners and clinical nurse specialists) use medical protocols and establish collaborative agreements with staff physicians.

Restorative Care

Patients recovering from acute illnesses or who have chronic illnesses or disabilities usually require services designed to restore their level of health. Care is necessary until patients return to their previous level of function or reach a new level of function limited by their illness or disability. The goals of restorative care are to help an individual regain maximal functional status, thereby enhancing his or her quality of life, and promote patient independence and self-care. With the emphasis on early discharge from hospitals, most patients require some level of restorative care. For example, some surgical patients require ongoing wound care and activity and exercise management until they have recovered to a point at which they are able to resume normal activities of daily living independently.

The intensity of care has increased in restorative care settings because patients leave hospitals earlier. It is common to have patients in a home or rehabilitation setting still receiving IV fluids (see Chapter 18), pain control (see Chapter 32), and enteral nutrition (see Chapter 33). The restorative health care team is an interprofessional health care team that includes the patient and family or significant others. In restorative settings nurses recognize that success depends on effective and early partnering with patients and their families. Patients and families require a clear understanding of goals for physical recovery, the rationale for any physical limitations, and the purpose and potential risks associated with therapies. The more that patients and families are involved in restorative care, the more likely it is that they will be motivated to follow treatment plans and be able to achieve optimal functioning.

Home Care. Home care is the provision of medically related professional and paraprofessional services and equipment to patients and families in their homes. Services provided include health maintenance, education, illness prevention, diagnosis and treatment of disease, palliation, and rehabilitation. Patients in home care use nursing services more than any other service. However, home care also includes medical and social services; physical, occupational, speech, and respiratory therapy; and nutritional therapy. A home care service coordinates the access to and delivery of home health equipment or durable medical equipment (DME), which is any medically related product adapted for home use.

Home care agencies provide almost every type of health care service in a patient's home. Health promotion and education traditionally are the primary objectives of home care, yet at present most patients receive professional services on the basis of some medically related need. The focus is on patient and family independence. Home care addresses recovery from and stabilization of illness in the home, where problems related to lifestyle, safety, environment, family dynamics, and health care practices are identified.

Home care agencies provide skilled and intermittent professional services and home care aide services. These services usually are delivered once or twice a day for as long as 7 days a week (Box 3-2). Approved home care agencies usually

BOX 3-2 HOME CARE SERVICES

WOUND CARE

Sterile dressing changes, debridement and irrigations, packing, and instruction of patients and family caregivers in wound care techniques

RESPIRATORY CARE

Oxygen therapy, mechanical ventilation, suctioning, and care of tracheostomies

VITAL SIGNS

Monitoring blood pressure and cardiopulmonary status; instructing patients and family caregivers in vital sign measurement

ELIMINATION

Ostomy care, appliance application, skin care, and irrigation; inserting indwelling and intermittent urinary catheters, irrigating, and instructing family caregivers in catheter management; home dialysis

NUTRITION

Administration of enteral feedings; assessment of nutrition and hydration status; instructing patients and family caregivers in tube feedings

REHABILITATION

Ambulation and gait training, using assistive devices, range-of-motion exercises, and instructing patients and family caregivers in transfer techniques

MEDICATIONS

Monitoring compliance; administering injections; and instructing patients and family caregivers in drug information, preparing medication, and steps to take in the event of side effects

INTRAVENOUS THERAPY

Administration of blood products, analgesic and chemotherapeutic agents; long-term hydration and instruction of patients and family caregivers in use of intravenous devices; steps to take in the event of disconnection or accidental fluid infusion; and side effects

LABORATORY STUDIES

Blood glucose monitoring (including patient and family caregiver instruction) and drawing blood for specific diagnostic purposes receive reimbursement for services from the government (such as Medicare and Medicaid in the United States), private insurance, and private payers. The government has strict regulations that govern reimbursement for home care services. An agency cannot simply charge whatever it wants for a service and expect to receive full reimbursement. Government programs set the cost for reimbursement of most professional services.

If you work as a home care nurse, you will have your own caseload and provide highly individualized nursing care, helping patients adapt to many permanent or temporary physical limitations so they are able to assume a more normal daily home routine. Home care requires a strong knowledge base in many areas such as family dynamics (see Chapter 24), cultural practices (see Chapter 20), spiritual values (see Chapter 21), and communication principles (see Chapter 11).

Rehabilitation. Rehabilitation is the use of multiple therapies such as physical, psychological, occupational, speech, and social services to help restore a person to the fullest physical, mental, social, vocational, and economic usefulness possible (Stanhope and Lancaster, 2012). Patients require rehabilitation after a physical or mental illness, injury, or chemical addiction. Rehabilitation was once available primarily for patients with illnesses or injury to the nervous or musculoskeletal system, but the health care delivery system has expanded its scope of such services. Today specialized rehabilitation services such as cardiovascular and pulmonary rehabilitation programs help patients and families adjust to necessary changes in lifestyle and learn to function with the limitations of their disease. Drug rehabilitation centers help patients become free from drug dependence and return to the community.

Ideally rehabilitation begins the moment a patient enters a health care setting for treatment. For example, some orthopedic programs now have patients undergo physical therapy exercises before major joint repair to enhance their recovery after surgery. Initially rehabilitation focuses on the prevention of complications related to an illness or injury. As the condition stabilizes, rehabilitation maximizes the patient's functioning and level of independence.

Rehabilitation occurs in many health care settings, including specific rehabilitation institutions, outpatient settings, and the home. Frequently patients needing long-term rehabilitation (e.g., patients who have had strokes and spinal cord injuries) have severe disabilities affecting their ability to carry out the activities of daily living. For rehabilitation services delivered in outpatient settings, patients get treatment at specified times during the week but remain at home the rest of the time. Specific rehabilitation strategies are applied to the home environment to help the patient achieve maximal levels of function and independence. Nurses and other members of the health care team visit homes and help patients and families learn to adapt to illness or injury.

Extended Care Facilities. An extended care facility provides intermediate medical, nursing, or custodial care for patients recovering from acute illness or patients with chronic illnesses or disabilities. Extended care facilities include intermediate care and skilled nursing facilities. Some include long-term care and assisted living facilities (see later discussion of continuing care). At one point extended care facilities primarily cared for older adults. However, because hospitals discharge their patients sooner, there is a greater need for intermediate care settings for patients of all ages. For example, a young patient who has experienced a traumatic brain injury resulting from a car accident typically transfers to an extended care facility for rehabilitative or supportive care until discharge to the home becomes a safe option. The growth of extended care facilities will increase as the number of older adults grows.

An intermediate care or skilled nursing facility offers skilled care from a licensed nursing staff. This often includes administration of IV fluids, wound care, long-term ventilator management, and physical rehabilitation. Patients receive extensive supportive care until they are able to move back into the community or into residential care.

Extended care facilities provide around-the-clock nursing coverage. If you work in this setting, you need nursing expertise that is similar to that of nurses working in acute care inpatient settings along with a background in gerontological nursing principles (see Chapter 22).

Continuing Care

Continuing care describes a variety of health, personal, and social services provided over a prolonged period to people who are disabled, who never were functionally independent, or who suffer a terminal disease. The need for continuing health care services is growing in the United States. People are living longer, and many of those with continuing health care needs have no immediate family members to care for them. A decline in the number of children families choose to have, the aging of care providers, and the increasing rates of divorce and remarriage complicate this problem. Continuing care is available within institutional settings (e.g., nursing centers or nursing homes, group homes, and retirement communities), communities (e.g., adult day care and senior centers), or the home (e.g., home care, home-delivered meals, and hospice) (Meiner, 2011). Elder care services that offer companionship, assistance with activities of daily living, and food preparation are another alternative for patients who do not need nursing care but need some assistance to stay independent.

Nursing Centers or Facilities. The language of long-term care is confusing and constantly changing. The nursing home has been the dominant setting for long-term care (Meiner, 2011). With the Omnibus Budget Reconciliation Act of 1987, the term *nursing facility* became the term for nursing homes and other facilities that provide long-term care. Now, *nursing center* is the most appropriate term. A nursing center typically provides 24-hour intermediate and custodial care for residents of any age with chronic or debilitating illnesses. Care provided usually includes nursing, rehabilitation, dietary, recreational, social, and religious services. In some cases patients stay in nursing centers for room, food, and laundry services only. Most people living in nursing centers are older adults. A nursing center is a resident's temporary or permanent home with surroundings made as homelike as possible (Sorrentino and Remmert, 2012). Residents receive a planned, systematic, and interdisciplinary approach to care to help them reach and maintain their highest level of function.

The nursing-center industry has become one of the most highly regulated industries in the United States. The Omnibus Budget Reconciliation Act of 1987, also known as the Nursing Home Reform Act, raised the standard of services provided by nursing centers. To receive payment from Medicare and Medicaid, nursing centers have to comply with the Act of 1987 and its minimal requirements for nursing homes. There currently are 18 requirements included in this law. Examples of the requirements include having sufficient nursing staff; developing a comprehensive plan of care for each resident; maintaining dignity and respect for each resident; and providing services needed to promote and/or maintain personal safety, quality of life, nutrition, grooming, and personal hygiene (Klauber and Wright, 2001).

Interdisciplinary functional assessment of residents is the cornerstone of clinical practice within nursing centers (Meiner, 2011). Government regulations require that staff in nursing centers assess each resident comprehensively, with care planning decisions made within a prescribed period. A resident's functional ability (e.g., ability to perform activities of daily living and instrumental activities of daily living) and long-term physical and psychosocial well-being are the focus. The facility needs to complete the Resident Assessment Instrument (RAI) on all residents. The RAI consists of the **Minimum Data Set (MDS)** (Box 3-3), Resident Assessment Protocols (RAPs), and utilization guidelines of each state. The RAI ultimately provides a national database for nursing facilities so policy makers will better understand the health care needs of the long-term care population. In addition, the MDS is a rich resource for nurses in determining the best type of interventions to support the health care needs of this growing population.

Assisted Living. **Assisted living** is one of the fastest-growing industries within the United States. It offers an attractive long-term care setting with a homier environment and greater resident autonomy. Patients require some assistance with activities of daily living but remain relatively independent within a partially protective setting. A group of residents live together, but each resident has his or her own room and shares dining and social activity areas. Usually people keep all of their personal possessions in their residences. Facilities range from hotel-like buildings with hundreds of units to modest group homes that house a handful of seniors. Assisted living provides independence, security, and privacy all at the same time (Ebersole et al., 2008). These facilities promote independence and physical and psychosocial health (Figure 3-2). Services in an assisted-living facility include medication management, exercise and educational activities, social activities, laundry, assistance with meals and personal care, 24-hour oversight, and housekeeping. Some facilities provide assistance with medication administration. Assisted-living facilities do not directly provide nursing care services, although a home care nurse is able to visit a patient in an assisted-living facility.

BOX 3-3 MINIMUM DATA SET AND EXAMPLES OF RESIDENT ASSESSMENT PROTOCOLS

MINIMUM DATA SET

- Resident's background
- Cognitive, communication/hearing, and vision patterns
- Physical functioning and structural problems
- Mood, behavior, and activity pursuit patterns
- Psychosocial well-being
- Bowel and bladder continence
- Health conditions
- Disease diagnoses
- Oral/nutritional and dental status
- Skin condition
- Medication use
- Special treatments and procedures

RESIDENT ASSESSMENT PROTOCOLS (EXAMPLES)

- Delirium
- Falls
- Pressure ulcers
- Psychotropic drug use

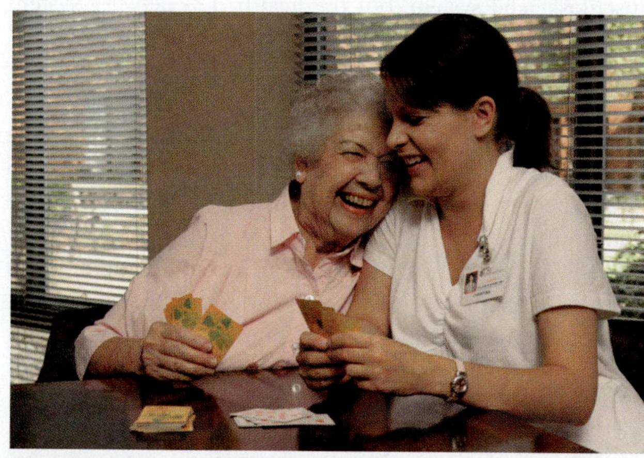

FIGURE 3-2 Providing nursing services in assisted-living facilities promotes physical and psychosocial health.

Unfortunately most residents of assisted-living facilities pay privately. The monthly payment varies according to services needed but is typically over $3000 per month (NCAL, 2012). With no government fee caps and little regulation, assisted living is not always an option for individuals with limited financial resources.

Respite Care. The need to care for family members within the home creates great physical and emotional burdens for adult caregivers, especially when the family member is physically or cognitively limited. The caregiver is usually an adult who not only has the responsibility for providing care to a loved one (e.g., spouse, parent, or sibling) but often maintains a full-time job, raises a family, and manages the routines of daily living as well. **Respite care** is a service that provides short-term relief or time off for people providing home care to an ill, disabled, or frail older adult (Meiner, 2011). Adult day care is one form of respite care. Trained volunteers in the home also provide respite care. The family caregiver is able to leave the home for errands or some social time while a responsible person stays in the home to care for the loved one. Alternatively some patients stay in a nursing center temporarily to provide the family relief.

Adult Day Care Centers. **Adult day care centers** provide a variety of health and social services to specific patient populations who live alone or with family in the community. Services offered during the day allow family members to maintain their lifestyles and employment and still provide home care for their relatives (Meiner, 2011). Day care centers are associated with a hospital or nursing home or exist as independent centers. Frequently the patients of such centers do not require hospitalization but need continuous health care services while their families or support people work. These patients include older adults needing daily physical rehabilitation, individuals with emotional illnesses needing daily counseling, and individuals with chemical dependence problems who are involved in rehabilitation programs. The centers usually operate 5 days per week during typical business hours and usually charge on a per-diem basis. Adult day care centers allow patients to retain more independence by living at home, thus potentially reducing the costs of health care by avoiding or delaying an older adult's admission to a nursing center.

Additional services offered in day care settings include transportation to and from the facility, assistance with personal care, nursing and therapeutic services (e.g., counseling and rehabilitation), meals, and recreational activities (Meiner, 2011). Nurses working in day care centers provide continuity between care delivered in the home and in the center. For example, nurses ensure that patients continue to take prescribed medication and receive treatments such as dressing changes. Knowledge of community needs and resources is essential in providing adequate support of patients, who often spend only a few hours a week in the day care setting (Ebersole et al., 2008).

Hospice. A **hospice** is a system of family-centered care that allows patients to live and remain at home with comfort, independence, and dignity while alleviating the strains caused by terminal illness. The focus of hospice care is palliative care, not curative treatment (see Chapter 26). A hospice benefits patients in the terminal phase of any disease such as cardiomyopathy, multiple sclerosis, acquired immunodeficiency syndrome (AIDS), or cancer.

A patient entering a hospice is at the terminal phase of illness; and the patient, family, and physician agree that no further treatment will reverse the disease process. Staff members collaborate to provide care that ensures death with dignity, usually in the patient's home. Hospice care is available 24 hours a day, 7 days a week; and services continue without interruption if the patient's care setting changes. Occasionally a patient is admitted to a hospice unit within a hospital or a freestanding hospice facility. The patient and family need to accept the fact that the hospice will not use emergency measures such as cardiopulmonary resuscitation to prolong life. The focus is on symptom management and ensuring the patient's comfort. The hospice multidisciplinary team works together continuously with the patient's health care provider to develop and maintain a patient-directed individualized plan of care.

If you decide to be a hospice nurse, you work in institutional and community settings. Hospice nurses are committed to the philosophy and objectives of the facilities for which they work. They provide care and support for a patient and family during the terminal phase and at the time of death and continue to offer bereavement counseling and follow-up to the family after the patient's death. Many hospice programs provide respite care, which is important in maintaining the health of the primary family caregiver.

Care Coordination

A problem that many patients face in today's complex health care delivery system is lack of coordination of care and services. Health care reform has stimulated the development of two systems that are focused on coordinating medical care for patients and families. Accountable care organizations (ACOs) were developed to coordinate medical care by primary care and specialty physicians, hospitals, and other health care providers, with the goal of providing high-quality coordinated care (Kovner and Knickman, 2011). An ACO works to make sure that patients receive the right care at the right time, without duplication of services or incidence of medical errors (CMS, 2012). In an ACO the health care providers are accountable for the quality and cost of care delivered to patients. A second model of care that was developed to improve coordination of care is the patient-centered medical home (PCMH). The goal of the PCMH is to make care for patients more efficient, effective, continuous, comprehensive, patient-centered, and coordinated (Kovner and Knickman, 2011; NCQA, 2011a). The PCMH uses technology, teamwork, and effective communication with patients to make care culturally sensitive and accessible, gather clinical data, and monitor patient outcomes (NCQA, 2011a). The primary care physician functions as the "hub" of the PCMH (Sultz and Young, 2011).

ISSUES IN HEALTH CARE DELIVERY

The climate in health care today influences health care professionals and consumers. As a nurse in the midst of an evolving health care system, be prepared to participate fully and effectively within the managed care environment. Those who provide patient care are the most qualified to make changes in the health care delivery system. As you face issues of how to maintain health care quality while reducing costs, you need to acquire the knowledge, skills, and values necessary to practice competently and effectively. It is also more important than ever to collaborate with your colleagues in health care in designing new approaches for patient care delivery.

BOX 3-4 INSTITUTE OF MEDICINE COMPETENCIES FOR THE TWENTY-FIRST CENTURY

PROVIDE PATIENT-CENTERED CARE
- Recognize and respect differences in patients' values, preferences, and needs.
- Relieve pain and suffering.
- Coordinate continuous care.
- Effectively communicate with and educate patients.
- Share decision making and management.
- Advocate for disease prevention and health promotion.

WORK IN INTERDISCIPLINARY TEAMS
- Cooperate, collaborate, and communicate.
- Integrate care to ensure that care is continuous and reliable.

EMPLOY EVIDENCE-BASED PRACTICE
- Integrate best research with clinical practice and patient values.
- Participate in research activities as possible.

APPLY QUALITY IMPROVEMENT
- Identify errors and hazards in care.
- Practice using basic safety design principles.
- Measure quality in relation to structure, process, and outcomes.
- Design and test interventions to change processes.

USE INFORMATICS
- Use information technology to communicate, manage knowledge, reduce error, and support decision making.

Modified from the Institute of Medicine: *Crossing the quality chasm: a new health system for the 21st century,* Washington, DC, 2001, National Academies Press; Institute of Medicine: *Health professions education: a bridge to quality,* Washington, DC, 2003, National Academies Press.

BOX 3-5 TEN RULES OF PERFORMANCE IN A REDESIGNED HEALTH CARE SYSTEM

1. Care is based on continuous healing relationships.
2. Care is individualized based on patient needs and values.
3. The patient is the source of control participating in shared decision making.
4. Knowledge is shared, and information flows freely.
5. Decision making is evidence based with care based on the best available scientific knowledge.
6. Safety is a system property and focused on reducing errors.
7. Transparency is necessary through sharing information with patients and families.
8. Patient needs are anticipated through planning.
9. Waste is continuously decreased.
10. Cooperation and communication among clinicians is a priority.

Modified from the Institute of Medicine: *Crossing the quality chasm: a new health system for the 21st century,* Washington, DC, 2001, National Academies Press; Institute of Medicine: *Health professions education: a bridge to quality,* Washington, DC, 2003, National Academies Press.

Competency

The Pew Health Professions Commission (1998) is a national and interdisciplinary group of health care leaders that recommended 21 competencies for health care professionals in the twenty-first century. These competencies emphasized the importance of public service, caring for the health of communities, and developing ethically responsible behaviors. In addressing the continued challenges facing the health care system, the Institute of Medicine (2001) identified five interrelated competencies that are essential for all health care workers in the twenty-first century (Box 3-4). The Institute of Medicine also identified 10 important rules of performance for a health care system to follow to better meet patient needs (Box 3-5) (IOM, 2003).

The health care practitioner competencies are an excellent tool for measuring how well you practice nursing. They also provide guidance as you grow within the nursing profession. A consumer of health care expects that the standards of nursing care and practice in any health care setting are appropriate, safe, and effective. Ongoing competency is your responsibility. Health care organizations ensure effective, quality care by establishing policies, procedures, and protocols that are scientifically valid and follow national accrediting standards. Your responsibilities are to follow policies and procedures and know the most current practice standards. As you progress in your career, it becomes your responsibility to obtain necessary continued education and earn certifications when you choose to practice in specialty areas.

Evidence-Based Practice

As you enter the nursing profession, it is a challenge to stay familiar with new information to provide the highest quality of patient care. Nursing practice is dynamic and always changing because of new information coming from research studies, practice trends, technological development, and social issues affecting patients. **Evidence-based practice** is a problem-solving approach to clinical practice that integrates the conscientious use of best evidence with a clinician's expertise and patient preferences and values in making decisions about patient care (Melnyk and Fineout-Overholt, 2010; Sackett et al., 2000). The goal of evidence-based practice is to apply evidence-based data when providing patient care to improve patient outcomes. Evidence-based practice helps you resolve problems that arise in the clinical setting and provide innovative health care that exceeds quality standards. Using evidence-based practice also helps you provide consistent patient care using effective and efficient decision-making processes (Melnyk and Fineout-Overholt, 2010) (see Chapter 7).

Quality Health Care

Quality health care is the "degree to which health services for individuals and populations increase the likelihood of desired health outcomes and are consistent with current professional knowledge" (IOM, 2001). Safety is a critical part of quality health care. For example, use of infection control standards and fall precautions reduces the incidence of infection and patient injury. Health care providers define the quality of their services by measuring health care outcomes that show how a patient's health status has changed. Examples of outcomes that are monitored are readmission rates for patients who have had surgery, functional health status of patients after discharge (e.g., ability and time frame for returning to work), and the rate of infection after surgery. As a nurse you play an important role in gathering and analyzing quality outcome data.

Health care agencies seek accreditation and certification as a way to demonstrate quality and safety in the delivery of care and evaluate the performance of an organization based on established standards. Accreditation is earned by an entire organization, whereas specific programs or services within an organization earn certifications (TJC, 2012b). The Joint Commission accredits health care organizations across the continuum of care, including hospitals and ambulatory care, long-term care, home care, and behavioral health agencies. Other accrediting agencies such as the Commission on Accreditation of Rehabilitation Facilities (CARF) and the Community Health Accrediting Program (CHAP) have a specific focus. Disease-specific certifications are available in most all chronic diseases (TJC, 2012b). Accreditation and certification survey processes help organizations identify problems and develop solutions to improve the quality and safety of delivered care and services.

More and more health care institutions are focused on improving processes as a way to improve. Many use strategies such as Six Sigma or value stream analysis. Six Sigma is a data-driven approach to process improvement that reduces variations in processes. It is a measure of quality (isixsigma, 2012b). For example, a nursing unit sets up a project to collect data on the process of administering the first dose of an ordered chemotherapy. The audit reveals delays from getting the drug from the pharmacy to the nursing unit. Using Six Sigma, the collected data are analyzed, and unnecessary steps in the process are identified. Based on this analysis the process is streamlined to decrease time from ordering to administration. Value stream mapping is another method that focuses on improvement of processes through studying each step of a process to determine if the step does not add value and costs the health care organization time and resources (isixsigma, 2012a). The aim is to eliminate unnecessary, costly steps.

Health plans throughout the United States rely on the Health Plan Employer Data and Information Set (HEDIS) as a quality measure. The National Committee for Quality Assurance (NCQA) created HEDIS as a tool to collect various data to measure the quality of care and services provided by different health plans. HEDIS compares how well health plans perform on 76 measures across five domains of care related to quality of care, access to care, and patient satisfaction (NCQA, 2011b). The Joint Commission (2012a) requires health care organizations to determine how well an organization meets patient needs and expectations. Organizations are using outcomes such as patient satisfaction as a basis to redesign how to manage and deliver care to improve quality.

Patient Satisfaction. Almost every major health care organization measures certain aspects of patient satisfaction. The Hospital Consumer Assessment of Healthcare Providers and Systems (HCAHPS) is a standardized survey developed to measure patient perceptions of their hospital experience (HCAHPS, 2012). HCAHPS was developed by the Centers for Medicare and Medicaid Services and the Agency for Healthcare Research and Quality (AHRQ) as a way for hospitals to collect and report data publicly for comparison purposes. The survey has 27 questions that ask patients to respond about communication with nurses and health care providers, responsiveness of hospital staff, pain management, communication about medications, discharge planning, cleanliness and quietness of the environment, overall satisfaction, and willingness to recommend the hospital (HCAHPS, 2012).

The Picker Institute (2012) identified eight dimensions of **patient-centered care** (Box 3-6) that most affect patients' experiences with health care. The eight dimensions cover much of the scope of nursing practice. This is no surprise because nurses are involved in almost every aspect of a patient's care in a hospital. When you look closely, you see that most of the dimensions reflected in patient satisfaction apply to almost any health care setting.

The Picker Institute surveys patient satisfaction in all eight dimensions. The survey looks globally at patient perceptions of care in an attempt to understand how all hospital departments influence patient satisfaction. Like other companies that distribute patient satisfaction surveys, the Picker Institute mails surveys to patients. Staff involved in patient care receive the satisfaction scores as feedback regarding their success in meeting patient expectations. It is the responsibility of staff to identify the unique issues that influence patient satisfaction for their area. For example, nurses working on an oncology unit have different patient satisfaction issues concerning physical comfort than nurses caring for new mothers. Patient satisfaction findings become the basis for many quality improvement studies.

It is important to identify patient expectations. The eight dimensions of care provide a useful guide. By learning early what a patient expects with regard to information, comfort, and availability of family and friends, you plan better patient care. When do you ask about a patient's expectations? It becomes a routine question when the patient first enters a health care setting, while care continues, and when a patient is ultimately discharged from your care. Patient expectations are an important measure of the evaluation of nursing care.

Magnet Recognition Program. The American Nurses Credentialing Center (ANCC) established the Magnet Recognition Program to recognize health care organizations that achieve excellence in nursing practice (ANCC, 2012b). Health care organizations that decide to apply for Magnet status must demonstrate quality patient care, nursing excellence,

BOX 3-6 PRINCIPLES OF PATIENT-CENTERED CARE

RESPECT FOR PATIENTS' VALUES, PREFERENCES, AND EXPRESSED NEEDS
- Patients expect you to treat them with dignity and respect.
- Patients want you to inform and involve them in decisions about their care.
- Patients' perceptions of needs should not be completely different from those identified by a care provider.
- A setting that respects the patient focuses on quality of life.

COORDINATION AND INTEGRATION OF CARE
- A competent and caring staff reduces patients' feelings of powerlessness.
- Patients look for someone to be in charge of care and communicate clearly with other health team members.
- Patients look to have services and procedures well-coordinated.
- Patients need to know at all times whom to call for help.

INFORMATION COMMUNICATION AND EDUCATION
- Patients expect to receive accurate and timely information about their clinical status, progress, or prognosis.
- Patients and families need to be informed of major changes in therapies or status.
- Patients need tests and procedures explained clearly in language they understand.
- Patients and family members want to know how to manage their own care.

PHYSICAL COMFORT
- Physical care that comforts patients is one of the most elemental services that caregivers provide.
- Nurses need to respond in a timely and effective way to any request for pain medication, to explain the extent of pain that patients can expect, and to offer alternatives for pain management.
- Patients expect privacy and to have their cultural values respected.
- Patients often need help to complete activities of daily living.
- The health care setting environment needs to be clean and comfortable.

EMOTIONAL SUPPORT AND ALLEVIATION OF FEAR AND ANXIETY
- Patients look to care providers to help reduce anxiety and concerns about health status, medical treatment, and prognosis of illness.
- Patients need to understand the impact that illness will have on their ability to care for themselves and their family.
- Patients worry about their ability to pay for their medical care. Are there staff members who will help with those concerns?

INVOLVEMENT OF FAMILY AND FRIENDS
- Care providers need to recognize, respect, and meet the needs of patients' family and friends.
- Patients have the right to determine if they want family members involved in decisions about their care.
- Patients expect you to properly inform family or friends who will provide physical support and care after discharge.

CONTINUITY AND TRANSITION
- Patients want information about which medications to take, dietary or treatment plans to follow, and danger signals for which to look after hospitalization or treatment.
- Patients expect to have their continuing health care needs met after discharge with well-coordinated services.
- Patients and family members expect access to any necessary health care resources (e.g., social, physical, financial) after discharge.

ACCESS TO CARE
- Patients want to get to hospitals, clinics, and physicians' offices easily and without hassle.
- Patients need to be able to find transportation when going to different health care settings.
- Patients want to schedule appointments at convenient times without difficulty.
- Patients want to be able to see a specialist when a referral is made.
- Patients expect to receive clear instructions on how to get referrals to other health care providers.

Data from Picker Institute: *Principles of patient-centered care,* 2012, http://pickerinstitute.org/about/picker-principles/. Accessed August 12, 2012.

and innovations in professional practice. The professional work environment must allow nurses to practice with a sense of empowerment and autonomy to deliver quality nursing care (Box 3-7). The newly developed Magnet model has five components that are affected by global issues that are challenging nursing today (ANCC, 2012a). The five components are Transformational Leadership; Structural Empowerment; Exemplary Professional Practice; New Knowledge, Innovation, and Improvements; and Empirical Quality Outcomes. Institutions achieve Magnet status by presenting evidence showing achievement of the 14 "Forces of Magnetism" (Box 3-8). Magnet status requires nurses to collect data on specific nursing-sensitive quality indicators or outcomes and compare their outcomes against a national, state, or regional database to demonstrate quality of care.

Nursing-Sensitive Outcomes. Nursing-sensitive outcomes are changes in patients' symptom experiences, functional status, safety, psychological distress, and costs as a result of nursing interventions. Nurses assume accountability and responsibility for the consequences of these outcomes. Examples include pressure ulcers, restraint prevalence, and falls. The American Nurses Association developed the National Database of Nursing Quality Indicators (NDNQI) (Box 3-9) to measure and evaluate nursing-sensitive outcomes with the purpose of improving patient safety and quality care (NDNQI, 2012). The NDNQI reports quarterly results on nursing outcomes at the nursing unit level. This provides a database for individual hospitals to compare their performance against nursing performance nationally (NDNQI, 2012).

BOX 3-7 EVIDENCE-BASED PRACTICE

PICO Question: Do nurses who work in Magnet hospitals experience a healthier work environment compared to nurses who work in non-Magnet hospitals?

SUMMARY OF EVIDENCE

Healthy work environments are a component of Magnet status. A healthy work environment has the characteristics of: nurse-physician collaboration, clinically competent peers, support for education, clinical autonomy, use of evidence-based practice, perception of adequate staffing, and supportive nurse manager-staff relationships (Kramer, Macquire, and Brewer, 2011). The literature supports that healthy work environments in Magnet hospitals contribute to higher job satisfaction and retention (Gokenbach and Drenkard, 2011; Ritter, 2011). Magnet hospitals were found to have nurses on the units with more years of experience and tenure on the nursing units (Kramer, Macquire, and Brewer, 2011). These experienced nurses can be a positive resource for newly hired nurses. An empowered, engaged workforce positively impacts patient satisfaction scores (Gokenbach and Drenkard, 2011). Research also found that nurses with Bachelor of Science in Nursing (BSN) degrees reported the more collegial and collaborative relationships with physicians (Kramer et al., 2011). The use of evidence-based practice strategies in Magnet hospitals contributes to improvement in patient outcomes in the nursing-sensitive indicators of falls, pressure ulcers, and use of restraints (Gokenbach and Drenkard, 2011).

APPLICATION TO NURSING PRACTICE

- Investigate returning to school for a BSN if not currently educated at this level (Kramer et al., 2011).
- Develop a relationship with an experienced nurse who can mentor you as you develop your professional career (Kramer et al., 2011).
- Become involved in unit activities related to shared governance and evidence-based practice (Gokenbach and Drenkard, 2011).

BOX 3-8 MAGNET MODEL AND FORCES OF MAGNETISM

MAGNET MODEL COMPONENTS	FORCES OF MAGNETISM
Transformational Leadership—A vision for the future and the systems and resources to achieve the vision are created by nursing leaders.	• Quality of Nursing Leadership • Management Style
Structural Empowerment—Structures and processes provide an innovative environment in which staff are developed and empowered and professional practice flourishes.	• Organizational Structure • Personnel Policies and Programs • Community and the Health Organization • Image of Nursing • Professional Development
Exemplary Professional Practice—Establishment of strong professional practice and demonstration of accomplishments of the practice	• Professional Models of Care • Consultation and Resources • Autonomy • Nurses as Teachers • Interdisciplinary Relationships
New Knowledge, Innovations, and Improvements—Contributions to the profession in the form of new models of care, use of existing knowledge, generation of new knowledge, and contributions to the science of nursing	• Quality Improvement
Empirical Quality Outcomes—Focus on structure and processes and demonstration of positive clinical, workforce, patient, and organizational outcomes	• Quality of Care

Modified from American Nurses Credentialing Center: *Magnet Recognition Program Model,* 2012, http://www.nursecredentialing.org/Magnet/ProgramOverview/New-Magnet-Model. Accessed August 18, 2012.

Nurses assume responsibility for a variety of outcomes that include individuals, family caregivers, the family, and the community. A research-based outcomes classification system, the Nursing Outcomes Classification (NOC), helps nurses better define and measure the impact of their interventions (Moorhead et al., 2008). NOC emphasizes patient outcomes that nursing interventions affect most, but all health care disciplines are able to use this system.

Because of the importance of nursing-sensitive outcomes, the AHRQ has funded several nursing research studies that looked at the relationship of nurse staffing levels to adverse patient outcomes. These studies found that higher levels of staffing by registered nurses (RNs) in hospitals were associated with fewer adverse patient outcomes. These studies also found that increased levels of nurse staffing positively affected nurse satisfaction. Future studies will evaluate the effect of nurse workload on patient safety and the relationship between nurses' working conditions and patient outcomes. Other studies are investigating how nurses' working conditions affect medication safety. Measuring and monitoring nursing-sensitive outcomes helps you improve your patients' outcomes. Nurses and health care facilities use nursing-sensitive

BOX 3-9 NDNQI NURSING QUALITY INDICATORS

- Patient falls
- Patient falls with injury
- Pressure ulcers—Community acquired, hospital acquired, unit acquired
- Staff mix
- Nursing hours per patient day
- RN surveys on job satisfaction and practice environment scale
- RN education and certification
- Pediatric pain assessment cycle
- Pediatric IV infiltration rate
- Psychiatric patient assault rate
- Restraint prevalence
- Nurse turnover
- Hospital-acquired infections of ventilator-associated pneumonia, central line–associated bloodstream infection, catheter-associated urinary tract infection

Data from National Database of Nursing Quality Indicators: *NDNQI: transforming data into quality care,* 2012, http://www.nursingquality.org. Accessed August 12, 2012.
IV, Intravenous; *RN,* registered nurse.

outcomes to improve nurses' workloads, enhance patient safety, and develop sensible policies related to nursing practice and health care.

Technology in Health Care

Technological advances continually influence health care organizations and change how nurses provide evidence-based care to patients (Simpson, 2012). Sophisticated equipment such as electronic IV infusion devices, cardiac telemetry equipment (devices that monitor a patient's heart rate wherever the patient is on a nursing unit), and electronic medical records are just a few examples changing the way providers deliver health care. In many ways technological systems make your work easier, but they do not replace your judgment. For example, when managing an IV infusion pump, it is your responsibility to monitor the device to be sure that it infuses on time and without complications. An electronic infusion device provides a constant rate of infusion, but you must be sure to calculate the rate correctly. The device sets off an alarm if the infusion slows, making it important for you to respond to the alarm and troubleshoot the problem. Technology does not replace a nurse's astute, critical eye and clinical judgment.

Telemedicine or telehealth is an emerging technology that is used to improve patient outcomes. In telemedicine electronic medical records and video teleconferencing are used by health care providers and nurses to provide care from a remote location (Mullen-Fortino et al., 2012). Vital signs and other types of physiological assessment findings are transmitted to monitor patient status (Radhakrishanan and Jacelon, 2012). Patient and family education and building the patient's self-care abilities are other interventions used in telehealth or telemedicine. Telehealth has been found to be an effective tool in promoting self-care in patients with heart failure (Radhakrishanan and Jacelon, 2012) and improved survival rates in patients in ICUs (Mullen-Fortino et al., 2012).

Computerized clinical information systems are replacing the traditional printed medical record. A comprehensive electronic record of a patient's medical problems, treatment, diagnostic procedures, and nursing care offers a rich source of information to health care providers. The health information system collects and organizes data, providing valuable information for research and quality improvement activities. For example, a nurse manager who wishes to track a nursing staff's progress in timely assessment of patients' pain is able to examine a database to review documented patient assessments and the time they occurred.

Documenting in a clinical information system minimizes free text entries and allows you to enter information quickly on specially designed flow sheets, pop-up screens, and nursing care plans. The computer displays important data in a way that allows you to follow your patient's progress easily. When using an electronic system, you need to document clinical information about a patient accurately and completely in a timely manner. All members of the health care team are able to gain access to the electronic record; thus you need to complete your documentation as soon as possible (see Chapter 10).

Globalization of Health Care

Globalization, the increasing interconnection of world economy, culture, and technology, is reshaping the health care delivery system (Oulton, 2012). Advances in communication, primarily through the Internet, allow nurses, patients, and other health care providers to talk with others worldwide about health care issues. Improved communication, easier air travel, and easing of trade restrictions are making it easier for people to engage in "health tourism." Health tourism is the travel to other nations to seek health care.

Many problems affect the health status of people around the world. For example, poverty is still deadlier than any disease and is the most frequently cited reason for death in the world today. It increases the disparities in health care services among **vulnerable populations** (Finkelman and Kenner, 2010). Nations and communities that experience poverty have limited access to vaccines, clean water, and standard medical care. The growth of urbanization also affects world health. As cities become more densely populated, problems with pollution, noise, crowding, inadequate water, improper waste disposal, and other environmental hazards become more apparent. Children, women, and older adults are vulnerable populations most threatened by poverty and urbanization. As a nurse you work toward improving the health of all populations. Although globalization of trade, travel, and culture improves the availability of health care services, the spread of communicable diseases such as tuberculosis and severe acute respiratory syndrome (SARS) has become more common. The results of global environmental changes and disasters also affect health. Changes in climate and natural disasters threaten food supplies and often allow infectious diseases to spread more rapidly.

As a nurse you must understand how worldwide communication and globalization of health care affect your practice. Health care consumers demand quality and service and have become more knowledgeable. They often search the Internet about their health concerns and medical conditions. They also use the Internet to select their health care providers. As a result of globalization, it is necessary for physicians and health care providers to make their services more accessible. Because of advances in communication, nurses and other health care providers practice across state and national boundaries. Furthermore, currently there is a nursing shortage in health care institutions across the United States. In an effort to provide high-quality care, health care institutions are recruiting nurses from around the world to work in the United States. This trend is expected to continue to fill vacant nursing positions (Buerhaus et al., 2009). The migration of nurses from their home countries to other countries often leaves the home country with insufficient resources to meet their own health needs (Nichols, Davis, and Richardson, 2010). The hiring of nurses from other nations has required American hospitals to better understand and work with nurses from different cultures and with different needs.

The International Council of Nurses (ICN), based in Switzerland, represents nursing worldwide. The purpose of the ICN is to advance professional nursing worldwide (ICN, 2011). ICN goals are focused on bringing nurses together, advancing nurses and the nursing profession, and influencing health policy worldwide (ICN, 2011). The unique focus of nursing on caring helps nurses address the issues presented by globalization. You help overcome these issues by working with other nurses to improve nursing education throughout the world, retaining nurses and recruiting people to be nurses, and being advocates for changes that will improve the delivery of health care.

THE FUTURE OF HEALTH CARE

Change threatens many of us, but it also opens opportunities for improvement. The ultimate issue in designing and delivering health care is the health and welfare of our population. Health care in the United States and around the world is not perfect. Many patients do not receive continuity of care when they see multiple health care providers. Many are uninsured or underinsured and unable to gain access to necessary services. However, health care organizations are striving to become better prepared to deal with the challenges in health care. Many are changing how they provide their services, reducing unnecessary costs, improving access to care, and trying to provide high-quality patient care. Finding the solutions necessary to improve the quality of health care depends on the active participation of nursing and the nursing community.

KEY POINTS

- Increasing costs and decreasing reimbursement are driving changes in health care, forcing health care institutions to deliver care more efficiently without sacrificing quality.
- In a managed care system the provider of care receives a predetermined capitated payment, regardless of services used by a patient.
- Levels of health care describe the scope of services and settings in which health care is offered to patients in all stages of health and illness.
- Occupational health nursing includes reducing exposure to environmental hazards, health education, and helping workers return to work safely.
- Successful community-based health programs involve building relationships with the community and incorporating cultural and environmental factors.
- Rehabilitation allows an individual to return to a level of normal or near-normal function after a physical or mental illness, injury, or chemical dependency.
- Nurse-managed clinics offer primary care delivered by advanced practice nurses with a focus on helping patients assume more responsibility for their health.
- Home care agencies provide almost every type of health care service, with an emphasis on patient and family independence.
- Discharge planning with coordination of services begins at admission to a health care facility and helps in the transition of a patient's care from one environment to another.
- Health care organizations are evaluated on the basis of outcomes such as prevention of complications, patients' functional outcomes, and patient satisfaction.
- Consumers of health care should be guaranteed that services are provided by competent health care professionals.
- Nurses need to remain knowledgeable and proactive about issues in the health care delivery system to provide quality patient care and positively affect health.

CLINICAL DECISION-MAKING EXERCISES

One day during gym class, Amy Sue starts to have more breathing problems than usual. Corrine, the school nurse, decides that Amy Sue needs to see her physician today. Corrine calls and notifies Anne, Amy Sue's mother, of the change in Amy Sue's health and the need for medical treatment.

1. On the phone Anne states, "We are now part of an accountable care organization. I am not sure what this means." How should Corrine explain an accountable care organization to Amy Sue's mother?

Anne's father Tony, age 72, came to the emergency department because he fell at the grocery store and was hospitalized for repair of his fractured left wrist. Tony had surgery and a cast applied to his left wrist. Tony is a widower who lives alone.

He has been told he will be discharged from the hospital after 2 days, and he wants to stay with Anne until he is ready to go home.

2. When does discharge planning need to be started for Tony? Explain.
3. Amy Sue's mother tells Corrine that she is very stressed with Amy Sue's and her father's health problems. Identify some health care services that Corrine can share with Anne to help her.

evolve

Answers to Clinical Decision-Making Exercises can be found on the Evolve website.

QSEN ACTIVITY: QUALITY IMPROVEMENT

Corrine's hours at the school have been decreased; thus she now leaves 2 hours before school is dismissed for the day. Since this change in hours started, more incidences of students getting the wrong medication have occurred.

Using your knowledge of quality improvement, explain how you would approach this problem.

evolve

Answers to QSEN Activities can be found on the Evolve website.

REVIEW QUESTIONS

1. Which health care activity is an example of preventive care?
   1. A patient visits the emergency department following a fall at home.
   2. The home care nurse visits the patient twice a week for wound care.
   3. An older couple visits their health care provider for their annual influenza vaccine.
   4. A patient makes an appointment for routine screening mammography.
2. Which of the following is an activity of patient-centered care focused on information communication and education?
   1. The nurse explains to the patient and family the surgical procedure and what to expect before and after surgery.
   2. The nurse provides privacy to the patient and family as they are talking with the health care provider about the treatment plan.
   3. The nurse sits and talks with the patient who is expressing fear about the diagnosis of cancer.
   4. The nurse responds promptly and brings the patient pain medication within 10 minutes of the patient's request.
3. Which of the following are true statements about Magnet recognition for hospitals? (Select all that apply.)
   1. The Magnet model is comprised of eight interrelated concepts focused on leadership competencies.
   2. Nurses within Magnet facilities collect data on nurse-sensitive outcomes.
   3. The work environment promotes a sense of empowerment and autonomy of nurses.
   4. Magnet recognition is a designation for hospitals that are able to maintain a low registered nurse (RN) vacancy rate.
4. Which of the following are examples of primary care health services? (Select all that apply.)
   1. Setting an appointment with the nurse practitioner after having pregnancy confirmed
   2. Outpatient surgery for repair of inguinal hernia
   3. Attending cardiac rehabilitation classes at the local hospital
   4. Attending exercise classes weekly at the local health fitness center
   5. Bringing in the newborn for well-baby visits
5. Which statement made by the patient about patient-centered medical homes shows the need for further teaching?
   1. "My doctor told me that participating in the patient-centered medical home will improve the coordination of all my specialists."
   2. "I will need to stay in the patient-centered medical home while I am getting my treatment for my leg infection."
   3. "My primary care doctor will coordinate all the care of all the specialists that I see."
   4. "My care seems to be more efficient and effective since I became part of the patient-centered medical home."
6. Which of the following people is most likely to benefit from participation in respite care?
   1. Mr. Wilson, who was discharged last week with repair of a fractured hip from a fall
   2. Mrs. Allen, who is the caregiver for her husband with Alzheimer's disease
   3. Mrs. Bradley, who is the mother of an 8-year-old child with chronic asthma
   4. Mr. Hilliard, who has diabetes mellitus and a left-heel pressure ulcer
7. Which of the following are examples of nursing-sensitive quality indicators or outcomes? (Select all that apply.)
   1. Nurse turnover rate
   2. Central line–associated bloodstream infections
   3. Pressure ulcers
   4. Influenza cases
   5. Patient falls with injury
   6. Postoperative respiratory infections
8. A patient is receiving health care by a health care provider using a traditional fee-for-service plan. Payment for the health care provider was computed after the patient

received services. Which type of health care plan does the patient have?

1. Health maintenance organization (HMO)
2. Preferred provider organization (PPO)
3. Private insurance
4. Medicaid

9. A patient asks you about Medicare coverage of home health nurse visits. To help explain this benefit, you provide the patient with an information handout on which Medicare part?
   1. Part A
   2. Part B
   3. Part C
   4. Part D

10. A nurse working in tertiary care would work in which of the following settings?
    1. Hospice unit
    2. Intensive care unit
    3. Occupational health clinic
    4. Cardiac rehabilitation center

evolve

Rationales for Review Questions can be found on the Evolve website.

1. 3; **2.** 1; **3.** 2, 3; **4.** 1, 4, 5; **5.** 2; **6.** 2; **7.** 1, 2, 3, 5; **8.** 3; **9.** 1; **10.** 2.

REFERENCES

Adashi EY, et al: Health care reform and primary care—the growing importance of the community health center, *N Engl J Med* 362(22):2047, 2010.

American Nurses Credentialing Center (ANCC): *Magnet Recognition Program Model*, 2012a, http://www.nursecredentialing.org/Magnet/ProgramOverview/New-Magnet-Model. Accessed August 18, 2012.

American Nurses Credentialing Center (ANCC): *Overview of ANCC Magnet recognition program*, 2012b, http://ancc.nursecredentialing.org/PromotionalMaterials/products/MAGBRO07V2.pdf. Accessed July 16, 2013.

Bobay KL, et al: Age-related differences in perception of quality of discharge teaching and readiness for hospital discharge, *Geriatr Nurs* 31(3):178, 2010.

Buerhaus PI, et al: The recent surge in nurse employment: causes and implications, *Health Affairs* 28(4):w657, 2009, published online 12 June 2009. DOI:10.1377/hlthaff.28.4.w657.

Burns HK, et al: Building an evidence-based practice infrastructure and culture: a model for rural and community hospitals, *J Nurs Admin* 39(7/8):321, 2009.

Centers for Medicare and Medicaid Services (CMS): *Accountable care organizations (ACOs)*, 2012, http://www.cms.gov/Medicare/Medicare-Fee-for-Service-Payment/ACO/index.html?redirect=/ACO/. Accessed July 16, 2013.

Department of Health and Human Services Centers for Medicare and Medicaid Services (DHHS CMS): *Critical access hospitals*, 2012, http://www.cms.gov/Outreach-and-Education/Medicare-Learning-Network-MLN/MLNProducts/downloads/CritAccessHospfctsht.pdf. Accessed July 2013.

Ebersole P, et al: *Toward healthy aging: human needs and nursing response*, ed 7, St Louis, 2008, Mosby.

Finkelman A, Kenner C: *Professional nursing concepts: competencies for quality leadership*, Sudbury, MA, 2010, Jones & Bartlett.

Gokenbach V, Drenkard K: The outcomes of magnet environments and nursing staff engagement: a case study, *Nurs Clin North Am* 46:89, 2011.

HCAHPS: *HCAHPS fact sheet (CAHPS Hospital Survey)*, 2012, http://www.hcahpsonline.org/facts.aspx. Accessed July 17, 2013.

Institute of Medicine (IOM): *Crossing the quality chasm: a new health system for the 21st century*, Washington, DC, 2001, National Academies Press.

Institute of Medicine (IOM): *Health professions education: a bridge to quality*, Washington, DC, 2003, National Academies Press.

International Council of Nurses (ICN): *Our mission*, 2011, http://www.icn.ch/about-icn/icns-mission/. Accessed July 17, 2013.

isixsigma: *Value stream mapping*, 2012a, http://www.isixsigma.com/dictionary/value-stream-mapping. Accessed July 17, 2013.

isixsigma: *What is Six Sigma?* 2012b, http://www.isixsigma.com/sixsigma/six_sigma.asp. Accessed July 17, 2013.

Klauber M, Wright B: *AARP Public Policy Institute: the 1987 Nursing Home Reform Act*, 2001, http://www.aarp.org/home-garden/livable-communities/info-2001/the_1987_nursing_home_reform_act.html. Accessed November 23, 2013.

Knickman JR, Kovner AR: Overview: the state of health care delivery in the United States. In Kovner AR, Knickman JR, editors: *Health care delivery in the United States*, ed 9, New York, 2009, Springer.

Kovner, AR, Knickman JR: *Jonas and Kovner's health care delivery in the United States*, ed 10, New York, 2011, Springer.

Kramer M, Macquire P, Brewer BB: Clinical nurses in Magnet hospitals confirm productive, healthy unit work environments, *J Nurs Manage* 19:5, 2011.

McDaniel G: *Integrated delivery network (IDN)*, 2011, http://www.glgresearch.com/Dictionary/HC-Integrated-Delivery-Network-(IDN).html. Accessed July 17, 2013.

Meiner SE: *Gerontologic nursing*, ed 4, St Louis, 2011, Mosby.

Melnyk BM, Fineout-Overholt E: *Evidence-based practice in nursing and healthcare: a guide to best practice*, ed 2, Philadelphia, 2010, Lippincott Williams & Wilkins.

Moorhead S, et al: *Nursing outcomes classification (NOC)*, ed 4, St Louis, 2008, Mosby.

Mullen-Fortino M, et al: Bedside nurses' perceptions of intensive care unit telemedicine, *Am J Crit Care* 21(1):24, 2012.

National Center for Assisted Living (NCAL): *Assisted living facility profile 2009*, 2012, http://www.ahcancal.org/ncal/resources/Pages/ALFacilityProfile.aspx. Accessed July 17, 2013.

National Committee for Quality Assurance (NCQA): *NCQA patient-centered medical home 2011*, 2011a, http://www.ncqa.org/

LinkClick.aspx?fileticket=ycS4coFOGnw%3d&tabid=631. Accessed July 17, 2013.

National Committee for Quality Assurance (NCQA): *What is HEDIS?* 2011b, http://www.ncqa.org/tabid/187/Default.aspx. Accessed July 17, 2013.

National Conference of State Legislatures: *Key provisions that take effect immediately*, 2010, http://www.ncsl.org/documents/health/factsheet_keyprov.pdf. Accessed November 21, 2013.

National Database of Nursing Quality Indicators (NDNQI): *NDNQI: transforming data into quality care*, 2012, http://www.nursingquality.org. Accessed July 17, 2013.

National Priorities Partnership: *Overview*, 2012, http://www.qualityforum.org/Topics/Overview.aspx. Accessed July 17, 2013.

Nichols BL, Davis CR, Richardson DR: An integrative review of global nursing workforce issues, *Annu Rev Nurs Res* 28:113, 2010.

Oulton J: Nursing in the international community: a broader view of nursing issues. In Mason DJ, et al, editors: *Policy and politics in nursing and health care*, ed 6, St Louis, 2012, Saunders.

Pew Health Professions Commission, The Fourth Report of the Pew Health Professions Commission: *Recreating health professional practice for a new century*, 1998, The Commission.

Picker Institute: *Principles of patient-centered care*, 2012, http://pickerinstitute.org/about/picker-principles. Accessed July 17, 2013.

Radhakrishanan K, Jacelon C: Impact of telehealth on patient self-management of heart failure: a review of the literature, *J Cardiovasc Nurs* 27(1):33, 2012.

Ritter D: The relationship between healthy work environments and retention of nurses in a hospital setting, *J Nurs Manage* 19:27, 2011.

Sackett DL, et al: *Evidence-based medicine: how to practice and teach EBM*, London, 2000, Churchill Livingstone.

Simpson RL: Technology enables value-based nursing care, *Nurse Admin Q* 36(1):85, 2012.

Singleton KA: Lead, follow, and get in the way: the medical-surgical nurse's role in health care reform, *Medsurg Nurs* 19(1):5, 2010.

Sorrentino SA, Remmert LN: *Mosby's textbook for nursing assistants*, ed 8, St Louis, 2012, Mosby.

Stanhope M, Lancaster J: *Public health nursing: population-centered health care in the community*, ed 8, St Louis, 2012, Mosby.

Sultz HA, Young KM: *Health care USA: understanding its organization and delivery*, ed 7, Sudbury, Mass, 2011, Jones & Bartlett Learning.

The Joint Commission (TJC): *2012 Comprehensive accreditation manual for hospitals*, Oakbrook Terrace, Ill, 2012a, The Commission.

The Joint Commission (TJC): *Facts about The Joint Commission*, 2012b, http://www.jointcommission.org/about_us/fact_sheets.aspx. Accessed July 17, 2013.

CHAPTER

4

Community-Based Nursing Practice

evolve WEBSITE

http://evolve.elsevier.com/Potter/essentials

- Crossword Puzzle
- Audio Glossary

OBJECTIVES

- Explain the relationship between public and community health nursing.
- Differentiate community health nursing from community-based nursing.
- Describe the role of the community health nurse.
- Discuss the role of the nurse in community-based practice.
- Explain the characteristics of patients from selected vulnerable populations that influence a nurse's approach to care.
- Describe selected competencies important for success in community-based nursing practice.
- Describe elements of a community assessment.

KEY TERMS

community-based nursing, p. 52
community health nursing, p. 51
incidence rate, p. 50
population, p. 51
public health nursing, p. 51
vulnerable populations, p. 53

CASE STUDY *Bosnian Community*

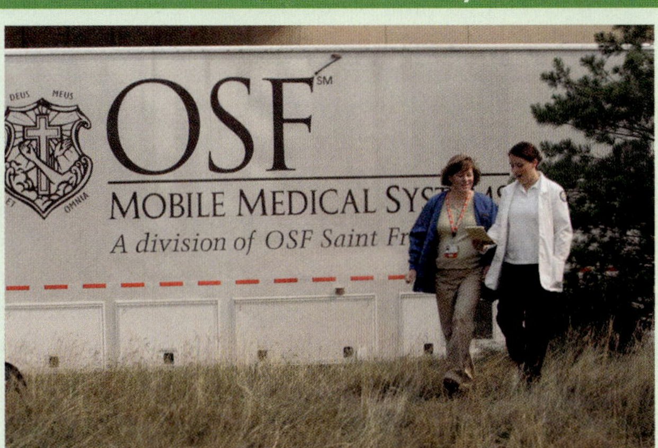

Kim Callahan is a student in a community health nursing course. She is working in a community nursing service within a large city. The majority of patients in this agency are Bosnian immigrants. A major care initiative in the agency is to provide well-child examinations and immunizations to prepare the children to enter the public school system.

In addition, Kim and her classmates conduct an assessment of the community health care needs and health care practices. This is a close community facing many challenges. Although chronic disease is absent, there is a lack of general preventive health care practices compounded by language barriers, including routine immunizations; dental health; well-baby examinations; well-women examinations; and basic screenings for diabetes, hypertension, and cholesterol.

Community-based care focuses on health promotion, disease prevention, and restorative care. Because patients stay in acute care settings for a short time, there is a growing need to organize health care delivery services where people live, work, socialize, and learn. One way to achieve this goal is through a community-based health care model. Community-based health care is a collaborative, evidence-based model designed to meet the health care needs of a community (Olson et al., 2011). A healthy community includes elements that maintain a high quality of life and productivity. For example, safety and access to health care services are elements that enable people to function productively in their community (USDHHS, 2011). As community health care partnerships develop, nursing is in a strategic position to play an important role in health care delivery and improve the health of the community.

The focus of health promotion and disease prevention is essential to the holistic practice of professional nursing. Throughout the history of nursing, many nurses have established and met the public health needs of their patients and their families. Within community health settings nurses are leaders in assessing, planning, implementing, and evaluating the types of public and community health services their communities need. Community health nursing and community-based nursing (see Chapter 3) are components or parts of health care delivery necessary to improve the health of the general public.

COMMUNITY-BASED HEALTH CARE

Community-based health care is a model of care that reaches everyone in the community, including the poor and underinsured. It focuses on primary prevention rather than acute care and provides knowledge about health and health promotion. It occurs outside traditional health care institutions such as hospitals and nursing homes. Community-based health care provides services for acute and chronic conditions to individuals and families within the community (Stanhope and Lancaster, 2014).

Today there are many challenges in community-based health. Social lifestyles, political policy, and economic ambitions have all influenced some of the major public health problems, including the following: lack of health care insurance, chronic illnesses such as diabetes and heart disease, and increases in sexually transmitted infections (USDHHS, 2011). In addition, underimmunization of infants and children and the appearance of pandemics or life-threatening diseases (e.g., swine flu, human immunodeficiency virus [HIV], and other emerging infections) continue to pose threats to populations and communities. More than ever before, the health care system needs a commitment to reform and bring attention to the health care needs of all communities.

Achieving Healthy Populations and Communities

The USDHHS Public Health Service designed a program to improve the overall health status of people living in this country (see Chapter 2). The *Healthy People Initiative* was first created to establish ongoing health care goals (Figure 4-1). The overall goals of *Healthy People 2020* are to increase the life expectancy and quality of life and eliminate health disparities through an improved delivery of health care services (USDHHS, 2011).

Improved delivery of health care occurs through the assessment of the health care needs of individuals, families, or members of the community; development and implementation of public health policies; and improved access to care. Assessment includes systematic data collection about the population, monitoring the health status of the population, and accessing information about the community (Stanhope and Lancaster, 2014). A systematic community assessment leads to community health promotion programs such as exercise programs for school-age children to reduce the risks for childhood obesity, nutrition education for expectant mothers, and smoking cessation for adolescents. In addition, the assessment helps to gather information on **incidence rates** such as identifying and reporting of new infections, determining adolescent pregnancy rates, and reporting the number of motor vehicle collisions by teenage drivers.

Community health professionals are involved in public policy development and implementation designed to improve the health of the community. Research-based findings help to design and implement health-related policies for the community. For example, data identify an increased incidence in motor vehicle collision fatalities when the driver is between 16 and 18 years old and driving after midnight. Community health professionals work with the legislature to develop driving restrictions for new teenage drivers to reduce motor vehicle fatalities.

Improved access to care ensures that essential community-wide health services are available and accessible to the total community (Stanhope and Lancaster, 2014). Examples include prenatal care coordination and well-baby immunization programs for the uninsured. Population-based public health programs focus on disease prevention, health protection, and health promotion. This focus provides the foundation for health care services at all levels (see Chapter 3).

The five-level health services pyramid is an example of how to provide community-based services within the existing health care services in a community (see Figure 3-1, Chapter 3). For example, a rural community has a hospital to meet the acute care needs of its patients. However, during a community assessment the nurse notices that there are few services to meet the needs of expectant mothers, reduce teenage smoking, or provide nutritional support for older adults. Community-based programs that provide these services improve the health of the specific populations and that of the population of the community. When the lower-level services are accessible and effective, there is a greater likelihood that the higher tiers will contribute to the total health of the community (Frieden, 2010). For example, when mosquito control is inadequate, it becomes more difficult to enforce health promotion efforts and prevent mosquito-borne diseases. On the other hand, when a community has the resources for providing childhood immunizations, primary preventive care

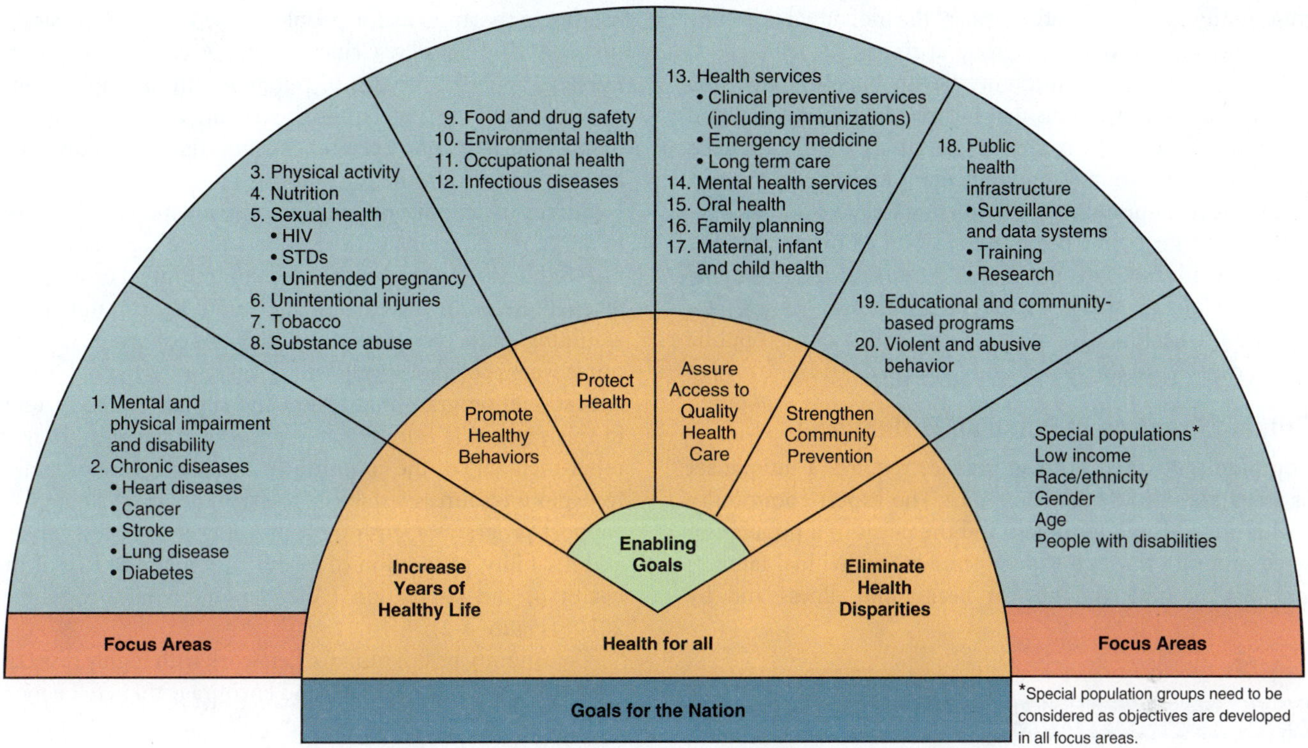

FIGURE 4-1 *Healthy People 2020:* Healthy people in healthy communities. (From Allender JA, Walton Spradley B: *Community health nursing: promoting and protecting the public's health,* ed 7, Philadelphia, 2010, Lippincott.)

services are able to focus on higher-tier services such as child developmental problems and child safety.

The principles of public health practice focus on achieving a healthy environment in which all individuals can live. These principles apply to individuals, families, and the communities in which they live. Nursing plays a role in all levels of the health services pyramid. By using public health principles, the nurse is able to better understand the types of environments in which patients live and the types of interventions necessary to help keep them healthy.

PUBLIC HEALTH NURSING

The terms *community health nursing* and *public health nursing* are frequently used interchangeably. A **public health nursing** focus requires understanding the needs of a **population,** or a collection of individuals who have in common one or more personal or environmental characteristics (Stanhope and Lancaster, 2014). Examples of populations include high-risk infants, older adults, and a cultural group such as Native Americans.

A public health nurse understands factors that influence health promotion and health maintenance of populations, trends and patterns influencing the incidence of disease within these populations, environmental factors contributing to health and illness, and the political processes used to affect public policy. For example, the public health nurse uses data regarding car accidents involving adolescents' use of cell phones or texting while driving to lobby for support of a policy ban on texting while driving.

Public health nursing requires preparation at the basic entry level, and sometimes a public health nurse requires a baccalaureate degree in nursing with supervised clinical practice in public health nursing. A specialist in public health is prepared at the graduate level with a focus in public health sciences (ANA, 2013).

COMMUNITY HEALTH NURSING

Community health nursing is nursing care provided in the community, with the primary focus on the health care of individuals, families, and groups in the community. The goal is to preserve, protect, promote, or maintain health (Stanhope and Lancaster, 2014). The emphasis is on improving the quality of health and life within that community. In addition, the community health nurse provides direct care services to subpopulations within that community. These subpopulations are often a clinical focus in which the nurse has gained expertise. For example, a case manager follows older adults recovering from stroke and sees the need for community rehabilitation services, or a nurse practitioner gives immunizations to patients with the objective of managing communicable disease within the community. By focusing on subpopulations, the community health nurse cares for the community as a whole and considers the individual or family to be only one member of a group at risk.

Competence as a community health nurse requires the ability to use interventions that include the broad social and political context of the community (Stanhope and Lancaster, 2014). The educational requirements for entry-level nurses practicing in community health nursing roles are not as clear-cut as those for public health nurses. Not all hiring agencies require an advanced degree. However, nurses with a graduate degree in nursing who practice in community settings are community health nurse specialists, regardless of their public health experience (Stanhope and Lancaster, 2014).

Nursing Practice in Community Health

Community-focused nursing practice requires a unique set of skills and knowledge (Box 4-1). The expert community health nurse comes to understand the needs of a population or community through experiences with individual families and clinical understanding of health and illness and by creating opportunities for people to live healthier physically, mentally, and socially. Critical thinking is essential for the nurse to apply knowledge of public health principles, community health nursing, family theory, and communication to identify the best approaches to collaborating with individuals and families within the population.

Successful community health nursing practice involves building relationships with members of the community and responding to changes within the community. For example, when there is an increase in the number of grandparents assuming child care responsibilities, the community health nurse works collaboratively with local schools to establish an educational program that assists and supports grandparents in this caregiving role. The nurse works in partnership with other members of the community and health care providers to explore resources; establish goals; and plan, evaluate, and support programs focusing on prevention of illness, injury, and disability, promotion of health, and maintenance of the health of the population (Allender and Walton Spradley, 2010) (Figure 4-2).

Community health nurses often work with highly resistant systems (e.g., welfare system) and encourage them to be more responsive to the needs of a population. Skills of patient advocacy, communicating people's concerns, and designing new systems in cooperation with existing systems help to make community nursing practice effective.

BOX 4-1 SYNTHESIS IN PRACTICE

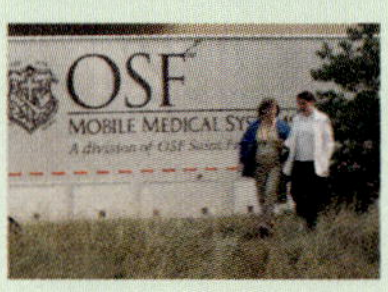

Many members of the Bosnian community are suspicious of the low cost and/or free care of the community agency and doubt that the examinations and results are confidential. One of the priorities of the community agency is to reach out to the community leaders to create an environment of trust and safety, which will hopefully lead to an increased use of the services. Kim is participating in community meetings with her community nurse preceptor. These meetings help explain the role of the community nurses in the delivery of care to the community and reinforce the privacy and confidentiality of the services provided.

Kim and her preceptor meet with community leaders to assess the beliefs and concerns of the community. Together they identify a lack of understanding in the community regarding health care practices in this country. In addition, the community has some misunderstandings and fear of health care services that the community agency and van provide.

Kim recognizes that members of this community came from a war-ravaged country where resources for health promotion were nonexistent. She understands the concerns and lack of understanding about community care and how this affects the use of services. Kim operates under the ethical principle of beneficence and wants to do the most good for the most people in this case. She respects the beliefs held by the community and their current level of health care knowledge.

If she views the community as a patient, Kim focuses her care on the total community. She continually assesses community knowledge and acceptance of the health care services provided. In addition, she identifies community leaders to serve as key people or contacts in educational programs designed to meet the health care needs of the community. These programs will also help to change community misconceptions and fear of the services provided.

COMMUNITY-BASED NURSING

Community-based nursing care takes place in community settings such as the home or a clinic where the focus is

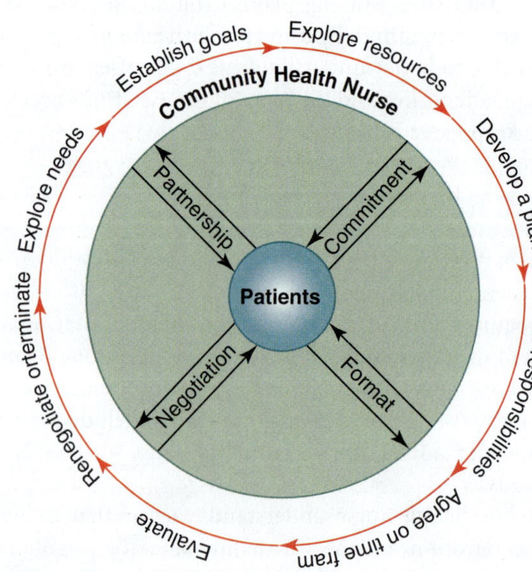

FIGURE 4-2 Nursing practice in community health. (From Allender JA, Walton Spradley B: *Community health nursing: promoting and protecting the public's health,* ed 7, Philadelphia, 2010, Lippincott.)

on the nursing care of the individual or family. It involves the safety needs of individuals and families and enhances their ability for self-care and independent decision making (Stanhope and Lancaster, 2014). A nurse uses critical thinking and decision making when caring for the individual patient and family—assessing health status, selecting nursing interventions, and evaluating outcomes of care. When providing direct care services where patients live, work, and play, it is important to be knowledgeable about the diverse needs of the individual and family and appreciate differences in style and ethnic and cultural practices. Through such knowledge, community-based nursing practice provides a means to partner with community leaders and improve the quality of health and well-being of all members in the community.

Community-based nursing centers are the first level of contact between members of a community and the health care delivery system. Ideally the health care providers are located within easy access to the residents in the community. This approach helps provide needed services and allows for the early detection and treatment of potential complex problems before costly hospital care becomes necessary. In addition, these centers offer direct access to multidisciplinary services such as maternal and child health, adult and adolescent health, sexual and reproductive health, and mental health. Community health centers often care for the most vulnerable populations, including the uninsured and underinsured (Olson et al., 2011).

Community-based nursing recognizes the interaction of the patient and family unit within the community, both of which operate within the sociopolitical system. The patient exists within the larger systems of family, community, and society. The nurse in a community-based practice setting is in the best position to understand the interaction of all of the units while caring for the patients and their families in the community. For example, the nurse works in a home health care setting with a patient who is newly diagnosed with diabetes. She or he works closely with the patient and family to create a comprehensive plan for the patient's health. As the nurse-patient relationship evolves, the nurse begins to understand the patient's habits or lifestyle patterns. She or he learns how these change when the patient is with friends and co-workers. Knowing the community and available resources (e.g., medical supply shops for glucose monitoring supplies and local diabetes association support groups) helps the nurse to provide comprehensive support for the patient's needs.

With the individual and family as patients, the context of community-based nursing is family-centered care within the community. This focus requires the nurse to be knowledgeable about family theory (see Chapter 24); principles of communication (see Chapter 11); and group dynamics and cultural awareness (see Chapter 20). This knowledge helps the nurse partner with patients and families and understand their health care needs. Ultimately the community-based nurse helps patients and their families assume responsibility for their health care decisions.

Vulnerable Populations

In the community setting nurses care for patients from diverse cultures and backgrounds and with various health conditions. However, changes in the health care delivery system have made high-risk groups the community health nurse's principal patients. For example, visiting low-risk mothers and babies is unlikely. Instead the nurse is more likely to make home visits to adolescent mothers or mothers with substance-abuse problems.

Vulnerable populations are groups of patients who are more likely to develop health problems as a result of excess risks, limited access to health care services, and dependency on others for care. Vulnerable populations include individuals living in poverty, the elderly, homeless individuals, people in abusive relationships, people with substance-abuse problems and/or mental illnesses, and new immigrants. Often vulnerable individuals belong to more than one group, with cumulative effects on their health. For example, many homeless individuals suffer from chronic physical conditions, mental illnesses, and substance abuse. These individuals typically have poorer outcomes than patients who have readily available access to resources and health care services.

The special needs of these groups create challenges for nurses in caring for increasingly complex acute and chronic health conditions. A community health nurse needs to determine community needs and appropriate interventions that will be successful in improving a community's level of health. Communication skills and caring practices are critical in identifying and understanding the patients' perceptions of their problems and planning successful health care strategies. Box 4-2 summarizes guidelines to follow when assessing members of vulnerable population groups.

Immigrant Populations. In the United States the immigrant population in 2010 exceeded 40 million (Camarota, 2012), representing a near 25% increase from the 2000 census report. This growth creates multiple health issues and many health care needs, which pose significant legal and health policy issues. For some immigrants access to health care is limited because of legal status; language barriers; and lack of benefits, resources, and transportation. In addition, some immigrant populations have specific health care risks such as for hepatitis B, tuberculosis, and dental problems (Stanhope and Lancaster, 2014). Frequently the immigrant population practices nontraditional healing practices. It is important that a nurse understands how these practices interfere with or complement traditional therapies. It is crucial that the nurse work collaboratively with the health care provider to listen to the patient, explain perceptions, and acknowledge differences. The nurse and health care provider need to work with the patient to recommend and negotiate a treatment plan that is sensitive to the physical, psychological, and safety needs of the patient, family, or community.

Poor and Homeless People. People who live in poverty are more likely to live in hazardous or dangerous environments, work at high-risk jobs, eat less-nutritious diets, and have multiple stressors in their lives (Box 4-3). Patients with

BOX 4-2 GUIDELINES FOR ASSESSING MEMBERS OF VULNERABLE POPULATION GROUPS

SETTING THE STAGE

- Create a comfortable, nonthreatening environment.
- Obtain information about the culture so the nurse has an understanding of their practices, beliefs, and values that affect their health care.
- Understand the meaning of the patient's language and nonverbal behavior to complete a culturally competent assessment (see Chapter 20).
- Be sensitive to the fact that patients often have priorities other than their health care. They include financial, legal, or social issues. Help them with these concerns before beginning a health assessment. If the patient needs financial assistance, consult a social worker. If there are legal issues, provide the patient with a resource. Do not attempt to provide financial or legal advice yourself.

NURSING HISTORY OF AN INDIVIDUAL OR FAMILY

- Because you often have only one opportunity to conduct a nursing history, it is necessary to obtain an organized history of all the essential information needed to help the individual or family during that visit.
- Collect data on a comprehensive form that focuses on the specific needs of the vulnerable population. However, be flexible so as not to overlook important health information. For example, when with an adolescent mother, obtain a nutritional history on both the mother and baby. Be aware of the developmental needs of the adolescent mom and listen to her social needs as well.
- Identify both developmental and health care needs. Remember, the goal is to collect enough information to provide family-centered care.
- Identify any risks to the patient's immune system. This is especially important for vulnerable patients who are homeless and sleep in shelters.

PHYSICAL EXAMINATION AND HOME ASSESSMENT

- Complete as thorough a physical and/or home assessment as possible. However, only collect data that will be important when providing care to the patient and family.
- Be alert for signs of physical or substance abuse (e.g., inadequately clothed to hide bruising, underweight, runny nose).
- When assessing the patient's home, observe: Is there adequate water and plumbing? What is the status of the utilities? Are foods and perishables stored properly? Are there signs of insects or vermin? Is the paint peeling? Are the windows and doors adequate? Are there water stains on the ceiling? Is there evidence of a leaky roof? What is the temperature? Is it comfortable? What does the outside environment look like: Are there vacant houses/lots nearby? Is there a busy intersection? What is the crime level?

Modified from Stanhope M, Lancaster J: *Foundations of nursing in the community: community oriented practice,* ed 4, St Louis, 2014, Mosby.

BOX 4-3 EVIDENCE-BASED PRACTICE

PICO Question: Do community health centers that provide community-centered care produce better patient outcomes compared with centers that do not provide community-centered care?

SUMMARY OF EVIDENCE

The populations of the poor and homeless are increasing, leading to an increase in their health care needs (Goodman et al., 2010; Prohaska et al., 2012). The health care needs of the poor and homeless include chronic illnesses, emerging infections, human immunodeficiency virus (HIV), cancer risks, physical abuse, substance abuse, and mental health disorders (Jacobson, 2011). The newly homeless are at greatest risk for changes in health status because of the struggle between residential instability and changes in their physical and/or mental status.

The homeless adolescent is usually without a nuclear family and has greater health care risks because of immaturity and risky behaviors. The adolescent alone has trouble coping with homelessness. However, newly homeless adolescents frequently maintain their prehomeless relationships. The continuation of these relationships is an important resource to maintain health and healthy practices, especially sexual practices, in this age-group. Females are at greater risk for threats to their physical safety. Males have more risky sexual behaviors and are less likely to use community health care resources (Tsemberis et al., 2012).

Effective community health centers provide a health safety net for the poor and homeless population, such as homeless adolescents (Tsemberis et al., 2012). Many centers provide primary and urgent care services. Within these centers there are resources to determine the health care needs of the community, identify health education needs, and provide child care and parenting classes. Highly successful centers assess for and respect the needs of the target community; provide safe, effective primary and urgent care services; and assist their patients to safe shelters or into transitional housing arrangements (Olson et al., 2011).

APPLICATION TO NURSING PRACTICE

- Promptly identify and assess the newly homeless to provide timely health and social interventions and enhance the chance for improved health status (Tsemberis et al., 2012).
- Obtain an ongoing, comprehensive listing of homeless shelters and transitional housing that is age and gender appropriate and know which resources to use to help a newly homeless person obtain placement in an appropriate residence.
- Provide access to "safe sex" behaviors (e.g., condom use, safe sex education, sexually transmitted infection, and HIV prevention) (Jacobson, 2011).
- Identify existing prehomeless social relationships and help the individual maintain them.
- Work with a patient to identify his or her personal and social resources (Olson et al., 2011; Prohaska et al., 2012).

low income levels not only lack financial resources but also sometimes live in poor environments and face practical problems such as poor or unavailable transportation.

Homeless patients have even fewer resources than the poor. They are usually jobless, do not have the advantage of shelter, and must cope with finding food and a place to sleep at night. Chronic health problems worsen because they do not get nutritious meals and do not have a place to store medications, if they can afford them. In addition, they lack a healthy balance of rest and activity because of walking throughout the day to meet basic needs. For many of these individuals the quickest access to health care is the emergency department to receive treatment for worsening conditions. In the community setting it is important that the nurse help these patients identify available resources, eligibility for assistance, and interventions to improve their health status.

People with Mental Illness. It is important to explore health and socioeconomic problems when caring for patients with mental illnesses such as depression, bipolar disorder, and personality disorders (e.g., schizophrenia, obsessive-compulsive, antisocial). When a patient suffers from a pervasive mental illness, the illness affects many aspects of the patient's life and requires medication therapy, counseling, housing, and vocational assistance. Many patients with pervasive mental illnesses are homeless or have poor housing. Others lack the ability to maintain employment or care for themselves on a daily basis (Prohaska, et al, 2012). In addition, these patients are at greater risk for abuse and assault.

Patients who are mentally ill are no longer routinely hospitalized in long-term psychiatric institutions. Instead the goal is to offer resources within their community. Although comprehensive service networks are in every community, many patients with mental illnesses still go untreated or they are left with fewer and more fragmented services, with little skill in surviving and functioning within the community. Collaboration with multiple community resources is a key to helping people with pervasive mental illnesses receive adequate health care (Allender and Walton Spradley, 2010).

Older Adults. Because people are living longer, there is an increase in the older-adult population. This means that more patients have chronic diseases such as hypertension, cancer, and substance abuse. There is a greater demand for health care services provided in a community setting (Table 4-1). Successful disease management and symptom control of chronic conditions help patients maintain or increase their quality of life. For the older-adult population it is important to view health promotion and disease management within a broad context. For example, in the United States nearly 25% of patients living with HIV are over the age of 50 and remain sexually active (Jacobson, 2011). You need to understand what health means to older adults and the steps they can take to promote healthy life styles and maintain their own health (see Chapter 22).

COMPETENCY IN COMMUNITY-BASED NURSING

A nurse in community-based practice needs a variety of skills and talents to be successful. In addition to helping patients with their health care needs and developing relationships within the community, the community health nurse needs skills in promoting health, preventing disease, and caring for the health of the community. The nurse uses the nursing process and critical thinking (see Chapters 8 and 9) to ensure individualized nursing care for specific patients and their families. Students' clinical practice in a community-based care setting will probably be in partnership with a community nurse. This section provides information about selected competencies such as caregiver, case manager, and educator, which are used in the community-based setting.

Caregiver

Most important is the caregiving role. Using the nursing process and critical thinking skills, you develop appropriate, individualized nursing care for specific patients and their families. In addition, you individualize care within the context of a patient's community to achieve long-term successful health outcomes. Work with the patient and family to develop a caring partnership to recognize actual and potential health care needs and identify community resources. As a caregiver, you build a healthier community that is safe and helps the population achieve and maintain an improved quality of life and optimal health status.

Case Manager

In community-based practice case management is an important competency. Case management means making an appropriate plan of care based on assessment of patients and families and coordinating needed resources and services for a patient's well-being across a continuum of care (see Chapter 3). Generally a community-based case manager assumes responsibility for the case management of multiple patients. This usually involves patients who need coordination of different health care services (e.g., patients with neurological disease, patients who have experienced trauma, patients with mental illnesses, and patients with complex medical conditions). The greatest challenge is coordinating the activities of many different providers and payers in different settings throughout a patient's continuum of care. An effective case manager anticipates obstacles and opportunities that exist within a community that will influence the ability to find solutions for the patient's and family's needs. Case management with individual patients and families reveals the overall picture of health services and the health status of a community.

Educator

Community-based nurses teach their patients individually or in groups. With the goal of helping patients assume responsibility for their own health care, the role of educator

TABLE 4-1 MAJOR HEALTH PROBLEMS IN OLDER ADULTS AND COMMUNITY HEALTH NURSING ROLES AND INTERVENTIONS

PROBLEM	COMMUNITY HEALTH NURSING ROLES AND INTERVENTIONS
Hypertension	Monitor blood pressure and weight; educate about nutrition and antihypertensive drugs; teach stress management techniques; promote a good balance between rest and activity; establish blood pressure screening programs; assess patient's current lifestyle and promote lifestyle changes; promote dietary modifications by using techniques such as a diet diary.
Cancer	Obtain health history; promote monthly breast self-examinations and annual Pap tests and mammograms for older women; promote regular physical examinations; encourage smokers to stop smoking; correct misconceptions about processes of aging; provide emotional support and quality of care during diagnostic and treatment procedures.
Arthritis	Educate adult about management of activities, correct body mechanics, availability of mechanical appliances, and adequate rest; promote stress management; counsel and assist the family to improve communication, role negotiation, and use of community resources; help adults avoid the false hope and expense of arthritis fraud.
Visual impairment (e.g., loss of visual acuity, eyelid disorders, opacity of the lens)	Provide support in a well-lighted, glare-free environment; use printed aids with large, well-spaced letters; help adult clean eyeglasses; help make arrangements for vision examinations and obtain necessary prostheses; teach adult to be cautious of false advertisements.
Hearing impairment (e.g., presbycusis)	Speak with clarity at a moderate volume and pace and face patient when performing health teaching; help make arrangements for hearing examination and obtain necessary prostheses; teach adult to be cautious of false advertisements.
Cognitive impairment	Provide complete assessment; correct underlying causes of disease (if possible); provide for a protective environment; promote activities that reinforce reality; assist with personal hygiene, nutrition, and hydration; provide emotional support to the family; recommend applicable community resources such as adult day care, home care aides, and homemaker services.
Alzheimer's disease	Maintain high-level functioning, protection, and safety; encourage human dignity; demonstrate to the primary family caregiver techniques to dress, feed, and toilet adult; provide frequent encouragement and emotional support to caregiver; act as an advocate for patient when dealing with respite care and support groups; protect patient's rights; provide support to maintain family members' physical and mental health; maintain family stability; recommend financial services if needed.
Dental problems	Perform oral assessment and refer to dentist as necessary; emphasize regular brushing and flossing, proper nutrition, and dental examinations; encourage patients with dentures to wear and take care of them; calm fears about dentist; help provide access to financial services (if necessary) and dental care facilities.
Substance and alcohol abuse	Get drug use history; educate adult about safe storage, risks for medication, drug-drug, drug-alcohol and drug-food interactions; give general information about drug (e.g., drug name, purpose, side effects, dosage); instruct adult about presorting techniques (using small containers with one dose of drug that are labeled with specific times to take drug). Counsel adults about substance abuse; promote stress management to avoid need for drugs or alcohol and arrange for and monitor detoxification if appropriate.
Sexually transmitted infections	Perform a full sexual risk assessment and bring awareness regarding risk factors and susceptibility to HIV/AIDS; educate about safe sexual practices such as abstinence and use of condoms and refer as necessary for HIV testing.

Data from Stanhope M, Lancaster J: *Foundations of nursing in the community: community oriented practice,* ed 4, St Louis, 2014, Mosby; Goodman C, et al: Activity promotion for community-dwelling older people: a survey of the contribution of primary care nurses, *Br J Community Nurs* 16(1):12–17, 2011; Baym-Williams J, Salyer J: Factors influencing the health-related lifestyles of community-dwelling older adults, *Home Healthc Nurse* 28:115–121, 2010; Jacobson SA: HIV/AIDS interventions in an aging US population, *Health Social Work* 36:2:149–156, 2011.

AIDS, Acquired immunodeficiency syndrome; *HIV,* human immunodeficiency virus.

is important in a community-based setting. Patients and families need to acquire certain knowledge and skills to care for themselves (see Chapter 12). When practicing in a community, you assess a patient's learning needs and readiness to learn, adapt teaching skills to instruct within the home setting, and make the learning process meaningful. Evaluate learning by reviewing a patient's level of knowledge and ability to perform specific skills, following up with phone calls, and referring the patient to community support and self-help groups. Evaluation of patient learning occurs over time and requires patience and commitment.

Epidemiologist

Community health nurses use basic principles of epidemiology such as tracking health problems; collecting and analyzing data to identify disease trends, outbreaks of illnesses, and disease incidence rates; and planning strategies to prevent or contain outbreaks. For example, several people in a community became ill with hepatitis A. The community health nurse conducted interviews with the people who became ill and identified an infected food handler at the restaurant where the food was consumed. In collaboration with the health department, the restaurant closed during a through sanitation of the kitchen. The nurse educated all employees about sanitation practices and coordinated postexposure immunization clinics. In addition, the nurse provided education about illness prevention to the community.

COMMUNITY ASSESSMENT

When practicing in a community setting, it is important to learn how to assess the community at large. Community assessment requires you to systematically collect data about a population to monitor the health status of the population and make information available about the health of the community (Stanhope and Lancaster, 2014). The community is the environment in which people live and work. Without an adequate understanding of that environment, any effort to promote community health and institute necessary change is unlikely to be successful. The community has three components or parts: structure or locale, the people or population, and the social systems. A complete assessment involves a careful look at each component to begin to identify needs for health policy, health program development, and service provision (Box 4-4).

When assessing the structure or locale, travel around a neighborhood or community and observe its design, location of services, and locations where residents meet. A public library or local health department is a great source for accessing statistics to assess the demographics of the community. Once you have a thorough understanding of the community structure or locale, perform individual patient assessments against that background (Box 4-5). For example, assess a patient's home for safety. Does he or she have secure locks on doors? Are windows secure and intact? Is lighting along walkways and entryways working? Be aware of the level of community violence and the resources that are available to the patient when help is necessary. No individual patient assessment should occur in isolation from the environment and conditions of the patient's community.

Finally investigate the social systems within a community. To get information about existing social systems such as schools or health care facilities, visit various sites and learn about their services. Which types of health promotion resources such as smoking cessation or weight watchers programs are available? Are any day care or adult day care resources available? Which types of health and wellness activities are active in the schools? Which types of safety programs

BOX 4-4 COMMUNITY ASSESSMENT

STRUCTURE
- Name of community or neighborhood
- Geographical boundaries
- Emergency services
- Water and sanitation
- Housing
- Economic status (e.g., average household income, number of residents on public assistance)
- Availability of public transportation system

POPULATION
- Age distribution
- Gender distribution
- Growth trends
- Density
- Educational level
- Predominant ethnic groups
- Predominant religious groups

SOCIAL SYSTEM
- Educational system
- Government
- Communication system
- Welfare system
- Volunteer programs
- Health system

BOX 4-5 EVALUATION

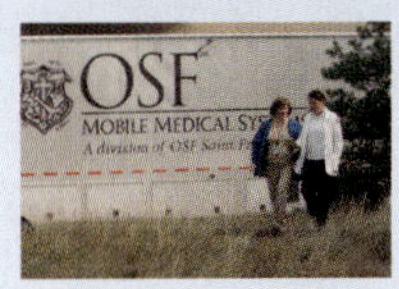

Kim spent the last 12 weeks working with the community agency and leaders in the Bosnian community. Her goal was to provide educational programs to explain how the clinic provides services, the confidentiality of the services, and the fact that the services were low cost and/or free to patients without adequate insurance or financial resources. Kim presented a series of three programs in the homes of four Bosnian leaders. She worked with the leaders on the design of the educational programs and continued to evaluate community response to the programs and health care needs. Throughout this period there was a gradual increase in the use of the services within the agency. In addition, young women within the community asked for prenatal classes.

Kim perceived a greater acceptance within the community. After the first 3 weeks following her class, there were fewer "missed" appointments, and the members of the community shared more relevant health care concerns with her. Finally Kim felt a sense of confidence and competence in developing community health care programs. She learned the importance of including the community and its leaders in all aspects of program building from the assessment of needs through program development and evaluation.

are sponsored by the police department? Knowing the social systems within a community increases your ability to help the community or individuals within that community improve their level of health. In addition, identifying the lack of these programs provides necessary data when advocating for resources for new social programs.

CHANGING PATIENTS' HEALTH

In community-based practice you care for patients from diverse backgrounds and in diverse settings. It is relatively easy over time to become familiar with the resources that are available within a particular community setting and identify the unique needs of individual patients. However, the challenge is how to promote and protect a patient's health within the context of the community. For example, can a patient with lung disease have the quality of life necessary when the patient's community has a serious environmental pollution problem? Likewise it is important to bring together the resources necessary to improve the continuity of care that patients receive. Be a leader in reducing the duplication of health care services and locating the best services for a patient's needs.

For effective community-based nursing, it is most important to understand patients' lives within the context of their communities. This begins when you are able to establish strong, caring relationships with patients and their families (see Chapter 19). Understanding the day-to-day activities of family life helps you adapt nursing interventions. Consider the time of day a patient goes to work, the availability of the spouse and patient's parents to provide child care, and the family values that shape views about health. Once you gain a picture of a patient's life, you develop patient-centered interventions to promote health and prevent disease.

KEY POINTS

- The principles of public health nursing practice focus on helping individuals and communities achieve a healthy living environment.
- The health of individuals and communities depends on access to quality health care. Community-based health centers are in an optimal position to provide comprehensive, culturally competent, quality primary care to underserved and vulnerable populations.
- Essential public health functions include assessment, policy development, and access to resources.
- When population-based health care services are effective, there is a greater likelihood that the higher tiers of services will contribute efficiently to health improvement of the population.
- The community health nurse considers the individual or family to be only one member of a group while providing care to the community as a whole.
- A successful community health nursing practice involves building relationships with the community and being responsive to changes within the community.
- The special needs of vulnerable populations form the backdrop for the challenges that nurses face in caring for patients' increasingly complex acute and chronic health conditions.
- Chronic health problems are common and worsen among the homeless because they have few resources.
- Essential competencies for a community-based nurse include caregiving, case management, patient education, and basic understanding of epidemiology.
- Assessment of a community includes three elements: structure or locale, the people, and the social systems.

CLINICAL DECISION-MAKING EXERCISES

Within the Bosnian community there are many single-parent families, usually widows with school-age children. One of the families that Kim meets is composed of Katrina Dudek, a 30-year-old widow, and her two children, a 6-month-old and a 3-year-old. Mrs. Dudek arrived in the community 5 months ago. Her husband was killed in a raid in their home in her native country. She is very fearful when anyone other than her close neighbors and friends enter her home. Kim and the community health nurse work with Mrs. Dudek to determine the health care needs of her children and herself. To date the community health agency has not been successful in providing well-child care or immunizations to a large part of the community or any care to Mrs. Dudek and her children. Kim and Mrs. Dudek talk about the need to have her children immunized and set that as a goal.

1. What information does Kim need about this Bosnian-community?
2. Identify three priorities that are important when initiating care for Mrs. Dudek's family.
3. Mrs. Dudek is fearful about providing an immunization history for her children. What should Kim do?
4. Which factors within her community increase Mrs. Dudek's vulnerability to health care problems?

evolve

Answers to Clinical Decision-Making Exercises can be found on the Evolve website.

QSEN ACTIVITY: PATIENT-CENTERED CARE

Kim participates with the public health nurse in a community-organized health clinic where immunizations, health promotion activities, and health education are provided. Using translation services, she learns that her patients want more information to be available in Bosnian regarding health education and are interested in how to obtain additional health care services. At the end of her day, Kim writes a reflective journal about her experiences with the Bosnian patients. She considers how diverse the Bosnian community is and whether their language barrier, cultural values, and social backgrounds affect their view of health.

Describe the effect that Kim's reflective practice can have on patient-centered care in the future.

evolve

Answers to QSEN Activities can be found on the Evolve website.

REVIEW QUESTIONS

1. When health care is provided in a community-based practice setting, what is (are) the overall goal(s) of *Healthy People 2020?*
   1. Assess the health care needs of individuals, families, and communities.
   2. Develop and implement public health policies and improve access to care.
   3. Gather information on incidence rates of certain diseases and social problems.
   4. Increase life expectancy and quality of life and eliminate health disparities.
2. A nursing student demonstrates correct understanding of community health nursing when explaining that a nursing approach merges knowledge from professional nursing theories and which of the following? (Select all that apply.)
   1. Population sciences
   2. Public health sciences
   3. Environmental sciences
   4. Mental health sciences
3. While assessing an immigrant community, the nurse identifies that the children are undervaccinated. In addition, she notes that there is a health clinic within a 3-mile radius. The nurse meets with the community leaders and explains the need for immunizations and educates them about the location of the clinic and the process for accessing health care resources. Together they develop a plan for improving the rate of vaccinations. Which of the following practices is the nurse providing? (Select all that apply.)
   1. Developing community resources
   2. Teaching the community about illnesses
   3. Promoting autonomy and decision making
   4. Improving the health care of the children in the community
4. An 82-year-old patient who experienced a stroke and will be using a wheelchair is being discharged home from the hospital. The family wants to care for the patient at home but does not have the resources for 24-hour care. The community-based nurse working as a case manager intervenes by:
   1. Telling the family that a long-term–care facility would be the best choice for a patient in a wheel chair.
   2. Making multiple referrals to a variety of community-based services.
   3. Organizing a community fund-raising event to pay for needed services.
   4. Contacting local nurses in the community to provide assistance to the family.
5. A community health nursing instructor and a group of students are organizing a health fair for the homeless population in a large urban setting. Funding is very limited and will not cover cost for space or transportation. Assuming that space is available at no cost at the following sites, where should the students suggest that the health fair be located?
   1. At the city's homeless shelter
   2. At the inner-city church
   3. At the largest inner-city police station
   4. At the local community college
6. What are the major health care problems in older adults in community settings?
   1. Chronic illness, sensory loss, substance abuse.
   2. Acute illness, sensory loss, and abandonment.
   3. Poverty, acute illness, and inadequate support systems.
   4. Acute illness, inadequate support systems, and substance abuse.
7. Which actions display effective nursing practice in the community? (Select all that apply.)
   1. Educating families of young children about the effects of lead paint in the home
   2. Conducting a blood pressure clinic at a senior health care center
   3. Prescribing treatments for patients when physicians are unable
   4. Forming partnerships with families in the community to share common goals
8. A high school in the community has an increase in the number of pregnant and new adolescent mothers. The community health nurse works with the school district to design and teach classes about nutrition during pregnancy, infant care, child safety, and time management. This an example of which community nursing competency?
   1. Caregiver
   2. Case manager
   3. Consultant
   4. Educator
9. The community health nursing student is correct when he states that the three key elements needed to be incorporated in a community assessment are:
   1. Individuals and families, community, and sociopolitical system.
   2. People, population growth, and health care systems.
   3. Geographical boundary, neighborhoods, and social systems.
   4. Geographical boundary, health care systems, and political systems.

10. Following a community assessment, the nurse identifies an area near an industrial park with increased respiratory illnesses. The community asks the nurse to come and speak about environmental trends associated with respiratory disease and how the community can reduce its risks. This is an example of which competencies? (Select all that apply.)
    1. Caregiver
    2. Case manager
    3. Epidemiologist
    4. Educator

evolve

Rationales for Review Questions can be found on the Evolve website.

1. 4; **2.** 2, 3; **3.** 2, 3, 4; **4.** 2; **5.** 1; **6.** 1; **7.** 1, 2, 4; **8.** 4; **9.** 1; **10.** 3, 4.

REFERENCES

Allender JA, Walton Spradley B: *Community health nursing: Promoting and protecting population's health*, ed 7, Philadelphia, 2010, Lippincott.

American Nurses Association (ANA): *Public health nursing scope and standards of practice*, ed 2, Washington, DC, 2013, The Association.

Camarota S: *Immigrants in the United States: a profile of America's foreign born population*, Center for Immigration Studies, 2012, http://www.cis.org/2012-profile-of-americas-foreign-born-population. Accessed March 20, 2013.

Frieden TR: A framework for public health action: the health impact pyramid, *Am J Public Health* 4(100):590–595, 2010.

Goodman C, et al: Activity promotion for community-dwelling older people: a survey of the contribution of primary care nurses, *Br J Community Health Nurs* 16(1):12–17, 2010.

Jacobson SA: HIV/AIDS interventions in an aging US population, *Health Social Work* (36):149–156, 2011.

Olson KL, et al: Cornerstones of public health nursing, *Public Health Nurs* 28(3):249–260, 2011.

Prohaska T, et al: *Public health for an aging society*, Baltimore, 2012, John Hopkins University Press.

Stanhope M, Lancaster J: *Foundations of nursing in the community: community-oriented practice*, ed 4, St Louis, 2014, Mosby.

Tsemberis S, et al: Housing stability and recovery among chronically homeless persons with co-occurring disorders in Washington, DC, *Am J Public Health* 102:1, 13–16, 2012.

US Department of Health and Human Services (USDHHS): *Healthy People 2020*, 2011, http://healthypeople.gov/2020/about/default.aspx. Accessed March 20, 2013.

CHAPTER

5

Legal Principles in Nursing

evolve WEBSITE

http://evolve.elsevier.com/Potter/essentials

- Crossword Puzzle
- Audio Glossary

OBJECTIVES

- Describe the legal obligations and role of nurses regarding federal and state laws that affect health care.
- Explain the legal concepts of standard of care and informed consent.
- List sources for standards of care for nurses.
- Explain the concept of negligence and identify the elements of professional negligence.
- Define the legal relationships of nurse-patient, nurse–health care provider, nurse-nurse, and nurse-employer.
- Identify nursing interventions to improve patient safety.

KEY TERMS

Safe and competent nursing care includes critical thinking skills and an understanding of the legal boundaries within which you practice. Frequently nurses practice under several sources and jurisdictions of health care law simultaneously. In addition to understanding the federal laws that apply to health care, it is also important to know the law and the rules and regulations of the regulatory agencies in your own state. An understanding of the law coupled with sound judgment helps to ensure safe and appropriate nursing care. You need to understand the legal limits of nursing and the standard of care that affects nursing practice to know your responsibilities as a patient advocate and protect patients from harm. If you have specific questions, consult with your own attorney or with the attorney for your employing institution.

LEGAL LIMITS OF NURSING

Sources of Law

Laws that apply to nursing practice today originally derived from two sources: common law and statutory laws. Common laws are based on judicial decisions or case law precedent, whereas statutory laws are rules codified by legislative bodies of government (Guido, 2010). An example of a judicial decision that guides health care practice is *Roe v. Wade*

CASE STUDY *Lynette Donovan*

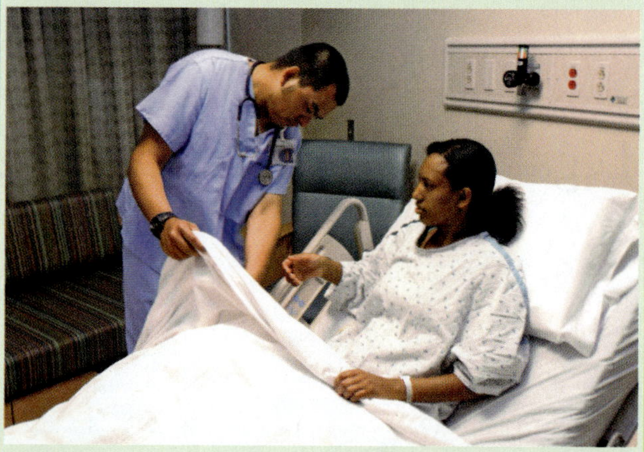

Lynette Donovan, a 15-year-old African-American female, was a passenger in a motor vehicle collision and is now admitted to the hospital with a fractured right femur. The emergency department health care provider applied a cast to the affected leg with insufficient padding. Lynnette told the nurses that her right leg felt numb, was swollen, and looked discolored. The nurses assessed Lynette's right leg and determined that these symptoms indicated impaired circulation in the extremity with the cast. The nurses were unable to reach Lynette's health care provider despite several calls. They did not notify the nursing supervisor of the patient's situation (Darling v. Charleston Community Memorial Hospital, 1965).

David Ortiz is a 23-year-old nursing student newly assigned to the nursing division and to Miss Donovan. His initial assessment notes that the patient's right leg is swollen, slightly blue, and slightly malodorous. Lynette seems very anxious and upset.

(410 U.S. 113, 1973), in which the U.S. Supreme Court identified time periods in which elective termination of a pregnancy is legal. Statutory laws are frequently made following judicial decisions at the federal or state level. An example of a federal statute that affects health care practice is the Americans With Disabilities Act (ADA), which protects the rights of individuals with disabilities (ADA, 1995) (Box 5-1). **Nurse Practice Acts** are examples of statutes enacted by state legislatures to regulate the practice of nursing. The Nurse Practice Acts of each state define the scope of nursing practice and expanded nursing roles, set educational requirements for nurses, and distinguish between nursing and medical practice. Nurse Practice Acts establish a regulatory agency such as a State Board of Nursing, which uses the principles of administrative law to guide the regulation of nursing practice (Guido, 2010). Nurse Practice Acts permit State Boards of Nursing to set rules, regulations, and guidelines that specifically define the standard of care in nursing practice. An example is the guidelines a nurse uses to avoid patient abandonment and sanctions for failure to follow the standard of care (Missouri State Board of Nursing Position Statement, 2007). To practice nursing you must be licensed by the State Board of Nursing of the state in which you wish to practice.

BOX 5-1 FEDERAL STATUTES IN NURSING PRACTICE

Americans With Disabilities Act (ADA) (1995)—A civil rights law protecting the disabled regarding access to public services, health care, and employment. Extended to include individuals with HIV infection

Emergency Medical Treatment and Active Labor Act (EMTALA) (1986)—"Antidumping" law that requires screening of patients in an emergency department and appropriate stabilization before transfer of the patient to another facility

Health Insurance Portability and Accountability Act (HIPAA) (1996)—Protects a patient from losing health insurance because of preexisting illnesses when changing jobs; also sets rules regarding release of a patient's protected health information and carries both civil and criminal penalties for violations

Patient Self-Determination Act (PSDA) (1991)—Requires health care facilities to provide information to all patients regarding advance directives and to document advance directives in the medical record

Federal Nursing Home Reform Act (1987)—Gives nursing home residents the right to be free of unnecessary and inappropriate restraints

National Organ Transplant Act (1984)—Prohibits purchase or sale of organs; provides immunity from civil and criminal actions against the hospital and health care providers and immunity from liability for the donor's estate

Mental Health Parity Act (1996)—Prohibits health plans from placing lifetime or annual limits on mental health benefits

HIV, Human immunodeficiency virus.

To be licensed in your state, you must have a passing score on the National Council Licensure Examination (NCLEX®) to obtain your initial license and meet the educational requirements set by the state. Many states require obtaining continuing education units for license renewal.

A State Board of Nursing has the power to suspend or revoke a nurse's license if the nurse's conduct violates provisions of the licensing statute. Criminal law violations, even if unrelated to nursing, may jeopardize your license status. Because the nursing license is a common law property right under the law, the State Board must fulfill the constitutional duty of **due process** in any disciplinary proceeding. Due process requires a State Board to notify the nurse of the listed charges or violations and conduct a hearing at which the nurse may hear the evidence of the charges and offer a defense with or without the assistance of legal counsel (Guido, 2010). In license hearings a panel of members of a State Board of Nursing conducts the hearing instead of a judge. Depending on your state administrative law rules, you may file an appeal of the State Board of Nursing judgment in a court of law. In any licensing proceeding nurses should exercise the right to legal counsel to ensure full protection of their rights.

Criminal Law

Criminal laws are federal or state statutory laws that define as a crime certain actions that inflict or threaten substantial harm to individuals or the public interest without justification (Guido, 2010). Criminal laws are separated into misdemeanors or felonies. A **misdemeanor** is a crime that, although injurious, does not inflict serious harm (Shilling, 2011). For example, parking your car in a designated no parking zone is a misdemeanor violation of a traffic law. A misdemeanor usually has a penalty of a monetary fine, forfeiture, or brief imprisonment. A **felony** is a serious offense that results in significant harm to another person or society in general. Felony crimes carry penalties of monetary restitution, imprisonment for greater than 1 year, or death (Guido, 2010). Examples of Nurse Practice Act violations that may carry criminal penalties include practicing nursing without a license and misuse of controlled substances.

Torts

Nursing practice is also regulated by common law or judicial case law of torts. **Torts** are civil wrongful acts or omissions against a person or a person's property that are compensated by awarding monetary damages to the individual whose rights were violated (Shilling, 2011). Torts are characterized as either intentional or unintentional.

Intentional torts are deliberate acts of wrongful conduct (Shilling, 2011). An example of an intentional tort in health care is assault and battery. Even though assault and battery can be criminal statutory violations, they may also be tort injuries in health care. The definitions of assault and battery are the same in both criminal and tort law. **Assault** is an intentional threat toward another person that places the person in reasonable fear of harmful, imminent, or unwelcome contact (Shilling, 2011). No actual contact is required for an assault to occur. An example of an assault in nursing practice is to threaten to restrain a patient for an x-ray procedure when the patient has refused consent. **Battery** is intentional offensive touching without consent or lawful justification (Shilling, 2011). The touching may be harmful to the patient by causing an injury, or it may be merely offensive to the patient's dignity. Battery generally always includes an assault. An example of a battery in health care is when a patient has consented to a right knee surgery and the surgeon performs surgery on the patient's left knee. An example of an assault and battery is to threaten to restrain a competent patient for an unconsented x-ray procedure and then to actually restrain him or her.

Negligence is an unintentional tort. **Negligence** is conduct that falls below the generally accepted standard of care of a reasonably prudent person (Karno, 2011). The definition of negligence has evolved over time through common law and case law to be the failure to use the degree of care that a reasonable person would use under the same or similar circumstances. An example of negligence is a driver's failure to stop at a clearly identified stop sign. Malpractice is an example of negligence, sometimes referred to as professional negligence. The law defines nursing **malpractice** as the failure to use that degree of care that a reasonable nurse would use under the same or similar circumstances. To establish the elements of malpractice, the patient/family or **plaintiff** must prove the following: (1) the nurse **defendant** owed a duty to the patient; (2) the nurse breached that duty; (3) the patient was injured because of the nurse's breach of duty; and (4) the patient has accrued damages as a result of the injury. Negligent acts may result in lawsuits against hospitals and nurses (Box 5-2). The negligent act may be as simple as failing to check a patient's armband and then administering medication to the wrong patient. Failure to monitor a patient's condition appropriately and communicate changes in the patient's condition to the health care provider that result in injury to the patient are examples of negligent acts that may result in malpractice. The best way to avoid being liable for malpractice is to give nursing care that meets the generally accepted standard of care. In a malpractice lawsuit the law uses nursing standards of care to measure nursing conduct and determine whether the nurse acted as any reasonably prudent nurse would act under the same or similar circumstances. Box 5-3 describes the steps of a typical malpractice lawsuit.

BOX 5-2 COMMON SOURCES OF NEGLIGENCE

Be aware of the common negligent acts that have resulted in lawsuits against hospitals and nurses:

1. Medication errors that result in injury to patients
2. Intravenous therapy errors resulting in infiltration or phlebitis
3. Burns to patients caused by equipment, bathing, or spills of hot liquids and foods
4. Falls resulting in injury to patients
5. Failure to use aseptic technique when required
6. Errors in sponge, instrument, or needle counts in surgical cases, meaning that an item was left in a patient
7. Failure to give a report or giving an incomplete report to oncoming shift personnel
8. Failure to adequately monitor a patient's condition
9. Failure to notify a health care provider of a significant change in a patient's status

STANDARDS OF CARE

Standards of care are legal guidelines for minimally safe and adequate nursing practice (Guido, 2010). They are defined by the following: (1) State Nurse Practice Acts, (2) state and federal hospital licensing laws and accreditation rules, (3) professional and specialty organizations (American Nurses Association [ANA], 2010), and (4) written policies and procedures of health care facilities. Written policies and procedures of a nurse's health care facility are specific guidelines and directions for nursing care and are usually found on every nursing unit in a policy and procedure manual. The procedure for following the "chain of command" to notify a health care provider of a serious change in patient status is frequently a part of the nursing unit policy and procedure manual. *In the case study the nursing staff caring for Lynette Donovan could have consulted the policy and procedure manual to determine who to contact if they were unable to reach her*

BOX 5-3 ANATOMY OF A LAWSUIT

Petition—Elements of the claim: The plaintiff outlines what the defendant nurse did wrong and how, as a result of that alleged negligence, the plaintiff was injured. In the case study the petition would state that the nurses failed to provide adequate care to the patient by failing to treat the changing condition appropriately.

Answer: The nurse admits or denies each allegation in the petition. Anything that is not admitted must be proved. The nurses admit or deny that they were able to provide further appropriate care to the patient to meet the standard of care during her change in condition.

Discovery: The process of uncovering all the facts of the case involves using interrogatories, full access to the medical records in question, and depositions. The patient and all health care staff are asked questions by counsel for the plaintiff and the defense. They answer under oath, and their testimony is recorded and kept for reference in the trial.

Interrogatories: Written questions requiring answers under oath usually concern witnesses, insurance experts, and which health care providers the plaintiff saw before and after the event.

Medical records: The defendant obtains all of the plaintiff's relevant medical records for treatment before and after the incident. Everything written by the nurses and the health care provider in the medical record is open to examination by both the plaintiff and the defendants.

Witnesses' depositions: Questions are posed to the witnesses under oath to obtain all relevant, nonprivileged information about the case.

Parties' depositions: The plaintiff and defendants (health care provider, nurse, and hospital personnel) are almost always deposed.

Other witnesses: Factual witnesses, both neutral and biased, are deposed to obtain information and their version of the case. They may include family members on the plaintiff's side and other medical personnel (e.g., nurses) on the defendant's side.

Treating health care providers' depositions: Before subsequent treating, health care providers' depositions may be taken to establish issues such as those concerning preexisting conditions, causation, the nature and extent of injuries, and permanency.

Experts: The plaintiff selects experts to establish the essential legal elements of the case against the defendant. The defendant selects experts to establish the appropriateness of the nursing care. Nursing experts are asked to testify to the reasonableness or inappropriate actions of the health care staff once the patient's condition began to change. The expert is asked to compare the actions of the nursing staff to the standard of care, which is what the reasonably prudent nurse in the same situation would have done.

Trial: The trial usually occurs at least 1 to 3 years after the filing of the petition. Approximately 5% of cases are actually tried before a judge. Most are dismissed or settled. Settlement means that compensation has been paid for the case to be dismissed.

PROOF OF NEGLIGENCE

- The nurse owed a duty to the patient.
- The nurse did not carry out the duty or breached it (failed to use that degree of skill and learning ordinarily used under the same or similar circumstances by members of the profession).
- The patient was injured.
- The patient's injury was caused by the nurse's failure to carry out that duty.
- The patient's injury resulted in compensable damages that can be quantified such as medical bills, lost wages, pain, and suffering.

health care provider in a timely manner. Standards of care change regularly to reflect current scientific or technological advances (DiMeo and Ballard, 2011).

It is important that you know the nursing scope of practice and the policies and procedures of your employing health care facility because these are the standards of care to which your actions will be compared if you are in a malpractice trial. If you become a specialized nurse such as a nurse anesthetist, intensive care nurse, certified nurse midwife, or operating room nurse, you are held to the standard of care and skill exercised by professionals in the specialty area. Nursing experts testify to the appropriate standard of care as indicated by the policy and procedure manual, your professional organization, or the State Nurse Practice Act and compare your conduct to these standards. A number of states have developed "apology statutes" that encourage a health care provider to disclose errors or unanticipated outcomes to a patient/family without admitting liability. These statutes are designed to improve communication and decrease litigation (Mastroianni et al., 2010). It is always important to be up to date regarding the policies and procedures of your agency and state and federal laws; current legal issues; and any new rules, regulations, or case law that affect your nursing practice.

Malpractice Insurance

Malpractice insurance provides you with an attorney, the payment of attorney's fees, and the payment of any judgment or settlement if a patient sues you for malpractice. If you work for a health care facility, the insurance of that facility covers you during your employment. If you plan on practicing nursing outside of your employing facility, you need to purchase additional malpractice insurance. For example, if a family friend asks you to provide nursing care in his or her home, the hospital malpractice insurance does not cover you if the family friend files suit against you. Malpractice insurance carriers are required by federal law to report all malpractice insurance verdicts and settlements made to the National Practitioner Data Bank (NPDB). The NPDB affects the professional practice of nursing when it compiles data on all advance practice nurses as health care practitioners (Guido, 2010). Registered nurse malpractice claims from 2006 through 2010 have maintained a stable liability cost pattern, averaging $250,000.00 total paid per claim (Nurses Service Organization, 2011).

Documentation

It is necessary to document patient assessments, interventions, and evaluations and develop a caring rapport with each patient to avoid liability. Frequently a nurse's notes are the first thing that an attorney reviews when a lawsuit is filed. As a nurse you chart facts, not assumptions, about patient behavior. In addition, you document as fully as possible the health care provider notifications made regarding a patient. Simply charting "physician notified" is insufficient information when presenting a chart in court. Your assessments and the reporting of significant changes in the assessments are very important factors in defending a lawsuit. Your documentation of your nursing care is your only record of what actually was done for a patient and serves as proof that you acted reasonably and safely. Trials over health care disputes that involve using the medical record as a source of factual information generally take 2 to 3 years to occur. Most individuals have flawed recall of events over a period of time. Therefore your nursing notes, written at the time of the event, are seen as better evidence of the facts of the event than any one person's memory. Nurses' notes written carelessly and without regard to detail or hospital standards of documentation do not reflect well on the health care provider's credibility or appearance of accountability to a judge or jury (Brous, Boulay, and Burger, 2011). Make sure that your documentation is thorough, accurate, and done in a timely manner (see Chapter 10).

When there is a deviation from the standard of care such as when a patient or visitor falls or an error is made, you document the event or incident in the form of an **occurrence report/incident report.** You complete an occurrence report when anything unusual happens that could potentially cause harm to a patient, visitor, or employee. Most health care facilities provide specific forms for this purpose (see Chapter 10). Objectively record the details of the event and any statements the patient makes. An example follows: "Patient found lying on floor on right side. Abrasion on right forehead. Patient stated, 'I fell and hit my head.'" At the time of the event, always assess the patient thoroughly; then contact the health care provider to examine him or her. After examining the patient, you and the health care provider document assessment findings in the progress notes. The health care provider orders follow-up care or treatment when necessary. Document any problematic effects caused by the event. Do not include subjective assumptions and statements assigning blame or fault in the nurses' notes or the occurrence report. Occurrence reports are not kept in patients' medical records, although they may be evidence in lawsuits in some jurisdictions (*In re Intracare Hospital*, 2007). ***Do not document in the nurses' notes that an occurrence report was completed.*** Follow the policy of your agency to determine what to do with the occurrence report after it is completed. Also be sure to report the occurrence to the appropriate person (e.g., the charge nurse, your manager).

Risk Management and Quality Assurance

The underlying rationale for quality improvement and risk-management programs is the development of an organizational system of ensuring appropriate, quality health care. **Risk management** involves several components, including identifying possible risks, analyzing them, acting to reduce them, and evaluating the measures taken to reduce them (Miller, 2011). The Joint Commission (TJC, 2013) requires the use of quality improvement and risk-management procedures. Both quality improvement and risk management require thorough documentation.

One documentation tool used in risk management is the occurrence report or incident report. By reviewing occurrence reports, administrators determine areas of patient risk. For example, if a certain kind of problem has occurred repeatedly such as patients falling when being transferred to stretchers, educational methods could be developed to help prevent the problem in the future.

Patient safety and improved care are the ultimate goals of risk management and quality assurance. Patient safety issues are the focus of attention by accrediting agencies such as The Joint Commission (TJC, 2013) and public interest groups such as the Institute of Medicine. **Never events** are preventable errors, which may include falls, urinary tract infections from improper use of catheters, and pressure ulcers (AHRQ, 2012). Recently the federal government and health care insurance companies developed policies to withhold reimbursement for preventable medical errors (CMS, 2008; AHRQ, 2012). Becoming involved in developing and monitoring the policies and procedures of the facility in which you work helps to develop a system and a culture of patient safety.

GOOD SAMARITAN LAWS

Good Samaritan laws exist in almost every state to encourage nurses and other health care providers to help in emergency situations. These laws limit liability and offer legal immunity if a nurse helps at the scene of an accident. For example, if you stop at the scene of an automobile accident and give appropriate emergency care such as applying pressure to stop hemorrhage, you are acting within accepted standards, even though proper equipment was not available. If the patient subsequently develops complications as a result of your actions, you are immune from liability as long as you acted without gross negligence. The statutes also provide that a nurse is able to assist a minor in an emergency at the scene of an accident or a competitive sports event before obtaining the parent's consent. Good Samaritan laws provide immunity to a nurse who does what is reasonable to save a person's life; however, if you perform a procedure for which you have no training, you are liable for any injury resulting from that act. Therefore provide only care that is consistent with your level of expertise (Guido, 2010). In addition, once you have committed to providing emergency care to a patient, you are responsible for following through (i.e., to safely transfer the care of the patient to someone who can provide needed care such as emergency medical technicians [EMTs] or emergency department staff).

CONSENT

A patient's signed consent form is necessary for admission to a health care facility, invasive procedures such as intravenous central line catheter insertion, surgery, some treatment programs such as chemotherapy, and participation in research studies (Guido, 2010). A patient signs a general consent form for treatment when he or she is admitted to the hospital or other health care facility. A patient or the patient's representative has to sign separate special consent forms before anyone performs specialized procedures. Box 5-4 outlines the general guidelines for legal consent to medical treatments. Take special consideration for and care of a patient who is deaf or illiterate or speaks a foreign language. In each instance take steps to ensure that the patient understands the document being signed (Guido, 2010). It is also important to be sensitive to the cultural issues of consent and understand the way in which patients and their families communicate to make important decisions. The cultural beliefs and values of your patients are sometimes very different from your own or the culture in which you are comfortable. Show respect by not imposing your cultural values on your patients or their families. For example, traditional Islamic and Jewish cultures have strict guidelines concerning consent for postmortem examinations and handling of the dead. In general, decision making by a member of a traditional Asian or Hispanic culture is done by the family together and not by the individual seeking treatment. However, remember that all patients are unique individuals; therefore it is necessary to assess their preferences for how to handle consent. When your patient refuses a treatment, it is necessary to make him or her aware of the consequences of his or her refusal.

When a competent patient refuses care or treatment, it is important to recognize that this act is legitimately his or her right. You should inform the health care provider of the patient's refusal to receive care and document the situation in the medical record.

BOX 5-4 STATUTORY GUIDELINES FOR LEGAL CONSENT FOR MEDICAL TREATMENT

Those who may consent to medical treatment are governed by state law but generally include the following:

I. Adults
   - A. Any competent individual 18 years of age or older for himself or herself
   - B. Any parent for his or her unemancipated minor
   - C. Any guardian for his or her ward
   - D. Any adult for the treatment of his or her minor brother or sister (if an emergency and parents are not present)
   - E. Any grandparent for a minor grandchild (if an emergency and parents are not present)

II. Minors (younger than 18 years of age)
   - A. Ordinarily minors may not consent to medical treatment without a parent. However, emancipated minors may consent to medical treatment without a parent. Emancipated minors include the following:
     1. Minors who are designated emancipated by a court order
     2. Minors who are married, divorced, or widowed
     3. Minors who are in active military service
   - B. Unemancipated minors may consent to medical treatment if they have specific medical conditions:
     1. Pregnancy and pregnancy-related conditions (Various states differ in characterizing a pregnant minor as either emancipated or unemancipated. Know the rules of your state in this matter.)
     2. A minor parent for his or her custodial child
     3. Sexually transmitted infection (STI) information and treatment
     4. Substance abuse treatment
     5. Outpatient and/or temporary sheltered mental health treatment
   - C. The issue of emancipated or unemancipated minor does not relieve the health care provider's duty to attempt to obtain meaningful informed consent (Guido, 2010).

Informed Consent

Informed consent is a patient's agreement to allow something such as surgery to happen based on a full disclosure of the risks, benefits, alternatives, and consequences of refusal (Brous, 2011). Informed consent requires that you ensure that a patient has all relevant information required to make a decision, that the patient is capable of understanding the relevant information, and that the patient actually gives consent. If you or a health care provider performs a procedure on a patient without informed consent, the person who performed the procedure can be liable for battery. You do not need to have written informed consent when performing most nursing care. However, it is important that you explain to a patient what you are going to do and ensure that the patient accepts the care you are going to provide. Written informed consent is needed when a patient is going to have an invasive medical procedure such as surgery. Documentation of written informed consent includes the following:

- The patient's signature
- The witnesses' signatures
- The date and time of signing
- Verification that the patient voluntarily signed the consent and discussed the risks, benefits, alternatives, and the right to refuse the procedure with the health care provider
- Verification that the patient understands the procedure and has had all questions answered satisfactorily

Because nurses do not perform surgery or direct medical procedures, providing information about the procedure and obtaining a patient's informed consent for it does not fall within a nurse's responsibility. Even though a nurse assumes the responsibility of witnessing a patient's signature on a consent form, he or she does not legally assume the duty of obtaining informed consent. The health care provider performing the procedure assumes that responsibility (Brous, 2011). When you provide consent forms for patients to sign, ask them if they understand the procedures for which they are giving consent. If patients deny any understanding or if you suspect that they do not understand, notify the health care provider and your nursing supervisor. A patient refusing surgery or other medical treatment must be informed about any harmful consequences of refusal. If a patient persists in refusing a treatment, make sure that the rejection is written, signed, and witnessed (Brous, 2011). Student nurses should always be aware of their school, facility, and/or state rules on whether or not the student can act as a witness of a patient's consent to treatment.

Parents are normally the legal guardians of pediatric patients; therefore they sign consent forms for treatment. If the parents are divorced, the parent with legal custody gives consent. When a parent refuses medically necessary treatment for a child, health care providers sometimes petition the court to intervene on the child's behalf. Using the standard known as "the best interests of the child," courts may overrule parental decisions (Child Welfare Information Gateway, 2010). Although there is no standard definition of the best interests of the child, courts generally consider the child's ultimate safety and well-being as the most important factors. Children, most often adolescents under the age of 16, may be characterized as emancipated or unemancipated minors. This characterization refers to their legal standing as competent adults. Even though an emancipated minor has not achieved the legal age of consent, he or she may give consent for procedures and treatment. Emancipation is certified by a legal document. Some states may characterize some adolescents as emancipated when certain conditions such as pregnancy exist. In this case the adolescent mother is considered competent to consent to treatment for herself and her child. When there is a question about an adolescent's capacity to consent to a procedure, contact the nursing supervisor for guidance (Guido, 2010).

If a patient is unconscious, you need to obtain consent from a person legally authorized to give consent on his or her behalf. In an emergency situation health care providers may provide care to patients without consent as long as it is presumed that a reasonable person would have agreed to the same or similar treatment (Brous, 2011). A patient who is legally incompetent needs to have the consent of a legal guardian, which is determined through a legal proceeding. If a mentally ill person refuses treatment, involuntary admission is limited to situations in which a patient is determined to be dangerous to himself or others (Guido, 2010). A patient's consent for voluntary psychiatric unit admission is also required. These patients retain the right to refuse treatment until a court has determined that they are incompetent to decide for themselves.

Restraints

A physical restraint is any manual method, physical or mechanical device, or material or equipment that immobilizes or reduces the ability of a patient to move freely (CMS, 2008). The use of restraints has been associated with serious complications and even death. It is imperative for you to know when and how to use and safely apply restraints. The Resident's Rights section of the Omnibus Budget Reconciliation Act (1988) regulates the use of physical or chemical restraints in long-term care nursing facilities. In addition, The Joint Commission (TJC, 2013) has set guidelines for the use of restraints in hospitals. These regulations set the standard that all patients have the right to be free from seclusion and physical or chemical restraints except to ensure the patient's safety in emergency situations. They further describe the procedures to follow to restrain any patient, including who orders restraints, when to write the order, and how often to renew the written order. The standards specifically prohibit restraining patients for staff convenience, punishment, or retaliation (Guido, 2010). The regulations also describe documentation of restraint use and follow-up assessments. In particular, the documentation needs to describe all of the less-restrictive interventions attempted before using a physical or chemical restraint (see Chapter 28). Liability for improper or unlawful restraint lies with the nurse and the health care facility.

Death and Dying

You also need to know your legal responsibilities concerning the care of patients during the process of death and dying. Carefully document all events that occur when you are caring for a dying patient. There are two standards for the determination of death: cardiopulmonary or whole brain (Uniform Determination of Death Act, 1980). The cardiopulmonary standard requires failure of a patient's circulatory and respiratory functions. The whole brain standard requires irreversible failure of all functions of the entire brain, including the brainstem. The reason for the development of the two definitions is to set the legal standard for determining death in all situations. The definitions are helpful when there is a question of whether to continue life support or when the discussion of organ donation is appropriate.

You are legally obligated to treat your deceased patient's remains with dignity and care (see Chapter 26). Wrongful handling causes emotional harm to survivors. In one litigated case survivors sued when a mislabeling of bodies led to an Orthodox Jewish person being prepared for a Roman Catholic funeral and a Roman Catholic person being prepared for an Orthodox Jewish burial (*In re Schiller,* 1977).

Advance Directives. You encounter legal issues associated with caring for patients who are terminally ill, severely debilitated, or in a persistent vegetative state (permanently comatose). One of these legal issues involves the right to refuse medical treatment and the withholding of food and nutrition. The doctrine of informed consent ensures that a patient has the right to refuse treatment. The Supreme Court has held that a competent person has the right to refuse medical treatment, including lifesaving food and nutrition (*Cruzan v. Director Missouri Department of Health,* 1990).

Many times the decision regarding lifesaving treatment is in writing in a patient's living will or advance directive. **Living wills** are documents instructing the health care provider to withhold or withdraw life-sustaining procedures in patients who are terminally ill. If a patient has executed a durable **power of attorney for health care,** the document designates an individual, also known as a **health care proxy,** who is able to give consent for health care treatment when the patient is no longer able. State law may designate a surrogate decision maker such as a spouse, who acts as a substitute when no documented preference exists. Each state providing for living wills or advance directives has its own requirements for executing them. In general you need two witnesses who are not relatives or the health care provider when a patient signs the document. Only a competent patient is able to revoke living wills, advance directives, and durable power of attorney for health care statements. Health care providers who ignore valid living wills, advance directives, or the directions of a health care power of attorney may be subject to civil liability. The Patient Self-Determination Act (1991) requires health care institutions to inquire whether a patient has created an advance directive, to give patients information on advance directives, and to document whether a patient states that he or she has an advance directive.

If a health care provider has documented in the progress notes that a patient is deteriorating and the health care provider and the patient have made the decision not to administer cardiopulmonary resuscitation, the health care provider should write a "do not resuscitate" (DNR) order. A DNR order is written, not given verbally. Health care providers need to regularly review DNR orders in case a patient's condition warrants a change. Be familiar with the policies of your institution and procedures concerning DNR orders.

Organ and Tissue Donation. A signed consent is necessary before donating a patient's body, tissues, or organs for medical use. In some states a patient signs the back of his or her driver's license in the presence of witnesses, indicating consent to having his or her body donated. Consent is valid unless the driver's license is revoked, canceled, or suspended; and the person has to give consent each time the license is renewed. Generally a hospital is not liable for honoring a patient's consent for organ donation despite the family's objection. However, in practice health care institutions honor a family's wishes even if they conflict with the patient's organ donation consent. State laws provide whether a nurse is able to witness the consent of an individual donating his or her body, organs, or tissues for medical use. Be aware of the policies and procedures of your employing institution and the laws in your state when someone asks you to serve as a witness for a person who is giving consent for organ donation.

In most states there is a law requiring that at the time of death a qualified health care provider ask a patient's family members to consider organ or tissue donation (National Organ Transplant Act, 1984). You approach individuals in the following order: (1) spouse, (2) adult son or daughter, (3) parent, (4) adult brother or sister, (5) grandparent, and (6) guardian. The person in the highest class makes the donation unless he or she knows of a refusal or contrary indication by the decedent (Uniform Anatomical Gift Act, 1987). In addition, the law also provides that the health care provider who certifies death shall not be involved in the removal or transplant of organs or tissues. The National Organ Transplant Act of 1984 prohibits selling or purchasing organs and regulates this area of medical and nursing practice. Organ and tissue donation remains voluntary. Consent forms are available for this purpose.

Autopsies. An autopsy requires consent by a patient before his or her death or by a close family member at the time of the patient's death (Autopsy Consent, 1998). The priority for giving consent for autopsies is (1) the patient, in writing before death; (2) durable power of attorney; (3) surviving spouse; and (4) surviving child, parent, brother, or sister in the order named. State statutes specify that, when there are reasonable grounds to believe that a patient died as a result of violence, homicide, suicide, accident, or death occurring in any unusual or suspicious manner, you need to notify the coroner. You also notify the coroner if a patient's death is unforeseen and sudden and a health care provider has not seen the patient in over 36 hours.

Confidentiality

The Health Insurance Portability and Accountability Act of 1996 (HIPAA, 1996) sets standards regarding the electronic exchange of private and sensitive health information. Known as the Privacy Standards (Carter, 2013), these rules create patient rights to consent to use and disclose protected health information, inspect and copy one's medical record, and amend mistaken or incomplete information. In addition, the standards require all hospitals and health agencies to have specific policies and procedures in place to ensure compliance with the standards. The policies and procedures need to provide reasonable safeguards to protect written and verbal communications about patients. Although HIPAA does not require such things as soundproof rooms in hospitals, it does mean that nurses and health care providers need to avoid discussing patients in public hallways and provide reasonable levels of privacy in communicating with and about patients in any matter. HIPAA violations have civil and criminal sanctions. Patient confidentiality is a right of all patients, and it is a privilege that a patient entrusts you with his or her personal health information. Dealing with deliberate violations of a patient's confidential personal health information by other staff members is a difficult situation. The best actions to take are to advise the staff members to stop, inform the nursing supervisor, and complete an occurrence report.

Issues of disclosure, privacy, and confidentiality are important concerns when working with patients or peers infected with bloodborne illnesses such as human immunodeficiency virus (HIV) or acquired immunodeficiency virus (AIDS), hepatitis, and sexually transmitted illnesses. You care for these patients in every segment of your nursing practice. Use Standard Precautions as a standard of care when caring for all patients (see Chapter 14). The Americans with Disabilities Act (ADA, 1995) applies to people with AIDS. This federal law protects the rights of disabled people and HIV-infected patients. Health care workers and other employees who refuse to work with HIV-infected people leave companies open to indirect charges of discrimination if the employer does not monitor the work environment. Several cases have held that the health care provider is obligated to disclose the fact that he or she is infected with HIV. The ADA regulations protect the privacy of infected people by giving individuals the opportunity to decide whether to disclose their disability. As a health care worker it is not a requirement for you to be tested for HIV as a condition of employment. If you are contaminated by a patient whose HIV status is unknown, you cannot check the patient's blood for HIV without the patient's consent.

Confidentiality and Social Media

Patient confidential information should only be shared with other health care providers within the confines of the provider-patient relationship. The act of keeping a patient's information confidential and safe forms the basis of the trust relationship between a patient and nurse. A patient also has an expectation to be treated with dignity and respect, which forms the basis of the patient's right to privacy. Whenever a nurse breaks a patient's trust by disclosing confidential information or violating a patient's right to privacy, the nurse-patient relationship is unalterably changed. This change affects not only that patient and that nurse but also the profession of nursing (ANA, 2011).

Journaling is a form of reflective practice, and it is important for any professional to collaborate and share professional development education and exchange ideas regarding the practice issues facing today's nurse professionals. However, when a professional fails to demonstrate a respect for the boundaries that must exist between a patient and a professional nurse or between professionals, the nursing profession loses credibility with the public it serves (NCSBN, 2011).

There is no expectation of privacy on social media sites. Posting on social media sites, even when patients or colleagues are not specifically described, breaches a patient's trust and may be a form of lateral violence with respect to co-workers (ANA, 2011). Inappropriate use of a patient's confidential information or image may be reported to the State Board of Nursing, and the nurse could face disciplinary charges (NCSBN, 2011). The ANA has developed a Social Media Policy (ANA, 2011), which recommends that, when using social media sites, a nurse should never name or describe a patient, never post an image of a patient, and never disparage a fellow employee or employer. In addition, the professional nurse has an obligation to report breaches of privacy and confidentiality. A nurse should become knowledgeable about his or her employer's policies on the use of social media. As a student nurse you should be aware of potential employers' use of social media. Many hospitals are now using social media as they hire new graduates. Even if there is not a breach of confidentiality, if the student has posted "unwisely," the employer may choose to use that information as a representation of the student's professional behavior.

OTHER LEGAL ISSUES IN NURSING PRACTICE

As a nurse you are faced with nursing issues that will become liability concerns. It is important for you to anticipate these issues so you are better prepared to deal with any problems that arise.

Health Care Provider Orders

A patient's physician or health care provider is responsible for directing the medical treatment of a patient. You are responsible for carrying out that medical treatment unless the order is in error, violates hospital policy, or is harmful to the patient. Therefore assess all physician or health care provider orders; if you determine that they are erroneous or harmful, obtain further clarification from that physician or health care provider (Figure 5-1). For example, if the written order indicates that a medication should be given but the nurse notes in the admission assessment that the patient reports that he or she has taken the medication in the past and developed a rash and a swollen neck afterward, the nurse is responsible to seek clarification from the health care provider. If the physician or health care provider confirms the order but you still believe that it is inappropriate, inform the nurse manager or the nursing supervisor. Do not carry out the order if there is a risk that harm will come to your patient. Your supervisor helps resolve the questionable order. If you knowingly carry out the questionable order without obtaining any supporting consultation from your supervisor or administrative staff, you are legally responsible for the harm suffered by your patient.

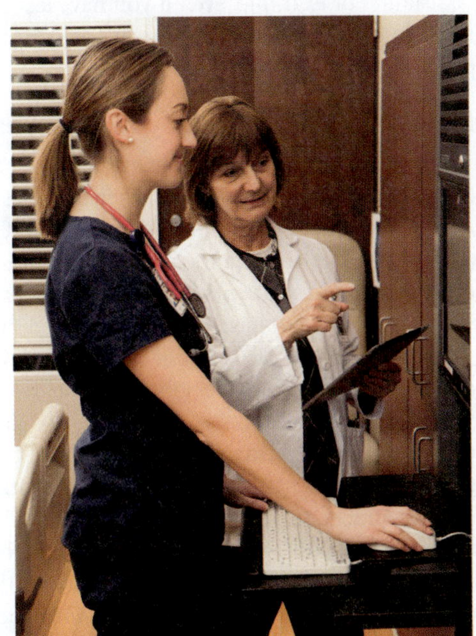

FIGURE 5-1 If an order creates questions, the nurse clarifies it with the physician or health care provider.

It is always important to put the patient's interests first while attempting to maintain a collegial approach in providing the ordered health care treatments. Notifying the appropriate health care provider through the chain of command is a long-standing and accepted practice when resolving an issue related to a questionable order (Karno, 2011).

Make sure that all physician or health care provider orders are in writing, dated and timed appropriately, and transcribed correctly. Verbal or telephone orders are not recommended because they leave possibilities for error. If a verbal or telephone order is necessary in an emergency, make sure that the physician or health care provider writes and signs it as soon as possible, usually within 24 hours (TJC, 2013).

Nursing Students

Nursing students are responsible for all of their actions that cause harm to patients (*Dimora v. Cleveland Clinics Foundation,* 1996). When a patient is injured as a direct result of your actions, you, your instructor, the staff nurses working with you, and the hospital or health care facility may all share the liability for the incorrect action. Faculty members are responsible for instructing and observing their students, but in some situations staff nurses also share these responsibilities. As a nursing student no one should assign you to perform tasks for which you are unprepared. Your instructors should carefully supervise you as you learn new procedures. Every nursing school should provide clear definitions of student responsibility. During the clinical rotation, generally the school liability insurance covers you; however, always check with your school as to the specific coverage.

Sometimes you are employed as a nursing assistant or a nurse's aide when you are not attending classes. When you work as an employee of a health care facility, perform only tasks that appear in a job description for a nurse's aide or nursing assistant. For example, even if you have learned how to administer intramuscular medications as a nursing student, do not perform this task as a nurse's aide.

Patient Abandonment and Delegation Issues

You encounter inadequate staffing during times of nursing shortages and staff downsizing periods when agencies seek to achieve cost containment. The Joint Commission (TJC, 2013) requires institutions to have guidelines for the number of staff needed to care for patients. Liability issues exist if a health care facility does not have enough registered nurses to provide competent and safe care and if a patient is injured as a result of negligent care by any personnel. If you are assigned to care for more patients than is reasonable for safe care, notify your nursing supervisor. If you are required to accept the assignment, document this information in writing and provide the document to nursing administrators. Although documentation does not relieve you of responsibility if patients suffer harm because of inattention, it shows that you attempted to act appropriately. Whenever you document information about short staffing, keep a copy of the document. Do not walk out when staffing is inadequate because this act could be regarded as patient abandonment. It is important to know the policies of your institution and procedures for handling inadequate staffing before such a situation arises. Registered nurses are always responsible for making nursing care judgments based on the nursing process. Even when a registered nurse delegates care to nursing assistive personnel or licensed practical nurses, the nurse maintains responsibility for patient outcomes (Box 5-5).

BOX 5-5 EVIDENCE-BASED PRACTICE

PICO Question: Which relational factors affect the safe delegation of patient care tasks between a registered nurse and a nursing assistant in the care of adults?

SUMMARY OF EVIDENCE

Increases in health care costs coupled with decreases in health care reimbursements and the overall nursing shortage require nurses to more frequently delegate tasks to nursing assistive personnel (NAP). Ambiguous understanding of what is required in appropriate delegation results in inadequate supervision of NAPs and lead to errors and negative patient outcomes.

Seventeen in-depth interviews with baccalaureate-prepared nurses from a variety of acute care settings were conducted to explore the nature and significance of delegation to NAPs (DiMeo and Ballard, 2011). The average number of years of experience in nursing was 8.8 years. Results showed that nurses define delegation in different ways. A racial difference between groups has implications for both relationships and communication between nurses and NAPs. Lack of trust and respect among members of the work group can affect the group process.

APPLICATION TO NURSING PRACTICE

- Delegation is defined as the transfer of responsibility for the performance of an activity from one individual to another while retaining accountability for the outcome.
- Trust and respect are important for nurse-NAP communication.
- Communication in the nurse-NAP relationship affects the quality of patient care.

Nurses within acute and long-term care facilities are often required to "float" from the area in which they normally practice to other nursing units. If you float, inform your supervisor if you lack experience in caring for the types of patients on the new nursing unit. Request an orientation to the unit. When you float you are held to the same standard of care as nurses who regularly work on that unit. A supervisor is liable if a staff nurse is assigned to a patient for whom he or she cannot safely care. In one case the court noted that, if employers float nurses out of their usual work area of practice, the employers need to provide training and education to prepare the nurses to work in the other areas (*Winkelman v. Beloit Memorial Hospital,* 1992).

Controlled Substances

The Comprehensive Drug Abuse Prevention and Control Act (1970) was initiated to control and regulate hospital drug distribution systems of narcotics, antidepressants, hypnotics, sedatives, stimulants, and hallucinogens. You administer controlled substances only under the direction of a licensed physician. However, several states allow advanced practice nurses to prescribe controlled substances.

Controlled substances are securely locked away, and only authorized personnel have access to them. Maintain precise records regarding the dispensing, wasting, and storage of controlled substances. There are criminal penalties for the misuse of controlled substances. There have been cases in which physicians have illegally prescribed and dispensed controlled substances. If you are employed by such a physician and fail to report these activities, you are legally accountable for aiding and abetting the physician.

Reporting Obligations

It is mandatory for health care providers to report incidents such as child, spousal, or elder abuse; rape; gunshot wounds; attempted suicide; and certain communicable diseases. To encourage reports of suspected cases, states provide legal immunity for the reporter if the person makes the report in good faith. Health care professionals who do not report suspected child abuse or neglect are liable for civil or criminal legal action. You are also required to report unsafe or impaired professionals. Because required reporting information varies among states, become familiar with the appropriate statutes in your state and the policies and procedures of your employing health care facility.

KEY POINTS

- Registered nurses are licensed by the state in which they practice.
- Under the law you are required to follow standards of care, which originate in Nurse Practice Acts, the guidelines of professional organizations, and written policies and procedures of employing institutions.
- You are responsible for performing procedures correctly and exercising professional judgment when you carry out physician or health care provider orders.
- All patients are entitled to confidential health care and freedom from unauthorized release of information.
- You are liable for malpractice if the following are established: (1) you (defendant) owed a duty to the patient (plaintiff), (2) you did not carry out or breached that duty, (3) the patient was injured, and (4) your failure to carry out that duty caused the patient's injury.
- Informed consent must meet the following criteria: (1) the person giving consent is competent and of legal age; (2) the consent is given voluntarily; (3) the person giving consent thoroughly understands the procedure, its risks and benefits, and alternative procedures; and (4) the person giving consent has a right to have all questions answered satisfactorily.
- You are obligated to follow a physician's or health care provider's order unless you believe that it is in error, violates hospital policy, or is possibly harmful to a patient, in which case you make a formal report explaining the refusal.
- You file an occurrence report in any unusual situation that will potentially cause harm to a patient; such reports are also for quality improvement and risk management.
- The civil law system is concerned with the protection of a person's private rights, and the criminal law system deals with the rights of individuals and society as defined by legislative statutes.
- Legal issues involving death include documenting all events surrounding the death, treating a deceased person with dignity, and obtaining timely consent for an autopsy from the decedent or close family member.
- A competent adult is able to legally give consent to donate specific organs, and nurses are sometimes able to serve as witnesses to this decision.
- You need to know the laws that apply to your specific area of practice.
- Depending on state laws, nurses are required to report possible criminal activities such as child abuse and certain communicable diseases.

CLINICAL DECISION-MAKING EXERCISES

Review the case study at the beginning of this chapter and answer the following questions. Remember that Lynette Donovan is legally a minor. She is hurt and afraid and in an unfamiliar setting. She may not be comfortable speaking with the health care providers who are present, and her expressions of pain may be modified by her circumstances.

1. Identify the elements of malpractice and how they apply to Lynette Donovan's case.
   a. Who owes a duty to Miss Donovan?
   b. Where would David Ortiz, the nursing student, look to determine whether he owes a duty to Miss Donovan?
   c. What is the standard of care owed to Miss Donovan?
   d. Was the duty to Miss Donovan met?

Lynette Donovan developed gangrene in the right leg. She requires a right below-the-knee amputation.

2. Is Miss Donovan capable of providing consent for this procedure? Which things should be included in the discussion to provide informed consent?
3. David Ortiz is returning from escorting Miss Donovan to the operating room for her procedure. He gets on the elevator, where there are several visitors and two nursing supervisors who are talking about the health care provider who "made Donovan lose her leg."
   a. What are the liability issues here?
   b. Are any laws broken?
   c. What should David Ortiz do?

evolve

Answers to Clinical Decision-Making Exercises can be found on the Evolve website.

QSEN ACTIVITY: SAFETY

David has completed his clinical experience for the day. As the circulation to Miss Donovan's right leg continued to worsen, an amputation of her leg was necessary. Mr. Ortiz observed the surgery and now returns to post-conference. The nursing instructor asks David to describe his experience. When he finishes relating the facts of the case, the instructor asks the group to describe which actions should have been taken by the nursing staff to have a better patient outcome.

If you were a nursing student in this post-conference, identify the actions that you think the nurses should have taken and place them in their order of priority.

evolve

Answers to QSEN Activities can be found on the Evolve website.

REVIEW QUESTIONS

1. Your adult patient is scheduled for an x-ray film of the head. He is refusing to go, despite the fact that the x-ray film will give vital information related to his chief complaint of a headache. The nurse learns of the patient's refusal and comes in to the patient's room saying, "If you don't go to this x-ray, I'll have to give you a shot to put you out." In your opinion, has the nurse committed a legal mistake?
   1. No, the nurse is acting in the best interests of the patient who needs the test to treat him.
   2. No, the nurse is merely trying to help the patient understand the necessity of cooperating with the ordered treatment regimen.
   3. Yes, the nurse may have committed an assault on the patient by verbally threatening him.
   4. Yes, the nurse may have committed malpractice by forcing the patient to do something against his will.
2. A nurse has received a letter from the State Board of Nursing in which he practices that he has been placed on probation and that his license is suspended. The nurse has received no other information about this action. What, if any, claims does this nurse have?
   1. The nurse has a claim against the State Board of Nursing for a violation of his right to privacy.
   2. The nurse has a claim against the State Board of Nursing for violating his rights to due process.
   3. The nurse has a claim against the hospital where he works for failing to represent him in a civil law suit.
   4. The nurse has no claim against the State Board of Nursing and the hospital.
3. A patient's daughter is speaking to the nurse caring for her father. The daughter has presented the nurse with a document identifying her as the spokesperson for the patient when he is no longer capable of speaking for himself. Which of the following best characterizes the daughter's legal relationship with her ailing father?
   1. Health care proxy
   2. Legal Samaritan
   3. Guardian ad litem
   4. Attorney
4. A patient is discussing her surgery with her surgeon. The physician leaves and asks you to have the patient sign the consent form in a few hours. Which statement made by the patient indicates that informed consent has likely been achieved?
   1. The patient states that the doctor has told her there is nothing more they can do and she is going home.
   2. The patient states that she has not spoken with her surgeon at all today.
   3. The patient states that her surgeon has told her that she doesn't need surgery.
   4. The patient states that she is having surgery on her leg in the morning and that she will have some pain and bleeding for a few days.
5. A nurse believes that a pediatric patient has been the victim of abuse based on verbal statements and scarring noted on the patient's abdomen and legs. Which of the following is the best action for the nurse to take?
   1. Do nothing but document the patient's condition
   2. Contact the patient's family
   3. Contact the patient's teacher
   4. Contact the Child Abuse Hotline
6. A health care provider has written an order for a patient to receive a medication every 6 hours for 7 days. You note that the patient has indicated that she is allergic to this medication (rash, shortness of breath). Which of the following should you do first?
   1. Contact the health care provider
   2. Contact the pharmacist
   3. Place a "hold" note on the medication administration record (MAR)
   4. Contact the nursing supervisor
7. A patient's visitor has fallen in the patient's room. Which of the following is the most appropriate action for the nurse to take?
   1. Call the nursing supervisor
   2. Assist the visitor and document with an occurrence report
   3. Assist the visitor and, if there is no injury, document nothing
   4. Assist the visitor and document the occurrence in the patient's chart
8. One of the elements of professional negligence is the failure to act according to the standard of care or breach of duty. Standard of care may best be defined as which of the following? (Select all that apply.)
   1. Nursing competence as defined by the State Nurse Practice Act
   2. Giving nursing care in the most expedient and timely way possible

3. The degree of nursing judgment and skill given by a reasonably prudent nurse under similar circumstances
4. Providing health services according to community expectations and ordinances

9. Although you normally work in a hospital setting, you have volunteered at a homeless shelter at a blood pressure clinic. If an incident occurs at the blood pressure clinic, what is your most likely liability protection provider?
   1. Your employer hospital malpractice insurance
   2. Your home insurance
   3. Your professional liability insurance
   4. No one (There is a small likelihood that a nurse will be sued in this type of situation.)
10. You are the night shift nurse for a hospital nursing division of 40 acutely ill postoperative patients. The staffing for the night shift is you plus two patient care technicians. Based on the end-of-shift report, the current staffing, and your assessment of the patients, you have determined that there is insufficient staff to safely take care of the patients on this nursing division. What is the best action for you to take?
    1. Leave the nursing division immediately and go home
    2. Contact the nursing supervisor, inform him or her of the situation, and leave the nursing division
    3. Contact the chief of medicine and inform her or him of the situation and document it
    4. Contact the nursing supervisor, inform him or her of the situation, and document it.

evolve

Rationales for Review Questions can be found on the Evolve website.

1. 3; **2.** 2; **3.** 1; **4.** 4; **5.** 4; **6.** 3; **7.** 2; **8.** 1, 3, 4; **9.** 3; **10.** 4.

REFERENCES

Agency of Healthcare Research and Quality (AHRQ): *Patient safety primers: never events*, 2012, US Department of Health and Human Services, http://psnet.ahrq.gov/primer.aspx?primerID=3. Accessed August 26, 2013.

American Nurses Association (ANA): *Scope and standards of practice*, ed 2, Silver Spring, MD, 2010, The Association.

American Nurses Association (ANA): *Principles for social networking and the nurse*, Silver Spring, MD, 2011, The Association.

Brous E: Patient rights and ethical considerations. In Grant PD, Ballard DC, editors: *Law for nurse leaders: a comprehensive reference*, New York, 2011, Springer

Brous E, Boulay D, Burger V: The nurse and documentation. In Grant PD, Ballard DC, editors: *Law for nurse leaders: a comprehensive reference*, New York, 2011, Springer.

Carter P: *HIPAA compliance handbook*, Austin, TX, 2013, Wolters Kluwer.

Centers for Medicare and Medicaid Services (CMS): *State Medicaid Director Letter*, SMDL#08-004, July 31, 2008, http://www.downloads.cms.gov/cmsgov/archived-downloads/SMDL/downloads/SMD073108.pdf. Accessed April 10, 2013.

Child Welfare Information Gateway: *2010 Determining the best interests of the child: summary of state laws*, 2010, US Department of Health and Human Services (USDHHS) Child Welfare Information Gateway, https://www.childwelfare.gov/systemwide/laws_policies/statutes/best_interest.cfm. Accesed August 16, 2013.

Grant PD, Ballard DC: *Law for nurse leaders: a comprehensive reference*, New York, 2011, Springer.

Guido G: *Legal and ethical issues in nursing*, ed 5, Upper Saddle River, NJ, 2010, Prentice Hall.

Karno S: Nursing malpractice/negligence and liability. In Grant PD, Ballard DC, editors: *Law for nurse leaders: a comprehensive reference*, New York, 2011, Springer

Mastroianni A, et al: The flaws in state apology and disclosure laws dilute their intended impact on malpractice suits, *Health Affairs* 29(9):1611, 2010.

Miller P: Risk management. In Grant PD, Ballard DC, editors: *Law for nurse leaders: a comprehensive reference*, New York, 2011, Springer.

Missouri State Board of Nursing: *Position statement: patient abandonment*, 2007, http://pr.mo.gov/nursing-focus-position.asp. Accessed August 13, 2013.

National Council of State Boards of Nursing (NCSBN): *White paper: a nurse's guide to the use of social media*, 2011, https://www.ncsbn.org/Social_Media.pdf. Accessed August 16, 2013.

Nurses Service Organization: *Understanding nurse liability, 2006-2010: a three-part approach*, 2011, http://www.nso.com/nurseclaimreport2011/nursing.resources/claim-studies.jsp?refID=nursesclaimreport2011. Accessed October 10, 2013.

Shilling D: *Lawyer's desk book*, Austin, TX, 2011, Wolters Kluwer.

The Joint Commission (TJC): *Standards, information, and requirements*, 2013, http://www.jointcommision.org/standards_information/joint_commission_requirements.aspx. Accessed August 16, 2013.

Statutes

Americans With Disabilities Act, 42 USC §121.010-12213 (1995).

Autopsy Consent, Mo Rev Stat, §194.115 (1998).

Comprehensive Drug Abuse Prevention and Control Act, Pub L No 91-513, 84 Stat §1236 (1970).

Emergency Medical Treatment and Active Labor Act (EMTALA) (1986).

Federal Nursing Home Reform Act (1987).

Health Insurance Portability and Accountability Act of 1996, Pub L No. 104 (1996).

Mental Health Parity Act (1996).

National Organ Transplant Act, Pub L No. 98-507 (1984).

Patient Self-Determination Act, 42 CFR 417 (1991).

Resident's Rights, Medicaid Statute, 42 USCA §1396R (1988).

Uniform Anatomical Gift Act (1987).

Uniform Determination of Death Act (1980).

Cases

Cruzan v. Director Missouri Department of Health, 497 US 261 (1990).

Darling v. Charleston Community Memorial Hospital, 33 Ill2d 326, 331, 211 NE2d 253 (1965).

Dimora v. Cleveland Clinics Foundation, 1996.

In re Intracare Hospital, 2007 WL 2682268 (Tex App, September 13, 2007).

In re Schiller, 148 NJ Super 168 (1977).

Roe v. Wade, 410 US 113 (1973).

Winkelman v. Beloit Memorial Hospital, 484 NW2d 211 (1992).

CHAPTER

6

Ethics

evolve WEBSITE

http://evolve.elsevier.com/Potter/essentials

- Crossword Puzzle
- Audio Glossary

OBJECTIVES

- Discuss the foundations of ethics and ethical practice in nursing.
- Describe and defend patient advocacy and the nurse's role.
- Describe the process for recognizing and resolving an ethical dilemma.

KEY TERMS

advocacy, p. 77
autonomy, p. 76
beneficence, p. 76
bioethics, p. 75
deontology, p. 79
ethical dilemma, p. 78
ethics, p. 74
ethics of care, p. 79
feminist ethics, p. 79
fidelity, p. 76
justice, p. 76
morals, p. 75
multidisciplinary ethics committee, p. 79
nonmaleficence, p. 76
principles of behavior, p. 76
utilitarianism, p. 79
value, p. 75

ETHICS

Nursing knowledge about patients uniquely positions nurses to contribute to patient care decisions, especially when the decisions are difficult or controversial. Your clinical practice is strengthened by your ongoing knowledge about professional standards of practice and the ethical principles that guide the navigation of difficult decisions in health care. Nursing excellence is comprised of elements greater than the sum of your clinical skills. In this chapter you review the ethical foundations that help to shape professional nursing practice.

Ethics refers to the consideration of standards of conduct, particularly the study of right and wrong behavior (*American Heritage Dictionary*, 2011). A fundamental concern of ethics is the effect of our actions on others. The study of ethics includes the study of personal behavior and issues of character such as kindness, tolerance, and generosity. In health care, ethical discourse provides a way to navigate difficult human issues such as suffering, futility, and respect for differences. Ethics helps us to navigate the application of new technologies that may trouble us or challenge our understanding of "normal" or "natural."

Basic Definitions

Ethical issues differ from legal issues. Legal issues are resolved by reference to laws that tend to be concrete and publicly determined. Breaking a law usually results in a public consequence such as a ticket for speeding or jail time for stealing. In Ms. Moreno's case (see the Case Study), age discrimination laws may guide the behavior of the librarians. If Ms. Moreno experiences age discrimination, the librarians could suffer the consequences of breaking a law.

CASE STUDY *Ms. Anna Moreno*

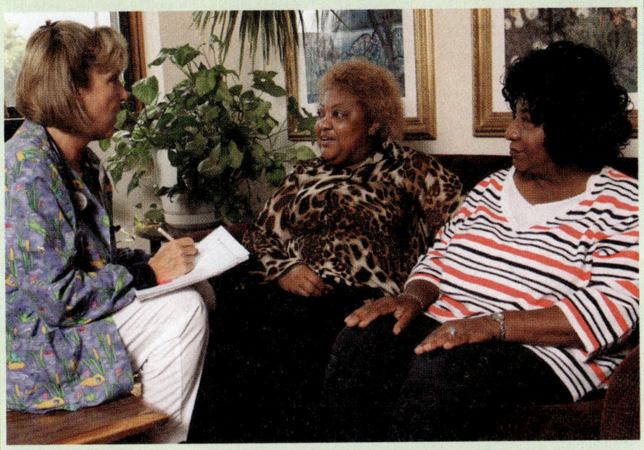

Ms. Anna Moreno is an 82-year-old retired schoolteacher who lives with her grown daughter, Lucille, and Lucille's three teenage children. Ms. Moreno helps with the care of Lucille's children when Lucille is at work. Ms. Moreno has well controlled diabetes and high blood pressure She maintains an active lifestyle; when she's not caring for the children, she volunteers at the library and at her church. However, 3 weeks ago Lucille received a call from the manager of the library where her mother volunteers. The manager described finding Ms. Moreno in the janitor's closet, confused and tearful. The manager also mentioned concerns about Ms. Moreno's diminishing ability to finish simple tasks such as shelving books and taking phone messages. During a recent clinic visit with her mother, Lucille asks the clinic nurse if she would write a letter to Ms. Moreno's manager stating that Ms. Moreno is in excellent health. The nurse asks why they need a letter. On learning more about the reason, the nurse suggests an evaluation of her mother's mental status just to be sure. Lucille becomes defensive and angry. She even accuses the library manager of discrimination against older adults, and she accuses the nurse of jumping to conclusions. She refuses offers of further evaluation for her mother or even to discuss the issues with her. After all, Lucille argues, her mother's blood pressure is normal, and her blood glucose remains well within normal limits. The nurse realizes that this situation is complicated. If Ms. Moreno's cognitive skills are indeed diminished, ethical issues such as privacy and autonomy need to be addressed. The nurse needs the help of others to sort out the best, most ethical response to the situation and to provide individualized patient care.

However, ethics has a broader base of interest than the law, referring more to issues of behavior and character. The terms *ethics* and *morals* sometimes are used interchangeably. **Morals** usually refer to judgment about behavior, and ethics refers to the study of the ideals of right and wrong behavior. In the case study the nurse uses ethical standards of practice to guide her decisions about how to proceed with the issues that she faces with this family.

Values play an important role in understanding ethics. A **value** is a personal belief about the worth a person holds for an idea, a custom, or an object. The values that he or she holds reflect cultural and social influences. For example, if his or her family makes a living in a rural place, the person may value the environment differently from someone who visits rural areas for recreation. Systems of ethics grow from shared values, negotiated and discussed over time through religious groups, ethnic groups, or work groups. As you enter the nursing profession, you undergo a similar process of learning shared values. Your understanding of nursing values and clarity about your own point of view supports you in making effective ethical decisions.

The study of **bioethics** represents a particular branch of ethics (i.e., the study of ethics within the field of health care). The field of bioethics has grown in the last four decades, beginning with the emergence of technologies related to organ transplant. When researchers perfected kidney transplant procedures in the early 1970s, the immediate ethical concern was the limited number of kidneys available compared with the greater number of patients in need of a transplant. The arrival of advanced medical technologies requires society to face difficult ethical questions. Who should get which resources? If quality of life should play a role in the decision, how shall we define it? Who should decide? In the study of bioethics health care professionals agree to negotiate these difficult and important questions (Box 6-1).

Nursing professionals play a vital role in the practice of bioethics since nurses bring a unique point of view into discussion about patient care. They participate in bioethical discussion as professionals and colleagues. As professionals

BOX 6-1 CARE OF THE OLDER ADULT

Protecting Privacy and Autonomy

- Efforts to help older adults remain independent are increasingly enhanced by new monitoring technologies. Devices that transmit clinical information such as blood sugar levels, nutritional intake, or patient distress, including falls, provide new opportunities to increase patient safety and decrease hospitalization or transfer to a nursing home.
- Technologies can impact patient privacy and autonomy. However, privacy concerns are driven ethically by the principal of respect for autonomy and legally by HIPAA statutes. If video images are transmitted to a distant location, is the image protected from public view at the destination? If laboratory results are transmitted digitally, can we ensure that the results are transmitted without risk to exposure to the general public?
- Providers should also consider issues of autonomy. Informed consent to allow electronic monitoring devices might protect patient autonomy but could be complicated by the presence of dementia.
- In an article exploring the use of technology, authors suggest that older adults may be more trusting in part because of a lack of a true understanding of how the technology can help or harm them (Kang et al., 2010). Providers will be able to advocate for patients beyond simply asking permission to use new monitoring devices in the home.

HIPAA, Health Insurance Portability and Accountability Act.

TABLE 6-1 PRINCIPLES OF HEALTH CARE ETHICS

PRINCIPLE	DEFINITION
Autonomy	Independence; self-determination; self-reliance
Justice	Fairness or equity
Fidelity	Faithfulness; striving to keep promises
Beneficence	Actively seeking benefits; promotion of good
Nonmaleficence	Actively seeking to do no harm

nurses abide by a professional code of ethics that reflects and defines practice. As colleagues in health, they bring a specific point of view to ethical discussions about health care issues.

Ethical Principles

Practitioners in health care delivery agree to a set of ethical principles that guide professional practice and decision making. These principles are common to all professions in health care. You will find these principles especially useful because they guide your commitment to advocacy, an important concept in caring for others (Table 6-1).

Autonomy refers to a person's independence. As a principle in bioethics, autonomy represents an agreement to respect a patient's right to determine a course of action. For example, before surgery a patient is required to sign a consent form. The purpose of the consent is to ensure in writing that the health care team respects the patient's independence by obtaining his or her permission to proceed. Respect for autonomy becomes complicated when the patient is a child or when he or she is cognitively impaired by disease, age, or trauma. Although the health care team turns to whoever is identified as legally responsible for the patient, the ethical goal remains to try to determine the best interests of the patient from the patient's point of view.

Justice refers to the principle of fairness. In health care the term reflects a commitment to fair treatment and fair distribution of health care resources. You may find reference to this principle during discussion about issues of access to care. It is not always clear just how to achieve a fair distribution of resources. Access to care remains uneven in the United States, with certain groups better able to find and afford health care than others. For example, according to the most recent National Healthcare Disparities report, poor people received worse care than high-income people for about 80% of core measures (AHRQ, 2011) (Box 6-2).

Fidelity refers to the agreement to keep promises and is based on the virtue of caring. The principle of fidelity also promotes your obligation as a nurse to follow through with the care offered to patients. For example, if you assess a patient for pain and then offer a plan to manage the pain, the principle of fidelity encourages you to do your best to provide follow-up that includes continuous reevaluation of pain levels. In this way you keep your promise to improve patient comfort.

The principle of **beneficence** promotes taking positive, active steps to help others. It encourages you to do good for a patient and guides decisions in which the benefits of a treatment pose a risk to the patient's well-being or dignity. A child's immunization causes discomfort during administration; but the benefits of protection from disease, for both the individual and society, outweigh the temporary discomforts. The agreement to act with beneficence shows compassion and requires that the best interest of a patient remains more important than self-interest. For example, you do not simply obey medical orders, but you also act thoughtfully to understand patient needs and then work actively to help meet those needs.

Nonmaleficence refers to the fundamental agreement to do no harm. It is closely related to the principle of beneficence. This principle is helpful in guiding your discussions about new or controversial technologies. For example, a bone marrow transplant procedure may promise a chance at cure, but what if the long-term prognosis is uncertain or the procedure requires long periods of pain and suffering? You consider these risks in relation to the potential good that may come from the procedure. The principle of nonmaleficence promotes a continuing effort to consider the potential for harm even when it is necessary to promote health.

Codes of Ethics

The American Nurses Association (ANA) and the International Council of Nurses (ICN) publish codes of ethics for nurses that set **principles of behavior** for them to embrace. They reflect common underlying principles (Box 6-3) that shape professional nursing practice, including responsibility, accountability, respect for confidentiality, competency, judgment, and advocacy.

Responsibility refers to the performance of duties associated with a nurse's role, including characteristics of reliability and dependability. For example, when administering a medication, you are responsible for assessing a patient's need for the medication, giving it safely and correctly, and evaluating the patient's response to it. By agreeing to act responsibly, you gain trust from patients, colleagues, and society.

Accountability refers to the ability to answer for your actions. You are accountable to yourself. You also balance accountability to patients, the profession, your employer, and society. You exercise moral accountability when making a reasoned judgment about what is right and then act accordingly. *For example, to best serve the interests of Ms. Moreno and her family, the nurse knows that she will need to do more than simply refuse to write a letter. The goal is the promotion of health and advocacy for Ms. Moreno.* The principle that guides the nurse is the principle of accountability.

A responsible nurse is competent in knowledge and skills. In the practice of nursing, competence ensures the provision of safe nursing care. The agreement to practice with competence is a common denominator for all state regulations and is in the nursing code of ethics. For example, you ensure that you are competent in your knowledge of the risks and

BOX 6-2 EVIDENCE-BASED PRACTICE

PICOT Question: For nonwhite or poor patients in the United States, is access to health care services compared to that for white or high-income patients getting better or worse over time?

In health care we commit to the principle of justice (i.e., to finding a way to ensure fair distribution of services). The commitment is clearly articulated in the American Nurses Association (ANA) code of ethics. The fact that access to care remains uneven in the United States presents us with an ethical problem. Although solutions may be complex and controversial, as members of the health care team we remain professionally committed to seeking a solution.

SUMMARY OF EVIDENCE

To help track the status of access to care in the United States, the federal Agency for Healthcare Research and Quality conducts an annual analysis of clinical outcomes in the United States. The report is mandated by the U.S. Congress. The results provide metrics for pilot programs and policy makers to measure effectiveness of efforts to resolve this ethical issue.

According to recent results (AHRQ, 2011), health care quality and access remain "unequal and suboptimal, especially for minority and low-income groups." Although overall quality is improving, access and disparities are not. As the report explains, "Urgent attention is warranted." The report highlights certain services, geographical areas, and populations that warrant immediate attention:

- Cancer screening and management of diabetes
- States in the central part of the country
- Residents of inner-city and rural areas
- Disparities in preventive services and access to care

Disparities in quality of care are common:

- Blacks, American Indians, and Alaska Natives received worse care than whites for approximately 40% of core measures.
- Asians received worse care than whites for approximately 20% of core measures.
- Hispanics received worse care than non-Hispanic whites for approximately 60% of core measures.
- Poor people received worse care than high-income people for approximately 80% of core measures.

Disparities in access are also common, especially among Hispanics and poor people:

- Blacks had worse access to care than whites for one third of core measures.
- Asians, American Indians, and Alaska Natives had worse access to care than whites for one of five core measures.
- Hispanics had worse access to care than non-Hispanic whites for five of six core measures.
- Poor people had worse access to care than high-income people for all six core measures.

APPLICATION TO NURSING PRACTICE

The Association of Black Nursing (ABNF) faculty provides a model for the application of this evidence to nursing practice.

- By means of its newsletter distributed broadly online encouraging nurses to promote the role of nurses in alleviating issues of access to care: "Professional nurses and nurse educators are uniquely qualified to address patient care effectiveness, patient safety, timeliness, patient-centered care, and access to care" (Edwards, 2011).
- Participate actively in health care reform: "ABNF members and its leadership are committed to eradicating health disparities in our respective communities and eliminating unequal treatment of minority nursing faculty and students in schools and colleges of nursing. With your participation and active involvement, we can make this dream of today a reality of tomorrow" (Edwards, 2011).
- Attend conferences to learn and discuss more about disparities in access to health care: "Teaching Clinical Nursing and Conducting Research in an Era of Healthcare Reform" (Edwards, 2011).

---

benefits of medications before you administer them. Because you are competent, the patient can trust that the medications you offer are safe.

Judgment refers to the ability to form an opinion or draw sound conclusions. To practice critical thinking, you learn to practice good judgment in nursing school (see Chapter 8). You continue to improve your judgment skills throughout your career.

Advocacy involves speaking up for patient care issues from your unique perspective and advocating for humane and dignified care. Patient care problems can arise from systems that affect your ability to deliver safe care or from specific clinical situations that affect patient outcomes. You can exercise advocacy in many ways, depending on your responsibilities and your relationship to patients. But the exercise of advocacy begins with your willingness to articulate your point of view. You get to know your patients while performing intimate tasks such as special procedures, teaching new skills, preparing for discharge. These activities allow you to witness patient characteristics unlike any other members of the health care team. As a result, you gain unique information about patients that can be essential to the success of the overall plan of care.

High on the list of elements in the ANA code of ethics is the promise to "promote, advocate for, and strive to protect the health, safety, and rights of the patient." A fundamental right of patients is the right to privacy. Privacy becomes a focus of increasing interest as health care becomes digitized. Federal legislation known as the Health Insurance Portability and Accountability Act of 1996, commonly called *HIPAA*, was designed in anticipation of electronic medical records and the resulting increased vulnerability of personal health information. HIPAA legislation requires that those with access to personal health information not disclose the information to a third party without patient consent, with few exceptions, and sets fines for violations (U.S. Department of

BOX 6-3 THE ICN CODE OF ETHICS FOR NURSES

PREAMBLE

Nurses have four fundamental responsibilities: to promote health, prevent illness, restore health, and alleviate suffering. The need for nursing is universal. Inherent in nursing is respect for human rights, including cultural rights and the right to life and choice, to dignity, and to be treated with respect. Nursing care is respectful of and unrestricted by considerations of age, colour, creed, culture, disability or illness, gender, sexual orientation, nationality, politics, race, or social status. Nurses render health services to the individual, the family, and the community and coordinate their services with those of related groups.

ELEMENTS OF THE CODE

1. Nurses and People

The nurse's primary professional responsibility is to people requiring nursing care. In providing care the nurse promotes an environment in which the human rights, values, customs, and spiritual beliefs of the individual, family, and community are respected. The nurse ensures that the individual receives sufficient information on which to base consent for care and related treatment. The nurse holds in confidence personal information and uses judgment in sharing this information. The nurse shares with society the responsibility for initiating and supporting action to meet the health and social needs of the public, in particular those of vulnerable populations. The nurse advocates for equity and social justice in resource allocation, access to health care, and other social and economic services. The nurse demonstrates professional values such as respectfulness, responsiveness, compassion, trustworthiness, and integrity.

2. Nurses and Practice

The nurse carries personal responsibility and accountability for nursing practice and for maintaining competence by continual learning. The nurse maintains a standard of personal health such that the ability to provide care is not compromised. The nurse uses judgment regarding individual competence when accepting and delegating responsibility. The nurse at all times maintains standards of personal conduct that reflect well on the profession and enhance public confidence. In providing care the nurse ensures that use of technology and scientific advances is compatible with the safety, dignity, and rights of people. The nurse strives to foster and maintain a practice culture promoting ethical behaviour and open dialogue.

3. Nurses and the Profession

The nurse assumes the major role in determining and implementing acceptable standards of clinical nursing practice, management, research, and education. The nurse is active in developing a core of research-based professional knowledge. The nurse is active in developing and sustaining a core of professional values. The nurse, acting through the professional organization, participates in creating and maintaining safe, equitable social and economic working conditions in nursing. The nurse practices to sustain and protect the natural environment and is aware of its consequences on health. The nurse contributes to an ethical organizational environment and challenges unethical practices and settings.

4. Nurses and Co-workers

The nurse sustains a collaborative and respectful relationship with co-workers in nursing and other fields. The nurse takes appropriate action to safeguard individuals, families, and communities when their health is endangered by a co-worker or any other person. The nurse takes appropriate action to support and guide co-workers to advance ethical conduct.

From International Council of Nurses: The *ICN code of ethics for nurses*, 2012, http://www.icn.ch/images/stories/documents/about/icncode_english. Accessed February 2013.
ICN, International Council of Nurses.

Health and Human Services, 1996). For example, sharing information is not prohibited when it is critical to the care of a patient and the recipient is another provider, a payer, or public health officer obligated to track public health concerns such as instances of tuberculosis or suspected child abuse. Even family members or friends of a patient are not permitted access to the patient's personal health information without the patient's consent. Frontline nurses are often called on to share clinical information with families and friends of patients. Therefore keeping track of patient preferences is critical to an ethical respect for privacy and confidentiality. Increasingly patients are queried on admission to a hospital about preferences for who can and cannot receive personal health information, and the responses are entered into the health record. Having this information in the medical record can be a great help to frontline nurses.

Developing a Personal Point of View

The ability to clarify and express your own point of view helps you to adhere to a professional code of ethics. Your point of view is shaped by your personal values. Values vary among people and change over time. Understanding your own values and acknowledging the values of others help to resolve conflict during decision making.

An **ethical dilemma** exists when the right thing to do is not clear or when members of the health care team cannot agree on the right thing to do. Ethical dilemmas require negotiation of differing points of view. Once you clarify your own point of view, you can turn to the patient and begin to clarify your understanding of the patient's point of view. If ethical problems arise, a clear understanding of the patient's point of view helps you speak for the patient even if your own point of view differs.

In the case study an ethical dilemma is taking shape. Ms. Moreno may be experiencing age discrimination at the library. But if declining health is the real cause of her problem, the daughter's hostility will delay proper evaluation. The clinic nurse is in a position to advocate for several competing points of view, including that of Ms. Moreno herself.

When the situation concerns issues of health, personal habits, and quality of life, all participants in a discussion benefit from clarity about personal values and a willingness to look beyond personal preferences for shared values. Your respect for the point of view of others, especially when it differs from your own, is a critical ingredient in the successful navigation of ethical deliberation.

ETHICAL SYSTEMS

Traditional theories of ethics provide a foundation for navigating ethical problems in health care (Beauchamp and Childress, 2008). This section contains descriptions of several common ethical philosophies that overlap in some areas and compete in others. In your everyday work as a nurse, you may encounter discussions that refer to one or another of these philosophies. Your personal values, personal experiences, and relationships with others influence which of these or which combination of them helps you to navigate ethical issues in your daily life.

Deontology

This system of ethics is perhaps most familiar to health care practitioners. **Deontology** defines actions as right or wrong based on "right-making characteristics" such as truth and justice (Beauchamp and Childress, 2008). It proposes that to evaluate an ethical situation we should determine the presence or absence of autonomy, justice, fidelity, beneficence, and nonmaleficence in a situation (see Table 6-1). We then use this determination as a guide for decisions about right action. If an act is just, respects autonomy, and provides good, the act is ethical. Difficulty arises when a person must choose between conflicting principles or when people do not agree on definitions of the principles.

Utilitarianism

You use a utilitarian ethic when determining the value of something based primarily on its usefulness. The greatest good for the greatest number of people is the guiding principle for action in this system. As with deontology, **utilitarianism** relies on the application of the principles of "good" and "greatest." Difficulties arise when people have conflicting definitions of "greatest good." The fundamental difference between utilitarianism and deontology lies in the focus on consequences or outcomes. Utilitarianism guides us to measure the effect, or consequences, that an act will have. By comparison, deontology focuses less on consequences and looks to the presence of pure principle.

Feminist Ethics

In the early 1980s prominent thinkers held that men more commonly reached higher stages of moral development than women (Kohlberg, 1981). He proposed that moral development occurs in measurable, predictable stages, reaching its highest stage with a sense of justice. Kohlberg's studies showed that young girls did not reach this stage as often as young boys. Carol Gilligan's groundbreaking work (1993) argued that Kohlberg's definitions were gender biased. She attempted to respect gender differences without valuing one gender over the other. She suggested that young girls pay more attention to community and young boys pay more attention to abstract ideals or principles. Her focus on community and women provided a foundation for the ethics of care that followed.

Feminist ethics proposes that we routinely ask how ethical decisions will affect women as a way to repair a history of inequality (Lindeman, 2005). For example, in a discussion regarding the ethics of fetal surgery (surgical intervention before birth of the child), feminist ethics proposes that we take into consideration the effect on both the mother and the fetus.

Ethics of Care

Proponents of ethics of care pay special attention to nursing practice. Pioneers in ethics of care included nursing scholars Jean Watson, Madeleine Leininger, and Sara Frys. As Leininger stated, caring is the "central and unifying domain for the body of knowledge and practices in nursing." (McCance, McKenna, and Boore, 1999). However, its principles apply to all members of a health care community, not just nurses (see Chapter 4). Nurses base their work in caring for patients, their families, and the maintenance of the institutions that provide health care services. **Ethics of care** suggest that health care workers resolve ethical dilemmas by paying attention to relationships and stories of the participants and by the promoting a fundamental act of caring. Attention to relationships distinguishes the ethics of care from other ethical viewpoints because it does not necessarily apply universal principles that are intellectual or analytical (McCance et al., 1999).

HOW TO PROCESS AN ETHICAL DILEMMA

Ethical problems are distressing for patients and caregivers. A guide for processing ethical dilemmas, based on ethical principles and shaped by the ANA code of ethics, serves to protect individual points of view while promoting resolution.

Most health care institutions establish a **multidisciplinary ethics committee** to process ethical dilemmas with representatives from nursing, medicine, and other professional disciplines and from the community. Ethics committees provide education, policy recommendation, and case consultation or review. Any involved person, including nurses or other health care providers, patients, and even families of patients, can request access to an ethics committee.

Ethical issues can be processed in settings other than by committee. Nurses provide insight about ethical problems at family conferences, staff meetings, or even in one-on-one meetings with patients.

Whether you resolve an ethical dilemma in a committee setting, at the bedside, or in a family conference, you apply a careful processing of the dilemma (Box 6-4). Resolving an ethical dilemma is similar to the nursing process because it requires systematic processing. The case study offers an illustration of a standardized process for resolving an ethical dilemma.

BOX 6-4 HOW TO PROCESS AN ETHICAL DILEMMA: MS. MORENO

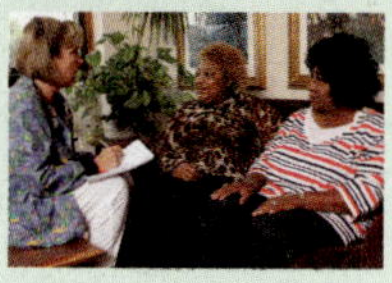

STEP 1. IS THIS AN ETHICAL DILEMMA?

- If a review of scientific data does not resolve the question, the question is perplexing, and an ethical dilemma exists.
- In the case study the nurse is perplexed. She cannot write a letter about Ms. Moreno's state of health without knowing more, but Ms. Moreno's daughter refuses to seek more information.

STEP 2. GATHER ALL INFORMATION RELEVANT TO THE CASE.

- Gathering facts is critical to an effective decision. An overlooked fact sometimes provides quick resolution or affects the options available. Patient, family, institutional, and social perspectives are important sources of relevant information.
- In the Ms. Moreno's case psychosocial information about her daughter and her daughter's children might shed important light.

STEP 3. EXAMINE AND DETERMINE YOUR OWN VALUES AND OPINIONS ABOUT THE ISSUES.

- Taking this step ensures that you can distinguish between your personal values and those of the other participants and allows you to become a more open listener.
- If you were the clinic nurse in the case study, how would you feel about elder care, child care, working mothers?

STEP 4. STATE THE PROBLEM CLEARLY.

- A clear, simple statement of the dilemma is not always easy but facilitates next steps.
- The immediate dilemma in the case study involves the need to validate Ms. Moreno's competence.

STEP 5. CONSIDER POSSIBLE COURSES OF ACTION.

- To respect all sides of an issue, it is helpful to list potential actions, especially when the list will reflect opinions that conflict.
- In the case study actions might include consulting with a social worker and a neurologist. Eventually the course of action will involve decisions about Ms. Moreno's ability to continue her work at the library.

STEP 6. NEGOTIATE THE OUTCOME.

- Sometimes courses of action that seem unlikely at the beginning of the process take on new possibility as they are put into consideration. Negotiation requires a confidence in your own point of view and a deep respect for the opinions of others.
- For Ms. Moreno and her family, effective negotiation with Ms. Moreno's daughter is critical to a positive outcome.

STEP 7. EVALUATE THE ACTION.

- The last step in resolving an ethical dilemma involves evaluating the outcomes. Do the interventions provide for compromise that is acceptable to all? An ethical dilemma is often complicated emotionally; thus it is helpful to review the original issues to ensure that the process has worked.
- For Ms. Moreno, even though the dilemma arose around the request for a letter, other issues were identified and addressed during the process: Ms. Moreno's possible mental decline, child care issues for Ms. Moreno's grandchildren, and the fact that her daughter Lucille was refusing outside help. Because the nurse gathered all the facts and included others in the process, the resolution was effective and satisfying both clinically and ethically.

Step 1: Is this an ethical dilemma?

The first step guides you to determine if the problem is an ethical one. You will learn to distinguish ethical problems from questions of procedure, legality, or medical diagnosis.

In the case study the nurse faces a difficult decision. She may share the daughter's concerns about age discrimination at the library, but at this point she cannot be sure about their accuracy. As the ANA code of ethics states, the nurse's primary commitment is to the patient. In keeping with that commitment, she wants to secure a proper evaluation for Ms. Moreno, but the daughter is adamantly against that. The situation is frustrating, and the right course of action is not immediately clear.

Step 2: Gather all relevant information.

Accurate and complete information is essential for the ethical process to go forward. Sometimes gathering information actually resolves the situation without further deliberation.

In this case the nurse already knows some information about Ms. Moreno, but what about the grandchildren? What about Lucille's job situation? Perhaps most important of all, what does Ms. Moreno understand about her situation, and what does she want to do about it?

Step 3: Examine and determine your own values and opinions about the issues.

The distinction between personal opinion and the opinions of others is essential to reach resolution. People reach different conclusions about the same situation with no malice intended toward other people. Remembering this helps you to be an effective participant.

Lucille could be correct about discrimination at the library. More likely she is overreacting to the situation. She may even be in denial about her mother's health because the loss of her mother's help with the children will affect her ability to keep her job. But the ability to process a dilemma requires that personal values be clear and that you strive to understand and accept the values of others, even when they differ from your own.

Step 4: State the problem clearly.

After reviewing relevant information, develop a statement of the problem. Discussions are more likely to remain focused and constructive when all parties agree on a statement of the problem.

In this case the problem is that Ms. Moreno is experiencing a loss of dignity for reasons that are not yet clear and the daughter is reluctant to pursue a clinical evaluation. What is the best thing to do to ensure Ms. Moreno's health and dignity?

Step 5: Consider possible courses of action.

In trying to resolve a dilemma, it can help to list the possible actions, even if you are not sure which is right.

In this case the nurse and Ms. Moreno's health care provider propose a meeting, seeking Lucille and Ms. Moreno's permission to include the librarian and a social worker. A representative from the clinic ethics committee offers to serve as a moderator. Lucille and her mother agree and request that their pastor also attend.

Step 6: Negotiate the outcome.

A constructive discussion unfolds. At one point Ms. Moreno asks about her husband. Lucille reminds her that her husband died 5 years ago. Ms. Moreno becomes agitated, confused by Lucille's comment. Later she falters speaking to the pastor, unable to recall his name. In the safe environment of the group meeting, Lucille begins to realize that her mother's condition is worse than she had understood. Tears fall, and she is practically unable to speak.

During the discussion that follows the group negotiates an agreeable outcome. The social worker and the health care provider will help Lucille obtain family leave from work so she can take care of the issues that affect her family situation: financial constraints, care of the children, care of Ms. Moreno, confidentiality, consent (how much does Ms. Moreno understand? can she realistically consent to medical procedures?).

The nurse creates a timeline of upcoming clinic visits. She includes family education about Ms. Moreno's diabetes and hypertension. The pastor ends the meeting with a prayer, which brings great comfort to the family.

Step 7: Evaluate the action.

The immediate issue of Ms. Moreno's clinical condition will be addressed, which is a successful outcome. The long range plan of care will require ongoing evaluation for its clinical and social effectiveness. In seeing this situation through to a positive outcome, the nurse has sustained her ethical commitment to "protect the health, safety, and rights of the patient" (ANA, 2001).

ETHICAL ISSUES IN NURSING

The following section describes examples of ethical dilemmas from a variety of health care settings.

End-of-Life Issues

Working with chronically ill or disabled patients involves decisions about quality of life such as a patient's ability to maintain independence and functional status. For example, you are assigned to care for a patient who is permanently disabled by a recent stroke, dependent on others for all his care, and unable to communicate meaningfully. During your shift as you are providing nourishment by mouth, he begins to aspirate, coughing and sputtering. The health care provider suggests a gastrostomy tube to prevent aspiration. The tube would probably diminish the aspiration risks, but you find that you are concerned that it would prolong the life of a patient who has no hope for recovery.

Step 1: Is this an ethical dilemma?

The decision about the gastrostomy tube is a difficult one, without an obvious right or wrong answer. The clinical issues about aspiration pneumonia may be clear, but they are not enough to help providers make a determination regarding suffering. What about the ethical issues concerning quality of life? How can the degree of suffering for both patient and family be measured? Since the patient is profoundly disabled by the stroke, the value and purpose of a gastrostomy tube becomes more complicated.

Step 2: Gather all the information relevant to the case.

What is the prognosis for this patient? What is the family perception of the prognosis? What are the religious or spiritual concerns of the family, and how do they describe the spiritual concerns of the patient? What are the surgical risks and benefits from placement of the gastrostomy tube? What is the medical risk for aspiration pneumonia in this patient before and after tube placement? Would pneumonia and the treatment represent an uncomfortable experience for the patient? Does the patient have a living will or advance directive, or has the patient assigned medical power of attorney to another person?

Step 3: Examine and determine your own values and opinions on the issues.

You could begin your examination by exploring personal feelings about the role of quality of life in medical decisions such as this one. Trying to understand the values of the patient and the patient's family is also important. What is your opinion about the competence of the patient? The competence of the family? If a decision is made with which you disagree, could you still participate in the care of the patient?

Step 4: State the problem clearly.

Will a gastrostomy tube improve the quality of this patient's life, or will it prolong suffering? How can the team best respect this patient's autonomy?

Step 5: Consider possible courses of action.

The first course of action entails further discussion to help answer these questions, since answers will be shaped by a blend of subjective and objective opinion. The outcome of the discussion would determine possible next steps. If the gastrostomy tube is placed, you would work to support the education of the family about care of the tube. If the patient and family decide against insertion of a gastrostomy tube, you might take this as a sign that end-of-life care is taking place and work to ensure that a referral to hospice care is made to provide continued support for the patient and family. In any case, your actions reflect a commitment for compassion for the patient unrestricted by the nature of the health problem (ANA, 2001).

Step 6: Negotiate the outcome.

Since the patient is not competent to participate, the health care team will have to rely on family members, significant others, or even legal documents to negotiate an outcome. Your role in the negotiations would include the contribution of your clinical assessment of the patient. You would also be able to provide insights about family dynamics based on your nursing observations.

Step 7: Evaluate the action.

Regardless of the decision, ongoing discussion with the family would ensure ongoing resolution to this difficult ethical situation.

Cultural and Religious Sensitivity

The professional standards of justice and beneficence require respect for cultural differences in the health care setting, regardless of your personal opinion or feeling. Occasionally you will face a situation in which religious beliefs precipitate an ethical dilemma. For example, you are taking care of a 15-year-old girl, admitted for management of her leukemia. Her religious beliefs do not allow her to receive blood transfusions, yet her condition will soon require a blood transfusion to prevent harmful consequences. Her parents share her religious convictions but are willing to compromise. The 15-year-old refuses to compromise.

Step 1: Is this an ethical dilemma?

The case is perplexing because respecting the patient's autonomy conflicts with the health care team's wish to do no harm and with the parents' willingness to compromise. The resolution of this dilemma will be difficult with profound consequences, regardless of the decision.

Step 2: Gather all the information relevant to the case.

How soon does the patient need the transfusion? Could her anemia be corrected by transfusion alternatives? What are the legal definitions of "minor" in your state? What are the specific religious constraints against blood transfusions that affect this case? Is the patient competent and fully aware of the consequences of her decision to refuse the transfusion?

Step 3: Examine and determine your own values and opinions about the issues.

How do you feel about this patient's religious beliefs? How close or distant are the patient's beliefs from your personal beliefs? What is your personal opinion about the ability of minors to understand and determine their medical course?

Step 4: State the problem clearly.

A patient who is a minor refuses a lifesaving transfusion on the grounds of religious belief. If she is forced to receive the transfusion, which might require restraints or physical force, her dignity will be compromised, and she will consider herself violated in the eyes of her God. If she does not receive the transfusion, she will probably not survive. Should the transfusion proceed in spite of the patient's refusal?

Step 5: Consider possible courses of action.

The health care team could respect the patient's wishes, in spite of the parents' position, by not giving the blood transfusion. The health care team could force the patient to receive a transfusion, with support from the parents, understanding that this act would likely require restraints or use of physical force. You could encourage the patient and her family to explore this dilemma with the guidance of a religious leader from their faith.

Step 6: Negotiate the outcome.

A patient care conference with the patient and her family is necessary. Your contribution, as this patient's nurse, would include your assessment of the patient's state of mind. If the medical team insists on the transfusion, they may decide to seek a court order, especially if the parents decide to support their daughter's wishes to refuse a transfusion. As advocate for the patient, even in the face of personal disagreement, you ensure that the patient's voice is fairly represented.

Step 7: Evaluate the action.

The outcome will depend on the agreement reached by conference participants. The goal will be to balance respect for autonomy with the principle of beneficence. In any case, in spite of the complexities of this case, you remain engaged with the resolution of the dilemma, guided by your commitment to "compassion and respect for the inherent dignity, worth, and uniqueness of every individual, unrestricted by considerations of social or economic status, personal attributes, or the nature of health problems" (ANA, 2001).

Social Networking Online

The development of online communication tools such as Facebook, Twitter, and LinkedIn provides great benefits for nurses; but the benefits exist alongside great risks. On one hand communication can be enhanced by online sites that promote messaging between nurses who work together but whose paths rarely cross. Socializing in this way can help to build unit cohesion. Researchers who work with clinical subjects are more likely to be able to track down people of interest to enrich a research project. Interactive online patient education can provide helpful links between patients and providers. Online sites can provide help for patients between hospitalizations or clinic visits, especially for patients who live long distances from their providers.

However, on the downside the risk of exposure of private information is tremendous. And perhaps even more important, professionalism itself can be jeopardized when nurses indiscriminately share their feelings and opinions in online public venues.

For example, you know about a Facebook site established for your work unit. You and your colleagues use it to post news about work-related classes, parties, and important social milestones such as marriages or births. At the end of a long shift during which a patient happened to die unexpectedly and two nurses called in sick, you notice that a colleague has posted a message describing the "terrible shift" she had to endure, including some details about the nurses who called in sick and the increased patient load. You realize that, since you have been "friended" by people outside the work area, these comments could also become visible to others who do not work on your unit and who are not nurses. You want to support your fellow nurses, but you worry that outsiders will have access to information that should remain private.

Step 1: Is this an ethical dilemma?

At this point, if your workplace does not have a policy that addresses online practices, a common understanding of right actions is lacking. Without common understanding you all remain perplexed. You and your colleagues will benefit from processing the situation as an ethical issue.

Step 2: Gather information relevant to the situation.

You could contact nurses at other facilities to learn about their policies for online social networking. You could conduct an Internet search for articles or other postings about health care providers and social networking. The ANA has published a position statement regarding social networking (ANA, 2011). In addition, the National Council for State Boards of Nursing has developed a white paper outlining suggested safe practices (NCSBN, 2011).

Step 3: Determine your own values about social networking among health care providers.

Issues of patient privacy are concerns that you will be eager to respect. But of equal concern is the issue of professionalism. On the one hand you may value a venue that allows for "venting" and team building. But what about patients who see the Facebook comments? Even if the comments are accurate and patient identifiers are eliminated, patients who see these comments will be affected, perhaps losing faith in the quality of nursing care on your unit or becoming concerned for favorite nurses and their well-being. These reactions to the online networking may be less visible to you at first, but a review of your own values will help to clarify the options and the resolution.

Step 4: State the problem clearly.

Is social networking that is safe and truly private a possibility in health care settings, or will guidelines that prohibit online networking become necessary to protect patient and workplace privacy?

Step 5: Consider possible course of action.

Upon researching the issue online and with other colleagues, you determine that your workplace will also benefit from clear, precise guidelines.

Step 6: Negotiate the outcome.

You offer to serve on a task force that will develop guidelines for your nursing colleagues and other providers in your workplace.

Step 7: Evaluate the action.

Since social networking remains an evolving technology, you might propose that nurses sponsor annual public discourse about the possibilities, risks, and benefits. By supporting open discussion about the issues, you ensure continuing evaluation of whatever guidelines you develop. Your actions are guided by your ethical responsibility for "articulating nursing values, for maintaining the integrity of the profession and its practice, and for shaping social policy" (ANA, 2001).

A systematic methodology for resolution of ethical dilemmas helps all participants gain a common understanding. Ethical dilemmas present great challenges. As a nurse you provide a unique, valuable voice to the process of resolution.

KEY POINTS

- Principles of ethics include autonomy, justice, fidelity, beneficence, and nonmaleficence.
- A professional code of ethics guides nursing practice.
- Professional nursing promotes accountability, responsibility, and advocacy.
- An ethical nurse maintains competence in practice and assumes responsibility for nursing judgments.
- The primary goal of advocacy is to support patient well-being.
- Professional nurses promote their commitment to patients, the profession, and society to provide high-quality health care.
- Ethical issues arise from differences in values, changing professional roles, and technological advances that challenge commonly held notions of health and well-being.
- A standardized structure for processing ethical dilemmas helps to resolve difficult situations.
- The nurse's point of view provides a unique and valuable voice in the resolution of ethical dilemmas.

CLINICAL DECISION-MAKING EXERCISES

In the case study at the beginning of this chapter, the patient's daughter asked the clinic nurse to protect her mother's library job by vouching for the patient's well-being. At the same time the daughter refused an assessment of her mother's cognitive condition.

1. The nurse decided to investigate further into the patient's situation, even though neither the patient nor the patient's daughter asked for further help. Describe the ethical and professional principles that justify the nurse's decision to take action.
2. If you were responsible for organizing a patient care conference or ethical consultation for Ms. Moreno, which disciplines besides your own would you consider including? List at least two and explain why you would include them.
3. Based on the case study concerning Ms. Moreno's care and the nurse's role in her care, list three basic principles of ethics that guided the nurse in this story. Show how the nurse's actions illustrate each principle.

evolve

Answers to Clinical Decision-Making Exercises can be found on the Evolve website.

QSEN ACTIVITY: INFORMATICS

Ms. Moreno's daughter, Lucille, is concerned that her mother does not always remember all the information and teaching given to her by her health care provider. Lucille accompanies her mother on her next visit to the health care provider. Ms. Moreno's health care provider's office just implemented an electronic health record. Lucille asks you if she can read her mother's health record to make sure she is knowledgeable about her mother's condition.

What is your best response for Lucille?

evolve

Answers to QSEN Activities can be found on the Evolve website.

REVIEW QUESTIONS

1. Ethical dilemmas often arise over a conflict of opinions. Each of the following steps constitutes a correct step to take toward resolution of an ethical dilemma. Indicate the order in which these steps should be taken.
   1. Clarify your own values about the issue.
   2. Call a meeting in which those involved in the dilemma can discuss (negotiate) the possible solutions to the dilemma.
   3. State the problem clearly in a way that all involved can understand.
   4. Gather all relevant information regarding the clinical, social, and spiritual aspects of the dilemma.
2. According to annual assessments performed by the Federal Government, certain groups of people in the United States have poor or no access to health care. You decide to write an editorial to your local newspaper expressing your opinion about this situation. Which ethical principle would you incorporate into your editorial?
   1. Accountability because as the nurse you are accountable for the well-being of all patient groups
   2. Respect for autonomy because autonomy is violated if care is not accessible
   3. Ethics of care because the caring action would be to provide resource access for all
   4. Justice since this concept addresses questions about the fair distribution of health care resources
3. You have agreed to serve on a Policy and Procedure committee at your hospital, representing the voice of bedside nurses from your unit. The committee is discussing a revision to the staffing ratio policy at your hospital by discussing these questions: How many patients can a nurse safely and effectively care for on your unit? Does the ANA professional code of ethics support your concerns about staffing ratios? Indicate the best answer.
   1. No, the code describes philosophical principles that are important to ethical discourse but unrelated to staffing ratios.
   2. Yes, the code supports nurses' participation in conditions of employment, including the promotion of quality health care using both individual and collective action.
   3. No, to support staffing ratio discussions the ANA publishes journals containing research about best practices in a variety of health care settings
   4. No, the code is not necessary for this discussion since historical foundations of nursing as defined by Florence Nightingale established staffing ratios before the ANA code of ethics.
4. You are working in an intensive care unit on the night shift. You have been caring for the same patient for three nights in a row. The patient's mother sleeps at the patient's bedside. Over time the mother has come to trust you, as evidenced by her long conversations with you while her child sleeps. Earlier in the week, in the presence of health care providers during morning rounds, she consented to an experimental surgical intervention for her child. But in conversation with you, she shares her doubts and confusions about the intervention. In the morning you ask the health care provider to consider an ethical consultation. What is the value of this nurse participating in discussions about ethical dilemmas? (Select all that apply.)
   1. Most state laws require that ethics committees include a nurse representative.
   2. The principal of beneficence promotes kindness in nurses.
   3. Nurses provide unique insight about patients that can be critical to the resolution of ethical dilemmas.
   4. Nurses can help articulate a patient's point of view based on specific nursing knowledge.
   5. Health care providers generally do not participate in ethical discourse.
5. Utilitarianism is a term commonly found in ethical discourse, but it stands for only one of several different approaches to ethical discourse. Which is a true statement about the ethical philosophy of utilitarianism?
   1. The value of an intervention is determined primarily by its usefulness to society.
   2. The value of an intervention is culturally established based on predetermined measures.
   3. The decision to provide medical care depends on a measure of the moral life of the patient.
   4. Attention to relationships provides resolution to ethical dilemmas.
6. Ethics of care suggests that you resolve an ethical dilemma by attention to relationships. As Madeleine Leininger described it, caring is the "central and unifying domain for the body of knowledge and practices in nursing." How does it differ from other approaches to ethical dilemmas? (Select all that apply.)
   1. Ethics of care applies exclusively to nursing practice.
   2. Ethics of care pays special attention to the stories of the people involved in an ethical issue.
   3. Ethics of care uses logic and intellectual analysis based on universal philosophical principles.
   4. Ethics of care depends less on universal principles than other approaches to analyze ethical dilemmas.
   5. Stories about relationships can be distracting when trying to resolve an ethical dilemma.

7. You are caring for a patient who will undergo a bone marrow aspiration, a difficult and painful procedure necessary to monitor the progress of recuperation after bone marrow transplantation. You are eager to minimize pain for this patient. You review the medical record for previous successful pain-management plans. You discuss the procedure with the patient. You advocate for the patient when the health care provider arrives to prepare for the procedure. Which ethical principle best describes the reasons for your actions?
   1. Beneficence
   2. Accountability
   3. Nonmaleficence
   4. Respect for autonomy
8. Which of the following actions is/are required of the nurse practicing advocacy? (Select all that apply.)
   1. Speak up for patient care issues even when others may disagree.
   2. Contribute money toward the patient's health care costs if the patient is indigent.
   3. Assess the patient's point of view and prepare to articulate it.
   4. Document all clinical changes in the medical record in a timely and legible way.
   5. Become an active member of professional nursing organizations.
9. At the hospital where you work, you care for a child admitted frequently for management of cystic fibrosis. The child's family has initiated a Cystic Fibrosis Support Group page on Facebook, and they invite you to "friend" their page. Which of the following justifications would you use to explain your decision to accept or not accept the invitation? (Select all that apply.)
   1. Nurse-patient boundaries may be violated, harming possibility for therapeutic relationship.
   2. By accepting you could share nursing information online about the patient as a way to educate the support group.
   3. Postings can easily spread to a wider audience with the potential for HIPAA violations.
   4. The law prohibits your use of social networking with patients.
10. Ethics in nursing practice includes an embrace of accountability or the ability to justify your actions. Even though your practice is defined in part by orders written by health care providers and policies enforced by administrators, you remain ethically accountable for your actions. Which of the following actions illustrates accountability? (Select all that apply.)
    1. Your patient receives a surgical procedure that is new to your facility. You ask your manager to provide an in-service about the procedure.
    2. A health care provider writes orders for pain-management medication even though the patient has been free of pain for 3 days. Out of respect for the health care provider's legal responsibilities, you administer the medications.
    3. During annual budget preparation at your facility, you advocate for annual pay increases for you and your peers.
    4. Your patient confides in you that she has recently lost her job and is anxious about her medical bills, including her ability to pay for medications after discharge. Health care coverage is not your area of expertise, but you know that the social worker might be able to help. You initiate a consultation request.

evolve

Rationales for Review Questions can be found on the Evolve website.

1. 4, 1, 3, 2; 2. 4; 3. 2; 4. 3, 4; 5. 1; 6. 2, 3; 7. 3; 8. 1, 3, 4; 9. 1, 3; 10. 1, 4.

REFERENCES

Agency for Healthcare Research and Quality (AHRQ): *National healthcare disparities report*, 2011, http://www.ahrq.gov/qual/nhdr10/Key.htm. Accessed July 31, 2013.

American Heritage Dictionary, ed 5, Boston, 2011, Houghton-Mifflin.

American Nurses Association (ANA): *Code of ethics for nurses with interpretative statements*, Washington, DC, 2001, The Association.

American Nurses Association (ANA): *Principles for social networking and the nurse*, Silver Spring, MD, 2011, The Association.

Beauchamp T, Childress J: *Principles of biomedical ethics*, ed 5, New York, 2008, Oxford University Press.

Edwards K: Inequality in Healthcare, *ABNF J* 22(4):83, 2011.

Gilligan C: *In a different voice*, Cambridge, Mass, 1993, Harvard University Press.

Kang HG, et al: In situ monitoring of health in older adults: technologies and issues, *J Am Geriatr Soc* 58(8):1579, 2010.

Kohlberg L: *Essays on moral development*, vols 1–3, San Francisco, 1981, Harper & Row.

Lindeman H: *An invitation to feminist ethics*, New York, 2005, McGraw-Hill Humanities.

McCance TV, McKenna HP, Boore JRP: Caring: theoretical perspectives of relevance to nursing, *J Adv Nurs* 30(6):1388, 1999.

National Council for State Boards of Nursing (NCSBN): *ANA and NCSBN unite to provide guidelines on social media and networking for nurses*, 2011 https://www.ncsbn.org/2927.htm. Accessed July 31, 2013.

US Department of Health and Human Services: *Health Information Privacy*, 1996, http://www.hhs.gov/ocr/privacy/. Accessed July 31, 2013.

CHAPTER 7

Evidence-Based Practice

evolve WEBSITE

http://evolve.elsevier.com/Potter/essentials

- Crossword Puzzle
- Audio Glossary

OBJECTIVES

- Discuss the relationship between evidence-based practice and the improvement of the safety and quality of nursing practice.
- Discuss the QSEN competencies for evidence-based practice.
- Describe the steps of evidence-based practice.
- Develop a PICO or PICOT question.
- Discuss the levels of evidence in the literature.
- Explain how critiquing the scientific literature leads to best evidence for practice changes.
- Discuss ways to apply evidence in nursing practice.
- Discuss ways to measure outcomes for an evidence-based practice change.
- Identify ways to sustain knowledge in evidence-based practice.
- Explain the relationship among nursing research, evidence-based practice, and quality improvement.

KEY TERMS

active error, p. 98
bias, p. 91
clinical guidelines, p. 90
evidence-based practice, p. 87
hypotheses, p. 92
latent error, p. 98
nursing-sensitive outcome, p. 95
peer-reviewed, p. 89
performance improvement (PI), p. 97
PICO, p. 89
quality improvement (QI), p. 97
reliable, p. 87
sentinel event, p. 98
valid, p. 91
variables, p. 92

Many nurses practice nursing according to what they learn in nursing school, their experiences in practice, and the policies and procedures of their institutions. This level of practice alone is not acceptable. Nursing practice is in an "age of accountability" in which quality, safety, and cost drive the direction of health care (Makadon et al., 2010; Moore et al., 2010; NQF, 2010). The general public is more informed about their own health and the incidence of medical errors within health care institutions. Health care organizations should show their commitment to each health care stakeholder (e.g., patients, insurance companies, government agencies) to reducing health care error and improving safety by putting into place evidence-based safe practices (National Quality Forum, 2010). Nurses and other health care providers can no longer accept and practice the status quo. Greater attention must be given to why certain health care approaches are used, which ones work, and which ones do not. EBP guides nurses and other health care providers in making effective, timely, and appropriate clinical decisions.

CASE STUDY *Amy and Nathan*

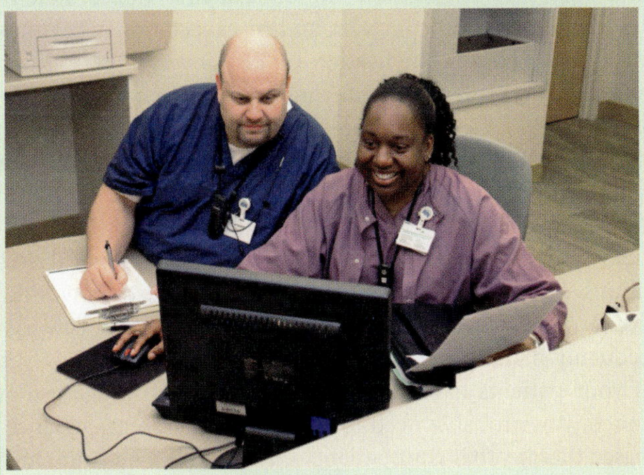

Amy and Nathan are two nurses who work in the surgical intensive care unit (ICU). They are members of the unit practice committee (UPC), which consists of a group of staff nurses, pharmacist, respiratory therapist, infection control practitioner, and physician. A UPC provides an ongoing forum for all clinicians in the department to discuss practice issues and explore ways to make improvements (Box 7-1). The committee meets monthly to discuss practice issues on the unit and has received a copy of the monthly report on the quality indicators for their unit. Amy notes that the incidence of central line–catheter-associated bloodstream infections (CLABSIs) has steadily increased during the last 3 months. Patients with central venous catheters (CVCs) used to deliver fluids and medications over extended periods of time (see Chapter 18) are becoming infected, but why? Nathan questions if the problem is related to the type of dressing placed over catheters or the way that sites are cleansed before insertion. The measurement of CLABSIs is considered a "Never Event," meaning that the hospital will not be reimbursed for the care of patients who have this hospital-acquired complication (Centers for Medicare and Medicaid Services, 2010). Thus it is important for UPC to find ways to prevent CLABSIs from occurring.

The UPC decides to explore these questions as part of its evidence-based practice (EBP) process. The first step is to develop a clinical question to efficiently search the scientific literature. Nathan volunteers to do the search with the aid of the hospital librarian. The aim is to determine what evidence is available so the committee can make an informed decision about standards needed to reduce CLABSIs in their patients.

BOX 7-1 EVIDENCE-BASED PRACTICE

PICO Question: Do nurse-led practice councils affect job satisfaction among staff nurses?

SUMMARY OF EVIDENCE

A study involving six hospitals evaluated the effects of nurse-led evidence-based practice (EBP) councils (Brody et al., 2012) in determining and disseminating EBP to improve the quality of patient care in the organizations. Staff involved in the councils received extensive education and training on EBP, performance improvement, and the change process. Qualitative data analysis indicated that staff became empowered as they participated in the councils. Another report in the literature addresses benefits derived from a clinical nurse specialist–led staff-represented clinical practice council for review of research to improve practice (Becker et al., 2012). The council program improved staff nurse's professionalism through increased use of leadership behaviors, autonomous practice, and the ability to influence patients' outcomes positively through EBP.

APPLICATION TO NURSING PRACTICE

- Involvement in EBP councils empowers staff to change standards of practice and improve quality of care.
- Council work helps staff believe that their work is meaningful.
- The EBP council process accelerates the growth of staff member's leadership skills.
- Teamwork between hospital departments improves from the EBP process.

A CASE FOR EVIDENCE-BASED PRACTICE

Evidence-based practice (EBP) is a problem-solving approach to clinical practice that combines the conscientious use of best evidence in combination with a clinician's expertise, patient preferences and values, and available health care resources in making decisions about patient care (Melnyk and Fineout-Overholt, 2011; Sackett et al., 2000). Put in simpler terms, EBP addresses a clinical problem by seeking the very best scientific and clinical evidence available for treating or managing the problem and implementing changes in practice. Using a sliding board to transfer a patient from bed to stretcher instead of lifting and using the research-based Braden scale (see Chapter 37) to routinely assess a patient's risk for skin breakdown are examples of using evidence at the bedside. Research shows that EBP improves patient outcomes (Bays and Hermann, 2010; Dammeyer et al., 2012; Heater, Becker, Olson, 1988).

Nurses regularly face important clinical decisions when caring for patients (e.g., Why do I use this approach in providing patient care? Is a change needed? Is there a way to improve patient outcomes?). Implementing health care processes or practices that are known to work (evidence based) in a **reliable** way is a feature of "quality care." Implementing new knowledge into practice requires a systematic approach that applies evidence to improve clinical and administrative practices (Newhouse and White, 2011). The Institute of Medicine in its report, "*The Future of Nursing*," recommends EBP as a nursing practice competency (IOM, 2010). EBP is also one of the Quality and Safety Education for Nurses' (QSEN) competencies, with the overall goal for the QSEN project being to meet the challenge of preparing future nurses to have the knowledge, skills, and attitudes (KSAs) necessary to continuously improve the quality and safety of the health care systems within which they work (QSEN, 2012). The QSEN competencies required for EBP include (QSEN, 2012):

- Demonstrating knowledge of basic scientific methods and processes.
- Describing EBP to include components of research evidence, clinical expertise, and patient/family values.
- Differentiating clinical opinion from research and evidence summaries.
- Describing reliable sources for locating evidence reports and clinical practice guidelines.
- Explaining the role of evidence in determining best clinical practice.
- Describing how the strength and relevance of available evidence influences the choice of interventions in providing patient-centered care.
- Discriminating between valid and invalid reasons for modifying evidence-based clinical practice based on clinical expertise or patient/family preferences.

As a nursing student you diligently read your textbooks and the assigned scientific articles. A good textbook incorporates current evidence into the practice guidelines and procedures it describes. Although a textbook relies on the scientific literature, sometimes information on a topic is outdated by the time a book is published. This is why it is important to also seek out scientific articles that are available on almost any topic involving nursing practice. However, not all articles present topics that are "research based." This means that some nursing practices are not based on findings from well-designed research studies because the findings are inconclusive or researchers have not yet studied the practices (Titler et al., 2001). Your challenge is to obtain the very best, most current information at the right time, when you need it for patient care.

The best scientific evidence comes from well-designed, systematically conducted research studies found in scientific, peer-reviewed journals. Researchers are usually able to conclude whether a new treatment or approach truly makes a difference at the completion of a research study. Unfortunately much of that evidence never reaches the bedside. Nurses in practice settings, unlike educational settings, do not have easy access to databases for scientific literature. Instead they often care for patients on the basis of tradition or convenience. Other sources of information from nonresearch evidence include:

- Performance-improvement and risk-management data.
- International, national, and local standards of care.
- Infection control data.
- Benchmarking.
- Retrospective or concurrent chart reviews.
- Clinicians' expertise.

It is important to always seek out research evidence rather than to depend solely on nonresearch-based evidence. When you face a clinical problem, ask yourself where the best evidence is to help you find the best solution in caring for patients.

Even when you use the best evidence available, application and outcomes differ based on your patients' values, state of health, preferences, concerns, and/or expectations (Layman, 2008). The correct application of EBP involves ethical and accountable professional nursing practice. In addition, EBP requires nurses to collaborate with interprofessional teams to seek the best evidence and ensure that it is relevant to their unique group of patients (Newhouse and White, 2011). As a nurse you use critical thinking skills to determine which evidence is appropriate and related to your patients' clinical situations. For example, a single research article involving older adults shows that the use of therapeutic touch is effective in reducing patients' perceptions of abdominal pain. However, if your patients have cultural beliefs that discourage use of touch, you probably need to search for a different evidence-based therapy that your patients will accept. Using your clinical expertise and considering patients' values and preferences ensure that you apply the evidence available in practice both safely and appropriately.

EVIDENCE-BASED PRACTICE STEPS

EBP is a systematic approach to rational decision making that aligns nursing practices with the best available scientific knowledge (Becker et al., 2012). A step-by-step approach ensures that you obtain the strongest available evidence to apply in patient care (Oh et al., 2010). Melnyk and Fineout-Overholt (2011) recommend a six-step process for EBP:

1. Ask a clinical question.
2. Collect the most relevant and best evidence.
3. Critically review and evaluate the evidence you gather.
4. Combine evidence with your clinical expertise and patient preferences and values in making a practice decision or change.
5. Evaluate the practice decision or change.
6. Communicate results of the change.

Newhouse and White (2011) note that a seventh and critical step is to sustain knowledge use. This means continuing practices or procedures within an organization that successfully lead to the routine use of evidence in practice.

Ask the Clinical Question

Always think about your practice when caring for patients. Question what does not make sense to you and what you think needs clarification. Think about a problem or area of interest that recurs, is time consuming, or is not logical. If you keep a clinical journal, your entries are a rich source for clinical questions.

Titler et al. (2001) suggest using problem- and knowledge-focused triggers to think critically about clinical and operational nursing-unit issues. A problem-focused trigger is one you face while caring for patients or a trend you see on a nursing unit. For example, Amy and Nathan identified from the quality indicator report that the trend in CLABSIs increased over each of the last 3 months. Data gathered from a health care setting allows you to examine clinical trends and form questions. Most hospitals keep monthly records on key quality or performance indicators such as medication errors or infection rates. All magnet-designated hospitals maintain the National Database of Nursing Quality Improvement (NDNQI). The database has information on falls, pressure ulcer incidence, and nurse satisfaction. Quality- and risk-management data do not give you evidence for finding a solution to a problem. Rather the data inform you about the nature or severity of problems, which then allows you to form practice questions. Other examples of problem-focused triggers include a patient injury following a fall or a postoperative patient who develops a stage III pressure ulcer.

A knowledge-focused trigger is a question that arises as a result of new information available on a topic. For example, "What is the current evidence for the best way to educate patients with low health literacy? Which approaches are effective in reducing delirium in the critical care unit?" Important sources of new scientific information include the standards and practice guidelines available from national agencies or organizations such as the Agency for Healthcare Research and Quality (AHRQ), the American Pain Society (APS), and the American Association of Critical Care Nurses (AACN). Other sources of knowledge-focused triggers include recent research publications and nurse experts within an organization.

When you ask a clinical question, you want to make it concise so it leads you to a reasonable number of scientific articles to review. You do not have time to read 100 articles to find the handful that are most helpful. You also do not want to make a practice change based on only one article. You want to be able to read the best four-to-six articles that specifically address your practice question. That is why it is best to use a **PICO** (or PICOT) format to state questions (Melnyk and Fineout-Overholt, 2011) (Box 7-2). Using a structured format for clinical questions helps you identify the key words that guide a successful literature search. *For example, Amy and Nathan first went to the literature with a general background question: "Which factors cause CLABSI in CVCs?" They were quickly frustrated when they found numerous articles about different factors that influence CLABSIs in CVCs. They decide to write two focused PICO questions: (1) "Does the use of 2% chlorhexidine (I) compared with alcohol (C) for cleansing central catheter insertion sites in hospitalized patients (P) reduce the incidence of CLABSI (O)?" (2) "Does the use of sterile barrier techniques during catheter insertion (I) compared with sterile gloving only (C) reduce the incidence of CLABSI (O) in postoperative surgical patients (P)?"* A well-designed PICO question does not have to follow the sequence of P, I, C, and O; but the aim is to ask a question that contains as many of the PICO elements as possible. Asking a PICOT question allows you to focus on the time frame for reaching outcomes from the interventions that pertain to your question.

> **BOX 7-2 DEVELOPING A PICO OR PICOT QUESTION**
>
> **P** = Patient population of interest
> Identify your patients by age, gender, ethnicity, disease, or health problem.
>
> **I** = Intervention of interest
> Which intervention do you want to use in practice (e.g., a treatment, diagnostic test, educational approach)?
>
> **C** = Comparison of interest
> What is the usual standard of care or current intervention that you now use in practice?
>
> **O** = Outcome
> What result do you wish to achieve or observe as a result of an intervention (e.g., change in patient behavior, physical finding, patient perception)?
>
> **T** = Time
> The time it takes to demonstrate an outcome (e.g., the time it takes for the intervention to achieve an outcome or how long participants are observed)

Less precise questions (e.g., What is the best way to reduce CLABSI? What is the best way to measure blood pressure?) are background questions that lead to many irrelevant articles and other sources of information, making it difficult to find the best evidence. However, it is sometimes necessary to begin with a background question if you do not have the knowledge yet as to how to form a more specific PICO(T) question. The PICO(T) format allows you to ask questions that are intervention focused. Some questions that arise in nursing practice do not always contain all of the PICO(T) elements. An example is a "meaning-focused" question such as, "How do women with breast cancer (P) rate their quality of life (O)?", which contains only a P and an O. These types of questions are frequently raised in daily nursing practice.

The questions you ask in a PICO(T) format identify knowledge gaps within a clinical situation. When you raise well–thought out questions, you discover evidence that is missing to guide clinical practice. Remember: do not be satisfied with clinical routines. Always question and use critical thinking to consider better ways to provide patient care.

Collect the Best Evidence

Once you have a clear and concise PICO(T) question, you are ready to search for evidence. Thousands of resources are available to aid in your search, including government and professional websites, agency procedure manuals, performance improvement data, existing clinical practice guidelines, and computerized bibliographical databases. Do not hesitate to ask for help to find appropriate evidence. Your faculty is always a key resource. When you are assigned to a health care setting, consider using experts such as advanced practice nurses, staff educators, risk managers, and infection control nurses.

When you go to the scientific literature for evidence, always seek the assistance of a medical librarian. A medical librarian knows the databases that are available to you (Box 7-3). The databases are repositories of published scientific studies, including peer-reviewed research. A **peer-reviewed** article is one submitted for publication and reviewed by a panel of experts familiar with the topic or subject matter of the article. The librarian is able to translate your PICO(T) question into the language or key words that yield the best evidence. When conducting a search, you enter and

BOX 7-3 SEARCHABLE SCIENTIFIC LITERATURE DATABASES AND SOURCES

CINAHL	Cumulative Index of Nursing and Allied Health Literature; includes studies in nursing, allied health, and biomedicine http://www.cinahl.com/
MEDLINE	Studies in medicine, nursing, dentistry, psychiatry, veterinary medicine, and allied health http://www.ncbi.nim.nih.gov
PsycINFO	Psychology and related health care disciplines http://www.apa.org/psycinfo/
Cochrane Database of Systematic Reviews	Full text of regularly updated systematic reviews prepared by the Cochrane Collaboration; includes completed reviews and protocols http://www.cochrane.org/reviews
National Guidelines Clearinghouse	Repository for structured abstracts (summaries) about clinical guidelines and their development; also includes condensed version of guideline for viewing http://www.guideline.gov/
PubMed	Health science library at the National Library of Medicine offers free access to journal articles http://www.nlm.nih.gov
Worldviews on Evidence-Based Nursing	Electronic journal containing articles that provide a synthesis of research and an annotated bibliography for selected references

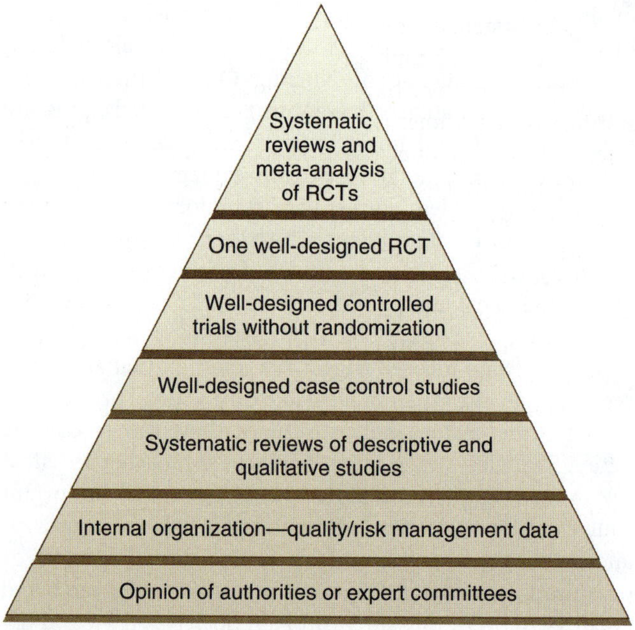

FIGURE 7-1 Hierarchy of evidence. *RCTs,* Randomized controlled trials. (Modified from Guyatt G, Rennie D: *Users' guides to the medical literature: a manual for evidence-based clinical practice,* Chicago, 2002, American Medical Association; Melnyk BM, Fineout-Overholt E: *Evidence-based practice in nursing and healthcare: a guide to best practice,* Philadelphia, 2005, Lippincott Williams & Wilkins.)

manipulate different key words until you get the combination that gives you the articles you want to read about your question. For example, Amy and Nathan's first PICO question includes the key words "catheter-associated bloodstream infection," "surgical patients," "chlorhexidine," and "alcohol." When you enter a word to search into a database, be prepared for some confusion with the evidence you obtain. The vocabulary in published articles is often vague. The word you select sometimes has one meaning to one author and a very different meaning to another. A medical librarian can help you learn how to choose alternative words (e.g., "surgery" versus "surgical patients") or terms that identify your PICO(T) question and thus ensure that you obtain evidence about your specific question.

MEDLINE and the Cumulative Index of Nursing and Allied Health Literature (CINAHL) are among the best-known comprehensive databases and represent the scientific knowledge base of health care (Melnyk and Fineout-Overholt, 2011). Some databases are available through vendors at a cost, whereas others are free of charge. As a student you have access to the databases purchased by your school. Vendors such as OVID usually offer several different databases. Databases are also available free on the Internet. The Cochrane Database of Systematic Reviews is a valuable resource of high-quality evidence. It includes the full text of regularly updated systematic reviews and protocols for reviews currently underway. Collaborative review groups prepare and maintain the reviews. The AHRQ supports the National Guidelines Clearinghouse (NGC) database. It contains **clinical guidelines** (i.e., systematically developed statements about a plan of care for a specific set of clinical circumstances involving a specific patient population). Examples of clinical guidelines on NGC include nursing care of dyspnea and treatment of adults with low back pain. The NGC is invaluable when you want to develop a plan of care for a patient (see Chapter 9).

The pyramid in Figure 7-1 represents one example of the hierarchy of available evidence. The level of rigor or the amount of confidence you have in the findings of a study decreases as you move down the pyramid. At this point in your nursing career you cannot be an expert on all aspects of the types of research studies conducted. But you can learn enough about the types of studies to help you know which ones have the best scientific evidence. Understanding the hierarchy of evidence helps you decide if evidence from a source is relevant, valid, and appropriate for use in practice. At the top of the pyramid are systematic reviews or meta-analyses, which are state-of-the-science summaries from an individual researcher or panel of experts. These research summaries are the perfect answers to PICO(T) questions because the researchers have rigorously summarized all current evidence on the question.

A good systematic review reports the findings from a literature search on a topic and tells you what evidence exists about your question. In a systematic review the researcher summarizes all studies conducted on a particular topic and reports if the current evidence supports a change in practice or if further study is needed. In the Cochrane Library all entries include information on meta-analyses or systematic reviews. A meta-analysis uses statistics to show the effect of an intervention on an outcome. A systematic review uses no statistics to draw conclusions.

A randomized controlled trial (RCT) is the highest level of experimental research. In an RCT a researcher tests an intervention (e.g., method for intravenous (IV) site care or patient education) against the usual standard of care. Researchers assign subjects in an experiment to either a control or a treatment group randomly. In other words all of the subjects have an equal chance to be in either group. The treatment group receives the experimental intervention, and the control group receives the usual standard of care. The researchers measure both groups for the same outcomes to see if the experimental intervention made a difference. When an RCT is completed, the researcher knows if the intervention leads to better outcomes than the standard of care.

A single RCT is not as conclusive as a review of several RCTs on the same question. However, a single RCT that tests the intervention included in your question yields very useful evidence. If an RCT is not available on your question, use results from other research studies such as descriptive or qualitative studies to answer your PICO(T) question (Box 7-4). The use of clinical experts may be at the bottom of the evidence pyramid, but do not consider clinical experts to be poor sources of evidence. Expert clinicians use evidence frequently as they build their own practice, and they are rich sources of information for clinical problems.

Health care agencies gather data about clinical practice trends such as NDNQI indicators. Typically quality- and risk-management data do not give you evidence for finding a solution to a problem, but the trending of the data (such as number of falls or type of medication errors over a period of 6 months) informs you about the nature or severity of problems occurring within the health care setting. Access to quality data helps you refine or redirect your PICO(T) question.

Critically Review and Evaluate the Evidence

With the help of the hospital librarian, Nathan searched three databases: PubMed, the CINAHL, and the Cochrane Database of Systematic Reviews. He found a systematic review summary on central line dressings from the Cochrane Data Base. An article from the highly regarded New England Journal of Medicine reported on a cohort study that showed a reduction in CLABSIs after use of a bundling of several interventions (including use of chlorhexidine and barrier precautions). Amy helped by searching the Centers for Disease Control and Prevention (CDC) website for clinical guidelines on central line catheters. Once they obtained the full text of all articles (not just the abstracts), Amy and Nathan distributed them to members of their UPC for critical review and evaluation.

BOX 7-4 TYPES OF RESEARCH STUDIES IN NURSING

Randomized Controlled Trial—Participants in a study are randomized to one of two groups and tested for the same outcome to determine if there is a difference in the effect of a treatment or intervention compared with a standard of care. It is the classic experiment and most rigorous level of research.

Quasi-experimental Study—Type of study that aims to determine whether a program or intervention has the intended effect on its participants. A true experiment includes (1) *pretest-posttest design*, (2) a *treatment group* and a *control group*, and (3) *random assignment* of study participants; however, quasi-experimental studies lack one or more of these design elements.

Descriptive—A researcher uses statistical measures to analyze data (e.g., survey responses, physical measures) to describe phenomena affecting patients or health care professionals.

Case Control Study—Study that compares patients who have a disease or outcome of interest with patients who do not have the disease or outcome. The researcher looks back (retrospectively) to compare how frequently the exposure to a risk factor is present in each group to determine the relationship between the risk factor and disease.

Cohort Study—Study that follows over time one or more populations (called *cohorts*) to determine which patient characteristics (risk factors) are associated with a disease or outcome.

Qualitative—Analysis of interviews, observations, and/or surveys to measure people's perceptions, feelings, or views of phenomena about which little is known.

Critically reviewing and analyzing the available evidence requires a systematic approach. Each source of evidence (article, clinical guideline, expert summary) must be reviewed to determine its value, feasibility, and utility of evidence for making a practice change. This requires you to review each source of evidence carefully to determine its scientific worth, identify the level of evidence from each source, summarize your findings, and determine if the evidence is conclusive regarding your practice question. The surgical ICU UPC committee reviews the articles and clinical guidelines on CLABSIs and decides if there is convincing evidence for the use of chlorhexidine instead of alcohol in cleansing catheter sites. They also determine if the use of barrier precautions during catheter insertion makes a difference in infection rates.

To begin it is important to understand basic research terminology such as sample, **bias,** dependent variable, and independent variable (Fineout-Overholt et al., 2010a). In addition, know the different types of study designs (see Box 7-4) to help explain how **valid** the findings of a study or information are in making conclusions about your PICO(T) question. The University of Pittsburgh (www.clinicalresearch.pitt.edu/docs/research-related_terms.pdfh) has a useful glossary of research terms.

BOX 7-5 RATING EVIDENCE

Evidence-based practice is ranked by the way the evidence was collected by the researcher or clinician. The following is an example of a rating system (Polit and Beck, 2008):

Level 1: Systematic reviews of randomized and nonrandomized clinical trials
Level 2: Single randomized and nonrandomized clinical trials
Level 3: Systematic review of correlational and observational studies
Level 4: Single correlational and observational studies
Level 5: Systematic review of descriptive, qualitative, and physiologic studies
Level 6: Single descriptive, qualitative, and physiological studies
Level 7: Opinions from authorities and expert committees

As a student new to nursing, it takes time to acquire the skills to critique research evidence. When you read an article from a scientific journal, do not let the statistics or technical wording cause you to put the article down and walk away. Your aim is to determine its worth to practice (Fineout-Overholt et al, 2010a):

- What is the level of evidence?
- How well was a study (if research article) conducted?
- How useful are the findings to practice?

When rating the evidence from a study, you determine the type of study based on an evidence hierarchy similar to the one in Figure 7-1. Then you use a numbering system (Box 7-5) for rating. For example, evidence from a systematic review would be rated a 1, evidence from a randomized trial is rated a 2, whereas published clinical articles are rated a lower level 6 (Oman, Duran, and Fink, 2008). Combining all articles gives you a sense of the highest level of evidence you have.

Read each article carefully to decide how well the study was conducted. When reading through a scientific study, summarize key elements. Many EBP committees use critical appraisal guides or useful checklists for evaluating studies (Fineout-Overholt et al., 2010a). A guide lists questions about essential elements of research (e.g., purpose, sample size, setting, method of study). It is important to know the elements of scientific articles to decide the value and relevance to your PICO(T) question. Evidence-based articles (research and clinical) include the following elements:

- *Abstract:* An abstract is a brief summary of the article that quickly tells you if the article is research or clinically based. An abstract summarizes the purpose of the study or clinical review, the type of study, major themes or findings, and the implications for nursing practice.
- *Introduction:* The introduction of a scientific article describes its purpose and the importance of the topic for the audience who reads it. There is usually brief supporting evidence as to why the topic is important from the author's point of view.

Together the abstract and introduction tell you if you want to continue to read the entire article. You know if the topic of the article is similar to your PICO(T) question or related closely enough to provide you useful information. Continue to read the next elements of the article.

- *Literature review or background:* A good author offers a detailed background of previous studies and the level of evidence or clinical information that exists about the topic of the article. The literature review explains what led the author to conduct a study or report on the clinical topic. This section of an article is very valuable. Perhaps the article itself does not address your specific PICO(T) question the way you want, but it can lead you to other more useful articles. Once you read the literature review, you should have a good idea of how past research led to the researcher's question. For example, a study designed to test the effects of aseptic practices on CLABSI reviews literature that describes the nature of CLABSI and the patients most at risk, the type of factors shown previously in the literature to contribute to CLABSI, and any previous interventions used to prevent CLABSI.
- *Manuscript narrative:* The "middle section" or narrative of a manuscript differs according to the type of evidence-based article it is (Melnyk and Fineout-Overholt, 2011). A clinical article describes a clinical topic, which often includes a description of a patient population, the nature of a certain disease or health problem, how patients are affected, and the appropriate nursing therapies. An author sometimes writes a clinical article to explain how to use a therapy or new technology. A research article contains several subsections within the narrative, including the following:
- *Purpose statement:* Explains the focus or intent of a study. It identifies which concepts are researched, including research questions (what the researcher intends to learn from the study) or **hypotheses** (predictions made about the relationship among study **variables**) (e.g., characteristics or traits that vary among subjects). An example of a research question is: Does the use of chlorhexidine 2% compared with povidone-iodine reduce CLABSI in patients with CVCs? Within that question the author is studying the variables (independent) of chlorhexidine and povidone-iodine solutions as they affect the outcome (dependent variable) of CLABSI in patients. In contrast, a hypothesis might state: Chlorhexidine 2% for site care reduces the incidence of CLABSI in patients with CVCs.
- *Methods or design:* Explains how researchers organize and conduct studies to answer research questions or test hypotheses. This is where you learn which type of study it is (e.g., RCT, case control, qualitative study). You also learn how many subjects (sample) or people are in a study. Generally the more subjects included in a study, the stronger the findings because a larger sample makes it easier to detect an effect from an intervention. However, in qualitative studies sample sizes are usually small. In health care studies subjects often include patients, family members, or health care staff.

The methods section also tells you the setting where a study was conducted, which may affect your interest in the findings. Remember, language in the methods section is sometimes confusing. Use a faculty member as a resource to help interpret this section.

- *Analysis:* This section explains how the data collected in a study are analyzed. If quantitative data such as physical measurements and scores on surveys are collected, statistical results from the study are explained. Statistics can be confusing. Focus on learning if the researcher found differences between groups or if an association was found between different variables. For example, if a researcher tests a new fall-prevention strategy, did the strategy reduce falls more so than the standard approach to care? The researcher statistically reports a "p value." The p value (usually set at 0.05) is a probability level that tells you whether the difference between two groups was likely related to the intervention or if it was simply a difference by chance (Burns and Grove, 2011). When the statistic shows that the value was less than the p value (<0.05), the result was likely the result of the intervention (less than 5% probability caused by chance). If a study involved collection of qualitative information such as audiotaped interviews or open-ended surveys, the analysis describes the major themes from the data. This section helps to determine if a study was conducted in a way that allows you to trust the results and use them to inform practice (Fineout-Overholt, et al., 2010b).
- *Results or conclusions*: Clinical and research articles have a summary section. In a clinical article the author explains the clinical implications for the topic presented. In a research article the author describes the findings from the study and explains whether a hypothesis is supported or how a research question is answered. Were the results clinically relevant (pertinent or connected to the clinical situation being studied)? A good author also discusses any limitations to a study in the results section. Study limitations are valuable in helping you decide if you want to apply the evidence with your patients.
- *Clinical implications*: A research article includes a section that explains if the findings from the study have clinical implications. The researcher explains how to apply findings in a practice setting for the type of subjects studied.

After you have critically reviewed each article for your PICO(T) question, combine the findings from all of the articles to determine the state of the evidence. If you used a critical appraisal guide for each article, summarize information in all of the forms into a final evaluation table. As you complete the evaluation table, use critical thinking to consider the scientific rigor or strength of the evidence and how well it answers your area of interest. Consider the evidence in light of your patients concerns, values, preferences, and available health care resources. Your review of articles offers a snapshot conclusion of the combined evidence on your PICO(T) question. As a new nurse you learn to judge whether to use the evidence for a particular patient or group of patients who usually have complex health care situations (Melnyk and Fineout-Overholt, 2011). Ethically it is important to consider evidence that benefits patients and does no harm.

After appraising all articles, the surgical ICU UPC focuses on the systematic review, cohort study, and CDC clinical guidelines as offering the most information about the use of chlorhexidine and other interventions for preventing CLABSI. The committee collaborates by discussing their conclusions, reviews the results of the final evaluation table, and also applies their clinical expertise. They consider the types of patients they see in the ICU and determine if the evidence is strong enough for use in practice. The systematic review article (evidence level 1) did not address chlorhexidine use but concluded that there is no definitive advantage of transparent IV dressings over gauze for preventing CLABSI. Although Level 7 evidence, the clinical guidelines from the CDC contained recommendations categorized on the basis of strength of existing scientific data and applicability. The CDC guidelines reported that research has shown no difference between transparent and gauze dressings in causing bloodstream infection (BSI) and highly recommends use of chlorhexidine for IV site care and the use of sterile barriers during catheter insertion. The cohort study (evidence level IV) showed a significant reduction in CLABSI in ICUs that used a bundle of interventions, including rigorous hand hygiene, chlorhexidine site care, and sterile barriers. The data from all studies were applicable to adult critically ill patients. The committee recommended adopting practice changes to include chlorhexidine site care, sterile barrier precautions for catheter insertion, and reinforcement of strict hand hygiene during all forms of central line site care.

Integrate the Evidence

Once you decide that the evidence is strong and applicable to your patients and clinical situation, incorporate it into practice. The easiest step is to take the evidence you find and apply it in your plan of care for a patient (see Chapter 9). Use the source of evidence as the scientific rationale for the intervention you plan to try. For instance, you are assigned to work in a long-term care nursing center, and you care for a patient with dementia who wanders. Your review of the literature offers strong evidence on techniques that can successfully reduce wandering. You decide to use several techniques from the articles you reviewed during your next clinical assignment to see if it reduces wandering in your assigned patient.

When you work as a part of a hospital committee or task force, sometimes EBP change occurs on a larger scale. Newhouse and White (2011) recommend that to be successful in changing practice within an organization, it is essential to *E*ngage, *E*ducate, *E*xecute, and *E*valuate. Once you have identified evidence to make a practice change, an organized collaborative effort is needed to bring appropriate administrators and staff all on board. Engagement involves bringing all stakeholders (individuals who have an interest or concern in the practice change) together to explain why the evidence-based interventions are important. For example, administrators want to know if the practice change improves patient outcomes and lowers costs. Staff nurses want to know if the practice change improves patient outcomes and how it will affect the way they provide care. Physicians also want to know how the practice change affects the way they provide care. To integrate evidence into practice, education of all those involved in the practice change must occur. This requires approaches such as teaching seminars, informational newsletters, and ongoing discussions during staff and UPC meetings.

The actual execution of a practice change requires planning, especially if it occurs on a large scale, involving more than one nursing unit or work area. The staff who are implementing a practice change must work closely with those who will be adopting the new practice to anticipate what will be needed to make a change successful. For example, new documentation forms, different types of supplies, or a change in the way information is communicated between disciplines may be needed. It is always best to trial a new practice change by conducting a 3-month pilot before implementing on a large scale. The results of the pilot tell you if the practice change can be implemented easily and if it results in desired outcomes.

A common approach used for integrating evidence into practice is to incorporate new evidence into policies and procedures (P&Ps). Many organizations have adopted an EBP approach when reviewing all P&Ps. A key feature of a practice environment that supports the use of best evidence is requiring clinical practice policies and procedures to be evidence based (Becker et al., 2012; Oman, Duran, and Fink 2008). Many organizations involve staff nurses and research-prepared advanced practice nurses to review scientific articles relevant to P&P and make appropriate revisions. P&P are important tools for supporting hospital-based nurses in using evidence in their everyday practice and promoting positive patient outcomes.

After reviewing the evidence on CLABSI, the surgical ICU UPC committee decides to revise the P&P for central catheter insertion and maintenance. Amy and Nathan recommend that the committee be responsible for conducting in-service sessions to educate all staff about the new P&P. A brief explanation about the change is also placed in the monthly newsletter of the unit. The bundle of interventions (hand hygiene, chlorhexidine use, and full barrier precautions) is implemented after the staff have the opportunity to ask questions about the new protocol in staff meetings. The ICU implements the new P&P with the UPC committee monitoring the monthly reports on CLABSI to determine if infection rates change. In addition, the UPC does spot audits of staff practices to be sure that the new interventions are being followed consistently to ensure that the change in practice is sustained.

You can use evidence in a variety of other ways through teaching tools, clinical practice guidelines, and new assessment or documentation tools. Depending on the amount of change needed to apply evidence in practice, it becomes necessary to involve a number of staff from a given nursing unit. It is important to consider the setting in which you want to apply the evidence. Is there support from all staff? Does/do the practice change(s) fit within the scope of practice in the clinical setting? Are there resources (time, equipment, staff) available to make a change? As a nursing student integrating evidence, your focus begins with searching for and applying best evidence to improve the care that you directly provide your patients. Using an EBP approach improves your skills and knowledge as a nurse and your patients' outcomes.

Evaluate the Practice Decision or Change

When you plan for the integration of evidence into practice, it is essential to decide how you will evaluate the outcomes. Remember the "O" in your PICO(T) question. It represents the outcomes you choose to measure as you integrate the evidence. These outcomes tell you how well the evidence-based intervention works. Sometimes your evaluation is as simple as determining if the expected outcome you set for a specific patient is met (see Chapter 9) after using a new evidence-based technique in care. For example, when using a new approach to preoperative teaching, does a patient learn what to expect after surgery?

When an EBP change occurs on a larger scale, an evaluation is more formal. For example, evidence of factors that reduce the incidence of CLABSI leads the surgical ICU to adopt the new P&P for central line catheter care. To evaluate the procedure the members of the EBP committee track the outcome of incidence of CLABSI over a course of time (e.g., 3 to 6 months). In this case the CLABSI measure is collected by the hospital on a monthly basis. In addition, the staff collects data to describe both the patients who develop CLABSI and those that do not. This comparative information is valuable in determining the effects of the procedure and whether modifications are necessary. Often outcome measures are not routinely collected, requiring staff to identify and then collect the outcomes required.

The evaluation of an EBP change determines if a practice change is desirable, if you need to modify your intervention, or if you need to discontinue a practice change. Unforeseen variables may lead to results that you do not anticipate. For example, the changes made in the protocol developed by Amy and Nathan might lead to an increase in CLABSIs. If this is not determined during evaluation, the practice would continue, and patients would suffer. *Never* implement a practice change without evaluating its effects. Often an EBP practice change must be stopped when the outcome measurements show poor outcomes.

Outcomes Measurement. An outcome is an observable effect of an intervention (see Chapter 9). Outcome measures determine if a patient progresses or if a practice change was beneficial or effective. In the example of the surgical ICU, the outcome measure is the incidence of CLABSI each month. This measure informs the ICU EBP committee if the new catheter-care procedure effectively reduces CLABSI.

Nurses work with many members of the health care team. As a result it is often difficult to associate an outcome with an intervention by a specific health care discipline. However, a **nursing-sensitive outcome** focuses on how patients and their health care problems are affected by nursing interventions (Oncology Nursing Society [ONS], 2004). Nursing-sensitive outcomes look at the effects of interventions within the scope of nursing practice. Examples of nursing-sensitive outcomes include:

- Symptoms (e.g., pain, fatigue, nausea).
- Functional status (e.g., activity tolerance, ability to perform activities of daily living).
- Safety (e.g., incidence of falls, infections, pressure ulcers).
- Psychological distress (e.g., anxiety, depression).

Patient education is a very common nursing intervention. Measuring educational outcomes occurs at several levels: reaction, learning, and behavior. When a nurse teaches a class to a group of patients or even one on one, a reaction outcome is one that evaluates how the learner feels about an educational activity. Did the patient enjoy the teaching experience? Did class members perceive that the nurse was competent in teaching? A learning outcome measures a patient's KSAs developed as a result of education. An example is a return demonstration. Perhaps the most important type of outcome resulting from patient education is a behavioral outcome, which evaluates the extent to which learners change their behavior as a result of education. Does a patient begin to follow the right meal plan at home or adhere to a medication schedule?

When identifying an outcome to evaluate a practice change, consider the type of measurement to use. Will you observe a patient behavior (taking a medication or performing an exercise or skill) or collect a physiological measure (e.g., weight or blood pressure)? Will measurement require you to conduct an interview, audit an existing medical record, or check results in a laboratory report? If you do not choose the correct measurement approach, you will not be certain if an outcome was met (Table 7-1). For example, if your practice change is a new relaxation technique for reducing patients' pain, your outcome of reduced pain is measured by using a pain-rating scale. If a practice change is a new type of breathing mask to reduce pressure ulcers on the face, the outcome of pressure ulcer incidence is measured using observation.

TABLE 7-1 OUTCOME MEASUREMENT

OUTCOME	MEASUREMENT APPROACH
Patient loses 10 lbs in 2 months.	Weight
Patient describes side effects of antihypertensive medication.	Patient interview
Patient is satisfied with nursing care.	Patient satisfaction survey
Patient expresses less fatigue after a 4-week exercise program.	Self-report fatigue scale
Incidence of methicillin-resistant *Staphylococcus aureus* drops among surgical patients.	Medical record laboratory reports

An outcome measure should be appropriate for patients or families. When you implement an EBP change, will you observe patients, or will you ask the patients to complete a survey or questionnaire? Consider if an outcome measure is too difficult for a patient to complete because of factors such as pain, fatigue, or level of consciousness.

You will be more successful in implementing EBP when outcome measurement plans are acceptable and important to the clinicians involved. This of course means including colleagues in any EBP project from the beginning when you select outcome measures. It is also important to be consistent and accurate when collecting outcome measures. Any clinicians who are involved in outcome measurement should receive proper training in data measurement and collection. For example, if outcome measurement involves a new device such as a pulse oximeter, each data collector must show competence in use of the oximeter. Those who collect outcome data must collect it in the same way. For example, if you decide to use a new patient satisfaction survey, EBP team members should practice administering the tool and use a single set of guidelines for administering it to patients. Competence and consistency in measurement help to ensure quality outcome data. Outcome measurement contributes to the body of evidence and strengthens the process of EBP.

Process Measurement. When you implement a practice change, you sometimes want to monitor whether or not the process or protocol was implemented. This requires a process measurement. For example, when the surgical ICU implements the use of chlorhexidine for central line catheter care, a process outcome is tracking documentation to see if chlorhexidine was used for site care. Process indicators (e.g., chart audit data or observations of staff using a protocol) simply tell you if an intervention was completed, but the information is useful in deciding if your approach to a practice change is working.

Communicate the Results

After collecting outcome measures to evaluate an EBP change, it becomes necessary to communicate results. If you implement an evidence-based intervention at an individual patient level, you let the patient know the results of your therapy. Is the patient's wound showing signs of healing? Has the patient correctly learned how to self-administer an injection? When your practice change occurs on a larger unit level, the first group to whom you communicate results is the clinical staff of a patient care unit. The EBP team should share results in a larger staff meeting or perhaps in a unit-based newsletter. Clinicians enjoy and appreciate seeing the results of a practice change. In addition, the practice change more likely is sustainable (i.e., remaining in place) when the staff are able to see that a change has been beneficial.

It is important for a health care agency to benefit as much as possible from EBP. A nursing unit or clinical area that makes an EBP change needs to communicate the results to the entire agency. Communication can occur by way of grand rounds or agency level committees. This increases the likelihood that nurses and other clinicians from different units will choose to make the same type of practice change. As a professional nurse it is critical for you to contribute to the growing knowledge of nursing practice. When you are involved in an EBP change, consider how you can communicate your results to the profession at large. Becoming involved in professional societies or organizations allows you to present EBP changes in scientific abstracts, poster presentations, or even podium presentations.

Sustain Knowledge Use

Sustaining change in practice as a result of the EBP process is a challenge. Health care institutions are bombarded by change from government and accrediting agencies, internal administrative initiatives, and the ongoing demands of delivering safe and effective patient care. When a new practice change is introduced, it is important that it be incorporated into the culture and practice environment of an organization. Once the surgical ICU adopts the new P&P for central line catheter care, they do not stop there. The committee posts the monthly CLABSI outcome measure on the conference room bulletin board for all staff to see. Members of the UPC conduct occasional audits to be sure that the processes of using chlorhexidine and sterile barriers are being followed by staff members. When the CLABSI measure trends back up, the UPC committee discusses the results and reviews the causes for each patient situation. Translating new knowledge into practice requires the collaboration of interprofessional teams that assume ownership of any change and encourage all those involved to adopt the change (Newhouse and White, 2011).

NURSING RESEARCH

After completing a thorough appraisal of the scientific literature, you sometimes find a gap in knowledge. If there is insufficient evidence to answer your PICO(T) question and make a practice change, the best way to answer your question is through the research process. At this time in your career you are not conducting research, but it is important for you to understand the process. Research is a systematic process that asks and answers questions to generate new knowledge. The new knowledge gained provides a scientific basis for nursing practice and validates the effectiveness of nursing interventions.

In the past much of the information used in nursing practice was borrowed from other disciplines such as biology, physiology, and psychology. Often this information was applied to nursing without testing or comparing ways of caring for patients. For example, nurses use several methods to help patients sleep. Interventions such as giving a patient a backrub, making sure that the bed is clean and comfortable, and preparing the environment by dimming the lights are frequently used and in general are logical, commonsense approaches. However, when you consider these measures in greater depth, questions arise about their applications. For example, are they the best methods to promote sleep? Do different patients in different situations require other interventions to promote sleep?

Research is an orderly series of steps that allow a researcher to move from asking a research question to finding the answer. It is more rigorous than EBP because a researcher must review all previous research related to his or her area of interest and select a relevant research question that can be studied. The aim of a study is to build on existing knowledge. A formal proposal is written to address the purpose of a study, the subjects, and the setting that are involved; how the subjects will be enrolled into the study; the actual methods for conducting the study; and the plan for analysis of study data. All researchers must conduct studies while protecting the rights of human subjects. An individual must know the purpose of any research, what it involves (time and activity), and all risks and benefits and be assured that participation is voluntary. Research studies must be approved by an institutional review board (IRB), also called a *human subjects committee.*

An actual research project takes time. The researcher and research team members follow an orderly and systematic process for enrolling subjects, obtaining their informed consent, administering any initial testing measures (e.g., physical measurements, observations, surveys, focus group discussions), applying any intervention (when appropriate to a study), collecting any final data, and analyzing the study results. Table 7-2 outlines briefly the elements of a research study that involves a pretest and posttest design. As in the case of EBP, a person conducting research disseminates or communicates the results of a research study by presenting at scientific conferences (poster or podium presentations) or publishing study results.

Once completed, the research process contributes new knowledge to the practice of nursing. A researcher attempts to design a study so the knowledge gained can later be applied repeatedly to other groups of patients. Nursing research creates the evidence for EBP. The highest level of evidence comes from well-designed experimental research studies (see Box 7-4). Nursing research improves nursing practice and raises the standards for the profession. Promoting EBP and research increases your scientific knowledge base for practice. The recipients of these improvements to practice are your patients, their families, and the communities in which they live.

QUALITY AND PERFORMANCE IMPROVEMENT

Near the bottom of the evidence pyramid (see Figure 7-1) is quality or performance data. Every health care organization gathers data on a number of health outcome measures as a way to determine their quality of care. Examples of quality data include fall rates, number of medication errors, incidence of pressure ulcers, and infection rates. Quality data trends can be an important trigger for the conduct of EBP projects and research.

TABLE 7-2 EXAMPLE OF A RESEARCH STUDY (PRETEST AND POSTTEST DESIGN)

Research Question: Does the use of a new bed sensor system reduce the number of falls and fall-related injuries in geriatric patients living in a nursing home?

TYPE OF STUDY	QUASI EXPERIMENTAL STUDY WITH PRETEST AND POSTTEST DESIGN
Study design	This study involved testing a new bed sensor system designed to alert staff when patients try to exit their bed. A group of 40 patients in a nursing home agreed to participate in the study. The outcome measures for the study were the number of falls and fall-related injuries.
Study procedure	Patients volunteered to participate and signed informed consents. A brief survey was collected to record the patients' ages, medical conditions, medications, and use of ambulatory devices. The patients' medical records provided pretest outcome data (i.e., the number of falls and fall-related injuries that the patients had experienced over the 3 months before the study). All patients were placed on beds with the new alarm system. Nursing home staff were trained on use of the sensors. The researcher collected data on any falls and fall-related injuries for 3 months (the length of the study).
Data analysis	The researchers ran statistical tests to learn if the patients fell less often or had fewer injuries after the sensor system was implemented. The researchers also analyzed if the patients who did fall had different characteristics (e.g., age, disease, medications) compared with those who did not fall.
Results	There were fewer patient falls during the 3 months after implementing the new sensor system compared with the 3 months before. The difference was statistically significant. The number of fall-related injuries also declined, but the result was not statistically significant. Adults with ambulatory deficits (unstable gait, balance) fell more often.
Implications	Sensor systems may help in the reduction of patient falls. More research is needed involving clinical trials with control and treatment groups.

Quality improvement (QI) and **performance improvement (PI)** are formal approaches for the analysis of health care–related processes. The two terms frequently are used interchangeably. An organization monitors specific quality outcomes and, when findings suggest potential problems, it institutes formal QI/PI initiatives. These projects usually occur more quickly than an EBP or research project. An organization analyzes and evaluates current performance data to solve system problems (e.g., supply delivery, appointment scheduling), people problems (e.g., staffing ratios, communication protocols) or clinical problems (e.g., surgical incision infection rates, patient injuries from falls). When interprofessional teams participate in PI activities, they may or may not use research findings; however, an evidenced-based approach is advised when dealing with clinical problems.

Health care organizations routinely promote efforts for improving patient care processes and outcomes, particularly with respect to reducing medical errors and enhancing patient safety. QI and PI are the continuous and ongoing efforts to achieve measurable improvements in the efficiency, effectiveness, performance, accountability, outcomes, and other indicators of quality services or processes.

Quality/Performance Improvement Programs

QI is a competency within the QSEN model. It begins with the use of data to monitor the outcomes of care processes (e.g., medication administration or surgical wound care). When problems are revealed, improvement methods are designed and tested to continuously improve the quality and safety of health care within a health care facility (QSEN, 2012). A well-organized QI/PI program focuses on processes or systems that significantly contribute to outcomes of an organization. Facilities need an organization-wide, systematic approach to ensure that everyone supports a continuous QI/PI philosophy. This begins with the organizational culture, in which all staff members understand their responsibility toward maintaining and improving quality. Typically in health care many people are involved in single processes of care. For example, medication delivery involves the health care provider who prescribes medications, the secretary who communicates new orders being written, the pharmacist who prepares the dosage, the transporter who delivers medications, and the nurse who prepares and administers the drugs. When an organization identifies a need to improve the medication administration process, all professions involved in medication administration need to be engaged in the QI/PI process. Because most health care processes are interprofessional, all members of the health care team collaborate together in QI/PI activities. As a member of the nursing team, you participate in recognizing trends in practice, identifying when recurrent problems develop, and initiating opportunities to improve the quality of care.

The QI/PI process begins at the staff level, where all disciplines become involved in identifying quality problems. This requires staff members to know the outcomes measured by the organization and the practice standards or guidelines that define quality. Unit QI/PI committees review quality data and the activities or services considered to be most important in providing quality care to patients. One way to identify the greatest opportunity for improving quality is to consider activities that are high volume (greater than 50% of the activity of a unit); high risk (potential for trauma or death); and problem areas for patients, staff, or the institution. For example, on an orthopedic nursing unit hip surgery volume

TABLE 7-3 EXAMPLES OF PERFORMANCE IMPROVEMENT MODELS

PERFORMANCE IMPROVEMENT MODEL	SUMMARY DESCRIPTION
1. Balanced scorecard	A multidimensional framework for managing strategy by linking objectives, initiatives, targets, and performance measures across key organization perspectives.
2. Root cause analysis (RCA)	A structured method used to analyze serious adverse events. A central tenet of RCA is to identify underlying problems that increase the likelihood of errors while avoiding the trap of focusing on mistakes by individuals.
3. Six Sigma	A disciplined methodology for process improvement that deploys a wide set of tools based on rigorous data analysis to identify sources of variation in performance and ways of reducing them.
4. *P*lan-*D*o-*S*tudy-*A*ct (PDSA)	An experiential learning method that involves analyzing a quality problem and testing a change by developing a plan to test the change (Plan), carrying out the test (Do), observing and learning from the consequences (Study), and determining which modifications should be made to the test (Act).

is high, older adults over 80 years of age have more postoperative complications, and family members are dissatisfied with patients' pain control. Any one of these factors could become the focus of a QI/PI project. Another example is The Joint Commission's annual patient safety goals (TJC, 2014), which provide an excellent focus for QI/PI initiatives (see Chapter 28). Sometimes a problem is presented to a committee in the form of a **sentinel event,** an unexpected occurrence involving death or serious physical or psychological injury of a patient. Once a committee defines the problem, it applies a formal model for exploring and resolving quality concerns. There are many models for QI and PI (Table 7-3).

Here is an example of a QI/PI process in response to a sentinel event:

On a 32-bed medicine oncology unit there has been an incident in which a patient received the incorrect blood type for a blood transfusion. The patient had an allergic reaction. Fortunately the nurse involved turned off the transfusion and initiated an emergency response. The patient survived; however, the incident raised serious questions about patient identification. One of The Joint Commission's patient safety goals for 2013 is identifying patients correctly (i.e., making sure that the correct patient gets the correct blood when getting a blood transfusion) (TJC, 2014). The UPC committee on the oncology unit is concerned since they administer blood transfusions frequently and this is the second incident in 12 months. The nurse manager on the oncology unit brings together an interprofessional team of nurses, physicians, laboratory personnel, and blood transporters. In addition, a member of the PI department joins the group to lead a root cause analysis (RCA). The process begins with the manager gathering data about the event (e.g., the patient's response to the blood, the transfusion order, staff on unit at time of incident, and interview of staff involved with transfusion). The UPC committee analyzes the sequence of events (i.e., physician order, obtaining a type-and-cross blood sample to determine patient's blood type, ordering the blood product, processing the order in the blood bank, delivering the unit of blood, and processing for checking patient identification). The goal of the RCA is to review all information and identify how the event occurred through identification of **active errors** *(i.e., the acts that personnel perform) and why it occurred through identification and analysis of* **latent errors** *(i.e., the organization or steps of the blood ordering and administration process). In this situation the UPC committee discovers the need for additional safeguards for checking patients' identifications at the bedside.*

QI combined with EBP is the foundation for excellent patient care and outcomes. Once a QI committee makes a practice change, it is important to communicate results to staff from all appropriate departments. Practice changes will likely not last when QI committees fail to report findings and the results of interventions. Regular discussions of QI activities through staff meetings, newsletters, and memos are good communication strategies. Often a QI study reveals information that prompts organization-wide change. An organization must be responsible for responding to the problem with the appropriate resources. Revision of P&Ps, modification of standards of care, and implementation of new support services are examples of ways an organization responds.

KEY POINTS

- EBP guides nurses and other health care providers in making effective, timely, and appropriate clinical decisions.
- The best scientific evidence comes from well-designed, systematically conducted research studies.
- Application and outcomes of EBP differ based on patients' values, state of health, preferences, concerns, and/or expectations.
- The steps of EBP include the following: Ask a clinical question, collect the most relevant and best evidence, critically appraise the evidence, integrate the evidence, evaluate the practice change, communicate results of the change, and sustain knowledge use.
- Using problem- and knowledge-focused triggers to think critically about clinical and operational nursing-unit issues helps you define a PICO(T) question.

- Using the PICO(T) format for clinical questions helps you identify key words that facilitate a successful literature search.
- Understanding the hierarchy of evidence helps you decide if evidence from a source is relevant, valid, and appropriate for use in practice.
- Critically appraising or analyzing the available evidence requires a systematic approach with each source of evidence to determine its value, feasibility, and usefulness of evidence for making a practice change.
- To make an EBP practice change it is necessary to Engage, Educate, Execute, and Evaluate.
- The use of outcome measurement to evaluate an EBP change determines if a practice change is desirable, if you need to modify your intervention, or if you need to discontinue a practice change.
- After appraising the evidence for a PICO(T) question, if the question is unanswered and there is a gap in knowledge, the research process is the next option for gaining new evidence.
- The aim of a research study is to build on existing knowledge.
- QI involves the review of quality data and identifies activities for improving the quality of a health care organization.

CLINICAL DECISION-MAKING EXERCISES

The surgical ICU where Amy and Nathan work has had an increased incidence of ventilator-associated pneumonia developing in their patients. Patients on ventilators have artificial airways and thus are at risk for aspirating mucus from their oral cavity into their trachea and lung. Secretions that commonly build up in the oral cavity of these patients contain infectious microorganisms. The aspiration of these secretions leads to pneumonia. The UPC believes that it is a clinical problem that warrants an EBP project. A physician on the committee reports that the medical ICU started to use an antiseptic mouthwash instead of a saline rinse for oral care. The UPC committee wonders if the development of a protocol for oral care is supported by the current literature.

1. Write a PICOT question for this clinical problem.

The UPC finds an article during the literature search that describes a study involving 112 patients in a cardiac ICU. All patients received a chlorhexidine oral care protocol during their ICU stay. Researchers compared the rate of ventilator-associated pneumonia before using chlorhexidine with the rate 3 months after using the protocol. Compared to the preintervention period, there was a significant reduction in ventilator-associated pneumonia in the postintervention period.

2. How would you describe this type of study?

A new nurse to the ICU tells Amy that she wants to use evidence she found in an article to reduce the time it takes for patients to get off ventilators. She sees it as a great opportunity to reduce complications and patients' length of stay. She says to Amy, "I want to get started on this. I would like to try it out on the patient I have today. What do you think?"

3. What is Amy's best response to this nurse?

evolve

Answers to Clinical Decision-Making Exercises can be found on the Evolve website.

QSEN ACTIVITY: EVIDENCE-BASED PRACTICE

A new nurse in the surgical ICU wants to join the UPC committee and be involved in EBP. She explains, "I believe the use of evidence from the literature is so important. In my last job, I found an article one time that had good information about pain management and I used it with all of my patients."

What should Amy explain to the nurse?

evolve

Answers to QSEN Activities can be found on the Evolve website.

REVIEW QUESTIONS

1. An oncology nurse is concerned about the number of patient falls occurring on the unit. The nurse observes that oncology patients who receive blood transfusions often receive Benadryl before a transfusion to reduce an allergic response. The drug Benadryl is an antihistamine that can cause drowsiness and dizziness. Which of the following is the best-worded PICO question for this practice issue?
    1. Do antihistamines lead to patient falls?
    2. Does the use of Benadryl before a transfusion compared to no antihistamine prevent falls?
    3. In oncology patients does the use of Benadryl reduce allergic responses from blood transfusions?
    4. Does the use of Benadryl before transfusions in oncology patients compared to no antihistamine affect the incidence of patient falls?
2. Number the following steps of EBP in the appropriate order.
    1. Critically appraise the evidence you gather.
    2. Sustain knowledge use.
    3. Evaluate the practice decision or change.
    4. Collect the most relevant and best evidence.
    5. Integrate the evidence.
    6. Communicate the results.
    7. Ask the clinical question.
3. While conducting a literature review, a nurse is seeking evidence in clinical guidelines developed for the clinical practice issue of pain management in the elderly. Which of the following is an example of a clinical guideline?

1. A summary of randomized clinical trials conducted to determine the effects of giving analgesics around the clock to older adults
2. A case study describing how an adult patient with dementia responded to pain-management approaches
3. A set of practice recommendations for pain management of patients in long-term care settings
4. A study of a cohort of elderly patients and their self-report of satisfaction with pain management in a hospital

4. A nurse working in a home health setting sees many patients who have asthma. The patients use inhalers that deliver prescribed medications to relieve airway obstruction. The nurse implements an EBP change that teaches patients the importance of taking their inhaler medications correctly and regularly on time using a new DVD program. The nurse measures the patients' behavior outcome of the practice change using which type of measurement?
   1. Measuring the patient's ability to breathe without distress
   2. Chart auditing teaching sessions
   3. Observing patient viewing the DVD
   4. Checking patients' inhaler for number of doses taken during a week's time
5. A nurse on an orthopedic unit is assigned to a patient in skeletal traction. The nurse has cared for similar patients in the past. In the staff room the nurse talks with other colleagues about what they know about pin-site care. The nurse asks a colleague, "What is the best practice for cleaning pin sites in skeletal traction?" This question is an example of a:
   1. Knowledge-focused trigger.
   2. Problem-focused trigger.
   3. PICO question.
   4. Hypothesis.
6. Which of the following is a process measurement?
   1. A nurse teaches a patient how to administer an injection and then observes the patient do a return demonstration.
   2. A nurse implements a new pain-management protocol and checks patients' charts to confirm if interventions are being provided.
   3. A nursing unit adopts a set of strategies for reducing pressure ulcers, and the UPC members use direct observation of the skin to measure incidence of pressure ulcers.
   4. A nursing unit implements a new fall-prevention protocol and checks the monthly performance data for incidence of falls on the unit.
7. The nurses on a medicine unit have seen an increase in the number of urinary tract infections (UTIs) developing in their patients. The nurses decide to initiate a quality improvement project using the PDSA model. Which of the following is an example of "Do" from that model?
   1. Implementing a new protocol for early removal of indwelling Foley catheters
   2. Reviewing the incidence of UTIs on patients cared for using the protocol
   3. Based on findings from patients who developed ulcers, implementing an evidence-based skin care protocol on all units
   4. Meeting with all disciplines to develop an approach for reducing UTIs
8. After a review of the literature regarding health literacy, the nurses in a diabetes outpatient clinic decide to revise the instructional manual on diabetes management to lower the reading level. Their hope is that by using the instructional materials over time they will see more patients being able to follow their medication regimens and better control their disease. Which of the following are outcome measures for this project? (Select all that apply.)
   1. Patients' reading level
   2. Patients' adherence to oral hypoglycemic medicines
   3. Patients' ability to plan a diabetes diet
   4. The number of patients who are given the new instructional manual
9. Consider the following clinical situation. A UPC committee is discussing the need to develop a new fever-management protocol for patients in their ICU. They want the protocol to be evidence based. In the past only the use of antipyretics has been the treatment approach. If the committee were to develop a PICOT question for this problem area, what would be the P?
   1. Fever
   2. Antipyretics
   3. Fever protocol
   4. Patients who are critically ill
10. During an EBP committee meeting, a nurse discusses the review of an article about the removal of nail polish before measuring pulse oximetry. The nurse reports that there is no conclusive evidence from the study that it is necessary to remove nail polish. A colleague on the committee asks the nurse, "Which level of evidence do you have?" The colleague's question is referring to:
    1. The scientific validity of the study findings.
    2. The number of articles that the nurse reviewed on the topic.
    3. Whether or not the pulse oximeter in the study is similar to the one used on the nurse's unit.
    4. The level in the hierarchy of evidence for the article that was reviewed by the nurse.

evolve

Rationales for Review Questions can be found on the Evolve website.

1. 4; **2.** 7, 4, 1, 5, 3, 6, 2; **3.** 3; **4.** 4; **5.** 1; **6.** 2; **7.** 1; **8.** 2, 3; **9.** 4;
10. 4

REFERENCES

Bays CL, Hermann CP: An evidence-based practice primer for infusion nurses, *J Infus Nurs* 33(4):220, 2010.

Becker E, et al: Clinical nurse specialists shaping policies and procedures via an evidence-based clinical practice council, *Clin Nurs Spec* 26(2):74, 2012.

Brody AA, et al: Evidence-based practice councils: potential path to staff nurse empowerment and leadership growth, *J Nurs Admin* 42(1):28, 2012.

Burns N, Grove SK: *Understanding nursing research: building an evidence-based practice*, St Louis, 2011, Elsevier, p 377.

Centers for Medicare and Medicaid Services: *Hospital-acquired conditions*, 2010, http://www.cms.gov/HospitalAcqCond/06_Hospital-Acquired_Conditions.asp. Accessed November 11, 2013.

Dammeyer JA, et al: Nurse-led change: a statewide multidisciplinary collaboration targeting intensive care unit delirium, *Crit Care Nurs Q* 35(1):2, 2012.

Fineout-Overholt E, et al: Evidence-based practice step by step: critical appraisal of the evidence: part 1, *Am J Nurs* 110(7):47, 2010a.

Fineout-Overholt E, et al: Evidence-based practice step by step: critical appraisal of the evidence: part II: digging deeper—examining the "keeper" studies, *Am J Nurs* 110(9):41, 2010b.

Heater BS, Becker AM, Olson RK: Nursing interventions and patient outcomes: a meta-analysis of studies, *Nurs Res* 37(5):303, 1988.

Institute of Medicine: *The future of nursing: leading change, advancing health*, Washington, DC, 2010, Institute of Medicine.

Layman EL: Implementing evidence-based nursing practice, *Nurse Leader* 2:15, 2008.

Makadon HJ, et al: Value management: optimizing quality, service and cost, *J Healthc Qual* 32(1):29, 2010.

Melnyk BM, Fineout-Overholt E: *Evidence-based practice in nursing and healthcare: a guide to best practice*, ed 2, Philadelphia, 2011, Lippincott Williams & Wilkins.

Moore CL, et al: Clinical process variation: effect on quality and cost of care, *Am J Managed Care* 16(5):385, 2010.

National Quality Forum (NQF): *Safe practices for better healthcare—2010 update: a consensus report*, Washington, DC, 2010, NQF.

Newhouse R, White KM: Guiding implementation: frameworks and resources for evidence translation, *J Nurs Admin* 41(12):513, 2011.

Oh EG, et al: Integrating evidence-based practice into RN-to-BSN clinical nursing education, *J Nurs Educ* 49(7):387, 2010.

Oman K, Duran C, Fink R: Evidence-based policy and procedures: an algorithm for success, *J Nurs Admin* 38(1):47, 2008.

Oncology Nursing Society (ONS): *Nursing-sensitive patient outcomes: description and framework*, 2004, http://www.ons.org/Research/NursingSensitive/Description. Accessed November 11, 2013.

Polit DF, Beck CT: *Nursing research: generating and assessing evidence for nursing practice*, ed 8, Philadelphia, 2008, Lippincott Williams & Wilkins.

Quality and Safety Education for Nurses (QSEN): *Quality and safety competencies*, 2012, Robert Wood Johnson Foundation, http://www.qsen.org/. Accessed November 11, 2013.

Sackett DL, et al: *Evidence-based medicine: how to practice and teach EBM*, London, 2000, Churchill Livingstone.

The Joint Commission (TJC): *National Patient Safety Goals*, Oakbrook Terrace, IL, 2014, The Commission. Available at http://www.jointcommission.org/standards_information/npsgs.aspx.

Titler MG, et al: The Iowa model of evidence-based practice to promote quality care, *Crit Care Nurs Clin North Am* 13(4):497, 2001.

CHAPTER 8

Critical Thinking

evolve WEBSITE

http://evolve.elsevier.com/Potter/essentials

- Crossword Puzzle
- Audio Glossary

OBJECTIVES

- Describe characteristics of a critical thinker.
- Discuss the nurse's responsibility in making clinical decisions.
- Describe how reflection improves clinical decision making.
- Describe the components of a critical thinking model for clinical decision making.
- Discuss critical thinking skills used in nursing practice.
- Explain the relationship between clinical experience and critical thinking.
- Discuss the critical thinking attitudes used in clinical decision making.
- Explain how professional standards influence a nurse's critical thinking.
- Discuss the relationship of the nursing process to critical thinking.

KEY TERMS

clinical decision making, p. 109
clinical inference, p. 108
critical thinking, p. 103
decision making, p. 107
diagnostic reasoning p. 107
intuition, p. 105
nursing process, p. 109
problem solving, p. 107
reflection, p. 104
scientific method, p. 107
workaround, p. 113

Every day you think critically without realizing it. If your computer flashes an error warning on the screen, you think about the steps you made before the error, consider the possible problem, and correct a key stroke or reboot the computer. If you decide to walk your dogs, go to the door, and notice that it is raining, you change into a different pair of walking shoes. These examples involve critical thinking as you face each day and prepare for all possibilities. As a professional nurse you care for patients with uniquely different types of health care problems. In each situation it is important to try to see the big picture and think smart. To think smart you need to develop critical thinking skills. This allows you to face each new experience and problem involving a patient's care with open-mindedness, creativity, confidence, and continual inquiry. *For example, when Marcy introduces herself to Ms. Logan, the patient is pleasant and easy to approach. But Marcy also notices that Ms. Logan grimaces as she sits down in the infusion chair and has difficulty moving about to find a comfortable position. Marcy's responsibility is to understand Ms. Logan's symptoms from her cancer and the effects of chemotherapy, which requires her to think critically and make sensible judgments so Ms. Logan receives the best nursing care possible. Marcy decides to assess the situation more thoroughly: "Ms. Logan, you look uncomfortable. Are you in pain? Where is the pain located? Is this the same pain you felt before?" Applying critical thinking to Ms. Logan's situation allows Marcy to recognize an emerging clinical pattern and know how and when to intervene.* Critical thinking is not a simple step-by-step,

CASE STUDY *Jennifer Logan*

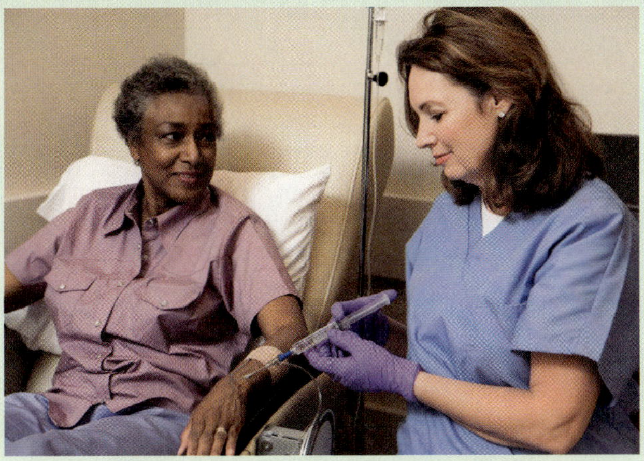

(Catherine Yeulet/Thinkstock)

Jennifer Logan is a 63-year-old woman who was first diagnosed with breast cancer 2 years ago. She comes to the outpatient infusion center to receive the start of a third course of chemotherapy. Her sister has come to the infusion center with her. Ms. Logan previously had radiation and surgery. Her disease is progressing, with the cancer now affecting her liver and bones. Marcy Thomas is the staff nurse caring for Ms. Logan. Marcy graduated from nursing school 4 months ago. She learned a great deal in orientation about the proper way to infuse chemotherapy and some of the side effects to expect from the treatment. Marcy is meeting Ms. Logan for the first time. She observes Ms. Logan walk into the infusion center with a slow gait, and she appears thin in comparison to her height. Her sister stays close to Ms. Logan as the two walk into the center.

linear process that you learn overnight. It is a process gained only through hard work, commitment, and an active curiosity about learning.

CLINICAL DECISIONS IN NURSING PRACTICE

When caring for patients, you are responsible for making accurate and appropriate clinical decisions. A clinical decision involves selecting appropriate treatments or interventions after determining a patient's health problems. Clinical decision making is a skill that separates professional nurses from nursing assistive personnel (NAP). To help patients maintain, regain, or improve their health you must think critically to problem solve and find solutions for their health problems. Good clinical decision making requires you to investigate and reflect on all aspects of a clinical situation or problem and to then apply nursing knowledge to choose the appropriate course of action (Guhde, 2010). Many patients have health care alterations that present clinical pictures that are not immediately clear and thus do not quickly reveal the actions you should take. Instead you must learn to question, wonder, and explore different interpretations. Then you try to find the set of actions that best helps your patients.

Because no two patients' health problems are the same, you always apply critical thinking differently. Observe patients closely, gather information about them, examine ideas and inferences about patient problems, recognize the problems, consider scientific principles relating to the problems, and develop an approach to nursing care. With experience you learn to creatively seek new knowledge, act quickly when events change, and make quality decisions for your patient's well-being. Although the responsibility for making clinical decisions seems challenging, it is what makes nursing a rewarding profession.

CRITICAL THINKING DEFINED

Thinking and learning are interrelated processes. The longer you practice as a nurse, the more your knowledge and practical experiences broaden your ability to make thoughtful observations, judgments, and decisions. **Critical thinking** is a continuous process characterized by open-mindedness, continual inquiry, and perseverance, combined with a willingness to look at each unique patient situation and determine which identified assumptions are true and relevant (Heffner and Rudy, 2008). Critical thinking involves recognizing that an issue (e.g., patient problem) exists, analyzing information related to the issue (e.g., clinical data about a patient), evaluating information (including assumptions and evidence), and drawing conclusions (Settersten and Lauver, 2004). To be an effective nurse you must engage in critical thinking. This requires you to fully assess a patient's health condition (see Chapter 9), meaning that you learn as much as possible about the patient from numerous sources to form a clear holistic view of his or her problems and approaches for resolving them. Critical thinking allows you to focus on the important issues at hand in any clinical situation and make decisions that provide desired outcomes (Raterink, 2011).

Marcy knows that, if Ms. Logan is undergoing a third course of chemotherapy, she likely has numerous side effects from her chemotherapy. If the cancer has spread to the liver and bones, numerous physical changes are likely affecting the patient. Marcy remembers her last instructor emphasizing the importance of seeing an illness "through the patient's eyes"; thus she wants to form a relationship with Ms. Logan and her sister to truly learn how the cancer is affecting both of them. Pain indeed may be a priority since it is easy to see. But Marcy knows that she needs a more in-depth understanding of Ms. Logan's condition to choose therapies that are not only effective but ones that the patient will likely accept.

You begin to learn critical thinking early in your practice. For example, when Marcy first learned about administering hygiene measures to patients, she read the nursing literature to learn more about the concept of comfort. What are the criteria for comfort? How do patients from other cultures perceive comfort? What are the different factors that contribute to comfort? The use of evidence-based knowledge (knowledge based on research or clinical expertise) (see Chapter 7) makes nurses more informed critical thinkers. Thinking critically and learning about the concept of comfort prepares

TABLE 8-1 CRITICAL THINKING SKILLS

SKILL	NURSING PRACTICE APPLICATION
Interpretation	Be orderly in data collection. For example, use a systematic approach to assess all characteristics of a patient's pain. Look for patterns to categorize data (e.g., defining characteristics of a nursing diagnosis [see Chapter 9]).
Analysis	Be open-minded as you look at information about a patient. Do not make careless assumptions. Does the information reveal what you believe is true, or are there other options?
Inference	Look at the meaning and significance of findings. Are there relationships between findings? Do the findings about a patient help you see that a problem exists?
Evaluation	Look at all situations objectively and systematically. Use criteria (e.g., expected outcomes, learning objectives, patient expectations) to determine results of nursing actions (see Chapter 9). Reflect on your own behavior and how it affects the evaluation process.
Explanation	Support your findings and conclusions. Use scientific knowledge and experience to choose strategies you use in the care of patients.
Self-regulation	Reflect on your experiences. Identify ways you can improve your own performance. What will make you believe that you have been successful?

Modified from Facione P: *Critical thinking: a statement of expert consensus for purposes of educational assessment and instruction. The Delphi report: research findings and recommendations prepared for the American Philosophical Association,* ERIC Doc No. ED 315-423, Washington, DC, 1990, ERIC.

TABLE 8-2 CONCEPTS FOR A CRITICAL THINKER

CONCEPT	COMPONENT
Truth seeking	Seek the true meaning of a situation. Be courageous, honest, and objective about asking questions.
Open-mindedness	Be tolerant of different views and be sure that you clearly know the views of your patients. Be sensitive to the possibility of your own biases and respect the right of others to have different opinions.
Analyticity	Be alert to potentially problematic situations; anticipate possible results or consequences (e.g., How should a patient respond to a certain treatment?); value reason; use evidence-based knowledge.
Systematicity	Be organized and focused and work hard in any inquiry. Organize inquiry based on priorities of care.
Self-confidence	Trust in your own reasoning processes.
Inquisitiveness	Be eager to acquire knowledge and learn explanations even when applications of the knowledge are not immediately clear. Value learning for learning's sake.
Maturity	Multiple solutions are acceptable. Reflect on your own judgments; have cognitive maturity.

Modified from Facione N, Facione P: Externalizing the critical thinking in knowledge development and clinical judgment, *Nurs Outlook* 44:129, 1996.

Marcy to better anticipate her patients' needs, identify comfort problems more quickly, and provide appropriate care. Critical thinking requires cognitive skills and the habit of asking questions, staying well informed, being honest in facing personal biases, and always being willing to reconsider and think clearly about issues (Facione, 1990). Table 8-1 summarizes core critical thinking skills that, when applied to nursing, show the complex nature of clinical decision making. Applying these skills takes practice. You need to have a sound knowledge base and thoughtfully consider the knowledge you gain during experiences with patients.

Learning to think critically helps you care for patients as their advocate and make informed choices about their care. Facione and Facione (1996) identified concepts for thinking critically (Table 8-2). Without these concepts, critical thinking skills are difficult to use. Critical thinking is more than just problem solving. It is an attempt to continually improve how you apply yourself when faced with patient care problems.

Reflection

When you care for patients, critical thinking begins by thinking about previous situations and considering relevant issues: How did I act? What could I have done differently? What should I do if I have the same opportunity in the future? **Reflection** is a part of critical thinking that involves the process of purposefully thinking back or recalling a situation to discover its purpose or meaning. *For example, before beginning care for Ms. Logan, Marcy thinks about a recent experience she had with a patient who suffered chronic pain from degenerative arthritis. Although the condition is different from that of Ms. Logan, the experience of caring for the patient is invaluable. Marcy goes through introspection or self-questioning to consider the approaches she used for her patient with arthritis. What might she have done differently when the patient reported little benefit from using relaxation exercises? Was her response appropriate when the patient said, "I don't know, I feel like I will never get any relief." How does this experience influence her ability to care for Ms. Logan, who is at risk for having chronic pain as long as she survives her cancer?* It is helpful for you as a nurse to think back on a patient situation to explore the

BOX 8-1 TIPS ON FACILITATING REFLECTION

- Stop and think about what is going on with your patient. What do your assessment findings mean? Which physical or behavioral changes are occurring? How do these changes compare with normal or baseline findings for the patient?
- Reflect carefully on any critical incidents (e.g., safety episodes, cardiac arrests, central events in the progression of a patient's disease, complex-care patients). What occurred? Which actions did you take? How did the patient respond? Did you think of taking any other options?
- Think about your feelings and the painful experiences you sometimes have. It helps to take any mixed emotions that you have and realize they are real.
- At the end of each day after caring for a patient, take time to reflect. Ask yourself whether you achieved your original plan of care. If you did, why were you successful? If you did not, what were the barriers or problems? What would you do differently or the same?
- Talk with a close friend who works with you and has observed your clinical work. Ask if the friend's observations are the same as yours.
- Keep all written care plans or clinical papers. Use them frequently as a resource for care of future patients.
- Take time to reflect, both after having cared for a patient and before caring for new patients with similar conditions. How is your current patient similar to or different from previous patients?

factors that influenced how you handled the situation. Reflection is like rewinding a videotape. It is not intuitive. It involves playing back a situation in your head and taking time to honestly review everything you remember about the situation. Research shows that reflective reasoning improves the accuracy of making diagnostic conclusions (Mamede et al., 2012). This means that, when you gather information about a patient, reflect on the meaning of your findings, and explore options about what the findings might mean, your ability to identify a patient's problem improves (see Chapter 9). It lessens the likelihood that reasoning is based on assumptions or guesswork. Reflection requires adequate knowledge; it is the ability to recreate ideas and experiences (Sewell, 2008). By reviewing your actions you see successes and opportunities for improvement. Always be cautious in using reflection. Too much emphasis on reflection can block thinking in the here and now because it often creates second-guessing. Learning from experience with patients can create an "aha" feeling because reflection reveals an awareness of how well you are performing as a professional. Box 8-1 lists tips on how to use reflection in your practice.

Language and Intuition

Use of language is another important aspect of critical thinking. Critical thinkers use language precisely and clearly. When language is unclear and inaccurate, it reflects sloppy thinking. It is important to communicate clearly with patients, their families, and health care professionals. When you use incorrect terminology and jargon or vague descriptions, communication is ineffective. If you do not obtain a professional interpreter when communicating with patients who speak a different language, you are taking the risk of miscommunicating important information. When you are vague or unclear with patients, families, and the nursing team, there are numerous implications. Your patients may be unable to cooperate with nursing care activities, families will perceive that you are insensitive to patient needs, and members of the nursing team will have difficulty following through on your recommendations because your communication was unclear. Always carefully frame your thoughts and send a clear message.

Intuition is an inner sensing or "gut feeling" that something is so. For example, you walk into a patient's room and, by looking at his or her appearance without the benefit of a thorough assessment, sense that he or she has worsened physically. Intuition is a common experience that many people have when interacting with their environments. Mothers develop an intuition about their children's behavior, especially after having had more than one child. Intuition is a component of clinical judgment and decision making, but it develops over time through clinical experience (Rew and Barrow, 2007). It acts as a trigger, leading you to consciously search for more data to confirm the sense of a change in a patient's status.

You cannot rely on intuition when caring for patients. Just as it is critical to know what knowledge you have, it is even more critical to know the knowledge you lack. Trust your intuition as a red flag that something is not quite right, but do not take it as an automatic fact. Always combine intuition with objective, scientific evidence (Rew and Barrow, 2007). Whenever you have an intuitive thought, look further to assess a patient's situation and consult with other professional colleagues. If you do not recognize what you do not know about patients, there is a risk for malpractice and even harming your patients. Thoughtful analysis of what you know and a review of the most current clinical data allow you to make accurate and sound clinical decisions.

THINKING AND LEARNING

Learning is a lifelong process. Your intellectual and emotional growth involves gaining new knowledge and refining the ability to think, problem solve, and make judgments. To learn, you must be flexible and always open to new information. The science of nursing is growing rapidly, and there will always be new evidence for you to apply in practice (see Chapter 7). As you have more clinical experiences and apply the knowledge gained, you become better at forming assumptions, presenting ideas, and making valid conclusions.

When you care for a patient, always think ahead and ask these questions: What is the patient's status now? How might it change and why? How do the patient's values and experiences affect the meaning of what I know? What do I know to improve the patient's condition? In what way will a specific therapy affect the patient? What should be my first action?

Do not allow your thinking to become routine or standardized. Instead learn to look beyond the obvious, explore each patient's response to health alterations, and recognize which actions are needed to benefit the patient. With experience you are able to recognize patterns of behavior, see commonalities in signs and symptoms, and anticipate reactions to therapies. Thinking about these experiences allows you to better anticipate each new patient's needs and recognize problems when they develop.

LEVELS OF CRITICAL THINKING IN NURSING

Your ability to think critically grows as you gain new knowledge and experience in nursing practice. Kataoka-Yahiro and Saylor (1994) developed a critical thinking model (Figure 8-1) that includes three levels of critical thinking in nursing: basic, complex, and commitment.

Basic Critical Thinking

As a beginning nursing student you make a more conscious effort to apply critical thinking because initially you are more task oriented and trying to learn how to organize nursing care activities. At the basic level of critical thinking a learner trusts that experts have the right answers for every problem. Thinking is concrete and based on a set of rules or principles. For example, as a nursing student you use a hospital procedure manual to confirm how to insert a feeding tube. You follow the procedure step-by-step without adjusting it to meet a patient's unique needs (e.g., positioning limitations or difficulty swallowing). You do not have enough experience to anticipate how to individualize the procedure. At this level answers to complex problems are either right or wrong (e.g., the tube will not advance because it is coiled in the throat), and one right answer usually exists for each problem. Basic critical thinking is an early step in the development of reasoning (Kataoka-Yahiro and Saylor, 1994). A basic critical thinker learns to accept the diverse opinions and values of experts (e.g., instructors and staff nurse role models). However, inexperience, weak competencies, and inflexible attitudes slow a person's ability to move to the next level of critical thinking.

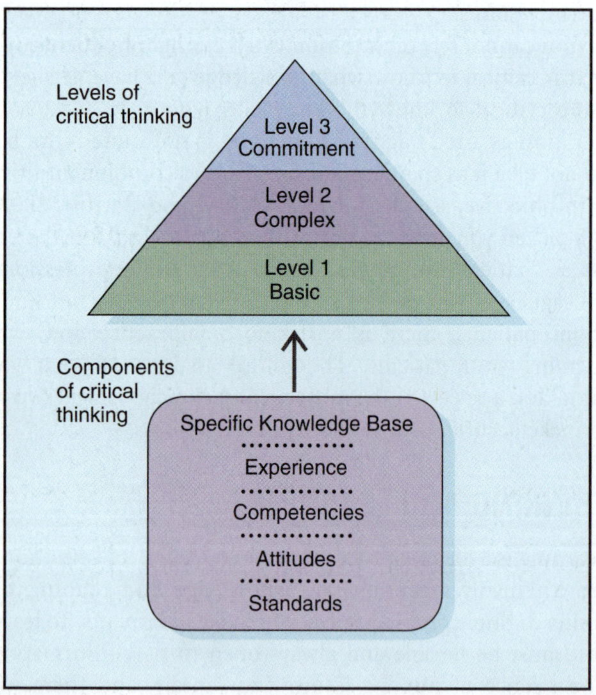

FIGURE 8-1 Critical thinking model for nursing judgment. (Redrawn from Kataoka-Yahiro M, Saylor C: A critical thinking model for nursing judgment, *J Nurs Educ* 33(8):351, 1994. Modified from Glaser E: *An experiment in the development of critical thinking*, New York, 1941, Bureau of Publications, Teachers College, Columbia University; Miller J, Malcolm N: Critical thinking in the nursing curriculum, *Nurs Health Care* 11:67, 1990; Paul R: *The art of redesigning instruction*. In Willsen J, Blinker AJA, editors: *Critical thinking how to prepare students for a rapidly changing world*, Santa Rosa, CA, 1993, Foundation for Critical Thinking.)

Complex Critical Thinking

Complex critical thinkers begin to separate themselves from experts. For example, you might try to insert a feeding tube and recognize that, when a patient has a swallowing problem, there is a need to adapt how you insert the tube. You learn to analyze and examine choices more independently. Your thinking abilities and initiative to look beyond expert opinion begin to change. As critical thinking skills grow, you learn that alternative and perhaps conflicting solutions exist.

Consider Ms. Logan, who expresses having sharp discomfort in her right hip as she sits in the infusion chair. She rates her pain at a level of a 7 on a scale of 0 to 10. Marcy notices that she is restless, cannot find a comfortable position, and begins to cry. She wonders if something else is contributing to the pain. Marcy takes a moment, sits down next to Ms. Logan, and says, "I can see that you're very uncomfortable. I'll call your doctor for medication to ease your pain, but can you tell me if anything else is bothering you? Ms. Logan looks toward her sister and then back at Marcy, "No one has asked recently. I haven't been sleeping because all of this has become too much. I believe that I can't get relief, and I'm just afraid of what will come next." Marcy has read how emotional factors can affect pain perception (see Chapter 32). She follows through in administering Ms. Logan a pain medication but asks if the patient would value talking with the cancer center psychologist. The patient sees this as a good suggestion.

In complex critical thinking you learn to synthesize knowledge. This means that you develop a new thought or idea based on your experience and knowledge over time. When you choose therapies for patients, each option has benefits and risks that you weigh in making a decision. Thinking becomes more creative and innovative. At this level you are more willing to consider deviations from standard protocols or procedures and provide more individualized care.

Commitment

The third level of critical thinking is commitment (Kataoka-Yahiro and Saylor, 1994). You anticipate the need to make choices without assistance from others. You accept accountability for whatever decisions you make. As a nurse you do more than just consider the complex alternatives that a problem poses. At the commitment level you choose an action or belief based on the alternatives available and stand by it. Sometimes an action is to not act or to delay an action until a later time. You choose to delay as a result of your experience and knowledge. Because you take accountability for the decision, you consider the results of the decision and determine whether it was appropriate.

CRITICAL THINKING COMPETENCIES

Kataoka-Yahiro and Saylor (1994) describe critical thinking competencies as the cognitive processes a nurse uses to make judgments about the clinical care of patients. There are three competencies: general critical thinking, specific critical thinking in clinical situations, and specific critical thinking in nursing. General critical thinking processes are not unique to the nursing profession. They include the **scientific method, problem solving,** and **decision making.** Specific critical thinking competencies in clinical health care situations include clinical inference, **diagnostic reasoning,** and clinical decision making. The specific critical thinking competency in nursing is the nursing process (see Chapter 9), which involves each of the other three specific critical thinking competencies.

General Critical Thinking

Scientific Method. The scientific method is a way to solve problems using reasoning. It is the systematic, ordered approach to gathering data and solving problems. It is used in nursing, medicine, and a variety of other health care disciplines. This approach looks for the truth or verifies that a set of facts agrees with reality. Nurse researchers use the scientific method when testing research questions in nursing practice situations. The scientific method has five steps:

1. Identifying the problem
2. Collecting data
3. Forming a question or hypothesis
4. Testing the question or hypothesis
5. Evaluating results of the test or study

The scientific method is one formal way to approach a problem, plan a solution, test the solution, and come to a conclusion. Table 8-3 provides an example of a nursing practice issue solved by applying the scientific method in a research study.

Problem Solving. You face problems every day, whether it is how to help a friend who has lost his or her job or how to operate a DVD player correctly. When a problem arises, you obtain information and apply it, together with what you already know, to find a solution. Patients routinely present problems in practice. *For example, Marcy learns that Ms. Logan has difficulty hearing explanations given by her health care provider. Her hearing has progressively worsened as she has undergone chemotherapy. Her sister accompanies her to the clinic as much as she can to help repeat and interpret her health care provider's explanations. However, Marcy learns that her sister is planning a vacation with her own family in the next 2 weeks. Marcy shares this information with the nurse coordinator in the health care provider's office. The nurse coordinator was not aware of the severity of Ms. Logan's hearing problem. She makes a note in the patient's record and plans to*

TABLE 8-3 USING THE SCIENTIFIC METHOD TO SOLVE NURSING PRACTICE QUESTIONS

Clinical Problem: The incidence of a health care–associated infection, *Clostridium difficile infection,* has increased on a hospital general medicine unit. The nursing staff on the unit practice committee, an infection control specialist, and a clinical nurse specialist in medicine have met to discuss factors that may be influencing the problem. They note that visitors are inconsistent in the use of antiseptic hand rubs. A staff member questions if use of hand rubs is the best approach for this type of infection.

Step	Application
Identify the problem.	• The incidence of *C. difficile* has increased among patients on a general medicine unit.
Collect data.	• Staff members review the literature about the nature of *C. difficile* infection and the hand antiseptic techniques that are recommended to prevent the infection. • Staff review the literature for any studies that have investigated hand-hygiene practices of visitors of hospitalized patients. • Staff review performance improvement reports for occurrence of *C. difficile* on the unit. • The infection control specialist is asked to discuss the trends being seen within the hospital regarding incidence of *C. difficile.*
Form a research question to study the problem.	• Does visitor use of antiseptic hand rub with chlorhexidine vs. hand washing with soap and water reduce incidence of *C. difficile* infection in medical patients?
Answer the question.	• The nurse specialist and a small team of staff plan a 4-month study approved by the hospital research board. • Patients' visitors are asked to use a chlorhexidine rub on their hands before entering and leaving patient rooms. • Visitors switch to performing hand washing with soap and water for the next 2 months. • Infection control tracks the incidence of *C. difficile* infection over the 4 months.
Evaluate the results of the study. Is the research question answered?	• Compare the incidence of *C. difficile* infection over 2 months for each of the two hand-hygiene methods.

be in attendance during the patient's next visit to the health care provider's office in case her sister cannot be there.

Problem solving represents a higher level of cognitive function. A traditional approach for solving problems is to clarify the problem, analyze possible causes, identify alternatives, assess each alternative, choose one, implement it, and evaluate whether the problem was solved. A systematic approach to problem solving makes it more likely that you will find an appropriate solution.

Effective problem solving also involves evaluating the solution over time to be sure that it is still effective. If a problem recurs, you try different options. Having solved a problem in one situation adds to your experience in your practice and allows you to apply the knowledge in future patient situations.

Decision Making. When you face a problem or situation and need to choose a course of action from several options, you are making a decision. Decision making focuses on resolving a problem. Following a set of criteria helps you make more thorough and thoughtful decisions. The criteria may be personal; based on an organizational policy; or, frequently in the case of nursing, a professional standard. For example, decision making occurs when a person decides on the choice of a health care provider. To make a decision, an individual has to recognize and define the problem or situation (need for a certain type of health care provider) and assess all options (consider recommended health care providers or choose one whose office is close to home). The person weighs each option against a set of personal criteria (experience, friendliness, and reputation), tests possible options (talks directly with the different health care providers), and makes a final choice. *In the case study Marcy notices a problem during her care of Ms. Logan: the patient's skin at the site where the intravenous (IV) needle is inserted into her implanted port (infusion port placed under the skin) appears inflamed. Marcy uses clinical criteria (e.g., presence of redness, tenderness, drainage, pain on palpation) that indicate a possible infection to more closely assess the insertion site, decide if infection is the problem, and determine if there is a need to report the problem to the health care provider.*

Although a set of criteria usually follows a sequence of steps, decision making involves moving back and forth when considering all criteria. It leads to informed conclusions that are supported by evidence and reason. It goes hand in hand with problem solving.

Specific Critical Thinking Competencies

Diagnostic Reasoning and Inference. Once you receive information about a patient in a clinical situation, diagnostic reasoning begins. It is the analytical process for determining a patient's health problems (Harjai and Tiwari, 2009). Accurate recognition of a patient's health problems is necessary before you decide on solutions and implement action. It requires you to assign meaning to the behaviors and physical signs and symptoms presented by a patient. Diagnostic reasoning begins when you interact with a patient or make physical or behavioral observations. An expert nurse sees the context of a patient situation (e.g., a patient who is feeling light-headed with blurred vision and who has a history of diabetes is possibly experiencing a problem with blood glucose levels), observes patterns and themes (e.g., symptoms that include weakness, hunger, and visual disturbances suggesting hypoglycemia), and makes decisions quickly (e.g., offers a food source containing glucose). The information a nurse collects and analyzes leads to a diagnosis of a patient's condition. Nurses do not make medical diagnoses; they make nursing diagnoses (see Chapter 9). They assess and monitor patients closely and compare patients' signs and symptoms with those that are common to a medical diagnosis. This type of diagnostic reasoning helps health care providers pinpoint the nature of a problem more quickly and select proper therapies.

Part of diagnostic reasoning is **clinical inference,** the process of drawing conclusions from related pieces of evidence and previous experience with the evidence. An inference involves forming patterns of information from data before making a nursing diagnosis. An example follows.

Marcy notices that Ms. Logan's recorded weight in the chart is 110 lbs (49.89 kg), and the patient is 5 ft 6 inches (167 cm) tall. The patient tells Marcy that she has not had an appetite for several months and eats small amounts of food during the day. The sister confirms that she has to come over to cook meals because Ms. Logan has little energy to prepare food. Seeing the pattern of assessment data, Marcy recognizes the clinical inference that Ms. Logan has a nutritional problem. An example of diagnostic reasoning is to then form a nursing diagnosis such as imbalanced nutrition: less than body requirements (see Chapter 9).

In diagnostic reasoning you use patient data that you gather or collect to logically identify a problem. As a student you confirm your judgments with more experienced nurses or your instructor. At times you can be wrong, but consulting with nurse experts gives you feedback to build on future clinical situations.

Often you cannot make a precise diagnosis during your first meeting with a patient. Sometimes you sense that a problem exists but do not have enough data to make a specific diagnosis. Some patients' physical conditions limit their ability to tell you about symptoms. Some choose to not share sensitive and important information during your initial assessment. Often patients' behaviors and physical responses become observable only under conditions not present during your initial assessment. When uncertain of a diagnosis, continue data collection using all sources of information. You need to critically analyze changing clinical situations until you are able to determine a patient's unique situation. Diagnostic reasoning is a continuous behavior in nursing practice. Any diagnostic conclusions that you make help in planning care for a nursing diagnosis. In addition, diagnostic conclusions about patients' medical problems help health care providers identify the nature of problems more quickly and select appropriate medical therapies.

Clinical Decision Making. Clinical decision making is a problem-solving activity that focuses on selecting appropriate treatment after forming diagnostic conclusions. When you face a clinical problem such as a patient who has an area of redness over the heel, you make a diagnostic conclusion that identifies the problem (impaired skin integrity in the form of a pressure ulcer); then you choose the best nursing interventions (skin care and turning). Nurses make clinical decisions to improve a patient's health or maintain wellness. This means minimizing the severity of the problem or resolving the problem completely. **Clinical decision making** requires careful reasoning so you choose the options for the best patient outcomes on the basis of a patient's condition and priority of the problem.

You develop expertise in clinical decision making by knowing your patients. Nurse researchers have found that expert nurses develop a level of knowing that leads to pattern recognition of patient symptoms and responses (White, 2003). This expertise begins with learning to assess patients thoroughly and actively engaging with them. You investigate and reflect on all aspects of a clinical observation or problem and then apply nursing knowledge to choose a course of action (Guhde, 2010). For example, an expert nurse who has worked on a general surgery unit for many years knows that when a patient's blood pressure falls, there is a need to assess the patient further. Thus, the nurse checks the patient's pulse and level of consciousness and quickly reviews any recent laboratory tests to eventually detect internal hemorrhage (fall in blood pressure, rapid pulse, change in consciousness, drop in blood count). The expert nurse is able to do this more quickly than a new nurse because of pattern recognition. Over time a combination of experience, time spent in a specific clinical area, and the quality of relationships formed with patients allow nurses to know clinical situations and quickly anticipate and select the right course of action. Spending more time during each patient encounter by thoroughly observing and measuring normal and abnormal findings is a way to know your patient better. In addition, consistently monitoring patients as problems develop helps you see how clinical changes evolve over time.

You base your selection of nursing interventions on clinical knowledge and specific information that you collect from your patients, including:

- Assessment data about a patient's status and situation, including data collected by actively listening to a patient discuss his or her health care needs.
- Knowledge about any clinical variables (e.g., age, severity of the problem, patient's preexisting disease conditions) involved in the situation and how the variables are linked together.
- A judgment about the likely course of events and outcomes of the diagnosed problem, considering any health risks a patient has.
- Additional relevant data about requirements in a patient's daily living, functional capacity, and social resources.
- Knowledge about the nursing intervention options available and the way in which specific interventions will predictably affect a patient's situation.

Always keep a patient your center of focus as you make clinical decisions. Making an accurate clinical decision allows you to set care priorities. Because different patients bring different variables to a situation, an activity is often a higher priority in one situation and less of a priority in another. For example, if a patient is physically dependent, unable to eat, and incontinent of urine, skin integrity is a greater priority than if the patient is immobile but continent of urine and able to eat a normal diet. Do not assume that a certain condition is an automatic priority. For example, you expect that a patient immediately out of surgery will experience a certain level of pain, which is often a priority of nursing care. However, if the patient is experiencing anxiety with heightened pain perception, it becomes necessary to focus on ways to relieve anxiety before pain-relief measures can be effective.

Critical thinking and clinical decision making are complicated because nurses care for multiple patients in fast-paced and unpredictable environments. When you work in a busy setting, use criteria such as the clinical condition of a patient, Maslow's hierarchy of needs (see Chapter 2), the risks involved in treatment delays, and patients' expectations of care to decide which patients have the greatest priorities. Critical thinking applied to clinical decision making allows you to attend to a patient whose condition is changing quickly and perhaps delegate less essential tasks to NAP. Skillful, prioritized clinical decision making allows you to manage the wide variety of problems associated with groups of patients.

The Nursing Process As a Competency. The critical thinking competency unique to nursing is the nursing process (Kataoka-Yahiro and Saylor, 1994). The **nursing process** is a five-step approach that incorporates diagnostic reasoning and clinical decision making (Figure 8-2). It includes assessment, diagnosis, planning, implementation, and evaluation (see Chapter 9). The purpose of the process is to diagnose and treat human responses to actual or potential health problems (ANA, 2010). Human responses include patient symptoms and physiological reactions to treatment, the need for knowledge, and a person's ability to cope with

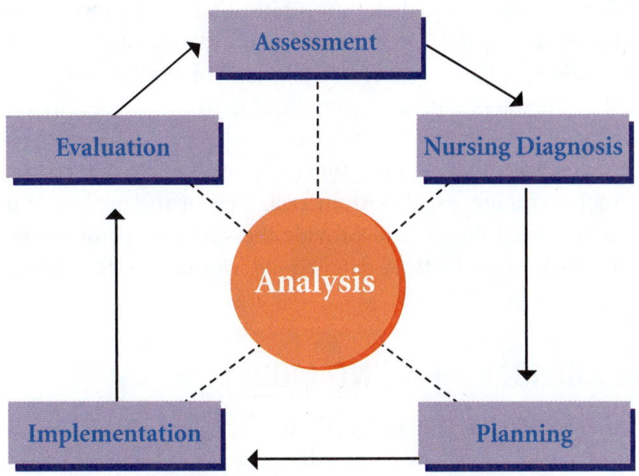

FIGURE 8-2 Five-step nursing process model.

TABLE 8-4 SUMMARY OF THE NURSING PROCESS

COMPONENT	PURPOSE	STEPS
Assessment	To gather, verify, and communicate data about a patient so a database is established	Collect nursing health history. Perform physical examination. Collect laboratory data. Validate or confirm that data are correct. Cluster data by common themes or problem areas. Document data.
Nursing Diagnosis	To identify a patient's health care needs in the form of nursing diagnoses	Analyze and interpret data. Identify patient problems. Form nursing diagnoses. Document nursing diagnoses.
Planning	Working with a patient, his or her family, and health care team members to set priorities of care, identify patient-centered goals and expected outcome, and prescribe an individualized approach to care	Identify patient goals mutually set with patient. Establish expected outcomes. Select nursing interventions. Document a nursing plan of care. Collaborate with other health care providers.
Implementation	To carry out nursing interventions necessary for accomplishing the plan of care	Perform nursing interventions. Reassess patient. Review and modify existing care plan.
Evaluation	To determine extent to which interventions helped achieve goals of care	Compare patient response with expected outcomes. Analyze reasons for results and conclusions. Modify care plan.

or adapt to health alterations and threats to their well-being. Use of the process allows nurses to identify patient problems accurately and meet agreed-on outcomes for better health. It requires a nurse to use the general and specific critical thinking competencies described earlier to focus on a specific patient's unique needs. The format for the nursing process offers a common language and process for nurses to "think through" patients' clinical problems (Kataoka-Yahiro and Saylor, 1994).

The nursing process is a blueprint or plan for patient care. It is flexible enough for you to use in all settings and with all patients. When you use it, you collect information about a patient, identify the patient's health care needs, determine priorities, and establish goals and expected outcomes of care. Then you develop and communicate a patient-centered plan of care, deliver nursing interventions, and evaluate the effectiveness of your care (Table 8-4). When you are competent in using the nursing process, you are able to focus not only on a single patient problem but also on multiple problems. As a nurse always think about and recognize which step of the process you are using. Within each step of the process you apply critical thinking to provide the very best professional care to your patients. A detailed description of the nursing process is in Chapter 9.

A CRITICAL THINKING MODEL

Models help explain concepts. Because critical thinking is complex, a model explains what is involved as you make clinical decisions and judgments about your patients. Kataoka-Yahiro and Saylor (1994) developed a model of critical thinking for nursing judgment based in part on previous works by Paul (1993), Glaser (1941), and Miller and Malcolm (1990) (see Figure 8-1). The model defines the outcome of critical thinking: nursing judgment that is relevant to nursing problems in a variety of health care settings. According to the model, there are five elements of critical thinking: knowledge base, experience, competence (e.g., problem solving or clinical decision making), attitudes, and standards. Nurses perform critical thinking within the competency of the nursing process. The elements of the model combine to explain how nurses make clinical decisions that are necessary for safe, effective nursing care (Box 8-2). Throughout this text the model shows you how to apply critical thinking as part of the nursing process.

Specific Knowledge Base

The first component of the critical thinking model is a nurse's specific knowledge base. Knowledge prepares you to better anticipate and identify patients' problems by understanding their origin and nature. Nurses' knowledge varies according to their educational experience (e.g., basic nursing education, continuing education courses, and additional college degrees). In addition, knowledge includes reading the nursing literature to remain current in nursing science. Your knowledge base will continually change as science progresses (Swinny, 2010). Your exposure to new knowledge comes directly from your educational experiences and when you collaborate and work side by side with knowledgeable colleagues. Your knowledge base includes information and theory from the basic

BOX 8-2 COMPONENTS OF CRITICAL THINKING IN NURSING

- I. Specific knowledge base in nursing
- II. Experience in nursing
- III. Critical thinking competencies
  - A. General critical thinking competencies
  - B. Specific critical thinking competencies in clinical situations
  - C. Specific critical thinking competency in nursing—the nursing process
- IV. Attitudes for critical thinking
  - A. Confidence
  - B. Independence
  - C. Fairness
  - D. Responsibility
  - E. Risk taking
  - F. Discipline
  - G. Perseverance
  - H. Creativity
  - I. Curiosity
  - J. Integrity
  - K. Humility
- V. Standards for critical thinking
  - A. Intellectual standards
    1. Clear—Plain and understandable (e.g., clarity in how one communicates)
    2. Precise—Exact and specific (e.g., focusing on a problem and possible solution)
    3. Specific—To mention, describe, or define in detail
    4. Accurate—True and free from error; getting to the facts (objective and subjective)
    5. Relevant—Essential and crucial to a situation (e.g., a patient's situation)
    6. Plausible—Reasonable or probable
    7. Consistent—Expressing consistent beliefs or values
    8. Logical—Engaging in correct reasoning from what one believes in a given instance to the conclusions that follow
    9. Deep—Containing complexities and multiple relationships
    10. Broad—Covering multiple viewpoints
    11. Complete—Thorough thinking and evaluation
    12. Significant—Focusing on what is important and not trivial
    13. Adequate (for purpose) —Satisfactory in quality or amount
    14. Fair—Being open-minded and impartial
  - B. Professional standards
    1. Ethical criteria for nursing judgment
    2. Criteria for evaluation
    3. Professional responsibility

Modified from Kataoka-Yahiro M, Saylor C: A critical thinking model for nursing judgment, *J Nurs Educ* 33(8):351, 1994. Data from Paul RW: The art of redesigning instruction. In Willsen J, Blinker AJA, editors: *Critical thinking: how to prepare students for a rapidly changing world,* Santa Rosa, CA, 1993, Foundation for Critical Thinking.

sciences, humanities, behavioral sciences, and nursing. You use your knowledge base in a different way from other health care professionals in regard to how you think about patient problems. This broad knowledge base gives you a holistic view of patients and their health care needs. The depth and extent of knowledge influence your ability to think critically about nursing problems. This is one reason why thoroughly knowing your patients is a vital part of critical thinking. *In the case study Marcy has graduated, but she enjoys learning. She decides to take a class in nursing informatics and participates in the monthly journal club held on her nursing unit. These experiences help her better understand the scientific articles she reads. Although she is new to nursing, her preparation and knowledge base help her make the clinical decisions necessary to care for Ms. Logan.*

Experience

Nursing is a practice discipline. You develop the knowledge of nursing through practice, or the hands-on care of patients. Experience, which is the second component of the critical thinking model, is the body of knowledge you gain from talking with patients and families, observing their courses of illness, providing interventions, and seeing the effects. Clinical learning is necessary for you to acquire clinical decision-making skills. You learn from your experiences in observing, sensing, and talking with patients and then reflecting actively on your experiences alone and with faculty and fellow students. Clinical experience is the laboratory for testing nursing knowledge. "Textbook" approaches and "simulation exercises" lay important groundwork for practice, but you need to adapt your practice to each setting, the unique qualities of each patient, and the experiences you gain from caring for previous patients. Benner (1984) notes that the expert nurse understands the context of a clinical situation, recognizes signs suggesting patterns, and interprets them as relevant or irrelevant. This level of competency comes with experience and a commitment to learning. Perhaps the best lesson you can learn is to value all patient experiences. Each clinical experience becomes a stepping stone to build new knowledge and stimulate innovative thinking.

Attitudes for Critical Thinking

To develop as a critical thinker you must be motivated to develop the attitudes and dispositions of a fair-minded thinker (i.e., you must be willing to suspend judgments until you truly understand another point of view and can articulate the position that another person holds on an issue [Heaslip, 2008]). Nurses make reasoned judgments in their application of the nursing process so they can act competently in practice. The fourth component of the critical thinking model is attitudes. Paul (1993) identifies 11 attitudes that are central features of a critical thinker (see Box 8-2). These attitudes define how a successful critical thinker approaches a problem. *For example, Marcy wants to understand the side effects of chemotherapy and*

TABLE 8-5 CRITICAL THINKING ATTITUDES AND APPLICATIONS IN NURSING PRACTICE

CRITICAL THINKING ATTITUDE	APPLICATION IN PRACTICE
Confidence	Learn how to introduce yourself to a patient: "Mrs. Tyms, I'm Chuck Lord, your nurse for this shift. I'll be responsible for your nursing care and will work with your doctor to make sure that you're comfortable." Speak with conviction when you begin a treatment or procedure. Do not let a patient think that you are unsure of performing care safely. Always be prepared (e.g., equipment organized, other patient needs met) before performing a nursing activity.
Thinking independently	Read the nursing literature, especially when there are different views on the same subject. Talk with colleagues and expert staff nurses to share ideas about nursing interventions.
Fairness	Listen to both sides in any discussion. If a patient or family member complains about a colleague, listen to the story and then speak with the colleague. Weigh all the facts.
Responsibility and accountability	Ask for help if you are not sure about how to perform an aspect of patient care. Report any problems immediately. Follow standards of practice in your care.
Risk taking	If your knowledge causes you to question a health care provider's order, do so. Offer alternative approaches to nursing care when colleagues are having little success with patients.
Discipline	Be thorough in whatever you do. Use known criteria for activities such as assessment and evaluation. Take time to be thorough.
Perseverance	Be wary of an easy answer. If colleagues give you information about a patient and some facts are missing, clarify the information or talk to the patient directly. If the same problems continue to occur on a nursing division, bring colleagues together, look for a pattern, and find a solution.
Creativity	Look for different approaches if interventions are not working. For example, a patient may need a different positioning technique or a different instructional approach that will suit his or her unique needs.
Curiosity	Always ask why. A clinical sign or symptom can indicate a variety of problems. Explore and learn more about the patient to make the right clinical judgments.
Integrity	Recognize when your opinions may conflict with those of a patient; review your position and decide how best to proceed to reach mutually beneficial outcomes.
Humility	Recognize when you need more information to make a decision. When you are new to a clinical division and unfamiliar with the patients, ask for an orientation to the area. Ask nurses regularly assigned to the area for assistance. Read the professional journals regularly to keep updated on new approaches to care.

symptoms of cancer that Ms. Logan is experiencing. Only then can she develop a relevant plan of care for her patient. She asks Ms. Logan to tell her about how the cancer and its treatment are affecting her and then asks if her sister can also share what she knows. Being able to listen to all sides of a story applies the critical thinking attitude of fairness. Marcy explores each symptom that Ms. Logan reveals and tries to learn how each symptom affects her ability to function in her home. This is the attitude of curiosity (i.e., exploring and learning as much as possible about patients). Critical thinking attitudes are guidelines for how to solve problems or make decisions. Table 8-5 summarizes how nurses use critical thinking attitudes in practice situations. A summary of each critical thinking attitude follows.

Confidence. To be confident is to feel certain in your ability to accomplish a task or goal such as performing a nursing procedure or making a diagnostic decision. Confidence grows with experience in recognizing your strengths and limitations. You gradually shift your focus from your own needs (e.g., remembering the steps to perform a procedure) to the patient's needs. When you are not confident in performing a nursing skill, you become anxious about not knowing what to do. This prevents you from attending to a patient. Always be aware of what you know and what you do not know. If you have a question about a procedure, discuss it with your nursing instructor or preceptor first before attempting it on a patient. Patient safety is always a priority. When you are confident, your patients recognize it by how you communicate and the way you perform nursing care. Confidence builds trust between you and your patients and conveys a sense of caring.

Thinking Independently. As you gain new knowledge, you learn to consider a wide range of ideas and concepts before forming an opinion or making a judgment. This does not mean that you ignore other people's ideas. Instead you learn to consider all sides of a situation. However, a critical thinker does not accept another person's ideas without question. When thinking independently, you challenge the ways others think and look for rational and logical answers to problems. An independent thinker applies evidence-based practice (see Chapter 7) when facing clinical decisions. You must be willing to try to seek answers to both difficult questions inherent in practice and the obvious (Heaslip, 2008). Independent thinking and reasoning improve and expand on nursing knowledge and practice.

Fairness. A critical thinker deals with situations justly. This means that bias or prejudice does not enter into a decision. For example, regardless of how you feel about obesity, you do not allow personal attitudes to influence the way you deliver care to patients who are overweight. Look at each situation objectively and analyze all viewpoints to understand the situation completely before arriving at a decision. Having a sense of imagination helps you develop an attitude of fairness. Imagining what it is like to be in your patient's situation helps you see it through his or her eyes and appreciate its complexity.

Responsibility and Accountability. When caring for patients, you are responsible for correctly performing nursing care activities based on standards of practice. Standards of practice are the minimum level of performance accepted to ensure high-quality care. For example, you do not take shortcuts or workarounds when you administer medications to a patient (e.g., failing to identify a patient or preparing medication doses for multiple patients at the same time). You are responsible for following the "six rights" of medication administration. A professional nurse is competent in performing nursing interventions. When you are competent, you make better clinical decisions about your patients. As a nurse you are answerable, or accountable, for your decisions and the outcomes of your actions. This means that you are accountable for recognizing when nursing care is ineffective and you know the limits and scope of your practice.

Risk Taking. People often associate taking risks with danger. Using your cell phone while driving 60 miles an hour down a highway is a risk that might result in injury to you and drivers around you. However, taking risks is not always negative. Risk taking is desirable, particularly when the result is a positive outcome. A critical thinker is willing to take certain risks in trying different ways to solve problems. The willingness to take risks comes from experience with similar problems. In nursing risk taking frequently results in patient care innovations. In the past nurses have taken risks in trying different approaches to skin and wound care and pain management, to name a few. As a result, they used more effective interventions than traditional approaches. When taking a risk, you consider all options; analyze any potential danger to a patient; and then act in a well-reasoned, logical, and thoughtful manner. In the end the evaluation of patient outcomes is critical.

Discipline. A disciplined thinker misses few details and follows an orderly or systematic approach when collecting information, making decisions, or taking action. *For example, Marcy asks Ms. Logan to rate her hip pain on a scale of 0 to 10. Instead of only asking that question, Marcy conducts a systematic pain assessment and also asks, "What makes the pain worse? Where does it hurt? Has anything helped to relieve the pain?"* Being disciplined helps you identify problems more accurately and select the most appropriate nursing interventions. Disciplined thinking does not lessen your creativity but instead ensures that your decision making is systematic, accurate, and comprehensive.

Perseverance. A critical thinker is determined to find effective solutions to patient care problems. This is especially important when problems remain unresolved or when they recur. You must learn as much as possible about a problem and try various approaches to care. Perseverance means to also keep looking for additional resources until you find a successful approach. A critical thinker who perseveres is not satisfied with minimal effort but constantly tries to achieve the highest level of quality care.

Creativity. Creativity involves original thinking. This means you find solutions outside of the standard routines of care while still following standards of practice. Creativity is a great motivator that helps you think of options and unique approaches. A patient's clinical problems, living environment, and social support systems are just a few examples of factors that can make the simplest nursing procedure more complicated. However, they can also become assets. *For example, Marcy talks with Ms. Logan and her sister to learn if the patient would be comfortable having the sister coach her through relaxation exercises. The exercises are a way to help Ms. Logan relax more fully and enhance the effects of her pain medications. The two agree and allow Marcy to instruct them on different relaxation exercise options.* Creativity involves tailoring unique approaches to a patient's specific needs.

Curiosity. A critical thinker's favorite question is, "Why?" In any clinical situation you learn a great deal of information about a patient. As you analyze patient information, data patterns emerge that are not always clear. Patterns may be new to you or very unusual. Curiosity motivates you to question further, investigate a clinical situation, and obtain all of the information needed to make a decision.

Integrity. Critical thinkers question and test their own knowledge and beliefs. Your personal integrity as a nurse builds trust from your co-workers. Nurses face many dilemmas or problems in everyday clinical practice (e.g., administering the wrong medicine to a patient, forgetting to check on a patient who falls in the bathroom). Everyone makes a mistake at times. A person of integrity is honest and willing to admit to any mistakes or inconsistencies in his or her own behavior, ideas, and beliefs. A professional always tries to follow the highest standards of nursing practice.

Humility. It is important for you to admit to your limitations in knowledge and skill. Critical thinkers admit what they do not know and try to find the knowledge needed to make proper decisions. It is very common for a nurse to be an expert in one area of clinical practice (e.g., general surgery) but a novice in another area (e.g., orthopedics). A patient's safety and welfare are at risk if you cannot admit your inability to deal with a practice problem. You must rethink a situation, seek out additional knowledge (e.g., colleagues, literature, clinical experts), and use the information to form an opinion and draw a conclusion.

Standards for Critical Thinking

The fifth component of the critical thinking model includes intellectual and professional standards (Kataoka-Yahiro and Saylor, 1994).

Intellectual Standards. Paul (1993) identified 14 intellectual standards (see Box 8-2) universal for critical thinking. An intellectual standard is a guideline or principle for rational thought. You apply these standards when you use the nursing process. When you consider a patient problem, apply intellectual standards such as precision, accuracy, and consistency to make sure that all clinical decisions are sound. A thorough use of the intellectual standards in clinical practice makes certain that you do not perform critical thinking haphazardly. When you reflect on your thinking, you can begin to recognize when you are unclear, imprecise, or inaccurate (Heaslip, 2008).

Marcy learns that the one symptom affecting Ms. Logan the most is fatigue. Marcy is precise when she asks Ms. Logan to rate her fatigue on a scale of 0 to 10, and she is specific when asking how fatigued she feels when she first awakens in the morning and just before taking a daytime nap. The standard of relevance applies when Marcy determines how Ms. Logan's fatigue affects her ability to prepare her own meals and perform daily hygiene. When asking Ms. Logan, "What bothers you the most from feeling fatigued?", Marcy is applying the intellectual standard of significance.

Professional Standards. Professional standards for critical thinking refer to ethical criteria for nursing judgments (e.g., advocacy, patient autonomy, and beneficence), evidence-based criteria used for assessment and evaluation (Box 8-3), and criteria for professional responsibility (Paul, 1993).

BOX 8-3 EXAMPLES OF OUTCOMES AND CORRESPONDING EVALUATION CRITERIA

OUTCOME: PAIN RELIEF

Evaluation Criteria: *Character of pain, including the following:* Onset (When did it first start?), duration (How long does it last during an episode? How long has the pain been bothering the patient?), location (Which area of body is involved?), severity (How intense is the pain based on objective measure using a visual analog scale?), type or description of pain (Is it aching, burning, cramping?), precipitating factors (What causes the pain to begin?), relieving factors (What helps to reduce or eliminate the pain?), other related symptoms (e.g., nausea, dizziness, blurred vision).

OUTCOME: IMPROVED PHYSICAL FUNCTION

Evaluation Criteria: *Ability to perform activities of daily living* (e.g., bathing, grooming, toileting) *or instrumental activities of daily living* (e.g., check writing, buying groceries, cleaning home).

OUTCOME: PATIENT LEARNING

Evaluation Criteria: *Patient recall of information* (e.g., Can patient describe how to perform a skill or discuss when to notify a health care provider about health changes?), *patient's ability to perform learned skill correctly* (Can patient demonstrate the skill learned?), *patient's success in adapting knowledge or skill in the home* (While visiting the home, does the patient apply knowledge correctly?).

Application of professional standards requires you to use critical thinking for the good of individuals or groups (Kataoka-Yahiro and Saylor, 1994). Standards of practice improve patient outcomes and thus maintain a high level of quality care.

Excellent nursing practice is a reflection of ethical standards (see Chapter 6). Patient care requires more than just the application of scientific knowledge. Being able to focus on a patient's values and beliefs helps you make clinical decisions that are just, faithful to the patient's choices, and beneficial to the patient's well-being. Critical thinkers maintain a sense of self-awareness through conscious awareness of their beliefs, values, and feelings and the multiple perspectives of their patients, family members, and professional peers.

Critical thinking also requires the use of evidence. Scientific knowledge is the framework for the evidence-based criteria used in making clinical judgments. Nurses routinely use evidence-based criteria to assess patients' conditions and determine the efficacy of nursing interventions. For example, the Infusion Nurses Society applied evidence in their development of criteria for a phlebitis scale used to assess for the presence of phlebitis at intravenous sites (see Chapter 18). Dr. Barbara Braden applied the evidence from her research to develop the Braden Scale, used to predict pressure ulcer risk. Evidence-based criteria for making clinical judgments are either scientifically based on research findings or practice based from standards developed by clinical experts or performance improvement initiatives. Examples of such standards are the clinical practice guidelines from the Agency for Healthcare Research and Quality (AHRQ) and the performance measures from the National Quality Forum (NQF) (e.g., asthma assessment and urinary incontinence management in older adults). The NQF performance measures offer a way to assess the performance of a health care institution against recognized standards. An NQF-endorsed performance measure reflects rigorous scientific and evidence-based review, input from patients and their families, and the perspectives of people throughout the health care industry (NQF, 2012).

The standards of professional responsibility that a nurse tries to achieve are the standards cited in Nurse Practice Acts, institutional practice guidelines, and professional organizations' standards of practice (e.g., The ANA Standards of Professional Performance [http://www.nursingworld.org/scopeandstandardsofpractice]). These standards "raise the bar" for the responsibilities and accountabilities that a nurse assumes in guaranteeing quality health care to the public.

DEVELOPING CRITICAL THINKING SKILLS

Enhancing critical thinking of nurse clinicians is a concern of health care leaders. Numerous factors exist within health care settings that often pose barriers to critical thinking (Box 8-4). Rising patient acuity and decreasing length of stay create an environment that challenges even experienced nurses who are adept at critical thinking. Berkow et al. (2011) argue that critical thinking is essential to nursing practice in that nurses must learn to readily see a holistic picture of their patients' conditions to recognize emerging clinical patterns. There are two useful tools in practice that can improve critical thinking skills: reflective journaling and concept mapping.

Purposeful reflection leads to a deeper understanding of issues and to the development of judgment and skill (Cirocco, 2007). One activity that helps you develop into a critical thinker is reflective journaling (see Box 8-1). Reflective writing requires you to record your clinical experiences in your own words in a personal journal. It is not simply a focus on nursing skills. Returning to the journal as a resource gives you the chance to explore personal perceptions that you had during patient care and develop the ability to apply theory in practice. Use of a journal also improves your observation and descriptive skills. Writing skills improve through the development of conceptual clarity. Sewell (2008) recommends that you answer the following questions in a journal entry:

- Did I respond appropriately in this situation? How should I have responded?
- Were there consequences to my actions? What were they, and whom did they affect?
- Why did I react like that? What was I thinking at that moment?
- Should I have reacted differently?
- Was I working from just instinct or evidence-based information?
- How did I feel about the experience when it happened? How do I feel now?

Keeping a journal of your patient care experiences helps you become aware of how you use clinical decision-making skills.

As a nurse you care for patients who have multiple health problems. In the beginning it is difficult to sort out the multiple problems of a given patient and how they are all interrelated. You learn how to assess each problem and develop a nursing diagnosis for it. However, it takes more complex critical thinking to see how the problems are related and conceptualize a holistic view of a patient. Concept maps help you to do that. A concept map is a visual representation of meaningful relationships between concepts (e.g., patient problems or nursing diagnoses and interventions), which then form propositions. Concept maps are visual road maps that highlight the meanings of these relationships (Hunter Revell, 2012). The primary purpose of a concept map is to synthesize relevant data about a patient such as assessment data, nursing diagnoses, health needs, nursing interventions, and evaluation measures. A concept map is a strategy for developing reflective thinking skills. Through a concept map you learn to organize or link information about a patient in a unique and meaningful way.

The concept map is a tool to link concepts learned in class to patients you actually care for in clinical courses (Hunter Revell, 2012). You learn to recognize how a patient's multiple problems are interrelated and that often a single nursing intervention is effective for more than one problem. Similarly, by focusing on a particular patient problem, this tool often helps you resolve associated problems. Concept maps come in many visual forms. You will see examples of them throughout this text. Chapter 9 offers actual examples of concept maps and provides details on their development.

BOX 8-4 EVIDENCE-BASED PRACTICE

PICO Question: For nurses who work in hospital settings, which factors create barriers to critical thinking compared with factors that enhance critical thinking?

SUMMARY OF EVIDENCE

Two studies examined work-related factors that influence critical thinking. One study used a survey that asked nurses to evaluate work-related conditions that enhance or pose barriers to critical thinking (Raterink, 2011). The second study involved direct observation of nurses working on medical-surgical and pediatric oncology units, with researchers conducting workflow analysis (Cornell et al., 2011). The studies revealed the complex world of nursing care, where critical thinking is conducted. Nurses find themselves working in very busy work environments, where they frequently switch from task to task across multiple patients. Conditions on a busy work unit do not consistently support thoughtful reflection and consideration (Cornell et al., 2011). Teamwork and staff support (e.g., positive role models) were found to be important enhancers to critical thinking (Raterink, 2011).

APPLICATION TO NURSING PRACTICE

Researchers recommend the following for support of critical thinking in health care settings:

- Teamwork
- Staffing patterns that allow for consistency in care (e.g., nurses assigned to same patients on consecutive days)
- Positive role models within the nursing unit staff
- Opportunity on units for reflection and consideration of clinical situations
- Quality time for care planning and managing priorities

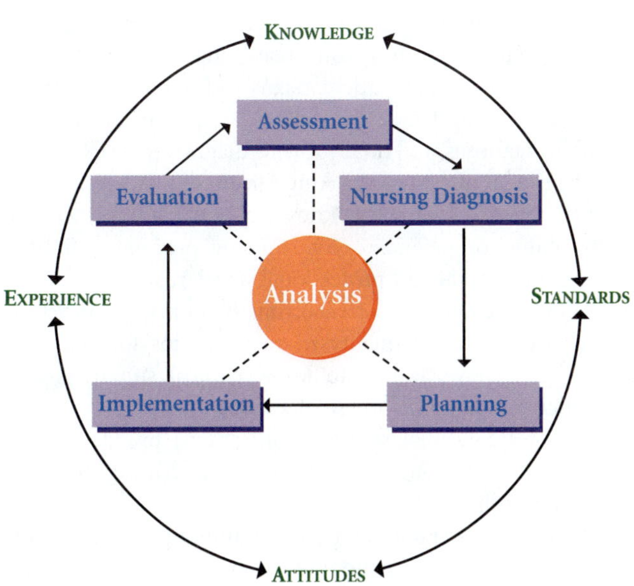

FIGURE 8-3 Synthesis of critical thinking with the nursing process competency.

CRITICAL THINKING SYNTHESIS

Critical thinking is a reasoning process by which you reflect on and analyze your own thoughts, actions, and knowledge and then make decisions about patient care. To be a good critical thinker requires dedication and a desire to grow intellectually. As a beginning nurse it is important to learn the steps of the nursing process and incorporate the elements of critical thinking (Figure 8-3). The two processes go hand in hand in making clinical decisions. This text provides a model to show you how important critical thinking is in nursing practice. Throughout the clinical chapters of this text, the components of critical thinking are emphasized to help you better understand their relationship to the nursing process.

KEY POINTS

- Clinical decision making requires you to investigate and reflect on all aspects of a clinical situation and then apply nursing knowledge to choose the appropriate course of action.
- Reflection is a process of purposefully thinking back on a situation to self-evaluate and review successes or opportunities for improvement.
- Intuition develops through clinical experience and acts as a trigger, leading a nurse to consciously search for data that confirm the sense of a change in a patient's status.
- Knowing patients begins with actively engaging them and learning to assess their situation thoroughly and actively.
- There are three levels of critical thinking in nursing: basic, complex, and commitment.
- In complex critical thinking you learn to analyze and examine alternatives more independently and take initiative to solve problems.
- The specific critical thinking competency in nursing is the nursing process, which involves clinical inference, diagnostic reasoning, and clinical decision making.
- The accuracy of diagnostic reasoning depends on how well you attend to a patient's signs and symptoms, identify patterns in the data, gather additional data to rule out possible diagnoses, and finally form a diagnostic conclusion.
- The model of critical thinking for nursing judgment consists of five elements: knowledge, experience, critical thinking competencies (e.g., nursing process), attitudes, and intellectual and professional standards.
- A combination of experience, time spent in a specific clinical area, and the quality of relationships formed with patients allows nurses to know clinical situations and anticipate the right course of action.
- Use of intellectual standards in clinical practice makes certain that you do not perform critical thinking haphazardly.
- Professional standards for critical thinking refer to ethical criteria for nursing judgments, evidence-based criteria used for assessment and evaluation, and criteria for professional responsibility.

CLINICAL DECISION-MAKING EXERCISES

Marcy has a discussion with Ms. Logan and her sister. She learns that Ms. Logan has problems sleeping.

1. What types of questions would Marcy ask if she wanted to apply the intellectual standard of being specific?

Marcy learns that Ms. Logan is concerned about her future and how long she will be able to live without becoming totally dependent on her sister. This is affecting her ability to sleep. Marcy encourages Ms. Logan and her sister to discuss feelings about their relationship and the sister's willingness to help as Ms. Logan's condition worsens.

2. Which critical thinking attitude is Marcy using in this situation?

The patient and sister are concerned about Ms. Logan's treatment plan. Both have questions for the oncologist that have as yet been unanswered.

3. How might the nurse demonstrate ethical standards in critical thinking? Explain.

evolve

Answers to Clinical Decision-Making Exercises can be found on the Evolve website.

QSEN ACTIVITY: PATIENT-CENTERED CARE

After completing her shift at the infusion center, Marcy reflects back on her day while completing her personal journal. She has two concerns about how she has approached Ms. Larson's care. Has she made too many assumptions about the sister's willingness to help? And how bothersome is the patient's fatigue? Fatigue can have a major impact on a patient's ability to manage self-care.

How might Marcy apply critical thinking attitudes in providing patient-centered care so she can communicate effectively with the sister and better understand Ms. Larson's beliefs about her fatigue?

evolve

Answers to QSEN Activities can be found on the Evolve website.

REVIEW QUESTIONS

1. A nurse prepares to insert a Foley catheter. The procedure manual calls for the patient to lie in the dorsal recumbent position. The patient complains of having back pain when lying on her back. Despite this, the nurse positions the patient supine with knees flexed to insert the catheter. This is an example of:
   1. Creativity in critical thinking.
   2. Intuition.
   3. Basic critical thinking.
   4. Complex critical thinking.

2. A nurse is preparing to administer a unit of blood. She follows the procedure for checking the patient's name on her armband against the name on the label of the blood unit. The bedside check is the final verification of the patient's identity. The nurse is following which critical thinking attitude?
   1. Accountability
   2. Conciseness
   3. Completeness
   4. Curiosity
3. A nurse is caring for an elderly male patient for the first time. The nurse notices in the patient's medical record that he has a history of a right-sided stroke. He has a cane leaning against the wall in his room. The nurse decides to assess his lower-extremity strength. Which of the following is an example of a clinical inference?
   1. Selecting a turning schedule for the patient
   2. Choosing to observe the patient walk
   3. Identifying that the patient has a mobility problem
   4. Measuring the patient's range of motion
4. The nurse enters the room of a patient with diabetes and heart disease. The nurse notes that the patient's color and facial expression suggest that something is not right. An assessment of vital signs, the patient's blood glucose level, and a review of the patient's diet intake this morning helps the nurse verify that the patient has a low blood glucose level. The nurse's choice of actions is an example of:
   1. Diagnostic reasoning.
   2. Intuition.
   3. Perseverance.
   4. Clinical inference.
5. A patient has been hospitalized for 2 weeks. The nurse calls a meeting of the social worker, physical therapist, and family to decide on whether to place the patient in a rehabilitation facility or home on discharge. Which step of the nursing process does this represent?
   1. Evaluation
   2. Assessment
   3. Intervention
   4. Planning
6. In which of the following examples is the nurse applying critical thinking skills in practice? (Select all that apply.)
   1. The nurse reflects on personal experience before inserting a urinary catheter in an older adult.
   2. The nurse uses a fall risk inventory scale to determine a patient's fall risk.
   3. The nurse explains the procedure step by step for giving an enema to a patient care technician.
   4. The nurse gathers data on a patient with a swallowing problem to identify a nursing diagnosis.
7. A nurse has been working on a medical unit for 3 weeks. A patient requires an intravenous catheter to be inserted, so the nurse refers to the policy and procedure manual to review how to perform the insertion. The level of critical thinking the nurse uses is:
   1. Commitment.
   2. Scientific method.
   3. Basic.
   4. Complex.
8. The nurse asks a patient how she feels about her impending heart surgery. The nurse reviewed a description of the surgery, the usual postoperative procedures, and complications to anticipate before the discussion. This is an example of which critical thinking component?
   1. Experience
   2. Curiosity
   3. Clinical decision making
   4. Knowledge application
9. Fill in the Blank. A patient returns from surgery following a knee replacement. The nurse asks the patient to rate his pain on a scale of 0 to 10. Use of the pain scale is an example of the intellectual standard of ______________.
10. Which of the following is unique to the commitment level of critical thinking?
    1. Weighs benefits and risks when making a decision
    2. Analyzes and examines choices more independently
    3. Requires concrete thinking
    4. Anticipates when to make choices without other's assistance

evolve

Rationales for Review Questions can be found on the Evolve website.

1. 3; 2. 1; 3. 3; 4. 1; 5. 4; 6. 1,2,4; 7. 3; 8. 4; 9. Precise; 10. 4.

REFERENCES

American Nurses Association (ANA): *Nursing's social policy statement: the essence of the profession*, Washington, DC, 2010, The Association.

Benner P: *From novice to expert*, Menlo Park, CA, 1984, Addison Wesley.

Berkow S, et al: Assessing individual frontline nurse critical thinking, *J Nurs Admin* 41(4):168, 2011.

Cirocco M: How reflective practice improves nurses' critical thinking ability, *Gastroenterol Nurs* 30(6):405, 2007.

Cornell P, et al: Barriers to critical thinking: Workflow interruptions and task switching among nurses, *JONA* 41(10):407, 2011.

Facione N, Facione P: Externalizing the critical thinking in knowledge development and clinical judgment, *Nurs Outlook* 44:129, 1996.

Facione P: *Critical thinking: a statement of expert consensus for purposes of educational assessment and instruction. The Delphi report: research findings and recommendations prepared for the American Philosophical Association*, ERIC Doc No. ED 315-423, Washington, DC, 1990, ERIC.

Glaser E: *An experiment in the development of critical thinking*, New York, 1941, Bureau of Publications, Teachers College, Columbia University.

Guhde J: Combining simulation, instructor-produced videos, and online discussions to stimulate critical thinking in nursing students, *Computers Informatics Nurs* 28(5):274, 2010.

Harjai PK, Tiwari R: Model of critical diagnostic reasoning: achieving expert clinician performance, *Nurs Educ Perspect* 30(5):305, 2009.

Heaslip P: *Critical thinking and nursing, the critical thinking community*, 2008, http://www.criticalthinking.org/pages/critical-thinking-and-nursing/834. Accessed November 11, 2013.

Heffner S, Rudy S: Critical thinking: what does it mean in the care of elderly hospitalized patients? *Crit Care Nurs Q* 31(1):73, 2008.

Hunter Revell SM: Concept maps and nursing theory: a pedagogical approach, *Nurse Educ* 37(3):131, 2012.

Kataoka-Yahiro M, Saylor C: A critical thinking model for nursing judgment, *J Nurs Educ* 33(8):351, 1994.

Mamede S, et al: Exploring the role of salient distracting clinical features in the emergence of diagnostic errors and the mechanisms through which reflection counteracts mistakes, *BMJ Qual Saf* 21(4):295, 2012.

Miller M, Malcolm N: Critical thinking in the nursing curriculum, *Nurs Health Care* 11:67, 1990.

National Quality Forum: *ABC's of measurement: How do we know? We measure*, 2012, NQF, http://www.qualityforum.org/Measuring_Performance/ABCs_of_Measurement.aspx. Accessed November 11, 2013.

Paul R: The art of redesigning instruction. In Willsen J, Blinker AJA, editors: *Critical thinking: how to prepare students for a rapidly changing world*, Santa Rosa, CA, 1993, Foundation for Critical Thinking.

Raterink G: Critical Thinking: Reported enhancers and barriers by nurses in long-term care: implications for staff development, *J Nurses Staff Dev* 27(3):136, 2011.

Rew L, Barrow EM: State of the science: intuition in nursing, a generation of studying the phenomenon, *ANS Adv Nurs Sci* 30(1):E15, 2007.

Settersten L, Lauver DR: Critical thinking, perceived health status, and participation in health behaviors, *Nurs Res* 53(1):11, 2004.

Sewell EA: Journaling as a mechanism to facilitate graduate nurses' role transition, *J Nurses Staff Dev* 24(2):49, 2008.

Swinny B: Assessing and developing critical thinking skills in the intensive care unit, *Crit Care Nurs Q* 33(1):2, 2010.

White AH: Clinical decision making among fourth year nursing students: an interpretive study, *J Nurs Educ* 42(3):113, 2003.

CHAPTER

9

Nursing Process

evolve WEBSITE

http://evolve.elsevier.com/Potter/essentials

- Glossary
- Crossword Puzzle

OBJECTIVES

- Describe each step of the nursing process.
- Explain the relationship between critical thinking and steps of the nursing process.
- Discuss approaches to data collection in nursing assessment.
- Differentiate between subjective and objective data.
- Explain the type of conclusions that result from data analysis.
- List the steps of the nursing diagnostic process.
- Describe the way in which defining characteristics and the etiological process individualize a nursing diagnosis.
- Discuss the process of priority setting.
- Describe goal setting.
- Discuss the difference between a goal and an expected outcome.
- Identify examples of nursing-sensitive outcomes.
- Develop a plan of care from a nursing assessment.
- Discuss the process of selecting nursing interventions.
- Describe how to evaluate nursing interventions selected for a patient.
- Describe how evaluation leads to revision or modification of a plan of care.

KEY TERMS

CASE STUDY ***Mrs. Tillman***

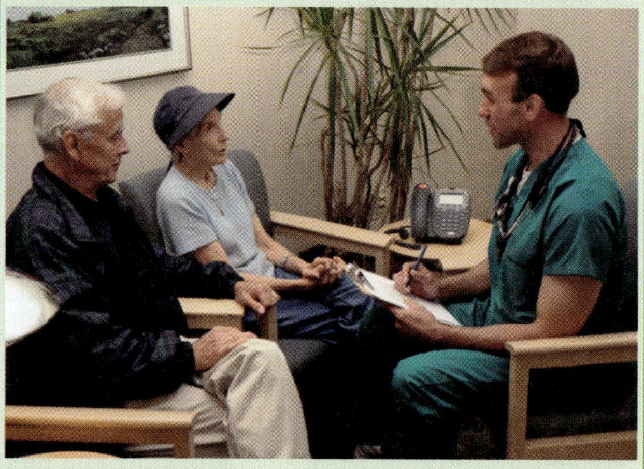

Rich is a nursing student who is assigned to care for Mrs. Jane Tillman, a 72-year-old woman with metastatic breast cancer. Mrs. Tillman recently retired after being a schoolteacher for 40 years. She had chemotherapy and radiation for her cancer, but magnetic resonance imaging (MRI) identified that the cancer spread to her lungs. Rich sees Mrs. Tillman and her husband Greg during the patient's visit to the outpatient cancer care clinic. He observes the patient sighing deeply and looking down as she talks with her husband. Rich knows from reading the medical record that the couple was told about Mrs. Tillman's prognosis during their last visit. He also reviewed information about chemotherapy and radiation therapy to learn about the various complications and health problems these therapies can cause. He prepares to use the nursing process to determine Mrs. Tillman's current health status and plan nursing therapies. His first step will be a thorough assessment, involving an interview with the patient and her husband and a health examination of the patient.

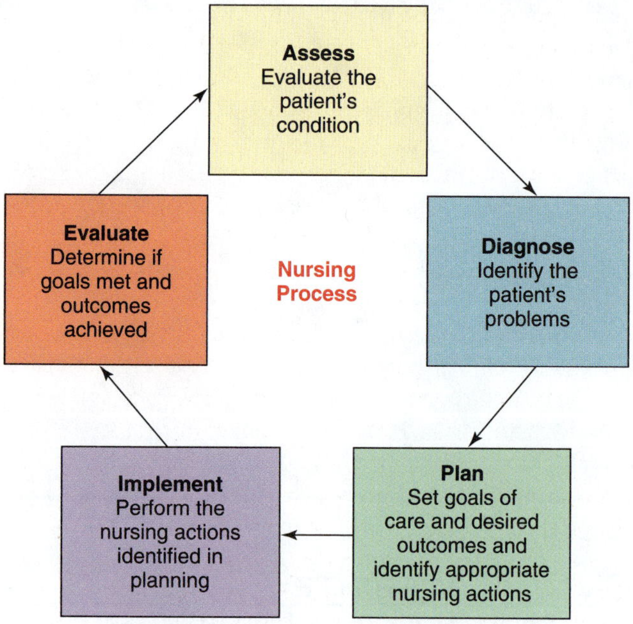

FIGURE 9-1 Five-step nursing process.

The **nursing process** is a critical thinking process that professional nurses use to apply the best available evidence to caregiving and the promotion of human functions and responses to health and illness (ANA, 2010). It is the fundamental blueprint for how to care for patients. A patient-centered care approach is essential in all steps of the nursing process. Patient-centered care enhances patient assessment, patient education, patient adherence to interventions, and patient outcomes (Bertakis and Azari, 2011).

The nursing process is also a standard of practice that, when followed correctly, protects nurses against legal problems related to nursing care. As a student you learn to integrate elements of critical thinking to form judgments and make safe and effective clinical decisions through the nursing process. The process includes five steps: assessment, nursing diagnosis, planning, implementation, and evaluation (Figure 9-1). Initially you learn how to apply the process step-by-step. However, as you gain more clinical experience and care for more than one patient, you learn to move back and forth through the steps of the process, critically making judgments about your patients' clinical situations and individualizing your approaches to care (O'Neill et al., 2011). The nursing process is central to your ability to provide timely and appropriate care to your patients.

The nursing process is a variation of scientific reasoning. Practicing the five steps of the nursing process helps you to be organized and conduct your practice in a systematic way. You learn to make inferences about the meaning of a patient's response to a health problem or generalize about the patient's functional state of health. Through assessment a pattern of a patient's health problems begins to form, and you gather more data to identify the patient's specific problems. Clearly defining your patient's problems provides a basis for planning and implementing relevant nursing interventions and evaluating the outcomes of care. Each time you meet a patient, you apply the nursing process as you see Rich do throughout this chapter.

ASSESSMENT

Assessment is the deliberate and systematic collection of data about a patient. The data reveal a patient's current and past health status, functional status, and present and past coping patterns (Carpenito-Moyet, 2013). Assessment requires you to apply critical thinking so in the end you have a clear picture of a patient's condition. There are two steps in nursing assessment:

1. Collection and verification of data from a primary source (the patient) and secondary sources (e.g., family, friends, health professionals, medical record)
2. Analysis of all data as a basis for the second step of the nursing process, developing nursing diagnoses and identifying collaborative problems

The purpose of the assessment is to establish a thorough **database** about a patient's perceived needs, health problems, and responses to these problems. In addition, the data reveal related experiences, health practices, goals, values, and expectations about the health care delivery system. To establish this database, you first apply knowledge that helps to identify what to assess. For example, your knowledge from the physical, biological, and social sciences allows you to ask relevant questions about a patient's health status and response to illness. You use this knowledge to collect relevant physical assessment data related to a patient's clinical condition. Critical thinking attitudes and intellectual standards allow you to direct questions expertly, clarify data, and gather further data for validation. Then you see the data patterns that reflect problems. Your experience allows you to recognize and anticipate what to assess. Experience leads you to ask the right questions, choosing only those that will give you the most relevant and useful information.

An assessment database includes a patient's comprehensive **health history,** which includes information about his or her physical and developmental status, emotional health, social practices and resources, goals, values, lifestyle, and expectations about the health care system. The database also includes physical examination findings and a summary of results from laboratory and diagnostic testing. The knowledge you gather about a patient's medical diagnosis and treatment from the literature and medical record is also part of the database that leads you to fully understand your patient's condition and health care needs. Critical thinking applied throughout the assessment process allows you to form conclusions or make decisions about a patient's health condition and direct assessment activities in a meaningful and purposeful way (see Chapter 8).

Rich introduces himself to Mrs. and Mr. Tillman and explains his role in the clinic. "I am a nursing student assigned to you today. I want to take some time to talk with you and ask you a few questions to see how you're doing. Then I will want to examine you by taking your blood pressure, listening to your lungs, and performing some other measures to get a good idea of your condition. I will be sharing what I find with your doctor. Then I want to work with you to put a plan together for your care. Is that okay with you?" Mrs. Tillman responds hesitantly, "Well, I guess so. I'm just not sure what to expect." Rich responds, "Well, let's start there. Tell me what you've been told by your doctor." Mrs. Tillman answers, "My breast cancer has spread; it's in my lungs." Rich notes, "I noticed you were sighing a minute ago. You look a bit down." Mrs. Tillman responds, "I'm so tired, and I've gone through two different courses of chemotherapy and then radiation; nothing has worked. Lately I just haven't had the energy to do what I like to do around the house. My husband and I are worn out." Mr. Tillman responds, "Yes, cancer is just exhausting." Rich replies, "It sounds as though this has been difficult for both of you. Mrs. Tillman, you say you're tired. Tell me how you spend a typical day. I want to learn about the symptoms you're having from your cancer and treatment." Rich reflects to himself and considers the physical examination techniques that he will want to use later to explore each symptom. He wants to be sure that he collects relevant assessment data without causing Mrs. Tillman unnecessary fatigue.

Rich has set the stage to begin an initial nursing assessment. He knows that a terminal disease can cause considerable grief and numerous physical changes. He wants to explore Mrs. Tillman's symptom experience and also learn her feelings about cancer so he can get a clearer sense of her emotional reaction. He applies critical thinking by asking relevant questions that will help reveal a clear picture of how cancer is affecting the patient on a daily basis. His knowledge base also leads him to direct the assessment of Mrs. Tillman's symptoms because cancer and cancer treatment cause a variety of physical and psychological changes. Good communication skills and critical thinking allow Rich to begin to gather information for a complete, accurate, and relevant database.

Prior clinical experience contributes to assessment skills. For example, if you cared for a patient with heart disease in the past, you know the type of factors that precipitate or signal chest pain. Thus you know how to thoroughly assess the types of factors that typically precede a patient's chest pain. You become competent in assessment through validation of abnormal assessment findings and personal observation of assessments performed by skilled nurses. You also learn to apply standards of practice and accepted standards of "normal" physical assessment data when assessing a patient. These standards help you collect the right kind of information and ensure that you have a standard against which to compare your findings. The use of attributes such as curiosity, perseverance, and risk taking ensures that your database is thorough and complete.

Data Collection

When you assess a patient, think critically about what to assess (i.e., what you need to know to provide safe, effective care). Determine which questions or measurements are appropriate based on your clinical knowledge and experience. Once you start, select additional questions and measurements based on your patient's responses. When you first meet a patient, make a quick observational overview or screening. Usually you base your overview on the treatment situation. For example, a community health nurse assesses a patient's neighborhood and community, a surgical nurse focuses on a patient's pain control and surgical wound healing, and a home care nurse focuses on a patient's environment and ways to cope with illness.

You learn to differentiate important data from the total data collected. A **cue** is information that you obtain through use of the senses. An **inference** is your judgment or interpretation of these cues (Figure 9-2). For example, the cue of Mrs. Tillman expressing a sense of feeling tired and not having energy for daily routines leads you to infer a problem with activity. Anything a patient says and any behaviors you observe are important cues. It is possible to miss cues when you conduct your initial overview. However, always be observant and try to interpret cues from the patient to know how in-depth your eventual assessment needs to be.

After your observational overview, you begin to focus on assessment cues and patterns of information that suggest

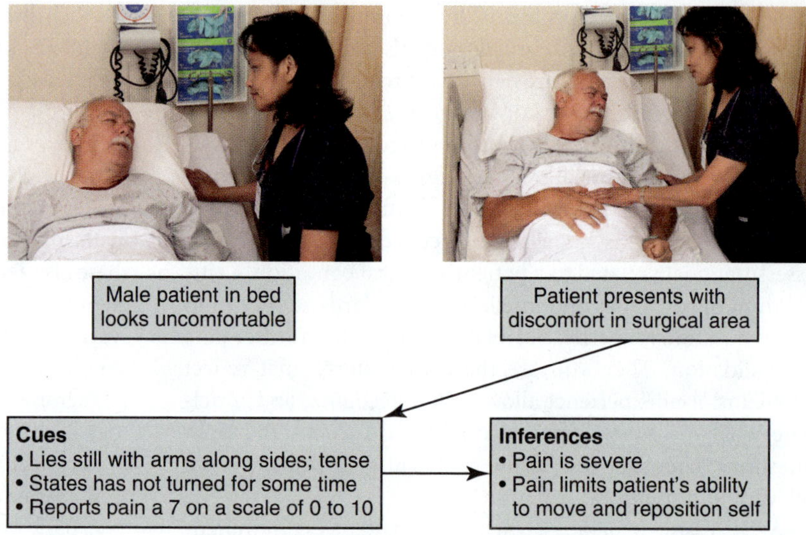

FIGURE 9-2 Observational overview using cues and forming inferences.

problem areas. However, it is essential to conduct a comprehensive assessment when you can. There are two approaches for a comprehensive assessment. One involves use of a structured database format, based on an accepted theoretical framework or practice standard. Gordon's 11 **functional health patterns** is a good example (Gordon, 1994). The theory or practice standard provides categories of information for you to assess. Gordon's model provides a holistic framework for assessment of a patient's health history, from which you derive a broad range of nursing diagnoses. Box 9-1 offers examples of the types of assessment data that you collect when using Gordon's functional health pattern model. An assessment moves from the general to the specific. For example, you assess all of Gordon's 11 functional health patterns to determine if any problems exist. The premise is that the categories lead you to perform the most comprehensive assessment of a patient's health care problems.

The second approach for conducting a comprehensive assessment is the problem-focused approach. You focus on a patient's situation and begin with problematic areas such as a patient's report of feeling tired. Then you ask the patient follow-up questions to clarify and expand. For example, Rich asks Mrs. Tillman how her lack of energy affects her ability to perform routine tasks and the extent to which it affects her physically (Table 9-1). Once he completes his initial assessment, he thoroughly analyzes the extent and nature of Mrs. Tillman's sense of feeling tired. This allows him to identify her health problem correctly so he can develop a comprehensive treatment plan.

Whichever approach you use for assessment, you begin to cluster cues, make inferences, and identify emerging patterns and potential problems. To do this well, you anticipate critically, which means that you always try to stay a step ahead of the assessment. For example, if you suspect that a patient has a certain type of health problem (e.g., fatigue), you pose questions that deal with responses typically seen with fatigue. Remember to always have supporting cues before you make an inference. Inferences lead you to further

BOX 9-1 TYPOLOGY OF 11 FUNCTIONAL HEALTH PATTERNS

Health perception–health management pattern: Describes patient's self-report of health and well-being; how health is managed (e.g., frequency of health care provider visits, adherence to prescribed therapies at home); knowledge of preventive health practices

Nutritional-metabolic pattern: Describes patient's daily/weekly pattern of food and fluid intake (e.g., food preferences, special diet, food restrictions, appetite); actual weight, weight loss or gain

Elimination pattern: Describes patterns of excretory function (bowel, bladder, and skin)

Activity-exercise pattern: Describes patterns of exercise, activity, leisure, and recreation; ability to perform activities of daily living

Sleep-rest pattern: Describes patterns of sleep, rest, and relaxation

Cognitive-perceptual pattern: Describes sensory-perceptual patterns; language adequacy, memory, decision-making ability

Self-perception–self-concept pattern: Describes patient's self-concept pattern and perceptions of self (e.g., self-concept/worth, emotional patterns, body image)

Role-relationship pattern: Describes patient's pattern of role engagements and relationships

Sexuality-reproductive pattern: Describes patient's patterns of satisfaction and dissatisfaction with sexuality pattern; patient's reproductive pattern; premenopausal and postmenopausal problems

Coping–stress-tolerance pattern: Describes patient's ability to manage stress; sources of support; effectiveness of the pattern in terms of stress tolerance

Value-belief pattern: Describes patterns of values and beliefs (including spiritual practices) and goals that guide the patient's choices or decisions

Data from Gordon M: *Nursing diagnosis: process and application,* ed 3, St Louis, 1994, Mosby; Carpenito-Moyet LJ: *Nursing diagnosis: application to clinical practice,* ed 14, Philadelphia, 2013, Lippincott Williams & Wilkins.

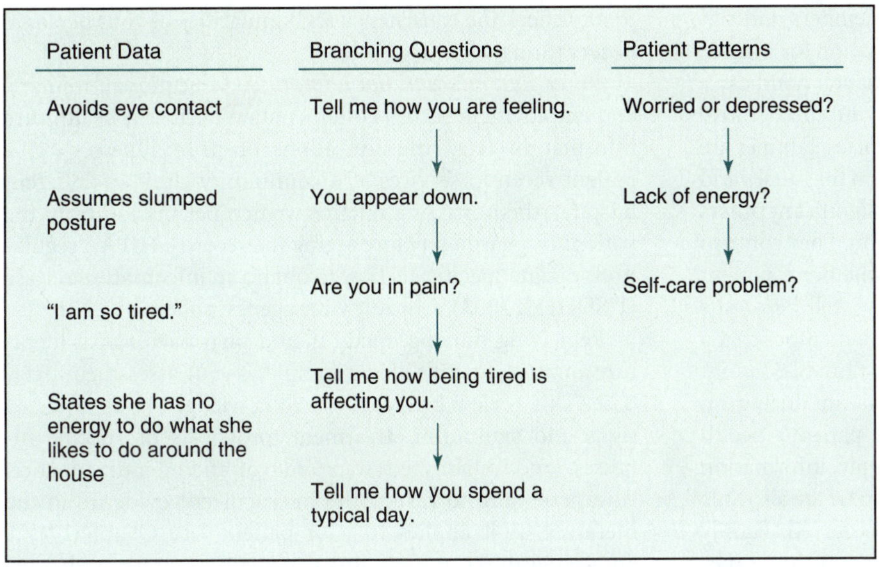

FIGURE 9-3 Example of branching logic for selecting assessment questions.

TABLE 9-1 FOCUSED PATIENT ASSESSMENT

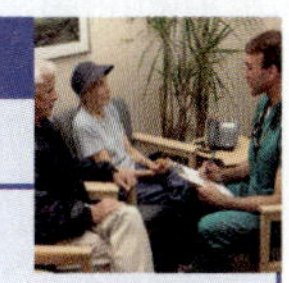

FACTORS TO ASSESS	QUESTIONS	PHYSICAL ASSESSMENT
Ability to perform routine tasks	Tell me how your fatigue affects how you do household activities. Describe what you did in a typical day before you had cancer. How has this changed?	Observe how quickly patient responds to questions. Observe posture and body movements.
Extent to which lack of energy affects her physically	Tell me how feeling tired affects your interest in social activities. Do you have more energy after you sleep or rest?	Observe facial and other nonverbal expressions.

questions. Once you ask a question or make an observation of a patient, the information branches to an additional series of questions or observations (Figure 9-3). You take a risk when you do not anticipate assessment questions. This can cause an incomplete assessment, or you might fail to recognize cues and dismiss relevant problems. Knowing how to probe and frame questions is a skill that grows with experience. You learn to decide which questions are relevant to a situation while at the same time making sure the assessment is complete.

Types of Data. There are two primary sources of data, subjective and objective. **Subjective data** are patients' verbal descriptions of their health problems. Only patients provide subjective data. For example, Mrs. Tillman's statements about being worn out and dealing with a difficult experience are subjective findings. Subjective data usually include feelings of anxiety, physical discomfort, or mental stress. Although only patients provide subjective data relevant to their health condition, be aware that the associated problems sometimes cause physiological changes, which you can further explore through objective data collection. For example, after listening to Mrs. Tillman describe her fatigue and its effects, Rich assesses her ability to walk a short distance.

Objective data are observations or measurements of a patient's health status. Inspection of the condition of a wound or observation of a patient's posture and gait are examples of objective data. You base your measurements of objective data on an accepted standard such as the Fahrenheit or Celsius measure on a thermometer, centimeters on a measuring tape, or known characteristics of behaviors. When you collect objective data, apply critical thinking intellectual standards (e.g., clear, precise, and consistent). Do not include your personal interpretive statements.

Sources of Data. You obtain data from a variety of sources. Each source of data provides information about the patient's level of wellness, risk factors, health practices and goals, and patterns of health and illness.

Patient. A patient is usually your best source of information. A patient who is alert and answers questions appropriately provides the most accurate information about health care needs, lifestyle patterns, present and past illnesses, perception of symptoms, and changes in activities of daily living (ADLs). Always consider the setting for your assessment. A patient experiencing acute pain in an emergency department will not offer the same depth of information as one who comes to an outpatient clinic for a routine checkup. Always be attentive and show a caring presence with patients (see Chapter 19). Patients are less likely to fully reveal the nature of their health care problems when you show little interest or are easily distracted by activities around them.

Family and Significant Others. Family members and significant others are primary sources of information for infants, children, critically ill adults, patients with mental handicaps, or patients who are unconscious or have reduced cognitive function. In cases of severe illness or emergencies, families are often the only available sources of information for nurses and other health care providers. The family and significant others are also good secondary sources of information. They confirm information that a patient provides (e.g., whether a patient takes medications regularly at home or how well he or she eats). Include the family when appropriate. Remember that a patient does not always want you to question the family. However, often spouses or close friends sit in during an assessment and provide their view of the patient's health problems or needs. Not only do they supply information about the patient's current health status, but they are also able to tell when changes in his or her status occurred. Family members are often very well informed because of their experiences living with the patient and observing how health problems affect ADLs. For example, Mr. Tillman is an excellent resource for describing how his wife's lack of energy affects her day to day.

Health Care Team. You frequently communicate with other health care team members when gathering information about patients. In the acute care setting, the change-of-shift report or patient hand-off is the way for nurses on one shift to communicate information to nurses or other health care providers on oncoming shifts (see Chapter 10). A hand-off is described as an interactive process of passing patient-specific information from one caregiver to another for the purpose of ensuring the continuity and safety of patient care (Wayne et al., 2008). Effective communication through hand-offs can improve care providers' perceptions of accuracy, completeness, and number of tasks transferred. Typically when nurses and other health care providers consult on a patient's condition, each contributes information about the patient. This includes how the patient is interacting within the health care environment, the patient's reactions to treatment, the results of diagnostic procedures or therapies, and how the patient responds to visitors. Every member of the health care team is a source of information for identifying and verifying information about the patient.

Medical Records. The medical record is a source for a patient's medical history, laboratory and diagnostic test results, current physical findings, and a health care provider's treatment plan. Data in the records offer baseline and ongoing information about a patient's response to illness and progress to date. The Health Insurance Portability and Accountability Act (HIPAA) of 1996 has a privacy rule that came into effect in 2003 to set standards for the protection of health information (U.S. Department of Health and Human Services [USDHHS], 2003). Information in a patient's record is confidential. Each health care agency has policies governing how health care providers can share information. A nurse can review a patient's medical record for assessment data but needs to know the agency policies governing how to share the information with other staff. The medical record is a valuable tool to check the consistency and similarities of your personal observations.

Other Records and the Literature. Educational, military, and employment records often contain pertinent health care information (e.g., immunizations or prior illnesses). If a patient received services at a community clinic or different hospital, the nurse first obtains written permission from the patient or guardian before seeing the records. HIPAA regulations dictate specifically how to obtain an information release (USDHHS, 2003). Consult your agency policies.

Reviewing nursing, medical, and pharmacological literature about a patient's illness completes your assessment database. This review increases your knowledge about expected signs and symptoms, treatment, prognosis of specific illnesses, and established standards of therapeutic practice. Always be sure to review the most current evidence in the literature as it applies to your patient (see Chapter 7). A knowledgeable nurse obtains pertinent, accurate, and complete information for the assessment database.

Methods of Data Collection. As a nurse you use the patient interview as the tool for assessing a patient's health history. Once you have collected data, you proceed to a physical examination.

Interview and Health History. The first step in establishing a database is to collect subjective information while interviewing a patient. An interview is an organized conversation with a patient (see Chapter 11). The initial interview involves assessing the patient's health history and obtaining information about the current illness. During the initial interview you have the opportunity to:

1. Introduce yourself to the patient, explain your role, and explain the role of others during care.
2. Establish a caring therapeutic relationship with the patient.
3. Explain how you will conduct the interview (e.g., first obtaining information about the patient's current concerns and then collecting other information).
4. Gain insight about the patient's concerns and worries.
5. Determine the patient's goals and expectations of the health care delivery system.
6. Obtain cues about which parts of the data collection phase require in-depth investigation.

Later interviews allow you to assess more about a patient's situation and focus on specific problem areas. An interview helps patients explain their own interpretations and understandings of their conditions. Therefore you and the patient are partners during the interview; you do not control it. An interview consists of three phases: orientation, working, and termination.

Always prepare for an interview. Collect any available information about a patient and create a favorable environment for the interview. For example, review the information you learn during any hand-off or change-of-shift report and plan to interview the patient during rounds and before you begin to deliver patient care. In a hospital setting you often need to provide measures for symptom relief before a patient is able to talk comfortably with you. In the home choose a location that is quiet and as free of interruptions as is possible.

Orientation Phase. The orientation phase begins with introducing yourself and your position and explaining the purpose of the interview. Explain to patients why you are collecting data and assure them that all the information and protected health information will remain confidential and be used only by health care professionals who provide his or her care (see Chapter 10). HIPAA regulations require patients to sign an authorization before you collect personal health data (USDHHS, 2003). This usually occurs in admitting or screening areas before you meet a patient.

During orientation you establish trust and confidence with a patient. One important goal for the initial interview is to lay the groundwork for understanding a patient's needs. In the initial discussion between Rich and Mrs. Tillman, Rich explains that he wants to put a plan together and to do so he wants to understand more about how Mrs. Tillman's cancer affects her during a typical day. He also tells the patient that he wants to learn more about the symptoms she is having.

Another goal for the interview is to begin a relationship that allows the patient to become an active partner in decisions about care. As the orientation phase proceeds, a patient usually begins to feel more comfortable speaking with you. Initially you gather demographic data (e.g., date of birth, gender, address, family members' names and addresses), as specified by the facility. Because this information is the least personal, it helps initiate development of the therapeutic relationship and eases transition into the working phase of the interview.

Working Phase. During the working phase you gather information about a patient's health status. Remember to stay focused, orderly, and unhurried. You begin by obtaining the patient's health history (Box 9-2). Use a variety of communication strategies such as active listening, paraphrasing, and summarizing to promote a clear interaction (see Chapter 11) and construct a thorough database. The use of open-ended questions in particular encourages patients to tell their story in detail.

Rich begins the working phase of his interview by focusing on Mrs. Tillman's sense of "feeling worn out." He attends to her concerns, immediately making her a partner in the interview, and then focuses on details that will reveal the extent to which cancer is affecting her life.

Rich: "You say you're worn out; tell me how you spend a typical day."

Mrs. Tillman: "When I first wake up, I actually feel pretty good. I'm able to get through breakfast and most of my bath before I start to feel tired."

Rich: "Uh-huh, go on." (active listening and probing)

Mrs. Tillman: "I used to do my errands midmorning, but I seem to lose energy. My husband decided to retire just this year. He helps me a great deal."

Rich: "You say you lose energy; tell me how you feel." (paraphrase and open-ended question)

Mrs. Tillman: "I just feel this sensation that I can't do any more. I'm too weak to move. I often have to take a nap midmorning. Isn't that ridiculous? The cancer has just weakened me so much."

Rich: "How you feel is not ridiculous; tell me how you feel after you nap." (open-ended question)

Rich explores in depth how Mrs. Tillman is physically affected by her cancer. He also gathers information from Mr. Tillman. The information ultimately directs him in identifying the patient's health problems and choosing appropriate nursing therapies.

The first interview with a patient is often the most extensive. Ongoing interviews, which occur each time you interact with your patient, do not need to be as extensive. They update a patient's status and focus more on changes in previously identified ongoing and new problems.

Termination Phase. As in the other phases of the interview, the termination phase requires skill on the part of the interviewer. Give your patient a clue that the interview is coming to an end. For example, you say, "There are just two more questions" or "We'll be finished in 5 to 6 minutes." This helps the patient maintain direct attention without being distracted by wondering when the interview will end. This approach also gives the patient a chance to ask questions. When ending the interview, summarize the important points and ask your patient if the summary is accurate. End the interview in a friendly manner, telling the patient when you will return to provide care. For example, "Thanks, Mrs. Tillman. You've given me a clear picture of your health and

BOX 9-2 BASIC COMPONENTS FOR A NURSING HEALTH HISTORY

Reasons for seeking health care: Goals of care, expectation of the services and care delivered, and expectations of the health care system

Present illness or health concern: Onset, symptoms, nature of symptoms (e.g., sudden or gradual), duration, precipitating factors, relief measures, and weight loss or gain

Health history: Prior illnesses throughout development; injuries and hospitalizations, surgeries; blood transfusions, allergies, immunizations; habits (e.g., smoking, caffeine intake, alcohol or drug abuse); prescribed and self-prescribed medications; work habits; relaxation activities; and sleep, exercise, and eating or nutritional patterns

Family history: Health status of immediate family and living relatives; cause of death of relatives; and risk factor analyses for cancer, heart disease, diabetes mellitus, kidney disease, hypertension, or mental disorders

Environmental history: Hazards, pollutants, and physical safety

Psychosocial and cultural history: Primary language, cultural group, community resources, mood, attention span, and developmental stage

Review of systems: Head-to-toe review of all major body systems and patient's knowledge of and compliance with health care (e.g., frequency of breast or testicular self-examination or last visual acuity examination) (Another option for an approach is to use *functional health patterns* as the method for organizing assessment data.)

how you've been affected. It's important for you to understand how we expect the cancer will affect you and how we can help you manage your symptoms. Is that OK? I hope to develop a plan of care that will manage your difficulty breathing and sense of fatigue. Do you have any questions?"

Interview Techniques. The way in which you conduct an interview is just as important as the questions you ask. Pay attention to the environment, patient comfort, and communication techniques (see Chapter 11) to be successful. During an interview direct the flow of conversation so you obtain adequate information and the patient has the chance to contribute freely. Ideally you want patients to tell their stories about their health problems so you can obtain as many details as possible.

Some interviews are focused, whereas others are comprehensive. Listen and consider the information shared. This helps you direct a patient to give more detail or to discuss a topic that probably reveals a possible problem. Because a patient's report includes subjective information, validate data from the interview later with objective data. For example, Mrs. Tillman reports that she often feels too weak to move. Rich later measures her muscle strength and tolerance to walking.

Remember that patients also obtain information during interviews. If you establish a positive nurse-patient relationship, the patient feels comfortable asking you questions about planned treatments, diagnostic procedures, and need for resources. Patients need this information to make decisions about their health care.

A good interview environment is free of distractions, unnecessary noise, and interruptions. A patient is more likely to be candid if an interview is private (i.e., out of earshot of other patients, visitors, and staff). Timing is important in avoiding interruptions. If possible, set aside a 15- to 30-minute period when no other activities are planned. Another option in a busy hospital setting is to set aside two 15-minute periods during your shift. Help the patient feel relaxed and unhurried. Before you begin the interview, be sure that the patient is comfortable. Comfort factors include toileting, providing adequate light and warmth, and positioning. Sit facing the patient to facilitate eye contact. During the interview observe your patient for signs of discomfort or fatigue.

When the interview involves a health history, try to find out, in the patient's own words, what the health problem is and what is likely causing it. Remember that patients are usually the best resources in explaining their health history. Begin by asking the patient a question to elicit his or her story. For example, say, "Tell me why you came to the hospital today" or "Tell me about the problems you're having." The use of **open-ended questions** prompts patients to describe a situation in more than one or two words. This technique leads to a discussion in which patients actively describe their health status. The use of open-ended questions strengthens the nurse-patient relationship because it shows that you want to invest time in hearing the patient's thoughts. Encourage the patient to tell the story all the way through. Reinforce your interest by using good eye contact and listening skills. Use **back-channeling,** which is the practice of giving positive comments such as "all right," "go on," or "uh-huh" to the speaker. These indicate that you have heard what the patient says and are interested in hearing the full story.

Once patients tell their story, use a problem-seeking interview technique. This approach takes the information provided in the patient's story and more fully describes and identifies specific problem areas. For example, focus on the symptoms that the patient identifies and ask **closed-ended questions** that limit his or her answers to one or two words such as "yes" or "no" or a number or frequency of a symptom. For example, ask, "How often do you feel really tired or fatigued?" or "After taking a nap, do you feel more rested?" As closed-ended questions reveal more information, you have the patient discuss historical information in more detail. A good interviewer leaves with a complete story that contains enough detail for understanding the patient's perceptions of his or her health status and the information needed to help identify nursing diagnoses and/or collaborative health problems. Always clarify or validate any information that is unclear.

Physical Examination. A physical examination allows a nurse to examine a patient's body to determine his or her state of health. It involves use of the techniques of inspection, palpation, percussion, auscultation, and smell. A complete examination includes a patient's height, weight, vital signs (see Chapter 15), general appearance and behavior, and a head-to-toe examination of all body systems (see Chapter 16).

Observation of Patient's Behavior. During an interview and physical examination it is important for you to closely observe a patient's verbal and nonverbal behaviors. This information adds depth to the objective database. You learn to determine whether data obtained by observation match what the patient states verbally. For example, if a patient expresses no concern about an upcoming diagnostic test but appears anxious and irritable, verbal and nonverbal data conflict. Observations lead you to gather the additional objective information to form accurate conclusions about a patient's condition.

An important aspect of observation includes a patient's level of function: the physical, developmental, psychological, and social aspects of everyday living. Observation of the level of function is different from what you learn about function during the interview. You observe what you see the patient doing such as self-feeding or making a decision rather than what the patient says he or she can do. Level of function differs from a physical assessment. The level of function involves a person's ability to perform during everyday activities. The hands-on physical examination measures the extent of function through measures such as range of motion and muscle strength.

Diagnostic and Laboratory Data. The results of diagnostic and laboratory tests identify or verify alterations questioned or identified during the nursing health history and physical examination. For example, during the health history the patient reports having had a bad cold for 6 days and at present has a productive cough with dark yellow sputum and mild shortness of breath. On physical examination you notice an elevated temperature, increased respirations, and decreased breath sounds in the right lower lobe. You review the results of an ordered complete blood count (CBC) and note that the white blood cell count is elevated (indicating an infection). In addition, the radiologist's report of a chest x-ray examination shows the presence of a right lower lobe infiltrate. Such findings combined suggest that the patient has the medical diagnosis of pneumonia and the associated nursing diagnosis of *Impaired Gas Exchange*. When a patient collects and monitors laboratory data at home such as with routine blood glucose monitoring for diabetes, ask him or her about the routine results to determine his or her response to illness and the effects of treatment measures. Compare laboratory data with the established norms for a particular test, age-group, and gender.

Cultural Considerations in Assessment

Good assessment techniques are important for patient-centered care, especially when caring for patients from cultural backgrounds different from your own (Box 9-3), such as ethnicity, sexual preference, or religious views. You must make a conscious effort to understand your patient's culture so you can provide better care within different value systems and act with respect and understanding without imposing your own attitudes and beliefs (see Chapter 20). These cross-cultural differences need to be addressed to obtain accurate assessment data (Suhonen et al., 2011). Communication and culture are interrelated in the way individuals express feelings verbally and nonverbally. When you learn the variations in how people of different cultural backgrounds communicate, you likely gather more accurate information from patients. Use the right approach, applying sensitive communication techniques such as speaking at eye level, using the proper distance, and listening to show respect for your patient. These techniques will likely result in the patient sharing more information. When you assess patients, consider the many factors that influence their health because of their cultural background.

BOX 9-3 PATIENT-CENTERED CARE

The nursing process is a good way to implement patient-centered care. To be effective, it is important during the assessment phase to ask a patient and family useful questions that begin to explore the patient's illness or health care problem in context of the patient's culture (Seidel et al., 2011).

IMPLICATIONS FOR PRACTICE

- When talking about a patient's illness:
  - What do you think is wrong with you?
  - What do you call your problem?
  - What worries you most about your illness?
- When talking about treatments:
  - What should be done to get rid of your problem?
  - Which types of treatments do you use?
  - Has anyone helped you with this problem?
  - What benefit do you expect from the treatment?
- When there are cross-cultural differences between health care professional and patient, ask yourself these questions (Suhonen, et al., 2011):
  - Learn what is unique to your patient's culture and its impact on the treatment plan.
  - Identify resources within the agency and community to help you to provide culturally competent care to the patient and family.
  - Recognize your own potential for cultural misunderstandings and strive to correct them.
  - Which types of treatments do you use?
  - Has anyone helped you with this problem?
  - What benefit do you expect from the treatment?

Data Validation

The ability to make accurate judgments on the basis of an assessment requires critical thinking. Once you have collected your data, validate the data you obtained. This helps you to more accurately analyze and interpret a patient's clinical picture. **Validation** of assessment data is the comparison of data with another source to confirm accuracy. For example, Rich observes Mrs. Tillman crying and logically infers that it is related to her cancer diagnosis. Making such an initial inference is not wrong, but problems result if you do not validate the inference with the patient. Rich should ask, "I notice that you've been crying. Can you tell me about it?" By doing so, Rich discovers the real reason for Mrs. Tillman's crying.

Ask your patient to validate the information you gather during the interview and health history. Validate findings from physical examination and observation of patient behavior by comparing data in the medical record and consulting with other health team members or even family members. Validation often leads you to gather more assessment data because it clarifies vague or ambiguous data. Occasionally you need to reassess previously covered areas of the nursing history or gather further physical examination data. A nurse continually analyzes and thinks about a patient's database, enabling him or her to fully understand the problems, judge their extent, and discover possible relationships between them.

Rich gathers initial data about Mrs. Tillman's physical health, having focused on her lack of energy and "feeling tired" and the effects it has on her ability to conduct daily activities. He applies critical thinking in his assessment to consider what he knew about the effects of cancer and the therapies Mrs. Tillman received, such as chemotherapy. The patient takes more frequent naps and reports little energy to do routine chores or engage in any social activities. Rich also learns a great deal about Mrs. Tillman's feelings about having advanced-stage cancer. He uses intellectual standards, being precise (specific feelings about prognosis), consistent, accurate (a self-report scale to measure her perceptions of her quality of life), and complete (probing to determine how her feelings affect her relationship with her husband). Rich learns that Mrs. Tillman worries about her husband. She tells Rich, "He means so much to me. The doctor has told me what to expect. I know this is going to be very hard for him." Rich could make several inferences from this comment, but he applies the critical thinking attitude of discipline and validates his inferences, "You sound worried about your husband. Describe what's bothering you." Mrs. Tillman confirms Rich's assessment, "I'm worried about Greg because he tries so hard to help me. I'm worried that he'll get worn out too."

Data Documentation and Communication

Communication of assessment findings, either verbally or through documentation, is the last step of a complete assessment. The timely, thorough, and accurate communication of facts is necessary to ensure continuity and appropriateness of patient care. If you do not report or record an assessment finding or problem interpretation, it is lost and unavailable to anyone else caring for the patient (see Chapter 10). If you do not give specific information, you leave another health care team member uninformed and often with only general impressions. Observation, reporting, and recording of a patient's status are legal and professional responsibilities. The Nurse Practice Acts in all states and the American Nurses Association policy statement (2010) require accurate data collection and recording as independent functions essential to the role of a professional nurse.

NURSING DIAGNOSIS

After reviewing and validating a patient's assessment, the next step of the nursing process is to form diagnostic conclusions to determine a patient's problems and level of care required. If a nurse forms an accurate diagnostic conclusion, nursing therapies will be appropriate and relevant. A nurse makes a diagnostic conclusion either in the form of a nursing diagnosis or a collaborative problem. A **nursing diagnosis** is a clinical judgment about individual, family, or community responses to actual and potential health problems or life processes that the nurse is licensed and competent to treat (NANDA-I, 2012). A nursing diagnosis provides the basis for the selection of nursing interventions to achieve outcomes for which the nurse is accountable (NANDA-I, 2012).

Never confuse a medical diagnosis with a nursing diagnosis. A **medical diagnosis** is the identification of a disease condition based on an evaluation of physical signs, symptoms, history, and diagnostic tests and procedures. Physicians and certified advanced practice nurses make medical diagnoses. Physicians are licensed to treat diseases or pathological processes described in medical diagnostic statements. For example, a physician treats a patient with the medical diagnosis of cancer through medications, radiation, and surgery. An advanced practice nurse can also treat medical diagnoses but does not perform surgery. In contrast, a patient's responses to cancer such as symptoms of pain and nausea and insufficient knowledge about treatment are nursing diagnoses that nurses manage. What makes a nursing diagnostic process unique is having patients involved in the process when possible.

A **collaborative problem** is an actual or potential physiological complication that nurses monitor to detect the onset of changes in a patient's status (Carpenito-Moyet, 2013). When collaborative problems develop, nurses intervene in collaboration with personnel from other health care disciplines such as social workers and dietitians. Nurses manage collaborative problems such as hemorrhage or infection using both physician-prescribed and nursing-prescribed interventions. For example, a patient who has a surgical wound is at risk for developing an infection; thus a physician prescribes antibiotics. The nurse monitors the patient for signs of infection, provides meticulous wound care, and administers the prescribed antibiotics.

Nurses use scientific and nursing knowledge and previous experience to analyze and interpret assessment data in identifying nursing diagnoses and collaborative problems unique for their patients. The remainder of this section focuses on the reasoning process for making a nursing diagnosis.

Critical Thinking and the Nursing Diagnostic Process

The nursing diagnostic process requires you to use critical thinking. This involves logically analyzing and interpreting assessment data about a patient to form a clinical judgment, in this case a nursing diagnosis. The **nursing diagnostic process** flows from the assessment process and includes data clustering, interpreting and analyzing, identifying patient needs, and formulating the nursing diagnosis or collaborative problem (Figure 9-4).

When you correctly analyze assessment data, you are able to identify patients' problems and make clinical decisions about their care. Analysis begins by organizing all of your data into meaningful and usable **data clusters.** A data cluster is a set of signs or symptoms gathered during assessment that you group together in a logical way. During clustering a cue or an individual sign, symptom, or finding alerts your thinking more than others. You begin to see how different data relate to one another. For example, Mrs. Tillman talks about not having any energy, taking frequent naps, and not being able to perform usual activities such as preparing meals. These cues show a pattern. **Data analysis** and interpretation involve recognizing patterns or trends in the clustered data, comparing them with standards, and coming to a reasoned conclusion about the patient's response to a health problem. Rich compares Mrs. Tillman's signs and symptoms with normal standards for a woman her age such as feeling rested, sleeping through the night, and being able to perform daily routines. Mrs. Tillman's clinical picture suggests that, as a response to her cancer, she is experiencing a pattern of fatigue that affects her activity level.

Through reasoning and judgment a nurse decides which assessment information explains a patient's health status. Often a patient presents multiple cues, suggesting more than one type of health problem or need. At times you have to gather additional data for clarification of your interpretation. *For example, Mrs. Tillman tells Rich that she has many*

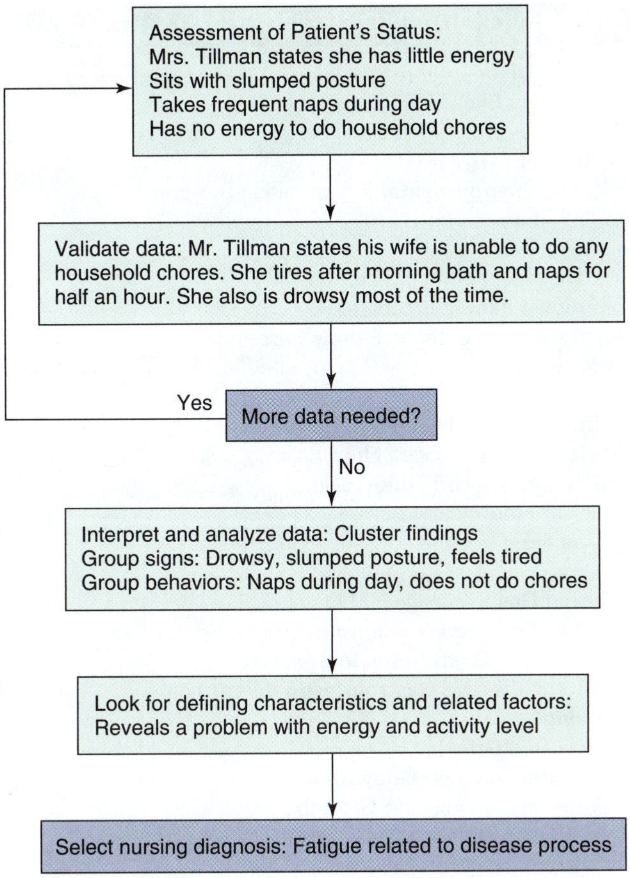

FIGURE 9-4 Nursing diagnostic process for Mrs. Tillman.

unanswered questions, even though her doctor has talked about how her cancer will progress. She says, "I hope I can just not wake up one morning." Rich infers that Mrs. Tillman dreads how the cancer will affect her. He seeks further information, "Let's talk about what your doctor said about the cancer." Mrs. Tillman relates, "He says that further chemotherapy likely will not be effective. I can expect to have trouble breathing and possibly pain, but he said he will be sure to give me what I need." Rich clarifies, "You sound a bit uncertain. Are you concerned that you'll suffer?" Mrs. Tillman begins to cry, "Yes, oh yes, that is my greatest fear. I really don't know what to expect." Rich further clarifies, "Have you received an explanation about palliative care?" Mrs. Tillman replies, "No, I haven't. What does that mean?" In looking for additional patterns of data, Rich decides that Mrs. Tillman is having a difficult time anticipating her impending death and has insufficient understanding of her health care options. These problems add to her pattern of fatigue.

Formulating the Nursing Diagnosis

Once a nurse sees how patterns of data point to a patient's health problems, it becomes important to identify these problems in a way that will be clear to all health care providers (Box 9-4). **NANDA International (NANDA-I)** has developed a model for organizing nursing diagnoses for documentation, auditing, and communication purposes. New diagnoses are continually developed through research and added to the NANDA-I listing. The use of standard formal nursing diagnoses serves several purposes:

- Provides a precise definition that gives all members of the health care team a common language for understanding patient needs
- Allows nurses to communicate what they do among themselves, with other health care professionals, and with the public
- Distinguishes the nurse's role from that of physicians and other health care providers
- Helps nurses focus on the scope of nursing practice
- Fosters the development of nursing knowledge

As a nurse reviews all assessment data, he or she compares the clusters and patterns of data with the clinical criteria for making a nursing diagnosis. **Defining characteristics** are the clinical criteria or assessment findings that support an actual nursing diagnosis. NANDA-I–approved nursing diagnoses have identified sets of defining characteristics that support identification of each nursing diagnosis (NANDA-I, 2012). Over time you become familiar with the defining characteristics for the more common nursing diagnoses in your practice. This makes recognition of nursing diagnoses easier. Box 9-5 shows an example of an approved nursing diagnosis and its associated defining characteristics and related factors. As you analyze clusters of data, you begin to consider various diagnoses that apply to your patient. For example, Rich reviews findings pertaining to Mrs. Tillman, who reported feeling tired and having a lack of energy. The defining characteristics of being tired and lacking energy apply to the nursing diagnoses of Fatigue and Activity Intolerance. However, Rich's assessment probed further to reveal Mrs. Tillman's inability to maintain usual levels of activity or routines, pointing his diagnostic conclusion toward Fatigue. It is important to learn that the absence of certain defining characteristics suggests that you reject a diagnosis under consideration. Carefully examine defining characteristics that support or eliminate a nursing diagnosis. To be more accurate, review all characteristics, eliminate nonrelevant ones, and confirm relevant ones.

While focusing on patterns of defining characteristics, you also compare a patient's pattern of data with data that are consistent with normal, healthful patterns. Use accepted norms as the basis for comparison and judgment. This includes using laboratory and diagnostic test values, professional standards, and normal anatomical or physiological limits. When comparing patterns, judge whether the grouped signs and symptoms are normal for the patient and within the range of healthful responses. As you isolate the defining characteristics that are not within healthy norms, you identify a patient need or problem. *For example, Rich assessed Mrs. Tillman's verbal report of feeling tired and lacking energy. These symptoms are not necessarily common for a 72-year-old and indicate a basic problem involving the patient's ability to participate in normal activity. He also learned that Mrs. Tillman has difficulty completing routine chores at times and requires frequent naps during the day. Rich recognized that Mrs. Tillman had a problem, but he reviewed the NANDA-I classifications to*

BOX 9-4 NANDA-INTERNATIONAL–APPROVED NURSING DIAGNOSES 2012-2014

Activity Intolerance
Risk for **Activity** Intolerance
Ineffective **Activity** Planning
Risk for Ineffective **Activity** Planning
Risk for **Adverse Reaction** to Iodinated Contrast Media
Ineffective **Airway** Clearance
Risk for **Allergy** Response
Anxiety
Risk for **Aspiration**
Risk for Impaired **Attachment**
Autonomic Dysreflexia
Risk for **Autonomic** Dysreflexia
Disorganized Infant **Behavior**
Readiness for Enhanced Organized Infant **Behavior**
Risk for Disorganized Infant **Behavior**
Risk for **Bleeding**
Risk for Unstable **Blood** Glucose Level
Disturbed **Body** Image
Risk for Imbalanced **Body** Temperature
Insufficient **Breast** Milk
Ineffective **Breastfeeding**
Interrupted **Breastfeeding**
Readiness for Enhanced **Breastfeeding**
Ineffective **Breathing** Pattern
Decreased **Cardiac** Output
Caregiver Role Strain
Risk for **Caregiver** Role Strain
Ineffective **Childbearing** Process
Readiness for Enhanced **Childbearing** Process
Risk for Ineffective **Childbearing** Process
Impaired **Comfort**
Readiness for Enhanced **Comfort**
Readiness for Enhanced **Communication**
Impaired **Verbal** Communication
Acute **Confusion**
Chronic **Confusion**
Risk for Acute **Confusion**
Constipation
Perceived **Constipation**
Risk for **Constipation**
Contamination
Risk for **Contamination**
Readiness for Enhanced Community **Coping**
Defensive **Coping**
Ineffective **Coping**
Readiness for Enhanced **Coping**
Ineffective Community **Coping**
Compromised Family **Coping**
Disabled Family **Coping**
Readiness for Enhanced Family **Coping**
Death Anxiety
Risk for Sudden Infant **Death** Syndrome
Decisional Conflict
Readiness for Enhanced **Decision-Making**
Ineffective **Denial**
Impaired **Dentition**
Risk for Delayed **Development**
Diarrhea
Risk for **Disuse** Syndrome
Deficient **Diversional** Activity
Risk for **Dry Eye**
Risk for **Electrolyte** Imbalance
Disturbed **Energy** Field
Impaired **Environmental** Interpretation Syndrome
Adult **Failure** to Thrive
Risk for **Falls**
Dysfunctional **Family** Processes
Interrupted **Family** Processes
Readiness for Enhanced **Family** Processes
Fatigue
Fear
Ineffective Infant **Feeding** Pattern
Readiness for Enhanced **Fluid** Balance
Risk for Imbalanced **Fluid** Volume
Deficient **Fluid** Volume
Excess **Fluid** Volume
Risk for Deficient **Fluid** Volume
Impaired **Gas** Exchange
Risk for Dysfunctional **Gastrointestinal** Motility
Dysfunctional **Gastrointestinal** Motility
Risk for Ineffective **Gastrointestinal** Perfusion
Grieving
Complicated **Grieving**
Risk for Complicated **Grieving**
Risk for Disproportionate **Growth**
Delayed **Growth** and Development
Deficient Community **Health**
Risk-Prone **Health** Behavior
Ineffective **Health** Maintenance
Impaired **Home** Maintenance
Readiness for Enhanced **Hope**
Hopelessness
Risk for Compromised **Human** Dignity
Hyperthermia
Hypothermia
Readiness for Enhanced **Immunization** Status
Ineffective **Impulse** Control
Functional Urinary **Incontinence**
Overflow Urinary **Incontinence**
Reflex Urinary **Incontinence**
Stress Urinary **Incontinence**
Urge Urinary **Incontinence**
Risk for Urge Urinary **Incontinence**
Bowel **Incontinence**
Risk for **Infection**
Risk for **Injury**
Insomnia
Decreased **Intracranial** Adaptive Capacity
Neonatal **Jaundice**
Risk for Neonatal **Jaundice**
Deficient **Knowledge**
Readiness for Enhanced **Knowledge**
Latex Allergy Response
Risk for **Latex** Allergy Response
Sedentary **Lifestyle**
Risk for Impaired **Liver** Function
Risk for **Loneliness**
Risk for Disturbed **Maternal-Fetal** Dyad

BOX 9-4 NANDA-INTERNATIONAL–APPROVED NURSING DIAGNOSES 2012-2014—cont'd

Impaired **Memory**
Impaired Bed **Mobility**
Impaired Physical **Mobility**
Impaired Wheelchair **Mobility**
Moral Distress
Nausea
Unilateral **Neglect**
Noncompliance
Readiness for Enhanced **Nutrition**
Imbalanced **Nutrition**: Less Than Body Requirements
Risk for Imbalanced **Nutrition**: More Than Body Requirements
Imbalanced **Nutrition**: More Than Body Requirements
Impaired **Oral** Mucous Membrane
Acute **Pain**
Chronic **Pain**
Impaired **Parenting**
Readiness for Enhanced **Parenting**
Risk for Impaired **Parenting**
Risk for Perioperative **Positioning** Injury
Risk for **Peripheral** Neurovascular Dysfunction
Disturbed **Personal** Identity
Risk for Disturbed **Personal** Identity
Risk for **Poisoning**
Post-Trauma Syndrome
Risk for **Post-Trauma** Syndrome
Readiness for Enhanced **Power**
Powerlessness
Risk for **Powerlessness**
Ineffective **Protection**
Rape-Trauma Syndrome
Ineffective **Relationship**
Readiness for Enhanced **Relationship**
Risk for Ineffective **Relationship**
Impaired **Religiosity**
Readiness for Enhanced **Religiosity**
Risk for Impaired **Religiosity**
Relocation Stress Syndrome
Risk for **Relocation** Stress Syndrome
Risk for Ineffective **Renal** Perfusion
Impaired Individual **Resilience**
Readiness for Enhanced **Resilience**
Risk for Compromised **Resilience**
Parental **Role** Conflict
Ineffective **Role** Performance
Bathing **Self-Care** Deficit
Dressing **Self-Care** Deficit
Feeding **Self-Care** Deficit
Toileting **Self-Care** Deficit
Readiness for Enhanced **Self-Care**
Readiness for Enhanced **Self-Concept**
Chronic Low **Self-Esteem**
Situational Low **Self-Esteem**
Risk for Chronic Low **Self-Esteem**
Risk for Situational Low **Self-Esteem**
Ineffective **Self-Health** Management
Readiness for Enhanced **Self-Health** Management
Risk for **Self-Mutilation**
Self-Mutilation
Self-Neglect
Sexual Dysfunction
Ineffective **Sexuality** Pattern
Risk for **Shock**
Impaired **Skin** Integrity
Risk for Impaired **Skin** Integrity
Sleep Deprivation
Readiness for Enhanced **Sleep**
Disturbed **Sleep** Pattern
Impaired **Social** Interaction
Social Isolation
Chronic **Sorrow**
Spiritual Distress
Risk for **Spiritual** Distress
Readiness for Enhanced **Spiritual** Well-Being
Stress Overload
Risk for **Suffocation**
Risk for **Suicide**
Delayed **Surgical** Recovery
Impaired **Swallowing**
Ineffective Family **Therapeutic** Regimen Management
Risk for **Thermal** Injury
Ineffective **Thermoregulation**
Impaired **Tissue** Integrity
Ineffective Peripheral **Tissue** Perfusion
Risk for Decreased Cardiac **Tissue** Perfusion
Risk for Ineffective Cerebral **Tissue** Perfusion
Risk for Ineffective Peripheral Tissue Perfusion
Impaired **Transfer** Ability
Risk for **Trauma**
Impaired **Urinary** Elimination
Readiness for Enhanced **Urinary** Elimination
Urinary Retention
Risk for **Vascular** Trauma
Impaired Spontaneous **Ventilation**
Dysfunctional **Ventilatory** Weaning Response
Risk for Other-Directed **Violence**
Risk for Self-Directed **Violence**
Impaired **Walking**

define her problem more specifically. He looked first at the domain of activity/rest. NANDA-I has a variety of nursing diagnoses that can apply to activity/rest (e.g., Activity Intolerance, Risk for Activity Intolerance, Fatigue, *and* Impaired Walking). *After carefully reviewing Mrs. Tillman's presenting symptoms, Rich selected* Fatigue. *The key to Rich's diagnosis was assessing how the patient's lack of energy affected her daily activities.*

It is critical for a nurse to eventually arrive at the correct diagnostic label for a patient's need. A nurse usually moves from general to specific. It helps to think of the problem

BOX 9-5 EXAMPLE OF A NANDA INTERNATIONAL–APPROVED NURSING DIAGNOSIS WITH DEFINING CHARACTERISTICS AND RELATED FACTORS

Diagnosis: Fatigue

DEFINING CHARACTERISTICS	RELATED FACTORS (EXAMPLES)
Inability to maintain usual level of physical activity	Psychological: Anxiety, stress, depression
Inability to maintain usual routines	Physiological: Poor physical condition, malnutrition
Lack of energy	Environmental: Humidity, lights, noise
Lethargy	
Increase in rest requirements	Situational: Negative life events, occupation

Used with permission from NANDA International: *NANDA-I nursing diagnoses: definitions and classification 2009-2011*, Oxford, UK, 2009, Wiley-Blackwell.

identification phase as the identification of a general health care problem and the formulation of the nursing diagnosis as the identification of a specific health problem. When you begin to identify a problem, review the NANDA-I domains to help you focus on nursing diagnoses pertinent to a particular domain.

Types of Nursing Diagnoses. NANDA-I has identified three types of nursing diagnoses: actual diagnoses, risk diagnoses, and health promotion diagnoses (NANDA-I, 2012). An actual nursing diagnosis describes human responses to health conditions or life processes that exist in an individual, family, or community. The selection of an actual diagnosis indicates that there are sufficient assessment data to support the nursing diagnosis. In Mrs. Tillman's case, *Fatigue* and *Death Anxiety* are actual nursing diagnoses.

A risk nursing diagnosis describes human responses to health conditions or life processes that may develop in a vulnerable individual, family, or community (NANDA-I, 2012). These diagnoses do not have related factors or defining characteristics because they have not occurred yet. Instead a risk diagnosis has risk factors. Risk factors are the environmental, physiological, psychosocial, genetic, and chemical elements that place a person at risk for a health problem. For example, with Mrs. Tillman having symptoms of fatigue, Rich would assess further for risk diagnoses such as *Risk for Falls.*

A health promotion nursing diagnosis is a clinical judgment of a person's, family's, or community's motivation and desire to increase well-being and actualize human health potential as expressed in the readiness to enhance specific health behaviors such as nutrition and exercise. Health promotion diagnoses can be used in any health state and do not require a patient to have a high level of wellness. This readiness is supported by defining characteristics (NANDA-I, 2012). *Readiness for Enhanced Comfort* is an example of a health promotion diagnosis.

TABLE 9-2 NANDA INTERNATIONAL NURSING DIAGNOSIS FORMAT

DIAGNOSTIC LABEL	RELATED FACTORS (EXAMPLES LISTED)
Fatigue	Psychological: Anxiety, depression, stress Physiological: Malnutrition, poor physical condition Environmental: Humidity, lights, noise Situational: Negative life events, occupation
Death anxiety	Perceived proximity of death Anticipating pain Anticipating suffering Discussions on topic of death

Components of a Nursing Diagnosis. The identification of a nursing diagnosis flows from the assessment and diagnostic process. Throughout this text nursing diagnoses are worded in a two-part format: the diagnostic label followed by a statement of a related factor (Table 9-2). It is this two-part form that provides a diagnosis with meaning and relevance for a particular patient.

Diagnostic Label. The diagnostic label is the name of the nursing diagnosis as approved by NANDA-I (see Box 9-4). It describes the essence of a patient's response to a health condition in as few words as possible. All NANDA-I approved diagnoses also have a definition. The definition describes the characteristics of the human response identified. Refer to these definitions to help you identify a patient's correct diagnoses. They help especially when selecting between two diagnoses with similar defining characteristics. The diagnostic labels include descriptors used to give additional meaning to the diagnosis. For example, the diagnosis *Impaired Physical Mobility* includes the descriptor *impaired.* The term *impaired* describes the nature of or change in mobility that best describes the patient's response. Examples of other descriptors are *compromised, decreased, delayed,* or *effective.*

Related Factor. The related factor of the nursing diagnosis is identified from the patient's assessment data and is the reason the patient is displaying the nursing diagnosis. The related factor is associated with a patient's actual or potential response to the health problem and can change by using specific nursing interventions (NANDA-I, 2012). It comes from the patient's assessment data; for this reason assessment data need to be accurate. A related factor provides context for the defining characteristics (see Box 9-5). It is a condition associated with or contributing to the diagnosis. For example, a nursing diagnostic statement applicable to Mrs. Tillman includes the diagnostic label (e.g., *Fatigue*) and the related factor (e.g., *the disease process of cancer*). Related factors include four categories: pathophysiological (biological or psychological), treatment-related, situational (environmental or personal), and maturational (Carpenito-Moyet, 2013). The "related to" phrase is not a cause-and-effect statement. It

TABLE 9-3 FORMULATION OF NURSING DIAGNOSES

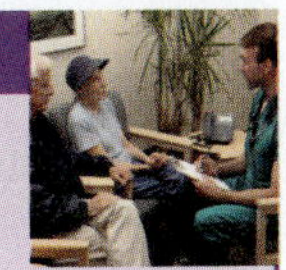

ASSESSMENT ACTIVITIES	DEFINING CHARACTERISTICS (CLUSTERING CUES)	NURSING DIAGNOSIS	ETIOLOGIES ("RELATED TO")
Ask patient to describe usual physical activity performed during the day.	Inability to maintain usual level of physical activity	Fatigue	Chronic disease process
Observe patient during care activities.	Lethargic Drowsy		
Question patient about frequency of rest periods.	Increase in rest requirements		
Ask patient to talk about any concerns or worries related to diagnosis of cancer.	Reports fear of suffering related to dying	Death anxiety	Anticipating suffering
Have patient describe her emotions.	Reports deep sadness		
Ask patient to discuss how she thinks her illness will affect her relationship with her husband.	Reports worry about impact of her own death on significant others		

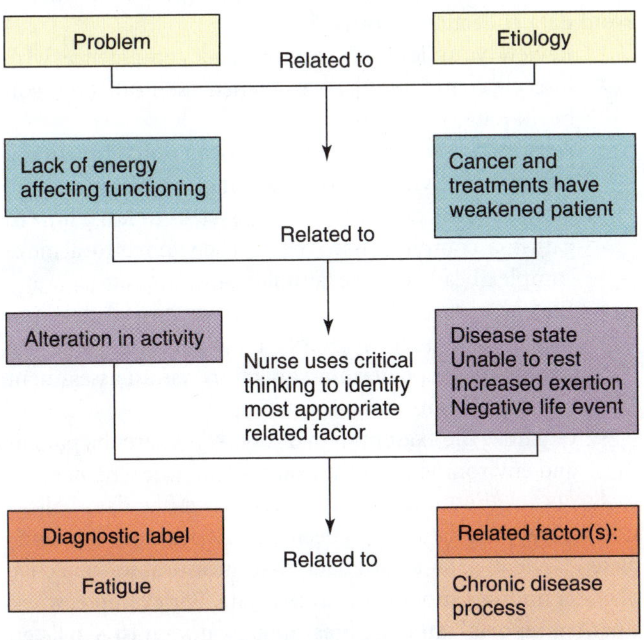

FIGURE 9-5 Relation between diagnostic label and etiology (related factor). (Redrawn from Hickey P: *Nursing process handbook*, St Louis, 1990, Mosby.)

indicates that the etiology contributes to or is associated with the problem (Figure 9-5). The "related to" phrase requires you to use critical thinking skills to individualize the nursing diagnosis and select subsequent nursing interventions.

Patients who have risk diagnoses (e.g., *Risk for Infection, Risk for Falls, Risk for Injury)* do not have related factors listed. A risk diagnosis is a clinical judgment about human experiences/responses to health conditions/life processes that have a high probability of developing in a vulnerable individual, family, group or community (NANDA-I, 2012). The diagnosis is supported by risk factors that contribute to the increased vulnerability. For example, Mrs. Tillman has sleeplessness, metastatic disease, and lack of strength. These risk factors all contribute to her increased vulnerability for a *Risk for Falls* nursing diagnosis.

The **etiology** is always within the domain of nursing practice and a condition that responds to nursing interventions. Sometimes nurses record medical diagnoses as the etiologies of nursing diagnoses. This is incorrect. Nursing interventions cannot change a medical diagnosis. For example, in Mrs. Tillman's case nursing interventions cannot change cancer. Thus the diagnosis of *Fatigue related to cancer* is incorrect. Instead, you direct nursing interventions at behavior or conditions that you can treat or manage. For example, the nursing diagnosis *Fatigue related to chronic disease process* is correct. Rich can develop interventions that are known to help manage fatigue related to the chronic and progressive nature of cancer.

Table 9-3 demonstrates the association between a nurse's assessment of a patient, the clustering of defining characteristics, and formulation of two different nursing diagnoses. The diagnostic process results in the formation of a total diagnostic statement that allows a nurse to develop an appropriate, patient-centered plan of care. The defining characteristics and relevant etiologies are from NANDA-I (2012).

Definition. NANDA-I approves a definition for each diagnosis following clinical use and testing. The definition describes the characteristics of the human response identified. For example, the definition of the diagnostic label *Fatigue* is an "overwhelming sustained sense of exhaustion and decreased capacity for physical and mental work at usual level" (NANDA-I, 2012). Always refer to a definition to help you identify a patient's diagnosis.

The PES Format. Some agencies prefer a three-part nursing diagnostic label. In this case the diagnostic label consists of the NANDA-I label, the related factor, and the defining characteristics (Ackley and Ladwig, 2011). This approach makes a diagnosis even more patient specific. The acronym PES stands for *p*roblem, *e*tiology, and *s*ymptoms. Using the nursing diagnosis in Mrs. Tillman's care plan as an example

- *P* (Problem) NANDA-I label: Death Anxiety
- *E* (Etiology or related factors): Anticipation of suffering
- *S* (Symptoms or defining characteristics): Increased expression of worries, difficulty breathing (examples)

PES diagnostic statement: Death Anxiety related to anticipation of suffering, evidenced by increased expression of worries, difficulty breathing.

Cultural Relevance of Nursing Diagnoses. When you select nursing diagnoses, always consider your patient's cultural background. It is important to see each patient as a unique person with cultural heritage, values, beliefs, and practices (Campinha-Bacote, 2011). Similarly consider your own cultural background. A patient's culture influences the type of health care problems that he or she experiences. When making a diagnosis, consider how culture influences the related factor for your diagnostic statement. For example, *Impaired Verbal Communication related to cultural differences* or *Noncompliance related to patient's value system* reflects diagnostic conclusions that consider a patient's unique cultural needs.

Knowledge Deficit is a common nursing diagnosis and is influenced by a patient's culture or a nurses' perception of the culture. Culture includes a patient's ethnicity, race, sexual preference, religious values, and socioeconomic status. For example, Chan et al. (2011) assessed the effects of a community-based intervention for Hispanic men to encourage informed decision making about prostate cancer screening. They noted that, once the men received information, they were more effective in informed decision making; as a result there was an increase in knowledge and an improved screening rate. When nurses are aware of the impact of culture on a patient's health care practices, they can identify individualized health-related problems and design culturally sensitive interventions, design appropriate patient education materials, and deliver patient-centered nursing care.

Concept Mapping Nursing Diagnoses. When you care for patients, it is a challenge to think about all of their needs and problems. This is especially true because of a nurse's holistic view of them. Few patients have only a single nursing diagnosis. Usually you care for patients with multiple nursing diagnoses. When you care for multiple patients, it becomes even more challenging to prioritize and focus on all patients' diagnoses. Developing a concept map helps you critically think about your patients' nursing diagnoses and how they relate to one another (Pilcher, 2011; Chabeli, 2010). Concept mapping helps you organize and link data about a patient's multiple diagnoses in a logical way. It graphically represents the connections between concepts (e.g., nursing diagnoses) that relate to a central subject (e.g., a patient's health problems). As you proceed in applying each step of the nursing process, your concept map expands with more detail about planned interventions (see Planning section). Concept mapping applied to nursing diagnoses encourages you to think critically, organize information, and understand complex relationships between patient assessment data and nursing diagnoses (Daley and Torre, 2010).

Figure 9-6 shows a concept map for Mrs. Tillman that includes the patient's assessment findings and four nursing diagnoses. As Rich forms the concept map, he begins to see relationships among the nursing diagnoses. For example, Mrs. Tillman's *Death Anxiety* makes it more difficult for her to sleep and results in *Fatigue,* which in turn is a factor for the *Risk for Falls.* Finally the diagnoses of *Deficient Knowledge* and *Death Anxiety* are also related. Having a poor understanding of her conditions heightens her anxiety, which can also worsen her ability to sleep. Through this concept map you are able to see how the diagnoses relate to one another.

Sources of Diagnostic Errors. Errors occur in the diagnostic process during data collection, data interpretation, clustering, and statement of the nursing diagnosis. Apply methodical critical thinking for an accurate nursing diagnostic process.

Errors in Data Collection. To avoid errors in data collection, be knowledgeable and skilled in all assessment techniques. Avoid inaccurate or missing data and collect data in an organized way. The following practice tips are essential to avoid data collection errors:

- Review your level of comfort and competence with interview and physical assessment skills before you begin data collection.
- Approach assessment in steps. Focus on completing a patient interview before starting an examination. Perhaps focus on only one body system to learn how to gather a complete assessment. Then move to a more complex head-to-toe examination.
- Review your clinical assessments in clinical or classroom settings, giving you a constructive learning opportunity to determine how to revise an assessment or gather additional information.
- Organize the examination. Properly prepare the patient and environment for the examination (see Chapter 16).

Errors in Interpretation and Analysis. After data collection review your database to decide if it is accurate and complete. Review data to validate that measurable, objective physical findings support subjective data. For example, when a patient reports "difficulty breathing," you want to also listen to lung sounds and assess respiratory rate and rhythm. When data are not validated, the result is an inaccurate match between clinical cues and the nursing diagnosis. Be careful to consider any conflicting cues or decide if there are insufficient cues to form a diagnosis. It is also important to consider a patient's cultural background or developmental stage when you interpret the meaning of cues. For example, a male patient may express pain very differently than a female patient. Misinterpreting how patients express pain could easily lead to an inaccurate diagnosis.

Errors in Data Clustering. Errors result when you cluster data prematurely, incorrectly, or not at all. Premature clustering occurs when you make the nursing diagnosis before grouping all data. For example, a patient has urinary incontinence and states that he has urgency and nocturia. You cluster the available data and identify *Impaired Urinary Elimination*

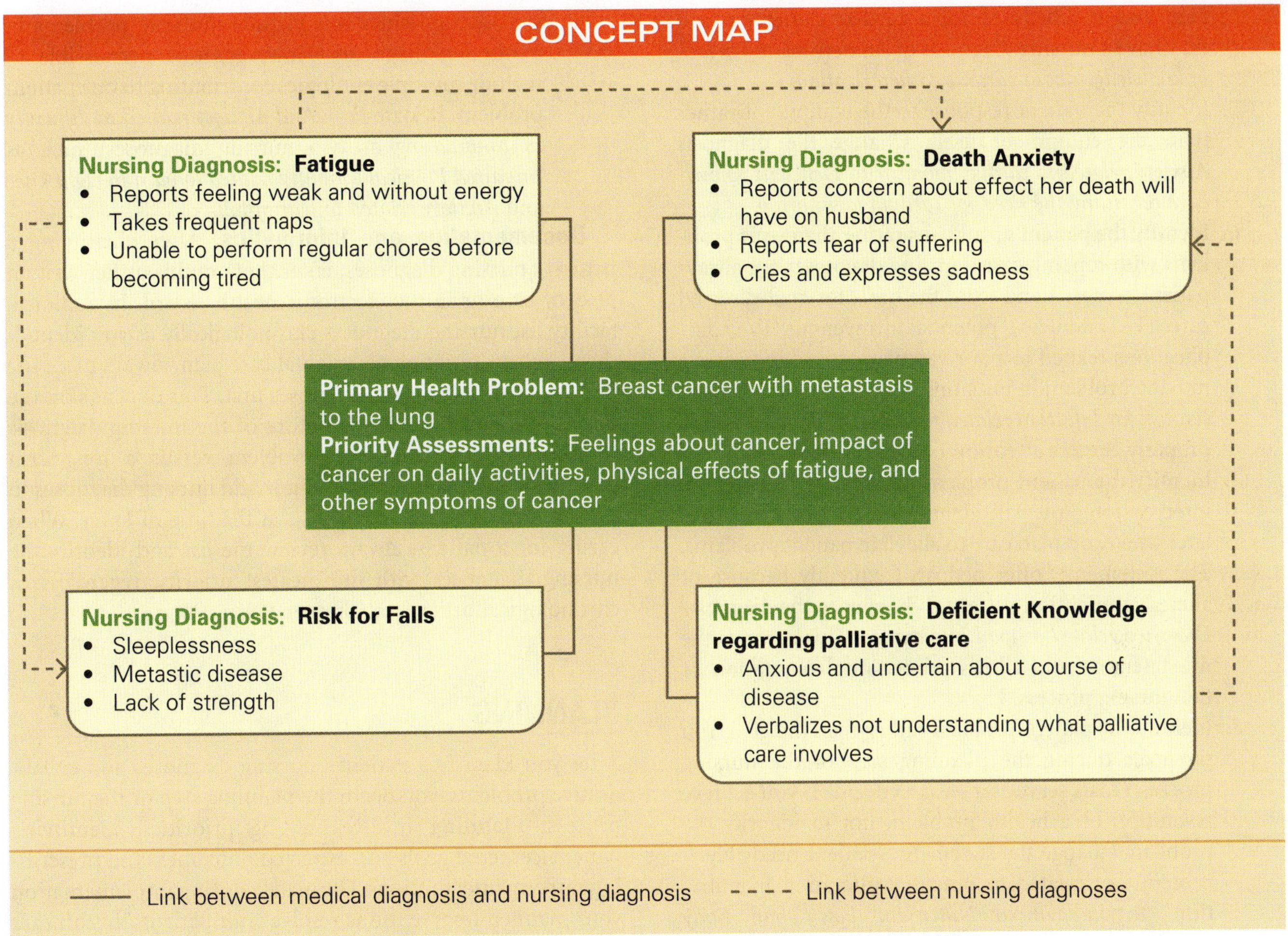

FIGURE 9-6 Concept map with nursing diagnoses.

as a probable nursing diagnosis. Incorrect clustering occurs when you try to make the nursing diagnosis fit the signs and symptoms obtained. In this example further assessment reveals that the patient also has bladder distention and dribbling; thus the correct diagnosis is *Urinary Retention.* The nursing diagnosis comes from the data, not the other way around. An incorrect nursing diagnosis affects the quality of nursing care.

Errors in the Diagnostic Statement. The correct selection of a diagnostic statement is more likely to result in the appropriate selection of nursing interventions and outcomes (NANDA-I, 2012). To reduce errors, word the diagnostic statement in appropriate, concise, and precise language. Use correct terminology reflecting a patient's response to the illness or condition. Use of standardized nursing language from NANDA-I ensures accuracy. Follow these guidelines:

1. Identify the patient's response, not the medical diagnosis (Carpenito-Moyet, 2013). Because the medical diagnosis requires medical interventions, it is legally inadvisable to include it in the nursing diagnosis. Change the diagnosis *Fatigue related to cancer* to *Fatigue related to chronic disease process.*
2. Identify a NANDA-I diagnostic statement, not a symptom. Identify nursing diagnoses from a cluster of defining characteristics that apply to a patient; one symptom is insufficient for problem identification. For example, shortness of breath alone does not identify a diagnosis. In contrast, shortness of breath, pain on inspiration, and productive cough in a postoperative patient form the cluster for *Ineffective Breathing Pattern related to increased airway secretions.*
3. Identify a treatable etiology, not a clinical sign or chronic problem. Select interventions to correct the etiology of the problem. A diagnostic test or chronic dysfunction is not an etiology that a nursing intervention is able to treat. A patient with cancer often develops anemia, reflected in low red blood cell counts. The diagnosis *Fatigue related to low red blood cell counts* is an incorrect diagnostic statement. *Fatigue related to the chronic disease process* is appropriate because it allows you to focus interventions on the physical responses common in chronic progressive disease.
4. Identify the problem caused by the treatment or diagnostic study rather than the treatment or study itself. Patients respond to diagnostic tests and medical treatment in many ways. These responses are the area of nursing concern. The patient who has severe chest

pain and is scheduled for a cardiac catheterization may have a nursing diagnosis of *Anxiety related to lack of knowledge about cardiac catheterization.*

5. Identify the patient response to the equipment rather than the equipment itself. Change the diagnosis *Anxiety related to cardiac monitor* to *Deficient Knowledge regarding the need for cardiac monitoring.*
6. Identify the patient's problems rather than your problems with nursing care. Nursing diagnoses are always patient centered and form the basis for goal-directed care. The statement, "potential intravenous (IV) complications related to poor vascular access" indicates a nursing problem in initiating IV therapy. The diagnosis *Risk for Infection related to presence of invasive lines* properly centers attention on patient needs.
7. Identify the patient problem rather than the nursing intervention. You will identify nursing interventions later when you plan care to alleviate patient problems. The statement, "offer bedpan frequently because of altered elimination patterns" changes to the diagnosis *Diarrhea related to food intolerance.* This corrects the misstatement and allows proper implementation of the nursing process.
8. Identify the patient problem rather than the goal. You set goals during the planning step of the nursing process. Goals serve as a basis to decide if you achieve resolution of a health problem, not to identify the problem. Change the statement, "patient needs high-protein diet related to potential alteration in nutrition" to *Imbalanced Nutrition: Less Than Body Requirements related to inadequate protein intake.* This diagnosis would allow you to then plan on the basis of the correct etiology.
9. Make professional rather than prejudicial judgments. Base nursing diagnoses on subjective and objective patient data and do not include your personal beliefs and values. Remove your judgment from *Risk for Impaired Skin Integrity related to poor hygiene habits* by changing the nursing diagnosis to *Risk For Impaired Skin Integrity related to lack of knowledge about perineal care.*
10. Avoid legally inadvisable statements that imply blame, negligence, or malpractice (Carpenito-Moyet, 2013). The diagnosis *Chronic Pain related to insufficient pain medication* implies that the health care provider gave an inadequate prescription. The correct way to identify the problem is to write *Chronic Pain related to improper use of medications.*
11. Identify the problem and etiology to avoid a circular statement. Such statements are vague and give no direction to nursing care. Change the diagnosis *Acute Pain related to alteration in comfort* to the specific patient problem and cause: *Acute Pain related to incisional trauma.*
12. Identify only one patient problem in a diagnostic statement. Every problem has different specific expected outcomes. Confusion during the planning step occurs when you include multiple problems in a nursing diagnosis. However, it is permissible to include multiple etiologies contributing to one patient problem. Restate *Pain And Anxiety related to difficulty in ambulating* as two nursing diagnoses, such as *Impaired Physical Mobility related to pain in right knee* and *Anxiety related to fear of fall.*

Documentation and Informatics. After identifying a patient's nursing diagnoses, enter them on his or her written plan of care or in the electronic health record. In a clinical facility list nursing diagnoses chronologically as you identify them. When initiating an original care plan, always place the highest-priority nursing diagnoses first. This depends on the patient's condition and the nature of the nursing diagnosis (e.g., acute physical health problem versus a long-term chronic health management issue). Add nursing diagnoses to the list. Date a nursing diagnosis at the time of entry. When caring for a patient, always review the list and identify the nursing diagnoses with the greatest priority, regardless of chronological order (see Chapter 10).

PLANNING

After you identify a patient's nursing diagnoses and collaborative problems, you begin the planning step of the nursing process. **Planning** involves setting priorities, identifying patient-centered goals and expected outcomes, and prescribing nursing interventions. Ultimately during implementation your planned interventions resolve your patients' health care problems. Perhaps the most important principle to learn about planning is the individualization of a plan of care for each patient's unique needs. Literature supports the impact of individualized compared with nonindividualized plans of care (Suhonen et al., 2008). The individualized nursing diagnoses and problems that you identify direct your selection of individualized nursing interventions and the goals and outcomes you hope to achieve (Suhonen et al., 2011).

Establishing Priorities

A single patient often has multiple diagnoses and collaborative problems. Eventually you will care for groups of patients. You must be able to set priorities for these patients carefully and wisely to ensure timely and effective care. Priority setting is the ordering of nursing diagnoses or patient problems using notions of urgency and importance to establish a preferential order for nursing actions. In other words, as you care for patients there are aspects of care that you need to deal with before others. By ranking nursing diagnoses in order of importance, you attend to your patient's most important needs and better organize ongoing care activities. Priorities help you anticipate and sequence nursing interventions when a patient has multiple problems. Together with your patients, you select mutually agreed-on priorities based on the urgency of the problem, the patient's safety and desires, the nature of the treatment indicated, and the relation among the diagnoses. Establishing priorities is not just a matter of numbering the nursing diagnoses on the basis of severity or physiological importance.

Classify priorities as high, intermediate, or low. Nursing diagnoses that, if untreated, result in harm to the patient or others have the highest priority. One way to consider diagnoses of high priority is to consider Maslow's hierarchy of needs. For example, you want to attend to a patient's oxygen, fluid, and nutrition needs before you focus on shelter or sexual needs. However, it is always important to consider each patient's unique case. High priorities are sometimes both psychological and physiological. Avoid classifying only physiological nursing diagnoses as high priority. Consider Mrs. Tillman's case study. The nursing diagnosis of *Death Anxiety* is a high-priority diagnosis because it has the potential to impair Mrs. Tillman's ability to become a participant in her own care and maintain a healthy relationship with her husband.

Intermediate-priority nursing diagnoses involve the nonemergent, nonlife-threatening needs of a patient. In Mrs. Tillman's case, *Fatigue* is an intermediate diagnosis. Mrs. Tillman's activity problem is linked to the progressive nature of her cancer and will be an ongoing challenge. Energy conservation and management therapies are important but not a life-threatening issue.

Low-priority nursing diagnoses are patient needs that are usually directly related to a specific illness or prognosis but also affect a patient's future well-being. Mrs. Tillman's nurse, Rich, knows that, as her disease progresses, Mrs. Tillman will have more health care needs. Her family may assume even more responsibility for in-home care. *Deficient Knowledge regarding palliative care related to inexperience* is a relevant diagnosis but of lower priority at this time compared with the other diagnoses. In future clinic visits Rich will plan when to begin discussion about palliative care with the Tillman family.

The order of priorities changes as a patient's condition changes. Each time you begin a sequence of care such as the beginning of a hospital shift or during a clinic visit, it is important to reorder priorities. Ongoing patient assessment is needed to determine the status of a patient's nursing diagnoses. The proper order of priorities ensures that you meet your patients' needs in a timely and effective way.

Priority setting also involves prioritizing specific interventions that you plan to use for a patient. For example, as Rich considers the high-priority diagnosis of *Death Anxiety,* he decides whether to complete individual counseling with Mrs. Tillman first or conduct a care conference with the patient, her husband, and the clinic nurse practitioner. Rich needs to prioritize interventions to be most effective in meeting desired goals and outcomes. It is always important to involve the patient in priority setting. In some situations you and the patient assign different priority rankings to nursing diagnoses and collaborative problems. If you each place a different value on health care needs and treatments, resolve these differences through open communication. However, when the patient's physiological and emotional needs are at stake, you need to assume primary responsibility for setting priorities.

Ethical care is part of priority setting. When ethical issues make priorities less clear, it is important to have open dialogue with the patient, family, and other health care providers. For example, when caring for patients with cancer and other disabling illnesses, it is important to discuss the situation with the patient and understand his or her expectations, understand your professional responsibility in providing care, know the health care providers' therapeutic and palliative goals, and then form a patient-centered care plan.

Critical Thinking in Setting Goals and Expected Outcomes

Once you identify a nursing diagnosis for a patient, ask yourself, what is the best approach to address and resolve the problem? What do you plan to achieve? Goals and expected outcomes are specific statements of patient behavior or physiological responses that you set to resolve a nursing diagnosis or collaborative problem. They serve two purposes: to provide clear direction for the selection and use of nursing interventions and to provide focus for evaluating the effectiveness of the interventions.

Goals of Care. A patient-centered goal is a broad statement that describes a desired change in a patient's condition or behavior. For Mrs. Tillman, who has a diagnosis of *Fatigue related to chronic disease process,* a goal of care would be "Patient will achieve improved energy level within 2 weeks." A goal is realistic and based on patient needs and resources. A patient goal represents predicted resolution of a problem, evidence of progress toward problem resolution, progress toward improved health status, or continued maintenance of good health or function (Carpenito-Moyet, 2013).

Each goal is time limited so the health care team has a common time frame for problem resolution. The time frame depends on the nature of the problem, etiology, overall condition of the patient, and treatment setting. A *short-term goal* is an objective behavior or response that you expect the patient to achieve in a short time, usually less than a week. In an acute care setting you may set goals for over a course of just a few hours. For example "Patient will maintain a balanced fluid status within the next 12 hours." A *long-term goal* is an objective behavior or response that you expect the patient to achieve over a longer period, usually over several days, weeks, or months. Goal setting establishes the framework for the nursing care plan. Table 9-4 shows the progression from nursing diagnoses to goals and expected outcomes, which you individualize to meet patient needs.

Goals are often based on standards of care or clinical guidelines established for minimal safe practice. For example, the Infusion Nurses Society (INS) has standards of care for prevention of the IV complication of phlebitis. When a nurse cares for a patient with a peripheral IV catheter, the goal "The IV site will remain free of phlebitis" is established on the basis of sound nursing practice standards.

Role of the Patient in Goal Setting. Always partner with your patients when setting goals. Mutual goal setting involves the patient and family (when appropriate) in prioritizing the goals of care and developing a plan of action to

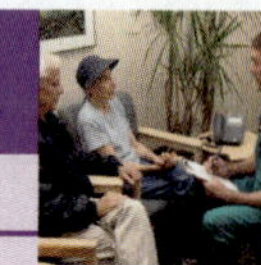

TABLE 9-4 EXAMPLES OF GOAL SETTING WITH EXPECTED OUTCOMES FOR MRS. TILLMAN

NURSING DIAGNOSES	GOALS	EXPECTED OUTCOMES
Fatigue related to chronic disease process	Mrs. Tillman will achieve an improved energy level within 2 weeks.	Patient's self-report of fatigue is 3 or less on a scale of 0 to 10 in 2 weeks. Patient is able to perform some household chores in 1 week.
Death Anxiety related to anticipation of suffering	Mrs. Tillman will express belief that she will achieve a comfortable death in 3 weeks.	Patient seeks information about palliative care treatment in 1 week. Patient reports acceptable comfort level in 2 weeks. Patient participates in health care decisions in 1 week.

achieve those goals. Unless goals are mutually set and there is a clear plan of action, patients will not participate. They need to understand and see the value of nursing therapies, even though they are often totally dependent on you as the nurse. When developing goals, act as an advocate or supporter for the patient to develop nursing interventions that promote his or her return to health or prevent further deterioration when possible.

Expected Outcomes. For Rich to evaluate if Mrs. Tillman has shown progress and achieved the goal of an improved energy level within 2 weeks, expected outcomes are necessary. **Expected outcomes** are measurable criteria to evaluate goal achievement. These measurable effects relate to a change in a patient's physical condition or behavior that results from individualized nursing interventions (Papastavrou et al., 2011). In Mrs. Tillman's case a measurable outcome for the goal of improved energy level includes "Patient's self-report of fatigue is 3 or less on a scale of 0 to 10" and "Patient is able to complete bathing without taking rest periods." The outcomes help Rich determine the success of selected interventions that effectively lessen Mrs. Tillman's fatigue. An outcome includes measurable criteria (e.g., 3 or less on a scale of 0 to 10, completes bathing without taking rest) to evaluate goal achievement (Table 9-5). Achieving outcomes means that a goal has been met. Expected outcomes provide a focus or direction for nursing care because they are the desired physical, psychological, social, emotional, developmental, or spiritual responses that show resolution of a patient's health problems.

Typically all health care providers contribute to achievement of patient outcomes. A **nursing-sensitive outcome** is a measurable patient or family state, behavior, or perception largely influenced by and sensitive to nursing interventions (Moorhead et al., 2012). Examples of nursing-sensitive outcomes include reduction in pain severity, incidence of pressure ulcers, and incidence of falls. In comparison, outcomes largely influenced by medical interventions include patient mortality and hospital readmission.

Outcomes are measurable, reliable, valid, suited to the patient, and sensitive to change (Moorhead et al., 2012). Consider the example of Mrs. Tillman's problem of fatigue. An outcome measure is a self-report fatigue scale. The scale provides a measurable way to objectively assess the patient's level of fatigue. Current evidence shows self-report scales are reliable (consistently measures an outcome) and valid (accuracy of a measure). A self-report scale is easy for a patient to complete without causing anxiety or physical distress as in the case of an exercise test for fatigue. The patient's perceptions of fatigue change over time and are reflected by differences in the fatigue scale.

TABLE 9-5 EXAMPLES OF NANDA INTERNATIONAL NURSING DIAGNOSES AND SUGGESTED NOC LINKAGES

NURSING DIAGNOSIS	SUGGESTED NOC OUTCOMES (EXAMPLES)	OUTCOME INDICATORS (EXAMPLES)
Fatigue	Activity tolerance	Walking pace Ease of performing activities of daily living Pulse rate with activity Ease of breathing with activity
	Energy conservation	Balances activity and rest Uses naps to restore energy Adapts lifestyle to energy level
Deficient Knowledge regarding palliative care	Knowledge of treatment regimen	Rationale for treatment Self-care responsibilities for ongoing treatment Expected effects of treatment

NOC, Nursing outcomes classification.

You normally develop several expected outcomes for each nursing diagnosis and goal. The reason for multiple outcomes is that sometimes one nursing action is not enough to resolve a patient problem. The listing of step-by-step expected outcomes gives you practical guidance in planning interventions. Always write expected outcomes sequentially with time frames. Time frames give you progressive steps in which to move a patient toward recovery. They also give an order for when to perform nursing interventions. In addition, time frames set limits for problem resolution.

Nursing Outcomes Classification. Health care agencies are very interested in measuring nursing-sensitive outcomes because of the effect they have on patient outcomes, quality of care, and health care costs. The *Nursing Outcomes Classification (NOC),* published by the Iowa Intervention Project, classifies, identifies, labels, and validates nursing-sensitive outcomes (Moorhead et al., 2012). NOC links evidence-based outcomes to every NANDA-I nursing diagnosis (Moorhead et al., 2012). NOC-suggested outcomes describe the focus of nursing care and provide ways to measure the success of nursing interventions (see Table 9-5). NOC helps you select appropriate nursing interventions to improve the quality of patient care for individuals, families, and communities in all health care settings (Moorhead et al., 2012). Using a common language allows nurses to plan effective patient care and provides a standardized way to measure the success of nursing interventions. In addition, the use of NOC facilitates the evaluation of the effects of nursing interventions over time and across a variety of health care settings.

Combining Goals and Outcome Statements. Many schools of nursing use a format for stating goals and outcomes as one statement. Staff in health care agencies often refer to the terms *goals* and *outcomes* interchangeably. This is acceptable as long as the criteria for writing goals and outcomes are met. The statement "Patient will experience an improved energy level as evidenced by a self-report of fatigue of 3 or less on a scale of 0 to 10 within 2 weeks" is acceptable. The goal portion of the statement broadly describes the desired patient status (improved energy level), and the outcome portion contains an observable criterion (3 on a scale of 0 to 10) to measure success. The documentation format used by health care agencies guides how nurses write goals and outcomes.

Guidelines for Writing Goals and Expected Outcomes. Follow these seven guidelines when writing goals and expected outcomes.

1. *Patient-centered:* Outcomes and goals reflect the patient behaviors or responses expected as a result of nursing interventions. Write the goal to reflect this, not to reflect your goals or interventions. A correct goal statement is, "Patient will ambulate independently in 3 days." A correct outcome statement: "Patient ambulates in the hall 3 times a day by 4/22." A common error is to write an outcome as an intervention, "Ambulate patient in the hall 3 times a day."
2. *Singular goal or outcome:* To ensure precise evaluation of care, each goal and outcome addresses only one behavior or response. If an outcome reads, "Patient's lungs are clear to auscultation, and respiratory rate is 22 breaths per minute by 8/22," consider the outcome when you evaluate that the lungs are clear but the respiratory rate is 28 breaths/min. It will be difficult to determine whether the expected outcome has been achieved. By splitting the statement into two parts, "Lungs are clear to auscultation by 8/22" and "Respiratory rate is 22 breaths per minute by 8/22," you determine specifically if the patient achieves each outcome. Singularity allows you to decide if there is a need to modify the plan of care.
3. *Observable:* You must be able to observe if change takes place in a patient's status. Observable changes occur in physiological findings and the patient's knowledge, perceptions, and behaviors. For example, you observe the goal, "Patient will achieve improved activity tolerance" through the outcome of, "Patient's heart rate remains within 10% of baseline following exercise." The outcome statement, "Patient appears less short of breath" is not a correct statement because there is no specific observable behavior for "appears less short of breath."
4. *Measurable:* You learn to write goals and expected outcomes that set standards against which to measure a patient's response to nursing care. Examples such as, "Body temperature remains 98.6° F" and "Apical pulse remains between 60 and 100 beats per minute" allow you to objectively measure changes in a patient's status. Do not use vague qualifiers such as "normal," "acceptable," "stable," or "sufficient" in the expected outcome statement. Vague terms make it difficult to determine a patient's response to care. Terms describing quality, quantity, frequency, length, or weight allow you to accurately evaluate if outcomes are met.
5. *Time limited:* The time frame for each goal and expected outcome indicates when you expect the response to occur. Time frames help you and the patient determine if progress is being made at a reasonable rate. If not, revision of the plan of care is necessary. Time frames also promote accountability in the delivery and management of nursing care.
6. *Mutual factors:* Mutually set goals and expected outcomes ensure that the patient and nurse agree on the direction and time limits of care. Mutual goal setting increases a patient's motivation and cooperation. As a patient advocate you apply standards of practice, patient safety, and basic human needs when helping patients set goals.
7. *Realistic:* Set goals and expected outcomes that the patient is able to reach. Achievable goals give patients a sense of accomplishment. This sense of accomplishment further increases a patient's motivation and cooperation. When establishing realistic goals, be sure to know the resources of the health care facility, family, and patient. For example, do a patient's cultural beliefs affect the goal you set? Does the patient have the necessary resources in the home to successfully meet goals?

Critical Thinking in Planning Nursing Care

During planning you make clinical decisions by choosing the nursing interventions most appropriate to your patient's nursing diagnoses and collaborative problems. The actual implementation of these interventions occurs during the implementation phase of the nursing process. Choosing suitable nursing interventions involves critical thinking applied in decision making. To select interventions you need to be competent in three areas: (1) knowing the scientific rationale, or reason, for the interventions; (2) possessing the necessary psychomotor and interpersonal skills to perform the interventions; and (3) being able to function within a particular setting to use the available health care resources effectively (Bulechek et al., 2012).

Types of Interventions. There are three categories of nursing interventions: nurse-initiated, physician-initiated, and collaborative interventions. Nurse-initiated interventions are the independent nursing interventions or actions that nurses initiate. These do not require direction or an order from another health care professional. Nurse-initiated interventions (independent nursing interventions) are autonomous actions based on scientific rationales. Examples include elevating an edematous extremity, offering counseling on coping, and instructing patients about medication side effects. These interventions benefit patients in a predicted way related to nursing diagnoses and patient goals (Bulechek et al., 2012). They require no supervision or direction from others. Each state within the United States has developed Nurse Practice Acts that define the legal scope of nursing practice (see Chapter 5). According to state Nurse Practice Acts, independent nursing interventions pertain to ADLs, health education and promotion, and counseling.

Physician-initiated interventions are dependent nursing interventions or actions that require an order from a physician or another health care professional. Such interventions are based on the health care provider's response to treat or manage a medical diagnosis. Advanced practice nurses who have collaborative agreements with physicians or who are licensed independently by state practice acts also write dependent interventions. As a nurse you intervene by carrying out the independent provider's written and/or verbal orders. Administering a medication, implementing an invasive procedure, and preparing a patient for diagnostic tests are examples of such interventions.

Each dependent nursing intervention involves specific nursing responsibilities and technical nursing knowledge. When you perform the intervention you must also know the types of observations and precautions to take for the intervention to be delivered safely and correctly. For example, when administering medications you are responsible for knowing the classification of the drug, its physiological action, normal dosage, side effects, and nursing interventions related to its action or side effects (see Chapter 17). When a physician orders diagnostic testing, you are responsible for scheduling the test, preparing the patient, and knowing the normal findings and associated nursing implications.

Collaborative interventions, or interdependent nursing interventions, are therapies that require the combined knowledge, skill, and expertise of multiple health care professionals. Typically when you plan care for a patient, you review the necessary interventions and determine if collaboration from other health care professionals is necessary. For example, in the case study Rich decides to have an interdisciplinary health care team conference to discuss a palliative care plan for Mrs. Tillman. Interdisciplinary conferences bring professionals from all disciplines involved in the patient's care to the table so together they can establish and execute the most appropriate plan of care.

Selection of Interventions. Never select interventions for a patient randomly. For example, patients with the diagnosis of *Anxiety* do not always need care in the same way with the same interventions. You treat *Anxiety related to the uncertainty of results from a diagnostic test* differently from *Anxiety related to a threat to loss of a loved one*. When choosing interventions, consider six factors: (1) characteristics of the nursing diagnosis, (2) expected outcomes and goals, (3) evidence base (research or clinical practice guidelines) for the intervention, (4) feasibility of the intervention, (5) acceptability to the patient, and (6) your own competency (Bulechek et al., 2012) (Box 9-6).

Literature supports that individualized or tailored nursing interventions achieve positive patient outcomes in areas of health promotion, supporting health behaviors, and reducing anxiety (Suhonen et al., 2011). In addition, individualized interventions are effective in improving a patient's functional status, increasing adherence to medication, and improving nutritional intake (Suhonen et al., 2008).

Review resources such as evidence in the literature, standard protocols or guidelines, the Nursing Interventions Classification (NIC), critical pathways, and current textbooks when choosing interventions. Collaboration with other health care professionals is also useful. As you select interventions, review your patient's needs, values, priorities, and previous experiences to select the nursing interventions that have the best potential for achieving the expected outcomes.

Nursing Interventions Classification. Just as with the standardized NOC, the Iowa Intervention Project developed a set of nursing interventions that provides a level of standardization to enhance communication of nursing care across all health care settings and to compare outcomes (Bulechek et al., 2012). The NIC model includes three levels: domains, classes, and interventions for ease of use. The domains (level 1) are the highest level, using broad terms (e.g., safety and basic physiological) to organize the more specific classes and interventions (Table 9-6). The second level of the model includes 30 classes, which offer useful clinical categories to which to refer when selecting interventions (Box 9-7). The third level includes interventions, defined as any treatment based on clinical judgment and knowledge that a nurse performs to enhance patient outcomes (Bulechek, et al., 2012). Each intervention has a variety of nursing activities from which to choose (see Box 9-7). The NIC interventions link with NANDA-I nursing diagnoses. For example, Mrs. Tillman has the problem of *Fatigue*, which falls under the domain of Physiological: Basic and the class of activity and exercise management. Under the class of activity and

BOX 9-6 SELECTING NURSING INTERVENTIONS

CHARACTERISTICS OF THE NURSING DIAGNOSIS
- Interventions should alter the etiological (related to) factor associated with the diagnostic label.
- When an etiological factor cannot change, direct interventions toward treating the signs and symptoms (e.g., NANDA-I defining characteristics).
- For potential or high-risk diagnoses, direct interventions at altering or eliminating risk factors for the nursing diagnoses.

EXPECTED OUTCOMES
- Specify expected outcomes before choosing interventions.
- Identify for each patient the outcomes that can be reasonably expected and attained as the result of nursing care.
- Use the Nursing Outcomes Classification to specify outcomes.

EVIDENCE BASE
- Know the research base for an intervention.
- Research will indicate the effectiveness of using an intervention with certain types of patients.
- When research is not available, use scientific principles (e.g., safety) or consult experts.

FEASIBILITY OF THE INTERVENTION
- A specific intervention has the potential for interacting with other interventions.
- Consider cost: Is the intervention clinically effective and cost efficient?
- Consider time: Are time and personnel resources available?

ACCEPTABILITY TO THE PATIENT
- An intervention must be acceptable to the patient and family and match a patient's goals, health care values, and culture.
- Promote informed choice; help a patient know how he or she is expected to participate.

CAPABILITY
- Be prepared to carry out the intervention.
- Be competent in knowing the scientific rationale for the intervention, possessing necessary psychomotor and interpersonal skills and being able to function in the particular setting.

Modified from Bulechek GM, et al: *Nursing interventions classification (NIC),* ed 6, St Louis, 2013, Mosby.

BOX 9-7 EXAMPLES OF LEVEL 3 INTERVENTIONS AND ACTIVITIES FOR ACTIVITY AND EXERCISE MANAGEMENT

A.ACTIVITY AND EXERCISE MANAGEMENT

Interventions to organize or assist with physical activity and energy conservation and expenditure

Level 3 Interventions
- Body Mechanics Promotion
  Examples of Nursing Activities for Body Mechanics Promotion: Instruct to use a firm mattress, assist to demonstrate appropriate sleeping positions, assist to avoid sitting in same position for prolonged periods.
- Energy Management
- Exercise Promotion
- Exercise Therapy: Ambulation
- Teaching Prescribed Activity/Exercise

Examples of Linked Nursing Diagnoses
- Activity Intolerance
- Fatigue
- Mobility, Impaired Physical

From Bulechek GM, et al: *Nursing interventions classification (NIC),* ed 6, St Louis, 2013, Mosby.

exercise management, there are a variety of interventions from which to choose (e.g., energy management, exercise therapy: ambulation). When you refer to an intervention within NIC such as energy management, there are numerous nursing activities or interventions from which to choose (see Mrs. Tillman's care plan). NIC is a valuable resource for you in selecting interventions for your unique patients.

Systems for Planning Nursing Care

In any health care setting a nurse is responsible for providing a plan of nursing care for each patient. The plan of care sometimes takes several forms (e.g., nursing Kardex, standardized care plans, and computerized plans). More hospitals today are adopting electronic health records (EHRs) and a documentation system that includes software programs for nursing care plans (Hebda and Czar, 2009). Generally a nursing care plan includes nursing diagnoses, goals and/or expected outcomes, and specific nursing interventions so any nurse is able to quickly identify a patient's needs and situation. Electronic care plans often follow a standardized format but allow you to individualize each plan to a unique patient's needs. In hospitals and community-based settings patients receive care from more than one nurse, physician, or allied health professional. Thus more institutions are developing **interdisciplinary care plans,** which include contributions from all disciplines involved in patient care. It improves the coordination of all patient therapies.

A nursing care plan reduces the risk for incomplete, incorrect, or inaccurate care. The plan is a guideline for coordinating nursing care, promoting continuity of care, and listing outcome criteria for the evaluation of care. It communicates nursing care priorities to other health care professionals and identifies and coordinates resources for delivering nursing care. For example, a plan might list the specific equipment and supplies necessary for nursing treatments (e.g., dressing change).

TABLE 9-6 NURSING INTERVENTIONS CLASSIFICATION (NIC) TAXONOMY

DOMAIN 1	DOMAIN 2	DOMAIN 3
Level 1 Domains		
1. Physiological: Basic Care that supports physical functioning	**2. Physiological: Complex** Care that supports homeostatic regulation	**3. Behavioral** Care that supports psychosocial functioning and facilitates lifestyle changes
Level 2 Classes		
A *Activity and Exercise Management:* Interventions to organize or assist with physical activity and energy conservation and expenditure	H *Drug Management:* Interventions to facilitate desired effects of pharmacological agents	O *Behavior Therapy:* Interventions to reinforce or promote desirable behaviors or alter undesirable behaviors
B *Elimination Management:* Interventions to establish and maintain regular bowel and urinary elimination patterns and manage complications caused by altered patterns	I *Neurologic Management:* Interventions to optimize neurologic functions	P *Cognitive Therapy:* Interventions to reinforce or promote desirable cognitive functioning or alter undesirable cognitive functioning
C *Immobility Management:* Interventions to manage restricted body movement and the sequelae	J *Perioperative Care:* Interventions to provide care before, during, and immediately after surgery	Q *Communication Enhancement:* Interventions to facilitate delivering and receiving verbal and nonverbal messages
D *Nutrition Support:* Interventions to modify or maintain nutritional status	K *Respiratory Management:* Interventions to promote airway patency and gas exchange	R *Coping Assistance:* Interventions to assist another to build on own strengths, adapt to a change in function, or achieve a higher level of function
E *Physical Comfort Promotion:* Interventions to promote comfort using physical techniques	L *Skin/Wound Management:* Interventions to maintain or restore tissue integrity	S *Patient Education:* Interventions to facilitate learning
F *Self-Care Facilitation:* Interventions to provide or assist with routine activities of daily living	M *Thermoregulation:* Interventions to maintain body temperature within a normal range	T *Psychological Comfort Promotion:* Interventions to promote comfort using psychological techniques
G *Electrolyte and Acid-Base Management:* Interventions to regulate electrolyte/acid-base balance and prevent complications	N *Tissue Perfusion Management:* Interventions to optimize circulation of blood and fluids to the tissue	

From Bulechek GM, et al: *Nursing interventions classification (NIC),* ed 6, St Louis, 2013, Mosby.

The nursing care plan enhances the continuity of nursing care by listing specific nursing actions necessary to achieve the goals of care. Nurses who care for the patient carry out the interventions throughout a given shift of care during a patient's length of stay. A correctly formulated nursing care plan makes it easy to continue care from one nurse to another. Care plans organize information exchanged by nurses in change-of-shift and hand-off reports (see Chapter 10). You learn to focus your reports on the nursing care, treatments, and expected outcomes documented in your care plans. At the end of a shift or during the transfer of a patient, you discuss the care plan and the patient's overall progress with the next caregiver. Thus all nurses are able to discuss current and relevant information about the patient's plan of care.

The care plan includes the patient's long-term needs. Incorporating the goals of the care plan into discharge planning is important. This is especially true for a patient undergoing long-term rehabilitation in the community who will require ongoing home care. Same-day surgeries and earlier discharges from hospitals require you as the nurse to begin planning discharge needs from the moment the patient enters a health care agency. The adaptation of the care plan enhances the continuity of nursing care between nurses working in hospital settings and those working in community agencies. Figure 9-7 provides an example of the care plan format used throughout this text.

Student Care Plans. Student care plans are useful for learning the problem-solving technique, the nursing process, skills of written communication, and organizational skills needed for nursing care. Most important, a student care plan helps you apply knowledge gained from the nursing and medical literature and the classroom to a practice situation. Students typically write care plans for each nursing diagnosis, using a columnar format that includes assessment findings, goals, expected outcomes, nursing interventions with supporting rationales, and evaluative outcome criteria. The student care plan is more elaborate than a care plan in a hospital or community health care agency because its purpose is to teach the process of planning care. Each nursing school uses a different format for student care plans. Some schools model the student care plan based on the format used by their related health care agencies.

Concept Mapping. In the nursing diagnosis section you were introduced to a concept map for Mrs. Tillman that displayed relevant assessment data and four interrelated nursing diagnoses. As you finalize Mrs. Tillman's concept map

DOMAIN 4	DOMAIN 5	DOMAIN 6	DOMAIN 7
4. Safety Care that supports protection against harm	**5. Family** Care that supports the family unit	**6. Health System** Care that supports effective use of the health care delivery system	**7. Community** Care that supports the health of the community
U *Crisis Management:* Interventions to provide immediate short-term help in both psychological and physiological crises V *Risk Management:* Interventions to initiate risk-reduction activities and continue monitoring risks over time	W *Childbearing Care:* Interventions to assist in understanding and coping with the psychological and physiological changes during the childbearing period Z *Childrearing Care:* Interventions to assist in rearing children X *Lifespan Care:* Interventions to facilitate family unit functioning and promote the health and welfare of family members throughout the lifespan	Y *Health System Mediation:* Interventions to facilitate the interface between patient/family and the health care system a *Health System Management:* Interventions to provide and enhance support services for the delivery of care b *Information Management:* Interventions to facilitate communication among health care providers	c *Community Health Promotion:* Interventions that promote the health of the whole community d *Community Risk Management:* Interventions that assist in detecting or preventing health risks to the whole community

you add individualized nursing interventions (Figure 9-8). When you care for a complex patient or several patients, it is a challenge to think about all of their needs and problems. This is especially true because of a nurse's holistic view of patients. Few patients have only a single nursing diagnosis. Usually you care for patients with multiple nursing diagnoses. When you care for multiple patients, it becomes even more challenging to prioritize and focus on all patients' diagnoses. Concept mapping is beneficial because of its ability to demonstrate visually how a patient's problems or nursing diagnoses are related. The ability to link these interrelated factors is an important aspect in clinical decision making (Pilcher, 2011). Concept mapping shows the connections between concepts (e.g., nursing diagnoses) that relate to a central subject (e.g., a patient's health problems). This method encourages you to think critically, organize information, understand complex relationships between nursing diagnoses and nursing interventions, and integrate theoretical knowledge into practice (Chabeli, 2010; Daley and Torre, 2010). A **concept map** provides a visual representation of the complex level of thinking that nursing care requires. It forms a picture of each patient's diagnoses and the interconnections between the assessment data and nursing interventions associated with the patient problems. The use of concept maps is a way for students to synthesize clinical experiences and prepare for preclinical and postclinical conferences (Chabeli, 2010).

Concept mapping is a way to develop reflective thinking skills (Box 9-8). If you consider what happens in the context of patient care, patient information, nursing diagnoses, interdisciplinary interventions, and patient outcomes are all interrelated and ordered to produce a plan of care. By using a concept map you create a visual representation of your patient's medical problems, nursing assessment data, nursing diagnoses, and their relationship to one another. As you proceed in applying each step of the nursing process, your concept map expands with more detail about planned interventions.

Rich's next step is to begin to plan interventions for each of Mrs. Tillman's nursing diagnoses while recognizing how the interventions can apply to more than one diagnosis (see Figure 9-8). Here are tips to help you develop a complete concept map:

1. Begin by collecting the patient's clinical assessment data.
2. Review all information about the patient's health problems, treatments, and medications in course textbooks, scientific literature, and other related resources.

CARE PLAN Death Anxiety

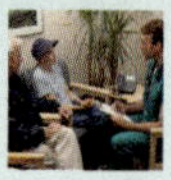

ASSESSMENT

Rich learns in his initial discussions with Mrs. Tillman that she feels a sense of dread and uncertainty about the course of cancer. Mrs. Tillman shares her emotions through crying and sadness in the way she looks down and has difficulty talking about her condition. She admitted to Rich that her greatest fear is not knowing if she might suffer from her disease. Rich knows from his review of pathophysiology the probable course of the patient's disease and the type of palliative care treatments her physician will recommend. He decides to assess further the extent of her death anxiety.

ASSESSMENT ACTIVITIES	FINDINGS/DEFINING CHARACTERISTICS*
Ask Mrs. Tillman to discuss her concerns about the effect her illness will have on her husband.	Patient is **concerned that husband will work too hard** and begin to have more physical problems.
Have Mrs. Tillman explain what she fears most about having a terminal illness.	Patient states that she **worries** she will have **difficulty getting her breath for a prolonged time.**
Question Mrs. Tillman about her desire to be able to make decisions regarding palliative care.	Patient expresses **concern about having little control** over what will happen.

NURSING DIAGNOSIS: Death Anxiety related to anticipation of suffering.

PLANNING

GOAL	EXPECTED OUTCOMES (NOC)†
Mrs. Tillman expresses belief that she will achieve a comfortable death within 3 weeks.	***Anxiety Level*** • Patient will verbalize feeling less anxious about the course of her disease in 1 week. • Patient uses relaxation techniques when anxiety heightens by 2 weeks. ***Participation in Health Care Decisions*** • Patient is able to specify her priorities in palliative care plan in 2 weeks. • Patient and husband establish end-of-life care plan in 3 weeks.

INTERVENTIONS (NIC)‡	RATIONALE
Anxiety Reduction	
• Plan a palliative care conference with patient, husband, and health care team and provide factual information on treatment options and availability of respite care for husband.	Information that helps patients understand their condition, disease course, and the benefits and burdens of treatment options reduces anxiety (Suhonen et al., 2008; Yancey, 2013). Interventions designed to meet individualized needs preserves autonomy and lessens uncertainty (Suhonen et al., 2011).
• Instruct patient in guided imagery and passive relaxation exercises.	Patients with advanced disease such as cancer require a moderate expenditure of energy to perform active progressive relaxation exercise. This can increase a person's existing fatigue. Passive relaxation and guided imagery are more appropriate options (Koithan, 2013).
• Explain specifically how palliative care measures will reduce symptoms patient is most anxious about.	You can lessen anxiety in terminally ill patients by explaining and managing underlying causes of anxiety (Weigel et al., 2007). for example, improving a patient's breathing and oxygenation helps to decrease anxiety (Yancey, 2013).

***Defining characteristics** are shown in **bold** type.
†Outcomes classification labels from Moorhead S, et al, editors: *Nursing outcomes classification (NOC)*, ed 5, St Louis, 2013, Mosby.
‡Intervention classification labels from Bulechek GM et al, editors: *Nursing interventions classification (NIC)*, ed 6, St Louis, 2013, Mosby.

FIGURE 9-7 Care plan for Mrs. Tillman.

CARE PLAN Death Anxiety—cont'd

INTERVENTIONS (NIC)‡	RATIONALE
Decision-Making Support	
• Provide information requested by patient, and help to identify advantages and disadvantages of all alternatives.	Respect for a patient's autonomy involves a commitment to support a patient's ability to make decisions in a well-informed way.
• Facilitate a discussion between patient and husband about end-of-life treatment preferences regarding life-extending treatment.	Difficult end-of-life decisions complicate the survivor's grief and create family divisions. When these decisions are handled well and patient's symptoms are controlled, families experience a meaningful conclusion to the loved one's death (Yancey, 2013).

EVALUATION

NURSING ACTIONS	PATIENT RESPONSE/FINDING	ACHIEVEMENT OF OUTCOME
Question Mrs. Tillman about level of anxiety she feels.	Patient states she feels less worried about suffering. "I know what I'm facing, and I know what they can give me when I have trouble breathing."	Patient obtaining control over anxiety; accepting course of her disease.
Ask Mr. Tillman if Mrs. Tillman practices guided imagery at home.	Husband reports patient uses guided imagery each afternoon for a period of 20 minutes.	Patient is applying anxiety control technique effectively in the home.
Have Mrs. Tillman discuss her feelings about an end-of-life care plan.	Patient is planning to discuss feelings with husband. Has not finalized plan yet. Wants to know more about respite care for husband.	Further discussion and support necessary to help patient and husband finalize an end-of-life care plan.

FIGURE 9-7, cont'd Care plan for Mrs. Tillman.

BOX 9-8 EVIDENCE-BASED PRACTICE

PICO Question: Does an educational program on concept mapping compared with standard lecture improve students' critical thinking competencies?

SUMMARY OF EVIDENCE

Concept mapping is a strategy for developing and improving critical thinking. A concept map has the potential to help a student develop self-appraisal and improve clinical decision making (Pilcher, 2011). Students developed concept maps for patients assigned during their clinical rotations. The concept maps encouraged students to apply six critical thinking competencies: interpretation, analysis, evaluation, inference, explanation, and self-regulation (Chabeli, 2010). As the students gained more clinical experience, they were able to draw on the knowledge acquired from previous concept maps to improve critical thinking and plan patient-centered care. The concept maps also helped students to identify multiple concerns affecting patients. They are appropriate with other health care disciplines and encourage interprofessional collaboration (Daley and Torre, 2010). Concept maps help students better understand how health care disciplines interact with one another to provide individualized patient care in a timely and cost-effective manner.

APPLICATION TO NURSING PRACTICE

- Use a concept map to improve preclinical preparation (Chabeli, 2010).
- Repeated practice and discussion with faculty facilitate the level of clinical decision making (Pilcher, 2011).
- Concept maps encourage understanding of complex relationships between patient's health care problems and nursing interventions (Chabeli, 2010).
- Use of concept maps between multiple health care disciplines fosters a holistic view of patients and better understanding of multiple concerns (Daley and Torre, 2010).

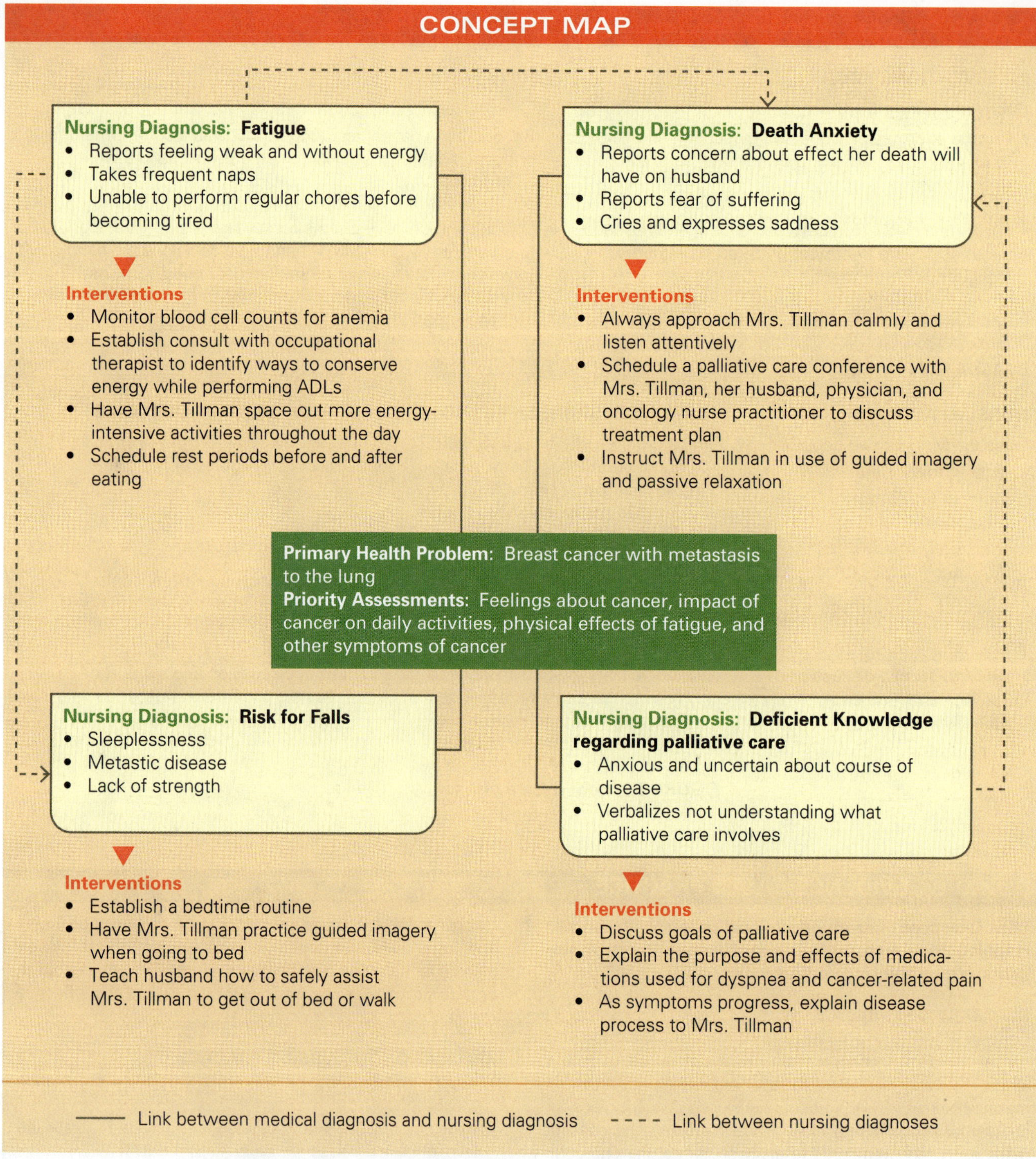
CONCEPT MAP
Nursing Diagnosis: Fatigue
• Reports feeling weak and without energy
• Takes frequent naps
• Unable to perform regular chores before becoming tired
Interventions
• Monitor blood cell counts for anemia
• Establish consult with occupational therapist to identify ways to conserve energy while performing ADLs
• Have Mrs. Tillman space out more energy-intensive activities throughout the day
• Schedule rest periods before and after eating
Nursing Diagnosis: Death Anxiety
• Reports concern about effect her death will have on husband
• Reports fear of suffering
• Cries and expresses sadness
Interventions
• Always approach Mrs. Tillman calmly and listen attentively
• Schedule a palliative care conference with Mrs. Tillman, her husband, physician, and oncology nurse practitioner to discuss treatment plan
• Instruct Mrs. Tillman in use of guided imagery and passive relaxation
Primary Health Problem: Breast cancer with metastasis to the lung
Priority Assessments: Feelings about cancer, impact of cancer on daily activities, physical effects of fatigue, and other symptoms of cancer
Nursing Diagnosis: Risk for Falls
• Sleeplessness
• Metastic disease
• Lack of strength
Interventions
• Establish a bedtime routine
• Have Mrs. Tillman practice guided imagery when going to bed
• Teach husband how to safely assist Mrs. Tillman to get out of bed or walk
Nursing Diagnosis: Deficient Knowledge regarding palliative care
• Anxious and uncertain about course of disease
• Verbalizes not understanding what palliative care involves
Interventions
• Discuss goals of palliative care
• Explain the purpose and effects of medications used for dyspnea and cancer-related pain
• As symptoms progress, explain disease process to Mrs. Tillman
Link between medical diagnosis and nursing diagnosis
Link between nursing diagnoses

FIGURE 9-8 Concept map with interventions. *ADLs,* Activities of daily living.

3. Review any standardized nursing care plans, clinical pathways, protocols, or patient education materials developed for patients on the nursing unit.
4. Prepare the concept map by first developing a skeleton diagram of the patient's health problems. Write the patient's primary health problems and key assessment priorities in the middle of the map. Next add boxes for the patient's nursing care needs like spokes on a wheel.
5. In each box identify and group clinical assessment data that seem to form patterns. Do not worry if you have difficulty labeling nursing diagnoses at first. It is important to first recognize the major nursing care focus for the patient. Remember that sometimes symptoms apply to more than one nursing diagnosis. Repeat symptoms under different categories when appropriate.

6. Analyze relationships among the nursing diagnoses. Draw lines between nursing diagnoses to show relationships. The links must be accurate, meaningful, and complete. You must be able to explain why nursing diagnoses are related. For example, Mrs. Tillman's' *Death Anxiety* and *Deficient Knowledge* are interrelated. In addition her *Fatigue* influences her *Risk for Falls.*
7. List on the map the nursing interventions that you select to attain the outcomes for each nursing diagnosis.
8. While caring for your patient, write down the patient's responses to each nursing activity. Also write your clinical impressions and inferences regarding his or her progress toward expected outcomes and the effectiveness of interventions. Use the concept map as a working tool and revise as needed.

Critical Pathways. Critical pathways are patient care-management plans that provide the interdisciplinary health team with the activities and tasks to be put into practice sequentially (over time). Their main purpose is to deliver timely care at each phase of the care process for a specific type of patient (Espinosa-Aguilar et al., 2008). A critical pathway clearly defines transition points in patient progress and draws a coordinated map of activities by which the health team can help to make these transitions as efficient as possible. A pathway allows staff from all disciplines such as medicine, nursing, and pharmacy to develop integrated care plans for a projected length of stay or number of visits. For example, a pathway for a surgical procedure recommends on a day-by-day basis a patient's activities, consultation, procedures, discharge planning activities, and educational topics expected for the patient's progression to discharge. It also includes outcomes such as the patient's ability to begin ambulation or to describe postoperative restrictions. A pathway ensures continuity of care because it maps out clearly the responsibility of each health care discipline. Well-developed pathways incorporate evidence-based protocols used in the care of the specific case type. You can use the pathway to monitor a patient's progress and as a documentation tool.

Consulting Other Health Care Professionals

Planning involves consultation with members of the health care team. Consultation occurs at any step in the nursing process, but you consult most often during planning and implementation. During these times you are more likely to identify a problem requiring additional knowledge, skills, or community or agency resources. Consultation is a process in which you seek the expertise of a specialist such as your nursing instructor or a clinical nurse specialist to identify ways to handle problems in patient care management or plan implementation of therapies. Consultation is based on the problem-solving approach, and the consultant is the stimulus for change. Often an experienced nurse is a valuable consultant when you face an unfamiliar patient care situation. Through consultation and collaboration you are able to use the best resources to individualize nursing actions to meet expected outcomes.

When to Consult. Consultation occurs when you identify a problem that you cannot solve using personal knowledge, skills, and resources. Consultation with other care providers increases your knowledge about a patient's problems and helps you learn skills and obtain resources. A good time to consult with another health care professional is when the exact problem remains unclear. An objective consultant enters a situation and more clearly assesses and identifies the nature of a problem.

How To Consult. Begin with your own understanding of a patient's clinical problems. The first step in arranging a consultation is to identify the general problem area. Second, direct the consultation to the appropriate professional such as another nurse, a social worker, or a dietitian. Third, provide the consultant with relevant information and resources about the problem area. Include a relevant, brief summary of the problem; methods used to resolve the problem so far; and outcomes of the methods. Share information from the patient's medical record and conversations with nurses, other members of the health team, and the patient's family.

Fourth, do not prejudice or influence consultants. Consultants are in the clinical setting to help identify and resolve a nursing problem. Biasing or prejudicing can block problem resolution. Avoid bias by not overloading consultants with subjective and emotional conclusions about a patient and problem.

Fifth, be available to discuss the consultant's findings and recommendations. When you request a consultation, provide a private, comfortable atmosphere for the consultant and the patient. However, this does not mean that you leave the environment. A common mistake is turning the whole problem over to the consultant. The consultant is not there to take over the problem but to help you resolve it. When possible, request the consultation for a day when both you and the consultant are working and during a time when there are few distractions.

Finally, include the consultant's recommendations in the care plan. The success of the advice depends on the implementation of the problem-solving strategies. Always give the consultant feedback about the outcomes.

IMPLEMENTATION

Implementation, the fourth step of the nursing process, begins after you develop the care plan. It involves providing care to patients. Implementation is the performance of nursing interventions necessary for achieving the goals and expected outcomes of nursing care. A nursing intervention is any treatment based on clinical judgment and knowledge that a nurse performs to enhance patient outcomes (Bulechek et al., 2012). Ideally the interventions a nurse uses are evidence based (see Chapter 7). Interventions include both direct and indirect care measures aimed at individuals, families, and the community.

Direct care interventions are treatments performed through interactions with patients. Examples are medication administration, insertion of an IV catheter, and counseling during a time of grief. **Indirect care interventions** are treatments performed away from but on behalf of the patient or group of patients (Bulechek et al., 2012). Examples are actions aimed at managing the patient's environment (safety and infection control), documentation, and interdisciplinary collaboration.

Implementation is continuous with all steps of the nursing process. Both direct and indirect care interventions fall under the categories discussed earlier: independent nursing (nurse-initiated), dependent nursing (physician-initiated), and collaborative interventions. For example, the direct care intervention of patient education is an independent nursing intervention. The indirect intervention of consultation is a collaborative intervention.

Standard Nursing Interventions

Health care settings offer various ways for nurses to create and individualize patient care plans. Although it is critical for each patient to have his or her own unique set of interventions, many health care systems have mechanisms for standardizing the more common types of interventions or approaches to care. Many patients have common health problems; thus standardized interventions make it quicker and easier for nurses to intervene. When these standardized interventions are evidence based, a nurse is more likely to deliver the most clinically effective care that will result in the best patient outcomes.

Clinical Practice Guidelines and Protocols. A **clinical practice guideline** or protocol is a systematically developed set of statements that helps nurses and other health care providers make decisions about appropriate health care for specific clinical situations (Manchikanti et al., 2010). A guideline establishes interventions for specific health care problems or conditions such as low back pain, dizziness, or deep vein thrombosis. A guideline is developed on the basis of an authoritative examination of current scientific evidence and helps health care providers make decisions about appropriate health care for specific clinical circumstances (NGC, 2010). Guidelines are key tools for improving the quality of patient care.

Clinicians within a health care agency review the scientific literature and their own standard of practice to create a clinical practice guideline. However, there are also guidelines already developed by national health groups such as the National Institutes of Health, the INS, and the National Guideline Clearinghouse. These clinical guidelines are available to any clinician or agency that wishes to adopt evidence-based guidelines in patient care. One valuable source for nursing practice guidelines is the Gerontological Nursing Interventions Research Center at the University of Iowa. The center has numerous clinical guidelines, including ones for acute confusion and delirium, bathing persons with dementia, and prevention of pressure ulcers (GNIRC, 2012).

In acute care settings it is common to find clinical protocols that outline independent nursing interventions for specific conditions. Examples are protocols for admission and discharge, pressure ulcer care, and fall prevention. Protocols are also used in interdisciplinary settings for diagnostic testing and physical, occupational, and speech therapies.

A **standing order** is a preprinted document containing orders for conducting routine therapies, monitoring guidelines, and/or diagnostic procedures for specific patients with identified clinical problems. A standing order directs the conduct of patient care in specific clinical settings. Licensed, prescribing health care providers in charge of care at the time of implementation approve and sign standing orders. These orders are common in critical care settings and other specialized practice settings in which patients' needs can change rapidly and require immediate attention. An example of a standing order is one specifying certain medications such as lidocaine or propranolol for an irregular heart rhythm. After assessing the patient and identifying the irregular rhythm, the critical care nurse gives the specified medication without first notifying the health care provider because his or her initial standing order covers the nurse's action. After completing a standing order, the nurse notifies the health care provider. Standing orders are also common in the community health setting, in which nurses face situations that do not permit immediate contact with a physician or health care provider. Standing orders give you the legal protection to intervene appropriately in the patient's best interest.

NIC Interventions. The NIC system developed by the University of Iowa differentiates nursing practice from that of other health care professionals by offering a language that nurses can use to describe sets of actions in delivering nursing care. The NIC interventions offer a level of standardization to enhance communication of nursing care across settings and compare outcomes. The NIC system has been incorporated into many health care information systems. By using NIC nurses learn the common interventions recommended for the various NANDA-I nursing diagnoses.

Critical Thinking in Implementation

The selection of nursing interventions for a patient is part of clinical decision making. Strong clinical reasoning and decision making help you accurately identify appropriate nursing interventions for a patient's specific nursing diagnoses and achieve appropriate patient outcomes (Muller-Staub et al., 2006; 2008). The critical thinking model discussed in Chapter 8 provides a framework for how to make decisions when implementing nursing care. Your knowledge about a patient's health problems leads you to select appropriate therapies. For example, knowledge of the disease course of metastatic cancer allows Rich to select interventions for pain relief, fatigue, and breathing alterations. His knowledge of the NIC classification directs him to select specific care activities for each of Mrs. Tillman's nursing diagnoses.

You also apply prior clinical experiences in performing specific interventions. Consider which interventions have worked before and which have not worked in previous clinical situations. Be aware of both professional and agency standards of practice. Standards of practice offer guidelines for selection of interventions, their frequency, and the determination of whether the procedures may be delegated. In Mrs.

Tillman's case the NGC has a guideline for cancer pain management that would be very helpful. As you perform any nursing intervention, apply intellectual standards. For example, when teaching patients be relevant, clear, and logical to promote patient learning (see Chapter 12). All critical thinking attitudes such as confidence, creativity, and discipline apply to implementation. A beginning student needs supervision from an instructor or experienced nurse to guide the decision-making process for implementation.

Implementation Process

Preparation for implementation ensures efficient, safe, and effective nursing care. Follow these five preparatory activities: reassess the patient, review and revise the existing nursing care plan, organize resources and care delivery, anticipate and prevent complications, and implement nursing interventions.

Reassessing the Patient. Patient assessment is a continuous process that occurs each time you interact with a patient. When you gather new data and identify a new patient need, you modify the care plan. You also modify a plan when you resolve a patient's health care need. Just before implementing a nursing activity, reassess your patient. This is a partial assessment and sometimes focuses on one dimension such as level of comfort or on one system such as the cardiovascular system. The reassessment helps you decide if the proposed nursing activity is still appropriate for the patient's level of wellness. For example, you planned to assist a patient with ambulation following lunch; however, a reassessment reveals shortness of breath and increased fatigue, which require you to help the patient back to bed.

Reviewing and Revising the Care Plan. After reassessing a patient, review the care plan and compare assessment data to validate the nursing diagnoses. Determine whether the nursing interventions are appropriate. If the patient's status has changed and the nursing diagnosis and related interventions are no longer appropriate, modify the nursing care plan. An out-of-date or incorrect care plan compromises the quality of nursing care. Review and modification enable you to provide timely nursing interventions to best meet a patient's needs. There are four steps to modifying the written care plan:

1. Revise data in the assessment section to reflect a patient's current status. Date any new data to inform other health team members of the time that the change occurred.
2. Revise nursing diagnoses. Delete diagnoses that are no longer relevant and add and date any new diagnoses. It is necessary to revise related factors and the patient's goals, outcomes, and priorities.
3. Revise specific interventions that correspond to the new nursing diagnoses and goals. This revision should reflect the patient's present status.
4. Determine the method of evaluation to achieve outcomes.

Rich prepares to have a discussion with Mrs. Tillman and her husband about palliative care. Before he begins, Rich reassesses Mrs. Tillman's level of anxiety to learn more specifically about what is contributing to her worry about suffering. She explains that she has a general sense of dread and does not want to have a lot of pain. Her worries keep her from sleeping at night on a regular basis. Rich probes this further and with new information identifies the nursing diagnosis of Disturbed Sleep Pattern. He revises his plan to focus instruction on planned comfort measures.

Organizing Resources and Delivering Care. Facility resources include equipment and skilled personnel. Organization of equipment and personnel makes timely, efficient, and skilled patient care possible. Preparation for care delivery also involves preparing the environment and patient for nursing interventions.

Equipment. Most nursing procedures require some equipment or supplies. Decide which supplies are necessary and determine their availability before you start implementation. Equipment should be in working order to ensure safe use. Place supplies in a convenient location to provide easy access during a procedure. Be sure extra supplies are available in case of errors or accidents, but do not take them into a patient's room or open them unless they are needed. Unused equipment left in rooms must be thrown away as a loss to an agency. Wise use of supplies controls health care costs. After a procedure return any unopened supplies.

Personnel. Nursing care delivery models vary among facilities (see Chapter 13). The model by which nursing is organized determines how nursing personnel deliver patient care. For example, a registered nurse's (RN's) accountabilities differ in a team nursing model from those in a primary nursing model. A primary nurse is accountable for the nursing care that a patient receives during his or her length of stay or course of visits. A team nurse is accountable for the specific shift in which he or she works. As a nurse you are responsible for determining whether to perform an intervention or delegate it to another member of the nursing team. Your assessment of a patient directs the decision about delegation and not the intervention alone. For example, you know nursing assistive personnel (NAP) can competently ambulate patients. However, you learn that a patient experienced an increased pulse rate after walking during the previous shift; thus you decide to personally assist the patient with ambulation and evaluate his or her cardiac status. In this case you redirect the NAP to perform an intervention for a more stable patient.

Nursing staff work together as patients' needs demand it. If a patient makes a request such as for use of a bedpan, position the patient on the pan if you have time rather than trying to find the NAP who is in a different room. When interventions are complex or physically difficult, you may need assistance from colleagues. For example, you are more effective in performing procedures when NAP help you position a patient and hand you supplies during the procedure.

Environment. A patient's care environment needs to be safe and conducive for implementing therapies. Patient safety is your first concern. If a patient has sensory deficits, physical disabilities, or an alteration in level of consciousness, arrange the environment to prevent injury (e.g., provide assistive devices [e.g., walkers or eyeglasses], rearrange furniture and equipment, and make rooms free of clutter). Patients benefit most from nursing interventions when surroundings are compatible with care activities. When you need to expose a patient's body parts, do so privately because the patient will be more relaxed. Reduce distractions to enhance learning opportunities. Make sure that lighting is adequate to perform procedures correctly.

Patient. Before you deliver interventions, be sure your patients are as physically and psychologically comfortable as possible. For example, symptoms such as nausea or pain interfere with a patient's full concentration and cooperation. Offer comfort measures before initiating interventions to help the patient participate more fully. If you need a patient to be alert, give a dose of pain medication to relieve discomfort but not impair mental faculties (e.g., ability to follow instruction, reasoning, and communication). If a patient is fatigued, delay ambulation until after he or she has had a chance to rest. Even if symptoms are not a factor, make the patient physically comfortable during interventions. Start any intervention by controlling environmental factors, positioning, and taking care of other physical needs (e.g., elimination). Also consider the patient's level of endurance and plan only the amount of activity that he or she can tolerate comfortably.

Awareness of a patient's psychosocial needs helps you create a favorable emotional climate. Some patients feel reassured by having a significant other present for encouragement and moral support. Other strategies include planning sufficient time or multiple opportunities for patients to work through and vent feelings and anxieties. Adequate preparation allows a patient to obtain maximal benefit from each intervention.

Anticipating and Preventing Complications. Risks to patients come from both illness and treatment. As a nurse look for and recognize these risks, adapt your choice of interventions to each situation, evaluate the relative benefit of the treatment versus the risk, and take risk-prevention measures. Many conditions place patients at risk for complications. For example, a patient who had a stroke has limited mobility and is at risk for developing pressure ulcers. Nurses are often the first ones to detect changes in patients' conditions. Your knowledge of pathophysiology and previous patient care experiences help identify possible complications that can occur. A thorough assessment reveals the level of a patient's current risk. Scientific rationales for how certain interventions (e.g., turning and use of pressure-relief devices) prevent or minimize complications help you select the preventive measures that will likely be most useful. Some nursing procedures pose risks for patients. Be aware of potential complications and take precautions. For instance, a patient who is to have a urinary catheter inserted is at risk for infection. In this situation thorough cleansing of the urethra before insertion reduces infection risk.

Identifying Areas of Assistance. Certain nursing situations require you to obtain assistance by seeking additional personnel, knowledge, and/or nursing skills. Before beginning care, review the plan to determine the need for assistance and the type required. Sometimes you need help to perform a procedure, provide comfort measures, or prepare a patient for a procedure. For example, when you care for a patient who is overweight and immobilized, you require additional personnel and transfer equipment to turn and position the patient safely. Be sure to determine in advance the number of additional personnel and when you need them. Discuss your need for assistance with potential resources such as other nurses or NAP.

You require additional knowledge and skills in situations in which you are less familiar or experienced. For example, seek additional knowledge when you give a new medication or implement a new procedure. You find such information in a hospital formulary or procedure book. If you are still uncertain about the new medication or procedure, ask other members of the health care team.

Because of the continual growth in health care technology, you may lack the skills needed to perform a new procedure. When this occurs, first locate information about the procedure in the literature and the agency procedures book. Next collect all equipment necessary for the procedure. Finally ask another nurse who is experienced in performing the procedure to provide assistance and guidance. The assistance can come from another staff nurse, supervisor, educator, or nurse specialist. Requesting assistance occurs frequently in practice and is a learning process that continues throughout educational experiences and into professional development.

Implementation Skills. Nursing practice includes cognitive, interpersonal, and psychomotor (technical) skills. You need each type of skill to implement direct and indirect nursing interventions. You are responsible for knowing when one type of implementation skill is preferred over another and for having the necessary knowledge and skill to perform each.

Cognitive Skills. Cognitive skills involve the application of critical thinking in the nursing process. Always use good judgment and sound clinical decision making when performing any intervention. This ensures that no nursing action is automatic. Always think and anticipate so you individualize patient care appropriately. Know the rationale for therapeutic interventions and understand normal and abnormal physiological and psychological responses. Know the evidence in nursing science to ensure that you deliver the most current and relevant nursing interventions.

Interpersonal Skills. Interpersonal skills are essential for effective nursing action. Develop a trusting relationship, express a level of caring, and communicate clearly with the patient and family (see Chapter 11). Effective communication is critical for keeping patients informed, providing effective teaching, and effectively supporting patients who have challenging emotional needs. Proper use of interpersonal skills enables you to perceive a patient's verbal and nonverbal communication accurately. As a member of the health care team, you communicate patient problems and needs clearly, intelligently, and in a timely manner.

Psychomotor Skills. Psychomotor skills require the integration of cognitive and motor activities. For example, when taking a pulse you need to understand anatomy and physiology (cognitive) and assume the proper positioning and use of touch to detect the pulse correctly (motor). With time and practice you learn to perform skills correctly, smoothly, and confidently. This is critical in establishing patient trust. You are responsible for acquiring necessary psychomotor skills. In the case of a new skill, assess your level of competency and obtain the necessary resources to ensure that the patient receives safe treatment.

Direct Care

Nurses provide a wide variety of direct care measures (i.e., activities that nurses perform with patient interaction). How a nurse interacts affects the success of any direct care activity. Remain sensitive to a patient's clinical condition, values and beliefs, expectations, and cultural views. All direct care measures require competent, safe practice. Show a caring approach when you provide direct care.

Activities of Daily Living. ADLs are activities usually performed during a normal day, including ambulation, eating, dressing, bathing, and grooming. A patient's need for assistance with ADLs may be temporary or permanent. A patient with impaired mobility because of bilateral arm casts has a temporary need for assistance. After the casts are removed, the patient gradually regains the strength and range of motion needed to perform ADLs. A patient with an irreversible injury to the cervical spinal cord is paralyzed and thus has a permanent need for assistance. Rehabilitation would not be realistic for such a patient. Instead through restorative care the patient learns new ways to perform ADLs so as to be less dependent on others.

When an assessment reveals that a patient is experiencing fatigue, a limitation in mobility, confusion, and/or pain, assistance with ADLs is likely needed. It can range from partial to complete care. Always consider a patient's preferences when assisting with ADLs. Consultation with physical or occupational therapy is also helpful. Involve the patient in planning the timing and types of interventions to enhance self-esteem and the willingness to become more independent.

Instrumental Activities of Daily Living. Illness or disability sometimes alters a patient's ability to be independent in society. **Instrumental activities of daily living (IADLs)** include skills such as shopping, preparing meals, writing checks, and taking medications. Nurses in home care and community nursing frequently help patients adapt ways to perform IADLs. Often family and friends are excellent resources for assisting patients. In acute care it is important for you to anticipate how patients' illnesses affect their ability to perform IADLs so you make the appropriate referrals.

Physical Care Techniques. You routinely use a variety of physical care techniques in patient care. Physical care techniques involve the safe and competent administration of nursing procedures (e.g., inserting a urinary catheter, performing range-of-motion exercises). The specific knowledge and skills needed to perform these procedures are in subsequent clinical chapters of this text. Common methods for administering physical care techniques appropriately include protecting you and the patient from injury, using proper infection control practices, staying organized, and positioning patients correctly. When you apply physical care during a procedure, know the clinical practice guidelines and how to perform the procedure, the standard frequency, and the expected outcomes.

Lifesaving Measures. A lifesaving measure is a physical care technique that you use when a patient's physiological or psychological state is threatened. The purpose of lifesaving measures is to restore physiological and psychological balance. Such measures include administering emergency medications, performing cardiopulmonary resuscitation, and protecting a violent patient. When an inexperienced nurse faces a situation requiring emergency measures, it is critical to obtain the assistance of an experienced professional.

Counseling. **Counseling** is a direct care method that helps patients use a problem-solving process to recognize and manage stress and facilitate interpersonal relationships. As a nurse you counsel patients to accept actual or impending changes resulting from stress. Counseling involves emotional, intellectual, spiritual, and psychological support (see Chapters 25 and 26). Examples of counseling strategies are behavior modification, bereavement counseling, biofeedback, and crisis intervention. A patient and family who need nursing counseling have normal adjustment difficulties and are upset or frustrated, but they are not necessarily psychologically disabled. A good example is the case of Mr. Tillman, who faces normal grief and the uncertainty of how cancer will affect his wife and his relationship with her. Nurse counseling encourages patients to examine available alternatives and decide which choices are useful and appropriate. When patients are able to examine alternatives, they develop a sense of control and are able to better manage stress. When patients have psychiatric diagnoses such as severe depression or schizophrenia, they require specialized therapy by mental health nurses or social workers, psychologists, or psychiatrists.

Teaching. Teaching is an important nursing responsibility. In teaching the focus of change is intellectual growth or the acquisition of new knowledge or psychomotor skills. As a nurse you teach correct principles, procedures, and techniques of health care to inform patients about their health status and prepare them for self-care (see Chapter 12). When patients are unable to assume self-care, nurses focus teaching efforts on family caregivers. Teaching takes place in all health care settings. As a nurse you are responsible for assessing the learning needs and readiness of patients and family caregivers, and you are accountable for the quality of education you deliver. Know your patients; be aware of the cultural and social factors that influence their willingness and ability to learn. It is also important to know your patient's health literacy level. Can he or she read directions or make calculations that are necessary with self-care skills? The teaching-learning process is an active interaction between the teacher and learner in which you, the teacher, address specific learning objectives. This process offers an organizational structure and framework for patient education.

Controlling for Adverse Reactions. An adverse reaction is a harmful or unintended effect of a medication, diagnostic test, or therapeutic intervention. Adverse reactions can follow any nursing intervention; thus learn to anticipate them and know which adverse reactions to expect. Nursing actions that control for adverse reactions reduce or counteract the reaction. For example, when applying a moist heat compress, you want to prevent burning the patient's skin. First assess the area requiring the compress. After application of the compress, check the area every 5 minutes for any adverse reaction such as excessive reddening of the skin from the heat. When administering a medication, understand the known and potential side effects of the drug. After administration of the medication, evaluate the patient's response for adverse effects. Also know the drugs that are available to counteract any side effects. Although adverse reactions are not common, they do occur. It is important that you recognize the signs and symptoms of an adverse reaction and intervene in a timely manner.

Preventive Measures. Preventive nursing actions promote health and prevent illness to avoid the need for acute or rehabilitative health care. Prevention includes promoting a patient's health potential, applying prescribed measures (e.g., immunizations), health teaching, and identifying risks for illness and/or trauma. Consider Mrs. Tillman's situation. Rich worries that, with her fatigue and the progressive nature of her cancer, she is likely to become weaker and less mobile. He recommends preventive measures to make the Tillman's home setting safer. He assesses their home environment and chooses the interventions (e.g., installing grab bars in the bath and rearranging furniture) that will improve Mrs. Tillman's safety and ability to move about comfortably in her home. All patients need nursing interventions aimed at promoting health and preventing illness. As changes in the health care system continue, there is and will be greater emphasis on health promotion and illness prevention.

Indirect Care

Indirect care measures are actions that support the effectiveness of direct care measures (Bulechek et al., 2012). Many indirect measures are managerial in nature such as documentation and medical order transcription. Others are environmental such as specimen and supply management. A good amount of a nurse's time is spent in indirect care activities. For example, communication of information about patients (e.g., change-of-shift report and consultation) is critical to ensure that direct care activities are planned and coordinated with proper resources. Delegation of care to NAP is another indirect care activity. Proper delegation ensures that the right care providers perform the right tasks so an RN and NAP work most efficiently for their patients.

Delegating, Supervising, and Evaluating the Work of Other Staff Members. Depending on the system of health care delivery, the nurse who develops the care plan frequently does not perform all of the nursing interventions. Some activities are coordinated and delegated to other members of the health care team (see Chapter 13). Remember that an RN delegates components of care but not the nursing process itself (ANA/NCBSN, 2012). Noninvasive and frequently repetitive interventions such as skin care, ambulation, grooming, and hygiene measures are examples of activities that you assign to NAP such as certified nurse assistants. Licensed practical nurses perform these measures in addition to medication administration and many invasive tasks (e.g., dressing care and catheterization). The nursing tasks or activities that members of the nursing team perform under the direction of an RN are identified according to legal parameters defined by each state in its Nurse Practice Act and by the scope of practice and standards established by professional nursing organizations (ANA, 2010).When you delegate aspects of care to another staff member, you are responsible for assigning the task and making sure that the staff member completes the task according to the standard of care. You are also responsible for delegating direct care interventions to personnel competent to provide the care.

EVALUATION

After a patient diagnosed with pneumonia has completed a 5-day pack of antibiotics, the health care provider has the patient return to the office to have a chest x-ray examination to determine if the pneumonia has cleared. When a nurse on a surgical unit provides wound care, he or she first assesses the appearance of the wound, applies the appropriate dressing, and returns later to inspect the wound to see if it has healed. These two scenarios depict the process of evaluation, the last step of the nursing process. The health care provider orders a chest x-ray examination, and the nurse reinspects the wound. Evaluation is the critical step of the nursing process that involves an examination of a condition or situation and then a judgment as to whether change has occurred.

Evaluation is crucial to deciding whether, after interventions have been delivered, a patient's condition or well-being improves (see Figure 9-7). You apply all that you know about a patient and the patient's condition together with experience with previous patients to evaluate if nursing care was effective. You conduct an evaluation to determine if expected outcomes are met, not if nursing interventions were completed. *For example, in Rich's plan of care for Mrs. Tillman, he has established the outcome of "The patient will verbalize feeling less anxious about the course of her disease within 1 week." Rich implements educational interventions to improve Mrs. Tillman's knowledge and anxiety-reduction exercises.* Evaluation *does* involve questioning Mrs. Tillman about her feelings toward her disease. Evaluation *does not* involve observation of her performing anxiety-reduction exercises. Expected outcomes are the standards against which you judge if goals have been met and care is successful.

Critical Thinking and Evaluation

Evaluation is an ongoing process that you conduct while caring for a patient. Once you deliver an intervention, you gather subjective and objective data from the patient, family, and health care team members. This includes reviewing knowledge about a patient's current condition, treatment, and resources available for recovery. By referring to previous experiences caring for similar patients, you are in a better position to know how to evaluate your patient. You then apply critical thinking attitudes and standards to determine whether outcomes of care are achieved. If outcomes are met, the overall goals for the patient are also met. You compare patient behavior and responses assessed before delivering nursing interventions with behavior and responses that occur after administering nursing care. For example, Rich's initial assessment revealed Mrs. Tillman's sense of anxiety about her impending death and uncertainty about her course of illness. On a subsequent clinic visit he considers the following questions: Has the patient's condition improved? Can the patient improve, or are there physical or psychological factors preventing recovery? To what degree does the patient's emotional health influence response to therapies? To evaluate Mrs. Tillman's progress, he asks her how she now feels about the cancer and its anticipated effects. She is able to talk about her cancer without crying. She also tells Rich, "I think I have a better idea of what to expect; but, more important, I know my doctor will do all he can to make me comfortable." The evaluation shows that the patient has accepted her prognosis and has a better sense of control over her condition.

In evaluation you make clinical decisions and continually redirect nursing care. For example, when evaluating a patient for a change in pain severity, you apply knowledge of disease processes, physiological responses to interventions, and the correct procedure for measuring pain severity to interpret whether a change has occurred and if it is desirable. If a patient continues to report pain at a higher level on a pain scale than expected, you consult with the health care provider to increase an analgesic dose or try different noninvasive approaches to help the patient relax and concentrate less on the pain. You continue to evaluate until the patient achieves pain relief.

Positive evaluations occur when you achieve expected outcomes that lead you to conclude that the nursing interventions effectively met the patient's goals. Negative evaluations or undesired results indicate that the interventions were not effective in minimizing or resolving the actual problem or avoiding a potential problem. Sometimes new data reveal that a patient's condition altered the patient's ability to meet the expected outcome. As a result, change the care plan and try different therapies or a different approach in administering existing therapies.

This sequence of critically evaluating and revising therapies continues until you and the patient appropriately resolve the problems. Outcomes must be realistic and adjusted based on the patient's prognosis and nursing diagnoses. Remember that evaluation is dynamic and ever changing, depending on a patient's nursing diagnoses and condition. A patient whose health status continuously changes requires more frequent evaluation. In addition, priority diagnoses are usually evaluated first. For example, you evaluate a patient's *Acute Pain* before evaluating the status of *Deficient Knowledge*.

The Evaluation Process

The evaluation process includes five elements: (1) identifying evaluative criteria and standards; (2) collecting data to determine if your patient met the criteria or standards; (3) interpreting and summarizing findings; (4) documenting findings; and (5) terminating, continuing, or revising the care plan.

Identifying Criteria and Standards. Your evaluative criteria include the goals and expected outcomes established during planning. Thus evaluation is most effective when you know what to observe or measure. During evaluation you compare your findings with the goals and expected outcomes set for your patient. Proper evaluation allows you to determine whether each patient reaches a level of wellness or recovery that is reflected in the goals of care.

Collecting Data. Evaluating a patient's response to nursing care requires the use of evaluative measures, which are simply assessment skills and techniques (e.g., auscultation of lung sounds, observation of a patient's skill performance, or discussion of the patient's feelings). In fact, evaluative measures are the same as assessment measures, but you perform them at the point of care when you make decisions about the patient's status and progress. The intent of assessment is to identify what if any problem exists. The intent of evaluation is to determine if the known problems have remained the same, improved, worsened, or otherwise changed.

In many clinical situations it is important to collect evaluative measures over a period of time to determine if a pattern of improvement or change exists. For example, a one-time observation of a pressure ulcer is insufficient to determine that the ulcer is healing. You want to see a consistency in change. For example, over a period of 2 days is the pressure ulcer decreasing in size? Is the amount of drainage declining? Recognizing a pattern of improvement or decline allows you to reason and decide if the patient's problems are resolved.

The primary source of data for evaluation is the patient. However, you also use input from the family and other caregivers. For example, you ask a family member to report on the amount of food a patient eats during a meal or how well the patient is able to sleep during the night. You sometimes consult with colleagues about how patients respond to therapies (e.g., pain medication) during a previous shift. In addition to outcomes, it is also important to evaluate if you met a patient's expectations of care. You evaluate patients about their perceptions of care such as, "Did you receive the type of pain relief you expected?" This level of evaluation is important to determine the patient's satisfaction with care and strengthen partnering between you and the patient.

Interpreting and Summarizing Findings. An expert nurse recognizes relevant evidence, even evidence that does not match clinical expectations, and makes judgments about a patient's condition. To develop clinical judgment you learn to match the results of evaluative measures with expected outcomes to determine whether or not a patient's status is improving. When interpreting findings you compare the patient's behavioral responses and physiological signs and symptoms that you expect to see with those actually seen during evaluation. To objectively evaluate the degree of success in achieving outcomes of care, use the following steps:

1. Examine the outcome criteria to identify the exact desired patient behavior or response.
2. Measure the patient's actual behavior or response.
3. Compare the established outcome criteria with the actual behavior or response.
4. Judge the degree of agreement between outcome criteria and the actual behavior or response.
5. If there is no agreement (or only partial agreement) between outcome criteria and patient response, why did they not agree? What barriers prevented achievement of outcomes?

Evaluation is easier to perform after you care for a patient over a period of time. You can then make subtle comparisons of patient responses and behaviors. When you have not had the chance to care for a patient over an extended time, evaluation improves by referring to previous experiences and asking colleagues familiar with the patient to confirm evaluation findings.

Remember to evaluate each expected outcome and its place in the sequence of care. If not, it is difficult to determine which outcome in the sequence was not met. This prevents you from revising and redirecting the plan of care at the most appropriate time.

Documenting Findings. Documentation and reporting are a part of evaluation. Accurate information needs to be present in a patient's medical record for nurses and other health care providers to make ongoing clinical decisions. When documenting a patient's response to interventions, always describe the same evaluative measures. Your aim is to present a clear argument from the evaluative data as to whether a patient is progressing or not. Communicate a patient's progress toward meeting outcomes and goals on assessment flow sheets and summary progress notes and by sharing information between nurses during change-of-shift reports (see Chapter 10).

Care Plan Revision. The result of interpreting evaluative data allows you to decide if you need to revise the plan of care. If your patient meets a goal successfully, discontinue that part of the care plan. Unmet and partially met goals require you to continue intervention. After you evaluate a patient, you often modify or add nursing diagnoses with appropriate goals and expected outcomes and then establish interventions. You must also redefine priorities. This is an important step in critical thinking (i.e., knowing how the patient is progressing and how problems either resolve or worsen).

Careful monitoring and early detection of problems are a patient's first line of defense. Base clinical judgments on your observations of what is occurring with a specific patient and not merely what happens to patients in general. Frequently changes are not very obvious. Evaluations are patient specific, based on a close familiarity with each patient's behavior, physical status, and reaction to caregivers.

Discontinuing a Care Plan. After you determine that expected outcomes and goals have been met, you confirm this evaluation with the patient when possible. If you and the patient agree, you discontinue that part of the care plan. Documentation of a discontinued plan ensures that other nurses will not unnecessarily continue interventions for that portion of the plan of care. Continuity of care assumes that care provided to patients is relevant and timely. You waste much time when you do not communicate achieved goals.

Modifying a Care Plan. When goals are not met, you identify the factors that interfere with goal achievement. Usually a change in a patient's condition, needs, or abilities makes alteration of the care plan necessary. For example, *while monitoring Mrs. Tillman's level of fatigue, Rich learns during a follow-up visit that Mrs. Tillman is now having difficulty breathing. Her breathing rate is elevated and shallower than her last visit. She confirms that she experiences shortness of breath, especially when climbing stairs at home. Her breathing difficulty has also aggravated her sense of fatigue. Mrs. Tillman explains, "I sometimes don't have the energy just to dress and eat." Rich knows that the breathing problem is related to progression of the cancer and thus establishes a new diagnosis, Impaired Gas Exchange related to damaged alveolar capillary membrane.*

At times a lack of goal achievement results from an error in nursing judgment or failure to follow each step of the nursing process. Patients often have multiple problems. Always remember the possibility of overlooking or misjudging something. When there is failure to achieve a goal, no matter what the reason, repeat the entire nursing process sequence for that nursing diagnosis to discover changes the plan needs. Reassess the patient, determine accuracy of the nursing diagnosis, establish new goals and expected outcomes, and select new interventions.

A complete reassessment of all patient factors relating to the nursing diagnosis and etiology is necessary when modifying a plan. Apply critical thinking as you compare new data about the patient's condition with previously assessed information. Knowledge from previous experiences helps you direct the reassessment process. Caring for patients who have had similar health problems gives you a strong background of knowledge to use for anticipating patient needs and knowing what to assess. Reassessment ensures that the database is accurate and relevant (standards for critical thinking). It also reveals any missing link or piece of information that was overlooked and perhaps responsible for preventing goal achievement. You sort, validate, and cluster all new data to analyze and interpret differences from the original database.

After reassessment determine which nursing diagnoses are accurate for the situation. Ask yourself whether you selected the correct diagnosis and whether the diagnosis and the etiological factor are current. Revise the problem list to reflect the patient's changed status. You may make a new diagnosis. You base nursing care on an accurate list of nursing diagnoses. Accuracy is more important than the number of diagnoses selected. As the patient's condition changes, the diagnoses do as well.

When you modify a care plan, also review the goals and expected outcomes for needed changes. Examine the goals for unchanged nursing diagnoses. Are they still appropriate? A change in one diagnosis may affect others. For example, if Mrs. Tillman now has *Impaired Gas Exchange*, it likely will require Rich to alter goals and outcomes with respect to her problem of *Fatigue*. It is also important to determine that each goal and expected outcome is realistic for the problem, etiology, and time frame. Unrealistic expected outcomes and time frames make goal achievement difficult.

Clearly document goals and expected outcomes for new or revised nursing diagnoses so all team members are aware of the revised care plan. When the goal is still appropriate but has not yet been met, you may change the evaluation date to allow more time. You may also decide at this time to change interventions. For example, when a patient's wound does not heal with a transparent dressing, you choose a different dressing material such as a colloid dressing. All goals and expected outcomes are patient centered, with realistic expectations for patient achievement.

The evaluation of interventions examines two factors: the appropriateness of the interventions selected and the correct application of the intervention. The appropriateness of an intervention is based on the standard of care for a patient's health problem. A **standard of care** is the minimum level of care accepted to ensure high quality of care to patients. Standards of care define the types of therapies typically administered to patients with specific problems or needs. If the patient who is receiving chemotherapy for leukemia has the nursing diagnosis *Nausea related to pharyngeal irritation*, the standard of care established by a nursing department for this problem includes pain-control measures, mouth-care guidelines, and diet therapy. The nurse reviews the standard of care to determine if the right interventions have been chosen or if additional ones are needed.

You may only need to increase or decrease the frequency of interventions when you revise a care plan. Use clinical judgment based on previous experience and a patient's actual response to therapy. For example, if a patient continues to have congested lung sounds, you increase the frequency of coughing and deep-breathing exercises to remove secretions.

During evaluation you may find that some planned interventions are designed for an inappropriate level of nursing care. If you need to change the level of care, substitute a different action verb, such as *assist* in place of *provide*, or *demonstrate* in place of *describe*. For example, assisting a patient with walking requires a nurse to be at the patient's side during ambulation, whereas providing an assistive device suggests that the patient is more independent. Sometimes the level of care is appropriate, but the interventions are unsuitable because of a change in the expected outcome. In this case discontinue the interventions and plan new ones.

Make any changes in the plan of care based on the nature of the patient's unfavorable response. Consulting with other health care providers often yields suggestions for improving the approach to care delivery. Practicing nurses are usually excellent resources because of their experience. Simply changing the care plan is not enough. Implement the new plan and reevaluate the patient's response to the nursing actions. Remember, *evaluation is continuous.*

KEY POINTS

- The nursing process has five steps: assessment, nursing diagnosis, planning, implementation, and evaluation.
- Use of the nursing process is the foundation for clinical decision making.
- When you first meet a patient, you conduct an initial assessment screening and then focus on cues and patterns of information to make a more comprehensive assessment.
- Attention to the environment, patient comfort, and communication techniques ensures a successful assessment interview.
- Data analysis involves recognizing patterns or trends, comparing data with standards, and forming a reasoned conclusion about the meaning of the data.
- Data clustering organizes assessment data into meaningful clusters of defining characteristics or sets of signs and symptoms.
- The diagnostic process includes analysis and interpretation of data, identification of patient and family needs, and formulation of nursing diagnoses and collaborative problems.
- Nursing diagnoses provide the basis for selection of nursing interventions to achieve outcomes for which a nurse is accountable.
- The absence of certain defining characteristics following a patient assessment suggests that you reject a nursing diagnosis under consideration.
- Nursing diagnostic errors may lead to inappropriate and/or inadequate nursing care.
- During the planning component you determine patient goals, establish priorities, develop expected outcomes of nursing care, and write a nursing care plan.
- The NOC has labels for describing the focus of nursing care and includes indicators for use in measuring success with interventions.
- A nurse begins a care plan by first addressing the nursing diagnoses that have the highest priority.
- The care plan is a guideline for patient care so all members of the health care team can quickly understand the care given.
- A concept map organizes and links data about a patient's multiple diagnoses in a logical way.
- There are three types of nursing interventions: nurse-initiated, physician-initiated, and collaborative.
- The NIC is a comprehensive standardized classification of the interventions that nurses use in the care of patients.
- Evaluation determines a patient's response to nursing actions and whether goals have been met.
- You evaluate by comparing the patient's response to nursing actions with expected outcomes established during planning.

- When goals of care are not met, you identify factors that interfere with goal achievement, reassess the patient's condition, revise existing or develop new nursing diagnoses, and select appropriate interventions.

CLINICAL DECISION-MAKING EXERCISES

Rich takes time to talk with Mr. Tillman and learns that he has been experiencing headaches for over 2 weeks and has difficulty falling asleep at night. Since taking on more responsibility for household chores, Mr. Tillman has little time for playing golf with friends. He worries about whether he will be able to support his wife as her cancer progresses. Rich notices frustration in Mr. Tillman's tone of voice. Mr. Tillman tells Rich, "I love my wife very much. I just think that she'll need a lot of care."

1. Identify the cues from which Rich infers that Mr. Tillman has a problem related to stress.
2. Identify a nursing diagnostic label appropriate to Mr. Tillman's situation and data that support this diagnosis.
3. Which interventions might you select for Mr. Tillman?

evolve

Answers to Clinical Decision-Making Exercises can be found on the Evolve website.

QSEN ACTIVITY: PATIENT-CENTERED CARE

Mrs. Tillman and her husband decide to use the facility hospice program. As part of this program, her acute care nurse Rich consults with the hospice nurse assigned to the Tillman family. Mrs. Tillman is dying and is no longer responsive; her husband is at her bedside. Although symptom management and skilled nursing care remain a care priority for Mrs. Tillman, Mr. Tillman's emotional and physical needs are now the top priority of care. Rich and the hospice nurse decide that they must assess Mr. Tillman's emotional status and support and his ability to meet his basic needs.

Which skills of assessment do they need to use to determine Mr. Tillman's needs?

How do Rich and the hospice nurse validate Mr. Tillman's needs and individualize a patient-centered plan of care?

evolve

Answers to QSEN Activities can be found on the Evolve website.

REVIEW QUESTIONS

1. A patient tells the nurse, "I have had this dull ache in my side now for 4 days; it really hurts when I bend over." The nurse responds, "All right, go on." The nurse's response is an example of:
   1. Inference.
   2. A cue.
   3. Back-channeling.
   4. Open-ended question.
2. A nurse working on a cardiac unit is assigned an 84-year-old patient who was just admitted with symptoms of lung infection. When the nurse enters the room, the nurse notices that the patient is short of breath, coughing, and has a respiratory rate of 36 breaths/min. The patient is anxious and states that she is "scared." The nurse does an initial preliminary assessment and follows up 30 minutes later. The nurse's knowledge about the patient results in which of the following assessment approaches? (Select all that apply.)
   1. A problem-focused approach
   2. A structured comprehensive approach
   3. Using multiple visits to gather a complete patient database
   4. Focusing on the functional health pattern of role-relationship
3. A patient has a pressure ulcer resulting from urine incontinence and sustained pressure over her coccyx. The nursing plan of care includes a goal of "Pressure ulcer heals in 3 weeks." Which of the following is an evaluative measure for this goal?
   1. Turn patient every 90 minutes.
   2. Measure the diameter of the ulcer.
   3. Measure the color of patient's urine.
   4. Determine patient's report of discomfort during turning.
4. A nurse has been interviewing a newly assigned patient. The cues from the assessment suggest that the patient has a problem breathing. The nurse does not validate the findings by doing a physical examination. This is an example of which type of error?
   1. Error in data clustering
   2. Error in data collection
   3. Error in diagnostic statement
   4. Error in interpretation and analysis
5. Which of the following are examples of data validation? (Select all that apply.)
   1. The nurse assesses the patient's heart rate and compares the value with the last value entered in the medical record.
   2. The nurse asks the patient if he is having pain and then asks him to rate the severity.
   3. The nurse observes a patient reading a teaching booklet and asks him if he has any questions about its content.
   4. The nurse obtains a blood pressure value that is abnormal and asks the charge nurse to repeat the measurement.
   5. The nurse asks the patient to describe a symptom by saying "go on."

6. Match the activity on the left with the source of diagnostic error. Sources of error may be used more than once.

Activity:	Source of error:
a. ___Nurse listens to lungs for first time and is not sure if abnormal lung sounds are present.	1. Collecting data
b. ___After reviewing objective data nurse selects diagnosis of *Pain* before asking patient to describe the sensation.	2. Interpreting
c. ___Nurse identifies an incorrect diagnostic label.	3. Clustering
d. ___Nurse does not consider the patient's cultural background when reviewing cues.	4. Labeling
e. ___Nurse prepares to complete decision on diagnosis and realizes that clinical criteria are grouped incorrectly to form a pattern.	

7. A nurse completes a respiratory assessment on a patient who had abdominal surgery 1 day ago. During the assessment she auscultates crackles in both lower lobes, and the patient coughs, producing light yellow sputum. The patient's body temperature is 37.0° C (98.6° F), pulse is 110, respiratory rate is 28 breaths/min, and blood pressure is 118/82. Pulse oximetry was 99% and is now 93%. The nurse identifies a nursing diagnosis of Impaired Gas Exchange. Which of the following goals are appropriate for this patient?
   1. Patient's pulse oximetry will be greater than 95%.
   2. Patient will deep breathe and cough every 2 hours.
   3. Patient's lungs will be clear to auscultation.
   4. Patient will be able to sleep through the night.
8. A nursing student is reporting off at the end of her shift to the RN. The student tells the RN that her patient has a priority nursing diagnosis of Pain. She tells the RN that the last time the ordered analgesic was given was 2 hours ago. The patient continues to report pain at a level of 4. The student also tried repositioning and distraction to reduce the patient's discomfort. She observed her patient grimace while turning. Which expected outcome measure did the student report to the RN?
   1. Administration of the analgesic as ordered
   2. The use of distraction as a pain-relief measure
   3. The reported pain level of 4 on a scale of 0 to 10
   4. Observation of the patient grimacing during turning
9. The nurse prepares to administer care to a patient by first positioning him more comfortably. She inspects his surgical wound and reinforces the dressing with extra tape. She explains the procedure that she will use for insertion of a urinary catheter. She prepares the patient and inserts the catheter. Which of the following steps is a dependent nursing intervention?
   1. Insertion of the urinary catheter
   2. Reinforcement of dressing with tape
   3. Instruction about the procedure for insertion of the urinary catheter
   4. Positioning the patient for comfort
10. During the implementation step of the nursing process, a nurse reviews and revises the nursing care plan. Place the following steps of review and revision in the correct order.
   1. Review the care plan.
   2. Decide if nursing interventions remain appropriate.
   3. Reassess the patient.
   4. Compare assessment findings to validate existing nursing diagnosis.

evolve

Rationales for Review Questions can be found on the Evolve website.

1. 3; 2. 1, 3; 3. 2; 4. 2; 5. 1, 4; 6. a=1, b=2, c=4, d=2, e=3; 7. 3; 8. 3; 9. 1; 10. 3, 4, 1, 2.

REFERENCES

Ackley BJ, Ladwig GB: *Nursing diagnosis handbook*, ed 9, St Louis, 2011, Mosby.

American Nurses Association (ANA): *Nursing's social policy statement: the essence of the profession*, ed 3, Washington, DC, 2010, The Association.

American Nurses Association (ANA) and the National Council of State Boards of Nursing (NCBSN): *Joint statement on delegation*, 2012, www.ncsbn.org/joint_statement.pdf. Accessed July 11 2012.

Bertakis KD, Azari R: Determinants and outcomes of patient-centered care, *Patient Educ Counsel* 85(10):46, 2011.

Bulechek GM, et al: *Nursing interventions classification (NIC)*, ed 6, St Louis, 2012, Mosby.

Campinha-Bacote P: Delivering patient-centered care in the midst of a cultural conflict: the role of cultural competence, *Online J Issues Nurs* 16(2):1, 2011.

Carpenito-Moyet LJ: *Nursing diagnosis: application to clinical practice*, ed 14, Philadelphia, 2013, Lippincott Williams & Wilkins.

Chabeli MM: Concept-mapping as a teaching method to facilitate critical thinking in nursing education: a review of the literature, *Health SA Gesondheid* 15(1):Art 432, 2010, DOI:10.4102/hsag.v15il.432.

Chan ECY, et al: A community-based intervention to promote informal decision making for prostate cancer screening among Hispanic American men: changed knowledge and role preferences: a cluster RCT, *Patient Educ Counsel* 84:e44, 2011.

Daley BJ, Torre DM: Concept maps in medical education: an analytical literature review, *Med Educ* 44:440, 2010.

Espinosa-Aguilar A, et al: Design and validation of a critical pathway for hospital management of patients with severe traumatic brain injury, *J Trauma* 64(5):1327, 2008.

Gerontological Nursing Intervention Research Center (GNIRC): *Evidence-based guidelines*, 2012, University of Iowa, http://www.nursing.uiowa.edu/excellence/gnirc. Accessed July 11, 2012.

Gordon M: *Nursing diagnosis: process and application*, ed 3, St Louis, 1994, Mosby.

Hebda T, Czar P: *Handbook of informatics for nursing and health care professionals*, ed 4, Upper Saddle, NJ, 2009, Pearson Prentice Hall.

Koithan MS: Complementary and alternative therapies. In Potter PA, et al, editor: *Fundamentals of nursing*, ed 8, St Louis, 2013, Mosby.

Manchikanti L, et al: A critical review of the American Pain Society clinical practice guidelines for interventional techniques. Part I, Diagnostic interventions, *Pain Physician* 13(3):E141, 2010.

Moorhead S, et al: *Nursing outcomes classification (NOC)*, ed 5, St Louis, 2012, Mosby.

Muller-Staub M, et al: Nursing diagnoses, interventions and outcomes—application and impact on nursing practice: systematic review, *J Adv Nurs* 56(5):514, 2006.

Muller-Staub M, et al: Implementing nursing diagnostics effectively: cluster randomized trial, *J Adv Nurs* 63(3):291, 2008.

NANDA International (NANDA-I): *NANDA International nursing diagnoses: definitions and classifications, 2012-2014*, Oxford, UK, 2012, Wiley-Blackwell.

National Guideline Clearinghouse (NGC): *Guidelines 2010*, 2010, Agency for Healthcare Research and Quality, http://www.guideline.gov. Accessed July 11 2012.

O'Neill S, et al: Nursing works: the application of lean thinking to nursing process, *J Nurs Admin* 41(12):546, 2011.

Papastavrou E, et al: Nurses' and patients' perceptions of caring behaviours: quantitate systematic review of comparative studies, *J Adv Nurs* 67(6):1191, 2011.

Pilcher J: Teaching and learning with concept maps, *Neonatal Network* 30(5):336, 2011.

Seidel HM, et al: *Mosby's guide to physical examination*, ed 7, St Louis, 2011, Mosby.

Suhonen R, et al: A review of outcomes of indivualised nursing interventions on adult patients, *J Clin Nurs* 17:843, 2008.

Suhonen R, et al: Nurses' perceptions of indivualised care: an international comparison, *J Adv Nurs* 67(9):1895, 2011.

US Department of Health and Human Services: *Standards for privacy of individually identifiable health information*, 2003, http://www.hhs.gov/ocr/privacy/hipaa/understanding/summary/guidanceallsections.pdf. Accessed September 10, 2013.

Wayne JD, et al: Simple standardized patient handoff system that increases accuracy and completeness, *J Surg Ed* 65(6):476, 2008.

Weigel X, et al: Apprehension among hospital nurses providing end-of-life care, *J Hospice Palliat Nurse* 9(2):86, 2007.

Yancey V: The experience of loss death and grief. In Potter PA, et al, editor: *Fundamentals of nursing*, ed 8, St Louis, 2013, Mosby.

CHAPTER

10

Informatics and Documentation

evolve WEBSITE

http://evolve.elsevier.com/Potter/essentials

- Crossword Puzzle
- Audio Glossary

OBJECTIVES

- Identify key reasons for reporting and recording patient care.
- Describe guidelines for effective documentation and reporting in a variety of health care settings.
- Describe methods for interdisciplinary communication within the health care team.
- Compare different methods used in documentation.
- Identify common record-keeping forms.
- Discuss advantages and disadvantages of standardized documentation forms.
- Discuss advantages of computerized documentation.
- Discuss the relationship between informatics and quality health care.

KEY TERMS

accreditation, p. 161
acuity recording, p. 168
case management plan, p. 167
change-of-shift report, p. 170
charting by exception (CBE), p. 167
clinical decision support system (CDSS), p. 175
computerized provider order entry (CPOE), p. 174
confidentiality, p. 175
diagnosis-related group (DRG), p. 163
documentation, p. 159
electronic health record (EHR), p. 165
firewall, p. 176
flow sheets, p. 168
focus charting, p. 167
graphic records, p. 168
hand-off report, p. 169
health care information system (HIS), p. 173
incident (occurrence or event) report, p. 172
informatics, p. 172
information technology (IT), p. 173
interdisciplinary care plan, p. 167
Kardex, p. 168
meaningful use, p. 166
nursing informatics, p. 174
password, p. 176
PIE note, p. 167
problem-oriented medical record (POMR), p. 166
record, p. 161
report, p. 161
SOAP note, p. 167
standardized care plans, p. 168
transfer report, p. 170

Documentation is a vital aspect of nursing practice. It is a key element of nursing practice and a key communication strategy between health care professionals (Pirie, 2011). It is defined as anything written or printed within a patient record, which may be paper, electronic, or a combination of both formats. The information you communicate about patient care reflects the type and frequency of care and provides accountability for each health care team member's care. The patient record provides evidence for credentialing, research, and reimbursement and a database for planning

CASE STUDY *Mrs. Smith*

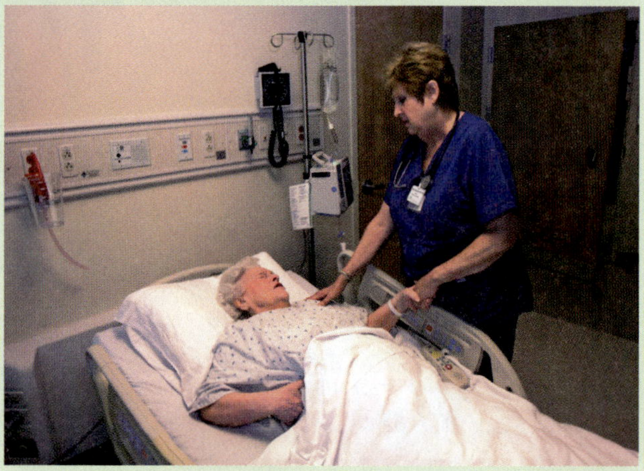

Mrs. Smith is a 93-year-old patient with a history of heart disease and chronic back pain. She lives alone and cares for herself. She typically deals with her back pain by going to a chiropractor. Recently, her pain became more severe and did not resolve with her usual treatments. On the morning of August 14, she was unable to get out of bed. Mrs. Smith was transported by ambulance to the nearest emergency department. She received intravenous pain medication and was admitted to a medical unit for further evaluation of her back pain, which she rated as a 10 on a scale of 0 to 10. After evaluating the results of diagnostic testing, her health care provider determined Mrs. Smith has fractures in her lower spine resulting from severe osteoarthritis. The orthopedic surgeon schedules surgery later in the day.

Jane is a nurse working on the medical unit. While completing Mrs. Smith's admission history, Jane finds out Mrs. Smith had a total knee replacement (TKR) at the same hospital 3 years ago. Jane pulls up Mrs. Smith's electronic record and finds her pain was not well controlled during that hospital stay. After Mrs. Smith's surgery, Jane collaborates with physical therapy to establish a plan of care that promotes pain control and helps Mrs. Smith return to the same level of independence she had before this hospitalization.

health care (ANA, 2010). In the patient's record document the nursing care you provide for a patient (e.g., assessments and interventions).

The health care environment creates many challenges for accurately documenting and reporting patient care. Quality nursing care depends on your ability to communicate effectively verbally and in writing, and you are held accountable for the accuracy of documentation you enter into the patient's record. Regulations from agencies such as The Joint Commission (TJC) and the Centers for Medicare and Medicaid Services (CMS) require health care institutions to monitor and evaluate the quality and appropriateness of patient care (ANA, 2010) (see Chapters 3 and 13). Typically such monitoring and evaluation occur through auditing information that health care providers document in patient records. As of October 1, 2008, Medicare no longer reimburses hospitals for certain preventable conditions such as hospital-acquired illnesses and injuries, (e.g., a urinary tract infection following catheterization or new pressure ulcers) (Geiger, 2012; Hellier, 2010). Thus it becomes even more important that your documentation accurately reflects the status of the patient, especially on admission, transfer, or discharge.

CONFIDENTIALITY

Nurses are legally and ethically obligated to keep information about patients confidential. Do not disclose information about a patient's status to other patients, family members (unless granted by the patient), or health care staff not involved in their care. Patients frequently request copies of their medical records, and they have the right to read them. Each institution has policies to control how medical records are shared. In most situations patients are required to give written permission for release of medical information.

The Health Insurance Portability and Accountability Act (HIPAA), which provides legislation to protect patient privacy for health information, governs all areas of health information management, including reimbursement, medical record coding, security, and patient record management. Under new regulations, to eliminate barriers that delay access to care, providers are required to notify patients of their privacy policy and make a reasonable effort to get written acknowledgment of this notification. HIPAA requires that disclosure or requests regarding health information be limited to the minimum necessary. This includes only the specific information required for a particular purpose. For example, if you need a patient's home telephone number to reschedule an appointment, access to the medical records is limited solely to telephone information.

Sometimes you have a reason for using health care records for data gathering, research, or continuing education. This is permitted if you use the records as specified and permission is granted. When you are a student in a clinical setting, confidentiality and compliance with HIPAA legislation are part of professional practice. You may review the medical record only for information needed to provide safe, efficient care. For example, when you are assigned to provide complete care for a patient, you need to review the current medical record and plan of care. However, you do not share this information with other classmates. In addition, never access the medical records of other patients on the specific clinical care area. Access to electronic health records (EHRs) is traced through the user log-in information. Not only is it unethical to view medical records of other patients, but breaches of confidentiality lead to disciplinary action by employers and even possible dismissal from work. To further maintain confidentiality and protect patient privacy, make sure that written materials used in your student clinical practice do not include patient identifiers such as room number, date of birth, medical record number, or other identifiable demographic information. Equally important, never print material from the EHR for personal use because it is a violation of HIPAA.

STANDARDS

Within a health care organization there are standards that govern the type of information you document. Institutional standards or policies often dictate the frequency of documentation such as how often you record a nursing assessment or a patient's level of pain. Know the standards of your health care organization to ensure complete and accurate documentation. Nurses are expected to meet the standard of care for every nursing task they perform. Patient records are used as evidence in a court of law if standards are not met (ANA, 2010).

In addition, your documentation must conform to the standards of the National Committee for Quality Assurance (NCQA) and accrediting bodies such as TJC to maintain institutional **accreditation** and minimize liability. Usually an organization incorporates accreditation standards into its policies and revises documentation forms to suit these standards. Current documentation standards require that all patients admitted to a health care facility have an assessment of physical, psychosocial, environmental, self-care, knowledge level, and discharge planning needs. TJC standard for record of care, treatment, and services requires that your documentation be within the context of the nursing process, including evidence of patient and family teaching and discharge planning (TJC, 2012). Other standards such as HIPAA include those directed by state and federal regulatory agencies and are enforced through the Department of Justice and the CMS (ANA, 2010).

INTERDISCIPLINARY COMMUNICATION WITHIN THE HEALTH CARE TEAM

The typical patient has many caregivers, including nurses, physicians, nursing assistive personnel, and therapists. To maintain quality care it is essential that effective communication occurs among all health team members. A documentation system that reflects interdisciplinary plans of care for a patient provides continuity of care and prevents fragmented and possibly dangerous care. Thus the medical record helps to ensure that all health team members are working toward a common goal of providing safe and effective care.

Patients' records and reports are two means for effective communication. A patient's **record** or chart is a confidential, permanent legal documentation of information relevant to that patient's health care. Information about the patient's health care is recorded after each patient contact. The record is a continuing account of the patient's health care status and is available to all members of the health care team. Records are either paper or digital, depending on the system used by the health care agency. Whichever format is used, each patient record includes the following:

- Patient identification and demographic data
- Informed consent for treatment or procedures
- Admission data
- Nursing diagnoses or problems and nursing or interdisciplinary care plan
- Record of nursing care treatment and evaluation
- Medical history and physical examination
- Medical diagnoses
- Therapeutic orders
- Medical and other health discipline progress notes
- Results of diagnostic and therapeutic tests and procedures
- Patient education
- Advance directives
- Summary of operative procedures
- Discharge diagnosis, plan and summary (TJC, 2012)

Reports are oral, written, or audiotaped exchanges of information between members of the health care team. Common reports given by nurses include change-of-shift reports, telephone reports, transfer reports, incident reports, and hand-off reports. Sometimes a physician or health care provider calls a nursing unit to receive a verbal report on a patient's condition and progress. The laboratory submits a written report providing the results of diagnostic tests. A transfer report informs the staff of a receiving health care setting about the type of care a patient will require.

PURPOSE OF RECORDS

A patient's record is a valuable source of data for all members of the health care team and the only permanent record documenting patient care from admission to discharge. Documentation serves multiple purposes, including communication, legal documentation, reimbursement, education, research, and quality process and performance improvement (ANA, 2010).

Communication

The record is a way for health care team members to provide continuity of care and communicate patient needs and progress toward meeting desired patient outcomes. TJC reports that poor communication, including verbal and written, among staff and with patients was one of the top ten reasons for sentinel events for 2011 (Sentinel events, 2012). The record includes the patient's assessment and responses to interventions and changes made in the plan of care. It is the most current and accurate source of information about a patient's health care status. The information communicated in a record prepares you to know a patient thoroughly so you make timely and appropriate care decisions. Base your communication on your assessment findings. It is best to document immediately following an assessment or intervention (ANA, 2010; Austin, 2011; Pirie, 2011).

Legal Documentation

Because jurors usually rely on information documented in the medical record to determine the patient care provided, effective documentation is one of the best defenses for legal claims associated with health care (Table 10-1). Record keeping is your professional responsibility; it is not an optional extra in your practice. To limit nursing liability your documentation must follow organizational standards for documentation,

TABLE 10-1 LEGAL GUIDELINES FOR RECORDING

GUIDELINES	RATIONALE	CORRECT ACTION
Do not erase, apply correction fluid, or scratch out errors made while recording.	Charting becomes illegible: it appears as if you were attempting to hide information or deface record.	Draw single line through error, write word *error* above it and sign your name or initials and title. Then record note correctly. Check agency policy (Austin, 2011; Pirie, 2011).
Do not write retaliatory or critical comments about patient or care by other health care professionals.	Statements can be used as evidence for nonprofessional behavior or poor quality of care.	Enter only objective descriptions of patient's behavior; patient comments should be quoted (Austin, 2011; Wood, 2010).
You need to add patient information.	New information is acquired.	If additional information is to be added to an existing entry, write the date and time of the new entry on the next available space and include and follow facility format (Austin, 2011).
	You forgot to chart during a shift.	Write the current date and time in the next available space and rationale for delay; label entry *late entry* and follow the format established by your facility (Austin, 2011). Check facility guidelines for late entries into an EMR. Facilities may limit the time period the entry can be made (Austin, 2011; Wood, 2010).
Correct all errors promptly.	Errors in recording can lead to errors in treatment.	Avoid rushing to complete charting; be sure that information is accurate (Austin, 2011).
Record all facts.	Record must be accurate and reliable.	Be certain that entry is factual; do not speculate or guess (Pirie, 2011).
Do not leave blank spaces in nurses' notes.	Another person can add incorrect information in space.	Chart consecutively, line by line; if space is left, draw line horizontally through it and sign your name at end (Austin, 2011).
Record all entries legibly and in black ink.	Illegible entries can be misinterpreted, causing errors and lawsuits; ink cannot be erased; black ink is more legible when records are photocopied or transferred to microfilm.	Never erase entries or use correction fluid and never use pencil or pens with erasable ink.
If order is questioned, record that clarification was sought.	If you perform an order known to be incorrect, you are just as liable for prosecution as the physician or health care provider is.	Do not record "physician made error." Instead chart that "Dr. Smith was called to clarify order for analgesic" (Nettina, 2010).
Chart only for yourself.	You are accountable for information you enter into chart.	Never chart for someone else. **Exception:** If caregiver has left unit for day and calls with information that needs to be documented, include name of source of information in entry and include that information was provided via telephone.
Avoid using generalized, empty phrases such as "status unchanged" or "had good day."	Specific information about patient's condition or case can be deleted accidentally if information is too generalized.	Use complete, concise descriptions of care.
Begin each entry with date and time and end with your signature and title.	This guideline ensures that correct sequence of events is recorded; signature documents who is accountable for care delivered.	Do not wait until end of shift to record important changes that occurred several hours earlier; be sure to sign each entry (Wood, 2010).
For computer documentation keep your password to yourself.	Maintains security and confidentiality.	Once logged onto computer, do not leave computer screen unattended and log out when you are finished charting (Wood, 2010).

EMR, Electronic medical record.

which include a clear indication of the individualized and goal-directed nursing care you provide. The best way to ensure that documentation meets legal standards is to record information timely, accurately, completely, legibly, and using standardized terminology as you provide care (ANA, 2010; Austin, 2011).

Reimbursement

Charting also determines the amount of reimbursement that a health care agency receives (Austin, 2011). **Diagnosis-related groups (DRGs)** are the basis for establishing reimbursement for patient care. A DRG is a classification based on patients' medical diagnoses. Under the prospective payment system, Medicare reimburses hospitals a set dollar amount for each DRG (see Chapter 3). Your nursing documentation verifies specific nursing care provided and thus supports the reimbursement that your health care agency receives.

A medical record verifies financial charges for equipment and services used in patient's care. Private insurance carriers and auditors from federal agencies review records to determine the reimbursement that a patient or a health care agency receives. Insurance companies do not reimburse for unskilled nursing care. They pay only for skilled medical and nursing care. Timely and accurate documentation of supplies and equipment used assists in accurate and timely reimbursement (ANA, 2010).

Education

A patient's record contains a variety of information (e.g., medical and nursing diagnoses, signs and symptoms of disease, successful and unsuccessful therapies, diagnostic findings, and patient behaviors). Reading the patient care record is an effective way to learn the nature of an illness and the patient's response to it. Review of patients with similar medical problems allows you to identify patterns and trends. Such information builds your clinical knowledge. As you identify patterns associated with specific diseases and conditions, you are able to anticipate the type of care your patients require and how patients respond to treatment.

Research

Statistical data are important elements of patient records, including the frequency of clinical disorders, complications, use of specific medical and nursing therapies, recoveries from illness, and mortality. After obtaining appropriate agency approvals, a nurse researcher reviews patients' records in a research study to collect information on a particular health problem. Analysis of the data collected contributes to evidence-based nursing practice and quality health care (ANA, 2010). For example, if a nurse researcher suspects that early ambulation decreases the complication rate in postoperative patients, the researcher reviews the records of select surgical patients to compare the rates of postoperative complications with early-versus-late ambulation.

Quality Process and Performance Improvement

TJC (2012) requires hospitals to establish quality improvement programs to conduct objective, ongoing reviews of patient care and asks institutions to establish standards for quality care. Audits help to determine whether standards of care are met. Audits assess the standard of records and identify areas for improvement and staff development. For example, nurses may monitor records to determine their success in documenting institution of fall precautions or evaluation of pain measures. The nurses then share any deficiencies identified during monitoring with all members of the nursing staff so corrections in policy or practice can be made. Auditing and monitoring programs keep you informed of the extent to which you meet standards of nursing practice and outcomes that patients experience (ANA, 2010) (see Chapter 3). Quality processes and performance improvement measures provide a method to evaluate quality of care to ensure the achievement of legislative mandates or address quality initiatives (ANA, 2010).

GUIDELINES FOR QUALITY DOCUMENTATION AND REPORTING

High-quality documentation and reporting are necessary to enhance efficient, safe, individualized patient care. Quality documentation and reporting have five important characteristics: factual, accurate, complete, current, and organized (ANA, 2010). Problems arise when a record is reviewed in a malpractice suit and there are time gaps, information is squeezed between lines or crossed out, or key facts are omitted (Austin, 2011; Glasper, 2011; Johnson and Nicholls, 2011).

In some settings agency policy requires a registered nurse to cosign documentation completed by licensed practical or vocational nurses, nursing students, or assistive personnel. A cosignature indicates that the supervising nurse reviewed the record entry and was aware of the care and patient status even though others delivered the care. Nurses must assess the patient themselves and read medical record entries before cosigning another health care provider's assessment record.

Factual

A factual record contains descriptive, objective information about what you see, hear, feel, and smell. Objective data are data that are measurable and observable such as the size of a wound or a patient's pulse oximetry reading. To be factual, avoid words such as *appears, seems,* or *apparently* because they are vague and lead to conclusions that you cannot support by objective information.

The only subjective data included in a record are what the patient says. Write subjective information with quotation marks, using the patient's own words. For example, the patient's statement, "*My lower back hurts*" is subjective and acceptable documentation. Another example is stated as follows: *Reports feeling a pressure in chest.* It is acceptable not to use quotation marks when you paraphrase the patient's words. When documenting subjective information, it is also important to include complementary objective findings so your database is as descriptive as possible (Austin, 2011).

Accurate

The use of precise measurements makes documentation more accurate. For example, documenting "Voided 450 mL clear urine" is more accurate than "Voided an adequate amount." To avoid misunderstandings and promote patient safety, write out any confusing abbreviations. The National Patient Safety Goals (NPSGs) require that health care institutions standardize abbreviations, acronyms, symbols, and dose designations throughout their system (TJC, 2012). The NPSGs also require institutions to identify a "do not use" list of abbreviations, acronyms, symbols, and dose designations (TJC, 2012) (see Chapter 17). It is important to know the acceptable and unacceptable abbreviation list of an institution to keep your documentation accurate and compliant with requirements.

Correct spelling demonstrates a level of competency and attention to detail. Misspelled words lead to confusion. For example, often words sound the same but have different meanings such as *accept* and *except* or *dysphagia* and *dysphasia.* Misspellings and incorrect use of terms alters the intended meaning.

TJC (2012) requires that all entries in medical records be dated and that there is a method to identify all authors' entries. Therefore any descriptive entry in a patient's record ends with the caregiver's identifiers (e.g., full name and status). Occasionally you include observations reported to another caregiver or interventions performed by someone else (e.g., "Patient suctioned by Judith Hill, RN.") As a nursing student you need to enter your full name and student nurse abbreviation (e.g., "Marianne Smith, SN [student nurse])." The abbreviation for *student nurse* often differs regionally, being either *NS,* which stands for *nursing student,* or *SN,* which stands for *student nurse.* Check with your educational institution for the preferred abbreviation. Your signature holds you accountable for information you record. Include your educational institution when required by agency policy.

Complete

The information within a recorded entry or a report needs to be clear, concise, and complete, containing appropriate and essential information. Criteria for thorough communication exist for certain health problems or nursing activities (Table 10-2). Make written entries in the patient's medical record describing nursing care that you administer and the patient's response. For example:

0845 Reports continuous throbbing pain on lateral aspect of left fractured femur increased with movement of the leg with a severity of 8 (scale 0-10). B/P: 132/74, T 37° C, P 92, R 18. Morphine sulfate 5 mg IV given for pain. Sue Jacobs, RN.

0915 Reports pain at 2 (scale 0-10) and able to turn in bed independently. States, "I feel much better now." Sue Jacobs, RN.

Include routine activities such as daily hygiene measures, vital signs, and pain assessment in flow sheets or graphic records according to agency policy. Describe these activities in detail when it is relevant because of a change in functional

TABLE 10-2 EXAMPLES OF CRITERIA FOR DOCUMENTATION AND REPORTING

TOPIC	CRITERIA TO DOCUMENT OR REPORT
Assessment	
Subjective data (patient behavior [e.g., anxiety, confusion, hostility])	• Description of episode in quotation marks • Onset, location, description of condition (severity, duration, frequency; precipitating, aggravating, and relieving factors) • Onset, behaviors exhibited, precipitating factors
Objective data (e.g., rash, tenderness, breath sounds)	• Onset, location, description of condition (severity, duration, frequency; precipitating, aggravating, and relieving factors) • Changes from baseline
Nursing Interventions and Evaluation	
Treatments (e.g., enema, bath, dressing change)	• Time administered, equipment used (if appropriate), patient's response (objective and subjective changes) compared with previous treatment (e.g., "rated pain 0 on a scale of 0 to 10 during dressing change" or "reported severe abdominal cramping during enema")
Medication administration	• Immediately after administration, document time medication given, dose, route, any preliminary assessments (e.g., pain level, vital signs), patient response or effect of medication; for example: • 0800 Pain reported at 6 (scale 0-10). Tylenol 500 mg given PO 1530: Patient reports pain level 2 (scale 0-10) • 1000: Pruritus and hives developed over lower abdomen 1 hour after penicillin was given
Patient teaching	• Information presented, method of instruction (e.g., discussion, demonstration, videotape, booklet), patient response, including questions and evidence of understanding such as return demonstration or change in behavior
Discharge planning	• Measurable patient goals or expected outcomes, progress toward goals, need for referrals

ability or status. For example, you have a patient who has previously required a total bath; and now the patient has improved and is able to wash his or her face, hands, and upper body. This change in patient activity warrants additional documentation.

Current

Making entries promptly is essential in effective documentation (TJC, 2012). Delays in documentation result in serious omissions, untimely delays, and possible errors in patient care. To increase timely documentation and decrease unnecessary duplication, many health care agencies keep records or computers near the patient's bedside to facilitate immediate documentation of care. You need to communicate the following nursing care at the time of occurrence:

1. Vital signs
2. Pain assessment
3. Administration of medications and treatments
4. Patient response to intervention
5. Preparation for diagnostic tests or surgery
6. Change in patient status and who was notified (e.g., physician, patient's family)
7. Treatment for sudden changes in patient status
8. Preoperative checklist
9. Admission, transfer, discharge, or death of patient

Most agencies use military time, a 24-hour time cycle. The military clock begins at 1 minute after midnight as 0001 and ends with midnight at 2400. For example, 10:22 AM is 1022 military time; 1:00 PM is 1300 military time. Figure 10-1 shows military time on a clock face. Use of military time helps to minimize errors in interpretation of AM and PM times.

Organized

Written communication is easier to understand when written in a logical, sequential order. For example, an organized note describes your assessment, interventions, and the patient's response in a sequence. It is also more effective when notes are concise, clear, and to the point. To make clear and organized entries it is often helpful to make a list of what you need to include before beginning to write in the permanent legal record. Organizing your information into categories minimizes frustration in trying to recall patient care activities provided. Suggested categories include what the patient tells you directly or from indirect sources if the patient is incapacitated; what you assess; what you do, including interventions performed in response to assessment findings; and what you teach the patient and family. Applying critical thinking skills along with the nursing process gives logic and order to nursing documentation.

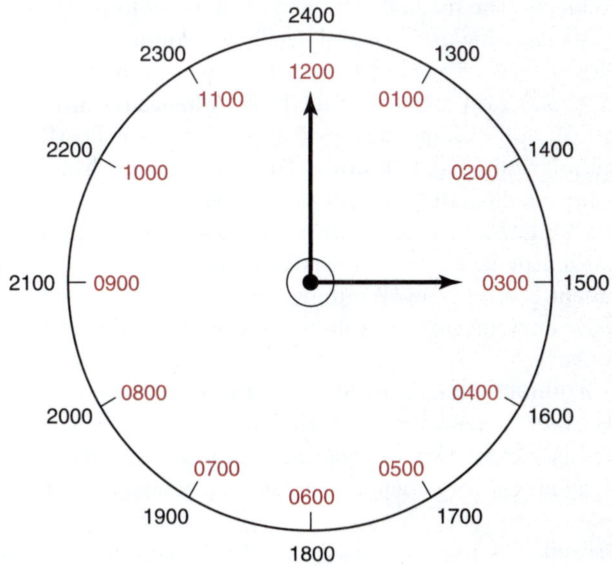

FIGURE 10-1 Comparison of 24 hours of military time with the hourly positions on the clock face for civilian time.

METHODS OF DOCUMENTATION

The documentation system selected by a nursing service reflects the philosophy of the department. Staff use the same documentation system throughout an agency. There are several acceptable methods for recording health care information (Table 10-3).

Paper and Electronic Documentation

Traditionally health care professionals documented on paper medical records. Paper records are episode oriented, with a separate record for each patient visit to a health care agency (Hebda and Czar, 2013). Key information such as patient allergies, current medications, and complications from treatment may be lost from one episode of care (e.g., hospitalization or clinic visit) to the next, jeopardizing a patient's safety. The need for patient safety has driven the increased usage of computerized documentation systems. The traditional paper medical record no longer meets the needs of today's health care industry. Thus hospitals and health care professionals are transitioning to use of EHRs.

The **electronic health record (EHR)** is a longitudinal electronic record of patient health information generated by one or more encounters in any care delivery setting (Healthcare Information and Management Systems Society [HIMSS], n.d.). It ensures coordination of care because all primary caregivers can view a common record of a patient's entire health care experience, including inpatient, outpatient, emergency care, and diagnostic studies. It integrates all pertinent patient information into one record, regardless of the number of times a patient enters a health care system. The EHR differs from the electronic medical record (EMR), although terms are used interchangeably. The EMR contains patient data gathered in a health care setting at a specific time and place and is part of the EHR. The EHR provides a more comprehensive picture of the clinical process (Brown et al., 2013).

In 2010 the Patient Protection and Affordable Care Act (ACA) mandated that health care agencies purchase a computerized information system and demonstrate "meaningful use." Reimbursement is provided to health care professionals

TABLE 10-3 FORMATS FOR DOCUMENTING

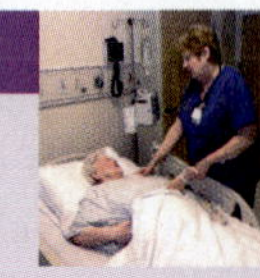

Case study continuation: Jane needs to record the information obtained from Mrs. Smith during the admission process. The following shows examples of various formats.

Narrative note	Stated: "I'm dreading surgery. Last time it hurt so much when I got out of bed." Discussed alternatives for pain control and importance of postoperative activity. Encouraged to ask for pain medication before pain is severe. Stated: "I feel better prepared now." Able to verbalize that activity enhances circulation and healing.
SOAP	***S*** (subjective data): "I'm dreading surgery. Last time it hurt so much when I got out of bed." ***O*** (objective data): Noted muscle tension and loud voice. ***A*** (assessment/analysis): Fear of postoperative pain. ***P*** (plan): Assess pain level every 2 hours. Provide comfort measures and give analgesics as needed.
PIE charting	***P*** (problem): "I'm dreading surgery. Last time it hurt so much when I got out of bed." ***I*** (intervention): Discussed alternatives for pain control and importance of postoperative activity. Encouraged to ask for pain medication before pain is severe. ***E*** (evaluation): "I feel better prepared now." Able to verbalize that activity enhances circulation and healing.
Focus charting	***D*** (data): "I'm dreading surgery. Last time it hurt so much when I got out of bed." ***A*** (action): Discussed alternatives for pain control and importance of postoperative activity. Encouraged to ask for pain medication before pain is severe. ***R*** (response): "I feel better prepared now." Able to verbalize that activity enhances circulation and healing. NOTE: Some agencies add ***P*** (plan). Example: ***P*** (plan): Assess pain level every 2 hours. Provide comfort measures and give analgesics as needed.

and hospitals that meet meaningful use benchmarks (Brown, et al., 2013). **Meaningful use** refers to the level with which information technology (IT) is available and used to support clinical decision making to improve quality, safety, and efficiency; reduce health disparities; engage patients and families in their health care; improve care coordination; improve population and public health; and maintain privacy and security. These benchmarks require health care providers to report certain data related to performance improvement and patient outcomes. Professional organizations and agencies also support the initiation of the EHR.

Guidelines are developed to assist you in safe computer charting.

1. Do not share your password with other caregivers. A good system requires frequent changes in personal passwords to prevent unauthorized persons from accessing and tampering with records.
2. Avoid leaving the computer terminal unattended when logged on.
3. Follow the correct protocol for correcting errors according to agency policy.
4. Software systems have a system for backup files. If you inadvertently delete part of the permanent record, follow agency policy. It is necessary to type an explanation into the computer file with the date, time, and your initials and to submit an explanation in writing to your manager (Sewell and Thede, 2013).
5. Avoid leaving information about a patient displayed on a monitor where others can see it. Keep a log that accounts for every copy of a computerized file that you have generated from the system.
6. Follow agency confidentiality procedures for documenting sensitive material such as a diagnoses, insurance coverage, or family status.
7. Protect printouts of computerized records. Shredding printouts and logging the number of copies generated by each caregiver are ways to minimize duplicate records and protect the confidentiality of patient information (Sewell and Thede, 2013).

Problem-Oriented Medical Records

The **problem-oriented medical record (POMR)** is a structured method of documentation that emphasizes the patient's problems. The method is organized in a way to correspond to the nursing process and facilitates communication of patient needs. Organization of data is by problem or diagnosis. Ideally each member of the health care team contributes to a single list of identified patient problems. The POMR has the following major sections: database, problem list, initial care plan, discharge summary, and progress notes.

Database. The database contains all available patient assessment data. This section is the foundation for identifying patient problems and planning care. The database remains active and current, and you make revisions as new data are available.

Problem List. The problem list is developed after a review of the patient data. You identify priority problems and list all problems in chronological order to serve as an organizing guide for the patient's care. Add new problems to the list as you identify them on the basis of your ongoing nursing assessment. Once problems are resolved, record the date and draw a line through the problem and its number.

Care Plan. TJC standards (2012) require that a care plan, also called a *plan of care,* be developed for all patients on admission to acute, subacute, rehabilitation, or extended care agencies. Disciplines involved in the patient's care develop a care plan, sometimes referred to as an **interdisciplinary care plan,** for each problem listed. For example, a physical therapist communicates a plan for increasing a patient's ambulation, whereas a speech therapist communicates a plan to improve the patient's swallowing. Nurses document a plan of care in a variety of formats. Generally these plans of care include nursing diagnoses, expected outcomes, and interventions (see Chapter 9).

Progress Notes. Health care team members use progress notes to monitor and record the progress of a patient's problems. Narrative notes, flow sheets, discharge summaries, and structured notes are formats you use to document the patient's progress.

Narrative Documentation. Narrative documentation is the traditional method for recording nursing care. However, in many settings other methods have replaced narrative charting. Narrative charting uses a storylike format to document information specific to patient conditions and nursing care. It is beneficial in emergency situations in which a chronological order of events is important. However, it does have some disadvantages, including the tendency to be repetitious and time consuming, and it requires the reader to sort through much information to locate the desired patient information (see Table 10-3).

SOAP Documentation. One format for entering a progress note is the **SOAP note.** SOAP is an acronym for the following:

S: Subjective data (verbalizations of the patient)

O: Objective data (data that are measured and observed)

A: Assessment (diagnosis based on the subjective and objective data)

P: Plan (what the caregiver plans to do)

An *I* and *E* are sometimes added (i.e., SOAPIE) in various institutions. The *I* stands for *intervention,* and the *E* represents *evaluation.* The logic for SOAP(IE) notes is similar to that of the nursing process: Collect data about each of your patient's problems, draw conclusions, and develop a plan of care. Number each SOAP note and title it according to the problem on the list (see Table 10-3).

PIE Documentation. The **PIE note** documentation format is similar to SOAP charting in its problem-oriented nature. However, it differs from the SOAP method in that PIE charting has a nursing origin, whereas SOAP originated from the medical model. PIE is an acronym for *p*roblem, *i*nterventions, *e*valuation as follows (see Table 10-3):

P: Problem or nursing diagnosis applicable to patient

I: Interventions or actions taken

E: Evaluation of the outcomes of nursing interventions

The PIE format simplifies documentation by unifying the care plan and progress notes into a complete record. It also differs from SOAP because the narrative note does not include assessment information. Your daily assessment data appear on special flow sheets, thus preventing duplication of information. You number or label the PIE notes according to the patient's problems. Once a patient's problem becomes resolved, you drop it from daily documentation. Continuing problems are documented daily.

Focus Charting. A third format is **focus charting.** It is a unique narrative format in that it places less emphasis on patient problems and instead focuses on patient concerns such as a sign or symptom, a condition, a behavior, or a significant event (Carpentino-Moyet, 2009). Each entry includes data (D), actions (A), and patient response (R). Focus charting combines a shorthand approach to documenting normal assessments and routine care with a concise longhand method for documenting exceptions to predetermined norms. In addition, focus charting saves time because it is easy for multiple caregivers to understand, it is adaptable to most health care settings, and it enables all caregivers to track the patient's condition and progress toward the outcomes of care. A disadvantage of focus charting is that it can be challenging to write accurate logical notes (see Table 10-3).

Charting by Exception

Charting by exception (CBE) is an innovative approach to reduce the time required to complete documentation. In a CBE system an agency defines criteria for nursing assessments and standards of practice for nursing interventions. CBE involves completing a flow sheet that incorporates these standard assessment criteria and interventions. You use a check mark on the flow sheet to indicate normal findings or routine interventions. You write narrative information only if findings are abnormal. You create problems if you chart normal findings along with the exceptions. By following the agency standards for charting in the CBE system, when you see any entries in the chart, you know that something out of the ordinary has occurred. This makes it easier to track unexpected changes in a patient's condition as they develop.

Case Management Plan and Critical Pathways

The **case management plan** of delivering care uses an interdisciplinary approach to document patient care and focuses on providing quality care in a cost-effective manner. The case management plan incorporates critical pathways, which standardize practice and improve interdisciplinary coordination (Cesta, 2012; Sewell and Thede, 2013). The concept refers to specific guidelines for care that describe patient treatment goals and outline the sequence and timing of interventions for meeting the goals efficiently. They are usually organized according to categories such as activity, diet, treatments, protocols, and discharge planning. Critical pathways are also referred to as clinical pathways, integrated care pathways, care maps, or care paths.

Advantages of case management plans include the ability for various health care team members to note variances in care, establish outcomes, identify potential problems, specify standards from the patient perspective, and know what to expect. Disadvantages focus on the need for acceptance of the recording form by all health care providers and individuals knowledgeable in the process to develop pathways.

COMMON RECORD-KEEPING FORMS

The patient chart includes a variety of forms to make documentation easy, quick, and comprehensive. When possible avoid duplication within the record.

Admission Nursing History Forms

Admission nursing history forms provide baseline data for later comparisons with changes in the patient's condition. The admitting nurse uses the form to document a thorough assessment (e.g., biographical data, physical and psychosocial/cultural assessment, and review of health risk factors) and identify relevant nursing diagnoses or problems for the patient's care plan. Each institution designs nursing history forms based on its standards of practice and philosophy of nursing care.

Flow Sheets and Graphic Records

Flow sheets and **graphic records** are part of the permanent health record and allow documentation of certain routine observations or specific measurements made repeatedly such as height and weight and activities of daily living such as the bath, vital signs, pain assessment, and intake and output. These provide a quick and easy reference for assessing changes in a patient's status. Critical care units commonly use flow sheets for many types of data. They are an effective way to record information so you are able to observe trends over time.

When documenting a significant change on a flow sheet, describe the change in the progress notes and nursing measures implemented in response to the change. For example, if a patient's blood pressure becomes dangerously high, record in the progress note the blood pressure; related assessments such as flushing and headache; and the medication administered to lower the pressure. Also include evaluation of the interventions (e.g., serial blood pressure and other pertinent evaluation measures).

Patient Care Summary or Kardex

Many hospitals now have computerized systems that provide certain basic information in the form of a patient care summary. Data automatically update as orders enter the system and as nurses make decisions. In some settings a **Kardex** (flip-over card file) kept at the nurses' station provides information for the daily care of a patient. It often has two parts: an activity and treatment section and a nursing care plan section. The updated information in the Kardex eliminates the need for you to refer repeatedly to the medical record. Information commonly found in the Kardex or patient care summary includes the following:

1. Basic demographic data (name, age, sex, date of birth)
2. Primary medical diagnosis and significant medical history
3. Current health care provider's orders (e.g., diet, activity, vital signs, blood tests, diagnostic tests), name of primary care and consulting providers
4. A nursing care plan or plan of care
5. Nursing orders or nursing interventions (e.g., intake and output, positioning, comfort measures, fall prevention, teaching)
6. Scheduled tests and procedures
7. Safety precautions used in the patient's care
8. Factors related to activities of daily living
9. Nearest relative/guardian or person to contact in an emergency
10. Emergency code status (e.g., "do not resuscitate" order)
11. Allergies, both food and medicine

Standardized Care Plans

Some institutions use **standardized care plans** to make documentation more efficient. The plans, based on institution standards of nursing practice, are preprinted established guidelines of care for patients with similar health problems. After completing a nursing assessment, place the appropriate standard care plans in your patient's record. It is very important that you make necessary modifications to individualize each care plan. Most standardized plans also allow the addition of specific desired outcomes and the target dates of achievement of these outcomes (see Chapter 9).

Discharge Summary Forms

Much emphasis is placed on preparing a patient for a timely discharge from a health care institution. Ideally you begin discharge planning on admission and in some cases even before admission, as is necessary with same-day surgery admissions and childbirth. When doing discharge planning, be responsive to changes in the patient's condition and involve the patient and family in the discharge planning process (see Chapter 3).

The primary goal of a discharge summary is to ensure the continuity of care, whether a patient is going home or transferring to another institution. A nursing discharge note needs to cover the reason for hospitalization; procedures performed; care, treatment, and services provided; patient's status at discharge; information provided to the patient and family; and provisions for follow-up care (TJC, 2012). Discharge summary forms make the summary concise and instructive. Many forms include copies that you give to the patient, family members, or home care nurses. Discharge summaries involve multiple disciplines and help to ensure that your patient leaves the hospital in a timely manner with the appropriate health care resources (Box 10-1).

Acuity Recording

An **acuity recording** system determines the hours of care for a nursing unit and the number of staff required to care for a given group of patients. Once a day staff nurses enter the

BOX 10-1 DISCHARGE SUMMARY INFORMATION

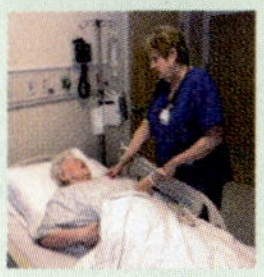

The physician discharges Mrs. Smith. The following are some of the key points that Jane considers when providing discharge information.

- Use clear, concise descriptions with words that Mrs. Smith understands.
- Provide step-by-step description of how to perform a procedure (e.g., home medication administration).
- Reinforce explanation with printed instructions.
- Identify precautions to follow when performing self-care or administering medications.
- Review signs and symptoms of complications that the patient needs to report to her health care provider.
- Obtain feedback from Mrs. Smith regarding discharge instructions.
- List names and phone numbers of health care providers and community resources for Mrs. Smith to contact.
- Identify any unresolved problem, including plans for follow-up and continuous treatment.
- List actual time of discharge, mode of transportation, and who accompanied Mrs. Smith.
- Document the patient encounter accordingly.

Example of a sample discharge note: Discharge teaching completed. Instructed when to return to the health care provider for follow-up care, restrictions on how much to lift at home (no more than 10 lbs), and how to best manage pain at home. Verbalized understanding of lifting techniques and pain medication action, side effects, and how often to take the medication. Informed to notify the health care provider if the pain does not subside with the prescribed pain medication dosage. Will make a follow-up appointment with the surgeon in 2 weeks. Phone 333-333-3333. Discharged via wheelchair at 1440 accompanied by daughter-in-law.

acuity scores of each of their patients into a computerized documentation system. Managerial and administrative staff gather the acuity data electronically to make staffing decisions. For example, an acuity system rates a patient's activity from 1 to 5 (1 requires the least amount of time, 5 requires the most amount of time). A patient returning from surgery who requires frequent assessments and interventions rates as an acuity level 4. On the same continuum, another patient awaiting discharge after an uneventful recovery from surgery rates as an acuity level 1.

HOME CARE DOCUMENTATION

Home care continues to grow as increasing numbers of older adults use home care services. Home health care services are reimbursed by Medicare, Medicaid, commercial insurance, and other managed care plans (ANA, 2008a; Nettina, 2010). Each payer has specific guidelines for establishing eligibility for home care reimbursement. When you provide home care, your documentation must specifically address the category of care and your patient's response to care. Home care agencies are evaluated for accurate, complete charting; adherence to standards that govern their reimbursement; and quality of care. Document all of your services for payment (e.g., direct skilled care, patient instructions, skilled observation, and evaluation visits) (TJC, 2012). Home care documentation includes the following: resource numbers in case of emergency; the ability of the patient or caregiver to perform needed home care procedures and troubleshoot equipment needs; and ability to recognize potential complications. Documentation also needs to show evidence that the home environment is safe for the treatment being received (ANA, 2008a).

LONG-TERM CARE DOCUMENTATION

The number of Americans needing long-term care (LTC) is expected to double by 2050 (Unwin et al., 2010). Documentation challenges in LTC are much different from those in the acute care setting. CMS established guidelines related to accidents and supervision of residents of long-term care facilities. Changes in the Medicare program in the form of the prospective payment system determine the standards and policies for reimbursement and documentation in long-term health care. Assess each resident in a long-term care agency receiving funding from Medicare and Medicaid programs using the Resident Assessment Instrument/Minimum Data Set (USDHHS, 2011). These tools provide standardized protocols for assessment and care planning and a minimum data set to promote quality improvement within and across facilities. When you review residents' records for reimbursement, there is an expectation that protocols such as skin assessments, wound care, and assisted ambulation are carried out. Quality documentation describes the services rendered and the patient's response to treatments, justifies the therapy services provided, and ensures that services are reimbursed by Medicare. The fiscal support for long-term care residents hinges on the justification of nursing care as demonstrated in sound documentation of the services rendered.

REPORTING

Reports are an exchange of information among health care team members. A report reflects a summary of activities or observations seen, performed, or heard by the health care provider. The types of reports most commonly used by nurses include the hand-off report; telephone report; and incident report; sometimes referred to as occurrence or event report.

Hand-Off Report

A **hand-off report** occurs any time one health care provider transfers care of a patient to another health care provider. The purpose of hand-off reports is to provide better continuity and individualized care for patients. A hand-off is the process of transferring responsibility for patient care from one provider to another. For example, if you find that a patient breathes better in a certain position, you relay that information to the next nurse caring for the patient. Examples of hand-off reports include change-of-shift reports and transfer reports (Staggers et al., 2011) (Figure 10-2).

Standardizing communication during hand-off reports helps ensure patient safety. Hand-off communication includes up-to-date information about a patient's condition, required care, treatments, medications, services, and any recent or anticipated changes (TJC, 2012). The average time spent by nurses in giving a hand-off report is 40 minutes (Staggers et al., 2011).

Regardless of the way hand-off reports are given, it is essential for staff to have an opportunity for last-minute updates, to clarify information, or to receive information on care events or changes in a patient's condition. Properly performed, a hand-off report provides an opportunity to share essential information to provide for patient safety and continuity of care.

An effective hand-off report is quick and efficient. Nurses give hand-off reports using paper, a voice recording, or an electronic method. Electronic hand-off reports are beneficial to improving patient safety and continuity of care (Govier and Medcalf, 2012). Nurses prefer the paper hand-off report over electronic reports (Staggers et al., 2011). Whichever format is used, a good report provides a baseline for comparisons and indicates the kind of care anticipated for the next nurse who will be caring for the patient. An organized and concise approach helps you set goals and anticipate patient needs and lessens the chance of overlooking important information. A sample format is as follows: background information (name, age, and medical diagnosis); primary health problem; unusual occurrences; discharge planning issues; identification of significant changes in measurable terms (e.g., pain scale); observations; findings; time when new, STAT, or prn medications were given; care required such as medications that need to be started, when to assess the effectiveness of STAT/prn medications, or when a dressing needs to be changed next; progress with teaching interventions; and family involvement. It is especially important to report any recent changes or priority situations concerning the patient's condition. Do not include normal findings or routine information retrievable from other sources or derogatory or inappropriate comments about a patient or family.

Change-of-Shift Report. The change-of-shift report is one type of hand-off report that occurs at the end of each shift. This report provides the transfer of relevant information from nurses who have completed a shift of care to nurses about to begin a shift of care. Shift reports happen in a variety of ways.

Sometimes nurses walk with each other from one patient's room to the next. This is called *walking rounds*. Walking reports given in person or during rounds allow you to obtain immediate feedback when questions arise about a patient's care. When you make rounds, the patient and family members also have the opportunity to participate in any discussions and care decisions. However, be careful about mentioning information that the patient should not hear (e.g., new laboratory or diagnostic reports not yet explained by the health care provider).

Nurses also give reports orally. Oral reports occur in person, with staff members from both shifts participating. They can also be audiotaped before the end of the shift by the nurse going off duty; the incoming staff listens to the report before assuming patient care. Recording reports often enhances efficiency and minimizes social interactions.

Transfer Reports. Patients frequently transfer from one unit to another or to another facility to receive different levels of care. For example, they transfer from intensive care units to general nursing units when the level of care no longer requires intense monitoring. A transfer report is another type of hand-off report that involves communication of information about patients from the nurse on the sending unit to the nurse on the receiving unit. Nurses usually give transfer reports by phone or in person. When giving a transfer report, include the following information:

1. Patient's name, age, date of birth, health care provider(s), and medical diagnosis
2. Summary of medical progress up to the time of transfer
3. Current health status (physical and psychosocial)
4. Allergies
5. Emergency code status
6. Family support
7. Current nursing diagnoses or problems and care plan
8. Any critical assessments or interventions to be completed shortly after transfer (helps receiving nurse establish priorities of care)
9. Up-to-date reconciled medication list (TJC, 2012)
10. Need for any special equipment such as isolation equipment, suction equipment, or traction

At the completion of the transfer report, the receiving nurse clarifies information by asking questions about the patient's status. Some institutions require a written transfer report sheet that includes information communicated in the transfer report.

Telephone Reports and Orders

Telephone Reports. A registered nurse makes a telephone report when significant events or changes in a patient's condition have occurred. A telephone report needs to include clear, accurate, and concise information. TJC reported that in 2011 communication such as verbal and written among staff and with patients was listed as one of the ten most frequently identified root causes of medical errors, also called *sentinel events* (Sentinel events, 2012). To help improve communication some institutions use SBAR, an acronym that stands for *s*ituation-*b*ackground-*a*ssessment-*r*ecommendation. SBAR standardizes telephone communication of significant events or changes in the patient's condition. It is a communication strategy designed to improve patient safety. For example, when describing the *situation*, you include the admitting and secondary diagnoses and the problem your patient is having

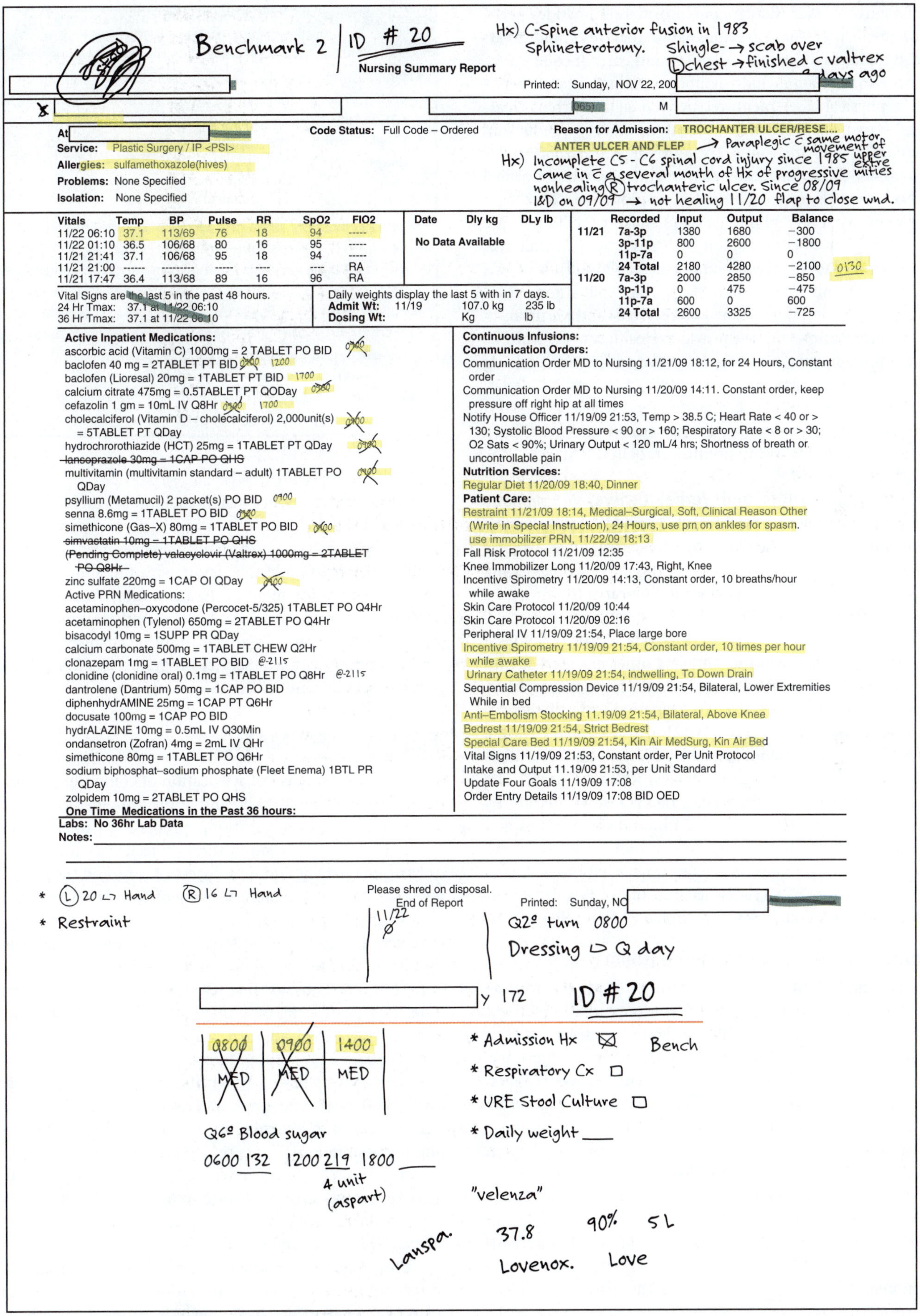

Benchmark 2 | ID # 20

Nursing Summary Report

Hx) C-Spine anterior fusion in 1983 Sphineterotomy. Shingle- → scab over Ⓛ chest → finished c valtrex 2 days ago

Printed: Sunday, NOV 22, 200

M

At

Code Status: Full Code – Ordered

Service: Plastic Surgery / IP <PSI>

Allergies: sulfamethoxazole(hives)

Problems: None Specified

Isolation: None Specified

Reason for Admission: TROCHANTER ULCER/RESE.... ANTER ULCER AND FLEP → Paraplegic c̄ same motor movement of upper extremities

Hx) Incomplete C5 - C6 spinal cord injury since 1985 Came in c̄ a several month of Hx of progressive nonhealing Ⓡ trochanteric ulcer. Since 08/09 I&D on 09/09 → not healing 11/20 flap to close wnd.

Vitals	Temp	BP	Pulse	RR	SpO2	FIO2
11/22 06:10	37.1	113/69	76	18	94	-----
11/22 01:10	36.5	106/68	80	16	95	-----
11/21 21:41	37.1	106/68	95	18	94	-----
11/21 21:00	-----	---------	-----	----	----	RA
11/21 17:47	36.4	113/68	89	16	96	RA

Vital Signs are the last 5 in the past 48 hours.
24 Hr Tmax: 37.1 at 11/22 06:10
36 Hr Tmax: 37.1 at 11/22 06:10

Date	Dly kg	DLy lb
No Data Available		

Daily weights display the last 5 with in 7 days.
Admit Wt: 11/19 107.0 kg 235 lb
Dosing Wt: Kg lb

	Recorded	Input	Output	Balance
11/21	7a-3p	1380	1680	−300
	3p-11p	800	2600	−1800
	11p-7a	0	0	0
	24 Total	2180	4280	−2100
11/20	7a-3p	2000	2850	−850
	3p-11p	0	475	−475
	11p-7a	600	0	600
	24 Total	2600	3325	−725

0130

Active Inpatient Medications:
ascorbic acid (Vitamin C) 1000mg = 2 TABLET PO BID 0900
baclofen 40 mg = 2TABLET PT BID 0900 1200
baclofen (Lioresal) 20mg = 1TABLET PT BID 1700
calcium citrate 475mg = 0.5TABLET PT QODay 0900
cefazolin 1 gm = 10mL IV Q8Hr 0900 1700
cholecalciferol (Vitamin D – cholecalciferol) 2,000unit(s) = 5TABLET PT QDay 0900
hydrochrorothiazide (HCT) 25mg = 1TABLET PT QDay 0900
~~lansoprazole 30mg = 1CAP PO QHS~~
multivitamin (multivitamin standard – adult) 1TABLET PO QDay 0900
psyllium (Metamucil) 2 packet(s) PO BID 0900
senna 8.6mg = 1TABLET PO BID 0900
simethicone (Gas–X) 80mg = 1TABLET PO BID 0900
~~simvastatin 10mg = 1TABLET PO QHS~~
~~(Pending Complete) valacyclovir (Valtrex) 1000mg = 2TABLET PO Q8Hr~~
zinc sulfate 220mg = 1CAP OI QDay 0900

Active PRN Medications:
acetaminophen–oxycodone (Percocet-5/325) 1TABLET PO Q4Hr
acetaminophen (Tylenol) 650mg = 2TABLET PO Q4Hr
bisacodyl 10mg = 1SUPP PR QDay
calcium carbonate 500mg = 1TABLET CHEW Q2Hr
clonazepam 1mg = 1TABLET PO BID @-2115
clonidine (clonidine oral) 0.1mg = 1TABLET PO Q8Hr @-2115
dantrolene (Dantrium) 50mg = 1CAP PO BID
diphenhydrAMINE 25mg = 1CAP PT Q6Hr
docusate 100mg = 1CAP PO BID
hydrALAZINE 10mg = 0.5mL IV Q30Min
ondansetron (Zofran) 4mg = 2mL IV QHr
simethicone 80mg = 1TABLET PO Q6Hr
sodium biphosphat–sodium phosphate (Fleet Enema) 1BTL PR QDay
zolpidem 10mg = 2TABLET PO QHS

Continuous Infusions:

Communication Orders:
Communication Order MD to Nursing 11/21/09 18:12, for 24 Hours, Constant order
Communication Order MD to Nursing 11/20/09 14:11. Constant order, keep pressure off right hip at all times
Notify House Officer 11/19/09 21:53, Temp > 38.5 C; Heart Rate < 40 or > 130; Systolic Blood Pressure < 90 or > 160; Respiratory Rate < 8 or > 30; O2 Sats < 90%; Urinary Output < 120 mL/4 hrs; Shortness of breath or uncontrollable pain

Nutrition Services:
Regular Diet 11/20/09 18:40, Dinner

Patient Care:
Restraint 11/21/09 18:14, Medical–Surgical, Soft, Clinical Reason Other (Write in Special Instruction), 24 Hours, use prn on ankles for spasm. use immobilizer PRN, 11/22/09 18:13
Fall Risk Protocol 11/21/09 12:35
Knee Immobilizer Long 11/20/09 17:43, Right, Knee
Incentive Spirometry 11/20/09 14:13, Constant order, 10 breaths/hour while awake
Skin Care Protocol 11/20/09 10:44
Skin Care Protocol 11/20/09 02:16
Peripheral IV 11/19/09 21:54, Place large bore
Incentive Spirometry 11/19/09 21:54, Constant order, 10 times per hour while awake
Urinary Catheter 11/19/09 21:54, indwelling, To Down Drain
Sequential Compression Device 11/19/09 21:54, Bilateral, Lower Extremities While in bed
Anti–Embolism Stocking 11.19/09 21:54, Bilateral, Above Knee
Bedrest 11/19/09 21:54, Strict Bedrest
Special Care Bed 11/19/09 21:54, Kin Air MedSurg, Kin Air Bed
Vital Signs 11/19/09 21:53, Constant order, Per Unit Protocol
Intake and Output 11.19/09 21:53, per Unit Standard
Update Four Goals 11/19/09 17:08
Order Entry Details 11/19/09 17:08 BID OED

One Time Medications in the Past 36 hours:
Labs: No 36hr Lab Data
Notes:

* Ⓛ 20 Hand Ⓡ 16 Hand
* Restraint

Please shred on disposal.
End of Report

Printed: Sunday, NO

11/22 ∅

Q2° turn 0800
Dressing ⇒ Q day

172 ID # 20

0800	0900	1400
MED	MED	MED

* Admission Hx ☒ Bench
* Respiratory Cx ☐
* URE Stool Culture ☐
* Daily weight ___

Q6° Blood sugar
0600 132 1200 219 1800 ___
4 unit (aspart)

"velenza"
37.8 90% 5 L
Lanspa. Lovenox. Love

FIGURE 10-2 Example of hand-off report sheet. (From Staggers N, et al: Nurses' information management and use of electronic tools during acute care handoffs, *West J Nurs Res* 34(2):153, 2011.)

as the current issue. *Background* information includes pertinent medical history, previous laboratory tests and treatments, psychosocial issues, allergies, and current code status. For *assessment* data include significant findings in your head-to-toe physical assessment, recent vital signs, current treatment measures, restrictions, recent laboratory results and diagnostics, and pain status. Then provide your *recommendation*, in which you suggest a plan of care and request orders and other needs to be addressed (Compton et al., 2012).

Document every phone call you make to a health care provider. Your documentation includes when the call was made, who made it (if you did not make the call), who was called, to whom information was given, what information was given, what information was received, and verification of the information with the provider. Health care institutions have a process for a verification "read-back" when receiving information or critical test results. An example follows: "Laboratory technician J. Ignacio reported a potassium level of 5.9. Information was transcribed and read back for verification. Dr. Wade notified at 2030. D. Markle, RN, read back."

Telephone Orders and Verbal Orders. A telephone order (TO) involves a health care provider stating a prescribed therapy over the phone to a registered nurse, whereas a verbal order (VO) involves a health care provider giving orders to a nurse while they are standing near each other. TOs and VOs frequently occur at night or during an emergency and frequently cause medical errors. The nurse receiving a VO or TO writes down the complete order or enters it into the computer as it is being given. Then the nurse reads it back, called *read-back,* and receives confirmation from the person who gave the order (TJC, 2012). An example follows: "4/16/2014: 0815, Tylenol 3, 2 tablets, every 6 hours for incisional pain. TO Dr. Knight/J. Woods, RN, read back." The health care provider later verifies the TO or VO legally by signing it within a set time (e.g., 24 hours) as set by hospital policy. Use TOs and VOs only when absolutely necessary and not for the sake of convenience. In some situations a second person listens to TOs (verify agency policy). Box 10-2 provides guidelines that promote accuracy when receiving TOs.

BOX 10-2 GUIDELINES FOR TELEPHONE AND VERBAL ORDERS

- Only authorized staff receive and record telephone or verbal orders. Hospital identifies in writing the staff that are authorized.
- Clearly identify the patient's name, room number, and diagnosis.
- Read back all orders to the health care provider (TJC, 2012).
- Use clarification questions to avoid misunderstandings.
- Write "TO" (telephone order) or "VO" (verbal order), including date and time, name of patient, complete order; sign the name of the health care provider and nurse.
- Follow agency policies; some institutions require documentation of the "read-back" or require two nurses to review and sign telephone (and verbal) orders.
- The health care provider cosigns the order within the time frame required by the institution (usually 24 hours—check agency policy).

Incident, Event, or Occurrence Reports

An incident is any event not consistent with the routine operation of a health care unit or routine care of a patient. Examples include patient falls, needlestick injuries, a visitor becoming ill, and medication errors. Completion of an **incident report,** also called either an **occurrence or event report,** occurs when there is an actual or potential injury; this report is not a part of the patient record (see Chapter 5).

Always contact the patient's health care provider when an incident happens. Note that you do not mention that an error occurred in the patient's medical record. Instead you document in the patient's medical record an objective description of what happened, what you observed, and which follow-up actions were taken. It is also important to evaluate and document the patient's response to the error or incident (Austin, 2011).

Follow agency policy when making an incident report. Incident reports are an important part of quality improvement. The overall goal is to identify changes needed to prevent future recurrence. File the report with the appropriate risk management department of the institution. Analysis of incident (or occurrence) reports helps identify trends within an organization to provide justification for changes in policies and procedures or for in-service programs. (See Chapter 5 for other examples and further discussion.)

HEALTH INFORMATICS

Health informatics is the application of computer and information science in all basic and applied biomedical sciences to facilitate the acquisition, processing, interpretation, optimal use, and communication of health-related data. The focus is the patient and the process of care, and the goal is to enhance the quality and efficiency of care provided (Hebda and Czar, 2013).

There is an increasing trend toward computerization of health care records in acute care, outpatient, home care, and long-term care settings (Box 10-3). Surveys show that approximately 27% of acute care hospitals and 12% of ambulatory care settings have adopted some form of EHRs (Moore and Fisher, 2012). Computerization of health care records provides a mechanism for identification, acquisition, manipulation, storage, and presentation of data so they can be transformed into information. The federal directive promoting the adoption of EMRs by 2014 mandates that nurses of the twenty-first century have broadened skill sets to deliver quality patient care (McBride et al., 2012; Walker, 2010). Today's nurses need to be knowledgeable in the science and application of nursing informatics.

Informatics is the science and art of turning data into information. It focuses on information and knowledge acquisition rather than the computer. All nurses deal with data,

BOX 10-3 EVIDENCE-BASED PRACTICE

PICO Question: Does the productivity of nurses and patient safety improve with health care agencies using electronic health records (EHRs) compared to those who do not use EHRs?

SUMMARY OF EVIDENCE

Diffusion of health information technologies (HITs) has the potential to increase productivity and improve patient safety by changing the workflow of nursing care and clinical decision making. As a result U.S. hospitals are increasingly adopting EHRs as a means to improve safety of the health care system. It is anticipated that hospitals who integrate various HIT options such as electronic medical records (EMRs), computerized provider order entry (CPOE), or bar-code medication administration (BCMA) will use fewer nurses, as measured by full-time equivalents (FTEs). However, results show that, in fact, more nurses are needed to oversee HIT applications and compensate for the temporary loss of productivity on EHR implementation (Abbass et al., 2012). Similarly changes in workflow resulting from EHR implementation do not always result in positive outcomes. For example, nurses' workflow changes resulted in a near-miss sentinel event as nurses used "work-arounds" to override the safety features of BCMA (Early et al., 2011). Both the perceptions of computers and attitudes toward EHRs held by nurses compromise the safety features of health information technology (Laramee et al., 2011). Nurses need to share what works best for the patient and clinician if the potential of HIT is to be realized.

APPLICATION TO NURSING PRACTICE

- When implementing EHR systems, clear processes with detailed instructions on how to use the EHR are needed to prevent nurses from creating work-arounds.
- Successful adaptation of EHR depends on sufficient preparation of staff about the benefits of technology in improving patient care safety.
- Set realistic expectations and assess user perceptions of the benefits of HIT to support nurses who have concerns about the benefit of EHR implementation.
- Successful infusion of technology relies on continual emphasis of the professional nurse's responsibility to patient safety. "Ongoing surveillance is needed to ensure that technology changes do not cause unwanted or unforeseen circumstances that could compromise patient safety" (Early et al., 2011).

information, and knowledge (Hebda and Czar, 2013). Informatics describes the study of the retrieval, storage, presentation, and sharing of data, information, and knowledge to provide quality, safe patient care (Sensmeier, 2011).

Informatics includes four key concepts. *Data* include numbers, characters, or facts that are collected according to a perceived need for analysis and possible action. Data have no significance beyond their existence. For example, what does the number 180 mean? It could be a laboratory value, a street number, or a secret code. By itself 180 means nothing. It represents data. *Information* is data that are interpreted, organized, or structured. Information provides the answers to "who, what, when, where" questions. If you take the blood pressure of a 57-year-old postoperative patient and the systolic blood pressure reading is 180 mm Hg and the diastolic blood pressure is 90 mm Hg, you have useful information. When the number 180 is combined with other data, it becomes meaningful. The data become information. The vital signs now have meaning when interpreted. *Knowledge* is the application of data and information. It answers the "how" question. You know that the patient just had surgery, has a history of high blood pressure, and did not receive the morning dose of antihypertensive medication. Using knowledge is essential in making decisions. You synthesized information (knowledge) from past experiences of caring for other postoperative patients with high blood pressure. Knowledge creates new questions and areas of research. *Wisdom* answers the "why" question and focuses on the appropriate application of that knowledge (Hebda and Czar, 2013). Wisdom comes with experience. In the above scenario, you report changes to the patient's health care provider. You also apply knowledge of pharmacology and intervene to manage the patient's blood pressure.

It is a challenge in health care settings to easily access data and information about patients. This is especially the case when you record information manually on printed forms. For example, a nurse working in risk management who is interested in investigating patient falls has to review page by page the records of patients who have fallen to identify the common factors contributing to falls. Remember that three important purposes of medical records are communication, education, and research. When health care organizations rely on handwritten patient records, the process of locating, summarizing, and comparing information is slow and difficult. Finding information for medical record purposes of health care education, research, audits, and reimbursement becomes cumbersome and inefficient. The Institute of Medicine (IOM) (2010) recognized that the only way to use data and information to improve care delivery and for quality improvement, research, and education is through IT.

Information technology (IT) refers to the management and processing of information, generally with the assistance of computers (Hebda and Czar, 2013). IT includes not only the use of computers, but also the knowledge of *how* to use computer technology such as databases, programming languages and tools, and communication protocols. Technology serves as the tool that allows transfer of the information that improves care. However, technology alone does not improve the efficiency and effectiveness of patient care. You are expected to understand the capabilities and limitations of technology. IT supports the process of synthesizing data and information into knowledge and wisdom (ANA, 2008b). IT is critical to all aspects of clinical decision making, consumer education, professional development, research, and the delivery of patient care.

A **health care information system (HIS)** is a group of systems used within a health care enterprise that support and enhance health care (Hebda and Czar, 2013). The role of HIS has grown more important because the public has a heightened awareness of reports of medical errors through public media and various initiatives implemented nationally such as HIPAA, personal health records, and EHRs. Increasing numbers of health care agencies are expanding the use and integration of EHR into their settings.

An HIS consists of two major types of information systems: administrative information systems and clinical information systems (CISs). The two systems operate together to improve the efficiency of data entry and communication. Administrative information systems include databases such as payroll, financial, and quality assurance systems.

CISs support activities are used to plan, implement, and evaluate patient care. All clinicians, including nurses, physicians, pharmacists, social workers, and therapists, use CISs. CISs include the EHR, monitoring systems and laboratory, radiology, and pharmacy systems. A monitoring system includes devices that automatically monitor and record biometric measurements (e.g., vital signs, oxygen saturation, cardiac index, and stroke volume) in critical care and specialty areas. The devices send measurements electronically and directly to the nursing documentation system.

The CIS also includes order entry systems, one of the most important systems in use today. They automate orders, eliminating written order forms and expediting the delivery of supplies to a nursing unit. The **computerized provider order entry (CPOE)** is one type of order entry system gaining popularity across the country, particularly with medication orders. Advantages of CPOE include reduced use of resources, quicker turnaround of orders, reduced length of stay, and an overall reduction in costs. More important, most CPOE systems have significant potential to reduce medication errors associated with illegibility and inappropriate drug use and dosing (Tschannen et al., 2011). CPOE refers to a process by which the health care provider directly enters orders for patient care into the hospital information system. In advanced systems, CPOE has built-in reminders and alerts that help the patient's provider select the most appropriate medication or diagnostic test. There are major initiatives from the IOM to improve the quality of care and reduce medication errors. Many believe CPOE is the answer. When a provider puts an order entry into the EHR, the order is sent immediately to the appropriate department. The direct order eliminates issues related to illegible handwriting and transcription errors. A CPOE system potentially speeds the implementation of the ordered diagnostic tests and treatments, which improves staff productivity and saves money (Tschannen et al., 2011).

Typically a health care agency uses one or several CISs and administrative information systems. For example, a small community hospital uses a nursing information system, an order entry system, and laboratory, radiology, and pharmacy systems to coordinate its core patient care services. A nurse documents nursing care on a computer, locates and reviews laboratory test results, orders sterile supplies, and enters health care provider orders for x-ray films and patients' medications. The billing of patient care services and payroll occurs through use of administrative information systems (Hebda and Czar, 2013).

Nursing Information Systems

Nursing information systems (NISs) are one of many subspecialties of CISs. Many hospitals now have NISs that support the documentation of nursing process activities and offer resources for managing nursing care delivery. A reliable NIS is the product of nursing informatics. **Nursing informatics** is a nursing specialty that manages and communicates data, information, knowledge, and wisdom by integrating nursing, computer, and information science (ANA, 2008b). Nursing informatics facilitates the integration of data, information, and knowledge to support patients, nurses, and other providers in decision making in all roles and settings. It supports new initiatives occurring within the health care arena such as CPOE, electronic medication administration records, and clinical documentation. The application of nursing informatics results in an efficient and effective NIS. Nursing informatics improves the health of individuals, families, communities, and populations by effectively managing information and enhancing communication (ANA, 2008b). Because of rapidly advancing emerging health care technologies, nursing practice of the future will not be the same as it is today. Nurses need knowledge and skills in computer literacy, information literacy, informatics, and the use of information technologies (Skiba, 2010; Sensmeier, 2011).

Numerous organizations, including the National League for Nursing (NLN), the American Nurses Association (ANA), the Technology Informatics Guiding Education Reform (TIGER), and the Robert Wood Johnson Foundation Quality and Safety Education for Nurses Initiative (QSEN), recommend that all nurses acquire a minimal level of awareness and competence in informatics and use of IT. Competence in informatics is not the same as computer competency. To become competent in informatics you need to be able to use evolving methods of discovering, retrieving, and using information in your practice (Hebda and Czar, 2013). This means that you learn to recognize when you need information and have the skills to find, evaluate, and use needed clinical information effectively.

An effective NIS incorporates principles of nursing informatics and supports the work you do. You need to be able to access a computer program easily, review the patient's medical history and orders, and go to the patient's bedside to conduct a comprehensive assessment. Once you have completed the assessment, you enter data into the computer terminal at the patient's bedside and develop a plan of care from the information gathered. The plan of care incorporates evidence-based practice guidelines, which you have found using your information science skills. The computer allows you to quickly share the plan of care with the patient. Periodically you return to the computer to check on laboratory test results and document the therapies you administer. The computer screens and optional pop-up windows make it easy to locate information, enter and compare data, and make changes. The NIS helps you determine diagnosis, prepare and implement nursing care plans, and evaluate care provided.

The transition from paper to online documentation systems presents both opportunities and challenges to nurses. Successful implementation of computer-based nursing process documentation requires a high level of acceptance of the nursing process, careful preparation of predefined care plans, organizational preparation, and inclusion of future users, including bedside nurses, in the development process. It is also essential to have sufficient technical equipment with integration into the hospital information system.

A barrier to the successful implementation of an NIS is the reluctance on the part of some nurses and other clinical staff to accept technological advances. Often clinicians fail to understand how technology can improve the way they deliver care and enhance clinical decision processes. Successful integration requires nurses to understand the potential of informatics and IT.

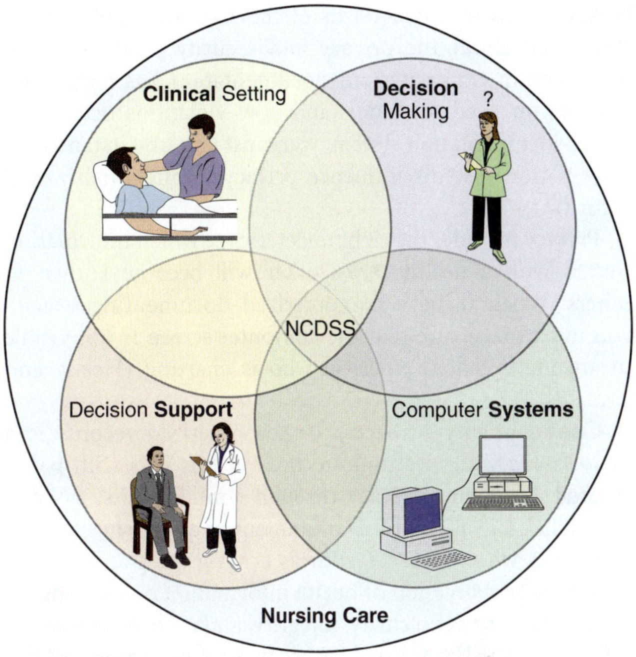

FIGURE 10-3 Model of a nursing clinical decision support system (NCDSS). (Courtesy Frank Lyerla.)

Clinical decision support systems (CDSSs) are computerized programs used within a health care setting to provide you with clinical knowledge and relevant patient information to help you improve patient care (Hebda and Czar, 2013). A CDSS uses a complex system of rules for analyzing data and presents information to support the decision-making process of the nurse (Figure 10-3). The information within a CDSS is current, is evidence based, and has the ability to be updated. The CDSS links a nurse to the latest evidence-based practice guidelines at the point of care (Dontje and Coenen, 2011). For example, CDSSs are used to improve glycemic control in hospitalized patients who have diabetes mellitus (Harrison et al., 2013). Information provided by a CDSS is given to the right person at the right time. For example, after a medication order is entered, the CDSS provides an alert to the provider if the dosage falls outside of the safe range. This enhances patient safety during the medication ordering process. CDSSs also improve nursing care. When patient assessment data are combined with patient care guidelines, nurses are better able to implement evidence-based nursing care, resulting in improved patient outcomes (Harrison and Lyerla, 2012; Sewell and Thede, 2013).

Privacy, Confidentiality, and Security Mechanisms

There are risks associated with the electronic system. The most common risks center on violations of patient privacy, patient **confidentiality,** and security. Privacy is the individual's right to limit access to his or her health care information. Confidentiality is the expectation that information shared with the health care provider will be used only for its intended purposes and not redisclosed unless medically necessary. Security protects the EHR from hackers who try to obtain confidential information (McGonigle and Mastrian, 2012). More health care organizations have computers linked together to maximize communication both inside and outside the facilities. These networks allow for efficiency and minimize fragmentation of health care. However, breaches of network security remain a concern (Carrington and Effken, 2011). Organizations have mechanisms in place to minimize security breaches. Such mechanisms include authentication of users, a strong password policy, and acceptable use policies of the network that indicate the type of activities allowed on the network. If you make an error within the electronic documentation system, you must follow agency policy for making corrections. There is always an audit trail with electronic documentation. In some situations, if the EHR is "down" for any reason, nurses maintain a paper record of the care provided. If the EHR system is down, the paper documentation remains a part of the legal record (Harrington et al., 2011). You must remember that charting factual, accurate, complete, and current guidelines also pertains to the electronic document. Just as in a paper documentation system, "if it's not documented" within the electronic record, "it's not done."

The implementation of HIPAA regulations heightened awareness about information security and privacy practices. HIPAA was the first federal legislation to protect automated patient records and provide uniform protection nationwide (Hebda and Czar, 2013). HIPAA regulations called for the establishment of an electronic patient records system and process to protect the privacy of individual health information. Electronic records facilitate efficient and effective sharing of information, but the ease of access raises concern among consumers. The California HealthCare Foundation (2010) survey found that two thirds of the American public were concerned about the privacy and security of their health information. Computerized documentation has legal risks. Just as you need to understand how violations occur in a paper documentation system, you must also understand how information systems influence privacy, confidentiality, and security.

Privacy includes the right to determine which information shared with a health care worker will become known to others. When using a computerized documenting system, you must make sure that the computer screen is not visible to anyone except the person who is charting (Hebda and Czar, 2013).

Confidentiality of access to computerized records is a major issue with electronic records just as it is with paper records. Protecting privacy through confidentiality policies and technology is a critical component of quality health care. Standards within HIPAA address criteria for standardizing electronic transmission of health information by focusing on the need to protect security, integrity, and authenticity of the information. HIPAA also requires institutions to protect the confidentiality of medical information stored in electronic records against reasonable and anticipated threats. The first line of maintaining patient confidentiality is achieved with a log-in process authenticating that the person is granted access. Authentication of the user is through an access code accompanied by a password.

A **password** is a collection of alphanumeric characters that a user types into the computer before accessing a program. A user is usually required to enter a password after the entry and acceptance of an access code or user name. A password does not appear on the computer screen when it is typed, nor should it be known to anyone but the user and information systems administrators (Hebda and Czar, 2013). Strong passwords use combinations of letters, numbers, and symbols that are not easy to guess. When using a health care agency computer system, it is essential that you do not share your computer password under any circumstances with anyone. A good system requires frequent and random changes in personal passwords to prevent unauthorized people from tampering with records. In addition, most staff have access only to patients in their work area. Select staff (e.g., administrators or risk managers) may be given authority to access all patient records. Most breaches of confidentiality come from inside the agency (Hebda and Czar, 2013).

Data security has three aspects: ensuring accuracy of data, protection of the data from unauthorized eyes inside or outside of the agency, and protection from data loss (Sewell and Thede, 2013). Data accuracy is ensured through mechanisms that check data during input and provide for correction of entries made in error. Accuracy of original data is the responsibility of the user.

Protection from inside intrusions occurs with audit trails. The trail reveals both unauthorized access and the identity of the person committing the violation. Keep in mind that audit trails are discoverable by a court of law. Another method to protect access to records from inside intrusions occurs with an automatic sign-off, a mechanism designed to log off a user from the computer system after a specified period of inactivity on the computer (Hebda and Czar, 2013). An automatic sign-off is often found in most patient care areas and other departments that handle sensitive data.

Protection from outside intrusions occurs with installation of firewalls and antivirus and spyware detection software. A **firewall** is a combination of hardware and software that protects private network resources (e.g., a hospital information system) from outside hackers, network damage, and theft or misuse of information. Computer data need protection from data loss resulting from either a system problem or a disaster (Sewell and Thede, 2013).

The data security process has taken on new meaning since the events of September 11, 2001. A disaster recovery plan must be in place. All agencies routinely create backup data and store the data off-site in a secure place (Hebda and Czar, 2013). Other considerations to maintain the security of the health care data include placing computers or file servers in restricted areas. Using a privacy shield on the computer screen helps to make information less visible. This form of security has limited benefit, especially if an organization uses mobile wireless devices such as notebooks, tablet personal computers (PCs), smartphones, and personal digital assistants (PDAs). These devices are easy to misplace or lose and can fall into the wrong hands. Some organizations use motion detectors or alarms with these devices to prevent theft. Password access with automatic logoff limits access to confidential information on these handheld devices.

Handling and Disposal of Information

Although it is important to keep medical records confidential, it is equally important to safeguard the information that is printed from the electronic record or extracted for report purposes. For example, a nurse prints a copy of a nursing activities work list to use as a day planner while administering care to patients. The nurse refers to information on the list and adds handwritten notes to enter later into the computer. Information on the list is considered personal health information (PHI). Thus the nurse must keep the information confidential and prevent unauthorized persons from viewing it. You destroy (e.g., shred) anything that is printed when the information is no longer needed.

The printing and faxing of information from a patient's record is a primary source for the unauthorized release of information. All papers containing PHI (e.g., Social Security number, date of birth or age, or patient's name or address) must be destroyed. Most agencies have shredders or locked receptacles for shredding and later incineration. Nurses also work in settings where they are responsible for erasing computer files from the hard drive containing calendars, surgery or diagnostic procedure schedules, or other daily records that contain PHI (Hebda and Czar, 2013). Be sure that you know the disposal policies for records in the institution where you work.

An institution needs to have sound policies for the use of fax machines, specifically which types of information you can send to which departments. You do not send more information by fax than what is needed or requested for immediate patient care needs. Take the following steps to enhance fax security (Hebda and Czar, 2013).

- Confirm that fax numbers are correct before sending to be sure that you direct information properly.
- Use a cover sheet, especially if a fax machine serves a number of different users.
- Authenticate at both ends of the transmission before data transmission to verify that source and destination are correct.
- Use programmed speed-dial keys to eliminate the chance of a dialing error and misdirected information.
- Use encryption to minimize ability to read confidential information.
- Use sealed envelopes for delivery.
- Place fax machines in a secure area.
- Limit machine access to designated individuals.
- Include a request to return documents by mail.
- Log fax transmissions. This feature is often available electronically on the machine.

KEY POINTS

- The record is a confidential, legal, and continuing account of the patient's health care status and is available to all members of the health care team. It facilitates communication with health care providers for continuity of patient care, maintains a legal and financial record of care, aids in clinical research, and guides professional and organizational performance improvement.
- Accurate and timely record keeping requires an objective interpretation of data with precise measurements, correct spelling, and proper use of abbreviations.
- Effective documentation verifies the specific nursing care provided, use of services and equipment, and medications administered and thus supports the reimbursement that your health care agency receives.
- To limit liability nursing documentation describes what happened to a patient and clearly indicates that individualized, goal-directed nursing care was provided based on the nursing assessment.
- Organize problem-oriented medical records by the patient's health care problems.
- Medicare guidelines for establishing a patient's home care reimbursement are the basis for documentation by home care nurses.
- Long-term care documentation is interdisciplinary and closely linked with fiscal requirements of outside agencies.
- Computerized information systems provide information about patients in an accessible and organized manner.
- The major purpose of hand-off reports is patient safety and to maintain continuity of care.
- When information relevant to care is communicated by telephone, verify the information by a "read-back" process.
- Incident (occurrence/event) reports objectively describe any event not consistent with the routine care of a patient.
- Nursing informatics facilitates the integration of data, information, knowledge, and wisdom to support patients, nurses, and other providers in decision making in all roles and settings.
- Protection of the confidentiality of patient's health information and the security of computer systems must remain a top priority.
- The computerized health record improves continuity of health care by providing the ability to compare data from various health care encounters and offering easily accessible data for purposes of communication, reducing liability, reimbursement, education, research, and auditing and monitoring.

CLINICAL DECISION-MAKING EXERCISES

You are caring for Mrs. Smith, who continues to have pain during the course of her postoperative stay in the hospital. Initially she received pain medication through her intravenous line. Now she is receiving oral pain medication, Ibuprofen one tab, on an as-needed basis. While you were at lunch, her roommate, Mrs. Jones, requested pain medication. The nurse covering for you inadvertently administered Vicodin one tab at 12:30 to Mrs. Smith instead of Mrs. Jones. When you return from lunch, you discover the medication error. You talk with the primary nurse about the current situation with Mrs. Smith. The EMR shows that Mrs. Smith has an allergy to acetaminophen (Tylenol). The nurse needs to contact Mrs. Smith's health care provider about the medication error.

1. Using the SBAR format, prepare the information that the nurse needs to provide to the health care provider about the medication error. Describe what each of the letters stand for in your description.
2. You note that the nurse who made the medication error charted the following in Mrs. Smith's medical record: *Vicodin one tab given to Mrs. Smith accidently at 1230. Health care provider notified of wrong medication. Incident report completed as per hospital policy and put into Mrs. Smith's medical record. Orders received to monitor patient for signs of allergic reaction.* Evaluate the documentation entry made by the nurse. Describe which parts of the documentation are recorded correctly and which part, if any, needs to be changed in the documentation?
3. Mrs. Smith is discharged. What information do you include in the discharge summary?

evolve

Answers to Clinical Decision-Making Exercises can be found on the Evolve website.

QSEN ACTIVITY: INFORMATICS

It is now 3 days after surgery for Mrs. Smith, and you are working the 3 to 11 PM *shift. You receive the hand-off report, which reports that Mrs. Smith has complaints of being "so weak" this afternoon. She refused to go to rehabilitation for her back strengthening exercises earlier in the day. You log into the EMR system and find Mrs. Smith's medical record. You review her recent laboratory data, including the complete blood count and earlier assessment information. You also note if any medications have been administered recently that might explain her weakness. The family is present and expresses concern over their mother's complaint of weakness. They note that it seems that the nursing staff spends much time on the computer. They ask how the EMR improves patient safety and quality care.*

How would you best respond to the family?

evolve

Answers to QSEN Activities can be found on the Evolve website.

REVIEW QUESTIONS

1. When taking a telephone order from a health care provider, it is common for most organizations to require the nurse to:
   1. Photocopy the order for your records.
   2. Write the order in its entirety and read it back to the health care provider for verification.
   3. Write the order but do not implement until it has been signed by the health care provider.
   4. Take the order from the health care provider but insist that the health care provider come to the patient care division to write the order himself or herself.
2. Which action is acceptable practice when documenting in an electronic health record (EHR)?
   1. Allowing a temporary staff member to use your computer user name and password
   2. Remaining logged in to a computer when you leave to administer a medication
   3. Allowing the health care provider covering your patient to quickly input an order using your computer password
   4. Preventing others from seeing a display monitor that contains patient information
3. You have been teaching a patient about a new medication for a recently diagnosed heart condition. To document this in the progress notes, you record the data, action, and evaluation of response to the teaching. This type of charting format is called:
   1. POMR.
   2. CBE.
   3. PIE.
   4. Focus charting.
4. Your facility has started to use military time. Your patient received a one-time dose of the diuretic furosemide (Lasix) 40 mg IV at 3 PM. How should you document the administration time?
   1. Patient received furosemide 40 mg IV at 1500 hours.
   2. Patient received furosemide 40 mg IV at 2100 hours.
   3. Patient received furosemide 40 mg IV at 1300 hours.
   4. Patient received furosemide 40 mg IV at 0300 hours.
5. You are giving a hand-off report to another nurse who will be caring for your patient at the end of your shift. Which of the following pieces of information do you include in the report? (Select all that apply.)
   1. The patient's name, age, and admitting diagnosis
   2. Allergies to food and medications
   3. Your evaluation that the patient is "grouchy"
   4. How much the patient has urinated
   5. That the patient's pain rating went from 6 to 3 on a scale of 0 to 10 after receiving 325 mg of Tylenol
   6. Did not receive dressing change because of inadequate staffing during the previous shift
6. What is an appropriate way for a nurse to dispose of printed patient information?
   1. Rip several times and place in a standard trash can
   2. Place in the patient's paper-based chart
   3. Place in a secure canister marked for shredding
   4. Burn the documents
7. A nurse caring for a patient who has hypertension documents a systolic blood pressure of 1200 mm Hg. Suddenly an alert warning appears on the screen warning the nurse that the number entered exceeds the range for human systolic blood pressure and that the value entered needs to be reviewed. This warning is known as what type of system?
   1. Electronic health record (EHR)
   2. Clinical documentation
   3. Clinical decision support system (CDSS)
   4. Computerized physician order entry (CPOE)
8. A group of nurses is discussing the advantages of using computerized provider order entry (CPOE). Which of the following statements best indicates that the nurses understand the major advantage of using it?
   1. "CPOE reduces transcription errors."
   2. "CPOE reduces the time necessary for health care providers to write orders."
   3. "Health care providers can write orders from any computer that has Internet access."
   4. "CPOE reduces the time nurses use to communicate with health care providers."
9. A patient had back surgery yesterday. During the dressing change you notice an increase in serosanguinous drainage from the incision. Because this is a deviation from the written assessment guidelines, you document this observation on the assessment flow sheet. This type of charting system is called:
   1. POMR.
   2. Charting by exception (CBE).
   3. Narrative.
   4. Focus.

10. Match the correct definition with the appropriate terminology related to electronic medical records.

1. Privacy	a. Expectation that information shared with health care provider(s) will be used only for its intended purposes
2. Security	b. Individual's right to limit access to one's health care information
3. Confidentiality	c. Protection from unauthorized access, malicious damage, and incidental and accidental damage

evolve

Rationales for Review Questions can be found on the Evolve website.

1. 2; **2.** 4; **3.** 4; **4.** 1; **5.** 1, 2, 4, 5; **6.** 3; **7.** 3; **8.** 1; **9.** 2; **10.** 1=b, 2=c, 3=a.

REFERENCES

Abbass I, et al: Impact of electronic health records on nurses' productivity, *CIN: Comput Inform Nurs* 30(5):237, 2012.

American Nurses Association (ANA): *Home health nursing: scope and standards of practice*, Silver Spring, MD, 2008a, nursesbooks.org.

American Nurses Association (ANA): *Nursing informatics scope and standards of practice*, Silver Spring, MD, 2008b, nursesbooks.org.

American Nurses Association (ANA): *Principles for documentation, principles for practice: a resource package for registered nurses*, Silver Spring, MD, 2010, nursesbooks.org.

Austin S: Stay out of court with proper documentation, *Nursing* 41(4):24, 2011.

Brown G, et al: *Health informatics: a systems perspective*, Chicago, IL, 2013, Health Administration Press.

California HealthCare Foundation: *Consumers Health Info Technology National Survey*, 2010, http://www.chcf.org/~/media/MEDIA%20LIBRARY%20Files/PDF/C/PDF%20ConsumersHealthInfoTechnologyNationalSurvey.pdf. Accessed August 20, 2012.

Carpenito-Moyet L: *Nursing care plans and documentation: nursing diagnosis collaborative problems*, ed 5, Philadelphia, 2009, Lippincott Williams & Wilkins.

Carrington J, Effken J: Strengths and limitations of the electronic health record for documenting clinical events, *CIN: Comput Inform Nurs* 29(6):360, 2011.

Cesta T: The case management process in effective and efficient action. *Hosp Case Manage* 20(4):55, 2012.

Compton J, et al: Implementing SBAR across a large multihospital health system, *Joint Commission J Qual Patient Safety* 38(6):261, 2012.

Dontje K, Coenen A: Mapping evidence-based guidelines to standardized nursing terminologies, *CIN: Comput Inform Nurs* 29(12):698, 2011.

Early C, et al: Scanning for safety, *CIN: Comput Inform Nurs* 29(3):157, 2011.

Geiger N: Viewpoint. On tying Medicare reimbursement to patient satisfaction surveys: a positive experience is not synonymous with quality of care, *Am J Nurs* 112(7):11, 2012.

Glasper A: Improving record keeping: important lessons for nurses, *Br J Nurs* 20(14):886, 2011.

Govier M, Medcalf P: Living for the weekend: electronic documentation improves patient handover, *Clin Med* 12(2):124, 2012.

Harrington L, et al: Documentation of others' work in the electronic health record, *Crit Care Nurse* 31(3):84, 2011.

Harrison R, Lyerla F: Using nursing clinical decision support systems to achieve meaningful use, *CIN: Computers Inform Nurs* 30:380, 2012.

Harrison R, et al: Use of a clinical decision support system to improve hypoglycemia, *Medsurg Nurs* 22(4):250, 2013.

Healthcare Information and Management Systems Society (HIMSS): *Electronic health record,* n.d., http://www.himss.org/ASP/topics_ehr.asp. Accessed August 1, 2012.

Hebda T, Czar P: *Handbook of informatics for nurses and healthcare professionals*, ed 5, Upper Saddle River, NJ, 2013, Pearson Prentice Hall.

Hellier S: Maybe someone should tell the nurses: pay-for-performance, *Health Care Manag* 29(2):172, 2010.

Institute of Medicine (IOM): *Future of nursing: leading change, advancing health*, Robert Wood Johnson Foundation Initiative on the Future of Nursing at the Institute of Medicine, Washington, DC, 2010, National Academies Press, http://iom.edu/Reports/2010/The-Future-of-Nursing-Leading-Change-Advancing-Health.aspx, 2010. Accessed August 1, 2012.

Johnson J, Nicholls M: Nursing documentation: how meaning is obscured by fragmentary language, *Nurs Outlook* 59(6):e6, 2011.

Laramee A, et al: Learning from within to ensure a successful implementation of an electronic health record, *CIN: Comput Inform Nurs* 29(8):468, 2011.

McBride S, et al: Health information technology and nursing, *Am J Nurs* 112(8):36, 2012.

McGonigle D, Mastrian K: *Nursing informatics and the foundation of knowledge*, ed 2, Burlington Mass, 2012, Jones & Bartlett Learning.

Moore A, Fisher K: Healthcare information technology and medical-surgical nurses, *CIN: Comput Inform Nurs* 30(3):157, 2012.

Nettina S, editor: *Lippincott manual of nursing practice*, ed 9, Philadelphia, 2010, Lippincott Williams & Wilkins.

Pirie S: Documentation and record keeping, *J Perioperative Practice* 21(1):22, 2011.

Sensmeier J: Transforming nursing practice through technology and informatics, *Nurs Manage* 42(11):20, 2011.

Sentinel events statistics for 2011, *Jt Comm Perspect* 32(5):5, 2012.

Sewell J, Thede L: *Informatics and nursing opportunities and challenges*, ed 4, Philadelphia, 2013, Lippincott Williams & Wilkins.

Skiba D: The future of nursing and the informatics agenda, *Nurs Educ Perspect* 31(6):390, 2010.

Staggers N, et al: Nurses' information management and use of electronic tools during acute care handoffs, *West J Nurs Res* 34(2):153, 2011.

The Joint Commission (TJC): *The Joint Commission comprehensive accreditation and certification manual*, eEdition, Oakbrook Terrace, IL, 2012, effective July 12, 2012, Author.

Tschannen D, et al: Nursing medication administration and workflow using computerized physician order entry, *CIN: Comput Inform Nurs* 29(7):401, 2011.

Unwin B, et al: Nursing home care. Part I. Principles and pitfalls of practice, *Am Fam Physician* 81(10):1219, 2010.

US Department Health & Human Services [USDHHS]: *CMS manual system* (Pub. 100-107 State Operations Provider Certification), 2011, http://www.cms.gov/Regulations-and-Guidance/Guidance/Transmittals/Downloads/R70SOMA.pdf. Accessed August 1, 2012.

Walker P: The TIGER initiative: a call to accept and pass the baton, *Nurs Econ* 28(5):352, 2010.

Wood S: Effective record keeping, *Pract Nurs* 39(4):20, 2010.

CHAPTER

11

Communication

evolve WEBSITE

http://evolve.elsevier.com/Potter/essentials

- Crossword Puzzle
- Audio Glossary

OBJECTIVES

- Describe the elements of the communication process.
- Describe the levels of communication and their uses in nursing.
- Differentiate aspects of verbal and nonverbal communication.
- Identify features and expected outcomes of the nurse-patient relationship.
- Describe a nurse's focus within each phase of a therapeutic nurse-patient relationship.
- Describe behaviors and techniques that affect communication.
- Discuss the principles of plain language for promoting health literacy.
- Explain the focus of communication within each phase of the nursing process.
- Discuss effective communication for patients of varying developmental levels.
- Explain techniques used to assist patients with special communication needs.

KEY TERMS

Communication is essential to achieve positive patient outcomes and is a deliberate nursing intervention that you use to engage patients and families in their own nursing care. Therapeutic communication conveys caring and allows you to perform nursing skills and demonstrate professional knowledge more effectively. Establishing competency in therapeutic communication supports quality and safety initiatives and enhances patient satisfaction. In today's complex practice environment it is more important than ever to communicate effectively to provide optimal patient care. Effective

CASE STUDY *Roberto Ruiz*

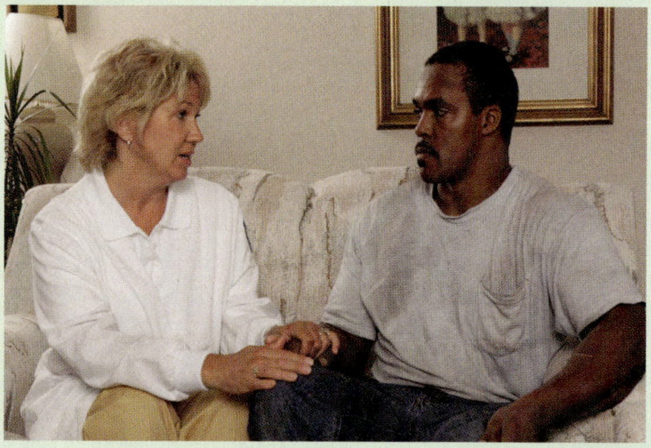

Roberto Ruiz is a 44-year-old man of Puerto Rican descent referred to hospice because he suffers from human immunodeficiency virus (HIV)/acquired immunodeficiency syndrome (AIDS). After being hospitalized in critical condition, Roberto has stabilized and returned home. He is weak and stays in most of the time because of his compromised immune system. He gave his beloved dog to a friend in case he did not survive his last hospitalization. Hospice goals were to support his medication regimen, manage his pain, and promote quality of life.

Roberto lives alone and has an established network of friends, having lived and worked in the community for over 10 years. His home is full of special art objects that he has collected. Roberto appears tired, speaks softly, and smiles frequently. He talks about how his quality of life is the best it has ever been. His home is the place he feels most peaceful.

Suzanne is a 54-year-old nurse whose mother died 10 years ago and received hospice care. This was a brief but significant experience that gave her a dedication to hospice and a commitment to maximizing quality of life in end-of-life care.

health care team communication strengthens nurses' engagement within their work units and organizations and improves nurse retention (Apker, Propp, and Ford, 2009).

You use nonverbal, verbal, and technological skills to communicate in both personal and professional situations. You send and receive information continually even through what is not said but implied by posture, tone of voice, or a facial expression. You communicate in person; in writing; over the telephone or by text; through fax and electronic mail; and with social media, including Facebook and Twitter. Communication in all of these modes is a dynamic and often complex process.

THE POWER OF COMMUNICATION

As with any aspect of treatment, communication may result in both harm and good. Your posture, your expressions and gestures, and every word you choose and phrase you speak can hurt or heal through the messages they send. Even techniques meant to be therapeutic can have unexpected negative effects. Failure to communicate leads to serious problems, increases liability, and threatens professional credibility. Inappropriate or missing communication causes delays in health care delivery and medical errors, increasing the cost to the patient, the health care agency, and society. Therapeutic communication empowers others and enables people to make health-promoting choices.

Self-awareness is important for effective communication (Arnold and Boggs, 2011). As you know more about yourself, you are able to relate to others more effectively. Reflection on your interactions increases your understanding of the communication process and improves your ability to communicate with your patients.

Suzanne reflects on her concerns when she first worked with patients who had HIV/AIDS. Now Suzanne has a very different perspective and is able to see Roberto as a person and not as a fearful disease. Roberto has introduced her to the healing power of music. Seeing how Roberto savors moments of each day, Suzanne begins to pay more attention to appreciating her own life and adds music and art to her daily routine.

BASIC ELEMENTS OF THE COMMUNICATION PROCESS

In your professional nursing role you learn to pay attention to each aspect of the communication process so interactions are purposeful and effective. The basic elements of the communication process are outlined below:

- The **sender** is the person who delivers the message. The roles of sender and receiver change back and forth as two persons interact.
- You send a message to the **receiver.** The message prompts a response. The more the sender and receiver have in common and the closer the relationship, the more likely it is that the receiver will accurately perceive the sender's meaning and respond appropriately.
- The **message** is the content of the conversation, including verbal and nonverbal information that the sender expresses. The most effective message is clear, organized, and expressed in a manner familiar to both the sender and the receiver.
- The message that the receiver returns to the sender is **feedback.** Feedback indicates whether the receiver understood the meaning of the sender's message. Your positive intent is not enough to ensure accurate reception of a message. Seek verbal and nonverbal feedback from the receiver to be sure that the receiver understands the message.
- The **channel** is the means of conveying and receiving messages through visual, auditory, and tactile senses. For example, your facial expression sends a visual message, and spoken words travel through auditory channels. Usually the more channels the sender uses to convey a message, the more clearly the receiver will understand the message.

- **Interpersonal variables** influence communication since the sender and receiver continually influence one another. A nurse may assume a complementary role when functioning as a clinical expert during health teaching and a symmetrical role when developing mutual health promotion goals with a patient.
- The **environment** is the physical and emotional climate in which an interaction takes place. Make the environment comfortable and suitable when sending a message to promote effective communication. The more appropriate the environment, the more successful the communication exchange.

LEVELS OF COMMUNICATION

As a nurse you communicate at different levels. You communicate with yourself, other individuals, and groups. Each level of communication is important and affects your nursing practice. Take advantage of opportunities to role play communication skills in nursing school and maximize continuing education and didactic instruction in your professional nursing role (Kesten, 2011).

Intrapersonal communication, also called *self-talk,* is a powerful form of communication that occurs within an individual. People "talk to themselves" by forming thoughts internally. These thoughts strongly influence perceptions, feelings, behavior, self-concept, and performance. Self-talk is a mental rehearsal for difficult tasks or situations so individuals deal with them more effectively. An example is reflection, which you can use to think back on previous patient care situations so you consider effective and ineffective approaches that you used previously (see Chapter 8). Be aware of the nature and content of your own thinking and try to replace negative, self-defeating thoughts with positive ones. Use positive self-talk to overcome obstacles and boost your confidence as a nurse.

Interpersonal communication is interaction that occurs between two people or within a small group. It refers to nonverbal and verbal behavior within a social context and includes the use of symbols and cues to give and receive meaning. Because messages received are sometimes different from messages intended, validate or mutually negotiate the meaning for all involved. Effective interpersonal communication includes idea and information sharing, problem solving, expressing feelings, making decisions, accomplishing goals, team building, and personal growth.

Public communication is the interaction of one individual with large groups of people. You may have opportunities to speak with groups of patients or consumers about health-related topics. You make special adaptations in eye contact, posture, gestures, voice inflection, and use of media materials to communicate messages effectively.

FORMS OF COMMUNICATION

You send messages in many different ways: verbally, nonverbally, concretely, and symbolically. People express themselves through language, movements, gestures, voice inflection, facial expressions, and use of space. Many forms of communication combine to create meaning in a sender's message.

Verbal Communication

Verbal communication involves the spoken or written word. Verbal language conveys specific meaning as you combine words. The following sections discuss the most important aspects of verbal communication.

Vocabulary. Communication is unsuccessful if a receiver cannot translate a sender's words and phrases. You work with people of various cultures who speak different languages. Even people who speak the same language use subcultural variations of words. For example, *dinner* means a midday meal for some, whereas others use *dinner* to mean the last meal of the day. Medical terms or jargon often sound like a foreign language to someone outside the health care field.

For many individuals with limited English proficiency (LEP), the inability to communicate in English is the primary barrier to accessing health information and services. These patients require you to use professional interpreters who are able to speak the person's primary language. Health information for people with LEP needs to be communicated plainly in their primary language, using words and examples that make the information understandable.

Denotative and Connotative Meaning. A single word sometimes has several meanings. Individuals who use a common language share the **denotative meaning** of a word. The word *baseball* has the same meaning for all individuals who speak English, but the word *code* denotes cardiac arrest primarily to health care providers. The **connotative meaning** is the shade or interpretation of the meaning of a word, which is influenced by the thoughts, feelings, or ideas that people have about the word. Families who are told that a loved one is in serious condition might believe that death is near, but to nurses the term *serious* may simply describe the nature of the illness and not the prognosis.

Pacing. Talking rapidly, using awkward pauses, or speaking extremely slowly and deliberately conveys an unintended message. Consider the following exchange:

> *Patient:* "Do you know if the doctor found anything wrong with me?"
> *Nurse:* "No … but I'm sure if he did … he would have come to explain things to you." (then very rapidly) "Now let's get back to what we were doing."

Long pauses and a rapid shift to another subject may give the impression that you are hiding the truth. Speak slowly, enunciate clearly, and use pauses to stress a particular point or give the listener time to understand.

Intonation and Volume. Tone of voice and volume dramatically affect the meaning of a message, and emotions directly influence tone of voice. A simple question or statement can express enthusiasm, anger, or concern. Be aware of your intonation and volume to avoid sending unintended messages. If a patient interprets your message as uncaring or condescending, communication is blocked. Pay attention to a patient's intonation and volume for information about his or her emotional state or energy level.

Clarity and Brevity. Effective communication is simple, short, and to the point to minimize confusion. Avoid phrases such as "you know" or "OK?" at the end of every sentence. Give examples to clarify messages for the receiver. Use short sentences and words that express an idea simply and directly.

Timing and Relevance. Timing is critical in communication. Even if a message is clear, poor timing prevents it from being effective. Do not begin routine teaching when a patient is in severe pain or emotional distress. The best time for interaction is when a patient expresses an interest in communicating because relevant messages are more effective. When a patient is facing emergency surgery, discussing the risks of smoking is less relevant than discussing what the staff will do to prepare the patient for surgery.

Nonverbal Communication

Nonverbal communication includes messages sent through body language without using words. Nonverbal forms of communication include facial expressions; vocal cues; eye contact; and cues such as gestures, posture, touch, odor, physical appearance, dress, silence, and the use of time (Arnold and Boggs, 2011). Nonverbal communication often accurately reveals true feelings because you may be less censored about nonverbal reactions. A patient who says he feels fine but frowns while moving and holds his body rigidly is probably in pain. Nonverbal cues add meaning to verbal communication and help you judge the reliability of verbal messages. Nonverbal behaviors vary in different cultures so gestures or expressions that are acceptable in one culture may have a different meaning and be considered rude in another culture (Arnold and Boggs, 2011).

Because nonverbal messages are usually not as obvious as verbal messages, it is important to become more aware of nonverbal behavior. Be sure that your nonverbal and verbal messages match. If you say that a patient is getting better but demonstrate an expression of doubt, you do not relieve a patient's anxiety.

Personal Appearance. Physical characteristics, manner of dress and grooming, and jewelry are indicators of well-being, personality, social status, occupation, religion, culture, and self-concept. First impressions are largely based on appearance (Figure 11-1). Your physical appearance influences a patient's perception of their care. You wear uniforms, scrubs, laboratory coats, business suits, or street clothes, depending on your role. Although your dress may not reflect your abilities, it takes longer to establish trust if your clothing differs from a patient's preconceived image.

Posture and Gait. The way people sit, stand, and move is a form of self-expression. Posture and gait reflect emotions, self-concept, and health status. An erect posture and a quick, purposeful gait communicate a sense of well-being and confidence. A slumped posture and slow, shuffling gait may indicate depression or fatigue. Leaning forward conveys attention.

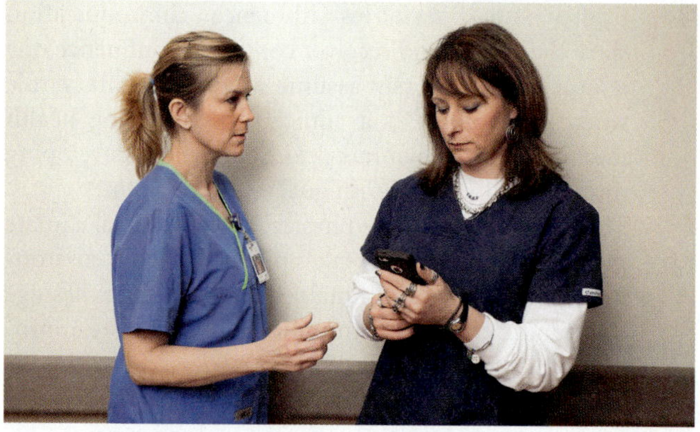

FIGURE 11-1 Contrast between two nurses.

Leaning backward in a more relaxed manner shows less interest or indicates caution.

Facial Expression. The face, the most expressive part of the body, reveals emotions such as surprise, fear, anger, happiness, and sadness. A sender's facial expressions often become the basis for judgments by the receiver. However, because of the diversity in facial expressions, meanings are often misunderstood. Facial expressions reveal, contradict, or suppress true emotions. People are often unaware of the messages their expressions send. When facial expressions are unclear, seek verbal feedback about the sender's intent. A patient who frowns after receiving information may be confused, angry, disapproving, or simply concentrating on a reply. In this case say, "I notice you're frowning," and have the patient clarify his or her response.

Patients watch nurses closely. Consider the effect that your facial expression has on a patient who asks, "Am I going to die?" The slightest change in the eyes, lips, or face reveals your true feelings. Learn to avoid showing overt shock, disgust, dismay, or other distressing reactions in a patient's presence.

Eye Contact. Many Americans, regardless of sociocultural differences, maintain eye contact during a discussion. By maintaining eye contact during conversation, you communicate respect and a willingness to listen. Eye contact allows you to observe another closely. Lack of eye contact may indicate anxiety, defensiveness, discomfort, or a lack of confidence in communicating. However, some cultures such as Asian and Native American consider eye contact to be intrusive or threatening and often avoid direct or prolonged eye contact (Stuart, Cherry, and Stuart, 2011). Always consider a person's culture when interpreting the meaning of eye contact.

Eye movements communicate feelings and emotions. Wide eyes express frankness, terror, and innocence. Downward glances show avoidance or modesty. Raised upper eyelids reveal displeasure, and a constant stare may be associated with hatred or coldness. Looking down on a person establishes authority, whereas interacting at the same eye level indicates equality in a relationship. You appear less dominant and less threatening when interacting at a patient's eye level. Equalizing the eye level with an angry person can diffuse a situation.

BOX 11-1 NURSING ACTIONS WITHIN THE ZONES OF PERSONAL SPACE AND TOUCH

ZONES OF PERSONAL SPACE

Intimate Zone (0 to 18 inches)
- Holding a crying infant
- Performing physical assessment
- Bathing, grooming, dressing, feeding, and toileting a patient
- Changing a patient's dressing

Personal Zone (18 inches to 4 feet)
- Sitting at a patient's bedside
- Taking the patient's nursing history
- Teaching an individual patient
- Exchanging hand-off communication at change of shift

Social Zone (4 to 12 feet)
- Making rounds with a health care provider
- Sitting at the head of a conference table
- Teaching a class for patients with diabetes
- Conducting a family support group

Public Zone (12 feet and greater)
- Speaking at a community forum
- Testifying at a legislative hearing
- Lecturing to a class of students

ZONES OF TOUCH

Social Zone (Permission Not Needed)
- Hands
- Arms
- Shoulders
- Back

Consent Zone (Permission Needed)
- Mouth
- Wrists
- Feet

Vulnerable Zone (Special Care Needed)
- Face
- Neck
- Front of body

Intimate Zone (Great Sensitivity Needed)
- Genitalia
- Rectum

Gestures. A salute, thumbs-up, fist bump, and tapping foot are types of gestures. Hands, shoulders, and feet emphasize, punctuate, and clarify the spoken word. Gestures alone carry specific meanings, or they may create messages with other communication cues. A finger pointed toward a person may communicate several different meanings; but if you frown and have a stern tone of voice, the gesture becomes a sign of accusation or threat.

Territoriality and Space. Territoriality is the need to gain, maintain, and defend one's exclusive right to space. *Territory* is separated and made visible to others such as a fence around a yard. *Personal space* is invisible, individual, and travels with a person. During interpersonal interaction people consciously maintain varying distances between themselves, depending on the nature of the relationship and situation. When personal space is threatened, people respond defensively and communicate less effectively. Examples of nursing actions within the four zones of personal space are listed in Box 11-1 (Kneisl and Trigoboff, 2013).

You must frequently move into patients' territory and personal space because of the nature of caregiving. Convey confidence, gentleness, and respect for privacy, especially when actions require intimate contact. Knock before you enter a room. As you leave, ask if the patient wants the door open or closed. Ask if you can reposition the bed table and clarify which items the patient wants within reach.

FACTORS INFLUENCING COMMUNICATION

Contextual factors influence the nature of communication and interpersonal relationships (Box 11-2). Awareness of these factors helps you to make sound decisions during the communication process.

Metacommunication is exploration of all factors that influence communication. Awareness of influencing factors helps you better understand what is communicated (Arnold and Boggs, 2011). *For example, Roberto smiles and states, "The pain isn't as bad as I thought it would be," but he has pursed lips and is grimacing while speaking.* Your nursing knowledge and experience with assessing a patient's pain makes you sensitive to cultural variations that affect communication. Awareness that a patient's verbal and nonverbal behaviors do not match prompts you to explore his or her feelings and concerns. This analysis of all aspects of communication is metacommunication.

Culture is an important factor influencing communication (see Chapter 20). Culture affects how people communicate, understand, and respond to health information (USDHHS, 2012). Your cultural and linguistic competence can contribute to patients' health literacy. Cultural competence is the ability of health organizations and practitioners to recognize the cultural beliefs, values, attitudes, traditions, language preferences, and health practices of diverse populations and to apply that knowledge to produce a positive health outcome (USDHHS, 2001). Whenever you communicate with patients, try to understand their situation through their eyes. This perspective makes communication more relevant and appropriate to each patient's situation and increases the likelihood of giving patients the information they need for desirable outcomes.

Health Literacy

The health of 90 million people in the United States may be at risk because of the difficulty some patients have in understanding and acting on health information (National Patient Safety Foundation, 2011). It is estimated that one out of five

BOX 11-2 FACTORS INFLUENCING COMMUNICATION

PSYCHOPHYSIOLOGICAL CONTEXT—*INTERNAL FACTORS* INFLUENCING COMMUNICATION

- Physical health (e.g., pain, hunger, weakness, dyspnea)
- Emotional status (e.g., anxiety, anger, depression)
- Growth and development status (e.g., age and developmental stage)
- Unmet needs (e.g., safety/security; love/belonging)
- Attitudes, values, and beliefs (e.g., confidence in health care providers; meaning of illness)
- Perceptions and personality (e.g., optimistic/pessimistic; trusting/nontrusting)
- Self-concept and self-esteem (e.g., positive/negative)

RELATIONAL CONTEXT—*NATURE OF THE RELATIONSHIP* BETWEEN THE PARTICIPANTS

- Social, helping, or working relationship
- Level of trust and self-disclosure between participants
- Degree of sharing among participants
- Shared history of participants
- Balance of power and control

SITUATIONAL CONTEXT—*REASON FOR* THE COMMUNICATION

- Information exchange
- Goal achievement
- Problem resolution
- Expression of feelings

ENVIRONMENTAL CONTEXT—*PHYSICAL SURROUNDINGS* IN WHICH COMMUNICATION TAKES PLACE

- Degree of privacy
- Comfort and safety level
- Noise level
- Presence of distractions

CULTURAL CONTEXT—*SOCIOCULTURAL ELEMENTS* THAT AFFECT THE INTERACTION

- Educational level of participants
- Language and self-expression patterns
- Customs and expectations

American adults reads at the fifth grade level or below, and the average American reads at the eighth to ninth grade level. The language that health care providers choose to use when communicating with patients can significantly impact whether they understand basic health information and the services needed to make appropriate health decisions. Follow these tips when communicating with patients whom you suspect have health literacy problems:

- Organize what you want to say so the most important points come first (e.g., when teaching about a medication, start with its purpose, the dose a patient is to take, and the time to take the medicine. Follow with information about side effects and what to report to a doctor).
- Break complex information into understandable chunks (e.g., "This medicine is for your heart. We want you to take a dose once a day. The best time is in the morning about an hour after you usually have breakfast.").
- Use simple language, avoiding jargon and defining technical terms (e.g., use the term *tablets* instead of medication)
- Use the active voice instead of passive (e.g., "One of the nurses will give you a prescription before you go home" [active]. "The prescription for your medicines is being prepared by one of the nurses" [passive].).

The Nurse-Patient Relationship

As Suzanne works with Roberto, she develops a therapeutic relationship. They work together to manage his pain. Roberto says, "I can stand some pain. I don't want to be 'out of it.' I want to feel alive." Suzanne sees Roberto as a courageous man. His passion for life is inspiring. She knows that posing questions for the patient's reflection helps her assess his needs and support his self-care strategies and end-of-life decision making. She asks, "What are your needs at this time?" and "Tell me about your concerns at this time and for the future." Roberto talks about wanting to get strong enough to have his dog again. He wants to make a trip home to New York to visit his family and make peace.

Helping relationships between you and your patients are created with care and skill and involve effective communication. The purpose of communication within the nurse-patient interaction is to influence a patient's health and well-being (Fleischer et al., 2009). Through **therapeutic communication,** an interactive dynamic process involving verbal and nonverbal exchanges between the nurse and patient, you develop a relationship with a patient to meet health-related goals (Arnold and Boggs, 2011). Box 11-3 summarizes the four phases of the nurse-patient relationship. Help your patients clarify needs and goals, solve problems, and cope with situational or maturational crises. You also help them explore the meaning of their illness experience and sort out responses to stressful situations to increase coping skills (Arnold and Boggs, 2011). Creating a therapeutic environment depends on your ability to communicate, provide comfort, and help patients meet their needs. Comforting strategies include gentle humor, physical comfort measures, emotionally supportive statements, and therapeutic touch. You provide information, support patients' active decision making, and offer opportunities for patients to engage in social exchange.

Nurse–Health Team Member Relationships

Effective communication with other members of the health care team positively influences teamwork and staff satisfaction and improves quality of patient care and safety (Beckett and Kipnis, 2009). To ensure quality and promote a culture of safety, health care organizations must address behaviors that threaten the performance of the health care team, including interpersonal skills and professionalism (TJC, 2008).

BOX 11-3 NURSING INTERVENTIONS DURING PHASES OF THE THERAPEUTIC RELATIONSHIP

PREINTERACTION PHASE—BEFORE MEETING THE PATIENT

- Review available data, including the medical and nursing histories.
- Talk to other caregivers who may have information about the patient.
- Anticipate health concerns or issues that may arise.
- Identify a location and setting that fosters comfortable, private interaction.
- Plan enough time for the initial interaction.

ORIENTATION PHASE—WHEN YOU AND THE PATIENT MEET AND GET TO KNOW ONE ANOTHER

- Set the tone for the relationship by adopting a warm, empathetic, caring manner.
- Recognize that the initial relationship may be casual, uncertain, and tentative.
- Expect the patient to test your competence and commitment.
- Closely observe and expect to be closely observed by the patient.
- Begin to make inferences and form judgments about patient messages and behavior.
- Assess the patient's health status.
- Prioritize patient problems and identify patient goals.
- Clarify the patient's and your roles.
- Form contracts with the patient to specify roles.
- Let the patient know when the relationship will end.

WORKING PHASE—WHEN YOU AND THE PATIENT WORK TOGETHER TO SOLVE PROBLEMS AND ACCOMPLISH GOALS

- Encourage and help the patient express feelings about his or her health.
- Encourage and help the patient with self-exploration.
- Provide information needed to understand and change behavior.
- Encourage and help the patient to set goals.
- Take actions to meet the goals set with the patient.
- Use therapeutic communication skills to facilitate successful interactions.
- Use appropriate self-disclosure and confrontation.

TERMINATION PHASE—DURING THE ENDING OF THE RELATIONSHIP

- Remind the patient that termination is near.
- Evaluate goal achievement with the patient.
- Reminisce about the relationship with the patient.
- Separate from the patient by relinquishing responsibility for his or her care.
- Achieve a smooth transition for the patient to other caregivers as needed.

Breakdown in communication among health care professionals is the most frequent cause of serious injuries and death in health care settings (Tschannen et al., 2011). Not surprisingly, each of the National Patient Safety Goals (TJC, 2014) is directly or indirectly related to communication. A risk for miscommunication exists when patients move from one nursing unit to another or from one provider to another. **Hand-off communication** is the verbal and written exchange of pertinent information during this transition of care (Ong and Coiera, 2011). Open and accurate communication, particularly during hand-offs, is essential to prevent errors.

Use of common language when communicating critical information helps prevent misunderstandings and creates a culture of safety. **SBAR** (pronounced S-BAR) has become a best practice for standardizing communication between health care providers. SBAR stands for *s*ituation, *b*ackground, *a*ssessment, and *r*ecommendation (Institute for Healthcare Improvement, 2011). *In the case study, when Roberto's pain is no longer adequately controlled, Suzanne communicates to Roberto's health care provider that he needs better pain control (situation) and gives the health care provider brief information about his history, noting that Roberto does not want to be "out of it" (background). She then gives an accurate description of his pain (assessment) and requests a modification of his pain regimen (recommendation).* Research indicates that effective communication with the health care provider and other health team members ensures patient safety and promotes optimal patient outcomes (Box 11-4).

Nurses work as a team. Effective communication and camaraderie among nurses in a work setting is essential for teamwork, which affects nurse recruitment and retention. Social, informational, and therapeutic interactions help team members build morale, accomplish goals, and strengthen working relationships. In fact, collegial relationships between all health care providers is characterized by communication elements of openness, accuracy, timeliness, and understanding are consistent with Magnet Hospital properties and support professional nursing practice (Manojlovich, Antonakos, and Ronis, 2009). Interprofessional collaboration is characterized by effective communication, respect, trust, and availability and is a key factor in reducing error and improving patient outcomes (Tschannen et al., 2011). Multidisciplinary care rounds or huddles improve teamwork by bridging the communication gap between care providers, reduce caregiver stress, facilitate the communication of consistent health information to patients and caregivers, and promote conflict resolution (Boos et al., 2010). Appropriate conflict-resolution strategies are essential in your professional nursing practice because conflict cannot be eliminated from the workplace; you should approach conflict as an opportunity for joint problem solving and personal and professional growth (Mahon and Nicotera, 2011).

Compassion fatigue is a relatively new term in the nursing literature. It is defined as a combination of secondary traumatic stress and burnout (Figley, 1995). Secondary traumatic stress occurs when you witness patients' experiences and stories of pain, fear, and suffering and you feel similar pain, fear, and suffering because you care (Figley, 1995). For example, an oncology nurse experiences secondary traumatic stress after observing over and over the disabling side effects that patients have from chemotherapy. Burnout occurs when your perceived demands of caregiving outweigh the resources

BOX 11-4 EVIDENCE-BASED PRACTICE

PICO Question: Do hand-off communication techniques compared with traditional end-of-shift report reduce sentinel events among acute care hospitalized patients?

SUMMARY OF EVIDENCE

Effective communication with a health care provider and other members of the health care team promotes optimal patient outcomes. The Joint Commission (TJC) (2008) reported that breakdown in communication was the root cause of sentinel events between 1995 and 2005. Sentinel events are unexpected occurrences that result in death or serious injury. Communication when the patient is handed over from one provider to another or from one setting to another is especially a problem. Hand-off communication occurs during nurse change-of-shift report, transfer of patients between units or facilities, report between departments such as from the emergency department to an inpatient unit and between disciplines such as physical therapy and nursing. Communication is also important when nurses are communicating changes in a patient's condition to other members of the health care team. Common language for communicating critical information can help prevent misunderstandings (Beckett and Kipnis, 2009). Health care providers need to allow sufficient time to ask and respond to questions. Reading back information also helps to identify any miscommunication and ensures that information received is accurate. Intimidating and disruptive behaviors affect communication and must not be tolerated in health care settings.

APPLICATION TO NURSING PRACTICE

- Develop common language for critical information for hand-off communications and communication of changes in a patient's condition (Beckett and Kipnis, 2009).
- Use a communication tool such as SBAR to standardize communication (IHI, 2011).
- Use a standardized format for change of shift report and hand-off communication.
- Use a standardized format for report when patients are transferred to other units or facilities (IHI, 2011).
- Provide the opportunity for questions and confirmation of understanding of communication.
- Have face-to-face communication when possible.
- Read back all health care provider orders or other pertinent information.
- Create a culture of patient safety that has zero tolerance for intimidating and disruptive behavior.
- Work in multidisciplinary teams to develop common language.
- Develop skills in assertive communication and conflict management.

you have available. For example, when you perceive that team members are not willing to work and collaborate together, it takes a toll on you and causes burnout. When a nurse experiences ongoing stressful patient relationships, he or she often disengages (Slatten, David Carson, and Phillips, 2011). This disengagement can also occur when perceived stress comes from nurse-physician relationships. It is not uncommon for nurses who are experiencing compassion fatigue to become angry, cynical, and have difficulty relating with patients and co-workers (Young et al., 2011). Although not yet established through research, compassion fatigue may be a condition leading to what is described as *lateral violence.*

Research confirms that health care providers do not always voice concerns about patients and actively avoid conflict in clinical settings (Lyndon, Zlatnik, and Wachter, 2011). **Lateral violence** (also called *horizontal violence*) sometimes occurs in nurse-nurse interactions and includes behaviors such as withholding information, making snide remarks, and demonstrating nonverbal expressions of disapproval such as raising eyebrows or making faces. New graduates and nurses new to a unit are most likely to face problems with lateral or horizontal violence. All nurses require resiliency skills to better manage the stressors that contribute to compassion fatigue and lateral violence, including skills in stress and conflict management, building connections with chosen colleagues to share difficult stories, and self-care to help them deal with difficult situations and be successful in providing safe and effective care (Mahon and Nicotera, 2011).

COMMUNICATION WITHIN CARING RELATIONSHIPS

Therapeutic communication strengthens all caring relationships established within the professional role. You create caring and helping relationships with the qualities and behavior explained in this section.

Establishing a Therapeutic Relationship

Professionalism. A patient's acceptance of you as a professional often depends on the manner in which you convey a professional and caring image. Verbal and nonverbal behaviors influence the helping relationship. Professional appearance, demeanor, and behavior are important in establishing trustworthiness and competence. When you act professionally, you communicate that you have assumed the professional helping role, you are clinically skilled, and your focus is on the patient. Inappropriate appearance and behavior in those who hold a professional role harm the image of nursing. Consider the level of trust a patient feels with each nurse in the following examples.

Annie Robbins is late for her shift. She walks on the unit chewing gum. She has a large chunky necklace and long dangling hair, and her underwear is visible beneath her uniform. Annie is wearing heavy makeup and perfume, has long painted fingernails, and her breath and clothing smell of smoke. Her name tag is not easily visible. She giggles, talks loudly, uses slang, rolls her eyes, grimaces, and writes vital signs on the skin of her hand. Annie reacts to problems by blaming others.

Mary Kline arrives at work on time and is organized, well prepared, and equipped for the responsibilities of her nursing role. She is clean and well-groomed, wears a clean pressed uniform, and is scent and odor free. She wears a simple pair of gold stud earrings. Her behavior reflects warmth, friendliness, confidence, and competence. She speaks clearly, uses good grammar, and listens to others. She helps and supports teammates, communicates effectively, and handles problems in a mature manner.

Courtesy. Professional courtesy conveys respect for others and oneself. It includes saying hello and goodbye, knocking on doors before entering, introducing oneself, and stating one's purpose. Other aspects of courtesy are addressing people by name, saying "please" and "thank you" to team members, and apologizing for making an error or causing someone distress. These are all parts of professional communication. When you are discourteous, patients and staff perceive you as rude or insensitive. This sets up barriers between you and your patients and causes friction or tension among team members.

Self-introduction is especially important. Failure to give your name, indicate your professional status, or acknowledge a patient creates uncertainty about an interaction and conveys an impersonal lack of commitment or caring. Make eye contact and smile. Initially acknowledge others by name to show your respect for the dignity and uniqueness of the other person. Begin initial interactions by including a title and the patient's last name to show respect. Ask others how they would like you to address them and let them know your personal preference as well. Using first names is appropriate for infants, young children, confused or unconscious patients, and close team members.

Showing genuine interest in a patient as a person is important in establishing a therapeutic relationship. As you get to know a patient and family, use limited social conversation to make connections. Commenting on a patient's choice of music, television show, reading materials, or personal items in the room can demonstrate interest; but you must move beyond social conversation to discuss issues or concerns affecting the patient's health.

Avoid Terms of Endearment and Excessive Socializing. Calling a patient "honey," "dear," "Grandpa," or "sweetheart" rather than by a personal name is inappropriate. Such casual familiarity from caregivers offends most people. Avoid referring to patients by diagnosis, room number, or other attribute. When you refer to them by characteristics rather than their names, it is demeaning and depersonalizing and sends the message that you do not care enough about the person to know him or her as an individual. Spending too much time socializing can undermine opportunities to establish a professional presence and a focus on meeting health-related goals.

Confidentiality. Always safeguard a patient's right to privacy by carefully protecting information of a confidential nature. Reassure patients that you will keep information private and keep that promise. Resist the temptation to share exciting or shocking information. Do not share information with people who are genuinely interested and concerned but have no legal right to the information.

Patient: "What's wrong with my roommate? She seems so sick."

Nurse: "I know you're concerned about Mrs. Hoover, but I can't share any personal information about a patient."

If you have to report information to others, tell the patient in advance, if possible. Sharing personal information or gossiping about others violates the ethical code and practice standards of nursing. It sends the message that you are not trustworthy and damages interpersonal relationships.

Trust. Trust is an essential building block of a therapeutic relationship. You foster trust when you communicate warmth and caring and demonstrate consistency, reliability, honesty, and competence. Trusting another person involves risk and vulnerability; but it also fosters open, therapeutic communication and enhances the expression of feelings, thoughts, and needs. Do not compromise trust by sending the message to patients that you are "too busy." Such a response becomes a protective excuse for not becoming involved with patients. It may also be a symptom of compassion fatigue.

Being untrustworthy or dishonest seriously damages relationships and violates legal and ethical standards of practice. Do not withhold key information, lie, or distort the truth. For example, a patient asks why the nurse is collecting his 24-hour urine sample again.

Nurse, lying: "The laboratory wants us to repeat the test because their machine broke down during the analysis and they need a fresh specimen."

A better response is, "I'm sorry, Mr. Rankins. We didn't send enough of your urine to the laboratory. We'll make every effort to ensure that enough is saved this time."

Acceptance and Respect. Conveying acceptance means that you are nonjudgmental and demonstrate unconditional respect. As a nurse you are expected to provide high-quality care regardless of social or economic status, personal attributes, or the nature of an illness. Acceptance includes giving positive feedback, making sure that verbal and nonverbal cues match, and using touch appropriately. Being empathetic, restating, and avoiding arguments also show acceptance and respect.

Presence. The concept of presence is an interpersonal process that is characterized by sensitivity, holism, intimacy, vulnerability, and adaptation to unique circumstances (Finfgeld-Connett, 2006). It involves conveying closeness and a sense of caring. By being present for another person when needed, you offer your presence even when the patient does not express the need verbally. You do this by showing a caring attitude, demonstrating your willingness to listen and talk, or just being physically present (see Chapter 19). Do not avoid patients whose behavior is troublesome. Such avoidance often increases the patient's negative behavior. Being *task oriented,* or making a technical procedure (e.g., administration of a medicine) your priority, is another way of not being emotionally available. You miss opportunities to assess patients, explore their concerns, calm anxiety, demonstrate empathy, teach, or involve patients in care. Patients perceive you as cold, uncaring, and unapproachable when you are task oriented. As a student it is difficult to integrate therapeutic communication when you perform technical skills because of the need to focus on the procedure. In time you learn to do both and promote more satisfactory interactions. Consider the quality of care given in each of the following scenarios.

> *Nurse A silently enters the patient's room:* "It's time for your pain shot."
>
> The patient, Mr. Stewart, is mildly startled and grimaces. Nurse A again tells him that she has a pain shot but does not offer further explanation. She quickly reaches for his arm, gives the injection, disposes of her supplies, and leaves the room without asking if the patient has other needs.
>
> *Nurse B, calling the patient's name as she enters the room:* "Mr. Stewart, I have your pain medication. Are you feeling as uncomfortable as you look?"
>
> *Patient:* "Yes, my back feels like a knife went through it. Will the pain ever go away?"
>
> *Nurse B lays syringe down and sits by patient:* "It's common to have some pain the first few days after surgery, but I'll work with you to keep you comfortable. This medicine should help. I'll give the shot and then show you how to move in bed so the pain won't get worse. I'll check back with you to confirm that you're more comfortable."

Nurse B assessed the patient's need for a caring presence, set aside her own task, and became available for the patient. Notice that this intervention was brief yet more effective than that of Nurse A. Question the assumption that nurses do not "have time" for caring connections. Caring is essential for effective care.

COMMUNICATION WITHIN THE NURSING PROCESS

In the nursing process you use communication to gather information for developing nursing diagnoses, planning your care, implementing nursing interventions, and evaluating your care (see Chapter 9). You also may use the nursing process to address patients' communication problems. Although the nursing process is a reliable framework for delivering comprehensive patient care, it does not work well unless you master the art of therapeutic communication. Successful communication occurs with knowledge acquired from books, experiences, and observation of others' communication skills. Communication techniques used within the nursing process are also applied during the problem-solving process with team members to resolve problems or accomplish goals within the clinical setting (Box 11-5).

BOX 11-5 COMMUNICATION EXAMPLES THROUGHOUT THE NURSING PROCESS

ASSESSMENT
- Verbal interviewing and history taking
- Visual observation of nonverbal behavior
- Visual, auditory, and tactile data gathering during physical examination
- Written medical records, diagnostic tests, and literature review

NURSING DIAGNOSIS
- Intrapersonal analysis of assessment findings
- Interpersonal validation of health care needs and priorities with patient and family
- Written and electronic documentation of nursing diagnosis

PLANNING
- Interpersonal team and interprofessional health planning sessions
- Interpersonal discussions with patient and family to determine methods of implementation
- Written or electronic documentation of expected outcomes and overall plan of care
- Written and/or verbal referrals to health care professionals

IMPLEMENTATION
- Verbal discussion with other health professionals
- Verbal, visual, auditory, and tactile health teaching
- Provision of support through therapeutic communication techniques
- Contact with other health resources
- Written and/or electronic documentation of patient's progress in medical record

EVALUATION
- Acquisition of verbal and nonverbal feedback
- Written analysis of actual and expected outcomes
- Identification of factors affecting outcomes
- Modification and update of written or electronic care plan
- Verbal and/or written explanation of revisions to patient

ASSESSMENT

Use communication during the assessment phase of the nursing process to gather information about a patient. The accuracy and completeness of the initial assessment can be compromised if patient and family communication needs are not identified and addressed (Walton, 2011). The time you spend assessing patients is a good time to establish the rapport needed for good communication. For example, through therapeutic communication techniques, you collect data about the patient's medical history and current problem or concern. *To learn more about Roberto's pain, Suzanne asks him several questions, including, "How is your pain different than it was last week?" "What has been most effective recently in managing your pain?" and "What concerns do you have about your pain?"* Systematically collect data and organize the data you collect. Document information you obtain from the patient, family, and significant others.

Physical and Emotional Factors. Assess physical or psychological factors that influence communication. Many altered health states limit communication, including facial trauma, cancer of the larynx or trachea, aphasia after a stroke, breathing problems, Alzheimer's disease, high anxiety, pain, and heavy sedation. Certain mental illnesses cause patients to have impaired communication such as pressured speech, constant verbalization of the same words or phrases, or a slow speech pattern. Review a patient's medical record for relevant information. The record describes any physical barriers to speech, neurological deficits, and pathophysiological conditions affecting hearing or vision. Also review the medication record. Opiates, antidepressants, antipsychotics, hypnotics, or sedatives cause patients to slur words or use incomplete sentences. Communicate directly with patients and family members to fully assess communication difficulties and build a plan to enhance communication.

Developmental Factors. Consider a patient's developmental level when assessing communication. An infant's self-expression is limited to crying, body movement, and facial expression. Older children express their needs more directly. Pay attention to your nonverbal behavior when working with children. Sudden movements, threatening gestures, and loud noises can be frightening. Include the parents as sources of information about the child's health.

Advancing age can influence communication. Problems with hearing, vision, or speech are barriers to communication. Assess the hearing ability and visual acuity of older adults (see Chapter 16). Get an older adult's attention before you begin your assessment questions. Face the patient and stand or sit on the same level so the patient can read your lips. Speak slowly and clearly. Give older adults enough time to ask questions. Remember, do not assume that an older adult has communication impairments.

Sociocultural Factors. When caring for patients from diverse cultural backgrounds, recognize how to adapt your communication approach. Show respect for all people regardless of their age, gender, religion, socioeconomic group, sexual orientation, or ethnicity. Recognize and attend to any personal biases or prejudices that might interfere with patients' care. Take cultural issues into account and work to be culturally sensitive. Accept patients' rights to adhere to cultural customs and norms. People of various cultures use different types of verbal and nonverbal cues to convey meaning. Make a conscious effort not to interpret messages through your own cultural perspective; instead consider the context of the other individual's background. Avoid stereotyping people from other cultures or making jokes about them (see Chapter 20). Consider the cultural sensitivity that the nurse demonstrates in our case study:

Suzanne arrives at Roberto's home for a visit. He offers her a snack and a beverage. She knows that Roberto has limited resources but graciously accepts the food and drink because she understands that in the Puerto Rican culture it would be insulting to refuse. Suzanne learns that Roberto wants to travel to New York to see his family. With further assessment she learns that he has several siblings living nearby and that the family in New York consists of two uncles and several cousins. Her understanding of the importance of the extended family in the Puerto Rican culture helps her appreciate the importance of the trip to New York. Expressing an understanding of the importance of the trip, even though he is in poor health, demonstrates cultural sensitivity.

Cultural insensitivity in communication takes many forms, including making fun of another's beliefs, practices, ethnicity, language, or dress. Telling jokes that make fun of ethnic groups, stereotyping obese patients, patronizing, and incorrectly interpreting culturally based behavior are examples of being culturally insensitive. Listen to patients' stories. Respect their views, opinions, and attitudes. Do not behave in ways that offend the cultural practices of others. In the previous example, Suzanne did not refuse her patient's offer of food and drink or question why he felt it important to see more distant relatives.

Language. Language barriers may exist with foreign-born patients and those who speak English as a second language. It is essential that you assess the patient's understanding of all communication and obtain a professional interpreter to ensure accurate communication. Do not allow family members to interpret important information that you need to obtain from patients.

Gender. Gender influences how we think, act, feel, and communicate. Being unaware of or insensitive to potential gender communication patterns can block the development of a therapeutic nurse-patient relationship. You need to assess communication patterns of each individual and not make assumptions simply based on gender. There may be differences in male and female communication patterns in health care settings, although gender does not need to be a barrier in developing therapeutic communication with patients (Arnold and Boggs, 2011).

NURSING DIAGNOSIS

After collecting assessment data from a patient, cluster pertinent defining characteristics for patterns and problems. Success in accurately identifying the patient's communication problem ensures the formulation of an accurate nursing diagnosis. Nursing diagnoses for patients with communication difficulties often include the following:

- *Compromised Family Coping*
- *Ineffective Coping*
- *Readiness For Enhanced Family Coping*
- *Powerlessness*
- *Impaired Social Interaction*

Impaired Verbal Communication is the nursing diagnosis to describe a patient who has limited or no ability to communicate verbally. It is defined as difficulty or inability to use or understand language in interpersonal reactions (Herdman, 2012). A patient with this diagnosis has defining characteristics such as the inability to articulate words, difficulty forming words, and difficulty understanding. This diagnosis is useful for a wide variety of patients with special problems and needs related to communication. The related factor for a diagnosis should focus on the cause of the communication disorder. In the case of impaired verbal communication, a related factor might be physiological, mechanical, anatomical, psychological, cultural, or developmental. Be accurate in choosing a related factor so the interventions you select will effectively resolve the patient's problem.

PLANNING

Once you identify the nature of a patient's communication problem, you must consider several factors to design a plan of care. For example, motivation improves communication. Patients often need encouragement to try different communication strategies. In addition, select interventions and communication techniques appropriate for the patient's age, cultural background, and practices. Give patients adequate time to practice new communication approaches. It also helps to plan practice sessions in a quiet, private environment. When possible, involve the family in selecting approaches that foster communication with the patient.

Goals and Outcomes. A plan of care supporting effective communication has the ultimate goal of enabling a patient to communicate his or her needs. Select expected outcomes that are specific and measurable. After you have implemented your interventions, outcomes allow you to determine if your goal was achieved. For example, the outcomes for Roberto include the following:

- Patient identifies two methods to maintain communication with family in New York.
- Patient verbalizes his concerns regarding his declining health.
- Patient initiates conversation about his preferences for care as he becomes weaker.

Sometimes you care for patients who have difficulty sending, receiving, and interpreting messages. This interferes with healthy interpersonal relationships. In this case impaired communication is a contributing factor to other nursing diagnoses such as *Impaired Social Interaction* or *Ineffective Coping*. Plan interventions that help patients improve their communication skills. For example, writing down key points or participating in role play helps patients rehearse situations in which they have difficulty communicating.

Setting Priorities. Always include a patient in setting goals and expected outcomes. You will not make any progress if a patient is not interested in achieving the goal you chose. You cannot address all problems at the same time; consider which is most important. Always maintain an open line of communication so a patient can express any immediate needs or problems. Keep a call light in reach for the patient restricted to bed or provide appropriate alternative communication devices such as a message board or Braille computer. If you plan to have a lengthy discussion with a patient, be sure to take care of his or her physical needs first to avoid interruptions. Make a patient comfortable by ensuring that any symptoms are under control.

Continuity of Care. Remember to include family caregivers during the planning and implementation phases of the nursing process. This collaboration supports the family and patient. When you use collaboration, patients are more likely to adhere to the treatment plan. Collaboration also promotes communication among family members to facilitate positive patient-family relationships. Encourage collaboration by asking others for ideas and suggestions about how to reach goals. It gives them the opportunity to express themselves and strengthens problem-solving ability.

In addition, collaborate with other health care providers who have expertise in communication strategies. Speech therapists help patients with aphasia. Professional interpreters are invaluable when a patient speaks a foreign language. Mental health advanced practice nurses help to communicate with angry or highly anxious patients.

IMPLEMENTATION

In carrying out any plan of care, nurses need to use communication techniques that are appropriate for patients' individual needs. Before learning how to adapt communication methods to help patients with serious communication impairments, it is necessary to learn therapeutic communication techniques that are the foundation of professional communication. It is also important to understand which communication techniques create barriers to effective interaction.

Therapeutic Communication Techniques. Therapeutic communication techniques are specific responses that encourage the expression of feelings and ideas and convey acceptance and respect (Box 11-6). By learning therapeutic communication techniques you become aware of the variety of nursing responses appropriate in different situations. Although some of the techniques may seem artificial or unnatural at first, your skill and comfort increase with practice and experience. Satisfaction results as you achieve outcomes using the therapeutic relationships you form.

Conveying Empathy. **Empathy** is the ability to understand and accept another person's perspective (Arnold and Boggs, 2011). You can never totally know another's experiences because you are not in that person's situation, but you can try to understand and acknowledge what the person is experiencing.

Empathic statements reflect an understanding of what a patient communicated and inform the patient that you heard both the feeling and the factual content of the communication. This allows a patient to validate or clarify feelings and perceptions. Empathic responses are neutral and nonjudgmental and foster shared respect. Use them to establish trust in very difficult situations. *In the case study Roberto stated that he did not want to be "out of it" and that he wanted to feel alive. An empathic response from Suzanne is, "It sounds like you don't like to take much pain medicine because feeling out of it makes it hard to do the things you want to do. I'm concerned that too much pain might also make it difficult for you to do what you want to do."*

Active Listening. **Active listening** means being attentive to what a patient is saying both verbally and nonverbally. Active listening facilitates patient communication. The ancient Greek philosopher Epictetus stated, "We have two ears and one mouth so we may listen more and talk less." That is good advice for nurses. Active listening enhances trust

BOX 11-6 THERAPEUTIC COMMUNICATION TECHNIQUES

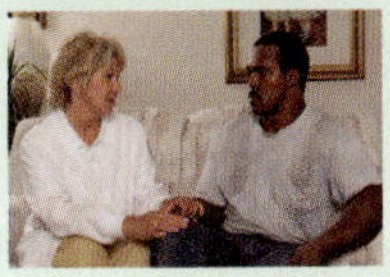

Roberto now expresses the desire to visit his family in New York and make peace with them. In one conversation about his relationship with his family, Suzanne demonstrates the use of several therapeutic communication techniques.

USING SILENCE

Suzanne sits quietly with Roberto and allows him time to collect his thoughts.

PARAPHRASING

Roberto: "I have some stuff I need to work out with my uncle, so I need to go see him."

Suzanne: "You feel it is important to go visit your uncle to address some unresolved issues."

CLARIFYING

Roberto: "Yeah, and I can't deal with the problems with my uncle when I'm out of it."

Suzanne: "When you say 'out of it,' do you mean the medication makes it hard to think straight?"

INSTILLING HOPE

Roberto: "I just don't know if I'll be able to make the trip to see my uncle, and it's really important to work things out with him."

Suzanne: "I believe you will find a way to make peace with your uncle."

because a nurse communicates acceptance and respect for a patient. Several nonverbal skills facilitate attentive listening. You identify them by the acronym SOLER (Townsend, 2009):

- **S**—*S*it facing the patient. This posture gives the message that you are there to listen and are interested in what the patient is saying.
- **O**—*O*bserve an open posture (e.g., keep arms and legs uncrossed). This posture suggests that you are open to what the patient says. A closed position conveys a defensive attitude, possibly provoking a similar response in the patient.
- **L**—*L*ean toward the patient. This posture conveys that you are involved and interested in the interaction.
- **E**—*E*stablish and maintain eye contact. This behavior conveys your involvement in and willingness to listen to what the patient is saying. Absence of eye contact or shifting the eyes gives the message that you are not interested in what the patient is saying. Be aware of cultural considerations regarding eye contact.
- **R**—*R*elax. It is important to communicate a sense of being relaxed and comfortable with the patient. Restlessness communicates a lack of interest and conveys a feeling of discomfort to the patient.

Sharing Observations. Nurses make observations by commenting on a patient's appearance and how he or she sounds or acts. Stating observations often helps a patient communicate without the need for extensive questioning, focusing, or clarification. This technique helps start a conversation with quiet or withdrawn persons. Do not state observations that will embarrass or anger a patient such as telling someone, "You're a mess!" Even if such an observation is made with humor, a patient can misinterpret the intent.

Sharing observations differs from making assumptions, which means drawing unnecessary conclusions about the other person without validating them. Making assumptions puts a patient in the position of having to contradict you. Examples include your interpretation of a patient's fatigue as depression and assuming that untouched food indicates lack of interest in meeting nutritional goals. Making observations is a gentler and safer technique: "I see you didn't eat any breakfast.," "You look tense.," or a positive observation such as, "I see you've been organizing your papers."

Using Silence. It takes time and experience to become comfortable with silence. Most people have a natural tendency to fill empty spaces with words, but sometimes silence is useful when they face decisions that require much thought. *For example, if Roberto and Suzanne were discussing the possibility of his needing to move out of his home to get the care he needs, silence could give him time to collect his thoughts and consider the alternatives.* Silence is especially therapeutic during times of sadness or grief.

Providing Information. Providing relevant information helps your patients make decisions, experience less anxiety, and feel safe and secure. Speak in simple language and translate medical terms. When offering options, stress that the patient has the right to make decisions. Provide information that enables others to understand what is happening and what to expect. *For example, Suzanne explains, "Roberto, this pain medicine may make you feel a little sleepy and groggy at first, but those side effects usually go away after 2 or 3 days."*

Clarifying. Clarifying validates whether the person interpreted the message correctly. Any time a message is unclear or ambiguous, try to restate it or ask the other person to restate it, explain further, or give an example of what he or she means. *For example, Suzanne says, "I'm not sure what you mean; when you say 'out of it,' do you mean that the medicine makes it difficult to think straight?"*

Focusing. Focusing directs conversation to a specific topic or issue when a discussion becomes unclear. It limits the area to which the sender can respond. Use it when the sender rambles or introduces many unrelated topics in the same conversation. *For example, if Roberto said, "I had a nice visit with my friend this morning. He's going to stop over tomorrow. I've been able to take care of my dog better. My medicines are doing okay, but the pain's still there. I've been looking at my art collection today, and I'm not sure what I want to do with it when I'm gone. You like art—I could recommend a good gallery if you want to buy some." Suzanne focuses the conversation by replying, "You've been thinking about what to do with your special belongings?"*

Paraphrasing. Paraphrasing is restating the sender's message in the receiver's own words to make sure that the receiver has received information accurately. Be careful not to change the meaning when you paraphrase. Confirm the meaning with the patient. *For example, Roberto states, "I've been walking more, and I'm able to do most of my housework. I don't need as much help around here now." Suzanne replies, "You feel you're getting stronger and more independent. Is that correct?"*

Summarizing. Summarizing is a concise review of main ideas from a discussion. It brings a sense of satisfaction and closure to an individual conversation or during the termination phase of a nurse-patient relationship. By reviewing a conversation, you focus on key issues and obtain additional relevant information as needed. *For example, after a session with much discussion about Roberto's plans and progress, Suzanne summarizes, "Today we talked about your plans to visit your family in New York and some things you can do to help increase your strength. You seem to understand the importance of eating right. Let me know if there is any other information I can get for you."*

Self-Disclosure. You may use self-disclosure during the working phase of a helping relationship. Self-disclosures are personal statements intentionally revealed to the other person. The purpose is to model and educate, foster a therapeutic alliance, validate reality, and encourage autonomy (Stuart, 2013). Keep self-disclosures relevant and appropriate. Make these statements to benefit the patient, not you, and use them sparingly so the patient remains the focus of the interaction. *Roberto's brother comes to visit and expresses how hard it is to make time for everything. An inappropriate response from Suzanne would be, "My mother had cancer and was in hospice too. It was so long and drawn out. I was so sad for so long. Even taking care of the kids was hard." An appropriate response is, "When my mother was dying, I was torn between wanting to stay with her every moment and trying to meet the needs of my family. Is that how it is for you?"*

Instilling Hope. Nurses recognize that hope is essential for healing and learn to communicate a "sense of possibility" to others (see Chapter 21). You give hope by commenting on the positive aspects of the other person's behavior, performance, or response. Sharing a realistic vision of the future and reminding others of their resources and strengths also strengthens hope. You can reassure patients that there are many kinds of hope and that meaning and personal growth can come from illness experiences.

Nontherapeutic Communication Techniques. Certain communication techniques hinder or damage professional relationships. These specific techniques are nontherapeutic and often cause recipients to use defenses to avoid being hurt or negatively affected. Nontherapeutic techniques discourage further expression of feelings and ideas and often result in negative responses or behaviors in others.

Inattentive Listening. Behaviors and nonverbal expressions such as fidgeting, breaking eye contact, daydreaming during conversation, and pretending to listen convey the message that what the sender has to say is not important. These behaviors discourage conversation and damage trust. Further examples are looking at your watch, tapping your foot impatiently, and documenting at the computer with your back to the patient.

Overusing Medical Vocabulary. Health care professionals have their own culture and language. Using technical words in discussions with patients can cause confusion and anxiety. Avoid excessive use of such terms or translate them into lay terms (e.g., medicine instead of medication, what you eat or drink instead of intake, get worse or better instead of progressive, shot instead of injection).

Prying or Asking Personal Questions. Asking irrelevant personal questions simply to satisfy your curiosity is inappropriate and invasive. Limit questions to health-related information.

Giving Approval or Disapproval. Do not impose your own attitudes, values, beliefs, and moral standards on others while in the professional helping role. People have the right to be themselves and make their own decisions. Avoid using terms such as *should, ought, good, bad, right,* or *wrong.* Agreeing, disagreeing, or sharing your personal opinion sends the subtle message that you are making value judgments about patient decisions. Instead offer options and help the other person anticipate the consequences of decisions. The problem and its solution belong to the patient, not you.

Roberto: "I really want to visit my uncles in New York, but I'm not sure I'm up for the trip."

Suzanne: "I don't think it's a good idea to try to travel that far."

A better response is, "It sounds like you want to see your family but are worried about your ability to travel right now. Let's talk about other ways you can stay in contact with them."

Changing the Subject. Changing the subject is a common problem when you are uncomfortable with a topic, but it is insensitive and tends to block further communication.

Automatic Responses. Clichés or stereotypical remarks such as, "You're never given more than you can handle," tend to belittle a patient's feelings and minimize the importance of his or her message. These automatic phrases communicate that you are not taking concerns seriously or responding thoughtfully.

False Reassurance. When a patient is seriously ill or distressed, you may be tempted to offer hope with statements such as, "I'm sure everything will be okay." Although you may be trying to be kind, false reassurance discounts the patient's concerns or situation and tends to block communication.

Asking for Explanations. Sometimes asking "why" implies an accusation and results in resentment, insecurity, and mistrust. Try to phrase questions without using "why." Rather than, "Why aren't you taking the medicines the doctor prescribed?" you could say, "Tell me about the problems you're having with your medicines."

Arguing. Challenging or arguing with someone's perception of a situation denies that his or her perceptions are real. It implies that they are lying, misinformed, or uneducated. *If Roberto tells Suzanne that he has no appetite and is not eating, her response of, "You must be eating; you haven't lost any weight" would block communication. Suzanne needs to present information in a way that avoids argument. A better response* *is, "I see that you've not lost any weight; tell me how you're meeting your nutritional needs since you don't have much of an appetite."*

Being Defensive. When patients express criticism, listen to what they have to say. Listening does not imply agreement. To discover reasons for a patient's anger or dissatisfaction, you need to listen uncritically. By avoiding defensiveness you are able to defuse anger and uncover deeper concerns. Rather than saying, "None of the nurses would intentionally ignore you," you respond, "You feel the nurses are ignoring you."

Sympathy. Sympathy is the concern, sorrow, or pity that you feel for a patient when you personally identify with his or her needs. Unlike empathy, which tries to understand a patient's experience, sympathy takes a subjective look at the patient's world. Sharing sympathy with another feels good, creates a bond, and minimizes differences; but it can prevent effective problem solving and impair good judgment. When you share a patient's needs, you are assuming that his or her feelings are similar to your own, and you are unable to help the patient select realistic solutions for problems. *For example, in the case study, if in response to Roberto's statement about his pain, Suzanne had said, "Oh, I know just what you mean. I hate feeling drugged," Roberto would not have had a chance to clarify his feelings, and Suzanne would miss an opportunity to get a deeper understanding of his perception of the situation.*

Decision Making and Communication. As a nurse you constantly make decisions about what, when, where, why, and how to send messages to others. Deciding which techniques best fit each unique nursing scenario is challenging. Many situations that arise in a complex and demanding practice environment challenge your decision-making skills and call for careful use of therapeutic techniques. Practice helps; therefore take the initiative to discuss and role play these scenarios before facing them in the clinical setting.

Assertiveness and Autonomy. Assertive communication is based on a philosophy of protecting individual rights and responsibilities. It includes the ability to be self-directive in acting to accomplish goals and advocate for others. An assertive response promotes self-esteem and upholds personal and professional rights. Feelings of security, competence, power, and professionalism characterize assertive responses. Assertive statements convey a message without resorting to sarcasm, whining, anger, blaming, or manipulation. Assertive responses are good tools to deal with criticism, change, negative conditions in personal or professional life, and conflict or stress in relationships. Negative interactions among nurses such as those that define horizontal or lateral violence adversely affect communication and collaboration (Longo and Smith, 2011).

Assertive responses often contain "I" messages, such as "I want," "I need," "I think," or "I feel." Simple assertive messages are usually stated in three parts, referencing the nurse, the other individual's behavior, and its effect.

> *Nurse to nurse:* "When you're late for work, I have to stay late, and that makes me late picking up my children from the babysitter."

> *Nurse to supervisor:* "I'm confused to hear you say I'm not performing well because I was told by my preceptor that I was meeting expectations. Please give me some examples of what you mean."

Avoiding Passive Responses. Passive responses avoid issues or conflict. Some characteristics are feelings of sadness, depression, anxiety, and hopelessness.

> *Nurse to loud and angry co-worker:* "I'm so frustrated; whatever you say."

A better response is, "This has been difficult. What can we do to make things better?"

Avoiding Aggressive Responses. Aggressive responses provoke confrontation at the other person's expense. Some characteristics of aggression are feelings of anger, frustration, resentment, and stress.

> *Nurse to angry patient:* "You can't talk to me that way."

A better response is, "I want to hear your concerns and help you have a positive experience. Can we talk about them now or should I come back later?"

Humor. Humor is a coping strategy that adds perspective and helps you and a patient adjust to stress. Laughter is a diversion from stress-related tension. It provides a sense of well-being and more of a feeling of control or mastery. Humor provides emotional support to patients and humanizes the illness experience. Laughter provides both a psychological and physical release for you and the patient; promotes open, relaxed interaction; and reinforces our shared experience in being human.

You assess whether humor is appropriate by noticing if patients use it in their conversations. Start with small examples to see if this is helpful. To offer positive humor, share humorous incidents or situations or share puns or simple jokes that are not offensive. Positive humor is associated with hope, love, and joy, with the intent to bring people closer. Avoid negative humor, which is inappropriate in a health care setting. Ethnic, religious, sexist, ageist, or put-down humor creates distance. Realize that humor sometimes backfires; not everyone appreciates a humorous approach because of negative moods, stress, or physical discomfort. Humor is often a signal for closer attention. When a patient preparing for surgery quips, "Well, I won't die from it," gently explore his or her concerns.

Sometimes health care providers use dark, negative humor after difficult or traumatic situations to survive a situation intact and relieve tension and stress. This "coping humor" may seem callous or uncaring by those not involved in the situation. Avoid using coping humor within earshot of patients or their loved ones. Understand that humor is a release; but timing, content, and receptivity are important in the use of therapeutic humor (Arnold and Boggs, 2011).

Touch. Touch is one of a nurse's most potent forms of communication. Nurses are privileged to experience more of this intimate form of personal contact than almost any other

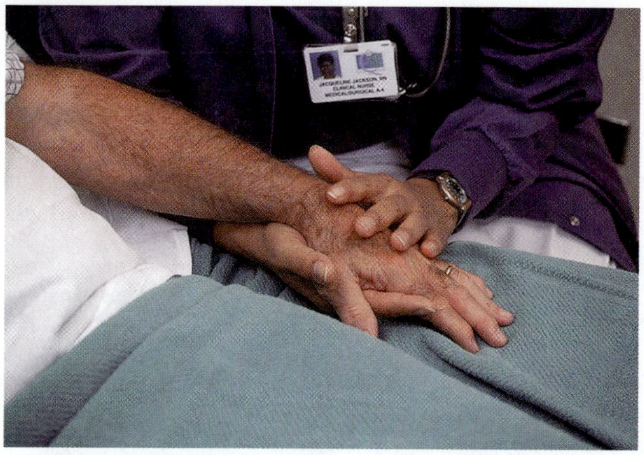

FIGURE 11-2 A nurse uses touch to communicate.

professional. Touch conveys affection, emotional support, encouragement, and personal attention (Figure 11-2). Therapeutic touch such as holding a hand is important for vulnerable patients who are experiencing severe illness with its accompanying physical and emotional losses. Sometimes touch is misinterpreted. Always be sensitive to a patient's response to touch. Following are examples of inappropriate and appropriate use of touch:

In a cancer support group the wife of a patient tearfully describes how overwhelmed she is feeling.

> *Inappropriate touch*: A nurse moves too quickly and tries to hug the wife without permission. The wife backs off and struggles to hold back more tears.
>
> *Appropriate touch*: A nurse says, "I see you're distressed (while placing her hand gently on the patient's shoulder)." The nurse attends to both the patient's verbal and nonverbal response to this touch.

Another concern is the confusion about the use of touch with culturally diverse patients (see Chapter 20). You must look for cues that a patient would welcome touch. We use touch to awaken patients, get their attention, or add emphasis to explanations. Touch may also convey understanding better than words or gestures, but is important to ask a patient what is culturally appropriate or forbidden.

Because much of what you do involves touching patients, learn to use touch wisely. The zones of touch are described in Box 11-1. Touch delivered in the social or consent zone is less anxiety producing than touch delivered in the vulnerable or intimate zone. Students initially find giving intimate care stressful, especially with patients of the opposite sex. Shift your focus from personal discomfort and focus on the intent to provide sensitive nursing care. Trust that you become more comfortable with experience. Remember that the patient who is ill and dependent must permit closer physical contact than is normally tolerated and may be uncomfortable with touch. Remain sensitive to your own responses and to patients' feelings. If a patient refuses to hold your hand while in pain or pulls away from physical contact, this signals that he or she is uncomfortable with being touched. People perceive touch negatively when it is given without consent; used within a hostile or mistrusting relationship; or delivered to a vulnerable, intimate, or painful area of the body. Your touch should never be angry, rough, violent, overly stimulating, threatening, overly tentative, sexual, or unnecessarily painful.

Communicating with Patients with Special Needs. Many health-related and developmental issues contribute to impaired communication. Promoting effective communication in nonvocal patients includes assessing communication needs, identifying alternative communication strategies, and creating an individualized plan of care (Grossbach, Stanberg, and Chlan, 2011). This includes a ventilator-dependent patient who cannot speak or an infant who is limited to crying, body movement, and facial expression. Others with special needs are patients who are hearing and visually impaired, people suffering from a stroke or late-stage Alzheimer's disease, and those on the autistic spectrum or with schizophrenia who respond to internal stimuli and misinterpret external stimuli. Patients who are deaf/hard of hearing or who have limited English proficiency require individualized communication approaches. People with limited English proficiency, including those who do not speak or understand English and patients with learning disabilities and limited vocal skills, challenge you to accommodate their special needs. In addition, unresponsive or heavily sedated patients are sometimes unable to send or receive verbal messages.

The patient who cannot communicate effectively has difficulty expressing needs and responding appropriately to the environment. Such people benefit greatly when you adapt communication techniques to their circumstances (Box 11-7). When caring for a patient with *Impaired Verbal Communication related to a language barrier, your first priority is to have a professional interpreter made available. If this cannot be achieved,* provide a list with pictures of simple words in the patient's language. The patient's use of these key images enables him or her to communicate basic needs such as food, water, toileting, rest, and pain relief. Collaborate with team members to design the best communication strategies.

Effective communication improves the quality of your patient's interpersonal relationships and well-being. If the patient uses ineffective communication techniques that interfere with coping or interpersonal relationships, intervene to help him or her send, receive, and interpret messages more effectively. Be a communication role model and teacher to help patients express needs, feelings, and concerns. Help patients develop social interaction skills and communicate thoughts and feelings clearly. This helps them interpret messages sent from others, increasing their autonomy and assertiveness. Methods such as role-playing allow patients to practice situations in which they have difficulty communicating.

Providing Alternative Communication Methods. Patients with physical communication barriers (e.g., those with a laryngectomy or endotracheal tube) may be unable to speak, or the clarity of speech may be so poor that they need alternative methods of communication (see Box 11-7). To decrease

BOX 11-7 COMMUNICATING WITH PATIENTS WHO HAVE SPECIAL NEEDS

PATIENTS WHO ARE HEARING IMPAIRED

- Ensure that patient has access to working hearing aids and glasses.
- Reduce environmental noise and distractions.
- Speak at a normal volume and avoid shouting.
- Rephrase vs. repeat if misunderstood.
- Punctuate speech with facial expression and gestures.
- Provide a sign language interpreter if needed.

PATIENTS WHO ARE VISUALLY IMPAIRED

- Ensure that patient has access to glasses, corrective lenses, and/or magnifying lenses.
- Communicate verbally before touching the patient.
- Orient the patient to sounds in the environment.
- Ensure that lighting is adequate for the patient to see the speaker.
- Identify yourself when entering the room and notify the patient when leaving the room.
- Modify written handouts to accommodate degree of visual impairment.
- Offer audio tapes for instructional information.

PATIENTS WHO ARE MUTE, UNABLE TO SPEAK, OR CANNOT SPEAK CLEARLY

- Answer call light in person.
- Listen attentively, be patient, and do not interrupt or finish patient's sentences.
- Ask simple questions that require "yes" or "no" answers.
- Allow time for understanding and responses.
- Use visual cues (e.g., words, pictures, objects) when possible.
- Allow only one person to speak at a time.
- Use normal volume and do not shout or speak too loudly.
- Let the patient know if you do not understand.
- Use communication aids as needed:
  - Pad and felt-tipped pen or Magic Slate
  - Flash cards
  - Communication board with words, letters, or pictures denoting basic needs
  - Computer toy ("speak and spell" type) for children
  - Call bells or alarms
  - Sign language
  - Use of eye blinks or movement of fingers for simple responses ("yes" or "no")
- Be attentive and responsive to restless physical movements (Grossbach, Stanberg, and Chlan, 2011).

PATIENTS WHO ARE COGNITIVELY IMPAIRED

- Reduce environmental distractions while conversing.
- Prioritize communication over other tasks (Hemsley, Balandin, and Worrall, 2011).
- Get the patient's attention before speaking.
- Use simple sentences and avoid long explanations.
- Avoid shifting from subject to subject.
- Ask one question at a time.
- Allow time for the patient to respond.
- Include family and friends in conversations when appropriate.

PATIENTS WHO ARE UNRESPONSIVE

- Call the patient by name during interactions.
- Communicate both verbally and by touch.
- Speak to the patient as though he or she could hear.
- Explain all procedures and sensations.
- Provide orientation to person, place, and time as needed.

PATIENTS WHO DO NOT SPEAK ENGLISH

- Speak to the patient in a normal tone of voice (shouting may be interpreted as anger).
- Establish a method for the patient to signal the desire to communicate (call light or bell).
- Avoid using family members, especially children, as interpreters.
- Provide a professional interpreter/translator as needed:
  - Use a person familiar with the patient's culture and with health care if possible.
  - Allow plenty of time for the interpreter to transmit messages.
  - Communicate directly to the patient and family rather than the interpreter.
  - Ask one question at a time.
  - Avoid making comments to the interpreter about the patient or family (they may understand some English).
- Develop a communication board, pictures, or cards using words translated into English for the patient to make basic requests (e.g., pain medication, water, elimination).
- Have a dictionary (e.g., English/Spanish) available if the patient can read.
- Provide written materials in English and in patient's primary language.

frustration, provide simple communication methods and allow the patient time to respond. The patient must be physically able to use the method you provide (e.g., communication boards or pencil and pad). Patients who are unable to speak are at risk for injury unless they are able to communicate personal needs quickly.

Communicating with Children. Communication with a child requires special considerations to develop a working relationship with the child and family. Confirm that information communicated by parents is consistent with other reports, including from the child. Offer a child toys or materials so the parent gives full attention to your information gathering. Give periodic attention to infants and younger children as they play to include them. An older child can be actively involved in communication. Consider the influence of development on language and thought processes.

Children, particularly the young, are especially responsive to nonverbal messages. Sudden movements or gestures can be frightening. Remain calm and gentle and, if possible, let a child make the first move. Use a quiet, friendly, confident tone of voice. A child feels helpless in most situations involving health care personnel, which makes it particularly important to facilitate the presence of parents. When giving explanations or directions, use simple, direct language and be honest.

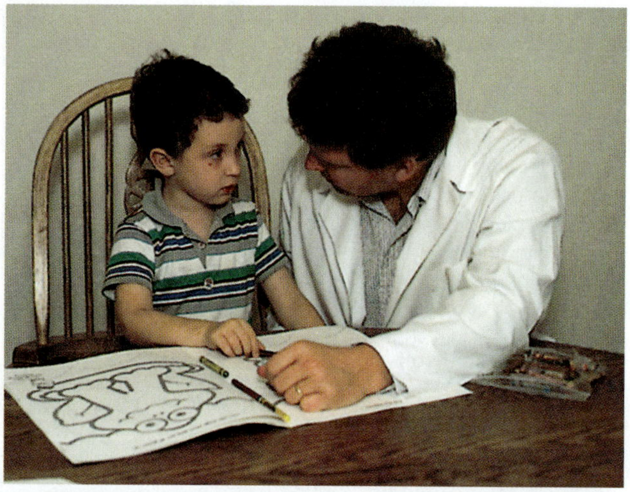

FIGURE 11-3 Drawing helps children communicate.

To minimize fear and anxiety, prepare a child by explaining what to expect and seeking input from parents when appropriate. Avoid staring and meet a child at eye level.

Drawing and playing with young children allows them to communicate nonverbally (making the drawing) and verbally (explaining the picture). Use a child's drawing as a basis for beginning a conversation (Figure 11-3).

Communicating with Older Adult Patients. Most older adults experience some loss of sensory function, which interferes with sending or receiving messages clearly. Many older adults adapt to sensory losses and learn to communicate effectively. When obvious deficits exist, maximize existing motor and sensory function to help patients communicate more effectively (see Box 11-7). You can make some simple modifications in your approach and the environment to improve communication with older adults (Box 11-8). Identify these challenges and work with patients to enhance effective communication.

EVALUATION

Together you and the patient determine the success of the plan of care by evaluating patient communication outcomes. Ask yourself if you understood what your patient communicated, if your patient had the opportunity to express feelings and concerns, and if your patient has unresolved needs.

Patient Care. Evaluate whether communication interventions were effective. Compare the expected outcomes you established in the plan of care with the actual outcomes you observe when interacting with patients. If you meet jointly established outcomes, you have resolved the goals of care and the nursing diagnosis. When outcomes remain unmet, you may revise the existing plan with new goals, outcomes, and/or interventions. For example, if using a pen and paper proves frustrating for a nonverbal patient whose handwriting is shaky, you revise the care plan to include use of a picture board instead. In this case observing the patient's handwriting and asking other caregivers about his or her success in communicating needs are your evaluation measures.

BOX 11-8 CARE OF THE OLDER ADULT

Improving Communication

In communicating with older adults the primary goal is to establish a reliable communication system that all health care team members easily understand. Ideally an interdisciplinary model delivers effective care for older adults. Communication with older adults requires special attention. Be aware of the physical, psychological, and social changes of aging. Use the following interventions to assist with impaired communication with older adults:

- During conversation maintain a quiet environment that is free from background noise.
- Avoid shifting from subject to subject; allow time for conversation.
- Be an attentive listener. Use explorative questions to facilitate conversation.
- Avoid long sentences to explain the subject. Try to keep it short, simple, and to the point.
- Allow older adults the opportunity to reminisce. Reminiscing has therapeutic properties that increase the sense of well-being.
- If you are experiencing problems understanding a patient, let the patient know and facilitate methods that help him or her speak more clearly. Consult with a speech therapist if necessary.
- Include a patient's family and friends in conversations, particularly in subjects known to the patient.
- Be aware of cultural differences among patients.

Remember that careful evaluation requires you to make observations similar to those in your original assessment. For example, after initially assessing the extent of a patient's ability to hear the spoken word and providing various interventions to promote hearing, you return to evaluate his or her ability to hear any interaction or instruction. It is also helpful to question the patient about whether needs were adequately met.

You should evaluate the effectiveness of your own communication by reflecting on the success of your verbal and nonverbal interactions with patients. This is useful in determining how your communication style might improve.

Patient Expectations. Review evaluation findings to decide if the patient's expectations of care were met. This is an important part of the evaluation process. Ask patients and their families for input about goal achievement, factors that affected outcomes, and suggestions for changes in the plan of care. *Suzanne consistently asked Roberto if the pain medications were relieving his discomfort. He was pleased that she was open to working with him to balance pain management with the clarity of his thinking.*

Avoiding patient input during evaluation and care plan modification leads to a task-oriented rather than a critical thinking, patient-centered approach to nursing. It denies the patient's right to see the total picture of care and be involved in all phases of the nursing process. *A goal of total pain relief for Roberto was incompatible with his own goals of being alert enough to care for his dog and interact with his extended family. Suzanne's willingness to consistently reevaluate the plan of care affected Roberto's quality of life. She used her therapeutic communication skills to engage the team in holistic care to address his goals for body, mind, and spiritual well-being. They focused on helping Roberto live every moment of his life the way he wanted to live it.*

KEY POINTS

- Communication is a powerful therapeutic tool and an essential nursing skill used to influence others and achieve positive health outcomes.
- Nurses consider many contexts and factors influencing communication when making decisions about what, when, where, how, why, and with whom to communicate.
- Communication is most effective when the receiver and sender accurately perceive the meaning of one another's messages.
- Effective verbal communication requires appropriate intonation, clear and concise phrasing, proper pacing of statements, and proper timing and relevance of a message.
- Effective nonverbal communication complements and strengthens the message conveyed by verbal communication.
- Strengthen helping relationships by establishing trust, empathy, autonomy, confidentiality, and professional competence.
- Effective communication techniques are facilitative and tend to encourage the other person to openly express ideas, feelings, or concerns.
- Ineffective communication techniques inhibit or block the other person's willingness to openly express ideas, feelings, or concerns.
- It is not uncommon for nurses who are experiencing compassion fatigue to have difficulty relating with patients and co-workers.
- A nurse blends social and informational interactions with therapeutic communication techniques so others explore feelings and manage health issues.
- The language that health care providers choose to use when communicating with patients can significantly impact whether patients understand basic health information.
- When using therapeutic humor, consider timing, receptivity, and content of the humorous intervention.
- Older adults with sensory, motor, or cognitive impairments require the adaptation of communication techniques to make up for their loss of function and special needs.

CLINICAL DECISION-MAKING EXERCISES

Roberto Ruiz developed pneumonia and became very weak. You are filling in for Suzanne while she is on vacation and come to check on him. You find him in bed, and he has not eaten since the evening before because he is too weak to fix a meal, his oxygen saturation level is low, and he is having pain with frequent coughing. It is apparent that he is not able to care for himself.

1. You believe that Roberto needs either hospitalization on a general medical floor or inpatient hospice care. Roberto is adamant that he will not leave his home. Which communication techniques would you use to address this concern?
2. You approach Roberto and put your hand on his shoulder. He responds angrily and tells you to leave him alone. What should you do?
3. Which factors are influencing Roberto's communication?
4. Roberto wants his pneumonia treated, but he does not want extraordinary measures taken. You call Roberto's primary health care provider, give an update on his condition, and determine the immediate plan of care. How could you best communicate with the health care provider?

evolve

Answers to Clinical Decision-Making Exercises can be found on the Evolve website.

QSEN ACTIVITY: PATIENT-CENTERED CARE

Roberto's condition has worsened, and he has reluctantly agreed to be admitted to an inpatient general medical unit participating in a Transforming Care at the Bedside (TCAB) initiative to promote a culture of quality and safety consistent with Quality and Safety Education for Nurses (QSEN). You understand that providing patient-centered care recognizes the patient as the source of control and as a full partner in providing compassionate and coordinated care (Cronenwett et al., 2007). The unit has identified several ways to improve communication among the health care team and with patients, including moving the location of the change-of-shift report to the bedside and establishing nurse-physician "intentional" rounds at the bedside (Chapman, 2009).

As the nurse caring for Roberto, state the plain language you will use with Roberto to describe the rationale behind conducting hand-off communication at the bedside.

How, if at all, do you adapt your communication with your co-workers since Roberto not only can hear everything you say but also is encouraged to participate in the exchange?

Describe how you communicate Roberto's values, preferences, and expressed needs to other members of the health care team who have never cared for Roberto, including his hospitalist, during morning huddle.

evolve

Answers to QSEN Activities can be found on the Evolve website.

REVIEW QUESTIONS

1. A patient states, "No one talked with me about a change in my medications, so just bring me what I take at home." Which of the following responses by the nurse is the best example of a therapeutic communication technique?
   1. "You must take your medications to get better and return home."
   2. "Your doctor wouldn't have prescribed these if you didn't need them."
   3. "Why don't you trust the care that you're receiving?"
   4. "I understand that you're concerned. Let me tell you about the medications."
2. A patient states, "I'm not sure my doctor has ordered the right medication for my hypertension." Which of the following responses is the most therapeutic as an immediate response?
   1. "So you're concerned that this medication may not be right for you?"
   2. "Why don't you think this is the right medication?"
   3. "I'll get some written information about this medication for you to read."
   4. Use silence and direct eye contact until the patient speaks again.
3. A nurse is attempting to establish a therapeutic relationship with an angry, depressed patient on a medical surgical unit. Which of the following is the best nursing intervention?
   1. Use humor to soften the intensity of the patient's anger.
   2. Establish a social friendship with the patient.
   3. Empathize with the patient as he describes current stressors.
   4. Establish daily time limits for the patient to talk negatively about his situation.
4. A nurse has a new surgical patient whose temperature spiked to 102.9° F. The nurse calls the health care provider using SBAR to structure the communication. List the order in which the nurse communicates the patient information.
   1. The surgical site is clean and dry.
   2. The patient has a history of systemic infections.
   3. The patient is febrile.
   4. The nurse requests an order for an antipyretic.
5. Which of the following nursing actions helps you establish a therapeutic relationship with a patient for whom English is not the primary language?
   1. Call all patients by first name unless they request otherwise.
   2. Provide the patient with a professional interpreter.
   3. Perform all care as quickly as possible and leave the room so the patient can rest.
   4. Engage in personal conversations with other members of the health care team while providing care.
6. A nursing professor overhears a nursing student say to a patient, "This is your third admission this month. Why did you stop taking your medication again?" Which of the following statement(s) would be most helpful for the student nurse to hear from her clinical instructor? (Select all that apply.)
   1. "Asking a why question could be interpreted as criticism. How could you have asked your question differently?"
   2. "Your question is good because it forced the patient to describe his thoughts and feelings about being medication noncompliant."
   3. "Your nonverbals showed genuine concern for your patient's readmission. It is important that your verbal statements and nonverbal messages match to avoid sending mixed messages."
   4. "I like the way you tied his readmission to his medication noncompliance. The confrontation sets the stage for the current hospitalization."
7. A female patient of Native American descent is upset and tells the nurse that the nursing assistant makes her feel uncomfortable when he looks into her eyes. Which of the following interventions is most appropriate for the nurse?
   1. Promote cultural sensitivity by teaching the nursing assistant that direct eye contact can be misinterpreted by some Native Americans.
   2. Ask the patient about a sexual abuse history.
   3. Assure the patient that the nursing assistant will be assigned to other patients.
   4. Inform the patient to use the Patient Satisfaction Survey to record her concerns anonymously.
8. An 84-year-old is admitted to a medical floor for severe malnutrition and dehydration. His wife, who has been the sole dependent care agent, appears tired, frail, and angry when she visits. She remarks, "Let's see what you can do with him." The nurse's most therapeutic response would be:
   1. "You must be relieved that your husband didn't die."
   2. "Tell me what you mean by, "Let's see what you can do with him."
   3. "We know how to care for patients like your husband."
   4. "It's too bad you didn't have any help to care for him at home."
9. You are caring for an 80-year-old woman, and you ask her a question while you are across the room washing your hands. She does not answer. What should you do next?
   1. Leave the room quietly because she evidently does not want to be bothered right now.
   2. Repeat the question in a loud voice, speaking very slowly.
   3. Move to her bedside, get her attention, and rephrase the question while facing her.
   4. Bring her a communication board so she can express her needs.
10. A 68-year-old man was diagnosed with Alzheimer's disease 4 years ago. The patient's cognitive abilities have since deteriorated, and the patient is withdrawn and frustrated. Which nursing intervention would be most helpful when communicating with this patient with a cognitive disorder?

1. Stand within 6 inches of the patient when providing direction.
2. Speak in a low monotone voice when communicating with the patient.
3. Ask only "yes" and "no" questions when talking to the patient.
4. Break tasks into small steps, giving one instruction at a time.

evolve

Rationales for Review Questions can be found on the Evolve website.

1. 4; **2.** 1; **3.** 3; **4.** 3, 2, 1, 4; **5.** 2; **6.** 1, 3; **7.** 1; **8.** 2; **9.** 3; **10.** 4.

REFERENCES

Apker J, Propp KM, Ford WS: Investigating the effect of nurse-team communication on nurse turnover: relationships among communication processes, identification, and intent to leave, *Health Commun* 24(2):106, 2009.

Arnold EC, Boggs KU: *Interpersonal relationships: professional communication skills for nurses*, ed 6, St Louis, 2011, Elsevier.

Beckett CD, Kipnis G: Collaborative communication: integrating SBAR to improve quality/patient safety outcomes, *J Healthc Qual* 31(5):19, 2009.

Boos VD, et al: The comprehensive care rounds: facilitating multidisciplinary communication among caregivers of complex patients in the neonatal intensive care unit, *Adv Neonatal Care* 10(6):301, 2010.

Chapman KB: Improving communication among nurses, patients, and physicians, *Am J Nurs* 109(11): 21, 2009.

Cronenwett L, et al: Quality and safety education for nurses, *Nurs Outlook* 55(3):122, 2007.

Figley C: *Compassion fatigue: coping with secondary traumatic stress disorder in those who treat the traumatized*, 1995, Psychology Press.

Finfgeld-Connett D: Meta-synthesis of presence in nursing, *J Adv Nurs* 55:708, 2006.

Fleischer S, et al: Nurse-patient interaction and communication: a systematic literature review, *J Public Health* 17:339, 2009.

Grossbach I, Stanberg S, Chlan L: Promoting effective communication for patients receiving mechanical ventilation, *Crit Care Nurse* 31(3):46, 2011.

Hemsley B, Balandin S, Worrall L: Nursing the patient with complex communication needs: time as a barrier and a facilitator to successful communication in hospital, *J Adv Nurs* 68(1):116, 2011.

Herdman TH, editor: *NANDA International: Nursing diagnoses: definitions and classification 2012-2014*, Oxford, 2012, Wiley Blackwell.

Institute for Healthcare Improvement (IHI): *SBAR technique for communication: a situational briefing model*, 2011, http://www.ihi.org/knowledge/Pages/Tools/SBARTechniqueforCommunication ASituationalBriefingModel.aspx. Accessed August 23 2013.

Kesten KS: Role-play using SBAR technique to improve observed communication skills in senior nursing students, *J Nurs Educ* 50(2):79, 2011.

Kneisl CR, Trigoboff E: *Contemporary psychiatric–mental health nursing*, ed 3, Boston, 2013, Pearson.

Longo J, Smith MC: A prescription for disruptions in care: community building among nurses to address horizontal violence, *ANS Adv Nurs Sci* 34(4):344, 2011.

Lyndon A, Zlatnik MG, Wachter RM: Effective physician-nurse communication: a patient safety essential for labor and delivery, *Am J Obstet Gynecol* 205(2):91, 2011.

Mahon MM, Nicotera AM: Nursing and conflict communication: avoidance as preferred strategy, *Nurs Admin Q* 35(2):152, 2011.

Manojlovich M, Antonakos CL, Ronis DL: Intensive care units, communication between nurses and physicians, and patients' outcomes, *Am J Crit Care* 18(1):21, 2009.

National patient safety foundation: *Health Literacy: statistics at-a-glance*, 2011, http://www.npsf.org/wp-content/uploads/2011/12/AskMe3_Stats_English.pdf. Accessed August 23, 2013.

Ong MS, Coiera E: A systematic review of failures in handoff communication during intrahospital transfers, *TJC J Qual Patient Saf* 37(6):274, 2011.

Slatten LA, David Carson K, Phillips P: Compassion fatigue and burnout: what managers should know, *Healthc Manager* 30(4):325, 2011.

Stuart B, Cherry B, Stuart J: *Pocket guide to culturally sensitive health care*, Philadelphia, 2011, FA Davis.

Stuart GW: *Principles and practice of psychiatric nursing*, ed 10, St Louis, 2013, Elsevier.

The Joint Commission (TJC): *Sentinel Event Alert*, Issue 40, 2008, http://www.jointcommission.org/sentinel_event_alert_issue_40_behaviors_that_undermine_a_culture_of_safety/. Accessed August 23, 2013.

The Joint Commission (TJC): *National Patient Safety Goals*, Oakbrook Terrace, IL, 2014, The Commission. Available at http://www.jointcommission.org/standards_information/npsgs.aspx.

Townsend MC: *Psychiatric mental health nursing: concepts of care*, Philadelphia, 2009, FA Davis.

Tschannen D, et al: Implications of nurse-physician relations: report of a successful intervention, *Nurs Econ* 29(3):127, 2011.

US Department of Health and Human Services (USDHHS): *National standards for culturally and linguistically appropriate services in health care*, Washington, DC, 2001, Office of Minority Health.

US Department of Health and Human Services (USDHHS): *Quick guide to health literacy*, 2012, http://www.health.gov/communication/literacy/quickguide/factsbasic.htm. Accessed August 23, 2013.

Walton MK: Communicating with family caregivers, *Am J Nurs* 111(12):47, 2011.

Young J, et al: Compassion satisfaction, burnout, and secondary traumatic stress in heart and vascular nurses, *Crit Care Nurs Q* 34(3):227, 2011.

CHAPTER 12

Patient Education

evolve WEBSITE

http://evolve.elsevier.com/Potter/essentials

- Crossword Puzzle
- Audio Glossary

OBJECTIVES

- Identify appropriate topics for a patient's health education needs.
- Describe the similarities and differences between teaching and learning.
- Identify the purposes of patient education.
- Describe the domains of learning.
- Differentiate factors that determine readiness to learn from those that determine ability to learn.
- Compare the nursing and teaching processes. Write learning objectives for a teaching plan.
- Describe the characteristics of an environment that promotes learning.
- Identify the principles of effective teaching and learning.
- Describe ways to adapt teaching for patients with different learning needs.
- Discuss ways to adapt teaching approaches for patients with low health literacy.
- Use the nursing process to make a teaching plan of care.
- Describe ways to incorporate teaching with routine nursing care.
- Identify methods for evaluating learning.
- Use the Teach Back method to confirm patient understanding and learning.
- Describe appropriate documentation of teaching and learning.

KEY TERMS

affective learning, p. 205
analogies, p. 218
attentional set, p. 206
cognitive learning, p. 205
health literacy, p. 211
learning, p. 204
learning objective, p. 204
motivation, p. 206
psychomotor learning, p. 206
reinforcement, p. 217
return demonstration, p. 218
Teach Back, p. 220
teaching, p. 204

Being a patient educator is one of the most important professional nursing roles because education is essential to patient safety, health, and well-being. Factors such as shorter hospital stays, the focus on reducing hospital readmissions within 30 days, and the increased demand on nurses' time complicate the ability to provide timely quality patient education. Nurses need to find the most effective way to educate patients because health care consumers continue to be more assertive in seeking information, understanding health, and finding resources available within the health care system. Providing patients with self-care information is necessary to ensure continuity of care from the hospital to the home. Patient education is important because the patient has a right to know and be informed about diagnosis and prognosis of illness, treatment options, how to perform care activities in the home, and risks associated with treatments. A

CASE STUDY *Latinka Drusko*

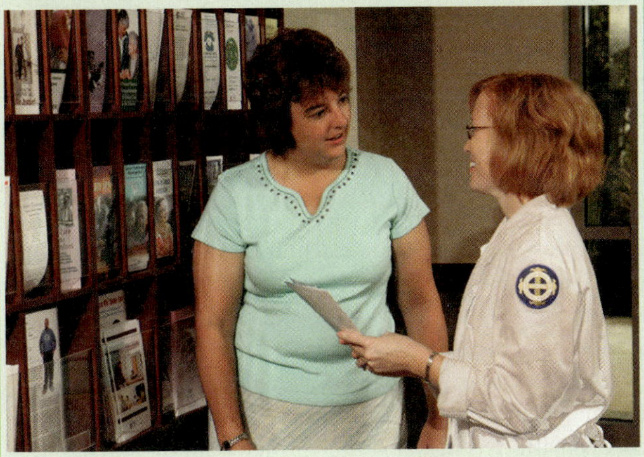

Latinka Drusko is a 55-year-old accountant. She immigrated to the United States from Bosnia in 1991 and has two grown sons who live close to her. Her husband died recently. Latinka is overweight and smokes 1 to 1½ packs of cigarettes a day. She is visiting her advanced practice nurse for her annual physical.

Ashley is a 23-year-old nursing student assigned to care for Latinka. During their first visit, Latinka states, "I'd like to get some information to help me become healthier. I would like to stop smoking and lose weight. Do you think you can help me?" Ashley gives Latinka some written material and sets up a time when they can meet later.

well-designed, comprehensive teaching plan that fits a patient's unique learning needs improves quality, reduces health care costs, helps patients make informed decisions about their health care, and allows them to become healthier and more independent.

STANDARDS FOR PATIENT EDUCATION

All state Nurse Practice Acts recognize that patient education is a professional responsibility of every nurse (Bastable, 2014; Redman, 2011). Patient education is considered a basic nursing competency by the American Association of Colleges of Nursing (AACN), National League for Nursing (NLN), The Quality and Safety Education for Nurses (QSEN) Institute, and the Institute of Medicine (IOM). In addition, health care accrediting organizations such as The Joint Commission (TJC), require that patients receive education and training specific to their needs (Funnell et al., 2011; Su et al., 2011). The nurses' role in patient education is becoming increasingly important because of the rapid changes in the health care system (Priharjo and Hoy, 2011). Nurses play an important role in providing information about illnesses and health and facilitating communication between the patient and the health care team to promote continuity of care (Vaartio-Rajalin and Leino-Kilpi, 2011). As a nurse you need to ensure that education takes place, evaluate if learning occurred, and document all steps of the process (Su et al., 2011).

PURPOSES OF PATIENT EDUCATION

Healthy People 2020 identifies patient education as a key intervention strategy to improve health behaviors (USDHHS, 2013). The goal of patient education is to promote optimal levels of health, safety, and independence for individuals, families, communities, and populations (McNeill, 2012). Patients often require information or skills to enhance or maintain health, prevent disease, restore health following illness, or establish a new level of optimal functioning as a result of illness or injury (Marbach and Griffie, 2011). To meet this need provide education to patients in convenient and familiar places (e.g., in their homes, churches, or schools).

Maintenance and Promotion of Health and Illness Prevention

As a nurse you are a resource for people who want to know more about their health. Patients engaged in their education are better prepared to make informed and personally significant choices and take care of themselves (Coulter, 2012). Self-care improves health outcomes, quality of life, mortality, and morbidity (Funnell et al., 2011; Mann, 2011). Many people participate in healthy activities such as regular exercise and health-screening programs to maintain or improve their health. You provide patient education in many places such as schools, homes, clinics, and the workplace to help patients adopt healthy behaviors (Box 12-1). For example, in childbearing classes expectant parents learn about physical and psychological changes in the woman and about fetal development. After learning about normal childbearing the mother is more likely to engage in physical exercise, and the father is more likely to support the mother during her pregnancy.

Restoration of Health

Injured or ill patients need information or skills to help improve or restore their level of health (see Box 12-1). Patients recovering from or adapting to illness or injury typically seek information about their condition. However, patients who find it difficult to adapt to illness may become passive and uninterested in learning. As a nurse you need to identify the patient's readiness to learn and try to motivate him or her to learn (Bastable, 2014). Family and friends frequently contribute to a patient's return to health and need to know as much as the patient. However, do not assume that you should involve them. Assess a patient's relationships with others before including family or friends in patient education.

Coping with Impaired Functioning

Not all patients fully recover from illness or injury. Many learn to cope with permanent health changes. In these cases patients need new knowledge and skills to continue activities of daily living (see Box 12-1). For example, a patient who loses the ability to speak after surgery of the larynx learns new ways of communicating. A patient with heart disease learns about diet, medication, and exercise to reduce further heart damage.

BOX 12-1 TOPICS FOR HEALTH EDUCATION

HEALTH MAINTENANCE AND PROMOTION AND ILLNESS PREVENTION

- First aid
- Avoidance of risk factors (e.g., smoking, alcohol)
- Growth and development
- Hygiene
- Immunizations
- Prenatal care and normal childbearing
- Nutrition
- Exercise
- Safety (e.g., in home, car, workplace, hospital)
- Screening (e.g., blood pressure, vision, cholesterol level)
- Lifestyle changes to reduce risk factors (e.g., smoking cessation, substance abuse treatment)

RESTORATION OF HEALTH

- Patient's disease or condition
  - Anatomy and physiology of body system affected
  - Cause of disease
  - Origin of symptoms
  - Expected effects on other body systems
  - Prognosis
  - Limitations on function
  - Rationale for treatment
  - Medications
  - Tests and therapies
  - Nursing measures
  - Surgical intervention
  - Expected duration of care
  - Hospital or clinic environment
  - Hospital or clinic staff
  - Long-term care
  - How patient can participate in care

COPING WITH IMPAIRED FUNCTION

- Home care
  - Medications
  - Diet
  - Activity
  - Self-help devices
- Rehabilitation of remaining function
  - Physical therapy
  - Occupational therapy
  - Speech therapy
- Prevention of complications
  - Knowledge of risk factors
  - Implications of noncompliance with therapy
  - Environmental alterations

Changes in function usually affect patients physically and psychosocially. In the case of serious illness or injury such as a heart attack or spinal cord injury, a patient's family often partners with the patient and learns how to help him or her manage health care needs. In these cases you include the family in patient education. Begin teaching as soon as you identify a patient's needs and determine that the family is willing to help. Provide information to help families cope with and adapt to emotional effects when your patients have long-term functional limitations. To be most effective you need to compare the desired level of health with your patient's actual state of health when planning and providing patient education.

TEACHING AND LEARNING

It is impossible to separate teaching from learning. **Teaching** is an interactive practice that results in an individual learning knowledge, new behaviors, or skills (Gilboy and Howard, 2009). A teacher provides information to encourage a learner to engage in activities that lead to a desired change. Effective teaching relies on effective and continuous communication between the teacher and the learner (Gilboy and Howard, 2009). The teaching process closely parallels the communication process (see Chapter 11). Effective nurses include patient-centered education in every patient encounter (e.g., when giving medications, discussing patient concerns, during hygiene care) and promote learning by communicating in a language recognized by the patient (Falvo, 2011).

Compare the steps of the teaching process with those of the communication process (Table 12-1). As a nurse you are the sender who wants to communicate a message to the receiver, your patient. Many interpersonal variables influence your style and approach. Attitudes, values, cultural preferences, emotions, and knowledge influence the way you send messages. Evaluating past experiences with teaching helps you choose the best way to present information (Bastable, 2014).

The receiver in the teaching-learning process is the learner. Interpersonal variables affect your patient's readiness and ability to learn. Language, attitudes, literacy level, cultural preferences, and values influence the ability to understand a message. The ability to learn depends on emotional and physical health, stage of development, and previous knowledge.

To be an effective teacher, be ready to evaluate the success of a teaching plan and provide positive reinforcement to your patient (Falvo, 2011). Examples of evaluating the effectiveness of your teaching include having your patients show you how to perform a newly learned skill (e.g., self-catheterization) and asking them to explain how they will incorporate newly ordered medications into their daily routines.

Learning is the purposeful acquisition of new knowledge, attitudes, behaviors, or skills (Bastable, 2014). Change occurs as a result of learning (McNeill, 2012). Learning is a complex process, especially if a patient is learning new skills, changing existing attitudes, transferring knowledge to new situations, or solving problems. Generally teaching and learning begin when a person identifies a need for knowing or acquiring an ability to do something. Teaching is most effective when it responds to a learner's immediate needs. The teacher identifies these needs by asking questions and determining the learner's interests. After you identify what you need to teach, consider developing specific learning objectives. A **learning objective** describes what the patient will be able to

TABLE 12-1 COMPARISON OF THE COMMUNICATION AND TEACHING PROCESS

COMMUNICATION	TEACHING
Referent	
Idea that initiates reason for communication	Perceived need to provide a person with information, establishment of relevant learning objectives by teacher
Sender	
Person who conveys message to another	Teacher who performs activities aimed at helping other person to learn
Intrapersonal Variables (Sender)	
Knowledge, values, emotions, and sociocultural influences that affect sender's thoughts	Teacher's philosophy of education (based on learning theory), knowledge of teaching content, teaching approach, experiences in teaching, emotions and values
Message	
Information expressed or transmitted by sender	Content or information taught
Channels	
Methods used to transmit message (visual, auditory, touch)	Methods used to present content (visual and auditory materials, touch, taste, smell)
Receiver	
Person to whom message is sent	Learner
Intrapersonal Variables (Receiver)	
Knowledge, values, emotions, and sociocultural influences that affect receiver's thoughts	Willingness and ability to learn (physical and emotional health, cultural background, education, experience, developmental level)
Feedback	
Information revealing that true meaning of message was received	Determination of whether learner achieved learning objectives

do after successful instruction. Learning objectives clearly state the purpose of the teaching and the expectations of the teaching sessions. Learning objectives focus on the learner, organize teaching, specify behavior or content, and provide the criteria for evaluation (Krau, 2011). It is especially helpful to develop objectives when you know you will be caring for a patient over time.

Role of the Nurse in Teaching and Learning

You have an ethical responsibility to teach your patients. This responsibility is outlined in the *Code of Ethics for Nurses* (Fowler, 2010) and the *Patient Care Partnership* (American Hospital Association, 2003). Both support patients' rights to make informed decisions about their care, which requires accurate, complete, and relevant information. Furthermore, TJC's *Speak Up Initiatives* (2013) help patients become more involved in their care and more aware of their right to know about the care they will receive in a language they can understand. You enhance patient safety by teaching patients their role in preventing medical errors.

Your responsibility is to provide information that your patients and their families need. To be successful:

- Answer patients' questions.
- Provide information based on each patient's health needs or treatment plans.
- Clarify information from a variety of sources (e.g., health care providers, newspapers, television, the Internet).

To be an effective educator, engage your patients as partners in learning. Do not merely pass on facts. For example, when Ashley considers her approaches for teaching Latinka, she individualizes her educational approach based on Latinka's desire and interest in making a behavior change, her existing knowledge about the effects of smoking, and her preferences for ways to learn. By engaging Latinka in the teaching and learning experience, Ashley achieves greater success in making her teaching relevant and meaningful to Latinka. Carefully determine what your patients need to know and provide education when they are ready to learn. Then evaluate the outcomes of teaching (i.e., Can they plan a medication schedule over 24 hours? Do they prepare the right foods for their prescribed diet? Do they know their activity restrictions?). When you value and tailor educational approaches, patients are better prepared to assume health care responsibilities.

DOMAINS OF LEARNING

Learning occurs in three domains or areas: (1) cognitive (understanding), (2) affective (attitudes), and (3) psychomotor (motor skills).

Cognitive learning includes what the patient knows and understands. All intellectual behaviors are in the cognitive domain. This includes the following:

- Acquisition of knowledge
- Comprehension (ability to understand)
- Application (using abstract ideas in concrete situations)
- Analysis (relating ideas in an organized way)
- Synthesis (recognizing parts of information as a whole)
- Evaluation (judging the worth of a body of information)

Affective learning includes a patient's feelings, attitudes, opinions, and values. The affective domain is sometimes hard to identify, but it greatly affects the success of education, either positively or negatively. Affective learning includes active listening and responding with a consistent value system.

Psychomotor learning occurs when patients acquire skills that require the integration of knowledge and physical skills. Examples of psychomotor learning are learning to walk with a walker and giving an insulin injection. As patients are able to complete psychomotor skills with more confidence, they are able to perform the behaviors in more complex or different situations (e.g., using a walker to walk across a street curb). Adaptation occurs when your patient changes a response as a result of unexpected problems. This results in originating, which involves creating new patterns of behavior.

Some learning topics involve all domains, whereas others involve only one. Patients often need to learn in each domain. For example, patients diagnosed with high blood pressure need to understand how their blood pressure affects the body and what they can do to lower it (cognitive domain). Patients begin to accept the chronic nature of high blood pressure by learning positive ways to cope with their illness (affective domain). Many patients learn to take their blood pressure at home. This requires them to learn how to use a sphygmomanometer for home use (psychomotor domain). When you understand each learning domain, you are better prepared to use appropriate teaching techniques and apply the basic principles of learning.

BASIC LEARNING PRINCIPLES

To teach effectively and efficiently you first need to understand how people learn. Learning depends on the motivation to learn, the ability to learn, learning styles, and the learning environment. The ability to learn depends on a patient's physical and cognitive characteristics, developmental level, physical wellness, and intellectual thought processes. Remember that people have different preferences for learning and that they learn information in different ways and at different speeds. Therefore to be most effective include a combination of teaching approaches that meet multiple learning preferences (McNeill, 2012).

Motivation to Learn

Motivation is an internal impulse such as an emotion or need that prompts, guides, and sustains human behavior (Miller and Stoeckel, 2011). A patient's situation, needs, previous knowledge, attitudes, and sociocultural factors influence the motivation to learn (Knoerl, Esper, and Hasenau, 2011). For example, patients who need knowledge for survival have a stronger motivation to learn than patients who need it for promoting health (Bastable, 2014). Patients who are motivated to learn are often actively involved in decisions about their care and thus are better able to manage their health care. If a person does not want to learn, it is unlikely that learning will occur. Some patients are motivated to learn so they can return to a previous level of functioning. For example, a patient with a lower-limb amputation is motivated to learn to walk with a prosthesis.

An **attentional set** is the mental state that allows a learner to focus on and understand the material. Before learning anything, patients must be able to pay attention to or concentrate on the information they will learn. Physical discomfort, anxiety, fatigue, nausea, and environmental distractions make it more difficult for patients to concentrate and interfere with learning. You determine a patient's level of comfort by assessing verbal and nonverbal cues before beginning a teaching plan. Teach only when your patient is able to focus on the information.

Anxiety, an uneasiness or uncertainty resulting from anticipating a threat or danger, decreases a patient's ability to pay attention. Learning requires a change in behavior, often leading to anxiety. A mild level of anxiety motivates learning. However, high levels of anxiety disable a person, creating an inability to attend to anything other than relieving the anxiety. Try strategies to manage your patient's anxiety (e.g., discussing concerns, using relaxation techniques) before providing education to improve comprehension and understanding of the information given.

Health education often involves changing attitudes and values that are not easy to change simply by teaching facts. You enhance learning by actively involving patients and allowing them to make decisions during an educational session (Edelman and Mandle, 2010). It becomes necessary to know how to help patients adapt what they need to learn to their day-to-day lifestyle. For example, to help a patient with diabetes learn to monitor blood glucose levels, you help the patient choose a blood glucose meter that is easy to use and then observe the patient use it. You also incorporate the patient's lifestyle into a schedule for blood glucose testing (Figure 12-1). In addition, knowing your patient's culture (see Chapter 20) and health beliefs (see Chapter 2) helps you develop patient-centered interventions to motivate your patients to learn (Box 12-2). Using a model such as the ACCESS model helps you to focus on cultural factors that influence patient education. The six aspects of the model are:

1. ***Assessment*** of a patient's lifestyle, health beliefs, cultural traditions, and health practices

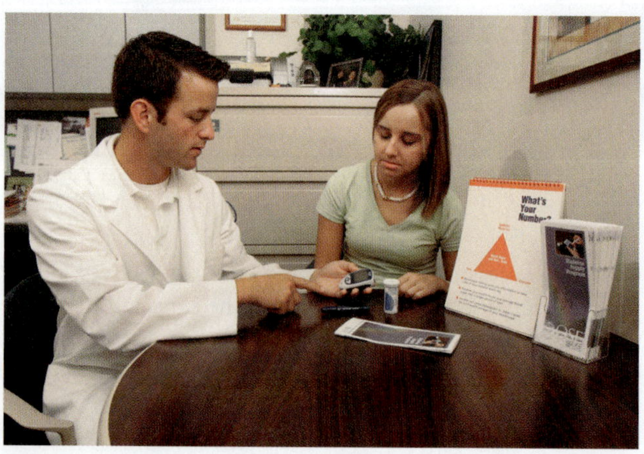

FIGURE 12-1 Nurse instructing patient with a glucose meter.

2. **Communication** with awareness of the many variations in verbal and nonverbal responses
3. **Cultural negotiation and compromise** that encourages awareness of various characteristics of a patient's culture and one's own biases
4. **Establishment** of respect for a patient's cultural beliefs and values; establishment of a caring rapport as the basis for a therapeutic relationship
5. **Sensitivity** to how patients from diverse backgrounds perceive their care needs and the various patterns of communications (terms, concepts, tone, and style of communication) they use.

BOX 12-2 PATIENT-CENTERED CARE

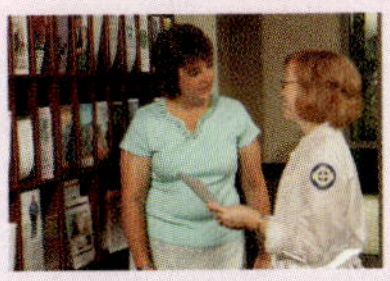

Ashley recognizes that she knows very little about Bosnian culture. Therefore, before she meets with Latinka, Ashley takes some time to read about it. She finds that during the 1990s about 300,000 people from Bosnia immigrated to the United States as a result of the Balkan wars. The immigrants were older and experienced significant trauma related to the war. Many women experienced violence personally or witnessed violence toward their family and friends. Thus they have a higher incidence of mental illnesses. People from Bosnia tend to have strong ties with their families and communities. Common values include hospitality, spontaneity, owning a home, and telling stories. Bosnians have unique health concerns. Researchers estimate that more than 60% of Bosnian refugees living in the United States smoke and they are much less likely to admit that they have a higher risk of developing long-term complications from smoking (Harris et al., 2012). Folk and family remedies are often passed down from mother to daughter. Common treatments include using herbal teas for colds or the flu. Bosnians who attend religious services tend to have lower levels of anxiety (Lavric and Flere, 2010); and those who participate in regular, moderate physical activity tend to have lower levels of depression (Gavric et al., 2012). Ashley uses this information about Bosnian culture to develop a culturally competent plan that focuses on helping Latinka lose weight and stop smoking.

IMPLICATIONS FOR PRACTICE

- Ashley has a better understanding of Bosnian culture, but she recognizes that not all Bosnian people are the same. Therefore she assesses Latinka's values and her beliefs about the American health care system.
- Ashley asks Latinka about her experiences with the war in Bosnia and is prepared to deal with sensitive issues related to mental health.
- Ashley uses her knowledge about Bosnian refugees and their attitudes about smoking to develop a patient-centered and culturally sensitive plan to help Latinka stop smoking (Harris et al., 2012).
- Ashley explores healthy coping strategies such as attending religious services and participating in regular exercise to help Latinka better deal with her feelings and fears (Gavric et al., 2012; Lavric and Flere, 2010).

6. **Safety** that enables patients to feel culturally secure and avoids disempowerment of their cultural identity; respecting and nurturing the unique cultural identity of the individuals is necessary (Knoerl et al., 2011, p. 336).

Readiness to Learn

Many factors affect readiness to learn. For example, your patients cannot learn when they are unwilling or unable to accept the reality of illness. A loss of health is usually very difficult for patients to accept. The stages of grieving (see Chapter 26) encompass a series of responses that patients experience during illness and affect readiness to learn. People experience these stages at different rates. It is important to properly time patient teaching to ease your patient's adjustment to illness or disability (Table 12-2). Introduce a teaching plan when your patient enters the stage of acceptance, which is most compatible with learning. Continue to teach as long as the patient remains in a stage conducive to learning. If a patient is not ready to learn, include family caregivers in teaching when appropriate and consider referring the patient to a home care nurse to ensure that patient needs are met.

A patient's health status also affects the readiness for education. Health status is affected by a patient's community and the accessibility, availability, and acceptability of health resources (Knoerl et al., 2011). A person who is acutely ill is concerned with survival. Conditions such as delirium, anxiety, fatigue, or pain interfere with his or her thinking. At these times the family often becomes the recipient of the education. The priority is to provide education to reduce the patient's or family's anxiety. Simple facts addressing immediate needs are most important. For example, a patient in pain is receptive to education about the use of a patient-controlled analgesia (PCA) pump but not how to use crutches.

Ability to Learn

Your patient's developmental level and cognitive and physical capabilities influence the ability to learn. Consider these important factors while developing a teaching plan.

Developmental Capability. Learning, like developmental growth, is an evolving process. Therefore consider your patient's stage of development and intellectual abilities so your teaching will be successful. Learning occurs more readily when new information complements existing knowledge. Assess the patient's level of knowledge, intellectual skills, and literacy level before beginning a teaching plan. For example, before reviewing a teaching booklet about healthy food choices, determine your patient's understanding of nutrition and his or her reading and comprehension skills.

Age-group. Age often reflects the developmental capability for learning and learning behaviors that a patient is able to acquire. Without proper biological, motor, language, and personal-social development, many types of learning cannot take place (see Chapter 22). Adapt your teaching approach based on the patient's developmental level (Box 12-3). When teaching a child it is very important to match the information you provide with the child's developmental stage. As people

TABLE 12-2 RELATIONSHIP BETWEEN PSYCHOSOCIAL ADAPTATION TO ILLNESS AND LEARNING

STAGE	PATIENT'S BEHAVIOR	LEARNING IMPLICATIONS	RATIONALE
Denial or disbelief	Patient avoids discussion of illness ("There's nothing wrong with me") and disregards physical restrictions. Patient suppresses and distorts information that has not been presented clearly.	Provide support, empathy, and careful explanations of all procedures while they are being done. Let patient know that you are available for discussion. Explain situation to family. Teach in present tense (explain current therapy).	Patient is not prepared to deal with problem. Any attempt to convince or tell patient about illness results in further anger or withdrawal. Provide only information patient pursues or absolutely requires.
Anger	Patient blames and complains and often directs anger at nurse.	Do not argue with patient but listen to concerns. Teach in present tense. Reassure family of patient's normality.	Patient needs opportunity to express feelings and anger. Patient is still not prepared to face future.
Bargaining	Patient offers to live better life in exchange for promise of better health. ("If God lets me live, I promise to be more careful.")	Continue to introduce only reality. Teach only in present tense.	Patient is still unwilling to accept limitations.
Resolution	Patient begins to express emotions openly, realizes that illness has created changes, and begins to ask questions.	Encourage expression of feelings. Begin to share information needed for future and set aside formal times for discussion.	Patient begins to perceive need for assistance and is ready to accept responsibility for learning.
Acceptance	Patient recognizes reality of condition, actively pursues information, and strives for independence.	Focus teaching on future skills and knowledge required. Continue to teach about present occurrences. Involve family in teaching information for discharge.	Patient is more easily motivated to learn. Acceptance of illness reflects willingness to deal with its implications.

BOX 12-3 TEACHING METHODS BASED ON PATIENT'S DEVELOPMENTAL CAPACITY

INFANT
- Keep routines (e.g., feeding, bathing) consistent.
- Hold infant firmly while smiling and speaking softly to convey sense of trust.
- Have infant touch different textures (e.g., soft fabric, hard plastic).

TODDLER
- Use play to teach a procedure or activity (e.g., handling examination equipment, applying bandage to doll).
- Offer picture books that describe story of children in hospital or clinic.
- Use simple words such as *cut* instead of *laceration* to promote understanding.

PRESCHOOLER
- Use role playing, imitation, and play to make it fun for preschoolers to learn.
- Encourage questions and offer explanations. Use simple explanations and demonstrations.
- Encourage children to learn together through pictures and short stories about how to perform hygiene.

SCHOOL-AGE CHILD
- Teach psychomotor skills needed to maintain health. (Complicated skills such as learning to use a syringe take considerable practice.)
- Offer opportunities to discuss health problems and answer questions.

ADOLESCENT
- Help adolescent learn about feelings and need for self-expression.
- Use teaching as collaborative activity.
- Allow adolescents to make decisions about health and health promotion (safety, sex education, substance abuse).
- Use problem solving to help adolescents make choices.

YOUNG OR MIDDLE ADULT
- Encourage participation in teaching plan by setting mutual goals.
- Encourage independent learning.
- Offer information so adult understands effects of health problem.

OLDER ADULT
- Teach when patient is alert and rested.
- Involve adult in discussion or activity.
- Focus on wellness and the person's strength.
- Use approaches that enhance reception of stimuli for patients with sensory alterations (see Chapter 38).
- Keep teaching sessions short.

mature into adulthood they often become more self-directed and are able to identify their own learning needs. Enhance learning by encouraging an adult learner to reflect on personal and life experiences. Assess what an adult patient knows, teach what the patient wants to know, and set mutual goals to improve educational outcomes (Coulter, 2012). Consider generational differences as well. For example, many baby boomers prefer visual aids and focusing on one topic at a time, whereas younger patients prefer using technology.

Physical Capability. The ability to learn depends on a person's level of physical development and overall physical health. To learn a psychomotor skill, your patient needs to have the necessary level of strength, coordination, and sensory acuity. For example, it is unrealistic for you to teach your patient to transfer from a bed to a wheelchair if he or she has insufficient upper body strength. Do not overestimate or underestimate a patient's physical abilities. To learn psychomotor skills, your patient requires the following characteristics:

1. Size (height and weight sufficient for the task to be performed or the equipment to be used [e.g., crutch walking])
2. Strength (ability of the patient to follow strenuous exercise program)
3. Coordination (ability to maintain balance, or having the dexterity needed for complicated motor skills such as using utensils or changing a bandage)
4. Sensory acuity (visual, auditory, tactile, gustatory, and olfactory: sensory resources needed to receive and respond to messages taught)

Any condition (e.g., fatigue, breathing difficulty, or depression) that drains a person's energy impairs the ability to learn. Postpone teaching when an illness becomes aggravated by complications such as pain, fever, or respiratory difficulty. While providing care assess a patient's energy level by noting his or her willingness to communicate, amount of activity initiated, and responsiveness toward questions. Stop teaching if a patient tires; resume teaching when the patient feels rested. Offer several short teaching sessions rather than one long session.

Learning Environment

Factors in the physical environment where teaching takes place make learning a pleasant or difficult experience. Choose settings that help patients focus attention on their learning task. Consider the number of people involved, need for privacy, room temperature and ventilation, room lighting, noise, and room furniture when choosing the setting.

The ideal environment that promotes learning is a room that has good lighting and ventilation, appropriate furniture, and a comfortable temperature (Figure 12-2). A darkened room interferes with a patient's ability to see the demonstration of a skill or visual aids such as posters or pamphlets. A room that is too cold, hot, or stuffy makes patients too uncomfortable to pay attention. Comfortable furniture eliminates distractions such as the need to change position or shift body weight. It is also important to choose a quiet setting that offers privacy and few interruptions. If a patient desires, include family members (especially the primary caregiver) in discussions. However, remember that some patients are reluctant to engage in discussions about their illnesses when family members are present.

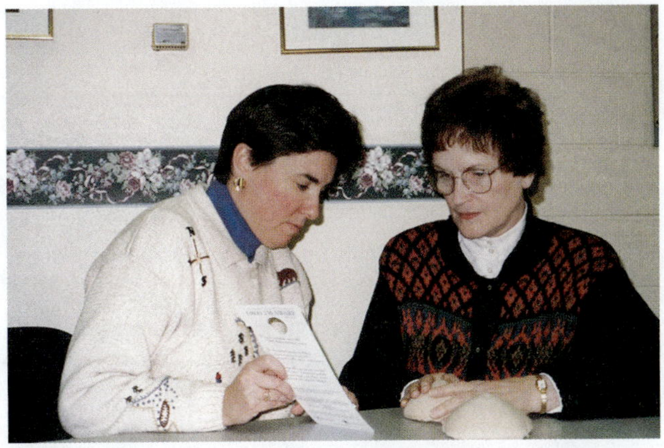

FIGURE 12-2 Choosing a comfortable, pleasant environment enhances the learning experience. Nurse is explaining breast self-examination procedure to patient.

Teaching a group of patients requires a room that allows everyone to be seated comfortably and within hearing distance of the teacher. The room needs to comfortably hold all members of the group. If the room is too large, participants are often tempted to sit outside the group along the perimeter. Arranging the group to allow participants to observe one another (e.g., in a circle) further enhances learning. More effective communication occurs as learners observe the verbal and nonverbal interactions of others.

INTEGRATING THE NURSING AND TEACHING PROCESSES

There are distinct similarities between the nursing process (see Chapter 9) and the teaching process (Table 12-3). Both processes require critical thinking (Box 12-4). Assessment reveals your patient's health care and learning needs. Use assessment data to determine nursing diagnoses unique to your patient's situation. Then develop and implement an individualized plan of care with appropriate interventions and evaluate the level of success in meeting the goals of care. Patient education is usually associated with individual learning needs or is the primary nursing diagnosis; thus you need to include patients when developing teaching plans. Learning needs specify the information or skills a patient requires. Nurses often collaborate with other health care professionals to identify learning objectives and implement a teaching plan. Use teaching and learning principles to ensure that your patient acquires knowledge and skills. Evaluate patient outcomes based on the learning objectives.

ASSESSMENT

An effective assessment provides the basis for individualized patient teaching. Assess the patient's learning needs to

TABLE 12-3 COMPARISON OF THE NURSING AND TEACHING PROCESSES

BASIC STEPS	NURSING PROCESS	TEACHING PROCESS
Assessment	Collect data about patient's physical, psychological, social, cultural, developmental, and spiritual needs from patient, family, all databases, medical record, nursing history, and literature.	Gather data about patient's learning needs, literacy level, motivation, ability to learn, and teaching resources from patient, family, learning environment, and all databases.
Nursing diagnosis	Identify appropriate nursing diagnoses.	Identify patient's learning needs on basis of three domains of learning.
Planning	Develop individualized care plan. Set diagnosis priorities based on patient's immediate needs.	Establish learning objectives stated in behavioral terms. Identify priorities regarding learning needs. Collaborate with patient on teaching plan.
Implementation	Collaborate with patient on care plan. Perform nursing care therapies. Include patient as active participant in care. Involve family in care as appropriate.	Identify type of teaching method to use. Implement teaching methods. Actively involve patient in learning activities. Include family participation as appropriate.
Evaluation	Identify success in meeting desired outcomes and goals of nursing care.	Determine outcomes of teaching-learning process. Measure patient's ability to achieve learning objectives. Reteach as needed.

BOX 12-4 SYNTHESIS IN PRACTICE

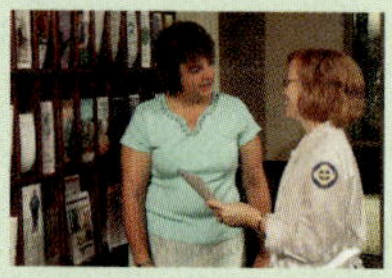

Ashley will be caring for Latinka during the rest of her clinical rotation. As Ashley begins to assess Latinka's educational needs, she reviews Latinka's health concerns and requests for information. Ashley knows that people learn best when you provide the information they want. She also wants to provide culturally competent patient education. Therefore she knows that assessing Latinka's perceptions of being overweight, being an immigrant in the United States, and how she is affected by the American health care system is a priority before she begins teaching about losing weight and smoking cessation.

Ashley's parents decided to stop smoking and have not smoked for 6 months. Ashley talks with her parents to find out which strategies were most helpful in their effort to quit smoking. She recalls that her mother gained about 10 lbs. She also read a research article that found that several women in the study gained weight after they quit smoking. Because Latinka expressed an interest in losing weight and quitting smoking, Ashley decides that she needs to help Latinka develop healthy strategies that do not involve food to cope with nicotine withdrawal symptoms.

Ashley knows that she has the ethical responsibility to provide culturally sensitive patient teaching. She needs to accept Latinka and respect her beliefs and attitudes when providing patient teaching. Ashley found patient education handouts about smoking cessation, but the handouts were designed for Caucasians and African-Americans, not for Bosnians. Therefore she decides to take the printed information home with her and make revisions so the information reflects Latinka's cultural preferences. Ashley also makes sure that the information is written in words that are easy to understand. She realizes that, if Latinka cannot read English well, she needs the printed information translated into Bosnian. Ashley is excited to learn more about Latinka and who she is as an individual. After establishing a caring relationship with Latinka, Ashley begins to assess her health needs and learning styles so she can put together an effective, individualized teaching plan.

determine what you need to teach and the patient's ability and motivation to learn. A thorough assessment helps you to identify available learning resources and choose the best teaching methods. Assessment also ensures a more individualized approach toward patient education (Table 12-4).

Patient Expectations. Together you and your patient identify critical information the patient needs to know. It is also essential to understand what your patient expects to learn. For example, if your patient is a teen-age boy newly diagnosed with type 1 diabetes mellitus, ask what he expects to learn about taking care of himself at home and while at school. Does he expect to self-administer the insulin, or is the expectation that a parent or school nurse will give the injections? Also assess your patient's expectations in all three learning domains. Questions such as, "What do you think is important for you to know to take care of yourself?" allow the patient to be an active participant in planning self-care. Learning needs change, depending on your patient's health status. Assessment of learning needs is an ongoing activity. Examples of key areas of assessment are (1) questions raised by the patient or family about health issues; (2) the patient's understanding of current health status, implications of illness, types of therapy, and prognosis; (3) information or skills needed to perform self-care; (4) experiences that influence the patient's need to learn; and (5) information necessary for family members to meet the patient's needs.

TABLE 12-4 FOCUSED PATIENT ASSESSMENT

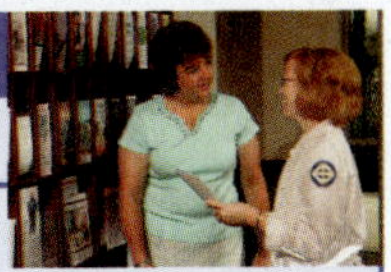

FACTORS TO ASSESS	QUESTIONS	PHYSICAL ASSESSMENT
Learning needs	Tell me what you know about your illness and its treatment. What would you like to know that would help you better manage your disease at home?	Observe expression on patient's face (e.g., puzzled, attentive, distracted).
Resources for learning	Who is the primary person who can help you at home? Will you have any trouble getting to the local health department to obtain teaching materials?	Observe for signs of anxiety when discussing home and transportation issues.
Ability to learn	Do you wear glasses or contacts? Do you have trouble seeing words printed in the newspaper? Do you have any difficulties hearing when someone speaks to you?	Observe where patient holds reading material and for squinting of eyes when reading. Observe whether patient turns head when attempting to listen.

Motivation to Learn. Ask questions to assess a patient's motivation to learn (i.e., is the severity or nature of a health problem one that the patient decides he or she is prepared and willing to learn). Ask questions that relate to a patient's learning behaviors, health beliefs, attitudes about health care providers, knowledge of health problem and information to be learned, physical symptoms that interfere with learning (e.g., fatigue, pain, or dizziness), sociocultural background, and learning-style preference (Inott and Kennedy, 2011).

Teaching Environment. Create an environment for a teaching session that is favorable to learning. Assess for distractions, noise, the patient's comfort level (e.g., sitting or lying, the need to use the toilet), and the availability of rooms and equipment. In the home setting you need to assess lighting, space, and the availability of equipment.

Learning Styles. Learning style preference is important to assess when helping patients learn. Current evidence shows that different people prefer different learning styles. The visual, auditory, kinesthetic/tactile (VAKT) learning style assessment provides a practical and useful way to determine a patient's learning style. To use this method you ask a patient informal questions such as, "When you need to learn to do something new, how do you go about it?" Use an evidence-based tool to assess learning styles when possible (McNeill, 2012).

There are two subsets of visual learning: linguistic and spatial. The linguistic learner prefers to use the written word. Computer-based instructions, books, articles, or other forms of written information best help a patient gain knowledge or skills. There are also spatial learners, and they prefer visual aids (e.g., pictures, models, demonstrations). Auditory learners favor listening and speaking. They often repeat back the information to themselves or to others. Kinesthetic/tactile learners are physically active and gain skills and knowledge through manipulation. They write, draw pictures, and manipulate models of information. Use strategies that incorporate all styles of learning to engage the learner and enhance learning (Duiveman and Bonner, 2012).

Resources for Learning. Identify resources for learning, which often include the support of family members or significant others. Assess how ready family and friends are to learn how to help care for a patient. Determine family perceptions of a patient's illness, a patient's willingness to involve family members in care, and a family's willingness to help provide care. Also determine the resources available in the home and the teaching tools needed. Ensure that teaching resources such as brochures, audiovisual materials, and posters are available when needed. Select the most appropriate teaching tool for the patient's needs and ability to learn. Teaching materials need to be current, presented logically, and written or presented in words that your learner can understand (Speros, 2011; Townsend, 2011).

Language and Cultural Factors. Assess the language the patient most commonly uses. Make sure that printed information is in the patient's native language if possible (Townsend, 2011). Hospitals are required by The Joint Commission to make translators available to patients. Do not use family members as interpreters. Determine the patient's role in the family and how his or her culture (educational background, occupation, ethnicity, religion) influences his or her perception of illness (Inott and Kennedy, 2011). For example, explore the significance prescribed medications and therapies has for a patient and consider alternative therapies he or she may use. Teaching that does not include cultural considerations is ineffective (Speros, 2011).

Health Literacy. Current evidence shows that health literacy is a strong predictor of health status and patient outcomes (Berkman et al., 2011; Townsend, 2011). Therefore you need to assess your patients' health literacy before providing instruction. **Health literacy** includes patients' reading and mathematics skills, comprehension, the ability to make health-related decisions, and successful functioning as a consumer of health care. It is influenced by individual, cultural, and social factors (Speros, 2011). Approximately 90 million people in the United States or about one-half of American adults lack the necessary health literacy and numeracy (ability to use numbers) skills necessary to obtain, process, and understand basic health information and services (Himmelfarb and Hughes, 2011; Townsend, 2011). Those with low health literacy are at greater risk for adverse health outcomes and come from all ages, races, and socioeconomic and educational backgrounds. Nurses and health care professionals have difficulty identifying patients with low health literacy because it is challenging to recognize (Himmelfarb and Hughes, 2011; Speros, 2011). Simply asking patients if they can read often does not work because they do not feel comfortable admitting that they cannot read. Adults with low literacy have found ways to respond without revealing their literacy limitations.

Current evidence supports using evidence-based assessment tools such as the Single-Item Literacy Screener (SILS). This tool asks questions such as, "How often do you have to have someone help you read instructions, pamphlets, or other written material from your doctor or pharmacy?" and "How confident do you feel in filling out medical forms by yourself?" (Speros, 2011). Incorporating questions such as these in your patient assessment helps you identify patients with low health literacy. Another assessment tool, the Newest Vital Sign (NVS) (http://pilot.train.hrsa.gov/uhc/pdf/module_02_job_aid_vital_sign.pdf), is available in English or Spanish; takes 3 minutes; and screens a patient's general literacy level, numeracy skills, and comprehension of health-related written materials. Other assessment data that indicate low health literacy include a patient's inability to complete forms, read a prescription label, or adhere to a treatment plan or a patient's displaying uncooperative behavior, asking no questions, or asking for help from the family (Himmelfarb and Hughes, 2011).

Special Needs of Children. Children pass through several developmental stages (see Chapter 22). You need to assess a child's cognitive and psychomotor abilities, physical strength, coordination, and reading level (see Box 12-3). Involve the parents during your assessment to better understand the child's needs, especially when children are very young and unable to care for themselves. Assess for pain, fatigue, anxiety, or any other symptoms that interfere with your patient's ability to pay attention to and participate in learning.

Older-Adult Considerations. The population of older adults continues to increase, and their care is becoming more complex. Thus use the best evidence when assessing an older adult's learning needs (Box 12-5). Older adults experience numerous physical and psychological changes as they age. These changes sometimes create barriers to learning. Assess sensory changes that require modification of teaching methods (Miller and Stoeckel, 2011). For example, if you assess decreased visual acuity in your patient, you need to use large-print materials to provide and reinforce patient teaching.

BOX 12-5 EVIDENCE-BASED PRACTICE

PICO Question: In older adults, do tailored instructions based on assessment of learning needs prevent hospital readmissions compared with standardized instruction?

SUMMARY OF EVIDENCE

The Affordable Care Act signed into law in 2010 required the Centers for Medicare & Medicaid Services to reduce payments to hospitals with excessive 30-day readmission rates (CMS, 2013). This refers to a patient being readmitted to the same or a different hospital for the same condition he or she was previously admitted, within 30 days of discharge. Readmission of elderly patients is related to many factors (e.g., the natural progression of chronic illnesses, poor continuity of care, limited financial resources, and ineffective patient education) (Linertova et al., 2011). The discharge needs of older adults are very complex, which requires nurses to carefully assess how to best meet their educational needs in the hospital and after discharge. Although no single intervention is effective, patient-centered education based on careful assessment that includes care after discharge has been shown to be effective in preventing readmissions in the older adult (Hansen et al., 2011; Linertova et al., 2011).

APPLICATION TO NURSING PRACTICE

- Collaborate with the entire health care team to understand the patient's treatment plan and ensure that patients have the information they need when they are discharged (Linertova et al., 2011).
- Include nutritional assessment and assess for depression when providing patient education. Meeting nutritional and psychosocial needs and providing individualized patient education about disease management is effective in preventing readmissions (Legrain et al., 2011).
- Engage older adults in their learning and ensure that they understand the information they need to communicate back to their health care provider on discharge (Hansen et al., 2011).
- Ensure that teaching materials are tailored to your patient's health literacy needs and socioeconomic factors and focus on the most important information your patient needs to know (Hansen et al., 2011).

NURSING DIAGNOSIS

After assessing information related to your patient's ability and need to learn, interpret data and cluster defining characteristics to form nursing diagnoses that reflect the patient's specific learning needs. This ensures that teaching will be goal directed and individualized. If a patient has several learning needs, the nursing diagnoses guide priority setting.

Several North American Nursing Diagnosis Association International (NANDA-I) nursing diagnoses apply to learning needs. When the diagnosis is *Deficient Knowledge,* the diagnostic statement describes the specific type of learning need and related factor (e.g., *Deficient Knowledge regarding psychomotor learning related to newly ordered injectable medication*). Some diagnoses are very similar to one another. Thus it is essential to identify the correct diagnosis based on the patient's defining characteristics to ensure effective nursing care. For example, when you care for a patient who is not physically active because the patient does not understand the importance of physical activity, the nursing diagnosis is *Sedentary Lifestyle related to deficient knowledge of health benefits of physical exercise.* However, if this same patient is having difficulty completing activities of daily living because of increased weight and the patient needs to know how to adapt activities to meet health needs, the nursing diagnosis is *Activity Intolerance related to generalized weakness,* and your plan of care would include patient education regarding how to improve endurance.

When you manage or eliminate health care problems through education, the related factor of the diagnostic statement refers to knowledge deficits. Include the specific type of learning need when possible. For example, when an older adult patient is not taking a medication at the appropriate time because she does not understand how the medication works (*Noncompliance with Medication Schedule related to deficient knowledge),* focus on explaining the action of the medication and its purpose. Other nursing diagnoses (e.g., *Acute Pain* or *Fear*) indicate that barriers to learning exist. In these situations you delay teaching until you resolve the priority nursing diagnosis. Other examples of nursing diagnoses that indicate learning needs include the following:

- *Ineffective Denial*
- *Ineffective Health Maintenance*
- *Ineffective Self-Health Management*
- *Risk-Prone Health Behavior*
- *Ineffective Family Therapeutic Regimen Management*

PLANNING

After determining nursing diagnoses, identify your patient's learning needs and develop a teaching care plan. When helping a patient change a health behavior, remember that knowledge alone does not change behavior. Discuss factors that facilitate and inhibit learning with your patient during planning. For the plan to be effective, collaborate with the patient, family, and other members of the health care team. The plan needs to include topics for instruction, teaching resources (e.g., equipment or booklets), recommendations for involving family, and teaching objectives. The setting influences the complexity of the plan. No matter what the length, the teaching plan provides continuity of instruction, especially when several nurses or disciplines share teaching responsibilities.

Goals and Outcomes. It is very important to set clear goals and measurable outcomes so you can effectively establish and later evaluate and revise a teaching plan as needed. Include the patient if possible when establishing learning goals and outcomes (see Care Plan). Expected outcomes guide the choice of teaching strategies and who is involved in the plan. Learning objectives are either short term (relating to immediate learning needs) or long term (relating to permanent adaptation to a health problem). Each objective is a statement of a single behavior that identifies a patient's ability to do something after a learning experience. The objective contains an active verb describing what the learner will do after the objective is met such as walk with crutches, administer an injection, or identify drug doses. Use a verb that has few interpretations and state the verb in terms of how the patient is to demonstrate learning (Krau, 2011).

In some health care settings you develop written teaching plans. In these cases include topics for instruction and resources, recommendations for involving family, and objectives of the teaching plan. Some plans are very detailed, whereas others are in an outline format (Box 12-6). Remember that the more specific your plan is, the easier it is to follow.

Setting Priorities. Learning objectives identify the expected outcomes of a planned learning experience, which help establish priorities for learning. Prioritize learning needs with your patient by focusing on what the patient needs to know, his or her nursing diagnoses, and previous knowledge (Figure 12-3). As the nurse you are ultimately responsible for ensuring that all teaching needs have been met. Therefore in

BOX 12-6 PATIENT TEACHING

Healthy Food Choices

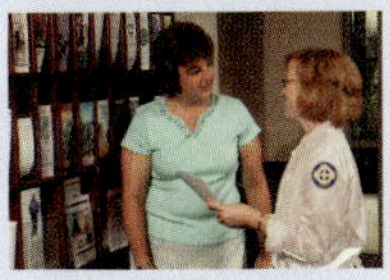

Before planning educational sessions, Ashley assesses what Latinka expects to learn while they are together. Latinka asks Ashley to help her make healthier food choices. Ashley begins by determining what Latinka normally eats. The Bosnian diet is high in animal fats and has a Turkish influence. Meat, bread, vegetables, stews, cheese, legumes, fish, eggs, coffee, sweetened fruit juices, and sweet cakes are common in the Bosnian diet. Using this information, Ashley develops the following teaching plan for Latinka.

OUTCOME

At the end of the teaching session, Latinka will identify three ways to make her diet lower in fat and calories.

TEACHING STRATEGIES

- Complete a diet history to explore what Latinka commonly eats.
- Review Latinka's favorite recipes and meals and make suggestions for food substitutions that make meals healthier (e.g., eat fruit instead of drinking sweetened fruit juice; use ground turkey, low-fat cheese, and margarine or vegetable oil; and decrease number of eggs used in recipes).
- Encourage Latinka to increase the number of legumes and fresh vegetables in her diet while decreasing the amount of sweet bread she eats.
- Provide Latinka with culturally sensitive teaching handouts on healthy food choices.
- Summarize what was taught.
- Make a follow-up appointment to reinforce teaching.

EVALUATION STRATEGIES

- Have Latinka complete a 3-day food diary and evaluate her food choices on her follow-up appointment.
- Ask Latinka to describe which substitutions to make in her favorite recipes to make them healthier.
- Ask Latinka to make a healthy menu for 2 days.

CARE PLAN

Readiness for Enhanced Knowledge

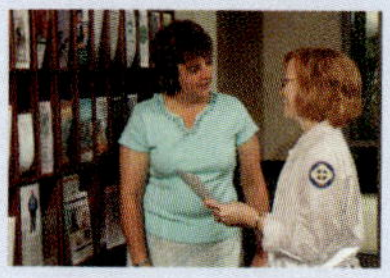

ASSESSMENT

Ashley knows that people who smoke are at risk for developing cancer. When Ashley met with Latinka last week, Latinka stated that she currently smokes 1-1½ packs of cigarettes a day and her husband recently died of bladder cancer. She mentioned that she was concerned about dying from cancer. After thinking about their previous meeting, Ashley plans to assess Latinka's willingness to stop smoking and potential barriers Latinka might experience if she decides to stop smoking.

ASSESSMENT ACTIVITIES	FINDINGS/DEFINING CHARACTERISTICS*
Assess how motivated Latinka is to stop smoking.	Latinka tried to quit smoking once before, but she states, "When my husband was diagnosed with cancer, the stress was too much, so I started smoking again. **I want to get control of my health now.** I just don't know how to do it."
Assess Latinka's readiness to learn about smoking cessation.	Latinka is **concerned about how smoking is affecting her health.** She knows that cigarette smoking is a risk factor for cancer and states that **she is ready to quit smoking for good.**

***Defining characteristics** are shown in **bold** type.

NURSING DIAGNOSIS: Readiness for Enhanced Knowledge related to desire to learn about smoking cessation

PLANNING

GOAL	EXPECTED OUTCOMES (NOC)†
	Knowledge: Health Promotion
• Latinka understands the effects of smoking on her health within 3 weeks.	• Latinka will read information about smoking cessation and the unhealthy effects of tobacco within 2 weeks. • Latinka will describe how smoking affects her health within 3 weeks.
	Risk Control: Tobacco Use
• Latinka quits smoking through the use of a smoking cessation plan within 6 months.	• Latinka will attend a community smoking cessation class within 2 weeks. • Latinka will describe strategies to use at home to quit smoking. • Latinka will follow strategies for smoking cessation within a month.

†Outcomes classification labels from Moorhead S et al.: *Nursing outcomes classification (NOC),* ed 5, St Louis, 2013, Mosby.

INTERVENTIONS (NIC)‡	RATIONALE
Health Education	
• Incorporate explanation of benefits of smoking cessation into Latinka's current knowledge and health beliefs.	Health care providers need to determine the health beliefs and perceived barriers to smoking cessation for teaching and smoking-cessation interventions to be successful (Kerr et al., 2011).
• Develop and/or find educational materials about smoking cessation that are based on assessment of Latinka's learning needs and readiness and motivation to change.	Educational materials designed for patient's unique needs and situations are effective in promoting smoking cessation (Kerr et al., 2011).
• Use group discussions and role playing to influence health beliefs, attitudes, and values.	Role playing and having patient perform behaviors enhance healthy behaviors (Bandura, 1997).
• Plan long-term telephone follow-up to reinforce healthy behavior.	Long-term follow-up and calling patients on the telephone while they are in the process of smoking cessation promote successful patient behaviors (Tzelepis et al., 2011).
Self-Modification Assistance	
• Encourage Latinka to identify small successes.	Relapses in smoking cessation are common. Helping patients see their successes encourages continued efforts to stop smoking and enhances patient's self-efficacy beliefs (Glasgow et al., 2009).

CARE PLAN—cont'd

Readiness for Enhanced Knowledge

Smoking Cessation Assistance

• Help Latinka set a definite quit date within the next 2 weeks.	Setting a specific quit date boosts the commitment to quit smoking (Balmford et al., 2010).
• Manage nicotine replacement therapy.	Using nicotine replacement therapy such as a transdermal nicotine patch promotes success with smoking cessation (Mahvan et al., 2011).

[‡]Intervention classification labels from Bulechek GM et al., editors: *Nursing interventions classification (NIC),* ed 6, St Louis, 2013, Mosby.

EVALUATION

NURSING ACTIONS	PATIENT RESPONSE/FINDING	ACHIEVEMENT OF OUTCOME
Ask Latinka to explain the effects of smoking on her health.	Latinka says she is embarrassed that she has not quit smoking sooner. She is able to explain how smoking affects breathing and the health of her lungs.	Latinka has a good working knowledge of the physical effects of smoking.
Ask Latinka to describe the strategies she has planned to quit smoking.	Latinka decided to quit smoking on her birthday. She states that her children call her once a day to check on her progress and provide support. She is using nicotine patches, but she admits that she forgets to change the patch "every now and then."	Latinka has developed and is implementing her smoking cessation plan. She needs further help identifying strategies that will help her remember to use her nicotine patches as ordered.
Ask Latinka to describe what she does whenever she is tempted to start smoking again.	Latinka states that she either chews sugar-free gum or calls one of her sons if she is tempted to smoke a cigarette.	Latinka implements healthy behaviors whenever she is tempted to smoke.

most situations it is not appropriate to delegate educational interventions to nursing assistive personnel (NAP). In some settings NAP may reinforce instruction but not initiate it. Usually patient safety is a teaching need that is most important. For example, a patient with newly diagnosed hypertension and angina needs to learn about newly prescribed medications, which typically include nitroglycerin spray for angina and a calcium channel blocker. In this situation knowledge regarding the early identification of chest pain and appropriate use of the nitroglycerin spray are the learning priorities.

Timing. When is the right time to teach? When a patient first enters a clinic or hospital? At discharge? At home? Each is appropriate because patients have learning needs as long as they stay in the health care system. Some times are not appropriate for teaching. For example, it is not appropriate to teach a patient who just received bad results about a diagnostic test. Plan to teach when a patient is most attentive, receptive, and alert. The frequency of sessions depends on the learner's abilities and the complexity of the material (McNeill, 2012).

The length of teaching sessions also affects learning. Prolonged sessions cause patients to lose concentration and attentiveness, especially older-adult patients. It is easier to maintain patients' interests when educational sessions are shorter (e.g., lasting 10 to 15 minutes) and more frequent. Nonverbal cues such as poor eye contact or slumped posture indicate that a patient has lost concentration. If you note a loss of concentration stop the session.

Organizing Teaching Material. Give careful consideration to the order of information presented. Organize material so it progresses from simple to complex because a person learns simple facts and concepts before learning how to make associations or complex interpretations of ideas. For example, to teach a woman how to feed her husband who has a gastric tube, first teach the wife how to measure the tube feeding and manipulate the equipment. Once you accomplish this, teach her how to administer the feeding.

Because patients are more likely to remember information taught in the beginning of a teaching session, present essential information first. Informative but less critical content follows the essential information. Other interventions that reinforce learning include using repetition and summarizing key points (Falvo, 2011).

Collaborative Care. Patients receive education in almost every health care setting. Although you are the primary member of the health care team responsible for patient education, often your patients' educational needs are highly complex. Collaboration with other health care professionals is required to successfully meet patient needs. Refer patients to appropriate multidisciplinary health care providers when

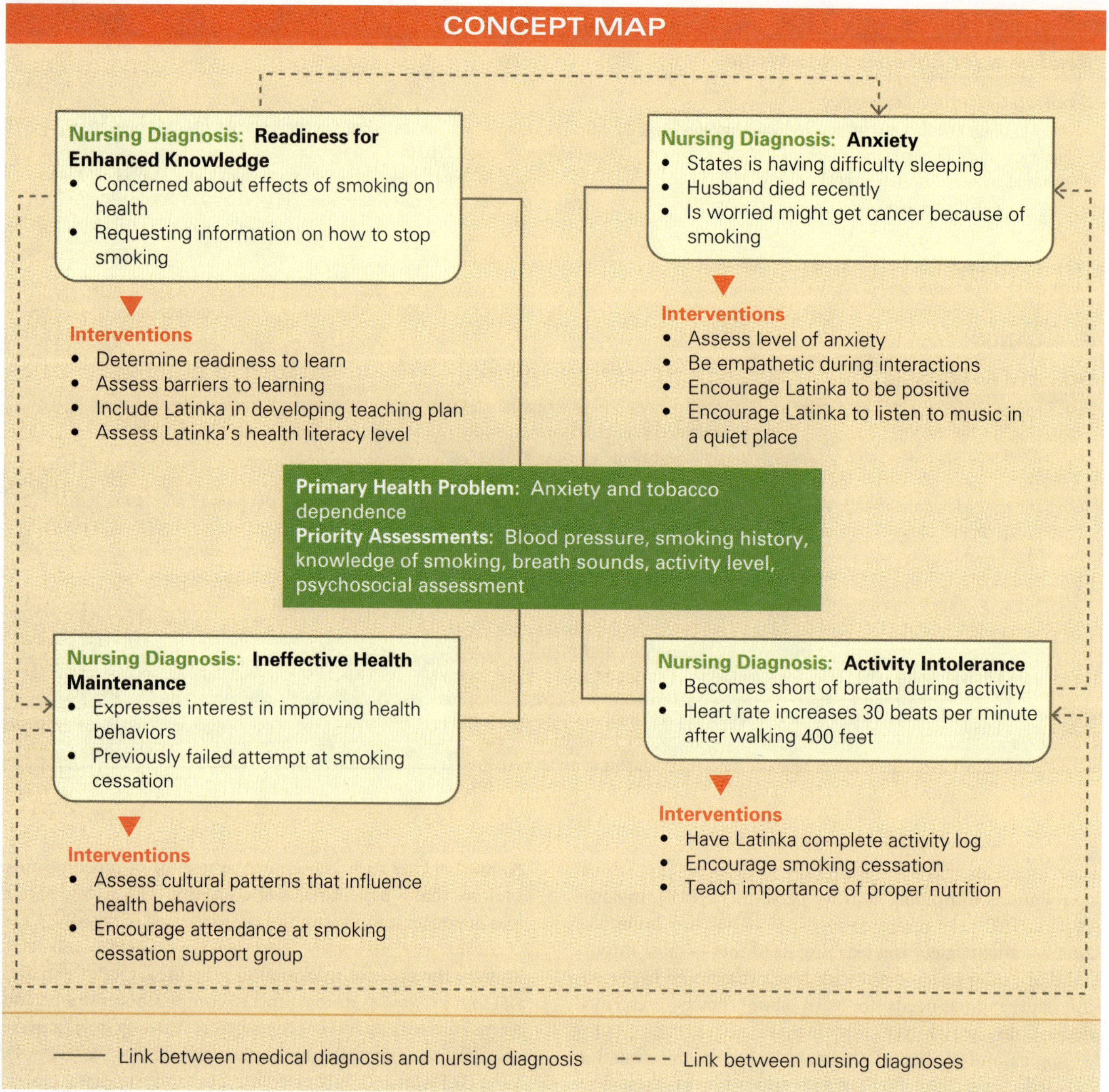

FIGURE 12-3 Concept map.

indicated. For example, refer a patient with a new diagnosis of chronic renal failure to a dietitian for dietary teaching. Patients in acute care settings often require assistance from discharge planners, case managers, and community agencies to be successfully discharged to home. It is your responsibility to collaborate with and include these interdisciplinary health care team members in the teaching plan. A variety of educational resources is available in the community, including diabetes education clinics, prenatal classes, and support groups. Be aware of potential resources and obtain consultations for your patients when needed. Encourage your patients to use these resources and reinforce information provided.

IMPLEMENTATION

Implementation of a teaching plan requires you to use critical thinking while you analyze assessment data and apply teaching and learning principles. Remember that each interaction with a patient is an opportunity to teach. Use evidence-based interventions to create an effective and active learning environment and maximize opportunities for learning. Because learning situations vary, there is no single correct way to teach. The principles of teaching are in effect techniques that incorporate the principles of learning.

Teaching Approaches. Teaching may be provided in a variety of ways, but it is important to choose a teaching approach that matches your patient's needs and learning style. A patient's learning needs change over time. Modify your teaching approach as you care for a patient over time.

Telling. Use the telling approach when teaching limited information such as when you are preparing a patient for an emergent diagnostic procedure. Outline the task a patient needs to do and give explicit instructions. There is no time for feedback with this method.

Participating. When using the participating approach, you and the patient set objectives and participate in the learning process together. The patient helps decide content, and you guide and counsel him or her. For example, a parent with a child diagnosed with sickle cell disease works with you to manage the child's pain. At the end of each teaching session you review the objectives with the parent and child and plan or revise what you will cover the next time you meet.

Entrusting. The entrusting approach gives patients the opportunity to manage their self-care. A patient accepts responsibilities and correctly performs a task while you observe his or her progress and remain available for assistance. For example, a patient who is receiving continuous intravenous pain medication at home for end-stage cancer requires a higher dose of pain medication. The patient understands the dosage of the medication and how the medication pump works. You help the patient determine an appropriate new pain medication dosage and allow him or her to adjust the settings on the medication pump.

Reinforcing. Reinforcement is using a stimulus that increases the probability of a response. A learner who receives reinforcement before or after a desired learning behavior will likely repeat the behavior. Feedback is a common form of reinforcement. Reinforcers are positive or negative. Positive reinforcement such as a smile or praise and support produces the desired responses. Although negative reinforcement (e.g., frowning) may work, people usually respond better to positive reinforcement.

Three types of reinforcers are social, material, and activity. Use social reinforcers (e.g., smiles, compliments, words of encouragement, or physical contact) to acknowledge a learned behavior. Examples of material reinforcers are food, toys, and music. These work best with young children. Activity reinforcers (e.g., physical therapy) rely on the principle that a person is motivated to engage in an activity if there is an opportunity to participate in more desirable activity on completion of this first activity. Choosing an appropriate reinforcer involves careful thought and attention to individual preferences. Never use reinforcers as threats. Reinforcement is not effective with every patient.

Incorporating Teaching with Nursing Care. As you gain confidence in your knowledge and clinical skills, you find that you are able to teach more effectively while you provide care to your patients. For example, you educate your patient on the actions of medications while you administer them. When you follow a teaching plan informally, your patient feels less pressure to perform, and learning becomes more of a shared activity. Teaching during routine care is efficient and cost-effective and makes the information more relevant.

Teaching Methods. Active participation is a key to learning. By actively experiencing a learning event, your patient is more likely to retain knowledge. A teaching method is the way you deliver information and is based on a patient's learning needs and preferences (Box 12-7). For example, older adults learn and remember more if the material is relevant to their needs and abilities and is provided at an appropriate pace (Box 12-8) (Miller and Stoeckel, 2011). The instructional method you choose depends on the time available for teaching, the setting, the resources available, and your comfort level with teaching. Skilled teachers are flexible and combine more than one method into a teaching plan.

One-on-One Discussion. Whenever you teach a patient at the bedside, in a health care provider's office, or in the home, you share information through one-on-one discussion. You provide information informally, allowing the patient to ask questions or share concerns. Use various teaching aids during the discussion, depending on the patient's learning needs.

Group Instruction. Group instruction offers an economical way to teach a number of patients at one time, and often the experience of being part of a group may provide the support necessary for patients to meet learning objectives (Redman, 2011). Group instruction often involves both lecture and discussion. Lectures are efficient in helping groups of patients learn about a subject. After hearing information from a lecture, learners need the opportunity to share ideas and seek clarification. Group discussions allow patients and families to learn from one another as they share common experiences.

Preparatory Instruction. Patients frequently face unfamiliar tests or procedures that create anxiety. Providing information about procedures helps them feel less anxious because they understand what to expect during a procedure. When preparatory instructions accurately describe actual experiences, patients are able to cope more effectively with the stress from the procedure and therapies. The following are guidelines for giving preparatory explanations:

1. Describe physical sensations during the procedure but do not evaluate them. For example, when drawing a blood specimen, explain that the patient will feel a sticking sensation as the needle punctures the skin.
2. Describe the cause of the sensation, preventing false impressions of the experience. For example, explain that a needle insertion burns because alcohol used to cleanse the skin enters the puncture site.
3. Prepare patients only for aspects of the experience that have commonly been noticed by other patients. For example, explain that it is normal for a tight tourniquet to cause a person's hand to tingle and feel numb.

Demonstrations. Demonstrations are useful methods for teaching psychomotor skills. An effective demonstration

BOX 12-7 TEACHING METHODS BASED ON PATIENT'S LEARNING NEEDS

COGNITIVE

Discussion (One-on-One or Group)

- Involves nurse and patient or nurse with several patients
- Promotes active participation and focuses on topics of interest to patient
- Allows peer support
- Enhances application and analysis of new information

Lecture

- More formal method of instruction because teacher controls it
- Helps learner acquire new knowledge and gain comprehension

Question-and-Answer Session

- Designed specifically to address patient's concerns
- Helps patient apply knowledge

Role-Play, Discovery

- Allows patient to actively apply knowledge in controlled situation
- Promotes synthesis of information and problem solving

Independent Project (Computer-Assisted Instruction), Field Experience

- Allows patient to assume responsibility for completing learning activities at own pace
- Promotes analysis, synthesis, and evaluation of new information and skills

AFFECTIVE

Role Play

- Allows expression of values, feelings, and attitudes

Discussion (Group)

- Allows patient to acquire support from others in group
- Permits patient to learn from others' experiences
- Promotes responding, valuing, and organization

Discussion (One-on-One)

- Allows discussion of personal, sensitive topics of interest or concern

PSYCHOMOTOR

Demonstration

- Provides presentation of procedures or skills by nurse
- Permits patient to incorporate modeling of nurse's behavior
- Allows nurse to control questioning during demonstration

Practice

- Gives patient opportunity to perform skills using equipment
- Provides repetition

Return Demonstration

- Permits patient to perform skills as nurse observes
- Is excellent source of feedback and reinforcement

Independent Project, Game

- Requires teaching method that promotes adaptation and origination of psychomotor learning
- Permits learner to use new skills

BOX 12-8 CARE OF THE OLDER ADULT

Effective Teaching Strategies for the Older Adult

- Provide individualized information that is based on what the patient needs to know (Legrain et al., 2011).
- Present information slowly in frequent sessions.
- Include family members when necessary.
- Repeat information frequently.
- Reinforce teaching with audiovisual material, written exercises, and practice.
- Emphasize the older adult's current concerns and past positive coping strategies (Touhy and Jett, 2012).
- Allow more time for learners to express themselves, demonstrate learning, and ask questions (Edelman and Mandle, 2010).
- Establish measurable and realistic short-term goals.
- Establish follow-up sessions (Legrain et al., 2011).
- Base new information on patients' previous level of learning.

requires advance planning. Include the following steps in a demonstration:

1. Assemble and organize equipment.
2. Perform each step in sequence while analyzing the knowledge and skills involved.
3. Determine when to give explanations, considering the patient's learning needs.
4. Judge the proper speed and timing of the demonstration based on the patient's cognitive abilities and anxiety level.

Demonstrate the procedure or skill under the same conditions that the patient will experience at home and in the same order in which the patient will perform it. Encourage the patient to ask questions so he or she clearly understands each step. To enable the patient to easily observe each step of the procedure, perform demonstrations slowly and avoid rushing. Give the patient the opportunity to practice the procedure under supervision. At the end of the session have the patient perform a **return demonstration.** During a return demonstration the patient completes the procedure independently to show competence.

Analogies. Learning occurs when a teacher translates complex language or ideas into words or concepts that a patient understands. **Analogies** add to verbal instruction by providing familiar images that make complex information more real and understandable (Miller and Stoeckel, 2011). For example, comparing arterial blood pressure to the flow of water through a hose is an analogy that is useful when explaining hypertension to a patient. When using analogies, know the concept; keep the analogy simple and clear; and be aware of the patient's background, experience, and culture.

Analogies work only if the other person understands the comparison.

Role Play. During role play your patients play themselves or someone else in the situation. Patients learn required skills and feel more confident in performing them independently following the role play. For example, you are teaching a family caregiver effective communication strategies to use with an older, confused parent. You pretend to be the parent who is having difficulty getting dressed. The caregiver responds to you in this situation. At the end of the session you help the caregiver evaluate the response and determine if an alternative approach would have been more effective.

Simulation. Simulation is a useful technique for teaching problem solving, application, and independent thinking. During individual or group discussion you present a problem or situation pertaining to the patients' learning for patients to solve. For example, you ask patients with heart disease to plan a meal low in cholesterol.

Use of Technology. Communication and patient teaching does not only happen in person; it also occurs electronically. The majority of Americans have access to the Internet, and almost half of U.S. adults own a smartphone (Pew Research Center, 2013). As technology continues to improve, more people are online and use online resources to enhance their health. When you use it appropriately, technology (e.g., online resources, apps, and social media) is a very effective teaching tool (Weaver, Lindsay, Gitelman, 2012). Help your patients who are interested in using technology to manage their health to find electronic patient education resources that help them better manage their health needs.

Maintaining Attention and Participation. All of the senses are channels for presenting information. Patients learn better when you stimulate multiple senses while you teach. In addition, your actions can increase learner attention and participation. When conducting a discussion with a patient, change the tone and intensity of your voice, make eye contact, and use gestures that accentuate key points of discussion. A learner remains interested in a teacher who is actively enthusiastic about the subject under discussion (Billings and Halstead, 2009).

Illiteracy and Other Disabilities. Medical terms are very confusing; thus you need to provide information in words that your patients are able to understand. People who have problems with illiteracy or other learning disabilities often have difficulty analyzing instructions and synthesizing information. They often also have limited problem-solving skills and do not ask questions to clarify information. Use a variety of interventions (e.g., audiotapes, videos, or drawing pictures) with patients who have low health literacy or other difficulties learning (Box 12-9).

Sometimes you provide education to patients who have sensory alterations (see Chapter 38). When caring for patients who are deaf, you may need to include a sign language interpreter to help implement your interventions. Visual impairments also affect the teaching strategy you use. Many times patients who are blind or have reduced vision have acute listening skills. To enhance communication and decrease anxiety, tell the patient that you are there and do not shout during teaching sessions.

Cultural Awareness. Health education materials often fail to address a patient's cultural beliefs, values, language, perceptions, and attitudes. Be aware of the patient's cultural background, beliefs, and ability to understand instructions. In some cases you need to provide information written in the patient's native language.

Cultural awareness poses a great challenge to provide culturally sensitive health care and patient education. For example, how you explain guidelines for safe sex might vary if a patient is heterosexual versus homosexual. A patient from a lower socioeconomic background will require nutritional education with a different focus on foods than a patient who has unlimited financial resources and able to purchase any type of food.

Effective educational strategies often require the use of different patterns of communication. When educating

BOX 12-9 PATIENT TEACHING STRATEGIES FOR THE PATIENT WITH LIMITED HEALTH LITERACY

- Make time for one-on-one educational sessions.
- Individualize teaching materials (e.g., reading level, use of graphics, photographs) to meet a patient's needs and match his or her reading level; if you do not know patient's reading level, provide information at a fifth-grade or lower level.
- Provide information in a variety of ways (e.g., written, on a computer, videotape, audiotape).
- Make teaching materials visually appealing.
- Use simple words that a patient can understand (e.g., shot instead of injection, walk instead of ambulate, medicine instead of medication).
- Use the active voice when providing instructions (e.g., tell patient to "take medicine before bedtime" instead of "medicine should be taken at bedtime").
- Use examples (e.g., what to do when feeling bad, how to set up a pill counter at home) to keep patient an active participant in learning.
- Present the most important information first and summarize it at the end of the session.
- Space out information to decrease intimidation.
- Use pictures or illustrations when possible.
- Encourage patients to ask questions during the teaching session.
- Ask specific questions (e.g., "When will you take this medicine each day?") and ask patient to "teach back" or "show back" what you have taught. For example, "We discussed the problems you need to call your doctor about, tell me what those are," or "I explained the type of foods that are high in salt; give me three examples" to evaluate learning.
- Observe patient's ability to perform any desired behaviors or self-care activities.

BOX 12-10 EVALUATION

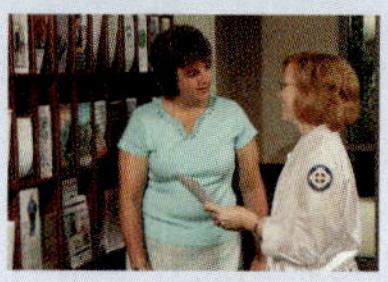

After Ashley and Latinka met for the first time, Latinka decided to quit smoking on her birthday, which was in 1½ weeks. During that time Ashley made an appointment for Latinka to see the advanced practice nurse at the health department so she could get a prescription for nicotine patches. Ashley and Latinka decided to meet 2 weeks after Latinka started her smoking cessation plan. In the meantime Ashley called Latinka on her birthday to provide encouragement and support.

Today Ashley and Latinka meet to evaluate how the teaching plan is going. Ashley completes a physical assessment and asks Latinka questions about her progress to date. Latinka states that she is less short of breath and has more energy now that she is not smoking. She feels better about herself and likes that her house does not smell like cigarette smoke as much anymore. Latinka's sons, who also smoked, decided to quit with their mom as a birthday present. Latinka states, "If one of us feels like smoking, we call one another for help. It's really nice that we can support one another." Ashley reinforces that having a good support system at home will help Latinka continue not to smoke. Latinka also relates that the nicotine patch is working well. She still suffers from nicotine withdrawal symptoms, but says, "They aren't that bad as long as I use my patches."

Because Ashley is also concerned about Latinka's weight-management plan, she asks her about her level of exercise and diet choices since the last time they met. Latinka says that she walks with her sons 2 days a week and with her neighbor another 2 days a week. She has also been experimenting with her recipes. She made her famous *burek*, which is a Bosnian meat pie. She used egg whites instead of egg yolks and ground sirloin instead of ground beef. She added more vegetables to her recipe and decreased the amount of butter she used. Latinka said, "I thought it was good, but I wasn't sure if it matched up to my old recipe. So I served it to my boys, and they didn't even notice the difference."

Ashley reviews healthy coping strategies with Latinka and provides reinforcement for all the positive changes made so far. They decide to meet again in 3 weeks. Ashley asks Latinka if there is anything that Latinka would like to review at their next appointment. Latinka says, "I want to review all the good things that will happen to me now that I'm not smoking. I also want to talk about what I'm going to do with all the money I'm saving now that I don't smoke. I might even bring you a sample from my new stew recipe." Latinka tells Ashley that she is so glad that Ashley is her nurse. Ashley feels a sense of satisfaction. She has helped Latinka make healthy changes, and she looks forward to learning more about Bosnian culture.

DOCUMENTATION NOTE

"Outcomes of education plan assessed. Reports quit smoking about 4 weeks ago on birthday. Sons have quit smoking also, providing support for one another. Has symptoms of nicotine withdrawal, but reports that nicotine replacement patch is helpful in minimizing symptoms. Verbalized increased feelings of energy and less shortness of breath. Walking 4 days a week with sons and neighbor. Is successfully experimenting with healthy substitutions in family recipes. Has asked to review short-term benefits associated with smoking cessation and will review diet information at next visit."

patients of different ethnic groups, do the following (Knoerl et al., 2011):

- Become aware of the distinctive aspects of each culture.
- If an interpreter is necessary, first determine your patient's beliefs about using an interpreter; in some cultures it is inappropriate to discuss private health-related issues with other people, people of other genders, or people who are younger. Always use a professional interpreter who understands medical terminology.
- Demonstrate respect for your patient and the family, address them using their appropriate titles, and pronounce their names correctly.
- Use culturally relevant teaching resources and approaches.

EVALUATION

Patient Care. Patient education is not complete until you evaluate the outcomes of the teaching-learning process (see Care Plan). During evaluation determine if your patient achieved learning objectives set during the planning stage (Box 12-10). Regardless of the method used to teach, use the **Teach Back** method (Box 12-11) to evaluate the patient's understanding of the material. The National Quality Forum recommends that nurses adopt this as part of "universal precautions" for patient education (Jager and Wynia, 2012). Sometimes you incorporate other methods of evaluation such as observing patient behaviors and return demonstration. For example, to evaluate learning in the patient who was taught how to use an asthma inhaler, have the patient demonstrate use of the inhaler (Sleath et al., 2011).

If evaluation indicates that a knowledge or skill deficit still exists, modify the teaching plan. Alternative teaching methods often help to clarify information or strengthen skills that the patient was unable to comprehend or perform originally. Evaluation reveals new learning needs or new factors that may interfere with the patient's ability to learn. Use this information to update the teaching plan and make it relevant to patient needs. Like the nursing process, the teaching process is continuous and ever changing.

Patient Expectations. After receiving education to manage health promotion activities, disease processes, and physical and functional limitations, patients return to their home and community. It is important to have a method for evaluating the patient's expectations regarding patient

BOX 12-11 TEACH BACK METHOD OF EVALUATION

Use the following questions to evaluate patient understanding of education. Ask the questions in an open-ended, respectful manner and modify them as needed (Himmelfarb and Hughes, 2011; Nigolian and Miller, 2011).

- "I want to be sure that I explained this clearly. When your family asks how you're supposed to take this medicine, what will you say?"
- "Let's review the main side effects of (insert name of medication). For what two things do you need to watch?"
- "We've talked a lot today about (insert appropriate topic). I want to be sure that I've explained everything clearly. What changes in (insert appropriate topic/condition/routine/person) will you call the health care provider about?"
- "On days when you and your wife (or husband) go out, what will you do about taking your (insert name of medication)?"
- "After talking today, what will your daily routine look like?"
- "Please use this model to show me how you'll do (procedure)?

education. Did the patient and family receive the education they expected? Were the expectations regarding self-care met? Are some education expectations remaining? Did the educational program increase a patient's ability to manage his or her health status at home? If your patients' expectations are not met, it is more likely that patients will not continue following the prescribed treatment plan, will be less independent, and perhaps will ignore signs and/or symptoms indicating a need to make an appointment with their health care provider.

DOCUMENTATION OF PATIENT TEACHING

Because patient teaching often occurs informally (e.g., during medication administration or physical examination), it is difficult to document it consistently. However, because nurses are professionally and legally responsible for providing accurate and timely information to patients, quality documentation is essential. Documentation also helps members of the health care team coordinate patient education. Document the following information about patient education:

1. *Assessment data and related nursing diagnoses:* Provide information and support for goals and outcomes.
2. *Interventions planned and used:* Planned education provides continuity of care. Specifically describe subject matter and what has been presented to so that other nurses can follow up and reinforce teaching (e.g., "verbalized side effects of digoxin").
3. *Evaluation of learning:* Document evidence of learning (e.g., a return demonstration of coughing and deep breathing). This informs staff about the patient's progress and determines material that you still need to teach. Always use the Teach Back method.
4. *Ability of patient and/or family to manage care:* Identify needs for outpatient or home care follow-up after discharge. Appropriate referrals meet the patient's needs better.

KEY POINTS

- Health education is aimed at the promotion, restoration, and maintenance of health.
- Teaching is most effective when it is responsive to a learner's needs and requires the learner's active involvement.
- Teaching is a form of interpersonal communication, with teacher and student actively involved in a process that increases the student's knowledge and skills.
- Teaching a patient a specific behavior involves incorporation of behaviors from all three learning domains.
- A person's health beliefs influence the willingness to gain the knowledge and skills necessary to maintain health.
- Patients of different age-groups require different teaching strategies as a result of developmental capabilities.
- Presentation of teaching content progresses from simple to more complex ideas.
- Assess the reading ability and the ability of the patient to understand health information before providing patient education.
- Patient teaching is culturally sensitive and individualized to meet the needs of each patient.
- A patient is an active participant in a teaching plan, agreeing to the plan, helping to choose instructional methods, and recommending times for instruction.
- A combination of teaching methods improves a learner's attentiveness and involvement.
- Teaching methodologies should match a patient's learning needs.
- Learning objectives describe what a person is to learn in behavioral terms.
- Evaluate a patient's learning by using the Teach Back method and observing the performance of expected learning behaviors under desired conditions.

CLINICAL DECISION-MAKING EXERCISES

Latinka and Ashley continue to meet to monitor Latinka's success with her smoking cessation plan. Overall Latinka is doing well with her plan, but she continues to forget to change her nicotine patch. As a result, Latinka's nurse practitioner decides to discontinue the nicotine patch and starts Latinka on a nonnicotine prescription medication used to help people stop smoking.

1. Reflect on the assessment data described here. How would the nurse revise existing nursing diagnoses for Latinka at this time? Why is it a priority?
2. When Ashley teaches Latinka about smoking cessation, her new medication, and when to take it, which of the domains of learning are involved?

3. As Ashley teaches Latinka about her new medication, she suspects that Latinka is experiencing difficulty understanding the written medication information provided by the manufacturer. Why do you think Latinka cannot understand the material? Describe the educational interventions Ashley needs to use at this time.

evolve

Answers to Clinical Decision-Making Exercises can be found on the Evolve website.

QSEN ACTIVITY: INFORMATICS

Latinka tells Ashley that she recently purchased a new smartphone and is excited about it. She asks Ashley if there are any apps that she can use to help her stop smoking, eat better, and manage her weight. Ashley knows that these apps help patients change their behaviors and better understand how to make positive changes at the same time.

Conduct a literature search and find at least one smartphone app that Ashley could suggest that Latinka use to stop smoking, improve her diet, and manage her weight. Why is it important for Ashley to evaluate these apps and help Latinka decide which ones to use?

evolve

Answers to QSEN Activities can be found on the Evolve website.

REVIEW QUESTIONS

1. A patient has been started on a diuretic for hypertension and needs to learn about the side effects of the medication. Understanding this information requires learning in the:
    1. Cognitive domain.
    2. Affective domain.
    3. Psychomotor domain.
    4. Attentional domain.
2. Which of the following are effective teaching-learning principles that a nurse uses when teaching a new mother how to breastfeed her baby? (Select all that apply.)
    1. Provide patient education when there are visitors in the room.
    2. Time teaching sessions to coincide with times when the patient's baby is hungry.
    3. Provide patient teaching when the patient is well rested and the baby is not crying.
    4. Include the patient's spouse in educational sessions if it is okay with her.
    5. Assess the patient's feelings about being a new mom and beliefs about breastfeeding at the end of the teaching session.
3. A nursing student is preparing to teach third-grade students about the importance of exercise. To achieve the best learning outcomes the nursing student:
    1. Provides information using a lecture.
    2. Provides several teaching handouts that the children can take home.
    3. Develops activities that involve the children in exercises they can do daily.
    4. Completes an extensive literature search focusing on prevention of childhood obesity.
4. An 86-year-old woman's priority nursing diagnosis is *Disturbed Sleep Pattern related to anxiety and lack of understanding of upcoming surgery.* The nurse teaches the patient what to expect before, during, and after surgery. The nurse knows that the patient understands the procedures to expect after surgery when the patient:
    1. Demonstrates how she will get out of bed following her surgery.
    2. States that she needs to ask her daughter to be at the hospital the day of her surgery.
    3. Needs reinforcement of information regarding pain management and activity following surgery.
    4. Calls her friends to tell them about the day of her surgery and how long she will be in the hospital.
5. A patient is being discharged in 2 days and will need to self-administer a medication subcutaneously. She has not had to take this medication in the past. The nurse allows the patient to prepare and administer her own injections. The teaching approach used in this situation is the:
    1. Telling approach.
    2. Selling approach.
    3. Entrusting approach.
    4. Participating approach.
6. A 68-year-old man needs to learn how to do self-catheterization. In teaching the patient about this, you need to:
    1. Speak loudly and clearly.
    2. Demonstrate the skill quickly and efficiently.
    3. Expect the patient to understand the information the first time you present it.
    4. Allow the patient time to express his feelings about catheterizing himself and ask questions.
7. A nurse is a preceptor for a nursing student who is caring for a 10-year-old boy with asthma. The nursing student needs to teach the child how to use an inhaler. The nurse intervenes when the student:
    1. Gives the child time to ask questions.
    2. Demonstrates how to use the inhaler step by step.
    3. Encourages the child to learn how to use the inhaler on his own.
    4. Assesses the child's hand strength and ability to administer the medication.
8. A nurse is preparing to teach a patient with poor health literacy about a new medication. What does the nurse do first?
    1. Schedules frequent teaching sessions
    2. Assesses patient's learning methods and needs

3. Asks the patient to explain what was taught and provide a return demonstration of skills learned
4. Includes the most important information about the medication at the beginning of the teaching session

9. A nurse wants to use individualized computer instruction with a group of low-income mothers at the public health department. Which of the following does the nurse do before using this instructional strategy?
   1. Assesses the patients' psychomotor skills
   2. Makes sure that the most important information is presented last
   3. Assesses the reading level of the information provided on the computer
   4. Ensures that there are photographs included in the computer program

10. Which of the following interventions implemented by the nurse when caring for a patient who recently had a stroke indicates that the nurse is incorporating teaching with nursing care?
    1. The nurse speaks clearly and develops alternative communication methods as needed.
    2. The nurse describes the importance of changing positions while turning the patient onto the side.
    3. The nurse determines the patient's reading level and ensures that teaching materials are written at the appropriate level.
    4. The nurse assesses the patient's culture and ensures that food delivered by the kitchen is consistent with the patient's cultural preferences.

evolve

Rationales for Review Questions can be found on the Evolve website.

1. 1; **2.** 2, 3, 4; **3.** 3; **4.** 1; **5.** 3; **6.** 4; **7.** 3; **8.** 2; **9.** 1; **10.** 2

REFERENCES

American Hospital Association (AHA): *The patient care partnership*, 2003, http://www.aha.org/advocacy-issues/communicatingpts/pt-care-partnership.shtml. Accessed May 19, 2013.

Balmford J, et al: The influence of having a quit date on smoking cessation, *Health Educ Res* 25(4):698, 2010.

Bandura A: *Self-efficacy: the exercise of control*, New York, 1997, WH Freeman.

Bastable S: *Nurse as educator: principles of teaching and learning for nursing practice*, ed 4, Sudbury, MA, 2014, Jones & Bartlett.

Berkman ND, et al: Low health literacy and health outcomes: an updated systematic review, *Ann Intern Med* 155(2):97, 2011.

Billings DM, Halstead JA: *Teaching in nursing: a guide for faculty*, ed 3, St Louis, 2009, Saunders.

Centers for Medicare & Medicaid Services (CMS): *Readmissions reduction program*, 2013, http://www.cms.gov/Medicare/Medicare-Fee-for-Service-Payment/AcuteInpatientPPS/Readmissions-Reduction-Program.html. Accessed July 3, 2013.

Coulter A: Patient engagement-what works? *J Ambulatory Care Manage* 35(2):80, 2012.

Duiveman T, Bonner A: Negotiating: experiences of community nurses when contracting with clients, *Contemp Nurse* 41(1):120, 2012.

Edelman CL, Mandle CL: *Health promotion throughout the life span*, ed 7, St Louis, 2010, Mosby.

Falvo DR: *Effective patient education: a guide to increased adherence*, ed 4, Sudbury, MA, 2011, Jones & Bartlett.

Fowler MDM: *Guide to the code of ethics for nurses: interpretation and application*, Silver Spring, MD, 2010, American Nurses Association.

Funnell MM, et al: National standards for diabetes self-management education, *Diabetes Care* 34(s1):s89, 2011.

Gavric Z, et al: Correlation between levels of physical activity and the occurrence of depression among patients in family medicine clinics, *Eur J Gen Med* 9(2):75, 2012.

Gilboy N, Howard PK: Research to practice: comprehension of discharge instructions, *Adv Emerg Nurs J* 31(1):4, 2009.

Glasgow RE, et al: Long-term results of a smoking reduction program, *Medical Care* 47(1):115, 2009.

Hansen LO, et al: Interventions to reduce 30-day rehospitalization: a systematic review, *Ann Intern Med* 155(8):520, 2011.

Harris J, et al: Perceptions of personal risk about smoking and health among Bosnian refugees living in the United States, *J Immigrant Minority Health* 14(3):413, 2012.

Himmelfarb CR, Hughes S: Are you assessing the communication "vital sign"? Improving communication with our low-health-literacy patients, *J Cardiovasc Nurs* 26(3):177, 2011.

Inott T, Kennedy BB: Assessing learning styles: practical tips for patient education, *Nurs Clin North Am* 46(3):313, 2011.

Jager AJ, Wynia MK: Who gets a teach-back? Patient-reported incidence of experiencing a teach-back, *J Health Communication: Int Perspect* 17(Suppl 3):294, 2012.

Kerr S, et al: A mixed-methods evaluation of the effectiveness of tailored smoking cessation training for healthcare practitioners who work with older people, *Worldviews Evidence-Based Nurs* 8(3):177, 2011.

Knoerl AM, Esper KW, Hasenau SM: Cultural sensitivity in patient health education, *Nurs Clin North Am* 46(3):335, 2011.

Krau SD: Creating educational objectives for patient education using the New Bloom's Taxonomy, *Nurs Clin North Am* 46(3):299, 2011.

Lavric M, Flere S: Trait anxiety and measures of religiosity in four cultural settings, *Mental Health Religion Cult* 13(7/8):667, 2010.

Legrain S, et al: A new multimodal geriatric discharge-planning intervention to prevent emergency visits and rehospitalizations of older adults: the optimization of medication in AGEd multicenter randomized controlled trial, *J Am Geriatr Soc* 59(11):2017, 2011.

Linertova R, et al: Interventions to reduce hospital readmissions in the elderly: in-hospital or home care: a systematic review, *J Eval Clin Pract* 17(6):1167, 2011.

Mahvan T, et al: Which smoking cessation interventions work best? *J Fam Pract* 60(7):430, 2011.

Mann KS: Education and health promotion for new patients with cancer: a quality improvement model, *Clin J Oncol Nurs* 15(1):55, 2011.

Marbach TJ, Griffie J: Patient preferences concerning treatment plans, survivorship care plans, education, and support services, *Oncol Nurs Forum* 38(3):335, 2011.

McNeill BE: You "teach" but does your patient really learn? Basic principles to promote safer outcomes, *Tar Heel Nurse* 74(1):9, 2012.

Miller MA, Stoeckel PR: *Client education: theory and practice*, Sudbury, MA, 2011, Jones & Bartlett.

Nigolian CJ, Miller KL: Teaching essential skills to family caregivers, *Am J Nurs* 111(11):52, 2011.

Pew Research Center: *Smartphone ownership 2013*, 2013, http://pewinternet.org/Reports/2013/Smartphone-Ownership-2013.aspx. Accessed August 15, 2013.

Priharjo R, Hoy G: Use of peer teaching to enhance student and patient education, *Nurs Stand* 25(20):40, 2011.

Redman BK: Ethics of patient education and how do we make it everyone's ethics, *Nurs Clin North Am* 46(3):283, 2011.

Sleath B, et al: Provider demonstration and assessment of child device technique during pediatric asthma visits, *Pediatrics* 127(4):642, 2011.

Speros CI: Promoting health literacy: a nursing imperative, *Nurs Clin North Am* 46(3):321, 2011.

Su WM, et al: Using a competency-based approach to patient education: achieving congruence among learning, teaching and evaluation, *Nurs Clin North Am* 46(3):291, 2011.

The Joint Commission (TJC): *Speak up initiatives*, 2013, http://www.jointcommission.org/speakup.aspx. Accessed May 19, 2013.

Touhy TA, Jett K: *Ebersole and Hess' toward healthy aging: human needs and nursing response*, ed 8, St Louis, 2012, Mosby.

Townsend MS: Patient-driven materials: low-literate adults increase understanding of health messages and improve compliance, *Nurs Clin North Am* 46(3):367, 2011.

Tzelepis F, et al: Proactive telephone counseling for smoking cessation: meta-analysis by recruitment channel and methodological quality, *J Natl Cancer Inst* 103(12):922, 2011.

US Department of Health and Human Services (USDHHS): *HealthyPeople.gov*, 2013, Available at http://www.healthypeople.gov/2020/default.aspx. Accessed August 14, 2013.

Vaartio-Rajalin H, Leino-Kilpi H: Nurses as patient advocates in oncology care: activities based on literature, *Clin J Oncol Nurs* 15(5):526, 2011.

Weaver B, Lindsay B, Gitelman B: Communication technology and social media: opportunities and implications for healthcare systems, *OJIN: Online J Issues Nurs* 17(3):3, 2012.

CHAPTER

13

Managing Patient Care

evolve WEBSITE

http://evolve.elsevier.com/Potter/essentials
- Crossword Puzzle
- Audio Glossary

OBJECTIVES

- Differentiate among the types of nursing care delivery models.
- Describe the elements of decentralized decision making.
- Discuss the ways in which a nurse manager supports staff involvement in a decentralized decision-making model.
- Discuss ways to apply clinical care coordination skills in nursing practice.
- Describe the process of interprofessional collaboration among nurses and health care providers.
- Discuss principles to follow in the appropriate delegation of patient care activities.

KEY TERMS

accountability, p. 229
authority, p. 229
autonomy, p. 229
decentralized management, p. 228
delegation, p. 234
primary nursing, p. 227
responsibility, p. 228
team nursing, p. 227
total patient care, p. 227

CASE STUDY *Jennifer*

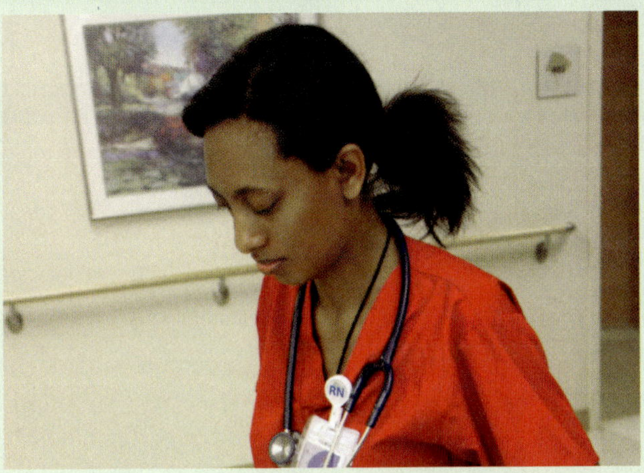

Jennifer is a nursing student assigned to care for three patients as part of her final clinical experience. Her first patient is Mrs. Sinclair, who will have surgery at 1 PM to repair her fractured right hip. It is the first time she has had surgery. It is now 11:30 AM. The operating room (OR) has notified Jennifer that OR staff will pick up Mrs. Sinclair in 30 minutes. Jennifer enters Mrs. Sinclair's room to complete the preoperative checklist and make final preparations for surgery. She finds Mrs. Sinclair moving about restlessly in bed and reluctant to talk. At the same time the call-light system at the bedside comes on, and the unit clerk notifies Jennifer that her second patient, Mr. Timmons, has finished his lunch and is ready for his pain medication so he can ambulate down the hall. Mr. Timmons had abdominal surgery 2 days ago for removal of a colon tumor. Her third patient, Mr. Dodson, has a postoperative wound infection. He is due for his next dose of antibiotic medication. Jennifer also knows that his wet-to-dry abdominal dressing is due to be changed.

As a nursing student, it is important for you to acquire the necessary knowledge, skills, and competencies that ultimately allow you to practice as an entry-level nurse. The National Council of State Boards of Nursing (NCSBN) identified competencies that registered nurses (RNs) and licensed practical and vocational nurses(LPN/LVNs) need on entry to practice (Kearney, 2009) (Box 13-1). Regardless of the type of setting in which you eventually choose to work as a nurse, you are responsible for practicing professional standards of care, using organizational resources, and participating in organizational routines. While doing this you provide direct patient care, use your time productively, collaborate with all members of the health care team, and use certain leadership characteristics to manage others on the nursing team. The delivery of nursing care within the health care system is a challenge because of the changes that are influencing health professionals, patients, and health care organizations (see Chapter 3). However, change offers opportunities. As you develop the knowledge and skills to become a nurse, you learn what it takes to effectively manage the patients for whom you care and to take the initiative in becoming a leader among your professional colleagues.

BUILDING A NURSING TEAM

Nurses want to work within an institutional culture that promotes autonomy and quality (Kramer, Maguire, and Brewer, 2011). Your education and the commitment you make to practice within established standards and guidelines ensure a rewarding professional career. It is also important to work as a member of a cohesive and strong nursing team that values mentoring, integrity, and respect for teamwork. An empowering work environment brings out the best in a professional. It concentrates on effective patient care systems (e.g., patient assessment, referral mechanisms, and collaboration among nurses and health care providers), supports risk taking and innovation, focuses on results and rewards, and offers professional opportunities for growth and advancement. Effective team development requires team building and training, trust, communication, and a workplace that facilitates collaboration (Huber, 2010).

One way of creating an empowering work environment is through the Magnet Recognition Program. The Magnet Recognition Program recognizes nursing services that build programs of excellence for the delivery of nursing care, promote quality in environments that support professional nursing practice, and promote achievement of positive patient outcomes (ANCC, 2012). A Magnet hospital has a culture that is dynamic and positive for nurses. Typically it has a system to recognize and reward nurses for clinical performance, has research programs, and uses evidence-based practice. The nurses have professional autonomy over their practice and control over the practice environment (Kramer, Schmalenberg, and Maguire, 2010). A Magnet hospital empowers the nursing team to make changes and be innovative. This culture produces a strong collaborative relationship among team members and improves patient quality outcomes (see Chapter 3).

The Institute of Medicine (IOM, 2004) called for health care to transform the work environment to focus on keeping patients safe. Because of their focus on patient assessment and evaluation, nurses are key team members to participate in transforming the health care environment. As a part of this transformation, the IOM (2001) called for all health care professionals to be educated to deliver patient-centered care using evidence-based practice, quality improvement approaches, and informatics. Nurses need to deliver safe, effective quality patient care through collaboration as a member of an interdisciplinary team (IOM, 2001).

It takes an excellent nurse manager and nursing staff to achieve an enriching work culture and environment. Together a manager and the nursing staff share a philosophy of care for their work unit. A philosophy of care incorporates the professional nursing staff's values and concerns for the way that they view and care for patients. For example, a philosophy addresses the purpose of the nursing unit, how staff will work with patients and families, and the standards of care for the work unit. It is a vision for how to practice nursing. Integral to the philosophy of care is the selection of a nursing care

BOX 13-1 ENTRY-LEVEL NURSE COMPETENCIES

- Able to understand the health care system and processes to see the big picture.
- Understand the environment of care
- Able to manage care of patients
- Able to critically think as demonstrated by assessment of a problem, identification of solution, implementation of solution, evaluation of care, and follow-up of care
- Communicate effectively with physicians and health care team members
- Demonstrate nursing knowledge and display confidence in knowledge base
- Work as a team member collaborating with health care team members
- Have a patient orientation and focus with actions focused on patient and patient needs
- Respect the rights, beliefs, wishes, and values of patients
- Be a patient advocate
- Recognize own limitations and see support of validation of decisions as needed
- Demonstrate knowledge of roles, responsibilities and functions of a nurse

Modified from Kearney MH: *Report of the findings from the post-entry competence study,* Chicago, 2009, National Council of State Boards of Nursing; National Council of State Boards of Nursing: *2009 tuning analysis: a comparison of U.S. and international nursing educational competences,* Chicago, 2010, National Council State Boards of Nursing.

delivery model and management structure that supports professional nursing practice.

NURSING CARE DELIVERY MODELS

A nursing care delivery model allows you to help your patients achieve desirable outcomes and satisfaction with care (Huber, 2010). Since Florence Nightingale, nurses have used a variety of nursing care delivery models to provide care. Nursing care delivery models contain the common components of nurse-patient relationship, clinical decision making, patient assignments and work allocation, interdisciplinary communication, and management of the environment of care (Huber, 2010). Team nursing, primary nursing, and total patient care models are most common in acute care settings. Case management and primary nursing are the common nursing care delivery models used in the home care setting (Table 13-1).

Team nursing was a response to the severe nursing shortage following World War II. By 2000 the interdisciplinary team was a more common model (Marriner Tomey, 2009). **Total patient care** delivery was the original care delivery model developed during Florence Nightingale's time. The model disappeared in the 1930s but can often be found today in critical care areas where nurses deliver total care to one or two patients (Yoder-Wise, 2011). The **primary nursing** model of care delivery was developed to place RNs at the

TABLE 13-1 NURSING CARE DELIVERY MODELS

NURSING MODEL	CHARACTERISTICS	ADVANTAGES	DISADVANTAGES
Team nursing	Registered nurse (RN) leads team of other RNs, practical nurses, and unlicensed assistive personnel (UAP). Team members provide direct patient care under supervision of RN. Team leader develops patient care plans, coordinates care among team members, and provides care requiring complex nursing skills. There is hierarchical communication from charge nurse to charge nurse, charge nurse to team leader, and team leader to team members.	Care is provided through a collaborative style that encourages each member of team to work with and help the other members. Team leader has a high level of autonomy. Decision making occurs at clinical level. Nursing care conferences help to solve patient problems. Patient care coordinator has time to manage unit issues.	RN team leader does not spend time with patients so patients may not see RN often. It takes time for team leader to delegate work. It is not effective if team leader has poor leadership skills.
Total patient care	RN is responsible for all aspects of care for one or more patients during a shift of care. Care is usually consistent, comprehensive, and holistic. Care can be delegated. RN works directly with patient, family, and health care team members.	Patient satisfaction with model is high. RNs plan care. RNs are required to collaborate frequently with other health care team members.	Continuity of care is a problem if RNs do not communicate patient needs to one another. It may not be cost-effective because of high number of RNs needed to provide care. There is lack of clarity on who is coordinating 24-hour care.
Primary nursing	One primary RN assumes responsibility for a caseload of patients. RN provides care for the same patients during their stay in the health care facility. RN assesses patient, develops plan of care, and delivers appropriate nursing interventions. Communication is lateral from nurse to nurse and caregiver to caregiver.	Model is flexible and uses a variety of staffing levels and mixes. It has a high level of autonomy and authority. It promotes collaboration with health care provider. It provides continuity of care. It reduces number of errors that occur when relaying orders.	RNs work with a limited number of patients, which limits knowledge and skill use. Other nurses cannot change care plan without discussing with primary nurse.

Modified from Marriner Tomey A: *Guide to nursing management and leadership,* ed 8, St Louis, 2009, Mosby; Yoder-Wise PS: *Leading and managing in nursing,* ed 5, St Louis, 2011, Elsevier.

bedside and improve nursing accountability for patient outcomes and the professional relationships among staff members (Marriner Tomey, 2009). The model became more popular in the 1970s and early 1980s as hospitals began to employ more RNs. Primary nursing supports a philosophy regarding nurse and patient relationships.

Case Management

Case management is a delivery of care approach that emerged in the 1980s as health care institutions needed to provide complex cost-effective care. The Case Management Society of America (2012) defines case management as "a collaborative process of assessment, planning, facilitation and advocacy for options and services to meet an individual's health needs. …" Case management coordinates and links health care services to patients and their families with the goal of promoting quality cost-effective outcomes (see Chapter 3). What is unique about case management is that clinicians, either as individuals or as part of a collaborative group, oversee the management of patients with specific case types, focusing on length of stay and improving clinical outcomes (e.g., patients with specific diagnoses presenting complex nursing and medical problems such as heart failure or diabetes mellitus) (Thomas, 2008). The case managers are usually held accountable for some standard of cost management and quality. In the hospital a case manager coordinates a patient's acute care and follows the patient after discharge home. For example, he or she calls a meeting of the patient, family, social services, dietitian, and physical therapist to plan the discharge of a patient following a stroke. Case managers do not provide direct care. Instead they collaborate with and supervise the care that other staff members deliver and actively coordinate patient discharge planning. Many organizations use critical pathways, which are multidisciplinary treatment plans, in a case-management delivery system as a mechanism to improve patient and institutional outcomes (Yoder-Wise, 2011). Advantages of case management include cost-effectiveness, focus on patients' complex health needs, efficiency in discharge planning, and multidisciplinary collaboration (Yoder-Wise, 2011).

DECISION MAKING

Decision making is a critical component of an effective manager and leader (Huber, 2010). It is the nursing manager who directs and supports staff in the realization of the established nursing philosophy of a facility. The nurse executive supports managers by establishing a nursing governance structure along with policies and procedures that help to achieve organizational goals and provide appropriate support to care delivery decisions. It takes a committed nurse executive, an excellent manager, and empowered nursing staff to create an enriching work environment.

Decentralized management, in which decision making is made at the staff level, is very common within health care organizations. It is clear that progressive health care organizations achieve more when they actively involve employees at all levels. Advantages of decentralization include increased morale and improved interpersonal relationships among staff. Staff members feel more important and are more willing to contribute. Decentralization also promotes creativity in problem solving (Marriner Tomey, 2009). As a result the role of a nurse manager has become critical in the management of effective nursing units or groups. Box 13-2 highlights the diverse responsibilities assumed by nursing managers. To make decentralized decision making work, managers need to move it down to the staff level. On a nursing unit it is important for all staff members (RNs, LPNs, and LVNs), nursing assistive personnel (NAP), and unit secretaries to feel involved, particularly with issues affecting their ability to care for patients. Decision making includes responsibility, autonomy, authority, and accountability (Marriner Tomey, 2009; Yoder-Wise, 2011).

Responsibility refers to the duties and activities that an individual is employed to perform. For professional nurses, a position description outlines a nurse's responsibilities in patient care and level of participation as a member of a nursing unit. Responsibility reflects ownership and obligation; the individual who oversees the employee gives responsibility, and the employee accepts it. For example, a staff nurse is responsible for completing a nursing assessment of all assigned patients, developing a plan of care that addresses each of the patient's nursing diagnoses, and implementing care strategies. The nurse is also responsible for making sure that other staff members know what care they are responsible for performing. As the staff delivers the plan of care, the nurse

BOX 13-2 RESPONSIBILITIES OF THE NURSE MANAGER

- Help staff establish annual goals for the unit and the systems needed to accomplish goals
- Monitor professional nursing standards of practice on the unit
- Develop an ongoing staff development plan, including one for new employees
- Recruit new employees (interview and hire)
- Conduct routine staff evaluations
- Establish self as a role model for positive customer service (customers include patients, families, and other health care team members)
- Serve as an advocate for the nursing staff to the administration of the institution
- Submit staffing schedules for the unit
- Conduct regular patient rounds and help to solve patient or family complaints
- Establish and implement a quality improvement (QI) plan for the unit
- Review and recommend new equipment needs for the unit
- Conduct regular staff meetings
- Conduct rounds with health care provider
- Establish and support necessary staff and interdisciplinary committees

is responsible for evaluating if the plan is successful and what to do when it is not successful. This responsibility becomes a work ethic for the nurse in delivering excellent patient care.

Autonomy is freedom of choice and responsibility for those choices (Marriner Tomey, 2009). Autonomy, consistent with the scope of professional nursing practice, maximizes your effectiveness as a nurse (Yoder-Wise, 2011). With clinical autonomy a professional nurse makes independent decisions about patient care. The nurse plans care for the patient within the scope of professional nursing practice and provides independent nursing interventions for the patient without physician permission (Skar, 2009). Another type of autonomy for nurses is work autonomy. In work autonomy a nurse makes independent decisions about the work of the unit such as scheduling or unit governance. Autonomy is not an absolute but occurs in degrees. For example, a nurse has the autonomy to develop and implement a discharge teaching plan based on specific patient needs for any hospitalized patient. He or she also provides nursing care that complements the prescribed medical therapy.

Authority refers to the official power to act in areas in which an individual has been given and accepts responsibility (Marriner Tomey, 2009). It provides a nurse power to make final decisions and give instructions related to the decisions. For example, a primary nurse managing a caseload of patients discovers that members of the nursing team did not follow through on a discharge teaching plan for an assigned patient. The primary nurse has the authority to consult other nurses to learn why they did not follow recommendations on the plan of care and to choose appropriate teaching strategies for the patient that all members of the team will follow. The primary nurse has the final authority in selecting the best course of action for a patient's care.

Accountability refers to liability or individuals being answerable for their actions. It involves follow-up and a reflective analysis of your decisions to evaluate their effectiveness. A staff nurse may delegate responsibility but is accountable for his or her patients' outcomes (Marriner Tomey, 2009). As another example, a nurse is accountable for ensuring that a patient learns the information necessary to improve self-care. By using authority in bringing the nursing team together, the nurse determines if collaboration was successful, if continuity in teaching occurred, and if the patient and family understood the information.

A successful decentralized nursing unit exercises these four elements on an ongoing basis. An effective manager sets expectations for the staff's ability to make decisions. Staff members need to feel comfortable in expressing differences of opinion and challenging ways in which the team functions. They do this while recognizing their own responsibility, autonomy, authority, and accountability. Ultimately decentralized decision making allows a nursing unit to achieve its vision of what professional nursing care should be.

Staff Involvement

With decentralized decision making on a nursing unit, all staff members actively participate in unit activities. Because the work environment promotes participation, all staff members benefit from the knowledge and skills of the entire work group. When staff members learn to value knowledge and the contributions of colleagues, better patient care is an outcome. The nursing manager supports staff involvement through a variety of ways:

1. *Establishment of nursing practice or problem-solving committees:* Staff committees establish and maintain professional nursing practice on a unit. Practice committees are involved in activities such as the review and revision of standards of care, development of policy and procedure, and resolution of repeated patient satisfaction issues. These activities ensure the delivery of quality care on the unit. A senior staff member usually chairs a committee. Managers do not always sit on the committee, but they receive regular reports of committee progress. The nature of work on the nursing unit determines committee membership. At times members of other disciplines (e.g., pharmacy, respiratory therapy, or clinical nutrition) participate on practice committees.
2. *Interprofessional collaboration among nurses and health care providers:* Interprofessional collaboration among nurses and health care providers is critical to the delivery of quality, safe patient care and creation of a work culture for practitioners (Andreatta, 2010; IECEP, 2011). Interprofessional collaboration involves bringing representatives of the various disciplines together to work with patients and families to deliver quality care (Figure 13-1) (IECEP, 2011). This brings different points of view to the table to identify, clarify, and solve complex patient problems. The nurse plays a unique role within the team and is often viewed as the team leader through coordination of communication and patient care (Burzotta and Noble, 2011; Halabisky et al., 2010). Open communication, cooperation, trust, mutual respect, and understanding of team member roles and responsibilities are critical for successful interprofessional collaboration (Andreatta, 2010; Burzotta and Noble, 2011). A change in education and team training of health care practitioners is needed to build effective teams to improve interprofessional collaboration (Andreatta, 2010; Halabisky et al., 2010).

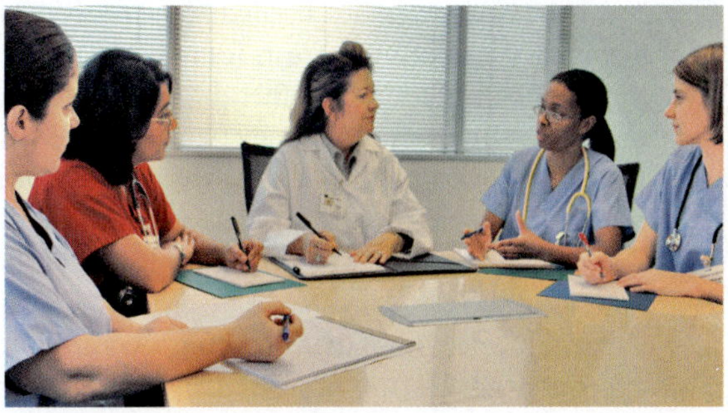

FIGURE 13-1 Interdisciplinary team collaborating on practice issues. (From Yoder-Wise P: *Leading and managing in nursing*, ed 5, St Louis, 2011, Mosby.)

BOX 13-3 EVIDENCE-BASED PRACTICE

PICO Question: Do simulations that include interprofessional education compared to other traditional learning activities improve nursing student learning of interprofessional collaboration skills?

SUMMARY OF EVIDENCE

A key component of delivery of high-quality, safe patient care is interprofessional collaboration (IPC) (Wagner, Liston, and Miller, 2011). Effective communication is a critical aspect of IPC. Simulation is a learning activity that provides students an opportunity to practice delivery of nursing care in a safe environment. Nursing students participating in simulation activities with medical students indicated that the simulation activities improved communication skills by providing opportunities to practice speaking to physicians, patients, and families (Wagner et al., 2011). Research shows that interprofessional education simulation activities in both live and virtual simulations are effective in improving the perceived need for collaboration, competency, and autonomy (Mohaupt et al., 2012; Riesen et al., 2012). Debriefing sessions after simulations offer another strategy to learn IPC (Mohaupt et al., 2012). Students enrolled in an interprofessional development course gained better understanding of roles of other team members, with some students showing an increased understanding of the purpose of IPC (Hylin, Lonka, and Ponzer, 2011).

APPLICATION TO NURSING PRACTICE

- Participate in simulation activities as available during and after graduation from nursing programs (Mohaupt et al., 2012).
- Work at understanding the roles of other interprofessional teams to improve your effectiveness as a member of the IPC team (Hylin et al., 2011).
- Actively participate in debriefing sessions after simulation activities as a strategy to improve your learning of IPC (Mohaupt et al., 2012).
- Observe other simulation teams completing the scenario as a learning activity (Wagner et al., 2011).

IECEP (2011) has identified four competencies that health care practitioners should bring to professional practice to be effective team members in interprofessional collaboration. The development of these competencies comes through interprofessional education (Box 13-3). Competencies needed for effective interprofessional collaboration are as follow:

a. Work with individuals of other professions to maintain a climate of mutual respect and shared values.
b. Use the knowledge of one's own role and those of other professions to appropriately assess and address the health care needs of patients and populations served.
c. Communicate with patients, families, communities, and other health care professionals in a responsive and responsible manner that supports a team approach to the maintenance of health and treatment of disease.
d. Apply relationship-building values and the principles of team dynamics to perform effectively in different team roles to plan and deliver patient-/population-centered care that is safe, timely, efficient, effective, and equitable.

3. *Interprofessional rounding:* Many institutions are conducting interprofessional rounding with the purpose of improving patient care coordination and communication among the health care team. During rounding members of the health care team round on patients and share patient information, answer questions asked by other team members, discuss patients' clinical progress, plan for discharge, and focus all team members on the same patient goals (Sharp, 2013). Interprofessional rounding has also been found to decrease medical errors and improve quality of care (Begue et al., 2012). For interprofessional rounding to be successful, health care team members need to be flexible.
4. *Staff communication:* In the present health care environment it is difficult for a manager to send a clear, accurate, and timely message to all members of a nursing staff. Staff members may become uneasy and distrusting if they fail to hear about planned changes on their unit. However, a manager does not assume total responsibility for all communication. Instead, she or he establishes a variety of approaches to ensure the quick and accurate communication of information to all staff members. For example, many managers distribute biweekly or monthly newsletters of ongoing unit or health care agency activities. They also post minutes of staff and practice committee meetings in an accessible location for all staff members to read. When the manager needs to discuss important issues regarding the operations of the unit or the organization with the staff, he or she conducts staff meetings. When the unit has practice or quality improvement committees, the manager assigns each member responsibility to communicate directly to a select number of staff members. In that way all staff members are contacted and have the opportunity to comment.
5. *Staff education:* A professional nursing staff always grows in knowledge. It is impossible to remain knowledgeable about current medical and nursing practice trends without ongoing education. The nurse manager is responsible for giving staff members the necessary opportunities to remain competent in their practice. This involves planning in-service training sessions, sending staff members to professional conferences, and having staff members present case studies or practice issues during staff meetings.

LEADERSHIP SKILLS FOR NURSING STUDENTS

As you begin to assume clinical assignments, it is important for you not only to learn how to care for patients but also to become a responsible and productive team member. Start by always being responsible and accountable for the care you provide your patients. Learn to become a leader by making good clinical decisions and learning from your mistakes. Seek help, collaborate closely with professional nurses, and strive to improve your performance during each patient interaction. Use the skills presented in the following paragraphs to become a competent professional. These skills require you to think critically and solve problems in the clinical setting. Thinking critically allows nurses to provide higher quality care, meet the needs of patients while considering the preferences, consider alternatives to problems, understand the rationale for performing nursing interventions, and evaluate the effectiveness of interventions. Clinical experiences help to develop these critical thinking skills (Benner et al., 2010).

Clinical Care Coordination

Learn to acquire the skills necessary to deliver patient care competently and in a timely and effective manner. In the beginning you may care for only one patient, but eventually you care for groups of patients. Clinical care coordination includes clinical decision making, priority setting, organizational skills, use of resources, time management, and evaluation. These activities of clinical care coordination require use of critical reflection, critical reasoning, and clinical judgment (Benner et al., 2010).

Clinical Decisions. When you begin a patient assignment, always conduct a focused but complete assessment of your patient's condition and ask what outcomes the patient expects in his or her care. This allows you to know your patient and the patient's situation and helps you to recognize his or her responses and patterns during care. Your assessment also directs you in making accurate clinical decisions about your patient's needs (see Chapter 8). Failing to make accurate clinical judgments about a patient has undesirable outcomes. The patient's condition worsens or remains the same when the potential for improvement is lost. An important lesson in clinical care is being thorough. Always attend to the patient, look for any cues (obvious or subtle) that point to a pattern of findings, and direct your assessment to explore the pattern further. Accurate clinical decision making keeps you focused on the proper course of action. Never hesitate to ask for assistance when a patient's assessment reveals a changing clinical condition.

Priority Setting. As you begin to make clinical judgments (including nursing diagnoses), a picture of the patient's total needs begins to form. While planning care, decide which patient needs or problems to address first (see Chapter 9). It is important to prioritize in all caregiving situations because it allows you to see relationships between patient problems and avoid delays in action (Hendry and Walker, 2004). When you have multiple tasks to perform for a single patient or a group of patients, you must integrate these tasks in your priority setting. To make this decision use Maslow's hierarchy of needs. According to Maslow, meet the patient's physiological needs such as oxygen, food, water, sleep, and elimination first. After meeting the physiological needs, meet the patient's higher-level needs of safety, security, belonging, esteem, and self-actualization (Marriner Tomey, 2009). Hendry and Walker (2004) classify patient problems in three priority levels:

- *High priority:* An immediate threat to a patient's survival or safety such as a physiological episode of obstructed airway, loss of consciousness, or a psychological episode of an anxiety attack
- *Intermediate priority:* Nonemergency, non–life-threatening actual or potential needs that a patient and family are experiencing (e.g., anticipating teaching needs of patients related to a new drug or taking measures to decrease postoperative complications)
- *Low priority:* Actual or potential problems that may not be directly related to a patient's illness or disease; often related to a patient's developmental and/or long-term health care needs (e.g., teaching for self-care in the home before discharge of a patient who has just been admitted to the hospital)

Many patients have all three types of priorities, requiring you to make careful judgments in choosing your course of action. Obviously high-priority needs demand your immediate attention. When a patient has diverse priority needs, sometimes it helps to focus on his or her basic needs. For example, you have a patient in traction who reports being uncomfortable from being in the same position. The dietary assistant arrives in the room to deliver a meal tray. Instead of immediately helping the patient with the meal, you reposition him or her and offer basic hygiene measures. The patient will likely become more interested in eating and more receptive to any instruction you provide after you make him or her feel comfortable.

Over time you will also be required to meet the priority needs of a group of patients. This requires you to know the priority needs of each patient within the group and assess each patient's needs as soon as possible while addressing high and intermediate needs in a timely manner. To identify which patients require assessment first, you rely on information from the change-of-shift report, the agency's classification system that identifies patient acuity, and information from each patient's medical record. Over time you learn to spontaneously rank patients' needs by priority or urgency. Remember to think about the resources that are available, be flexible in recognizing that priority needs change, and consider how to use your time wisely. The case study provides an example of how to prioritize your patient care (Box 13-4).

You also need to set priorities on the basis of patient expectations. Sometimes you establish an excellent plan of care; but if your patient is resistant to certain therapies or disagrees with your approach, you have very little success. Working closely with the patient and family is important. Share the priorities you define with the patient to establish a level of agreement and cooperation.

Organizational Skills. Implementing a plan of care requires you to be effective and efficient. Effective use of time entails doing the right things, whereas efficient use of time entails doing things right. As you address your patient's priorities, certain organizational skills ensure that you become

BOX 13-4 CASE STUDY: PRIORITY SETTING—JENNIFER

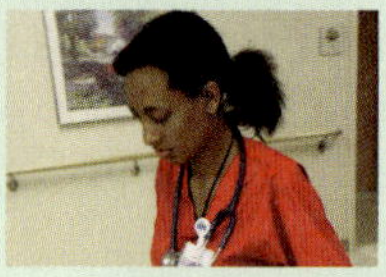

In setting her priorities, Jennifer remembers the categories of priority needs that she learned in school and prioritizes her care according to these. Jennifer asks the unit clerk to send John, another nursing student, to Mr. Timmons' room to check on him and tell him that Jennifer is preparing a patient for surgery and will be with him as soon as she finishes. Jennifer stays with Mrs. Sinclair and begins an assessment to determine the cause of the restlessness. She also asks Mrs. Sinclair if she has any questions or concerns about surgery. Mrs. Sinclair voices her concerns about pain after surgery. Jennifer reinforces the earlier teaching that she did on patient-controlled analgesia pumps. This seems to relax Mrs. Sinclair. Jennifer completes her preoperative preparation and checklist. She tells Mrs. Sinclair that the operating room staff will be here in 15 minutes to get her. Jennifer then goes to assess Mr. Timmons' pain. She prepares and verifies Mr. Timmons' identification using two acceptable identifiers and administers the prescribed pain medication. Jennifer asks Tina, the nursing assistant, to help him with his walk. Jennifer gathers the supplies for the dressing change. On the way to the room she obtains and verifies the antibiotic for Mr. Dodson. In Mr. Dodson's room she first verifies Mr. Dodson's identification using two acceptable identifiers and administers the antibiotic. After Mr. Dodson takes his antibiotic, Jennifer sets up and then completes the dressing change. She finishes caring for Mr. Dodson by documenting the care she performed.

more efficient. Efficient care conserves effort and minimizes interruptions. One way to be efficient is by combining various nursing activities (i.e., doing more than one thing at a time). This takes practice. For example, during medication administration or while obtaining a specimen, combine therapeutic communication skills, teaching interventions, and assessment and evaluation. Try to establish and strengthen relationships with patients and use any patient contact as an opportunity to teach or give important information. Always attend to a patient's behaviors and responses to therapies to assess if any new problems are developing and to evaluate responses to interventions.

A nursing procedure is easier to perform if you are well organized. Prepare in advance by having all necessary equipment and supplies available and making sure to prepare the patient. Be sure that the patient is comfortable, positioned correctly for the procedure, and well informed to increase the likelihood that the procedure will go smoothly. Sometimes you need the assistance of colleagues to perform or complete a procedure (e.g., helping to turn a patient for an enema or handing supplies during a dressing change). It is always wise to have the work area organized and preliminary steps completed before asking colleagues for assistance.

When you deliver care based on established priorities, events sometimes occur that interfere with your plans. For example, just as you begin to provide a patient's bath, the x-ray film technician enters to obtain a portable chest film. Once the technician completes the x-ray film procedure, the phlebotomist arrives to draw a sample of blood. Your priorities seem to conflict with the priorities of other health care personnel. It is important to always keep the patient's needs as the center of attention. The patient experienced symptoms earlier that required a chest film and laboratory work. In such a case it is important to be sure to complete the diagnostic tests. In another example a patient is waiting to visit family, and the chest film was a routine order from 2 days ago. The patient's condition has since stabilized, and the x-ray technician is willing to return later to shoot the film. Attending to the patient's hygiene and comfort so the family is able to visit is more of a priority at this time.

Use of Resources. Another important aspect of clinical care coordination is appropriate use of resources. Resources in this case include members of the health care team. In any setting the administration of patient care occurs more smoothly when staff members work together. As a student always look for opportunities to help other staff members. For example, answer a call light, help a staff member make a bed, or offer to sit and talk with another nurse's patient. Never hesitate to ask staff members to help you, especially when there is the opportunity to make a procedure or activity more comfortable and safer for the patient. For example, assistance in turning, positioning, and ambulating patients is frequently necessary when patients experience impaired mobility. Have a staff member help with handing you equipment and supplies during a more complicated procedure such as a blood draw or a dressing change to make the procedure more efficient. This is an excellent way for you to learn how to delegate aspects of care activities and work with NAP.

In many instances you recognize personal limitations and use professional resources for assistance. For example, you assess a patient and find relevant clinical signs and symptoms but are unfamiliar with the patient's underlying physical condition. You then consult with an RN who confirms your findings and helps you take the proper course of action for the patient. Throughout your professional career there are always new experiences. A leader knows his or her limitations and seeks professional colleagues for guidance and support.

Time Management. Changes in health care and increasing complexity of patients create stress for nurses as they work to meet patient needs (Marriner Tomey, 2009). One way to manage this stress is through the use of time-management skills. These skills involve learning how, where, and when to use your time. Managing yourself better leads to better management of your time (see Chapter 25). Because you have a limited amount of time with patients, it is essential to remain goal oriented and focused on your patients' priorities. For example, priorities of care help you determine which procedures you perform first, patient assessments that you will do on an ongoing basis, and the anticipated response of your patient to care activities.

One useful time-management skill involves making a priority to-do list (Thomack, 2012). When you first begin working with a patient or group of patients, make a list that sequences the nursing activities that you will perform. The change-of-shift report helps you prioritize activities based on what you learn about your patients' conditions and the care provided before your arrival to the unit. Consider activities that have specific time limits in terms of addressing patient needs such as administering a pain medication before a scheduled procedure or instructing a patient before discharge home. Analyze the items on your list that agency policies or routines will schedule. Note which activities need to be done on time and which you are able to do at your discretion. For instance, you need to administer medications within a specific schedule, but you can also perform other activities while you are in the patient's room. Finally estimate the amount of time needed to complete the various activities. Activities requiring the assistance of other staff members usually take longer because you plan around their schedule.

Effective time management also involves setting goals and developing a plan to help you complete one task before starting another (Thomack, 2012). Complete the activities that you begin with one patient before moving on to the next if possible. Your care then becomes less fragmented, and you can better focus on what you are doing for each patient. As a result it is less likely that you will make errors in your care. Other strategies to help you manage your time are keeping a time log to determine where time is currently spent, keeping your work area clean and clutter free, delegating tasks as possible, and trying to decrease interruptions as you are completing tasks (Thomack, 2012).

Evaluation. One of the most important aspects of clinical care coordination is evaluation (see Chapter 9). It is a mistake to think that evaluation occurs at the end of an activity. It is an ongoing process. Once you assess a patient's needs and begin therapies directed at a specific problem area, immediately evaluate if therapies are effective and the patient's response. The process of evaluation compares actual patient outcomes with expected outcomes. When expected outcomes are not being met, evaluation reveals the need to continue current therapies for a longer period, revise approaches to care, or introduce new therapies. Throughout the day as you care for a patient, anticipate when you need to return to the bedside to evaluate your care. For example, you decide to return 30 minutes after you administered a medication, 15 minutes after an intravenous (IV) line has begun infusing, or 60 minutes after discussing discharge instructions with the patient and family.

Keeping a focus on evaluation of a patient's progress lessens the chance of becoming distracted by the tasks of care. It is common to assume that staying focused on planned activities ensures that you perform care appropriately. However, task orientation does not guarantee positive patient outcomes. The competent nurse learns that at the heart of good organizational skills is the constant inquiry into the patient's condition and progress toward an improved level of health.

BOX 13-5 SBAR AS COMMUNICATION TOOL

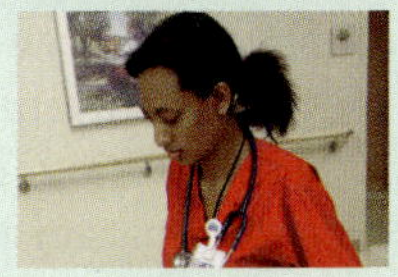

Thirty minutes after Jennifer administered 1 tablet of Percodan 20 mg PO to Mr. Timmons she evaluates its effect. Mr. Timmons rates his pain is an 8 on a scale of 0 to10. Jennifer prepares an SBAR to contact the health care provider.

Situation: Thirty minutes after Mr. Timmons received his pain medication, he continues to rate his pain as an 8 on a pain scale of 0 to 10.

Background: Mr. Timmons had abdominal surgery 2 days ago for removal of a colon tumor. He had his patient-controlled analgesia (PCA) pump with intravenous (IV) morphine removed 4 hours ago. He has one tablet of Percodan 20 mg PO ordered every 6 hours. This is the first dose of the oral medication that was administered.

Assessment: One tablet of Percodan 20 mg PO is not sufficient to manage Mr. Timmons' pain on the second postoperative day. He does not want to walk with the level of pain he is experiencing.

Recommendation: Request a change of the pain medication order to an increase in dose or a different medication every 4 hours for Mr. Timmons.

Team Communication

As a part of a nursing team, each nurse is responsible for open and professional verbal and electronic communication. Structured communication techniques used by health care teams that improve communication include briefings or short discussions among team members, group rounds on patients, and use of Situation-Background-Assessment-Recommendation (SBAR) when sharing information (see Chapter 11) (Nadzam, 2009). Regardless of the setting, nurses learn that an enriching, professional environment is one in which staff members respect one another's ideas, share information, and keep one another informed. On a busy nursing unit this means keeping the nurse in charge of the unit and colleagues informed about patients with emerging problems (Box 13-5). This also includes informing health care providers who have been called for consultation. Strategies you can use to improve your communication with health care providers include addressing the health care provider by name, having the patient and chart available when discussing patient issues, focusing on the patient problem, and being professional but not aggressive (Nadzam, 2009).

In a clinic setting it means sharing unusual diagnostic findings or conveying important information regarding a patient's source of family support. One way of fostering good team communication is by setting expectations of one another. An efficient team counts on all members when needs arise. Sharing expectations of what, when, and how to communicate is a step toward establishing a strong work team. Always treat colleagues with respect. Listen to the ideas of other staff members without interruption. Be honest and direct in what you say. Clarify what others are saying and build on the merits of co-workers' ideas (Marriner Tomey, 2009). When using electronic communication, be open and courteous, summarize issues, and send messages with only necessary details. When using electronic communication, it is important to communicate the appropriate information to the correct person, always maintaining patient privacy and confidentiality (NCSBN, 2011).

Delegation

The art of effective delegation is a skill that you as a student need to observe and practice to improve your management skills. **Delegation** is the process of assigning part of one person's responsibility to another qualified person in a specific situation (NCSBN, 1995). The Nurse Practice Act of your state, along with authority, accountability, and responsibility, is the basis for effective delegation (Plawecki and Amrhein, 2010; Weydt, 2010). Delegation results in achievement of quality patient care, improved efficiency, increased productivity, empowerment of staff, and development of others (Huston, 2009; Marriner Tomey, 2009). For example, asking a staff member to obtain an ordered specimen while you attend to a patient's pain medication request effectively prevents a delay in the patient's gaining pain relief. Delegation also provides job enrichment. A nurse shows trust in colleagues by delegating tasks to them and showing staff members that they are important players in the delivery of care. Successful delegation is important to the quality of the RN-NAP relationship and their willingness to work together (Gravlin and Bittner, 2010; Potter, Deshields, and Kuhrik, 2010). Never delegate a task that you dislike doing or would not do yourself because this creates negative feelings and poor working relationships. Remember that, even though the delegation of a task transfers the responsibility and authority to another person, you are still accountable for the delegated tasks.

Professional nurses are finding themselves in situations in which they need more support to do the daily, repetitive tasks of care such as basic hygiene, specimen collection, and feeding patients. The RN needs time to coordinate care delivery for groups of patients, conduct individual assessments, and make professional judgments about a patient's health and therapeutic needs. She or he also needs time to deliver complex therapies and provide patient counseling and education. An LPN/LVN in acute care benefits from acquiring support to deliver care to a group of patients whose needs are complex. In long-term care settings the LPN/LVN directs care and relies on NAP to provide basic care measures. A nurse is simply not able to do all the work necessary to care for groups of patients.

To be able to perform your professional responsibilities as a nurse, learn how to work effectively with other staff members. Each health care team member has a set of job responsibilities that contribute to the overall care of patients. As a nurse your job is to help the care team work efficiently. Because you oversee the care of groups of patients, it sometimes is necessary for you to delegate work to others.

As a nurse you transfer or assign the responsibility to complete a task to others, but you retain accountability for the outcome. For example, you delegate catheter care to competent and trained NAP after you have assessed the condition of the patient's catheter and perineal tissues. However, you are ultimately accountable for having the patient receive catheter care. As the RN you remain accountable for the overall nursing care of the patient when you delegate responsibilities to a competent individual (Marriner Tomey, 2009). Because the steps of the nursing process of assessment, diagnosis, planning, implementation, and evaluation require you to use nursing judgment, you do not delegate these activities (ANA and NCSBN, 2006). Thus exercise good judgment at all times in deciding which tasks to delegate and in which situations. The National Council of State Boards of Nursing offers guidelines for delegation of tasks in accordance with an RN's legal scope of practice (Box 13-6).

BOX 13-6 THE FIVE RIGHTS OF DELEGATION

RIGHT TASK

The right task is one that you can delegate for a specific patient such as tasks that are repetitive, require little supervision, are relatively noninvasive, have results that are predictable, and have minimal potential risk.

RIGHT CIRCUMSTANCES

Consider the patient setting, available resources, and other relevant factors before delegating. In an acute care setting patients' conditions can change quickly. Good clinical decision making and critical thinking are needed to ensure that the nursing assistive personnel has the appropriate resources, equipment, and supervision to provide safe and effective care.

RIGHT PERSON

The right person is delegating the right tasks to the right person to be performed on the right person.

RIGHT DIRECTION/COMMUNICATION

Give a clear, concise description of the task, including its objective, limits, and expectations. Communication must be ongoing between the nurse and nursing assistive personnel during a shift of care.

RIGHT SUPERVISION

Provide appropriate monitoring, evaluation, intervention as needed, and feedback. Nursing assistive personnel should feel comfortable asking questions and seeking assistance.

Data from National Council of State Boards of Nursing: *Delegation: concepts and decision-making process,* Chicago, 1995, The Council; National Council of State Boards of Nursing, *The five rights of delegation,* Chicago, 1997, The Council; American Nurses Association (ANA) and National Council of State Boards of Nursing (NCSBN): *Joint statement on delegation,* http://www.ncsbn.org/pdfs/joint_statement.pdf, 2006; and Plawecki LH, Amrhein DW: A question of delegation: unlicensed assistive personnel and the professional nurse, *J Gerontol Nurs* 36(8):18, 2010.

It is important to recognize that, regarding delegation to NAP, you delegate tasks, not patients. Further do not automatically delegate a task because it is a task; rather delegate it because it is appropriate for someone else to perform it. For example, as the nurse you are always responsible for the assessment of a patient's ongoing status; but, if a patient is stable, you delegate vital sign monitoring to NAP. It is important for you to collaborate with NAP and ask them to take on tasks that you determine are safe and appropriate for them to provide.

Effective delegation requires constant communication (i.e., sending clear messages and listening so all participants understand expectations regarding patient care) (Gravlin and Bittner, 2010). Know how to give clear instructions, effectively prioritize patient needs and therapies, and be able to give staff members timely and meaningful feedback. Make sure to listen so all participants understand expectations regarding patient care. You need to communicate when and what information to report such as expected observations and specific patient outcomes (NCSBN, 2005). During delegation communication is a two-way process. Therefore allow NAP the chance to ask questions and have your expectations made clear (ANA and NCSBN, 2006). Conflict may occur between RNs and NAP when there is little or poor communication (Potter et al., 2010). Handoff disconnects, lack of knowledge about the workload of team members, and difficulty dealing with conflict are examples of communication failures that result in delegation ineffectiveness and omissions of nursing care (Gravlin and Bittner, 2010).

The final steps in delegation are evaluation of the staff member's performance, achievement of the patient's outcomes, the communication process used, and any problems or concerns that occurred (NCSBN, 2005). Provide praise and recognition when the staff member performs the task correctly and does a good job. If the staff member's performance is not satisfactory, give constructive and appropriate feedback. Feedback given should be specific regarding any mistakes that staff members make, explaining how to avoid the mistake or a better way to handle the situation. Give feedback in private to preserve the staff member's dignity. When you give feedback, make sure to focus on things that are changeable, choose only one issue at a time, and give specific details. Frequently when the performance of NAP does not meet expectations, it is because of inadequate training or assignment of too many tasks. You discover the need to review a procedure with staff and offer demonstration or even recommend that additional training be scheduled with the education department. If too many tasks are being delegated, this might be a nursing practice issue. All staff should discuss the appropriateness of delegation on their unit. Sometimes NAP need help in learning how to prioritize. In some cases you need to learn that you are overdelegating.

Clear directions and statement of desired outcomes increase the likelihood of successful completion of a task. If you observe a change in patient status, that the task is not being performed as directed or by agency policy and procedures, or that the NAP is having difficulty completing the task, you need to intervene and follow up as needed (ANA and NCSBN, 2006). It is your responsibility to complete documentation of the delegated task. Here are a few tips on appropriate delegation (Huston, 2009):

- *Assess the knowledge and skills of the person to whom you are delegating:* Determine what NAP knows and what he or she is able to do by asking open-ended questions that elicit conversation and details. For example, ask, "How do you usually put the cuff on when you measure a blood pressure?" or "Tell me how you prepare the tubing before you give an enema."
- *Match tasks to the assistant's skills:* Know which skills the training program includes for NAP at your facility. Determine if personnel have learned critical thinking skills such as knowing when a patient is in danger or what changes to report.
- *Communicate clearly:* Always provide complete, accurate, and clear directions by describing a task, the desired outcome, and the time period within which the person is to complete the task. Never give instructions through another staff member. Make the person feel as though he or she is part of the team. For example, "I'd like you to help me by getting Mr. Floyd up to ambulate before lunch. Be sure to check his blood pressure before he stands and write your finding on the graphic sheet. OK?"
- *Listen attentively:* Listen to the NAP's response after you provide directions. Does the NAP feel comfortable in asking questions or requesting clarification? If you encourage a response, listen to what the person has to say. Be especially attentive if the staff member has been given a deadline to meet by another nurse. Help sort out priorities.
- *Provide feedback:* Always give NAP feedback regarding performance, regardless of outcome. Let him or her know when a job was well done. If an outcome is undesirable, find a private place to discuss what occurred, any miscommunication, and how to achieve a better outcome in the future.

KEY POINTS

- A manager sets a philosophy for a work unit, ensures appropriate staffing, and mobilizes staff and institutional resources to achieve objectives. A manager also motivates staff members to carry out their work, sets standards of performance, and makes the right decisions to achieve objectives.
- Empowering staff members brings out the best in a manager and allows him or her to concentrate on effective patient care systems, support risk taking and innovation, and focus on results and rewards.
- Nursing care delivery models vary by the responsibility of the RN in coordinating care delivery and the roles that other staff members play in helping with care.
- Critical to the success of decentralized decision making is making staff members aware that they have responsibility,

authority, and accountability for the care they give and the decisions they make.

- A nurse manager fosters decentralized decision making by establishing nursing practice committees and supporting interdisciplinary collaboration between nurses and health care providers.
- Clinical care coordination involves accurate clinical decision making, establishing priorities, efficient organizational skills, appropriate use of resources and time management skills, and an ongoing evaluation of care activities.
- Each member of a nursing work team is responsible for open, professional communication.
- When done correctly, delegation improves job efficiency and job enrichment.
- Exercise good judgment at all times in deciding which tasks to delegate and in which situations.

CLINICAL DECISION-MAKING EXERCISES

During her final week on clinical, Jennifer is assigned to Mr. Simon and Mrs. Burns. Mr. Simon was admitted 2 days ago for an exacerbation of his heart failure. He tells Jennifer that he is ready to ambulate in the hall for his evening walk. Mr. Simon's health care provider ordered a urine specimen to be collected today. Mrs. Burns was admitted earlier in the morning through the emergency department following an episode of chest pain. Jennifer finds that Mr. Simon is resting comfortably and visiting with his daughter. He is eager to go for his walk. Mrs. Burns is very restless and experiencing chest discomfort. Her blood pressure is decreased, and her pulse is increased from her admission baseline vital signs.

1. As Jennifer assesses Mr. Simon and Mrs. Burns, she identifies multiple needs for both patients. On which patient does Jennifer need to focus first? Explain your answer.
2. Which tasks are appropriate for Jennifer to delegate to the nurse technician, Linda? Explain your answer.
3. Jennifer is preparing a presentation on delegation for her nursing management class. Explain the five rights of delegation that Jennifer should discuss during the presentation. Provide an example for each of the rights.

evolve

Answers to Clinical Decision-Making Exercises can be found on the Evolve website.

QSEN ACTIVITY: TEAMWORK AND COLLABORATION

Jennifer participates in the interdisciplinary conference that was scheduled on the unit to plan for the discharge of Mrs. Sinclair following the repair of her hip fracture. She observes the conference and notes that, over the course of the 20-minute meeting, the team effectively develops a discharge plan for Mrs. Sinclair. During her observation she notes that the team recognizes the expertise of the various disciplines, displays behaviors and characteristics that foster effective interdisciplinary teamwork.

Describe the behaviors and characteristics needed for effective interdisciplinary teamwork.

evolve

Answers to QSEN Activities can be found on the Evolve website.

REVIEW QUESTIONS

1. The nurses on a clinical unit voted to trial self-scheduling for 6 months. After the 6-month period, an evaluation will be completed with one component being to evaluate nurses' satisfaction with the process. Which component of decision making are the nurses practicing?
   1. Authority
   2. Responsibility
   3. Accountability
   4. Autonomy
2. The nurse received report on the patients to whom she is assigned during the shift. Which patient should the nurse see first?
   1. The patient who had a hysterectomy 2 days ago and is scheduled for discharge later this morning
   2. The patient who is scheduled for a colonoscopy in 2 hours
   3. The patient 2 days following gastric surgery who is complaining of shortness of breath
   4. The patient who is complaining of nausea but has not vomited
3. The registered nurse (RN) checks her patient, a 62-year-old man admitted to the hospital with pneumonia. The patient has been coughing profusely and requires nasotracheal suctioning. He also has an intravenous (IV) infusion of antibiotics. He is febrile with a temperature of 38.3° C (101° F). He asks the RN if he can have a bed bath because he has been perspiring profusely. The task for the RN to delegate to the nursing assistive personnel working with her today is:
   1. Teaching the use of incentive spirometer.
   2. Changing the IV dressing.
   3. Nasotracheal suctioning.
   4. Administering a bed bath.
4. The nurse completed morning rounds on her assigned patients and is giving the nursing assistant directions for what needs to be done in the next hour. Which statements are examples of appropriate ways to communicate directions when delegating nursing care? (Select all that apply.)
   1. "Please go to room 20A and see what the patient needs."
   2. "I would like you to take all the vital signs for rooms 12 and 13 and let me know if there are any problems."

3. "Would you start the patient's bath while I check on the IV line in room 14? I'll help you with turning her so I can assess her skin and decide on the turning schedule we'll need to follow."
4. "I want you to help the patient in room 16B off the bedpan and get the stool specimen if he passed any stool. I left the specimen container in the bathroom."
5. "Thank you for walking the patient down the hallway this morning. You did a good job assisting him and then documenting his vital signs in the medical record."

5. The patient for whom you are caring on the cardiac unit stops breathing. You start cardiopulmonary resuscitation (CPR). You recognize that this is classified as which type of priority?
   1. High
   2. Direct
   3. Intermediate
   4. Low
6. The nurse asks the nursing assistive personnel (NAP) to take the patient's blood pressure with the patient in a lying, sitting, and standing position. The NAP asks the nurse why the blood pressure needs to be taken 3 times. The nurse explains the reasons for taking the blood pressure in 3 positions. The nurse's interaction with the NAP is an example of which of the five rights of delegation?
   1. Right supervision
   2. Right task
   3. Right communication
   4. Right circumstances
7. Which task is appropriate for the RN to delegate to the nursing assistive personnel (NAP)?
   1. Assessing the vital signs on a patient who is experiencing chest pain
   2. Explaining to a patient how to change the dressing on the abdominal incision
   3. Providing patient teaching on a newly prescribed medication
   4. Administering a soap-suds enema to a patient per order
8. A registered nurse (RN) is responsible for a caseload of patients during their stay in the hospital. Communication is lateral from RN to RN, and the RN has a degree of autonomy and authority. Which care delivery model is the nurse practicing within?
   1. Total patient care
   2. Primary nursing
   3. Team nursing
   4. Case management
9. Which activity by the nursing student shows a strategy for effective organizational skills?
   1. The student makes two trips to the supply room to gather materials for a dressing change.
   2. The student stopped twice while setting up her medications to help another student.
   3. The student commented on how unorganized she felt and stated that she would do better next week.
   4. As the student is bathing the patient, she teaches interventions for good foot care to the patient.
10. The nurse delegated the task of taking a patient to the bathroom to the nursing assistive personnel (NAP). Which activities by the nurse indicate that appropriate delegation was practiced? (Select all that apply.)
   1. The nurse mentally reviewed the patient's condition and determined that she could ambulate to the bathroom with the assistance of one person.
   2. The nurse instructed the NAP to take the patient to the bathroom as soon as possible.
   3. The nurse told the NAP that she would answer her question about whether the patient has activity limitations later because she had to administer a STAT medication.
   4. The nurse asked the NAP if she thought that she could get the patient out of bed on her own and walk her to the bathroom.
   5. The nurse told the NAP in the break room that she did not save the patient's urine for the 12-hour urine collection that was in progress.
   6. The nurse told the NAP that she would come in and see if she needed assistance with the patient right after she administered a medication.

evolve

Rationales for Review Questions can be found on the Evolve website.

1. 4; 2. 3; 3. 4; 4. 3, 4, 5; 5. 1; 6. 3; 7. 4; 8. 2; 9. 4; 10. 1, 4, 6

REFERENCES

American Nurses Association (ANA) and National Council of State Boards of Nursing (NCSBN): *Joint statement on delegation*, 2006, https://www.ncsbn.org/Delegation_joint_statement_NCSBN-ANA.pdf. Accessed September 9, 2013.

American Nurses Credentialing Center (ANCC): *Overview of ANCC Magnet recognition program*, 2012, http://ancc.nursecredentialing.org/PromotionalMaterials/products/MAGBRO07V2.pdf. Accessed August 18, 2012.

Andreatta PB: A typology for health care teams, *Health Care Manage Rev* 35(4):345, 2010.

Begue A, et al: Retrospective study of multidisciplinary rounding on a thoracic surgical oncology unit, *Clin J Oncol Nurs* 16(6):E198, 2012.

Benner P, et al: *Educating nurses: a call for radical transformation*, San Francisco, CA, 2010, Jossey-Bass.

Burzotta L, Noble H: The dimensions of interprofessional practice, *Br J Nurs* 20(5):310, 2011.

Case Management Society of America: *What is a case manger?* 2012, http://www.cmsa.org/Home/CMSA/WhatisaCaseManager/tabid/224/Default.aspx. Accessed September 9, 2013.

Gravlin G, Bittner NP: Nurses' and nursing assistants' reports of missed care and delegation, *J Nurs Admin* 40(7/8):329, 2010.

Halabisky B, et al: eLearning, knowledge brokering and nursing: strengthening collaborative practice in long-term care, *CIN: Comput Informat Nurs* 28(5):264, 2010.

Hendry C, Walker A: Priority setting in clinical nursing practice: literature review, *J Adv Nurs* 47(4):427, 2004.

Huber DL: *Leadership and nursing care management*, ed 4, St Louis, 2010, Elsevier.

Huston CJ: 10 tips for successful delegation, *Nursing* 39(3):54, 2009.

Hylin U, Lonka K, Ponzer S: Students' approaches to learning in clinical interprofessional context, *Med Teacher* 33:e204, 2011.

Interprofessional Education Collaborative Expert Panel (IECEP): *Core competencies for interprofessional collaborative practice: report of an expert panel*, Washington, DC, 2011, Interprofessional Education Collaborative.

Institute of Medicine (IOM): *Crossing the quality chasm: a new health system for the twenty-first century*, Washington, DC, 2001, National Academies Press.

Institute of Medicine (IOM): *Keeping patients safe: transforming the work environment*, Washington, DC, 2004, National Academies Press.

Kearney MH: *Report of the findings from the post-entry competence study*, Chicago, 2009, National Council of State Boards of Nursing.

Kramer M, Maguire P, Brewer BB: Clinical nurses in Magnet hospitals confirm productive, healthy unit work environments, *J Nurs Manage* 19:5, 2011.

Kramer M, Schmalenberg C, Maguire P: Nine structures and leadership practices essential for a magnetic (healthy) work environment, *Nurs Admin Q* 34(1):4, 2010.

Marriner Tomey A: *Guide to nursing management and leadership*, ed 8, St Louis, 2009, Mosby.

Mohaupt J, et al: Understanding interprofessional relationships through the use of contact theory, *J Interprof Care* 26(5):370, 2012.

Nadzam DM: Nurses' role in communication and patient safety, *J Nurs Care Qual* 24(3):184, 2009.

National Council of State Boards of Nursing (NCSBN): *Delegation: concepts and decision-making process*, Chicago, 1995, The Council.

National Council of State Boards of Nursing (NCSBN): *Working with others: a position paper*, Chicago, 2005, The Council.

National Council of State Boards of Nursing (NCSBN): *White Pater: a nurse's guide to the use of social media*, Chicago, 2011, National Council of State Boards of Nursing. https://www.ncsbn.org/Social_media_guidelines.pdf. Accessed September 13, 2013.

Plawecki LH, Amrhein DW: A question of delegation: unlicensed assistive personnel and the professional nurse, *J Gerontol Nurs* 36(8):18, 2010.

Potter PA, Deshields T, Kuhrik M: Delegation practices between registered nurses and nursing assistive personnel, *J Nurs Manage* 18:157, 2010.

Riesen E, et al: Improving interprofessional competence in undergraduate students using a novel blended learning approach, *J Interprof Care* 26(4):312, 2012.

Sharp H: Multidisciplinary team rounding: engaging patients and improving communication at the bedside, *New Hampshire Nursing News* January, February, March:14, 2013.

Skar R: The meaning of autonomy in nursing practice, *J Clin Nurs* 19:2226, 2009.

Thomas PL: Case manager role definitions: do they make an organizational impact? *Prof Case Manage* 13(2):61, 2008.

Thomack B: Time management for today's workplace demands, *Workplace Health Safety* 60(5):201, 2012.

Wagner J, Liston B, Miller J: Developing interprofessional communication skills, *Teach Learn Nurs* 6:97, 2011.

Weydt A: Developing delegation skills, *Online J Issues Nurs* 15(2):1, 2010.

Yoder-Wise PS: *Leading and managing in nursing*, ed 5, St Louis, 2011, Elsevier.

CHAPTER

14

Infection Prevention and Control

evolve WEBSITE

http://evolve.elsevier.com/Potter/essentials

- Crossword Puzzle
- Audio Glossary

OBJECTIVES

- Identify the normal defenses of the body against infection.
- Discuss the development of the inflammatory response.
- Describe the signs and symptoms of a localized and a systemic infection.
- Describe characteristics of each link of the infection chain.
- Assess patients at risk for acquiring an infection.
- Explain conditions that promote development of health care–acquired infections (HCI).
- Describe strategies for Standard Precautions.
- Identify principles of medical and surgical asepsis.
- Describe nursing interventions designed to break each link in the infection chain.
- Perform proper barrier isolation techniques.
- Perform proper procedures for hand hygiene.
- Apply and remove a surgical mask and gloves using correct technique.

KEY TERMS

Airborne Precautions, p. 254
antibody, p. 242
antigen, p. 243
asepsis, p. 243
aseptic technique, p. 243
asymptomatic, p. 240
carriers, p. 240
colonization, p. 240
communicable disease, p. 240
Contact Precautions, p. 254
disinfection, p. 250
Droplet Precautions, p. 254
endogenous infection, p. 243
exogenous infection, p. 243
flora, p. 243
health care–acquired infection (HAI), p. 243
immunity, p. 242
infection, p. 240
inflammation, p. 243
inflammatory response, p. 243
medical asepsis, p. 243
microorganisms, p. 240
necrotic, p. 243
pathogenicity, p. 242
pathogens, p. 240
reservoir, p. 240
Standard Precautions, p. 249
sterilization, p. 250
suprainfection, p. 243
surgical asepsis, p. 243
symptomatic, p. 240
transmission-based precautions, p. 249
virulence, p. 240

Current trends, public awareness, and rising costs of health care have increased the importance of infection prevention and control. Increases in drug-resistant microorganisms, health care–acquired infections (HAIs), and concern about occupational exposure to tuberculosis (TB), human immunodeficiency virus (HIV), and hepatitis have increased concern about transmission of infections within health care settings. As a nurse you participate in cost-effective, quality health care by using strategies that prevent or reduce the risk for infections. This chapter emphasizes techniques for

CASE STUDY *Mrs. Eldredge*

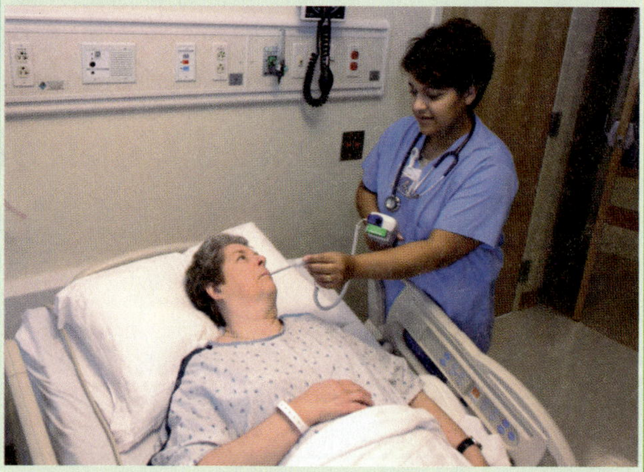

Mrs. Eldredge is a 63-year-old woman who lives alone and enjoys an active social life. She has diabetes that is well controlled with oral hypoglycemic medications and diet. She had a total hip replacement and went home as expected on her fourth postoperative day. Two weeks after her surgery, Mrs. Eldredge was readmitted to the hospital because she started having increased pain in her hip.

Kathy Jackson is a nursing student who is caring for Mrs. Eldredge in the hospital. Kathy assesses Mrs. Eldredge's incision and notes that is red, swollen, and warm. Mrs. Eldredge has a low-grade fever (37.6° C [99.8° F]). Mrs. Eldredge states, "I am not sure what is wrong with me, but my hip really hurts." Kathy talks with Mrs. Eldredge's nurse and orthopedic surgeon to discuss the situation. The orthopedic surgeon determines Mrs. Eldredge has an infection, opens her hip incision, and orders wound irrigation with dressing changes three times a day.

prevention and control of infections and the critical thinking skills necessary to achieve these goals.

SCIENTIFIC KNOWLEDGE BASE

Nature of Infection

An infection is the invasion of a susceptible host (e.g., a patient) by potentially harmful microorganisms (pathogens), resulting in disease. The principal infecting agents are bacteria, viruses, fungi, and protozoa (Table 14-1). It is important to know the difference between an infection and colonization. Colonization is the presence and growth of microorganisms within a host but without tissue invasion or damage (Tweeten, 2009). All people have microorganisms on their skin, but usually no disease results. Disease or infection results only if the pathogens grow or multiply and alter normal tissue function. An infectious disease transmitted directly from one person to another is considered a contagious or communicable disease (Tweeten, 2009). If the pathogens multiply and cause clinical signs and symptoms, the infection is symptomatic. If clinical signs and symptoms are not present, the illness is termed asymptomatic. For example, hepatitis C is most efficiently transmitted through the direct entry of blood into the skin through a percutaneous exposure, even if the source (patient) is asymptomatic (Ghany et al., 2009).

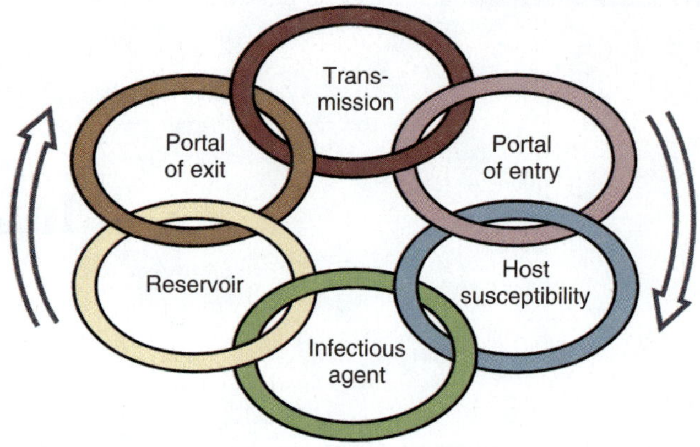

FIGURE 14-1 Chain of infection.

Chain of Infection

The presence of a pathogen does not mean that an infection will begin. The process resulting in an infection is referred to as the *chain of infection*. Components of the chain include the infectious agent or pathogen, reservoir or place for pathogen growth, portal of exit from the reservoir, mode of transmission or vehicle, portal of entry into the reservoir, and a susceptible host (Figure 14-1). Infection develops if the links in this chain remain intact. Preventing infections involves breaking the chain of infection.

Infectious Agent. The development of an infection depends on the number of microorganisms present; their virulence, or the ability to produce disease; their ability to enter and survive in a host; and the susceptibility of the host. Resident skin microorganisms are not virulent. However, they can cause serious infection when surgery or an invasive procedure allows them to enter deep inside tissues or when a patient is severely immunocompromised. Patients become immunocompromised when their immune system is impaired. Some factors that increase a patient's risk for immunocompromise include cancer chemotherapy, organ antirejection medication, or acquired immunodeficiency syndrome (AIDS).

Reservoir. A place where microorganisms survive, multiply, and wait to transfer to a susceptible host is called a reservoir. Common reservoirs are humans and animals (hosts), insects, food, water, and organic matter on inanimate surfaces (fomites). Frequent reservoirs for HAIs include health care workers (especially their hands), patients' body excretions and secretions, equipment, and the health care environment. There are two types of human reservoirs: those with acute or symptomatic disease and those who show no signs of disease but are carriers of it. Humans can transmit microorganisms in either case.

Portal of Exit. After microorganisms find a site in which to grow and multiply, they must find a portal of exit if they are to enter another host and cause disease. They exit through a variety of sites such as the skin and mucous membranes,

TABLE 14-1 COMMON PATHOGENS AND SOME INFECTIONS OR DISEASES THEY PRODUCE

ORGANISM	MAJOR RESERVOIR(S)	MAJOR DISEASES/INFECTIONS
Bacteria		
Escherichia coli	Colon	Gastroenteritis, urinary tract infection
Staphylococcus aureus	Skin, hair, upper respiratory tract	Wound infection, abscess, cellulitis, osteomyelitis, bacteremia, pneumonia, food poisoning, toxic shock syndrome
Streptococcus (beta hemolytic group A) organisms	Oropharynx, skin, perianal area	"Strep throat," rheumatic fever, scarlet fever, impetigo, wound infection
Streptococcus (beta hemolytic group B) organisms	Adult genitalia	Urinary tract infection, wound infection, postpartum sepsis, neonatal sepsis
Mycobacterium tuberculosis	Droplet nuclei from lungs	Tuberculosis
Neisseria gonorrhoeae	Genitourinary tract, rectum, mouth	Sexually transmitted infection, pelvic inflammatory disease, septic arthritis, newborn ophthalmitis
Rickettsia rickettsii	Wood tick	Rocky Mountain spotted fever
Staphylococcus epidermidis	Skin	Wound infection, bacteremia
Viruses		
Hepatitis A virus	Feces	Hepatitis A
Hepatitis B virus	Blood, certain body fluids, tissues involved in sexual contact	Hepatitis B
Hepatitis C virus	Blood, certain body fluids, tissues involved in sexual contact	Hepatitis C
Herpes simplex virus (type I)	Lesions of mouth, skin, genitals	Cold sores, herpetic whitlow, sexually transmitted disease
Human immunodeficiency virus (HIV)	Blood, semen, vaginal secretions via sexual contact	Acquired immunodeficiency syndrome (AIDS)
Fungi		
Aspergillus organisms	Soil, dust, mouth, skin, colon, genital tract	Aspergillosis, pneumonia, sepsis
Candida albicans	Skin, mouth, genital tract	Candidiasis, pneumonia, sepsis
Protozoa		
Plasmodium falciparum	Blood	Malaria

Modified from Ritter H: Clinical microbiology. In Carrico R, editor: *APIC text of infection control and epidemiology,* Washington, DC, 2009, Association for Professionals in Infection Control and Epidemiology.

respiratory tract, gastrointestinal (GI) tract, urinary tract, reproductive tract, and blood.

Modes of Transmission. Many times there is little that you are able to do about the infectious agent or the susceptible host; however, by practicing infection prevention and control techniques such as hand hygiene, you interrupt the mode of transmission (Box 14-1). The same microorganism is sometimes transmitted by more than one route. For example, the virus that causes chickenpox spreads by airborne route in droplet nuclei and also by direct contact with vesicle fluid. Hands of health care workers often transmit microorganisms. This mode of transmission is called *direct transmission*. Indirect transmission occurs when microorganisms are transferred to health care worker's hands from contaminated items that are part of patient care such as a blood pressure cuff or a bedside table (WHO, 2009).

Portal of Entry. Organisms are able to enter the body through the same routes that they use for exiting. Common portals of entry include broken skin, mucous membranes, genitourinary (GU) tract, GI tract, and respiratory tract. For example, obstruction to the flow of urine caused by the presence of a blocked urinary catheter allows organisms to go up into the urethra.

Susceptible Host. Susceptibility to an infection depends on an individual's degree of resistance to pathogens. Although everyone is constantly in contact with large numbers of microorganisms, an infection does not develop until an individual becomes susceptible to the strength and numbers of these microorganisms. The more virulent an organism, the greater the dose, the more likely it is that a person will develop an infection. Some of the factors that influence a person's susceptibility (degree of resistance) include age, nutritional

BOX 14-1 MODES OF TRANSMISSION

ROUTES AND MEANS

Contact

- *Direct:* Person-to-person or physical contact between source and susceptible host (e.g., touching patient feces and then touching own face or mouth or consuming contaminated food)
- *Indirect:* Personal contact of susceptible host with contaminated inanimate object (e.g., needles or sharps, dressings)
- *Droplet:* Large particles that travel up to 3 feet and come in contact with susceptible host (e.g., from coughing, sneezing, talking)
- *Airborne:* Droplet nuclei, residue or evaporated droplets suspended in air (e.g., from coughing, sneezing, talking)

Vehicles

- Contaminated items
- Water
- Drugs, solutions
- Blood
- Food (improperly handled, stored, cooked; fresh or thawed meats)

Vector

- External mechanical transfer (flies)
- Internal transmission such as with parasitic conditions between vector and host, for example:
  - Mosquito
  - Louse
  - Tick
  - Flea

Modified from Tweeten S: General principles of epidemiology. In Carrico R, editor: *APIC text of infection control and epidemiology,* Washington, DC, 2009, Association for Professionals in Infection Control and Epidemiology.

status, presence of chronic disease, trauma, and smoking. Organisms with resistance to key antibiotics are becoming more common in all health care settings, but especially acute care. This is associated with the frequent and sometimes inappropriate use of antibiotics over the years in all settings (i.e., acute care, ambulatory care, clinics, and long-term care). A person's natural defenses against infection and certain risk factors affect susceptibility (see Assessment section).

A host is not considered susceptible if it has acquired **immunity** through either a natural or an artificially induced event. Natural active immunity results from having a certain disease such as measles and mounting an immune response that usually lasts a lifetime. Active immunity also results from the administration of a vaccine. Natural passive immunity is the acquisition of an **antibody** by one person from another such as a baby born with its mother's antibodies. The baby acquires these antibodies through the placenta during the last months of pregnancy. This type of immunity is of short duration, usually lasting only a few weeks to months (Palmeira et al., 2012).

Course of Infection

Infections follow a progressive course (Figure 14-2). The severity depends on the extent of the infection, the **pathogenicity** and virulence of the causative microorganism, and the susceptibility of the host. If the infection is localized such as in a wound, antibiotic therapy and proper wound care control the spread of the infection and minimize the illness. The patient usually experiences only localized symptoms such as pain, tenderness, and swelling at the wound site. An infection that affects the entire body instead of just a single organ or part is systemic, characterized by a fever and increase in white blood cells (WBCs). Often systemic infections are fatal.

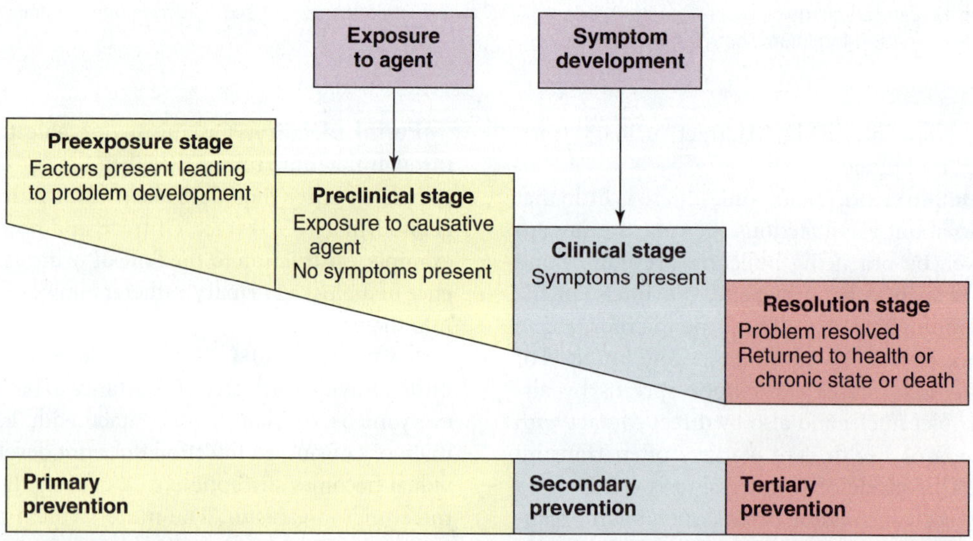

FIGURE 14-2 Stages of the natural history of a condition and their relationship to primary, secondary, and tertiary levels of prevention. (From Clark MJ: *Community health nursing: caring for populations,* ed 4, Upper Saddle River, NJ, 2003, Pearson Education.)

Defenses Against Infection

The body has normal defenses against infection, including normal flora, body system defenses, and the immune system. Intact skin protects from pathogens, and linings of the nasal passages act to prevent organisms from entering the lungs. Each organ system has defense mechanisms to prevent exposure to infection. In addition, the inflammatory response of the body is a protective reaction that neutralizes pathogens and repairs body cells.

Normal Flora. The normal flora of the body is made up of a large numbers of microorganisms residing on the surface and deep layers of the skin, in the saliva, and on the oral mucosa and intestinal walls. Normal flora usually does not cause disease but instead helps to maintain health. For example, skin flora reduces multiplication of organisms landing on the skin. The number and variety of flora maintain a sensitive balance with other microorganisms to prevent infection. Any factor that disrupts this balance places a person at increased risk for infection. For example, the use of broad-spectrum antibiotics for the treatment of infection eliminates or changes normal bacterial flora, often leading to suprainfection. Microorganisms resistant to antibiotics cause serious infection (Lehne, 2013).

Body System Defenses. Microorganisms are able to easily enter the skin, respiratory tract, and GI tract. However, these body systems also have unique defenses against infection that are physiologically suited to their structure and function (Table 14-2). Any condition that impairs the specialized defenses of an organ increases susceptibility to infection.

Inflammation. The cellular response of the body to injury or infection is inflammation. Inflammation is a protective vascular reaction that delivers fluid, blood products, and nutrients to interstitial tissues in an area of injury. This process neutralizes and eliminates pathogens or necrotic tissues and establishes a means of repairing body cells and tissues (Table 14-3). Signs of inflammation include swelling, redness, heat, pain or tenderness, and loss of function in the affected body part. When inflammation becomes systemic, signs and symptoms usually include fever, leukocytosis (increased number of WBCs), malaise, anorexia, nausea, vomiting, and lymph node enlargement. Many physical agents (e.g., temperature extremes and radiation), chemical agents (e.g., gastric acid or poisons), and microorganisms trigger the inflammatory response.

Immune Response. When a foreign material (antigen) enters the body, a series of responses changes the biological makeup of the body. The next time that antigen enters the body, antibodies bind to the antigens they find and neutralize, destroy, or eliminate them.

Health Care–Acquired Infection

Patients in health care settings, especially hospitals and long-term care facilities, are at a higher risk for infection than patients seen in the home. Patients in health care settings often have multiple illnesses, are older adults, and are often poorly nourished. These factors make them more susceptible to infection. In addition, many patients have a lowered resistance to infection because of underlying medical conditions (e.g., HIV, diabetes mellitus, autoimmune disorders, or malignancies) that impair or damage the immune responses of the body. Invasive treatment devices such as intravenous (IV) catheters or indwelling urinary catheters impair or bypass the natural defenses of the body against microorganisms. Treatments with multiple antibiotics for long periods of time are also associated with an increased risk for certain infections (Lehne, 2013).

When a patient develops an infection that was not present or incubating at the time of admission to a health care setting, it is called a health care–acquired infection (HAI). A community-acquired infection is one that was present at the time of admission to a health care setting. The conscientious practice of hand hygiene and aseptic technique reduces the risk for HAIs. The Joint Commission lists prevention of infection as one of its National Patient Safety Goals, with a focus on infections that are difficult to treat and on infections involving central intravenous access, postoperative conditions, and the urinary tract (TJC, 2014).

HAIs are exogenous or endogenous. An exogenous infection comes from microorganisms found outside the individual such as *Salmonella, Clostridium tetani,* and *Aspergillus.* They do not exist as normal flora. An endogenous infection occurs when part of a patient's flora becomes altered and overgrowth results (e.g., staphylococci, enterococci, yeasts, and streptococci). This often happens when a patient receives broad-spectrum antibiotics that alter normal flora. When sufficient numbers of microorganisms normally found in one body site move to another site, an endogenous infection develops. The number of microorganisms needed to cause an HAI depends on the virulence of the organism, the susceptibility of the host, and the body site affected (Box 14-2).

Asepsis. Efforts to minimize the onset and spread of infection are based on the principles of aseptic technique. Aseptic technique is an effort to keep patients as free from exposure to infection-causing pathogens as possible. The term asepsis means the absence of disease-producing microorganisms. The two types of aseptic technique are medical asepsis and surgical asepsis.

Medical asepsis, or clean techniques, includes procedures used to reduce the number and prevent the spread of microorganisms. Hand hygiene, barrier techniques, and routine environmental cleaning are examples of medical asepsis.

Surgical asepsis, or sterile technique, includes procedures to eliminate all microorganisms from an area. Sterilization destroys all microorganisms and their spores (CDC, 2008b; Spratt et al., 2012). Nurses in the operating room, in labor and delivery, and at the bedside practice sterile technique when using sterile instruments and supplies for patient care. Surgical asepsis demands the highest level of aseptic technique and requires that all areas be kept free of infectious microorganisms (AORN, 2013).

Health care workers are responsible for providing a safe environment for patients. It is easy to forget key procedural

TABLE 14-2 NORMAL BODY SYSTEM DEFENSE MECHANISMS AGAINST INFECTION

DEFENSE MECHANISMS	ACTION	FACTORS THAT MAY ALTER DEFENSE
Skin		
Intact multilayered surface, first line of defense of body against infection	Provides mechanical barrier to microorganisms and antibacterial activity	Cuts, abrasions, puncture wounds, areas of maceration
Shedding of outer layer of skin cells	Removes organisms that adhere to outer layers of skin	Failure to bathe regularly, improper hand-hygiene techniques
Sebum	Contains fatty acid that kills some bacteria	Excessive bathing
Mouth		
Intact multilayered mucosa	Provides mechanical barrier to microorganisms	Lacerations, trauma, extracted teeth
Saliva	Washes away particles containing microorganisms Contains microbial inhibitors (e.g., lysozyme)	Poor oral hygiene, dehydration
Eye		
Tearing and blinking	Provides mechanisms to reduce entry (blinking) or help wash away (tearing) particles containing pathogens	Injury, exposure-splash, splatter of blood or other potentially infectious material into the eye
Respiratory Tract		
Cilia lining upper airways, coated by mucus	Trap inhaled microbes and sweep them outward in mucus to be expectorated or swallowed	Smoking, high concentration of oxygen and carbon dioxide, decreased humidity, cold air
Macrophages	Engulf and destroy microorganisms that reach alveoli of lung	Smoking immunosuppression
Urinary Tract		
Flushing action of urine flow	Washes away microorganisms on lining of bladder and urethra	Obstruction to normal flow by urinary catheter placement, obstruction from growth or tumor, or delayed micturition
Intact multilayered epithelium	Provides barrier to microorganisms	Introduction of urinary catheter, continual movement of catheter in urethra
Gastrointestinal Tract		
Acidity of gastric secretions	Chemically destroys microorganisms incapable of surviving low pH	Administration of antacids, histamine-2 blockers
Rapid peristalsis in small intestine	Prevents retention of bacterial contents	Delayed motility from fecal impaction in large bowel or mechanical obstruction by masses
Vagina		
At puberty normal flora cause vaginal secretions to achieve low pH	Inhibits growth of many microorganisms	Antibiotics and birth control pills that disrupt normal flora

steps or take shortcuts that break aseptic procedures when rushed. Failure to follow proper technique places patients at risk for infections that can seriously impair their recovery and may even lead to death.

NURSING KNOWLEDGE BASE

Body substances such as feces, urine, and wound drainage contain potentially infectious microorganisms. For this reason health care workers are at risk for exposure to microorganisms in the hospital, long-term care, and home settings (Fauerbach, 2009). Nursing science has contributed to identifying specific infection prevention practices for health care workers. These practices reduce the risk for cross-contamination and transmission to other patients when caring for a patient with a known or suspected infection (CDC, 2007).

The experience of having a serious infection creates feelings of anxiety, frustration, and loneliness in patients and/or

TABLE 14-3 INFLAMMATION

PHYSIOLOGICAL RESPONSE	SIGNS AND SYMPTOMS
Vascular and Cellular Response	
Arterioles supplying infected or injured area dilate, delivering blood and leukocytes.	Redness
Tissue necrosis causes release of histamine, bradykinin, prostaglandin, and serotonin, which increase blood vessel permeability.	Warmth, edema
Fluid, protein, and cells enter interstitial spaces to cause swelling.	Pain
White blood cells (WBCs) enter tissues and phagocytose microorganisms. More WBCs are released into bloodstream.	WBC count normally 5000-10,000/mm^3; value increased with infection, inflammation, stress, trauma
Phagocytic release of pyrogens from bacteria occurs.	Fever
Inflammatory Exudate	
Fluid, dead cells, and WBCs form exudate at inflammatory site that later clears with lymphatic drainage.	Purulent drainage Serous or sanguineous exudates
Tissue Repair	
Healthy new cells replace damaged cells. Cells mature to take on structural characteristics and appearance of injured cells.	Tissue defects heal and close

BOX 14-2 EXAMPLES OF SITES FOR AND CAUSES OF HEALTH CARE–ACQUIRED INFECTIONS

Improperly performing hand hygiene increases patient risk for all types of health care–acquired infections.

URINARY TRACT
- Unsterile insertion of urinary catheter
- Improper positioning of drainage tubing
- Open drainage system
- Disconnection of catheter and tube
- Contact between drainage bag port and contaminated surface
- Improper specimen collection technique
- Obstruction or interference with urinary drainage
- Urine in catheter or drainage tube being allowed to reenter bladder (reflux)
- Repeated catheter irrigations

SURGICAL OR TRAUMATIC WOUNDS
- Improper skin preparation before surgery (i.e., shaving vs. clipping hair; not performing a preoperative bath or shower)
- Failure to cleanse skin surface properly
- Failure to use aseptic technique during dressing changes
- Use of contaminated antiseptic solutions

RESPIRATORY TRACT
- Contaminated respiratory therapy equipment
- Failure to use aseptic technique while suctioning airway
- Improper disposal of secretions

BLOODSTREAM
- Contamination of IV fluids by tubing
- Adding medications to IV fluid
- Addition of connecting tube or stopcocks to IV system
- Improper care of needle insertion site
- Contaminated needles or catheters
- Failure to change IV access site when inflammation first appears
- Improper technique during administration of multiple blood products
- Improper care of peritoneal or hemodialysis shunts
- Improperly accessing an IV port

IV, Intravenous.

their families (Zastrow, 2011). These feelings worsen when patients are isolated to prevent transmission of a microorganism to other patients or health care staff. Isolation disrupts normal social relationships with visitors and caregivers. Patient safety is often an additional risk for the patient on isolation precautions (Zastrow, 2011). For example, a patient with dementia is at increased risk for falling when confined in a room with the door closed. Family members sometimes fear the possibility of developing the infection and avoid contact with the patient. Some patients perceive the simple procedures of proper hand hygiene and gown and glove use as evidence of rejection. Help patients and families reduce some of these feelings by discussing the disease process; explaining isolation procedures, and maintaining a friendly, understanding manner.

Cultural, religious, or social beliefs influence how a patient reacts to an infectious disease and also influence infection prevention. Increasing information improves patients' health outcomes when you provide culturally relevant care. Social support for patients promotes their adherence to treatment. How a patient reacts to an infection or infectious disease is important for you to know in establishing a plan of care. The challenge is to identify and support behaviors that maintain human health or prevent infection.

NURSING PROCESS

ASSESSMENT

Assess all risk factors for a patient's susceptibility to infection and his or her current clinical status (Box 14-3). A review of the medical history with a patient and family sometimes reveals a recent exposure to a communicable disease. By assessing existing signs and symptoms (e.g., the condition of a wound, the presence of fever), you determine whether a patient's clinical condition indicates the onset or extension of an infection. During the interview process assess the patient's and family's knowledge of a known infection or disease to determine the course of the condition and their level of knowledge of infection control practices.

Because a patient's nutritional health directly influences susceptibility to infection, a thorough diet history is necessary. Determine a patient's normal daily nutrient intake and whether preexisting problems such as impaired swallowing or oral pain alter food intake.

Review laboratory data as soon as they are available (Table 14-4). Laboratory values such as increased WBCs and/or a positive blood culture often indicate infection. Consider the patient's age when assessing laboratory data. For example, in

BOX 14-3 FACTORS AFFECTING SUSCEPTIBILITY TO INFECTION

AGE
- Infants have immature immune systems.
- Children acquire more immunity but are susceptible to infectious diseases such as mumps and measles if unvaccinated.
- Young and middle-age adults have refined body system defenses and immunity.
- Older adults' immune responses decline, and the structure and function of major organs change (see Box 14-4).

HEREDITY
- Some congenital and genetic chromosome disorders have an effect on humoral or cellular immunity.
- Patients with diabetes and those with a hereditary predisposition to diabetes are at increased risk for infections and delayed wound healing.

CULTURAL PRACTICES
- Various cultural or religious beliefs or practices influence patients' decisions to seek treatment for an infection or use methods to prevent infections. For example, a Native American or Latino patient seeks treatment from a "healer" rather than a health care provider, or a patient does not use a condom because of religious beliefs.

NUTRITIONAL STATUS
- A reduction in protein, carbohydrates, and fats as a result of illness, inadequate diet, or debility increases a patient's susceptibility to infection and delays wound repair.

STRESS
- Increased stress elevates cortisone levels, causing decreased resistance to infection.
- Continuous stress exhausts energy stores.

REST AND EXERCISE
- Inadequate rest and exercise increase stress and decrease bodily functions such as elimination and circulation.

INADEQUATE DEFENSES
- Primary and secondary defenses are altered (e.g., broken skin or mucosa, traumatized tissue, suppressed immune response).

PERSONAL HABITS
- Smoking reduces respiratory ciliary action and decreases resistance to respiratory infections.
- Alcohol ingestion impairs the effect of antibiotics.
- Risky sexual behavior such as multiple sex partners increases the chance for exposure to HIV and agents of other sexually transmitted diseases.

ENVIRONMENTAL FACTORS
- Crowded living conditions and adequacy and safety of water supply influence the patient's susceptibility to infections.
- Inadequate refrigeration and cooking facilities increase a patient's exposure to foodborne illness such as salmonellosis or campylobacteriosis.

IMMUNIZATION/DISEASE HISTORY
- Patients who have not received recommended immunizations are at risk for vaccine-preventable diseases such as measles, mumps, and rubella.
- Older adults with underlying medical conditions decrease their susceptibility to influenza and pneumococcal pneumonia when they receive immunizations.

MEDICAL THERAPIES
- Certain drugs such as cortisone and certain invasive therapies such as intravenous catheters or surgeries increase the risk for infection.

CLINICAL APPEARANCE AND DATA
- Localized infections usually present with redness, swelling, and pain or tenderness. There is sometimes a purulent drainage from wounds or lesions.
- Systemic infections present with fever, chills, nausea and vomiting, loss of appetite, or lymph node enlargement.
- Clinical data may show an increase in white blood cells, a positive culture, or an abnormal x-ray film examination.

HIV, Human immunodeficiency virus.

the older adult bacterial growth in urine without clinical symptoms does not always indicate the presence of a urinary tract infection (Beverage et al., 2011).

Early recognition of infection helps you make the correct nursing diagnosis and establish a treatment plan. In addition, alert other members of the health care team to the need for further investigation of the patient's condition, facilitating initiation of prompt therapy and barrier protection (i.e., use of gloves, masks, and gowns). Because of increased attention to the prevention of infection, the Centers for Disease Control and Prevention (CDC, 2007) and the Occupational Safety and Health Administration (OSHA, 1991) have stressed the importance of barrier protection.

Also assess the effects that an infection has on a patient and family. Some patients with chronic or serious infections such as TB or AIDS experience psychological and social problems from self-imposed isolation or rejection by friends and family. Provide education related to the infection and ask the patient how the infection is affecting his or her ability to maintain relationships and perform activities of daily living. Determine whether chronic infection has drained the patient's financial resources.

Patient Expectations. Identify patients' expectations about their care during your assessment. Some patients and their families wish to know more about the disease process, whereas others only want to know the interventions necessary to treat the infection and prevent future infections. Encourage patients to verbalize their expectations so you are able to establish interventions to meet their priorities.

Older Adult Considerations. When a person ages, normal physiological changes occur that influence susceptibility to infection. These changes include decreased immunity, dry mucous membranes, decreased secretions, and decreased elasticity in tissues. As a result of these changes, older adults are predisposed to infections (Box 14-4).

NURSING DIAGNOSIS

Following assessment, review all of your findings, analyze clusters of defining characteristics, and select accurate and relevant nursing diagnoses. For the nursing diagnosis *Risk for Infection,* examples of defining characteristics include risk factors such as inadequate primary defenses (e.g., broken skin or stasis of body fluids), inadequate secondary defenses (e.g., decreased hemoglobin and WBCs), and chronic disease.

Clusters of defining characteristics lead to the selection of a nursing diagnosis. The related factors, revealed in the assessment, ensure individualization of the diagnosis. An accurate related factor ensures a more relevant and thorough care plan. For example, you have a patient with a decreased WBC count, multiple IV catheters, and inflammation around a single catheter site. You diagnose the patient as being at *Risk for Infection.* The risk factor, *IV catheter placement,* directs you

TABLE 14-4 LABORATORY TESTS TO SCREEN FOR INFECTION

LABORATORY VALUE	NORMAL (ADULT) VALUES	INDICATION OF INFECTION
White blood cell (WBC) count	5,000-10,000/mm^3	Increased in acute infection; decreased in certain viral or overwhelming infections
Erythrocyte sedimentation rate	Up to 15 mm/hr for men and 20 mm/hr for women	Elevated in presence of inflammatory process
Iron level	Male 80-180 mcg/dL; female 60-160 mcg/dL	Decreased in chronic infection
Blood cultures	Normally sterile, without microorganism growth	Presence of microorganism growth may indicate infection
Wound, sputum, or throat cultures	Possible normal flora	Presence of microorganism growth may indicate infection
Urinalysis	Nitrite and leukocyte negative	Nitrite and leukocyte positive; WBC count greater than 20/mm^3
Differential Count (Percentage of Each Type of WBC)		
Neutrophils	55%-70%	Increased in acute infection; may be decreased in overwhelming bacterial infection (older adult)
Lymphocytes	20%-40%	Increased in chronic bacterial and viral infection; decreased in sepsis
Monocytes	2%-8%	Increased in protozoal, rickettsial, and tuberculosis infections
Eosinophils	1%-4%	Increased in parasitic infection
Basophils	0.5%-1%	Normal during infection

BOX 14-4 CARE OF THE OLDER ADULT

Infection Control Considerations

- There are fewer tears to flush and remove debris from the eye and a decrease in lysozymes that affect certain microorganisms. A decreased blink reflex leads to corneal dryness. Caution patients and families to observe for eye infections and use artificial tears when necessary.
- Drying of the oral mucosa and recession and weakening of gingival tissues require frequent oral hygiene and regular dental care.
- Increased chest diameter and rigidity, weakened cough, decreased ability to swallow, and decreased elastic tissue surrounding alveoli predispose older adults to ventilatory problems and difficulty handling lung secretions. Good pulmonary hygiene (frequent coughing and deep-breathing exercises, positioning to enhance ventilatory movement, early ambulation, and oral hygiene with chlorhexidene reduce risk of aspiration and postoperative pneumonia).
- Decreased production of digestive juices and a reduction in intestinal motility affect removal of potential pathogens in the bowel. Patients and families should learn about safe food preparation and eat foods that are nutritionally good and easy to digest. Provide smaller meals more frequently.
- Thinning of the dermal and epidermal skin layers, along with a decrease in skin elasticity, predisposes older adults to skin tearing. Meticulous nursing care is necessary to prevent pressure ulcers in bedridden patients (see Chapter 36).
- Decreased production of T and B lymphocytes. With reduced immunity it is important for older adults to receive regular immunizations and medical checkups.

Modified from Gantz M: Geriatrics. In Carrico R, editor: *APIC text of infection control and epidemiology,* Washington, DC, 2009, Association for Professionals in Infection Control and Epidemiology.

to change the catheter regularly and take measures to minimize microorganism transfer through the IV system such as scrubbing the hub of the catheter before accessing the IV line to give medication (O'Grady et al., 2011).

Infection or its associated treatment is the related factor for a number of nursing diagnoses. In the case of the diagnosis *Social Isolation,* the related factor is sometimes the isolation precautions used for infection control. Direct nursing interventions in these situations at minimizing the effect that isolation has on the patient's ability to socialize. Nursing diagnoses that you use with patients susceptible to or affected by infection include the following:

- *Disturbed Body Image*
- *Risk for Falls*
- *Risk for Infection*
- *Imbalanced Nutrition: Less Than Body Requirements*
- *Acute Pain*
- *Impaired Skin Integrity*
- *Social Isolation*
- *Impaired Tissue Integrity*

The presence of an actual infection poses a collaborative problem requiring your intervention. Objective data such as an elevated temperature, open draining wound, inflammation of a wound site, and laboratory values revealing an increased WBC count indicate an actual infection. Subjective findings include the patient's complaint of chills, malaise, or tenderness at the wound site. Work with health care providers, registered dietitians, and other team members in monitoring the infection, providing therapies such as antibiotic administration and wound care, and implementing appropriate infection prevention and control measures.

PLANNING

Develop a patient's care plan based on each nursing diagnosis. For each diagnosis identify specific goals and outcomes, set priorities, and plan for continuing care after discharge.

Goals and Outcomes. You determine patient goals and outcomes based on your patient's preferences and identified nursing diagnoses. For example, if your patient has the diagnosis *Risk for Infection,* then you set a goal of "Patient will remain free from infection during hospitalization." A related outcome is "Patient will change own dressing using sterile technique in 2 days." You plan to involve other members of the health care team, such as a wound care nurse, in your patient's care.

Setting Priorities. Set the priorities for care based on a patient's nursing diagnoses. Give special attention to any urgent needs that an infection creates. For example, if a patient's infection becomes systemic, you need to manage fever and prevent dehydration. Once the infection begins to resolve, focus priorities on patient education and emotional support.

Collaborative Care. It is important that a patient's required level of care be maintained after discharge. Assess the patient, family, and other caregivers for their ability to provide care at home. For example, assess whether the patient or a family member is able to perform necessary dressing changes. Involve other members of the health care team such as the discharge planner or social services as necessary.

IMPLEMENTATION

Your nursing interventions control and prevent infection. These interventions are applicable for all types of health care settings, including a patient's home.

Health Promotion. Prevention is key to reducing infections in all health care settings. Review with and teach patients and their family caregivers measures that strengthen the host's defenses such as nutrition, recommended immunizations, personal hygiene, and regular rest and exercise (Box 14-5). In addition, explain infection prevention and control principles such as hand hygiene and methods for disposing of medical waste that are designed to prevent infections from occurring. Based on your assessment of a patient's cultural views and preferences, integrate infection prevention and

BOX 14-5 PATIENT TEACHING

Infection Prevention and Control

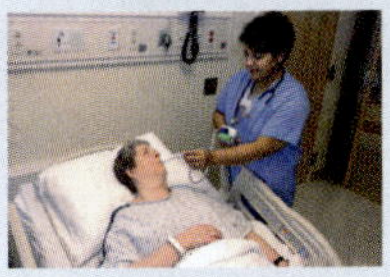

Mrs. Eldredge is nearing discharge. Kathy develops a teaching plan to help Mrs. Eldredge understand how to change her dressing and prevent further infection at home.

OUTCOME

Mrs. Eldredge changes her dressing using proper infection prevention and control techniques.

TEACHING STRATEGIES

- Demonstrate proper hand hygiene. Instruct Mrs. Eldredge to perform hand hygiene before and after all wound care and after touching infected body fluids.
- Instruct Mrs. Eldredge about the signs and symptoms of wound infection and when to notify the health care provider.
- Instruct Mrs. Eldredge to place contaminated dressings and other disposable items containing infectious body fluids in impervious plastic or brown paper bags.
- Instruct Mrs. Eldredge to clean noticeably soiled linen separate from other laundry. Wash in warm water with detergent. There are no special recommendations for setting dryer temperature.

EVALUATION STRATEGIES

- Ask Mrs. Eldredge to describe techniques used to reduce transmission of infection and the signs and symptoms of infection.
- Have Mrs. Eldredge demonstrate dressing change, including hand hygiene and disposal of contaminated dressings.

control measures into the patient's daily lifestyle and cultural practices.

Nutrition. Nutrition has a major influence on resistance to infection. Nutritional requirements vary, depending on age, health status, and other variables. A proper diet helps the immune system function and consists of a variety of foods from all food groups (see Chapter 33). Design education programs specific to patients' learning needs. Collaborate with registered dietitians as needed. Cultural considerations such as food selection and method of preparation are critical in influencing a patient's nutritional status. Teach the patient the importance that a proper diet plays in maintaining immunity and preventing infection. Incorporate the patient's food preferences when possible.

Hygiene. One infection prevention and control goal of personal hygiene is to reduce microorganisms on the skin and maintain the well-being of mucous membranes such as the mouth and vagina (Fauerbach, 2009). Patients need to understand the techniques for cleansing the skin and how to avoid spread of microorganisms in body secretions or excretions. For example, teach patients how to wash their perineum from clean to dirty, from the urethra down toward the rectum, using a clean washcloth (see Chapter 29). Also encourage patients to maintain good oral hygiene.

Immunization. Immunization programs for infants and children have decreased the occurrence of many childhood diseases such as diphtheria, whooping cough, and measles. More recently developed vaccines for hepatitis A and chickenpox (varicella) provide immunity to both adults and children for highly communicable diseases (Haiduven and Poland, 2009). In addition, specific vaccines such as influenza and pneumococcal vaccines have decreased the mortality and morbidity previously seen in older adults or patients with underlying medical problems such as chronic lung disease (CLD). Advise patients about the advantages of immunizations; but also make them aware of the contraindications for certain vaccines, especially in pregnant or lactating women. You can access the most current immunization schedule at www.cdc.gov/vaccines/recs/acip.

Adequate Rest and Regular Exercise. Adequate rest (see Chapter 31) and regular exercise help prevent infection. Physical exercise increases lung capacity, circulation, energy, and endurance. It also decreases stress and improves appetite, sleeping, and elimination. Balance the need for regular exercise with the need for rest and sleep. Some patients need education about the importance of sleep and rest for infection prevention.

Acute Care. A patient with an infection has many needs. By monitoring the course of an infection carefully, you choose the most appropriate measures to maintain or restore the patient's health. Disinfection and sterilization of supplies and good hand hygiene are examples of aseptic methods used to control the spread of microorganisms.

When a patient develops an infection, continue preventive care to reduce the risk for transmission to health care workers and other patients. Good hand hygiene and use of barriers such as gloves or masks minimize exposure to infection. These measures are known as **Standard Precautions**, which you use routinely with every patient, regardless of diagnosis. Patients with communicable diseases and infections that are easily transmissible to others require special precautions called **transmission-based precautions** (CDC, 2007). Isolation precautions involve control of a patient's environment by forming barriers against bacterial spread.

Treatment of an infection includes identification and elimination of the organism and support of a patient's defenses. Nurses collect specimens of body fluids or drainage from infected body sites and send the specimens to the laboratory for cultures. When the causative organism is identified, the health care provider usually prescribes an antimicrobial. Administer antibiotics carefully, watching for allergic reactions and assessing the effect on the patient's infection. It is important to teach patients the importance of taking all of their antibiotics as ordered when discharged home.

Systemic infections (i.e., those that affect the body as a whole) require measures to manage or prevent the complications of fever (see Chapter 15). Drinking fluids regularly prevents dehydration resulting from diaphoresis. Increased metabolism requires an adequate nutritional intake. Rest preserves energy for the healing process.

Localized infections often require measures to facilitate removal of infectious organisms such as using moist-to-dry dressings or irrigating wounds (see Chapter 37) to remove infected drainage from wound sites. Applying warm compresses helps blood flow to an infected site, thus delivering components of the blood needed to fight an infection. Use medical and surgical aseptic techniques to manage wounds and handle infected drainage or body fluids correctly.

During any infection support the patient's body defense mechanisms. For example, when a patient has diarrhea, cleanse the skin promptly and dry it thoroughly to prevent breakdown.

Medical Asepsis. Basic medical aseptic techniques break the infection chain. Use these techniques for all patients, even when no infection is diagnosed. Aggressive preventive measures are highly effective in reducing HAIs.

Control or Elimination of Infectious Agents. With the increased use of disposable equipment, nurses are sometimes less aware of disinfection and sterilization procedures. The proper cleaning, disinfection, and sterilization of contaminated objects significantly reduce and/or eliminate microorganisms (CDC, 2008b, Rutala and Weber, 2009).

Cleaning. Cleaning involves removing organic material such as blood or inorganic material such as soil from objects. Generally this involves the use of water, a detergent/disinfectant, and proper mechanical scrubbing action. Cleaning occurs before disinfection and sterilization procedures (CDC, 2008b; Rutala and Weber, 2009). Check the policy of the health care facility before cleaning. In most institutions technicians clean equipment. When cleaning objects soiled with blood or body fluids, use personal protective equipment (PPE) such as gloves, goggles, and mask to protect yourself from splashing fluids.

Disinfection and Sterilization. Disinfection and sterilization use both physical and chemical processes. Both processes disrupt the internal functioning of microorganisms by destroying cell proteins. **Disinfection** eliminates almost all pathogenic organisms, with the exception of bacterial spores. **Sterilization** eliminates or destroys all forms of microbial life, including spores (Rutala and Weber, 2009). Sterilization methods include processing items using steam, dry heat, hydrogen peroxide plasma, or ethylene oxide (ETO). The level of disinfection and sterilization required depends on the type and use of the contaminated item (Box 14-6). You are responsible for checking package integrity and/or expiration dates before using an object designated as sterile. Dispose of items not meeting the criteria for being sterile or return them to the sterilization-processing department (CDC, 2008b).

Control or Elimination of Reservoirs. To control or eliminate infection in reservoir sites, eliminate sources of body fluids, drainage, or solutions that possibly harbor microorganisms. For example; carefully discard disposable articles that become contaminated with infectious material (Box 14-7).

Control of Portals of Exit. It is important to avoid talking, sneezing, or coughing directly over a surgical wound or sterile dressing field to control organisms exiting through the respiratory tract. Also teach patients to protect others when they sneeze or cough and give patients disposable wipes or tissues to control spread of microorganisms. Try not to work with patients who are highly susceptible to infection if you have a cold or other communicable infection.

Another way of controlling the exit of microorganisms is by using Standard Precautions when handling body fluids such as urine, feces, and wound drainage. Wear clean gloves if there is a chance of contact with any blood or body fluids and perform hand hygiene after providing care. Be sure to bag contaminated items appropriately.

BOX 14-6 CATEGORIES OF ITEMS REQUIRING STERILIZATION, DISINFECTION, AND CLEANING

CRITICAL ITEMS

Items that enter sterile tissue or the vascular system present a high risk for infection if they are contaminated with microorganisms, especially bacterial spores. *Critical* items must be *sterile.* Some of these items include:

- Surgical instruments
- Cardiac or intravascular catheters
- Urinary catheters
- Implants

SEMICRITICAL ITEMS

Items that come in contact with mucous membranes or nonintact skin also present a risk. These objects must be free of all microorganisms (except bacterial spores). *Semicritical items* must be *high-level disinfected (HLD)* or *sterilized.* Some of these items include:

- Respiratory and anesthesia equipment
- Endoscopes
- Endotracheal tubes
- Gastrointestinal endoscopes
- Diaphragm fitting rings

After rinsing, items must be dried and stored in a manner to protect from damage and contamination

NONCRITICAL ITEMS

Items that come in contact with intact skin but not mucous membranes must be clean. *Noncritical items* must be *disinfected.* Some of these items include:

- Bedpans
- Blood pressure cuffs
- Bed rails
- Linens
- Stethoscopes
- Bedside trays and patient furniture
- Food utensils

BOX 14-7 INFECTION PREVENTION AND CONTROL TO REDUCE RESERVOIRS OF INFECTION

BATHING

- Use soap and water to remove drainage, dried secretions, or excess perspiration.

DRESSING CHANGES

- Change dressings that become wet and/or soiled (see Chapter 37).

CONTAMINATED ARTICLES

- Place tissues, soiled dressings, or soiled linen in fluid-resistant bags for proper disposal.

CONTAMINATED SHARPS

- Place all needles—safety needles and needleless systems—into puncture-proof containers located at the site of use. Federal law requires use of needle safety technology. Blood tube holders are single use only (OSHA, 2001).

BEDSIDE UNIT

- Keep table surfaces clean and dry.

BOTTLED SOLUTIONS

- Do not leave bottled solutions open.
- Keep solutions tightly capped.
- Date bottles when opened and discard in 24 hours.

SURGICAL WOUNDS

- Keep drainage tubes and collection bags patent to prevent accumulation of serous fluid under skin surface.

DRAINAGE BOTTLES AND BAGS

- Wear gloves and protective eyewear if splashing or spraying with contaminated blood or body fluids is anticipated.
- Empty and dispose of drainage suction bottles according to facility policy.
- Empty all drainage systems on each shift unless otherwise ordered by health care provider.
- Never raise drainage system (e.g., urinary drainage bag) above level of site being drained unless it is clamped off.

Control of Transmission. Effective infection prevention and control requires that you know the modes of transmission of microorganisms and the methods of control. In any health care setting a patient usually has a personal set of care items. Sharing graduated containers for measuring urine, bath basins, and eating utensils among patients create routes for transmission of infection. When using a stethoscope, always wipe off the bell, diaphragm, and ear tips with a disinfectant such as an alcohol wipe before proceeding to the next patient. Ear tips are a common location for staphylococcal organisms (Whittington et al., 2009).

Because certain microorganisms travel easily through the air, do not shake linens or bedclothes. Dust with a treated or dampened cloth to prevent dust particles from entering the air.

To prevent transmission of microorganisms through indirect contact, do not allow soiled items and equipment to touch your clothing. A common error is to carry dirty linen in the arms against the uniform. Use special linen bags or carry soiled linen with the hands held out from the body. Never put clean or soiled linens on the floor.

Hand Hygiene. The most effective basic technique in preventing and controlling transmission of infection is hand hygiene (Box 14-8). Hand hygiene is a general term that applies to four techniques: handwashing, antiseptic hand wash, antiseptic hand rub, or surgical hand antisepsis. Handwashing is defined by the CDC (2009) as the vigorous, brief rubbing together of all surfaces of lathered hands, followed by rinsing under a stream of warm water. The fundamental principle behind handwashing is removal of microorganisms mechanically from the hands and rinsing with water. Handwashing does not kill microorganisms. An antiseptic hand wash means washing hands with warm water and soap or other detergents containing an antiseptic agent. Some antiseptics kill bacteria and some viruses. An antiseptic hand rub means applying an antiseptic hand-rub product to all surfaces of the hands to reduce the number of microorganisms present. Ethanol-based hand antiseptics containing 60% to 90% alcohol appear to be the most effective against common pathogens found on the hands (CDC, 2009). Alcohol-based products are more effective for standard handwashing or hand antisepsis (nonsoiled hands) by health care workers than regular soap or antimicrobial soaps (CDC, 2008a). Surgical hand antisepsis is an antiseptic hand-wash or hand-rub technique that surgical personnel perform before surgery to eliminate transient and reduce resident hand flora. Antiseptic detergent preparations have persistent antimicrobial activity (CDC, 2008a; WHO, 2009).

Alcohol-based hand antiseptics are not effective on hands that are visibly dirty or are contaminated with organic materials (CDC, 2013). Thus when hands are visibly dirty or contaminated with proteinaceous material or visibly soiled with blood or other body fluids, wash them with either a plain soap or an antimicrobial soap and water. Handwashing is also indicated before eating and after using the toilet. Wash hands if they are exposed to spore-forming organisms such as *Clostridium difficile* or *Bacillus anthracis* (CDC, 2008b) (Box 14-9).

If hands are not visibly soiled, you may use an alcohol-based hand rub to decontaminate the hands in the following situations:

1. Before, after, and between direct patient contact (e.g., taking a pulse, lifting a patient, performing a procedure)
2. Before putting on sterile gloves and before inserting invasive devices such as indwelling urinary catheters and peripheral vascular catheters
3. After contact with body fluids or excretions, mucous membranes, nonintact skin, and wound dressings (even if gloves were worn)

BOX 14-8 PROCEDURAL GUIDELINE

Hand Hygiene

DELEGATION CONSIDERATIONS

The skill of hand hygiene is performed by all caregivers. *Hand hygiene is not optional.*

EQUIPMENT

Alcohol-based waterless antiseptic containing emollients, easy-to-reach sink with warm running water, antimicrobial or nonantimicrobial soap, paper towels or air dryer, and disposable nail cleaner *(optional)*

STEPS

1. Inspect surface of hands for breaks or cuts in skin or cuticles.
2. Note condition of nails. Nail tips need to be less than ¼ inch long and free of artificial nails or extenders or polish, especially cracked polish. Avoid artificial nails and long or unkempt nails, which harbor microorganisms (CDC, 2008a). Agency policies frequently ban artificial nails and nail polish. Check agency policy. Report and cover any skin lesions before providing patient care.
3. Inspect hands for visible soiling.
4. Push wristwatch and long uniform sleeves above wrists. Avoid wearing rings. If worn, remove during washing (check agency policy). Be sure that fingernails are short, filed, and smooth.
5. Hand antisepsis using an instant alcohol waterless antiseptic rub:
   a. **Following manufacturer directions,** dispense ample amount of product into palm of one hand (see illustration).
   b. Rub hands together, covering all surfaces of hands and fingers with antiseptic (see illustration).
   c. Rub hands together until alcohol is dry. Allow hands to completely dry before applying gloves.

Clinical Decision Point: If hands feel dry after rubbing hands together for 10-15 seconds, an insufficient volume of product likely was applied (Boyce et al., 2002).

6. Handwashing using regular lotion soap or antimicrobial soap and water:
   a. Stand in front of sink, keeping hands and uniform away from sink surface. (If hands touch sink during handwashing, repeat.)
   b. Turn faucet on or push knee pedals laterally or press pedals with foot to regulate flow and temperature (see illustration).
   c. Avoid splashing water against uniform.
   d. Regulate flow of water so temperature is warm.
   e. Wet hands and wrists thoroughly under running water. Keep hands and forearms lower than elbows during washing.
   f. Apply 3 to 5 mL of antiseptic soap and rub hands together, lathering thoroughly (see illustration). Soap granules and leaflet preparations may be used.

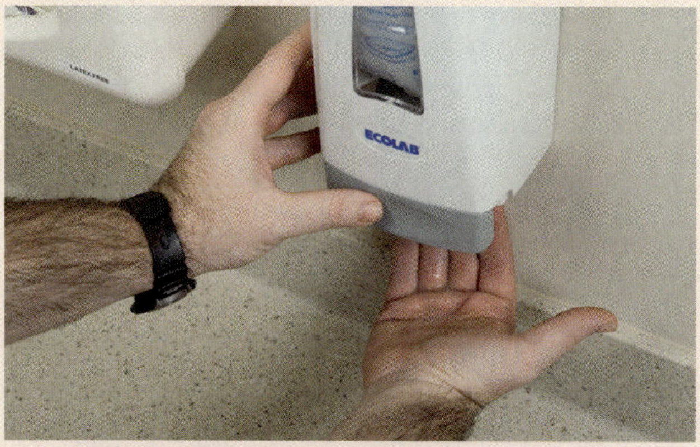

STEP 5a Apply waterless antiseptic to hands.

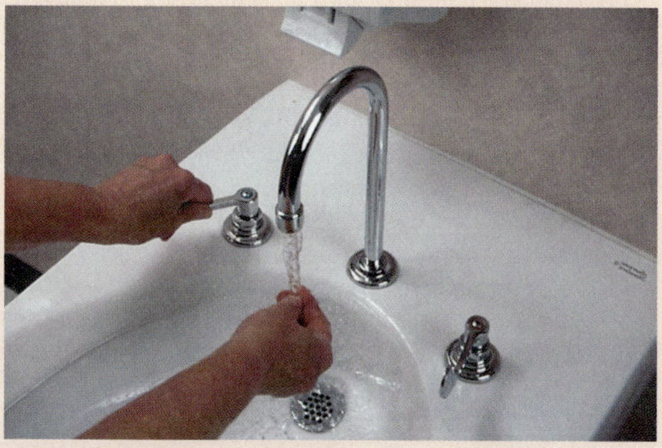

STEP 6b Regulate flow of water.

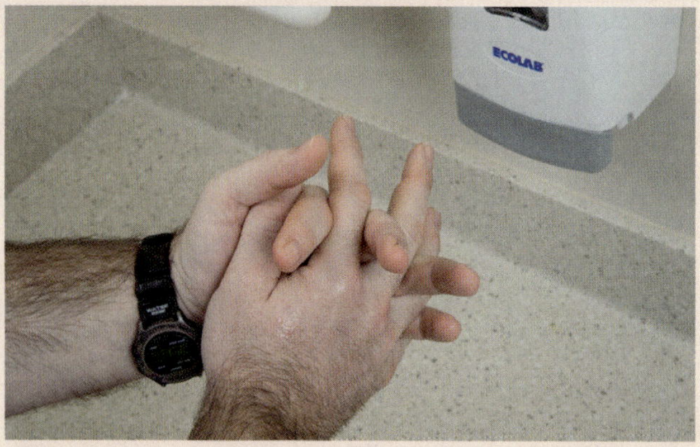

STEP 5b Rub hands thoroughly, making sure to cover all surfaces of the fingers and hands.

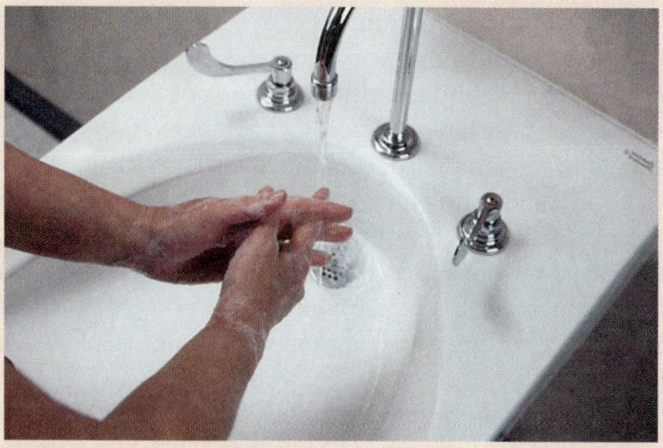

STEP 6f Wet hands; apply soap and lather hands thoroughly.

BOX 14-8 PROCEDURAL GUIDELINE—cont'd

Hand Hygiene

Clinical Decision Point: The decision whether to use an antiseptic soap or alcohol-based hand sanitizer depends on whether the hands are visibly soiled, the procedure you will perform, and the patient's immune status.

g. Wash hands using plenty of lather and friction for at least 15 to 20 seconds (Boyce et al., 2002; CDC, 2013). A tip is to sing the Happy Birthday song twice. Interlace fingers and rub palms and back of hands with circular motion at least 5 times each. Keep fingertips down to facilitate removal of microorganisms.

h. Areas under fingernails are often soiled. Clean them with the fingernails of other hand and additional soap or clean with a disposable nail cleaner.

i. Rinse hands and wrists thoroughly, keeping hands down and elbows up (see illustration).

j. Dry hands thoroughly from fingers to wrists and forearms with paper towel, single-use cloth, or warm air dryer.

k. If used, discard paper towel in proper receptacle.

l. To turn off hand faucet, use clean, dry paper towel. Avoid touching handles with hands (see illustration.). Turn off water with foot or knee pedals (if applicable).

7. Apply lotion to hands. Use facility-provided lotion if available. Avoid petroleum-based lotions.

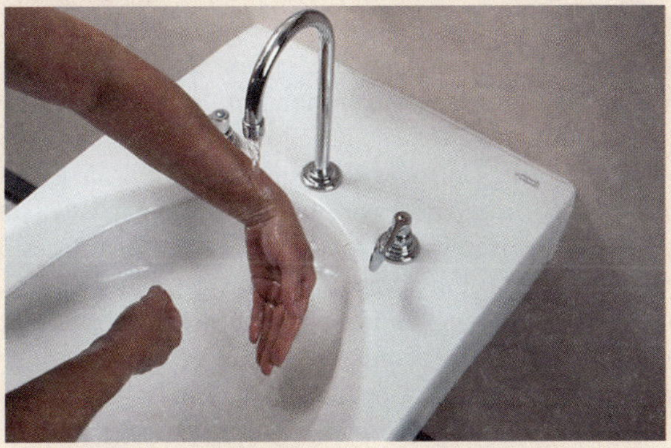

STEP 6i Rinse hands.

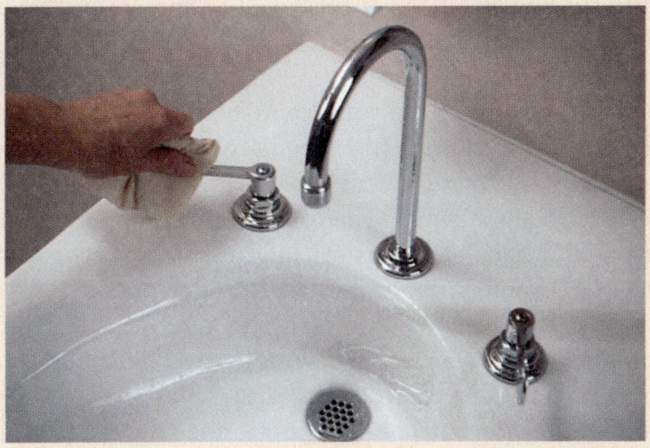

STEP 6l Turn off faucet with clean, dry paper towel.

BOX 14-9 EVIDENCE-BASED PRACTICE

PICO Question: With hospitalized patients diagnosed with *Clostridium difficile,* does the use of soap and water before and after patient care compared with the use of alcohol-based hand gels before and after patient care decrease the transmission of *C. difficile* to other patients cared for by the same health care personnel?

SUMMARY OF EVIDENCE

Although many types of health care–associated infections (HAIs) are declining, an infection caused by *C. difficile* remains at historically high levels. *C. difficile* is a spore-forming, gram-positive anaerobic bacillus that produces two exotoxins: toxin A and toxin B. It is a common cause of antibiotic-associated diarrhea and is linked to 14,000 American deaths each year (Cohen et al., 2010). Those most at risk are people, especially older adults, who take antibiotics and also receive medical care. When a person takes antibiotics, normal flora that protect against infection are destroyed for several months. During this time patients can get sick from *C. difficile* picked up from contaminated surfaces or spread from a health care provider's hands. Evidence shows alcohol is ineffective in killing *C. difficile* spores. Handwashing with soap and water has the greatest efficacy in removing spores from hands. Thus evidence supports the use of soap and water over the use of alcohol-based hand rubs when contact with *C. difficile* is suspected or likely (Cohen et al., 2010; Jabbar et al., 2010). The use of gloves by health care workers prevents the contamination of hands with *C. difficile* spores. If gloves are removed properly to prevent hand contamination, any potential benefit of using soap and water over alcohol based hand hygiene products is likely negated (Dubberke & Gerding, 2011).

APPLICATION TO NURSING PRACTICE

- Use soap and water for hand hygiene when caring for a patient diagnosed with *C. difficile* to remove organisms from the hands.
- Apply gloves prior to entering the room of a patient with *C. difficile* and remove gloves properly after care.
- Perform hand hygiene before and after wearing gloves.
- Proper hand hygiene helps to prevent transmission of infections to health care workers' other patients.

4. When moving from a contaminated to a clean body site during care
5. After contact with surfaces or objects in the patient's room (e.g., overbed table, bed linen, IV pump)
6. After removing gloves (CDC, 2008a, 2009)

You may also wash hands with an antimicrobial soap and water in these situations.

Isolation and Barrier Protection. In 2007 the Hospital Infection Control Practices Advisory Committee (HICPAC) of the CDC published revised guidelines for isolation precautions. HICPAC recommends that facilities modify these guidelines according to need and as dictated by federal, state, or local regulations. The guidelines contain recommendations for respiratory hygiene/cough etiquette as part of Standard Precautions. The CDC recommendations contain two tiers of precautions (Table 14-5). The first and most important tier is called *Standard Precautions;* the CDC designed it to be used for care of all patients, in all settings, regardless of risk or presumed infection status. Standard Precautions are the primary strategies for prevention of infection transmission and apply to contact with blood, body fluids, nonintact skin, mucous membranes, and equipment or surfaces contaminated with these potentially infectious materials. The strategy of respiratory hygiene/cough etiquette applies to any person with signs of respiratory infection, including cough, congestion, rhinorrhea, or increased production of respiratory secretions when entering a health care site. Educating health care staff, patients, and visitors to cover the mouth and nose with a tissue when coughing, dispose properly of used tissues, and perform hand hygiene is among the elements of respiratory hygiene. These precautions protect patients and health care workers (Box 14-10).

Assess the need for Standard Precautions based on the potential for transmission of infection, regardless of a patient's diagnosis. For example, when suctioning a patient with a tracheostomy, wearing gloves, eyewear, and a mask is appropriate protection, regardless of the presence of known respiratory infection.

The second tier of precautions (see Table 14-5) includes precautions designed for the care of patients who are known or suspected to be infected or colonized with microorganisms transmitted by the droplet, airborne, or contact route (CDC, 2007; Brisko, 2009). There are three types of transmission-based precautions: **Airborne, Droplet,** and **Contact Precautions.** They are used singly or in combination for diseases that have multiple routes of transmission (e.g., chickenpox). Use them in addition to Standard Precautions.

One important aspect of care for patients on isolation is compliance with hand hygiene and changing gloves between exposure to body sites and patient equipment. Inadequate glove changes and hand hygiene often lead to contamination of previously colonized sites (Haas, 2009). Noncompliance with glove changing and hand hygiene increases the risk of HAIs.

Because of the resurgence of TB, the CDC (2005) developed guidelines to prevent its transmission to health care workers and stresses the importance of isolation for the patient with known or suspected TB in a special negative-pressure room. Close the doors to the patient's room to control direction of airflow. Wear a special high-filtration particulate respirator on entering a respiratory isolation room. Make sure that respirators are able to fit health care workers with different facial sizes and characteristics. When worn correctly, particulate respirators and masks (Figures 14-3 and 14-4) have a tighter face seal and filter at a higher level than routine surgical masks (OSHA, 1995).

Multidrug-resistant organisms (MDROs) such as methicillin-resistant *Staphylococcus aureus* (MRSA) and vancomycin-resistant enterococcus (VRE) have become more common as a cause of colonization and HAIs. MDROs are organisms that have developed a resistance to one or more broad-spectrum antibiotics, making the organism hard to treat effectively. MRSA is frequently associated with increased patient death and causes close to 19% of health care–associated bloodstream infections (Becker and Kahl, 2009). VRE poses a risk to patients who are immune-compromised and debilitated (Archibald, 2009). *Clostridium difficile* infection is one of the most common and costly HAIs. Patient susceptibility to *C. difficile* usually requires prior treatment with antibiotics. Unlike MRSA and VRE, *C difficile* is harder to eliminate from the environment because it is a spore-forming organism, meaning it can remain on surfaces in a dormant state for long periods of time. To reduce the risk of cross-contamination among patients, use Contact Precautions in addition to Standard Precautions when caring for patients with multidrug-resistant organisms.

Regardless of the type of isolation or barrier protection used, follow certain basic principles when delivering care in a patient's room. Understand how certain diseases are transmitted and which barriers you need to prevent transmission. For example, you do not routinely need to wear a gown or gloves when giving oral medications, but you do need these barriers when changing a dressing from a draining wound. Gloves are appropriate when helping a patient with an oral medication if the patient needs assistance putting the medication in the mouth.

Take care to avoid exposing an article brought into a patient's room to any infectious material. Bag or decontaminate any contaminated article (e.g., blood pressure cuff) according to agency policy. Decontaminate equipment that is shared among patients.

Before you institute isolation measures, explain to the patient and family the nature of the patient's condition, the purpose of the isolation barriers, and ways to carry out specific precautions. Teach them the proper way to perform hand hygiene and apply gloves, masks, or gowns. Demonstrate each procedure and give the patient and family an opportunity to practice.

Explain methods of transmission of infectious organisms so patients and family members understand the difference between contaminated and clean objects. Provide for a patient's sensory stimulation during isolation. Encourage the family to bring the patient reading materials, puzzle books, and similar items. Take the opportunity to listen to the

TABLE 14-5 CENTERS FOR DISEASE CONTROL AND PREVENTION ISOLATION GUIDELINES

Standard Precautions (Tier 1) for Use with All Patients

- Standard Precautions apply to blood, blood products, all body fluids, secretions, excretions (except sweat), nonintact skin, and mucous membranes.
- Perform hand hygiene before, after, and between direct contact with patients. (Examples of between contact: Cleaning hands after a patient care activity, moving to a non–patient care activity, then cleaning hands again before returning to perform patient contact).
- Perform hand hygiene after contact with blood, body fluids, secretions, and excretions; after contact with surfaces or articles in a patient's room; and immediately after gloves are removed.
- When hands are visibly soiled or contaminated with blood or body fluids, wash them with either a nonantimicrobial soap or an antimicrobial soap and water.
- When hands are not visibly soiled or contaminated with blood or body fluids, use an alcohol-based hand rub to perform hand hygiene.
- Wash hands with antimicrobial soap and water if contact with spores (e.g., *Clostridium difficile*) is likely to have occurred.
- Do not wear artificial fingernails or extenders if duties include direct contact with patients at high risk for infection and associated adverse outcomes.
- Wear gloves when touching blood, body fluids, secretions, excretions, nonintact skin, mucous membranes, or contaminated items or surfaces. Remove gloves and perform hand hygiene between patient care encounters and when going from a contaminated to a clean body site.
- Wear PPE when the anticipated patient interaction indicates that contact with blood or body fluids may occur.
- A private room is unnecessary unless the patient's hygiene is unacceptable (e.g., uncontained secretions, excretions, or wound drainage).
- Discard all contaminated sharp instruments and needles in a puncture-resistant container. Health care facilities must make available needleless devices. Any needles should be disposed of uncapped, or a mechanical safety device is activated for recapping.
- Respiratory hygiene/cough etiquette: Have patients cover the nose/mouth when coughing or sneezing; use tissues to contain respiratory secretions, and dispose of in nearest waste container; perform hand hygiene after contacting respiratory secretions and contaminated object/materials; contain respiratory secretions with procedure or surgical masks; sit at least 3 feet away from others if coughing.

Transmission-Based Precautions (Tier 2) for Use with Specific Types of Patients

CATEGORY	DISEASE	BARRIER PROTECTION
Airborne Precautions (Droplet nuclei smaller than 5 microns)	Measles, chickenpox (varicella), disseminated varicella-zoster, pulmonary or laryngeal tuberculosis	Private room, negative-pressure airflow of at least 6-12 exchanges per hour via HEPA filtration Mask or respiratory protection device, n95 respirator (depending on condition)
Droplet Precautions (Droplets larger than 5 microns; being within 3 feet of the patient)	Examples include *B. pertussis,* influenza virus, adenovirus, rhinovirus, *N. meningitides,* Group A streptococcus (until first 24 hours of antimicrobial therapy); refer to agency policy	Private room or cohort patients Mask or respirator required depending on condition (refer to agency policy)
Contact Precautions (Direct patient or environmental contact)	Colonization or infection with multidrug-resistant organisms such as VRE and MRSA, *Clostridium difficile,* shigella, and other enteric pathogens; major wound infections; herpes simplex; scabies; varicella zoster (disseminated); respiratory syncytial virus in infants, young children, or immunocompromised adults	Private room or cohort patients (see agency policy), gloves, gowns
Protective environment	Allogeneic hematopoietic stem cell transplants	Private room; positive-pressure airflow with 12 or more air exchanges per hour; HEPA filtration for incoming air Mask to be worn by patient when out of room during times of construction in area.

Modified from Centers for Disease Control and Prevention, Hospital Infection Control Practice Advisory Committee: Guidelines for isolation precautions in hospitals, *MMWR Morb Mortal Wkly Rep* 57(RR-16):39, 2007.

HEPA, High efficiency particulate air; *MRSA,* methicillin-resistant *Staphylococcus aureus; PPE,* personal protective equipment; *VRE,* vancomycin-resistant enterococci.

BOX 14-10 PROCEDURAL GUIDELINES

Caring for a Patient on Isolation Precautions

DELEGATION CONSIDERATIONS

The skill of caring for patients on isolation precautions can be delegated to nursing assistive personnel (NAP). However, it is the nurse who assesses the patient's status and isolation indications. Instruct NAP about:

- Reason patient is on isolation precautions.
- Special precautions regarding individual patient needs such as transportation to diagnostic tests.

EQUIPMENT

Personal protective equipment (PPE) determined by type of isolation: gowns, gloves, mask, protective eyewear or face shield; supplies necessary for procedures performed in room; soiled linen and trash receptacles, sharps container, disposable blood pressure (BP) cuff

STEPS

1. Assess isolation indications (e.g., patient's medical history for exposure, laboratory tests, wound drainage).
2. Review laboratory test results to identify type of microorganism for which patient is isolated and if patient is immunosuppressed.
3. Review agency policies and precautions necessary for the type of isolation ordered and consider care measures that you will perform while in patient's room.
4. Review nurses' notes or speak with colleagues regarding patient's emotional state and adjustment to isolation.
5. Assess whether patient has a known latex allergy to avoid sensitivity or allergic reaction.
6. Perform hand hygiene and prepare all equipment that you will need to take into patient's room. In some cases equipment remains in the room (e.g., stethoscope or BP cuff). Decide which isolation equipment is necessary before entering a patient's room. For example, decide whether you will need a gown and gloves for a patient on Contact Precautions or if you will need a special respirator mask for a patient on Airborne Precautions.
7. Prepare for entrance into isolation room:
   a. Apply cover gown, being sure that it covers all outer garments. Pull sleeves down to wrist. Tie securely at neck and waist (see illustration).
   b. Apply either surgical mask or fitted respirator around mouth and nose. (Type and fit-testing depends on type of precautions and facility policy.) The nurse must have a medical evaluation and be fit tested before using a respirator.
   c. If needed, apply eyewear or goggles snugly around face and eyes. If prescription glasses are worn, side shield may be used.
   d. Apply clean gloves. (**Note:** Wear unpowdered, latex-free gloves.) If gloves are worn with gown, bring glove cuffs over edge of gown sleeves (see illustration).
8. Enter patient's room. Arrange supplies and equipment. (If equipment will be removed from room for reuse, place on clean paper towel.)
9. Explain purpose of isolation and necessary precautions to patient and family. Offer opportunity to ask questions. Assess for evidence of emotional problems that can occur from isolation.
10. Assess vital signs (see Chapter 15).
    a. If patient is infected or colonized with a resistant organism (e.g., vancomycin-resistant enterococci [VRE], methicillin-resistant *Staphylococcus aureus* [MRSA]), equipment remains in room. This includes the stethoscope and BP cuff (CDC, 2011).
    b. If stethoscope is to be reused, clean diaphragm or bell with alcohol. Set aside on clean surface.
    c. Use individual electronic or disposable thermometer and blood pressure cuffs when available.

Clinical Decision Point: If disposable thermometer indicates a fever, assess for other signs/symptoms of infection. Confirm fever using an alternative thermometer. Do not use electronic thermometer if patient is suspected or confirmed to have *C. difficile* (Cohen et al., 2010).

11. Administer medications (see Chapter 17):
    a. Give oral medication in wrapper or cup.
    b. Dispose of wrapper or cup in plastic-lined receptacle.

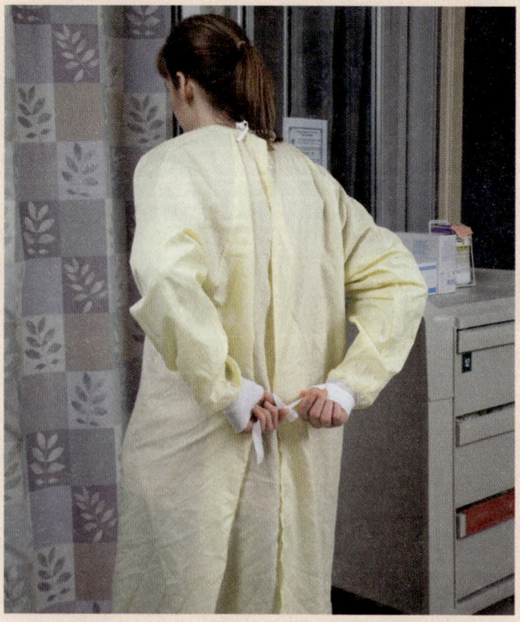

STEP 7a Tie gown at waist and neck.

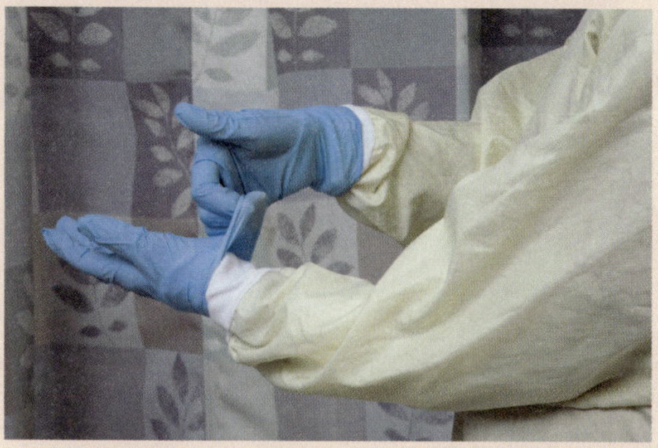

STEP 7d Apply gloves over gown sleeves.

BOX 14-10 PROCEDURAL GUIDELINES—cont'd

Caring for a Patient on Isolation Precautions

c. Wear gloves when administering an injection.
d. Discard safety needle and syringe or uncapped needle into the sharps container.
e. Place a reusable syringe (e.g., Carpuject) on clean towel for eventual removal and disinfection.
f. If you are not wearing gloves and hands contact a contaminated article or body fluids, perform hand hygiene as soon as possible.

12. Administer hygiene, encouraging patient to ask questions or express concerns about isolation. Provide informal teaching at this time.
    a. Avoid allowing gown to become wet. Carry washbasin out away from gown; avoid leaning against any wet surface.
    b. Remove linen from bed; avoid contact with your gown. Place in leak-proof linen bag.
    c. Provide clean bed linen and set of towels.
    d. Change gloves and perform hand hygiene if they become excessively soiled and further care is necessary.
13. Collect specimens:
    a. Place specimen containers on clean paper towel in patient's bathroom. Follow agency procedure for collecting specimen of body fluids.
    b. Transfer specimen to container without soiling outside of container. Place container in plastic bag and place label on outside of bag or per facility policy. Label specimen in front of patient (TJC, 2014).
    c. Perform hand hygiene and reglove if additional procedures are needed.
    d. Check label on specimen for accuracy. (Warning labels are often used, depending on agency policy.) Send to laboratory. Label containers with a biohazard label (see illustration).
14. Dispose of linen, trash, and disposable items.
    a. Use sturdy, moisture-resistant single bags to contain soiled articles. Use double bag if necessary for heavily soiled linen or heavy, wet trash.
    b. Tie bags securely at top in knot (see illustration).

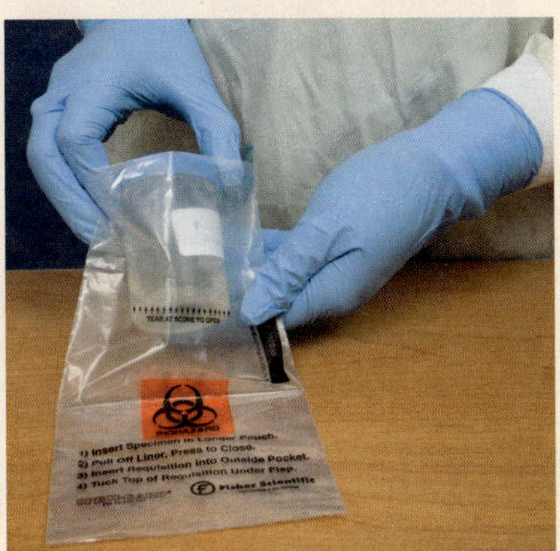

STEP 13d Specimen container placed in biohazard bag and sealed.

15. Remove all reusable equipment. Clean any contaminated surfaces with agency-approved disinfectant (see agency policy).
16. Resupply room as needed. Have a staff member outside the isolation room hand you new supplies.
17. Explain to patient when you plan to return to room. Ask whether patient requires any personal care items, books, or magazines.
18. Leave isolation room. The order for removing PPE depends on what was needed for the type of isolation. The sequence listed is based on full PPE being required.
    a. Remove gloves. Remove one glove by grasping cuff and pulling glove inside out over hand. Hold removed glove in gloved hand. With ungloved hand, slide finger inside cuff of remaining glove at wrist. Pull glove off over first glove. Discard gloves in proper container (see illustration).

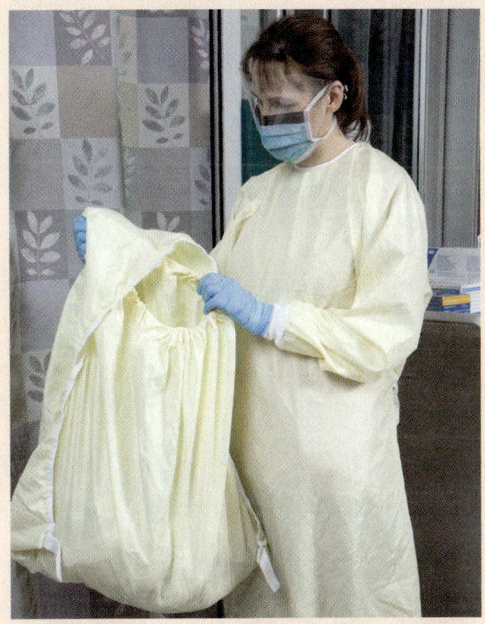

STEP 14b Tie trash bag securely.

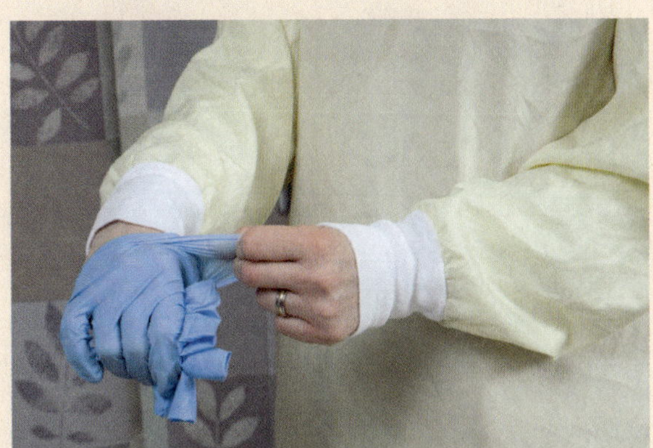

STEP 18a Remove gloves.

Continued

BOX 14-10 PROCEDURAL GUIDELINES—cont'd

Caring for a Patient on Isolation Precautions

b. Remove eyewear/face shield or goggles by handling at headband or earpieces. Discard in proper container.
c. Untie neck strings and then back strings of gown. Allow gown to fall from shoulders (see illustration). Remove hands from sleeves without touching outside of gown. Hold gown inside at shoulder seams and fold inside out. Discard in laundry bag if gown is made of fabric or in trash can if gown is disposable.
d. Remove mask—If mask secures over your ears, remove elastic from ears and pull away from face. For a tie-on mask, untie *bottom* mask strings and then top strings. Hold top strings and pull mask away from face; drop into trash receptacle. Do not touch outer surface of mask.
e. Perform hand hygiene.
f. Retrieve wristwatch and stethoscope (unless items must remain in room) and record vital signs on note paper.
g. Leave room and close door if necessary. (Make sure that door is closed if patient is on Airborne Precautions.)
h. Dispose of all contaminated supplies and equipment in a manner that prevents spread of microorganisms to other people (check health care facility or agency policy). Perform hand hygiene.

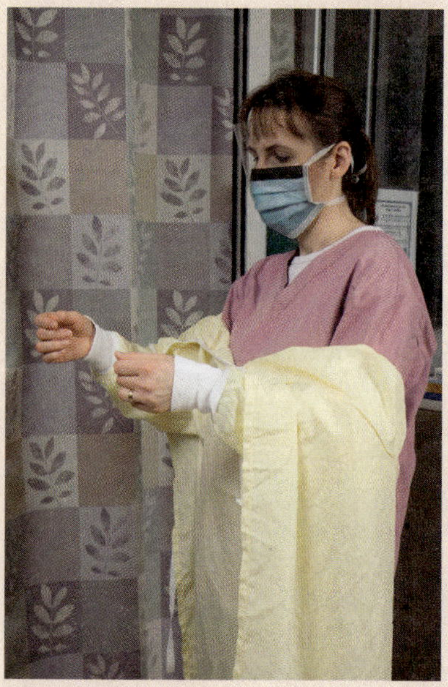

STEP 18c Remove gown by allowing it to fall from shoulders and remove so outside of gown is now inside.

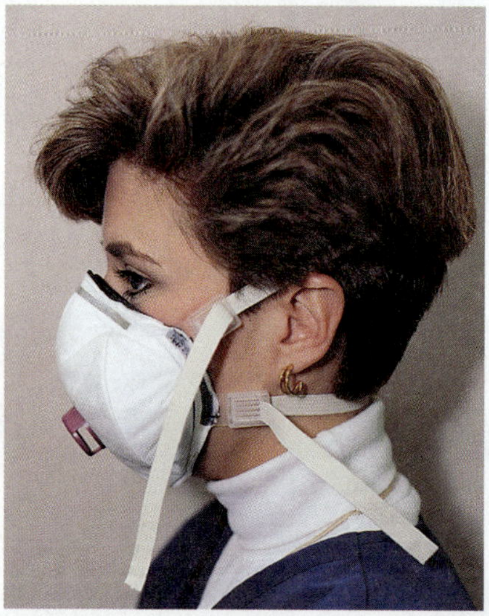

FIGURE 14-3 Disposable high-efficiency particulate air (HEPA)–purifying respirator.

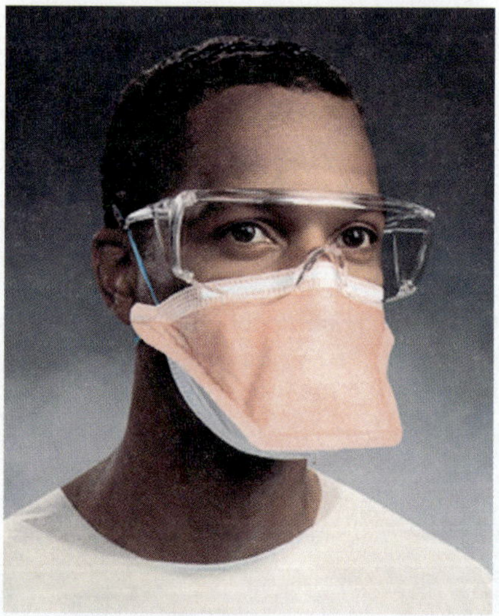

FIGURE 14-4 N95 respirator mask with protective eyewear. (Courtesy Kimberly-Clark Healthcare, Roswell, GA.)

patient's concerns or interests. If you rush care or show a lack of interest in the patient's needs, he or she will feel rejected and even more isolated. Explain the patient's potential risk for depression or loneliness to family members. Encourage visitors to avoid negative expressions or actions concerning isolation. Advise family members on ways to provide meaningful stimulation.

Protective Environment. In some situations you use special rooms for highly susceptible patients such as transplant recipients and patients with neutropenia (low WBC count). Post a card on the patient's room door with a list of the precautions in use when a private room is recommended (check agency policy). The card is a handy reference for health care workers and visitors and alerts all who enter the room of any special precautions in use. Each facility is different; therefore make sure that you follow facility policies on isolation practice (Seigel et al., 2007).

The isolation room or an adjoining anteroom, if present, needs to contain hand-hygiene supplies, bathing, and toilet facilities. Personnel and visitors need to perform hand hygiene before entering and on exiting a patient's room. If toilet facilities are unavailable, there are special procedures for handling portable commodes, bedpans, or urinals (check agency policy). Store PPE in an anteroom between the room and hallway or in a location convenient to where the PPE is going to be used for patient care. Resupply PPE as needed.

Each patient care room, including those used for isolation, contains a trash container with plastic liners. Rooms used for isolation also contain a soiled linen hamper. These containers prevent transmission of microorganisms by preventing leakage and waste from contaminating the outside surface. Have a disposable, rigid container available in the room to discard used needles, sharps, and syringes.

Depending on the microorganisms identified and the mode of transmission, critically evaluate which articles or equipment to take into an isolation room. For example, the Hospital Infection Control Practices Advisory Committee (HICPAC) of the CDC recommends taking only dedicated articles into an isolation room of a patient infected or colonized with VRE (CDC, 2007).

Personal Protective Equipment. Gowns or cover-ups protect health care workers from coming in contact with infected blood and body fluids or materials. Gowns used for barrier protection are made of a fluid-resistant material, and you need to change the gown immediately if it is damaged or heavily contaminated.

You wear gowns when soiling the skin or clothing is likely from contact with blood or body fluids or when a patient has uncontained secretions. Isolation gowns usually open at the back and have ties or snaps at the neck and waist to keep the gown closed and secure. A gown is long enough to cover all outer garments. Long sleeves with tight-fitting cuffs provide added protection.

Wear a mask or respirator if you anticipate splashing or spraying of blood or body fluids. The mask also protects you from inhaling microorganisms from a patient's respiratory tract and prevents the transmission of pathogens from your respiratory tract. Occasionally a patient who is susceptible to infection wears a mask to avoid inhaling pathogens. Patients requiring respiratory precautions wear surgical masks when ambulating or being transported outside of their room to protect other patients and personnel.

Masks prevent the transmission of infections caused by direct contact with mucous membranes. A mask discourages the wearer from touching the nose or mouth. A properly applied mask fits snugly over the mouth and nose so the pathogens and body fluids cannot enter or escape through the sides (Box 14-11). If the person wears glasses, the top edge of the mask fits below the glasses so they do not cloud over as the person exhales. Keep talking to a minimum while wearing a mask. Discard a mask that has become moist because it is ineffective. Discard the mask when leaving a patient's room. Warn patients and family members that a mask sometimes causes a sensation of smothering. If family members become uncomfortable, have them leave the room and discard their masks.

BOX 14-11 PROCEDURAL GUIDELINES

Applying a Surgical Type of Mask

DELEGATION CONSIDERATIONS

The skill of applying a surgical mask can be delegated when NAP are trained in required sterile procedure. The nurse informs NAP to:

- Put on the mask following the appropriate steps.
- Change the mask if it becomes moist or contaminated.
- Remove the mask when leaving the patient's room.

EQUIPMENT

Disposable mask

STEPS

1. Find top edge of mask (usually has thin metal strip along edge). Pliable metal fits snugly against bridge of nose.
2. Hold mask by top two strings or loops. Tie two top ties at top of back of head (see illustration), with ties above ears. (*Alternative:* Slip loops over each ear.)

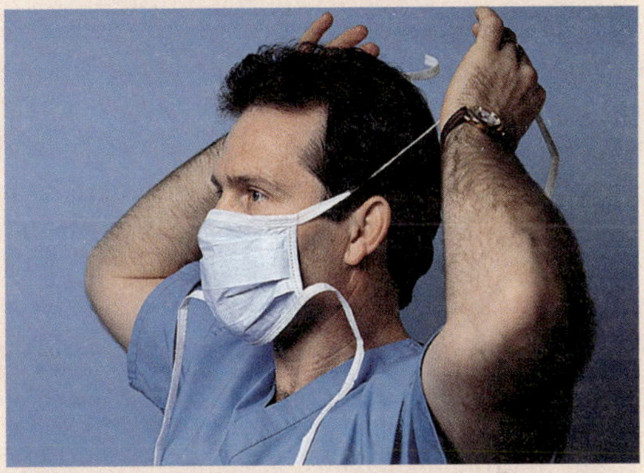

STEP 2 Attaching top two ties of a tie-on mask.

3. Tie two lower ties snugly around neck with mask well under chin (see illustration).

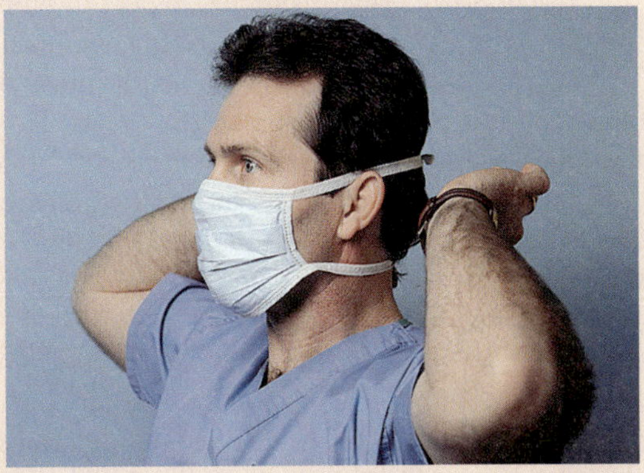

STEP 3 Securing bottom two ties of a tie-on mask.

4. Gently pinch upper metal band around bridge of nose. **NOTE:** Change mask if wet, moist, or contaminated.
5. Remove mask by untying *bottom* mask strings and then top strings; pull mask away from face and drop into trash receptacle. (Do not touch outer surface of mask.)

Apply disposable gloves when there is a risk for exposing the hands to blood, body fluids, mucous membranes, nonintact skin, or potentially infectious material on objects or surfaces. In addition, use gloves when you have scratches or breaks in the skin and when performing venipuncture, fingersticks, or heelsticks. You wear gloves alone or in combination with other PPE. When other PPE is necessary, first put on a mask and eyewear (if required), apply a gown (if required), and then apply gloves. Pull the glove cuffs up over the wrists or cuffs of a gown.

After contacting infectious material, change gloves and perform hand hygiene even if you have not finished caring for the patient. If your actions do not involve more patient contact, it is not necessary to reapply gloves. Teach patients and their families the reasons for wearing gloves and the correct method for applying them.

Many gloves used for barrier protection or surgical asepsis are made of latex. Before applying latex gloves, assess a patient's potential for having a latex allergy. Individuals most at risk include those with a history of spina bifida, congenital or urogenital defects, indwelling urinary catheterization, use of condom catheters, multiple childhood surgeries, and food allergies. A history of occupational exposure to latex is another risk for a patient. The symptoms of latex allergy range from mild dermatitis to severe anaphylactic shock. Latex sensitivity results from repeated contact or by inhaling aerosolized latex allergens contained in the glove powder.

The Association of PeriOperative Registered Nurses (AORN, 2013) provides the following suggestions for nurses to avoid becoming allergic to latex:

1. Whenever possible wear powder-free gloves (they are lower in protein allergens).
2. Wear gloves only when indicated.
3. Wash with a pH-balanced soap immediately after removing gloves.
4. Apply only non–oil-based hand care products (oil-based products break down latex allergens).
5. If a reaction or dermatitis occurs, report to employee health service and/or seek medical treatment immediately.

Wear eyewear and face shields properly fitted during procedures in which it is possible to splatter the eyes or face with blood or other infectious material (see Figure 14-4). In many instances caregivers purchase their own eyewear with prescription lenses. Regular glasses are insufficient. Glasses need to have side shields to prevent material from entering the eye between the glasses and face.

Specimen Collection. A patient with a suspected or actual infectious disease sometimes has many laboratory studies. Body fluids and materials suspected of containing infectious organisms are collected for culture and sensitivity tests. In the laboratory the specimen is placed in a special medium that promotes the growth of organisms. A laboratory technologist then identifies the type of microorganisms growing in the culture. Additional sensitivity test results indicate the antibiotics to which the organisms are resistant or sensitive. This helps the health care providers choose the proper medications to use in a patient's treatment.

Obtain all culture specimens with sterile equipment. Collecting fresh material from the site of infection, as in the case of wound drainage, ensures that resident flora do not contaminate the specimen. Seal all specimen containers tightly to prevent spillage and contamination of the outside of the containers (Box 14-12). After you transfer specimens to containers, label each specimen properly with the patient's name, patient identifier, date and time, and type of specimen. Label specimens in the presence of the patient (TJC, 2014). Place specimen containers in labeled leak-proof biohazard bags before transporting them to the laboratory. Follow facility policy to transport laboratory specimens.

Bagging. In general, bagging articles is the same for all patients regardless of whether they are on isolation or not. Bagging articles prevents accidental exposure of personnel to contaminated articles and contamination of the surrounding environment. Specific procedures for specimen transport are institution dependent (Ritter, 2009).

Place all soiled linen in a designated waterproof bag in the patient's room. Do not overfill the bag. Handle, transport, and process linen soiled with blood or body fluids in a way that prevents exposure of skin or mucous membrane and/or contamination of the health care worker's clothing. Some hospitals still require double bagging. A standard-size linen bag, not overfilled, tied securely and intact is adequate to prevent infection transmission. Consult agency policy and any applicable regulations for the proper procedure.

Biohazardous waste includes both infectious and medical waste that must be disposed of in special red bags or per facility policy. These disposal procedures are a high expense for health care facilities. Consider the following waste materials to be infectious or medical waste (Hedrick and Wideman, 2009):

- Cultures, including discarded cultures of infectious organisms
- Pathological waste such as discarded human tissue, organs, and body parts
- Blood and blood products, including discarded serum or plasma and materials containing free-flowing blood
- Sharps, including discarded needles, syringes, scalpels, blood vials, broken or unbroken glass, and pipettes
- Selected isolation material; discarded waste material from patients with highly communicable diseases

Removal of Protective Equipment. The method of removing protective clothing, gloves, eyewear, gown, and mask before leaving an isolation room depends on the protective equipment worn at the time. If you wear all four protective items, first remove the gloves because they are most likely to be contaminated. If you untie a gown while wearing gloves, there is a chance of contaminating your hair or a portion of your uniform. The procedural guidelines for isolation precautions review steps for removing PPE (see Box 14-10).

Transporting Patients. Patients infected with highly communicable organisms such as the TB bacillus may leave their rooms only for essential purposes such as diagnostic

BOX 14-12 SPECIMEN COLLECTION TECHNIQUES*

Ensure that each specimen containers or the bag in which it is placed has a biohazard symbol on the outside.

WOUND SPECIMEN

Perform hand hygiene and apply clean gloves. Clean area around wound edges with antiseptic swab. Wipe from edges outward to remove old exudate (see Chapter 37). Remove gloves, perform hand hygiene, and reapply gloves. Use a cotton-tipped swab or syringe to collect as much drainage as possible. Have clean test tube or culture tube ready on clean paper towel. After swabbing center of wound site, grasp collection tube with paper towel. Carefully insert swab without touching outside of tube and secure top of tube. For some specimens you need to crush end of tube and push swab into fluid. Transfer tube into biohazard bag for transport and perform hand hygiene.

BLOOD SPECIMEN CULTURE (this procedure is usually performed by the laboratory technician)

Wearing gloves, clean venipuncture site with antiseptic swab, with first swab moving back and forth on horizontal plane, another swab on vertical plane, and last swab in a circular motion from site outward for 5 cm (2 inches) lasting a total of 30 seconds. Allow to dry. Clean tops of culture bottles for 15 seconds with agency-approved cleansing solution. Use 20 mL needle-safe syringe and collect 10 to 15 mL of blood per culture bottle (check health care facility or agency policy). Perform venipuncture at two different sites to decrease likelihood of both specimens being contaminated with skin flora. Place blood culture bottles on clean paper towel on bedside table or other surface; swab off bottle tops with alcohol. Inject appropriate amount of blood into each bottle. Transfer specimen into clean, labeled biohazard bag for transport. Remove gloves and perform hand hygiene.

STOOL SPECIMEN

Wearing gloves, use clean cup with seal top (need not be sterile) and tongue blade to collect small amount of stool, approximately 2 to 3 cm (approximately 1 inch). Place cup on clean paper towel in patient's bathroom. Using tongue blade, collect needed amount of feces from patient's bedpan. Transfer feces to cup without touching outside surface of cup. Dispose of tongue blade and place seal on cup. Transfer specimen into clean biohazard bag for transport. Remove gloves and perform hand hygiene.

URINE SPECIMEN

Apply gloves; cleanse needleless port on urinary catheter and use needleless syringe to collect 1 to 5 mL of urine. Fill sterile specimen cup or specimen tube and place on clean towel in patient's bathroom. Have patient follow procedure to obtain clean voided specimen (see Chapter 34) if not catheterized. Secure top of transfer container, label for transport, and place in biohazard bag. Remove gloves and perform hand hygiene.

From Pagana KD, Pagana TJ: *Mosby's diagnostic and laboratory test reference,* ed 11, St Louis, 2012, Mosby.
*Health care facility or agency policies may differ on type of containers and amount of specimen material required.

procedures or surgery. Before transferring a patient to a wheelchair or stretcher, give him or her appropriate barrier protection. For example, patients infected by an organism transmitted by the respiratory tract need to wear surgical masks. Personnel transporting patients practice the appropriate precautions while in a patient's room and remove PPE when leaving the room. Notify personnel in diagnostic areas or the operating room that the patient is on isolation precautions. Record the type of isolation on the patient's chart and explain ways to avoid transmitting infection during transport (Seigel et al., 2007).

Control of Portals of Entry. Many measures that control the exit of microorganisms also control the entrance of pathogens. Provide interventions to control and prevent organisms from gaining a portal of entry (Box 14-13).

Protection of the Susceptible Host. A patient's resistance to infection improves by using measures that protect normal body defense mechanisms. In the acute care setting many of the interventions either promote existing body defense mechanisms or control exposure to microorganisms. For example, regular bathing removes transient microorganisms from the skin. Lubrication helps to keep the skin hydrated and intact. Regular oral hygiene removes proteins in the saliva that attract microorganisms. Flossing removes tartar and plaque that cause infection. An adequate fluid intake promotes normal urine formation and a resultant outflow of urine to flush the bladder and urethra of microorganisms. For patients who are immobilized or dependent, regular coughing and deep-breathing exercises remove mucus from lower airways.

Role of the Infection Prevention and Control Department. Most health care facilities employ health professionals who are specially trained in the area of infection prevention and control. Their responsibilities include collection and analysis of data on HAIs, surveillance of multidrug-resistant organisms, and providing consultation and education to staff and others about infection prevention and control.

Health Promotion in Health Care Workers and Patients. A health care worker who becomes ill exposes susceptible patients to infectious diseases. Agencies typically offer employee health services to assist in infection prevention and control such as immunization programs, recommendations for work restrictions, and protocols for management of job-related exposures to infectious diseases (Haiduven and Poland, 2009).

Surgical Asepsis. Surgical asepsis, or aseptic technique, is designed to eliminate all microorganisms, including spores and pathogens, from an object and to protect an area from these microorganisms. Surgical asepsis requires more precautions than medical asepsis. Breaks in technique result in contamination, thus increasing a patient's risk for infection (Church, 2009).

BOX 14-13 INFECTION CONTROL OF PORTALS OF ENTRY

INTACT SKIN AND MUCOSA

- Keep skin clean and well lubricated.
- Avoid positioning patients on tubes or objects that might cause breaks in skin.
- Use dry, wrinkle-free linen.
- Offer frequent oral hygiene (see Chapter 29).
- Provide frequent position changes for patients with impaired mobility.
- Clean skin of patients who are incontinent with nonabrasive agent; avoid drying with abrasive towel or tissue.

URINARY TRACT

- Teach women to clean rectum and perineum by wiping from area of least contamination (urinary meatus) toward area of most contamination (rectum).
- Do not allow urine in drainage bags and tubes to flow back into bladder. Never raise drainage system above level of bladder.
- Keep points of connection between catheter or drain and tubing closed.

INVASIVE TUBES AND LINES

- When obtaining specimens from drainage tubes or inserting safety needles into intravenous lines, disinfect tube ports by wiping them liberally with disinfectant solution before entering system. Scrub hub before accessing site. Before inserting an intravenous line, cleanse the skin with antiseptic. Cleansing the skin and tubing removes and, in some cases, kills microorganisms.

WOUND CARE

- Keep draining wounds covered to contain drainage.
- Clean outward from wound site using clean swab for each application (see Chapter 37).

Although you commonly practice surgical asepsis in the operating room, labor and delivery area, and major diagnostic or procedural areas, you also use surgical aseptic techniques at a patient's bedside (e.g., when inserting IV or urethral catheters). Use surgical asepsis during procedures that require intentional perforation of a patient's skin (e.g., surgical incision), when the integrity of the skin is broken from trauma or burns, and during procedures that involve insertion of a catheter or surgical instruments into sterile body cavities (AORN, 2013; Church, 2009).

Multiple steps involving sterile technique are used in the operating room such as applying a mask, protective eyewear, and a cap; performing a surgical scrub; and applying a sterile gown and gloves. In contrast, performing a sterile dressing change at a patient's bedside requires only hand hygiene and putting on sterile gloves (Box 14-14). Regardless of the procedures followed in different settings, the use of surgical asepsis depends on developing an aseptic conscience. Always recognize the importance of strict adherence to aseptic principles. In addition, be an excellent role model and patient advocate, reinforcing proper practice for other caregivers (AORN, 2013).

Preparation for Sterile Procedures. In treatment rooms and at the bedside it is important to have a patient's full cooperation in maintaining aseptic technique. Therefore assess the patient's understanding of sterile procedure and the reasons for not moving or interfering with the procedure. Special precautions such as masking the patient or changing his or her position are sometimes necessary to prevent contamination during procedures. Determine whether a patient has undergone a sterile procedure in the past. Explain how you will perform the procedure and what the patient can do to avoid contaminating sterile objects:

1. Avoid sudden movements of body parts covered by sterile drapes.
2. Do not touch sterile supplies, drapes, or your sterile gloves and gown.
3. Avoid coughing, sneezing, or talking over a sterile area.

Certain sterile procedures last for an extended time. Assess each patient's needs (e.g., pain control or elimination) in advance and anticipate factors that will disrupt a procedure. If a patient is in pain, administer analgesics no more than 30 minutes before a sterile procedure begins. Patients often are placed in relatively uncomfortable positions during sterile procedures. Help the patient assume the most comfortable position possible. Finally the patient's condition sometimes results in events that contaminate a sterile field. For example, a patient with a respiratory infection coughs, transmitting organisms that contaminate the sterile field. Anticipate such a problem and have a solution ready such as offering a mask to the patient before the procedure begins.

Principles of Surgical Asepsis. Principles of surgical asepsis include the following:

1. *A sterile object remains sterile only when touched by another sterile object.* The following principles guide you in placement and handling of sterile objects:
   - Sterile touching sterile remains sterile (e.g., wear sterile gloves to handle objects on a sterile field).
   - Sterile touching clean becomes contaminated (e.g., if the sterile tip of a syringe touches the surface of a clean disposable glove, the syringe is contaminated).
   - Sterile touching contaminated becomes contaminated (e.g., when you touch a sterile object with an ungloved hand, the object is contaminated).
   - Sterile touching questionable is contaminated (e.g., when you find a tear or break in the covering of a sterile object, discard or reprocess it, regardless of whether the object appears untouched).
2. *Place only sterile objects on a sterile field.* Be sure the item is sterile before use. The package or container holding a sterile object must be intact and dry. A package that is torn, punctured, wet, or open is unsterile. When placing sterile items on sterile field (e.g., sterile drape), do not reach over the field (Figure 14-5).
3. *A sterile object or field out of the range of vision or an object held below a person's waist is contaminated.* Never turn your back on a sterile tray or leave it unattended. Any

BOX 14-14 **PROCEDURAL GUIDELINES**

Putting on Sterile Gloves

DELEGATION CONSIDERATIONS

The skill of sterile glove application can be delegated to NAP if NAP are qualified to perform sterile glove procedure. The nurse guides NAP to:

- Stop and reapply gloves if they become contaminated.

EQUIPMENT

Pair of proper-sized sterile gloves (latex or synthetic neolatex)

NOTE: Hypoallergenic, low-powder, and low-protein latex gloves may contain enough latex protein to cause an allergic reaction (Molinari and Harte, 2009).

STEPS

1. Consider procedure you will perform and consult agency policy on use of gloves.
2. Inspect hands for cuts, open lesions, or abrasions. Cover with occlusive dressing before gloving.
3. Assess whether patient or health care worker has a known allergy to latex.
4. Determine correct glove size and type of glove material that you will use.
5. Examine glove package to ensure that package is not wet, torn, or discolored.
6. **Apply Sterile Gloves**
   a. Perform thorough hand hygiene.
   b. Remove outer glove package wrapper by carefully separating and peeling apart sides.
   c. Grasp inner package and lay it on clean, flat surface just above waist level. Open package, keeping gloves on inside surface of wrapper.
   d. Identify right and left glove. Each glove has a cuff approximately 5 cm (2 inches) wide. Glove dominant hand first. In illustrations the left hand is dominant.
   e. With thumb and first two fingers of nondominant hand, grasp edge of cuff of glove for dominant hand. Touch only inside surface of glove.
   f. Carefully pull glove over dominant hand (see illustration 1), leaving a cuff and being sure that cuff does not roll up wrist. Be sure that thumb and fingers are in proper spaces (see illustration 2).
   g. With gloved dominant hand, slip fingers underneath cuff of second glove (see illustration).
   h. Carefully pull second glove over nondominant hand (see illustration). Do not allow fingers and thumb of gloved dominant hand to touch any part of exposed nondominant hand. Keep thumb of dominant hand abducted.
   i. After second glove is on, interlock hands and keep above waist level (see illustration). Cuffs usually fall down after application. Be sure to touch only sterile sides.
7. Dispose of gloves
   a. Follow steps for glove removal (see Box 14-10, Step 18a).

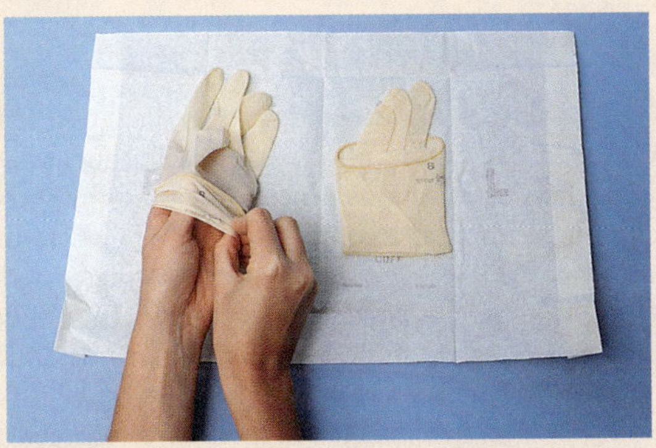

STEP 6f(1) Pull glove over dominant hand; touch only turned-up cuff.

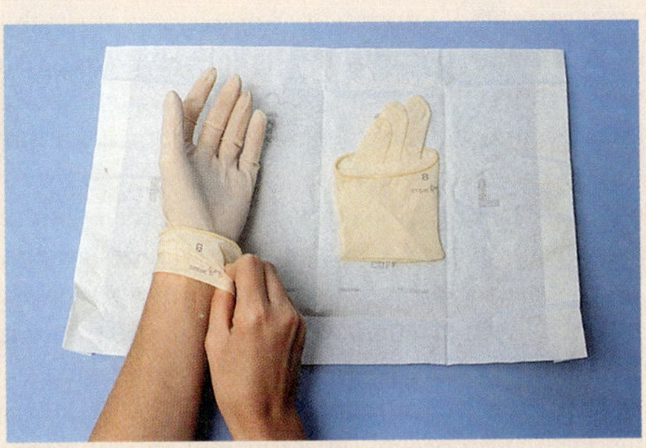

STEP 6f(2) Ensure that thumb and fingers are in proper spaces.

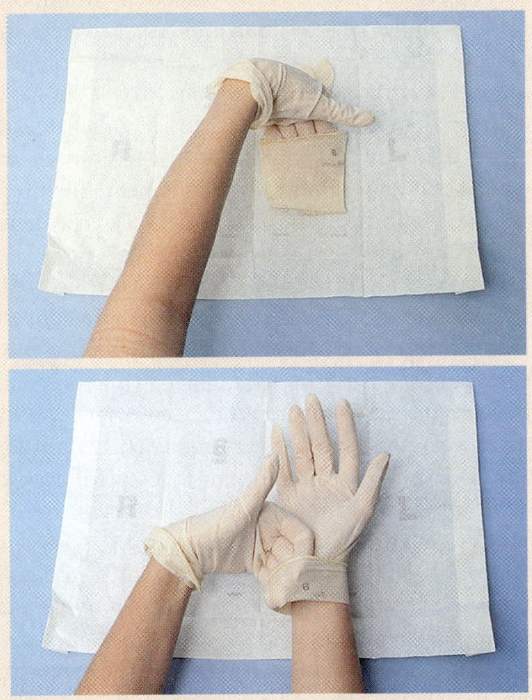

STEPS 6g and h Use gloved dominant hand to pull glove onto nondominant hand.

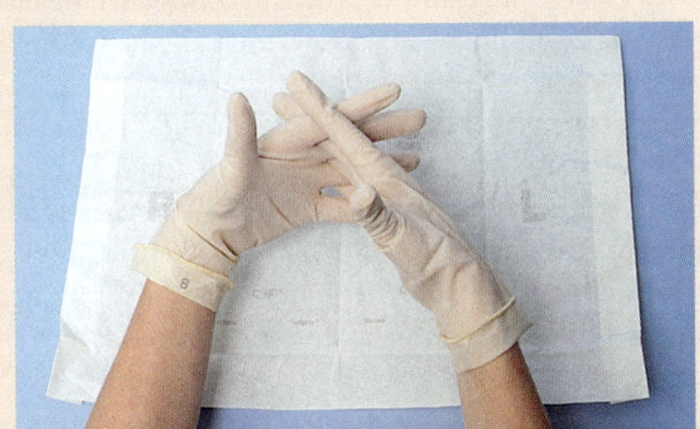

STEP 6i Interlock hands, touching only sterile sides.

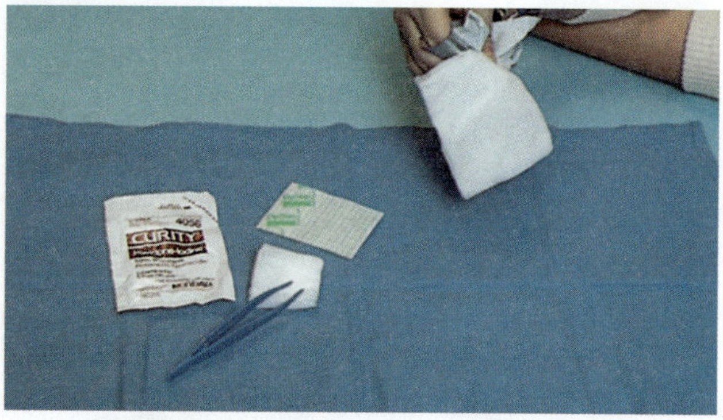

FIGURE 14-5 Adding item to a sterile field.

object held below waist level is considered contaminated because you cannot view it at all times. Keep sterile objects either on or out over the sterile field.

4. *A sterile object or field becomes contaminated by prolonged exposure to the air.* Avoid activities that create air currents such as excessive movements or rearranging linen after a sterile object or field becomes exposed. Minimize the number of individuals walking into an area where sterile packages are being opened or are open. Microorganisms also travel by droplet through the air. No one should talk, laugh, sneeze, or cough over a sterile field or when gathering and using sterile equipment. Wear a mask when opening a tray and adding sterile equipment. Microorganisms traveling through the air can fall on sterile items or fields if you reach over the work area (Box 14-15).
5. *A sterile object or field becomes contaminated by capillary action when a sterile surface comes in contact with a wet contaminated surface.* Moisture seeps through the protective covering of a sterile package, allowing microorganisms to travel to the sterile object. When stored sterile packages become wet, discard the objects immediately or send the equipment to be sterilized again. Spilling solution over a sterile drape contaminates the field unless the drape cannot be penetrated by moisture.
6. *Because fluid flows in the direction of gravity, a sterile object becomes contaminated if gravity causes a contaminated liquid to flow over the surface of an object.* To avoid contamination during a surgical hand scrub, hold your hands above the elbows. This allows water to flow downward without contaminating your hands and fingers. Because gravity makes water flow downward, this is also the reason for drying from fingers to elbows with the hands held up after the scrub.
7. *The edges of a sterile field or container are contaminated.* A 2.5-cm (1-inch) border around a sterile towel or drape is considered contaminated (Box 14-16). The edges of sterile containers become exposed to air after they are open and are thus contaminated. After you remove a sterile needle from its protective cap or after you remove forceps from a container, the objects must not touch the edge of the container. The lip of an opened bottle of solution also becomes contaminated after it is exposed to air. When pouring a sterile liquid, first pour a small amount of solution and discard it. The solution washes away any microorganisms on the bottle lip. Then pour the liquid a second time to fill a sterile container with the amount of solution you need.

Restorative and Continuing Care. The need for infection prevention and control is also present when patients are in the restorative phase of their care. Nurses in long-term care settings contribute to high-quality health care by practicing skills and techniques necessary to prevent infections.

Long-Term Care. Some of the same risks for infections that are present in acute care apply in long-term care facilities (LTCF) such as skilled nursing homes (Rosenbaum et al., 2009). Risks for HAIs increase because most residents are elderly and are dealing with age-associated physical changes that alter the natural barriers to infection (see Box 14-4). In addition, the population in these facilities is requiring more complex medical care as a result of increased transitions between health care settings. Infections are among the most frequent causes of transfer from LTCFs to acute care hospitals and 30-day hospital readmissions (CDC, 2013). Increasing the influenza vaccination rates of personnel who work in LTCFs helps reduce this problem.

Pneumonia, urinary tract infections, and pressure ulcer infections are the three most common infections in LTCFs. You play an important role in the control of these infections by using critical thinking skills and knowledge of how to prevent these infections. See Chapters 30, 34, and 37 for additional information on approaches for preventing and managing these infections.

EVALUATION

Patient Care. The evaluation of a patient's status is important in preventing infection or caring for a patient's local infection or infectious process. Measure the success of infection prevention and control techniques by determining whether you achieved the goals for preventing or reducing infection. Compare a patient's response such as a decline in fever or decreased wound drainage. In some situations you evaluate a patient's response to proposed environmental changes. For example, when a patient is discharged home with a draining wound, medical asepsis in the home is important. The patient and family members need to practice proper hand-hygiene techniques when interacting with the patient or any care-related equipment. You evaluate their ability to follow medical asepsis through direct observation. Another example is observing if items in the patient's living area (e.g., bed linen, nightstand, or personal bathroom) are properly cleaned.

Patients with surgical or traumatic wounds require extensive management (see Chapter 37). You design infection control practices to either prevent or control spread of wound infection and then evaluate the patient's response to nursing interventions by noting fever, wound pain or drainage, swelling around the wound, decreased energy, and increased fatigue. Evaluation of wound status and patient response to wound healing are priorities. You cannot always use fever as

BOX 14-15 PROCEDURAL GUIDELINES

Opening Wrapped Sterile Items

DELEGATION CONSIDERATIONS

The skill of opening wrapped sterile items can be delegated to nursing assistive personnel (NAP) if NAP are qualified to perform the procedure. Guide the NAP to:

- Start procedure over with new equipment if contamination occurs at any point.

EQUIPMENT

Sterile kit or package, waist-high countertop or table surface

STEPS

1. Place sterile kit or package containing sterile items on clean, dry, flat work surface above waist level.
2. Open outside cover and remove kit from dust cover. Place on work surface.
3. Grasp outer surface of tip of top outermost flap.
4. Open outermost flap away from body, keeping arm outstretched and away from sterile field (see illustration).
5. Grasp outside surface of edge of first side flap.
6. Open side flap, pulling to side, allowing it to lie flat on table surface. Keep your arm to the side and not over sterile surface (see illustration). Do not allow flaps to spring back over sterile contents.
7. Repeat steps for second side flap (see illustration).
8. Grasp outside border of last and innermost flap.
9. Stand away from sterile package and pull flap back, allowing it to fall flat on table (see illustration).
10. Use inner surface of package (except for 1-inch border around edges) as a field to add items because it is sterile. Grasp the 1-inch border to move field over work surface.

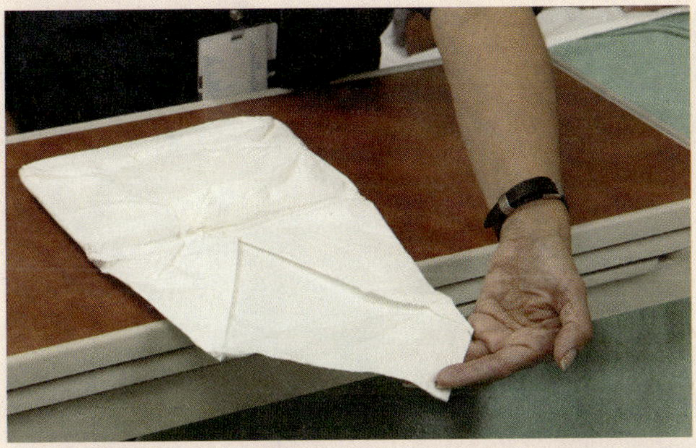

STEP 4 Open top flap away from body.

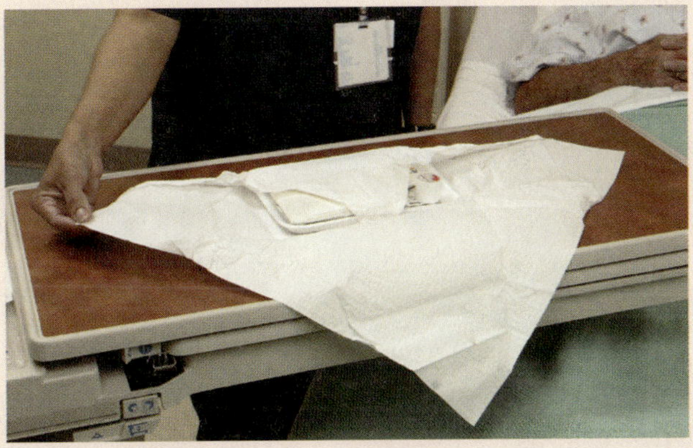

STEP 7 Open second side flap.

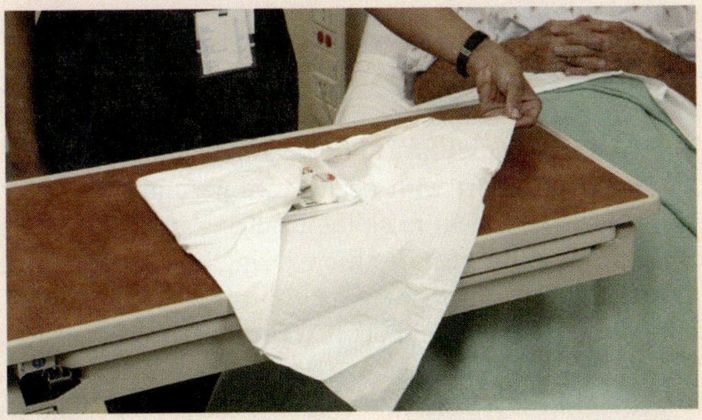

STEP 6 The nurse's arm is kept out away from the sterile field while opening a side flap.

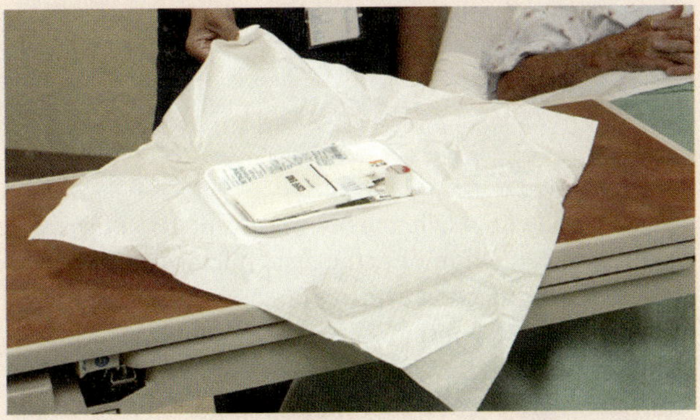

STEP 9 Open back flap.

a sole measure because a fever may appear later in the wound infection process, especially with chronic wounds.

Patient Expectations. When providing patient care, routinely review whether you are meeting the patient's expectations. Ask your patient if he or she perceives that the symptoms of an infection are under control (e.g., the pain of a healing wound, the dysuria of a urinary infection). If your patient is going to be discharged home with an open wound or with a urinary catheter or an intravenous access device in place, help him or her identify concerns and determine what he or she needs to ease the transition to care in the home.

Attentive listening to your patients and their families helps you determine their level of satisfaction with care and if the plan of care met their expectations. Maintain open communication and give your patients an opportunity to express new expectations, their satisfaction, and care concerns as they transition from your care to their home or another care setting.

BOX 14-16 PROCEDURAL GUIDELINES

Preparation of a Sterile Field

DELEGATION CONSIDERATIONS

The skill of preparing a sterile field may be delegated to nursing assistive personnel (NAP) if NAP are qualified to perform the procedure. Guide the NAP to:

- Start procedure over with new equipment if contamination occurs at any point.

EQUIPMENT

Sterile pack, sterile gloves *(optional)*

STEPS

1. Perform hand hygiene.
2. Place pack containing sterile drape on work surface and open as described in Box 14-15.
3. Apply sterile gloves *(optional;* check agency policy).
4. With fingertips of one hand, pick up folded top edge of sterile drape along the 1-inch border.
5. Gently lift drape up from its outer cover and let it unfold by itself without touching any object. Keep it above waist. Discard outer cover with other hand.
6. With other hand grasp an adjacent corner of drape and hold it straight up and away from body (see illustration).
7. Holding drape, first position and lay bottom half over intended work surface (see illustration).
8. Allow top half of drape to be placed over work surface last (see illustration).
9. Grasp 1-inch border around edge to position as needed.

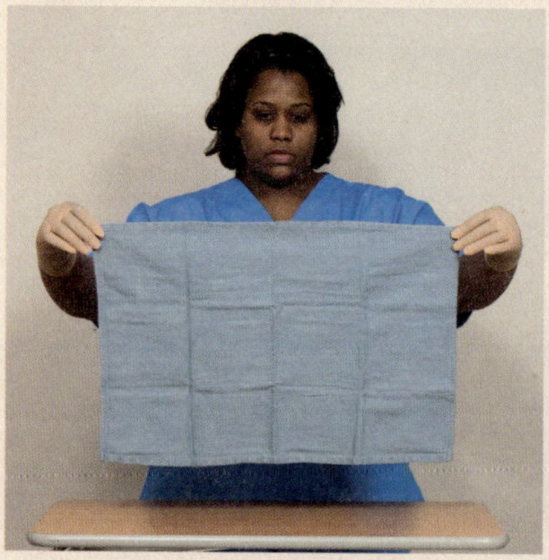

STEP 6 Hold corners of sterile drape up and away from body.

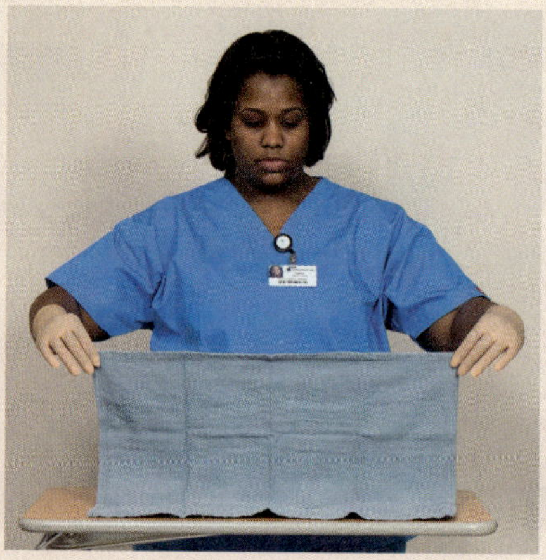

STEP 7 Position bottom half of sterile drape over top half of work surface.

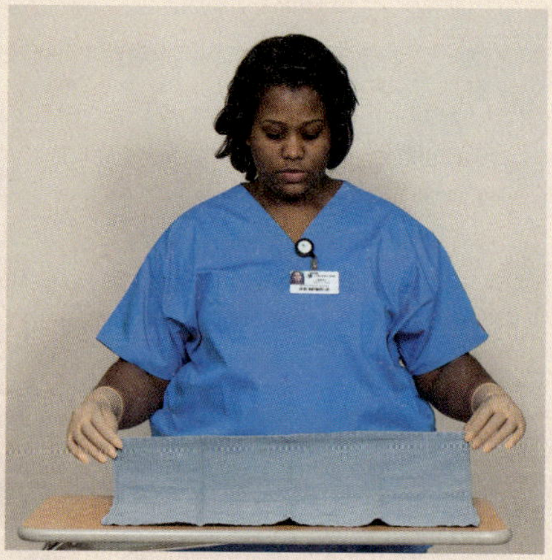

STEP 8 Allow top half of drape to be placed over bottom half of work surface.

KEY POINTS

- Normal body flora help the body resist infection by reducing the reproduction of pathogenic microorganisms.
- Immunity to infection depends on the capacity to produce antibodies in response to exposure to an antigen.
- An infection can develop if the six elements of the infection chain are present and uninterrupted.
- The virulence of a microorganism depends on its ability to resist attack by normal bodily defenses.
- Increasing age, poor nutrition, stress, inherited conditions, chronic disease, and treatments or conditions that compromise the immune response increase susceptibility to infection.
- Wear gloves when in contact with blood or potentially infectious material. Wear a gown and mask in combination with an eye protection device such as goggles or glasses with solid side shields whenever you anticipate splashes or spray of blood or potentially infectious material.
- The main cause of health care–associated infections is nonadherence to hand hygiene.
- Invasive procedures, medical therapies, long hospitalization, and contact with health care personnel increase a hospitalized patient's risk for acquiring an HAI.
- Surgical asepsis requires more stringent techniques than medical asepsis.
- The CDC recommends that you consider all patients as potentially infected with HIV and other bloodborne pathogens; therefore health care workers reduce the risk for exposure to blood and body fluids by following Standard Precautions using appropriate barrier protection with all patients.
- Following aseptic principles is the key to your success in preventing patients from acquiring infections.
- A patient on isolation precautions is subject to sensory deprivation because of the restricted environment.
- If the skin is broken or if you perform an invasive procedure into a body cavity normally free of microorganisms, use surgical aseptic practices.
- A sterile object becomes contaminated by direct contact with a clean or contaminated object, exposure to airborne microorganisms, or contact with a wet surface.

CLINICAL DECISION-MAKING EXERCISES

Kathy hands off Mrs. Eldredge's care to Carman Hernandez. Carman assesses Mrs. Eldredge's incision and observes warmth, edema, and redness, with a small amount of yellow drainage coming from the incision. Mrs. Eldredge also has a temperature of 38.9°C (102°F), a pulse of 104, blood pressure of 124/68 mm Hg, and respirations of 16 breaths/min. Carman and the registered dietitian complete a nutritional assessment on Mrs. Eldredge and note that she had poor nutritional intake 1 month before her surgery because of hip pain and an inability to stand to prepare meals. When she came home after her surgery, her incisional pain increased, and she developed a fever; thus she did not feel like eating. Her weight loss is minimal—3 lbs. However, her nutritional laboratory test results note that she is anemic and her serum protein levels are decreased. In addition, her blood glucose is also slightly elevated. Mrs. Eldredge's health care provider orders a wound culture. In addition, Mrs. Eldredge is receiving wound care, antibiotic therapy, and supportive care, including nutrition and progressive exercise.

1. List three assessment findings that indicate that Mrs. Eldredge's surgical site is infected.
2. Mrs. Eldredge's wound culture grew a resistant strain of *Staphylococcus aureus*. Carman checked the facility policy for isolation precautions and found that Mrs. Eldredge needs to be on Contact Precautions. What are Carman's next steps?
3. What personal protective equipment does Carman need to wear to change Mrs. Eldredge's dressing? Explain your answer.

evolve

Answers to Clinical Decision-Making Exercises can be found on the Evolve website.

QSEN ACTIVITY: QUALITY IMPROVEMENT

Carman Hernandez, the nurse caring for Mrs. Eldredge, notices that more patients have been readmitted with surgical site infection (SSI) over the past few months. Carman shares her observation with her manager and the infection control and prevention (ICP) practitioner who covers her surgical nursing unit. After the unit data related to readmissions are reviewed, Carman and her manager put together a quality improvement group with other unit staff and meet with the ICP practitioner to determine if any variables are common to all the cases and which types of interventions would be appropriate.

What is a good first step for Carman before attending the meeting?

What actions might the group take?

evolve

Answers to QSEN Activities can be found on the Evolve website.

REVIEW QUESTIONS

1. What is the *most* effective action the nurse takes to break the chain of infection?
    1. Perform hand hygiene
    2. Wear gloves
    3. Provide education on infection prevention
    4. Provide private rooms for all patients
2. An older patient is obese and is being treated with chemotherapy for colon cancer. Which of the following nursing diagnoses is the highest priority based on these data?
    1. Acute Pain
    2. Anticipatory Grieving
    3. Risk for Infection
    4. Impaired Tissue Integrity
3. Which nursing intervention decreases the risk for urinary tract infection when placing an indwelling urinary catheter into a patient?
    1. Encourage the patient to drink additional fluids immediately before the insertion
    2. Wear a mask, gown, and sterile gloves during the procedure
    3. Maintain strict surgical asepsis during the entire procedure
    4. Have the patient void before the insertion
4. A nurse discovers that there is a large amount of drainage on a surgical dressing and the bed linens when attempting to insert a new peripheral intravenous (IV) catheter. The nurse performs hand hygiene, puts on clean gloves, and assesses the wound beneath the dressing to be sure that the situation is not emergent. Which action should the nurse take next?
    1. Remove gloves and perform hand hygiene before changing the bed linen
    2. Remove gloves and perform hand hygiene before regloving and applying a clean dressing
    3. Call for someone else to insert the IV line
    4. Immediately apply new dressing and notify the health care worker
5. Why is it important for the nurse to use appropriate skin antisepsis before insertion of any invasive device?
    1. Inserting a device such as an intravenous line or drainage tube bypasses the skin as a natural barrier to infection.
    2. It enhances the effect of antibiotics administered at the same time.
    3. The sterility of the inserted device is not always certain.
    4. The patient may have poor personal hygiene or some type of infectious skin condition.

6. A patient diagnosed with a multidrug-resistant organism in the surgical wound asks the nurse what this means. What is the nurse's best response?
   1. There is more than one organism in the wound that is causing the infection.
   2. The antibiotics the patient has received are not strong enough to kill the organism.
   3. The patient needs more than one type of antibiotic to kill the organism.
   4. The organism has developed a resistance to one or more broad-spectrum antibiotics, indicating that the organism is hard to treat effectively.
7. Which are effective ways to prevent transmission of microorganisms between patients? (Select all that apply.)
   1. Following isolation precautions correctly when caring for a patient in transmission-based precautions
   2. Cleaning hands before and after each patient encounter with soap and water or hand gel containing alcohol
   3. Cleaning hands before and after wearing personal protective equipment such as gloves, gowns, masks, and goggles
   4. Providing all patients with private rooms
8. When is it recommended by the CDC that you use soap and water instead of an alcohol-based hand cleaner?
   1. When ungloved hands are visibly soiled
   2. When caring for a patient with a diagnosis of *Clostridium difficile*
   3. Before eating and after toileting
   4. All of the above
9. A patient is placed on Airborne Precautions for a confirmed tuberculosis respiratory infection. The nurse notices that the patient seems to be depressed and withdrawn. Which are the best interventions that the nurse takes to help the patient? (Select all that apply.)
   1. Encourage the patient to voice his or her feelings and concerns regarding the diagnosis and isolation precautions.
   2. Consider making a social services consultation if patient continues to display symptoms of depression.
   3. Explain the reason for Airborne Precautions and answer the patient's questions, giving him or her reassurance that you will respond promptly when needed.
   4. Remove your respirator mask intermittently so the patient can see your face.
10. Infection prevention precautions are not needed with patients who are in the hospital for other reasons besides infection.

    True

    False

evolve

Rationales for Review Questions can be found on the Evolve website.

1. 1; **2.** 3; **3.** 3; **4.** 2; **5.** 1; **6.** 4; **7.** 1, 2, 3; **8.** 4; **9.** 1, 2, 3; **10.** False.

REFERENCES

Archibald L: Enterococci. In Carrico R, et al, editors: *APIC text of infection control and epidemiology*, ed 3, Washington, DC, 2009, Association for Professionals in Infection Control and Epidemiology (APIC).

Association of periOperative Nurses (AORN): *Perioperative standards and recommended practices*, Denver, 2013, The Association.

Becker K, Kahl B: Staphylococci. In Carrico R, et al, editors: *APIC text of infection control and epidemiology*, Washington, DC, 2009, Association for Professionals in Infection Control and Epidemiology (APIC).

Beverage LA, et al: Optimal management of urinary tract infections in older people, *Clin Interv Aging* 6:173, 2011.

Boyce JM, et al: Guideline for hand hygiene in health-care settings: recommendations of the Healthcare Infection Control Practices Advisory Committee and the HICPAC/SHEA/APIC/IDSA Hand Hygiene Task Force, *MMWR Recomm Rep* 51(RR-16):1, 2002.

Brisko V: Isolation precautions. In Carrico R, et al, editors: *APIC text of infection control and epidemiology*, ed 3, Washington, DC, 2009, Association for Professionals in Infection Control and Epidemiology (APIC).

Centers for Disease Control and Prevention (CDC): Guidelines for preventing the transmission of *Mycobacterium tuberculosis* in health care facilities, *MMWR Recomm Rep* 54:RR-17, 2005.

Centers for Disease Control and Prevention (CDC), Hospital Infection Control Practice Advisory Committee: Guidelines for isolation precautions in hospitals, *MMWR Recomm Rep* 57(RR-16):39, 2007.

Centers for Disease Control and Prevention (CDC), Hospital Infection Control Practice Advisory Committee, and the HICPAC/SHEA/APIC/IDSA Hand Hygiene Task Force: *Guideline for hand hygiene in health-care settings*, Atlanta, 2008a, Centers for Disease Control and Prevention.

Centers for Disease Control and Prevention (CDC) and the Hospital Infection Control Practice Advisory Committee, Rutala W, Weber D, and the Healthcare Infection Control Practices and Advisory Committee: *Guidelines for disinfection and sterilization in healthcare facilities*, 2008b, http://www.cdc.gov/ncidod/eid/vol7no2/rutala.htm. Accessed February 15, 2009.

Centers for Disease Control and Prevention (CDC): *OPRP: general information on hand hygiene*, 2009. Accessed August 7, 2013.

Centers for Disease Control and Prevention (CDC): *Precautions to prevent the spread of MRSA in healthcare settings*, 2011, http://www.cdc.gov/mrsa/prevent/healthcare.html. Accessed August 10, 2013.

Centers for Disease Control and Prevention: *Wash your hands*, 2013, http://www.cdc.gov/features/handwashing/. Accessed August 10, 2013.

Cohen S, et al: Clinical practice guidelines for *Clostridium difficile* infection in adults: 2010 update by the Society for Healthcare Epidemiology of America (SHEA) and the Infectious Diseases Society of America (IDSA), *Infect Control Hosp Epidemiol* 31(5):431, 2010.

Church NB: Surgical services. In Carrico R, editor: *APIC text of infection control and epidemiology*, Washington, DC, 2009, Association for Professionals in Infection Control and Epidemiology.

Dubberke ER, Gerding DN: *Rationale for hand hygiene recommendations after caring for a patient with* Clostridium difficile *infection*, 2011, http://www.shea-online.org/Portals/0/CDI%20hand%20hygiene%20update.pdf. Accessed August 11, 2013.

Fauerbach L: Risk factors for infection transmission. In Carrico R, editor: *APIC text of infection control and epidemiology*, Washington, DC, 2009, Association for Professionals in Infection Control and Epidemiology.

Ghany M, et al: Diagnosis, management, and treatment of hepatitis C: an update, *Hepatology* 49(4):1335, 2009.

Haas J: Hand hygiene. In Carrico R, et al, editors: *APIC text of infection control and epidemiology*, ed 3, Washington, DC, 2009, Association for Professionals in Infection Control and Epidemiology (APIC).

Haiduven D, Poland G: Immunization in the healthcare worker. In Carrico R, editor: *APIC text of infection control and epidemiology*, Washington, DC, 2009, Association for Professionals in Infection Control and Epidemiology.

Hedrick E, Wideman JM: Waste management. In Carrico R, editor: *APIC text of infection control and epidemiology*, Washington, DC, 2009, Association for Professionals in Infection Control and Epidemiology.

Jabbar U, et al: Effectiveness of alcohol-based hand rubs for removal of *Clostridium difficile* spores from hands, *Infect Control Hosp Epidemiol* 31(6):565, 2010.

Lehne RA: *Pharmacology for nursing care*, ed 8, St Louis, 2013, Saunders.

Molinari J, Harte J: Dental services. In Carrico R, et al, editors: *APIC text of infection control and epidemiology*, ed 3, Washington, DC, 2009, Association for Professionals in Infection Control and Epidemiology (APIC).

Occupational Safety and Health Administration (OSHA): Occupational exposure to bloodborne pathogens: final rule, 29 CFR 1919:1130, *Fed Reg* 56:64175, 1991.

Occupational Safety and Health Administration (OSHA): Respiratory protective devices: final rules and notice, *Fed Reg* 60:30336, 1995.

Occupational Safety and Health Administration (OSHA): Needlestick Safety Prevention Act of 2000, 29CFR part 1910, *Fed Reg* 66:5317, 2001, updated April 2007, http://www.osha.gov/SLTC/bloodbornepathogens/index.html. Accessed August 3, 2012.

O'Grady NP, et al: Guidelines for the prevention of intravascular catheter-related infections, *Am J Infect Control* 39(4 suppl):S1, 2011.

Palmeira P, et al: IgG placental transfers in healthy and pathological pregnancies, *Clin Dev Immunol* 2012:985646, 2012.

Ritter H: Clinical microbiology. In Carrico R, editor: *APIC text of infection control and epidemiology*, Washington, DC, 2009, Association for Professionals in Infection Control and Epidemiology.

Rosenbaum P, et al: Long-term care. In Carrico R, editor: *APIC text of infection control and epidemiology*, Washington, DC, 2009, Association for Professionals in Infection Control and Epidemiology.

Rutala WA, Weber DJ: Cleaning, disinfection, and sterilization in healthcare facilities. In Carrico R, editor: *APIC text of infection control and epidemiology*, Washington, DC, 2009, Association for Professionals in Infection Control and Epidemiology.

Seigel JD, et al: *Guideline for isolation precautions: preventing transmission of infectious agents in healthcare settings*, 2007, Centers for Disease Control and Prevention, http://www.cdc.gov/ncidod/dhqp/pdf/guidelines/Isolation2007.pdf. Accessed August 10, 2012.

Spratt D, et al: The role of healthcare professions in preventing surgical site infections, *AORN J* 95(4):425, 2012.

The Joint Commission (TJC): *National Patient Safety Goals*, Oakbrook Terrace, IL, 2014, The Commission. Available at http://www.jointcommission.org/standards_information/npsgs.aspx.

Tweeten S: General principles of epidemiology. In Carrico R, editor: *APIC text of infection control and epidemiology*, Washington, DC, 2009, Association for Professionals in Infection Control and Epidemiology.

Whittington AM, et al: Bacterial contamination of stethoscopes on the intensive care unit, *Anesthesia* 64:620, 2009.

World Health Organization (WHO): *WHO guidelines on hand hygiene in health care*, Geneva Switzerland, 2009, Author.

Zastrow RL: Emerging infections: the contact precautions controversy, *Am J Nurs* 111(3):47, 2011.

CHAPTER 15

Vital Signs

evolve WEBSITE

http://evolve.elsevier.com/Potter/essentials

- Video Clips
- Crossword Puzzle
- Audio Glossary

OBJECTIVES

- Explain the principles and mechanisms of thermoregulation.
- Describe nursing interventions that promote heat loss and heat conservation.
- Discuss physiological changes associated with fever.
- Accurately assess body temperature, pulse, respiration, oxygen saturation, and blood pressure.
- Describe factors that cause variations in vital signs.
- Identify ranges of acceptable vital sign values for an infant, child, and adult.
- Explain variations in techniques used to assess vital signs in an infant, a child, and an adult.
- Correctly delegate vital sign measurement to nursing assistive personnel.

KEY TERMS

afebrile, p. 273
antipyretic, p. 274
apical pulse, p. 281
apnea, p. 290
auscultatory gap, p. 286
bradycardia, p. 281
bradypnea, p. 290
core temperature, p. 272
diaphoresis, p. 273
diastolic pressure, p. 282
digital thermometers, p. 278
dysrhythmia, p. 281
end tidal CO_2 monitoring, p. 290
eupnea, p. 289
febrile, p. 273
fever, p. 273
heat stroke, p. 275
hemoglobin, p. 290
hypertension, p. 282
hyperthermia, p. 275
hypotension, p. 282
hypothermia, p. 275
infrared thermometer, p. 277
Korotkoff sound, p. 285
nonshivering thermogenesis, p. 272
orthostatic hypotension, p. 282
oxygen saturation, p. 290
perfusion, p. 289
pulse deficit, p. 281
pulse pressure, p. 282
pyrexia, p. 273
sphygmomanometer, p. 284
systolic pressure, p. 282
tachycardia, p. 281
tachypnea, p. 290
vasoconstriction, p. 272
vasodilation, p. 272
ventilation, p. 288
vital signs, p. 270

The cardinal vital signs are temperature, pulse, respiration, blood pressure, and oxygen saturation. Another vital sign, pain, is a standard of care in health care settings (see Chapter 32). Frequently pain and discomfort are the problems that lead a patient to seek health care. Therefore assessing your patient for pain helps you understand the patient's clinical status and progress.

Many factors such as the temperature of the environment, physical exertion, and the effects of illness cause vital signs to change, sometimes outside the acceptable range. Accurately

CASE STUDY *Ms. Coburn*

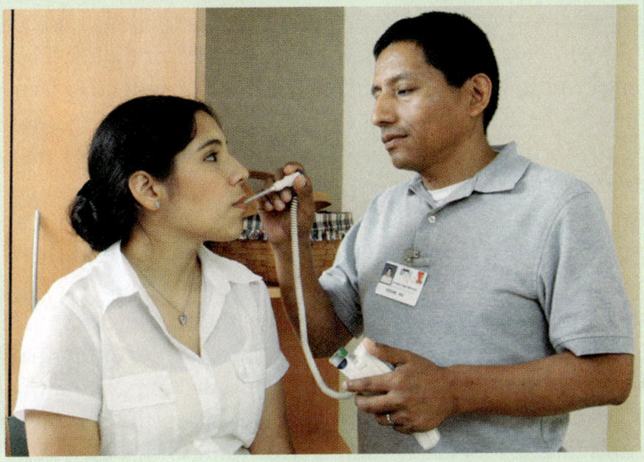

Ms. Coburn is a 26-year-old school teacher who is 20 lbs overweight. Her maternal grandparents immigrated to America from Brazil. She lives alone in an apartment building. She has smoked one pack of cigarettes a day since she was 16 years old. Ms. Coburn made an appointment with her health care provider because she started having headaches and frequently felt tired.

Miguel is a 42-year-old Latino nurse who enjoys providing health-related teaching to the patients at the clinic and has provided nursing care for Ms. Coburn for the past 2 years. During Ms. Coburn's visit Miguel assesses her symptoms. He asks her about her headache and fatigue. After interviewing Ms. Coburn, Miguel takes her vital signs. Her temperature is 36.7° C (98° F), respiratory rate is 14 breaths/min, pulse is 86 beats/min, and blood pressure is 164/98 mm Hg. Ms. Coburn asks Miguel, "So does this mean I'm healthy?" Miguel responds, "Ms. Coburn, your blood pressure is pretty high right now. After you see the nurse practitioner today, I am going to take your blood pressure again. We're also going to talk about the changes you can begin to make to help you be healthier and feel better."

measuring vital signs and assessing pain provide data to determine a patient's usual state of health (baseline data), the response to physical and psychological stress, and medical and nursing therapies. A change in vital signs indicates a change in physiological functioning or a change in comfort, signaling the necessity for medical or nursing intervention.

Measurement of vital signs is a quick and efficient way of monitoring your patient's condition, identifying problems, and evaluating a patient's response to intervention. You need to take vital signs accurately because the data you obtain from a patient provides a wealth of information. Vital signs and other physiological measurements are the backbone for clinical problem solving.

GUIDELINES FOR MEASURING VITAL SIGNS

Initial vital sign assessment occurs when patients enter a health care agency. A complete set of vital signs is included in a complete physical assessment (see Chapter 16). Sometimes you take vital signs individually to assess a patient's condition. Likewise, a patient's needs and conditions determine when, where, how, and by whom vital signs are measured. Correctly obtaining vital signs, interpreting values, beginning interventions, communicating findings appropriately, and recognizing the need for reevaluation are essential nursing skills. Use the following guidelines to help incorporate vital sign measurements into your nursing practice:

1. Measuring vital signs is your responsibility. You may delegate this duty in certain situations (e.g., stable patients) to nursing assistive personnel (NAP). However, it is your responsibility to review vital sign data, interpret their significance, and critically think through decisions regarding interventions.
2. Assess equipment to ensure that it is working correctly and provides accurate findings.
3. Select equipment based on a patient's condition and physical characteristics (e.g., do not use a regular adult-size blood pressure cuff for an obese patient).
4. Know your patient's normal vital signs range. A patient's usual values sometimes differ from the standard range because of age or physical state. Use a patient's usual values as a baseline comparison.
5. Know a patient's medical history, therapies, and prescribed medications. Some illnesses or treatments cause predictable vital sign changes.
6. Control or minimize environmental factors that affect vital signs. A patient's heart rate taken immediately after exercising does not provide accurate data or a true picture of the patient's condition.
7. Use an organized, systematic approach when measuring vital signs.
8. Based on a patient's condition, collaborate with the health care provider to decide the frequency of vital sign assessment. In the hospital the health care provider orders a minimum frequency of vital sign measurements for each patient. After surgery or treatment intervention, you obtain vital signs frequently to detect complications. If a patient's physical condition worsens, it is necessary to monitor vital signs as often as every 5 to 10 minutes. You also use vital sign assessment before or during medication administration. For example, a health care provider orders cardiac medications to be given if a patient's pulse or blood pressures are within a certain range. Outside of the hospital vital sign assessment happens whenever a patient seeks care from a health care provider. In either environment you are responsible for judging whether a patient needs more frequent assessments (Box 15-1).
9. Analyze the results of vital sign measurement based on a patient's condition and past medical history (PMH).
10. Verify and communicate significant changes in vital signs. Baseline measurements provide a starting point for identifying and accurately interpreting possible changes. When vital signs appear abnormal, have another nurse repeat the measurement. Inform the charge nurse or health care provider of abnormal vital

BOX 15-1 WHEN TO MEASURE VITAL SIGNS

- On admission to a health care facility
- When assessing patients during home care visits
- In a hospital on a routine schedule according to a health care provider's order or standards of practice
- Before, during, and after a surgical procedure or invasive diagnostic procedure
- Before, during, and after the transfusion of blood products
- Before, during, and after the administration of medications or applications of therapies that affect cardiovascular, respiratory, or temperature-control functions
- When a patient's general physical condition changes (e.g., loss of consciousness or increased intensity of pain)
- Before, during, and after nursing interventions influencing a vital sign (e.g., before and after a patient currently on bed rest ambulates, before and after a patient performs range-of-motion exercises)
- When a patient reports nonspecific symptoms of physical distress (e.g., feeling "funny" or "different")

signs immediately, document findings in your patient's record, and report vital sign changes to nurses during hand-off communications (TJC, 2012).

BODY TEMPERATURE

Body temperature is the difference between the amount of heat produced by body processes and the amount lost to the external environment.

Heat produced − Heat lost = Body temperature

Despite environmental temperature extremes and physical activity, temperature-control mechanisms of human beings keep body **core temperature,** or temperature of deep tissues, relatively constant during sleep, exposure to cold, and strenuous exercise. However, surface temperature fluctuates, depending on blood flow to the skin and the amount of heat lost to the external environment. Bodily tissues and cells function efficiently within a relatively narrow temperature range, from 36° to 38° C (96.8° to 100.4° F), but no single temperature is normal for all people. For healthy young adults the average oral temperature is 37° C (98.6° F). In the elderly population the average core temperature ranges from 35° to 36.1° C (95° to 97° F) as a result of decreased immunity (Touhy and Jett, 2014). Time of day also affects body temperature, with the lowest body temperature at 6 AM and the at 4 PM in healthy people. The circadian rhythm alters body temperature about 0.5° C (0.9° F) throughout each day. An acceptable temperature range for adults depends on age, gender, range of physical activity, and state of health.

Women generally experience greater fluctuations in body temperature than men. Hormonal variations during the menstrual cycle cause body temperature fluctuations. Progesterone levels rise and fall cyclically during menstruation. When progesterone levels are low, the body temperature is a few tenths of a degree below baseline. The lower temperature persists until ovulation occurs. During ovulation greater amounts of progesterone enter the circulation and raise the body temperature to previous baseline levels or higher. These temperature variations help to predict a woman's most fertile time to become pregnant. Body temperature changes also occur during menopause. Women who have stopped menstruating often experience periods of intense body heat and sweating lasting from 30 seconds to 5 minutes. During these periods there are often intermittent increases in skin temperatures of up to 4° C (7.2° F).

Temperatures vary, depending on the measurement site. Sites reflecting core temperature such as the pulmonary artery are more reliable indicators of body temperature than sites reflecting surface temperature such as the armpit or axilla. Pulmonary artery temperature monitoring, used in the critically ill patient, offers accurate readings because of the blood mix from all regions of the body (Schey et al., 2010). If a patient has decreased tissue perfusion, the pulmonary artery temperature remains accurate because it measures internal body temperature.

Body Temperature Regulation

Physiological and behavioral mechanisms precisely regulate and control body temperature mechanisms. For the body temperature to stay constant and within an acceptable range, the body needs to maintain the relationship between heat production and heat loss.

Neural and Vascular Control. The hypothalamus, located between the cerebral hemispheres of the brain, controls body temperature by attempting to maintain a comfortable temperature or "set point." When the hypothalamus senses an increase in body temperature, it sends impulses out to reduce body temperature by sweating and **vasodilation** (widening of blood vessels). The increased blood flow to the skin enables heat loss through radiation. If the hypothalamus senses that body temperature is lower than the set point, it sends signals out to increase heat production by muscle shivering or heat conservation by **vasoconstriction** (narrowing of surface blood vessels). Disease or trauma to the hypothalamus or spinal cord, which carries hypothalamic messages, decreases the ability of the body to control body temperature.

Heat Production. Temperature regulation relies on normal heat production processes. Heat is produced as a by-product of metabolism. As metabolism increases the body produces additional heat. When metabolism decreases the body produces less heat. Heat production occurs during rest, voluntary movement, involuntary shivering, and **nonshivering thermogenesis.** The voluntary movement of muscular activity during exercise requires additional energy. Metabolism increases during activity, resulting in an increased heat production up to 50 times normal. Shivering is an involuntary body response to temperature differences in the body. Shivering can increase heat production 4 to 5 times higher than normal. However, in the neonate the immature temperature regulation system does not allow for shivering.

Instead the neonate metabolizes vascular brown adipose tissue for heat production. This process is called *nonshivering thermogenesis*.

Heat Loss. Heat loss and production occur at the same time. The exposure of the skin to the environment results in constant, normal heat loss through radiation, conduction, convection, and evaporation. Infants and young children have a greater ratio of surface area to body weight; thus they lose more heat to the environment than adults.

Radiation is the transfer of heat between two objects without physical contact. Heat radiates from the skin to any surrounding cooler object. Up to 85% of the surface area of the human body radiates heat to the environment. During surgery patients often lose excessive amounts of heat in the cool environment of the operating room; thus you need to closely monitor your patient's temperature during and after surgery.

A small amount of heat loss occurs through conduction, which is the transfer of heat from one object to another with direct contact. When warm skin touches a cooler object, heat transfers from the skin to the object until temperatures equalize. Heat conducts through solids, gases, and liquids. In patients with fevers, increasing conductive heat loss occurs through application of ice packs or bathing with tepid water. Applying several layers of clothing reduces conductive loss. The body gains heat by conduction when it contacts materials warmer than skin temperature such as prewarmed blankets.

Convection is the transfer of heat away from the body by air movement. Fans promote heat loss through convection. The rate of heat loss increases when moist skin comes into contact with slightly moving air. Heat energy transfers from a liquid to a gas state by evaporation. The body continuously loses heat by evaporation; approximately 600 to 900 mL of water evaporates daily from the skin and lungs. Through perspiration or sweating the body promotes additional evaporative heat loss. **Diaphoresis** (i.e., excessive sweating) drastically lowers body temperature and typically presents on the forehead, upper chest, and arms.

Skin in Temperature Regulation. Skin, subcutaneous tissue, and fat help to maintain body temperature through insulation. Therefore people with more body fat have more natural insulation than slim or muscular individuals. The skin, or integumentary system (along with neural control), regulates body temperature similar to the way a car radiator controls engine temperature. The car engine generates a great deal of heat. Water pumps through the engine to collect the heat and carry it to the radiator, where a fan transfers the heat from the water to the outside air. The internal organs of the body produce heat, and during exercise or increased sympathetic stimulation the amount of heat produced is greater than the usual core temperature. Blood flows from the internal organs, carrying heat to the body surface. There blood passing through the vascular areas of the hands and feet varies from minimal flow to as much as 30% of the blood pumped from the heart. Heat transfers from the blood through vessel walls to the surface of the skin and is lost to the environment through heat loss mechanisms.

Behavioral Control. When the environmental temperature falls, a person adds clothing, moves to a warmer place, raises the thermostat setting on a furnace, increases muscular activity by running in place, or sits with arms and legs tightly wrapped together. In contrast, when the temperature becomes hot, a person removes clothing, stops activity, lowers the thermostat setting on an air conditioner, seeks a cooler place, or takes a cool shower.

Considerations for Older Adults. The elderly do not maintain a constant body temperature in stressful situations because of neurosensory changes that occur in their thermoregulation, leaving them sensitive to hyperthermia and hypothermia (Amoore, 2010). Likewise, decreased immune function results in an inability to mount an effective initial response to infection. Consequently older adults often present with a normal to only slightly elevated temperature. Therefore it is important for you to recognize that elderly patients who have low-grade fevers may be sicker than they appear.

Temperature Alterations

Body temperature changes are related to excess heat production, heat loss, too little heat production, or any combination of these alterations. The nature of the change affects the type of clinical problems experienced by a patient.

Fever. The condition of **pyrexia** or **fever** occurs because heat loss mechanisms are unable to keep pace with excess heat production, resulting in an abnormal rise in body temperature. A fever is usually not harmful if it stays below 39° C (102.2° F) in adults or 40° C (104° F) in children. A single temperature reading does not always indicate a fever and often results from outside influences such as a recent increase in physical activity or environmental changes. You determine your patient's fever by taking several temperature readings at different times during the day and comparing them to their usual values.

A true fever results from an alteration in the hypothalamic set point. Substances that trigger the immune system such as bacteria or viruses stimulate the release of hormones in an effort to promote bodily defense against infection. These hormones also trigger the hypothalamus to raise the set point, inducing a **febrile** episode. To reach the new set point the body produces and conserves heat. The patient experiences chills, shivers, and feels cold, even though the body temperature is rising. If the set point has been "overshot" or if the immune triggers are removed, the skin becomes warm and flushed because of vasodilation. Diaphoresis results in evaporative heat loss. When a fever "breaks," the temperature returns to an acceptable range, and the patient becomes **afebrile.** A fever pattern is present when a febrile episode recurs (Box 15-2).

Fever serves as an important defense mechanism. Therefore most health care providers do not treat an adult's fever until it is over 39° C (102.2° F). Mild temperature elevations enhance the immune system of the body by stimulating white blood cell production. Increased temperature reduces the concentration of iron in the blood plasma, causing bacterial growth to slow. Fever also fights viral infections by

BOX 15-2 PATTERNS OF FEVER

Sustained	A constant body temperature continuously above 38° C (100.4° F) that demonstrates little fluctuation
Intermittent	Fever spikes mixed with usual temperature levels; temperature returns to acceptable value at least once in 24 hours
Remittent	Fever spikes and falls without a return to acceptable temperature levels
Relapsing	Periods of febrile episodes mixed with acceptable temperature values; febrile episodes and periods of normothermia sometimes longer than 24 hours

stimulating interferon, the natural virus-fighting substance of the body.

Fevers also serve a diagnostic purpose. Fever patterns differ, depending on the causative pyrogen (i.e., the substance such as bacteria that causes the fever). The duration and degree of fever depend on the strength of the pyrogen and the ability of the individual to respond. The term *fever of unknown origin (FUO)* refers to a fever the cause of which cannot be determined.

Treatment for a fever depends on its cause; adverse effects; and the strength, intensity, and duration of the elevated temperature. You play a key role in assessing fever and implementing temperature-reducing strategies (Box 15-3). The goal is a "safe" rather than a "low" temperature. Health care providers determine the cause of fever by isolating the causative bacterium or virus. In this case you get culture specimens for laboratory analysis such as urine, blood, sputum, and wound drainage. If the culture is bacterial in origin, the health care provider orders appropriate antibiotics to be given to effectively destroy bacteria and eliminate body stimulus for fever.

Most fevers in children are of viral origin, lasting only briefly, and have limited effects (Jhaveri et al., 2011). However, children have immature temperature control mechanisms; therefore temperatures sometimes rise rapidly. Dehydration and febrile seizures occur during rising temperatures in children between 6 months and 3 years of age. Febrile seizures are unusual in children over 5 years of age. The extent of the temperature change, often exceeding 38.8° C (102° F), seems to be a more important factor than the rapidity of the temperature increase. Interventions for children's fevers are based on their response to the illness and not on the temperature level itself.

Sometimes a fever results from a hypersensitivity response to a medication, especially when the medication is taken for the first time. These fevers are often accompanied by other allergy symptoms such as rash, hives, or itching. Treatment involves stopping the medication responsible for the reaction.

The objective of fever therapy is to increase heat loss, reduce heat production, and prevent complications. Nondrug

BOX 15-3 NURSING MANAGEMENT OF PATIENTS WITH A FEVER

ASSESSMENT

- Obtain frequent temperature readings (i.e., tympanic, rectal) during a fever.
- Assess for contributing factors such as dehydration, infection, or environmental temperature.
- Identify physiological response to fever (e.g., diaphoresis, tachycardia, hypotension).
- Obtain all vital signs.
- Assess skin color and temperature, presence of thirst, anorexia, and malaise; observe for shivering and diaphoresis.
- Assess patient comfort and well-being.

INTERVENTIONS (UNLESS CONTRAINDICATED)

- Before antibiotic therapy obtain blood cultures when ordered (see Chapter 14). Obtain blood specimens at the same time as a temperature spike, when the causative organism is most prevalent.
- Minimize heat production: reduce the frequency of activities that increase oxygen demand such as excessive turning and ambulation; allow rest periods; limit physical activity.
- Maximize heat loss: reduce external covering on patient's body without causing shivering; keep clothing and bed linen dry.
- Satisfy requirements for increased metabolic rate: provide supplemental oxygen therapy as ordered to improve oxygen delivery to body cells; provide measures to stimulate appetite, and offer well-balanced meals; provide fluids (at least 3 L/day for a patient with normal cardiac and renal function) to replace fluids lost through insensible water loss and sweating.
- Promote patient comfort: encourage oral hygiene because oral mucous membranes dry easily from dehydration and have increased potential for bacterial invasion; control temperature of the environment without inducing shivering; apply cool, damp cloth to patient forehead.
- Identify onset and duration of febrile episode phases: examine previous temperature measurements for trends.
- Initiate health teaching as indicated.
- Maintain environmental temperature at 21° to 27° C (70° to 80° F).

therapies (see Box 15-3) for fever increase heat loss by evaporation, conduction, convection, or radiation. Use caution when implementing nursing interventions and think about heat production and heat loss mechanisms. For example, when using nursing interventions to enhance body cooling, make sure to avoid stimulating shivering. Shivering is counterproductive because of the heat produced by muscle activity. Physical cooling, including regulating room temperature and using fans (as appropriate) and water-cooled blankets, are appropriate when a patient's own thermoregulation fails or in patients with neurological damage (e.g., spinal cord injury).

Antipyretics are medications that reduce fever. Nonsteroidal drugs such as acetaminophen, salicylates, indomethacin, ibuprofen, and ketorolac reduce fever by increasing heat loss.

Health care providers order antipyretics if a fever is over 39° C (102.2° F). Although not used to treat fever, corticosteroids reduce heat production by interfering with the hypothalamic response. It is important to note that these drugs mask signs of infection by suppressing the immune system. Therefore patients on steroids need to be observed closely, especially if they are at risk for infection.

Hyperthermia. An elevated body temperature related to the inability of the body to promote heat loss or reduce heat production is **hyperthermia.** Fever is an upward shift in the set point, whereas hyperthermia is caused by an overload on the temperature release mechanisms (McCance and Huether, 2010). Any injury to the hypothalamus impairs heat loss mechanisms. Educate patients at risk for hyperthermia to:

- Avoid strenuous exercise in hot, humid weather.
- Avoid exercising in areas with poor ventilation.
- Drink fluids such as water and clear fruit juices before, during, and after exercise.
- Wear light, loose-fitting, light-colored clothing.
- Wear a protective covering over the head when outdoors.
- Expose themselves to hot climates gradually.

Prolonged exposure to the sun or high environmental temperatures overwhelms the heat loss mechanisms of the body. Heat also depresses hypothalamic function. These conditions cause **heat stroke,** a dangerous heat emergency, defined as a body temperature of 40.2° C (104.4° F) or more (Mattis and Yates, 2011). Signs and symptoms of heat stroke include giddiness, confusion, delirium, excess thirst, nausea, muscle cramps, visual disturbances, and incontinence. The most important sign of heat stroke is hot, dry skin. Heat stroke can be fatal. Call 9-1-1 for emergency assistance as you begin cooling the person:

- Move the person out of the sun to the shade or a shelter.
- Cool the person quickly. Ways to cool include placing wet towels over the skin, placing the person in a tub of tepid water or into a tepid shower, spraying the person with cool water from a garden hose, and placing oscillating fans in the room.
- If the person can drink, give cool nonalcoholic liquids.
- Continue to take the temperature until it drops to 38.3° to 38.8° C (101° to 102° F).

Emergency medical treatment includes applying hypothermia blankets, giving intravenous (IV) fluids, and irrigating the stomach and lower bowel with cool solutions.

Hypothermia. Heat loss during prolonged exposure to cold overwhelms the ability of the body to produce heat, causing **hypothermia.** Hypothermia is classified by core temperature measurements as mild, moderate, or severe (Table 15-1). It is either intentional or accidental. During prolonged neurological or cardiac surgery, surgeons use intentional hypothermia to reduce body needs for oxygenated blood.

Accidental hypothermia usually develops gradually and may go unnoticed for several hours. A patient experiences uncontrolled shivering, loss of memory, depression, and poor judgment. As the body temperature falls below 34° C (93.2° F), heart and respiratory rates and blood pressure decrease.

TABLE 15-1 CLASSIFICATION OF HYPOTHERMIA

	C	F
Mild	34°-36°	93.2°-96.8°
Moderate	30°-34°	86°-93.2°
Severe	<30°	<86°

The priority treatment for hypothermia is prevention of a further decrease in body temperature. Removing wet clothes, replacing them with dry ones, and wrapping a patient in blankets are key nursing interventions (Davis, 2012). In emergencies, when a patient is not in a health care setting, place the patient under blankets next to a warm person. A conscious patient benefits from drinking hot liquids such as soup while avoiding alcohol and caffeinated fluids. Keeping the head covered, increasing room temperature, or placing heating pads next to areas of the body (head and neck) that lose heat the quickest helps. The severity of the hypothermia dictates the treatments performed.

Prevention is the key for patients at risk for hypothermia. It involves educating patients, family caregivers, and friends. Patients most at risk include the very young; the very old; and people debilitated by trauma, stroke, diabetes, drug or alcohol intoxication, sepsis, and Raynaud's disease (Davis, 2012). Patients with mental illness or handicaps are at risk for developing hypothermia because they are unaware of the dangers of cold conditions. People without adequate home heating, shelter, diet, or clothing are also at risk.

Measurement of Temperature

Assessment of temperature regulation requires you to make judgments about the site for temperature measurement, type of device, and frequency of measurement.

Sites. You measure body temperature by using core or body surface sites. The core temperatures of the pulmonary artery, esophagus, and urinary bladder are often used in critical care settings and require continuous invasive monitoring devices placed in arteries or internal orifices. The most common sites for intermittent temperature measurements are surface sites such as the tympanic membrane, temporal artery, mouth, rectum, and axilla. You can also take your patient's temperature by applying noninvasive, chemically prepared thermometer patches to the skin as long as a patient is not critically ill (Schey et al., 2010).

To ensure accurate temperature readings, measure each site correctly (see Skill 15-1). Depending on the site used, temperatures normally vary between 36° C (96.8° F) and 38° C (100.4° F). Medical consensus accepts that rectal temperatures are usually 0.5° C (0.9° F) higher than oral temperatures, whereas tympanic and axillary temperatures are usually 0.5° C (0.9° F) lower than oral temperatures. Sites reflecting core temperatures are more reliable than sites reflecting surface temperature. Each temperature measurement site has advantages and disadvantages (Box 15-4). Choose the safest

BOX 15-4 ADVANTAGES AND LIMITATIONS OF SELECT TEMPERATURE MEASUREMENT SITES

SITE ADVANTAGES	SITE LIMITATIONS
ORAL	
Easily accessible—requires no position change Comfortable for patient Provides accurate surface temperature reading Reflects rapid change in core temperature Shown to be a reliable route to measure temperature for intubated patients	Causes delay in measurement if patient recently ingested hot/cold fluids or foods, smoked, or chewed gum Not used with patients who have had oral surgery, trauma, shaking or chills, or history of seizures Not used with infants; small children; or confused, unconscious, or uncooperative patients Risk for body fluid exposure
TYMPANIC MEMBRANE	
Easily accessible site Minimal patient repositioning required Can be obtained without disturbing or waking patient Used for patients with tachypnea without affecting breathing Very rapid measurement (2 to 5 seconds) Unaffected by oral intake of food or fluids or by smoking Best to use in children age 2 and older Technique does not require the removal of clothing Easy to use without the risk of cross-infection between patients Not influenced by environmental temperature (Sener et al., 2012)	Susceptible to user error (Amoore, 2010) Has a low sensitivity for detecting fever in comparison with standard core temperature measurement methods (i.e., rectal, bladder) (Kimberger et al., 2007) Requires removal of hearing aids before measurement Requires disposable sensor cover with only one size available Otitis media and cerumen impaction distort readings Not used with patients who have had surgery of the ear or tympanic membrane Does not accurately measure core temperature changes during and after exercise Affected by ambient temperature devices such as incubators, radiant warmers, and facial fans Anatomy of ear canal makes it difficult to position correctly in neonates, infants, and children younger than 3 years old
RECTAL	
Considered gold standard for estimating core temperature Argued to be more reliable than alternative sites when oral temperature is difficult or impossible to obtain	Lags behind core temperature during rapid temperature changes Not used for patients with diarrhea or patients who have had rectal surgery, rectal disorders, bleeding tendencies, or neutropenia Requires positioning and is a source of patient embarrassment and anxiety Risk for body fluid exposure Requires lubrication Not used for routine vital signs in newborns Readings sometimes influenced by impacted stool
AXILLA	
Safe and inexpensive Used with newborns, children of any age, and unconscious patients	Long measurement time Requires continuous positioning Measurement lags behind core temperature during rapid temperature changes Not recommended to detect fever in infants and young children Requires exposure of thorax, which results in temperature loss, especially in newborns Affected by exposure to environment, including time to place thermometer and between axilla used (Amoore, 2010). Underestimates core temperature

BOX 15-4 ADVANTAGES AND LIMITATIONS OF SELECT TEMPERATURE MEASUREMENT SITES—cont'd

SITE ADVANTAGES	SITE LIMITATIONS
SKIN	
Inexpensive Provides continuous reading Safe and noninvasive	Measurement lags behind those obtained at other sites during temperature changes, especially during hyperthermia Diaphoresis or sweat impairs adhesion Affected by environmental temperature Cannot be used on patients with adhesive allergy
TEMPORAL ARTERY	
Easy to access without position change Useful for screening body temperature Very rapid measurement No risk for injury to patient or nurse Eliminates need to disrobe or unbundle Comfortable for patient Used in premature infants, newborns, and children Reflects rapid change in core temperature Sensor cover not required	Does not provide information that is an adequate substitute for core temperature measurement (Kimberger et al., 2007) Inaccurate with head covering or hair on forehead Affected by skin moisture such as diaphoresis or sweating Research has shown temporal artery temperatures to be sometimes inaccurate because they are prone to user error (Bahr et al., 2010).

and most accurate site for each patient. Use the same site when repeated measurements are needed.

Thermometers. Four types of thermometers are commonly available for measuring body temperature: electronic, infrared, digital, and disposable chemical dot. The mercury-in-glass thermometers are obsolete in the health care setting because of the environmental hazards of mercury. However, some patients may still use mercury-in-glass thermometers at home. If you find a mercury-in-glass thermometer in the home, teach the patient about safer temperature devices and encourage him or her to take the thermometer to a neighborhood hazardous disposal location.

Each device measures temperature in either the Celsius or Fahrenheit scale. Electronic thermometers allow you to convert scales by activating a switch. Use the following formulas for manual conversion:

To convert Fahrenheit to Celsius, subtract 32 from the Fahrenheit reading and multiply the result by $\frac{5}{9}$.

$$\text{Example: } (104°\text{ F} - 32°\text{ F}) \times \frac{5}{9} = 40°\text{ C}$$

To convert Celsius to Fahrenheit, multiply the Celsius reading by $\frac{9}{5}$ and add 32 to the product.

$$\text{Example: } \left(\frac{9}{5} \times 40°\text{ C}\right) + 32 = 104°\text{ F}$$

Electronic Thermometers. Electronic thermometers have a rechargeable battery-powered display unit, a thin wire cord, and a temperature-processing probe or sensor covered by a disposable probe cover (Figure 15-1). Separate probes are available for oral (blue tip) and rectal (red tip) use. You obtain axillary temperatures with the oral probe. Electronic thermometers provide two modes of operation, 4-second predictive temperatures and 3-minute standard temperatures (Amoore, 2010). In daily clinical situations the 4-second predictive is more common.

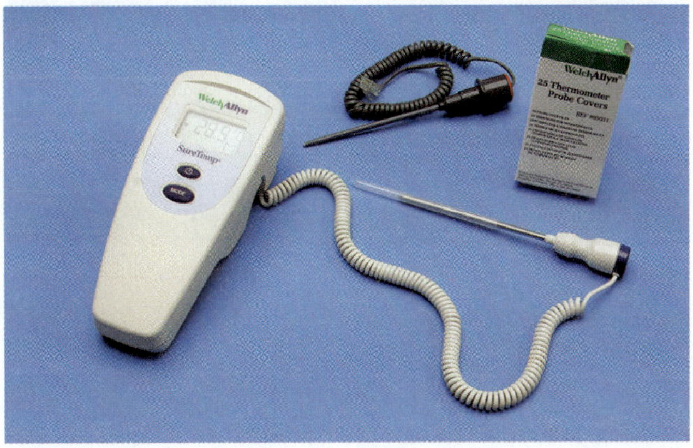

FIGURE 15-1 Electronic thermometer used for oral, rectal, and axillary measurements.

Infrared thermometers rely on thermal radiation from the ear canal, tympanic membrane, axilla, and temporal artery to measure body temperature. The tympanic membrane thermometer has an otoscope-like speculum with an infrared sensor tip that detects heat radiated from the tympanic membrane of the ear (Figure 15-2). Within seconds after placement in the ear canal and pressing the scan button, a sound signals when the peak temperature has been measured, and a reading appears on the display unit. The temporal artery thermometer measures blood flow through the superficial temporal artery. Proper technique involves sweeping an infrared handheld scanner across the forehead or just behind the ear (Figure 15-3). After scanning is complete, a reading appears on the display unit. Oral Tympanic temperatures are considered reliable noninvasive measures of core temperature within the febrile range if used appropriately

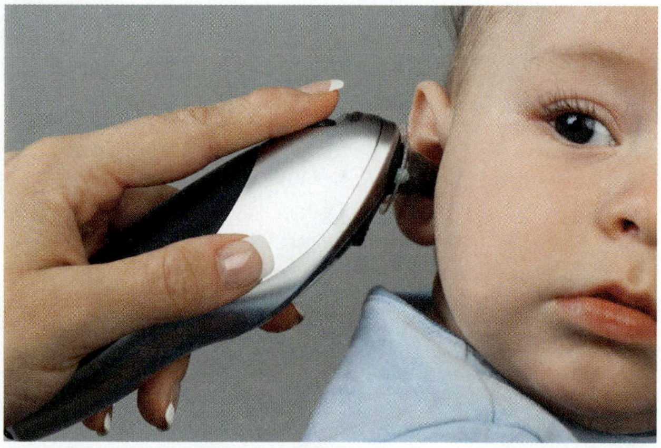

FIGURE 15-2 Tympanic membrane thermometer. (Courtesy Welch Allyn.)

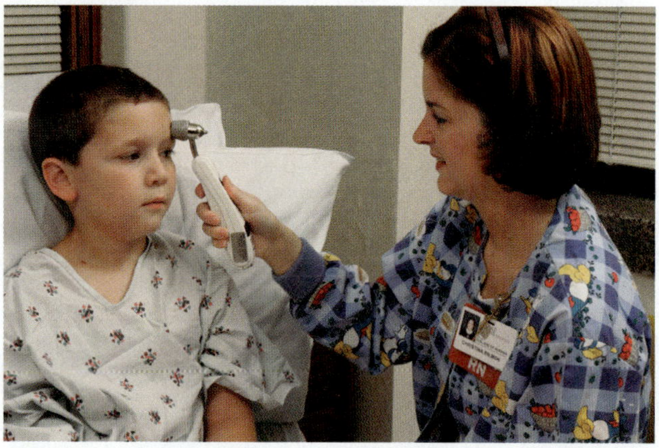

FIGURE 15-3 Temporal artery thermometer scanning forehead.

(Jefferies et al., 2011) (see Box 15-4). There is inadequate evidence to support the use of a temporal artery thermometer for acutely ill hospitalized patients because of reported problems with consistency in measurement techniques and resultant inaccuracies of readings (Box 15-5). The temporal artery thermometer is likely appropriate for screening for fever, but further research is needed.

Digital thermometers contain a probe connected to a microprocessor chip, which translates signals into degrees and sends a temperature measurement to a digital display. You use a digital thermometer for oral, rectal, and axillary measurements. The rectal temperature is still the gold standard for estimating core body temperature, but the thermometer is difficult to use in older adults.

Chemical Thermometers. Single-use or reusable chemical thermometers are thin strips of plastic with a temperature sensor on one end. The sensor consists of chemically impregnated dots that change color at different temperatures. In the Celsius version there are 50 dots, each representing temperature increments of 0.1° C over a range of 35.5° C to 40.4° C. The Fahrenheit version has 45 dots with increments of 0.2° F over a range of 96° F to 104.8° F. Chemicals on the thermometer change color to reflect temperature reading; 3 minutes for axilla and 1 minute for oral (Amoore, 2010). Most are designed for single use (Figure 15-4). For that reason they are useful in caring for patients in emergency departments or in protective isolation (see Chapter 14). In addition, chemical thermometers are useful for screening temperatures, especially in infants and young children. You need to confirm readings with electronic thermometers when treatment decisions must be made.

Another form of disposable thermometer is a temperature-sensitive patch or tape. Applied to the forehead or abdomen, temperature-sensitive areas of the patch change color at different temperatures.

BOX 15-5 EVIDENCE-BASED PRACTICE

PICO Question: Among hospitalized patients with fevers, does the use of electronic temporal artery thermometers compared with electronic rectal thermometers provide accurate temperature readings?

SUMMARY OF EVIDENCE

Accurately monitoring a patient's body core temperature is a crucial part of nursing care. Both hypothermia and hyperthermia have adverse effects on patient outcomes. Without accurate methods for obtaining body temperature, a delay in diagnosing and treatment often occurs (Barnason et al., 2011). Health care agencies use noninvasive measuring techniques because they are quick and safe. Many types of noninvasive electronic instruments are used in the health care setting for measuring temperature, including temporal artery thermometers (TATs). Research studies evaluating the effectiveness of the TAT found evidence that in febrile patients improper technique often results in inaccurate readings. Some researchers recommend that TATs be discontinued in the hospital setting because of the high incidence of user error (Bahr et al., 2010). However, a recent study conducted in an emergency department found that if properly used by ED staff, temporal artery thermometers can be used to reliably obtain temperature in pediatric patients younger than 4 years (Reynolds et al., 2014). In a study involving an obese population (body mass index [BMI] >30), accuracy of the TAT was compromised because of insulation of the patients' temporal artery (Marable et al., 2009).

APPLICATION TO NURSING PRACTICE

- You need to use the correct technique to ensure accuracy, regardless of the electronic device you use to take a patient's temperature.
- Know your patients' baseline temperature and medical history to enable accurate interpretation of temperature variations.
- If you get a temperature reading that is outside of the normal temperature for your patient, repeat the measurement. Use a different device if possible to ensure the accuracy of your reading.

PULSE

The pulse represents the number of cardiac cycles per minute and is the palpable rhythm of blood flow in a peripheral

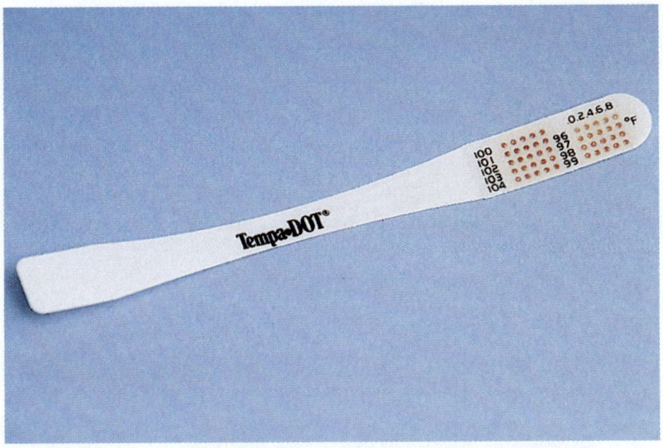

FIGURE 15-4 Disposable, single-use thermometer strip.

artery (Seidel et al., 2011). The ejection of blood from the left ventricle during systole enters the aorta through the aortic valve. The ejected blood moves through the major and peripheral arteries (e.g., in the wrist); thus it feels like a tap when you lightly palpate the artery against underlying bone or muscle. The number of pulsing sensations occurring in 1 minute is the pulse rate. An adult's normal heart rate ranges from 80 to100 beats/min. In children the average heart rate is significantly increased and varies by age (McCance and Huether, 2010).

Locating a Peripheral Pulse

You assess any accessible artery for pulse rate (Figure 15-5), but the radial and apical locations are the most common sites for pulse rate assessment because each is easy to locate and palpate. When a patient's condition deteriorates suddenly, use the carotid site to quickly locate a pulse. Use the radial or carotid pulse when teaching patients how to monitor their own heart rates (e.g., athletes or patients using heart medications). If the radial pulse is abnormal, difficult to palpate, or inaccessible because of a dressing or cast, assess the apical pulse for 1 minute. When a patient takes medication that affects the heart rate, the apical pulse provides a more accurate assessment. Table 15-2 summarizes pulse sites and criteria for measurement. Skill 15-2 outlines radial and apical pulse rate assessment.

Using a Stethoscope

You use a stethoscope to auscultate the sound waves created by an apical pulse (Figure 15-6). The five major parts of the stethoscope are the earpieces, binaurals, tubing, bell chest piece, and diaphragm chest piece.

Make sure that the plastic or rubber earpieces fit snugly in the ear canal and that the binaurals are angled and strong enough so the earpieces stay firmly in place without causing discomfort. The earpieces follow the contour of the ear canal, pointing toward the face when the stethoscope is in place.

The polyvinyl tubing is flexible and 30 to 45 cm (12 to 18 inches) in length. Longer tubing decreases sound-wave transmission. The tubing is thick walled and moderately rigid to eliminate transmission of environmental noise and prevent kinking, which distorts the sound. Stethoscopes have one or two tubes.

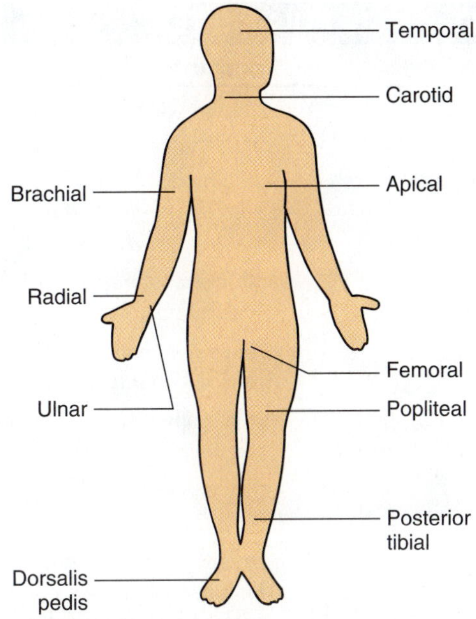

FIGURE 15-5 Location of peripheral pulses.

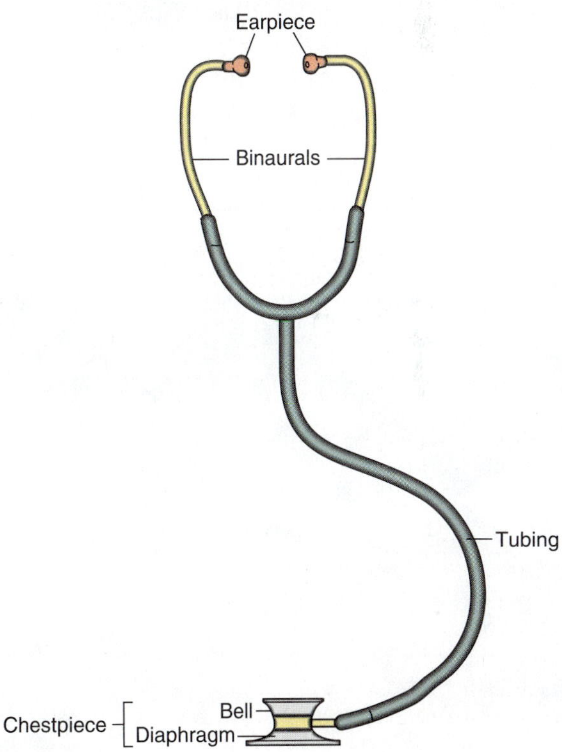

FIGURE 15-6 Parts of a single-tubing stethoscope.

The chest piece consists of a bell and diaphragm that rotates into position, depending on which part you chose to use. Lightly tap each surface to determine which side is functioning. The diaphragm is the circular, flat-surfaced portion of the chest piece covered with a thin plastic disk. It transmits high-pitched sounds created by the high-velocity movement of air and blood. Use it to auscultate bowel, lung, and heart sounds. Always place the stethoscope directly on the skin

TABLE 15-2 PULSE SITES

SITE	LOCATION	ASSESSMENT CRITERIA
Temporal	Over temporal bone of head, above and lateral to eye	Easily accessible site used to assess pulse in children
Carotid	Along medial edge of sternocleidomastoid muscle in neck	Easily accessible site used in patient with physiological shock or during adult CPR when other sites are not palpable
Apical	Fifth intercostal space at left midclavicular line	Site used to auscultate for apical pulse
Brachial	Groove between biceps and triceps muscles at antecubital fossa	Site used to assess upper-extremity blood pressure; used during infant CPR
Radial	Radial or thumb side of forearm at the wrist	Common site used to assess character of pulse peripherally; assesses status of circulation to hand
Ulnar	Ulnar side of forearm at wrist	Site used to assess status of circulation to ulnar side of hand; used to perform Allen's test
Femoral	Below inguinal ligament, midway between symphysis pubis and anterior superior iliac spine	Site used to assess character of pulse in patient with physiological shock or during CPR when other pulses are not palpable; assesses status of circulation to leg
Popliteal	Behind knee in popliteal fossa	Site used to auscultate lower-extremity blood pressure; assesses status of circulation to lower leg
Posterior tibial	Inner side of ankle, below medial malleolus	Site used to assess status of circulation to foot
Dorsalis pedis	Along top of foot, between extension tendons of great and first toe	Site used to assess status of circulation to foot

CPR, Cardiopulmonary resuscitation.

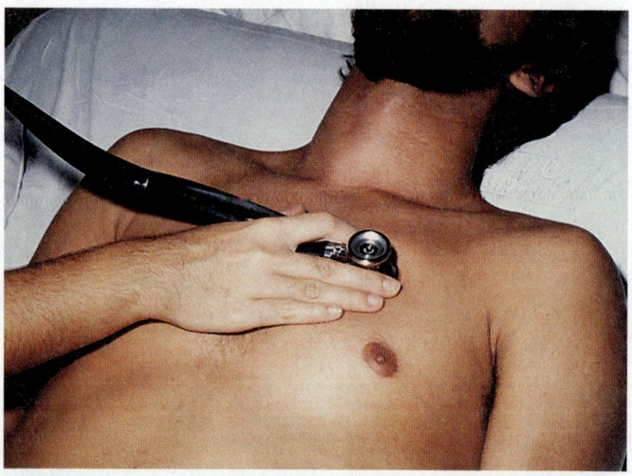

FIGURE 15-7 Positioning the diaphragm of the stethoscope.

because clothing obscures the sound. Position the diaphragm to make a tight seal against the patient's skin (Figure 15-7). Exert enough pressure on the diaphragm to leave a temporary red ring on the patient's skin when it is removed.

The bell is the cone-shaped chest piece usually surrounded by a rubber ring to avoid chilling the patient. It transmits low-pitched sounds created by the low-velocity movement of blood. Use it to auscultate heart and vascular sounds. Apply the bell lightly, resting the chest piece on the skin (Figure 15-8). Compressing the bell against the skin reduces low-pitched sounds.

One type of stethoscope has one chest piece that combines the bell and diaphragm together. When you use light pressure, the chest piece becomes the bell; when you press the chest piece slightly harder, the bell converts to a diaphragm. The size of the stethoscope chest piece varies from small (used for infants and young children) to large. Determine the appropriate chest piece to use by assessing the surface area being auscultated.

The stethoscope is a delicate instrument and requires proper care for optimal function. Remove the earpieces regularly and clean them of cerumen (earwax). Inspect the bell and diaphragm for dust, lint, and body oils. Clean with either alcohol or mild soap and water between patients. Routinely cleaning the diaphragm and bell with alcohol pads reduces bacterial colonization and potentially decreases hospital-acquired infections (Schroeder et al., 2009). Do not use fabric stethoscope covers. They present a potential infection control problem because they are often contaminated with bacteria.

Assessment of Pulse

Pulse Rate. Before measuring a pulse you need to review a patient's medical record to obtain a baseline rate. Remember, pulse rates vary with a patient's age. Compare your patient's actual pulse rate with the expected usual values (Table 15-3). When assessing the pulse, consider the variety of factors influencing pulse rate (Table 15-4). A combination of these factors often causes significant changes. If you detect

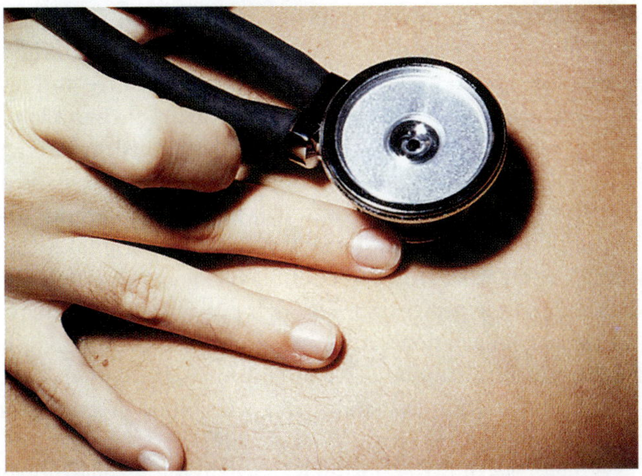

FIGURE 15-8 Positioning the bell of the stethoscope.

TABLE 15-3 ACCEPTABLE RANGES OF HEART RATE FOR AGE

AGE	HEART RATE(BEATS/MIN)
Infant	120-160
Toddler	90-140
Preschooler	80-110
School-ager	75-100
Adolescent	60-90
Adult	60-100

TABLE 15-4 FACTORS INFLUENCING PULSE RATES

FACTOR	INCREASE PULSE RATE	DECREASE PULSE RATE
Exercise	Short-term exercise	Long-term exercise conditions the heart, resulting in lower rate at rest and quicker return to resting level after exercise
Temperature	Fever, heat, hyperthermia	Hypothermia
Emotions	Acute pain and anxiety increase sympathetic stimulation, affecting heart rate	Unrelieved severe pain increases parasympathetic stimulation, affecting heart rate; relaxation
Medications	Positive chronotropic medications such as epinephrine	Negative chronotropic medications such as digitalis, beta-adrenergic blockers
Hemorrhage	Loss of blood increases sympathetic stimulation	
Postural changes	Standing or sitting	Lying down
Pulmonary conditions	Diseases causing poor oxygenation such as asthma and chronic obstructive pulmonary disease (COPD)	

an abnormal rate while palpating a peripheral pulse, the next step is to auscultate the apical pulse for 1 minute to obtain a more accurate assessment of cardiac contractility.

Assess the **apical pulse** by listening for heart sounds (see Chapter 16). After properly positioning the bell or the diaphragm of the stethoscope on the chest, try to identify the first and second heart sounds (S_1 and S_2). At normal slow rates S_1 is low pitched and dull, sounding like a "lub." S_2 is a higher pitched, shorter sound and creates the sound "dub." Count each set of "lub-dub" as one heartbeat. Count the number of "lub-dubs" occurring in 1 minute.

Pulse rate assessment often reveals variations in heart rate. Two common abnormalities in heart rate are **tachycardia** and **bradycardia.** Tachycardia is an abnormally elevated heart rate, more than 100 beats/min in adults. Bradycardia is a slow rate, less than 60 beats/min in adults.

Pulse Rhythm. Normally a regular interval of time occurs between each pulse or heartbeat. A regular interval interrupted by an early beat, late beat, or missed beat indicates an abnormal rhythm or **dysrhythmia.** A dysrhythmia alters cardiac function, particularly if it occurs repetitively. If your patient has a dysrhythmia, you need to assess how often it is occurring. Dysrhythmias are regularly irregular or irregularly irregular. The health care provider sometimes orders additional tests to evaluate the occurrence of dysrhythmias (see Chapter 27).

An inefficient contraction of the heart that fails to transmit a pulse wave to the peripheral pulse site creates a **pulse deficit.** To assess a pulse deficit, ask another nurse to assess the radial pulse rate while you assess the apical rate. If you discover a difference between the apical and radial pulse rates, a pulse deficit exists. Pulse deficits are frequently associated with dysrhythmias.

Strength and Equality. The strength or amplitude of a pulse reflects the volume and pressure of the blood ejected against the arterial wall with each heart contraction and the condition of the arterial vascular system leading to the pulse site. Normally the pulse strength remains the same with each heartbeat. Assess both radial pulses at the same time to compare the characteristics of each. Pulse strength or amplitude is assigned a number grade and described as increased, full, or bounding (+3); normal, easily palpable (+2); thready, weak, barely palpable (+1); or absent (0) (Seidel et al., 2011). Evaluate pulse strength and equality during assessment of the vascular system (see Chapter 16).

BLOOD PRESSURE

Blood pressure is the force exerted on the walls of an artery created by the pulsing blood under pressure from the heart. Blood flows throughout the circulatory system because of pressure changes, moving from an area of high pressure to an area of low pressure. Under high pressure the left ventricle ejects blood into the aorta; the peak pressure is known as **systolic pressure.** When the ventricles relax, the blood remaining in the arteries exerts a minimum or **diastolic pressure.** Diastolic pressure is the minimal pressure exerted against the arterial wall at all times.

The standard unit for measuring blood pressure is millimeters of mercury (mm Hg). The measurement indicates the height to which the blood pressure raises a column of mercury. You record blood pressures as a ratio with the systolic reading before the diastolic (e.g., 120/80 mm Hg). The difference between systolic and diastolic pressure is the **pulse pressure.** For a blood pressure of 120/80 mm Hg, the pulse pressure is 40.

Physiology of Arterial Blood Pressure

Blood pressure depends on the interrelationships of cardiac output, peripheral vascular resistance, blood volume, blood viscosity, and artery elasticity. An increase in cardiac output is usually the result of greater heart muscle contractility, an increase in heart rate, or an increase in blood volume. An increase in cardiac output increases blood pressure. When peripheral arteries constrict such as during periods of stress, peripheral vascular resistance increases, which results in an increase in blood pressure. As vessels dilate and resistance falls, blood pressure drops. When blood is forced through the rigid arteries, blood pressure rises. If the blood volume decreases such as during dehydration or hemorrhage, less pressure is exerted against arterial walls, and blood pressure falls. When the percentage of red blood cells increases, the blood viscosity increases, causing the heart to contract more forcefully to move the blood through the circulatory system, resulting in an increased blood pressure.

Blood Pressure Variations

Many factors during the day continually influence blood pressure. A single measurement does not adequately reflect a patient's blood pressure. Blood pressure trends, not individual measurements, guide your nursing interventions. Understanding the factors that cause alterations in blood pressure helps you to accurately interpret blood pressure measurements. Box 15-6 summarizes factors affecting blood pressure.

Hypertension. The most common alteration in blood pressure is **hypertension,** an often asymptomatic disorder characterized by persistently elevated blood pressure. Hypertension is defined as systolic blood pressure (SBP) greater than 140 mm Hg, diastolic blood pressure (DBP) greater than 90 mm Hg, or the need for antihypertensive medication (Bertoia et al., 2011). The Joint National Committee on Prevention, Detection, Evaluation, and Treatment of High Blood Pressure (JNC) (NHBPEP, 2004) set criteria for determining categories of hypertension (Table 15-5). Hypertension is a known risk factor for cardiovascular morbidity and mortality. Obesity, cigarette smoking, excessive alcohol intake, elevated blood cholesterol, and continued exposure to stress are also linked to hypertension. For high-risk groups the American Heart Association (AHA) recommends maintaining a blood pressure less than 130/80 and for patients with ventricular dysfunction the treatment goal is blood pressure less than 120/80 mm Hg (Aronow et al., 2011).

A diagnosis of hypertension is based on the average of two or more seated blood pressure measurements, properly measured with well-maintained equipment, at each of two or more visits to an office or clinic after an initial screening (Pickering et al., 2005). Thus, one blood pressure recording revealing a high SBP or DBP does not qualify as a diagnosis of hypertension. However, if you assess a high reading (e.g., 150/90 mm Hg), encourage the patient to return for another checkup within 2 months (Table 15-6). Recently the AHA published specific parameters for elderly patients. When an SBP less than 150 mm Hg is achievable on one or two antihypertensive medications, the health care provider needs to try to safely lower the SBP to less than 140 mm Hg. However, health care providers do not need to prescribe any further antihypertensive medication if an elderly patient's SBP is greater than or equal to 150 mm Hg while on four or more prescribed antihypertensive medications and the patient experiences undesirable side effects when more medication is prescribed or the DBP is less than 65 mm Hg (Aronow et al., 2011).

Hypotension. **Hypotension** is an SBP less than 90 mm Hg or a DBP less than 60 mm Hg. Although some adults have low blood pressure normally, for a majority hypotension is an abnormal finding associated with an illness (e.g., hemorrhage or myocardial infarction). Hypotension occurs when arteries dilate; the peripheral vascular resistance decreases, the circulating blood volume decreases, or the heart fails to provide adequate cardiac output. Signs and symptoms associated with hypotension include pallor, skin mottling, clamminess, confusion, dizziness, chest pain, increased heart rate, and decreased urine output. Hypotension is usually life threatening and needs to be reported immediately to the patient's health care provider.

Orthostatic hypotension, also referred to as postural hypotension, is a reduction of SBP of at least 20 mm Hg or a reduction of DBP of at least 10 mm Hg within 3 minutes of quiet standing (Lanier et al., 2011). It occurs when patients with normal blood pressure experience a drop in blood pressure on rising to an upright position and is associated with symptoms of light-headedness or dizziness. In severe cases loss of consciousness occurs. When a healthy person changes from a lying to sitting to standing position, the peripheral blood vessels in the legs constrict, preventing the pooling of

BOX 15-6 FACTORS INFLUENCING BLOOD PRESSURE

AGE

Blood pressure (BP) tends to rise with advancing age:

AGE	AVERAGE ARTERIAL PRESSURE (mm Hg)
Newborn (3000 g [6.6 lbs])	65/41
1 month	85/54
1 year	86/40
6 years	94/56
10-13 years	103/62
14-17 years	110/65

Assess the level of a child's or adolescent's BP with respect to sex, body size, and age. Larger children have higher BPs than smaller children of the same age (Hockenberry and Wilson, 2011).

GENDER

- There is no clinically significant difference in BP levels between boys and girls before puberty.
- After puberty males have higher readings.
- During and after menopause women have higher BPs than men of the same age.

ETHNICITY

- The incidence of hypertension is higher in African-Americans than in European Americans.
- African-Americans tend to develop more severe hypertension at an earlier age and have twice the risk for complications of hypertension such as stroke and heart attack. Hypertension-related deaths are also higher among African-Americans.

SYMPATHETIC STIMULATION

- Pain, anxiety, and fear stimulate the sympathetic nervous system, causing BP to rise. A full bladder can increase sympathetic stimulation, elevating BP (Ogedegbe and Pickering, 2010).

DAILY VARIATION

- BP varies throughout the day with lower blood pressure during sleep, increasing during the day (Ogedegbe and Pickering, 2010).
- BP can drop 10% to 20% during nighttime sleep (Ogedegbe and Pickering, 2010).

MEDICATION AND TREATMENT

- Some medications directly or indirectly affect BP. Opioids, sedatives, general anesthetics, antihypertensives, and vasodilators lower pressure, whereas vasoconstrictors, blood, and IV fluid infusion raise blood pressure.

ACTIVITY

- Older adults often experience a 5- to 10-mm Hg fall in BP about 1 hour after eating.
- BP falls as a person moves from lying to sitting or standing position; normal postural variations are minimal.
- Increase in oxygen demand by the body during activity increases BP.

WEIGHT

- Obesity is a risk factor for hypertension (Falkner et al., 2010).
- In school-age children the higher their body mass index (BMI), the greater the risk for developing hypertension at an early age (Meininger et al., 2010).

DIET

- A diet low in sodium and high in potassium can reduce BP. Vegetarian diets and limited alcohol consumption (fewer than two drinks per day for men and one per day for women) are associated with low BP (Appel et al., 2009). BP reductions are greater among older adults implementing dietary modifications.

SMOKING

- Smoking results in vasoconstriction, a narrowing of blood vessels. BP rises when a person smokes and returns to baseline about 15 minutes after stopping smoking (NHBPEP, 2004).

TABLE 15-5 CLASSIFICATION OF BLOOD PRESSURE FOR ADULTS 18 YEARS AND OLDER

CATEGORY	SYSTOLIC (mm Hg)*		DIASTOLIC (mm Hg)*
Normal	<120		<80
Prehypertension†	120-139	or	80-89
Stage 1 hypertension	140-159	or	90-99
Stage 2 hypertension	≥160	or	≥100

Data from National High Blood Pressure Education Program: *Seventh report of the Joint National Committee on prevention, evaluation, and treatment of high blood pressure (JNC 7)*, 2004, http://www.nhlbi.nih.gov/guidelines/hypertension/. Accessed October 13, 2013.

*Based on the average of two or more readings taken at each of two or more visits after an initial screening. Patient should not be taking antihypertensive drugs and not be acutely ill. When systolic and diastolic blood pressures fall into different categories, select the higher category to classify the individual's blood pressure status. For example, classify 160/92 mm Hg as stage 2 hypertension.

†Based on average of two or more readings.

TABLE 15-6 RECOMMENDATIONS FOR BLOOD PRESSURE FOLLOW-UP

INITIAL BLOOD PRESSURE	FOLLOW-UP RECOMMENDED*
Normal	Recheck in 2 years.
Prehypertension	Recheck in 1 year.†
Stage 1 hypertension	Confirm within 2 months.†
Stage 2 hypertension	Evaluate or refer to source of care within 1 month. For those with higher pressure (e.g., >180/110 mm Hg), evaluate and treat immediately or within 1 week, depending on clinical situation and complications.

Data from National High Blood Pressure Education Program: *Seventh report of the Joint National Committee on prevention, evaluation, and treatment of high blood pressure (JNC 7)*, 2004, http://www.nhlbi.nih.gov/guidelines/hypertension/. Accessed October 13, 2013.
*Modify the scheduling of follow-up according to reliable information about past blood pressure measurements, other cardiovascular risk factors, or target organ damage.
†Provide advice about lifestyle modifications.

blood in the legs caused by gravity. Orthostatic hypotension occurs when the peripheral blood vessels in the legs are already constricted or are unable to constrict in response to a change in position. Fluid volume deficit from decreased blood volume, dehydration, or recent blood loss; prolonged bed rest; anemia; or antihypertensive medications place patients at risk for orthostatic hypotension. Assess for orthostatic hypotension by obtaining pulse and blood pressure readings with the patient supine, sitting, and standing (Box 15-7).

Measurement of Blood Pressure

You measure arterial blood pressure either directly (invasively) or indirectly (noninvasively). The direct method requires the insertion of a thin catheter into an artery. Risks associated with continuous invasive blood pressure monitoring require the use of an intensive care setting. The more common noninvasive method requires use of the **sphygmomanometer** and stethoscope. You measure blood pressure indirectly by palpation or auscultation (see Skill 15-3).

Blood Pressure Equipment. Before assessing blood pressure, you need to become comfortable using a sphygmomanometer and stethoscope. A sphygmomanometer includes a pressure manometer, an occlusive cloth or disposable vinyl cuff that encloses an inflatable rubber bladder, and a pressure bulb with a release valve that inflates the bladder. The aneroid manometer has a glass-enclosed circular gauge containing a needle that registers millimeter calibrations. Aneroid manometers are safe, lightweight, portable, and compact (Figure 15-9). Before using a manometer, be sure that the needle points to zero. Metal parts in the aneroid manometer are subject to temperature variations and need to be checked every 6 months to verify their accuracy. Mercury manometers are prohibited in health care settings because of the hazard of mercury.

The release valves of the sphygmomanometer must be clean and freely movable in either direction. The valve, when closed, should hold the pressure constant. Frequent calibration is necessary to ensure accuracy. A sticky valve makes

BOX 15-7 PROCEDURAL GUIDELINES

Measuring Orthostatic Blood Pressure

DELEGATION CONSIDERATIONS

The skill of measuring orthostatic blood pressure (BP) cannot be delegated to nursing assistive personnel (NAP).

EQUIPMENT

Sphygmomanometer, stethoscope

STEPS

1. Determine if it is appropriate to measure patient's orthostatic blood pressure. Orthostatic vital signs are not indicated in patients who (Agency for Healthcare Research and Quality, 2013):
   - Have supine hypotension.
   - Have a sitting blood pressure ≤90/60 mm Hg.
   - Have acute deep vein thrombosis.
   - Exhibit the clinical syndrome of shock.
   - Have severely altered mental status.
   - Have possible spinal injuries.
   - Have lower extremity or pelvic fractures.
   - Are not mobile enough to get out of bed.
2. Perform hand hygiene.
3. Have patient lie in bed with head of bed flat for a minimum of 3 minutes, preferably 5 minutes (Agency for Healthcare Research and Quality, 2013). With patient supine, take BP reading in each arm. Select arm with highest systolic reading for subsequent measurements.
4. Leaving BP cuff in place, help patient to sitting position. Take BP at 1 minute. If orthostatic signs or symptoms occur, such as dizziness, weakness, light-headedness, feeling faint, sudden pallor, or a sitting BP ≤90/60 mm Hg, put patient back to bed in the supine position.
5. Leaving BP cuff in place, help patient to standing position. Take BP at 1 minute and 3 minutes with patient in standing position (CDC, 2013). If orthostatic signs or symptoms occur (as previously noted), stop BP measurement and help patient to supine position. In most cases you detect orthostatic hypotension within 1 minute of standing.
6. If patient is unable to stand, sit patient upright with legs dangling over the edge of the bed.
7. Record patient's BP in each position (e.g., "140/80 supine, 132/72 sitting, 108/60 standing"). Note any additional symptoms or complaints. A drop in systolic BP of ≥20 mm Hg, a drop in diastolic BP of ≥10 mm Hg, or an experience light-headedness or dizziness is considered abnormal (CDC, 2013).
8. Report findings of orthostatic hypotension or orthostatic signs or symptoms to nurse in charge or health care provider. Instruct patient to ask for assistance when getting out of bed if orthostatic hypotension is present or orthostatic signs or symptoms occur.
9. Perform hand hygiene.

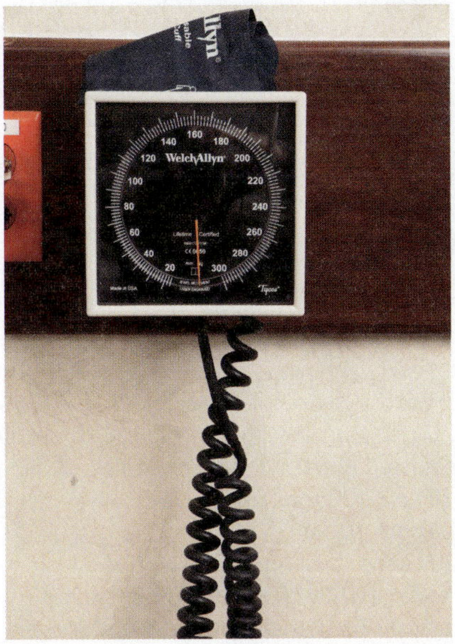

FIGURE 15-9 Wall-mounted aneroid sphygmomanometer.

pressure cuff deflation hard to regulate. The pressure bulb and tubing should be airtight.

Cloth or disposable vinyl compression cuffs contain an inflatable bladder and come in several different sizes. The size selected is proportional to the circumference of the limb being assessed. Ideally you select a cuff that is at least 40% greater than the arm circumference (or 20% wider than the diameter) of the midpoint of the limb being used to obtain measurements. The bladder, enclosed by the cuff, encircles at least 80% of the arm of an adult and the entire arm of a child. The lower edge of the cuff is above the antecubital fossa, allowing room for placement of the stethoscope. An improperly placed or fitted cuff causes inaccurate blood pressure measurement (Table 15-7).

TABLE 15-7 COMMON MISTAKES IN BLOOD PRESSURE ASSESSMENT

ERROR	EFFECT
Bladder or cuff too wide	False-low reading
Bladder or cuff too narrow too short	False-high reading
Cuff wrapped too loosely or unevenly	False-high reading
Deflating cuff too slowly	False-high diastolic reading
Deflating cuff too quickly	False-low systolic and false-high diastolic reading
Arm below heart level	False-high reading
Arm above heart level	False-low reading
Arm not supported	False-high reading
Stethoscope that fits poorly or impairment of the examiner's hearing, causing sounds to be muffled	False-low systolic and false-high diastolic reading
Stethoscope applied too firmly against antecubital fossa	False-low diastolic reading
Inflating too slowly	False-high diastolic reading
Repeating assessments too quickly	False-high systolic reading
Inadequate inflation level	False-low systolic reading
Multiple examiners using different Korotkoff sounds for diastolic readings	False-high systolic and false-low diastolic reading

Auscultation. The best environment for blood pressure measurement by auscultation is in a quiet room at a comfortable temperature. Although a patient is able to lie or stand, sitting is the best position. It is best to have a patient assume the same position during each blood pressure measurement to permit a meaningful comparison of values. Before assessment, control factors responsible for artificially high readings such as pain, anxiety, or exertion. *As an example, in the case study Ms. Coburn was anxious when first entering the examination room. After she sees the nurse practitioner, Miguel retakes her blood pressure. Her blood pressure this time is 146/94 mm Hg (1st reading 164/98 mm Hg).*

A patient's perception that the physical or interpersonal environment is stressful affects blood pressure. Measurements taken at home are sometimes different from those taken at a patient's place of employment or health care provider's office.

During the initial assessment you obtain and record blood pressures in both arms. Normally there is a difference of 5 to 10 mm Hg between the right and left arms. In subsequent assessments measure the blood pressure in the arm with the higher pressure. Pressure differences between extremities greater than 20 mm Hg indicate vascular problems and need to be reported to the charge nurse or health care provider.

Indirect measurement of arterial blood pressure works on a basic principle of pressure. Blood flows freely through an artery until an inflated cuff applies pressure to tissues and causes the artery to collapse. When the cuff slowly deflates, the point at which blood flow returns and sound appears through auscultation is the SBP.

In 1905 Nikolai Korotkoff, a Russian surgeon, first described the sounds heard over an artery during cuff deflation. The first **Korotkoff sound** is a clear, rhythmic tapping series that corresponds to the pulse rate and gradually increases in intensity. Onset of the sound corresponds to the systolic pressure. A murmur or swishing sound appears as the cuff continues to deflate, which is the second Korotkoff sound. As the artery distends, blood flow becomes turbulent. The third Korotkoff sound is a crisper and more intense tapping. The fourth Korotkoff sound becomes muffled and low pitched as the cuff is further deflated. The onset of the fourth Korotkoff sound is the diastolic pressure in infants and children, pregnant women, and patients with elevated cardiac output or peripheral vasodilation. The fifth Korotkoff sound

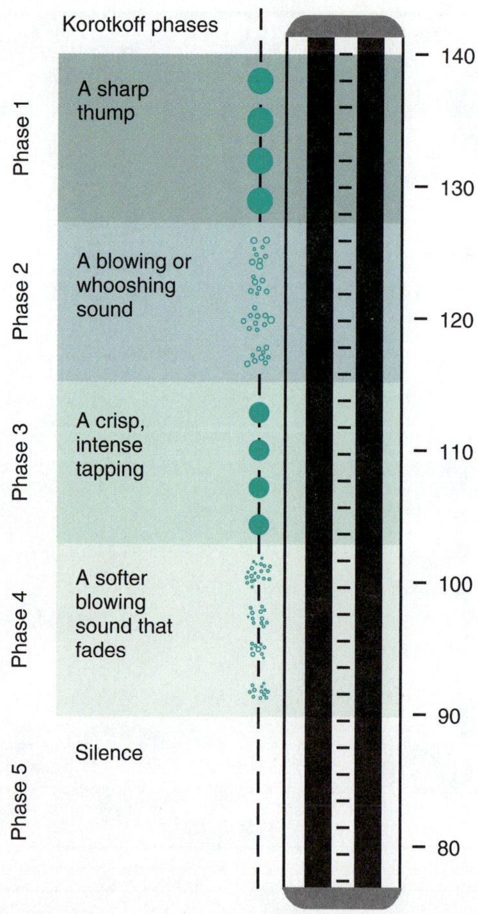

FIGURE 15-10 Sounds auscultated during blood pressure measurement can be differentiated into five Korotkoff phases. In this example the blood pressure is 140/90.

is the disappearance of sound; in adolescents and most adults this sound corresponds with the DBP (Figure 15-10). In some patients the sounds are clear and distinct, whereas in others only the beginning and the ending sounds are heard. Research has focused on whether the bell or the diaphragm more accurately auscultates the fifth Korotkoff sound. Although the bell auscultates lower-pitched sounds, research shows no significant difference in using the diaphragm or bell (Kantola et al., 2005).

The AHA recommends recording two numbers for a blood pressure measurement: the point on the manometer when the first sound is heard for SBP and the point on the manometer when the fifth sound (disappearance of sound) is heard for DBP (Pickering et al., 2005). Some institutions recommend recording the point when you hear the fourth sound, especially for patients with hypertension. You divide the numbers by slashed lines (e.g., 120/80, 120/100/80), note the arm used to measure the blood pressure, and record the patient's position (e.g., LA 158/78, sitting).

You base decisions about patient care and implementing nursing interventions on the blood pressure measurements in combination with other findings. Obtaining an accurate blood pressure is critical. There are several possibilities for error if the auscultation procedure is not followed correctly

BOX 15-8 PROCEDURAL GUIDELINES

Palpating the Systolic Blood Pressure

DELEGATION CONSIDERATIONS

The skill of obtaining blood pressure (BP) by palpation cannot be delegated to nursing assistive personnel (NAP).

EQUIPMENT

Sphygmomanometer

STEPS

1. Perform hand hygiene.
2. Apply BP cuff to extremity selected for measurement.
3. Continually palpate the brachial, radial, or popliteal artery of the selected extremity with fingertips of one hand.
4. Inflate BP cuff 30 mm Hg above point at which you no longer palpate pulse.
5. Slowly release valve and deflate cuff, allowing manometer needle to fall at rate of 2 mm Hg per second.
6. Note point on manometer when pulse is again palpable; this is the systolic BP.
7. Deflate cuff rapidly and completely. Remove cuff from patient's extremity unless you need to repeat the measurement.
8. Perform hand hygiene.

(see Table 15-7). If you are unsure of a reading, ask another nurse to reassess the blood pressure.

Ultrasonic Stethoscope. If you are unable to auscultate Korotkoff sounds because of a weak arterial pulse, use an ultrasonic stethoscope (see Chapter 16). This stethoscope allows you to hear low-frequency systolic sounds and is commonly used in infants and children and for investigating low blood pressure in adults.

Palpation. Indirect measurement of blood pressure by palpation is useful for patients whose arterial pulsations are too weak to create Korotkoff sounds. Severe blood loss and weakened heart contractility are examples of conditions that result in blood pressures too low to auscultate accurately. In this case you assess the SBP by palpation (Box 15-8). DBP is difficult to determine by palpation. When using the palpation technique, you record the systolic value only and the location and manner in which it was measured (e.g., RA 78/–, palpated).

Sometimes you use palpation techniques with auscultation. In some patients with hypertension the sounds usually heard over the brachial artery when the cuff pressure is high disappear as pressure is reduced and then reappear at a lower level. This temporary disappearance of sound is the **auscultatory gap.** It typically occurs between the first and second Korotkoff sounds. The gap in sound sometimes covers a range of 40 mm Hg, possibly causing an underestimation of SBP or an overestimation of DBP. Be certain to inflate the cuff high enough to hear the true SBP before the auscultatory gap. Palpation of the radial artery helps to determine how high to inflate the cuff. Inflate the cuff 30 mm Hg above the pressure at which the palpated radial pulse disappears and slowly release the cuff until the radial pulse returns. This correlates

BOX 15-9 ADVANTAGES AND LIMITATIONS OF AUTOMATIC BLOOD PRESSURE MACHINES

ADVANTAGES
- Ease of use
- Efficient when frequent repeated measurements are indicated
- Ability to use a stethoscope not required
- Allows you to record blood pressure (BP) more frequently, as often as every 15 seconds with accuracy

LIMITATIONS
- Expensive
- Requires source of electricity
- Requires space to position machine
- Sensitive to outside motion interference; not used in patients with seizures, tremors, or shivers or patients unable to cooperate
- Not accurate for hypotensive patients or in conditions with reduced blood flow (e.g., hypothermia)
- Systolic readings by automated wrist manometers are the most unreliable, and automated arm monitors tend to provide higher measures than the mercury standard on average (Nelson et al., 2008)
- Adherence to accuracy standards for electronic BP machine manufacturers is voluntary
- Vulnerable to error in patients with irregular heart rate and obese extremities
- Systolic BP possibly overestimated
- Multiple readings are essential to provide clinicians and patients with accurate information on which to base diagnostic and treatment decisions (Wan et al., 2010)

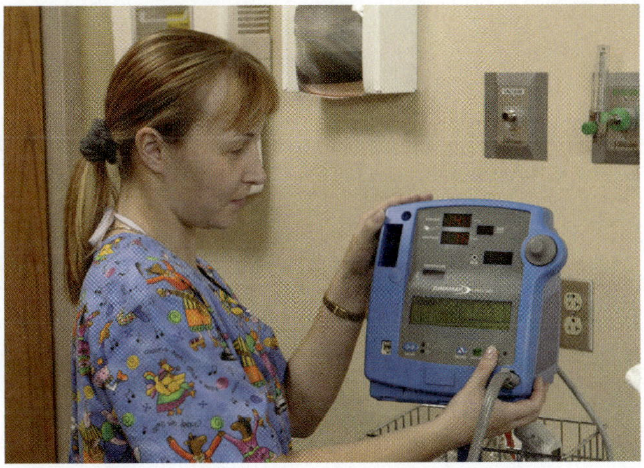

FIGURE 15-11 Electronic blood pressure machines vary in appearance.

with the systolic pressure. Document the blood pressure reading with an auscultatory gap (e.g., "BP RA 180/94 with an auscultatory gap from 180 to 160").

Electronic Blood Pressure Machines. Many different styles of electronic blood pressure machines are available to determine blood pressure automatically (Figure 15-11). Electronic blood pressure machines rely on an electronic sensor to detect the vibrations caused by the rush of blood through an artery. When the cuff deflates, one style of blood pressure machine determines the initial burst of oscillations and translates the information to a systolic pressure reading. The machine records a diastolic measurement when the oscillations are lowest, just before they stop. Although electronic blood pressure machines are fast and free the care provider for other activities, it is necessary to consider their advantages and limitations (Box 15-9). Use the devices when frequent assessment is necessary such as in potentially hemodynamically unstable patients, during or after invasive procedures, or when therapies require frequent monitoring (Box 15-10).

Blood Pressure Assessment in Lower Extremities. If your patient has dressings, casts, IV catheters, or arteriovenous fistulas or shunts in the upper extremities, measure blood pressure in a lower extremity. Comparing upper-extremity blood pressure with the blood pressure in the legs is also necessary for patients with certain cardiac and blood pressure abnormalities. The popliteal artery, palpable behind the knee in the popliteal space, is the site for auscultation. Position the cuff with the bladder over the posterior aspect of the midthigh, 2.5 cm (1 inch) above the popliteal artery. Make sure that the cuff is wide enough and long enough to allow for the larger girth of the thigh. For most measurements place the patient in a prone position. If such a position is impossible, flex the knee slightly for easier access to the artery (Figure 15-12). The procedure is identical to brachial artery auscultation. SBP in the legs is usually higher by 10 to 40 mm Hg than in the brachial artery, but the DBP is the same.

Assessment of Blood Pressure in Children. All children 3 years of age through adolescence should have blood pressure checked at least annually. Blood pressure in children changes with growth and development. You need to help parents understand the importance of this routine screening to detect children who are at risk for hypertension. Measuring blood pressure in infants and children is difficult for several reasons:

1. Smaller cuff size is required.
2. Readings are difficult to obtain in restless or anxious infants and children.
3. Placing stethoscope too firmly on the antecubital fossa causes errors in auscultation.
4. Korotkoff sounds are difficult to hear in children because of low frequency and amplitude; a pediatric stethoscope bell is helpful.

BOX 15-10 PROCEDURAL GUIDELINES

Automatic Blood Pressure Measurement

DELEGATION CONSIDERATIONS

The skill of blood pressure (BP) measurement using an electronic BP machine can be delegated to nursing assistive personnel (NAP) unless patient is considered unstable. The nurse instructs the NAP to:

- Obtain BP measurements at appropriate times as determined by agency policy, health care provider's order, or patient condition such as frequent postoperative measurements.
- Consider patient-specific factors that affect the patient's usual values.
- Select appropriate limb for BP measurement.
- Select appropriate-size BP cuff for designated extremity and appropriate cuff for the machine.
- Immediately report any abnormalities, which the nurse confirms.

EQUIPMENT

Electronic BP machine, BP cuff of appropriate size as recommended by manufacturer, source of electricity

STEPS

1. Determine the appropriateness of using electronic BP measurement. Patients with irregular heart rate, peripheral vascular disease, seizures, tremors, and shivering are not candidates for this device.
2. Perform hand hygiene.
3. Determine best site for cuff placement (see Skill 15-3, Assessment Step 4).
4. Help patient to comfortable position, either lying or sitting. Plug in device and place it near patient, ensuring that connector hose between cuff and machine reaches.
5. Locate on/off switch and turn on machine to enable device to self-test computer systems.
6. Select appropriate cuff size for patient extremity and appropriate cuff for machine. Electronic BP cuff and machine are matched by manufacturer and are not interchangeable.
7. Expose extremity for measurement by removing constricting clothing to ensure proper cuff application. Do not place BP cuff over clothing.
8. Prepare BP cuff by manually squeezing all air out of cuff and connecting cuff to connector hose.
9. Wrap flattened cuff snugly around extremity, verifying that only one finger fits between cuff and patient's skin. Make sure that "artery" arrow marked on outside of cuff is correctly placed (see illustration for Skill 15-3, Implementation Step 5, illustration *B*).
10. Verify that connector hose between cuff and machine is not kinked. Kinking prevents proper inflation and deflation of cuff.
11. Following manufacturer directions, set frequency control of automatic or manual; press start button. The first BP measurement pumps the cuff to a peak pressure of about 180 mm Hg. After this pressure is reached, the machine begins a deflation sequence that determines the BP. The first reading determines peak pressure inflation for additional measurements.
12. When deflation is complete, digital display provides the most recent values and flash time in minutes that have elapsed since the measurement occurred.

Clinical Decision Point: **If unable to obtain BP with electronic device, verify machine connections (e.g., plugged into working electrical outlet, hose-cuff connections tight, machine on, correct cuff). Repeat electronic BP; if unable to obtain, use auscultatory technique (see Skill 15-3).**

13. Set frequency of BP measurements, upper and lower alarm limits for systolic, diastolic, and mean BP readings. Intervals between BP measurements are set from 1 to 90 minutes. You determine frequency and alarm limits based on patient's acceptable range of BP, nursing judgment, agency standards, or health care provider's order.
14. You are able to obtain additional readings at any time by pressing the start button. (Sometimes you need these for unstable patients.) Pressing the cancel button immediately deflates cuff.
15. If frequent BP measurements are required, leave cuff in place. Remove it every 2 hours to assess underlying skin integrity and, if possible, alternate BP sites. Patients with abnormal bleeding tendencies are at risk for microvascular rupture from repeated inflations. When you are finished using the electronic BP machine, clean BP cuff according to facility policy to reduce transmission of microorganisms.
16. Compare electronic BP readings with auscultatory BP measurements to verify accuracy of electronic BP device.
17. Record BP and site assessed on vital sign flow sheet, nurses' notes, or electronic medical record. Record any signs of BP alterations in nurses' notes. Report abnormal findings to nurse in charge or health care provider.
18. Perform hand hygiene.

The same auscultation method used with adults is appropriate for children. An infant or child younger than 5 years of age lies supine with the arm supported at heart level. Older children sit. It is important for the child to be relaxed and calm. Allow at least 15 minutes for children to recover from recent activity or excitement before taking a reading. It helps to have a parent nearby. Prepare the child for the unusual sensation of the blood pressure cuff during inflation. Most children understand the analogy of a "tight hug on your arm" and will be more cooperative. Do not choose a cuff based on the name of the cuff (e.g., "infant"). Average width of a cuff bladder for an infant is 2½ to 3¼ inches; average width of a cuff bladder for a child is 4¾ to 5½ inches.

RESPIRATION

Respiration is the mechanism the body uses to exchange gases between the atmosphere, blood, and cells. It involves three processes: **ventilation** (the mechanical movement of gases into and out of the lungs), diffusion (the movement of oxygen

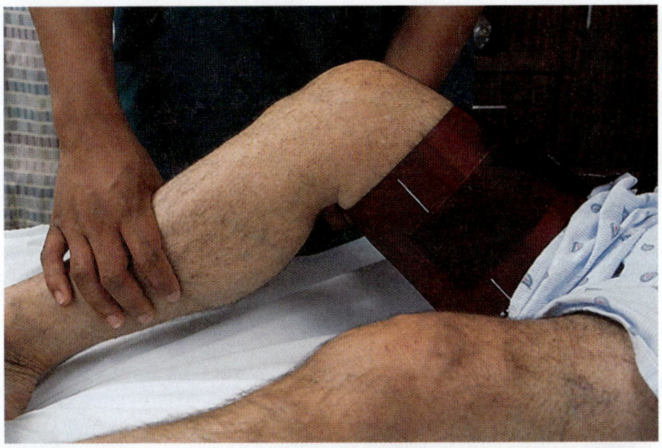

FIGURE 15-12 Lower-extremity blood pressure cuff positioned above popliteal artery at midthigh with knee flexed.

[O_2] and carbon dioxide [CO_2] between the alveoli and the red blood cells), and **perfusion** (the distribution of red blood cells to and from the pulmonary capillaries). Analyzing respiratory ability requires integrating assessment data from all three processes. Assess ventilation by determining respiratory rate, depth, and rhythm. You assess diffusion and perfusion by evaluating oxygen saturation.

Assessment of Ventilation

Adults normally breathe in a smooth, uninterrupted pattern of 12 to 20 breaths/min. Levels of CO_2 in the arterial blood normally regulate ventilation by stimulation of chemoreceptors in the carotid and heart bodies. The normal rate and depth of ventilation, **eupnea,** is interrupted by sighing. The sigh, a prolonged deeper breath, is a protective physiological mechanism for expanding small airways and alveoli not ventilated during a normal breath.

Accurate assessment of ventilation depends on recognizing normal thoracic and abdominal movements. During quiet breathing the chest wall gently rises and falls. When breathing requires greater effort, the intercostal and accessory muscles work actively to move air in and out. The shoulders sometimes rise and fall, and the accessory muscles of ventilation in the neck visibly contract. Diaphragmatic movement becomes less noticeable as costal breathing increases.

Measurement of Respiration

Accurate measurement of respiration requires observation and palpation of chest wall movement. A sudden change in the character of respirations is an important assessment finding. For example, slow respirations in your patient with head trauma can indicate a brainstem injury. Likewise, increased respirations can be seen in a patient experiencing pain or anxiety.

When assessing respiration, keep in mind your patient's usual respiratory rate, his or her breathing pattern, and the influence that any disease or illness has on respiratory function. In addition, consider the relationship between respiratory and cardiovascular function and the influence of therapies on respiration. Box 15-11 summarizes factors influencing respiration. The objective measurement of respiration includes the rate and depth of breathing and the rhythm of ventilatory movements (see Skill 15-4).

BOX 15-11 FACTORS INFLUENCING CHARACTER OF RESPIRATIONS

EXERCISE
- Exercise increases respiratory rate and depth to meet the need of the body for additional oxygen and to rid the body of CO_2.

ACUTE PAIN
- Pain alters rate and rhythm of respirations; breathing becomes shallow.
- Patient inhibits or splints chest wall movement when pain is in area of chest or abdomen.

ANXIETY
- Anxiety increases respiratory rate and depth as a result of sympathetic stimulation.

SMOKING
- Chronic smoking changes pulmonary airways, resulting in increased respiratory rate at rest when not smoking.

BODY POSITION
- Standing or sitting erect promotes full ventilatory movement and lung expansion; stooped or slumped position impairs ventilatory movement; lying flat prevents full chest expansion.

MEDICATIONS
- General anesthetics, sedative-hypnotics, and excessive doses of opioid analgesics depress respiratory rate and depth.
- Amphetamines and cocaine may increase rate and depth; bronchodilators cause airway dilation that can ultimately slow respiratory rate.

NEUROLOGICAL INJURY
- Damage to brainstem impairs the respiratory center and inhibits respiratory rate and rhythm.

HEMOGLOBIN FUNCTION
- Decreased hemoglobin levels (anemia) reduce oxygen-carrying capacity of blood, which increases respiratory rate.
- Increased altitude lowers amount of saturated hemoglobin, which increases respiratory rate and depth.
- Abnormal blood cell function (e.g., sickle cell disease) reduces ability of hemoglobin to carry oxygen, which increases respiratory rate and depth.

CHEST WALL MOVEMENT
- Constrictive chest or abdominal dressings limit chest wall movement.
- Presence of abdominal incisions limit chest wall movement.

Respiratory Rate. Observe a full inspiration and expiration when counting respirations. The respiratory rate varies with age (Table 15-8). A respiratory rate less than 12 per

TABLE 15-8 ACCEPTABLE RANGE OF RESPIRATORY RATES FOR AGE

AGE	RATE (BREATHS/MIN)
Newborn	35-40
Infant (6 months)	30-50
Toddler (2 years)	25-32
Child	20-30
Adolescent	16-20
Adult	12-20

minute or lower than acceptable limits is **bradypnea,** whereas a rate over 20 or greater than the acceptable limits is **tachypnea. Apnea** is the lack of respiratory movements. A respiratory monitoring device that helps assess respiratory rate is the apnea monitor. This noninvasive device uses electrodes attached to a patient's chest wall to sense movement. An absence of chest wall movement triggers the apnea alarm. Apnea monitoring is used frequently in the hospital and home to observe for prolonged apneic events in infants.

Ventilatory Depth. Assess the depth of respirations by observing the degree of movement in the chest wall. Ventilatory movements are deep, normal, or shallow. A deep respiration involves a full expansion of the lungs with obvious movement of the rib cage and full exhalation. A normal respiration is relaxed, automatic, and silent. Respirations are shallow when only a small quantity of air passes through the lungs and ventilatory movement is difficult to see. Implement more objective techniques such as lung excursion when chest wall movement is unusually shallow or not symmetrical (see Chapter 16).

Ventilatory Rhythm. Respiratory rhythm or breathing pattern is either regular or irregular. While assessing respiration, observe the interval between each respiratory cycle. With normal breathing a regular interval occurs between each respiratory cycle. In the presence of irregular ventilatory rhythm such as periods of apnea with shallow or deep breathing, a more detailed physical assessment is imperative (see Chapter 30). Infants tend to breathe less regularly. Young children sometimes breathe slowly for a few seconds and suddenly breathe more rapidly.

MEASUREMENT OF OXYGEN SATURATION (PULSE OXIMETRY)

Pulse oximetry is the indirect measurement of **oxygen saturation** and is the fifth vital sign (see Skill 15-5). The pulse oximeter is a photosensor with two light-emitting diodes (LEDs) of differing wavelengths that measures the combined absorption of oxygenated and deoxygenated **hemoglobin** (Miner and Mathews, 2012) (Figure 15-13). Oxygen saturation is computed and displayed as a percentage. The more hemoglobin that is saturated by oxygen, the higher the oxygen saturation. Normally SpO_2 is between 95% and 100%, however, in patients with extensive respiratory disease such as chronic obstructive pulmonary disease (COPD), a SpO_2 greater than 90% may be acceptable.

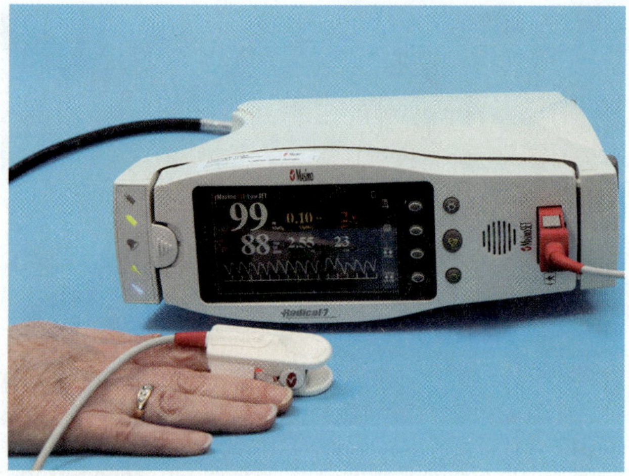

FIGURE 15-13 Pulse oximeter connected to finger sensor.

The measurement of SpO_2 is simple and painless and carries fewer risks than those associated with invasive measurements of SaO_2 such as arterial blood gas sampling. A vascular, pulsatile area (e.g., fingertip or earlobe) is needed to detect the degree of change in the transmitted light. Factors that affect light transmission (such as sensor movement or fingernail polish) or peripheral arterial pulsations (such as hypotension or anemia) also affect the measurement of SpO_2. An awareness of these factors allows for accurate interpretation of abnormal SpO_2 measurements. Measuring SpO_2 can be conducted intermittently or continuously to assess ongoing therapies.

MEASUREMENT OF END-TIDAL CARBON DIOXIDE

End-tidal carbon dioxide ($ETCO_2$) values are important to assess when caring for seriously ill patients when monitoring lung ventilation and perfusion is essential. The special noninvasive $ETCO_2$ monitor attaches directly into the ventilator system and measures the exhaled carbon dioxide through sensors in the ventilator. **$ETCO_2$ monitoring** benefits a patient because it is noninvasive and painless and provides an accurate assessment of arterial carbon dioxide retention values (Cinar et al., 2012). Commonly used in mechanically ventilated patients, $ETCO_2$ monitoring can also be implemented with nonintubated patients.

SPECIAL CONSIDERATIONS

Physiological changes caused by aging influence the measurement and interpretation of older adults' vital signs (Box 15-12). You often provide patient teaching to patients of all ages related to vital sign results (Box 15-13). For example, patients with hypertension require education on risk-factor modification. Teach your patients taking cardiac medications

BOX 15-12 CARE OF THE OLDER ADULT

Considerations When Obtaining Vital Sign Measurements

TEMPERATURE

- The normal temperature of older adults is at the lower end of the acceptable temperature range, 36° C (96.8° F). Therefore temperatures considered normal for an adult may represent a fever in an older adult.
- Older adults are very sensitive to slight changes in environmental temperature because their thermoregulatory systems are not as efficient (Touhy and Jett, 2014).
- A decrease in sweat gland reactivity in the older adult results in a higher threshold for sweating at high temperatures, which leads to hyperthermia and heatstroke.
- With aging, loss of subcutaneous fat reduces the insulating capacity of the skin; older men are at especially high risk for hypothermia.

PULSE RATE

- It is often difficult to palpate the pulse of an older adult. A Doppler device provides a more accurate reading.
- The older adult typically has a decreased heart rate at rest (Touhy and Jett, 2014).
- It takes longer for the heart rate to rise in the older adult to meet sudden increased demands that result from stress, illness, or excitement. Once elevated, the pulse rate of an older adult takes longer to return to normal resting rate.
- When assessing the apical rate of an older woman, lift the breast tissue gently and place the stethoscope at the fifth intercostal space (ICS) or the lower edge of the breast.
- Heart sounds are sometimes muffled or difficult to hear in older adults because of an increase in air space in the lungs.

BLOOD PRESSURE

- The normal range for blood pressure is the same for older adults and younger adults (NHBPEP, 2004).
- Older adults often have decreased upper arm mass, which requires special attention to selection of blood pressure cuff size.
- Skin of older adults is more fragile and susceptible to cuff pressure injury when blood pressure measurements are frequent.
- Older adults sometimes have an increase in systolic pressure related to decrease in vessel elasticity, whereas the diastolic pressure remains the same, resulting in a wider pulse pressure.
- Instruct older adults to change positions slowly and wait after each change to avoid orthostatic hypotension and prevent injuries.

RESPIRATION

- Aging causes ossification of costal cartilage and downward slant of ribs, resulting in a more rigid rib cage, which reduces chest wall expansion. Kyphosis and scoliosis, which may occur in older adults, also restrict chest expansion and decrease tidal volume.
- The respiratory system matures by the time a person reaches 20 years of age and begins to decline in healthy people after the age of 25. Despite this decline, older adults are able to breathe effortlessly as long as they are healthy. However, sudden events that require an increased demand for oxygen (e.g., exercise, stress, illness) can create shortness of breath in the older adult (Touhy and Jett, 2014).
- Identifying an acceptable pulse oximeter sensor site is difficult with older adults because of the likelihood of peripheral vascular disease, decreased cardiac output, cold-induced vasoconstriction, and anemia, which decrease pulsatile flow.

BOX 15-13 VITAL SIGN PATIENT TEACHING CONSIDERATIONS

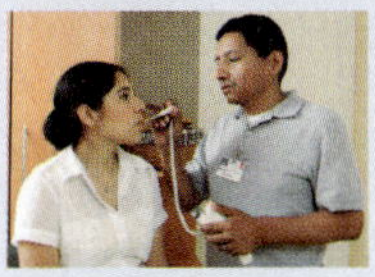

After caring for Ms. Coburn, Miguel sees the need to educate her about the different types of vital signs. Based on Ms. Coburn's current problems, Miguel determines that the priority is to focus on hypertension and ways to prevent or control elevated blood pressure (BP). Miguel states, "We need to watch your BP closely over the next few weeks. In the meantime, remember that you decided that you are going to walk for at least 15 minutes 3 days a week, try to eat foods with less salt, and think about not smoking anymore. To maintain your overall health, you also need information about temperature, pulse, respirations, and BP." Miguel then implements a teaching plan.

OUTCOME

Ms. Coburn verbalizes understanding of how temperature, pulse, BP, and respirations relate to her health status.

TEACHING STRATEGIES

When educating Ms. Coburn about vital sign measurement, Miguel considers the following issues and implements appropriate teaching strategies.

Temperature

- Identify Ms. Coburn's ability to initiate preventive health measures and recognize alteration in body temperature. Educate Ms. Coburn and her family about measures to prevent body temperature alterations.
- Explain the risk factors for hypothermia: fatigue; malnutrition; cold, wet clothing; alcohol intoxication.
- Educate about the risk factors for heat stroke: strenuous exercise in hot, humid weather; tight-fitting clothing in hot environments; exercising in poorly ventilated areas; sudden exposure to hot climates; poor fluid intake before, during, and after exercise.

Continued

BOX 15-13 VITAL SIGN PATIENT TEACHING CONSIDERATIONS—cont'd

- Educate Ms. Coburn about the importance of taking and continuing antibiotics as directed until course of treatment is completed if she ever needs antibiotic therapy.

Pulse Rate

- Teach Ms. Coburn how to take her carotid pulse. Patients taking certain cardiac and antihypertensive medications need to learn to assess their own pulse rates to detect side effects and the safety of taking these medications.
- Explain the need to take pulse before, during, and after exercise. Patients who exercise or are in cardiac rehabilitation programs need to learn to assess their own pulse to determine their response to the exercise.

Blood Pressure

- Educate Ms. Coburn about her risk factors for hypertension. People with family history of hypertension are at significant risk. Obesity, cigarette smoking, heavy alcohol consumption, high blood cholesterol and triglyceride levels, and continued exposure to stress are factors linked to hypertension (McCance and Huether, 2010).
- Ensure that Ms. Coburn understands her own blood BP values, long-term follow-up care and therapy, the usual lack of symptoms, ability of therapy to control but not cure hypertension, and benefits of a consistently followed treatment plan.
- Explain the importance of an appropriate-size BP cuff for home use. Demonstrate how to use the BP cuff, and have Ms. Coburn perform a return demonstration.
- Instruct the patient or the caregiver to take BP readings at the same time each day and after patient has had a brief rest. Instruct to take measurements while patient is sitting or lying down and to use same position and arm each time BP is taken.
- Describe how to determine the size of BP cuff needed. If the BP is difficult to hear, it is possible that the cuff is too loose, not big enough, or too narrow. Other possible problems include that the stethoscope is not over the arterial pulse, the BP cuff was deflated too quickly or too slowly, or it was not pumped high enough for systolic readings.

Respiration

- Explain the effect of high-risk behaviors such as cigarette smoking on oxygen saturation.
- Instruct Ms. Coburn or her family to contact home care nurse or health care provider if unusual fluctuations in respiratory rate or rhythm occur.
- Educate Ms. Coburn about the signs and symptoms of hypoxemia: headache, somnolence, confusion, shortness of breath, dyspnea.

EVALUATION STRATEGIES

- Have Ms. Coburn describe her normal vital sign values.
- Ask Ms. Coburn to state three risk factors for hypertension.
- Observe Ms. Coburn take her temperature and BP with the equipment she will use at home. Evaluate her technique and provide guidance as needed.
- Have Ms. Coburn take her carotid pulse while you take her radial pulse. Determine her accuracy in pulse taking by comparing the pulse rate that she measured with the one you obtained.

that they affect pulse rate and how to check their own pulse.

DOCUMENTING VITAL SIGNS

Specific graphic flow sheets exist for recording vital signs. However, more and more institutions are using electronic medical records, which require you to enter data directly into a computerized patient record (see Chapter 10). Identify and use your agency policy for documenting vital signs. In a community-based setting, record vital signs in the appropriate document for that particular clinic or home visit. Record any patient teaching regarding vital signs. When a vital sign is above or below the expected value, enter a note in the patient's chart regarding the finding and related interventions.

SAFETY GUIDELINES FOR NURSING SKILLS

Ensuring patient safety is an essential role of the professional nurse. To ensure patient safety, communicate clearly with members of the health care team, assess and incorporate the patient's priorities of care and preferences, and use the best evidence when making decisions about your patient's care. When performing the skills in this chapter, remember the following points to ensure safe, individualized patient care:

- Vital sign measurement devices are often shared among patients. Clean each device carefully between patients to decrease risk for infection.
- Blood pressure cuffs and pulse oximetry sensors can apply excessive pressure on fragile skin. Rotating sites during repeated measurements decreases risk for skin breakdown.
- Analyze the trends of vital sign measurement and report abnormal findings to the health care provider.
- Determine vital sign frequency based on the patient's condition.

SKILL 15-1 MEASURING BODY TEMPERATURE

View Video!

DELEGATION CONSIDERATIONS

The skill of temperature measurement can be delegated to nursing assistive personnel (NAP). The nurse informs the NAP to:

- Select the appropriate route and device to measure temperature.
- Take appropriate precautions when properly positioning the patient for rectal temperature measurement.
- Consider patient-specific factors that falsely raise or lower temperature.
- Obtain temperature measurements at appropriate times as determined by agency policy, health care provider's orders, or patient condition such as when a patient is shivering or feels warm.
- Know the usual temperature values for the patient.
- Immediately report any abnormal temperatures, which you need to confirm.

EQUIPMENT

- Appropriate thermometer
- Soft tissue or wipe
- Alcohol swab
- Water-soluble lubricant (for rectal measurements only)
- Pen, vital sign flow sheet or record, or patient's electronic medical record
- Clean gloves, plastic thermometer sleeve, disposable probe or sensor cover
- Towel

STEP	RATIONALE
ASSESSMENT	
1. Assess for signs and symptoms that accompany temperature alterations. *Hyperthermia:* Decreased skin turgor; tachycardia; hypotension; concentrated urine *Heatstroke:* Hot, dry skin; tachycardia; hypotension; excessive thirst; muscle cramps; visual disturbances; confusion or delirium *Hypothermia:* Pale skin; skin cool or cold to touch; bradycardia and dysrhythmias; uncontrollable shivering; reduced level of consciousness; shallow respirations	Physical signs and symptoms indicate abnormal temperature, indicating need for temperature measurement. You accurately assess nature of variations.
2. Consider normal daily fluctuations in temperature.	Body temperature tends to be lowest in early morning, peak in late afternoon, and gradually decline during the night. Fever is more accurately identified if you take a temperature between 5 and 7 PM.
3. Determine any activity that interferes with accuracy of temperature measurement. When taking oral temperature, wait 15 minutes before measuring temperature if patient has smoked, chewed gum, or ingested hot or cold liquid or food.	Smoking, chewing gum, and ingesting hot or cold substances may cause false temperature readings in oral cavity.
4. Assess pertinent laboratory values, including complete blood count (CBC).	A white blood cell (WBC) count greater than 12,000/mm^3 in a nonpregnant adult suggests the presence of infection, which can lead to hyperthermia; a WBC count less than 5000/mm^3 suggests that the ability of the body to fight infection is compromised, which can lead to ineffective thermoregulation.
5. Identify medications or treatments that may influence temperature.	Antiinflammatory drugs, steroids, and warming or cooling blankets affect body temperature.
6. Determine appropriate site and measurement device you will use.	Chosen on basis of preferred site for temperature measurement and patient contraindications (see Box 15-4).
7. Determine previous baseline temperature and measurement site from patient's record.	Allows for assessment of change in patient's condition with future measurements.
PLANNING	
1. Identify patient using two identifiers (e.g., name and birthday or name and account number) according to agency policy.	Ensures correct patient. Complies with The Joint Commission requirements for patient safety (TJC, 2014).
2. Explain to patient how you will take temperature and importance of maintaining proper position until reading is complete.	Patients are often curious about their temperatures and may remove thermometer prematurely to read results.

SKILL 15-1 MEASURING BODY TEMPERATURE—cont'd

STEP	RATIONALE
IMPLEMENTATION	
1. Perform hand hygiene.	Reduces transmission of microorganisms.
2. Explain route by which you will take temperature and importance of maintaining proper position until reading is complete.	Patients are often curious about such measurements and prematurely remove thermometer to read results.
3. Help patient to a comfortable position that provides easy access to temperature measurement site.	Ensures patient comfort and accuracy of temperature reading.
4. Obtain temperature reading.	
A. Oral Temperature Measurement With Electronic Thermometer	
Option: Apply clean gloves when there are respiratory secretions or facial or mouth wound drainage.	Use of oral probe cover, which is removable without physical contact, minimizes need to wear gloves.
(1) Remove thermometer pack from charging unit. Attach oral thermometer probe stem (blue tip) to thermometer unit. Grasp top of probe stem, being careful not to apply pressure on ejection button.	Charging provides battery power. Ejection button releases plastic cover from probe stem.
(2) Slide disposable plastic probe cover over thermometer probe stem until cover locks in place (see illustrations).	Soft plastic cover will not break in patient's mouth and prevents transmission of microorganisms between patients.
(3) Ask patient to open mouth; gently place thermometer probe under tongue in posterior sublingual pocket lateral to center of lower jaw (see illustration).	Heat from superficial blood vessels in sublingual pocket produces temperature reading. With electronic thermometer temperatures in right and left posterior sublingual pocket are significantly higher than in area under front of tongue.
(4) Ask patient to hold thermometer probe with lips closed.	Maintains proper position of thermometer during recording.
(5) Leave thermometer probe in place until audible signal indicates completion and patient's temperature appears on digital display; remove thermometer probe from under patient's tongue.	Makes sure that probe stays in place until signal occurs to ensure accurate reading.
(6) Push ejection button on thermometer probe stem to discard plastic probe cover into appropriate receptacle.	Reduces transmission of microorganisms.
(7) Return thermometer probe stem to storage position of recording unit.	Returning probe stem automatically causes digital reading to disappear. Storage position protects stem.
B. Rectal Temperature Measurement With Electronic Thermometer	
(1) Draw curtain around bed and/or close room door. Help patient to side-lying or Sims' position with upper leg flexed. Move aside bed linen to expose only anal area. Keep patient's upper body and lower extremities covered with sheet or blanket.	Maintains patient's privacy, minimizes embarrassment, and promotes comfort.

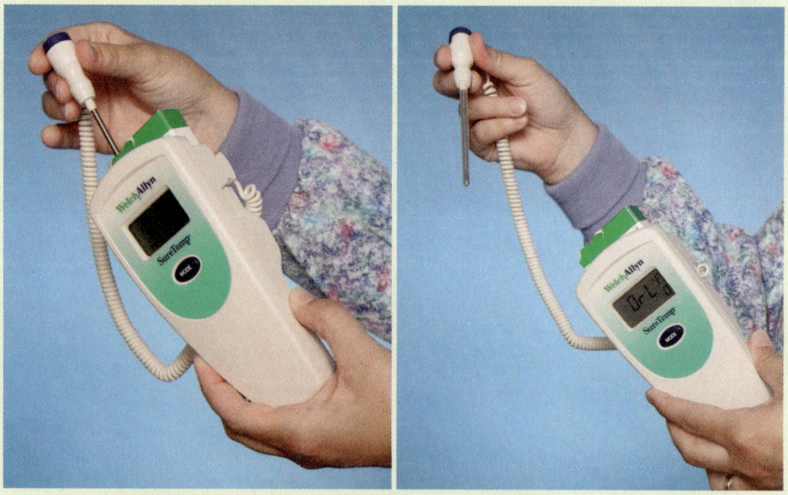

STEP 4A(2) Disposable plastic cover placed over probe.

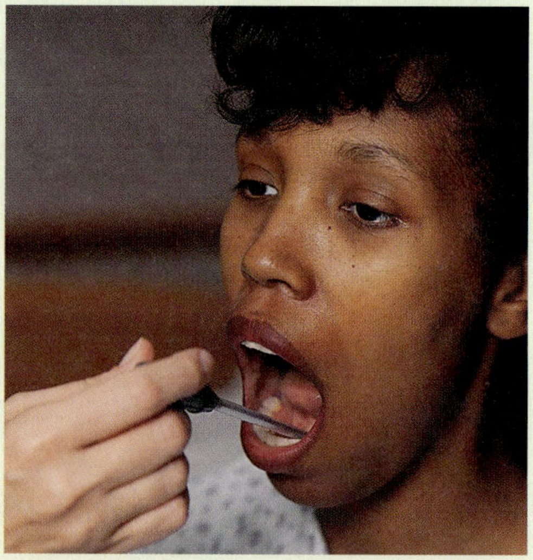

STEP 4A(3) Probe under tongue in posterior sublingual pocket.

STEP	RATIONALE
(2) Apply clean gloves. Cleanse anal region when feces and/or secretions are present. Remove soiled gloves and reapply clean gloves.	Maintains Standard Precautions when exposed to items soiled with body fluids (e.g., feces).
(3) Remove thermometer pack from charging unit. Attach rectal thermometer probe stem (red tip) to thermometer unit. Grasp top of probe stem, being careful not to apply pressure on ejection button.	Charging provides battery power. Ejection button releases plastic cover from probe stem.
(4) Slide disposable plastic probe cover over thermometer probe stem until cover locks in place.	Probe cover prevents transmission of microorganisms between patients.
(5) Squeeze liberal portion of lubricant onto tissue. Dip blunt end of thermometer probe into lubricant, covering 2.5 to 3.5 cm (1 to 1½ inch) for adult.	Lubrication minimizes trauma to rectal mucosa during insertion. Tissue avoids contamination of remaining lubricant in container.
(6) With nondominant hand, separate patient's buttocks to expose anus. Ask patient to breathe slowly and relax.	Fully exposes anus for thermometer insertion. Relaxes anal sphincter for easier thermometer insertion.
(7) Gently insert thermometer probe into anus in direction of umbilicus 2.5 to 3.5 cm (1 to 1½ inch) for adult. If resistance is felt during insertion, withdraw immediately. Do not force thermometer.	Ensures adequate exposure against blood vessels in rectal wall.

***Clinical Decision Point:* If you cannot insert thermometer into rectum adequately, remove thermometer and consider alternative method for obtaining temperature.**

STEP	RATIONALE
(8) Once positioned, hold thermometer probe in place until audible signal indicates completion and patient's temperature appears on digital display; remove thermometer probe from anus (see illustration).	Probe needs to stay in place until signal occurs to ensure accurate reading.
(9) Push ejection button on thermometer stem to discard plastic probe cover into appropriate receptacle. Wipe probe stem with alcohol swab, paying particular attention to ridges where probe stem connects to probe.	Reduces transmission of microorganisms.
(10) Return thermometer stem to storage position of recording unit.	Returning thermometer stem to storage position automatically causes digital reading to disappear. Storage position protects stem.
(11) Wipe patient's anal area with tissue or soft wipe to remove lubricant or feces and discard tissue. Help patient assume a comfortable position.	Provides for comfort and hygiene.

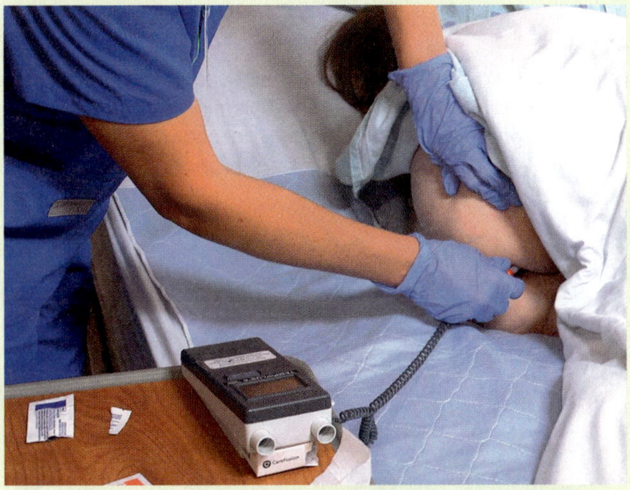

STEP 4B(8) Probe removed smoothly from anus.

SKILL 15-1 MEASURING BODY TEMPERATURE—cont'd

STEP	RATIONALE
C. Axillary Temperature Measurement With Electronic Thermometer	
(1) Draw curtain around bed and/or close room door. Help patient to supine or sitting position. Move clothing or gown away from shoulder and arm.	Maintains patient's privacy, minimizes embarrassment, and promotes comfort. Exposes axilla for correct thermometer probe placement.
(2) Remove thermometer pack from charging unit. Attach oral thermometer probe stem (blue tip) to thermometer unit. Grasp top of thermometer probe stem, being careful not to apply pressure on ejection button.	Ejection button releases plastic cover from probe.
(3) Slide disposable plastic probe cover over thermometer stem until cover locks in place.	Probe cover prevents transmission of microorganisms between patients.
(4) Raise patient's arm away from torso. Inspect for skin lesions and excessive perspiration. Insert thermometer probe into center of axilla, lower arm over probe, and place arm across patient's chest.	Maintains proper position of probe against blood vessels in axilla.

Clinical Decision Point: **Do not use axilla if skin lesions are present because local temperature may be altered and area may be painful to touch.**

STEP	RATIONALE
(5) Once positioned, hold thermometer probe in place until audible signal indicates completion and patient's temperature appears on digital display; remove thermometer probe from axilla.	Thermometer probe needs to stay in place until signal occurs to ensure accurate reading.
(6) Push ejection button on thermometer stem to discard plastic probe cover into appropriate receptacle.	Reduces transmission of microorganisms.
(7) Return thermometer stem to storage position of recording unit.	Returning thermometer stem to storage position automatically causes digital reading to disappear. Storage position protects stem.
(8) Help patient assume a comfortable position, replacing linen or gown.	Restores comfort and sense of well-being.
D. Tympanic Membrane Temperature Measurement With Infrared Thermometer	
(1) Help patient into comfortable position with head turned toward side, away from you. If patient has been lying on one side, use upper ear. Obtain temperature from patient's right ear if you are right-handed. Obtain temperature from patient's left ear if you are left-handed.	Ensures comfort and exposes auditory canal for accurate temperature measurement. Heat trapping in ear facing down causes false-high readings. Using the appropriate hand reduces the angle of approach. The less acute the angle, the better the probe seal.
(2) Note if there is obvious earwax present in patient's ear canal. If so, switch to other ear or select alternative measurement site.	Earwax on lens cover of speculum blocks a clear optical pathway. Earwax can lower tympanic temperature by 0.3°C (0.6°F).
(3) Remove thermometer handheld unit from charging base, being careful not to apply pressure to the ejection button.	Base provides battery power. Removal of handheld unit from base prepares it to measure temperature. Ejection button releases plastic probe cover from thermometer tip.
(4) Slide disposable speculum cover over otoscope-like tip until it locks into place. Be careful not to touch lens cover.	Soft plastic probe cover prevents transmission of microorganisms between patients. Lens cover must be free of dust, fingerprints, and earwax to ensure clear optical path.

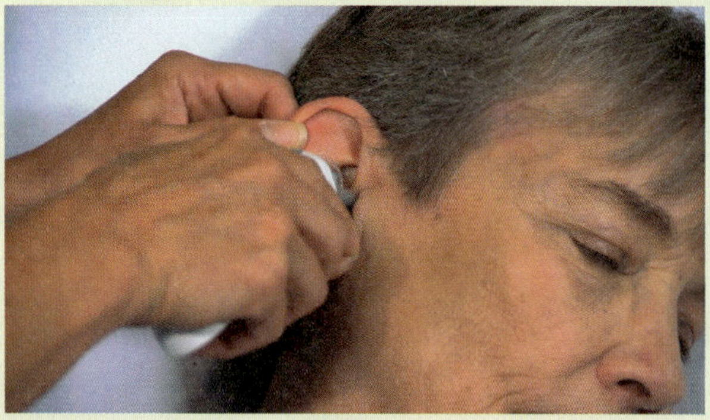

STEP 4D(5) Tympanic membrane thermometer with probe cover placed in patient's ear.

STEP	RATIONALE
(5) Insert infrared speculum into ear canal following manufacturer instructions for tympanic probe positioning (see illustration).	Correct positioning of speculum probe tip with respect to ear canal allows maximum exposure of tympanic membrane.
(6) For children younger than 3 years of age, point covered probe toward midpoint between eyebrow and sideburns.	Ear tug straightens external auditory canal, allowing maximum exposure of tympanic membrane.
(7) Fit speculum tip snugly into canal and do not move, pointing speculum tip toward nose.	Gentle pressure seals ear canal from ambient air temperature, which alters readings as much as 2.8° C (5° F). Operator error leads to false-low temperature readings.
(8) Once positioned, press scan button on handheld unit. Leave speculum in place until audible signal indicates completion and patient's temperature appears on digital display.	Pressing scan button causes detection of infrared energy. Speculum probe tip needs to stay in place until signal indicating device has detected infrared energy.
(9) Carefully remove speculum from auditory canal.	Prevents rubbing of sensitive outer ear lining.
(10) Push ejection button on handheld unit to discard speculum cover into appropriate receptacle.	Reduces transmission of microorganisms. Automatically causes digital reading to disappear.
(11) If temperature is abnormal or second reading is necessary, replace speculum cover and wait 2 to 3 minutes before repeating measurement in same ear or repeat measurement in other ear. Consider trying an alternative temperature site or instrument.	Time allows ear canal to regain usual temperature readings.
(12) Return handheld unit to thermometer base.	Protects sensor tip from damage.
(13) Help patient back to comfortable position.	Restores comfort and sense of well-being.
E. **Temporal Artery Temperature Measurement With Infrared Thermometer**	
(1) Ensure that forehead is dry; wipe with towel if needed.	Thermometer sensor is distorted by moist skin.
(2) Place sensor flush on patient's forehead.	Contact avoids measurement of ambient temperature.
(3) Press red scan button with your thumb. Slowly slide thermometer straight across forehead while keeping sensor flush on skin (see Figure 15-3).	Continuous scanning for highest temperature continues until you release scan button.
(4) Keeping scan button pressed, lift sensor from forehead and touch it to skin on neck, just behind earlobe. Peak temperature occurs when clicking sound during scanning stops. Read digital display; release scan button.	Sensor confirms highest temperature behind earlobe.
(5) Clean sensor with alcohol swab.	Prevents transmission of microorganisms.
5. If gloves worn, remove and dispose of in appropriate receptacle. Perform hand hygiene.	Reduces transmission of microorganisms.
6. Return thermometer to charger or thermometer base.	Maintains battery charge of thermometer unit.
7. Inform patient of temperature reading and document measurement.	Promotes participation in care and understanding of health status.
EVALUATION	
1. If you are assessing temperature for the first time, establish temperature as baseline if it is within acceptable range.	Used to compare future temperature measurements.
2. Compare temperature reading with patient's previous temperature and acceptable temperature range for patient's age-group.	Body temperature fluctuates within narrow range; comparison reveals presence of abnormality. Improper placement or movement of thermometer causes inaccuracies.
3. If patient has fever, take temperature approximately 30 minutes after administering antipyretics and every 4 hours until temperature stabilizes.	Determines if temperature begins to fall in response to therapy.
4. Use Teach Back—State to the patient, "I want to be sure I explained to you clearly the factors that can influence body temperature and ways to prevent your temperature from going too high or too low. Can you tell me what you could do to reduce your temperature on a hot day?" Revise your instruction now or develop plan for revised patient teaching to be implemented at an appropriate time if patient is not able to teach back correctly.	Evaluates what the patient is able to explain or demonstrate.

SKILL 15-1 MEASURING BODY TEMPERATURE—cont'd

RECORDING AND REPORTING

- Record temperature and route in nurses' notes, vital sign flow sheet, or electronic medical record. Record in nurses' notes any signs or symptoms of temperature alterations.
- Document measurement of temperature after administration of specific therapies in narrative form in nurses' notes.
- Document your evaluation of patient learning.
- Report abnormal findings to nurse in charge or health care provider immediately.

UNEXPECTED OUTCOMES AND RELATED INTERVENTIONS

- Temperature is 1°C or more *above* usual range.
  - Assess possible sites for localized infection and for related data suggesting systemic infection.
  - Follow interventions listed in Box 15-3.
  - If fever persists or reaches unacceptable level as defined by health care provider, administer antipyretics as ordered.
- Temperature is 1°C or more *below* usual range.
  - Initiate measures to increase body temperature.
  - Remove any wet clothing or linen and cover patient with warm blankets.
  - Monitor apical pulse rate and rhythm (see Skill 15-2) because hypothermia causes bradycardia and dysrhythmias.

SKILL 15-2 ASSESSING THE RADIAL AND APICAL PULSES

View Video!

DELEGATION CONSIDERATIONS

The skill of pulse measurement can be delegated to nursing assistive personnel (NAP) if the patient is stable and not at high risk for acute or serious cardiac problems. The nurse instructs the NAP to:

- Consider factors related to the patient's history, usual values, or risk for abnormally slow or irregular pulse.
- Obtain appropriate pulse measurement frequency at appropriate times as determined by agency policy, health care provider's orders, or patient condition such as the presence of chest pain or dizziness.
- Immediately report any changes or abnormalities to the nurse.

EQUIPMENT

- Wristwatch with second hand or digital display
- Pen, pencil, vital sign flow sheet or record or patient's electronic medical record
- Stethoscope (apical pulse only)
- Alcohol swab

STEP	RATIONALE
ASSESSMENT	
1. Determine need to obtain radial and/or apical pulse:	
a. Assess risk factors for pulse alterations. • History of heart disease • Cardiac dysrhythmia • Onset of sudden chest pain or acute pain from any site • Invasive cardiovascular diagnostic tests • Surgery • Sudden infusion of large volume of intravenous (IV) fluid • Internal or external hemorrhage, dehydration • Medications that alter cardiac function (e.g., antiarrhythmics, antihypertensives, vasodilators, and vasoconstrictors)	These conditions place patients at risk for pulse alterations. A history of peripheral vascular disease often alters pulse rate and quality.
b. Assess for signs and symptoms of altered cardiac function: dyspnea, fatigue, chest pain, orthopnea, syncope, palpitations (person's unpleasant awareness of heartbeat), dependent edema, cyanosis or pallor of skin (see Chapter 30).	Physical signs and symptoms indicate alteration in cardiac function, which affects pulse rate and rhythm.
c. Assess for signs and symptoms of peripheral vascular disease: pale, cool extremities; thin, shiny skin with decreased hair growth; thickened nails.	Physical signs and symptoms indicate alteration in local arterial blood flow.

STEP	RATIONALE
2. Assess for factors influencing pulse rate and rhythm: age, exercise, recent caffeine or nicotine intake, position changes, fluid balance, medications, temperature, sympathetic stimulation from stress (e.g., fear or anxiety).	Allows you to accurately assess presence and significance of pulse alterations. Acceptable range of pulse rate changes with age (see Table 15-3). Caffeine and nicotine increase pulse rate. Pulse rate is increased immediately by smoking; this lasts as long as 15 minutes (NHBPEP, 2004).
3. Assess pertinent laboratory values, including serum potassium and complete blood count (CBC).	Low values for hemoglobin are associated with decreased oxygen transport, which can increase pulse rate. Low potassium or high potassium can cause arrhythmias.
4. Determine patient's previous baseline pulse rate (if available) from patient's record.	Allows you to assess for change in condition. Provides comparison with future pulse measurements.
5. Determine if patient has latex allergy.	If patient has latex allergy, verify that stethoscope is latex-free.
PLANNING	
1. Identify patient using two identifiers (e.g., name and birthday or name and account number) according to agency policy.	Ensures correct patient. Complies with The Joint Commission requirements for patient safety (TJC, 2014).
2. Explain to patient that you will assess pulse or heart rate. Encourage him or her to relax and not speak. If patient has been active, wait 5 to 10 minutes before assessing pulse.	Activity and anxiety elevate heart rate. Patient's voice interferes with ability to hear sound when measuring apical pulse. Obtaining pulse rates at rest allows for objective comparison of values.
IMPLEMENTATION	
1. Perform hand hygiene.	Reduces transmission of microorganisms.
2. Draw curtain around bed and/or close door.	Maintains privacy.
3. Obtain pulse measurement.	
A. **Radial Pulse:**	
(1) Help patient into supine or sitting position.	Provides easy access to pulse sites.
(2) If supine, place patient's forearm straight alongside or across lower chest or upper abdomen with wrist extended straight (see illustration). If sitting, bend patient's elbow 90 degrees and support lower arm on chair or on your arm.	Relaxed position of lower arm and extension of wrist permit full exposure of artery to palpation.
(3) Place tips of first two or middle three fingers over groove along radial or thumb side of patient's inner wrist (see illustration). Slightly extend wrist with palm down until strongest pulse is felt.	Fingertips are most sensitive parts of hand to palpate arterial pulsation. Thumb has pulsation that interferes with accuracy.
(4) Lightly compress against radius, obliterate pulse initially, and relax pressure so pulse becomes easily palpable.	Pulse is more accurate with moderate pressure. Too much pressure occludes pulse and impairs blood flow.
(5) Determine strength of pulse. Note whether thrust of vessel against fingertips is bounding (+4); full/strong (+3), normal/expected (+2); diminished or barely palpable (+1); or absent (0).	Strength reflects volume of blood ejected against arterial wall with each heart contraction. Accurate description of strength improves communication among nurses and other health care providers.

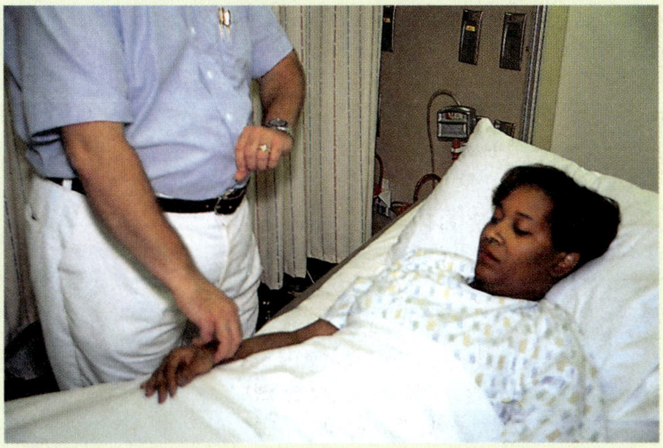

STEP 3A(2) Pulse check with patient's forearm at side with wrist extended.

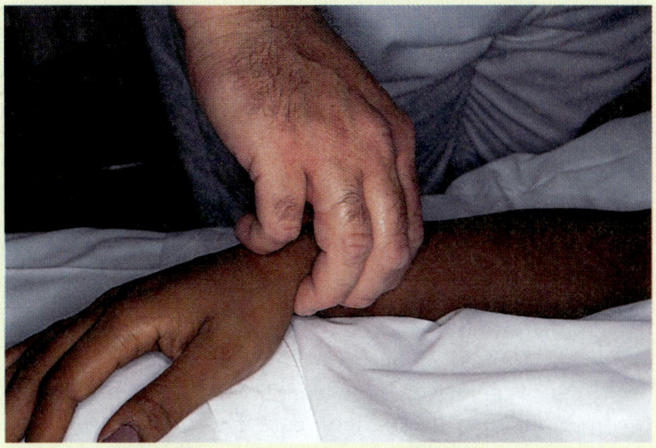

STEP 3A(3) Hand placement for pulse checks.

SKILL 15-2 ASSESSING THE RADIAL AND APICAL PULSES—cont'd

STEP	RATIONALE
(6) After feeling pulse, look at second hand of watch and begin to count rate: when sweep hand hits number on dial, start counting with zero, one, two, and so on.	Rate is accurate only after making sure that pulse can be palpated. Timing begins with zero. Count of one is first beat palpated after timing begins.
(7) If pulse is regular, count rate for 30 seconds and multiply total by 2.	A 30-second count is accurate for rapid, slow, or regular pulse rates.
(8) If pulse is irregular, count rate for 60 seconds. Assess frequency and pattern of irregularity.	Inefficient contraction of heart fails to transmit pulse wave, resulting in irregular pulse. Longer time period promotes accurate count.
(9) When pulse is irregular, compare radial pulses bilaterally.	Marked inequality indicates compromised arterial flow to one extremity, and you need to take action.

Clinical Decision Point: **If pulse is irregular, assess for pulse deficit. Count apical pulse (Step 3B) while a colleague counts radial pulse. Begin pulse count by calling out loud simultaneously when to begin measuring pulses. If pulse count differs by more than 2, a pulse deficit exists, which sometimes indicates alterations in cardiac function.**

STEP	RATIONALE
B. **Apical Pulse:**	
(1) Clean earpieces and diaphragm of stethoscope with alcohol swab. Perform hand hygiene.	Reduces transmission of microorganisms.
(2) Draw curtain around bed and/or close door.	Maintains privacy and minimizes embarrassment.
(3) Help patient to supine or sitting position. Move bed linen and gown to uncover sternum and left side of chest.	Exposes portion of chest wall for selection of auscultatory site.
(4) Locate anatomical landmarks for identifying apical impulse ([point of maximal impulse [PMI]) (see illustrations for Step 3B[4], *A* to *D*). The heart is located behind and to left of sternum with base at top and apex at bottom. Find angle of Louis just below suprasternal notch between sternal body and manubrium (feels like a bony prominence). Slip finger down each side of angle to find second intercostal space (ICS). Carefully move fingers down left side of sternum to fifth ICS and laterally to left midclavicular line (MCL). A light tap felt within area 1 to 2 cm (½ to 1 inch) of apical impulse is reflected from apex of heart.	Using anatomical landmarks allows correct placement of stethoscope over apex of heart to auscultate heart sounds clearly. If unable to palpate apical impulse, reposition patient on left side. In presence of serious heart disease, locate apical impulse to left of MCL or at sixth ICS.
(5) Place diaphragm of stethoscope in palm of hand for 5 to 10 seconds.	Warming metal or plastic diaphragm prevents patient from being startled and promotes comfort.
(6) Place diaphragm of stethoscope over apical impulse at the fifth ICS at left MCL and auscultate for normal S_1 and S_2 heart sounds (heard as "lub-dub") (see illustrations).	Allow stethoscope tubing to extend straight without kinks so it does not distort sound transmission. Normal sounds S_1 and S_2 are high pitched and best heard with diaphragm.
(7) When you hear S_1 and S_2 with regularity, use second hand of watch or digital display and begin to count rate: when sweep hand hits number on dial, start counting with zero, then one, two, and so on.	Apical rate is accurate only after you are able to hear sounds clearly. Timing begins with zero. Count of one is first sound auscultated after timing begins.
(8) If apical rate is regular, count for 30 seconds and multiply by 2.	Assess regular apical rate for 30 seconds.

Clinical Decision Point: **If heart rate is irregular or patient is receiving cardiovascular medication, count for 1 minute (60 seconds). Irregular rate is more accurately assessed when measured over longer interval.**

STEP	RATIONALE
(9) Note if heart rate is irregular and describe pattern of irregularity (S_1 and S_2 occurring early or later after previous sequence of sounds [e.g., every third or every fourth beat is skipped]).	Irregular heart rate indicates dysrhythmia. Regular occurrence of dysrhythmia within 1 minute indicates inefficient contraction of heart and alteration in cardiac function.
(10) Replace patient's gown and bed linen; help patient return to comfortable position.	Restores comfort and promotes sense of well-being.

STEP	RATIONALE
(11) Perform hand hygiene.	Reduces transmission of microorganisms.
(12) Clean earpieces and diaphragm of stethoscope with alcohol swab routinely after each use.	Stethoscopes are frequently contaminated with microorganisms. Regular disinfection controls health care–acquired infections.
4. Discuss findings with patient as needed and document measurement.	Promotes participation in care and understanding of health status.

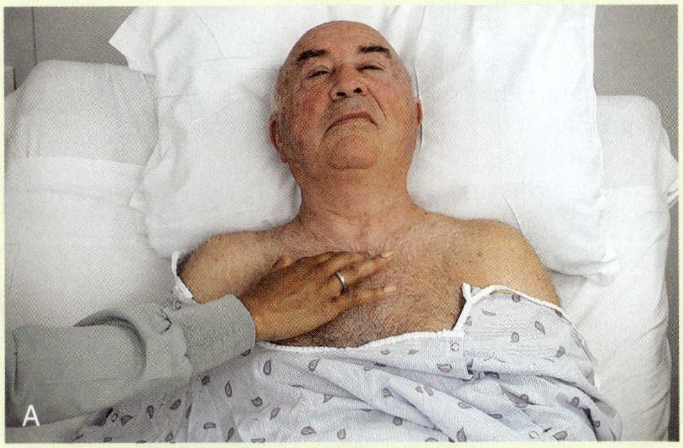

STEP 3B(4)A Locating angle of Louis.

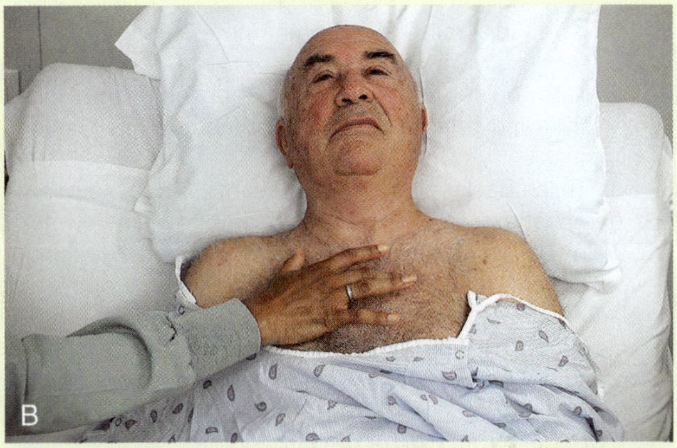

STEP 3B(4)B Locating left second intercostal space (2ICS).

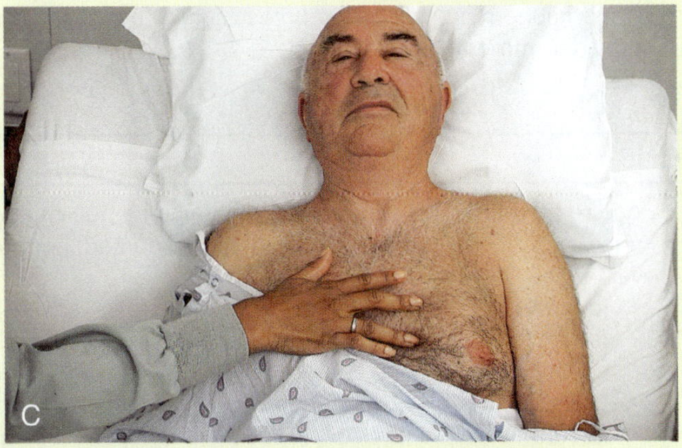

STEP 3B(4)C Moving down left side of the sternum to fifth intercostal space (5ICS).

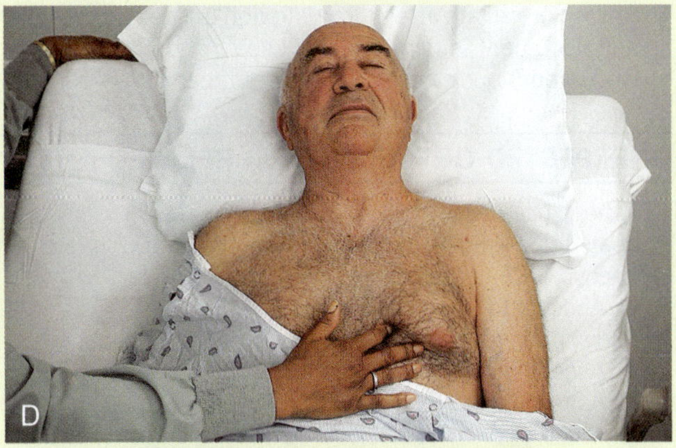

STEP 3B(4)D Locating apical impulse.

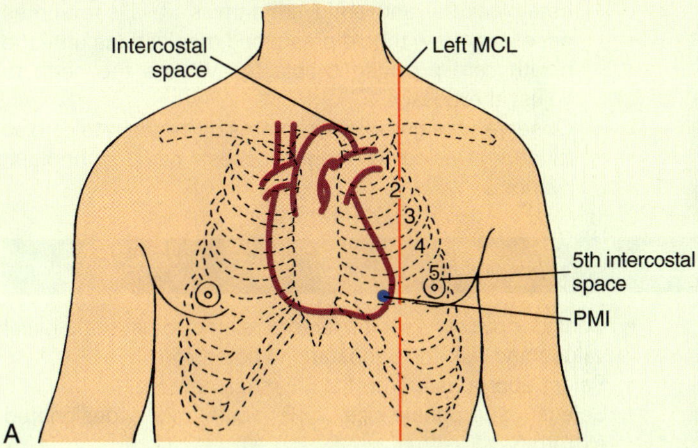

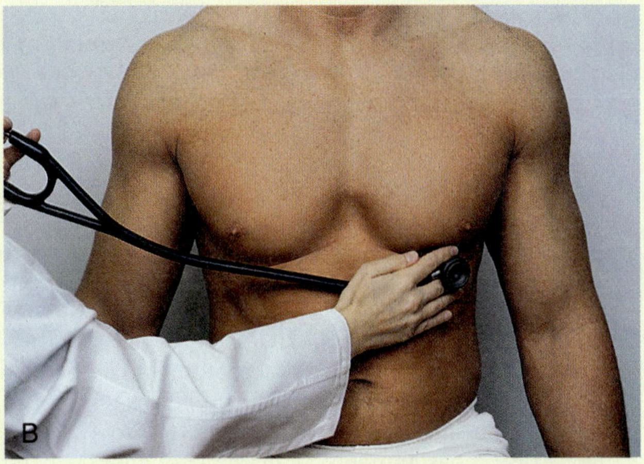

STEP 3B(6) A, Location of apical impulse in adults. **B,** Stethoscope over apical impulse.

SKILL 15-2 ASSESSING THE RADIAL AND APICAL PULSES—cont'd

STEP	RATIONALE
EVALUATION	
1. Compare readings with previous baseline and/or acceptable range of heart rate for patient's age (see Table 15-3).	Evaluates for change in condition and presence of cardiac alterations.
2. Compare peripheral pulse rate with apical rate and note any discrepancy.	Differences between measurements indicate pulse deficit and warn of cardiovascular compromise. Some abnormalities require therapy.
3. Compare radial pulse equality and note any discrepancy.	Differences between radial arteries indicate compromised peripheral vascular system.
4. Correlate pulse rate with data obtained from blood pressure and related signs and symptoms (palpitations, dizziness).	Pulse rate and blood pressure are interrelated; synthesis of information may assist in identification of an abnormality.
5. Use Teach Back—State to the patient, "I want to be sure I demonstrated and explained clearly how and when to obtain your own pulse rate. Can you show me by counting your pulse rate?" Revise your instruction now or develop plan for revised patient teaching to be implemented at an appropriate time if patient is not able to teach back correctly.	Evaluates what the patient is able to explain or demonstrate.

RECORDING AND REPORTING

- Record pulse rate and assessment site in nurses' notes, vital signs flow sheet, or electronic medical record.
- Record pulse rate after administration of specific therapies and document in narrative in nurses' notes.
- Document your evaluation of patient learning.
- Record any signs and symptoms of alteration in cardiac function in nurses' notes.
- Report abnormal findings to nurse in charge or health care provider immediately.

UNEXPECTED OUTCOMES AND RELATED INTERVENTIONS

- Patient has irregular radial pulse or a pulse less than 60 beats/min (bradycardia) or greater than 100 beats/min (tachycardia) beats per minute.
  - Auscultate the apical pulse.
- Radial pulse is weak, thready, or difficult to palpate.
  - Assess both radial pulses and compare findings.
  - Assess for swelling in surrounding tissues or other cause of decreased blood flow (e.g., dressing or cast).
  - Perform complete assessment of all peripheral pulses (see Chapter 16).
  - Observe for signs and symptoms associated with altered tissue perfusion, including pallor and cool skin temperature of tissue distal to the weak pulse.
  - Auscultate apical pulse to determine pulse rate and identify if pulse deficit exists.
  - Have a second nurse assess pulses.
- Adult patient has an apical pulse greater than 100 beats/min (tachycardia) or greater than the expected normal value (see Table 15-3).
  - Identify related data, including pain, fear, anxiety, recent exercise, hypotension, blood loss, fever, or inadequate oxygenation.
  - Observe for signs and symptoms associated with abnormal cardiac function, including fatigue, chest pain, orthopnea, cyanosis.
- Apical pulse is less than 60 beats/min (bradycardia) in an adult or less than the expected normal value (see Table 15-3).
  - Observe for factors that alter heart rate such as digoxin, beta-blockers, and antidysrhythmias; it is sometimes necessary to withhold prescribed medications until the health care provider is able to evaluate the need to adjust the dosage.
  - Observe for signs and symptoms of inadequate cardiac function, including fatigue, chest pain, orthopnea, cyanosis.

SKILL 15-3 BLOOD PRESSURE MEASUREMENT

DELEGATION CONSIDERATIONS

The skill of blood pressure (BP) measurement can be delegated to nursing assistive personnel (NAP) unless the patient is considered unstable. The nurse directs NAP to:

- Obtain BP measurements at appropriate times as determined by agency policy, health care provider's order, or patient condition.
- Consider patient-specific factors related to patient's usual values and risk for orthostatic hypotension.
- Select appropriate limb for BP measurement.
- Select appropriate-size BP cuff for designated extremity.
- Immediately report any abnormalities, which the nurse confirms.

EQUIPMENT

- Calibrated aneroid sphygmomanometer
- Cloth or disposable vinyl pressure cuff of appropriate size for patient's extremity
- Stethoscope
- Alcohol swab
- Pen, vital sign flow sheet or record, or patient's electronic medical record

STEP	RATIONALE
ASSESSMENT	
1. Assess for medical conditions that potentially may alter blood pressure: • History of cardiovascular disease • Renal disease • Diabetes • Circulatory shock (hypovolemic, septic, cardiogenic, or neurogenic) • Acute pain • Increased intracranial pressure • Postoperative conditions • Toxemia of pregnancy	Conditions place patients at risk for BP alterations.
2. Assess for signs and symptoms of BP alterations:	Physical signs and symptoms sometimes indicate alterations in BP.
• Hypertension: Assess for headache (usually occipital), flushing of face, nosebleed, and fatigue in older adults. • Hypotension: Dizziness; confusion; restlessness; pale, dusky, or cyanotic skin and mucous membranes; cool, mottled skin over extremities.	Hypertension is often asymptomatic until pressure is very high.
3. Assess for factors that influence BP (see Box 15-6).	Allows you to control for factors to measure BP accurately.
4. Determine best site for BP assessment. Avoid applying cuff to extremity when IV fluids are infusing; an arteriovenous shunt or fistula is present; breast or axillary surgery has been performed on that side; extremity has been traumatized or diseased or requires a cast or bulky bandage. Use lower extremities when brachial arteries are inaccessible.	Inappropriate site selection results in poor amplification of sounds, causing inaccurate readings. Application of pressure from inflated bladder temporarily impairs blood flow and further compromises circulation in extremity that already has impaired blood flow.
5. Determine previous baseline BP (if available) from patient's record. Determine if patient has a latex allergy.	Allows you to assess for change in condition. Provides comparison with future BP measurements. If patient has latex allergy, verify that stethoscope and BP cuff are latex free.
PLANNING	
1. Communicate with patient about assessing BP. Have patient rest at least 5 minutes before measuring lying or sitting BP and 1 minute when standing (NHBPEP, 2004). Ask patient not to speak while measuring BP.	Reduces anxiety, which can falsely elevate readings. BP readings taken at different times are more objective to compare when assessed with patient always at rest. Exercise causes false elevations in BP. A recent study found systolic and diastolic pressure increased during talking by 5 and 6 mm Hg compared with the resting measurement (Zheng et al., 2012).
2. Be sure that patient has not ingested caffeine or smoked for 30 minutes before BP assessment (NHBPEP, 2004).	Caffeine or nicotine causes false elevations in BP. Smoking increases BP immediately and lasts up to 15 minutes. Caffeine increases BP up to 3 hours.
3. Have patient assume sitting position with feet flat on the floor. Be sure that room is warm, quiet, and relaxing.	Maintains patient's comfort during measurement. Sitting is preferred to lying. Leg crossing at knee increases systolic and diastolic BP. Patient's perceptions that physical or interpersonal environment is stressful affect BP measurement. Talking and background noise result in inaccurate readings (Ogedegbe and Pickering, 2010).
4. Select cuff of appropriate size.	Improper cuff size results in inaccurate readings (see Table 15-7). If cuff is too small, it tends to come loose as it is inflated or results in false-high readings. If the cuff is too large, false-low readings result.
5. Clean stethoscope earpieces and diaphragm with alcohol swab. Perform hand hygiene.	Reduces transmission of microorganisms.

SKILL 15-3 BLOOD PRESSURE MEASUREMENT—cont'd

STEP	RATIONALE
IMPLEMENTATION	
1. Identify patient using two identifiers (e.g., name and birthday or name and account number) according to agency policy.	Ensures correct patient. Complies with The Joint Commission requirements for patient safety (TJC, 2014).
2. Perform hand hygiene.	Reduces transmission of microorganisms.
3. Assess BP by auscultation. With patient sitting or lying, position patient's forearm, supported with a pillow (if needed) so it is at heart level, with palm turned up (see illustration); for thigh, position with knee slightly flexed. If sitting, instruct patient to keep feet flat on floor without legs crossed. If supine, support patient's arm with pillow so cuff is at level of right atrium.	If arm is extended and not supported, patient performs isometric exercise that increases diastolic pressure. Placement of arm above level of heart causes false-low reading 2 mm Hg for each inch above heart level (Ogedegbe and Pickering, 2010). Even in the supine position, a diastolic pressure effect up to 3 to 4 mm Hg occurs for each 5 cm change in heart level. If the arm is resting on the bed, it will be below heart level. For this reason, when measurements are taken in the supine position the arm should be supported with a pillow (Pickering et al., 2005). Crossing the legs may raise systolic pressure by 2 to 8 mm Hg (Pickering et al., 2005).
4. Expose extremity (arm or leg) fully by removing constricting clothing. A sleeve should not be rolled up such that it has a tourniquet effect above the blood pressure cuff (Pickering et al., 2005). Do not place BP cuff over clothing.	Ensures proper cuff application.
5. Palpate brachial artery (arm) or popliteal artery (leg). With cuff fully deflated, apply bladder of cuff above artery by centering arrows marked on cuff over artery. If there are no center arrows on cuff, estimate center of bladder and place this center over artery. Position lower end of cuff 2.5 cm (1 inch) above site of pulsation (antecubital or popliteal space). With cuff fully deflated, wrap it evenly and snugly around extremity (see illustrations).	Inflating bladder directly over artery ensures that proper pressure is applied during inflation. Loose-fitting cuff causes false-high readings. . Allows room for placement of the stethoscope.
6. Position manometer vertically at eye level. Make sure that observer is no farther than 1 m (approximately 1 yard) away.	Looking up or down at scale results in inaccurate readings.

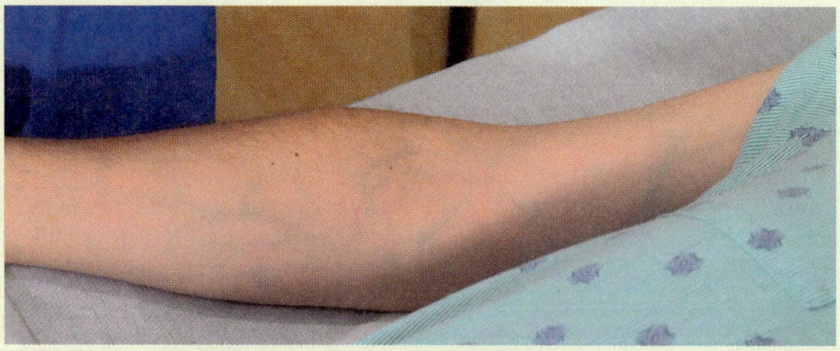

STEP 3 Patient's forearm supported on bed.

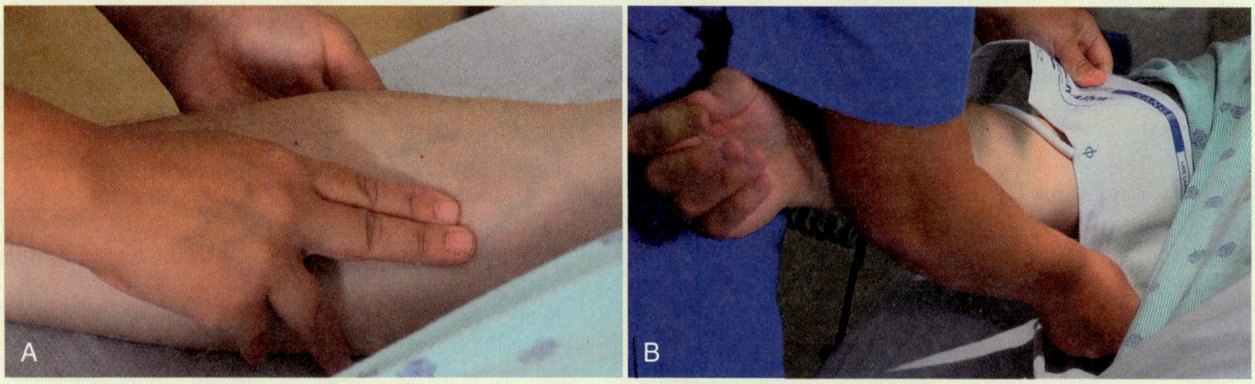

STEP 5 **A,** Palpate patient's brachial artery. **B,** Center bladder of cuff above artery.

STEP	RATIONALE
7. Measure BP.	
A. Two-Step Method:	
(1) Relocate pulse. Palpate artery distal to cuff with fingertips of nondominant hand while inflating cuff rapidly to pressure 30 mm Hg above point at which pulse disappears. Slowly deflate cuff and note point when pulse reappears. Deflate cuff fully and wait 30 seconds.	Estimating systolic pressure prevents false-low readings, which result in presence of auscultatory gap. Palpation determines maximal inflation point for accurate reading. If unable to palpate artery because of weakened pulse, use ultrasonic stethoscope (see Chapter 16). Completely deflating cuff prevents venous congestion and false-high readings.
(2) Place stethoscope earpieces in ears and be sure that sounds are clear, not muffled.	Ensures that each earpiece follows angle of ear canal to facilitate hearing.
(3) Relocate artery and place bell or diaphragm of stethoscope over it. Do not allow chest piece to touch cuff or clothing (see illustration).	Proper stethoscope placement ensures best sound reception. Bell provides better sound reproduction, whereas diaphragm is easier to secure with fingers and covers larger area. Stethoscope improperly positioned causes muffled sounds that often result in false-low systolic and false-high diastolic readings.
(4) Close valve of pressure bulb clockwise until tight.	Tightening valve prevents air leak during inflation.
(5) Quickly inflate cuff to 30 mm Hg above patient's estimated systolic pressure (see illustration).	Rapid inflation ensures accurate measurement of systolic pressure.
(6) Slowly release pressure bulb valve and allow manometer needle gauge to fall at rate of 2 to 3 mm Hg per second.	Too-rapid or too-slow decline in pressure release causes inaccurate readings.
(7) Note point on manometer when you hear first clear sound. The sound slowly increases in intensity.	First Korotkoff sound reflects systolic BP.
(8) Continue to deflate cuff gradually, noting point at which sound disappears in adults. Note pressure to nearest 2 mm Hg. Listen for 20 to 30 mm Hg after last sound and allow remaining air to escape quickly.	Fourth Korotkoff sound involves distinct muffling and is indication of diastolic pressure in children. Beginning of fifth Korotkoff sound is indication of diastolic pressure in adults (NHBPEP, 2004; Pickering et al., 2005).
B. One-Step Method:	
(1) Place stethoscope earpieces in ears and be sure that sounds are clear, not muffled.	Earpiece should follow angle of ear canal to facilitate hearing.
(2) Relocate artery and place diaphragm of stethoscope over it. Do not allow chest piece to touch cuff or clothing.	Proper stethoscope placement ensures optimal sound reception.
(3) Close valve of pressure bulb clockwise until tight.	Tightening valve prevents air leak during inflation.
(4) Quickly inflate cuff to 30 mm Hg above patient's usual systolic pressure.	Inflation above systolic level ensures accurate measurement of systolic pressure.
(5) Slowly release pressure bulb valve and allow manometer needle to fall at rate of 2 to 3 mm Hg per second. Note point on manometer when you hear first clear sound. The sound slowly increases in intensity.	Too-rapid or too-slow decline in pressure release causes inaccurate readings. First Korotkoff sounds reflect systolic pressure.
(6) Continue to deflate cuff gradually, noting point at which sound disappears in adults. Note pressure to nearest 2 mm Hg. Listen for 20 to 30 mm Hg after last sound and allow remaining air to escape quickly.	Fourth Korotkoff sound is indication of diastolic pressure in children. Beginning of fifth Korotkoff sound is indication of diastolic adult pressure (NHBPEP, 2004; Pickering et al., 2005).

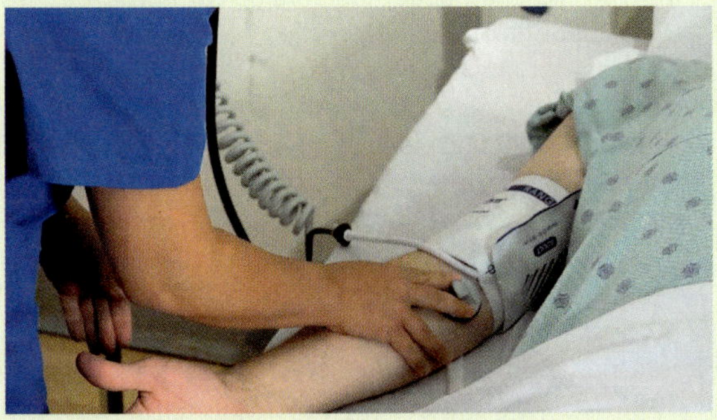

STEP 7A(3) Stethoscope placed over brachial artery to measure blood pressure.

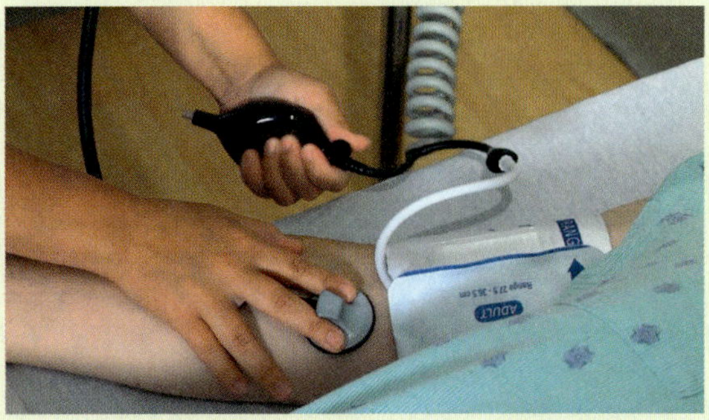

STEP 7A(5) Inflate the blood pressure cuff.

SKILL 15-3 BLOOD PRESSURE MEASUREMENT—cont'd

STEP	RATIONALE
8. The American Heart Association recommends average of two sets of BP measurements 2 minutes apart. Use second set as patient's baseline.	Two sets of BP measurements help to prevent false positives based on a patient's sympathetic response (alert reaction). Averaging minimizes effect of anxiety, which often causes first reading to be higher than subsequent measurements (NHBPEP, 2004; Pickering et al., 2005).
9. Remove cuff from patient's extremity unless you need to repeat measurement. If this is first assessment of patient, repeat procedure on other extremity.	Comparison of BP in both extremities detects circulatory problems. (Normal difference of 5 to 10 mm Hg exists between extremities.)
10. Help patient return to comfortable position and cover arm or leg if previously clothed.	Restores comfort and promotes sense of well-being.
11. Discuss findings with patient as needed.	Promotes participation in care and understanding of health status. Makes patient accountable for follow-up assessment.
12. Clean earpieces, bell, and diaphragm of stethoscope with alcohol swab. Perform hand hygiene.	Reduces transmission of microorganisms from patient to patient and nurse to patient.
EVALUATION	
1. Compare reading with previous baseline and/or acceptable value of BP for patient's age.	Evaluates for change in condition and alterations.
2. Compare BP in both arms or both legs.	If using upper extremities, use arm with higher pressure for subsequent assessments unless contraindicated.
3. Correlate BP with data obtained from pulse assessment and related cardiovascular signs and symptoms (e.g., dizziness, chest pain or excess fatigue).	BP and heart rate are interrelated.
4. Use Teach Back: State to the patient "I want to be sure I explained clearly the factors that increase blood pressure and ways you can reduce your personal risk. Can you tell me what ways you can reduce your risk of high blood pressure?" Revise your instruction now or develop plan for revised patient teaching to be implemented at an appropriate time if patient is not able to teach back correctly.	Evaluates what the patient is able to explain or demonstrate.

RECORDING AND REPORTING

- Record BP and site assessed on vital sign flow sheet, nurses' notes, or patient's electronic medical record.
- Record any signs and symptoms of BP alterations in narrative form in nurses' notes.
- Document measurement of BP after administration of specific therapies in narrative form in nurses' notes.
- Document your evaluation of patient learning.
- Report abnormal findings to nurse in charge or health care provider immediately.

UNEXPECTED OUTCOMES AND RELATED INTERVENTIONS

- Unable to obtain BP reading.
  - Determine presence of signs and symptoms of altered cardiac function; if present, notify nurse in charge or health care provider.
  - Use alternative sites or procedures to obtain BP: auscultate BP in different extremity, use ultrasonic stethoscope, implement palpation method to obtain systolic BP.
  - Repeat any electronic BP measurement with sphygmomanometer. Electronic BP measurements are less accurate in low blood flow conditions.
- BP is above acceptable range.
  - Repeat BP measurement in other extremity and compare findings.
  - Observe for related symptoms, although symptoms are sometimes not apparent until BP is extremely elevated.
  - Report elevated BP to nurse in charge or health care provider to initiate appropriate evaluation and treatment.
- BP is not sufficient for adequate perfusion and oxygenation of tissues.
  - Compare BP value to baseline. A systolic reading of 90 mm Hg is an acceptable value for some patients.
  - Place patient in supine position to enhance circulation and restrict activity that may decrease BP further.
  - Assess for signs and symptoms associated with hypotension, including tachycardia; weak, thready pulse; weakness; dizziness; confusion; cool, pale dusky, or cyanotic skin. Assess for factors that would contribute to a low BP, including hemorrhage and dilation of blood vessels resulting from hypothermia, anesthesia, or medication side effects.
- Patient has a difference of more than 20 mm Hg systolic or diastolic when comparing BP measurements on upper extremities.
  - Report abnormal findings to nurse in charge or health care provider.

SKILL 15-4 ASSESSING RESPIRATION

View Video!

DELEGATION CONSIDERATIONS

The skill of respiration assessment can be delegated to nursing assistive personnel (NAP) unless the patient is considered unstable. The nurse instructs the NAP to:

- Obtain respiration measurements at appropriate times as determined by agency policy, health care provider's order, or patient condition such as onset of labored breathing or complaints of breathing difficulty.
- Consider specific patient factors related to history or risk for increased or decreased respiratory rate or irregular respiration.
- Immediately report any confirmed abnormalities in respiratory rate or rhythm.

EQUIPMENT

- Wristwatch with second hand or digital display
- Pen, pencil, vital sign flow sheet, or patient's medical record

STEP	RATIONALE
ASSESSMENT	
1. Assess for conditions that increase risk for respiratory alterations: • Fever • Pain and anxiety • Diseases of chest wall or muscles • Constrictive chest or abdominal dressings • Presence of abdominal incisions • Gastric distention • Chronic pulmonary disease (emphysema, bronchitis, asthma) • Traumatic injury to chest wall • Presence of a chest tube • Respiratory infection (pneumonia, acute bronchitis) • Pulmonary edema and emboli	Conditions that place patient at risk for respiratory/ventilatory alterations are detected by changes in respiratory rate, depth, and rhythm; head injury with damage to brainstem; and anemia.
2. Assess for signs and symptoms of respiratory alterations: restlessness; irritability; confusion; reduced level of consciousness; pain during inspiration; labored or difficult breathing; orthopnea; use of accessory muscles; adventitious breath sounds; bluish or cyanotic appearance of nail beds, lips, mucous membranes, and skin (see Chapter 16); inability to breathe spontaneously; thick, frothy, blood-tinged, or large amounts of sputum produced on coughing.	Physical signs and symptoms that indicate alterations in respiratory status and/or ventilation.
3. Assess pertinent laboratory values (if available):	
a. Arterial blood gases (ABGs) (values vary slightly within institutions). Normal values are: • pH 7.35 to 7.45 • $PaCO_2$ 35 to 45 mm Hg • Hg PaO_2 80 to 100 mm Hg • SaO_2 95% to 100%	Arterial blood gases measure arterial blood pH, partial pressure of O_2 and CO_2, and arterial O_2 saturation, which reflect patient's oxygenation status.
b. Pulse oximetry (SpO_2): Usual value of SpO_2 95% to 100%; value less than 90% is considered hypoxemia; values below 90% are acceptable only in certain chronic disease conditions.	SpO_2 less than 90% is often accompanied by changes in respiratory rate, depth, and rhythm.
c. Complete blood count (CBC): Normal CBC for adults (values may vary within institutions): hemoglobin: 14 to 18 g/100 mL, males; 12 to 16 g/100 mL, females; hematocrit: 42% to 52%, males; 37% to 47%, females; red blood cell count: 4.7 to 6.1 million/mm^3, males; 4.2 to 5.4 million/mm^3, females (Pagana and Pagana, 2011).	CBC measures red blood cell count; volume of red blood cells; and concentration of hemoglobin, which reflects patient's blood capacity to carry O_2.
4. Assess for factors that influence respirations (see Box 15-11).	Allows you to control for factors that might alter findings.
5. Determine previous baseline respiratory rate (if available) from patient's record.	Allows you to assess for change in condition. Provides value for comparison with future respiratory measurements.
6. Assess respirations after measuring pulse in adult.	Inconspicuous assessment of respirations immediately after pulse assessment prevents patient from consciously or unintentionally altering rate and depth of breathing.

SKILL 15-4 ASSESSING RESPIRATION—cont'd

STEP	RATIONALE
PLANNING	
1. Assist patient to comfortable position, preferably sitting or lying with head of bed elevated 45 to 60 degrees. If patient has been active, wait 5 to 10 minutes before assessing respirations.	Sitting erect promotes full ventilatory movement. Position of discomfort causes patient to breathe more rapidly. Exercise increases respiratory rate and depth. Assessing respirations while patient rests allows for objective comparison of values.

Clinical Decision Point: **Assess patients with difficulty breathing (dyspnea) such as those with heart failure or abdominal ascites or in late stages of pregnancy in the position of greatest comfort. Repositioning increases the work of breathing, which increases respiratory rate.**

STEP	RATIONALE
IMPLEMENTATION	
1. Identify patient using two identifiers (e.g., name and birthday or name and account number) according to agency policy.	Ensures correct patient. Complies with The Joint Commission requirements for patient safety (TJC, 2014).
2. Draw curtain around bed and/or close door. Perform hand hygiene.	Maintains privacy. Prevents transmission of microorganisms.
3. Be sure that patient's chest is visible. If necessary move bed linen or gown.	Ensures clear view of chest wall and abdominal movements.
4. Place patient's arm in relaxed position across abdomen or lower chest or place your hand directly over patient's upper abdomen.	A similar position used during pulse assessment allows you to assess respiratory rate subtly. Patient's hand or your hand rises and falls during respiratory cycle.
5. Observe complete respiratory cycle (one inspiration and one expiration).	You determine an accurate rate only after viewing the entire respiratory cycle.
6. After observing cycle, look at second hand of watch and begin to count rate: when sweep hand hits number on dial, begin time frame, counting one with first full respiratory cycle.	Timing begins with count of one. Respirations occur more slowly than pulse; thus timing does not begin with zero.
7. If rhythm is regular, count number of respirations in 30 seconds and multiply by 2. If rhythm is irregular, less than 12, or greater than 20, count for 1 full minute.	Respiratory rate is equivalent to number of respirations per minute. Suspected irregularities require assessment for at least 1 minute.
8. Note depth of respirations, subjectively assessed by observing degree of chest wall movement while counting rate. Also assess depth by palpating chest wall excursion (see Chapter 16) after counting rate. Describe depth as shallow, normal, or deep.	Character of ventilatory movement reveals specific disease state that is restricting volume of air moving into and out of the lungs.
9. Note rhythm of ventilatory cycle. Normal breathing is regular and uninterrupted. Do not confuse sighing with abnormal rhythm.	Character of ventilations reveals specific types of alterations. Periodically people unconsciously take single deep breaths or sighs to expand small airways prone to collapse.

Clinical Decision Point: **An irregular respiratory pattern or occurrence of periods of apnea (cessation of respiration for several seconds) is a symptom of underlying disease in the adult; you need to report this finding to the nurse in charge or health care provider immediately. The patient requires further assessment (see Chapter 30) and immediate intervention. An irregular respiratory rate and short apneic spells are normal for newborns.**

STEP	RATIONALE
10. Replace bed linen and patient's gown.	Restores comfort and promotes sense of well-being.
11. Perform hand hygiene.	Reduces transmission of microorganisms.
12. Discuss findings with patient as needed.	Promotes participation in care and understanding of health status.
EVALUATION	
1. If assessing respirations for first time, establish rate, rhythm, and depth as baseline if within acceptable range.	Used to compare future respiratory assessment.
2. Compare respiration with patient's previous baseline and usual rate, rhythm, and depth.	Allows you to assess for changes in patient's condition and for presence of respiratory alterations.
3. Correlate respiratory rate, depth, and rhythm with data obtained from pulse oximetry (see Skill 15-5) and arterial blood gas measurements if available.	Ventilation, perfusion, and diffusion are interrelated.

RECORDING AND REPORTING

- Record respiratory rate and character in nurses' notes, vital sign flow sheet, or electronic medical record.
- Record abnormal depth and rhythm in narrative form in nurses' notes.
- Document measurement of respiratory rate after administration of specific therapies in narrative form in nurses' notes.
- Document type and amount of oxygen therapy if used by patient during assessment.
- Report abnormal findings to nurse in charge or health care provider immediately.

UNEXPECTED OUTCOMES AND RELATED INTERVENTIONS

- Respiratory rate is below 12 (bradypnea) or above 20 (tachypnea). Breathing pattern is irregular. Depth of respirations may be increased or decreased; patient complains of feeling short of breath.
  - Observe for related factors, including obstructed airway, noisy respirations, cyanosis, restlessness, irritability, confusion, productive cough, use of accessory muscles, and abnormal breath sounds (see Chapter 16).
  - Help patient to supported sitting position (semi-Fowler's or high-Fowler's) unless contraindicated.
  - Provide oxygen as ordered (see Chapter 30).
  - Assess for environmental factors that influence patient's respiratory rate such as secondhand smoke, poor ventilation, or gas fumes.

SKILL 15-5 MEASURING OXYGEN SATURATION (PULSE OXIMETRY)

View Video!

DELEGATION CONSIDERATIONS

The skill of oxygen saturation measurement can be delegated to nursing assistive personnel (NAP) unless patient is unstable. The nurse instructs the NAP to:

- Obtain oxygen saturation measurements at appropriate times as determined by agency policy, health care provider's order, or patient condition such as onset of labored breathing or cyanosis.
- Select appropriate sensor site, probe, and patient position for measurement of oxygen saturation.
- Immediately report any reading lower than 90%, which the nurse needs to confirm.
- Refrain from using pulse oximetry as an assessment of heart rate because the oximeter does not detect an irregular pulse.

EQUIPMENT

- Oximeter
- Oximeter probe appropriate for patient and recommended by oximeter manufacturer
- Acetone or nail polish remover if needed
- Pen, vital sign flow sheet, or record or patient's medical record

STEP	RATIONALE
ASSESSMENT	
1. Assess for conditions that decrease oxygen saturation: acute or chronic compromised respiratory function, recovery from general anesthesia or conscious sedation, traumatic injury to chest wall with or without collapse of underlying lung tissue, ventilator dependence, and changes in supplemental oxygen therapy or activity intolerance.	Certain conditions place patients at risk for decreased oxygen saturation.
2. Assess for signs and symptoms of alterations in oxygen saturation such as altered respiratory rate, depth, or rhythm; adventitious breath sounds (see Chapter 16); restlessness; irritability; confusion; reduced level of consciousness; labored or difficult breathing; cyanotic appearance of nail beds, lips, mucous membranes, skin.	Physical signs and symptoms indicate abnormal oxygen saturation. SpO_2 generally must fall below 85% before any changes in skin color are noted.
3. Assess for factors that normally influence measurement of SpO_2 such as oxygen therapy, respiratory therapy (e.g., postural drainage and percussion), hypotension, hemoglobin level, body temperature, and medications (e.g., bronchodilators).	Allows control for factors that might alter findings and accurate assessment of oxygen saturation variations. Peripheral vasoconstriction related to hypothermia interferes with SpO_2 determination.
4. Determine previous baseline SpO_2 (if available) from patient's record.	Baseline information provides basis for comparison and assists in assessment of current status and evaluation of interventions.

SKILL 15-5 MEASURING OXYGEN SATURATION (PULSE OXIMETRY)—cont'd

STEP	RATIONALE
5. Determine most appropriate patient-specific site (e.g., finger, earlobe, bridge of nose, forehead) for sensor probe placement by measuring capillary refill (see Chapter 16). If capillary refill time is more than 2 seconds, select alternative site.	Changes in SpO_2 are reflected in circulation of finger capillary bed within 30 seconds and earlobe capillary bed within 5 to 10 seconds. Blanch times that are greater than 2 seconds may indicate (U.S. National Library of Medicine, 2013): • Dehydration • Shock • Peripheral vascular disease (PVD) • Hypothermia
a. Site must have adequate local circulation and be free of moisture.	Finger and earlobe sensors require pulsating vascular bed to identify hemoglobin molecules that absorb emitted light. Moisture impedes ability of sensor to detect SpO_2 levels.
b. Determine if nails are polished.	Research shows that nail polish can falsely lower SpO_2 (Cicek et al., 2010).
c. If patient has tremors or is likely to move, use earlobe or forehead.	Motion artifact is common cause of inaccurate readings.
d. If patient is obese, clip-on probe may not fit properly; obtain disposable (tape-on) sensor.	
6. Determine if patient has latex allergy.	If patient has latex sensitivity or latex allergy, do not use adhesive sensors.
PLANNING	
1. Obtain oximeter and appropriate probe for patient and place at bedside.	Mixing probes from different manufacturers results in burn injury to patient.
2. Identify patient using two identifiers (e.g., name and birthday or name and account number) according to agency policy.	Ensures correct patient. Complies with The Joint Commission requirements for patient safety (TJC, 2014).
3. Explain purpose of procedure to patient and how you will measure oxygen saturation. Instruct patient to breathe normally.	Promotes patient cooperation and increases compliance. Prevents large fluctuations in minute ventilation and possible error in SpO_2 readings.
IMPLEMENTATION	
1. Perform hand hygiene.	Reduces transmission of microorganisms.
2. Position patient comfortably. If finger monitoring site is chosen, support lower arm.	Ensures probe positioning and decreases motion artifact that interferes with SpO_2 determination.
3. Remove fingernail polish from digit with acetone or polish remover if necessary. Acrylic nails without polish do not interfere with SpO_2 determination.	Opaque coatings can decrease light transmission. Nail polish containing blue pigment absorbs light emissions and may falsely alter saturation.
4. Attach sensor to monitoring site. Instruct patient that clip-on sensor will feel like tight elastic band on finger or ear but will not hurt.	Patient may not expect pressure of spring tension of sensor on finger or earlobe. Select sensor site based on peripheral circulation and extremity temperature. Peripheral vasoconstriction alters SpO_2.

Clinical Decision Point: **Do not attach sensor to finger, ear, or bridge of nose if area is edematous or skin integrity is compromised. Do not attach sensor to hypothermic finger. Select ear or bridge of nose if adult patient has a history of peripheral vascular disease. Do not place sensor on same extremity as used for electronic blood pressure cuff because blood flow to finger is temporarily interrupted when cuff inflates, resulting in inaccurate reading that triggers alarms. Do not use earlobe and bridge of nose sensors for infants and toddlers because their skin is fragile.**

STEP	RATIONALE
5. Once sensor is in place, turn on oximeter by activating power. Observe pulse waveform/intensity display and audible beep. Correlate oximeter pulse rate with patient's radial pulse.	Pulse waveform/intensity display enables detection of valid pulse or presence of interfering signal. Pitch of audible beep is proportional to SpO_2 value. Double-checking pulse rate ensures oximeter accuracy. Oximeter pulse rate, patient's radial pulse, and apical pulse rate should be the same.

Clinical Decision Point: **If oximeter pulse rate, patient's radial pulse, and apical pulse are different, reevaluate oximeter probe placement and reassess pulse rates.**

STEP	RATIONALE
6. Inform patient that oximeter will alarm if sensor falls off or if patient moves sensor.	Prepares patient to be a participant in care.
7. Leave sensor in place until oximeter readout reaches constant value and pulse display reaches full strength during each cardiac cycle. Read SpO_2 on digital display.	Readings take 10 to 30 seconds, depending on site selected.
8. If patient requires continuous monitoring, verify SpO_2 alarm limits and volume, which are preset by manufacturer at low of 85% and high of 100%. Determine limits for SpO_2 and pulse rate alarms based on each patient's condition. Verify that alarms are on. Assess skin integrity under sensor every 2 hours. Relocate sensor at least every 24 hours or more frequently if skin integrity is altered or tissue perfusion is compromised.	Ensures that alarms are set at appropriate limits and volumes to avoid frightening patients and visitors. Spring tension of sensor or sensitivity to disposable sensor adhesive causes skin irritation and leads to disruption of skin integrity.
9. Discuss findings with patient as needed.	Promotes participation in care and understanding of health status.
10. If intermittent or spot-checking SpO_2 measurements are planned, remove sensor and turn oximeter power off. Store sensor in appropriate location.	Batteries drain if oximeter is left on. Oximeter sensors are expensive and vulnerable to damage.
11. Help patient return to comfortable position.	Restores comfort and promotes sense of well-being.
12. Perform hand hygiene.	Reduces transmission of microorganisms.
EVALUATION	
1. Compare SpO_2 readings with patient baseline and acceptable values.	Comparison reveals presence of abnormality.
2. Compare SpO_2 with SaO_2 obtained from arterial blood gas measurements (see Chapter 30) if available.	Documents reliability of noninvasive assessment. Pulse oximetry only warns of dangerous low levels of oxygen saturation. Values are not accurate under 80%.
3. Correlate SpO_2 reading with data obtained from respiratory rate, depth, and rhythm assessment (see Skill 15-4). Note use of oxygen therapy.	Measurements assessing ventilation, perfusion, and diffusion are interrelated.
4. During continuous monitoring assess skin integrity underneath probe at least every 2 hours, based on patient's peripheral circulation.	Prevents tissue ischemia.

RECORDING AND REPORTING

- Record SpO_2 value on nurses' notes, vital sign flow sheet, or electronic medical record.
- Record type and amount of oxygen therapy used by patient during assessment.
- Record any signs and symptoms of reduced oxygen saturation in narrative form in nurses' notes.
- Document measurement of SpO_2 after administration of specific therapies in narrative form in nurses' notes.
- Report abnormal findings to nurse in charge or health care provider immediately.

UNEXPECTED OUTCOMES AND RELATED INTERVENTIONS

- SpO_2 is less than 90%.
  - Evaluate for additional signs and symptoms of decreased oxygenation, including anxiety, cyanosis, restlessness, and tachycardia.
  - Help patient to a position that maximizes ventilatory effort (e.g., place obese patient in a high-Fowler's position).
  - Notify nurse in charge or health care provider.

KEY POINTS

- Vital sign measurement includes the physiological measurements of temperature, pulse, blood pressure, respiration, and oxygen saturation.
- You measure vital signs as part of a complete physical examination or in a review of a patient's condition.
- Measure vital signs when your patient is at rest and the environment is controlled for comfort.
- Evaluate vital sign changes with other physical assessment findings using clinical judgment to determine measurement frequency.
- Knowledge of the factors influencing vital signs helps to determine and evaluate abnormal values.

- Changes related to aging influence the vital sign measurement and nursing interventions for older adults.
- Vital signs provide a basis for evaluating response to nursing interventions.
- Changes in one vital sign often influence characteristics of the other vital signs.
- Maintain a patient's body temperature by initiating interventions that promote heat loss, production, or conservation.
- Respiratory assessment includes determining the effectiveness of ventilation, perfusion, and diffusion.
- Assessment of respiration involves observing ventilatory movements throughout the respiratory cycle.
- Hypertension is diagnosed only after an average of readings made during two or more subsequent visits reveals an elevated blood pressure.
- Selecting and applying the blood pressure measurement cuff improperly results in errors in blood pressure measurement.

CLINICAL DECISION-MAKING EXERCISES

Ms. Coburn, the 26-year-old schoolteacher, is taken to the emergency department with difficulty breathing and feeling "sick." Her skin is hot to touch and she has labored, shallow breathing. Ms. Coburn stated at the time of admission that she has not been drinking much lately because she has become nauseated. She complains of being tired and irritable. When her vital signs are taken 30 minutes later, the results display an oral temperature of 38.4° C (101.2° F), pulse 110, RR 20, BP 96/56, SpO_2 on room air is 92%. Ms. Coburn is lying on her right side with the head of the bed flat.

1. List the priority interventions that you need to implement at this time. Provide rationale.
2. Which vital signs can you delegate to the nursing assistive personnel (NAP) at this time?
3. Intravenous fluids are started, and Ms. Coburn is placed on 2L oxygen per nasal cannula. An hour after admission, Ms. Coburn's vital signs are as follows: right arm BP 136/92 mm Hg; left arm BP 132/64 with the head of bed at 30 degrees; right radial pulse 114, +4 strength; respiratory rate 26 and regular; SpO_2 93%; tympanic temperature 39.2° C (102.6° F). Ms. Coburn states, "I've been coughing up thick tan mucus."
   a. List the priority interventions you need to implement at this time.
   b. Is Ms. Coburn experiencing hyperthermia or pyrexia? Explain your answer.

evolve

Answers to Clinical Decision-Making Exercises can be found on the Evolve website.

QSEN ACTIVITY: EVIDENCE-BASED PRACTICE

Ms. Coburn has been admitted to the hospital. You are caring for her and decide to verify her temporal temperature reading of 39.2° C (102.6° F) with a tympanic membrane thermometer. Because you are interested in evidence-based practice (see Chapter 7), you recently conducted a literature search pertaining to temperature accuracy in the hospitalized patient, and you know that obtaining accurate temperature readings is sometimes problematic. Your literature search showed that nurses who do not use temporal artery thermometers correctly often have inaccurate readings in patients who are febrile. Out of the six articles you reviewed, four were randomized control trials involving use of the temporal thermometer compared with standard electronic thermometers. Three of the four articles did not recommend the temporal thermometer for definitive temperature determination, but stated it can be used in screening. Two of the articles were systematic reviews. Neither review supported use of the temporal thermometer for anything other than screening. You will present your information at your next unit meeting.

Regarding the evidence you found, which types of research evidence have greater strength in their findings than others?

Based on the research articles you collected, do you think you are ready to recommend to your co-workers a change in practice? Explain your answer.

evolve

Answers to QSEN Activities can be found on the Evolve website.

REVIEW QUESTIONS

1. A male patient is in the emergency department with nausea and vomiting. His vital signs are HR 116, BP 92/62, respiratory rate 20, pulse oximeter 94%, and tympanic membrane temperature 36.2° C (97.2° F). He is pale and diaphoretic. Which nursing interventions are appropriate in the care of this patient? (Select all that apply.)
   1. Provide the patient water to prevent dehydration
   2. Dry off the skin and provide warming blanket
   3. Raise the head of bed to promote oxygenation
   4. Check the ear canal for cerumen (earwax) and retake temperature
   5. Ask the nursing assistive personnel (NAP) to retake the patient's blood pressure
2. Your patient had an oral temperature of 38.3° C (101° F) 30 minutes ago. When you go into the room to recheck the temperature, you discover that the patient just drank a glass of cold water. What is the most appropriate action to take at this time?
   1. Take the patient's temperature by the rectal route.
   2. Wait 15 minutes before retaking the patient's oral temperature.
   3. Come back in 2 hours so you can stay on schedule.
   4. Go ahead and take the patient's oral temperature.

3. You are caring for a patient admitted to the medical floor 2 hours ago for dizziness and confusion. The patient took the first dose of a new blood pressure medication that lowers the heart rate. Which vital signs can you delegate to the nursing assistive personnel (NAP)? (Select all that apply.)
   1. Temperature
   2. Heart rate
   3. Oxygen saturation
   4. Respirations
   5. Blood pressure
4. A patient has the following vital signs: heart rate 52 beats/min, BP 80/52, respirations 14 breaths/min, oral temperature 37.1°C (98.8°F), and SpO_2 98%. What is the appropriate interpretation of these vital signs?
   1. Tachycardia with hypertension
   2. Bradycardia with hypertension
   3. Tachycardia with hypotension
   4. Bradycardia with hypotension
5. A patient who had surgery 8 hours ago has a blood pressure (BP) of 126/84 while lying down. The BP is 94/54 when sitting up at 1 minute. The patient states that he is light-headed, and you see that he has become pale. What is the most likely cause for the change in blood pressure?
   1. Normal hypotension following surgery
   2. Side effect of fluid shifts in the body following surgery
   3. Orthostatic hypotension
   4. Normal response to repositioning to a sitting position
6. When choosing the correct blood pressure cuff for an adult patient, the nurse would take into consideration ________________ and ________________.
7. A newly admitted patient has a tympanic temperature of 38.8°C (102°F). What is the priority nursing intervention?
   1. Obtain blood cultures after you give the first dose of antibiotic
   2. Remove all the patient's blankets and sheets and the patient's shirt
   3. Turn down the room thermostat until the patient starts shivering
   4. Monitor temperature for trends in elevation
8. You just started your shift and are reviewing your four patients' vital signs that were taken by the nurse assistive personnel (NAP). You note that the NAP documented lower-than-expected blood pressure (BP) readings on all your patients. When you retake the BP, what is the most likely reason you will find for the low pressures that were obtained previously?
   1. BP cuffs were too wide for the patients' arm circumference.
   2. Bladder of BP cuff was inflated and deflated too slowly.
   3. BP cuffs were too narrow for the patients' arm circumference.
   4. BP cuff was not wrapped evenly around the patients' arms.
9. When you are palpating your patient's pulse, you note an irregular rhythm. You review the patient's electronic health record and find that before this the patient's pulse was regular. What is your priority action?
   1. Assess your patient for a pulse deficit
   2. Take an apical pulse for 15 seconds
   3. Document your finding and notify the health care provider the next day if the pulse remains irregular
   4. Assess your patient's temperature
10. When assessing a patient, you find that the patient is alert and oriented but the pulse obtained by the pulse oximeter is significantly less than the pulse you just took. What do you need to do first?
    1. Notify the health care provider or the nurse in charge
    2. Provide supplemental oxygen
    3. Check that the oximeter is intact
    4. Assess your patient for signs and symptoms of decreased oxygenation

evolve

Rationales for Review Questions can be found on the Evolve website.

1. 2, 3, 4; 2. 2; 3. 1, 3, 4; 4. 4; 5. 3; 6. Width of the blood pressure cuff and circumference of the patient's arm; 7. 4; 8. 1; 9. 1; 10. 3

REFERENCES

Agency for Healthcare Research and Quality: *Preventing falls in hospitals: a toolkit for improving quality of care: orthostatic vital sign measurement*, 2013, http://www.ahrq.gov/legacy/research/ltc/fallpxtoolkit/fallpxtool3f.htm. Accessed November 15, 2013.

Amoore DJ: Best practice in the measurement of body temperature, *Nurs Stand* 24(42):42, 2010.

Appel LJ, et al: Dietary approaches to prevent and treat hypertension, *Hypertension* 47:296, 2009.

Aronow WS, et al: ACCF/AHA 2011 expert consensus document on hypertension in the elderly: a report of the American College of Cardiology Foundation Task Force on clinical expert consensus documents, *J Am Coll Cardiol* 57(20):2037, 2011.

Bahr SJ, et al: Clinical nurse specialist–led evaluation of temporal artery thermometers in acute care, *Clin Nurse Specialist* 24(5):238, 2010.

Barnason S, et al; Emergency Nursing Resources Development Committee: *Clinical practice guideline: non-invasive temperature measurement in the emergency department*, 2011, http://www.ena.org/practice-research/

research/CPG/Documents/TemperatureMeasurementCPG.pdf. Accessed October 13, 2013.

Bertoia ML, et al: Implications of new hypertension guidelines in the United States, *Hypertension* 58(3):361, 2011.

Centers for Disease Control and Prevention: *Measuring orthostatic blood pressure*, 2013, http://www.cdc.gov/homeandrecreationalsafety/pdf/steadi/measuring_orthostatic_bp.pdf. Accessed November 15, 2013.

Cicek HS, et al: Effect of nail polish and henna on oxygen saturation determined by pulse oximetry in healthy young adult females, *Emerg Med* 28(9):783, 2010.

Cinar O, et al: Can mainstream end-tidal carbon dioxide measurement accurately predict the arterial carbon dioxide level of patients with acute dyspnea in ED, *Am J Emerg Med* 30(2):358, 2012.

Davis RA: The big chill: accidental hypothermia, *Am J Nurs* 112(1):38, 2012.

Falkner B, et al: High blood pressure in children: clinical and health policy implications, *J Clin Hypertens* 12(4):261, 2010.

Hockenberry MJ, Wilson D: *Wong's nursing care of infants and children*, ed 9, St Louis, 2011, Mosby.

Jefferies S, et al: A systematic review of the accuracy of peripheral thermometry in estimating core temperatures among febrile critically ill patients, *Crit Care Resusc* 13(3):194, 2011.

Jhaveri R, et al: Management of the non-toxic appearing acutely febrile child: a 21st century approach, *J Pediatr* 159(2):181, 2011.

Kantola I, et al: Bell or diaphragm in the measurement of blood pressure? *J Hypertens* 23(3):499, 2005.

Kimberger O, et al: Temporal artery versus bladder thermometry during perioperative and intensive care unit monitoring, *Anesth Analg* 105(4):1042, 2007.

Lanier JB, et al: Evaluation and management of orthostatic hypotension, *Am Fam Physician* 84(5):527, 2011.

Marable K, et al: Temporal artery scanning falls short as a secondary, noninvasive thermometry method for trauma patients, *J Trauma Nurs* 16(1):41, 2009.

Mattis JG, Yates AM: Heat stroke: helping patients keep their cool, *Nurse Pract* 36(5):48, 2011.

McCance KL, Huether SE: *Pathophysiology: the biological basis for disease in adults and children*, ed 6, St Louis, 2010, Mosby.

Meininger JC, et al: Overweight and central adiposity in school-age children and links with hypertension, *J Pediatr Nurs* 25(2):119, 2010.

Miner QJ, Mathews GR: An assessment of the accuracy of pulse oximeters, *Anaesthesia* 67(4):396, 2012.

National High Blood Pressure Education Program (NHBPEP): *Seventh report of the Joint National Committee on prevention, evaluation, and treatment of high blood pressure (JNC 7)*, 2004, http://www.nhlbi.nih.gov/guidelines/hypertension/. Accessed October 13, 2013.

Nelson D, et al: Accuracy of automated blood pressure monitors, *J Dent Hygiene* 82(4):35, 2008.

Ogedegbe G, Pickering T: Principles and techniques of blood pressure measurement, *Cardiol Clin* 20(2):571, 2010.

Pagana KD, Pagana TK: *Mosby's diagnostic and laboratory test reference*, ed 10, St Louis, 2011, Mosby.

Pickering TG, et al; Subcommittee of Professional and Public Education of the American Heart Association Council on High Blood Pressure Research: Recommendations for blood pressure measurement in humans and experimental animals: Part 1: blood pressure measurement in humans: a statement for professionals from the Subcommittee of Professional and Public Education of the American Heart Association Council on High Blood Pressure Research, *Hypertension* 45:142, 2005.

Reynolds M, et al: Are temporal artery temperatures accurate enough to replace rectal temperature measurement in pediatric ED patients? *J Emerg Nurs* 40(1):46, 2014.

Schey BM, et al: Skin temperature and core-peripheral temperature gradient as markers of hemodynamic status in critically ill patients: a review, *Heart Lung* 39(1):27, 2010.

Schroeder A, et al: What's growing on your stethoscope? *J Fam Pract* 58(8):404, 2009.

Seidel HM, et al: *Mosby's physical examination*, ed 7, St Louis, 2011, Mosby.

Sener S, et al: Agreement between axillary, tympanic, and mid-forehead body temperature measurements in adult emergency department patients, *Eur J Emerg Med* 19(4): 252, 2012.

The Joint Commission (TJC): *Joint Commission introduces new, customized tool to improve hand-off communications*, 2012, http://www.jointcommission.org/issues/article.aspx?Article=RZlHoUK2oak83WO8RkCmZ9hVSIJT8ZbrI4NznZ1LEUk%3D. Accessed October 13, 2013.

The Joint Commission (TJC): *National Patient Safety Goals*, Oakbrook Terrace, IL, 2014, The Commission. Available at http://www.jointcommission.org/standards_information/npsgs.aspx.

Touhy TA, Jett KF: *Ebersole and Hess' gerontological nursing healthy aging*, ed 4, St Louis, 2014, Mosby.

US National Library of Medicine: *Medline Plus: capillary nail refill test*, 2013, http://www.nlm.nih.gov/medlineplus/ency/article/003394.htm. Accessed November 11, 2013.

Wan Y, et al: Determining which automatic digital blood pressure device performs adequately: a systematic review. *J Hum Hypertens* 24(7):431, 2010.

Zheng D, et al: Effect of respiration, talking and small body movements on blood pressure measurement, *J Hum Hypertens* 26:458, 2012.

CHAPTER

16

Health Assessment and Physical Examination

evolve WEBSITE

http://evolve.elsevier.com/Potter/essentials

- Video Clip
- Crossword Puzzle
- Audio Glossary

OBJECTIVES

- Discuss the purposes of health assessment.
- Describe the techniques used with each physical assessment skill.
- Discuss how cultural awareness influences health assessment.
- Describe proper patient positioning during each phase of the examination.
- List techniques to promote a patient's physical and psychological comfort during an examination.
- Prepare a therapeutic environment before the physical examination.
- Identify data to collect from the nursing history before an examination.
- Discuss ways to incorporate health promotion and health teaching into an assessment.
- Discuss normal physical findings for patients across the life span.
- Identify self-screening assessments commonly performed by patients.
- Use physical-assessment techniques and skills during routine nursing care.
- Document assessment findings on appropriate forms.
- Communicate abnormal findings to appropriate personnel.

KEY TERMS

adventitious sounds, p. 343
arcus senilis, p. 333
atrophy, p. 329
auscultation, p. 318
bruit, p. 349
cerumen, p. 334
costovertebral angle, p. 357
crackles, p. 344
cyanosis, p. 325
dorsum, p. 327
dyspnea, p. 341
edema, p. 325
erythema, p. 326
indurated, p. 328
inspection, p. 317
integument, p. 325
intercostal space, p. 341
jaundice, p. 326
olfaction, p. 319
orthopnea, p. 341
pallor, p. 325
palpation, p. 317
percussion, p. 317
petechiae, p. 328
phlebitis, p. 352
thrill, p. 349
turgor, p. 328

Nurses obtain information important to planning patient care in a variety of settings. To gather this information, nurses conduct health assessments at health fairs or screening clinics, in health care providers' offices, in patients' homes, or in acute care settings. Depending on the circumstances, you will use either a complete or a focused health assessment to gather patient information. A complete health assessment involves a nursing history, behavioral assessment, and physical examination. You will use focused health assessments to gather information related to a specific body system, such as

CASE STUDY *Mr. Neal*

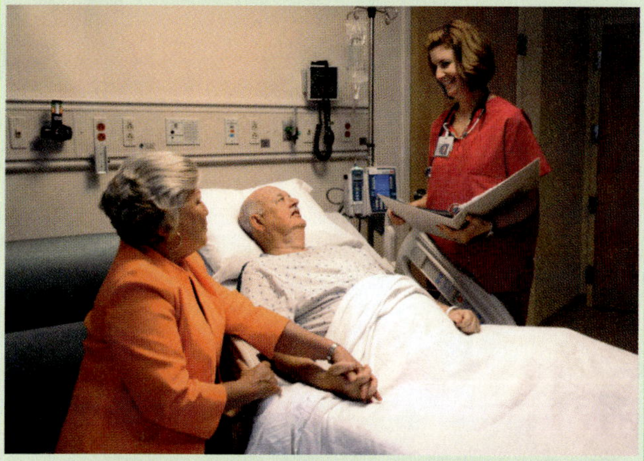

Mr. Neal, a 76-year-old retired college professor, has a history of rectal bleeding and change in bowel habits. He has a history of a high-fat diet and mild hypertension and smokes two packs of cigarettes a day. He denies any family history of colon cancer. Mr. Neal is being admitted to the surgical floor for bowel surgery. His wife is with him when he is admitted.

Jane is the nursing student assigned to care for Mr. Neal during the day shift. She begins her assessments with a review of chart and the health care provider's orders.

when a patient first presents to the hospital or comes for cholesterol and blood glucose screening. Continuity in health care improves when you make ongoing, objective, and comprehensive assessments.

PURPOSES OF HEALTH ASSESSMENT AND PHYSICAL EXAMINATION

Gather information about the patient's health status from the health history. Unless the physical examination is performed as a regular component of daily care in an acute setting, you or a health care provider begins by determining why a patient is seeking health care. This is commonly called the *chief concern.* Ask questions about any signs or symptoms that are associated with the concern. In addition, ask about the patient's complete past medical history or current concerns. Since many conditions are familial, ask the patient about family history. In clinics or other settings, a patient often completes written forms before being seen by a health care provider.

Think critically about the information the patient provides, apply knowledge from previous clinical care, and methodically conduct the examination to create a clear picture of the patient's status. You need to complete a thorough assessment to accurately identify a nursing diagnosis and construct a plan of care. Learn to group significant findings into patterns of data that reveal actual or "risk for" nursing diagnoses (see Chapter 9). Gather information obtained during the initial physical examination to provide a baseline of the patient's functional abilities. Use this baseline as a comparison for future assessment findings. Subsequent physical examinations can reveal information that confirms, refutes, or adds to the history.

A physical examination is patient centered. In an acutely ill patient you first assess only the involved body system(s). Afterwards, you conduct a more comprehensive examination so you are able to learn more about the patient's total health status. A complete physical examination is conducted for routine screening to promote wellness behaviors and preventive health care measures; determine eligibility for health insurance, military service, or a new job; and admit a patient to a hospital setting or long-term care facility. Use a physical assessment to:

1. Gather baseline information about a patient's health status.
2. Supplement, confirm, or refute information learned during the history taking.
3. Identify or confirm nursing diagnoses.
4. Make clinical judgments about a patient's current or changing health status and ability to manage it.
5. Evaluate the outcomes of care.

CULTURAL SENSITIVITY

Respect the cultural differences of patients when completing an examination (see Chapter 20). Remember that cultural differences influence a patient's behavior. Consider the patient's health beliefs, use of alternative therapies, nutritional habits, relationships with family, and comfort with your physical closeness during the examination and history taking. If your patient does not speak English, obtain a medical translator who can interpret your questions and the patient's responses correctly. Consider cultural or social norms when performing an examination of the opposite gender; another person of the patient's gender or culturally approved family member needs to be in the room when this situation occurs.

Improved patient outcomes result from recognition of and respect for cultural differences. Avoid stereotyping on the basis of gender or race. There are differences between cultural and physical characteristics. Learn to recognize common disorders for ethnic populations within the local community. Assess a patient's ability to get, process, and understand health care information and how he or she makes health care decisions based on cultural beliefs (Ingram, 2012). Recognition of cultural differences helps you provide higher-quality care.

INTEGRATION OF PHYSICAL ASSESSMENT WITH NURSING CARE

Learn to integrate an examination during routine patient care. For example, assess the condition of the skin during a bed bath or observe a patient's gait, range of motion (ROM), or muscle strength as the patient ambulates. This practice makes efficient use of time and conserves a patient's energy.

SKILLS OF PHYSICAL ASSESSMENT

A comprehensive physical assessment involves the use of five skills: inspection, palpation, percussion, auscultation, and olfaction.

Inspection

Inspection is the use of vision to distinguish normal from abnormal findings. It is important to know what to consider normal for patients of different age, gender, or cultural group. With experience you are better able to recognize normal variations among patients. Inspection is a simple technique, and the quality of an inspection depends on your willingness to be thorough and systematic. To inspect body parts accurately, follow these principles:

1. Make sure that adequate lighting is available.
2. Position and expose body parts so you can view all surfaces.
3. Inspect each area for size, shape, color, symmetry, position, and abnormalities.
4. When possible, compare each area inspected with the same area on the opposite side of the body.
5. Use additional light (e.g., a penlight) to inspect skin surfaces or body cavities.
6. Do not hurry inspection. Pay attention to detail.

After inspection of a body part, findings sometimes indicate the need for further examination. Use palpation with or after visual inspection.

Palpation

Palpation involves the use of the hands to touch body parts and make sensitive assessments. It typically occurs right after inspection. However, when examining the abdomen, palpation occurs after auscultation. Use palpation to examine all accessible parts of the body. For example, palpate the skin for temperature, moisture, texture, turgor, tenderness, and thickness. Palpate the abdomen for tenderness, distention, or masses. Use different parts of the hand to detect characteristics such as texture, temperature, and perception of movement. Use Standard Precautions if any body fluids are present.

Assist the patient with relaxing and positioning comfortably because muscle tension during palpation impairs your ability to interpret physical findings. Asking the patient to take slow, deep breaths enhances muscle relaxation. Be sure to instruct the patient to point out more sensitive or tender areas and observe for any nonverbal signs of discomfort. *Palpate tender areas last.*

To palpate you need warm hands, short fingernails, and a gentle approach. After washing hands, perform palpation slowly, gently, and deliberately. Light palpation of structures such as the abdomen determines areas of irregularity or tenderness (Figure 16-1, *A*). Place your hand on the area you are examining and depress about 1 cm (½ inch). Examine tender areas further for potentially serious abnormalities. Light intermittent pressure is best when palpating; heavy prolonged pressure causes loss of sensitivity in the hand. If a patient

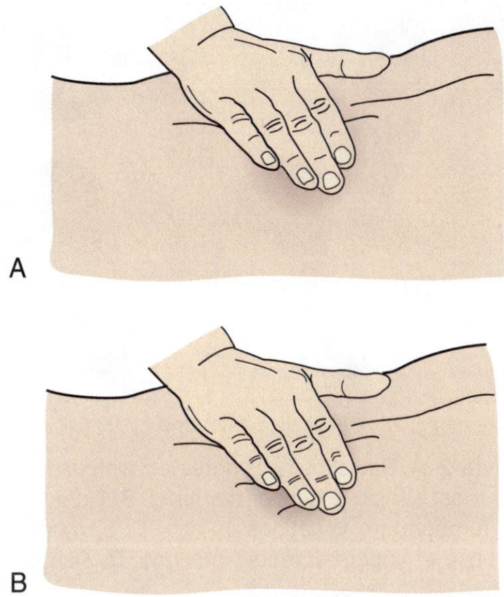

FIGURE 16-1 A, During light palpation gentle pressure against underlying skin and tissues can detect areas of irregularity and tenderness. **B,** During deep palpation depress tissue to assess condition of underlying organs.

reports pain, do not proceed to deep palpation in the area of concern.

After light palpation use deeper palpation to examine the condition of organs (Figure 16-1, *B*). Depress the area that you are examining deeply and evenly (Seidel et al., 2011). Caution is the rule. To avoid injuring a patient do not try deep palpation without clinical supervision. Apply deep palpation with one or both hands (bimanually). Bimanual palpation involves one hand placed over the other while applying pressure. The upper hand exerts downward pressure as the other hand feels the subtle characteristics of underlying organs and masses.

Use the most sensitive parts of the hand (i.e., the palmar surface of the fingers and finger pads) to determine position, texture, size, consistency, masses, fluid, and pulsation (Figure 16-2, *A*). Assess temperature with the dorsal surface, or back, of the hand (Figure 16-2, *B*). The palm of the hand is more sensitive to vibration (Figure 16-2, *C*). Measure position, consistency, and turgor by lightly grasping the body part with the fingertips (Figure 16-2, *D*).

Do not palpate without considering a patient's condition. For example, if a patient has a fractured rib, use extra care to locate the painful area. Do not palpate a vital artery with pressure that obstructs blood flow.

Percussion

Percussion involves tapping the body with the fingertips to produce a vibration that travels through body tissues. This vibration is transmitted through the body tissues, and the character of the sound heard depends on the density of the underlying tissue. The resulting sounds determine the location, size, and density of underlying structures and help verify abnormalities assessed by palpation and auscultation. By

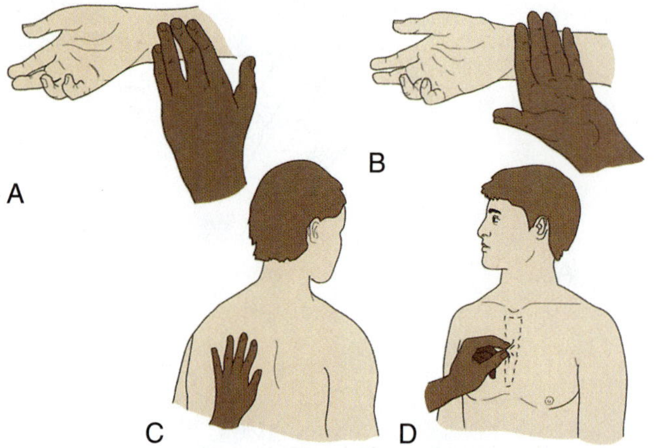

FIGURE 16-2 **A,** Radial pulse is detected with pads of fingertips, the most sensitive part of the hand. **B,** Dorsum of hand detects temperature variations in skin. **C,** Bony part of the palm at base of fingers detects vibrations. **D,** Skin is grasped with fingertips to assess turgor.

knowing the way various densities influence sound, you can locate organs or masses, map their boundaries, and determine their size. Percussion is usually reserved for advanced practitioners who are able to use findings to make clinical decisions.

Auscultation

Auscultation is listening for sounds produced by the body. Some sounds such as voice sounds are audible to the human ear. Other sounds such as those made by the cardiovascular, respiratory, and gastrointestinal (GI) systems require use of a stethoscope. Recognize abnormal sounds after learning normal variations. Become more proficient at auscultation by learning the type of sounds that each body structure makes and the location in which you hear the sounds best. Also learn which areas do not normally produce sounds.

To auscultate you need good hearing acuity, a good stethoscope, and knowledge of how to use the stethoscope properly. If you have a hearing disorder, use a stethoscope with additional sound amplification. Chapter 15 describes the parts of the stethoscope and its general use. The bell is best for low-pitched sounds such as vascular and certain heart sounds, and the diaphragm is best for high-pitched sounds such as bowel and lung sounds. Practice using the stethoscope. Extraneous sounds created by movement of the tubing or chest piece interfere with auscultation of body organ sounds. By deliberately producing these sounds, you learn to recognize and disregard them during the actual examination (Box 16-1). Learn to recognize the following characteristics of sounds:

- *Pitch:* How frequently sound wave cycles are generated per second by a vibrating object (The higher the frequency, the higher the pitch of a sound and vice versa.)
- *Intensity:* Amplitude of a sound wave (Auscultated sounds are described as loud or soft.)
- *Quality:* Sounds of similar frequency and loudness from different sources (Terms such as *blowing* or *gurgling* describe quality of sound.)
- *Duration:* Length of time that sound vibrations last (Duration of sound is short, medium, or long. Layers of soft tissue dampen the duration of sounds from deep internal organs.)

Auscultation requires concentration and practice. Always consider the part of the body auscultated and the cause of the sounds. For example, the sounds heard over the abdomen are caused by intestinal peristalsis and are heard over all four

BOX 16-1 USING A STETHOSCOPE

1. Place earpieces in both ears with tips of earpieces turned toward the face. *Lightly* blow into the diaphragm. Again place earpieces in your ears, this time with ends turned toward the back of the head. *Lightly* blow into the stethoscope diaphragm. You find that you hear clearer sounds with the earpiece turned toward the face. After you have learned the right fit for the loudest sound, wear the stethoscope the same way each time.
2. Put the stethoscope on and *lightly* blow into the diaphragm. If sound is barely audible, *lightly* blow into the bell. Sound is carried through only one part of the chest piece at a time. If the sound is greatly amplified through the diaphragm, the diaphragm is in position for use. If sound is barely audible through the diaphragm, the bell is in position for use.
3. Place the diaphragm over the anterior part of your chest. Ask a friend to speak in a normal conversational tone. Environmental noise seriously detracts from hearing the noise created by body organs. When using a stethoscope, the patient and the examiner need to remain quiet.
4. Put the stethoscope on and gently tap the tubing. It is often difficult to avoid stretching or moving the stethoscope tubing. Position yourself so the tubing hangs free. Moving or touching the tubing creates extraneous sounds.
5. *Care of the stethoscope:* Remove earpieces regularly and clean or remove cerumen (earwax). Keep the bell and diaphragm free of dust, lint, and body oils. Keep the tubing away from your body oils. Avoid draping the stethoscope around the neck next to the skin. To clean, wipe the entire stethoscope (e.g., diaphragm, tubing) with alcohol or soapy water. Be sure to dry all parts thoroughly. Follow manufacturer recommendations.
6. *Infection control:* Harmful bacteria, even antibiotic-resistant microorganisms, transfer from patient to patient when using portable equipment such as stethoscopes. Follow institution infection control guidelines, especially Contact Precautions, to decrease this risk. Clean the stethoscope (diaphragm/bell) with a disinfectant before reuse on another patient. Using a disinfectant such as isopropyl alcohol (with or without chlorhexidine), benzalkonium, and sodium hypochlorite is effective in reducing the number of bacterial colonies. Earpieces of stethoscopes are sources of transferable bacteria as well when you inadvertently touch your ears and then care for the patient. Potential pathogens could contaminate earpieces. Using hand hygiene before and after patient contact decreases the risk for transmitting microorganisms from your ear to your patient. Do not use cloth stethoscope covers because these have been shown to easily become contaminated.

TABLE 16-1 ASSESSMENT OF CHARACTERISTIC ODORS

ODOR	SITE OR SOURCE	POTENTIAL CAUSES
Alcohol	Oral cavity	Ingestion of alcohol, diabetes
Ammonia	Urine	Urinary tract infection, renal failure
Body odor	Skin, particularly in areas where body parts rub together (e.g., under arms and breasts) Wound site Vomitus	Poor hygiene, excess perspiration (hyperhidrosis), foul-smelling perspiration (bromhidrosis) Wound abscess Abdominal irritation, contaminated food
Feces	Vomitus/oral cavity (fecal odor) Rectal area	Bowel obstruction Fecal incontinence
Foul-smelling stools in infant	Stool	Malabsorption syndrome
Halitosis	Oral cavity	Poor dental and oral hygiene, gum disease
Sweet, fruity ketones	Oral cavity	Diabetic ketoacidosis
Stale urine	Skin	Uremic acidosis
Sweet, heavy, thick odor	Draining wound	*Pseudomonas* (bacterial) infection
Musty odor	Casted body part	Infection inside cast
Fetid, sweet odor	Tracheostomy or mucus secretions	Infection of bronchial tree (*Pseudomonas* bacteria)

abdominal quadrants as intermittent "tinkling" sounds. After understanding the cause and character of normal auscultated sounds, it becomes easier to recognize abnormal sounds and their origins.

Olfaction

While assessing a patient become familiar with the nature and source of body odors (Table 16-1). **Olfaction,** or smelling, helps to detect abnormalities not recognized by other means. Unusual smells lead to detection of serious abnormalities.

PREPARATION FOR ASSESSMENT

Proper preparation of the environment, equipment, and patient ensures a smooth examination. A disorganized approach when preparing for a physical examination causes errors and incomplete findings. Always use Standard Precautions throughout the examination (see Chapter 14). It is necessary to wear gloves during palpation and percussion when there is a possibility of coming in contact with body fluids to reduce contact with microorganisms.

Environment

A physical examination requires privacy. A well-equipped examination room is preferable, but often the examination occurs in the patient's room. In the home you may perform the examination in the patient's bedroom. Adequate lighting is necessary for proper illumination of body parts. Ideally an examination room is soundproof so patients feel comfortable discussing their conditions. Be sure to eliminate other sources of noise, take precautions to prevent interruptions, and ensure that the room is warm enough to maintain comfort.

Sometimes it is difficult to perform a complete examination when patients are in beds or on stretchers. A special examination table makes it easier for you to reach the patient and eases patient movement into specific positions. Carefully assist patients so they do not fall when getting on and off the table. Patients with mobility impairments require safe transfer to an examination table. The patient is the expert; thus you need to ask for the patient's input when moving him or her from the bed to the table safely, either with a standing assisted transfer or by being lifted, as with a child or small adult.

Consider patient comfort while on the examination table. When a patient lies supine, raise the head of the table about 30 degrees, using a small pillow if needed. When examining a patient in bed, raise the bed to reach the patient's body parts more easily. Do not leave a confused, combative, or uncooperative patient unsupervised on an examination table.

Equipment

Perform hand hygiene before equipment preparation and the examination. Have equipment readily available and arranged in order for easy use (Box 16-2). It should be as warm as appropriate. Rub the diaphragm of the stethoscope briskly against one hand before applying it to the skin. Check all equipment to ensure that it functions properly. The ophthalmoscope and otoscope require batteries and light bulbs.

Physical Preparation of a Patient

A patient's physical comfort is vital for a successful examination. Before starting ask if the patient needs to use the restroom. An empty bladder and bowel make examination of the abdomen, genitalia, and rectum easier. If needed collect urine or fecal specimens at this time. Be sure to explain the proper method for collecting specimens and make sure to label each specimen properly.

Physical preparation involves being sure that a patient is dressed or covered properly. A patient in the hospital wears a simple gown. A patient at an office visit or screening event might have to undress and wear a light cover, depending on

BOX 16-2 EQUIPMENT AND SUPPLIES FOR PHYSICAL ASSESSMENT

- Cervical brush or broom (if needed)
- Cotton applicators
- Disposable pad/paper towels
- Drapes
- Eye chart (e.g., Snellen chart)
- Flashlight and spotlight
- Forms (e.g., physical, laboratory)
- Gloves (sterile or clean)
- Gown for patient
- Ophthalmoscope
- Otoscope
- Papanicolaou (Pap) liquid preparation (if needed)
- Percussion (reflex) hammer
- Pulse oximeter
- Ruler
- Scale with height measurement rod
- Specimen containers, slides, wooden or plastic spatula, and cytologic fixative (if needed)
- Sphygmomanometer and cuff
- Sterile swabs
- Stethoscope
- Tape measure
- Thermometer
- Tissues
- Tongue depressors
- Tuning fork
- Vaginal speculum (if needed)
- Water-soluble lubricant
- Wristwatch with second hand or digital display

the body part involved. Cover sheets and gowns are made of disposable paper, cotton, or linen. Provide a patient privacy and plenty of time during undressing, avoiding unnecessary embarrassment. After patients have undressed and put on a gown, they sit or lie down on the examination table with a sheet over the lap or lower trunk. Make sure that the patient stays warm by eliminating drafts, controlling room temperature, and providing warm blankets. Routinely ask if the patient is comfortable.

Positioning. During the examination ask the patient to assume proper positions so body parts are accessible and the patient stays comfortable. Table 16-2 lists and shows the preferred positions for each part of the examination. Patients' abilities to assume positions depend on their physical strength, mobility, ease of breathing, age, and degree of wellness. Explain the positions and help patients assume them. Adjust the sheets or drapes so the area examined is accessible, making sure not to unnecessarily expose a body part. A patient may need to assume more than one position during the examination. To decrease the number of times a patient changes positions, organize the examination so you perform all techniques requiring a sitting position first, those that require a supine position next, and so forth. Use extra care when positioning older adults or patients with weak muscles because they are more prone to having limitations.

Psychological Preparation of a Patient

Many patients find an examination tiring or stressful, or they experience anxiety about possible findings. A thorough, simple, and clear explanation of the purpose and steps of each assessment lets patients know what to expect and helps them cooperate with each step. As you examine each body system give a detailed explanation. Convey an open, professional, and relaxed approach. A stiff, formal approach inhibits a patient's ability to communicate, but being too casual does not give the patient confidence in your ability (Seidel et al., 2011).

Use a medical interpreter for patients who do not speak or understand English. If a patient is hearing or speech impaired, identify the communication system that will be used (sign language interpreter, word board, or talk box). If necessary, use Braille, audiotaped information, or three-dimensional anatomic models to help a patient with visual impairments understand information (Seidel et al., 2011).

When a patient and nurse are of opposite gender, it helps to have a third person of the patient's gender in the room. The presence of a third person assures the patient that you will behave ethically. This person is also a witness to the conduct of the examiner and the patient.

During the examination watch the patient's emotional responses. Observe whether his or her facial expression shows fear or concern. Watch if body movements appear stiff from anxiety. Remain calm and explain each step clearly. It is sometimes necessary to stop the examination and ask how the patient feels. Do not force a patient to continue. Findings are more accurate if you postpone until the patient can cooperate and relax.

Assessment of Different Age-Groups

Different interview styles and approaches are needed to perform a health history and examine patients of different age-groups. When assessing children be sensitive and anticipate a child's reaction to the examination as a strange and unfamiliar experience. Routine pediatric examinations focus on health promotion and illness prevention, particularly for the care of well children who receive competent parenting and have no serious health problems (Hockenberry and Wilson, 2011). The examination focuses on growth and development, sensory screening, dental examination, and behavioral assessment. Children who are chronically ill or disabled, foster children, foreign born, or adopted sometimes require additional assessments because of their unique health risks. When examining children the following tips help in data collection:

1. Gain a child's trust before doing any type of an examination. Talk and play with the child first. It also helps to perform parts of the examination that you can do visually before actually touching the child.
2. Children feel safer during an examination if it is initiated from the periphery and then moves to the center. For example, examine the extremities before moving to the chest.
3. When obtaining histories of infants and children, gather all or part of the information from parents or guardians.
4. Because parents sometimes think they are being tested or judged by the examiner, offer support during examination and do not pass judgment.

TABLE 16-2 POSITIONS FOR EXAMINATION

POSITION	AREAS ASSESSED	RATIONALE	LIMITATIONS
Sitting 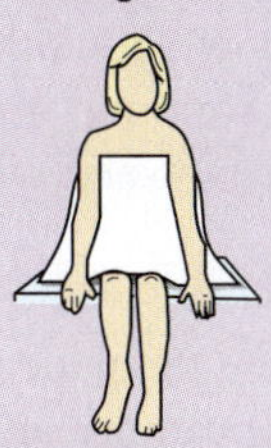	Head and neck, back, posterior thorax and lungs, anterior thorax and lungs, breasts, axillae, heart, vital signs, and upper extremities	Sitting upright provides full expansion of lungs and better visualization of symmetry of upper body parts.	Physically weakened patient is sometimes unable to sit. Use supine position with head of bed elevated instead.
Supine 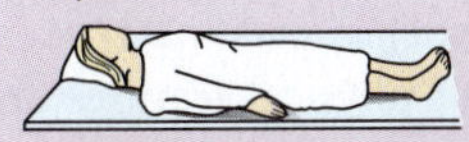	Head and neck, anterior thorax and lungs, breasts, axillae, heart, abdomen, extremities, pulses	This is most normally relaxed position. It provides easy access to pulse sites.	If patient becomes short of breath easily, raise head of bed.
Dorsal recumbent 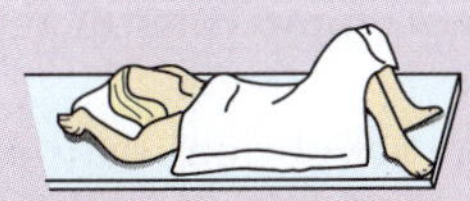	Head and neck, anterior thorax and lungs, breasts, axillae, heart, abdomen	This position is for abdominal assessment because it promotes relaxation of abdominal muscles.	Patients with painful disorders are more comfortable with knees flexed.
Lithotomy* 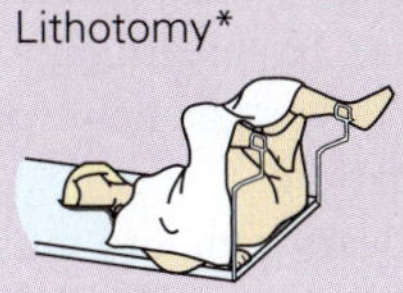	Female genitalia and genital tract	This position provides maximal exposure of genitalia and facilitates insertion of vaginal speculum.	Lithotomy position is embarrassing and uncomfortable; examiner minimizes time that patient spends in it. Keep patient well draped.
Sims'* 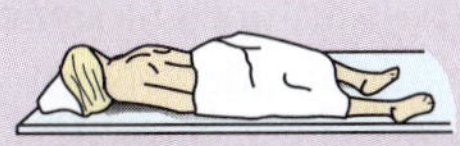	Rectum and vagina	Flexion of hip and knee improves exposure of rectal area.	Joint deformities hinder patient's ability to bend hip and knee.
Prone 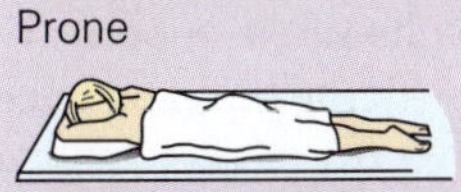	Musculoskeletal system	This position is only for assessing extension of hip joint, skin, and buttocks.	Patients with respiratory difficulties do not tolerate this position well.
Lateral recumbent 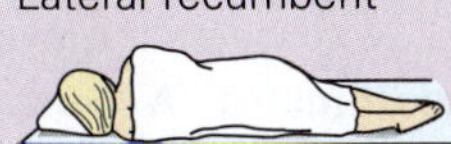	Heart	This position helps to detect murmurs.	Patients with respiratory difficulties do not tolerate this position well.
Knee-chest* 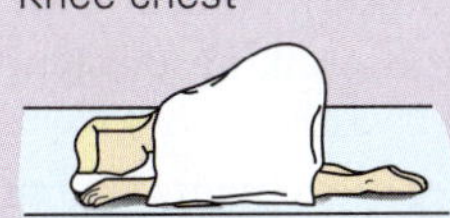	Rectum	This position provides maximal exposure of rectal area.	This position is embarrassing and uncomfortable.

*Patients with arthritis or other joint deformities may be unable to assume this position.

5. Call children by their preferred name and address parents formally (e.g., as "Mr. and Mrs. Brown") rather than by first names.
6. Open-ended questions often allow parents to share more information and describe more of the child's problems.
7. Older children and adolescents tend to respond best when treated as adults and individuals and often can provide details about their health history and severity of symptoms.
8. Remember, an adolescent has a right to confidentiality. After talking with parents about historical information, arrange to speak privately with the adolescent.

A comprehensive health assessment and examination of older adults includes physical data, developmental stage, family relationships, group involvement, and religious and occupational pursuits. An important part of health assessment involves analysis of basic activities of daily living (ADLs) (e.g., dressing, bathing, toileting, feeding, and continence) that are fundamental to independent living. In addition, assess the more complex instrumental ADLs (e.g., using the telephone, preparing meals, and managing money). Any examination of an older adult also includes an evaluation of mental status.

During the examination recognize that with advancing age the body does not respond vigorously to injury or disease. Therefore older people do not always exhibit the expected signs and symptoms. Characteristically older adults have blunted or atypical signs and symptoms. Follow these principles described by Touhy and Jett (2014) during examination of an older adult:

1. Do not assume that aging is always accompanied by illness or disability. Older adults are able to adapt to change and maintain functional independence.
2. Allow extra time; be patient, relaxed, and unhurried with older adults.
3. Provide adequate space for an examination, particularly if a patient uses a mobility aid.
4. Plan the history and examination, taking into account an older adult's energy level, physical limitations, pace, and adaptability. More than one session is sometimes necessary to complete the assessment.
5. Measure performance under the most favorable conditions. Take advantage of natural opportunities for assessment (e.g., during bathing, grooming, mealtime).
6. Sequence an examination to keep position changes to a minimum. Be efficient throughout the examination to limit patient movement.
7. Be sure that an examination of an older adult includes review of mental status.

ORGANIZATION OF THE EXAMINATION

A health assessment follows the completion of the health history (see Chapter 9). Your health assessment documentation needs to include each body system, including which subjective data to collect. Electronic or paper physical assessment documentation forms allow you to record objective and subjective data in the same sequence that it was gathered. Use common and accepted medical abbreviations to keep documentation accurate and concise. Information from the health history focuses your attention on specific parts of the examination. For example, if a patient shares recent experiences with difficulty in breathing, conduct a careful examination of the thorax and lungs. New objective data supplement information from the history to confirm or refute the data.

Be systematic and well organized about the examination so you do not miss important assessments. A complete head-to-toe approach includes all body systems and helps you anticipate each step. In an adult begin by assessing the head and neck, progressing methodically down the body to include all body systems. Compare both sides of the body for symmetry. If a patient is seriously ill, examine the body system most at risk for being abnormal. If a patient becomes fatigued, provide rest periods. Perform any painful procedures near the end of the examination.

General Survey

Before meeting a patient, review the health record to determine his or her primary health problems or concerns and the reason that he or she is seeking health care. Begin your assessment with a general survey when you first meet your patient. Make mental notes of your patient's behavior and appearance. The survey includes assessments about characteristics of an illness; a patient's hygiene, skin condition, and body image; emotional state; recent changes in weight; and developmental status. Be alert for any signs of physical or psychological abuse. The survey reveals important information about the patient's behavior that influences how you communicate instructions to the patient and continue the assessment.

General Appearance and Behavior

Assess appearance and behavior while preparing the patient for the examination. The review of general appearance and behavior includes the following:

1. *Gender and race:* A person's gender affects the type of examination necessary. Different physical features are related to gender and race.
2. *Age:* Age influences normal physical characteristics and a person's ability to participate in some parts of the examination.
3. *Signs of distress:* Sometimes there are obvious signs or symptoms indicating pain (grimacing, splinting painful area), difficulty in breathing (ease of breathing or shortness of breath), or anxiety. These signs help you determine the order of the examination.
4. *Body type:* Observe if a patient appears trim and muscular, obese, or excessively thin. Body type reflects level of health, age, and lifestyle.
5. *Posture:* Normal standing posture is an upright stance with parallel alignment of hips and shoulders. Normal sitting posture involves some degree of rounding of the shoulders. Changes in older adults often appear as a stooped, forward-bent posture, with the hips and knees somewhat flexed and arms bent at the elbows.
6. *Gait:* Observe the patient walking into the room or along the bedside (if ambulatory). Note whether movements are coordinated or uncoordinated. A person normally walks with arms swinging freely at the sides, with the head and face leading the body. Note how well the patient who uses a wheelchair or walking assistance is able to move.
7. *Body movements:* Observe whether movements are purposeful. Note any tremors involving the extremities. Determine if any body parts are immobile.
8. *Hygiene and grooming:* Note the patient's level of cleanliness by observing the appearance of the hair, skin, and fingernails. Note if the patient's clothes are clean. Grooming depends on both the activities being performed just before the examination and the patient's occupation or socioeconomic level. Note the use of hygiene products or excessive use of cosmetics.
9. *Dress:* Culture, lifestyle, socioeconomic level, and personal preference affect clothing choices. Note whether clothing is appropriate for temperature and weather conditions. Depressed or mentally ill people may be unable to choose proper clothing. Some older adults wear extra clothing because of sensitivity to cold.
10. *Body or breath odor:* Unpleasant odors result from physical exercise, poor hygiene, or certain disease states.

11. *Affect, mood, and behavior:* Affect is a person's feelings as they appear to others. Patients express mood or emotional state verbally and nonverbally. Note if verbal expressions match nonverbal behavior and whether or not mood is appropriate for the situation. Observe facial expressions while asking questions.
12. *Speech:* Normal speech is understandable and moderately paced; speech patterns are associated with the patient's thoughts. Note if the patient talks rapidly or slowly. Emotions or neurological impairment may cause an abnormal speech pace. Observe if the patient speaks in a normal tone with clear inflection of words.
13. *Patient abuse:* Child maltreatment, intimate partner violence, and elderly abuse are growing health problems. You need to assess for psychological abuse and obvious physical injury or neglect (e.g., evidence of malnutrition or presence of bruising on the extremities or trunk) (WHO, 2012). If you suspect abuse find a way to interview the patient privately. If you are inexperienced seek another health care provider's assistance. Patients are more likely to reveal problems when the suspected abuser is not present. Assess for the patient's fear of the spouse or partner, caregiver, parent, or adult child. Note if the partner or caregiver has a history of violence, alcoholism, or drug abuse. Identify if the partner or caregiver is unemployed, ill, or frustrated in caring for the patient. *If you assess a pattern of findings indicating abuse, most states mandate a report to a social service center (refer to state guidelines). Obtain immediate consultation with a health care provider, social worker, and other support staff to facilitate placement in a safer environment.* Table 16-3 summarizes clinical indicators of abuse.
14. *Drug use:* Drug abuse and addiction result from excessive use of alcohol, nicotine, illegal substances, or prescription drugs used for nonmedical reasons. Drug abuse and addiction affect all socioeconomic groups. A single visit with a health care provider does not always

TABLE 16-3 CLINICAL INDICATORS OF ABUSE

PHYSICAL FINDINGS	BEHAVIORAL FINDINGS
Child Sexual Abuse	
Vaginal or penile discharge Blood on underclothing Pain, itching, or unusual odor in genital area Genital injuries Difficulty sitting or walking Pain while urinating; recurrent urinary tract infections Foreign bodies in rectum, urethra, or vagina Sexually transmitted diseases Pregnancy in young adolescent	Problem sleeping or eating; anxiety, depression Fear of certain people or places Play activities recreate the abuse situation Regressed behavior Sexual acting out or knowledge of explicit sexual matters Preoccupation with others' or own genitals Profound and rapid personality changes Poor school performance Poor relationship with peers
Intimate Partner Violence	
Injuries and trauma inconsistent with reported cause Multiple injuries involving head, face, neck, breasts, abdomen, and genitalia (black eyes, orbital fractures, broken nose, fractured skull, lip lacerations, broken teeth, strangulation marks) X-ray films show old and new fractures in different stages of healing Abrasions, lacerations, bruises, welts Burns Human bites Stress-related disorders such as irritable bowel syndrome, exacerbation of asthma, or chronic pain	Attempted or thoughts of suicide Emotional distress Anxiety and phobias Posttraumatic stress disorder Pattern of substance abuse (follows physical abuse) Low self-esteem Depression and problems with eating or sleeping Physical inactivity Smoking Unsafe sexual behavior Stress-related complaints (headache, anxiety)
Older Adult Abuse	
Injuries and trauma are inconsistent with reported cause (e.g., cigarette burn, scratch, bruise, bite) Hematomas Bruises at various stages of resolution Bruises, chafing, excoriation on wrist or legs (restraints) Burns Fractures inconsistent with cause described Dried blood	Dependent on caregiver Physically and/or cognitively impaired Combative Wandering Verbally belligerent Minimal social support Prolonged interval between injury and medical treatment

Data from Cooper C, et al: The prevalence of elder abuse and neglect: a systematic review, *Age Aging* 37(2):151, 2008; Hockenberry MJ, Wilson D: *Wong's nursing care of infants and children,* ed 9, Mosby, 2011, WHO, *Intimate partner violence,* 2012. Accessed at http://www.who.int/reproductivehealth/publications/violence.

BOX 16-3 RED FLAGS FOR SUSPICION OF SUBSTANCE ABUSE

- Patients who frequently miss appointments
- Patients who frequently request written excuses for absence from work
- Patients who have chief complaints of insomnia, "bad nerves," or pain that does not fit a particular pattern
- Patients who often report lost prescriptions (e.g., tranquilizers, pain medications) or ask for frequent refills
- Patients who make frequent emergency department visits
- Patients who have a history of changing health care providers or bring in medication bottles prescribed by several different providers
- Patients with histories of gastrointestinal bleeds, peptic ulcers, pancreatitis, cellulitis, or frequent pulmonary infections
- Patients with frequent sexually transmitted diseases, complicated pregnancies, multiple abortions, or sexual dysfunction
- Patients who complain of chest pains or palpitations or who have a history of admissions to rule out myocardial infarctions
- Patients who give histories of activities that place them at risk for human immunodeficiency virus (HIV) infections (multiple partners, multiple rapes)
- Patients with family history of addiction; history of childhood sexual, physical, or emotional abuse or social and financial or marital problems

Data from American Psychiatric Association: *Diagnostic and statistical manual of mental disorders,* ed 4, Washington, DC, 2000, The Association; Ries R, Wilford B: *Principles of addiction medicine,* ed 4, Chevy Chase, MD, 2009, Lippincott Williams & Wilkins.

reveal the problem, but after several visits one may be able to confirm signs or behaviors with a well-focused history and physical examination. Establish trust with the patient, remaining nonjudgmental, because substance abuse involves both emotional and lifestyle issues. Box 16-3 lists indicators that should lead to further assessment for alcohol abuse. When you suspect abuse or addiction among those ages 18 or older, a tool such as the NIDA Quick Screen V1.0 helps to identify the level of risks associated with substance abuse (NIDA, 2012). If alcohol abuse is the major problem, assess adult risk by using the CAGE questions (an acronym for the following): Have you ever felt the need to *Cut down* on your drinking or drug use? Have people *Annoyed* you by criticizing your drinking or drug use? Have you ever felt bad or *Guilty* about your drinking or drug use? Have you ever used or had a drink first thing in the morning as an *Eye-opener* to steady your nerves or feel normal? For adolescents use the T-ACE modification to assess a patient's degree of tolerance (e.g., how many drinks does it take to make you feel high?) (Burns, Gray, and Smith, 2010).

Vital Signs

Assessment of vital signs (see Chapter 15) is the first part of the physical examination. Positioning or moving a patient can result in inaccurate values. Be sure to recheck and report any vital signs outside of normal ranges to the primary health care provider.

Height and Weight

Height and weight reflect a patient's general level of health. This information may also be important for diagnostic testing and dosing of medications. Weight is routinely measured during health screenings and visits to health care providers' offices or clinics and when patients are admitted to a health care setting. Measuring an infant's or child's height and weight provides data about his or her growth and development. In older adults height and weight coupled with a nutritional assessment help to identify dietary problems or other functional deficits. Be sure to recognize overall trends in height and weight changes. Frequently adults become shorter with vertebral changes related to aging.

Daily variation in a patient's weight normally occurs as a result of fluid loss or retention. Health assessments screen for abnormal weight changes, using the nursing history data to focus on possible causes for weight changes. Determine the patient's current height and weight, noting weight gains or losses. Assess changes in diet habits, appetite, prescription or over-the-counter drugs, or physical symptoms. Standardized tables provide normal expected weights for a patient at a given height.

Several types of scales are available, including built-in hospital bed scales, wheelchair scales, and digital or mechanical standing scales. Mechanical scales need to be calibrated regularly. To ensure accurate clinical decisions, weigh patients at the same time of day, on the same scale, and in the same clothes (Byrd et al., 2011). Patients capable of bearing their own weight use a standing scale. The scale measures in weight increments to the nearest 0.1 kg or 0.1 lb depending on if the scale is set to weigh the patient in kilograms or pounds (Seidel et al., 2011). The patient stands on the scale platform and remains still. Electronic scales automatically display weight within seconds. Electronic scales are automatically calibrated each time they are used.

Weigh infants in baskets or on platform scales. Remove the infant's clothing, keeping the room warm to reduce heat loss. A light cloth or paper placed on the scale prevents surface contamination from urine or feces. Hold a hand lightly above the infant to prevent accidental falls. Measure the weight of an infant in ounces, grams, and kilograms.

To measure the height of a weight-bearing patient, have the patient remove his or her shoes. When needed place a paper towel on the scale platform so the patient's feet remain clean. The platform scale has a metal rod attached to the back of the scale; this swings out and over the crown of the patient's head. Have the patient stand erect. Measure his or her height in centimeters or inches.

Place an infant in the supine position on a firm surface, shoes removed (Figure 16-3). Portable devices are available

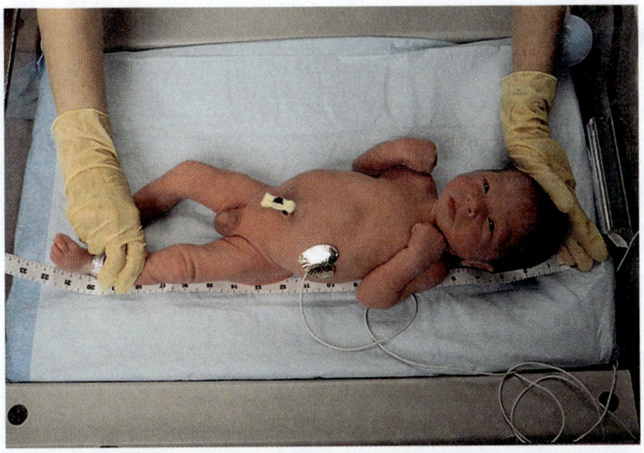

FIGURE 16-3 Measuring infant length. (From Murray SS, McKinney ES: *Foundations of maternal-newborn and women's health nursing*, ed 5, St Louis, 2010, Saunders.)

that provide a reliable means to measure height. While the caregiver holds the infant's head against the headboard, straighten the legs at the knees and place the footboard against the bottom of the infant's feet. Record the infant's length to the nearest 0.5 cm or ¼ inch.

SKIN, HAIR, AND NAILS

The **integument** consists of the skin, hair, scalp, and nails. First inspect all skin surfaces or assess the skin gradually while examining other body systems. Use the skills of inspection, palpation, and olfaction to assess the function and integrity of the integument.

Skin

Skin assessment reveals changes in oxygenation, circulation, nutrition, local tissue damage, and hydration. In a hospital setting many patients are older adults, debilitated patients, or young but seriously ill patients. Such patients may be at risk for skin lesions resulting from trauma to the skin during administration of care, prolonged pressure during immobilization, or reactions to medications. Patients at high risk are the neurologically impaired, chronically ill, and orthopedic patients. Others include those with diminished mental status, poor tissue oxygenation, low cardiac output, or inadequate nutrition. In nursing homes and extended care facilities some patients are at risk for many of the same problems, depending on their level of mobility and the presence of chronic illness. Routinely assess the skin to look for primary or initial lesions that develop. Without proper care primary lesions often deteriorate to become secondary lesions that require more extensive nursing care.

Be alert for any lesions that show evidence of cancer. Melanoma, an aggressive form of skin cancer, is 10 times more common in Caucasians than African-Americans or Hispanics and those who engage in high-risk behaviors such as frequent use of tanning beds (ACS, 2013a). Approximately 76,250 new cases of melanoma and 2.2 million cases of the highly curable basal cell and squamous cell cancers are diagnosed in the United States every year (ACS, 2013a). Cutaneous malignancies are the most common neoplasms seen in patients. Make sure to perform a thorough skin assessment for all patients and educate them about self-examination (Box 16-4).

The condition of the patient's skin reveals the need for nursing intervention. Use assessment findings to determine the type of hygiene measures required to maintain integrity of the integument (see Chapter 29). Adequate nutrition and hydration become goals of therapy if an alteration in the status of the integument is identified. Identify risk for poor skin integrity, including use of soap and water. Vigorous towel drying significantly affects the barrier function of the skin among adults, whereas using no-rinse cleansers and cleaning cloths leads to less damage to skin (Cowdell, 2011).

You need adequate lighting and comfortable temperatures when assessing the skin. The recommended light is natural sunlight; halogen lighting is another option. Sunlight is the best choice for detecting skin changes in patients with darker skin (Newson, 2008). A room that is too warm causes superficial vasodilation, resulting in increased skin redness. Patients who are sensitive to cold develop **cyanosis** (bluish color) around the lips and nail beds.

You inspect all skin surfaces during an examination; begin with a brief overall visual review of the entire body. The examination includes inspecting skin color, moisture, temperature, texture, and turgor, vascular changes, **edema,** phlebitis, and lesions. Wear clean gloves when any moisture is present. Carefully palpate any abnormalities. Skin odors are usually noted in skinfolds such as the axillae or under the female patient's breasts.

Nursing History. Ask the patient about history of skin changes, including dryness, pruritus, sores, rashes, lumps, color, odor, and nonhealing lesions. Localized changes in skin color are sometimes the first indicators of skin cancer. Inquire about the patient's history of sun exposure, use of sunscreen, and predisposition to develop skin cancer (fair, freckled, light-colored hair or eyes, family history). Assess for use of topical medications, sun lamps, or tanning beds and exposure to creosote, coal, tar, or radium. Ask if the patient has noticed any changes in skin coloring; then proceed with inspection.

Color. Skin color varies by body part and person. Despite individual variations, skin color is usually uniform over the body. Table 16-4 lists common variations in skin color. Normal skin pigmentation ranges from ivory or light pink to ruddy pink in light skin and from light to deep brown or olive in dark skin. In older adults pigmentation increases unevenly, causing discolored skin. While inspecting the skin, be aware that cosmetics or tanning agents sometimes mask color.

The assessment of color first involves areas of the skin not exposed to the sun. Usually you see color hues best on the palms of the hands, soles of the feet, lips, tongue, and nail beds. Note if the skin is unusually pale or dark. Areas of increased color (hyperpigmentation) and decreased color (hypopigmentation) are common. Skin creases and folds are darker than the rest of the body.

Inspect sites where you can more easily identify abnormalities. For example, you can see **pallor** (unusual paleness)

BOX 16-4 EVIDENCE-BASED PRACTICE

PICO Question: In individuals who practice high-risk behaviors or have a familial tendency for skin cancers, does monthly systematic skin inspection result in earlier diagnosis of skin cancers than annual examinations with the health provider?

SUMMARY OF EVIDENCE

The American Cancer Society (ACS) estimates that there were 12,190 deaths from skin cancers in 2012 (ACS, 2013a). A melanoma is a cancerous (malignant) tumor that begins in the cells that produce the skin coloring (melanocytes). Melanoma is almost always curable in its early stages. However, it is likely to spread, and once it has spread to other parts of the body, the chances for a cure are much less. There are several risk factors for melanoma: major factors are positive family history of melanoma, a prior melanoma, and multiple or unusual moles (nevi). Other factors include fair skin, freckling, and light hair; immune suppression; age under 30; excessive exposure to the sun (especially before age 18); and the use of tanning beds/booths.

The ACS (2013a) outlines the warning signs of skin cancer using the ABCD mnemonic: A is for *A*symmetry—look for uneven shape; B is for *B*order irregularity—look for edges that are blurred, notched, or ragged; C is for *C*olor—pigmentation is not uniform; blue, black, brown variegated, tan, or areas of unusual colors such as pink, white, gray, blue, or red are abnormal; and D is for *D*iameter, greater than the size of a typical pencil eraser.

Research has indicated that skin cancer, when detected early and treated properly, is highly curable. Overall survival rates for melanoma at the 5-year mark are 92%, with 99% for localized melanoma; when grouped in regional and distant stages the survival rates dramatically decrease (ACS, 2013a). Therefore early intervention is of utmost importance.

The results from the research studies have made it a nursing responsibility to provide skin screening and intervention for all patients and families, especially those who have been identified as melanoma prone. Research has shown that educating children about sun-protective behaviors is difficult because children seem to possess strong attitudes against sun protection (DeMarco, 2008).

APPLICATION TO NURSING PRACTICE

- Instruct patients to conduct a complete monthly self-examination of the skin and scalp, noting moles, blemishes, and birthmarks.
- Perform the examination after a bath or shower, including a head-to-toe check.
- Use a well-lit room and mirrors to examine all skin surfaces. If necessary have the patient ask a family member/significant other to aid in the investigation.
- Teach your patients to contact their health care provider if a skin lesion or mole starts to bleed or ooze or feels different (swollen, hard, lumpy, itchy, or tender to the touch). Especially instruct older adults, who tend to have delayed wound healing.
- Inform your patients of ways to prevent skin cancer by avoiding overexposure to the sun:
  - Wear sunglasses, wide-brimmed hats, and long sleeves and long pants.
  - Apply broad-spectrum sunscreens with SPF 15 or greater to protect against ultraviolet B (UVB) and ultraviolet A (UVA) rays approximately 15 minutes before going into the sun and after swimming, perspiring, or bathing.
  - Avoid tanning under the direct sun at midday (10 am to 4 pm).
  - Do not use indoor sunlamps, tanning parlors, or tanning pills.
  - Inform patients who are on medications that make the skin more sensitive to the sun (e.g., oral contraceptives, statins, antiinflammatories, antihypertensives, immunosuppressives) to take extra precautions when spending time in the sun.
  - Provide children with a sun protection educational program with a diversified curriculum taught over an extended period of time (DeMarco, 2008).
  - Inform patients to protect their children from the sun. Severe sunburns in childhood greatly increase melanoma risk later in life (ACS, 2013a).

more easily in the face, buccal mucosa (mouth), conjunctivae, and nail beds. Observe for cyanosis (bluish discoloration) in the lips, nail beds, palpebral conjunctivae, and palms. To recognize pallor in the dark-skinned patient, observe that normal brown skin appears to be yellow-brown and normal black skin appears to be ashen gray. Also assess the lips, nail beds, and mucous membranes for generalized pallor that causes them to appear ashen gray. Assessment of cyanosis in darker-skinned patients requires that you observe areas where pigmentation occurs the least (conjunctivae, sclera, buccal mucosa, tongue, lips, nail beds, and palms and soles). In addition, verify findings with clinical manifestations (Newson, 2008). A bluish-tint of the lips and gums may be a normal finding in darker-skinned patients (Seidel et al., 2011).

The best site to inspect for **jaundice** (yellow-orange discoloration) is the patient's sclera. You can see normal reactive hyperemia, or redness, most often in regions exposed to pressure such as the sacrum, heels, and greater trochanter (see Chapter 37). Inspect for any patches or areas of skin color variation. Localized skin changes such as pallor or **erythema** (red discoloration) often indicate circulatory changes or are caused by localized vasodilation resulting from sunburn or fever. To help identify erythema in the dark-skinned patient, palpate the area for heat and warmth to note the presence of skin inflammation. An area of an extremity that appears unusually pale results from an arterial occlusion or edema.

There is a pattern of findings associated with patients who are chemically dependent and intravenous (IV) drug abusers (Table 16-5). It is sometimes difficult to recognize signs and symptoms with just one examination. Edematous, reddened, and warm areas along the arms and legs suggest a pattern of

TABLE 16-4 SKIN COLOR VARIATIONS

COLOR	CONDITION	CAUSES	ASSESSMENT LOCATIONS
Bluish (cyanosis)	Increased amount of deoxygenated hemoglobin (associated with hypoxia)	Heart or lung disease, cold environment	Nail beds, lips, base of tongue, skin (severe cases)
Pallor (decrease in color)	Reduced amount of oxyhemoglobin	Anemia	Face, conjunctivae, nail beds, palms of hands
	Reduced visibility of oxyhemoglobin resulting from decreased blood flow	Shock	Skin, nail beds, conjunctivae, lips
Loss of pigmentation	Vitiligo	Congenital or autoimmune condition causing lack of pigment	Patchy areas on skin over face, hands, arms
Yellow-orange (jaundice)	Increased deposit of bilirubin in tissues	Liver disease, destruction of red blood cells	Sclera, mucous membranes, skin
Red (erythema)	Increased visibility of oxyhemoglobin caused by dilation or increased blood flow	Fever, direct trauma, blushing, alcohol intake	Face, area of trauma, sacrum, shoulders, other common sites for pressure ulcers
Tan-brown	Increased amount of melanin	Suntan, pregnancy	Areas exposed to sun: face, arms; areolae, nipples

TABLE 16-5 PHYSICAL FINDINGS OF THE SKIN INDICATIVE OF SUBSTANCE ABUSE

PHYSICAL FINDING	COMMONLY ASSOCIATED DRUG
Diaphoresis	Sedative-hypnotic (including alcohol)
Spider angiomas	Alcohol, stimulants
Burns (especially fingers)	Alcohol
Needle marks	Opioids
Contusions, abrasions, cuts, scars	Alcohol, other sedative hypnotics
"Homemade" tattoos	Cocaine, intravenous opioids (prevents detection of injection sites)
Increased vascularity of face	Alcohol
Red, dry skin	Phencyclidine (PCP)

Modified from Lehne RA: *Pharmacology for nursing care,* ed 8, St Louis, 2013, Mosby; Ries R, Wilford B: *Principles of addiction medicine,* ed 4, Chevy Chase, MD, 2009, Lippincott Williams & Wilkins.

recent repeated IV injections. Evidence of old injection sites appears as hyperpigmented and shiny or scarred areas.

Moisture. The hydration of skin and mucous membranes helps to reveal body fluid imbalances, changes in skin environment, and regulation of body temperature. Moisture refers to wetness and oiliness. The skin is normally smooth and dry, whereas areas such as the axillae are normally moist; minimal perspiration or oiliness is present (Seidel et al., 2011). Increased perspiration is associated with activity, warm environments, obesity, anxiety, or excitement. Use ungloved fingertips to palpate skin surfaces and observe for dullness, dryness, crusting, and flaking. Flaking is the appearance of dandruff when the skin surface is rubbed lightly. Scaling involves fishlike scales that are easily rubbed off the surface of the skin. Both flaking and scaling indicate abnormally dry skin. Excessively dry skin is common in older adults and people who use skin-drying soaps during bathing (Cowdell, 2011). Other factors causing dry skin include lack of humidity, exposure to sun, smoking, stress, excessive perspiration, and dehydration. Excessive dryness worsens existing skin conditions. Bariatric patients with large abdominal skinfolds are at high risk for moisture that encourages the growth of bacteria and fungi, which contribute to rashes and infection (Rush and Muir, 2012).

Temperature. The temperature of the skin depends on the amount of blood circulating through the dermis. Increased or decreased skin temperature reflects an increase or decrease in blood flow. An increase in skin temperature often accompanies localized erythema or redness of the skin. A reduction in skin temperature reflects a decrease in blood flow. Remember that a cold examination room affects the patient's skin temperature and color.

Accurately assess temperature by palpating the skin with the dorsum or back of the hand. Compare symmetrical body parts. Normally the skin temperature is warm and consistent throughout the body. Always assess skin temperature for patients at risk for impaired circulation, such as when skin temperature varies in one area or after a cast application or vascular surgery. You can identify a stage I pressure ulcer early by noting warmth and erythema on an area of the skin (see Chapter 37).

Texture. The character of the surface of the skin and the feel of deeper portions are its texture. Determine whether the

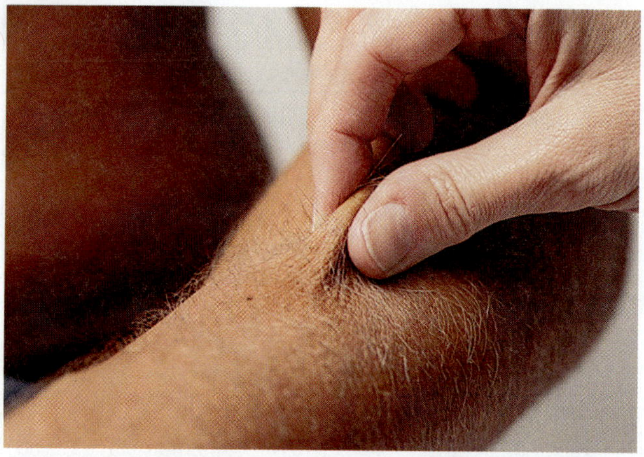

FIGURE 16-4 Assessment of skin turgor.

patient's skin is smooth or rough, thin or thick, tight or supple, or indurated (hardened) or soft by stroking it lightly with the fingertips. The texture of the skin is normally smooth, soft, and flexible in children and adults. However, it is usually not uniform. The palms of the hands and soles of the feet tend to be thicker. In older adults the skin becomes wrinkled and leathery because of a decrease in collagen, subcutaneous fat, and sweat glands.

Localized changes result from trauma, surgical wounds, or lesions. If you find irregularities in texture such as scars or induration, ask the patient if there has been recent skin injury. Deeper palpation sometimes reveals irregularities such as tenderness or localized areas of induration commonly caused by repeated injections.

Turgor. Turgor is the elasticity of the skin. Normally the skin loses its elasticity with age. Edema or dehydration diminishes turgor. To assess skin turgor grasp a fold of skin on the back of the forearm or sternal area with the fingertips and release (Figure 16-4). Normally the skin lifts easily and snaps back immediately to its resting position. It stays pinched or tented when turgor is poor. A decrease in turgor predisposes a patient to skin breakdown.

Vascularity. Skin circulation affects color in localized areas and the appearance of superficial blood vessels. With aging capillaries become fragile. Localized pressure areas, found after a patient has remained in one position, appear reddened, pink, or pale (see Chapter 37). Petechiae are pinpoint-size red or purple spots on the skin caused by small hemorrhages in the skin layers. They do not blanch but may indicate serious blood-clotting disorders, drug reactions, or liver disease.

Edema. Areas of the skin become swollen or edematous from fluid buildup in the tissues. Direct trauma and impairment of venous return are two common causes of edema. Inspect edematous areas for location, color, and shape. The formation of edema separates the surface of the skin from the pigmented and vascular layers, masking skin color. Edematous skin also appears stretched and shiny. Palpate edematous areas to determine mobility, consistency, and tenderness. When pressure from your finger leaves an indentation in the edematous area, it is called *pitting edema.* To assess pitting edema press the edematous area firmly with the thumb for several seconds and release. The depth of pitting, recorded in millimeters, determines the degree of edema (Seidel et al., 2011). For example, +1 edema equals 2 mm depth, and +2 edema equals 4 mm (see Figure 16-35).

Lesions. The skin is normally free of lesions, except for common freckles or age-related changes such as skin tags or senile keratosis (thickening of skin), cherry angiomas (ruby red papules), and atrophic warts. Primary lesions occur as initial spontaneous manifestations of a pathological process such as an insect bite or are secondary and result from later formation of trauma to a primary lesion such as a pressure ulcer. When you detect a lesion, inspect it for color, location, texture, size, shape, type (Box 16-5), grouping (e.g., clustered or linear), and distribution (localized or generalized). Observe any exudate for color, odor, amount, and consistency. Measure the size of the lesion by using a small, clear, flexible ruler divided in centimeters. Measure lesions in height, width, and depth.

Palpation determines the mobility, contour (flat, raised, or depressed), and consistency (soft or indurated) of the lesion. Palpate gently, covering the entire area of the lesion. If the lesion is moist or has draining fluid, wear clean gloves during palpation. Note if the patient complains of tenderness during palpation. Cancerous lesions frequently undergo changes in color and size. Report abnormal lesions that have changed in character (e.g., color or size) to a health care provider for further examination.

Hair and Scalp

Inspecting the condition and distribution of body hair and integrity of the scalp requires good lighting. Hair assessment occurs during all portions of the examination. Assess its distribution, thickness, texture, lubrication, and grooming.

Nursing History. Assess if the patient has noticed a change in growth or loss of hair or change in texture. Determine if the patient wears a wig or hairpiece and ask if he or she is comfortable with it being removed briefly to examine the skin underneath. Determine if the patient is on a medication or has any medical conditions that possibly alter hair texture or growth (e.g., chemotherapy or vasodilator).

During inspection explain that it is necessary to separate parts of the hair to detect abnormalities. Wear clean gloves to avoid possible infection from lesions or lice. First inspect the color, distribution, quantity, thickness, texture, and lubrication of body hair. It is normally distributed evenly, is neither excessively dry nor oily, and is pliant or flexible. While separating sections of scalp hair, observe for characteristics of color and coarseness. Normal terminal hair (long, coarse, thick hair on the scalp, axillae, and pubic areas) varies in color from light blond to black to gray. In older adults the hair becomes dull gray, white, or yellow. It also thins over the scalp, axillae, and pubic areas. Older men lose facial hair, whereas older women sometimes develop hair on the chin and upper lip.

Changes occur in the thickness, texture, and lubrication of scalp hair. Disturbances such as a febrile illness or scalp

BOX 16-5 TYPES OF PRIMARY SKIN LESIONS

Macule: Flat, nonpalpable change in skin color, smaller than 1 cm (e.g., freckle, petechia)

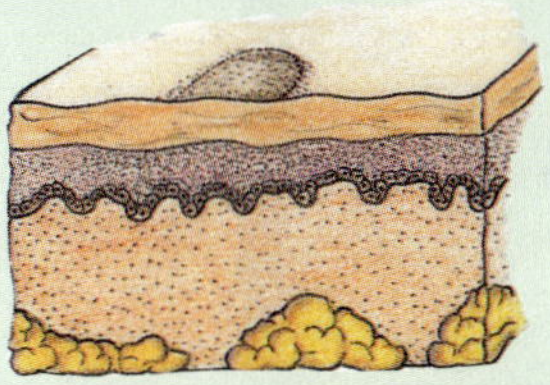

Papule: Palpable, circumscribed, solid elevation in skin, smaller than 0.5 cm (e.g., elevated nevus)

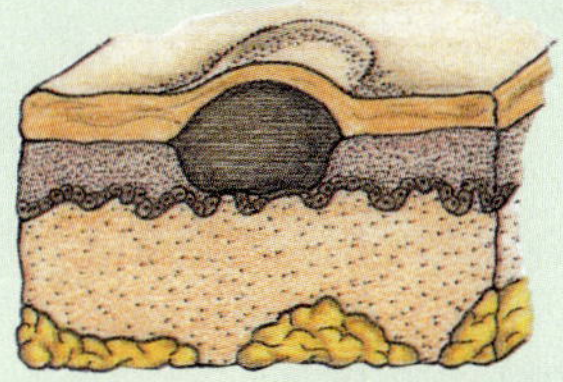

Nodule: Elevated solid mass, deeper and firmer than papule, 0.5 to 2 cm (e.g., wart)

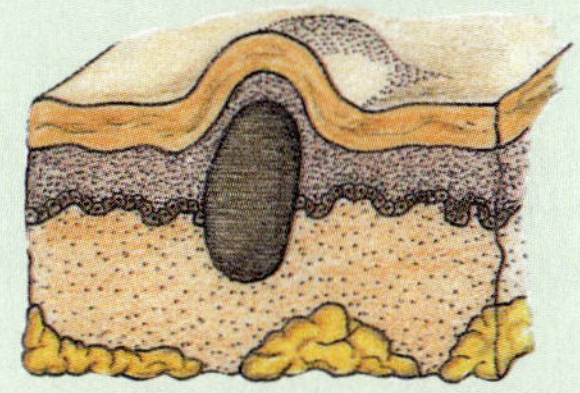

Tumor: Solid mass that extends deep through subcutaneous tissue, larger than 1 to 2 cm (e.g., epithelioma)

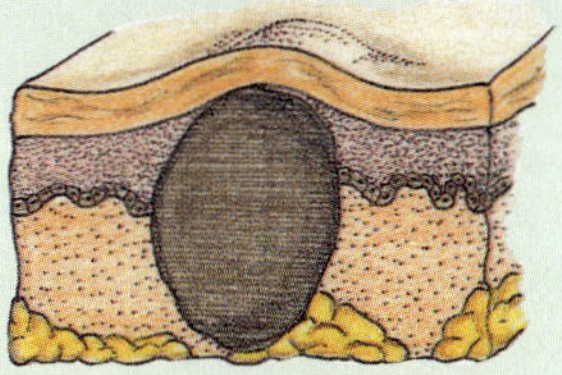

Wheal: Irregularly shaped, elevated area or superficial localized edema, varies in size (e.g., hive, mosquito bite)

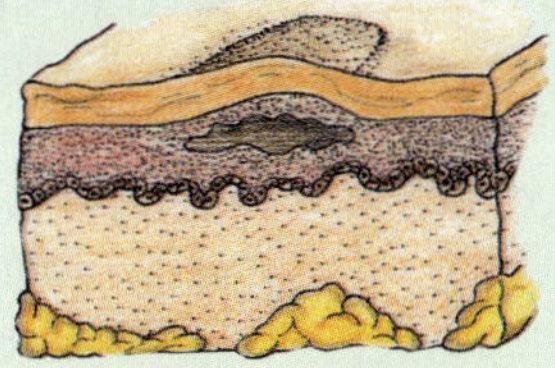

Vesicle: Circumscribed elevation of skin filled with serous fluid, smaller than 1 cm (e.g., herpes simplex, chickenpox)

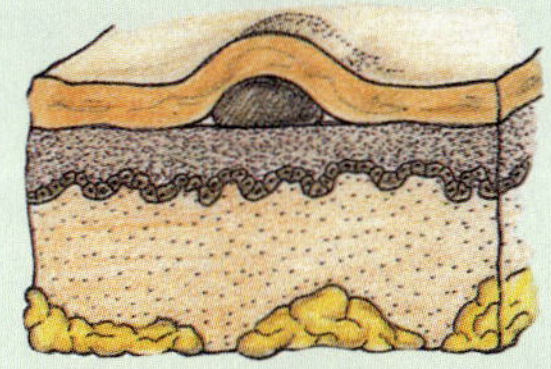

Pustule: Circumscribed elevation of skin similar to vesicle but filled with pus; varies in size (e.g., acne, staphylococcal infection)

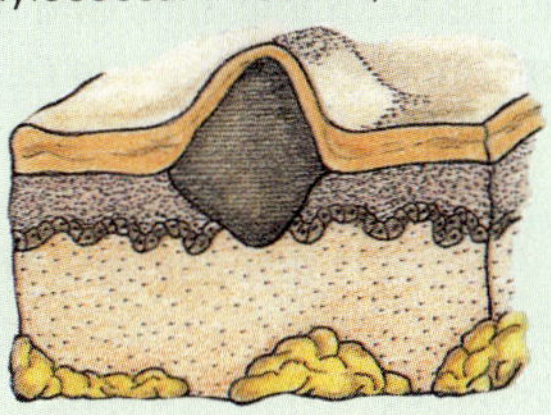

Ulcer: Deep loss of skin surface that sometimes extends to dermis and frequently bleeds and scars; varies in size (e.g., venous stasis ulcer)

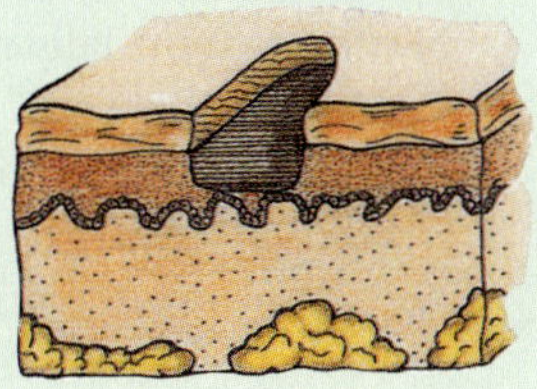

Atrophy: Thinning of skin with loss of normal skin furrow with skin appearing shiny and translucent; varies in size (e.g., arterial insufficiency)

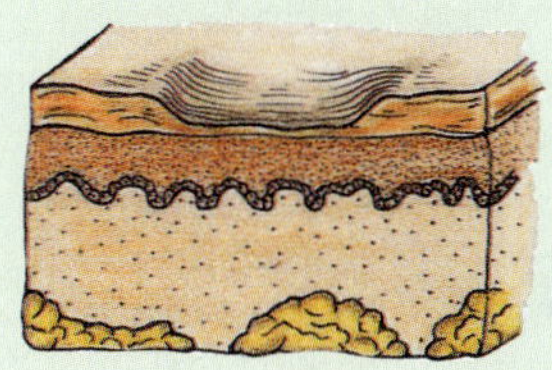

disease sometimes result in hair loss. Conditions such as thyroid disease alter the condition of the hair, making it fine and brittle. Hair loss (alopecia) or thinning of the hair is usually related to genetic tendencies and endocrine disorders such as diabetes and menopause. Poor nutrition causes stringy, dull, dry, and thin hair. The hair is lubricated from the oil of sebaceous glands. Excessively oily hair is associated with androgen hormone stimulation. Dry, brittle hair occurs with aging and excessive use of chemical agents.

The amount of hair covering the extremities is sometimes reduced as a result of aging or a disease process such as arterial insufficiency, most common over the lower extremities. In women do not confuse a loss of hair with shaved legs.

Inspect the scalp for lesions, which are not easily noticed in thick hair. The scalp is normally smooth and inelastic with even coloration. By carefully separating strands of hair, thoroughly examine the scalp for lesions. Note the characteristics of any scalp lesions. If you find lumps or bruises, ask if the patient has experienced recent head trauma. Moles on the scalp are common. Warn the patient that combing or brushing sometimes causes a mole to bleed. Dandruff or psoriasis frequently causes scaliness or dryness.

Careful inspection of hair follicles on the scalp and pubic areas may reveal lice or other parasites. There are head lice, body lice, and crab lice. Head and crab lice attach their eggs to hair. Lice eggs look like oval particles of dandruff. The lice themselves are difficult to see. Observe for bites or pustular eruptions in the follicles and areas where skin surfaces meet such as behind the ears and in the groin. The discovery of lice requires immediate treatment and family education (Box 16-6).

Nails

The condition of the nails reflects general health, state of nutrition, a person's occupation, and level of self-care. The most visible portion of the nails is the nail plate, the transparent layer of epithelial cells covering the nail bed. The vascularity of the nail bed creates the underlying color of the nail. The semilunar, whitish area at the base of the nail bed is called the *lunula,* from which the nail plate develops.

Nursing History. Ask the patient if there have been any recent changes in the nails (e.g., splitting, breaking, or thickening) or recent trauma. Determine the patient's nail care practices such as use of acrylic nails or risk for exposure to fungi at nail salons. Determine any physiologic risk factors for nail problems (e.g., diabetes mellitus, peripheral vascular disease, or older age).

BOX 16-6 PATIENT TEACHING

Hair and Scalp Assessment

OUTCOME

Patient performs proper hygiene practices for care of the hair and scalp.

TEACHING STRATEGIES

- Instruct in basic hygiene practices for care of the hair and scalp (see Chapter 29).
- Instruct patients who have head lice to shampoo thoroughly with pediculicide (shampoo available at drug stores) in cold water, comb thoroughly with fine-tooth comb (following product directions), and discard comb. Caution against use of products containing lindane, a toxic ingredient known to cause adverse reactions. Repeat shampoo treatment 12 to 24 hours later.
- After combing remove any detachable nits or nit cases with tweezers or between the fingernails. A dilute solution of vinegar and water helps loosen nits.
- Instruct patients and parents about ways to reduce transmission of lice:
  - Do not share personal-care items with others.
  - Vacuum all rugs, car seats, pillows, furniture, and flooring thoroughly and discard vacuum bag.
  - Seal nonwashable items in plastic bags for 14 days if parents are unable to dry-clean or vacuum.
  - Use thorough hand-hygiene practices.
  - Launder all clothing, linen, and bedding in hot soap and water and dry in a hot dryer for at least 20 minutes. Dry-clean nonwashable items.
  - Do not use insecticide.
  - Instruct patient to notify his or her partner if lice were sexually transmitted.
  - Avoid physical contact with infested individuals and their belongings, especially clothing and bedding.
  - Soak combs, brushes, and hair accessories in lice-killing products for 1 hour or in boiling water for 10 minutes.

EVALUATION STRATEGIES

- Have patient describe methods used to care for the hair and scalp.
- Have patient explain the steps to reduce lice transmission.

Inspect the nail bed color, cleanliness, and length; the thickness and shape of the nail; the texture of the nail; the angle between the nail and the nail bed; and the condition of tissue around the nail. The nails are normally transparent, smooth, well rounded, and convex, with surrounding cuticles smooth, intact, and without inflammation. In light-skinned patients nail beds are pink with translucent white nail tips. In dark-skinned patients they are darkly pigmented, have a blue or reddish hue, and have yellow-tinged nail tips. A brown or black pigmentation is normal with longitudinal streaks (Figure 16-5). Trauma, cirrhosis, diabetes mellitus, and hypertension cause splinter hemorrhages. Vitamin, protein, and electrolyte changes cause various lines or bands to form on nail beds.

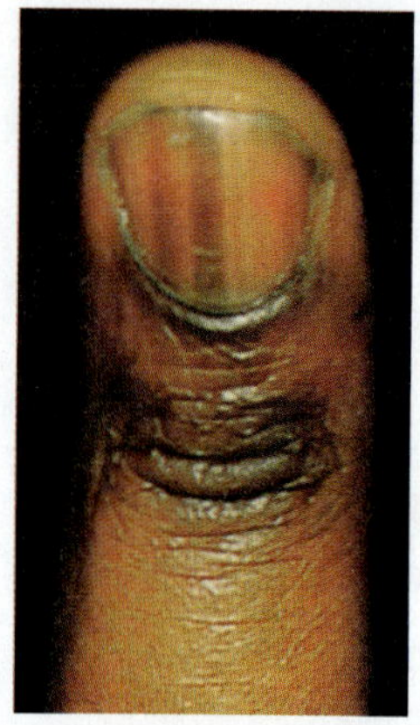

FIGURE 16-5 Pigmented bands in nail of patient with dark skin. (From Seidel HM, et al: *Mosby's guide to physical examination,* ed 7, St Louis, 2011, Mosby.)

Nails normally grow at a constant rate, but direct injury or generalized disease impairs growth. With aging the nails of the fingers and toes become harder and thicker. Longitudinal striations develop, and the rate of nail growth slows. Nails become more brittle, dull, and opaque and turn yellow in older adults because of insufficient calcium. Also with age the cuticle becomes less thick and wide.

Inspection of the angle between the nail and nail bed normally reveals an angle of 160 degrees (Box 16-7). A larger angle and softening of the nail bed indicate chronic oxygenation problems.

Palpate the nail base to determine firmness and condition of circulation. It is normally firm. To palpate gently grasp the patient's finger and observe its color. An ongoing bluish or purplish cast to the nail bed occurs with cyanosis. A white cast or pallor results from anemia. Observe for jaundice (yellow-orange), which indicates liver disease.

Calluses and corns often occur on the toes or fingers. A callus is flat and painless, resulting from thickening of the epidermis such as the finger that supports a pencil or pen or on the bottom of the feet. Friction and pressure from shoes cause corns, usually over bony prominences. During the examination instruct the patient in proper nail care (Box 16-8).

HEAD AND NECK

An examination of the head and neck includes assessment of the head, eyes, ears, nose, mouth, pharynx, and neck (lymph nodes, carotid arteries, thyroid gland, and trachea). During assessment of peripheral arteries also assess the carotid arteries. Assessment of the head and neck uses inspection, palpation, and auscultation.

Head

Nursing History. Determine if your patient has a recent history of head trauma or neurological symptoms such as headache, dizziness, seizures, poor vision, or loss of consciousness. Review the patient's occupation, participation in contact sports, and use of protective head gear.

BOX 16-7 ABNORMALITIES OF THE NAIL BED

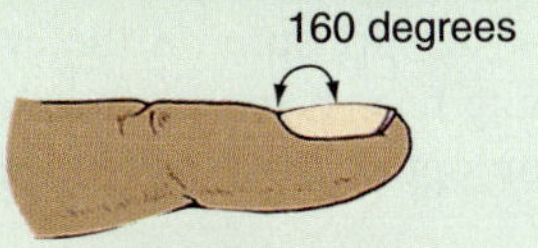

Normal nail: Approximately 160-degree angle between nail plate and nail

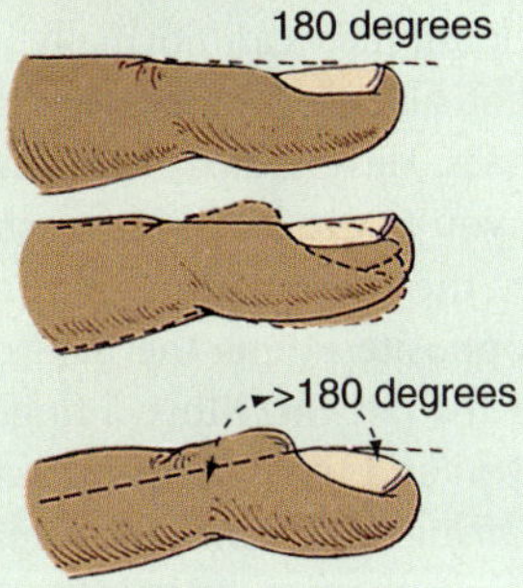

Clubbing: Change in angle between nail and nail base (eventually greater than 180 degrees); nail bed softening with nail flattening; often enlargement of fingertips
Causes: Chronic lack of oxygen: heart or pulmonary disease

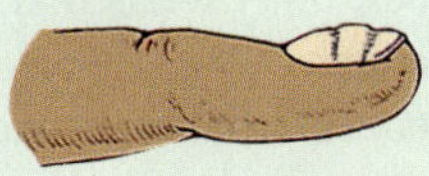

Beau's lines: Transverse depressions in nails indicating temporary disturbance of nail growth (nail grows out over several months)
Causes: Systemic illness such as severe infection; nail injury

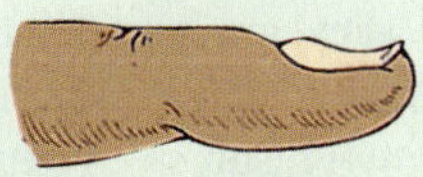

Koilonychia (spoon nail): Concave curves
Causes: Iron deficiency anemia, syphilis, use of strong detergents

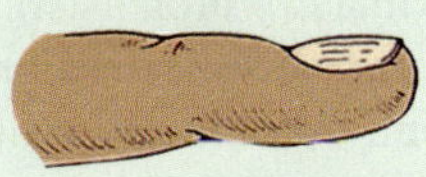

Splinter hemorrhages: Red or brown linear streaks in nail bed
Causes: Minor trauma, subacute bacterial endocarditis, trichinosis

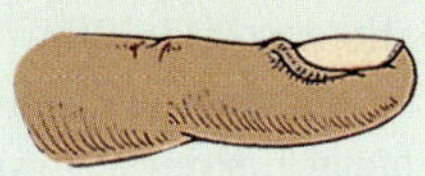

Paronychia: Inflammation of skin at base of nail
Causes: Local infection, trauma

Inspect the patient's head, noting the position, size, shape, and contour. The head is normally held upright and midline to the trunk. Holding the head tilted to one side is an indication of unilateral hearing or visual loss. A horizontal jerking or bobbing indicates a tremor.

Note facial features, looking at the eyelids, eyebrows, nasolabial folds, and mouth for shape and symmetry. It is normal for slight asymmetry to exist. If there is facial asymmetry, note if all features on one side of the face are affected or if only part of the face is involved. Various neurological disorders such as a facial nerve paralysis affect different nerves that innervate muscles of the face.

Examine the size, shape, and contour of the skull. Generally it is round with prominences in the frontal area anteriorly and the occipital area posteriorly. Trauma typically causes local skull deformities. Palpate the skull for nodules or masses. Gently rotate the fingertips down the midline of the scalp and then along the sides of the head to identify abnormalities.

BOX 16-8 PATIENT TEACHING

Nail Assessment

OUTCOME

Patient properly cares for fingernails, feet, and toenails.

TEACHING STRATEGIES

- Instruct patient to cut nails only after soaking them about 10 minutes in warm water. (Exception: Patients with diabetes are warned against soaking nails because this dries the hands and feet; dry skin leads to infection.)
- Caution patient to avoid using over-the-counter preparations to treat corns, calluses, or ingrown toenails.
- Tell patient to cut nails straight across and even with tops of fingers or toes. If patient has diabetes, tell him or her to file rather than cut nails (see Chapter 29).
- Instruct patient to shape nails with file or emery board.
- If patient has diabetes:
  - Wash feet daily in warm water and carefully dry them, especially between toes. Inspect feet each day in good lighting, looking for dry places and cracks in skin. Soften dry feet by applying cream or lotion such as Nivea, Eucerin, or Alpha Keri.
  - Do not put lotion between toes; moisture between toes promotes growth of microorganisms, leading to infection.
  - Caution patient against using sharp objects to poke or dig under toenail or around cuticle.
  - Have patient see a podiatrist for treatment of ingrown toenails and nails that are thick or tend to split.

EVALUATION STRATEGIES

- Inspect nails during next home visit.
- Have patient explain steps to avoid injury to the fingernails, feet, and toenails.

In infants a large head results from congenital anomalies or the accumulation of cerebrospinal fluid in the ventricles (hydrocephalus). Acromegaly causes an enlarged jaw and facial bones in affected adults.

Eyes

Examination of the eye includes assessment of visual acuity, visual fields, and external and internal eye structures. Figure 16-6 shows a cross section of the eye. The assessment detects visual alterations and determines the level of assistance that patients require when ambulating or performing self-care activities. Patients with visual problems need special aids for reading educational materials or instructions.

Nursing History. Review with the patient any history of partial or complete vision loss from eye disease (e.g., glaucoma or cataracts), eye trauma, diabetes, hypertension, or eye surgery. Assess for common symptoms of eye disease such as eye pain, photophobia (sensitivity to light), burning, itching, excessive tearing, diplopia (double vision), blurred vision, or visual disturbances (e.g., flashing lights, halos, or "film" over vision field). Review the patient's occupational history, use of glasses or contact lenses, use of safety glasses, and visits to

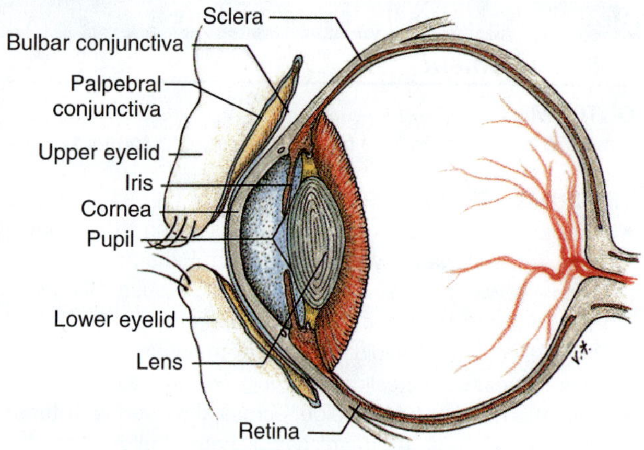

FIGURE 16-6 Cross section of eye.

BOX 16-9 PATIENT TEACHING

Eye Assessment

OUTCOME

Patient follows recommendations for preventive eye care, including regular eye care examinations and protection from injury.

TEACHING STRATEGIES

- Tell patient that people under age 40 need to have a complete eye examination every 3 to 5 years (or more often if family histories reveal risks such as diabetes or hypertension).
- Teach patients that people over age 40 need to have a complete eye examination every 2 years to screen for conditions that may develop without patient awareness (e.g., glaucoma), which increases to annual examinations after 65.
- Describe the typical symptoms of eye disease (see Chapter 38).
- Instruct older adults to take the following precautions because of normal vision changes: avoid or use caution while driving at night, increase lighting in the home to reduce risk for falls, and paint the first and last steps of a staircase and the edge of each step in between a bright color to aid in depth perception.

EVALUATION STRATEGIES

- Ask the patient and family member to report the most recent ophthalmologist visit and plans for future visits.
- Ask patient to describe common symptoms of eye disease.
- Have patient describe safety measures for eye protection when working at home or with tools and equipment.

optometrist (Box 16-9). Determine the patient's current medication use, including any eye medication.

Visual Acuity. The assessment of visual acuity (i.e., the ability to see small details) tests central vision. The easiest way to assess visual acuity is to ask the patient to read printed material or a Snellen chart under adequate lighting. Patients need to wear prescription glasses or contact lenses during the assessment. Identify the language the patient speaks and reading ability. Asking the patient to read aloud helps determine literacy. Position the patient 6 m (20 feet) away from the chart. Test each eye separately by covering one eye with a card or gauze square, careful to avoid pressure on the eye. A patient who has difficulty reading related to vision needs to consult an ophthalmologist or optometrist for further evaluation.

Visual Fields. Objects in the periphery can normally be seen when a person looks straight ahead. To assess visual fields, remove the patient's eyeglasses. Have the patient stand or sit 60 cm (2 feet) away, facing you at eye level. He or she gently closes or covers one eye (e.g., the left) and looks at your eye directly opposite. Close the opposite eye as the field of vision is superimposed on that of the patient. Move a finger equidistant at arm's length from you and the patient outside the field of vision and then slowly bring it back into the visual field. Ask the patient to tell you when the finger is visible. If you see the finger before the patient does, this reveals that a portion of the patient's visual field is reduced.

External Eye Structures. To inspect external eye structures, stand directly in front of the patient at eye level and ask him or her to look at your face. Ask patients to remove glasses or contacts for the remainder of the examination.

Position and Alignment. Assess the position of the eyes in relation to one another. Normally they are parallel to one another. Bulging eyes (exophthalmos) usually indicate hyperthyroidism. Crossed eyes (strabismus) result from neuromuscular injury or inherited abnormalities. A tumor or inflammation of the orbit causes abnormal eye protrusion.

Eyebrows. Inspect the eyebrows for size, extension, texture of hair, alignment, and movement. Coarseness of hair and failure to extend beyond the temporal canthus may reveal hypothyroidism. If the brows are thinned, identify if the patient plucks or waxes the hair. Aging causes loss of the lateral third of the eyebrows. Have the patient raise and lower the eyebrows. They normally raise and lower symmetrically. An inability to move them indicates a facial nerve paralysis (cranial nerve VII).

Eyelids. Inspect the eyelids for position, color, condition, and direction of lashes; assess the patient's ability to open, close, and blink. When the eyes are open in a normal position, the lids do not cover the pupil, and you cannot see the sclera above the iris. The lids are also close to the eyeball. An abnormal drooping of the lid over the pupil is called *ptosis,* caused by edema or impairment of the third cranial nerve. In the older adult ptosis results from a loss of elasticity that accompanies aging. An older adult frequently has lid margins that turn out (ectropion) or in (entropion). An entropion sometimes leads to the lashes of the lid irritating the conjunctiva and cornea, increasing risk for infection. Normally the eyelashes are distributed evenly and curved outward away from the eye.

The lids close symmetrically. Ask the patient to open the eyes, and observe the blink reflex, during which the cornea is lubricated. Normally a patient blinks involuntarily and bilaterally as many as 20 times a minute. Report absent, infrequent, rapid, or monocular (one-eyed) blinking. Failure of

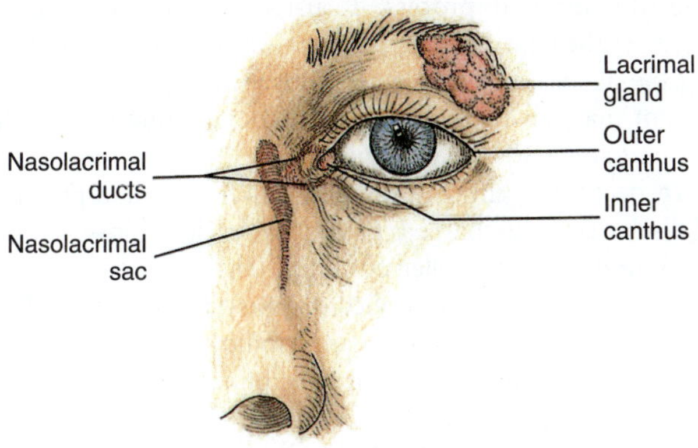

FIGURE 16-7 Lacrimal apparatus.

lids to close exposes the cornea to drying. This condition happens in unconscious patients or those with facial nerve paralysis.

Lacrimal Apparatus. The lacrimal gland (Figure 16-7), located in the upper, outer wall of the anterior part of the orbit, is responsible for tear production. Tears flow from the gland across the surface of the eye to the lacrimal duct, which is in the nasal corner or inner canthus of the eye. Inspect the lacrimal gland for edema and redness. Palpate the gland area gently to detect tenderness. Normally the gland cannot be felt. The nasolacrimal duct may become obstructed, blocking the flow of tears. Observe for evidence of excess tearing or edema in the inner canthus. Gentle palpation of the duct at the lower eyelid just inside the orbital rim causes a regurgitation of tears.

Conjunctivae and Sclerae. The bulbar conjunctiva covers the exposed surface of the eyeball up to the outer edge of the cornea. Observe the sclera under the bulbar conjunctiva; it normally has the color of white porcelain in Caucasians and light yellow in darker-skinned patients. To view both structures gently retract both lids simultaneously with thumb and index finger pressed against the lower and upper bony orbits. For adequate exposure retract the eyelids without placing pressure directly on the eyeball. Ask the patient to look up, down, and side to side. Inspect for color, texture, and the presence of edema or lesions.

Normally the conjunctivae are free of erythema. The presence of redness indicates allergic or infectious conjunctivitis. Conjunctivitis is a highly contagious infection, and the crusty drainage that collects on eyelid margins easily spreads from one eye to the other. Perform proper hand hygiene (see Chapter 14) before and after the examination. Wear clean gloves during the examination.

Corneas. The cornea is the transparent, colorless portion of the eye covering the pupil and iris. From a side view it looks like the crystal of a wristwatch. While the patient looks straight ahead, inspect the cornea for clarity and texture while shining a penlight obliquely across its surface. Normally the cornea is shiny, transparent, and smooth. In older adults it loses its luster. Any irregularity in the surface indicates an abrasion or tear that requires further examination by a health care provider. Both conditions are very painful. To test for the

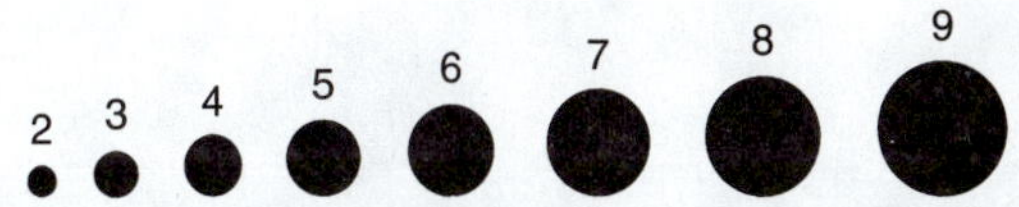

FIGURE 16-8 Chart depicting pupillary size in millimeters.

corneal blink reflex, see the cranial nerve function section of this chapter.

Pupils and Irises. Observe the pupils for size, shape, equality, accommodation, and reaction to light. They are normally black, round, regular, and equal in size (3 to 7 mm in diameter) (Figure 16-8). The iris should be clearly visible. Note the color and details of the iris. In an older adult it becomes faded. A thin white ring along the margin of the iris, called an **arcus senilis,** is common with aging but abnormal in anyone under age 40.

Cloudy pupils indicate cataracts. Continuous dilation of pupils results from neurological disorders, glaucoma, trauma, eye medication, or withdrawal from opioids. Pinpoint pupils are a common sign of opioid intoxication. When shining a beam of light through the pupil and onto the retina, the third cranial nerve is stimulated, causing the muscles of the iris to constrict. Any abnormality along the nerve pathways from the retina to the iris alters the ability of the pupils to react to light. Changes in intracranial pressure, lesions along the nerve pathways, locally applied ophthalmic medications, and direct trauma to the eye alter pupillary reaction.

Test pupillary reflexes (to light and accommodation) in a dimly lit room. Instruct the patient to look straight ahead, bring a penlight from the side of the patient's face, and direct the light onto the pupil (Figure 16-9, *A* and *B*). A directly illuminated pupil constricts, and the opposite pupil constricts consensually. Observe the quickness and equality of the reflex. Repeat the examination for the opposite eye.

To test accommodation ask the patient to gaze at a distant object (the far wall) and then at a test object (finger or pencil) held approximately 10 cm (4 inches) from the bridge of the patient's nose. The pupils normally converge and accommodate by constricting when looking at close objects. The pupil responses are equal. If assessment of pupillary reaction is normal in all tests, record the abbreviation PERRLA (pupils equal, round, reactive to light and accommodation).

Internal Eye Structures. An advanced nurse practitioner or other health provider usually performs examination of the internal eye structures through the use of an ophthalmoscope.

Ears

The ear assessment determines the integrity of ear structures and hearing acuity. Inspect and palpate external ear structures, inspect middle ear structures with the otoscope, and test the inner ear by measuring the patient's hearing acuity. Assessment of patients with hearing impairment provides useful data in planning effective communication techniques.

Nursing History. Review risk factors for hearing problems with the patient (e.g., intake of aspirin or noise

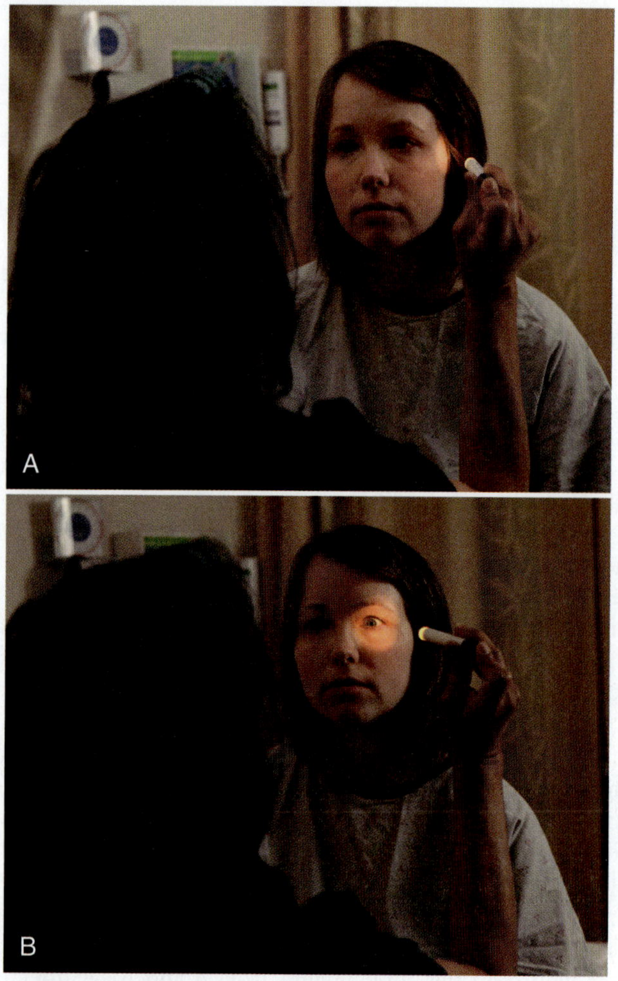

FIGURE 16-9 **A,** To check pupillary reflexes, the nurse first holds the penlight to the side of patient's face. **B,** Illumination of pupil causes pupillary constriction.

exposure) and assess for history of ear trauma or surgery. Determine if the patient has ear pain, itching, discharge, tinnitus (ringing in ears), vertigo (loss of balance), or change in hearing. Note behavior that indicates hearing loss such as leaning forward to hear, inattentiveness to speech, and requests to repeat comments. Determine the onset and contributing factors to the hearing problem. Assess if the patient wears a hearing aid and how he or she normally cleans the ears.

Auricles. With the patient sitting inspect the size, shape, symmetry, flexibility, landmarks, position, and color of the auricle. The auricles are normally of equal size and level with one another. The upper point of attachment to the head is normally in a straight line with the outer canthus, or corner of the eye. Ears that are low set or at an unusual angle may indicate a chromosome abnormality or renal disorders. Ear color is the same as the face without moles, cysts, deformities, or nodules. Redness is a sign of inflammation or fever.

Palpate the auricles for texture, tenderness, swelling, and skin lesions. Auricles are normally smooth, firm, mobile, and without lesions. If the patient complains of pain, gently pull the auricle, press on the tragus, and palpate behind the ear over the mastoid process. If palpating the external ear increases the pain, an external ear infection is likely. If palpating the auricle and tragus does not influence the pain, the patient may have a middle ear infection. Tenderness in the mastoid area indicates mastoiditis.

Inspect the opening of the ear canal for size and presence of discharge. If discharge is present, wear clean gloves during the examination. A swollen or occluded meatus is not normal. A yellow, waxy substance called **cerumen** is common. Yellow or green foul-smelling discharge indicates infection or a foreign body in the canal. The color of cerumen is darker in dark-skinned patients.

Ear Canals and Eardrums. Observe the deeper structures of the external and middle ear with the use of an otoscope. A special ear speculum attaches to the handle of the ophthalmoscope. For best visualization select the largest speculum that fits comfortably in the patient's ear. Before inserting it, check for foreign bodies in the opening of the auditory canal.

Make sure that the patient avoids moving the head during the examination to avoid damage to the canal and tympanic membrane. Hold the head of moving infants and young children. Lie infants supine with their heads turned to one side and their arms held securely at their sides or snuggly wrap them in a blanket. Have young children sit on their parents' laps with their legs held between the parents' knees.

Turn on the otoscope by rotating the dial at the top of the handle. To insert the speculum properly, ask the patient to tip the head slightly to the opposite shoulder. Hold the handle of the otoscope in the space between the thumb and index finger, supported on the middle finger. This leaves the ulnar side of your hand to rest against the patient's head, stabilizing the otoscope as it is inserted into the canal (Seidel et al., 2011). Insert the scope while pulling the auricle upward and backward in the adult and older child (Figure 16-10). This maneuver straightens the ear canal. In children under 3 years of age, pull the auricle down and back.

Insert the speculum slightly down and forward, 1 to 1.5 cm (½ to ¾ inch) into the ear canal. Take care not to scrape the sensitive lining of the ear canal, which is painful. The ear canal normally has little cerumen and is uniformly colored with tiny hairs in the outer third of the canal. Observe for color, discharge, scaling, lesions, foreign bodies, and cerumen. Normally cerumen is dry (light brown to gray and flaky) or moist (dark yellow or brown) and sticky. Dry cerumen occurs more often in Asians and Native Americans (Seidel et al., 2011). A reddened canal with discharge is a sign of inflammation or infection. In older adults accumulated cerumen is a common cause of mild hearing loss. During the examination ask the patient how he or she normally cleans the ear canal (Box 16-10). Caution the patient on the danger of inserting pointed objects into the canal. Avoid the use of cotton-tipped applicators to clean the ears because this causes impaction of cerumen deep in the ear canal.

The light from the otoscope allows visualization of the eardrum (tympanic membrane). Know the common anatomical landmarks and their appearance (Figure 16-11).

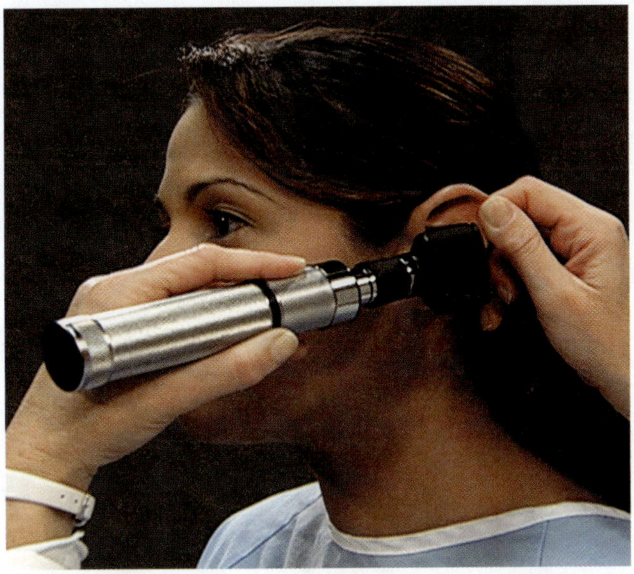

FIGURE 16-10 Otoscopic examination. (From Seidel HM, et al: *Mosby's guide to physical examination,* ed 7, St Louis, 2011, Mosby.)

BOX 16-10 PATIENT TEACHING

Ear Assessment

OUTCOME

Patient follows preventive guidelines for screening hearing loss of voice and environmental sounds.

TEACHING STRATEGIES

- Encourage patients over age 65 or with noticeable change in hearing to have regular hearing checks. Explain that a reduction in hearing is a normal part of aging (see Chapter 38).
- Instruct family members of patients with hearing losses to avoid shouting, speaking instead with low tones while directly facing the patient.

EVALUATION STRATEGIES

- In future visits question patient about frequency of hearing checks.
- Observe patient with hearing loss interacting with family members.

Move the auricle to see the entire drum and its periphery. Because the eardrum is angled away from the ear canal, the light from the otoscope appears as a cone shape rather than a circle. The umbo is near the center of the drum, behind which is the attachment of the malleus. The underlying short process of the malleus creates a knoblike structure at the top of the drum. Check carefully to be sure that there are no tears or breaks in the membrane of the eardrum. The normal eardrum is taught, translucent, shiny, and pearly gray. It is free from tears or breaks. A pink or red bulging membrane indicates inflammation. A white color reveals pus behind it. If cerumen is blocking the tympanic membrane, warm water irrigation safely removes the wax.

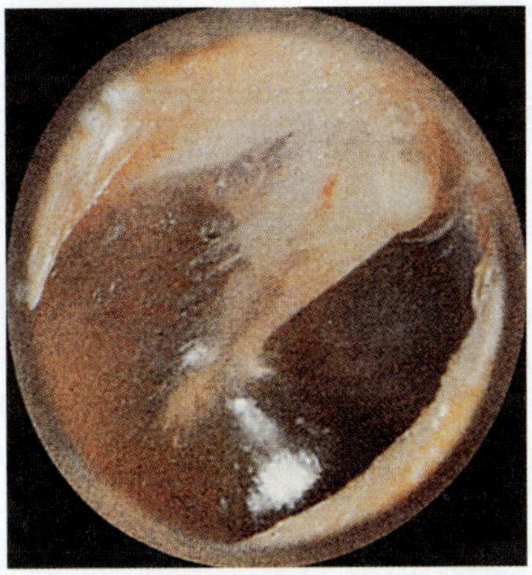

FIGURE 16-11 Normal tympanic membrane. (Courtesy Dr. Richard A. Buckingham, Abraham Lincoln School of Medicine, University of Illinois, Chicago.)

Hearing Acuity. A patient with hearing loss often fails to respond to conversation. The three types of hearing loss are conduction, sensorineural, and mixed. A conduction loss interrupts sound waves as they travel from the outer ear to the cochlea of the inner ear because they are not transmitted through the outer and middle ear structures. A sensorineural loss involves the inner ear, auditory nerve, or hearing center of the brain. In this instance sound is conducted through the outer and middle ear structures, but the continued transmission of sound becomes interrupted at some point beyond the bony ossicles. A mixed loss involves a combination of conduction and sensorineural loss.

Patients working or living around loud noises are at risk for hearing loss. Adolescents are at risk for premature hearing loss from continued exposure to loud music through earbuds connected to electronic music devices or loud concerts. Deterioration of the cochlea and thickening of the tympanic membrane cause older adults to gradually lose hearing acuity. Older adults experience an inability to hear high-frequency sounds and consonants (e.g., *s, z, t,* and *g*). They are especially at risk for hearing loss caused by ototoxicity resulting from high maintenance doses of antibiotics (e.g., aminoglycosides).

To conduct a hearing assessment, have the patient remove any hearing aid, if worn. Note the patient's response to questions. Normally he or she responds without excess requests to have the questions repeated. If you suspect a hearing loss, check the patient's response to the whispered voice. Test one ear at a time while the patient occludes the other ear with a finger. Ask the patient to gently move the finger up and down during the test. While standing 30 to 60 cm (1 to 2 feet) from the testing ear, cover your mouth so the patient is unable to read lips. After exhaling fully, whisper softly toward the non-occluded ear, reciting random numbers with equally accented syllables such as *nine-four-ten.* Ask the patient to repeat what was heard. If necessary gradually increase voice intensity until the patient repeats the numbers correctly. Then test the other ear for comparison. If a hearing loss is present, further testing

BOX 16-11 PATIENT TEACHING

Nose and Sinus Assessment

OUTCOME

Patient follows good preventive practices to ensure against loss of olfaction, injury to olfactory organs, or safety when there is decreased olfaction.

TEACHING STRATEGIES

- Caution patients against overuse of over-the-counter nasal sprays, which can injure nasal olfactory organs.
- Instruct older adults to install smoke detectors on each floor of their home.
- Instruct older adults to always check dated labels on food to ensure against spoilage.

EVALUATION STRATEGIES

- Have patient explain proper use of over-the-counter nasal sprays.
- Inspect patient's home during visit and look for smoke detectors.
- Ask to check food items in the refrigerator.

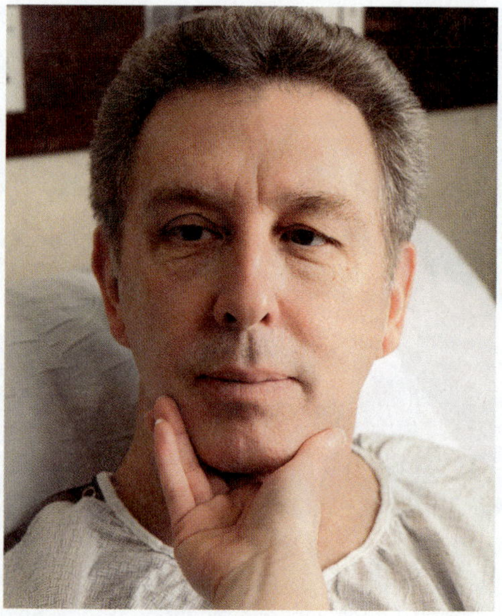

FIGURE 16-12 Inspection of nose and facial features for symmetry.

should be recommended with experienced practitioners using a tuning fork or audiometry.

Nose and Sinuses

Assess the integrity of the nose and sinuses by inspection and palpation. The patient sits during the examination. A penlight allows for gross examination of each naris. A more detailed examination requires using a nasal speculum to inspect deeper nasal turbinates. Do not use a speculum unless a qualified practitioner is present.

Nursing History. Determine if the patient has a history of exposure to dust or pollutants, allergies, nasal obstruction, recent trauma, discharge, frequent infections, headaches, or postnasal drip. Assess for any history of nosebleed (epistaxis) or use of nasal sprays, including frequency and duration (Box 16-11). Ask if there are any breathing difficulties or snoring.

Nose. When inspecting the external nose, observe the shape, size, skin color, and presence of deformity or inflammation. The nose is normally smooth and symmetrical and is the same color as the face (Figure 16-12). Recent trauma causes edema and discoloration. If swelling or deformities exist, gently palpate the ridge and soft tissue of the nose by placing one finger on each side of the nasal arch and gently moving fingers from the nasal bridge to the tip. Note any tenderness, masses, and underlying deviations. Nasal structures are usually firm and stable.

When a person breathes, air normally passes freely and noiselessly through the nose. To assess patency of the nares, place a finger on the side of the patient's nose and occlude one naris. Ask the patient to breathe with the mouth closed. Repeat the procedure for the other naris.

While illuminating the anterior nares, inspect the mucosa for color, lesions, discharge, swelling, and evidence of bleeding. If discharge is present apply clean gloves. Normal mucosa is pink and moist without lesions. Pale mucosa with clear discharge indicates allergy. A mucoid discharge indicates rhinitis. A sinus infection results in yellowish or greenish discharge. Habitual use of intranasal cocaine and opioids causes puffiness and increased vascularity of the nasal mucosa. For the patient with a nasogastric tube, check for local skin breakdown (excoriation) of the naris, characterized by redness and skin sloughing.

To view the septum and turbinates, have the patient tip the head back slightly to provide a clear view. Illuminate the septum and look for alignment, perforation, or bleeding. Normally it is close to the midline and thicker anteriorly than posteriorly. Normal mucosa is pink and moist without lesions. A deviated septum obstructs breathing and interferes with passage of an enteral nasal tube. Perforation of the septum often occurs after repeated use of intranasal cocaine. Note any polyps (tumorlike growths) or purulent drainage.

Sinuses. Examination of the sinuses involves palpation. In cases of allergies or infection, the interior of the sinuses becomes inflamed and swollen. The most effective way to assess for tenderness is by externally palpating the frontal and maxillary facial areas. Palpate the frontal sinus by exerting pressure with the thumb up and under the patient's eyebrow. Gentle, upward pressure easily elicits tenderness if sinus irritation is present. Do not apply pressure to the eyes. If tenderness of sinuses is present, ask a nurse or health care provider with advanced experience to transilluminate the sinuses.

Mouth and Pharynx

Assess the mouth and pharynx to detect signs of overall health; determine oral hygiene needs; and develop therapies for patients with dehydration, restricted intake, oral trauma, or oral airway obstruction. To assess the oral cavity use a penlight and tongue depressor or single gauze square. Wear clean gloves and have the patient sit or lie during the examination. Assess the oral cavity while administering oral hygiene.

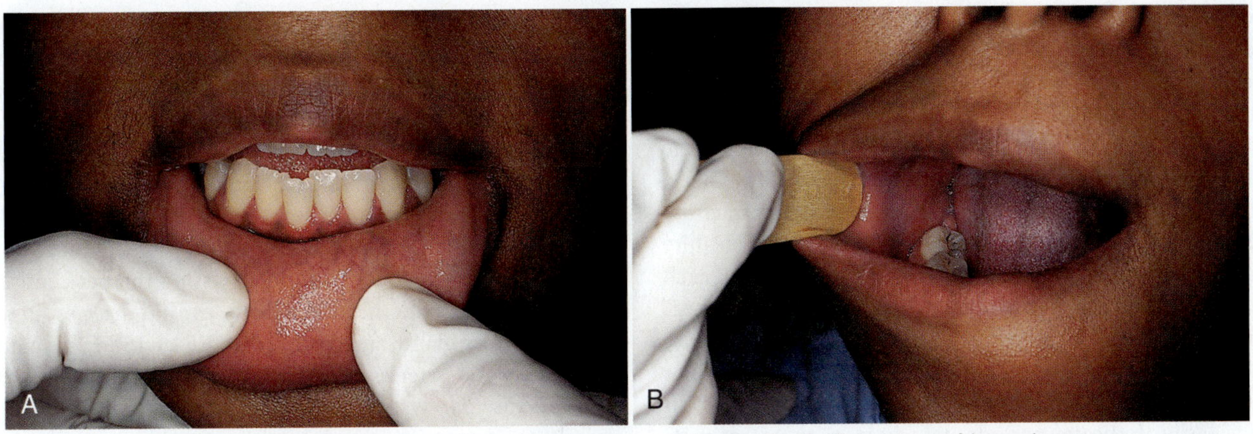

FIGURE 16-13 **A,** Inspection of inner oral mucosa of lower lip. **B,** Retraction of buccal mucosa allows for clear visualization.

Nursing History. Determine if the patient wears dentures or retainers and how they fit. Assess for any recent changes in appetite or weight, which indicate problems with chewing and swallowing. Assess the patient's dental hygiene practices. To identify cancer risks determine if the patient smokes, chews tobacco, or consumes alcohol. Identify if he or she still has his or her tonsils and adenoids.

Lips. Inspect the lips for color, texture, hydration, contour, and lesions. With the patient's mouth closed, view the lips from end to end. Normally they are pink, moist, symmetrical, smooth, and without lesions. Lip color in the dark-skinned patient varies from pink to plum. Have female patients remove their lipstick before the examination. Anemia causes pallor of the lips, with cyanosis caused by respiratory or cardiovascular problems. Any lesions such as nodules or ulcerations can be related to infection, irritation, or skin cancer.

Buccal Mucosa, Gums, and Teeth. Ask the patient to clench the teeth and smile to observe teeth occlusion. The upper molars normally rest directly on the lower molars, and the upper incisors slightly override the lower incisors. Assess for symmetry.

Inspect the teeth to determine the quality of a patient's dental hygiene (Box 16-12). Note the position and alignment of the teeth. To examine the posterior surface of the teeth, have the patient open the mouth with lips relaxed. Use a tongue depressor to retract the lips and cheeks, especially when viewing the molars. Note the color of teeth and the presence of dental caries, tartar, and extraction sites. Normal healthy teeth are smooth, white, and shiny. A chalky white discoloration of the enamel is an early sign of caries formation. Brown or black discolorations indicate the formation of caries. An older adult's teeth often feel rough when tooth enamel calcifies, and there may be loose or missing teeth because of increased bone resorption. Yellow and darkened teeth are also common in the older adult because of general wear and tear that exposes the darker, underlying dentin.

To view the inner oral mucosa, ask the patient to remove any dental appliance. View the inner oral mucosa by having the patient open the mouth slightly and gently pull the lower lip away from the teeth (Figure 16-13, *A*). Repeat this process for the upper lip. Inspect the mucosa for color, hydration, texture, and lesions such as ulcers, abrasions, or cysts. Normally the mucosa is a glistening pink, smooth, and moist. Palpate any lesions with a gloved hand for tenderness, size, and consistency.

To inspect the buccal mucosa, ask the patient to open the mouth and gently retract the cheeks with a tongue depressor or gloved finger covered with gauze (Figure 16-13, *B*). View the surface of the mucosa from right to left and top to bottom. A penlight illuminates the most posterior portion of the mucosa. For patients with normal pigmentation the buccal

BOX 16-12 PATIENT TEACHING

Mouth and Pharyngeal Assessment

OUTCOME

Patient follows good preventive practices to ensure oral and dental health.

TEACHING STRATEGIES

- Discuss proper techniques for oral hygiene, including brushing and flossing (see Chapter 29).
- Explain the early warning signs of oral cavity and pharynx cancer, including a sore that bleeds easily and does not heel, a lump or thickening, and red or white patch on the mucosa that persists. Difficulty chewing, swallowing, and moving the tongue or jaw are late symptoms (ACS, 2013a).
- Encourage regular dental examinations every 6 months for children, adults, and older adults.
- Identify older patients who have difficulty chewing and changes in the teeth. Teach patients to eat soft foods; cut food into small pieces; and eat more frequent, smaller meals.

EVALUATION STRATEGIES

- Ask patient to demonstrate brushing.
- Have patient identify when to have regular dental checkups.
- Have patient identify the warning signs of oral cavity and pharynx cancer.
- Ask older adult to keep a diet record for 3 days.

mucosa is a good site to inspect for jaundice and pallor. In older adults it is normally dry because of reduced salivation. Thick white patches (leukoplakia) are often a precancerous lesion seen in heavy smokers and alcoholics. Palpate for any buccal lesions by placing the gloved index finger within the buccal cavity and the thumb on the outer surface of the cheek.

Examine the gums (gingivae) for color, edema, retraction, bleeding, and lesions while retracting the cheeks. Healthy gums are pink, moist and smooth and fit tightly around each tooth. Dark-skinned patients often have patchy pigmentation. In older adults the gums are usually pale. With clean gloves palpate the gums to assess for lesions, thickening, or masses. Normally there is no tenderness. Spongy gums that bleed easily indicate periodontal disease or vitamin C deficiency.

Tongue and Floor of Mouth. Carefully inspect the tongue on all sides and the floor of the mouth. Have the patient relax the mouth and stick the tongue out halfway. The gag reflex is elicited if the patient protrudes the tongue too far. Using the penlight examine the tongue for color, size, position, texture, movement, and coating or lesions. A normal tongue appears medium or dull red in color, moist, slightly rough on the top surface, and smooth along the lateral margins. When the tongue protrudes it remains at midline. To test the tongue for mobility, ask the patient to raise it and move it from side to side. It should move freely.

The undersurface of the tongue and floor of the mouth are highly vascular. Take extra care to inspect this area, a common site of origin for oral cancer lesions. The patient lifts the tongue by placing its tip on the palate behind the upper incisors. Inspect for color, swelling, and lesions such as cysts. The ventral surface of the tongue is pink and smooth, with large veins between the frenulum folds.

Palate. Have the patient extend the head backward, holding the mouth open to allow you to inspect the hard and soft palates. The hard palate, or roof of the mouth, is located anteriorly. The whitish hard palate is dome shaped. The soft palate extends posteriorly toward the pharynx. It is normally light pink and smooth. Observe the palates for color, shape, texture, and extra bony prominences or defects.

Pharynx. Perform an examination of the pharyngeal structures to rule out infection, inflammation, or lesions. Have the patient tip the head back slightly, open the mouth wide, and say "Ah" while you place the tip of a tongue depressor on the middle third of the tongue. Take care not to press the lower lip against the teeth (Figure 16-14). By placing the tongue depressor too far anteriorly, the posterior part of the tongue mounds up, obstructing the view. Placing the tongue depressor on the posterior tongue elicits the gag reflex.

With a penlight, first inspect the uvula and soft palate. Both structures, which are innervated by the tenth cranial nerve (vagus), rise centrally as the patient says "Ah." Examine the anterior and posterior tonsillar pillars and note the presence or absence of tonsillar tissue. The posterior pharynx is behind the pillars. Normally pharyngeal structures are smooth, pink, and well hydrated. Small irregular spots of lymphatic tissue and small blood vessels are normal. Note edema, petechiae, lesions, or exudate. Patients with chronic sinus problems frequently exhibit a clear exudate that drains along the wall of the posterior pharynx. Yellow or green exudate indicates infection. A patient with a typical sore throat has a reddened and edematous uvula and tonsillar pillars with possible presence of yellow exudate.

Neck

Assessment of the neck includes assessing the neck muscles, lymph nodes of the head and neck, carotid arteries, jugular veins, thyroid gland, and trachea (Figure 16-15). Examination of the carotid arteries and jugular veins is addressed as part of the vascular system assessment. Inspect and palpate the neck to determine the integrity of neck structures and examine the lymphatic system. An abnormality of superficial lymph nodes sometimes reveals the presence of infection or malignancy. Examination of the thyroid gland and trachea also helps to rule out malignancies. Perform this examination with the patient sitting.

Nursing History. Determine if the patient has a history of a recent cold or infection, enlarged lymph nodes, or exposure to radiation or toxic chemicals. If there is a history of enlarged lymph nodes, inquire about any past history of IV drug use, hemophilia, and risk factors for human immunodeficiency virus (HIV) infection. Learn if the patient takes thyroid medication for a history of hypothyroidism or hyperthyroidism; ask about a family history of thyroid disease. Ask the patient to describe any head or neck injury or pain of head and neck structures.

Neck Muscles. First inspect the gross neck structures with the neck in the usual anatomical position. Observe for symmetry of neck muscles. Ask the patient to flex the neck with the chin to the chest, hyperextend the neck backward, and move the head laterally to each side and then sideways with the ear moving toward the shoulder. This tests the sternocleidomastoid and trapezius muscles. The neck normally moves freely without discomfort.

Lymph Nodes. An extensive system of lymph nodes collects lymph from the head, ears, nose, cheeks, and lips (Figure 16-16). With the patient's chin raised and head tilted slightly

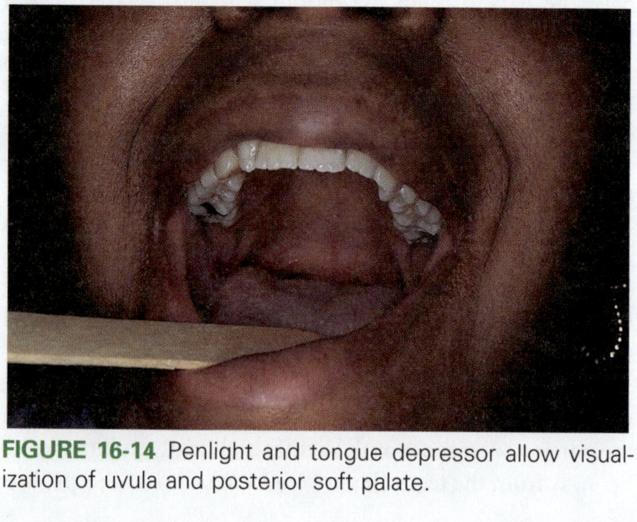

FIGURE 16-14 Penlight and tongue depressor allow visualization of uvula and posterior soft palate.

back, first inspect the area where lymph nodes are distributed and compare both sides. This position stretches the skin slightly over any possible enlarged nodes. Inspect visible nodes for edema, erythema, or red streaks. Nodes are not normally visible.

Use a methodical approach to palpate the lymph nodes to avoid overlooking any single node or chain. The patient relaxes with the neck flexed slightly forward. Inspect and palpate both sides of the neck for comparison. During palpation either face or stand to the side of the patient for easy access to all nodes. Using the pads of the middle three fingers of each hand, gently palpate in a rotary motion over the nodes. Check each node methodically in the following sequence: occipital nodes at the base of the skull, postauricular nodes over the mastoid, preauricular nodes just in front of the ear, retropharyngeal nodes at the angle of the mandible, submandibular nodes, and submental nodes in the midline behind the mandibular tip. Try to detect enlargement and note the location, size, shape, surface characteristics, consistency, mobility, tenderness, and warmth of the nodes. If the skin is mobile, move it over the area of the nodes (Figure 16-17). It is important to press underlying tissue in each area and not simply move the fingers over the skin.

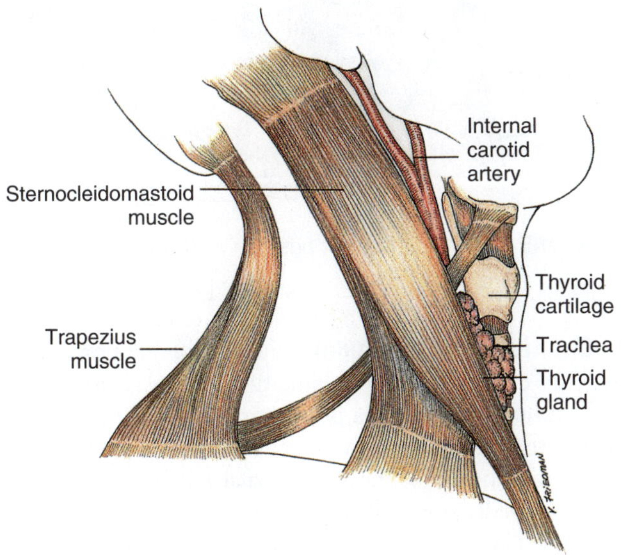

FIGURE 16-15 Anatomical position of major neck structures. Note triangles formed by muscles.

To palpate supraclavicular nodes ask the patient to bend the head forward and relax the shoulders. Palpate these nodes by hooking the index and third finger over the clavicle, lateral to the sternocleidomastoid muscle. Palpate the deep cervical nodes only with the fingers hooked around the sternocleidomastoid muscle.

Normally lymph nodes are not easily palpable. Lymph nodes that are large, fixed, inflamed, or tender indicate a problem such as local infection, systemic disease, or neoplasm (Seidel et al., 2011). Tenderness almost always indicates inflammation (Box 16-13). A problem involving a lymph node of the head and neck means an abnormality in the mouth, throat, abdomen, breasts, thorax, or arms. These are the areas drained by the head and neck nodes.

Thyroid Gland. The thyroid gland lies in the anterior lower neck, in front of and to both sides of the trachea. The

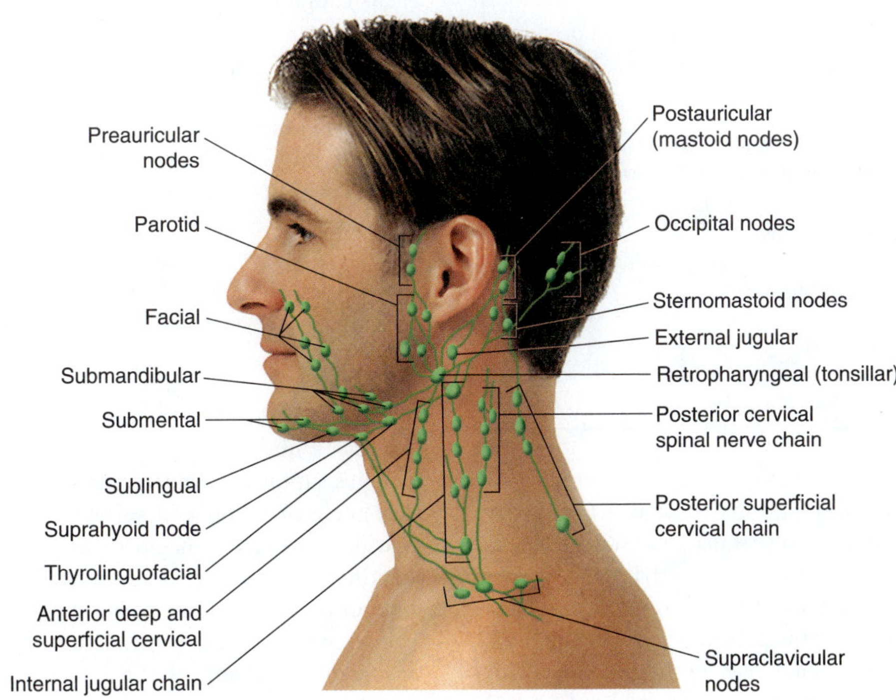

FIGURE 16-16 Palpable lymph nodes in head and neck. (From Seidel HM, et al: *Mosby's guide to physical examination,* ed 7, St Louis, 2011, Mosby.)

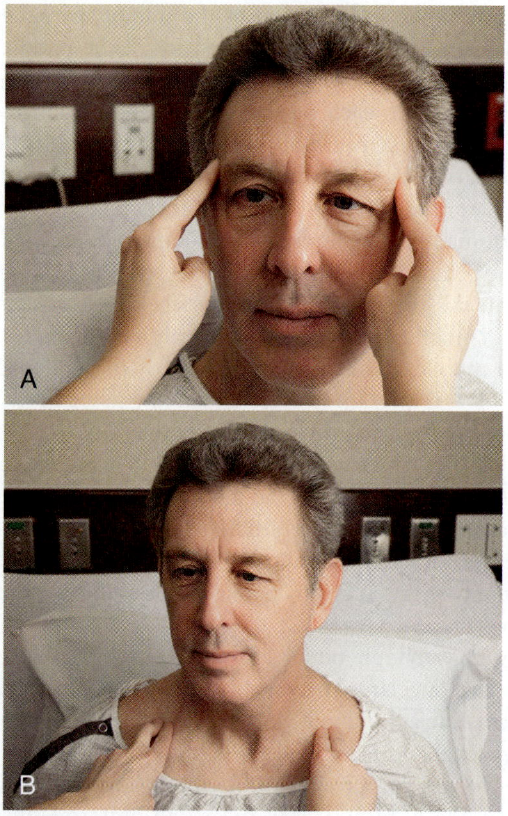

FIGURE 16-17 **A,** Palpation of preauricular lymph nodes. **B,** Palpation for supraclavicular lymph nodes.

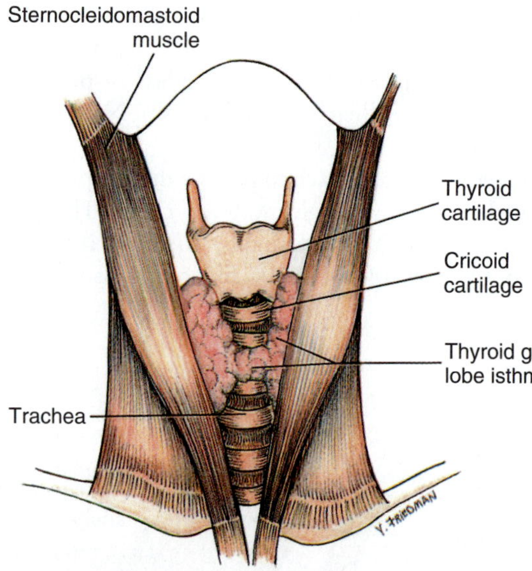

FIGURE 16-18 Anatomical position of the thyroid gland.

BOX 16-13 PATIENT TEACHING

Neck Assessment

OUTCOME

Patient takes proper preventive action if a mass is noticed in the neck.

TEACHING STRATEGIES

- Stress the importance of regular compliance with medication schedule to patients with thyroid disease.
- Instruct patients about the lymph nodes and how infection commonly causes node tenderness.
- Instruct patients to call a health care provider when they notice a lump or mass in the neck.

EVALUATION STRATEGIES

- Have patient explain when to notify health care provider about a neck mass.

gland is fixed to the trachea with the isthmus overlying the trachea and connecting the two irregular, cone-shaped lobes (Figure 16-18). Inspect the lower neck overlying the thyroid gland for obvious masses, symmetry, and any subtle fullness at the base of the neck. Offer the patient a glass of water and, while observing the neck, have him or her swallow. This maneuver helps to visualize an abnormally enlarged thyroid gland. More experienced nurses examine the thyroid by palpating for more subtle masses.

Carotid Artery and Jugular Vein. Examination of these vessels is discussed under examination of the vascular system.

Trachea. The trachea is a part of the upper respiratory system that requires direct palpation. It is normally located in the midline above the suprasternal notch. Masses in the neck or mediastinum and pulmonary abnormalities cause lateral displacement. Have the patient sit or lie down during palpation. Determine the position of the trachea by palpating at the suprasternal notch, slipping the thumb and index fingers to each side. Note if your finger and thumb shift laterally. Do not apply forceful pressure to the trachea because this elicits coughing.

THORAX AND LUNGS

Physical assessment of the thorax and lungs requires an in-depth review of the ventilatory and respiratory functions of the lungs. If disease is affecting the lungs, it affects other body systems as well. For example, reduced oxygenation causes changes in mental alertness because of the sensitivity of the brain to lowered oxygen levels. You use data from all body systems to determine the nature of pulmonary alterations.

Before assessing the thorax and lungs, be familiar with the landmarks of the chest (Figure 16-19). These landmarks help you locate findings and use assessment skills correctly. The patient's suprasternal notch, manubrium, costal angle, clavicles, angle of Louis, and vertebrae are key landmarks that provide a series of imaginary lines for sign and symptom identification. Keep a mental image of the location of the lobes of the lung and the position of each rib (Figure 16-20). The proper orientation to anatomical structures ensures a thorough assessment of the anterior, lateral, and posterior thorax.

Locating the position of each rib is critical to visualizing the lobe of the lung being assessed. To begin, locate the angle

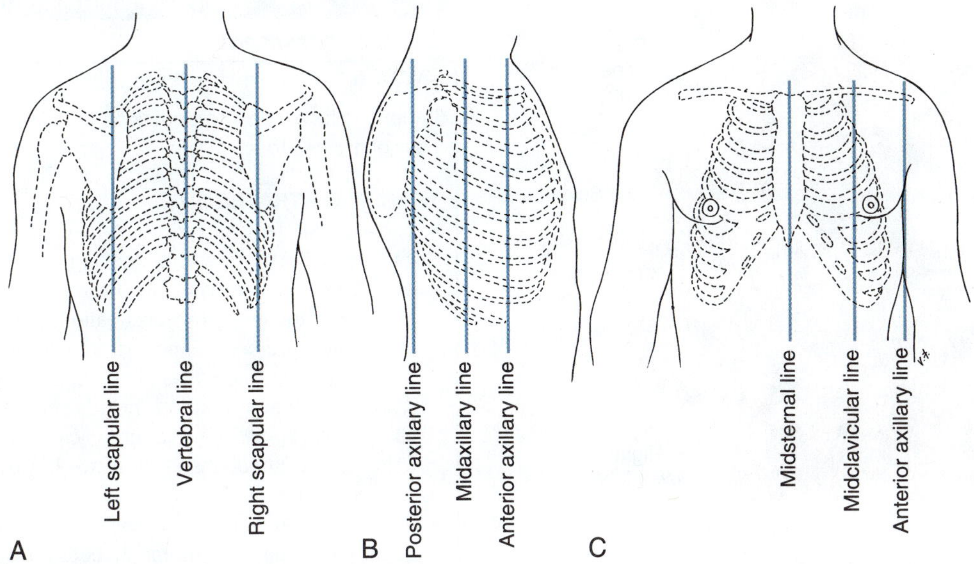

FIGURE 16-19 Anatomical chest wall landmarks. **A,** Posterior chest. **B,** Lateral chest. **C,** Anterior chest.

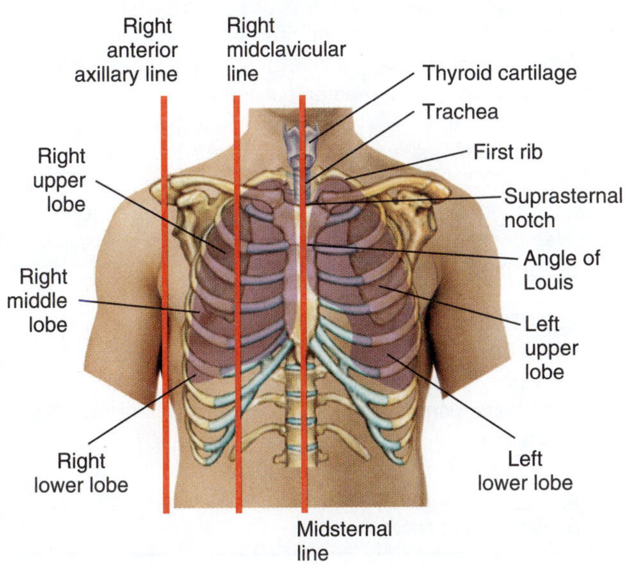

FIGURE 16-20 Anterior position of lung lobes in relation to anatomical landmarks. (From Seidel HM, et al: *Mosby's guide to physical examination,* ed 7, St Louis, 2011, Mosby.)

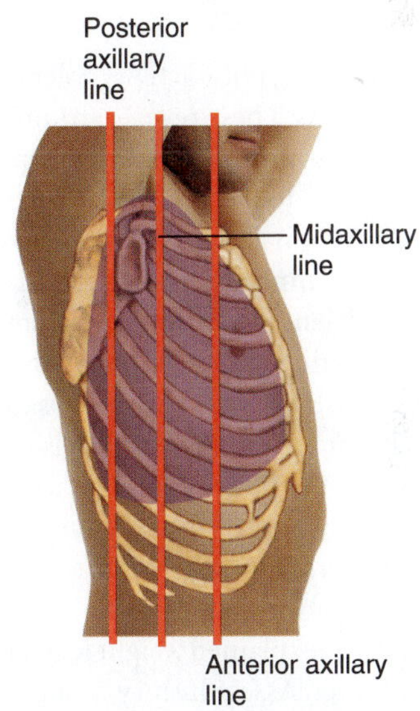

FIGURE 16-21 Lateral position of lung lobes in relation to anatomical landmarks. (From Seidel HM, et al: *Mosby's guide to physical examination,* ed 7, St Louis, 2011, Mosby.)

of Louis at the junction between the manubrium and the body of the sternum. Knowing that the second rib extends from the angle makes it easy to locate and palpate the **intercostal spaces** (between the ribs) in succession. The spinous process of the third thoracic vertebra and the fourth, fifth, and sixth ribs serves to locate the lobes of the lung laterally (Figure 16-21). The lower lobes project laterally and anteriorly.

Posteriorly the tip or inferior margin of the scapula lies approximately at the level of the seventh rib. Identify the seventh rib, count upward to locate the third thoracic vertebra, and align it with the inner borders of the scapula to locate the posterior lobes (Figure 16-22).

Examination of the lungs and thorax is most effective when the patient is undressed to the waist. Begin with the patient sitting for assessment of the posterior and lateral chest and sitting or lying down for examination of the anterior chest. A female patient may keep a gown draped loosely over her chest while you examine the posterior chest.

Nursing History

First interview the patient for any recent problems of increased work of breathing. Ask the patient about *persistent cough* (productive or nonproductive), *blood-streaked sputum, voice change, chest pain,* shortness of breath, **orthopnea** (must be in upright position to breathe), **dyspnea** (breathlessness)

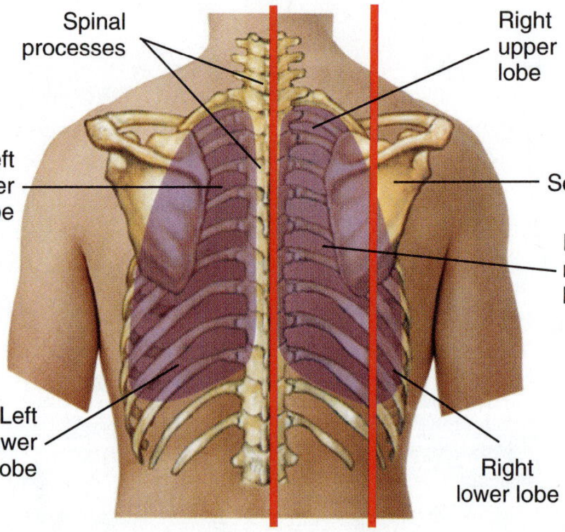

FIGURE 16-22 Posterior position of lung lobes in relation to anatomical landmarks. (From Seidel HM, et al: *Mosby's guide to physical examination,* ed 7, St Louis, 2011, Mosby.)

during exertion or at rest, poor activity tolerance, or *recurrent pneumonia or bronchitis.* These reveal cardiopulmonary problems or warning signs for lung cancer (symptoms in italics). Assess for a history of tobacco or marijuana use, including type of tobacco, duration and amount (pack-years = number of years smoking × number of packs per day), age started, efforts to quit, and length of time since smoking stopped. Determine if your patient works in an environment containing pollutants (e.g., asbestos or coal dust), is exposed to radiation, or resides in an area with high levels of particulate air contaminants. Teach the patient about warning signs of lung disease (Box 16-14).

Review risk factors for tuberculosis (TB) and/or HIV infection and assess for symptoms, including persistent cough, hemoptysis, unexplained weight loss, fatigue, anorexia, night sweats, and fever. Assess history of allergies to airborne irritants, foods, drugs, or chemical substances. Ask if the patient has had pneumonia or influenza vaccine and a TB test. Review the patient's family history for cancer, TB, allergies, or chronic obstructive pulmonary disease.

Posterior Thorax

Begin examination of the posterior thorax by observing for any signs or symptoms in other body systems that indicate pulmonary problems. Reduced mental alertness, nasal flaring, somnolence (sleepiness), and cyanosis are examples of symptoms or findings that indicate oxygenation problems. Inspect the posterior thorax by observing the shape and symmetry of the chest from the patient's back and sides. Pay close attention to the position of the scapula bilaterally. Note the anteroposterior (AP) diameter. Body shape or posture significantly affects ventilatory movement. Normally the chest contour is symmetrical, with the AP diameter ⅓ to ½ the size of the transverse or side-to-side diameter. Infants have an almost round shape with a 1:1 ratio between the AP and transverse diameters. In adults a barrel-shaped chest (AP diameter = transverse) characterizes chronic lung disease. A more rounded chest is also associated with older age. Congenital and postural alterations cause abnormal contours. Patients with breathing problems may lean over a table or splint the side of the chest. Splinting or holding the chest wall because of pain causes a patient to bend toward the affected side, which impairs ventilatory movement.

With the patient sitting or standing, position yourself at a midline position behind the patient, look for deformities, position of the spine, slope of the ribs, retraction of the intercostal spaces during inspiration, and bulging of the intercostal spaces during expiration. The scapulae are normally symmetrical and closely attached to the thoracic wall. The normal spine is straight without lateral deviation. Posteriorly the ribs tend to slope across and down. The ribs and

BOX 16-14 PATIENT TEACHING

Lung Assessment

OUTCOME

Patient follows recommendations that improve and protect pulmonary health.

TEACHING STRATEGIES

- Explain risk factors for chronic lung disease and lung cancer, including cigarette smoking; history of smoking for over 20 years; exposure to environmental pollution; and radiation exposure from occupational, medical, and environmental sources. Exposure to residential radon and asbestos also increases risk, especially for cigarette smokers. Other risk factors include certain metals (arsenic, cadmium), some organic chemicals, and tuberculosis. Exposure to secondhand cigarette smoke increases risk for nonsmokers (ACS, 2013a).
- Share brochures on lung cancer from the American Cancer Society with patient and family before discharge from the hospital (see Case Study).
- Discuss with patient the warning signs of lung cancer such as a persistent cough, blood-streaked sputum, chest pains, and recurrent attacks of pneumonia or bronchitis.
- Counsel elderly patients and their partners as appropriate on benefits of receiving influenza and pneumonia vaccinations because of a greater susceptibility to respiratory infection.
- Instruct patients with chronic obstructive pulmonary disease (COPD) or other respiratory illnesses in coughing and pursed lip–breathing exercises (see Chapter 30).
- Refer people at risk for tuberculosis who visit clinics or health care centers for skin testing.

EVALUATION STRATEGIES

- Patient describes risk factors for lung disease and cancer, identifying any known risks for cancer.
- Patient lists warning signs for lung cancer.
- Patient maintains up-to-date immunizations for influenza and pneumonia and is regularly tested for tuberculosis.
- Patients with chronic illnesses demonstrate breathing and coughing exercises.

intercostal spaces are easier to see in a thin person. Normally no bulging or active movement occurs within the intercostal spaces during breathing. Bulging or retraction indicates that the patient is using great effort to breathe.

Also assess the rate and rhythm of breathing at this time (see Chapter 15). Observe the thorax as a whole. It normally expands and relaxes with equality (symmetry) of movement bilaterally. In healthy adults the normal respiratory rate varies from 12 to 20 respirations/min.

Palpate the posterior thorax beginning with the thoracic muscles and skeleton for lumps, masses, pulsations, and unusual movement. Use caution if you note pain or tenderness. Fractured rib fragments could be displaced against vital organs. If you find a suspicious mass or swollen area, lightly palpate it for size, shape, and typical qualities of a lesion.

To measure chest excursion or depth of breathing, stand behind the patient and place the thumbs along the spinal processes at the tenth rib, with the palms lightly contacting the posterior lateral surfaces. Place thumbs about 5 cm (2 inches) apart pointing toward the spine and fingers pointing laterally (Figure 16-23). Press the hands toward the spine so a small skinfold appears between the thumbs. Do not slide the hands over the skin. Instruct the patient to take a deep breath after exhaling. Note movement of the thumbs. Expect chest excursion to be symmetrical, separating the thumbs 3 to 5 cm (1¼ to 2 inches). Reduced chest excursion is caused by pain, postural deformity, or fatigue. In older adults chest excursion normally declines because of costal cartilage calcification and respiratory muscle atrophy.

Auscultation assesses the movement of air through the tracheobronchial tree and detects mucus or obstructed airways. Normally air flows through the airways in an unobstructed pattern. Recognizing the sounds created by normal airflow allows for detection of sounds caused by airway obstruction. The patient sits during auscultation of the lungs.

Place the diaphragm of the stethoscope firmly on the skin, over the posterior chest wall between the ribs. The patient folds the arms in front of the chest and keeps the head bent forward while taking slow, deep breaths with the mouth slightly open. Listen to an entire inspiration and expiration at each position of the stethoscope (Figure 16-24, *A*). If sounds are faint, as in an obese patient, ask the patient to breathe harder and faster temporarily. Breath sounds are much louder in children because of their thin chest walls. In small children listen through the bell of a pediatric stethoscope because of their small chest. Use a systematic pattern comparing the sounds in one region on one side of the body with sounds in the same region on the opposite side.

Auscultate for normal breath sounds and abnormal or **adventitious sounds.** Normal breath sounds differ in character, depending on the area you auscultate. Bronchovesicular and vesicular sounds normally are heard over the posterior thorax. Bronchovesicular sounds are medium-pitched blowing sounds normally heard between the scapulae. The sounds have equal inspiratory and expiratory phases. The character of bronchovesicular sounds is created by air moving through large airways. Vesicular sounds are normally heard over the periphery of the lungs. Air moving through the smaller airways creates these sounds. Vesicular sounds are soft, breezy, and low pitched; and the inspiratory phase is about 3 times longer than the expiratory phase.

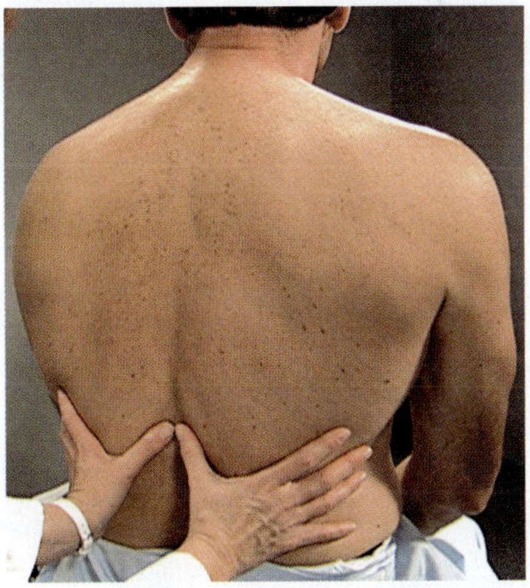

FIGURE 16-23 Palpating thoracic expansion by placing thumbs at the level of the tenth rib. As patient inhales, movement of chest excursion separates thumbs. (From Seidel HM, et al: *Mosby's guide to physical examination,* ed 7, St Louis, 2011, Mosby.)

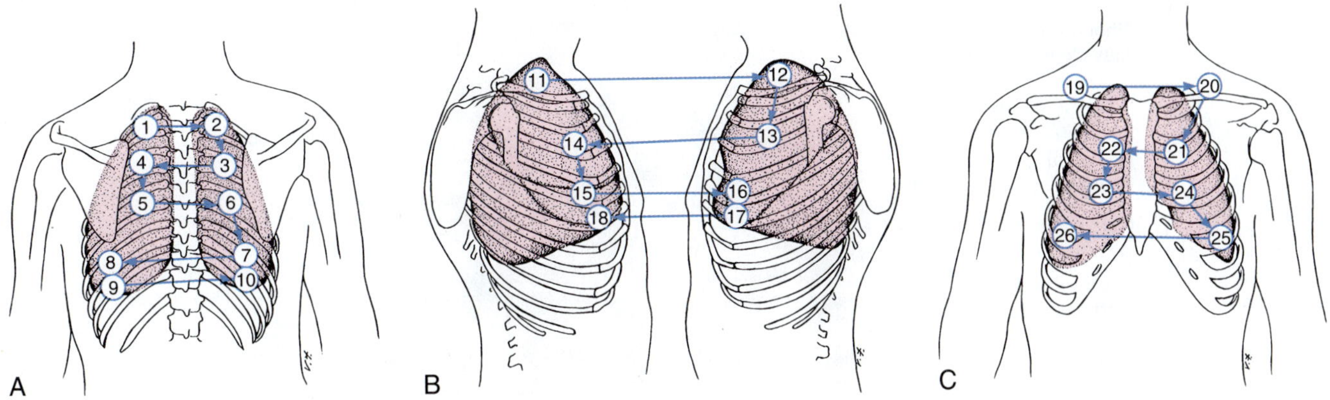

FIGURE 16-24 **A** to **C,** Systematic pattern (posterior-lateral-anterior) is followed for palpating and auscultating the thorax.

Abnormal sounds result from air passing through moisture, mucus, or narrowed airways. They also result from alveoli suddenly reinflating or from an inflammation between the pleural linings of the lung. Adventitious sounds often occur superimposed over normal sounds. The four types of adventitious sounds are **crackles,** rhonchi, wheezes, and pleural friction rub. Each sound has its own cause and is characterized by typical auditory features (Table 16-6 and Figure 16-25). During auscultation note whether the sound is on inspiration, expiration, or both and the location and characteristics of the sounds. Listen for the absence of breath sounds (found in patients with collapsed or surgically removed lobes).

Lateral Thorax

Extend the assessment of the posterior thorax to the lateral sides of the chest (Figure 16-24, *B*). Have the patient raise the arms to improve access to lateral thoracic structures. Use inspection, palpation, and auscultation skills to examine the lateral thorax. Normally the breath sounds you hear are vesicular.

TABLE 16-6 ADVENTITIOUS BREATH SOUNDS

SOUND	SITE AUSCULTATED	CAUSE	CHARACTER
Crackles	Most common in dependent lobes: right and left lung bases	Random, sudden reinflation of groups of alveoli; disruptive passage of air through small airways	Fine crackles: High-pitched fine, short, interrupted crackling sounds heard during end of inspiration; usually not cleared with coughing Moist crackles: Lower, more moist sounds heard during middle of inspiration; not cleared with coughing Coarse crackles: Loud, bubbly sounds heard during inspiration; not cleared with coughing
Rhonchi (sonorous wheeze)	Primarily heard over trachea and bronchi; if loud enough, can be heard over most lung fields	Muscular spasm, fluid, or mucus in larger airways, new growth or external pressure causing turbulence	Loud, low-pitched, rumbling coarse sounds heard either during inspiration or expiration; may be cleared by coughing
Wheezes (sibilant wheeze)	Heard over all lung fields	High-velocity airflow through severely narrowed or obstructed airway	High-pitched, continuous musical sounds such as a squeak heard continuously during inspiration or expiration; usually louder on expiration
Pleural friction rub	Heard over anterior lateral lung field (if patient is sitting upright)	Inflamed pleura, parietal pleura rubbing against visceral pleura	Has dry, grating quality heard during inspiration; does not clear with coughing; heard loudest over lower lateral anterior surface

Data from Seidel HM, et al: *Mosby's guide to physical examination,* ed 7, St Louis, 2011, Mosby.

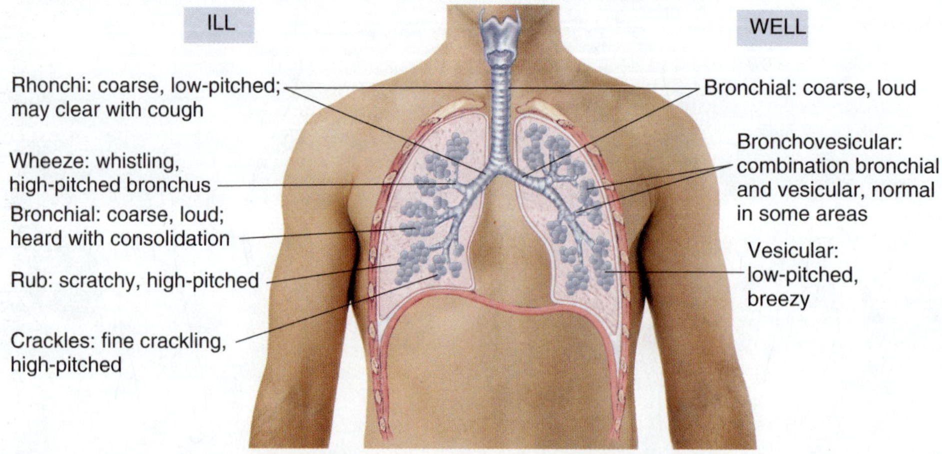

FIGURE 16-25 Schema of breath sounds in the ill and well patient. (From Seidel HM et al: *Mosby's guide to physical examination,* ed 7, St Louis, 2011, Mosby.)

Anterior Thorax

Inspect the anterior thorax for the same features as the posterior thorax. Have the patient sit upright if possible to maximize chest expansion. Observe the accessory muscles of breathing: sternocleidomastoid, trapezius, and abdominal muscles. The accessory muscles move minimally with normal passive breathing. The accessory and abdominal muscles contract when a patient requires effort to breathe as a result of strenuous exercise or disease. Some patients produce a grunting sound.

Observe the width of the costal angle. It is usually larger than 90 degrees between the two costal margins. Observe the breathing pattern. Assess respiratory rate and rhythm anteriorly (see Chapter 15). The male patient's respirations are usually diaphragmatic, whereas the female's are more costal.

Auscultation of the anterior thorax follows a systematic pattern (Figure 16-24, *C*). Pay special attention to the lower lobes, where mucus secretions commonly gather. Listen for bronchovesicular and vesicular sounds above and below the clavicles and along the lung periphery. Auscultate for bronchial sounds, which are loud, high pitched, and hollow sounding with expiration lasting longer than inspiration (3:2 ratio). You normally hear this sound over the trachea.

HEART

Compare your assessment of heart function with findings from the vascular assessment. Alterations in either system sometimes manifest as changes in the other. Some patients with signs and symptoms of heart (cardiac) problems have a life-threatening condition requiring immediate attention. In this case act quickly and conduct only the parts of the examination that are absolutely necessary. When a patient is more stable, conduct a more thorough assessment.

Assess cardiac function through the anterior thorax. Form a mental image of the exact location of the heart (Figure 16-26). In the adult the heart is located in the center of the chest (precordium) behind and to the left of the sternum, with a small section of the right atrium extending to the right of the sternum. The base of the heart is the upper portion, and the apex is the bottom tip. The surface of the right ventricle constitutes most of the anterior surface of the heart. A section of the left ventricle shapes the left anterior side of the apex. The point of maximal impulse (PMI) is palpable at the fifth intercostal space at the left midclavicular line in adults and children older than 7 years of age. In children younger than age 7 the PMI is at the fourth intercostal space at the left midclavicular line (Hockenberry and Wilson, 2011).

To assess heart function you need to understand the cardiac cycle and associated physiological events (Figure 16-27). The heart normally pumps blood through its four chambers in a methodical, even sequence. Events on the left side occur just before those on the right. As the blood flows through each chamber, valves open and close, pressures within chambers rise and fall, and chambers contract. Each event creates a physiological sign. Both sides of the heart function in a coordinated fashion.

There are two phases to the cardiac cycle: systole and diastole. During systole the ventricles contract and eject blood from the left ventricle into the aorta and from the right ventricle into the pulmonary artery. During diastole the ventricles relax, and the atria contract to move blood into the ventricles and fill the coronary arteries.

Heart sounds occur in relation to physiological events in the cardiac cycle. As systole begins, ventricular pressure rises and closes the mitral and tricuspid valves. Valve closure causes the first heart sound (S_1), often described as "lub." The ventricles then contract, and blood flows through the aorta and pulmonary circulation. After the ventricles empty, ventricular pressure falls below that in the aorta and pulmonary artery. This allows the aortic and pulmonic valves to close, causing the second heart sound (S_2), described as "dub." As ventricular pressure continues to fall, it drops below that of the atria. The mitral and tricuspid valves reopen to allow ventricular filling. Rapid ventricular filling may create a third heart sound (S_3), heard more often in children and young adults. An S_3 is an abnormal finding in adults over 30 years of age. A fourth

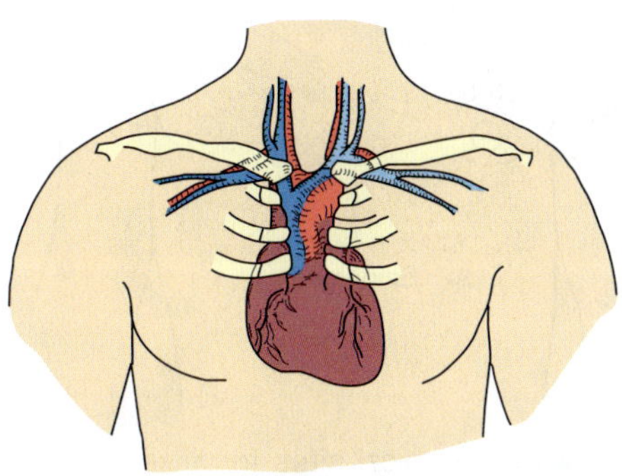

FIGURE 16-26 Anatomical position of the heart.

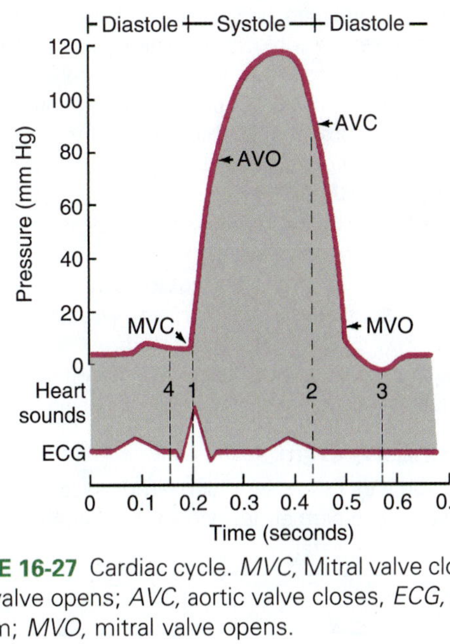

FIGURE 16-27 Cardiac cycle. *MVC,* Mitral valve closes; *AVO,* aortic valve opens; *AVC,* aortic valve closes, *ECG,* electrocardiogram; *MVO,* mitral valve opens.

heart sound (S_4) occurs when the atria contract to enhance ventricular filling. An S_4 may be heard in healthy older adults, children, and athletes; but it is not normal in adults. An S_4 needs to be reported to a health care provider.

Nursing History

The nursing history focuses on risk factors for cardiovascular disease (Box 16-15). Determine the patient's history of smoking; alcohol intake; caffeine intake; use of prescriptive and recreational drugs; exercise habits; and dietary patterns, including fat and sodium intake. Ask if the patient is taking medications for cardiovascular function (e.g., antidysrhythmics or antihypertensives) and if he or she knows their purpose, dosage, and side effects. Assess for chest pain or discomfort, palpitations, excess fatigue, cough, dyspnea, edema of the feet, cyanosis, fainting, or orthopnea. These are key symptoms of heart disease. If the patient reports chest pain, determine if it is cardiac in nature; anginal pain is usually a deep pressure or ache that is substernal and diffuse, radiating to one or both arms, the neck, or the jaw. Determine if the patient has a stressful lifestyle. Assess for personal or family history of heart disease, diabetes, high cholesterol, hypertension, stroke, or rheumatic heart disease.

BOX 16-15 PATIENT TEACHING

Heart Assessment

OUTCOME

Patient chooses healthy heart practices, noting personal risk factors for heart disease.

TEACHING STRATEGIES

- Explain risk factors for heart disease, including high dietary intake of saturated fat or cholesterol, lack of regular aerobic exercise, smoking, excess weight, stressful lifestyle, hypertension, and family history of heart disease.
- Refer patient to appropriate available resources for controlling or reducing risks (e.g., nutritional counseling, exercise class, stress-reduction programs).
- Explain that research shows clinical benefit from reducing dietary intake of cholesterol and saturated fats. Teach patient that approximately 70% to 75% of saturated fatty acids come from meats, poultry, fish, and dairy products. The American Heart Association (AHA, 2013) recommends a diet that includes an intake of total fat less than 35% of calories, saturated fatty acids less than 10% of calories, and cholesterol level less than 200 mg/dL (Moore, 2009).
- Encourage regular measurement of total blood cholesterol levels and triglycerides. Desirable levels are less than 200 mg/dL. More than one cholesterol measurement is needed to assess the blood cholesterol level accurately. Since low-density lipoprotein (LDL) cholesterol is the major component of atherosclerotic plaques, tests should include separate measurement of LDL cholesterol. An LDL cholesterol level of 160 mg/dL or higher indicates high risk for heart disease (AHA, 2013).
- Advise patients to avoid secondhand cigarette smoke since nicotine causes vasoconstriction.
- Advise patients to quit smoking to lower the risk for coronary heart disease and coronary vascular disease (AHA, 2013).
- Have patient consult with health care provider regarding the benefit of taking a daily low dose of aspirin.

EVALUATION STRATEGIES

- Patient identifies risk factors for heart disease.
- Have patient and partner develop a meal plan low in saturated fat and cholesterol.
- Check patient's cholesterol level during follow-up appointments.

Inspection and Palpation

Ensure that the patient is comfortable and not anxious. Anxiety and discomfort may cause tachycardia, which produces inaccurate findings. Use the skills of inspection and palpation simultaneously. The examination begins with the patient supine and the upper body elevated 45 degrees because patients with heart disease frequently suffer shortness of breath while lying flat. Stand at the patient's right side. Discourage him or her from talking, especially when auscultating heart sounds. Good lighting in the room is essential.

Direct your attention to the anatomical sites best suited for assessment of cardiac function. Inspect the angle of Louis; feel the ridge in the sternum approximately 5 cm (2 inches) below the sternal notch. Slip the fingers along the angle on each side of the sternum to feel the adjacent ribs. The intercostal spaces are just below each rib. The second intercostal space allows for identification of each of the six anatomical landmarks (Figure 16-28). The second intercostal space on the right is the aortic area, and the left second intercostal space is the pulmonic area. You need deeper palpation to feel the spaces in obese or heavily muscled patients. After locating the pulmonic area, move the fingers down the patient's left sternal border to the third intercostal space, called the *second pulmonic area*. The tricuspid area is located at the fourth or fifth intercostal space along the sternum. To find the apical or mitral area, locate the fifth intercostal space

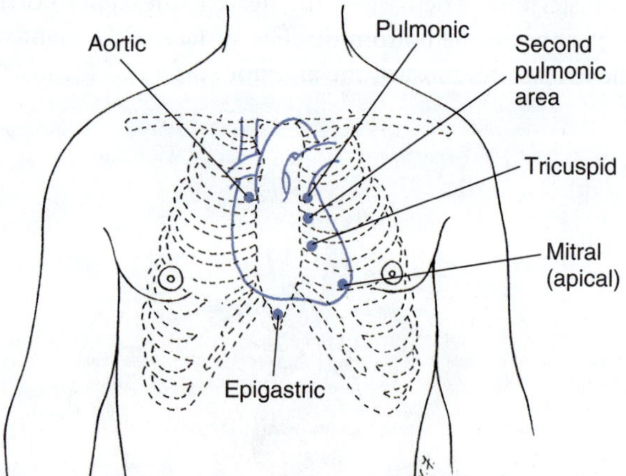

FIGURE 16-28 Anatomical sites for assessment of cardiac function.

just to the left of the sternum and move the fingers laterally to the left midclavicular line. Locate the apical area with the palm of the hand or the fingertips. Normally you feel the apical impulse as a light tap in an area 1 to 2 cm (½ to ¾ inch) in diameter at the apex. Another landmark is the epigastric area at the tip of the sternum where you palpate for aortic abnormalities.

Locate the six anatomical landmarks of the heart; inspect and palpate each area. Look for the appearance of pulsations, viewing each area over the chest at an angle to the side. Normally you do not see pulsations, except perhaps at the PMI in thin patients or the epigastric area as a result of abdominal aortic pulsation. Use the proximal halves of the four fingers together and alternate with the ball of the hand to palpate for pulsations. Touch the areas gently to allow movements to lift the hand. Normally you do not feel any pulsations or vibrations in the second, third, or fourth intercostal spaces. Loud murmurs cause a vibration. Time palpated pulsations or vibrations and their occurrence in relation to systole or diastole by auscultating heart sounds simultaneously.

You should feel the apical impulse or PMI easily. If not, have the patient turn onto the left side, moving the heart closer to the chest wall. Estimate the size of the heart by noting the diameter of the PMI and its position relative to the midclavicular line. In cases of serious heart disease the cardiac muscle enlarges, with the PMI found to the left of the midclavicular line. The PMI is sometimes difficult to find in older adults because the chest deepens in its AP diameter. It is also difficult to find in muscular or overweight patients. You usually find an infant's PMI at the third or fourth intercostal space more easily because of the child's thin chest wall.

Auscultation

Auscultation of the heart detects normal heart sounds, extra heart sounds, and murmurs. Concentrate on detecting low-intensity sounds caused by valve closure. To begin auscultation eliminate all sources of room noise and explain the procedure to reduce the patient's anxiety. Follow a systematic pattern beginning at the aortic area and inching the stethoscope across each of the anatomical sites. Listen for the complete cycle ("lub-dub") of heart sounds clearly at each location. If you suspect a problem, repeat the sequence using the bell of the stethoscope. Sometimes the patient assumes three different positions during the examination (Figure 16-29):

- Sitting up and leaning forward (good for all areas and to hear high-pitched murmurs)
- Supine (good for all areas)
- Left lateral recumbent (good for all areas; best position to hear low-pitched sounds in diastole)

Learn to identify the first (S1) and second (S2) heart sounds. At normal rates S1 occurs after the long diastolic pause and before the short systolic pause. S1 is high pitched, dull in quality, and heard best at the apex. If it is difficult to hear S1, time it in relation to the carotid pulse. S2 follows the short systolic pause and precedes the long diastolic pause; you hear it best at the aortic area.

Auscultate for rate and rhythm after hearing both sounds clearly. Each combination of S_1 and S_2 or "lub-dub" counts as one heartbeat. Count the rate for 1 minute and listen for the interval between S_1 and S_2 and then the time between S_2 and the next S_1. A regular rhythm involves regular intervals of time between each sequence of beats. There is a distinct silent pause between S_1 and S_2. Failure of the heart to beat at regular successive intervals is a **dysrhythmia.** Some dysrhythmias are life threatening.

When assessing an irregular heart rhythm, compare apical and radial pulse rates simultaneously to determine if a pulse deficit exists. Auscultate the apical pulse first and then immediately assess the radial pulse (one-examiner technique). Assess the apical and radial rates at the same time when two examiners are present. When a patient has a pulse deficit, the radial pulse is slower than the apical because ineffective contractions fail to send pulse waves to the periphery. Report a

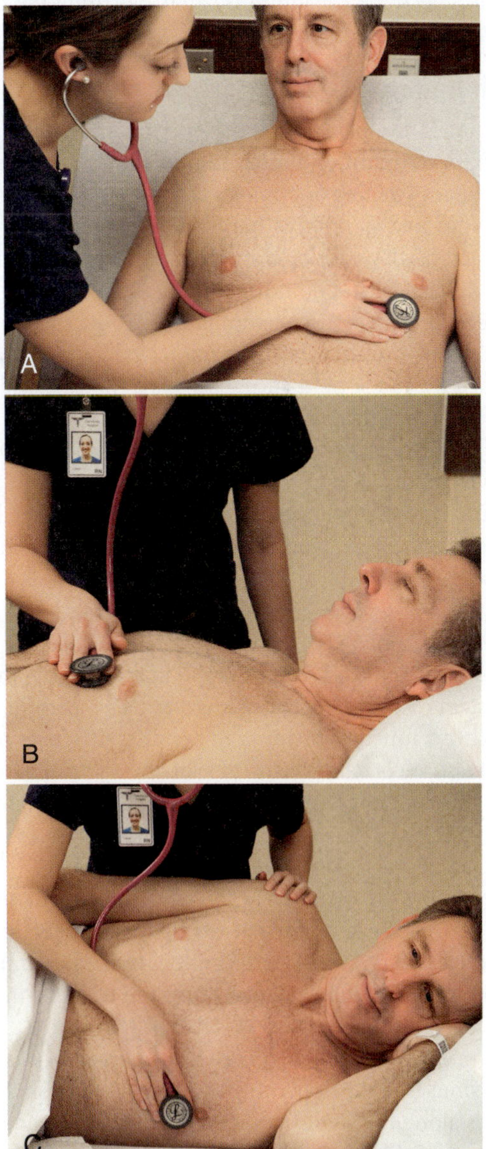

FIGURE 16-29 Sequence of patient positions for heart auscultation. **A,** Sitting. **B,** Supine. **C,** Left lateral recumbent.

difference in pulse rates to the health care provider immediately.

Assess extra heart sounds and murmurs at each auscultatory site. Use the bell of the stethoscope and listen for low-pitched extra heart sounds such as S_3 and S_4 gallops, clicks, and rubs. Presence of extra heart sounds or murmurs sometimes indicates a pathological condition; therefore such sounds should be reported to the health care provider immediately. Typically advanced practice nurses perform this part of the examination.

VASCULAR SYSTEM

Examination of the vascular system includes measuring the blood pressure (see Chapter 15) and assessing the integrity of the peripheral vascular system. Use the skills of inspection, palpation, and auscultation. Perform portions of the vascular examination during other body system assessments. For example, check the carotid pulse after palpating the cervical lymph nodes.

Health History

Determine if the patient has leg cramps; numbness or tingling in the extremities; sensation of cold hands or feet; pain in the legs; or swelling or cyanosis of the feet, ankles, or hands. These signs and symptoms may indicate vascular disease. If the patient has leg pain or cramping in the lower extremities, ask if walking or standing for long periods or during sleep aggravates or relieves the symptoms. This question helps to clarify if the problem is musculoskeletal or vascular. Ask patients if they wear tight-fitting garters or hosiery and if they sit or lie in bed with legs crossed. These activities impair venous return. Consider previous cardiac risk factors that may predispose to vascular disease (e.g., smoking or nutritional problems). Assess the patient's medical history for heart disease, hypertension, phlebitis, diabetes, or varicose veins.

Carotid Arteries

When the left ventricle pumps blood into the aorta, the arterial system transmits pressure waves. The carotid artery reflects heart function better than peripheral arteries because their pressure correlates with that of the aorta. The carotid artery supplies oxygenated blood to the head and neck (Figure 16-30). The overlying sternocleidomastoid muscle protects it.

To examine the carotid arteries have the patient sit or lie supine with the head of the bed elevated 30 degrees. Examine one carotid artery at a time. If both arteries are simultaneously occluded during palpation, the patient loses consciousness as a result of inadequate circulation to the brain. Do not palpate or massage the carotid arteries vigorously because the carotid sinus is in the upper third of the neck. The sinus sends impulses along the vagus nerve. Stimulating the vagus nerve causes a reflex drop in heart rate and blood pressure, which causes syncope (light-headedness) or circulatory arrest. This is a particular problem for older adults.

Begin inspection of the neck for obvious pulsation of the artery. Have the patient turn the head slightly away from the artery being examined. Sometimes the wave of the pulse is visible. Absence of a pulse wave may indicate arterial occlusion (blockage) or stenosis (narrowing).

To palpate the pulse ask the patient to look straight ahead or turn the head slightly toward the side being examined. Turning relaxes the sternocleidomastoid muscle. Slide the tips of your index and middle fingers around the medial edge of the sternocleidomastoid muscle. Gently palpate to avoid occlusion of circulation (Figure 16-31).

The normal carotid pulse is localized rather than diffuse. As a strong pulse the carotid has a thrusting quality. As the patient breathes no change occurs. Rotation of the neck or a shift from a sitting to a supine position does not change the

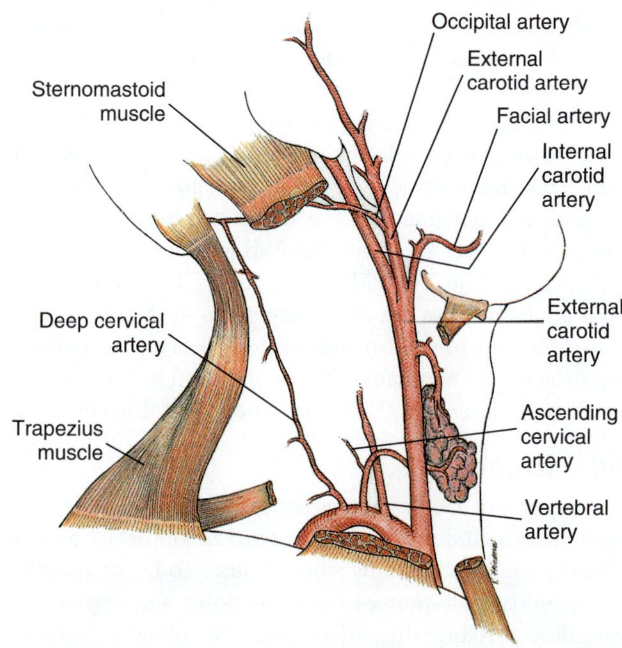

FIGURE 16-30 Anatomical position of carotid artery.

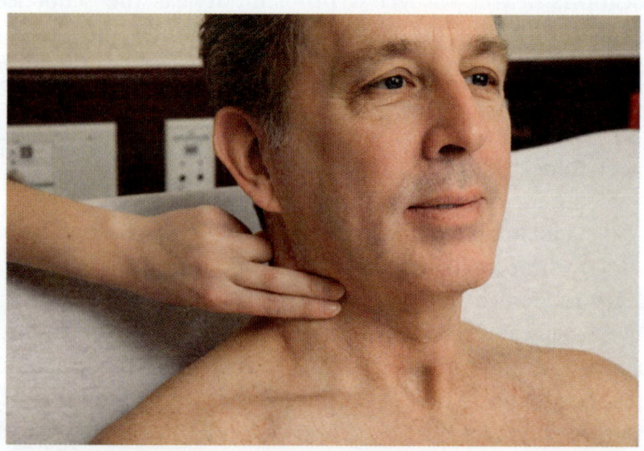

FIGURE 16-31 Palpation of internal carotid artery along margin of sternocleidomastoid muscle.

quality of the carotid artery. Both carotid arteries normally are equal in pulse rate, rhythm, and strength and are equally elastic. Diminished or unequal carotid pulsations indicate atherosclerosis (plaque buildup in arteries) or other forms of arterial disease.

The carotid is the most commonly auscultated pulse. Auscultation is especially important for middle-age or older adults or patients suspected of having cerebrovascular disease. When the lumen of a blood vessel is narrowed, blood flow is disturbed. As blood passes through the narrowed section, this creates turbulence, causing a blowing or swishing sound. The blowing sound is called a **bruit** (pronounced "brew-ee"). Place the bell of the stethoscope over the carotid artery at the base of the neck and move it gradually toward the jaw. Ask the patient to hold his or her breath for a few heartbeats so respiratory sounds do not interfere with auscultation. Normally you do not hear any sound during carotid auscultation. Palpate the artery lightly for a **thrill** (palpable bruit) if you hear a bruit.

Jugular Veins

The most accessible veins for examination are the internal and external jugular veins in the neck. Both veins drain bilaterally from the head and neck into the superior vena cava. The external jugular lies superficially and is just above the clavicle. The internal jugular lies deeper, along the carotid artery (Figure 16-32). Normally when a patient lies in the supine position, the external jugular distends and becomes easily visible. In contrast the jugular veins normally flatten when the patient is in a sitting or standing position. However, some patients with heart disease have distended jugular veins when sitting.

To measure venous pressure inspect the jugular veins with the patient in the supine position (normally veins protrude), when standing (normally veins are flat), and when sitting at a 45-degree angle (jugular veins are distended only if patient has right-sided heart failure). An advanced practice nurse completes the specific measurement of jugular venous pressure.

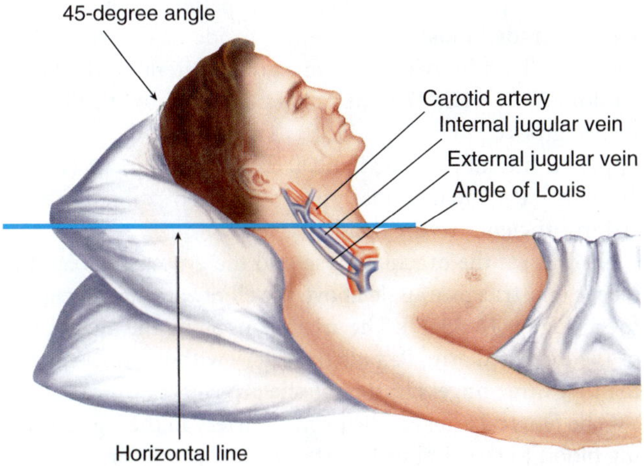

FIGURE 16-32 Position of patient to assess jugular vein distention. (From Thompson JM, et al: *Mosby's clinical nursing*, ed 4, St Louis, 1997, Mosby.)

Peripheral Arteries and Veins

To examine the peripheral vascular system, begin by assessing the adequacy of blood flow to the extremities by measuring arterial pulses and inspecting the skin and nails. Then assess the integrity of the venous system. Assess the arterial pulses in the extremities to determine sufficiency of the entire arterial circulation. Factors such as coagulation disorders, local trauma or surgery, constricting casts or bandages, and systemic diseases impair circulation to the extremities. Discuss risk factors for circulatory problems with the patient (Box 16-16).

Peripheral Arteries. Examine each peripheral artery using the distal pads of the second and third fingers. The thumb helps anchor the brachial and femoral arteries. Apply firm pressure but avoid occluding a pulse. When a pulse is difficult to find, it helps to vary pressure and feel all around the pulse site.

Routine vital signs usually include assessment of the rate and rhythm of the radial artery because it is easily accessible (see Chapter 15). Count the pulse for either 30 seconds or a full minute, depending on the character of the pulse. Always count an irregular pulse for 60 seconds. With palpation you normally feel the pulse wave at regular intervals. When an interval is interrupted by an early, late, or missed beat, the

BOX 16-16 PATIENT TEACHING

Vascular Assessment

OUTCOME

Patient chooses activities that maintain or improve peripheral vascular status.

TEACHING STRATEGIES

- Explain the effects of high-fat diet choices, discussing how cholesterol and transfats contribute to the development of atherosclerosis and lead to hypertension.
- Explain high risks for peripheral artery disease, including smoking, hypertension, diabetes, stroke, kidney disease with hemodialysis, or heart disease.
- Explain the benefit of regular monitoring of blood pressure (BP) (daily, weekly, or monthly) with available home BP monitors.
- Instruct patients with risk or evidence of vascular insufficiency in the lower extremities to avoid tight clothing over the lower body or legs, avoid sitting or standing for long periods, walk regularly, and elevate the feet when sitting.

EVALUATION STRATEGIES

- Patient identifies when blood pressure reading is within normal limits for age.
- Patient and partner demonstrate self-monitoring of blood pressure.
- Patient discontinues or decreases smoking activity, controls diabetes, and follows treatment for other chronic diseases.

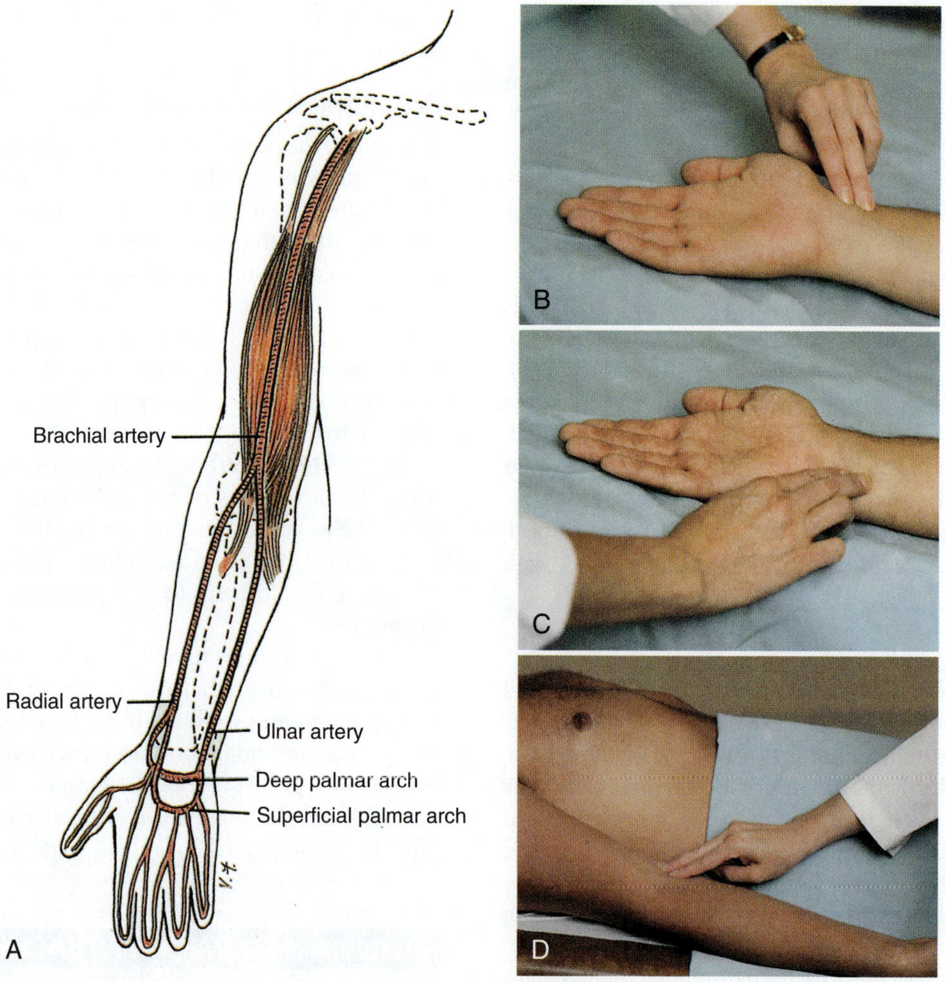

FIGURE 16-33 A, Anatomical positions of brachial, radial, and ulnar arteries. **B,** Palpation of radial pulse. **C,** Palpation of ulnar pulse. **D,** Palpation of brachial pulse.

pulse rhythm is irregular. In emergencies health care providers usually assess the carotid artery because it is accessible and most useful in evaluating heart activity. To check local circulatory status of tissues, palpate the peripheral arteries long enough to note that a pulse is present.

Assess each peripheral artery for elasticity of the vessel wall, strength, and equality. Normally the arterial wall is elastic, making it easily palpable. Depress the artery; it springs back to shape when pressure is released. An abnormal artery is described as hard, inelastic, or calcified.

The strength of a pulse is a measurement of the force with which blood is ejected against the arterial wall. Some examiners use a rating from 0 (absent, not palpable) to 4 (bounding) (Seidel et al., 2011).

Measure all peripheral pulses for equality and symmetry. Compare pulses on each side of the body. Lack of symmetry indicates impaired circulation such as a localized obstruction or an abnormally positioned artery.

In the upper extremities the brachial artery channels blood to the radial and ulnar arteries of the forearm and hand. If circulation in this artery becomes blocked, the hands do not receive adequate blood flow. If circulation in the radial or ulnar artery becomes impaired, the hand still receives adequate perfusion. An interconnection between the radial and ulnar arteries guards against arterial occlusion (Figure 16-33, *A*).

To locate pulses in the arm have the patient sit or lie down. Find the radial pulse along the radial side of the forearm at the wrist. Thin individuals have a groove lateral to the flexor tendon of the wrist. Feel the radial pulse with light palpation in the groove (Figure 16-33, *B*). The ulnar pulse is on the opposite side of the wrist and feels less prominent (Figure 16-33, *C*). Palpate the ulnar pulse only when evaluating arterial insufficiency to the hand.

To palpate the brachial pulse find the groove between the biceps and triceps muscle above the elbow at the antecubital fossa (Figure 16-33, *D*). The artery runs along the medial side of the extended arm. Palpate the artery with the fingertips of the first three fingers in the muscle groove.

The femoral artery is the primary artery in the leg, delivering blood to the popliteal, posterior tibial, and dorsalis pedis arteries (Figure 16-34, *A*). An interconnection between the posterior tibial and dorsalis pedis arteries guards against local arterial occlusion. Wearing disposable gloves, find the femoral

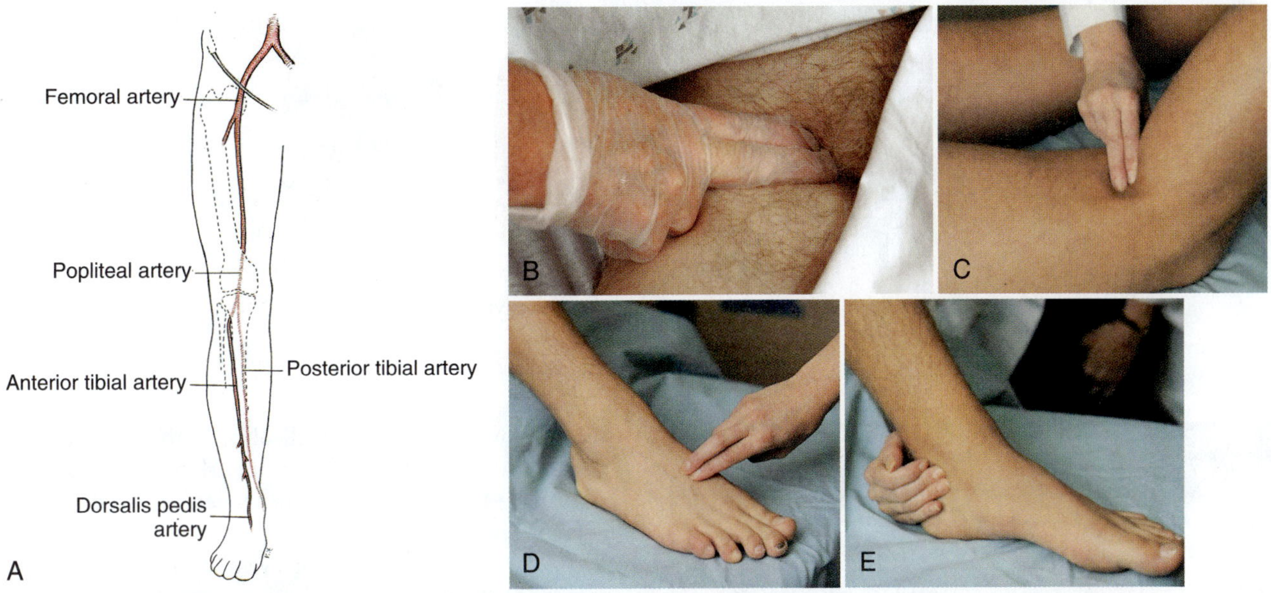

FIGURE 16-34 **A,** Anatomical position of femoral, popliteal, dorsalis pedis, anterior tibial, and posterior tibial arteries. **B,** Palpation of femoral pulse. **C,** Palpation of popliteal pulse. **D,** Palpation of dorsalis pedis pulse. **E,** Palpation of posterior tibial pulse.

pulse with the patient lying down with the inguinal area exposed (Figure 16-34, *B*). The femoral artery runs below the inguinal ligament, midway between the symphysis pubis and the anterosuperior iliac spine. Sometimes you use deep palpation to feel the pulse. Bimanual palpation is effective in obese patients. Place the fingertips of both hands on opposite sides of the pulse site. Feel a pulsatile sensation when the arterial pulsation pushes the fingertips apart.

The popliteal pulse runs behind the knee (Figure 16-34, *C*). Have the patient slightly flex the knee with the foot resting on the examination table or assume a prone position with the knee slightly flexed. Instruct the patient to keep leg muscles relaxed. Palpate with the fingers of both hands deeply into the popliteal fossa, just lateral to the midline. The popliteal pulse is difficult to locate.

With the patient's foot relaxed locate the dorsalis pedis pulse. The artery runs along the top of the foot in a line with the groove between the extensor tendons of the great and first toes (Figure 16-34, *D*). To find the pulse place the fingertips between the great and first toe and slowly move up the dorsum of the foot. This pulse is sometimes congenitally absent.

Find the posterior tibial pulse on the inner side of each ankle (Figure 16-34, *E*). Place the fingers behind and below the patient's medial malleolus (ankle bone). With the patient's foot relaxed and slightly extended, palpate the artery.

Ultrasound Stethoscopes. If a pulse is difficult to palpate, an ultrasound (Doppler) stethoscope is a useful tool that amplifies sounds of a pulse wave. Apply a thin layer of transmission gel to the patient's skin at the pulse site or directly onto the transducer tip of the probe. Turn on the volume control and place the tip of the probe at a 45- to 90-degree angle on the skin. Move the transducer until you hear a pulsating "whooshing" sound, which indicates that arterial blood flow is present. Document in the patient's record that the pulse was "doppled" and at what location.

Tissue Perfusion. The condition of the skin, mucosa, and nail beds offers useful data about the status of circulatory blood flow. Examine the face and upper extremities, looking at the color of skin, mucosa, and nail beds. The presence of cyanosis requires special attention. Heart disease sometimes causes central cyanosis (bluish discoloration of the lips, mouth, and conjunctivae), indicating poor arterial oxygenation. Blue lips, earlobes, and nail beds are signs of peripheral cyanosis, which indicates peripheral vasoconstriction. When cyanosis is present, consult with a health care provider to have laboratory testing of oxygen saturation to determine the severity of the problem. Examination of the nails involves inspection for clubbing (a bulging of the tissues at the nail base), resulting from insufficient oxygenation at the periphery.

Inspect the lower extremities for changes in color, temperature, and condition of the skin indicating either arterial or venous alterations (Table 16-7). This is a good time to ask the patient about history of pain in the legs. If an arterial occlusion is present, the patient has signs resulting from absence of blood flow. Pain is distal to the occlusion. The *5 Ps* characterize an occlusion: *p*ain, *p*allor, *p*ulselessness, *p*aresthesias, and *p*aralysis. Venous congestion causes tissue changes indicating inadequate circulatory flow back to the heart.

During examination of the lower extremities also inspect skin and nail texture; hair distribution on the lower legs, feet, and toes; venous pattern; and scars, pigmentation, or ulcers. Palpate the legs for color and temperature. Assess for capillary refill.

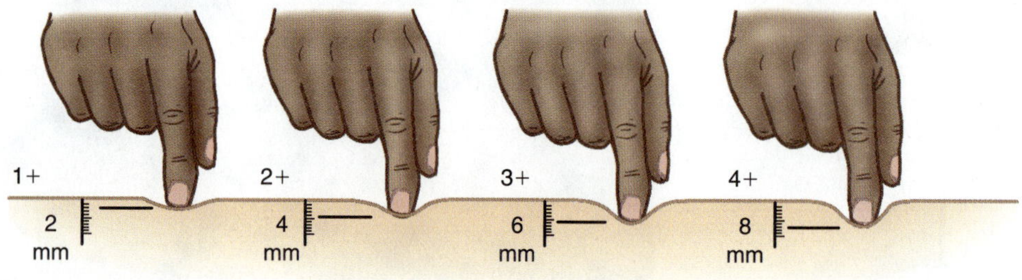

FIGURE 16-35 Assessing for pitting edema. (From Seidel HM, et al: *Mosby's guide to physical examination,* ed 7, St Louis, 2011, Mosby.)

TABLE 16-7 SIGNS OF VENOUS AND ARTERIAL INSUFFICIENCY

ASSESSMENT CRITERION	VENOUS	ARTERIAL
Color	Normal or cyanotic	Pale; worsened by elevation of extremity; dusky red when extremity lowered
Temperature	Normal	Cool (blood flow blocked to extremity)
Pulse	Normal	Decreased or absent
Edema	Often marked	Absent or mild
Skin changes	Brown pigmentation around ankles	Thin, shiny skin; decreased hair growth; thickened nails

The absence of hair growth over the legs indicates circulatory insufficiency. Do not confuse an absence of hair on the legs with shaved legs. Many men have less hair around the calves because of tight-fitting dress socks or jeans. Chronic recurring ulcers of the feet or lower legs are a serious sign of circulatory insufficiency and require a health care provider's intervention.

Peripheral Veins. Assess the status of the peripheral veins by asking the patient to assume sitting and standing positions. Assessment includes inspection and palpation for varicosities, peripheral edema, and phlebitis. Varicosities are superficial veins that become dilated, especially when legs are in a dependent position. They are common in older adults because the veins normally fibrose, dilate, and stretch. They are also common in people who stand for prolonged periods. Varicosities in the anterior or medial part of the thigh and the posterolateral part of the calf are abnormal.

Dependent edema around the feet and ankles is a sign of venous insufficiency or right-sided heart failure. It is common in older adults and people who spend a lot of time standing (e.g., nurses, waitresses, and security guards). To assess for pitting edema, use your thumb to press firmly for several seconds over the medial malleolus or the shins and then release. A depression left in the skin indicates edema. Grading +1 through +4 characterizes the severity of the edema (Figure 16-35).

Phlebitis (inflammation of a vein) occurs commonly after trauma to the vessel wall, infection, immobilization, or prolonged insertion of IV catheters (see Chapter 18). To assess for phlebitis inspect the calves for localized redness, tenderness, and swelling over vein sites. Gentle palpation of calf muscles reveals warmth, tenderness, and firmness of the muscle. Unilateral edema of the affected leg is one of the most reliable findings of phlebitis. A Doppler study is a noninvasive test that examines venous blood flow and is commonly done if deep vein thrombosis is suspected. Another method is to perform the Homans' sign test by slightly flexing the patient's knee and dorsiflexing the foot. A complaint of calf pain with the procedure is a positive sign and may indicate venous thrombosis. Using the Homans' sign test is contraindicated in patients with known deep vein thrombosis because part of the clot may become dislodged from its original site during this test, resulting in a pulmonary embolism.

Lymphatic System

Assess the lymphatic drainage of the lower extremities during examination of the vascular system or during the female or male genital examination. Superficial and deep lymph nodes drain the legs, but only two groups of superficial nodes are palpable. With the patient supine palpate the area of the superior superficial inguinal nodes in the groin area (Figure 16-36). Then move your fingertips toward the inner thigh, feeling for any palpable inferior nodes. Use a firm but gentle pressure when palpating over each lymphatic chain. Multiple nodes are not normally palpable, although a few soft, nontender nodes are not unusual. Enlarged, hardened, tender nodes reveal potential sites of infection or metastatic disease.

BREASTS

It is important to examine the breasts of female and male patients. Males have a small amount of glandular tissue, a potential site for the growth of cancer cells, in the breast. In contrast the majority of the female breast is glandular tissue.

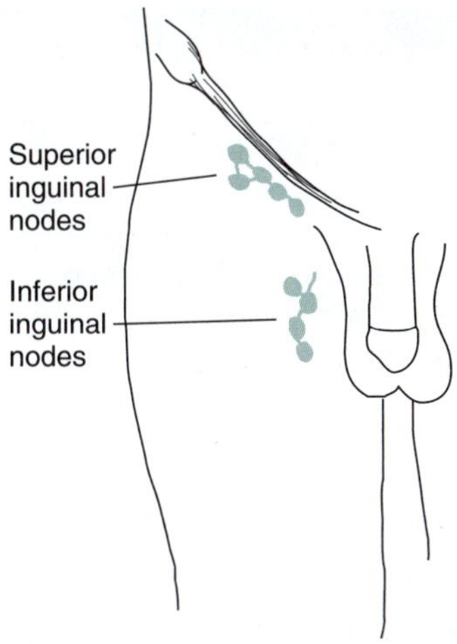

FIGURE 16-36 Inguinal lymph nodes.

Female Breasts

Among women an estimated 230,480 new cases of invasive breast cancer will be diagnosed, with 2140 new cases expected among men (1% of all cancer cases) in the United States. In addition, more than 57,000 cases of in situ breast cancer will be diagnosed (ACS, 2013a). Breast cancer is second to lung cancer as the leading cause of death in women with cancer. Early detection is the key to cure. A responsibility for you is to teach patients health behaviors such as breast self-examination (BSE) (Box 16-17).

Women need to be taught to know how their breasts usually look and feel and report changes to a health care professional. In addition, they need to know about the benefits and limitations of performing a systematic BSE. Once thought essential for early breast cancer detection, BSEs are now considered optional (ACS, 2013b). If a patient performs BSE, assess the method she uses and the time that she does the examination in relation to her menstrual cycle. The best time for BSE is when the breasts are not tender or swollen, usually a few days after a menstrual period ends. If a woman is postmenopausal advise her to check her breasts on the same day each month. A pregnant woman should also check her breasts on a monthly basis. A clinical breast examination should be part of a regular health examination by a health professional.

Older women require special attention when reviewing the need for BSE. Fixed incomes limit many older women; thus they often do not have regular clinical breast examination and mammography. Unfortunately many older women ignore changes in their breasts, assuming that they are a part of aging. In addition, physiological factors affect the ease with which older women can perform BSE. Musculoskeletal limitations, diminished peripheral sensation, reduced eyesight, and changes in joint ROM limit palpation and inspection abilities. Find resources for older women, including free screening programs. Teach family members to perform the patient's examination.

The American Cancer Society (2013b) recommends the following guidelines for the early detection of breast cancer:

1. Monthly BSE is an option for women in their 20s and 30s.
2. Women 20 years of age and older need to report any breast changes to a health care provider immediately.
3. Women need a clinical breast examination by a health care provider every 3 years from ages 20 to 40 and annually over age 40.
4. Women with a family history of breast cancer need an annual examination by a health care provider.
5. Asymptomatic women need a screening mammogram by age 40; women age 40 and over need an annual mammogram.
6. For women with an increased risk, the ACS recommends discussion of screening options and additional testing with a health care provider.

The patient's history reveals normal development changes and signs of breast disease. Because of this glandular structure, the breast undergoes changes during a woman's life. Knowledge of these changes (Box 16-18) allows you to complete an accurate assessment.

Nursing History. The nursing history reveals risk factors for breast cancer, such as being a woman over age 40 or a personal or family history of breast cancer, especially with the BRCA1 and BRCA2 inherited gene mutations. Also early-onset menarche (before age 12) or late-age menopause (after age 55) affects risk. Other risk factors include never having children, giving birth to the first child after age 30, recent use of oral contraceptives, previous chest radiation, alcohol use, and being overweight. Ask if the patient (both genders) has noticed a lump, thickening, pain, or tenderness of the breast; discharge, distortion, retraction, or scaling of the nipple; or change in breast size. Determine the patient's use of medications that increase risk (oral contraceptives, steroids, or estrogen). Determine caffeine intake to review risk factors for fibrocystic breast changes. Determine activity level, alcohol intake, and current weight. Ask if the patient performs monthly BSE. If so, determine the time of month she performs the examination in relation to menstrual cycle. Have the patient describe or demonstrate the method used. If the patient reports a breast mass, assess for related symptoms.

Inspection. Have the patient remove the top gown or drape to allow simultaneous visualization of both breasts. Have her stand or sit with her arms hanging loosely at her sides. If possible, place a mirror in front of her during inspection so she sees what to look for when performing BSE. To recognize abnormalities the patient needs to be familiar with the normal appearance of her breasts. Describe observations or findings in relation to imaginary lines that divide the breast into four quadrants and a tail. The lines cross at the center of the nipple. Each tail extends outward from the upper outer quadrant (Figure 16-37).

Inspect the breasts for size and symmetry. Normally they extend from the third to the sixth ribs, with the nipple at the level of the fourth intercostal space. It is common for one breast to be smaller. However, inflammation or a mass can cause a difference in size. With age the ligaments supporting

BOX 16-17 PATIENT TEACHING

Female Breast Assessment

OUTCOME

Patient performs activities to ensure breast health or provide early identification of breast disease.

TEACHING STRATEGIES

- Women who are 20 years of age and over should be told about the benefits and limitations of breast self-examination (BSE) (ACS, 2013d). Emphasize the importance of prompt reporting of any new breast symptoms to a health care professional. Women who choose to do BSE should receive instruction and have their technique reviewed. Provide the following information about breast self-examination (BSE):
  1. BSE should be done once a month so the woman becomes familiar with the usual appearance and feel of her breast. Familiarity makes it easier to notice any changes in the breast from one month to another. Early discovery of a change from "normal" is the main idea behind BSE.
  2. For women who menstruate, the best time to do BSE is the fourth through the seventh day of the menstrual cycle or right after the menstrual cycle ends, when the breasts are least likely to be tender or swollen. Women who no longer menstruate should pick a day such as the first day of the month to remind them to do BSE.
  3. Males should also examine their breasts, areolas, nipples, and axillae for any swelling, nodules, or ulcerations.
  4. When a woman has breast implants, it might be helpful for the surgeon to identify the edges of the implant. Women who are pregnant or breastfeeding should also do a breast self-examination (ACS, 2013d).
- Teach the steps for performing BSE:
  1. Lie down on your back and place your right arm behind your head. The examination is completed lying down, not standing up (ACS, 2013d). The reasoning is when you lie down the breast tissue spreads evenly over the chest wall and is as thin as possible, making it much easier to feel all the breast tissue.
  2. Use the finger pads of the three middle fingers on your left hand to feel for lumps in the right breast. Use overlapping, dime-sized, circular motions of the finger pads to feel the breast tissue. Use three different levels of pressure to feel all the breast tissue. Light pressure is needed to feel the tissue closest to the skin, medium pressure to feel a little deeper, and firm pressure to feel the tissue closest to the chest and ribs. It is normal to feel a firm ridge in the lower curve of each breast, but you should tell your doctor if you feel anything else out of the ordinary. If you are not sure how hard to press, discuss this with your health care provider. Use each pressure level to feel the breast tissue before moving on to the next spot.
  3. Move around the breast in an up-and-down pattern starting at an imaginary line drawn straight down your side from the underarm and moving across the breast to the middle of the chest (sternum, or breastbone). Be sure to check the entire breast area going down until you feel only ribs and up to the neck or collar bone (clavicle). There is some evidence that the up-and-down pattern is the most effective pattern for covering the entire breast.
  4. Repeat the self-examination in the left breast, putting your left arm behind your head and examining the right breast as noted in Steps 1 to 3.
  5. While standing in front of a mirror with your hands pressing firmly down on your hips, look at your breasts, observing for any changes in size, shape, contour, dimpling, or redness or scaliness of the nipple or breast tissue. Pressing down on your hips contracts the chest wall muscles and enhances any breast changes.
  6. Examine each underarm while sitting or standing and with your arm only slightly raised so you can easily feel in this area for any lumps or changes. Raising your arm straight tightens the tissue in this area, making it harder to examine.
  7. Call your health care provider if you find a lump or other abnormality.
- Have the patient perform return demonstration of BSE and offer the opportunity to ask questions.
- Explain recommended frequency of mammography and assessment by a health care provider.
- Discuss signs and symptoms of breast cancer and differentiate them from the symptoms of benign (fibrocystic) disease.
- Inform a woman who is obese or has a family history of breast cancer that she is at higher risk for the disease (ACS, 2013a). Encourage following low-fat diet, including limiting meat consumption to well-trimmed, lean beef, pork, or lamb; removing skin from cooked chicken before eating it; selecting tuna and salmon packed in water and not oil; and using low-fat dairy products.
- Encourage the patient to reduce intake of caffeine. Although this is controversial, many believe that decreasing caffeine intake reduces symptoms of benign (fibrocystic) breast disease.

EVALUATION STRATEGIES

- Patient demonstrates BSE.
- During future visits determine if patient has had screening mammography.
- Have patient describe signs and symptoms of breast cancer compared with benign (fibrocystic) breast disease.

BOX 16-18 NORMAL CHANGES IN THE BREAST DURING A WOMAN'S LIFE SPAN

PUBERTY (8 TO 20 YEARS)*

Breasts mature in five stages. One breast may grow more rapidly than the other. The ages at which changes occur and rate of developmental progression vary.

Stage 1 (Preadolescent)

This stage involves elevation of the nipple only.

Stage 2

The breast and nipple elevate as a small mound, and the areolar diameters enlarge.

Stage 3

There is further enlargement and elevation of the breast and areola, with no separation of contour.

Stage 4

The areola and nipple project into the secondary mound above the level of the breast (does not occur in all girls).

Stage 5 (Mature Breast)

Only the nipple projects, and the areola recedes (varies in some women).

YOUNG ADULTHOOD (20 TO 30 YEARS)

Breasts reach full (nonpregnant) size. Shape is generally symmetrical. Breasts are sometimes unequal in size.

PREGNANCY

Breast size gradually enlarges to 2 to 3 times the previous size. Nipples enlarge and become erect. Areolae darken, and diameters increase. Superficial veins become prominent. The nipples expel a yellowish fluid (colostrum).

MENOPAUSE

Breasts shrink. Tissue becomes softer, sometimes flabby.

OLDER ADULTHOOD

Breasts become elongated, pendulous, and flaccid as a result of glandular tissue atrophy. The skin of the breasts tends to wrinkle, appearing loose and flabby.

Nipples become smaller and flatter and lose erectile ability.†

Nipples invert because of shrinkage and fibrotic changes.‡

Data from: *Hockenberry MJ, Wilson D: *Wong's nursing care of infants and children,* ed 9, St Louis, 2011, Mosby; †Seidel HM, et al: *Mosby's guide to physical examination,* ed 7, St Louis, 2011, Mosby; ‡Touhy TA, Jett KF: *Ebersole & Hess' Toward healthy aging,* ed 8, St Louis, 2012, Mosby.

the breast tissue weaken, causing the breasts to sag and the nipples to lower.

Observe the contour or shape of the breasts and note masses, flattening, retraction, or dimpling. Breasts vary in shape from convex to pendulous or conical. Retraction or dimpling results from invasion of underlying ligaments by tumors. The ligaments fibrose and pull the overlying skin inward toward the tumor. Edema also changes the contour of the breasts. To bring out the presence of retraction or changes in the shape of the breasts, ask the patient to assume three positions: raise arms above the head, press hands against the hips, and extend arms straight ahead while sitting and leaning forward. Each maneuver causes a contraction of the pectoral muscles, which accentuate the presence of any retraction.

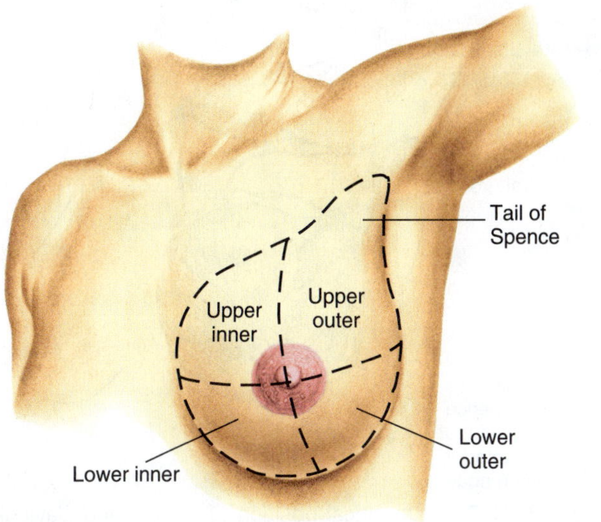

FIGURE 16-37 Quadrants of the left breast and axillary tail of Spence. (From Seidel HM, et al: *Mosby's guide to physical examination,* ed 7, St Louis, 2011, Mosby.)

Carefully inspect the skin for color; venous pattern; and presence of edema, lesions, or inflammation. Lift each breast when necessary to observe lower and lateral aspects for color and texture changes. The breasts are the color of neighboring skin, and venous patterns are the same bilaterally. Venous patterns are easily visible in thin or pregnant women. Women with large breasts often have redness and excoriation of the undersurface caused by rubbing of skin surfaces.

Inspect the nipple and areola for size, color, shape, discharge, and the direction the nipples point. The normal areolae are round or oval and nearly equal bilaterally. Color ranges from pink to brown. In light-skinned women the areola turns brown during pregnancy and remains dark. In dark-skinned women the areola is brown before pregnancy (Seidel et al., 2011). Normally the nipples point in symmetrical directions, are everted, and have no drainage. If the nipples are inverted, ask if this has been present since birth. A recent inversion or inward turning of the nipple indicates an underlying growth. Rashes or ulcerations are not normal on the breast or nipples. Note any bleeding or discharge from the nipple. Clear yellow discharge 2 days after childbirth is common. While inspecting the breasts, explain the characteristics you see. Teach the patient the significance of abnormal signs or symptoms.

Palpation. Palpation assesses the condition of underlying breast tissue and lymph nodes. Breast tissue consists of glandular tissue, fibrous supportive ligaments, and fat. Glandular tissue is organized into lobes that end in ducts opening onto the surface of the nipple. The largest portion of glandular tissue is in the upper outer quadrant and tail of each

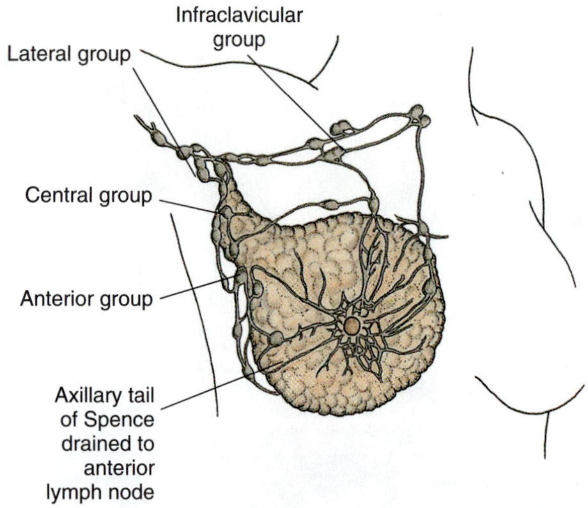

FIGURE 16-38 Anatomical position of axillary and clavicular lymph nodes.

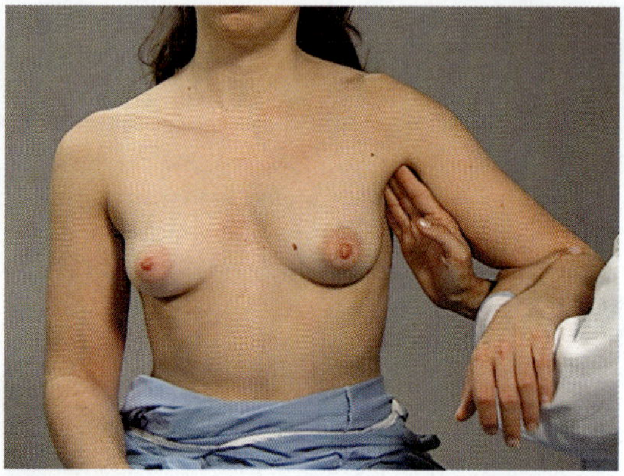

FIGURE 16-39 Support patient's arm and palpate axillary lymph nodes. (From Seidel HM, et al: *Mosby's guide to physical examination,* ed 7, St Louis, 2011, Mosby.)

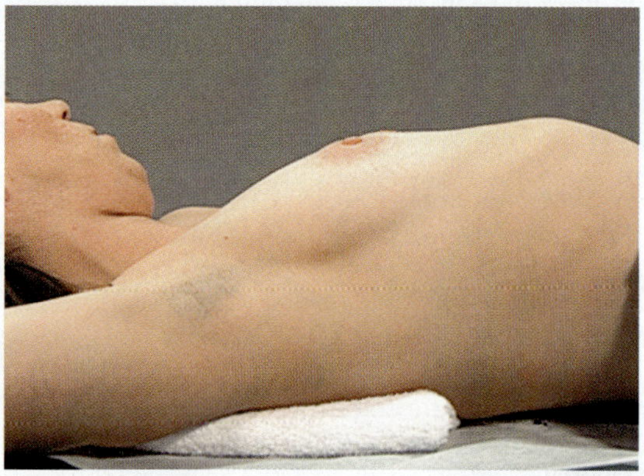

FIGURE 16-40 Patient lies flat with arm abducted and hand under head to help flatten breast tissue evenly over the chest wall. (From Seidel HM, et al: *Mosby's guide to physical examination,* ed 7, St Louis, 2011, Mosby.)

breast. Suspensory ligaments connect to skin and fascia underlying the breast to support the breast and maintain its upright position. Fatty tissue is located superficially and to the sides of the breast.

A large proportion of lymph from the breasts drains into axillary lymph nodes. Learn the location of supraclavicular, infraclavicular, and axillary nodes (Figure 16-38). The axillary nodes drain lymph from the chest wall, breasts, arms, and hands. A tumor of one breast sometimes involves nodes on both sides of the body.

To palpate lymph nodes have the patient sit with arms at her sides and muscles relaxed. While facing the patient and standing on the side you are examining, support her arm in a flexed position and abduct the arm from the chest wall. Place the free hand against her chest wall and high in the axillary hollow (Figure 16-39). With your fingertips press gently down over the surface of the ribs and muscles. Palpate the axillary nodes with the fingertips gently rolling soft tissue. Palpate four areas of the axilla: the edge of the pectoralis major muscle along the anterior axillary line, the chest wall in the midaxillary area, the upper part of the humerus, and the anterior edge of the latissimus dorsi muscle along the posterior axillary line. Normally lymph nodes are not palpable. Note the number, consistency, mobility, and size of palpable nodes. A palpable node feels like a small mass that is hard, tender, and immobile. Also palpate along the upper and lower clavicular ridges. Perform the procedure for the patient's other side.

Perform palpation of breast tissue with the patient lying supine. This position allows the breast tissue to flatten evenly against the chest wall. The patient raises her hand and places it behind the neck to further stretch and position breast tissue evenly. Place a small pillow or towel under her shoulder blade to further position breast tissue (Figure 16-40).

If the patient complains of a mass, examine the opposite breast first to ensure an objective comparison of normal and abnormal tissue. Use the pads of the first three fingers to compress breast tissue gently against the chest wall, noting tissue consistency. During a clinical breast examination, perform palpation systematically in one of three ways: (1) using a vertical technique with the fingers moving up and down each quadrant; (2) clockwise or counterclockwise, forming small circles with the fingers along each quadrant and the tail; or (3) palpating from center of the breast in a radial fashion, returning to the areola to begin each spoke (Figure 16-41). Whatever approach you use, be sure to cover the entire breast and tail, directing attention to any areas of tenderness. When palpating large, pendulous breasts, use a bimanual technique. Support the inferior portion of the breast in one hand while using the other hand to palpate breast tissue against the supporting hand.

During palpation note the consistency of breast tissue. The breasts of a young patient are firm and elastic. In an older patient the tissue may feel stringy and nodular. The patient's familiarity with the texture of her own breasts is most important. The lobular feel of glandular tissue is normal. The lower edge of each breast feels firm and hard and indicates the normal inframammary ridge, not a tumor. It helps to move the patient's hand so she feels normal tissue variations. Palpate abnormal masses to determine location in relation to

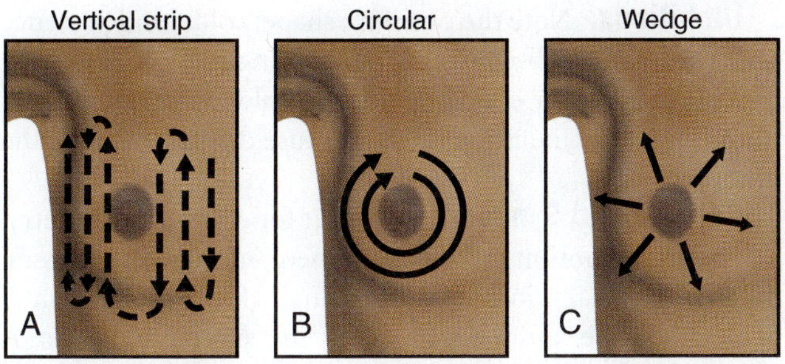

FIGURE 16-41 Various methods for breast palpation. **A,** Palpate from top to bottom in vertical strips. **B,** Palpate in concentric circles. **C,** Palpate out from the center in wedge sections. (From Seidel HM, et al: *Mosby's guide to physical examination,* ed 7, St Louis, 2011, Mosby.)

quadrants, diameter in centimeters, shape (e.g., round or discoid), consistency (soft, firm, or hard), tenderness, mobility, and discreteness (clear or unclear borders). Cancerous lesions are hard, fixed, nontender, irregular in shape, and usually unilateral.

Give special attention when palpating the nipple and areola. Palpate the entire surface gently. Use the thumb and index finger to compress the nipple and note any discharge. During the examination of the nipple and areola the nipple may become erect with wrinkling of the areola. These changes are normal.

After completing the examination have the patient demonstrate self-palpation. Observe her technique and emphasize the importance of a systematic approach. Urge the patient to see her health care provider if she discovers an abnormal mass during monthly self-examination (see Box 16-17).

Male Breasts

Examination of the male breast is relatively easy. Inspect the nipple and areola for nodules, edema, and ulceration. An enlarged male breast results from obesity or glandular enlargement. Steroid use contributes to breast enlargement in young males. Fatty tissue feels soft, whereas glandular tissue is firm. Use the same techniques to palpate for masses used in examination of the female breast. Because male breast cancer is relatively rare, routine self-examinations are unnecessary. However, men with a first-degree relative (e.g., mother) with breast cancer are at increased risk for the development of breast cancer and should perform regular breast self-examinations.

ABDOMEN

The abdominal examination is complex because of the number of organs located within and near the abdominal cavity. It includes an assessment of structures of the lower GI tract in addition to the liver, stomach, uterus, ovaries, kidneys, and bladder. Abdominal pain is a common reason that patients report when seeking health care. An accurate assessment requires matching patient history data with an assessment of the location of physical symptoms.

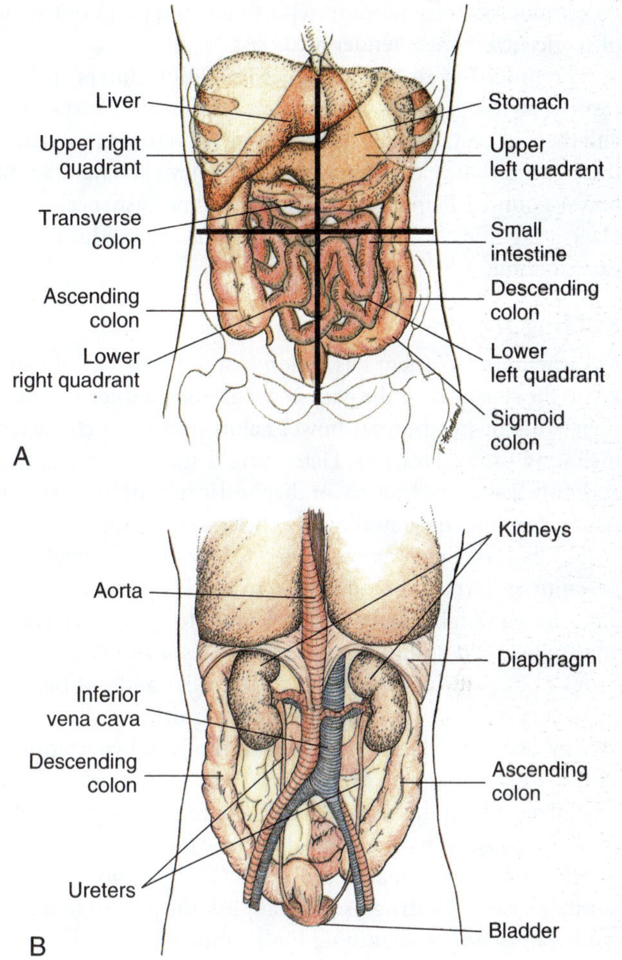

FIGURE 16-42 A, Anterior view of abdomen divided by quadrants. **B,** Posterior view of abdominal sections.

Assess the organs anteriorly and posteriorly. A system of landmarks helps to map out the abdominal region. The xiphoid process (tip of the sternum) is the upper boundary of the anterior abdominal region. The symphysis pubis is the lower boundary. Divide the abdomen into four imaginary quadrants to refer to assessment findings (Figure 16-42, *A*) and record them in relation to each quadrant. Posteriorly the lower ribs and heavy back muscles protect the kidneys, which are located from the T12 to L3 vertebrae (Figure 16-42, *B*). The costovertebral angle formed by the last rib and vertebral column is a landmark used during palpation of the kidney.

During the abdominal examination the patient needs to relax. Tight abdominal muscles make palpation difficult. Ask the patient to void before beginning. Be sure that the room is warm and cover the patient's upper chest and legs. The patient lies supine or in a dorsal recumbent position with the arms at the sides and knees slightly bent. Place small pillows beneath the knees. If the patient places the arms under the head, the abdominal muscles tighten. Proceed calmly and slowly, being sure that there is adequate lighting. Expose the abdomen from just above the xiphoid process down to the symphysis pubis. Warm hands and stethoscope promote relaxation. Ask the patient to report pain and point out areas of tenderness. Assess tender areas last.

The order for an abdominal examination differs slightly from that for previous assessments. Begin with inspection and then auscultation. By using auscultation before palpation there is less chance of altering the frequency and character of bowel sounds. Palpation could falsely increase peristalsis. Have a tape measure and marking pen available during the examination.

Nursing History

Ask whether the patient has abdominal or low back pain and assess the character of the pain in detail (see Chapter 32). Also review his or her normal bowel habits and stool character, including use of laxatives. Determine if the patient has had abdominal surgery, trauma, or diagnostic tests of the GI tract. Assess for difficulty swallowing, belching, flatulence (gas), bloody emesis (hematemesis), black or tarry stools (melena), heartburn, diarrhea, or constipation. Assess if the patient has had a recent weight change or intolerance to diet (e.g., nausea, vomiting, or cramping). If the patient takes antiinflammatory drugs (e.g., aspirin, ibuprofen, or steroids) and antibiotics, there is risk for GI upset or bleeding. Inquire about a family history of cancer, kidney disease, alcoholism, hypertension, or heart disease. Assess the patient's usual intake of alcohol. Also determine if the female patient is pregnant and note the date of her last menstrual period. Review the patient's history for risk factors for hepatitis B virus (HBV) exposure (e.g., hemodialysis or IV drug use). Finally ask the patient to locate tender areas before beginning the examination.

Inspection

Always observe the patient during routine care activities. Note his or her posture and look for evidence of abdominal splinting, lying with the knees drawn up, or moving restlessly in bed. A patient free from abdominal pain does not guard or splint the abdomen. To inspect the abdomen for abnormal movement or shadows, stand on the patient's right side and inspect the abdomen from above. By sitting down to look across the abdomen, you assess abdominal contour. Direct the examination light over the abdomen. Inspect it for continuity, any retractions, bulging, and symmetry.

Skin. Inspect the skin over the abdomen for color, scars, venous patterns, lesions, and striae (stretch marks). The skin is subject to the same color variations as the rest of the body. Venous patterns are normally faint, except in thin patients. Artificial openings indicate drainage sites resulting from surgery (see Chapter 39) or an ostomy (see Chapters 34 and 35). Scars reveal evidence of past trauma or surgery that created permanent changes in underlying organ anatomy. Bruising indicates accidental injury, physical abuse, or a type of bleeding disorder. Ask if the patient self-administers injections (e.g., insulin or anticoagulants). Unexpected findings include generalized skin color changes such as jaundice or cyanosis. A glistening taut (tight) appearance indicates ascites.

Umbilicus. Note the position; shape; color; and presence of inflammation, discharge, or protruding masses. A normal umbilicus is flat or concave with the color the same as surrounding skin. Underlying masses cause displacement of the umbilicus.

Contour and Symmetry. Inspect for contour, symmetry, and surface motion of the abdomen, noting any masses, bulging, or distention. A flat abdomen forms a horizontal plane from the xiphoid process to the symphysis pubis. A round abdomen protrudes in a convex sphere from a horizontal plane. A concave abdomen appears to sink into the muscular wall. Each of these findings is normal if the shape of the abdomen is symmetrical. In older adults there is often an overall increased distribution of adipose tissue. The presence of masses on only one side, or asymmetry, indicates an underlying pathological condition.

Intestinal gas, tumor, or fluid in the abdominal cavity causes distention (swelling). When distention is generalized, the entire abdomen protrudes. The skin often appears taut, as if it were stretched over the abdomen. When gas causes distention, the flanks do not bulge. However, if fluid is the source of the problem such as in ascites, the flanks bulge. Ask the patient to roll onto one side. A protuberance forms on the dependent side if fluid is the cause of the distention. Ask the patient if the abdomen feels unusually tight. Be careful not to confuse distention with obesity. In obesity the abdomen is large, rolls of adipose tissue are often present along the flanks, and the patient does not complain of tightness in the abdomen. If abdominal distention is expected, measure the abdomen by placing a tape measure around it at the level of the umbilicus. Consecutive measurements show any increase or decrease in distention. Use a marking pen to indicate where you applied the tape measure.

Enlarged Organs or Masses. Observe the contour of the abdomen while asking the patient to take a deep breath and hold it. Normally the contour remains smooth and symmetrical. To evaluate abdominal musculature, have the patient raise his or her head. This position causes superficial abdominal wall masses, hernias, and muscle separations to become more apparent.

Movement or Pulsations. Inspect for movement. A patient with severe pain has diminished respiratory movement and tightens abdominal muscles to guard against the pain. Observe for peristaltic movement and aortic pulsation by looking across the abdomen from side to side. These movements are visible in thin patients; otherwise no movement is present.

Auscultation

The abdominal examination is one exception when you auscultate before palpation to reduce the risk for altering the frequency and intensity of bowel sounds. Ask the patient not to speak. Patients with GI tubes connected to suction need them temporarily turned off before beginning the examination.

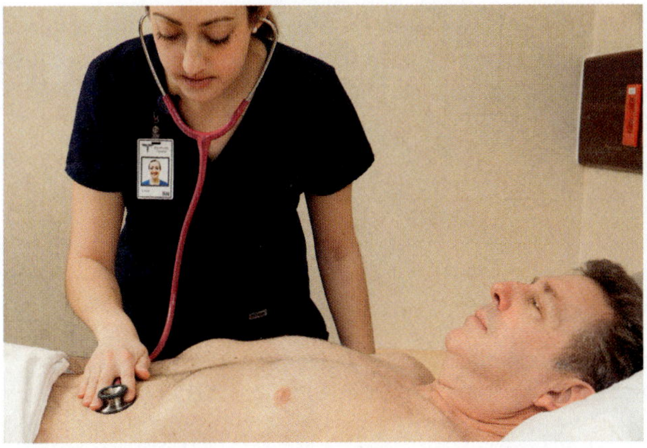

FIGURE 16-43 Auscultation of abdomen using diaphragm of stethoscope.

Bowel Motility. Bowel sounds are the audible passage of air and fluid that normal intestinal contractions (peristalsis) create. Place the warmed diaphragm of the stethoscope lightly over each of the four quadrants (Figure 16-43). Normally air and fluid move through the intestines, creating soft gurgling or clicking sounds that occur irregularly 5 to 35 times per minute (Seidel et al., 2011). Sounds may last ½ second to several seconds. It normally takes 5 to 20 seconds to hear a bowel sound. However, it takes 5 minutes of continuous listening before determining that bowel sounds are absent. Auscultate all four quadrants to be sure that you do not miss any sounds. The best time to auscultate is between meals. Sounds are generally described as normal, audible, absent, hyperactive, or hypoactive.

Absent sounds indicate a lack of peristalsis, possibly caused by bowel obstruction, paralytic ileus (decreased or absent peristalsis), or peritonitis (inflammation of the peritoneum). Hyperactive sounds are loud, "growling" sounds (borborygmi) that indicate increased GI motility. Inflammation of the bowel, anxiety, bleeding, excess ingestion of laxatives, and reaction of the intestines to certain foods cause increased motility (Box 16-19).

Vascular Sounds. Bruits auscultated in affected blood vessels indicate narrowing of the blood vessels and turbulent disrupted blood flow. Presence of bruits in the abdominal area reveals aneurysms or stenotic vessels. Use the bell of the stethoscope to auscultate in the epigastric region and each of the four quadrants. Normally there are no vascular sounds over the aorta (midline through the abdomen) or femoral arteries (lower quadrants). Report a bruit immediately to a health care provider.

Palpation

Palpation primarily detects areas of abdominal tenderness, distention, or masses. As assessment skills improve, learn to palpate for specific organs such as the liver, using light and deep palpation.

Use light palpation over each abdominal quadrant. Initially avoid areas previously identified as problem spots. Lay the palm of the hand with fingers extended and approximated lightly on the abdomen. Explain the maneuver to the patient; with the palmar surface of the fingers depress 1.3 cm (½ inch) in a gentle dipping motion (Figure 16-44, *A*). Avoid quick jabs and use smooth, coordinated movements. For ticklish patients first place the patient's hand on the abdomen with your hand on the patient's hand; continue until the patient tolerates palpation. Assess for muscular resistance, tenderness, distention, and superficial organs or masses. Observe for signs of discomfort. The abdomen is normally smooth with consistent softness and nontender without masses. The older adult often lacks abdominal tone.

With experience perform deep palpation (Figure 16-44, *B* and *C*) to assess abdominal organs and detect less obvious masses. You need short fingernails. It is important for the patient to be relaxed while the hands depress approximately 2.5 to 7.5 cm (1 to 3 inches) into the abdomen. Never use

BOX 16-19 PATIENT TEACHING

Abdominal Assessment

OUTCOME

Patient experiences regular digestion and elimination.

TEACHING STRATEGIES

- Explain factors that promote normal bowel elimination such as diet, regular exercise, limited use of over-the-counter drugs causing constipation, establishment of a regular elimination schedule, and adequate fluid intake (see Chapter 35).
- Caution patient about dangers of excessive use of laxatives or enemas.
- Instruct patient to have new onset of abdominal pain or discomfort evaluated by a health care provider.
- If patient has chronic pain, explain measures used for pain relief (e.g., relaxation exercises, positioning) (see Chapter 32).
- Instruct patient about warning signs of colon cancer, including rectal bleeding, cramping pain in lower abdomen, black or tarry stools, blood in the stool, and a change in bowel habits (constipation or diarrhea).
- Instruct patient to report any noticeable yellowing of eyes, mucous membranes, or skin.
- If patient is a health care worker or has contact with blood or body fluids of affected people, encourage him or her to receive series of three hepatitis B (HBV) vaccine doses.

EVALUATION STRATEGIES

- Reassess patient's bowel elimination pattern and stool characteristics after therapy begins.
- Observe patient's use of pain-relief measures and reassess character of pain.
- Patient obtains early treatment for abdominal discomfort or jaundice.
- During future visits check patient's compliance with HBV vaccine schedule.
- Ask patient to state signs and symptoms of colon cancer.

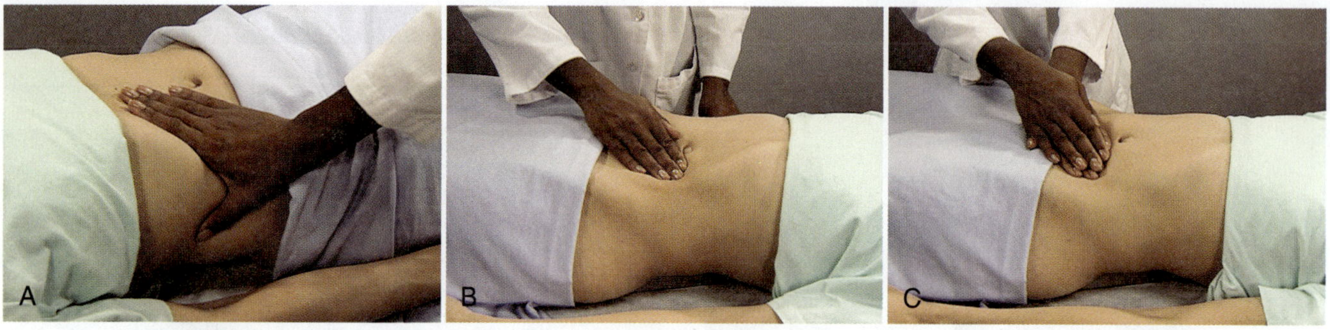

FIGURE 16-44 A, Light palpation of abdomen. **B**, Deep palpation of abdomen. **C,** Deep bimanual palpation. (From Seidel HM, et al: *Mosby's guide to physical examination,* ed 7, St Louis, 2011, Mosby.)

deep palpation over a surgical incision or over extremely tender organs. It is also unwise to use deep palpation on abnormal masses. Deep pressure causes tenderness in the healthy patient over the cecum, sigmoid colon, and aorta and in the midline near the xiphoid process (Seidel et al., 2011).

Assess each quadrant systematically. Palpate masses for size, location, shape, consistency, tenderness, pulsation, and mobility. Test for rebound tenderness by pressing a hand slowly and deeply into the involved area and then letting go quickly. The test is positive if the patient feels pain when the hand is released. Rebound tenderness occurs in patients with peritoneal irritation such as in appendicitis; pancreatitis; or any peritoneal injury causing bile, blood, or enzymes to enter the peritoneal cavity.

Aortic Pulsation. To assess aortic pulsation palpate with the thumb and forefinger of one hand deeply into the upper abdomen just left of the midline. Normally a pulsation is transmitted forward. If the aorta is enlarged from an aneurysm (localized dilation of a vessel wall), the pulsation expands laterally. Do not palpate a pulsating abdominal mass. In obese patients it is often necessary to palpate with both hands, one on each side of the aorta.

FEMALE GENITALIA AND REPRODUCTIVE TRACT

Examination of the female genitalia requires a calm, relaxed approach. The gynecological examination is one of the most difficult experiences for adolescents. Cultural background further adds to apprehension. For example, in some cultural groups women allow only a female health care provider to perform a physical assessment. Other cultures have a strong social value for modesty. Provide a thorough explanation as to the reason for the procedures used in the examination and ask the patient if there is a need for a chaperone during the examination. The lithotomy position assumed during the examination is often a source of embarrassment. Make the patient feel comfortable by correctly positioning and draping her. Be sure to explain each portion of the examination in advance so patients anticipate each action. Adolescents sometimes choose to have a female parent present in the examination room.

Sometimes a patient requires a complete examination, including assessing external genitalia and performing a vaginal examination. The nurse examines external genitalia while performing routine hygiene measures or preparing to insert a urinary catheter. An examination is a part of each woman's preventive health care because ovarian cancer causes more deaths than any other cancer of the female reproductive system; the risk of having ovarian cancer during a lifetime is 1 in 71 (ACS, 2013e).

Adolescents and young adults are examined because of the growing incidence of sexually transmitted infections (STIs). The average age of menarche among young girls has declined, and the majority of male and female teenagers are sexually active by age 19 (Hockenberry and Wilson, 2011). Since the patient assumes a lithotomy or dorsal recumbent position, rectal and anal assessments are combined with this examination.

Nursing History

Begin by asking what the patient hopes to learn or do as a result of the examination. Establish rapport with her to increase her comfort level, focusing on her feelings about exposing herself to a health care provider. Next the nursing history reviews the patient's previous illness or surgeries involving reproductive organs, including STIs. A review of the menstrual history includes age at menarche, frequency and duration of menstrual cycle, character of flow, presence of dysmenorrhea (painful menstruation), pelvic pain, dates of last two menstrual periods, and premenstrual symptoms. Ask if the patient has had signs of bleeding, vaginal discharge, or pain outside the normal menstrual period or after menopause. Ask if she has symptoms or history of genitourinary problems such as burning during urination, frequency, urgency, nocturia, hematuria, incontinence, or stress incontinence.

Ask the patient to describe her obstetrical history, including each pregnancy and history of abortions or miscarriages. Also question her about current and past contraceptive practices and problems encountered. It is important to determine if the patient uses safe sex practices. Discuss risks of STIs and HIV infection. Also review a patient's risk for developing cervical, endometrial, or ovarian cancer (Box 16-20).

BOX 16-20 **PATIENT TEACHING**

Female Genital and Reproductive Tract Assessment

OUTCOME

Patient follows routine preventive and safety measures for gynecological health.

TEACHING STRATEGIES

- Instruct patient in the purpose and recommended frequency of Papanicolaou (Pap) tests and gynecological examinations. Explain that the Pap test is needed annually for women who are sexually active or over age 21. Patients are screened more often if certain risk factors exist such as a weak immune system, multiple sex partners, smoking, and a history of infections (e.g., human papillomavirus [HPV]).
- Counsel females about genital HPV infection and the need to receive the HPV vaccine before becoming sexually active. The vaccine is ideally recommended for 11- and 12-year-old girls. Females who are already sexually active may benefit from the vaccine, but it may not be as effective if already exposed to HPV. It is also recommended for females age 13 through 26 who have not yet been vaccinated.
- Counsel patients with sexually transmitted infections (STIs) about diagnosis and treatment.
- Instruct in genital self-examination: Using a mirror, position self to examine the area covered by the pubic hair. Spread the hair apart, looking for bumps, sores, or blisters, Also look for any warts, which appear as small, bumpy spots and enlarge to fleshy, cauliflower-like lesions. Next spread the outer vaginal lips apart and look at the clitoris for bumps, blisters, sores, or warts. Also look at both sides of the inner vaginal lips. Inspect the area around the urinary and vaginal openings for bumps, blisters, sores, or warts.
- Explain warning signs of STIs: pain or burning on urination, pain during sex, pain in the pelvic area, bleeding between menstrual periods, an itchy rash around the vagina, and vaginal discharge.
- Teach measures to prevent STIs: male partner's use of condoms, restricting number of sexual partners, avoiding sex with people who have several other partners, and perineal hygiene measures.
- Tell patients with STIs to inform their sexual partner(s) of the need for an examination.
- Reinforce the importance of perineal hygiene (as appropriate).

EVALUATION STRATEGIES

- Ask patient to explain the need for routine gynecological examination and Pap test.
- Have patient describe ways to prevent transmission of STIs.
- Ask patient to describe safe sex practices.

Preparation of the Patient

As a nursing student your responsibility is to assist the patient's primary health care provider with the examination. For a complete examination you need the following special equipment: examination table with stirrups, vaginal speculum of correct size, adjustable light source, sink, clean gloves, plastic or wooden spatula, cervical brush or broom device, glass slides and cytologic fixative, culture plates or media, and deoxyribonucleic acid (DNA) probe kits for chlamydia and gonorrhea (Seidel et al., 2011).

Make sure that equipment is ready before the examination begins. Ask the patient to empty her bladder; often it is necessary to collect a urine specimen. For an external genitalia assessment, help the patient to the lithotomy position in bed or on an examination table. On the table place and stabilize her feet into stirrups for a speculum examination and have her slide the buttocks down to the edge of the table. Place a hand at the edge of the table and instruct the patient to move until touching the hand. Her arms should be at her sides or folded across the chest to prevent tightening of abdominal muscles.

Provide a drape or sheet for the patient. A good method is to cover the knees and symphysis, depressing the drape between her knees (Seidel et al., 2011). After the examination begins, lift the drape over the perineum. The male examiner always needs to have a female in attendance during the examination. A female examiner may prefer to work alone but should have a female attendant if the patient is particularly anxious, is emotionally unsteady, or has requested one.

External Genitalia

Make sure that the perineal area is well illuminated. Apply clean gloves on both hands. The perineum is extremely sensitive and tender; do not touch the area suddenly without warning the patient. It is best to touch the neighboring thigh first before advancing to the perineum.

While sitting at the end of the examination table or bed, inspect the quantity and distribution of hair growth. Preadolescents have no pubic hair. During adolescence hair grows along the labia, becoming darker, coarser, and curlier. In an adult hair grows in a triangle over the female perineum and along the medial surface of the thighs. Normally it is free of nits and lice.

Inspect surface characteristics of the labia majora. The skin of the perineum is smooth, clean, and slightly darker than other skin. The mucous membranes appear dark pink and moist. The labia majora are gaping or closed and appear dry or moist. They are usually symmetrical. After childbirth the labia majora separate, causing the labia minora to become more prominent. When a woman reaches menopause, the labia majora become thinned. With advancing age they become atrophied (decrease in size). The labia majora are normally without inflammation, edema, lesions, or lacerations.

To inspect the remaining external structures, use your nondominant hand and gently place the thumb and index finger inside the labia minora and retract the tissues outward (Figure 16-45). Be sure to have a firm hold to avoid repeated retraction against the sensitive tissues. Use the other hand to palpate the labia minora between the thumb and second finger. On inspection the labia minora are normally thinner than the labia majora, and one side is sometimes larger. The

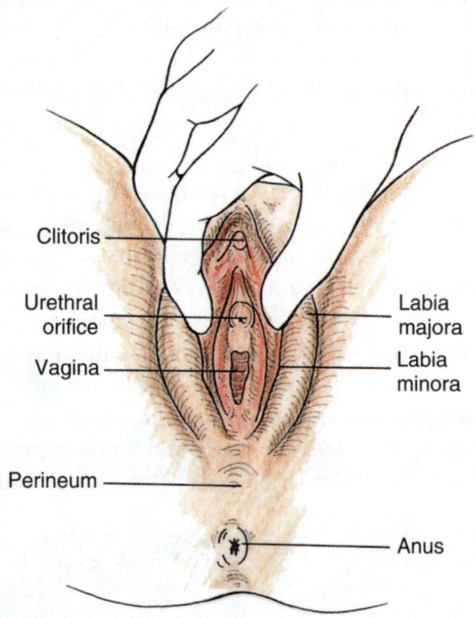

FIGURE 16-45 Female external genitalia.

tissue feels soft on palpation and without tenderness. The size of the clitoris varies, but it normally does not exceed 2 cm (¾ inch) in length and 0.5 cm (¼ inch) in diameter. Look for atrophy, inflammation, or adhesions. If inflamed the clitoris is a bright cherry red. In young women it is a common site for syphilitic lesions or chancres, which appear as small open ulcers that drain serous material. Some older women have malignant changes that result in dry, scaly, nodular lesions.

Inspect the urethral orifice carefully for color and position. Normally it is intact and without inflammation. The urethral meatus is anterior to the vaginal orifice and pink. It appears as a small slit or pinhole opening just above the vaginal canal. Note any discharge, polyps, or fistulas.

Inspect the vaginal orifice (introitus) for inflammation, edema, discoloration, discharge, and lesions. Normally the introitus is a thin vertical slit or large orifice. The tissue is moist. While inspecting the vaginal orifice or introitus, notice the condition of the hymen, which is just inside the introitus. In the virgin female the hymen restricts the opening of the vagina. Only remnants of the hymen remain after sexual intercourse.

Inspect the anus looking for lesions and hemorrhoids (see rectal examination). After completion of the external examination, dispose of examination gloves, offer the patient perineal hygiene, and perform hand hygiene.

Patients who are at risk for contracting STIs need to learn to perform a genital self-examination (see Box 16-20). The purpose of the examination is to detect signs or symptoms of STIs. Many people do not know that they have an STI (e.g., chlamydial infection), and some STIs (e.g., syphilis) can remain undetected for years. Therefore it is essential to stress the importance of regular screening for STIs in sexually active individuals.

Speculum Examination of Internal Genitalia

An examination of internal genitalia requires much skill and practice. Advanced practice nurses and primary care providers perform this examination. Beginning students more than likely only observe the procedure or assist the examiner by helping the patient with positioning, handing off specimen supplies, and comforting the patient.

The examination involves use of a plastic or metal speculum consisting of two blades and an adjustable thumbscrew. The examiner inserts the speculum into the vagina to assess the vaginal walls and cervix for cancerous lesions and other abnormalities. During the examination the examiner collects a Papanicolaou (Pap) test to test for cervical and vaginal cancer.

MALE GENITALIA

An examination of the male genitalia assesses the integrity of the external genitalia, inguinal ring, and canal. Because the incidence of STIs in adolescents and young adults is high, an assessment of the genitalia needs to be a routine part of any health maintenance examination for this age-group. Use a calm, gentle approach to lessen the patient's anxiety. Offer the patient the option of having a companion or parent available during the examination. Have him void and then lie supine with the chest, abdomen, and lower legs draped or stand during the examination. Apply clean gloves.

Nursing History

Begin by explaining the purpose of the genital examination. Especially for adolescents, discuss the components of the male examination. Review the patient's normal urinary elimination pattern, including frequency of voiding; history of nocturia; character and volume of urine; daily fluid intake; and symptoms of burning, urgency and frequency, difficulty starting stream, and hematuria. The history also includes a review of previous surgery or illness involving urinary or reproductive organs, including STIs. The patient's sexual history and use of safe sex habits identifies any risks for HIV infection or other STIs. Patients at risk require extensive education. Ask if the patient has difficulty achieving erection or ejaculation and review medications that influence sexual performance, including diuretics, sedatives, antihypertensives, and tranquilizers. Ask if the patient has noted penile pain or swelling, genital lesions, or urethral discharge, which indicate signs and symptoms of STIs. The patient's knowledge of testicular self-examination provides a guide for health teaching (Box 16-21). Determine if the patient has noticed heaviness or painless enlargement of a testis or irregular lumps (warning signs of testicular cancer). If he reports an enlargement in the inguinal area, assess if it is intermittent or constant; associated with straining or lifting; or painful; and whether coughing, lifting, or straining at stool increases the pain. These are all signs and symptoms that indicate an inguinal hernia.

BOX 16-21 PATIENT TEACHING

Male Genitalia Assessment

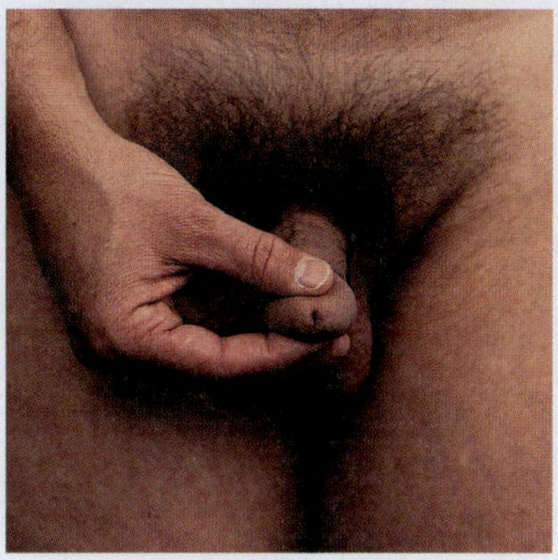

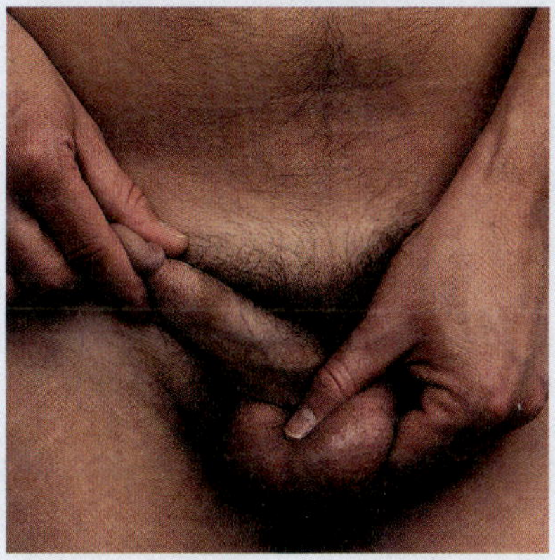

OUTCOME

Patient follows routine preventive and safety measures for genital and testicular health.

TEACHING STRATEGIES

- **Provide the following information about genital self-examination to all male patients 15 years and older:**
  - Perform the examination monthly after a warm bath or shower when the scrotal sac is relaxed and less thick.
  - Stand naked in front of a mirror, hold the penis in your hand, and examine the head. Pull back the foreskin if uncircumcised to expose the glans.
  - Inspect and palpate the entire head of the penis in a clockwise motion, looking carefully for any bumps, sores, blisters, or unusual discharge. Blisters and bumps may be light colored or red and resemble pimples.
  - Look for genital warts.
  - Look at the opening (urethral meatus) at the end of the penis for discharge.
  - Look along the entire shaft of the penis for the same signs.
  - Be sure to separate pubic hair at the base of the penis and carefully examine the skin underneath.
- **Provide the following information about testicular self-examination (TSE) to all men 15 years and older:**
  - Look for swelling or lumps in the skin of the scrotum while looking in the mirror.
  - Use both hands, placing the index and middle fingers under the testicles and the thumb on top (see illustration).
  - Gently roll the testicle, feeling for lumps, swelling, soreness, or change in consistency (hardening).
  - Find the epididymis (a cordlike structure on the top and back of the testicle; it is not a lump).
  - Feel for small, pea-size lumps on the front and side of the testicle. The lumps are usually painless and are abnormal.
  - Call your health care provider about abnormal findings.
- Counsel patients with sexually transmitted infections (STIs) about diagnosis and treatment.
  - Explain warning signs of STIs: Pain on urination and during sex, abnormal penile discharge (different from usual), swollen lymph nodes, or rash or ulcer on skin or genitalia.
  - Teach measures to prevent STIs: Use of condoms, avoiding sex with infected partners, restricting number of sexual partners, avoiding sex with people who have multiple partners, using regular perineal hygiene.
- Tell patients with an STI to inform sexual partner(s) of the need to have an examination.
- Instruct patient to seek treatment as soon as possible if partner becomes infected with an STI.

EVALUATION STRATEGIES

- Observe patient demonstrate genital self-examination and testicular self-examination.
- Ask patient to describe methods for preventing and treating STIs.

Illustrations from Seidel HM, et al: *Mosby's guide to physical examination,* ed 7, St Louis, 2011, Mosby.

Sexual Maturity

First note the sexual maturity of the patient by observing the size and shape of the penis and testes; the size, color, and texture of scrotal skin; and the character and distribution of pubic hair. The testes first increase in size in preadolescence. By the end of puberty the testes and penis enlarge to adult size and shape, and scrotal skin darkens and becomes wrinkled. With puberty hair growth occurs and is coarse and abundant in the pubic area. The penis has no hair, and the scrotum has very little hair. Also inspect the skin covering the genitalia for lice, rashes, excoriations, or lesions. Normally the skin is clear, without lesions.

Penis

To inspect penile surfaces thoroughly, manipulate the genitalia or have the patient help. Inspect the corona, prepuce (foreskin), glans, urethral meatus, and shaft (Figure 16-46). In uncircumcised males retract the foreskin to reveal the glans and urethral meatus. The foreskin usually retracts easily. A small amount of white, thick smegma sometimes collects

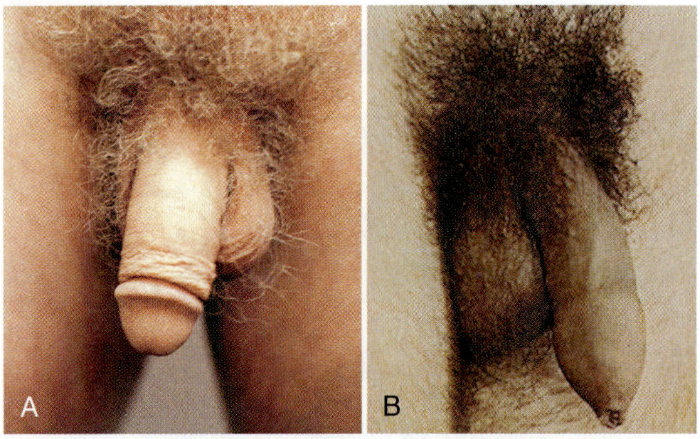

FIGURE 16-46 Normal male genitalia. **A,** Circumcised. **B,** Uncircumcised. (From Seidel HM, et al: *Mosby's guide to physical examination,* ed 7, St Louis, 2011, Mosby.)

under this foreskin. In the circumcised male the glans is exposed. It should look smooth and pink along all surfaces. The urethral meatus is slitlike and normally positioned at the tip of the glans. In some congenital conditions the meatus is displaced along the penile shaft. The area between the foreskin and glans is a common site for venereal lesions.

Gently compress the glans between your thumb and index finger; this opens the urethral meatus for inspection of discharge, lesions, and edema. Normally the opening is glistening and pink without discharge. Palpate any lesion gently to note tenderness, size, consistency, and shape. When inspection and palpation of the glans are complete, pull the foreskin down to its original position. Continue by inspecting the entire shaft of the penis, including the undersurface, looking for any lesions, scars, or edema. Palpate the shaft between the thumb and first two fingers to detect localized areas of hardness or tenderness. A patient who has lain in bed for a prolonged time may develop dependent edema in the penile shaft.

It is important for all male patients to learn to perform a genital self-examination to detect signs and symptoms of STIs. Many people who have an STI do not know it. Self-examination is a routine part of self-care (see Box 16-21).

Scrotum

Be especially cautious while inspecting and palpating the scrotum because the structures that lie within the scrotal sac are very sensitive. The scrotum is divided internally into two halves. Each half contains a testicle, epididymis, and the vas deferens, which travels upward into the inguinal ring. Normally the left testicle is lower than the right. Inspect the size, color, shape, and symmetry of the scrotum while observing for lesions or edema.

Gently lift the scrotum to view the posterior surface. The scrotal skin is usually loose, and the surface is coarse. The skin color is often more deeply pigmented than body skin. Tightening or loss of wrinkling reveals edema. The size of the scrotum normally changes with temperature variations, contracting in cold and relaxing in warm temperature. Lumps in the scrotal skin are commonly sebaceous cysts.

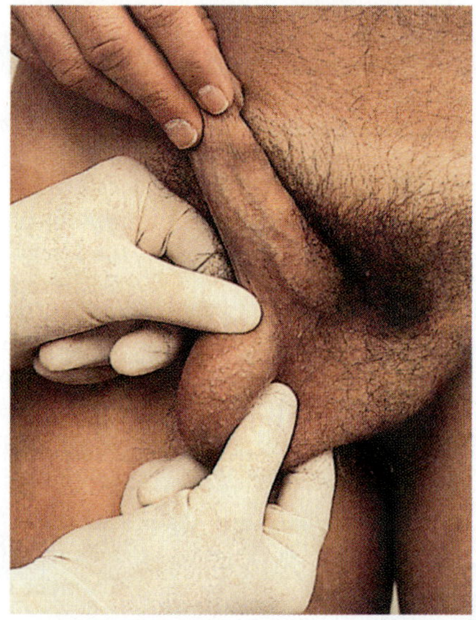

FIGURE 16-47 Palpating contents of scrotal sac. (From Seidel HM, et al: *Mosby's guide to physical examination,* ed 7, St Louis, 2011, Mosby.)

Testicular cancer is a solid tumor commonly found in young men ages 18 to 34 years. Early detection is critical. Explain testicular self-examination while examining the patient. The testes are normally sensitive but not tender. The underlying testicles are normally ovoid and approximately 2 by 4 cm ($\frac{3}{4}$ by $1\frac{5}{8}$ inches) in size. While the patient retracts the penis upward, gently palpate the testes and epididymis between the thumb and first two fingers (Figure 16-47). Note the size, shape, and consistency of tissue and ask if the patient feels any tenderness. The testes feel smooth and rubbery and are free from nodules. The epididymis is resilient. In the older adult the testicles decrease in size and are less firm during palpation. The most common symptoms of testicular cancer are a painless enlargement of one testis and appearance of a palpable small, hard lump about the size of a pea on the front or side of the testicle. Continue to palpate the vas deferens separately as it forms the spermatic cord toward the inguinal ring, noting nodules or swelling. It normally feels smooth and discrete.

Inguinal Ring and Canal

The external inguinal ring provides the opening for the spermatic cord to pass into the inguinal canal. The canal forms a passage through the abdominal wall, a potential site for hernia formation. A hernia is a protrusion of a portion of intestine through the inguinal wall or canal. Sometimes an intestinal loop enters the scrotum. The patient stands during this portion of the examination.

During inspection ask the patient to strain or bear down. The maneuver helps to make a hernia more visible. Look for obvious bulging in the inguinal area. Complete the examination by palpating for inguinal lymph nodes. Normally small, nontender, mobile horizontal nodes are palpable. Any abnormality indicates local or systemic infection or malignant disease.

RECTUM AND ANUS

A good time to perform the rectal examination is after the genital examination. Usually you do not perform the examination in young children or adolescents. The examination detects colorectal cancer in its early stages. In men the rectal examination also detects prostatic tumors. The rectal examination is uncomfortable; thus explaining all steps helps the patient relax.

Nursing History

The nursing history reviews a patient's risk factors for colorectal cancer, including personal and family history of colorectal cancer, polyps, or inflammatory bowel disease (ACS, 2013c). Determine if the patient has experienced bleeding from the rectum, black or tarry stools (melena), rectal pain, or change in bowel habits, all of which are warning signs of colorectal cancer. Assess dietary habits, including intake of high-fat foods, diet high in processed or red meats, or deficient fiber content, which are linked to colon cancer. Determine whether the patient has undergone screening for colorectal cancer (digital examination, fecal occult blood test, flexible sigmoidoscopy, and colonoscopy). Ask male patients if they have experienced weak or interrupted urine flow, an inability to urinate, or difficulty starting or stopping the urine flow. In addition, ask if they have had polyuria; nocturia; hematuria; dysuria; or continuing pain in the lower back, pelvis, or upper thighs. These all are warning signs of prostate cancer. Also review the patient's use of laxatives, cathartics, codeine, or iron preparations, which can cause elimination problems (Box 16-22).

Inspection

Female patients remain in the dorsal recumbent position following genitalia examination, or they assume a side-lying (Sims') position. The best way to examine men is to have the patient stand and bend over forward with the hips flexed and upper body resting across the examination table. Examine a nonambulatory patient in Sims' position.

Using the nondominant hand gently retract the buttocks to view the perianal and sacrococcygeal areas. Perianal skin is smooth and more pigmented and coarser than skin overlying the buttocks. Inspect anal tissue for skin characteristics, lesions, external hemorrhoids (dilated veins that appear as reddened skin protrusions), ulcers, inflammation, rashes, or excoriation. Anal tissues are moist and hairless, and the anus is held closed by the voluntary external sphincter. Next ask the patient to bear down as though having a bowel movement. Any internal hemorrhoids or fissures appear at this time. Use clock referents (e.g., 12 o'clock or 5 o'clock) to describe the location of findings. There normally is no protrusion of tissue.

Digital Palpation

Examine the anal canal and sphincters with digital palpation. In male patients palpate the prostate gland to rule out enlargement. Usually advanced practitioners perform this part of the examination.

BOX 16-22 PATIENT TEACHING

Rectal and Anal Assessment

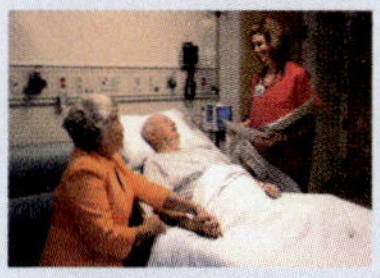

OUTCOME

Mr. Neal follows recommended guidelines for early detection of colorectal cancer and prostate screenings.

TEACHING STRATEGIES

- Discuss the American Cancer Society (ACS) guidelines (ACS, 2013f) for early detection of colorectal cancer. Beginning at age 50 both men and women at average risk should use one of these screening tests:
  - Fecal occult blood test (FOBT) or fecal immunochemical test (FIT) annually.
  - Flexible sigmoidoscopy (FSIG): Visual inspection of the rectum and lower colon with a hollow, lighted tube performed by a health care provider every 5 years.
  - Annual FOBT and FSIG every 5 years (preferred).
  - Double-contrast barium enema every 5 years if recommended by health care provider.
  - Colonoscopy every 10 years if recommended.
  - Computed tomography (CT) colonoscopy every 5 years if recommended.
- Individuals at increased risk need to discuss options with their health care provider.
- Discuss warning signs of colorectal cancer.
- Discuss dietary planning and healthy lifestyle choices to maintain or improve colon health.
- Warn patients about problems caused by overuse of laxatives, cathartic medications, codeine, or enemas.
- Discuss with male patients the ACS guidelines (ACS, 2013f) for early detection of prostatic cancer:
  - The ACS does not support routine testing at this time.
  - Health care professionals should discuss potential benefits and limitations of prostate cancer early-detection testing with men before any testing begins. This discussion should include an offer for testing with the prostate specific antigen (PSA) blood test and digital rectal examination annually beginning at age 50.
  - This discussion should start at age 45 for men at high risk, including African-American men and men who have a first-degree relative diagnosed with prostate cancer at an early age (before 65).
- Discuss with male patients the warning signs of prostate cancer.

EVALUATION STRATEGIES

- During future visits ask if Mr. Neal has had a rectal examination performed.
- Have Mr. Neal explain the warning signs of colorectal and prostate cancer.
- Ask Mr. Neal to describe lifestyle and food choices that maintain colon health.

MUSCULOSKELETAL SYSTEM

The assessment of the musculoskeletal system focuses on determining ROM, muscle strength and tone, and joint and muscle condition. The examination is conducted as a separate examination as for a sports physical or integrated into other parts of the total physical examination. Assess this system while performing other nursing care measures such as bathing or positioning. Muscular disorders often result from neurological disease. For this reason health care providers often conduct a neurological assessment simultaneously.

While examining the patient's musculoskeletal function, visualize the anatomy of bone and muscle placement and joint structure (see Chapter 36). Joints vary in their degree of mobility. Some, as in the knee, are freely movable. The spinal vertebrae are examples of slightly movable joints. For a complete examination you uncover the limb or area being examined so the muscles and joints are free to move. Have the patient sit, lie supine or prone, or stand while assessing muscle groups.

Nursing History

Determine the patient's history of musculoskeletal injury or trauma that resulted from sports, employment, exercise, or chronic illnesses. Assess for osteoporosis risk factors, including the following: use of alcohol/caffeine; cigarette smoking; constant dieting; calcium intake less than 500 mg daily; thin and light body frame; nulliparous status; menopause before age 45; estrogen deficiency; postmenopause status; family history of osteoporosis; Caucasian, Asian, Native American, or Northern European ancestry; advanced age; history of fractures/falls; sedentary lifestyle; chronic diseases (e.g., Cushing's disease, hyperthyroidism and hypothyroidism, malabsorption/malnutrition disorders, and neoplasms); long-term use of corticosteroids, methotrexate, phenytoin, and aluminum-containing antacids; lack of exposure to sunlight.

The nursing history includes a patient's description of problems with bone, muscle, or joint function, including history of recent falls, trauma, lifting heavy objects, fractures, and bone or joint disease. It is useful to assess a patient's normal activity pattern, including the type of exercise routinely performed (Box 16-23). Also assess the nature and extent of pain or stiffness and determine if alterations affect the patient's ability to perform ADLs and participate in social activities.

General Inspection

Observe the patient's gait and posture when entering the examination room. When a patient is unaware that he or she is being observed, gait is more natural. Later a more formal test has the patient walk in a straight line away, turn, and return to the origin point. Note how the patient walks, sits, and rises from a sitting position. Normally patients walk with arms swinging freely at the sides and the head leading the body. Older adults walk with smaller steps and a wider base of support. Note foot dragging, limping, shuffling, and the position of the trunk in relation to the legs. Be sure to compare extremities bilaterally. Patients in wheelchairs or who use walking assistance are assessed for smooth movements and stability.

Observe the patient from the side in a standing position. The normal standing posture is an upright stance with parallel alignment of the hips and shoulders (Figure 16-48). There should be an even contour of the shoulders, level scapulae and iliac crests, alignment of the head over the gluteal folds, and symmetry of extremities. With the patient standing sideways note the normal cervical, thoracic, and lumbar curves. Holding the head erect is normal. As the patient sits, some degree of rounding of the shoulders is normal. Older adults tend to assume a stooped, forward-bent posture, with hips and knees somewhat flexed and arms bent at the elbows, raising the level of the arms.

BOX 16-23 PATIENT TEACHING

Musculoskeletal Assessment

OUTCOME

Patient follows measures to prevent or minimize osteoporosis.

TEACHING STRATEGIES

- Instruct patient in correct postural alignment. Consult with a physical therapist to provide patient with exercises for improving posture.
- For women age 65 and older recommend routine screening for osteoporosis (Prihar and Katz, 2008). Recommend men for screening as well; they are equally at risk for development of osteoporosis as they age.
- To reduce bone demineralization instruct older adults in a proper exercise program (e.g., weight-bearing, muscle-strengthening exercise) to be followed 3 or more times a week.
- Encourage intake of calcium and vitamin D to meet the recommended daily allowance. Increased vitamin D aids calcium absorption.
- Recommendation for calcium supplements for adults over age 25 is 1000 to 1500 mg/day. For vitamin D supplements, instruct patients to take no more than 500 mg of calcium at one time.
- Explain to patients with low back pain that they will benefit from modification of worker risk factors (e.g., lifting heavy weights, use of protective equipment), regular aerobic exercise, exercises that strengthen the back and increase trunk flexibility, and learning how to lift properly.
- Instruct patient in use of assistive devices (e.g., zippers on clothing instead of buttons, elevation of chairs to minimize bending of knees and hips) when patient is unable to perform activities of daily living.
- Instruct older adults and those with osteoporosis in proper body mechanics and range-of-motion and moderate weight-bearing exercises (e.g., swimming, walking) to minimize trauma and subsequent bone fractures.
- Instruct older patients to pace activities to compensate for loss in muscle strength.

EVALUATION STRATEGIES

- Observe patient's posture for shortening or increase in curvature.
- Have patient describe methods to prevent osteoporosis.
- Observe patient perform range-of-motion exercises.
- Have patient or family member describe use of self-care aids.

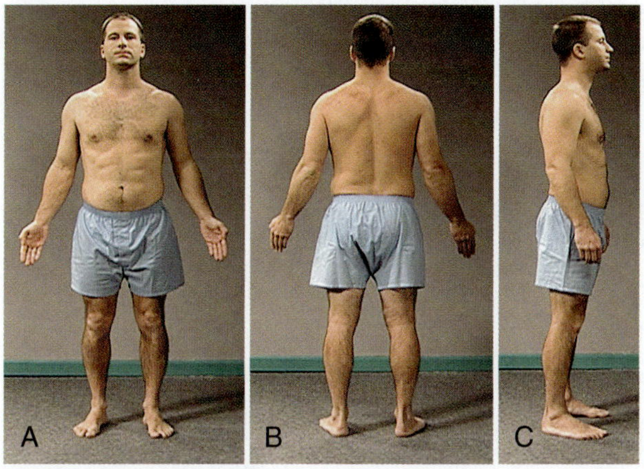

FIGURE 16-48 Inspection of overall body posture. **A,** Anterior view. **B,** Posterior view. **C,** Lateral view. (From Seidel HM, et al: *Mosby's guide to physical examination,* ed 7, St Louis, 2011, Mosby.)

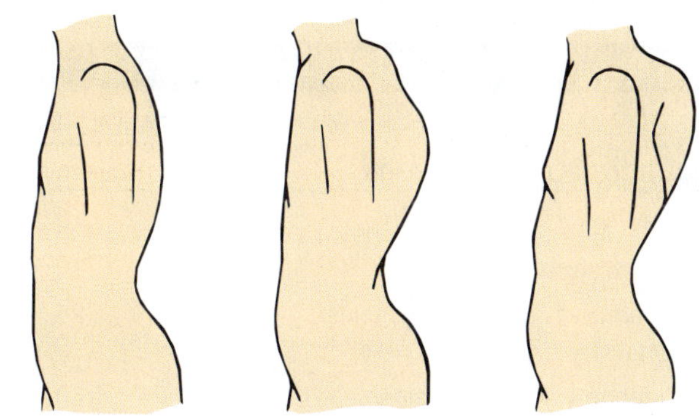

FIGURE 16-49 Common postural abnormalities. **A,** Lordosis. **B,** Kyphosis. **C,** Scoliosis.

Common postural abnormalities include, lordosis, kyphosis, and scoliosis (Figure 16-49). Lordosis, or swayback, is an increased lumbar curvature. Kyphosis, or hunchback, is an exaggeration of the posterior curvature of the thoracic spine. This postural abnormality is common in the older adult. A lateral spinal curvature is called *scoliosis.* Loss of height is frequently the first clinical sign of osteoporosis, in which height loss occurs in the trunk as a result of vertebral fracture and collapse. Osteoporosis is a metabolic bone disease that causes a decrease in quality and quantity of bone. It affects 10 million Americans, and another 34 million are diagnosed with osteopenia, the majority of which are women (Silverman, 2008). This disease now affects 1 to 2 million men, and it will affect another 6 million women (Liu et al., 2008). Although a small amount of height loss is expected with aging, if the amount of loss is great, osteoporosis is likely. As men and women age, they are more likely to have osteoporotic fractures of the forearm/wrists, hips, and vertebrae.

During general inspection look at the extremities for overall size, gross deformity, bony enlargement, alignment, and symmetry. Normally there is bilateral symmetry in length, circumference, alignment, and position and number of skinfolds (Seidel et al., 2011). A general review pinpoints areas requiring specialized assessment.

Palpation

Apply gentle palpation to all bones, joints, and surrounding muscles during a complete examination. In the case of a focused assessment, examine only the involved area. Note any warmth, tenderness, edema, or resistance to pressure. The patient should feel no discomfort when you apply palpation. Muscles should be firm. When assessing the vertebrae, ask the patient to bend at the waist, arms hanging down. Bimanually palpate either side of the spinal column to note any deviations or curvatures.

Range of Joint Motion

The examination includes comparison of both active and passive full ROM. Ask the patient to put each major joint and its muscle groups through full ROM. Learn the terminology for each joint movement (Table 16-8) and teach the patient how to move through each ROM. To assess passive ROM ask the patient to relax and then passively move the joints through their ROM. Compare the same body parts for equality in movement. Do not force a joint into a painful position. Know the normal range of each joint and the extent to which you can move the patient's joints. Ideally assess the patient's normal range to determine a baseline for assessing later change. Joints are typically free from stiffness, instability, swelling, or inflammation. There normally is no discomfort when applying pressure to bones and joints. In older adults joints often become swollen and stiff, with reduced ROM resulting from cartilage erosion and fibrosis of synovial membranes. If a joint appears swollen and inflamed, palpate it for warmth.

Muscle Tone and Strength

Assess muscle strength and tone during ROM measurement. Note muscle tone (i.e., the slight muscular resistance felt as you move the relaxed extremity passively through its ROM). Ask the patient to allow an extremity to relax or hang limp, sometimes difficult if the patient feels pain in the extremity. Support the extremity and grasp each limb, moving it through the normal ROM. Normal tone causes a mild, even resistance to passive movement through the entire range.

If a muscle has increased tone, or hypertonicity, you meet considerable resistance with sudden passive movement of a joint. Continued movement eventually causes the muscle to relax. A muscle that has little tone (hypotonicity) feels flabby. The involved extremity hangs loosely in a position determined by gravity.

For assessment of muscle strength the patient assumes a stable position. He or she performs maneuvers demonstrating strength of major muscle groups (Table 16-9). Compare symmetrical muscle pairs for strength, based on a grading scale of 0 to 5 (Table 16-10). The arm on the dominant side is normally stronger than the arm on the nondominant side. In the older adult a loss of muscle mass causes bilateral

TABLE 16-8 TERMINOLOGY FOR NORMAL RANGE-OF-MOTION POSITIONS

TERM	RANGE OF MOTION	EXAMPLES OF JOINTS
Flexion	Movement decreasing angle between two adjoining bones; bending of limb	Elbow, fingers, knee
Extension	Movement increasing angle between two adjoining bones	Elbow, fingers, knee
Hyperextension	Movement of body part beyond its normal resting extended position	Head
Pronation	Movement of body part so front or ventral surface faces downward	Hand, forearm
Supination	Movement of body part so front or ventral surface faces upward	Hand, forearm
Abduction	Movement of extremity away from midline of body	Leg, arm, fingers
Adduction	Movement of extremity toward midline of body	Leg, arm, fingers
Internal rotation	Rotation of joint inward	Knee, hip
External rotation	Rotation of joint outward	Knee, hip
Eversion	Turning of body part away from midline	Foot
Inversion	Turning of body part toward midline	Foot
Dorsiflexion	Flexion of toes and foot upward	Foot
Plantar flexion	Bending of toes and foot downward	Foot

TABLE 16-9 MANEUVERS TO ASSESS MUSCLE STRENGTH

MUSCLE GROUP	MANEUVER
Neck (sternocleidomastoid)	Place hand firmly against patient's upper jaw. Ask patient to turn head laterally against resistance.
Shoulder (trapezius)	Place hand over midline of patient's shoulder, exerting firm pressure. Have patient raise shoulders against resistance.
Elbow	
Biceps	Pull down on forearm as patient attempts to flex arm.
Triceps	As you flex patient's arm, apply pressure against forearm. Ask patient to straighten arm.
Hip	
Quadriceps	When patient is sitting, apply downward pressure to thigh. Ask patient to raise leg up from table.
Gastrocnemius	Patient sits while examiner holds shin of flexed leg. Ask patient to straighten leg against resistance.

weakness, but muscle strength remains greater in the dominant arm or leg.

Examine each muscle group. Ask the patient first to flex the muscle to be examined and then to resist when you apply opposing force against that flexion (Figure 16-50). It is important to not allow the patient to move the joint. Gradually increase pressure to a muscle group (e.g., elbow extension). Have the patient resist the pressure applied by attempting to move against resistance (e.g., elbow flexion).

TABLE 16-10 MUSCLE STRENGTH

MUSCLE FUNCTION LEVEL	SCALES: GRADE	SCALES: % NORMAL
No evidence of contractility	0	0
Trace of movement	1	10
Full range of motion, not against gravity*	2	25
Full range of motion against gravity but not against resistance	3	50
Full range of motion against gravity; some resistance but weak	4	75
Full range of motion against gravity; full resistance	5	100

From Seidel HM, et al: *Mosby's guide to physical examination,* ed 7, St Louis, 2011, Mosby.
*Passive movement.

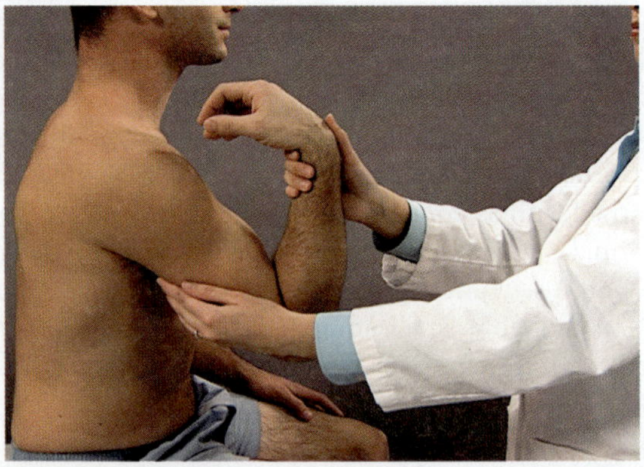

FIGURE 16-50 Assess muscle strength: flexion of elbow against opposing force. (From Seidel HM, et al: *Mosby's guide to physical examination,* ed 7, St Louis, 2011, Mosby.)

The patient resists until instructed to stop. Vary the amount of pressure applied and observe the joint move. If you identify a weakness, compare the size of the muscle with its opposite counterpart by measuring the circumference of the muscle body with a tape measure. A muscle that has atrophied (reduced in size) feels soft and baggy when palpated.

NEUROLOGICAL SYSTEM

An assessment of neurological function alone is quite time consuming. For efficiency integrate neurological measurements with other parts of the physical examination. For example, test cranial nerve function while assessing the head and neck. Observe mental and emotional status during the initial interview.

Consider many variables when deciding the extent of the examination. A patient's level of consciousness influences the ability to follow directions. General physical status influences tolerance to assessment. A patient's description of signs and symptoms helps to determine the need for a thorough neurological assessment. If a patient complains of headache or a recent loss of function in an extremity, he or she needs a complete neurological assessment. For a complete examination you need the following special equipment:

- Reading material
- Vials of aromatic substances (e.g., orange, peppermint extract, and coffee)
- Opposite tip of cotton swab broken in half or paper clip for testing ability to distinguish sharp from dull
- Snellen eye chart
- Penlight
- Vials containing sugar, salt, lemon with applicators
- Tongue blade
- Two test tubes hot and cold water for temperature sensation testing
- Cotton balls or cotton-tipped applicators
- Tuning fork
- Reflex hammer
- Familiar objects such as coins, keys, paperclips

Nursing History

Review the patient's use of analgesics, alcohol, sedative-hypnotics, antipsychotics, antidepressants, nervous system stimulants, or recreational drugs. Determine if he or she has a recent history of seizures/convulsions and screen for symptoms of headache, tremors, dizziness, vertigo, numbness or tingling of body parts, visual changes, weakness, pain, or changes in speech. The presence of any symptom requires a more detailed review (e.g., onset, severity, precipitating factors, or sequence of events). Discuss with the patient's family any recent changes in the patient's behavior (e.g., increased irritability, mood swings, memory loss, or change in energy level). Ask the patient for a history of changes in vision, hearing, smell, taste, and touch. A history of head or spinal cord trauma, meningitis, congenital anomalies, neurological disease, or psychiatric counseling focuses your assessment of select findings. If an older-adult patient displays sudden acute confusion (delirium), review history for drug toxicity, serious infections, metabolic disturbances, heart failure, and severe anemia.

Mental and Emotional Status

You learn about mental capacities and emotional state by interacting with a patient. Ask questions during an examination to gather data and observe the appropriateness of emotions and thoughts. There are special assessment tools designed to assess a patient's mental status. For example, the Mini-Mental State Examination (MMSE) measures patient's orientation and cognitive function. It asks questions such as "What is the date?"

To ensure an objective assessment consider a patient's cultural and educational background, values, beliefs, and previous experiences. An alteration in mental or emotional status reflects a disturbance in cerebral functioning. The cerebral cortex controls and integrates intellectual and emotional functioning. Primary brain disorders, medications, and metabolic changes are examples of factors that change cerebral function.

Level of Consciousness

A person's level of consciousness exists along a continuum from being fully awake, alert, and cooperative to unresponsiveness to any form of external stimuli. Talk with the patient, asking questions about events involving him or her or concerns about health problems. A fully conscious patient responds to questions quickly and expresses ideas logically. As a patient's consciousness lowers, use the Glasgow Coma Scale (GCS) for an objective measurement of consciousness on a numerical scale (Table 16-11). The patient needs to be as alert as possible before testing. Use caution when using the scale if a patient has sensory losses (e.g., vision or hearing). The GCS allows evaluation of a patient's neurological status over time. The higher the score, the better the patient's neurological function. Ask short, simple questions, such as "What

TABLE 16-11 GLASGOW COMA SCALE

ACTION	RESPONSE	SCORE
Eyes open	Spontaneously	4
	To speech	3
	To pain	2
	None	1
Best verbal response	Oriented	5
	Confused	4
	Inappropriate words	3
	Incomprehensible sounds	2
	None	1
Best motor response	Obeys commands	6
	Localized pain	5
	Flexion withdrawal	4
	Abnormal flexion	3
	Abnormal extension	2
	Flaccid	1

Patient's total score ranges from 3 to 15.

is your name?" or "Where are you?" Also ask the patient to follow simple commands, such as "Move your toes."

If a patient is not conscious enough to follow commands, try to elicit a pain response. Apply firm pressure with the thumb over the root of the patient's fingernail. The normal response to painful stimuli is withdrawal of the body part from the stimulus.

Behavior and Appearance

Behaviors, moods, hygiene, grooming, and choice of dress reveal pertinent information about mental status. Assess the patient's mannerisms and actions during the entire physical assessment. Note both nonverbal and verbal behaviors. Does the patient respond appropriately to directions? Does his or her mood vary with no apparent cause? Does he or she show concern about appearance? Is the patient's hair clean and neatly groomed, and are the nails trimmed and clean? The patient should behave in a manner expressing concern and interest in the examination. He or she should make eye contact and express appropriate feelings that correspond to the situation. Normally a patient's appearance shows some degree of personal hygiene.

Choice and fit of clothing reflect socioeconomic background or personal taste rather than deficiency in self-concept or self-care. Avoid being judgmental and focus assessments on the appropriateness of clothing for the weather. Older adults sometimes neglect their appearance because of a lack of energy, financcs, or reduced vision.

Language

Normal cerebral function allows a person to understand spoken or written words and express the self through written words or gestures. Assess the patient's voice inflection, tone, and manner of speech. Normally a patient's voice has inflections, is clear and strong, and increases in volume appropriately. Speech is fluent. When communication is clearly ineffective (e.g., omission or addition of letters and words, misuse of words, or hesitations), assess the patient for aphasia. Injury to the cerebral cortex results in aphasia.

The two types of aphasia are sensory (or receptive) and motor (or expressive). With receptive aphasia a person cannot understand written or verbal speech. With expressive aphasia a person understands written and verbal speech but cannot write or speak appropriately when attempting to communicate. A patient sometimes suffers from a combination of receptive and expressive aphasia. When communication is ineffective, assess language capabilities with simple assessment techniques. Ask the patient to name familiar objects when pointing at them. Ask him or her to respond to simple verbal commands such as "Stand up." Finally ask him or her to read a simple sentence out loud. Normally a patient names objects correctly, follows commands, and reads sentences correctly.

Intellectual Function

Intellectual function includes memory, knowledge, abstract thinking, and judgment. Testing each aspect of function involves a specific technique. However, because cultural and educational background influences the ability to respond to test questions, do not ask questions related to concepts or ideas with which the patient is unfamiliar. Validate information with a family member if appropriate.

Memory. Assess immediate recall and recent and remote memory. Patients demonstrate immediate recall by repeating a series of numbers in the order they are presented or reverse order. Patients normally recall five to eight digits forward or four to six digits backward.

First explain that you will test the patient's memory. Then state clearly and slowly the names of three unrelated objects. After stating all three, ask the patient to repeat each. Continue until the patient is successful. Later in the assessment ask the patient to repeat the three words again. The patient should be able to identify the three words. Another test for recent memory involves asking the patient to recall events occurring during the same day (e.g., what was eaten for breakfast).

To assess past memory ask the patient to recall the maiden name of the patient's mother, a birthday, or a special date in history. Compare the response to recorded data from the health record. It is best to ask open-ended questions rather than simple yes/no questions. A patient usually has immediate recall of such information. With older adults do not interpret a hearing loss as confusion.

Knowledge. Assess knowledge by asking how much the patient knows about his or her illness or the reason for hospitalization. You can also ask questions about basic facts (e.g., who is the president?). By assessing a patient's knowledge you can determine his or her ability to learn or understand. If there is an opportunity to teach, test the patient's mental status by asking for feedback during a follow-up visit.

Abstract Thinking. Interpreting abstract ideas or concepts reflects the capacity for abstract thinking. For an individual to explain common sayings such as "A stitch in time saves nine" or "Don't count your chickens before they're hatched," requires a higher level of intellectual functioning. Note whether the patient's explanations are relevant and concrete. The patient with altered mental state probably interprets the phrase literally or merely rephrases the words.

Judgment. Judgment requires a comparison and evaluation of facts and ideas to understand their relationships and form appropriate conclusions. Attempt to measure the patient's ability to make logical decisions with questions such as "Why did you decide to seek health care?" or "What would you do if you suddenly became ill at home?" Normally a patient makes logical decisions.

Cranial Nerve Function

Although cranial nerve function is not commonly completed as part of the bedside assessment, you may test all 12 cranial nerves or a single nerve or related group of nerves to determine function. A dysfunction in one nerve reflects an alteration at some point along the distribution of the cranial nerve. Measurements used to assess the integrity of organs within the head and neck also assess cranial nerve function. A complete assessment involves testing the 12 cranial nerves in order of their numbers. To remember the order of the nerves, use this simple phrase: "On old Olympus' towering tops a Finn and German viewed some hops." The first letter of each word in the phrase is the same as the first letter of the names of the cranial nerves listed in order (Table 16-12).

Sensory Function

The sensory pathways of the central nervous system conduct the sensations of pain, temperature, position, vibration, and crude and finely localized touch. Different nerve pathways relay the sensations. Most patients require only a quick screening of sensory function unless there are symptoms of reduced sensation, motor impairment, or paralysis.

Normally a patient has sensory responses to all stimuli tested. He or she feels sensations equally on both sides of the body in all areas. Perform all sensory testing with the patient's eyes closed so he or she is unable to see when or where a stimulus strikes the skin (Table 16-13). Then apply stimuli in a random, unpredictable order to maintain the patient's attention and prevent detection of a predictable pattern. Ask the patient to describe when, what, and where each stimulus is felt. Compare symmetrical areas of the body while applying stimuli to the arms, trunk, and legs.

Motor Function

An assessment of motor function includes measurements made during the musculoskeletal examination. In addition, you assess cerebellar function. The cerebellum coordinates

TABLE 16-12 CRANIAL NERVE FUNCTION AND ASSESSMENT

CRANIAL NERVE	NAME	TYPE	FUNCTION	ASSESSMENT METHOD
I	Olfactory	Sensory	Sense of smell	Ask patient to identify different aromas in each nostril such as coffee and vanilla.
II	Optic	Sensory	Visual acuity and visual fields	Use Snellen chart or ask patient to read printed material while wearing glasses.
III	Oculomotor	Motor	Pupil constriction and dilation	Assess directions of gaze.
			Extraocular eye movement	Measure pupil reaction to light reflex and accommodation.
IV	Trochlear	Motor	Upward and downward movement of eyeball	Assess directions of gaze.
V	Trigeminal	Sensory and motor	Sensory nerve to skin of face	Lightly touch cornea with wisp of cotton. Assess corneal reflex. Measure sensation of light pain and touch across skin of face.
			Motor nerve to muscles of jaw	Palpate temples as patient clenches teeth; observe chewing.
VI	Abducens	Motor	Lateral movement of eyeballs	Assess directions of gaze.
VII	Facial	Motor and sensory	Facial expression	Look for asymmetry as patient smiles, frowns, puffs out cheeks, and raises and lowers eyebrows.
			Taste	Have patient identify salty or sweet taste on front of tongue.
VIII	Auditory	Sensory	Hearing and equilibrium	Assess ability to hear spoken word.
IX	Glossopharyngeal	Sensory and motor	Taste	Ask patient to identify sour or sweet taste on back of tongue.
			Ability to swallow and speak	Use tongue blade to elicit gag reflex; have person swallow.
X	Vagus	Sensory and motor	Sensation of pharynx and behind ear	Ask patient to say "Ah." Observe movement of palate and pharynx.
			Movement of vocal cords	Assess speech for hoarseness.
XI	Spinal accessory	Motor	Movement of head and shoulders	Ask patient to shrug shoulders and turn head against passive resistance.
XII	Hypoglossal	Motor	Position of tongue	Ask patient to stick out tongue to midline and move it from side to side.

muscular activity, maintains balance and equilibrium, and helps to control posture. Patients with any degree of motor dysfunction are at risk for injury (Box 16-24).

Coordination. To avoid confusion, demonstrate each maneuver and have the patient repeat it while you observe for smoothness and balance in the patient's movement. In older adults normally slow reaction time causes movements to be less rhythmical.

To assess fine-motor function, have the patient extend the arms out to the sides and touch each forefinger alternately to the nose, first with eyes open, then with eyes closed (Figure 16-51). Performing rapid, rhythmical, alternating movements demonstrates coordination in the upper extremities. While sitting, the patient begins by patting the knees with both hands. Then he or she alternately turns up the palm and back of the hands while continuously patting the knees

TABLE 16-13 ASSESSMENT OF SENSORY NERVE FUNCTION

FUNCTION	EQUIPMENT	METHOD	PRECAUTIONS
Pain	End of paper clip or wooden end of cotton applicator	Ask patient to voice when he or she feels dull or sharp sensation. Alternately apply sharp and blunt ends of paper clip or broken cotton swab to surface of skin. Note areas of numbness or increased sensitivity.	Remember that areas where skin is thickened such as heel or sole of foot are less sensitive to pain.
Temperature	Two test tubes, one filled with hot water, one with cold	Touch skin with tube. Ask patient to identify hot or cold sensation.	Omit test if pain sensation is normal.
Light touch	Cotton ball or cotton-tipped applicator	Apply light wisp of cotton to different points along surface of skin. Ask patient to voice when he or she feels sensation.	Apply at areas where skin is thin or more sensitive (e.g., face, neck, inner aspect of arms, top of feet and hands).
Vibration	Tuning fork	Apply stem of vibrating fork to distal interphalangeal joint of fingers and interphalangeal joint of great toe, elbow, and wrist. Have patient voice when and where he or she feels vibration.	Be sure that patient feels vibration and not merely pressure.
Position		Grasp finger or toe, holding it by its sides with thumb and index finger. Alternate moving finger or toe up and down. Ask patient to state when finger is up or down. Repeat with toes.	Avoid rubbing adjacent appendages as you move finger or toe. Do not move joint laterally; return to neutral position before moving again.
Two-point discrimination	Two ends of paper clip	Lightly apply one or both ends of paper clip or broken cotton swab simultaneously to surface of skin. Ask patient whether he or she feels one or two pricks. Find the distance at which patient can no longer distinguish two points.	Apply paper clip tips to same anatomical site (e.g., fingertips, palm of hand, upper arms). Minimum distance at which patient discriminates two points varies (2 to 8 mm on fingertips).

BOX 16-24 PATIENT TEACHING

Neurological Assessment

OUTCOME

Patient makes good decisions and follows safety measures to maintain neurological function: cognition, reflexes, sensation, or motor function.

TEACHING STRATEGIES

- Teach patient to seek emergency care to rule out stroke with any of these symptoms: any sudden visual changes; sudden confusion; change in speech; weakness, sudden numbness, tingling, or loss of movement, especially on one side of the body.
- Teach patient to immediately seek emergency treatment for a sudden, severe headache that is different from past headaches.
- Explain to family or friends the implications of any behavioral or mental impairment shown by the patient.
- If patient has sensory or motor impairments, explain measures to ensure safety (e.g., use of ambulation aids, use of safety bars in bathrooms or on stairways).
- Teach older adults to plan enough time to complete tasks because their reaction time is slow.

EVALUATION STRATEGIES

- Ask family to discuss patient behaviors that result from neurological impairments.
- Have patient explain safety measures used to prevent injury from sensory or motor limitations.

(Figure 16-52). Test low-extremity coordination with the patient lying supine, legs extended. Place your hand at the ball of the patient's foot. The patient taps the hand with the foot as quickly as possible, alternating feet. The feet do not normally move as rapidly or evenly as the hands.

Balance. Assess balance and gross-motor function by asking the patient to stand with feet together, arms at the sides, both with eyes open and closed. Protect the patient's safety by standing at the side and observe for swaying. Expect slight swaying of the body in the Romberg's test. A loss of balance (positive Romberg) causes a patient to fall to the side.

Reflexes. Eliciting reflexes demonstrates integrity of sensory and motor pathways. Deep tendon reflexes are elicited by mildly stretching a muscle and tapping a tendon and cutaneous reflexes are elicited by stimulating the skin superficially.

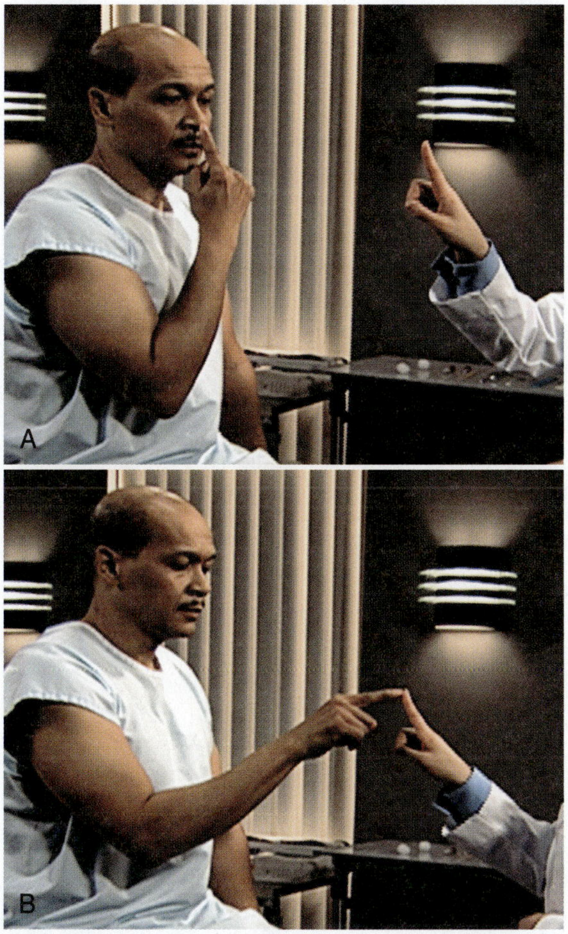

FIGURE 16-51 Examination of fine motor function. (From Seidel HM, et al: *Mosby's guide to physical examination*, ed 7, St Louis, 2011, Mosby.)

AFTER THE EXAMINATION

Record findings from the physical assessment during the examination or at the end. Specific forms are available to record data. Review all findings before helping the patient dress in case of a need to recheck any information or gather additional data. Integrate physical assessment findings into the plan of care.

After completing the assessment, give the patient time to dress. A hospitalized patient often needs help with hygiene and returning to bed. When the patient is comfortable, share a summary of the assessment findings. If the findings show serious abnormalities such as an irregular heart rate, consult the patient's health care provider before revealing any findings. It is the health care provider's responsibility to make definitive medical diagnoses. Explain the type of abnormality found and the need for the health care provider to conduct an additional examination.

The examination space needs to be cleaned when you are finished. Use infection control practices to remove materials or instruments soiled with potentially infectious wastes. If the patient's bedside was the site for the examination, clear away soiled items from the bedside table and make sure the bed linen is dry and clean. The patient will appreciate a clean gown and the opportunity to wash the face and hands. Afterward be sure to perform hand hygiene.

If necessary arrange for further ancillary examinations such as x-ray film examinations, laboratory tests, or ultrasonography after a physical examination. The tests provide additional screening information to rule out and help diagnose specific abnormalities found during the examination. Explain the purpose of these tests and the sensations that the patient will experience.

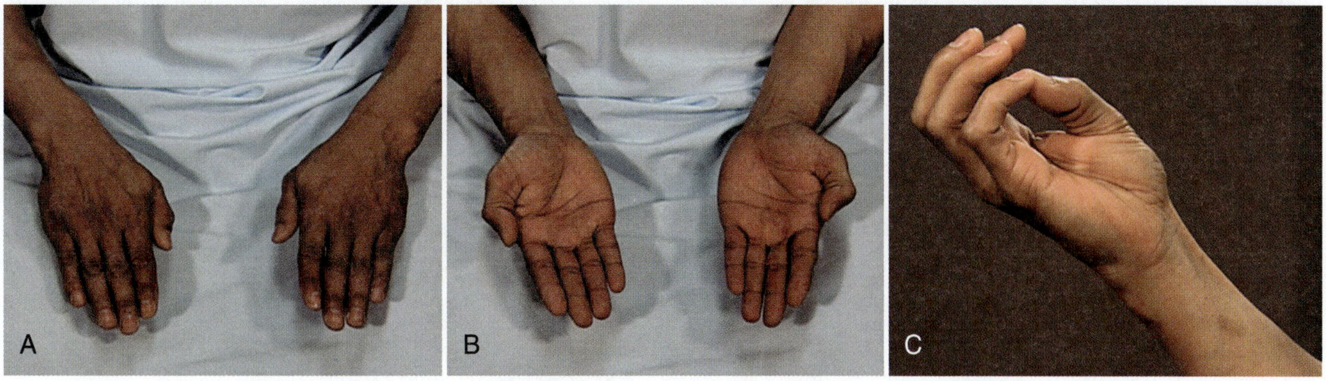

FIGURE 16-52 Examination of coordination with rapid alternating movements. **A** and **B,** Alternatively pat knees with back and then palm of both hands. **C,** Touch thumb to each finger in sequence, increasing in speed. (From Seidel HM, et al: *Mosby's guide to physical examination*, ed 7, St Louis, 2011, Mosby.)

KEY POINTS

- Baseline assessment findings reflect a patient's functional abilities and serve as the basis for comparison with subsequent assessment findings.
- Physical assessment of a child or infant requires the application of the principles of growth and development.
- Recognize that the normal process of aging affects physical findings collected from an older adult.
- Be alert for any signs or indicators of intimate partner violence or elderly abuse.
- If you suspect substance abuse, conduct a Quick Screen to determine the patient's need for further intervention.
- Integrate patient teaching throughout the examination to help patients learn about health promotion and disease prevention.
- Inspection requires good lighting, full exposure of the body part, and a careful comparison of the part with its counterpart on the opposite side of the body.
- Palpation involves the use of parts of the hand to detect different types of physical characteristics.
- Use auscultation to assess the character of sounds created in various body organs.
- Perform a physical examination only after properly preparing the environment and equipment and preparing the patient physically and psychologically.
- Throughout the examination keep the patient warm, comfortable, and informed of each step of the assessment process. Ensure confidentiality and maintain privacy of the patient.
- A competent examiner learns to be systematic while combining assessments of different body systems simultaneously.
- Information from the history helps to focus on body systems likely to be affected.
- Creating a mental image of internal organs in relation to external anatomical landmarks enhances accuracy in assessing the thorax, heart, and abdomen.
- When assessing heart sounds, imagine events occurring during the cardiac cycle.
- Never palpate the carotid arteries simultaneously.
- When examining a woman's breasts, explain the techniques for BSE.
- The abdominal assessment differs from other parts of the examination in that auscultation follows inspection.
- During assessment of the genitalia explain the technique for genital self-examination.
- Conduct an assessment of musculoskeletal function when observing the patient ambulate or participate in other active movements.
- Assess mental and emotional status by interacting with the patient throughout the examination.
- At the end of the examination provide for the patient's comfort and document a detailed summary of physical assessment findings.

CLINICAL DECISION-MAKING EXERCISES

Jane continues to care for Mr. Neal. He had a colon resection for cancer 2 days ago. The morning shift has just started, and on walking rounds the nurse reports that he slept well and denied any problems. His pain is being managed with an intravenous (IV) pump. Mr. Neal is allowed nothing by mouth (NPO) and has an IV line for parenteral fluids, a nasogastric (NG) tube connected to low intermittent suction, and an abdominal dressing.

1. a. To what general survey information does Jane pay particular attention as she greets Mr. Neal in the morning?
   b. Which assessments should be done while Mr. Neal is supine? Sitting on the side of the bed?
2. On auscultation of the lateral and posterior lung fields, Jane hears a crackling noise on inspiration. What is this sound and what does it indicate? Jane instructs Mr. Neal to cough, but on reauscultation the sounds do not disappear. Respiratory rate is 20 and unlabored. What should Jane do next?
3. Jane next assesses Mr. Neal's cardiac status. His apical heart rate is 84 beats/min, rhythm regular. Based on this finding, what skin color should Jane expect to find when inspecting fingertips and mucous membranes?

evolve

Answers to Clinical Decision-Making Exercises can be found on the Evolve website.

QSEN ACTIVITY: PATIENT-CENTERED CARE

After surgery the surgeon informs Mr. Neal of the diagnosis of bowel cancer. As she plans discharge teaching, Jane considers Mr. Neal's habits and current health practices that are high risk not only for bowel cancer but also for lung and heart disease. Mrs. Neal stated that she was primarily responsible for menu planning and food preparation. Jane considers which information to emphasize, while recognizing the importance of teaching both the patient and his wife.

Which patient-centered approach should Jane use when selecting teaching materials? Give examples of effective questions that can be used to learn more about the Neals' current knowledge and preferences. Identify which level of evidence provides the strongest background information and teaching resources on which to base teaching plans.

evolve

Answers to QSEN Activities can be found on the Evolve website.

REVIEW QUESTIONS

1. At the urgent care clinic the nurse observes a patient walk to the treatment room, turn, and step up to sit on the examination table. This is a way to obtain data related to which areas of the general survey? (Select all that apply.)
   1. Body type
   2. Hygiene and grooming
   3. Signs of physical distress
   4. Body movements and gait
   5. Drug or substance abuse
2. A patient with a diagnosis of diabetes mellitus is admitted to the hospital for an infected toe. The nurse detects unpleasant, musky odors during the general assessment. Which technique of assessment is being used?
   1. Auscultation
   2. Inspection
   3. Olfaction
   4. Palpation
3. How should a nurse apply Standard Precautions when assessing a patient's hair after noting an open, draining wound at the hair line near the right temple?
   1. Apply gloves before handling the hair
   2. Ask the patient to wash the hair before continuing the examination
   3. Have the patient part and move the hair when instructed to do so
   4. Comb the patient's hair with a fine-tooth comb
4. During a health screening sports clinic, a high-school student states that it is difficult to bend the knee. Which movement of the knee joint is necessary to perform this action?
   1. Extension
   2. Lateral flexion
   3. Rotation
   4. Flexion
5. A patient is recovering from right hip surgery 2 days ago. Which patient finding should be immediately reported to the health care provider?
   1. Grimacing when moving right leg
   2. Inability to palpate a right foot dorsalis pedal pulse
   3. Coarse breath sounds that clear with coughing
   4. Kyphosis of the posterior curvature of the thoracic spine
6. Which of the following carotid artery assessment techniques is incorrect?
   1. Compressing the right and left carotid arteries simultaneously
   2. Asking the patient to flex the neck to better view the arteries
   3. Performing the examination while the patient is supine
   4. Listening with the bell over the carotid artery
7. A nurse assesses the abdomen for bowel sounds. The nurse would listen to the abdomen with the patient in which of the following positions?
   1. Supine with knees slightly flexed
   2. Prone position
   3. Sitting in bed at a 45-degree angle
   4. Lying in a left lateral position
8. The nurse explains steps of the breast examination to a group of college-age women. Which position should the nurse instruct the women to use to allow the best palpation of breast tissue?
   1. Sitting upright with hands clasped just above the umbilicus
   2. Lying supine with a small folded towel under the shoulder, arm flexed behind head
   3. Upright with arm opposite of the side being examined flexed at the waist
   4. Leaning forward with breasts hanging freely
9. A child who has asthma is having respiratory distress. The nurse auscultates high-pitched, continuous musical sounds bilaterally over the lung fields. How should the sounds be documented?
   1. Crackles
   2. Rhonchi
   3. Wheezes
   4. Pleural friction rub
10. A patient sustained a head injury after falling on the sidewalk while walking the dog. Which assessments would indicate a change in neurologic function? (Select all that apply.)
    1. Visual changes
    2. Ability to follow verbal commands
    3. Uncoordinated movements and loss of balance
    4. Glasgow Coma Scale score of 15
    5. Inability to understand verbal speech

evolve

Rationales for Review Questions can be found on the Evolve website.

1. 1, 2, 3, 4; **2.** 3; **3.** 1; **4.** 4; **5.** 2; **6.** 1; **7.** 1; **8.** 2; **9.** 3; **10.** 1, 3, 5

REFERENCES

American Cancer Society (ACS): *Cancer facts and figures 2013*, 2013a, http://www.cancer.org/research/cancerfactsstatistics/cancerfactsfigures2013/index. Accessed November 23, 2013.

American Cancer Society (ACS): *Breast cancer early detection, diagnosis, and staging*, 2013b, http://www.cancer.org/cancer/breastcancer/detailedguide/breast-cancer-detection. Accessed November 23, 2013.

American Cancer Society (ACS): *Colorectal cancer: what are the risk factors for colorectal cancer?* 2013c, http://www.cancer.org/cancer/colonandrectumcancer/detailedguide/colorectal-cancer-risk-factors. Accessed November 24, 2013.

American Cancer Society (ACS): *Learn about cancer: American Cancer Society recommendations for early breast cancer detection*, 2013d, http://www.cancer.org/Cancer/BreastCancer/DetailedGuide/breast-cancer-detection. Accessed February 6, 2014.

American Cancer Society (ACS): *Ovarian cancer*, 2013e, http://www.cancer.org/cancer/ovariancancer/detailedguide/ovarian-cancer-key-statistics. Accessed November 24, 2013.

American Cancer Society (ACS): *American Cancer Society guidelines for the early detection of cancer*, 2013f, http://www.cancer.org/healthy/findcancerearly/cancerscreeningguidelines/american-cancer-society-guidelines-for-the-early-detection-of-cancer. Accessed November 24, 2013.

American Heart Association (AHA): *Getting healthy*, 2013, http://www.heart.org/HEARTORG/GettingHealthy/GettingHealthy_UCM_001078_SubHomePage.jsp. Accessed July 12, 2013.

Burns E, Gray R, Smith LA: Brief screening questionnaires to identify problem drinking during pregnancy: a systematic review, *Addiction* 105:601, 2010.

Byrd J, et al: Research corner. Scale consistency study: how accurate are inpatient hospital scales? *Nursing* 41(11):21, 2011.

Cowdell F: Older people, personal hygiene, and skin care, *Medsurg Nurs* 20(5):235, 2011.

DeMarco R: Primary prevention of skin cancer in children and adolescents: a review of the literature, *J Pediatr Oncol Nurs* 25(2):67, 2008.

Hockenberry MJ, Wilson D: *Wong's nursing care of infants and children*, ed 9, 2011, Mosby.

Ingram RR: Using Campinha-Bacote's process of cultural competence model to examine the relationship between health literacy and cultural competence, *J Adv Nurs* 68(3):695, 2012.

Liu H, et al: Screening for osteoporosis in men: a systematic review for an American College of Physicians Guideline, *Ann Intern Med* 148(9):685, 2008.

Moore MC: *Pocket guide to nutritional care*, ed 6, St Louis, 2009, Elsevier.

National Institute on Drug Abuse (NIDA): *Screening for drug use in general medical settings, resource guide*, 2012, http://www.drugabuse.gov/publications/resource-guide. Accessed November 24, 2013.

Newson P: Knowledge for practice: observations and assessment, *Nurs Residential Care* 10(4):165, 2008.

Prihar B, Katz S: Patient education as a tool to increase screening for osteoporosis, *J Am Geriatr Soc* 56(5):961, 2008.

Rush A, Muir M: Maintaining skin integrity in bariatric patients, *Br J Community Nurs* 17(4):154, 2012.

Seidel HM, et al: *Mosby's guide to physical examination*, ed 7, St Louis, 2011, Mosby.

Silverman S: Osteoporosis and the new absolute risk algorithm, *Future Rheumatol* 3(1):15, 2008.

Touhy T, Jett K: *Ebersole and Hess' Gerontological nursing & healthy aging*, ed 4, St Louis, 2014, Mosby.

World Health Organization (WHO): *Intimate partner violence*, 2012, http://www.who.int/reproductivehealth/publications/violence/rhr12_36/en/index.html. Accessed November 24, 2013.

CHAPTER

17

Administering Medications

evolve WEBSITE

http://evolve.elsevier.com/Potter/essentials

- Video Clips
- Crossword Puzzle
- Audio Glossary

OBJECTIVES

- Discuss legal responsibilities in medication prescription and administration.
- Describe the physiological mechanisms of medication action.
- Compare and contrast the different types of medication effects and reactions.
- Discuss factors that influence medication actions.
- Describe factors to consider when choosing routes of medication administration.
- Calculate prescribed medication dosages correctly.
- Describe the roles and responsibilities of the prescriber, pharmacist, and nurse in medication administration.
- Identify and implement nursing actions that prevent medication errors.
- Describe the role of informatics in the promotion of medication safety.
- List the six rights of medication administration and implement their use in clinical practice.
- Discuss factors to include in assessing a patient's needs for and response to medication therapy.
- Discuss developmental factors that influence pharmacokinetics.
- Describe safety measures used in medication administration.
- Discuss methods used to teach patients about prescribed medications.
- Integrate patient-centered care while correctly and safely preparing and administering medications.

KEY TERMS

absorption, p. 380
adverse effects, p. 382
allergic reactions, p. 383
anaphylactic reactions, p. 383
apothecary system, p. 387
biological half-life, p. 384
biotransformation, p. 381
buccal, p. 386
detoxify, p. 381
idiosyncratic reaction, p. 383
infusions, p. 387
injections, p. 387
intradermal (ID), p. 386
intramuscular (IM), p. 386
intraocular, p. 386
intravenous (IV), p. 386
medication abuse, p. 379
medication allergy, p. 383
medication dependence, p. 379
medication error, p. 393
medication interaction, p. 383
medication reconciliation, p. 394
metric system, p. 387
ophthalmic medications, p. 409
opioids, p. 378
parenteral administration, p. 386
peak, p. 384
pharmacokinetics, p. 380
polypharmacy, p. 403
prescriptions, p. 387
pressurized metered-dose inhalers (pMDIs), p. 412
side effect, p. 382
solution, p. 387
subcutaneous, p. 386
sublingual, p. 385
synergistic effect, p. 383
therapeutic effect, p. 382
toxic effects, p. 382
transdermal disk, p. 386
trough, p. 384
Z-track injection, p. 422

CASE STUDY *Esther Simmons*

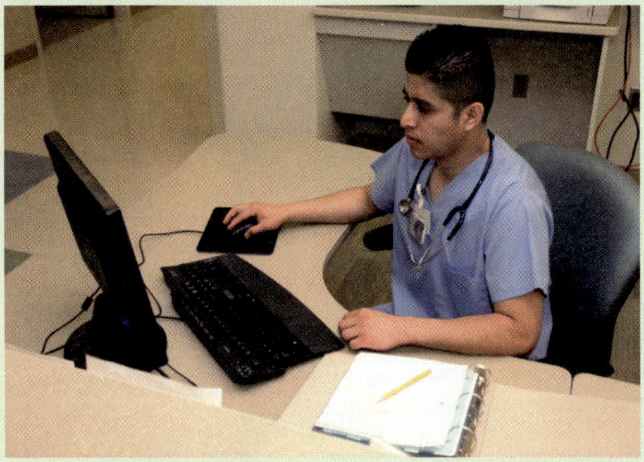

Esther Simmons is an 85-year-old African-American woman who lives in her home. She is on a skilled care floor in a hospital following hip replacement surgery. Her strength and mobility are improving, and she is planning to return home with home care nursing within the week.

Emilio Fernandez is a 31-year-old nursing student who is assigned to care for Esther today. While reviewing the medical record, Emilio finds that Esther has several chronic illnesses, including diabetes, heart disease, hypertension, and arthritis. To manage these illnesses successfully, Esther needs to take many medications on a routine basis. Several of her medications have changed, and several have been added since she was admitted. Based on this assessment, Emilio determines that Esther needs to learn how to administer her medications safely at home.

Patients with acute or chronic health problems use different tools to manage their health. One tool they often use is medication, a substance used in the diagnosis, treatment, relief, or prevention of health problems. No matter where patients receive their health care, you as the nurse play an essential role in medication administration and teaching. You also evaluate the effectiveness of medications in restoring or maintaining health.

As a nurse you are responsible for evaluating the effects of medications on a patient's health status and teaching a patient about medications and their side effects. You are also responsible for ensuring that patients follow medication regimens and evaluating patients' medication administration techniques. In the acute care setting you spend much time administering medications. Before discharge, make sure that patients are adequately prepared to administer their medications at home. When patients cannot administer their own medications, family caregivers or home care personnel are usually responsible for medication administration. In this situation you provide education to the patient and/or caregiver in all aspects of medication administration.

SCIENTIFIC KNOWLEDGE BASE

Because medication administration is essential to nursing practice, you need to be knowledgeable about the actions and effects of the medications you give to patients. To safely and accurately administer medications, you need to have an understanding of legal aspects of medication administration, pharmacokinetics (the movement of drugs in the human body), life sciences, anatomy, pathophysiology, and mathematics.

Medication Legislation and Standards

Governmental Regulation of Medications. The role of the U.S. government in regulation of the pharmaceutical industry is to protect the health of the people by ensuring that medications are safe and effective. The Pure Food and Drug Act requires that all medications to be free of impure products. Subsequent legislation sets standards related to safety, potency, and effectiveness. Enforcement of medication laws rests with the U.S. Food and Drug Administration (FDA). The FDA ensures that all medications on the market undergo rigorous review before allowing manufacturers to distribute them to the public. State and local medication laws must comply with federal laws. Some individual states have stricter controls than the federal government.

In 1993 the FDA instituted the MedWatch program. This voluntary program encourages nurses and other health care professionals to report when a medication, product, or medical event causes serious harm to a patient. Mandatory reporting is required for medication manufacturers, distributors, and packers. MedWatch forms are available to report such events (USFDA, 2013).

Health Care Institutions and Medication Laws. Health care institutions establish individual policies to meet federal, state, and local regulations. The size of an institution, the types of services it provides, and the types of personnel it employs influence these policies. Institutional policies are often more restrictive than governmental controls. For example, an institutional policy requires the automatic discontinuation of opioid analgesics after a set number of days. Although a prescriber may reorder a medication, this policy helps to control unnecessarily prolonged medication therapy and requires the prescriber to frequently review a patient's need for the medication.

Medication Regulations and Nursing Practice. State Nurse Practice Acts have the most influence over nursing practice because they define the scope of nurses' professional functions and responsibilities. In general most practice acts are purposefully broad so as not to limit nurses' professional responsibilities. Institutions and agencies interpret specific actions allowed under the act; but they are not able to modify, expand, or restrict the intent of the act. The primary intent of state Nurse Practice Acts is to protect the public from unskilled, undereducated, and unlicensed nurses.

You are responsible for following legal provisions when administering controlled substances such as **opioids,** which are controlled through federal and state guidelines. Nurses who violate the Controlled Substances Act face fines, imprisonment, and loss of nurse licensure. Hospitals and other health care institutions have policies for the proper storage and distribution of opioids (Box 17-1).

BOX 17-1 GUIDELINES FOR SAFE OPIOID ADMINISTRATION AND CONTROL

- Keep all opioids in a locked, secure place (e.g., cabinet or computerized medication cart).
- Keep a running count of opioids by counting them whenever dispensing them. If you find a discrepancy, correct and report the discrepancy immediately.
- Keep a record each time someone dispenses an opioid. The record includes the patient's name, date, time of drug administration, name of drug, and dosage. If the facility keeps a paper record, the nurse dispensing the drug signs the record. If the facility uses a computerized system, the computer records the nurse's name.
- Keep an ongoing record of opioids used and the number remaining.
- If you have to waste part of a controlled substance, a second nurse witnesses the disposal of the unused portion. Both nurses record their names on the controlled substance record.

Nontherapeutic Medication Use. Medication misuse includes overuse, underuse, erratic use, and contraindicated use of medications. Patients of all ages misuse medications. Some people use them for purposes other than their intended effect. Factors such as peer pressure, curiosity, and the pursuit of pleasure are some motivators for nontherapeutic medication use. Problems with medication use are not limited to heroin, cocaine, and other illegal drugs. The incidence of prescription and over-the-counter (OTC) drug misuse and abuse is also on the rise. The most commonly abused prescription medications include opioids, stimulants, tranquilizers, and sedatives. Common OTC medications that patients misuse or abuse include cough syrup and cold medication containing dextromethorphan (NIH NIDA, 2013).

You are ethically and legally responsible for understanding the problems of people who use medications improperly. **Medication abuse** happens when patients repeatedly use an addictive substance (e.g., opioids or alcohol). **Medication dependence** happens when a patient experiences withdrawal symptoms when the medication is stopped abruptly. When caring for patients with medication abuse or dependence, be aware of your values and attitudes about the willful use of potentially harmful substances. Therapeutic relationships develop when your personal values do not interfere with the acceptance or understanding of your patients' needs. Knowing the physical, psychological, and social changes resulting from medication abuse allows you to identify patients with medication problems.

Stress in the workplace, personal problems, and the strong desire to perform well are some factors that cause nurses and other health care professionals to misuse medications. Recognize and understand the problems of colleagues who abuse medications. A wide variety of programs to help people are offered through an institution employee assistance program (EAP), the State Board of Nursing, and community agencies.

Pharmacological Concepts

Medication Names. Medications have three different names. The chemical name is an exact description of the composition and molecular structure of a medication. In clinical practice health care workers rarely use chemical names. The United States Adopted Names Council assigns the generic name of a medication. Generic names are not as complex as chemical names. The generic name becomes the official name that is listed in publications such as the *United States Pharmacopeia* (USP). The trade, proprietary, or brand name of a medication is the name under which a manufacturer markets a medication. The trade name has the symbol ® at the upper right of the name, indicating that the manufacturer has registered the medication name. Because a medication can be made in different formulations and marketed by different companies, one medication can have many trade names. The following is an example of the different names of a common medication,

- Chemical name: *N*-acetyl-*para*-aminophenol
- Generic name: Acetaminophen
- Trade Names: APAP, Tylenol, Acephen, Panadol

Some medications have similar spellings and sound similar (e.g., Cedax and Cidex). Medication errors frequently occur with medications that look alike and sound alike. Therefore The Joint Commission (TJC) requires hospitals and other health care organizations to implement safety measures to prevent errors associated with medications that are often confused with one another (TJC, 2013a), which includes maintaining a list of look-alike, sound-alike medications such as the one published by The Institute of Safe Medication Practices [ISMP] (2011a) (http://www.ismp.org/Tools/confuseddrugnames.pdf).

Classification. Medications with similar characteristics are grouped into classifications. Medication classification indicates the effect of a medication on a body system, the symptoms that a medication relieves, or its desired effect. Sometimes the last syllables of the generic name indicate the classification of a medication. For example, the syllables *olol* at the end of *propranolol* tell you that this medication is in the beta-adrenergic blocker classification. Usually each class contains more than one medication that health care providers can prescribe for a type of health problem. For example, some patients with Alzheimer's dementia take five different medications to improve their cognitive impairment. These drugs are separated into two different classifications: cholinesterase inhibitors and *N*-methyl-d-aspartate (NMDA) antagonists (Lehne, 2013). Some medications are in more than one class. For example, aspirin is an analgesic, antipyretic, and antiinflammatory medication.

Medication Forms. Medications are available in a variety of forms or preparations. The form of a medication determines its route of administration. Manufacturers make many medications in several forms such as tablets, capsules,

TABLE 17-1 FORMS OF MEDICATION BY ROUTE OF ADMINISTRATION

Medication Forms Commonly Prepared for Administration by Oral Route	
Solid Forms	
Caplet	Solid dosage form for oral use; shaped like a capsule and coated for ease of swallowing
Capsule	Medication encased in a gelatin shell
Tablet	Powdered medication compressed into hard disk or cylinder
Enteric coated	Tablet that is coated so it does not dissolve in stomach; meant for intestinal absorption
Liquid Forms	
Elixir	Clear fluid containing water and alcohol; designed for oral use; usually has sweetener added
Extract	Concentrated medication form made by removing the active portion of medication from its other components
Aqueous solution	Substance dissolved in water and syrups
Aqueous suspension	Finely dissolved particles in liquid medium; when left standing, particles settle to bottom of container
Syrup	Medication dissolved in concentrated sugar solution
Other Oral Forms and Terms Associated with Oral Preparations	
Troche (lozenge)	Flat, round dosage form containing medication that dissolves in mouth; not meant for ingestion
Aerosol	Aqueous medication sprayed and absorbed in mouth and upper airway; not meant for ingestion
Sustained release	Tablet or capsule that contains small particles of a medication coated with material that requires varying amount of time to dissolve
Medication Forms Commonly Prepared for Administration by Topical Route	
Ointment (salve or cream)	Semisolid, externally applied preparation, usually containing one or more medications
Liniment	Usually contains alcohol, oil, or soapy emollient
Lotion	Semiliquid suspension often used to cool, protect, or clean skin
Paste	Thick ointment; absorbed through skin more slowly than ointment; often used for skin protection.
Transdermal patch	Medicated disk or patch; medication absorbed through skin over designated period of time (e.g., 24 hours)
Medication Forms Commonly Prepared for Administration By Parenteral Route	
Solution	Sterile preparation that contains water with one or more dissolved compounds
Powder	Sterile particles of medication that are dissolved in sterile solution (e.g., water, normal saline) before administration
Medication Forms Commonly Prepared for Instillation into Body Cavities	
Intraocular disk	Medicated disk (similar to a contact lens) that is inserted into eye; medication absorbed over designated period of time.
Suppository	Solid dosage form mixed with gelatin and shaped in form of a pellet for insertion into body cavity (rectum or vagina); melts when it reaches body temperature, allowing medication to be absorbed

elixirs, and suppositories. When administering a medication, be certain to use the proper form (Table 17-1).

Pharmacokinetics as the Basis of Medication Actions

For a medication to be therapeutically useful, it is taken into a patient's body; is absorbed and distributed to cells, tissues, or a specific organ; and alters physiological functions. **Pharmacokinetics** is the study of four major processes: medication absorption, distribution, metabolism, and excretion (Lehne, 2013). You use knowledge of pharmacokinetics to time medication administration, select the route of administration, predict patients' risks for alterations in medication action, and evaluate patients' responses to medications.

Absorption. **Absorption** refers to passage of medication molecules from the site of administration into the blood. Factors that influence medication absorption are the route of administration, ability of a medication to dissolve, blood flow to the site of administration, body surface area, and lipid solubility of a medication.

Route of Administration. Each route has a different rate of absorption. When you place medications on the skin, absorption is slow because of the physical makeup of the skin. The body also absorbs oral medications at a slow rate because these medications have to pass through the gastrointestinal (GI) tract. The body absorbs medications through the mucous membranes and respiratory airways quickly because these tissues contain many blood vessels. Intravenous (IV) injection produces the most rapid absorption because medications given by this route are absorbed into the systemic circulation immediately.

Ability of a Medication to Dissolve. The ability of an oral medication to dissolve depends largely on its formulation or preparation. Acidic medications are absorbed in the gastric mucosa rapidly, whereas medications that are alkaline are not absorbed until reaching the small intestine. Solutions and suspensions are already in a liquid state and are easier for the body to absorb than tablets or capsules.

Blood Flow to the Area of Absorption. The blood supply to the site of administration determines how quickly the body absorbs a drug. Sites with rich blood supplies absorb medications more quickly. For example, the body absorbs a medication administered in the muscle (intramuscular [IM] route) faster than a medication administered in the subcutaneous tissue (subcutaneous route) because the blood supply to muscle is richer than the blood supply to subcutaneous tissue.

Body Surface Area. The size of the surface with which the medication comes in contact affects how quickly the body absorbs the medication. If the surface area is large, the medication is absorbed more quickly; thus its effects occur more quickly. This explains why many medications are absorbed more quickly and take effect faster when they are absorbed in the small intestine rather than the stomach (Lehne, 2013). An inhaled medication absorbs more quickly than an oral medication because of the large surface are of the lung.

Lipid Solubility of the Medication. Highly soluble medications are easier for the body to absorb because they readily cross the cell membrane, which is made of a lipid layer. Another factor that affects absorption of a medication is the presence of food in the stomach. Some oral medications are absorbed more quickly on an empty stomach, whereas others are unaffected by gastric contents. In addition, some medications interfere with the absorption of one another if given at the same time.

Distribution. After a medication is absorbed, it moves throughout the body. The rate and extent of distribution depend on the physical and chemical properties of medications and the physiology of the person taking the medication.

Circulation. Once a medication enters the bloodstream, the blood carries it throughout the tissues and organs of the body. How fast it gets there depends on the vascularity of the various tissues and organs. The distribution of a medication is inhibited when medical conditions limit blood flow or intended sites of action have a poor blood supply. For example, solid tumors have poor blood supply and therefore are resistant to therapy intended to destroy them (Lehne, 2013).

Membrane Permeability. To be distributed to an organ, a medication needs to pass through all the biological membranes of that organ. Some membranes serve as barriers to the passage of medications. For example, the blood-brain barrier allows only lipid-soluble medications to pass into the brain and cerebrospinal fluid. Therefore central nervous system (CNS) infections sometimes require treatment with antibiotics injected directly into the subarachnoid space in the spinal cord. Older patients often experience adverse effects (e.g., confusion) because they experience a change in the permeability of the blood-brain barrier, which enhances the passage of fat-soluble medications into the brain. The placental membrane is a nonselective barrier to medications. Lipid-soluble, nonionized drugs easily cross the placenta and can cause serious harm to the fetus (Lehne, 2013).

Protein Binding. The degree to which medications bind to serum proteins such as albumin affects medication distribution. Most medications bind to protein to some extent. When medications bind to albumin, they do not exert pharmacological activity. The unbound, or "free," medication is its active form. Older adults or patients with liver disease or malnutrition have decreased albumin in the bloodstream. Because more medication is unbound in these patients, they are at risk for an increase in medication activity, toxicity, or both.

Metabolism. After a medication reaches its site of action, it is metabolized. **Biotransformation** occurs when enzymes **detoxify** (remove toxic qualities), degrade (break down), and remove biologically active chemicals. Most biotransformation occurs within the liver, although the lungs, kidneys, blood, and intestines also metabolize medications. The liver is especially important because its specialized structure oxidizes and transforms many toxic substances. The liver degrades many harmful chemicals before they become distributed to the tissues. If a decrease in liver function occurs such as with aging or liver disease, the body slowly eliminates a medication, resulting in a buildup of the medication. When organs that metabolize medications do not function correctly, patients are at risk for medication toxicity.

Excretion. After medications are metabolized, they exit the body through the kidneys, liver, bowel, lungs, and exocrine glands. The chemical makeup of a medication determines which organ excretes the medication. The kidneys are the main organs that excrete medications. Some medications escape extensive metabolism and exit unchanged in the urine. Others undergo biotransformation in the liver before the kidneys excrete them. If renal function declines, a patient is at risk for medication toxicity. If the kidney cannot adequately excrete a medication, it is necessary to reduce the dose. Maintenance of an adequate fluid intake (50 mL/kg/day) promotes proper elimination of medications for the average adult.

Gaseous and volatile compounds such as nitrous oxide and alcohol exit through the lungs. Deep breathing and coughing (see Chapter 39) help a patient eliminate anesthetic gases more quickly following surgery. The exocrine glands excrete lipid-soluble medications. When medications exit through sweat glands, the skin sometimes becomes irritated. The nurse helps the patient with good hygiene practices (see Chapter 29) to promote cleanliness and skin integrity.

The GI tract is another route for medication excretion. Many medications enter the hepatic circulation to be broken down by the liver and excreted into the bile. After they enter the intestines through the biliary tract, the intestines resorb them. Factors that increase peristalsis (e.g., laxatives or enemas) accelerate medication excretion through the feces, whereas factors that slow peristalsis (e.g., inactivity or improper diet) prolong the effects of a medication.

Medications are often excreted through the mammary glands. In these cases there is a risk that a nursing infant will ingest the chemicals. Teach mothers to check the safety of any medication used while breastfeeding.

Types of Medication Action

Medications vary considerably in the way they act. A patient does not always respond in the same way to each successive dose of a medication. Sometimes the same medication dosage causes very different responses in different patients. Box 17-2 lists important variables that influence medication action.

Therapeutic Effects. Each medication has a **therapeutic effect,** the intended or desired physiological response of a medication. For example, you administer nitroglycerin to reduce cardiac workload and increase myocardial oxygen supply, which eliminates chest pain. Sometimes a single medication has many therapeutic effects. For example, aspirin is an analgesic, antipyretic, and antiinflammatory; and it reduces platelet aggregation (clumping of blood platelets). It is important to know what is wrong with your patient and the expected therapeutic effect for each medication that your patient receives. This knowledge allows you to teach a patient about the intended effect of each medication and evaluate its effectiveness.

Adverse Effects. Every medication has the ability to harm a patient. Undesired, unintended, and often unpredictable responses to medication are referred to as **adverse effects.** Adverse drug effects range from mild to severe. Some happen immediately, whereas others develop over time. Be alert and assess unusual individual responses to drugs, especially with newly prescribed medications. Patients most at risk for adverse medication reactions include the very young and older adults, women, patients taking multiple medications, patients extremely underweight or overweight, and patients with renal or liver disease. If adverse effects are mild and tolerable, patients often remain on the medications. However, if they are not tolerated and are potentially harmful, stop giving the medication immediately. Report all adverse reactions to a patient's health care provider and record the adverse effects in the patient's medical record. Health care providers report the occurrence of adverse effects to the FDA through the MedWatch program (USFDA, 2013).

A **side effect** is a predictable and often unavoidable adverse effect produced at a usual therapeutic dose. For example, some antihypertensive medications and antidepressants cause impotence in male patients. Some side effects are harmless, and some cause injury. If the side effects are serious enough to cancel the beneficial effects of the therapeutic action of a medication, health care providers usually discontinue the medication. Patients often stop taking medications because of side effects, the most common of which are anorexia, nausea, vomiting, constipation, drowsiness, and diarrhea.

Toxic effects are capable of causing injury or death. They often develop after prolonged intake of a medication or when it accumulates in the blood because of impaired metabolism or excretion. Excess amounts of a medication within the body have lethal effects, depending on its action. Do not give the

BOX 17-2 FACTORS INFLUENCING MEDICATION ACTIONS

GENETIC DIFFERENCES

- A person's genetic makeup influences drug metabolism. Members of a family sometimes have similar reactions to the same medication.

PHYSIOLOGICAL VARIABLES

- Gender, age, body weight, nutritional status, and illnesses all affect drug actions.
- Hormonal differences between men and women affect drug metabolism.
- Children usually require lower drug doses than adults. However, sometimes they need larger doses, depending on the medication. The changes accompanying aging alter the influence of drugs.
- There is a direct relationship between the concentration of a medication administered and how quickly it is absorbed by body tissues.
- Diseases that impair the function of an organ responsible for normal pharmacokinetics also impair drug action (e.g., if a patient has liver failure, the metabolism of medications is slower).

ENVIRONMENTAL CONDITIONS

- Stress and the exposure to heat and cold affect drug actions. For example, patients receiving vasodilators require lower drug dosages in warm weather.
- The setting in which a person takes a drug influences a patient's reaction. When patients are alone or isolated, they may need more pain medication than if they were in a room with other patients or if their families visit them frequently.

PSYCHOLOGICAL FACTORS

- A patient's attitude, his or her reaction to the meaning of a drug, and a nurse's behavior affect drug actions. To enhance the effect of a medication, ensure that patient understands and accepts the need for the drug and administer it with supportive behavior.

DIET

- Medication and nutrient interactions alter the action of a drug or the effect of a nutrient. For example, mineral oil decreases the absorption of fat-soluble vitamins.
- Proper drug metabolism requires healthy nutritional levels.

TABLE 17-2 MILD ALLERGIC REACTIONS

SYMPTOM	DESCRIPTION
Urticaria (hives)	Raised, irregularly shaped skin eruptions with varying sizes and shapes; have reddened margins and pale centers
Eczema (rash)	Small, raised vesicles that are usually reddened; often distributed over entire body
Pruritus	Itching of skin; accompanies most rashes
Rhinitis	Inflammation of mucous membranes lining nose; causes swelling and clear, watery discharge
Wheezing	Constriction of smooth muscles that surround bronchioles; occurs mainly on inspiration and can lead to airway obstruction
Angioedema	Short-term subcutaneous or submucosal swellings of face, neck, lips, larynx, hands, feet, genitalia, or viscera

medication if a patient experiences toxic effects and report the effects to the patient's health care provider immediately. Sometimes antidotes are available to treat specific types of medication toxicity. For example, if a patient experiences severe respiratory depression after receiving morphine sulfate, you administer naloxone (Narcan) to reverse the toxic effects of the morphine.

Some medications cause unpredictable effects such as **idiosyncratic reactions,** in which a patient overreacts or underreacts to a medication or has a reaction different from that which is expected. For example, a child receiving an antihistamine (e.g., Benadryl) becomes extremely agitated or excited instead of drowsy. Stop giving the patient the medication if idiosyncratic reactions occur and consult with the health care provider to determine if the patient needs to stop taking the drug.

When patients become immunologically sensitized to a medication after taking at least one dose, **allergic reactions** occur. With repeated administration a patient develops an allergic response to the medication, its chemical preservatives, or a metabolite. The medication or chemical acts as an antigen, triggering the release of antibodies. When a patient's immune system causes abnormal reactions to a medication, the patient has a **medication allergy.** Allergic symptoms vary, depending on an individual and the medication; they range from mild to severe. Table 17-2 summarizes common, mild allergy symptoms. Sudden constriction of bronchiolar muscles, edema of the pharynx and larynx, and severe wheezing and shortness of breath all characterize severe or **anaphylactic reactions.** In anaphylaxis a patient becomes severely hypotensive, necessitating emergency resuscitation measures. A patient with a known history of an allergy to a medication

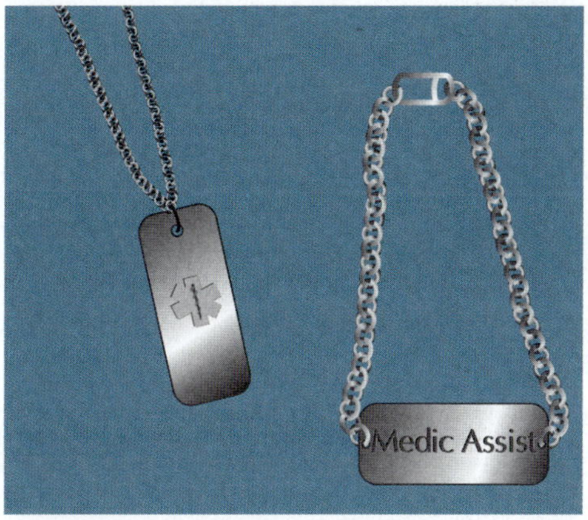

FIGURE 17-1 Identification bracelet and medal.

should not take the medication again. The patient also needs to wear a medical identification bracelet or medal (Figure 17-1) that alerts health care providers to the allergy in case he or she is unconscious when receiving medical care. Notify a patient's health care provider immediately if you suspect that your patient is having an allergic reaction to a medication. Antihistamines, epinephrine, and bronchodilators are prescribed to treat anaphylactic reactions. Document all medication allergies in the patient's medical record.

Medication Interactions. A **medication interaction** occurs when one medication modifies the action of another. A medication sometimes enhances or diminishes the action of other medications and alters the way in which the body absorbs, metabolizes, or eliminates another medication. Know the medications that your patients take and be aware of and assess for potential medication interactions. When two medications have a **synergistic effect,** their combined effect is greater than their effects when given separately. For example, alcohol is a CNS depressant that has a synergistic effect on antihistamines, antidepressants, barbiturates, and opioids.

When a medication interaction is desirable, a health care provider orders a combination of medications to create this interaction for the patient's benefit. For example, a patient with moderate hypertension typically receives several medications such as diuretics and vasodilators that act together to control blood pressure. Consult with your patient's health care provider when medication interactions are undesirable. Sometimes the timing of the medications needs to be changed, whereas other times one or both of the medications need to be changed or stopped.

Medication Dose Responses. A medication undergoes absorption, distribution, metabolism, and excretion after it enters the body. Except when administered intravenously, medications take time to enter the bloodstream. The minimum effective concentration (MEC) is the plasma level below which a patient does not experience the effect of a medication. The toxic concentration is the plasma level at which a patient experiences toxic effects of a medication. The goal of medication therapy is to achieve a constant therapeutic level, which falls between the MEC and the toxic concentration. As patients take medication doses over time, the

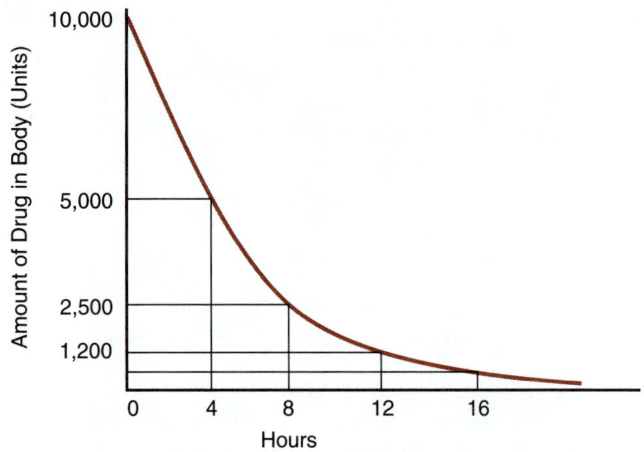

FIGURE 17-2 Biological half-life (t½). (From McKenry L, Tessier E, Hogan M: *Mosby's pharmacology in nursing*, ed 22, St Louis, 2006, Mosby.)

plasma level of the medication fluctuates constantly between doses. The **peak** concentration is the highest plasma level, whereas the **trough** concentration is the lowest level. Sometimes health care providers prescribe medications (e.g., vancomycin) based on peak and trough levels. You usually draw trough levels 30 minutes before administering the medication, and you draw the peak whenever the medication is expected to reach its peak concentration based on the pharmacokinetics of the medication.

All medications have a **biological half-life,** which is the time it takes for the body to lower the amount of unchanged medication by half. A drug with a short half-life (e.g., 2 to 3 hours) needs to be given more frequently than a drug with a longer half-life (e.g., 10 to 12 hours). The half-life of a medication does not change with the dose; its half-life is always the same no matter how much medication is administered. For example, if you give 10,000 units of a medication and the medication has a half-life of 4 hours, your patient will excrete 5000 units of the medication in 4 hours. In the next 4 hours your patient will eliminate 2500 units. This process continues until the medication is totally eliminated from the patient's body (Figure 17-2). The goal of medication administration is to achieve a therapeutic plateau (i.e., a point at which the blood level of a medication remains consistent). To maintain a therapeutic plateau, a patient receives regular fixed doses at specific intervals that correspond with their half-life. For example, research has shown that pain medications are most effective when they are given "around the clock" rather than when the patient intermittently complains of pain. This results in a constant serum level of pain medication. After an initial medication dose, the patient receives each successive dose when the previous dose reaches its half-life.

You and your patient follow prescribed doses and dosage intervals (Table 17-3). Health care agencies usually set schedules for medication administration. However, you can change this schedule based on your knowledge about a medication. For example, you work at an agency where medications ordered once a day are given at 0800. Your patient has a medication ordered once a day that works better when given before bedtime; therefore you adjust the time to give the medication accordingly. Acute care agencies also follow guidelines from the ISMP to determine safe, effective, and timely administration of medications (CMS, 2011; ISMP, 2011b). According to the guidelines, hospitals determine if medications are time critical. Medications that are time critical most likely cause harm or have subtherapeutic effects if they are not administered on time (usually 30 minutes before or after the scheduled dose). Non–time-critical medications most likely do not cause harm if they are given within 1 to 2 hours before or after the scheduled time. Thus you need to administer time-critical medications at a precise time, within 30 minutes before or after their scheduled time. You administer non–time-critical medications within 1 to 2 hours of their scheduled time. Ensure that you follow your agency medication policies about the timing of medications to ensure that your patients receive their medications at the right time (CMS 2011; ISMP, 2011b).

TABLE 17-3 COMMON DOSAGE ADMINISTRATION SCHEDULES

ABBREVIATION	MEANING
AC, ac	Before meals
ad lib	As desired
BID, bid	Twice each day
Daily	Every day
PC, pc	After meals
prn	Whenever there is a need
qAM	Every morning, every AM
qh	Every hour
q4h	Every 4 hours
q6h	Every 6 hours
q8h	Every 8 hours
QID, qid	4 times per day
STAT	Give immediately
TID, tid	3 times per day

When you teach patients about dosage schedules, use familiar language. For example, when teaching a patient about twice-daily medication dosing, instruct him or her to take the medication in the morning and again in the evening. Knowledge of the time intervals of medication action help you anticipate the effect of the medication. With this knowledge, instruct the patient when to expect a response.

Routes of Administration

The route prescribed for administering a medication depends on its properties and desired effect (Table 17-4). It also depends on the patient's physical and mental condition.

TABLE 17-4 **FACTORS INFLUENCING CHOICE OF ADMINISTRATION ROUTES**

ADVANTAGES BY ROUTE	DISADVANTAGES/CONTRAINDICATIONS
Oral, Buccal, Sublingual Routes	
Convenient and comfortable Economical Sometimes produce local or systemic effects Rarely cause anxiety	Avoided when patient has alterations in GI function (e.g., nausea, vomiting), reduced GI motility (after general anesthesia or bowel inflammation), gastric suction, surgical resection of portion of GI tract, and reduced ability to swallow Sometimes irritate lining of GI tract, discolor teeth, or have unpleasant tastes
Parenteral (Subcutaneous, IM, IV, ID, Epidural)	
Can be used when oral drugs are contraindicated	Risk for introducing infection Some medications more expensive Risk for tissue damage
More rapid absorption occurs than with topical or oral routes IV infusion provides drug delivery for critically ill patients; if peripheral perfusion is poor, IV route preferred over injection Epidural provides excellent pain control	Subcutaneous, IM, and ID not used in patients with bleeding tendencies IM and IV absorbed quickly, increasing risk for drug reactions Can cause considerable anxiety in many patients, especially children Some patients experience pain with repeated needlesticks
Topical	
Skin	
Primarily provides local effect Painless Limited side effects	Absorption too rapid if applied over skin abrasions, increasing systemic effects Medications slowly absorbed through skin
Transdermal	
Prolonged systemic effects with limited side effects.	Leaves oily or pasty substance on skin and soils clothing
Mucous Membranes*	
Local application to involved sites provides therapeutic effects Aqueous solutions readily absorbed and capable of causing systemic effects Potential route of administration when oral drugs contraindicated	Mucous membranes highly sensitive to some drug concentrations Insertion of rectal and vaginal medication often causes embarrassment Patient with ruptured eardrum cannot receive irrigations Rectal suppositories contraindicated if patient has active rectal bleeding or history of rectal surgery
Inhalation	
Provides rapid relief for local respiratory problems Easily used for introduction of general anesthetic gases.	Some local agents cause serious systemic effects
Intraocular Disk	
Route advantageous in that it does not require frequent administration as eyedrops do	Local reactions possible Patient must be taught how to insert and remove disk Expensive Contraindicated with eye infections

GI, Gastrointestinal; *ID*, intradermal; *IM*, intramuscular; *IV*, intravenous.
*Includes eyes, ears, nose, vagina, rectum, and ostomy.

Collaborate with the prescriber to determine the best route for a patient's medication. For example, you are caring for a patient who has 650 mg of acetaminophen ordered by mouth every 4 hours as needed for a temperature greater than 38° C (100.4° F). Your patient has a temperature of 38.5° C (101.2° F), is vomiting, and is unable to tolerate oral fluids. You consult with the prescriber and have the medication changed to a rectal suppository because the patient cannot tolerate oral medications at this time.

Oral Routes. The oral route is the easiest and the most commonly used. Medications are given by mouth and swallowed with fluid. Oral medications have a slower onset of action and a more prolonged effect than parenteral medications. Patients generally prefer the oral route.

Sublingual Administration. A sublingual medication is readily absorbed after being placed under the tongue to dissolve (Figure 17-3). If patients chew or swallow medications given by the sublingual route, they do not experience the

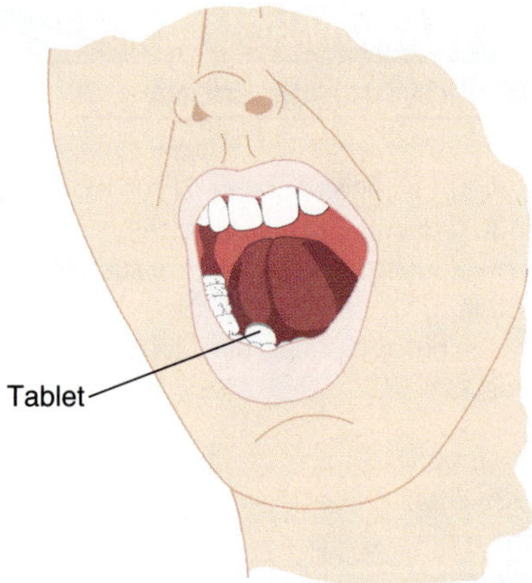

FIGURE 17-3 Sublingual administration of tablet.

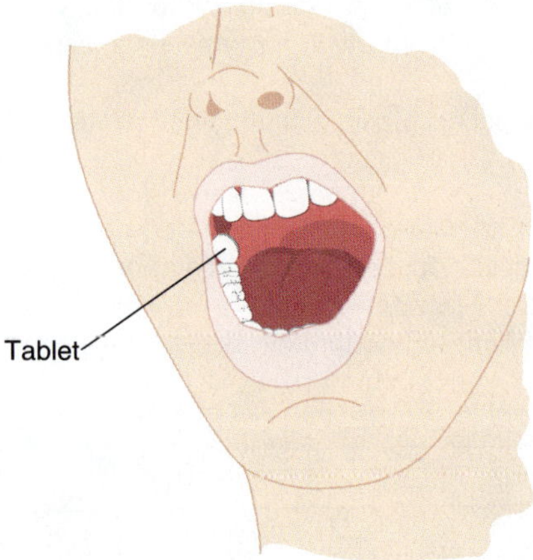

FIGURE 17-4 Buccal administration of tablet.

desired effect. Nitroglycerin is commonly given sublingually. Tell your patient not to take a drink, eat, or chew gum until the medication is completely dissolved.

Buccal Administration. Administration of a medication by the **buccal** route involves placing the solid medication in the mouth between the gums and mucous membranes of the cheek until it dissolves (Figure 17-4). Teach patients to place medication against alternate cheeks with each dose to avoid mucosal irritation. Also teach them not to chew or swallow the medication or take any liquids with it. A buccal medication acts locally on the mucosa or systemically as it is swallowed in a person's saliva.

Parenteral Routes. **Parenteral administration** involves injecting a medication into body tissues. The four major parenteral routes are as follows:

1. **Subcutaneous:** Injection into tissues just below the dermis of the skin
2. **Intramuscular (IM):** Injection into a muscle
3. **Intravenous (IV):** Injection into a vein
4. **Intradermal (ID):** Injection into the dermis just under the epidermis

Some medications are administered into body cavities through other routes, including epidural, intraperitoneal, intrathecal or intraspinal, intracardiac, intrapleural, intraarterial, intraosseous, and intraarticular routes. Nurses usually do not administer medications through these routes. Regardless of who actually administers the medication, you are responsible for monitoring the integrity of the system of medication delivery, understanding the therapeutic value of the medication, and evaluating the patient's response to the therapy.

Topical Administration. Medications applied to the skin and mucous and respiratory membranes generally have local effects. A topical medication is applied to the skin by spreading it over an area, applying moist dressings, soaking body parts in a solution, or giving medicated baths. Systemic effects occur if a patient's skin is thin, if the medication concentration is high, or if contact with the skin is prolonged.

Some topical medications (e.g., nitroglycerin, clonidine [Catapres], estrogens) have systemic effects when you give them topically by a **transdermal disk** or patch. The disk firmly holds the medicated ointment to the skin. Patients wear these topical applications for as little as 12 hours or as long as 7 days.

You can apply topical medications to mucous membranes in a variety of other ways, including the following:

1. By directly applying a liquid or ointment (e.g., eyedrops, gargling, swabbing the throat)
2. By inserting a medication into a body cavity (e.g., placing a suppository in the rectum or vagina, inserting medicated packing into the vagina)
3. By instilling fluid into a body part or cavity (e.g., eardrops, nose drops, bladder or rectal instillation [fluid is retained])
4. By irrigating a body cavity (e.g., flushing eye, ear, vagina, bladder, or rectum with medicated fluid [fluid is not retained])
5. By spraying a medication into a body cavity (e.g., instillation into nose and throat)

Inhalation Route. The deeper passages of the respiratory tract provide a large surface area for inhaled medications to be absorbed, resulting in local or systemic effects. You administer inhaled medications into nasal passages, in oral passages, or through tubes that go from the patient's mouth to the trachea. Medications given by the inhalation route are readily absorbed and work quickly because of the rich vascular alveolar-capillary network in the pulmonary tissue.

Intraocular Route. **Intraocular** medication delivery involves administering medication into the eye. One kind of intraocular route involves inserting a medication disk similar to a contact lens into the patient's eye. The eye medication disk has two soft outer layers that have medication enclosed in them. You insert the disk into the patient's eye, much like a contact lens. The disk remains in the patient's eye for up to 1 week (Lavik et al., 2011). Pilocarpine, a medication used to treat glaucoma, is the most common medication disk used.

Systems of Medication Measurement

Safely administering medications requires the ability to compute medication doses accurately and measure medications correctly. A careless mistake in placing a decimal point or adding a zero to a dose can lead to a fatal error. Check every dose carefully before giving a medication.

The health care industry uses the metric, apothecary, and household systems of measurement for medication therapy. Globally most nations use the metric system as their standard of measurement. Although the U.S. Congress has not officially adopted the metric system, most health professionals in the United States use it. Health care providers usually write **prescriptions,** or orders for medications, that are to be self-administered at home by patients in household measures. Prescribers rarely use the **apothecary system,** a measurement system that includes ounces, pounds, and pints.

Metric System. As a decimal system the **metric system** is the most logically organized. Metric units are easy to convert and calculate using simple multiplication and division. Each basic unit of measurement is organized into units of 10. Multiplying or dividing by 10 forms secondary units. In multiplication the decimal point moves to the right; in division the decimal moves to the left. For example:

$$10\text{ mg} \times 10 = 100\text{ mg}$$

$$10\text{ mg} \div 10 = 1\text{ mg}$$

The basic units of measurement in the metric system are the meter (length), liter (volume), and gram (weight). For medication calculations use only the volume and weight units and use lowercase or uppercase letters to designate units:

Gram = g or Gm

Liter = l or L

Milligram = mg

Milliliter = mL

A system of Latin prefixes designates subdivision of the basic units: deci- (1/10 or 0.1), centi- (1/100 or 0.01), and milli- (1/1000 or 0.001). Greek prefixes designate multiples of the basic units: deka- (10), hecto- (100), and kilo- (1000). Use fractions or multiples of a unit when writing medication doses in metric units. Always give fractions in decimal form:

$$500\text{ mg or } 0.5\text{ g, not } \tfrac{1}{2}\text{ g}$$

$$10\text{ mL or } 0.01\text{ L, not } \tfrac{1}{100}\text{ L}$$

Many actual and potential medication errors occur with the use of fractions. Follow practice standards when medications are ordered in fractions to prevent medication errors. For example, to make the decimal point more visible, a leading zero is always placed in front of a decimal (e.g., use 0.5, not .5). On the other hand, do not use a trailing zero (i.e., a zero after a decimal point) because, if a health care worker does not see the decimal point, the patient may end up receiving 10 times more medication than that which is prescribed (e.g., use 5 not 5.0) (TJC, 2014).

Household Measurements. Household units of measurement are familiar to most people. Their disadvantage is their inaccuracy. Household utensils such as teaspoons and cups often vary in size. Scales to measure pints or quarts are often not well calibrated. Household measures include drops, teaspoons, tablespoons, and cups for volume and pints and quarts for weight. The advantages of household measurements are their convenience and familiarity. When the accuracy of a medication dose is not critical, it is safe to use household measures. For example, you can safely measure many OTC medications by this method. Table 17-5 gives common equivalents from each measurement unit.

TABLE 17-5 EQUIVALENTS OF MEASUREMENT

METRIC	APOTHECARY	HOUSEHOLD
1 mL	15-16 minims*	15 drops (gtt)
5 mL	1 dram*	1 teaspoon (tsp)
15 mL	4 drams*	1 tablespoon (tbsp)
30 mL	1 fluid ounce	2 tablespoons (tbsp)
240 mL	8 fluid ounces	1 cup (c)
480 mL (approximately 500 mL)	1 pint (pt)	1 pint (pt)
960 mL (approximately 1 L)	1 quart (qt)	1 quart (qt)
3840 mL (approximately 5 L)	1 gallon (gal)	1 gallon (gal)

*Minims and drams are no longer acceptable units of measure for medication administration, although some medication cups and syringes list them. Use mL for safe medication preparation (Gray Morris, 2010).

Solutions. As a nurse you use solutions of various concentrations for **injections,** irrigations, and **infusions.** A **solution** is a given mass of solid substance dissolved in a known volume of fluid or a given volume of fluid dissolved in a known volume of another fluid. When a solid is dissolved in a fluid, the concentration is in units of mass per units of volume (e.g., g/mL, g/L, or mg/mL). Sometimes you also express a concentration of a solution as a percentage. For example, a 10% solution is 10 g of solid dissolved in 100 mL of solution. A proportion also expresses concentrations. A 1/1000 solution represents a solution containing 1 g of solid in 1000 mL of liquid or 1 mL of liquid mixed with 1000 mL of another liquid.

NURSING KNOWLEDGE BASE

In 1999 the Institute of Medicine (IOM) published the book *To Err Is Human: Building a Safer Health System.* This book created national awareness about the effect of medical errors within the health care system. For example, approximately 98,000 people die in any given year as a result of medical errors that happen in hospitals. This means that more people die from medical errors than from motor vehicle accidents, breast cancer, acquired immunodeficiency syndrome (AIDS), and workplace injuries.

Nurses play an important role in patient safety, especially when it comes to medication administration. The safe administration of medications and prevention of medication errors are national patient safety concerns (NQF, 2013). To safely administer medications to patients, it is essential that you calculate dosages accurately. You also need to understand the roles that different health care providers play in prescribing and administering medications. Your previous learning is important. Apply what you know and do not be afraid to ask questions when administering medications. Use the nursing process as a framework to organize your thoughts and actions.

Clinical Calculations

To administer medications safely, use your mathematics skills to calculate dosages and mix solutions. This is important because you do not always dispense medications in the unit of measure in which they are ordered and delivered. Medication companies package and bottle medications in standard dosages. For example, the patient's health care provider orders 1 g of a medication that is available only in milligrams. You are responsible for converting available units of volume and weight to the desired doses. Know the approximate equivalents in all major measurement systems.

Conversions Within One System. When converting measurements within the metric system, you use division or multiplication. For example, to change milligrams to grams, divide by 1000 or move the decimal three points to the left:

$$1000\text{ mg} = 1\text{ g}$$

$$350\text{ mg} = 0.35\text{ g}$$

To convert liters to milliliters, multiply by 1000 or move the decimal three points to the right:

$$1\text{ L} = 1000\text{ mL}$$

$$0.25\text{ L} = 250\text{ mL}$$

To convert units of measurement within the household system, you need to know the equivalent. For example, when converting fluid ounces to quarts, you know that 32 ounces is the equivalent of 1 quart. To convert 8 ounces to a quart measurement, divide 8 by 32 to get the equivalent, $\frac{1}{4}$ or 0.25 quart.

Conversion Between Systems. Frequently you calculate the correct dose of a medication by converting weights or volumes from one system of measurement to another. For example, metric units are converted to equivalent household measures to ease medication administration at home. To convert from one measurement system to another, always use equivalent measurements. Tables of equivalent measurements are available in all health care institutions. The pharmacist is also a good resource.

Before making a conversion, compare the measurement system available with what was ordered. For example, a health care provider orders 10 mL of Robitussin (guaifenesin) for your patient. To provide proper instruction to the patient, you convert "mL" to a common household measurement. By referring to a table such as Table 17-5, you determine that 10 mL = 2 tsp. Therefore you instruct the patient to take 2 tsp of Robitussin.

Dosage Calculations. Dosage calculation methods include the ratio and proportion method, the formula method, and dimensional analysis. Use the method that is the most logical to you. Before you begin any calculation, make a mental estimate of the approximate and reasonable dosage. If your estimate does not closely match the answer you calculate, you need to recheck your math before preparing and administering the medication. Many nursing students feel uncomfortable or anxious when they have to do medication calculations (Wright, 2010). To enhance accuracy and decrease your anxiety, think critically about the steps you go through in calculating medications and practice doing calculations to feel more confident about your math skills (Walsh, 2008). In addition, choose a method of calculation with which you are most comfortable and use it consistently (Gray Morris, 2010).

Most health care agencies require a nurse to double-check calculations with another nurse before giving medications, especially when the risk for giving the wrong medication dose is high (e.g., heparin or insulin). *Always* have another nurse or health care professional double-check your work if the answer to a medication calculation seems unreasonable or inappropriate.

The Ratio and Proportion Method. A ratio indicates the relationship between two numbers. The numbers in a ratio are separated by a colon (:). The colon in the ratio indicates that you need to use division. Think of a ratio as a fraction; the number to the left is the numerator and the number to the right is the denominator. For example, the ratio 1:2 is the same as $\frac{1}{2}$. A proportion is an equation that has two ratios of equal value. Write a proportion in one of three ways:

Example 1: $1:2 = 5:10$

Example 2: $1:2::5:10$

Example 3: $1/2 = 5/10$

In a proportion the first and last numbers are called the *extremes* and the second and third numbers are called the *means*. If you multiply the extremes, you get the same result as if you multiplied the means. For example, in the preceding proportions, if you multiply the means and extremes, you end up with the following equations: $1 \times 10 = 10$ and $2 \times 5 = 10$. Because the numbers in a proportion are in a specific relationship with one another, if you know three of the numbers in the proportion, it is easy to calculate the unknown number. To use this method, you first need to make sure that all terms are in the same unit and system of measurement. After estimating the correct dose in your mind, set up the proportion, labeling all terms in the proportion. Place the ratio that you know (e.g., information on the drug label) first. Put the terms of the ratio in the same sequence (e.g., mg:mL = mg:mL).

Cross multiply the means and the extremes and then divide both sides by the number before the × to obtain the dosage. Always remember to label your answer. If your answer is not close to your estimate, recheck your math.

Example: A patient's health care provider ordered 100 mg of phenytoin (Dilantin) to be administered in a gastric tube. The solution comes in a bottle labeled phenytoin 125 mg/5 mL. To calculate how much you need to give, you use the following steps:

1. Estimate the answer: The amount you have to give is a little less than the amount that is provided in the solution. Therefore the patient needs a little less than 5 mL of medication.
2. Set up the proportion:

$$\frac{125\text{ mg}}{5\text{ mL}} = \frac{100\text{ mg}}{x\text{ mL}}$$

3. Cross multiply the means and the extremes:

$$125x = 100 \times 5$$

$$125x = 500$$

4. Divide both sides by the number before *x*:

$$\frac{125x}{125} = \frac{500}{125}$$

$$x = \frac{500}{125}$$

$$x = 4\text{ mL}$$

5. Compare your estimate from Step 1 with your answer in Step 4: The answer (4 mL) is close to the estimated amount (a little less than 5 mL). Therefore your answer is correct; prepare and administer 4 mL in the patient's gastric tube.

The Formula Method. When using the formula method to calculate medication dosages, you memorize the formula and substitute information from the medication order into the formula. Estimate what you think the answer should be; then place and label all the information from the medication order into the formula. Ensure that all measures in the formula are in the same units and system of measurement before calculating the dosage. If the measures are not in the same measurement system, convert the numbers to the same system before calculating the dosage. Calculate and label your answer. Compare your answer to your estimated answer; if your estimate is not similar to your answer, recheck your math. Use the following basic formula when using the formula method:

$$\frac{\text{Dose ordered}}{\text{Dose on hand}} \times \text{Amount on hand} = \text{Amount to administer}$$

The dose ordered is the amount of medication prescribed. The dose on hand is the weight or volume of medication available in units supplied by the pharmacy. It is expressed on the medication label as the contents of a tablet or capsule or as the amount of medication dissolved per unit volume of liquid. The amount on hand is the basic unit or quantity of the medication that contains the dose on hand. For solid medications the amount on hand is usually one capsule or tablet. The amount of liquid on hand depends on the container (e.g., 1 mL or 1 L). The amount to administer is the actual amount of available medication that you will administer. You always express your answer in the same unit as the amount on hand.

Example: Your patient needs to receive Demerol (meperidine), 50 mg IM (dose ordered). The medication is available only in ampules containing 100 mg (dose on hand) in 1 mL (amount on hand). You apply the formula method as follows:

1. Estimate the answer: The medication is a liquid; thus you need to figure out the answer in milliliters. The amount that you need to give is ½ of what the dose is, so your answer is going to be about a ½ mL.
2. Set up the formula:

$$\frac{\text{Dose ordered}}{\text{Dose on hand}} \times \text{Amount on hand} = \text{Amount to administer}$$

$$\frac{50\text{ mg}}{100\text{ mg}} \times 1\text{ mL} = \text{Amount to administer}$$

3. Calculate your answer:

$$\frac{50\text{ mg}}{100\text{ mg}} \times 1\text{ mL} = 0.5\text{ mL}$$

4. Compare your estimate from Step 1 with your answer in Step 3: both your estimate and your answer are the same; prepare 0.5 mL in a syringe and administer it to your patient.

Dimensional Analysis. Dimensional analysis is also known as the factor-label method or the unit factor method. Because only one equation is needed and the same steps are used in solving every medication problem, you do not have to memorize formulas. Dimensional analysis requires you to use your critical thinking skills. Some nursing students who use dimensional analysis calculate medications more accurately than when they use the formula method (Koohestani and Baghcheghi, 2010). Use the following steps to solve medication problems using dimensional analysis:

1. Identify the unit of measure that you need to administer. For example, if you are giving a pill, you are usually giving a tablet or a capsule; for parenteral or oral medications the unit is milliliters.
2. Estimate the answer in your mind.
3. Place the name or appropriate abbreviation for *x* on the left side of the equation (e.g., *x* tab, *x* mL).
4. Place available information from the problem in a fraction format on the right side of the equation. Place the abbreviation or unit that matches what you are going to administer (determined in Step 1) in the numerator.

5. Look at the medication order and add other factors into the problem. Set up the numerator so it matches the unit in the previous denominator.
6. Cancel out like units of measurement on the right side of the equation. You should end up with only one unit left in the equation, and it should match the unit on the left side of the equation.
7. Reduce to the lowest terms if possible and solve the problem or solve for *x*. Label your answer.
8. Compare your estimate from Step 1 with your answer in Step 2.

Example: A patient's health care provider orders 0.5 g of ampicillin to be given IM q8h. You have a vial of ampicillin that says 250 mg/mL. Calculate the dose to administer using dimensional analysis by following these steps:

1. *Identify the unit of measure that you need to administer:* This medication is given intramuscularly, which is a parenteral medication. Therefore your answer will be in milliliters (mL).
2. *Estimate the answer in your mind:* The medication order of 0.5 g is larger than 250 mg. Because the medication is in a vial of 250 mg in 1 mL, you will need to give more than 1 mL. Based on your knowledge about converting in the metric system, you convert 0.5 g to milligrams by moving the decimal point three places to the right. Therefore 0.5 g is the same as 500 mg. The number 500 is 2 times 250; thus the answer is about 2 mL.
3. *Place the name or appropriate abbreviation for x on the left side of the equation:*

$$x \text{ mL} =$$

4. *Place available information from the problem in a fraction format on the right side of the equation:* You are going to administer the medication in milliliters, so place the milliliter in the numerator.

$$x \text{ mL} = \frac{1 \text{ mL}}{250 \text{ mg}}$$

5. *Look at the medication order and add other factors into the problem. Set up the numerator so it matches the unit in the previous denominator:* The order is for 0.5 g, and the medication is available in 250-mg vials. You know that 1 g = 1000 mg; add this conversion to your calculation.

$$x \text{ mL} = \frac{1 \text{ mL}}{250 \text{ mg}} \times \frac{1000 \text{ mg}}{1 \text{ g}} \times \frac{0.5 \text{ g}}{1}$$

6. *Cancel out like units of measurement on the right side of the equation.*

$$x \text{ mL} = \frac{1 \text{mL}}{250 \cancel{\text{mg}}} \times \frac{1000 \cancel{\text{mg}}}{1 \cancel{\text{g}}} \times \frac{0.5 \cancel{\text{g}}}{1}$$

7. *Reduce to the lowest terms if possible and solve the problem or solve for* x. *Label your answer.*

$$x = \frac{1000 \times 0.5}{250}$$

$$x = \frac{500}{250}$$

$$x = 2 \text{ mL}$$

8. *Compare your estimate from Step 1 with your answer in Step 2:* Your answer is 2 mL, which matches the estimate you made in Step 2. Prepare and administer 2 mL of the medication as calculated.

Pediatric Calculations. Current evidence shows that children are 3 times more at risk for experiencing a medication error than adults. Medication errors involving children usually happen because a child received either the wrong dose or wrong amount of medication (TJC, 2008a). The risk for medication errors in children is especially high because medication dosages are often weight-based and many medications are packaged for adults.

Calculating children's medications dosages requires caution (Hockenberry and Wilson, 2011). Even small discrepancies or errors in medication amounts can negatively affect a child's health status (Gray Morris, 2010). A child's age, weight, and maturity of body systems affect the ability to metabolize and excrete medications. For example, premature infants have underdeveloped livers and kidneys, which make them especially susceptible to the harmful effects of medications. As children develop out of the newborn period, they metabolize medications quicker, resulting in the need for more frequent dosing of medications to achieve the desired effect of the medication. You sometimes have difficulty evaluating a child's response to medications, especially when he or she cannot communicate with you verbally. For example, a side effect of vancomycin, an antibiotic, is ototoxicity. If a child taking vancomycin cannot talk yet, assessing for ototoxicity is challenging.

Different methods are used to calculate children's medication dosages. Most of the time you use a child's weight to calculate the dose. You can use the ratio and proportion method, the formula method, or dimensional analysis to calculate a pediatric dose using body weight. Body surface area (BSA) is used in rare situations (e.g., determining chemotherapy doses). Refer to a pediatric or pharmacology resource and consult with a patient's health care provider or pharmacist if you have to calculate medications doses for a child.

Administering Medications

In addition to nurses, a prescriber and pharmacist also help to ensure that the right medication gets to the right patient. You are responsible to know which health care providers are able to prescribe medications. Examples of prescribers include physicians, advanced practice nurses, and physician's assistants. Practice acts vary by state, and policies vary by agency. Be sure that you are familiar with your Nurse Practice Act and agency policies when taking prescriptions and administering medications to protect your patient and yourself. In addition, you are accountable for knowing which medications are prescribed, their therapeutic and nontherapeutic effects, and a patient's needs and abilities related to medication administration. You also are responsible for evaluating the desired effects of a patient's medications.

Prescriber's Role. A health care provider prescribes a patient's medications by writing an order on a form in the patient's medical record, in an order book, or on a legal prescription pad. Prescribers sometimes use computers or handheld electronic devices (e.g., smart phones, tablets) when ordering medications. Many health care settings use computerized physician order entry (CPOE) to enter medication orders. CPOE requires a prescriber to enter essential information about the medication order, preventing incomplete and illegible orders, enhancing communication, and decreasing medication errors.

In some situations a prescriber talks directly with the nurse and gives a verbal order. Other times the prescriber gives the nurse an order over the telephone; this is known as a *telephone order*. To ensure safety, telephone and verbal orders are only given when written or electronic communication between a prescriber and nurse is not possible. When receiving a verbal or telephone order, a nurse writes the order and the name of the prescriber, signs the order, and follows agency policy to indicate that the order was verified by reading the order back to the prescriber. The prescriber countersigns the order at a later time, usually within 24 hours after making it. Follow guidelines when taking verbal orders (NCCMERP, 2006). Agency policies vary regarding who can take verbal orders and when they can be taken. Generally nursing students cannot take medication orders, and verbal orders should be taken only in emergency situations. You cannot give any medication without an order.

Prescribers often use abbreviations when writing orders. The abbreviations indicate dosage frequencies or times, routes of administration, and special information for giving medications (see Table 17-3). Many medication errors occur because of the use of abbreviations. The ISMP maintains a list of abbreviations that are associated with a high incidence of medication errors (ISMP, 2011a). *Do not use these abbreviations* when documenting medication orders or other information about medications (ISMP, 2011a; TJC, 2013b). Abbreviations often vary; check agency policy to determine which abbreviations you can use and what they mean.

Some conditions change the status of a patient's medication orders. For example, surgery automatically cancels all of a patient's preoperative medications (see Chapter 39). A transfer from a general medical unit to an intensive care unit also cancels all of a patient's medication orders, requiring the health care provider to write new orders. When a patient is transferred to another health care agency or to a different unit within a hospital or is discharged, the health care provider reviews the medications and writes new orders as indicated.

Types of Orders in Acute Care Agencies. You need to have an order for a medication before you can administer it to your patient. Five common types of medication orders are based on the frequency and/or urgency of medication administration.

Standing Orders. You carry out a standing order until the health care provider cancels it by another order or until a prescribed number of days elapses. A standing order sometimes indicates a final date or number of dosages. Many institutions have policies for automatically discontinuing standing orders. The following are examples of standing orders:

quinapril, 20 mg PO q12h

azithromycin, 500 mg PO IV daily for 2 days, then 500 mg PO daily for 7 days

prn Orders. A health care provider sometimes orders a medication to be given only when a patient requires it. This is a prn order. You use objective and subjective assessment and nursing discretion to determine whether the patient needs the medication. Often the health care provider sets minimum intervals for the time of administration. This means that you cannot give the medication any more frequently than when it is prescribed. An example of a prn order is:

magnesium hydroxide, 30 mL PO prn for constipation

When administering prn medications, you need to document the assessment data you used to decide to give the medication and the time of medication administration. Frequently evaluate the effectiveness of the medication and record findings in the appropriate record.

prn medication orders that include ranges (e.g., morphine sulfate 2-4 mg IV push q 2-4h prn for pain) are often unclear and frequently cause medication errors. If a prescriber writes an order with a range, ensure that the order follows agency policies. An example of a safer range order is: increase morphine dosage 50% to 100% if pain is moderate to severe.

Single (One-Time) Orders. A prescriber often orders a medication to be given only once at a specified time. This is common for preoperative medications or medications given before diagnostic examinations. For example:

Versed, 6 mg IM on call to OR

STAT Orders. A STAT order means that you give a single dose of a medication immediately and only once. Health care providers usually write STAT orders for emergencies when the patient's condition changes suddenly. For example:

Apresoline, 10 mg IV STAT

NOW Orders. A NOW order is more specific than a one-time order and is used when a patient needs a medication quickly but not right away, as in a STAT order. Verify your agency policy to determine how much time you have to administer a NOW medication after it is ordered. Only administer medications ordered NOW one time. For example:

Give vancomycin 1 g IV piggyback NOW

Prescriptions. Prescriptions are written for patients who are to take medications outside the hospital. The

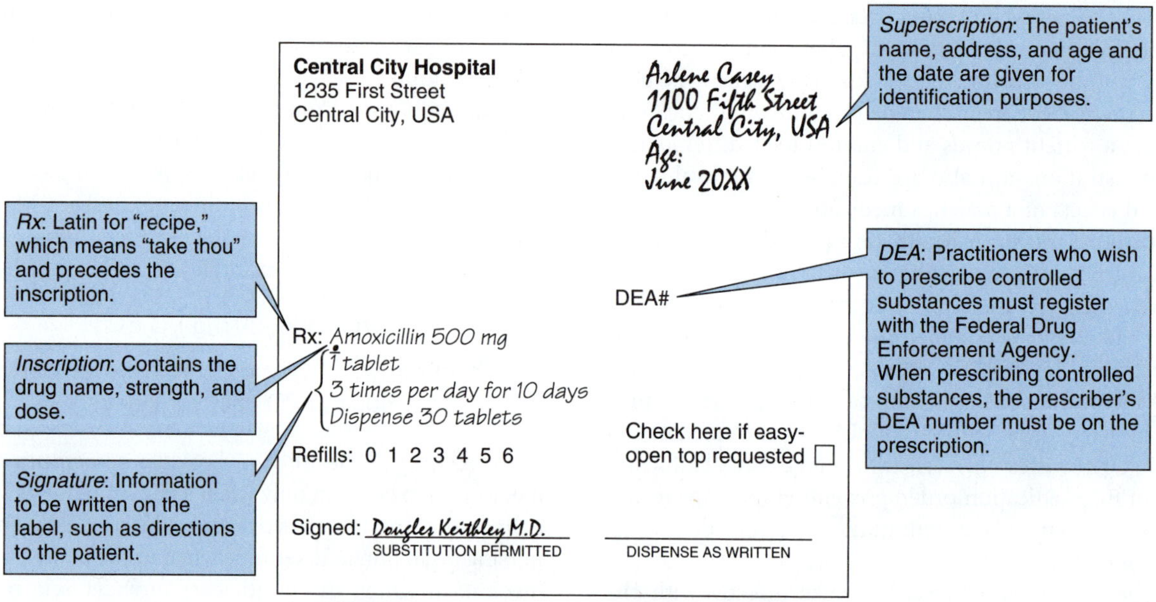

FIGURE 17-5 Example of medication prescription.

prescription includes more detailed information than a regular order because the patient needs to understand how to take a medication and when to refill the prescription if necessary. The parts of a prescription are included in Figure 17-5.

Pharmacist's Role. Pharmacists prepare and distribute prescribed medications. They work with nurses, physicians, and other health care providers to evaluate the effectiveness of medication therapy. Pharmacists assess the medication plan and evaluate a patient's medication-related needs. Pharmacists are responsible for filling prescriptions accurately and for being sure that prescriptions are valid. They rarely mix compounds or solutions except in the case of IV medications because most medication companies deliver medications in a form ready for use. Pharmacists are responsible for ensuring the dispensation of the right medication, in the right dosage and amount, and with an accurate label. Pharmacists also provide information about medications, including actions, side effects, interactions, and incompatibilities.

Distribution Systems. Systems for storing and distributing medications vary. Pharmacists provide the medications, but nurses distribute them to patients. Institutions providing nursing care have special areas for stocking and dispensing medications such as special medication rooms, portable locked carts, computerized medication cabinets, and individual storage units in patients' rooms. Medication storage areas need to be locked when unattended.

Unit Dose. The unit-dose system uses portable carts containing a drawer with a 24-hour supply of medications for each patient. The unit dose is the ordered dose of medication that a patient receives at one time. Each tablet or capsule is wrapped separately. At a designated time each day, the drawers in the cart are refilled. The cart also contains limited amounts of prn and stock medications for special situations. The unit-dose system is designed to reduce the number of medication errors and saves steps in dispensing medications.

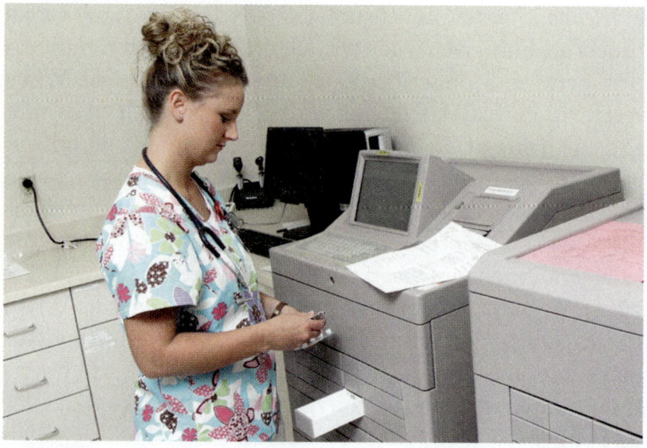

FIGURE 17-6 Computer-controlled medication dispensing system.

Automated Medication Dispensing Systems. Automated medication dispensing systems (AMDSs) are used successfully throughout the United States (Figure 17-6). The systems within a health care agency are networked with one another and with other computer systems in the agency (e.g., the computerized medical record). AMDSs control the dispensing of all medications, including opioids and other controlled substances. Each nurse has a security code that allows access to the system. If your agency uses a system that requires bioidentification, you have to place your finger on a screen to access the computer. Once logged onto the AMDS, you select the patient's name and his or her medication profile. Then you select the medication, dosage, and route from a list on the computer screen. The system opens the medication drawer or dispenses the medication, records the event, and charges it to the patient. If the system is connected to the patient's medical record, it records information about the medication (e.g., name, dose, and time) and the name of the nurse who retrieved the medication from the AMDS in

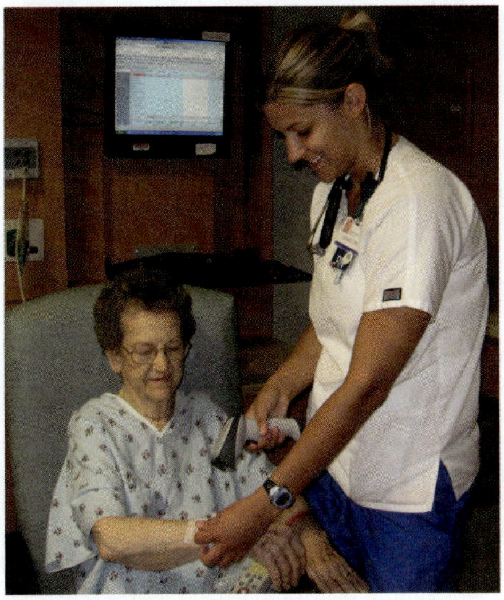

FIGURE 17-7 Nurse using bar-code scanner during medication administration.

the patient's medical record. Some systems require nurses to scan bar codes before recording this information in the patient's computerized medical record (Figure 17-7). AMDS and bar-code scanning often reduce the chance of medication errors (Mandrack et al., 2012).

Nurse's Role. When you administer medications to patients, you need knowledge and a set of skills that are unique to nursing. Responsibilities of medication administration include administering medications correctly, monitoring their effects, assessing a patient's ability to self-administer medications, and determining whether a patient should receive a medication at a given time. Patient and family education about proper medication administration and monitoring is an integral part of your role. Never delegate this to nursing assistive personnel (NAP). Use the nursing process to integrate medication therapy into care.

Medication Errors

A **medication error** can cause or lead to inappropriate medication use or patient harm. Medication errors include inaccurate prescribing; administering the wrong medication, dose, route, and time interval; and administering extra doses or failing to administer a medication. A patient death or serious injury because of a medication administration error is now a serious reportable event (NQF, 2013), which makes the prevention of medication errors a national priority (see Chapter 28). The process of administering medications is very complex; thus it is highly prone to errors. As a nurse it is essential to be vigilant in prevention of medication errors during preparation and administration (Box 17-3). Advances in technology and informatics help decrease the occurrence of medication errors (Box 17-4).

Medication errors are often related to miscommunication among the members of the health care team, product design, or procedures and systems such as product labeling and distribution. When an error occurs, a patient's safety and well-being become the top priority. As a nurse, assess and examine a patient's condition and notify the health care provider of an incident as soon as possible. Report the incident to the appropriate person in the institution (e.g., manager or supervisor) once the patient is stable.

When a medication error occurs and you are involved, you are responsible for preparing a written occurrence or incident report within 24 hours of the incident. The report includes patient identification information; the location and time of the incident; an accurate, factual description of what occurred and what was done; and your signature. The incident report is not a permanent part of the medical record and should not be referred to in the patient's medical record (see Chapters 5 and 10). This legally protects the health care professional and agency. Agencies use occurrence reports to track incident patterns and initiate quality improvement programs as needed.

BOX 17-3 STEPS TO TAKE TO PREVENT MEDICATION ERRORS

- Prepare medications for only one patient at a time.
- Follow the six rights of medication administration.
- Be sure to read labels at least 3 times (comparing MAR with label) before administering a medication.
- Use at least two patient identifiers every time you administer a medication.
- Do not allow any other activity to interrupt your administration of medication to a patient (e.g., phone call, pager, discussions with other staff).
- Double-check all calculations and verify with another nurse.
- Do not interpret illegible handwriting; clarify with prescriber.
- Question unusually large or small doses.
- Document all medications as soon as they are given.
- When you have made an error, reflect on what went wrong; ask how you could have prevented the error. Complete an occurrence report per agency policy.
- Evaluate the context or situation in which a medication error occurred. This helps to determine if nurses have the necessary resources for safe medication administration.
- Attend in-service programs that focus on the medications that you commonly administer.
- Ensure that you are well rested when you are caring for patients. Current evidence shows that nurses make more errors when they are fatigued.
- Involve patient when administering medications and address all your patient's concerns before administering them.
- Follow agency policies and protocols during medication administration; do not take short cuts.

Data from Fallis WM, et al: Napping during night shift: practices, preferences, and perceptions of critical care and emergency department nurses, *Crit Care Nurse* 31(2):e1, 2011; Mandrack M, et al: Nursing best practices using automatic dispensing cabinets: nurses' key role in improving medication safety, *Medsurg Nurs* 21(3):134, 2012; NCCMERP: *Reducing medication errors associated with at-risk behaviors by healthcare professionals,* 2007, http://www.nccmerp.org/council/council2007-06-08.html. Accessed August 1, 2012.
MAR, Medication administration record.

BOX 17-4 INFORMATICS AND MEDICATION SAFETY

Medication errors frequently happen when a nurse incorrectly administers medications at a patient's bedside. Innovations in technology and informatics have reduced the number of medication errors in nursing practice:

- Networked computers allow health care providers to see a current list of ordered and discontinued medications.
- Internet and intranet access allows nurses and other health care providers to access current information about medications (e.g., indications, desired effects, adverse effects) and specific agency policies that address medication administration (e.g., how fast to administer an intravenous push [IVP] medication).
- Some agencies have prescribers directly enter medication orders into a computer system or personal handheld computer.
- Automated medication dispensing systems, bar-coding technology, and electronic medication administration records (MARs) help with medication reconciliation, administration, and documentation.

APPLICATION TO NURSING PRACTICE

- Actively participate in the evaluation and selection of advanced technologies. Also participate in the development of nursing policies and protocols used for medication administration.
- Always follow agency policies when administering medications.
- Implement agency policies when technology cannot be used (e.g., during downtime or power outages).
- Follow manufacturer guidelines for care of electronic equipment and report problems with technology immediately.

Report all medication errors, including mistakes that do not cause obvious or immediate harm or near misses. You need to feel comfortable in reporting an error and not fear repercussions from managerial staff (NCCMERP, 2012). Many hospitals are adopting a "just culture" environment. A fair and just culture is one that learns and improves by openly identifying and examining its own weaknesses (Frankel, Leonard, and Denham, 2006). These organizations create an open, fair, and just culture to learn from errors and then adopt improved systems and processes that minimize risk of human error. Even if patients suffer no harm from medication errors, agencies benefit from learning why mistakes occurred and what can be done to avoid similar errors in the future (Popescu et al., 2011).

Medication errors frequently occur when a patient is transferred (e.g., to another health care agency or another unit within the hospital) or discharged. Therefore reconciling a patient's list of medications during the transfer or discharge process is a National Patient Safety Goal (TJC, 2014). You play an important role in **medication reconciliation** (Box 17-5). Medication reconciliation is a process in which you compare the medications that your patient took in the previous setting (e.g., home or another nursing unit) with the current

BOX 17-5 PROCESS FOR MEDICATION RECONCILIATION

1. Obtain a current list of the patient's medications.
2. Develop an accurate list of new medications to be prescribed.
3. Compare new medication orders with the current list.
4. Make clinical decisions based on the comparison (e.g., investigate any discrepancies with the patient's health care provider).
5. Communicate the updated and verified list to health care team members, caregivers, and the patient.

Data from Barnsteiner JH: Medication reconciliation. In *Patient safety and quality: an evidence-based handbook for nurses,* AHRQ Publication No. 08-0043, April 2008, Agency for Healthcare Research and Quality, Rockville, MD, http://www.ahrq.gov/professionals/clinicians-providers/resources/nursing/resources/nurseshdbk/index.html. Accessed September 4, 2013.

medication orders whenever you admit a patient to a new health care setting (Alexander et al., 2012). When the patient leaves that setting for another setting (e.g., skilled care facility or intensive care unit), you communicate your patient's current medications with the health care providers in the new setting. You also need to reconcile your patient's medications if your patient is discharged from the agency. Most health care agencies have computerized or written forms used to facilitate medication reconciliation. Reconciling medications is challenging and requires a great deal of concentration and time. Eliminate distractions and take your time when reconciling your patient's medications. Always clarify information whenever needed. You often need to consult with your patient, the patient's caregivers, family members, and the interdisciplinary health care team (e.g., physicians, advanced practice nurses, pharmacists) when reconciling a patient's medications (Balon and Thomas, 2011).

CRITICAL THINKING

Synthesis

You apply elements of critical thinking whenever you perform the nursing process with patients. Consider the scientific knowledge that you have learned, your experiences, critical thinking attitudes, and standards to ensure an individualized approach to patient care.

Knowledge. You use knowledge from many disciplines when administering medications. Knowledge of physiology and pathophysiology helps you understand why a particular medication has been prescribed for a patient and how it will alter the patient's physiology as it exerts its therapeutic effect. Knowledge about medications is also important. You need advanced knowledge about medications because of the growing number of medications readily available to patients, the acute and complex nature of patient problems, and higher acuity levels in acute care settings. Use knowledge about growth and development principles in medication administration. For example, knowledge about older adults indicates that some elderly patients have difficulty with medication self-administration because of sensory changes and lack of knowledge. Use growth and development principles to ensure that elderly patients take their medications as ordered (Edelman and Mandle, 2010).

Experience. As a nursing student you have limited experience with medication administration as it applies to professional practice. However, clinical experiences provide you with the opportunity to apply the nursing process to medication administration. As you gain experience in medication administration, cognitive skills (e.g., medication calculations and recognizing side effects) and psychomotor skills (e.g., the preparation and actual administration of a medication) become more refined. As you continue to observe patients' responses to medications, you increase your ability to anticipate and evaluate the effects of medications.

Attitudes. To administer medications safely to patients, several critical thinking attitudes are essential. For example, you show discipline when you take adequate time to prepare and administer medications. You take the time to read your patient's history and physical, review your patient's orders, look up medications that you do not know in a medication reference book, and determine why your patient is taking each prescribed medication. Every step of safe medication administration requires a disciplined attitude and a comprehensive, systematic approach.

Responsibility is another critical thinking attitude that is essential to medication administration. When you administer a medication to a patient, you accept the responsibility that the medication or the nursing actions in administering it will not harm the patient in any way. You are responsible for knowing that the medication that is ordered for the patient is the correct medication and the correct dose. You are ultimately accountable for administering an ordered medication that is obviously inappropriate for the patient. Therefore be familiar with the therapeutic effect, usual dosage, anticipated changes in laboratory data, and side effects of all medications that you administer.

Standards. Professional standards guide medication administration. The American Nurses Association (ANA, 2010) *Standards of Nursing Practice* (see Chapters 5 and 13), based on the nursing process, apply to the activity of medication administration. To ensure safe medication administration, be aware of the six rights of medication administration:

1. The right medication
2. The right dose
3. The right patient
4. The right route
5. The right time
6. The right documentation

Right Medication. A medication order is required for any medication that you administer. Sometimes prescribers write orders by hand in a patient's chart. Alternatively some agencies use CPOE. CPOE allows a prescriber to electronically enter ordered medications. This eliminates the need for written orders. Regardless of how the order for the medication is received, you compare the written orders with the medication administration record (MAR) when health care providers first order medications. In addition, verify medication information whenever new MARs are written or distributed or when patients transfer from one nursing unit or health care setting to another (TJC, 2013a).

Once you determine that the information on a MAR is accurate, use the MAR to prepare and administer medications. When preparing medications in bottles or containers, compare the label of the medication container with the medication administration order 3 times: (1) while removing the container from the drawer or shelf, (2) as you remove the amount of medication ordered from the container, and (3) at the bedside before administering the medication to the patient. Never prepare medications from unmarked containers or containers with illegible labels (TJC, 2013a). With unit-dose packaged medications, you check the medication label and dosage when you take it out of the medication dispensing system. Finally you verify all medications at the patient's bedside with the patient's MAR, using at least two patient identifiers before giving the patient any medications (TJC, 2014).

Because a nurse who administers medications is responsible for any errors related to those medications, only administer medications that you prepare. If a patient questions a medication, it is important not to ignore these concerns. An alert patient knows whether a medication is different from that normally taken. Sometimes when a patient notices a medication discrepancy, you find that his or her medication order has been changed; however, other times the patient's questions reveal an error. Never give a medication until you investigate the patient's concerns and recheck it against the prescriber's orders. If a patient refuses a medication, discard it rather than returning it to the original container. You can save unit-dose medications if they are not opened.

When caring for patients at home, teach them to keep medications in their original labeled containers. Offer patients a written schedule to help them remember which medications they need to take. Advise them to bring their medication list with them whenever entering the health care system.

Right Dose. The unit-dose system is designed to minimize errors. When you prepare a medication from a larger volume or strength than needed or when a health care provider orders a system of measurement different from that which the pharmacy supplies, the chance for error increases. Have another nurse check your work when performing medication calculations or conversions.

After calculating dosages, prepare medications using standard measurement devices. Use graduated cups, syringes, and scaled droppers to measure them accurately. At home, have patients use kitchen measuring spoons or commercially available medication measuring devices rather than teaspoons and tablespoons, which vary in volume.

Medication errors often occur when pills need to be split. To promote patient safety in inpatient settings, pharmacists split the medications, label and package them, and send them to the nurse for administration. If your patient needs to split medications at home, provide clear instructions, and ensure that the patient has a pill-splitting device at home (ISMP, 2006).

Right Patient. An important step in administering medications safely is being sure that you give the medication to the right patient. It is difficult to remember every patient's name and face. Therefore, before giving a medication to a patient, you need to use at least two patient identifiers *every time* you administer medications, even if you know the patient (TJC, 2014). Acceptable patient identifiers include a patient's name on an armband, a patient stating his or her name, or an identification number assigned by a health care agency. Do not use a patient's room number as an identifier. To identify a patient correctly in an acute care setting, compare the patient identifiers on the MAR with the patient's identification bracelet while at his or her bedside. If an identification bracelet becomes illegible or is missing, get a new one for the patient. In health care settings that are not acute care settings, TJC (2008b) does not require the use of armbands for identification. However, you still need to use a system that verifies the patient's identification with at least two identifiers before administering medications.

Implementing the required identification process requires you to collect patient identifiers reliably when the patient is admitted to a health care agency. Once the identifiers are assigned to a patient (e.g., putting identifiers on an armband and placing the armband on the patient), you use them to match the patient with the MAR, which lists the correct medications.

In addition to using two identifiers, some agencies use a wireless bar-code scanner to help identify the right patient. This system requires you to scan a personal bar code that is commonly placed on your name tag, a bar code on the single-dose medication package, and the patient's armband (see Figure 17-7). A computer stores this information for documentation purposes. This system helps eliminate medication errors because it provides another step to ensure that the right patient receives the right medication (Hook et al., 2008).

Right Route. Always consult the prescriber when an order does not specify a route of administration. Likewise, if the specified route is not the recommended route or an appropriate route, alert the prescriber immediately.

Recent evidence shows that medication errors involving the wrong route are common (Kuitunen et al., 2008; Teunissen et al., 2013). For example, enteral and parenteral medications are at risk for confusion in the pediatric population because liquid medications are frequently given orally. Therefore, when you prepare liquid medications, whether they are enteral or parenteral, take precautions to ensure that you prepare and give them correctly. Prepare injections only from preparations designed for parenteral use. The injection of a liquid designed for oral use produces local complications such as sterile abscess or fatal systemic effects. Medication companies label parenteral medications "for injectable use only." Some agencies now use different syringes for enteral and parenteral medication administration. The enteral syringes are a different color than the parenteral syringes and are clearly labeled for oral or enteral use only. In addition, the syringe tips of these enteral syringes are incompatible with parenteral medication administration systems. Needles do not attach to the syringes, and the syringes cannot be inserted into any type of IV line (ISMP, 2012).

Right Time. Know why a medication is ordered for certain times of the day and whether you can alter the time schedule. For example, two medications are ordered, one q8h (every 8 hours) and the other 3 times a day. You give both medications 3 times within a 24-hour period. The prescriber intends for you to give the q8h medication every 8 hours around the clock to maintain therapeutic blood levels of the medication. In contrast, you give the 3 times per day medication at 3 different times during the waking hours. Each agency has a recommended time schedule for medications ordered at frequent intervals. Use your nursing judgment to alter the recommended times if necessary or appropriate.

A prescriber often gives specific instructions about when to administer a medication. A preoperative medication to be given "on call" to surgery means that you give the medication when the operating room staff tell you that they are coming to get the patient for surgery. You give a medication ordered pc (after meals) within 30 minutes after a meal when the patient has a full stomach. You give a STAT medication immediately.

Give priority to medications that must act and be given at certain times. Hospitals determine which medications are time critical and which are non–time critical (CMS, 2011; ISMP, 2011b). You administer time-critical medications within 30 minutes before or after they are scheduled around the clock to maintain therapeutic blood levels. Examples of time-critical medications include antibiotics, anticoagulants, insulin, anticonvulsants, and immunosuppressive agents. Give all routinely ordered non–time-critical medications within 1 to 2 hours before or after the scheduled time or per agency policy (CMS, 2011; ISMP, 2011b).

Some medications require your clinical judgment when determining the proper time for administration. Administer a prn sleeping medication when the patient is prepared for bed. In addition, use nursing judgment when giving prn analgesics. For example, you sometimes need to obtain a STAT order from the health care provider if the patient requires a medication before the prn interval has elapsed. Document whenever you call the patient's health care provider to obtain a change in a medication order.

Before discharge from a health care setting, evaluate a patient's need for home care, especially if the patient was admitted because of problems related to self-medication administration. At home some patients have to take many medications throughout the day. Help plan schedules based on recommended medication intervals and a patient's daily schedule. For patients who have difficulty remembering when to take medications, make a chart that lists the times when to take each one or prepare a special container that organizes and stores them according to when the patient needs to take them (Figure 17-8).

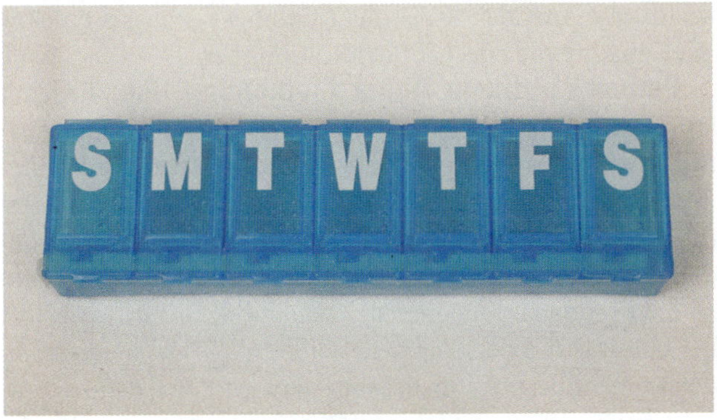

FIGURE 17-8 Medication organization container to help patients remember to take medications.

Right Documentation. Nurses and other health care providers rely on accurate documentation to communicate with one another. Many medication errors result from inaccurate documentation. Therefore ensure that accurate and appropriate documentation exists before and after giving medications.

Before you administer medications be sure that the MAR indicates the patient's full name; the name of the ordered medications written out in full (no medication name abbreviations); the time the medication is to be administered; and the dose, route, and frequency of the medication. Common problems with medication orders include incomplete information, inaccurate dosage form or strength, illegible orders or signature, incorrect placement of decimals, and nonstandard terminology. If you ever have questions about a medication order, contact the health care provider immediately to verify the order *before* giving your patient the medication. It is the prescriber's responsibility to provide accurate information about medication orders. If you are unable to contact the prescriber or resolve confusion about the medication, follow your agency policy, usually called a *chain-of-command* policy, to determine who you need to contact next. Follow your agency chain-of-command policy until you resolve issues related to your patient's medications.

Some medications require you to assess the patient before administration (e.g., taking a patient's blood pressure before administering an antihypertensive medication). Ensure that you document all preassessment data in a patient's medical record before administering a medication. Record the administration of each medication on the MAR immediately after administration. Never document that you have given a medication until you have actually given it. Inaccurate documentation such as failing to document giving a medication or documenting an incorrect dose leads to errors in subsequent decisions about your patient's care. Consider the following situation: A patient receives an antihypertensive medication before breakfast, but the nurse fails to document it. The nurse caring for the patient goes home, and the patient has a new nurse for the day. The new nurse notices that the antihypertensive medication is not documented and assumes that the previous nurse did not give the medication. Therefore the new nurse gives the patient another dose of the antihypertensive drug. Approximately 2 hours later the patient experiences hypotension, causing him or her to fall and break a hip when getting out of bed. Accurate documentation would have prevented this situation from happening.

You need to document the name of the medication, the dose, the time of administration, and the route on the MAR. Also document the site of any injections you give. Document a patient's responses to medications, either positive or negative, in the nursing notes. Notify a patient's health care provider of any negative responses to medications; and document the time, date, and name of the health care provider you notified in the patient's chart. The efforts you make in ensuring the right documentation helps you provide safe care to your patients.

Maintaining Patients' Rights. In accordance with *The Patient Care Partnership* (AHA, 2003) and because of the potential risks related to medication administration, a patient has the right to:

1. Be informed of medication name, purpose, action, and potential undesired effects.
2. Refuse a medication, regardless of the consequences.
3. Have qualified nurses and other health care providers assess a medication history, including allergies and use of herbals.
4. Be properly advised of the experimental nature of medication therapy and to give written consent for its use.
5. Receive labeled medications safely without discomfort in accordance with the six rights of medication administration (see section on medication delivery).
6. Receive appropriate supportive therapy in relation to medication therapy.
7. Not receive unnecessary medications.
8. Be informed if prescribed medications are a part of a research study.

Know your patients' rights and handle all your patients' and families' questions respectfully and professionally. Do not become defensive if a patient refuses medication therapy; all patients of consenting age have the right to refuse care.

NURSING PROCESS

ASSESSMENT

You assess many factors to determine a patient's need for and potential response to medication therapy. Perform a thorough assessment on all your patients to help ensure safe medication administration.

History. Before administering medications, obtain or review the patient's medical history, which provides indications or contraindications for medication therapy. Disease or illness places patients at risk for adverse medication effects. For example, if a patient has a gastric ulcer, compounds containing aspirin increase the likelihood of bleeding. Long-term health problems require specific medications. This knowledge helps you anticipate the medications that your patient requires. A patient's surgical history sometimes indicates use of medications. For example, after a thyroidectomy a patient requires thyroid hormone replacement.

Allergies. All members of the health care team need to know a patient's history of allergies to medications, foods, and latex. Many medications have ingredients found in food sources. For example, propofol, which is used for anesthesia and sedation, contains inactive ingredients of egg lecithin and soybean oil. Therefore patients who have an egg or soy allergy should not receive propofol (Skidmore-Roth, 2013). If a patient has a latex allergy, then latex-free gloves are applied when administering parenteral or topical medications. In an acute care setting patients wear identification bands that list medication allergies. All allergies and the types of reactions are noted on the patient's admission notes, medication records, and history and physical.

Medication History. When taking a medication history, assess which medications a patient takes, including prescription and nonprescription drugs and herbal supplements. Include the length of time the patient has taken each drug, current dosage schedule, and whether the patient has experienced adverse effects to any of the medications. If it is possible, assess if the patient takes medications correctly (e.g., count doses or have the patient keep a diary to track when medications are taken). Review information about the medications, including action, purpose, normal dosages, routes, side effects, and nursing implications for administration and monitoring. Be sure that the prescriber has ordered a safe dose, especially in the case of older adults or children. In addition, be aware of medication interactions and special nursing interventions needed for medication administration. Often you need to consult several references. Pharmacology textbooks and handbooks; electronic medication manuals available on a desktop, laptop, or handheld computer; nursing journals; the *Physicians' Desk Reference* (PDR); medication package inserts; and pharmacists are valuable resources. You are responsible for knowing as much as possible about each medication that your patients receive.

Diet History. Collect a diet history of a patient's normal eating patterns and food preferences so you can plan an effective dosage schedule (e.g., important when patients take medications around meal times). Some medications interact with food. In these cases assess when patients take these medications to determine if they avoid foods that interact with their medications.

Patient's Perceptual or Coordination Problems. For a patient with visual, muscle strength, or coordination limitations, self-administration is sometimes difficult. Assess a patient's ability to prepare doses (e.g., open containers or fill syringes) and take medications (e.g., perform self-injection or instill eyedrops) correctly. If a patient is unable to self-administer medications, you need to assess whether family or friends are available to assist.

Patient's Current Condition. The ongoing physical or mental status of a patient affects whether you give a medication and how you administer it. Assess a patient carefully before giving any medication. For example, check the patient's blood pressure before giving an antihypertensive. If the blood pressure is unusually low (e.g., systolic pressure below 100 mm Hg), hold the medication and notify the patient's health care provider. Assessment findings serve as a baseline in evaluating the effects of medication therapy.

Patient's Attitude About Medication Use. Patients' attitudes about medications affect their adherence to medication therapy. Sometimes their attitudes reveal medication dependence or avoidance. Patients do not usually express their feelings about taking a medication, especially if dependence is a problem. Observe a patient's behavior for evidence of medication dependence or avoidance. Also assess his or her cultural and personal beliefs about Western medicine to determine if his or her beliefs interfere with medication compliance (Box 17-6 and Chapter 20).

Older Adult Considerations. Adherence is the degree or extent that a patient follows the recommendations about day-to-day treatment by a health care provider with respect to the timing, dosage, and frequency of therapies (Cramer et al., 2008). Nonadherence with medications affects the health and safety of all patients and is common in older adults because they often take many medications and have complex medication administration schedules (Touhy and Jett, 2012). Medication adherence rates among patients range from 10% to 100%, depending on the type of therapy and the measurement and/or definition of adherence (Foulon et al., 2011; Kripalani, Yao, and Haynes, 2007). A patient's risk for nonadherence increases with the number of medications that he or she takes and the amount of times in a day that he or she has to take them (Bae et al., 2012; Saini et al., 2009). Poor patient education, fear of addiction, or the perception that a medication is not needed also cause nonadherence. Other factors contributing to nonadherence in older adult populations include depression, problems with cognitive or functional abilities, dislike for medication side effects, a busy and active lifestyle, and inability to afford medications. Carefully assess the medications that your patients take and compare what your patients tell you they take with what their health care provider prescribed. If you suspect nonadherence, investigate contributing factors and work with the patient to develop a medication schedule that the patient will follow. Implement interventions that help promote medication adherence. Because of the negative outcomes associated with nonadherence, determining how to better help older adults comply with medication schedules and other associated therapies has recently been a major focus of research (Box 17-7).

Patient's Knowledge and Understanding of Medication Therapy. Ask assessment questions to assess your patient's knowledge of medications (Table 17-6). A patient's knowledge and understanding of medication therapy influence the willingness or ability to follow a medication regimen. Unless a patient understands the purpose of a medication, the importance of regular dosage schedules and proper administration methods, and the possible side effects, adherence is unlikely. If a patient is having trouble adhering to medication therapy, be sure to discuss financial resources and transportation issues as well. During assessment you discover that some patients do not understand their medications. When this happens, you need to determine your patient's readiness to learn, what he or she expects to learn, his or her

BOX 17-6 PATIENT-CENTERED CARE

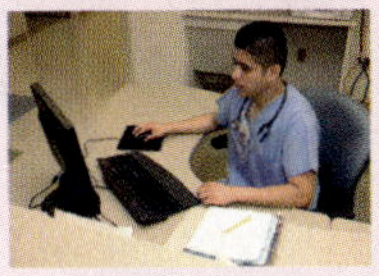

Emilio is worried that Esther will have trouble managing her medications at home because she takes so many. He knows that to help Esther manage her medications at home he needs to learn more about her culture, her attitudes about medication use, and factors that affect medication adherence. When compared with the general population, African-Americans have a greater chance of dying from heart disease, cancer, stroke, and diabetes. It is important for Emilio to assess Esther's socioeconomic status and determine if she has difficulty accessing resources such as a pharmacy or transportation to her physician. Many African-Americans have large social networks and a strong religious faith; both can be very helpful in managing illness (Giger, 2013).

Elderly patients often have many chronic illnesses. Patients with chronic illnesses often take multiple medications multiple times of the day, putting them at a greater risk for having trouble adhering to their medication schedules at home (Saini et al., 2009). In addition, the more medications a patient takes, the greater the risk of experiencing drug interactions and side effects. Sensory changes (e.g., decreased visual acuity) and changes in motor ability (e.g., fine-motor skills) also frequently affect an elderly patient's ability to self-administer medications (Touhy and Jett, 2012).

IMPLICATIONS FOR PRACTICE

- Emilio knows that not all elderly African-American people are the same. To provide quality individualized care, he assesses Esther's cultural beliefs and determines which factors affected her ability to manage her medications before she entered the hospital.
- Emilio asks Esther about her relationships with family and friends and assesses her spiritual and religious preferences. He asks her to identify family and friends who can help her when she goes home.
- Because Esther had a hip replacement, Emilio anticipates that she will have difficulty getting her medications from the pharmacy. After discovering that Esther is active in her church, Emilio gets permission from her to contact the minister at her church. He asks the minister to identify church members who are able to help Esther get to the pharmacy or go to the pharmacy for her so she can obtain her medications at home.
- Because she was so independent before her surgery, Emilio knows that Esther may become discouraged when she gets home because she will need help at home until she completely heals from her surgery. Emilio finds out that Esther has a strong sense of spirituality. Therefore he encourages her to use spirituality-based coping methods (e.g., praying, quiet reflection) when she goes home.

BOX 17-7 EVIDENCE-BASED PRACTICE

PICO Question: Do patient education interventions enhance an older adult's ability to accurately self-administer medications at home?

SUMMARY OF EVIDENCE

When older adults transition from the hospital to home, they often experience difficulty managing their home medications. This is usually because the medication routines change, they often suffer from information overload, and they are unsure about the side effects they will experience (Barnason et al., 2010). In addition, elderly patients often have difficulty affording their medications. Although the factors contributing to nonadherence in older adults have been well studied, research evaluating nursing interventions to help patients better manage their medications at home is not as plentiful (Ruppar et al., 2008). Current evidence shows that nursing interventions need to include more than just patient education (Lam et al., 2011). Effective interventions include providing individualized telephone follow-up at home (Barnason et al., 2010), allowing patients to self-administer their medications under a nurse's supervision in the hospital (Lam et al., 2011), and reducing the number of medications and frequency of doses (Saini et al., 2009). Other effective interventions include collaborating with physicians and pharmacists; providing written information about medications, medication schedules, and diseases; symptom monitoring; and motivational counseling (Ruppar et al., 2008).

APPLICATION TO NURSING PRACTICE

- Assess an older adult's learning preferences before implementing interventions to enhance medication adherence.
- Include older adults and their family caregiver when planning care for medication preparation and administration.
- Ensure that interventions include a variety of approaches, including written and verbal patient education, counseling, simplifying medication schedules when possible, and allowing the patient to self-administer medications under supervision.
- Frequently evaluate an older adult's ability to self-administer medications; if changes in orientation or ability to manage medications at home occur, evaluate the older adult for the presence of medication interactions or new side effects.

ability to learn, and what he or she understands about prescribed medications (see Chapter 12).

Patient Expectations. In assessing patients' expectations about medication administration, determine their perceptions about their illnesses and their medications. Their expectations and beliefs and their perceptions and preferences influence their adherence. Do your patients believe that their medications will be helpful? How do they feel about their adverse effects? Do they believe that they will be able to afford the medications? It is your responsibility to monitor your patients' medication adherence. To facilitate adherence develop a trusting relationship with your patients that is open, ongoing, and collaborative.

NURSING DIAGNOSIS

Assessment provides data about a patient's condition, ability to self-administer medications, and medication adherence, which you use to determine actual or potential problems with medication therapy. As you review assessment data, you see

TABLE 17-6 FOCUSED PATIENT ASSESSMENT

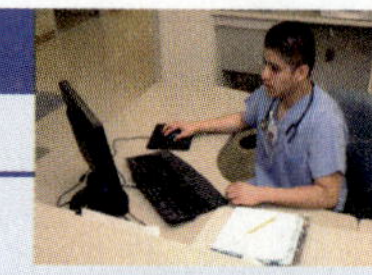

FACTORS TO ASSESS	QUESTIONS	PHYSICAL ASSESSMENT
Understanding of medication	Explain which medications you are taking and why you are taking them. How frequently and what times of the day do you take your medications?	Assess nonverbal communication to help determine if patient understands medications. Assess content of answers for accuracy in responses.
Medication side effects	How do you feel after you take your medications? Are there any symptoms that bother you?	Assess for side effects based on medications that patient is taking (e.g., if patient is on antihypertensive medication, assess blood pressure for orthostatic hypotension).
Medication adherence	Have you ever not taken all your medications as ordered? Why? Do you ever have difficulties paying for your medications? Which pharmacy do you use to fill your prescriptions? How do you get there?	Assess for expected desired effects of medications (e.g., if patient is on antidepressant, assess for signs and symptoms of depression).

clusters or patterns that reveal defining characteristics for nursing diagnoses. For example, if a patient admits to missing a medication dose and has difficulty remembering when to take medications, these data often indicate the diagnosis of *Ineffective Self-Health Management* regarding a medication schedule. Once you select a diagnosis, you need to identify the appropriate related factor. For example, the related factors of inadequate resources versus lack of knowledge require different interventions. If the patient's ineffective medication management is related to inadequate finances, collaborate with family members, social workers, or community agencies to help the patient receive necessary medications. If the related factor is lack of knowledge, implement a teaching plan with follow-up. The following is a list of nursing diagnoses that you sometimes use when administering medications to patients:

- *Anxiety*
- *Ineffective Health Maintenance*
- *Readiness for Enhanced Self-Health Management*
- *Deficient Knowledge (Medications)*
- *Noncompliance*
- *Ineffective Family Therapeutic Regimen Management*

PLANNING

During planning organize nursing activities to ensure the safe administration of medications. Current evidence shows that distractions or hurrying during medication preparation and administration increases the risk for medication errors (Haw and Cahill, 2011; Hewitt, 2010). Give yourself adequate time and avoid interruptions and distractions while preparing and administering medications. Some agencies have quiet zones in medication rooms so nurses do not interrupt their colleagues during preparation. Another way to avoid medication errors is to have all the equipment you need available before you start. Be diligent in planning and following a safe routine every time you prepare and administer medications.

Goals and Outcomes. Goals of medication administration include better control of a patient's disease, improved health, and adherence to a medication regimen. Work closely with your patients to set goals, outcomes, and appropriate nursing interventions. Whether a patient attempts self-administration or you assume responsibility for administering medications, you set goals and expected outcomes to use time wisely during medication administration. For example, if you are caring for a patient with newly diagnosed hypertension, you establish the following goal and expected outcomes:

Goal: The patient will verbalize a plan to safely self-administer all medications before discharge.

Outcomes:

1. The patient verbalizes understanding of desired and adverse effects of medications before discharge.
2. The patient describes doses and administration schedule for ordered medications before discharge.

Setting Priorities. You frequently need to set priorities during medication administration, especially when you care for multiple patients at the same time. Assess your patient's clinical condition on an ongoing basis to determine which nursing diagnosis takes the greatest priority and which medications you need to administer first. Medications that are to be administered around the clock (e.g., antibiotics) need to be given in a timely manner to maintain therapeutic serum levels. Frequently medications given for pain or to prevent serious harm to a patient such as antihypertensives, cardiac medications, and antiseizure drugs are of a higher priority than other medications. The priorities for every patient are different. It is your responsibility to know your patients and prioritize their needs appropriately.

In addition to administering medications, teaching patients about their medications is another priority. Plan to teach patients about their medications while you administer them. Family members usually reinforce the importance of medication regimens. Therefore collaborate with the patient's family or friends when you provide instruction. When patients are hospitalized, begin teaching when the patient is admitted; do not postpone instruction until the day of discharge. In outpatient or community settings, ensure that patients know where and how to obtain medications and that they are able to read medication labels.

Collaborative Care. As patients move from one health care setting to another, it is essential to establish a plan for continuity of care. Reconcile your patients' medications every time you admit, transfer, or discharge them. Communicate the patients' medication lists to appropriate members of the health care team. Collaboration with other health care team members (e.g., health care providers, pharmacists, social workers, and dietitians) plays an essential role in administering medications safely and effectively.

IMPLEMENTATION

Health Promotion. In promoting or maintaining patients' health, remember that health beliefs, personal motivation, socioeconomic factors, and habits (e.g., excessive alcohol intake) influence their adherence with medication schedules. Several nursing interventions promote adherence. These include teaching patients and their families about the benefits of medications and how and why to take them correctly. It is important to integrate a patient's health beliefs and cultural practices into the treatment plan. Make referrals to community resources if a patient is unable to afford or cannot arrange transportation to obtain necessary medications.

Patient and Family Teaching. If you do not inform patients properly about medications or if your patients have problems with health literacy, it is possible that they will take their medications incorrectly or not take their medications at all. Adapt your approaches so patients understand all medication instructions. Provide information about the purpose of medications and their actions and effects. Many health care agencies offer easy-to-read patient education sheets on specific types of medications. A patient needs to know how to take a medication properly and what will happen if he or she fails to do so. For example, after receiving a prescription for an antibiotic, a patient needs to understand the importance of taking the full prescription. Failure to do this leads to a worsening of the condition and the development of bacteria resistant to the medication. Also teach patients ways to change medication schedules to fit into their lifestyles. Patients who are placed on newly prescribed medications may need more involved instruction (Box 17-8). Ensure that everything you teach the patient and all teaching materials that you provide match a patient's health literacy level (see Chapter 12).

When your patients depend on daily injections, teach them how to prepare and administer an injection correctly using aseptic technique. Teach family members or friends these instructions in case the patient becomes ill or physically unable to handle a syringe or complete the injection. Provide specially designed equipment such as syringes with enlarged calibrated scales for easier reading or braille-labeled medication vials for patients with visual alterations.

BOX 17-8 PATIENT TEACHING

Preparing for Home Medication Administration

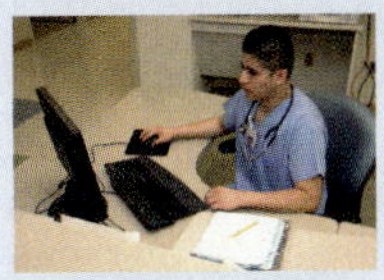

Emilio finds out that Esther will be going home at the end of the week. Before she can leave, she needs to learn how to self-administer her medications safely. Older-adult patients often have difficulty with medication adherence because they have difficulty affording medications. They also often take medications out of their normal containers, have difficulties opening medication packages, and have problems related to health literacy. Based on this information, Emilio develops the following teaching plan for Esther.

OUTCOME

At the end of the teaching session, Esther is able to self-administer her medications safely and correctly.

TEACHING STRATEGIES

- Sit with Esther at a table in a room that is well lit and has limited distractions (e.g., television off).
- Include Esther's family caregivers in educational sessions (Ownby et al., 2012).
- Have Esther's caregiver bring all of her medications from home to the hospital. Compare the medications Esther has at home with the medications that she is going to take at home. Determine which medications she understands.
- Assess Esther's health literacy by determining her ability to understand what she reads and do simple medication calculations. If she has poor health literacy, ensure that information is presented at a level that she can understand and arrange for help from family, friends, and/or home care nurses to help her when she goes home (Cornett, 2009).
- Review information about medications, including desired effect, dose, frequency, and adverse effects with Esther. Show her how to use a medication organizer. Encourage her to leave medications not in the organizer in their original containers.
- Provide patient teaching materials that include helpful pictures to enhance Esther's understanding of prescribed medications. Ensure that the print and pictures on the teaching sheets are large enough for her to see.

EVALUATION STRATEGIES

- Ask Esther questions about her medications (e.g., "Why are you taking these medications?" "When do you take your medications?").
- Ask Esther to write out a medication schedule that includes how much of each medication she should take and when she should take it.
- Have Esther verbalize the symptoms related to the possible adverse effects of medications that she is taking and identify what to report to her health care provider.
- Have Esther set up her own medications for 1 day and evaluate her accuracy.

Patients need to be aware of the symptoms of medication side effects or toxicity. Inform family members of medication side effects such as changes in behavior because they often recognize these effects first. Your patients are better able to

BOX 17-9 COMPONENTS OF MEDICATION ORDERS

A medication order needs to have the following:

Patient's full name: The patient's full name distinguishes the patient from other people with the same last name.

Date and time that the order is written: Include the day, month, year, and time. Designating the time that an order is written clarifies when certain orders are to stop automatically. If an incident occurs involving a medication error, it is easier to document what happened when this information is available.

Drug name: The physician or advanced practice nurse orders a generic or trade-name drug. Correct spelling is essential to prevent confusion with drugs with similar spellings.

Dosage: Include the amount or strength of the medication.

Route of administration: Drug route is important because you administer some drugs by more than one route. Be sure to clarify unsafe or illegible abbreviations with the prescriber to avoid medication errors.

Time and frequency of administration: You need to know when to initiate drug therapy. Orders for multiple doses establish a routine schedule for drug administration.

Signature of prescriber: The signature makes the order a legal request.

cope with problems caused by medications if they understand what to observe for and how and when to act. All patients need to learn the basic guidelines for medication safety. These guidelines ensure the proper use and storage of medications in the home.

Acute Care Activities. In the acute care setting expert nursing interventions, timely observation, and documentation of patient responses to medications are essential. Several nursing interventions are critical to providing safe and effective medication administration.

Receiving, Transcribing, and Communicating Medication Orders. A medication order is required to administer any medication to a patient. The medication order needs to contain all the elements in Box 17-9. The process of verification of medications varies among health care agencies. During the transcription process a nurse and pharmacist check all medication orders for accuracy and thoroughness several times. They also verify that a patient's ordered medications are appropriate, taking into consideration the patient's current health problems, treatments, laboratory values, and other prescribed medications. Once they determine that the medication is appropriate, it is added to the MAR. The MAR is either printed on paper, or it is available electronically. When it is electronic, it is called an *eMAR*. Regardless of the type of MAR your agency uses, it includes a patient's name, medical record number, room, and bed number; medical and food allergies; other patient identifiers (e.g., birthdate); and the name, dosage, frequency, time, and route of administration for each medication.

For patient safety it is essential that you refer to the MAR each time you prepare a medication and have it available at the patient's bedside when administering medications. Verify the accuracy of every medication you give to a patient with the patient's orders. If the medication order is incomplete, incorrect, or inappropriate or if there is a discrepancy between the written order and what is on the MAR, consult with the prescriber. Do not give the medication until you are certain that you are able to follow the six rights of medication administration. When you give the wrong medication or an incorrect dose, you are legally responsible for the error.

Accurate Dosage Calculation and Measurement. You calculate each dose when preparing medications. To avoid calculation errors pay close attention to the process of calculation and avoid interruptions from other people or nursing activities. Ask another nurse to double-check your calculations against the prescriber's order if you are in doubt about the accuracy of your calculation or if you are calculating a new or unusual dose.

Correct Administration. Before administering a medication, verify the patient's identity by using at least two patient identifiers (TJC, 2014). Identifiers are usually on a patient's armband. Compare the two identifiers with the MAR to ensure that you are giving the medications to the correct patient. You also can ask the patient to state his or her name as a third identifier. Use aseptic technique and proper procedures when handling and giving medications. Some medications require an assessment before administration (e.g., assessing heart rate before giving a cardiac glycoside).

Recording Medication Administration. After administering a medication, you record it immediately on the appropriate record form. Never chart a medication before administering it. Recording immediately after administration prevents errors. The recording of a medication includes the name of the medication, dosage, route, and exact time of administration. Some agency policies require that you record the location of an injection.

If a patient refuses a medication or is undergoing tests or procedures that result in a missed dose, explain why you did not give the medication in the nurses' notes. Some agencies require that you circle the prescribed administration time on the medication record when a patient misses a dose. Be sure to follow all agency policies when documenting medication administration.

Restorative and Continuing Care. Because of the numerous types of restorative care settings, medication administration activities vary. In the home care and rehabilitation settings, patients usually administer their own medications. However, patients with functional limitations often need help from caregivers. Provide education to patients and/or caregivers to help them administer medications accurately and safely.

Special Considerations for Administering Medications to Specific Age-Groups. A patient's developmental level affects how you administer medications. Knowledge of your patient's developmental needs helps you anticipate responses to medication therapy.

Infants and Children. Children vary in age; weight; surface area; and the ability to absorb, metabolize, and excrete medications. Children's medication dosages are usually lower than

BOX 17-10 TIPS FOR ADMINISTERING MEDICATIONS TO CHILDREN

ORAL MEDICATIONS

- Liquids are safer and easier to swallow than pills to avoid aspiration.
- Use droppers for administering liquids to infants; straws often help older children swallow pills.
- Offer juice, a soft drink, or a frozen juice bar after child swallows a drug.
- When mixing drugs with foods or liquids use only a small amount. Children sometimes refuse to take all of a larger mixture.
- Avoid mixing medications in a child's favorite foods or liquids because the child may later refuse them.
- Use a plastic, disposable oral syringe to prepare liquid doses, especially those less than 10 mL (cups, teaspoons, and droppers do not provide accurate measures).

INJECTIONS

- Be very careful when selecting IM injection sites. Infants and small children have underdeveloped muscles.
- Children can be unpredictable and uncooperative. Have someone available to hold a child if needed.
- Always awaken a sleeping child before giving him or her an injection.
- Distracting a child with conversation or a toy reduces pain perception.
- Give the injection quickly and do not fight with the child.
- Apply a lidocaine ointment to an injection site per protocol before the injection to reduce the pain perception during the injection.

IM, Intramuscular.

those of adults, but children require higher dosages of some medications than adults. Therefore take special caution when preparing medications for children (Box 17-10). Medications are not always prepared and packaged in standardized dose ranges for children and often require careful calculations. In many pediatric settings it is standard practice to have a second nurse verify all dose calculations to ensure safe medication administration. A child's parents often are valuable resources for determining the best way to give the child medications. Sometimes it is less traumatic for the child if a parent gives the medication while you supervise.

Older Adults. Older adults also require special consideration during medication administration (Box 17-11). In addition to physiological changes of aging (Figure 17-9), behavioral and economic factors influence an older person's use of medications.

Polypharmacy. Polypharmacy happens when a patient uses two or more medications to treat the same illness, takes two or more medications from the same chemical class, or uses two or more medications with the same or similar actions to treat different illnesses. It also occurs when the patient mixes nutritional supplements or herbal products with medications (Touhy and Jett, 2012). Because many older adults suffer chronic health problems, polypharmacy is common (Zwicker and Fulmer, 2012). When patients experience polypharmacy, there is a high risk for medication interactions with other medications and with foods that patients eat. There is also an increased risk for adverse drug reactions (ADRs).

Sometimes polypharmacy happens when multiple drugs are needed to treat a patient's illnesses. For example, an older adult needs to take a diuretic, a beta-blocker, and an angiotensin-converting enzyme (ACE) inhibitor to control her blood pressure. However, polypharmacy becomes harmful when a patient takes more medications than needed. Many factors contribute to polypharmacy. Taking OTC medications frequently, lack of knowledge about medications, incorrect beliefs about medications, and visiting several health care providers to treat different illnesses increase the risk for polypharmacy. Implement the following nursing interventions to decrease the risks associated with polypharmacy and ADRs (Zwicker and Fulmer, 2012):

- Complete a comprehensive medication assessment any time the older adult enters the health care system, focusing on:
  - Prescribed and OTC medications, vitamins, supplements, and herbal remedies.
  - Use of alcohol and illicit drugs.
  - Symptoms of and/or risks for ADRs.
- Collaborate and communicate frequently with the interdisciplinary team about your patient's medications.

BOX 17-11 CARE OF THE OLDER ADULT

Special Considerations for Administering Medication to Older Adults

- Involve patients in decision making about their medications as much as possible; empowering and educating patients allows older adults to make educated decisions and reduces chances of experiencing adverse drug reactions (Zwicker and Fulmer, 2012).
- Have patient take medications in a comfortable setting that is free from distractions.
- Include a family member or caregiver when providing education about medications (Touhy and Jett, 2012).
- If the patient has difficulty swallowing a large capsule or tablet, ask the health care provider to substitute a liquid medication if possible. Remember that crushing a tablet and placing it in applesauce or fruit juice distorts the action of some medications, reduce the dose, or cause choking or aspiration of particles of medication or applesauce.
- Provide memory aids in print large enough for the patient to see (Touhy and Jett, 2012).
- Watch the patient remove the caps from pill bottles and prepare medications to ensure that he or she is preparing and taking medications accurately.
- Try alternatives to medications when appropriate such as proper diet instead of vitamins, exercise instead of laxatives, bedtime snacks instead of hypnotics, weight reduction, and limited salt or fats in diet instead of antihypertensive agents (Zwicker and Fulmer, 2012).

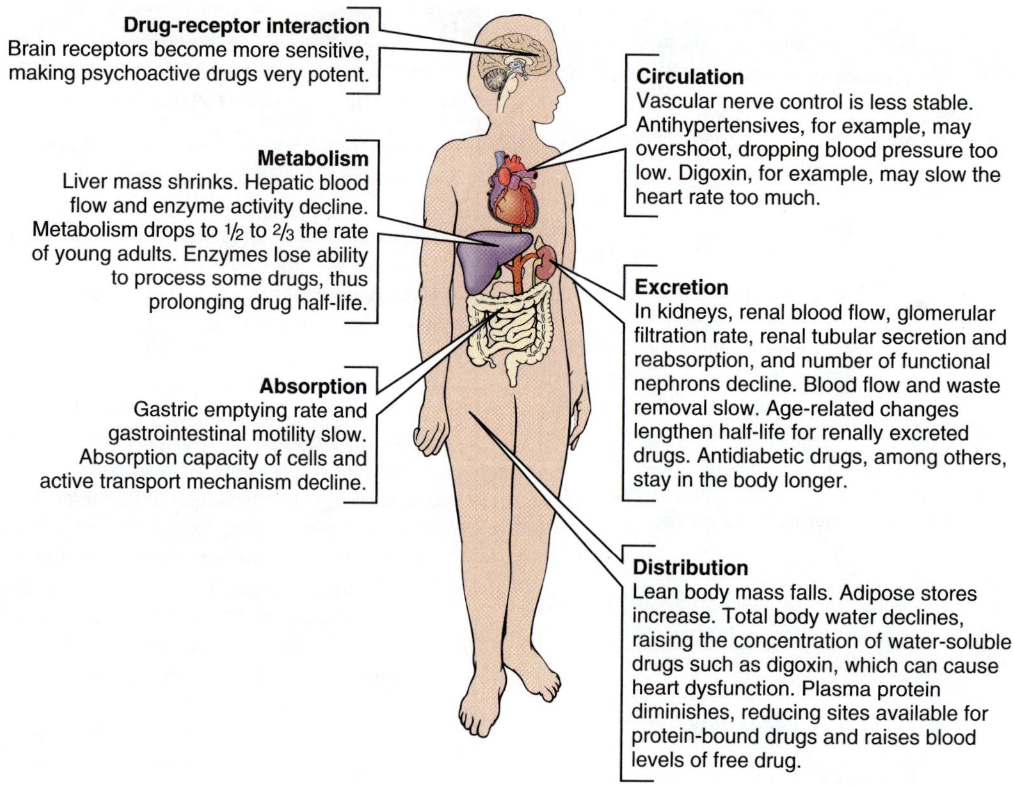

FIGURE 17-9 Effects of aging on drug metabolism. (From Lewis SL et al: *Medical-surgical nursing,* ed 8, St Louis, 2011, Mosby.)

- When reviewing your patient's medications, consider:
  - Is this the lowest and most effective dose possible?
  - Do any of the medications need to be discontinued?
  - Are there safer medications that would be just as effective?
  - What is your patient's renal function?
- If your patient develops new symptoms, determine if they are a cause of an ADR before asking for or administering a new medication to treat the symptoms.
- Keep your patient's medication list up-to-date.
- Encourage patients to only go to one pharmacy for prescriptions.

EVALUATION

Evaluation of medication administration is an essential role of professional nursing that requires critical thinking skills and knowledge of medications, physiology, and pathophysiology (Box 17-12). Thoroughly and accurately gather data and complete a holistic evaluation of your patients. Their clinical condition can change minute by minute. Compare expected and actual findings and determine if predicted changes have occurred in their response to their medications. When patients do not experience the expected outcomes of their medication therapy, investigate possible reasons and determine appropriate revision of the patient's care plan.

Patient Care. The goal of safe and effective medication administration involves careful evaluation of the patient's response to therapy and ability to assume responsibility for self-care. Constantly ask questions and use your knowledge of each of your patients' medications to evaluate their responses to them on an ongoing basis. Is the change in your patient's condition related to a change in health status, does it result from medications, or both? Ask your patients questions and evaluate a variety of data to determine if they are experiencing the desired effects of their medications. Also determine if your patients are experiencing any ADRs.

You use many different measures to evaluate patient responses to medications: direct observation of physiological measures (e.g., blood pressure or laboratory values), behavioral responses (e.g., level of agitation), and rating scales (e.g., pain scale). Also use patient statements and responses to questions you ask as evaluative measures (e.g., "I slept better last night"). Review your patients' goals, expected outcomes, and corresponding evaluative measures when determining effects of medication therapy.

Patient Expectations. When evaluating the effectiveness of medications, it is also essential to determine if your patients are experiencing the outcomes of the medications that they desire. Select an evaluation method based on your patients' expectations, knowledge level, and cognitive and psychomotor abilities. For example, when caring for patients who are in pain, ask if their medications are effective in relieving their pain. When caring for patients who take eyedrops, it is important to watch them instill the drops into their eyes. When patients have to prepare and administer injections

BOX 17-12 EVALUATION

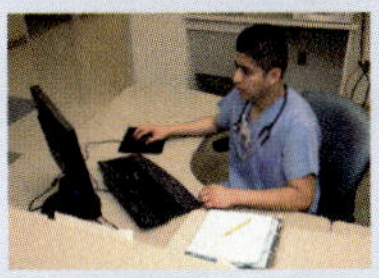

Emilio continues to care for Esther and learns that she will be going home soon. He knows from the preparation that he did before caring for Esther that older-adult African-American women often have trouble adhering to their medications when they are discharged from the hospital. He knows that issues related to poor knowledge about the medications, transportation, and cost often prohibit patients from taking their medications. Therefore he asks Esther to explain the purpose, dosage, and adverse effects of each medication. As Esther describes her medications, Emilio reinforces information as needed and gives her medication teaching sheets. He asks her if she thinks she is going to have any difficulty getting her medications. Esther tells Emilio that she knows she will be able to afford her medications but she is worried because she is not going to be able to drive when she goes home. Together they decide that Emilio will call her pastor to see if there is anyone in her church who can help her get to the pharmacy.

DOCUMENTATION NOTE

"Provided patient education and teaching sheets for all medications. Verbalizes understanding of medications and was able to teach back all information except for information about treatment of hypoglycemia related to glyburide. States does not anticipate financial difficulties in paying for medications but is concerned about transportation issues on discharge. Will reinforce signs, symptoms, treatment, and prevention of hypoglycemia and contact pastor per patient's request to determine availability of transportation assistance."

BOX 17-13 INTERVENTIONS TO PREVENT ASPIRATION OF MEDICATIONS IN PATIENTS WITH DYSPHAGIA

- Allow patient to self-administer medications if possible.
- Position patient in an upright, seated position with feet flat on the floor, hips and knees at 90 degrees, head midline, and back erect if possible.
- When patient puts the medication in the mouth, make sure that chin is tucked or tilted down slightly. When patient swallows, the chin can be lifted, and the head tilted back to help the medication get into the stomach.
- If patient has unilateral weakness, place the medication in the stronger side of the mouth. Turning the head toward the weaker side helps the medication move down the stronger side of the esophagus.
- Administer medications one at a time, ensuring that patient swallows each medication before introducing the next one.
- Thicker liquids are often easier to tolerate. Thicken regular liquids or offer fruit nectars to enhance swallowing.
- You can crush some medications and place them into pureed foods if necessary. Refer to a medication reference to verify which medications are safe to crush.
- Straws decrease the amount of control that patient has over the amount of fluid taken into the mouth. Therefore do not have patient use a straw.
- Time medications to coincide with meals if appropriate.
- Give medications at times when patient is well rested and awake.
- Minimize distractions during medication administration times.
- If dysphagia is severe, explore alternative routes of administration (e.g., intravenous).

(e.g., insulin), you need to watch them prepare the medication in the syringe and administer the injection. To determine if your patients adhere to and understand their medication schedules, ask them to verbalize when they take their medications and how much they take or ask them to write out their schedule for you on a piece of paper. Ask your patients to describe how they feel about taking their medications and if they are experiencing any difficulties with or unexpected reactions to them. Involving patients in the evaluation of their medications communicates that you respect their preferences and values and view them as the experts in the management of their health and their health care needs.

ORAL ADMINISTRATION

The easiest and most desirable way to administer medications is by mouth (see Skill 17-1). Patients usually are able to ingest or self-administer oral medications with a minimum of problems. Food sometimes affects the absorption of medications. Give medications on an empty stomach if absorption is decreased by food. Likewise give medications with meals if absorption is enhanced by food (Lehne, 2013). Most tablets and capsules need to be swallowed and administered with approximately 60 to 240 mL of fluid as allowed. However, some situations contraindicate the patient's ability to receive medications by mouth (see Table 17-4). Many medications interact with food and herbal supplements. You are responsible for knowing about these interactions. Understanding how food and herbals affect medication absorption helps you determine the best time to give oral medications.

An important precaution to take when administering any oral preparation is to protect patients from aspiration. Aspiration occurs when food, fluid, or medication intended for GI administration goes into the respiratory tract. Evaluate your patient's ability to swallow before administering oral medications. When there is a risk for aspiration, use certain interventions (Box 17-13). Properly positioning a patient is essential in preventing aspiration. When possible place the patient in a seated or Fowler's position. If your patient has difficulty swallowing, consult appropriate personnel (e.g., speech therapist) for a swallow evaluation before administering oral medications and use other routes of medication administration (e.g., IV or subcutaneous). Sometimes you give medications through a nasogastric or feeding tube when the patient cannot swallow. Box 17-14 summarizes guidelines for administering medications through gastric tubes.

BOX 17-14 PROCEDURAL GUIDELINES

Administering Medications Through an NG Tube, G-Tube, J-Tube, or Small-Bore Feeding Tube

DELEGATION CONSIDERATIONS

The skill of administering medications through an enteral tube cannot be delegated to nursing assistive personnel (NAP). The nurse informs NAP to:

- Watch for the potential side effects of medications and report their occurrence.

EQUIPMENT

60-mL syringe (catheter tip for large-bore tubes; Luer-Lok tip for small-bore tubes), gastric pH test tape (scale of 0 to 11.0), graduated container, water or sterile water for immunocompromised patients, medication to be administered, pill crusher if medication is in tablet form, MAR (electronic or printed), clean gloves

STEPS

1. Check accuracy and completeness of each MAR with prescriber's written medication order. Check patient's name, drug name and dosage, route of administration, and time for administration. Clarify incomplete or unclear orders with health care provider before administration.
2. Assess patient's knowledge about medication. Assess medical history and history of allergies to medications and food. Ensure that patient's food and drug allergies are listed on the MAR and prominently displayed on the medical record per agency policy.
3. Avoid complicated medication schedules that frequently interrupt enteral feedings. Investigate and use alternative routes of medication administration if possible (e.g., transdermal, rectal, intravenous).
   a. Determine where medication is absorbed and ensure that point of absorption is not bypassed by feeding tube. For example, some medications such as antacids are absorbed in the stomach. If the patient's tube is in the intestines, these medications are not absorbed because the tube bypasses the stomach (Williams, 2008).
   b. Determine if medication interacts with enteral feeding. If interaction occurs, hold the feeding for at least 30 minutes before giving the medication (see agency policy or consult with pharmacist or drug reference).
4. Perform hand hygiene and prepare medication (see Skill 17-1, Implementation Step 1). Fill graduated container with 50 to 100 mL of tepid water. Use sterile water for immunocompromised or critically ill patients (Bankhead et al., 2009). Check label of medication with MAR two times for accuracy. *This is the first and second accuracy check.*
   a. Prepare medications in a liquid form (suspension, elixir, or solution) when possible to prevent tube obstruction (Bankhead et al., 2009).
   b. Before crushing tablets, be sure that they can be crushed. Buccal, sublingual, enteric coated, or sustained-release medications cannot be crushed (Williams, 2008).
5. *Never* add a medication directly to the tube feeding (Bankhead et al., 2009). Sometimes the feeding needs to be held before and/or after medication administration. Verify this and the amount of time that you hold a feeding with your agency policy, a pharmacist, or a medication reference manual before administering the medication to maximize the therapeutic effect of the medication (Bankhead et al., 2009; Williams, 2008).
6. Take medications to patient at correct time (see agency policy). Give STAT, first time or loading doses, and single-order medications at time ordered. Give time-critical medications no later than 30 minutes before or after scheduled dose. Give non–time-critical scheduled medications within a range of either 1 or 2 hours of scheduled dose (ISMP, 2011b). Perform hand hygiene.
7. Identify the patient using two identifiers (i.e., name and birthday or name and account number) according to agency policy. Compare identifiers with information on MAR or medical record.
8. Compare label of medications against MAR one more time at patient's bedside. *This is the third accuracy check.*
9. Explain procedure to patient and educate patient about medications.
10. Elevate head of bed to minimum of 30 degrees and preferably 45 degrees (unless contraindicated) or sit patient up in a chair (Bankhead et al., 2009).
11. Grind simple compressed tablets to a fine powder. Open hard gelatin capsules and pour powder into a medication cup. Dissolve crushed tablets, contents of capsules, and powders in 15 to 30 mL of sterile water. Dissolve each medication separately (Bankhead et al., 2009).
12. Do not give whole or undissolved medications through the feeding tube (Williams, 2008).
13. Put on clean gloves. **NOTE:** If patient has a latex allergy, use latex-free gloves.
14. If continuous enteral tube feeding is infusing, adjust infusion pump to hold tube feeding. Verify placement of any tube that enters mouth or nose using pH testing (see Chapter 33).
15. Assess gastric residual (see Chapter 33).
16. Pinch or clamp enteral tube and remove syringe. Draw up 30 mL of water into syringe. Reinsert tip of syringe into tube, release clamp, and flush tubing. Clamp tube again and remove syringe.
17. Draw up medication in syringe. Do *not* mix medications together (Bankhead et al., 2009).
18. Connect syringe with medication to NG tube, G-tube, J-tube, or small-bore feeding tube. Do not use pigtail vent.
19. Administer medication either by pushing medication through tube with syringe or by allowing medication to flow into body freely by using gravity. Administer each medication separately. If resistance is felt when pushing medication through tube, stop medication administration and contact patient's health care provider.
20. Flush tube with at least 15 to 30 mL of sterile water between each medication (Bankhead et al., 2009; Boullata, 2009).
21. Once you have given all medications, flush tube once more with 30 to 60 mL of water (Bankhead et al., 2009; Boullata, 2009).
22. Restart tube feeding if appropriate. Hold feeding for 30 minutes or longer if needed to avoid changes in bioavailability of medications (Bankhead et al., 2009).
23. Clean area and put supplies away. Remove gloves and perform hand hygiene.

BOX 17-14 PROCEDURAL GUIDELINES—cont'd

Administering Medications Through an NG Tube, G-Tube, J-Tube, or Small-Bore Feeding Tube

24. Document name of medications, dose, route, and time on MAR.
25. Evaluate patient's response to medication therapy at times that correspond with onset, peak, and duration of medication. If patient does not achieve the desired effect, a different medication or route of administration is possibly indicated because of problems with drug bioavailability when given by the enteral route.
26. Use Teach Back—State to the patient, "I want to be sure I explained your medications correctly. Can you tell me the name of each of your medications, why you are taking them, how much to take, when to take them, and which side effects you may experience?" If patient self-administers medications, state, "Show me how you are going to take your medications at home." Evaluate what the patient is able to explain or demonstrate. Revise your instruction now or develop plan for revised patient teaching to be implemented at an appropriate time if patient is not able to teach back correctly.

G-tube, Gastrostomy tube; *J-tube,* jejunostomy tube; *MAR,* medication administration record; *NG* tube, nasogastric tube.

TOPICAL MEDICATION APPLICATIONS

Topical medications are applied locally, most often to intact skin. They come in many forms (see Table 17-1). They are also applied to mucous membranes.

Skin Applications

Before and during any application assess the skin thoroughly. Because many locally applied medications such as lotions, pastes, and ointments create systemic and local effects, wear gloves and use applicators when administering them. Use sterile technique if the patient has an open wound. Skin encrustation and dead tissues harbor microorganisms and block contact of medications with the tissues to be treated. Therefore clean the skin thoroughly before applying topical medications.

Apply each type of medication according to directions to ensure proper penetration and absorption. When applying ointments or pastes, spread the medication evenly over the skin and cover the involved area well without applying an overly thick layer. Apply a gauze dressing if ordered over the area to prevent soiling the clothes and wiping away the medication. Spread lotions and creams evenly onto the surface of skin; rubbing causes irritation. Apply a liniment by rubbing it gently but firmly into the skin. Dust a powder lightly to cover the affected area with a thin layer. Note the area applied and condition of skin in the patient's chart and document the name and administration of the medication on the MAR.

Some medications are given by a transdermal patch that delivers a timed-release dose for a significant amount of time (e.g., 12 hours or 24 hours). Before applying a new patch remove the old one because medication remains on the patch even after its recommended duration of use. Harmful adverse effects often occur when a patch is not removed. For example, patients who use fentanyl patches for pain management sometimes experience respiratory depression, coma, and death when they are not removed. Transdermal patches are often transparent and are difficult to find. To remind nurses to remove the patch before applying a new one, many health care agencies include an order for removal of the patch on the MAR. When you apply a transdermal patch, document that you removed the old patch and indicate where you placed the new one on the MAR. Additional safeguards include asking patients if they use transdermal patches, applying a visible label to the patch, and never assuming that an old patch has fallen off if you cannot find it; instead fully inspect the patient's skin before applying a new patch. Because patients sometimes forget to mention topical medications, make sure that you ask patients if they take any medications other than by the oral route (e.g., topical, transdermal, or cream) whenever taking a medication history (ISMP, 2007a). Be sure to remove a patch before a patient has magnetic resonance imaging (MRI) to prevent serious patient burns (Hong et al., 2010). Provide appropriate patient education. For example, current evidence shows that the absorption of medications through transdermal patches increases significantly during exercise (Lenz and Gillespie, 2011). Therefore teach patients to exercise at a lower intensity for 1 to 2 weeks when starting to take a transdermal patch to determine which side effects will most likely occur and to exercise when it is cooler and there is less direct exposure to the sun. Because of the potential for serious injury, provide thorough patient teaching to patients who use fentanyl patches; consider referring them to the teaching brochure provided online by the ISMP (2011c).

Mucous Membrane Applications

Nasal Instillation. Patients with nasal sinus alterations often receive medications by spray, drops, or tampons (Box 17-15). The most commonly administered form of nasal instillation is decongestant spray or drops, used to relieve symptoms of sinus congestion and colds. Caution patients to avoid abuse of nose drops and sprays because overuse leads to rebound nasal congestion. In addition, when patients swallow excess decongestant solution, serious systemic effects develop, especially in children. Saline drops are safer as a decongestant for children than nasal preparations that contain sympathomimetics (e.g., Afrin or Neo-Synephrine).

It is easier to have a patient self-administer sprays because the patient can control the spray and inhale as it enters the nasal passages. If patients use nasal sprays repeatedly, observe the nares for irritation. Severe nosebleeds are usually treated by the patient's health care provider with packing or nasal tampons that contain epinephrine to reduce blood flow.

BOX 17-15 PROCEDURAL GUIDELINES

Administering Nasal Instillations

DELEGATION CONSIDERATIONS

The skill of administering nasal instillations cannot be delegated to nursing assistive personnel (NAP). Instruct the NAP to:

- Watch for the potential side effects of medications and report their occurrence.

EQUIPMENT

Prepared medication with clean dropper or spray container, penlight, facial tissue, small pillow *(optional)*, washcloth *(optional)*, clean gloves (if patient has nasal drainage), medication administration record (MAR) (electronic or printed)

STEPS

1. Check accuracy and completeness of each MAR with prescriber's original medication order. Check patient's name, drug name and dosage, route of administration, and time for administration. Clarify incomplete or unclear orders with health care provider before administration.
2. Determine which sinus is affected by referring to medical record if giving nasal drops.
3. Assess patient's medical history (e.g., history of hypertension, heart disease, diabetes mellitus, and hyperthyroidism) and allergies to medications and foods. Make sure that patient's drug and food allergies are listed on the MAR and prominently displayed on the patient's medical record per agency policy.
4. Perform hand hygiene. Using a penlight, inspect condition of nose and sinuses. Palpate sinuses for tenderness (see Chapter 16).
5. Assess patient's knowledge regarding use of and technique for instillation and willingness to learn self-administration.
6. Perform hand hygiene and prepare medication: See Skill 17-1, Implementation Steps 1a-g, k, l. Be sure to compare label of medication against MAR at least two times while preparing medication for accuracy. *This is the first and second accuracy check.*
7. Take medications to patient at correct time (see agency policy). Give STAT, first-time or loading doses, and single-order medications at time ordered. Give time-critical medications no later than 30 minutes before or after scheduled dose. Give non–time-critical scheduled medications within a range of either 1 or 2 hours of scheduled dose (ISMP, 2011b). Perform hand hygiene.
8. Identify patient using two identifiers (i.e., name and birthday or name and account number) according to agency policy. Compare identifiers with information on MAR or medical record.
9. Compare MAR with medication labels one more time at patient's bedside. *This is the third accuracy check.*
10. Explain procedure to patient regarding positioning and sensations to expect such as burning or stinging of mucosa or choking sensation as medication trickles into throat.
11. Arrange supplies and medications at bedside. Apply clean gloves if patient has nasal drainage. **NOTE:** If patient has a latex allergy, use latex-free gloves.
12. Gently roll or shake container.
13. Instruct patient to clear or blow nose gently unless contraindicated (e.g., risk for increased intracranial pressure or nosebleeds).
14. *Administer nasal drops:*
    a. Help patient to supine position and position head properly:
        (1) For access to posterior pharynx, tilt patient's head backward.
        (2) For access to ethmoid or sphenoid sinus, tilt head back over edge of bed or place small pillow under patient's shoulder and tilt head back (see illustration).

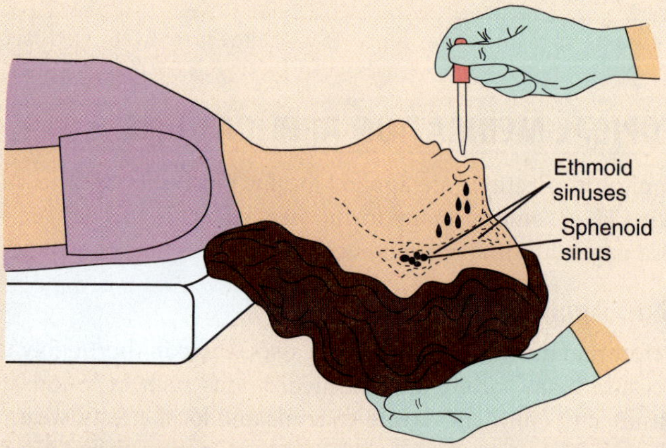

STEP 14a(2) Position for instilling nose drops into ethmoid or sphenoid sinus.

        (3) For access to frontal or maxillary sinus, tilt head back over edge of bed or pillow with head turned toward side to be treated (see illustration).

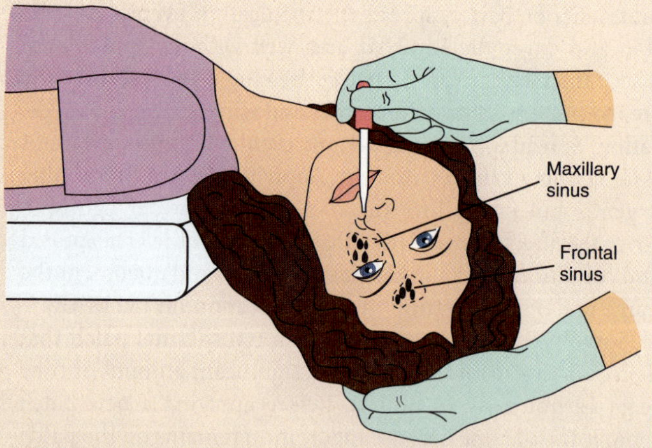

STEP 14a(3) Position for instilling nose drops into frontal and maxillary sinus.

    b. Support patient's head with nondominant hand.
    c. Instruct patient to breathe through mouth.
    d. Hold dropper 1 cm (½ inch) above nares and instill prescribed number of drops toward midline of ethmoid bone.
    e. Have patient remain in supine position 5 minutes.
    f. Offer facial tissue to blot runny nose but caution patient against blowing nose for several minutes.

BOX 17-15 PROCEDURAL GUIDELINES—cont'd

Administering Nasal Instillations

15. *Administer nasal spray:*
    a. Help patient to supine position and position head slightly tilted forward.
    b. Help patient place spray nozzle into appropriate nares, pointing nozzle to side and away from center of nose.
    c. Have patient spray medication into nose while inhaling.
    d. Help patient take nozzle out of nose and instruct him or her to breathe out through mouth.
    e. Offer facial tissue but caution patient against blowing nose for several minutes.
16. Help patient to comfortable position after drug is absorbed.
17. Dispose of soiled supplies in proper container and perform hand hygiene.
18. Document name of medication, dose, route, and time on MAR.
19. Observe patient for onset of side effects 15 to 30 minutes after administration. Ask if patient is able to breathe through nose after decongestant administration. May be necessary to have patient occlude one nostril at a time and breathe deeply.
20. Evaluate patient's response to medications at times that correlate with onset, peak, and duration of medication. Evaluate patient for both desired effect and adverse effects.
21. Use Teach Back—State to the patient, "I want to be sure I explained your medications correctly. Can you tell me the name of your medications, why you are taking them, how much to take, when to take them, and which side effects you may experience? Also, please describe what could happen if you use decongestants too frequently." If patient self-administers medications, state, "Show me how you are going to take your medications at home." Evaluate what the patient is able to explain or demonstrate. Revise your instruction now or develop plan for revised patient teaching to be implemented at an appropriate time if patient is not able to teach back correctly.

Eye Instillation. **Ophthalmic medications** are given for eye conditions such as glaucoma. Common medications used by patients are eyedrops and ointments. Some eyedrops are prescribed, and others are available OTC (e.g., Visine or Murine). Many patients who receive eye medications are older adults. Age-related problems, including poor vision, hand tremors, and difficulty grasping or manipulating small containers, affect the ability of older adults to self-administer eye medications. Educate your patients and their family members about the proper techniques for administering eye medications (see Skill 17-2). Evaluate the patient's and family's ability to self-administer through a return demonstration of the procedure. Showing patients each step of the procedure for instilling eyedrops improves their adherence. Apply the following principles when administering eye medications:

1. Avoid instilling any form of eye medication directly onto the cornea. The cornea of the eye has many pain fibers and is thus very sensitive to anything applied to it.
2. Avoid touching the eyelids or other eye structures with eyedroppers or ointment tubes. The risk for transmitting infection from one eye to the other is high.
3. Use eye medication only for a patient's affected eye.
4. Never allow a patient to use another patient's eye medications.

You administer some medications using an intraocular disk (see Skill 17-2). The disk remains in place for up to 1 week. Teach your patient receiving medications in this way to monitor for adverse reactions to the disk and explain methods of insertion and removal.

Ear Instillation. Internal ear structures are very sensitive to temperature extremes. Instill eardrops at room temperature to prevent vertigo (severe dizziness) or nausea. Although the structures of the outer ear are not sterile, you use sterile drops and solutions in case the eardrum is ruptured. The entrance of nonsterile solutions into middle ear structures can result in infection. If a patient has ear drainage, check with the health care provider to be sure that the patient does not have a ruptured eardrum before instilling eardrops. Never occlude the ear canal with the dropper or irrigating syringe. Forcing medication into an occluded ear canal creates pressure that will injure the eardrum. When administering medications into the ear, straighten the ear canal properly to allow medications to reach the deeper, external ear structures. Box 17-16 provides guidelines for administering eardrops and ear irrigations and describes how to straighten the ear canal for children and adults.

Vaginal Instillation. Vaginal medications are available as suppositories, foams, jellies, or creams. Suppositories come individually packaged and are stored in a refrigerator to prevent them from melting. After inserting a suppository into the vaginal cavity, body temperature causes it to melt and be distributed and absorbed. Administer foams, jellies, and creams with an applicator or inserter and give a suppository with a gloved hand in accordance with Standard Precautions (Box 17-17). Patients often prefer administering their own vaginal medications. Give the patient privacy to do this. After instillation of the medication, some patients wish to wear a perineal pad to collect drainage. When you give vaginal medications to treat infection, discharge is usually foul smelling. Follow aseptic techniques and offer your patient frequent opportunities to maintain perineal hygiene (see Chapter 29).

Rectal Instillation. Rectal suppositories are thinner and more bullet-shaped than vaginal suppositories. The rounded end prevents anal trauma during insertion. Rectal suppositories contain medications that exert local effects such as promoting defecation or systemic effects such as reducing nausea. They are often stored in the refrigerator until administered.

BOX 17-16 PROCEDURAL GUIDELINES

Administering Ear Medications

DELEGATION CONSIDERATIONS

The skill of administering ear medications cannot be delegated to nursing assistive personnel (NAP). Inform the NAP to:

- Watch for the potential side effects of medications and report their occurrence.

EQUIPMENT

Drops: Medication bottle with dropper, cotton-tipped applicator, cotton ball (optional), clean gloves if patient has drainage from ear; *irrigation:* irrigating solution and syringe, kidney basin, towel; medication administration record (MAR) (printed or electronic)

STEPS

1. Check accuracy and completeness of each MAR with prescriber's written medication order. Check patient's name, drug name and dosage, route of administration, and time for administration. Clarify incomplete or unclear orders with health care provider before administration.
2. Assess patient's medical history (e.g., history of dizziness, hearing loss) and allergies to medications, food, and latex.
3. Perform hand hygiene and prepare medication (see Skill 17-1, Implementation Steps 1a-g, k, l). Be sure to compare the label of the medication with the MAR at least two times during medication preparation. *This is the first and second accuracy check.*
4. Take medications to patient at correct time (see agency policy). Give STAT, first-time or loading doses, and single-order medications at time ordered. Give time-critical medications no later than 30 minutes before or after scheduled dose. Give non–time-critical scheduled medications within a range of either 1 or 2 hours of scheduled dose (ISMP, 2011b). Perform hand hygiene.
5. Identify patient using two identifiers (i.e., name and birthday or name and account number) according to agency policy. Compare identifiers with information on MAR or medical record.
6. Compare the label of the medication with the MAR one more time at patient's bedside. *This is the third accuracy check.* Hold medication container in your hands for a few minutes to bring medication to body temperature.
7. Explain procedure to patient regarding positioning and sensations to expect such as hearing bubbling or a feeling of water in ear as medication trickles into ear.
8. Teach patient about medication.
9. *Administer eardrops:*
   a. Put on clean gloves if patient has ear drainage. **NOTE:** If patient has a latex allergy, use latex-free gloves. Gently clean outer ear with washcloth if drainage is present.
   b. Place patient in side-lying position if not contraindicated by his or her condition, with ear to be treated facing up. Patient may also sit in a chair or at the bedside. If the eardrops are in a cloudy suspension, shake them for about 10 seconds.
   c. Straighten ear canal by pulling auricle down and back for children younger than 3 years or upward and outward for patients 3 years of age and older.
   d. Instill prescribed drops holding dropper 1 cm (½ inch) above ear canal (see illustration).

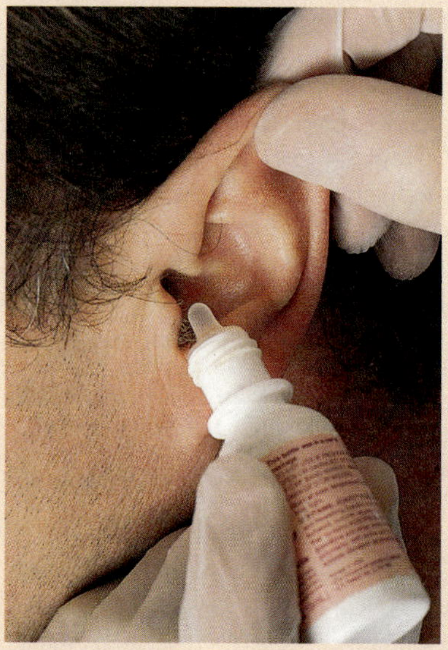

STEP 9d Instill prescribed drops holding dropper above ear canal.

   e. Ask patient to remain in side-lying position for 2 to 3 minutes. Apply gentle massage or pressure to tragus of ear with finger.
   f. If cotton ball is needed, place it into the outermost part of ear canal; do not press it into the canal. Remove cotton after 15 minutes.
10. *Administer ear irrigations:*
   a. Assess the tympanic membrane or review medical record for history of eardrum perforation, which contraindicates ear irrigation.
   b. Help patient into sitting or lying position with head tilted or turned toward affected ear. Place towel under patient's head and shoulder and have patient hold basin under affected ear.
   c. Fill irrigating syringe with solution (approximately 50 mL) at room temperature.
   d. Gently grasp auricle and straighten ear by pulling it down and back for children younger than 3 years or upward and outward for patients 3 years of age and older.
   e. Slowly instill irrigating solution by holding tip of syringe 1 cm (½ inch) above opening of ear canal. Allow fluid to drain out during instillation. Continue until you use all solution.
11. Clean area and put supplies away.
12. Remove gloves and perform hand hygiene.
13. Document name of medication, dose, route, and time on MAR.
14. Evaluate patient's response to medication at times that correspond with its onset, peak, and duration.
15. Use Teach Back—State to the patient, "I want to be sure I explained your ear drops correctly. Can you tell me the name of your ear drops, why you are taking them, how much to take, when to take them and which side effects you may experience?" If patient self-administers medications, state, "Show me how you are going to take your ear drops at home." Evaluate what the patient is able to explain or demonstrate. Revise your instruction now or develop plan for revised patient teaching to be implemented at an appropriate time if patient is not able to teach back correctly.

BOX 17-17 **PROCEDURAL GUIDELINES**

Administering Vaginal Medications

DELEGATION CONSIDERATIONS

The skill of administering vaginal medications cannot be delegated to nursing assistive personnel (NAP). Inform the NAP to:

- Report new or increased vaginal discharge or bleeding and occurrence of potential side effects of medication.
- Offer to provide perineal care following medication administration.

EQUIPMENT

Vaginal cream, foam, jelly, or suppository with applicator (if required); clean gloves; towels and/or washcloth; perineal pad; drape or sheet; water-soluble lubricating jelly; medication administration record (MAR) (electronic or printed)

STEPS

1. Check accuracy and completeness of each MAR with prescriber's written medication order. Check patient's name, drug name and dosage, route of administration, and time for administration. Clarify incomplete or unclear orders with health care provider before administration.
2. Assess patient's medical history (e.g., history of vaginal drainage) and allergies to medications, food, and latex.
3. Perform hand hygiene and prepare medication (see Skill 17-1, Implementation Steps 1a-g, k, l). Compare the label of the medication with the MAR two times while preparing the medication. *This is the first and second accuracy check.*
4. Take medications to patient at correct time (see agency policy). Give STAT, first-time or loading doses, and single-order medications at time ordered. Give time-critical medications no later than 30 minutes before or after scheduled dose. Give non–time-critical scheduled medications within a range of either 1 or 2 hours of scheduled dose (ISMP, 2011b). Perform hand hygiene.
5. Identify patient using two identifiers (i.e., name and birthday or name and account number) according to agency policy. Compare identifiers with information on MAR or medical record.
6. Compare label of medication against the MAR one more time at patient's bedside. *This is the third accuracy check.*
7. Explain procedure to patient regarding positioning and sensations to expect such as feelings of moisture or wetness in the vaginal area. Be sure that patient understands the procedure if he or she plans to self-administer medication. Teach patient about the medication.
8. Close room door or pull curtain to provide privacy.
9. Put on clean gloves. **NOTE:** If patient has a latex allergy, use latex-free gloves.
10. Be sure that there is adequate lighting to visualize vaginal opening. Assess vaginal area, noting the appearance of any discharge and the condition of the external genitalia. Cleanse area with towel or washcloth if needed (see Chapters 16 and 29).
11. Help patient into dorsal recumbent position and keep abdomen and lower extremities draped.
12. *Administer vaginal suppository:*
    a. Remove suppository from wrapper and apply liberal amount of sterile water-based lubricating jelly to smooth or rounded end. Lubricate gloved index finger of dominant hand.
    b. With nondominant gloved hand gently separate and hold labial folds.
    c. With dominant gloved hand gently insert rounded end of suppository along posterior wall of vaginal canal entire length of finger (7.5 to 10 cm or 3 to 4 inches) (see illustration).

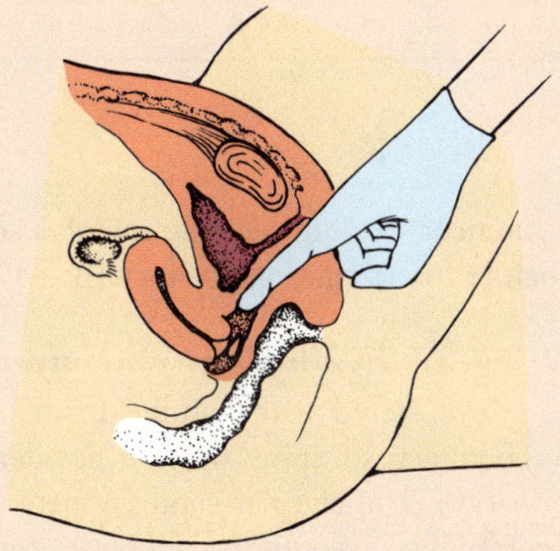

STEP 12c Insertion of suppository into vaginal canal.

    d. Withdraw finger and wipe away remaining lubricant from around vaginal opening and labia.
13. *Administer cream or foam:*
    a. Fill cream or foam applicator following package directions.
    b. With nondominant gloved hand gently separate and hold labial folds.
    c. With dominant gloved hand gently insert applicator about 5 to 7.5 cm (2 to 3 inches). Push applicator plunger to deposit medication into vagina (see illustration).

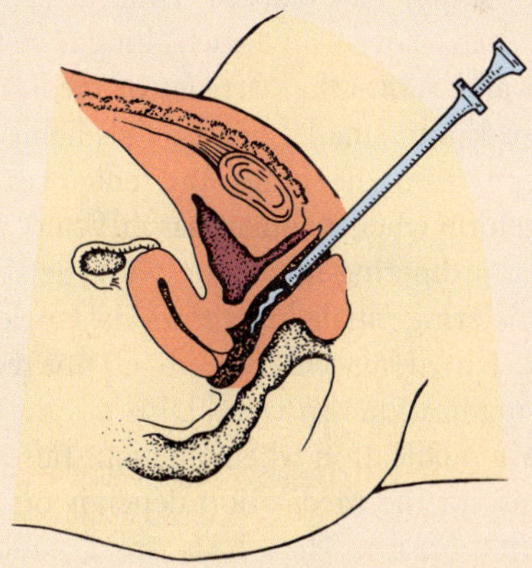

STEP 13c Instillation of medication in vaginal canal.

    d. Withdraw applicator and place on paper towel. Wipe off residual cream from labia or vaginal opening.
14. Dispose of supplies, remove gloves, and perform hand hygiene.
15. Instruct patient to remain on back for at least 10 minutes to allow for distribution and absorption of medication throughout vaginal cavity.
16. Document medication administration on MAR.
17. If applicator is used, reapply gloves. Wash applicator with soap and warm water, rinse, and store for future use.

Continued

BOX 17-17 PROCEDURAL GUIDELINES—cont'd

Administering Vaginal Medications

18. Offer perineal pad to patient when she begins to ambulate.
19. Evaluate patient's response to medication and ability to administer it.
20. Use Teach Back—State to the patient, "I want to be sure I explained your vaginal medication correctly. Can you tell me the name of your medication, why you are taking it, how much to take, when to take it, and which side effects you may experience?" If patient self-administers medication, state, "Show me how you are going to take your vaginal medication at home." Evaluate what the patient is able to explain or demonstrate. Revise your instruction now or develop plan for revised patient teaching to be implemented at an appropriate time if patient is not able to teach back correctly.

Sometimes you need to clear the rectum with a small cleansing enema before inserting a suppository (Box 17-18).

Administering Medications by Inhalation

Medications administered with handheld inhalers are dispersed through an aerosol spray, mist, or powder that penetrates lung airways. The alveolar-capillary network absorbs medications rapidly. **Pressurized metered-dose inhalers (pMDIs),** breath-actuated metered-dose inhalers (BAIs), and dry powder inhalers (DPIs) deliver inhaled medications that produce local effects in the airway such as bronchodilation. Some medications create serious systemic side effects.

pMDIs use a chemical propellant to push the medication out of the inhaler, requiring a patient to apply about 5 to 10 pounds of pressure to the top of the canister to administer the medication. Children and older adults with chronic lung diseases often use pMDIs. Because of their diminished hand strength, be sure to assess if patients have enough strength to use the pMDI.

Sometimes patients use a spacer with the pMDI. A spacer is a 10.16- to 20.32-cm (4- to 8-inch) long tube that attaches to the pMDI and allows the particles of medication to slow down and break into smaller pieces. This helps the medication get deeper into the lungs and enhances absorption. Spacers are helpful when a patient has difficulty coordinating the steps or coordinating inhalation with the steps involved in self-administering inhaled medications. However, patients who do not use their spacers correctly do not receive the full effect of the medication. BAIs and DPIs do not use spacers.

BAIs release medication when a patient raises a lever and inhales. Release of the medication depends on the strength of the patient's breath. Thus BAIs are a good choice for patients who have difficulty using pMDIs (Restrepo and Gardner, 2010).

DPIs hold dry powder medication and create an aerosol when a patient inhales through a reservoir. The reservoir holds a dose of the medication. When DPIs are unit dosed, a patient loads a single dose of medication into the inhaler with each use. Other DPIs hold enough medication to last for a month. DPIs require less manual dexterity. There is no need to coordinate puffs with inhalation because the device is activated when a patient breathes. However, the medication sometimes clumps when a patient is in a humid environment, and some patients cannot inspire fast enough to administer the entire medication dosage.

Patients who receive medications by inhalation frequently have a chronic respiratory disease such as chronic asthma, emphysema, or bronchitis. Some inhaled medications are described as *rescue* medications, whereas others are called *maintenance* medications. Rescue medications are short-acting; thus patients take them to relieve acute respiratory distress immediately. Patients need to be cautioned not to overuse their rescue medications. If respiratory distress increases, instruct the patient to contact his or her health care provider and not to overuse the rescue mediations. He or she may need an adjustment of the maintenance medication.

Patients take maintenance medications on a daily schedule to prevent acute respiratory distress; thus their effects start within hours of administration and last for a longer period of time than rescue inhalers. Some inhalers combine rescue and maintenance medications. Proper use of inhalers improves patient outcomes and decreases mortality associated with chronic airway diseases. However, current evidence shows that many patients do not use their inhalers correctly (Restrepo and Gardner, 2010). Patient education is essential (see Skill 17-3).

Help your patients determine when inhalers are empty and need to be replaced. Do not float the pMDI in water to determine how much medication is left because the container floats even if it is empty. Devices that attach onto the MDI and count down the number of remaining doses are available for MDIs. Some DPIs have an indicator that shows how many doses are left. However, these are not always accurate. Therefore the best way to calculate how long medication in an inhaler will last is to divide the number of doses in the container by the number of doses that your patient takes per day. For example, your patient is to take albuterol, a beta-adrenergic agonist bronchodilator. The ordered dose is 2 puffs 4 times a day (qid). The canister has a total of 200 puffs. You complete the following calculations to determine how long the MDI will last:

$$2 \text{ puffs} \times 4 \text{ times a day} = 8 \text{ puffs per day}$$

$$200 \text{ puffs} \div 8 \text{ puffs per day} = 25 \text{ days}$$

BOX 17-18 PROCEDURAL GUIDELINES

Administering Rectal Suppositories

DELEGATION CONSIDERATIONS

The skill of administering rectal medications cannot be delegated to nursing assistive personnel (NAP). Inform the NAP to:

- Watch for and report fecal discharge or bowel movement and the potential side effects of medications.
- Offer to provide perineal care following medication administration.

EQUIPMENT

Rectal suppository, clean gloves, drape or sheet, water-soluble lubricating jelly, tissue, medication administration record (MAR) (electronic or printed)

STEPS

1. Check accuracy and completeness of each MAR with prescriber's written medication order. Check patient's name, drug name and dosage, route of administration, and time for administration. Clarify incomplete or unclear orders with health care provider before administration.
2. Assess patient's medical history (e.g., hemorrhoids, anal fissures, rectal surgery or bleeding) and allergies to medications, food, and latex.
3. Perform hand hygiene and prepare medication (see Skill 17-1, Implementation Steps 1a-g, k, l). Be sure to compare the label of the medication with the MAR two times during medication preparation. *This is the first and second accuracy check.*
4. Take medications to patient at correct time (see agency policy). Give STAT, first-time or loading doses, and single-order medications at time ordered. Give time-critical medications no later than 30 minutes before or after scheduled dose. Give non–time-critical scheduled medications within a range of either 1 or 2 hours of scheduled dose (ISMP, 2011b). Perform hand hygiene.
5. Identify patient using two identifiers (i.e., name and birthday or name and account number) according to agency policy. Compare identifiers with information on MAR or medical record.
6. Compare the label of the medication with the MAR one more time at patient's bedside. *This is the third accuracy check.*
7. Explain procedure to patient regarding positioning and sensations to expect such as feelings of needing to defecate. Be sure that patient understands the procedure if he or she plans to self-administer medication. Teach patient about the medication.
8. Close room door or pull curtain to provide privacy.
9. Put on clean gloves. **NOTE:** If patient has a latex allergy, use latex-free gloves.
10. Help patient to the Sims' position. Keep patient draped with only anal area exposed.
11. Be sure that there is adequate lighting to visualize anus. Assess external condition of anus and palpate rectal walls as needed (see Chapters 16 and 35). Dispose of gloves in proper receptacle if soiled.
12. Apply new pair of clean gloves if gloves were discarded in previous step. **NOTE:** If patient has a latex allergy, use latex-free gloves.
13. Remove suppository from wrapper and lubricate rounded end with sterile water-soluble lubricating jelly (see illustration). Lubricate index finger of dominant hand with water-soluble jelly.

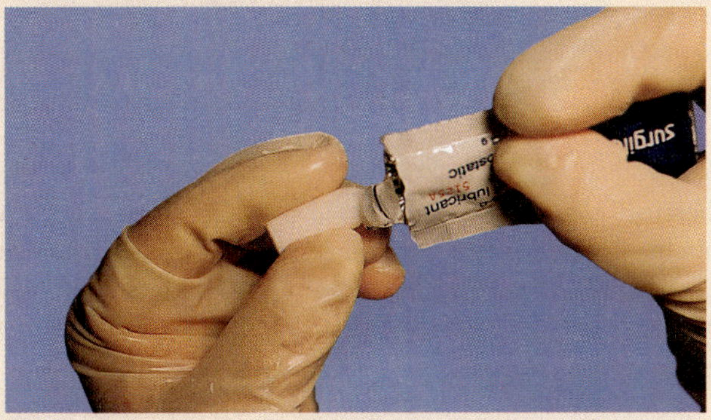

STEP 13 Lubricate tip of rectal suppository with water-soluble jelly.

14. Ask patient to take slow deep breath through mouth and relax anal sphincter.
15. Retract buttocks with nondominant hand. With dominant hand insert suppository gently through anus, past internal sphincter and against rectal wall, 10 cm (4 inches) in adults or 5 cm (2 inches) in children and infants (see illustration). You may need to apply gentle pressure to hold buttocks together momentarily to keep medication in place.

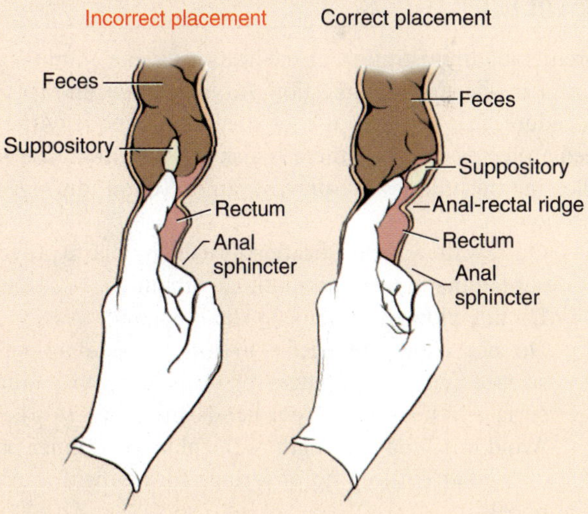

STEP 15 Inserting rectal suppository. (From deWit S: *Fundamental concepts and skills for nursing,* ed 3, Philadelphia, 2009, Saunders.)

16. Withdraw finger and wipe anal area with tissue.
17. Dispose of supplies, remove gloves, and perform hand hygiene.
18. Instruct patient to remain on side for at least 5 minutes.
19. If suppository is a laxative or stool softener, place call light within reach of patient.

Continued

BOX 17-18 PROCEDURAL GUIDELINES—cont'd

Administering Rectal Suppositories

20. Document name of medication, dose, route, and time on MAR.
21. Evaluate patient's response to medication at times that correlate with the onset, peak, and duration of the medication.
22. Use Teach Back—State to the patient, "I want to be sure I explained your rectal medication correctly. Can you tell me the name of your medication, why you are taking it, how much to take, when to take it, and which side effects you may experience?" If patient self-administers medication, state, "Show me how you are going to take your rectal medication at home." Evaluate what the patient is able to explain or demonstrate. Revise your instruction now or develop plan for revised patient teaching to be implemented at an appropriate time if patient is not able to teach back correctly.

Therefore the canister will last 25 days. To ensure that the patient does not run out of medication, teach him or her to refill the medication at least 7 to 10 days before it runs out.

Administering Medications by Irrigation

You use some medications to irrigate or wash out body cavities. Irrigations deliver a stream of solution. Sterile water, saline, or antiseptic solution irrigations of the eye, ear, throat, vagina, and urinary tract are common. If there is a break in the skin or mucosa, use aseptic technique. When the cavity to be irrigated is not sterile, as is the case with the ear canal or vagina, clean technique is acceptable. Irrigations cleanse an area, instill a medication, or apply hot or cold to injured tissue (see Chapter 37).

PARENTERAL ADMINISTRATION OF MEDICATIONS

Parenteral administration of medications is the administration of medications by injection. An injection is an invasive procedure that requires use of aseptic technique. After a needle pierces the skin, there is risk for infection. Use the following techniques to prevent an infection during an injection:

- Quickly draw the medication into the syringe to prevent contamination of solution in an ampule.
- Do not allow the ampule to stand open.
- Do not allow the needle to touch a contaminated surface (e.g., outer edges of ampule or vial, outer surface of needle cap, your hands, the countertop).
- Avoid touching the length of the plunger or inner part of the barrel. Keep tip of syringe covered with cap or needle.
- Wash skin soiled with dirt, drainage, or feces with soap and water. Use friction and a circular motion while cleaning with an antiseptic swab. Swab from center of site and move outward in a 5 cm (2-inch) radius.

Each type of injection requires certain skills to ensure that the medication reaches the proper location. The effects of a parenterally administered medication develop rapidly, depending on the rate of medication absorption. Therefore you need to observe the patient's response to the medication closely.

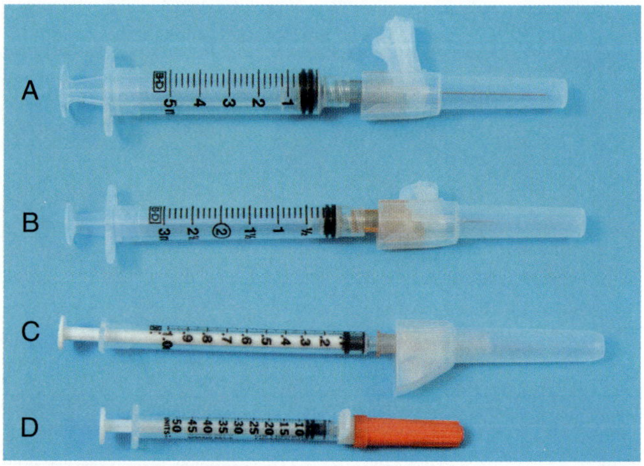

FIGURE 17-10 Types of syringes. **A,** 5-mL syringe. **B,** 3-mL syringe. **C,** Tuberculin syringe marked in 0.01 (hundredths) for doses less than 1 mL. **D,** Insulin syringe marked in units (50).

Equipment

A variety of syringes and needles are available, each designed to deliver a certain volume of a medication to a specific type of tissue. Use nursing judgment when determining the syringe or needle that is most appropriate.

Syringes. Syringes have a cylindrical barrel with a close-fitting plunger and a tip designed to fit the hub of a hypodermic needle. Syringes are single use, disposable, and classified as being Luer-Lok or non–Luer-Lok. Luer-Lok syringes (Figure 17-10, *A* and *B*) have needles that are twisted onto the tip to lock themselves in place. This design prevents the inadvertent removal of a needle. The needles on non–Luer-Lok syringes (Figure 17-10, *C* and *D*) slip onto the tip.

All syringes have safety devices to prevent needlestick injuries.

Syringes come in a number of sizes, ranging from 0.5 to 60 mL. It is unusual to use a syringe larger than 5 mL for an injection. A 1- to 3-mL syringe is usually adequate for IM and subcutaneous injections. You use large syringes to administer certain IV medications and irrigate wounds or drainage tubes. Some syringes are prepackaged with a needle attached. However, sometimes you need to change the needle based on the route of administration and the size of the patient.

The tuberculin syringe (see Figure 17-10, *C*) is calibrated in sixteenths of a minim and hundredths of a milliliter and

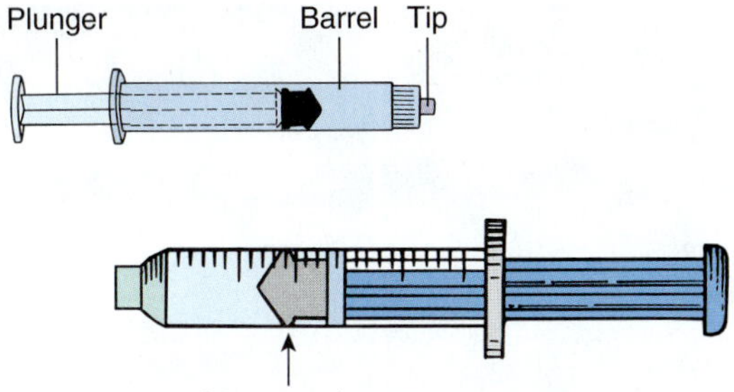

FIGURE 17-11 Parts of a syringe.

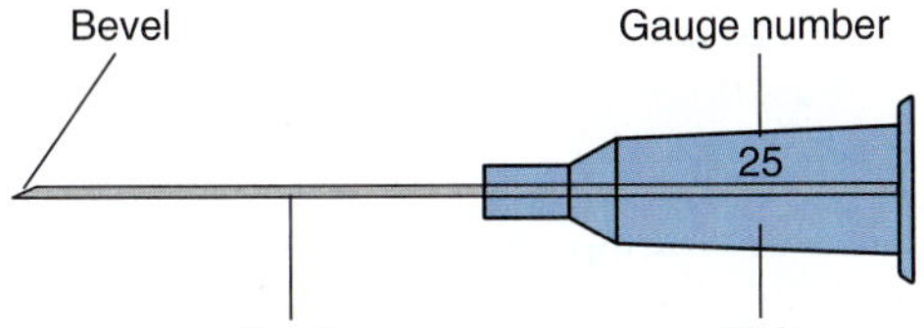

FIGURE 17-12 Parts of a needle.

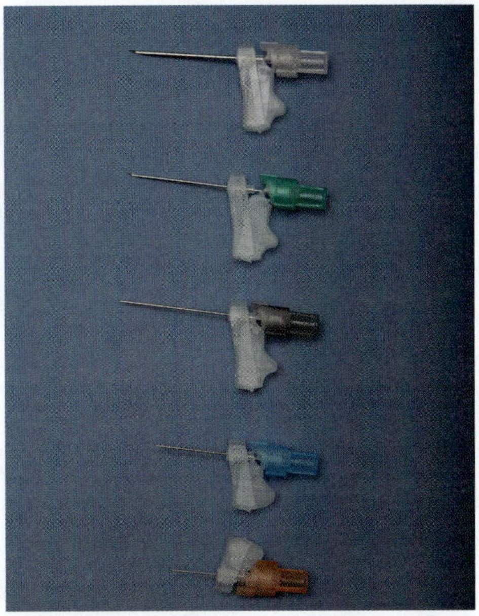

FIGURE 17-13 Hypodermic needles *(top to bottom):* 18 gauge, 1½-inch length; 21 gauge, 1½-inch length; 22 gauge, 1½-inch length; 23 gauge, 1-inch length; and 25 gauge, ⅝-inch length.

has a capacity of 1 mL. You use tuberculin syringes to prepare small amounts of medications (e.g., ID and subcutaneous injections). You also use a tuberculin syringe when you need to prepare small, precise doses for infants or young children.

Insulin syringes (see Figure 17-10, *D)* hold 0.3 to 1 mL and are calibrated in units. Most insulin syringes are U-100s, designed for use with U-100 strength insulin. Each milliliter of solution contains 100 units of insulin.

To fill a syringe, pull the plunger outward while the needle tip remains immersed in the prepared solution. To maintain sterility, touch the outside of the syringe barrel and the handle of the plunger; but do not touch the tip or inside of the barrel, the hub, the shaft of the plunger, and the needle (Figure 17-11).

Needles. Some needles come attached to syringes. Others come packaged individually to allow flexibility in selecting the right needle for a patient. Needles are disposable, and most are made of stainless steel. A needle has three parts: the hub, which fits onto the tip of a syringe; the shaft, which connects to the hub; and the bevel, or slanted tip (Figure 17-12). The tip of a needle, or the bevel, is always slanted. When injected into tissue, the bevel creates a narrow slit that quickly closes when you remove the needle. This prevents leakage of medication, blood, or serum. Long, beveled tips are sharp and narrow, which minimizes discomfort when entering tissue used for subcutaneous or IM injections.

Most needles vary in length from ¼ to 3 inches (Figure 17-13). The needle length you choose depends on a patient's size and weight and the route of administration. A child or slender adult generally requires a shorter needle. Use longer needles (1 to 1½ inches) for IM injections and shorter needles (⅜ to ⅝ inch) for subcutaneous injections. Needles also vary in gauge or circumference. As a needle gauge gets smaller, its diameter becomes larger. The selection of a gauge depends on the length of the needle and the viscosity of fluid that you inject or infuse.

Disposable Injection Units. Disposable, single-dose, prefilled syringes are available for some medications. Check the medication and concentration carefully because prefilled syringes look very similar. With these syringes you do not need to prepare medication dosages, except perhaps to expel portions of unneeded medications.

The Tubex and Carpuject systems include reusable plastic syringe holders and disposable, sterile cartridge units (Figure 17-14). When using this system, load the cartridge Luer tip first into the plastic syringe holder, secure it (following package directions), and check for air bubbles in the syringe. Advance the plunger to expel air and excess medication, as with a regular syringe. You can use the glass cartridge with needleless systems or safety needles. After giving the medication, dispose of the glass cartridge safely in a puncture-proof and leakproof receptacle.

Preparing an Injection From an Ampule

Ampules contain single doses of medication in a liquid. They are available in many sizes, from 1 mL to 10 mL or more (Figure 17-15, *A*). An ampule is made of glass with a constricted, prescored neck that you snap off to allow access to the medication. A colored ring around the neck indicates where the ampule is prescored. Aspirate the medication into a syringe using a filter needle to prevent glass particles from being drawn into the syringe with the medication (Cocoman and Murray, 2008; Nicoll and Hesby, 2002). Replace the filter needle with an appropriate-size safety needle or needleless access device before administering the medication.

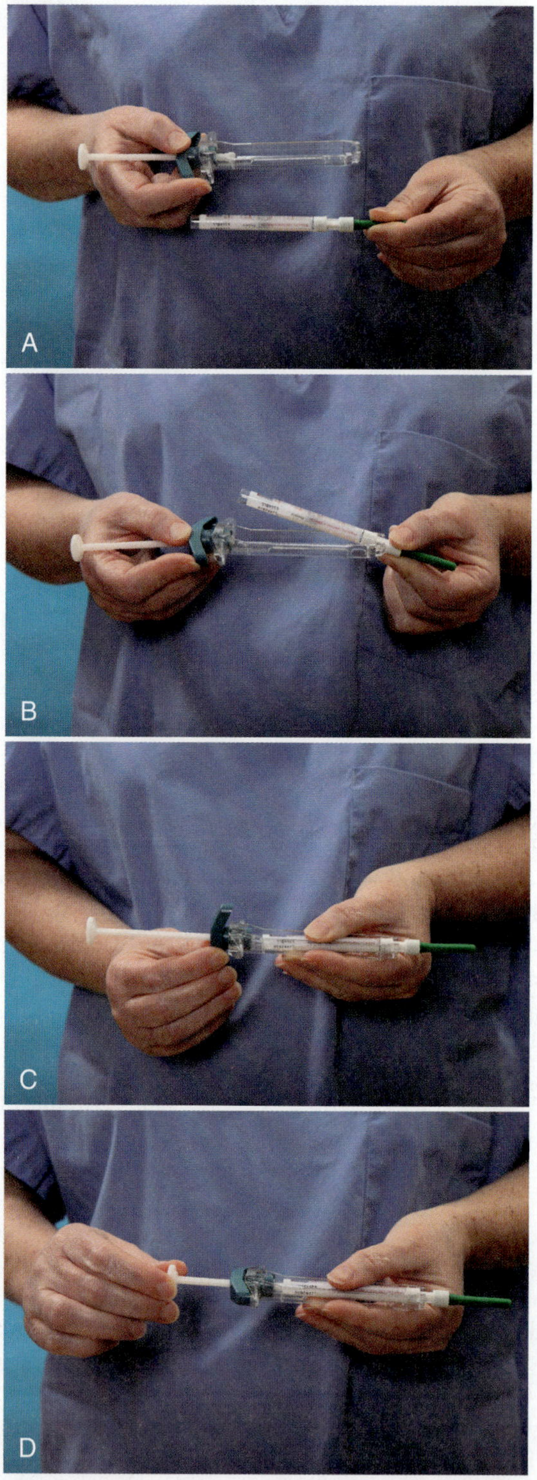

FIGURE 17-14 **A,** Carpuject syringe and prefilled sterile cartridge with needle. **B,** Assembling Carpuject. **C,** Cartridge slides into syringe barrel, turns, and locks at needle end. **D,** Plunger then screws into cartridge end. Expel excess medication to obtain accurate dose *(not pictured).*

Preparing an Injection From a Vial

A vial is a single-dose or multidose container with a rubber seal at the top (Figure 17-15, *B*). A cap protects the seal until it is ready to use. Vials contain liquid or dry forms of medications. Medications that are unstable in solution are packaged dry. The vial label specifies the solvent or diluent used to dissolve the medication and the amount of diluent needed to prepare a desired medication concentration. Normal saline and sterile distilled water are commonly used to dissolve medications.

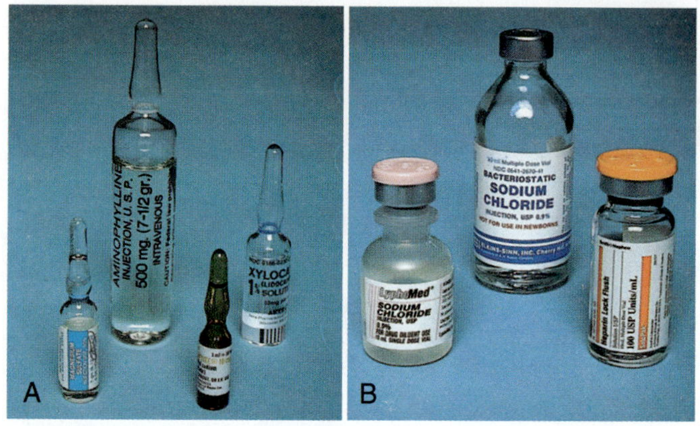

FIGURE 17-15 **A,** Medication in ampules. **B,** Medication in vials. Rubber top must be cleansed with alcohol when vial is opened or reused.

Unlike an ampule, a vial is a closed system. Thus you need to inject air into it to withdraw the solution. A vacuum develops within a vial if you fail to inject air when withdrawing solution, making withdrawal of medication difficult (see Skill 17-4). Although not necessary, you may decide to use a filter needle when preparing medication from a vial, especially if you are concerned that you will draw parts of the rubber stopper or other particles into the syringe (Cocoman and Murray, 2008; Nicoll and Hesby, 2002).

To prepare a powdered medication, first draw up the amount and type of diluent or solvent recommended on the vial label in a syringe. Inject the diluent into the vial in the same manner as injecting air into the vial. Most powdered medications dissolve easily. You have to withdraw the needle or the needleless access device from the vial when mixing the contents. Gently shake or roll the vial between your hands to thoroughly dissolve the powdered medication. Reinsert the needle or the needleless access device to draw up the dissolved medication. After mixing multidose vials, place a label that includes the date and time of mixing and the concentration of medication per milliliter on the vial. Multidose vials sometimes require refrigeration after they are diluted.

Mixing Medications

If two medications are compatible, it is possible to mix them in one injection. Most nursing units have charts that list common compatible medications. If you are uncertain about medication compatibilities, consult a pharmacist or a medication reference.

Mixing Medications from a Vial and an Ampule. When you mix two medications and one is in a vial and the other is in an ampule, prepare the medication from the vial first. Then withdraw the medication from the ampule using the same syringe and a filter needle. Follow this order because

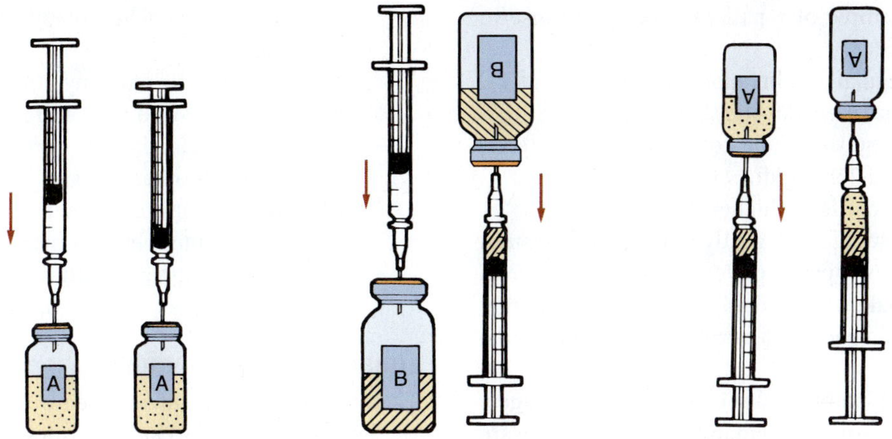

FIGURE 17-16 Steps in mixing medications from two vials.

it is not necessary to add air to withdraw the medication from an ampule.

Mixing Medications from Two Vials. Use the following principles when mixing medications from two vials:

1. Do not contaminate one medication with another.
2. Ensure that the final dosage is accurate.
3. Maintain aseptic technique.

You need only one syringe to mix medications from two vials (Figure 17-16). Aspirate the volume of air equivalent to the first medication dose (vial A) into the syringe. Inject the air into vial A, making sure that the needle does not touch the solution. Withdraw the needle or the needleless access device from vial A and aspirate air that is equivalent to the second medication dose (vial B) into the syringe. Inject the volume of air into vial B and immediately withdraw the medication in vial B into the syringe. Insert the needle or needleless access device into vial A, being careful not to push the plunger and expel the medication within the syringe into the vial. Withdraw the desired amount of medication from vial A into the syringe. After preparing the correct dose, withdraw the needle or needleless access device from vial A and apply a new safety needle suitable for injection.

Insulin Preparation

Insulin is the hormone used to treat diabetes mellitus. You administer it by injection because the GI tract breaks down an oral form and destroys it. In the United States and Canada health care providers usually prescribe U-100 insulin, which contains 100 units of insulin per milliliter of solution. You must use a 100-unit, scaled syringe to safely prepare and administer 100-unit insulin.

Insulin is also commercially available in concentrations of 500 units per milliliter, which is called U-500 insulin. Because there is no insulin syringe currently designed to prepare U-500 insulin, many medication errors have resulted with use of this type of insulin. Thus you need to use extreme caution when administering U-500 insulin. When ordering U-500 insulin, ensure that prescribers specify units and volume (e.g., 150 units, 0.3 mL of U-500 insulin). When preparing the dose, use tuberculin syringes to draw up the doses and verify dosages with another nurse or a pharmacist before you administer a dose of U-500 insulin. Additional safeguards when using U-500 insulin include having the insulin listed as concentrated in computerized medication dispensing systems, making prescribers and pharmacists verify that a patient is to receive U-500 insulin when it is ordered, stocking it on patient care units only when it is ordered for a specific patient, and removing it from the nursing unit when the patient is no longer on the unit. In addition, some health care institutions require nurses and pharmacists to participate in a safety time-out to review the order and discuss safe administration guidelines (ISMP, 2007b; Samann et al., 2011).

Insulin is classified by rate of action, including rapid-acting, short-acting, intermediate-acting, and long-acting. To provide safe care you need to know the onset, peak, and duration of each of your patient's ordered insulin doses. Refer to a medication reference or consult with a pharmacist if you are unsure of this information. Regular insulin is the only type that you can give intravenously.

Orders for insulin attempt to mimic the normal pattern of insulin release from the pancreas. Thus a patient with diabetes sometimes requires more than one type of insulin. In addition, a patient may receive several injections in a day. For example, in a two-dose protocol a combination of short- and intermediate-acting insulin is injected twice daily. Other insulins come in a premixed solution (e.g., 70/30 insulin is 70% NPH [intermediate] and 30% regular), eliminating the need to mix insulins in a syringe. Some patients use an insulin pen. The pen provides multiple doses and allows you or the patient to dial in the dose and attach a needle for insulin administration, avoiding the need for a syringe during insulin preparation.

Health care providers usually order insulin by specific dosages at select times. Correction insulin, sometimes called *sliding-scale insulin,* provides an insulin dose based on the patient's blood glucose level. The term *correction* insulin indicates that patients need small amounts of rapid- or short-acting insulin to correct their elevated blood sugars. Reliance on correction insulin is unlikely to achieve glucose control; thus it should only be ordered on a temporary basis

(ADA, 2012). An example of a patient's correction insulin order reads as follows:

Give 5 units of regular insulin subcutaneously for blood glucose levels between 150 and 200 mg/dL.

Give 10 units of regular insulin for blood glucose levels between 201 and 275 mg/dL.

Call for blood glucose levels higher than 275 mg/dL.

Before drawing up insulin doses, gently roll all cloudy insulin preparations between the palms of your hands to resuspend the insulin. Do not shake insulin vials. Shaking causes bubbles to form and take up space in a syringe, thus altering the dosage.

If more than one type of insulin is required to manage a patient's diabetes, you can mix them in one syringe *if* they are compatible (Box 17-19). If regular and intermediate-acting insulin are ordered, prepare the regular insulin first to prevent contamination with the intermediate-acting insulin. Use the following principles when mixing insulins (ADA, 2004; Novo Nordisk, 2013):

- Patients whose blood glucose levels are well controlled on a mixed-insulin dose need to maintain their individual routine when preparing and administering their insulin.
- Do not mix insulin with any other medications or diluents unless approved by the prescriber.
- Never mix insulin glargine (Lantus) or insulin detemir (Levemir) with other types of insulin.
- Inject rapid-acting insulins mixed with NPH insulin within 15 minutes before a meal.
- Verify insulin dosages with another nurse while you prepare them if required by agency policy.

Administering Injections

Each injection route differs based on the type of tissues the medication enters. The characteristics of the tissues influence the rate of medication absorption, which affects the onset of medication action. Before injecting a medication, know the volume of the medication to administer, characteristics and viscosity of the medication, and the location of anatomical structures underlying injection sites (see Skill 17-5).

Failure to select an injection site in relation to anatomical landmarks results in nerve or bone damage during needle

BOX 17-19 PROCEDURAL GUIDELINES

Mixing Two Types of Insulin in One Syringe

DELEGATION CONSIDERATIONS

The skill of mixing two kinds of insulin in one syringe cannot be delegated to nursing assistive personnel (NAP).

EQUIPMENT

Insulin vials, insulin syringe, alcohol swab, medication administration record (MAR) (printed or electronic)

STEPS

1. Check accuracy and completeness of each MAR with prescriber's medication order. Check patient's name, drug name and dosage, route of administration, and time for administration. Clarify incomplete or unclear orders with health care provider before administration.
2. Review medical history (e.g., type of diabetes, reason for elevated blood sugars) and allergies to medications, food, and latex.
3. Verify insulin labels carefully against the MAR before preparing the dose to ensure that you give the correct type of insulin. *This is the first accuracy check.*
4. Perform hand hygiene.
5. If patient takes insulin that is cloudy, roll the bottle of insulin between the hands to resuspend the insulin preparation.
6. Wipe off tops of both insulin vials with alcohol swabs and allow to dry.
7. Verify insulin dosages against MAR a second time. *This is the second accuracy check.*
8. If mixing rapid- or short-acting insulin with intermediate-acting insulin, take insulin syringe and aspirate volume of air equivalent to dose to be withdrawn from intermediate-acting insulin first. If two intermediate-acting insulins are mixed, it makes no difference which vial you prepare first.
9. Insert needle and inject air into vial of intermediate-acting insulin. Do not let the tip of the needle touch the insulin.
10. Remove the syringe from the vial of intermediate-acting insulin without aspirating medication.
11. With the same syringe, inject air equal to the dose of rapid- or short-acting insulin into the vial and withdraw the correct dose into the syringe.
12. Remove the syringe from the rapid- or short-acting insulin and get rid of air bubbles to ensure accurate dosing.
13. After verifying insulin dosages with MAR a third time, show insulin prepared in syringe to another nurse to verify that you prepared correct dosage of insulin. *This is the third accuracy check.* Determine which point on syringe scale combined units of insulin measure by adding the number of units of both insulins together (e.g., 5 units regular + 10 units NPH = 15 units total).
14. Place the needle of the syringe back into the vial of intermediate-acting insulin. Be careful not to push plunger and inject insulin in syringe into the vial.
15. Invert the vial and carefully withdraw the desired amount of insulin into syringe.
16. Withdraw needle and check fluid level in syringe. Keep needle of prepared syringe sheathed or capped until ready to administer medication. Show another nurse the syringe to verify that you prepared the correct dose.
17. Dispose of soiled supplies in proper receptacle. Place empty vials in puncture-proof and leak-proof container and perform hand hygiene.
18. Because rapid- or short-acting insulin binds with intermediate-acting insulin, which reduces the action of the faster-acting insulin, administer mixture within 5 minutes of preparing it.

Modified from American Diabetes Association (ADA): Insulin administration: position statement, *Diabetes Care* 27(1S):S106, 2004.

insertion. If you do not aspirate the syringe before injecting an IM medication, you may accidentally inject the medication directly into an artery or vein. Injecting too large a volume of medication for the site selected causes extreme pain and results in local tissue damage.

Many patients, particularly children, fear injections. You give some patients with serious or chronic illnesses several injections daily. You minimize the patient's discomfort in the following ways:

1. Use a sharp-beveled needle in the smallest suitable length and gauge.
2. Position a patient as comfortably as possible to reduce muscular tension.
3. Select the proper injection site, using anatomical landmarks.
4. Apply a vapocoolant spray (e.g., Fluori-Methane spray or ethyl chloride) or topical anesthetic (e.g., EMLA cream) to the injection site before giving the medication when possible.
5. Divert a patient's attention from the injection through conversation.
6. Insert the needle quickly and smoothly to minimize tissue pulling.
7. Hold the syringe steady while the needle remains in tissues.
8. Inject the medication slowly and steadily.

Subcutaneous Injections. Subcutaneous injections involve injecting medications into the loose connective tissue under the dermis (see Skill 17-5). Because subcutaneous tissue is not as richly supplied with blood as the muscles, medication absorption is somewhat slower than with IM injections. The body absorbs medications completely if a patient's circulatory status is normal. Because subcutaneous tissue contains pain receptors, patients often experience slight discomfort. Injection into blood vessels is rare; thus you do not need to aspirate when giving subcutaneous injections (Lilley et al., 2011). You only give small subcutaneous doses (0.5 to 1.5 mL) of water-soluble medications to adults because subcutaneous tissue is sensitive to irritating solutions and large volumes of medications. In children give smaller volumes, less than 0.5 mL (Hockenberry and Wilson, 2011). Collection of medications within the tissues causes sterile abscesses, which appear as hardened, painful lumps under the skin.

The best subcutaneous injection sites include the outer posterior aspect of the upper arms, the abdomen from below the costal margins to the iliac crests, and the anterior aspect of the thighs (Figure 17-17). The site most frequently recommended for heparin injections is the abdomen (Figure 17-18). Subcutaneous sites for other medications include the scapular areas of the upper back and the upper ventral or dorsal gluteal areas. Choose an injection site that is free of skin lesions, bony prominences, and large underlying muscles or nerves.

The site used for enoxaparin (low-molecular-weight heparin [LMWH]) is on the right or left side of the abdomen at least 2 inches from the umbilicus. This area is often called the patient's *love handles.* Pinch the site as you insert the needle. Administer LMWH in its prefilled syringe with the attached needle and do not expel the air bubble in the syringe before giving the medication (Sanofi-Aventis, 2012).

You inject subcutaneous insulin injection sites preferably into the upper arm and the anterior and lateral portions of the thigh, buttocks, and abdomen. Rotating injections within the same body part for a sequence of injections provides more consistency in the absorption of insulin. For example, if you inject the morning insulin into a patient's arm, give the next injection in a different place in the same arm, at least 2.5 cm away from the previous site. Avoid using the same site for at least 1 month. The rate of absorption is another factor in site selection for insulin administration. The abdomen has the quickest absorption rate, followed by the arms, thighs, and buttocks (ADA, 2004).

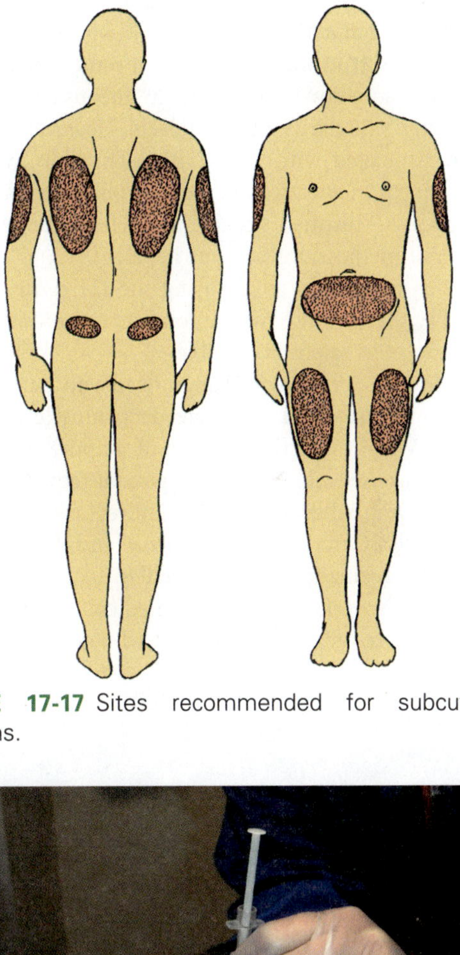

FIGURE 17-17 Sites recommended for subcutaneous injections.

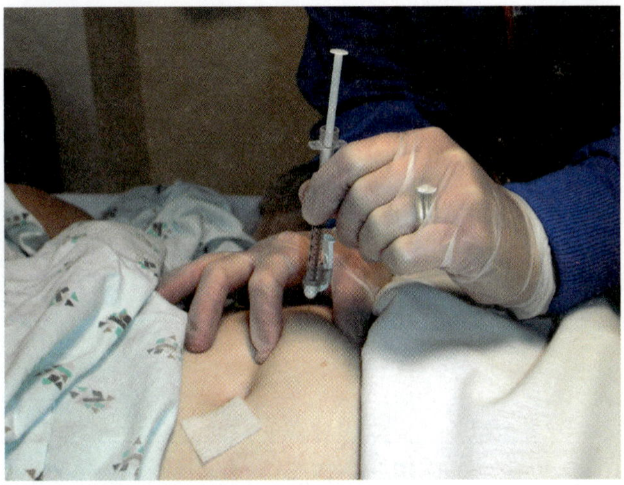

FIGURE 17-18 Giving subcutaneous heparin in abdomen.

A patient's body weight indicates the depth of the subcutaneous layer. Therefore base the needle length and angle of insertion on the patient's weight (Annersten and Willman, 2005). Generally a 25-gauge ⅝-inch needle inserted at a 45-degree angle or a ½-inch needle inserted at a 90-degree angle deposits medications into the subcutaneous tissue of a normal-size patient (Figure 17-19). Some children require only a 1.25-cm (½-inch) needle. If a patient is obese, pinch the tissue and use a needle long enough to insert through fatty tissue at the base of the skinfold. Thin patients sometimes have insufficient tissue for subcutaneous injections. The upper abdomen is the best site for injection with this type of patient. To ensure that a subcutaneous medication reaches the subcutaneous tissue, you use the following rule to determine the appropriate angle of injection: if you are able to grasp 5 cm (2 inches) of tissue, insert the needle at a 90-degree angle; if you are able to grasp 2.5 cm (1 inch), insert the needle at a 45-degree angle.

Intramuscular Injections. The IM route provides faster medication absorption than the subcutaneous route because of the greater vascularity of the muscle. However, IM injections are associated with many risks. Therefore, whenever administering a medication by the IM route, first verify that the injection is justified (Nicoll and Hesby, 2002; WHO, 2006). Some medications such as hepatitis A and influenza vaccinations need to be given using the IM route. In these cases ensure that you use the appropriate technique to inject the medication as safely as possible.

Use a longer and heavier-gauge needle to pass through subcutaneous tissue and penetrate deep muscle tissue (see Skill 17-5). Weight and the amount of adipose tissue influence needle size selection. An obese patient requires a needle 2 to 3 inches long, whereas a thin patient requires only a ½- to 1-inch needle (Camden, 2009; Nicoll and Hesby, 2002). Because most agencies only have needles that range from ⅜ to 1½ inches, investigate different medication routes when IM injections are ordered for patients who are obese (TCHP Education Consortium, 2005).

Administer IM injections so the needle is perpendicular to the patient's body and as close to a 90-degree angle as possible (Nicoll and Hesby, 2002) (see Figure 17-19). Muscle is less sensitive to irritating and viscous drugs. A normal, well-developed adult safely tolerates 2 to 5 mL of medication in a larger muscle without much pain (Nicoll and Hesby, 2002; Prettyman, 2005). However, the body does not absorb larger medication volumes (4 to 5 mL) well. Children, older adults, and thin patients tolerate only 2 mL of an IM injection. Give no more than 1 mL of medication in one injection to small children and older infants and do not give more than 0.5 mL to smaller infants (Hockenberry and Wilson, 2011).

Assess the muscle before giving an injection. Make sure that it is free of tenderness. Repeated injections in the same muscle cause severe discomfort. With a patient relaxed, palpate the muscle to rule out any hardened lesions. Help a patient assume a comfortable position to minimize discomfort during an injection.

Sites. When selecting an IM site, consider the following: Is the area free of infection or necrosis? Are there local areas of bruising or abrasions? What is the location of underlying bones, nerves, and major blood vessels? What volume of medication will you administer? Each site has certain advantages and disadvantages.

Ventrogluteal. The ventrogluteal site is the preferred and safe site for all adults, children, and infants, especially for medications that have larger volumes and are more viscous and irritating (Hockenberry and Wilson, 2011; Nicoll and Hesby, 2002). This site involves the gluteus medius muscle, which is situated away from major nerves and blood vessels. Research shows that injuries such as fibrosis, nerve damage, abscess, tissue necrosis, muscle contraction, gangrene, and pain are associated with all of the common IM sites *except* the ventrogluteal site (Nicoll and Hesby, 2002).

To locate the ventrogluteal muscle, have your patient lie in a supine or lateral position. Flexing the knee and hip helps the patient relax this muscle. Place the palm of your hand against the greater trochanter of the patient's hip with the

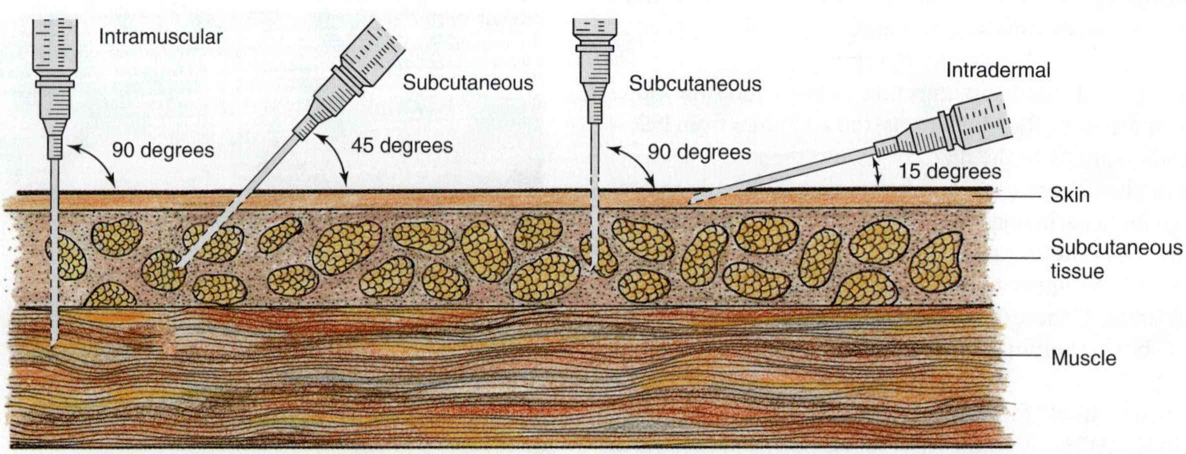

FIGURE 17-19 Comparison of angles of insertion for IM (90 degrees), subcutaneous (45 and 90 degrees), and ID (15 degrees) injections.

wrist perpendicular to the femur. Use the right hand for the left hip and the left hand for the right hip. Point your thumb toward the patient's groin with your index finger placed on the anterosuperior iliac spine. Point your middle finger back along the iliac crest toward the buttock. Your index finger, the middle finger, and the iliac crest form a V-shaped triangle (Nicoll and Hesby, 2002). The injection site is the center of the triangle (Figure 17-20).

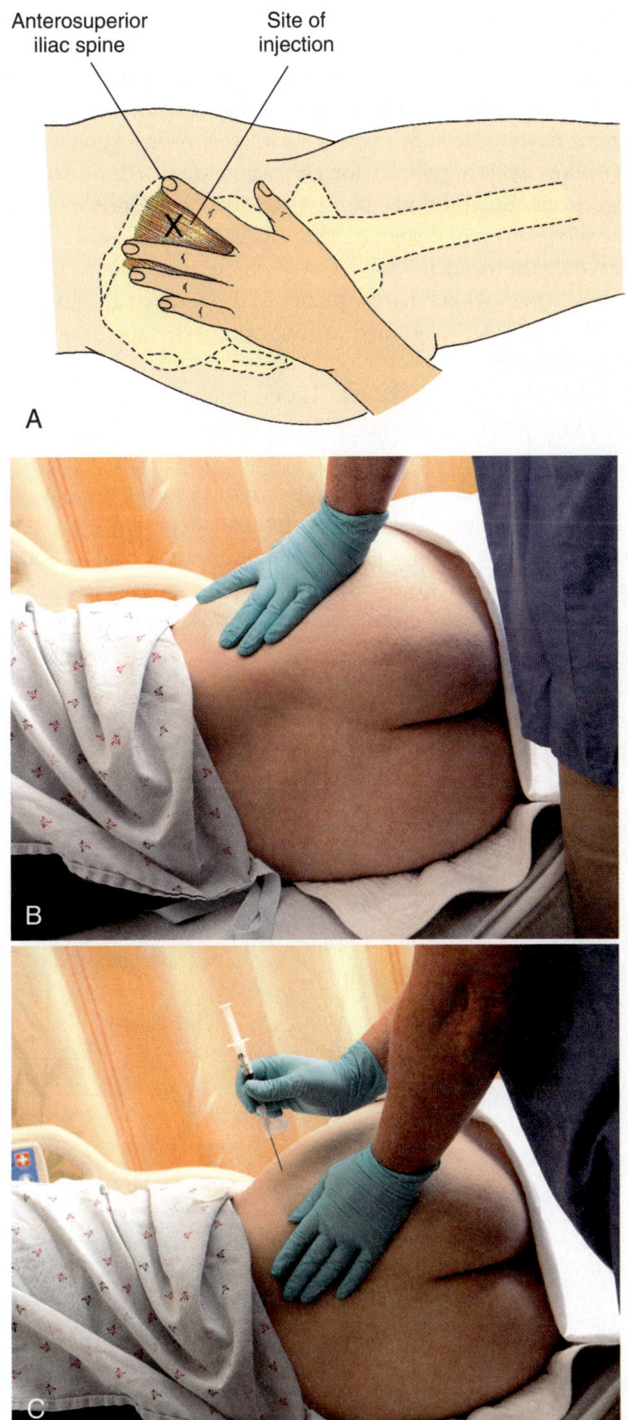

FIGURE 17-20 **A,** Landmarks for ventrogluteal site. **B,** Locating ventrogluteal site in patient. **C,** Giving intramuscular injection in ventrogluteal muscle using Z-track method.

Vastus Lateralis. The vastus lateralis muscle is another injection site used in adults and children. The muscle is thick and well developed and is located on the anterior lateral aspect of the thigh. It extends in an adult from a hand breadth above the knee to a hand breadth below the greater trochanter of the femur (Figure 17-21). Use the middle third of the muscle for injection. The width of the muscle usually extends from the midline of the thigh to the midline of the outer side of the thigh. With young children or patients who are cachectic, grasp the body of the muscle during injection to be sure that you deposit the medication in muscle tissue. Ask the patient to lie flat with the knee slightly flexed or assume a sitting position to relax the muscle. The vastus lateralis site is preferable for infants, toddlers, and children receiving biologicals (e.g., immunoglobulins, vaccines, or toxoids) (Nicoll and Hesby, 2002).

Deltoid. Although the deltoid site is easily accessible, the muscle is not usually well developed. There is a risk for injury because the radial and ulnar nerves and brachial artery lie within the upper arm along the humerus. Carefully assess the muscle, consult medication references to ensure that this is a safe site for the medication, and carefully locate the site using anatomical landmarks. Use this site only for small medication volumes (2 mL or less), when giving immunizations (e.g.,

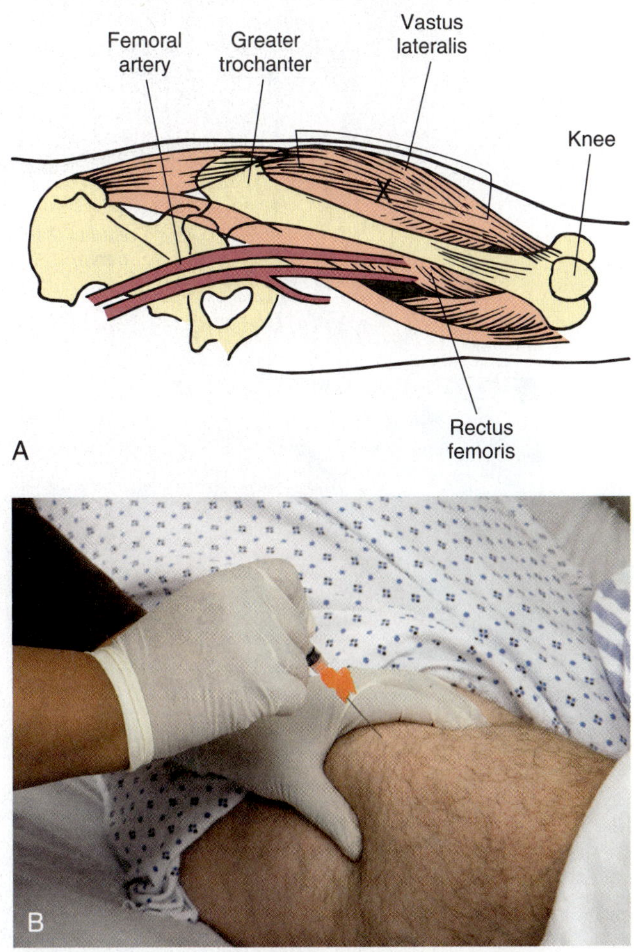

FIGURE 17-21 **A,** Landmarks for vastus lateralis site. **B,** Giving IM injection in vastus lateralis muscle.

influenza, tetanus, and diphtheria), or when other sites are inaccessible because of dressings or casts (Nicoll and Hesby, 2002). To locate the muscle, fully expose a patient's upper arm and shoulder and have the patient relax the arm at the side and flex the elbow (Figure 17-22). Do not roll up a tight-fitting sleeve. Have the patient sit, stand, or lie down. Palpate the lower edge of the acromion process, which forms the base of a triangle in line with the midpoint of the lateral aspect of the upper arm. The injection site is in the center of the triangle, about 3 to 5 cm (1 to 2 inches) below the acromion process. You also can locate the site by placing four fingers across the deltoid muscle, with the top finger along the acromion process. The injection site is then three finger widths below the acromion process.

Z-Track Method. It is recommended that you use the **Z-track injection** method when giving IM injections to minimize irritation by sealing the medication in muscle tissue (Nicoll and Hesby, 2002). To use the Z-track method, apply a new needle to the syringe after preparing the medication so no solution remains on the outside needle shaft. Then choose an IM site, preferably in a larger, deeper muscle such as the ventrogluteal muscle. Place the ulnar side of the nondominant hand just below the site and pull the overlying skin and subcutaneous tissues approximately 2.5 to 3.5 cm (1 to 1½ inches) laterally or downward. Hold the skin in this position until you administer the injection. After preparing the site with an antiseptic swab, inject the needle deep into the muscle. Grasp the barrel of the syringe with the thumb and index finger of the nondominant hand. Slowly inject the medication if there is no blood return on aspiration. The CDC (2012) states you no longer need to aspirate when *giving immunizations* to reduce discomfort. It is your responsibility to follow agency policies for aspiration when administering injections. Keep the needle inserted for 10 seconds to allow the medication to disperse evenly. Release the skin after withdrawing the needle. This leaves a zigzag path that seals the needle tract where tissue planes slide across one another (Figure 17-23). The medication cannot escape from the muscle tissue.

Intradermal Injections. ID injections are usually used for skin testing (e.g., tuberculin screening or allergy tests). Because these medications are potent, you inject them into the dermis, where blood supply is reduced and medication absorption occurs slowly. Some patients experience a severe anaphylactic reaction if medications enter the circulation too rapidly. You need to assess the injection site for changes in color and tissue integrity. Therefore choose an ID site that is

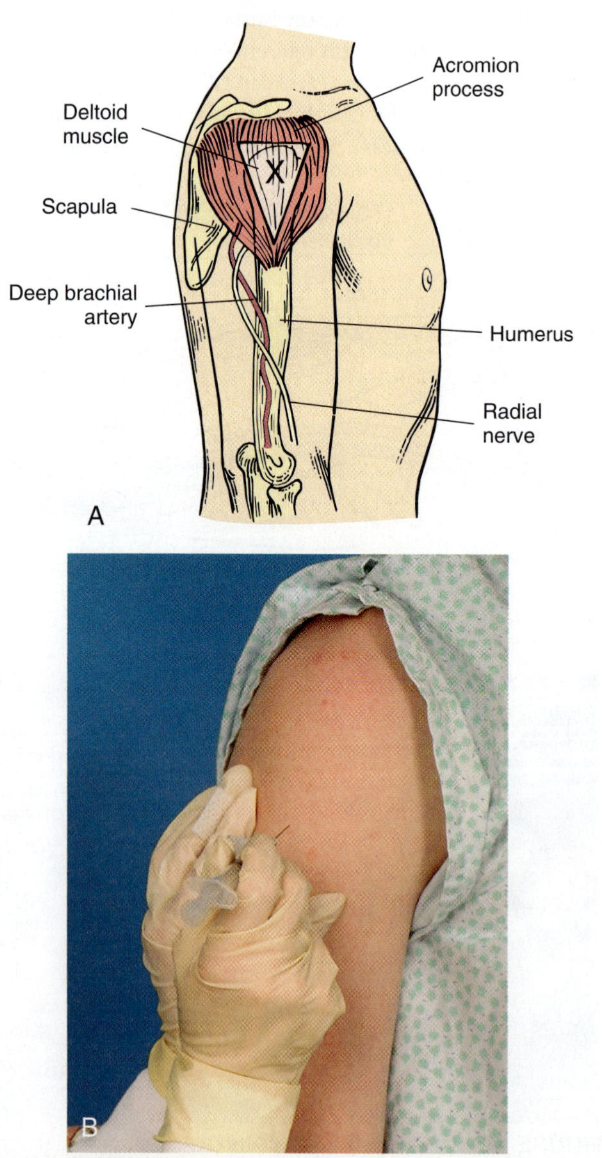

FIGURE 17-22 **A,** Landmarks for deltoid site. **B,** Giving IM injection in deltoid muscle.

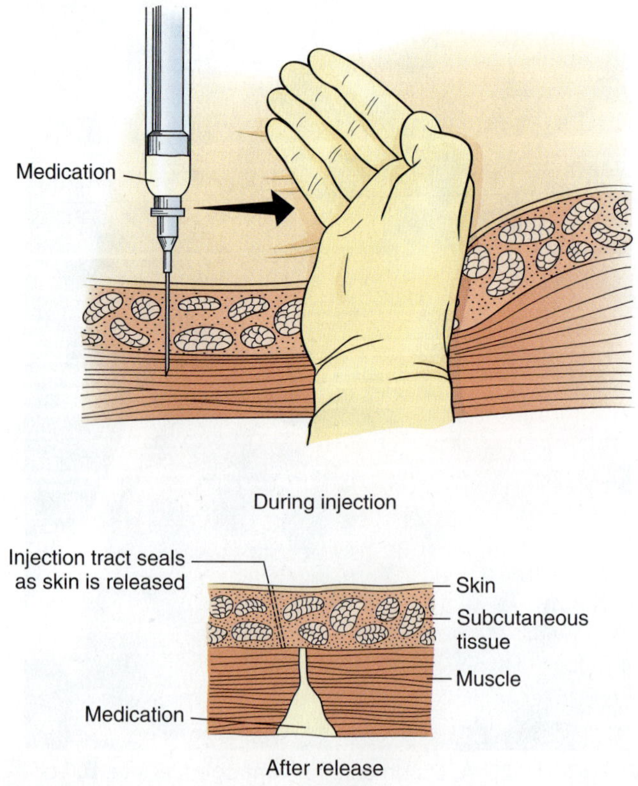

FIGURE 17-23 Z-Track method of injection prevents deposit of medication into sensitive tissues.

lightly pigmented, free of lesions, and relatively hairless. The inner forearm and upper back are ideal locations.

To administer an injection intradermally, use a tuberculin or small syringe. The angle of insertion for an ID injection is 5 to 15 degrees (see Figure 17-19). As you inject the medication, a small bleb resembling a mosquito bite appears on the surface of the skin (see Skill 17-5). If a bleb does not appear or if the site bleeds after needle withdrawal, there is a good chance that the medication entered subcutaneous tissues. In this case test results will not be valid.

Intravenous Administration. You administer IV medications by the following methods:

1. As mixtures within large volumes of IV fluids
2. By injection of a bolus, or small volume, of medication through an existing IV infusion line or intermittent venous access
3. By "piggyback" infusion of a solution containing the prescribed medication and a small volume of IV fluid through an existing IV line

In all three methods the patient has either an existing IV infusion line or an IV site that is accessed intermittently for infusions. In most institutions policies and procedures identify who is able to give IV medications and the situations in which they can be given. These policies are based on the medication, capability and availability of staff and type of monitoring equipment available.

Chapter 18 describes the technique for performing venipuncture and establishing continuous IV fluid infusions. Medication administration is only one reason for supplying IV fluids. You use IV fluid therapy primarily for fluid replacement in patients unable to take oral fluids and as a means of supplying electrolytes and nutrients.

Administering medications by the IV route has advantages. You use the IV route in emergencies when you need to deliver a fast-acting medication quickly. The IV route is also best when it is necessary to establish constant therapeutic blood levels. Some medications are highly alkaline and irritating to muscle and subcutaneous tissue. These medications cause less discomfort when given intravenously.

Safe Intravenous Medication Administration Principles. When using any method of IV medication administration, observe patients closely for symptoms of adverse reactions. After a medication enters the bloodstream, it begins to act immediately, and there is no way to stop its action. Therefore avoid errors in dose calculation and preparation. Follow the six rights of safe medication administration, double-check medication calculations with another nurse, and understand the desired action and side effects of every medication that you administer. If a medication has an antidote, have it available during administration. When administering potent medications, assess vital signs before, during, and after the infusion. Verify the prescribed rate of infusion with a medication reference or pharmacist before administering an IV medication to ensure that you give the medication safely over the appropriate amount of time. Patients experience severe adverse reactions when IV medications are given too quickly.

Large-Volume Infusions. Medications can be mixed in large volumes (500 mL or 1000 mL) of compatible IV fluids such as normal saline or lactated Ringer's solution. Because the medication is not in a concentrated form, the risk for side effects or fatal reactions is lessened when infused over the prescribed time frame. Vitamins and potassium chloride are two types of medications commonly added to IV fluids. However, there is a danger with continuous infusion. If the IV fluids infuse too rapidly, patients suffer circulatory fluid overload.

Although nurses mixed medications in IV fluids in the past, this practice is no longer supported on a routine basis (ASHP, n.d.). Many safety risks such as inaccurate calculations, nonaseptic preparation, and incorrect labeling occur when nurses have to prepare these medications on patient care units. Thus current best practices include using IV medications that come in standardized concentrations and dosages; standardized procedures for IV medication ordering, preparation, and administration; and use of ready-to-administer doses when possible (ASHP, 2008). Nurses only mix medications into IV fluids in emergency situations and *never* prepare high-alert medications (e.g., heparin, dopamine, dobutamine, nitroglycerin, potassium, antibiotics, or magnesium) on a patient care unit. If you have to mix a medication in a bag of IV fluids, first verify that you have to do this with the pharmacist. If the pharmacist confirms that you need to mix the medication, ask another nurse to verify your medication calculations and have that nurse watch you during the entire procedure to ensure safe medication administration. First you need to ensure that the medication is compatible with the IV fluids. Then prepare the medication in a syringe (see Skill 17-4) using strict aseptic technique. Clean the injection port of the IV container with an antiseptic swab, take the sheath off the syringe, and stick the needle through the injection port. Push the medication into the IV fluid and mix the solution by turning the IV container gently end to end. Finally attach a label following the ISMP safe IV label guidelines (2013b) and administer the medication to the patient at the ordered rate (see Chapter 18). *Do not* add medications to IV bags that are already hanging because there is no way to determine the exact concentration of the medication. *Only* add medications to new IV fluid containers.

To administer medications in large IV infusions, regulate the IV rate according to the prescriber's order. Monitor patients closely for adverse reactions to the medications and fluid volume overload. Also check the IV site frequently for signs of infiltration and phlebitis (see Chapter 18).

Intravenous Bolus. An IV bolus involves introducing a concentrated dose of a medication directly into the systemic circulation (see Skill 17-6). Because a bolus requires only a small amount of fluid to deliver a medication, it is an advantage when a patient's fluid intake is restricted. The IV bolus, or "push," is the most dangerous method for administering medications because the body absorbs medications as soon as you administer them; thus there is no time to correct errors. In addition, a bolus sometimes causes direct irritation to the lining of blood vessels. Before administering a bolus, confirm placement of the IV line. Never give an IV medication if the insertion site appears puffy or red or the IV fluid does not flow at the proper rate. Accidental injection of a medication into the tissues around a vein often causes pain, sloughing of tissues, and abscesses.

Determine the rate of administration of an IV bolus medication by the amount of medication that can be given each minute. For example, if a patient is to receive 5 mL of a medication over 5 minutes, give 1 mL of the IV bolus medication every minute or give 0.5 mL every 30 seconds. Look up each medication to determine the recommended concentration and rate of administration. Consider the purpose for which a medication is prescribed and any potential adverse effects related to the rate or route of administration when giving a medication by IV push.

Volume-Controlled Infusions. Another way to give IV medications is through small amounts (25 to 100 mL) of compatible IV fluids (see Skill 17-7). The fluid is in a secondary fluid container separate from the primary fluid bag. The container connects directly to the primary IV line or to separate tubing that inserts into the primary line. Different types of containers used include volume-control administration sets (e.g., Volutrol or Pediatrol), piggyback sets (Figure 17-24), and mini-infusers. Using volume-controlled infusions has the following advantages:

1. Volume-controlled infusions dilute and infuse medications over longer time intervals (e.g., 30 to 60 minutes), reducing risks to the patient associated with IV push.
2. You can administer medications (e.g., antibiotics) that are stable for a limited time in solution.
3. They control IV fluid intake.

Piggyback. A piggyback is a small (25- to 250-mL) IV bag or bottle connected to a short tubing line that connects to the *upper* Y-port of a primary infusion line or to an intermittent venous access (see Figure 17-24). The IV container that holds the medication is labeled following the ISMP (2013b) IV piggyback medication format (Figure 17-25). The piggyback tubing is a microdrip or macrodrip system (see Chapter 18). The set is called a *piggyback* because the small bag or bottle is set higher than the primary infusion bag or bottle. In the piggyback setup the main line does not infuse when the

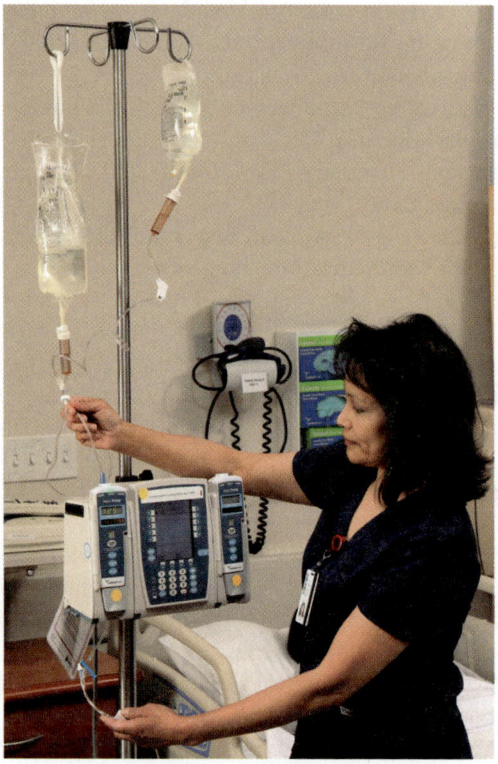

FIGURE 17-24 Piggyback setup.

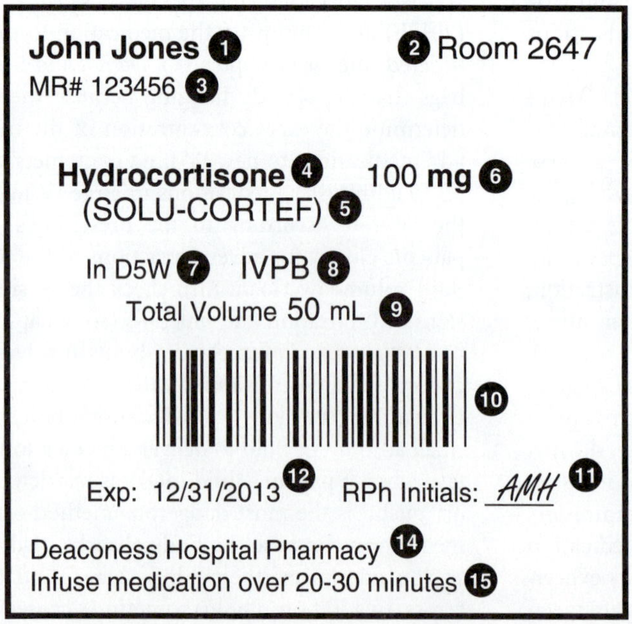

1. **Patient name**
2. Location
3. Second identifier (Date of birth, financial #, Encounter #, Medical Record #)
4. **Generic name**
5. BRAND name
6. **Patient dose**
7. Diluent
8. Route
9. Total volume
10. Bar code
11. Initials as needed
12. Expiration Date as needed in a MM/DD/YYYY format
13. Other information as required by state or federal law
14. Pharmacy information if required
15. Comments

FIGURE 17-25 IV piggyback medication with label following ISMP safe labeling.

piggybacked medication is infusing. The port of the primary IV line contains a back-check valve that automatically stops flow of the primary infusion once the piggyback infusion flows. After the piggyback solution infuses and the solution within the tubing falls below the level of the primary infusion drip chamber, the back-check valve opens, and the primary infusion begins to flow again.

Volume-Control Administration. Volume-control administration sets (e.g., Volutrol, Buretrol, or Pediatrol) are small (150-mL) containers that attach just below the primary infusion bag or bottle. The set is attached and filled in a manner similar to that used with a regular IV infusion. However, the priming of the set is different, depending on the type of filter (floating valve or membrane) within the set. Follow package directions for priming sets (see Chapter 18).

Mini-infusion Pump. The mini-infusion pump is battery operated and delivers medications in very small amounts of fluid (5 to 60 mL) within controlled infusion times. It uses standard syringes.

Intermittent Venous Access. An intermittent venous access device (commonly called a *saline lock*) is an IV catheter with a small "well" or chamber covered by a rubber cap. You insert special rubber-seal injection caps into most IV catheters (see Chapter 18). Advantages to intermittent venous access include the following:

1. Cost savings resulting from the omission of continuous IV therapy
2. Saving nurses' time by eliminating constant monitoring of IV flow rates
3. Increased mobility, safety, and comfort for patients by eliminating the need for a continuous IV line

Assess the patency and placement of your patient's IV site before giving an IV bolus or piggyback medication. After you administer the medication through an intermittent venous access device, flush it with a solution to keep it patent. Generally normal saline is effective as a flush solution for peripheral catheters. Some institutions require the use of heparin. Be sure to check and follow institutional policies regarding the care and maintenance of the IV site.

Safety in Administering Medications by Injection

Needleless Devices. The most frequent route of exposure to bloodborne disease is from needlestick injuries. These injuries commonly occur when health care workers recap needles, mishandle IV lines and needles, or leave needles at a patient's bedside. Exposure to bloodborne pathogens is one of the deadliest hazards to which nurses are exposed on a daily basis. However, over 80% of needlestick injuries are preventable with the implementation of safe needle devices. The Needlestick Safety and Prevention Act requires health care facilities to use safe needle devices to reduce the frequency of needlestick injury (OSHA, n.d.b).

Safety syringes have a sheath or guard that covers a needle immediately after it is withdrawn from the skin, eliminating the chance for a needlestick injury (Figure 17-26). Dispose of the syringe and sheath together in a receptacle. Use "needleless" devices whenever possible to reduce the risk for needlestick injuries (OSHA, n.d.b). Always dispose of needles and other instruments considered "sharps" into clearly marked puncture-proof and leakproof containers (Figure 17-27). Never force a needle into a full needle disposal receptacle and never place used needles and syringes in a wastebasket, in your pocket, on a patient's meal tray, or at the patient's bedside. Health care agencies have staff whose job it is to dispose of full containers. Box 17-20 lists recommendations for the prevention of needlestick injuries.

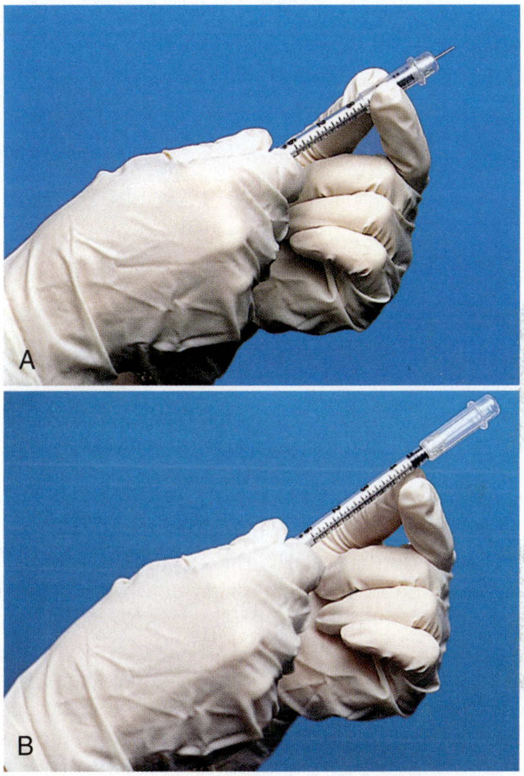

FIGURE 17-26 Needle with plastic guard to prevent needlesticks. **A,** Position of guard before injection. **B,** After injection the nurse locks guard in place, covering needle.

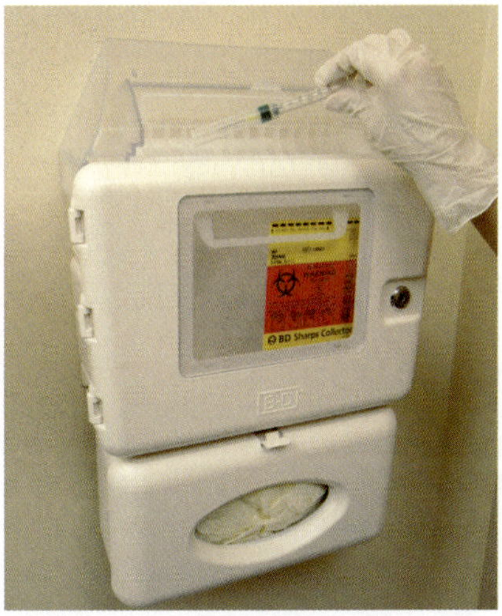

FIGURE 17-27 Sharps disposal using only one hand.

BOX 17-20 RECOMMENDATIONS FOR THE PREVENTION OF NEEDLESTICK INJURIES

- Avoid using needles when effective needleless systems or sharps with engineered sharps injury protection (SESIP) safety devices are available.
- Do not recap needles of any kind.
- Plan safe handling and disposal of needles before beginning a procedure.
- Immediately dispose of needles, needleless systems, and SESIP into puncture-proof and leak-proof sharps disposal containers.
- Review new technology and safer devices designed to eliminate or reduce needlesticks at least annually.
- Obtain feedback from employees who deliver patient care and are at risk for needlestick injuries.
- Agencies maintain sharps injury logs as part of employee health programs that include:
  - Type and brand of device involved with the needlestick.
  - Where the needlestick occurred.
  - A description of how the needlestick occurred.
  - A way to protect the confidentiality of injured employees.

From Occupational Safety and Health Administration (OSHA): *Bloodborne pathogens and needlestick prevention: OSHA standards,* n.d.b, http://www.osha.gov/SLTC/bloodbornepathogens/standards.html. Accessed November 11, 2012.

SAFETY GUIDELINES FOR NURSING SKILLS

Ensuring patient safety is an essential role of the professional nurse. To ensure patient safety, communicate clearly with members of the health care team, assess and incorporate the patient's priorities of care and preferences, and use the best evidence when making decisions about your patient's care. When performing skills in this chapter, remember the following points to ensure safe, individualized patient care.

- Be vigilant during the entire process of medication administration and make sure that your patients receive the appropriate medications. Know why your patient is receiving each medication; know what you need to do before, during, and after medication administration; and evaluate the effectiveness and assess for adverse effects after your patients take medications.
- Take care of yourself. Ensure that you are as healthy as possible to allow yourself the ability to think as clearly and critically as possible. Healthy behaviors such as getting adequate sleep, making healthy food choices, and coping with stress in positive ways help you better process information and make safe decisions during the process of medication administration.
- Prepare medications in areas that are free from distractions and verify that they have not expired while preparing them.
- Use at least two identifiers before administering medications to your patients.
- Clarify unclear orders and ask for help whenever you are uncertain about a medication order or calculation. Consult with your peers, pharmacists, and other health care providers and be sure that you resolve all concerns related to medication administration before preparing and giving medications.
- Use technology (e.g., bar scanning, electronic MARs) that is available in your agency when preparing and giving medications. Follow all policies related to use of the technology and do not use "work arounds." Nurses who use work arounds fail to follow agency protocols, policies, or procedures during medication administration in an attempt to administer medications to patients in a more timely fashion. Failing to follow the standard of care greatly increases the risk for making a medication error and impairs patient safety. It also places you at risk for malpractice and disciplinary action (see Chapter 5).
- Educate your patients about each medication they take while you are administering medications.
- Most of the time you cannot delegate medication administration. Ensure that you follow standards set by your state's Nurse Practice Act and guidelines established by your health care agency. Licensed practical nurses (LPNs) or licensed vocational nurses (LVNs) usually can administer medications via the oral (PO), subcutaneous, IM, and ID routes. Sometimes they can give medications intravenously if they have had special training and if the medications are not high-alert. Some states also allow certified medical assistants (CMAs) to administer some types of medications (e.g., oral medications) in some health care settings (e.g., long-term care facilities). The skills in this chapter assume that you are not in a setting where you can delegate medication administration to NAP. If you are in a state and a health care setting that allow you to delegate medication administration, make sure that you follow guidelines for safe delegation (see Chapter 13), your agency policies, and the standards outlined in your state Nurse Practice Act.

SKILL 17-1 ADMINISTERING ORAL MEDICATIONS

View Video!

DELEGATION CONSIDERATIONS

The skill of administering oral medications cannot be delegated to nursing assistive personnel (NAP). The nurse informs NAP about:

- Potential side effects of medications and to report their occurrence.
- Informing nurse if patient condition changes or worsens (e.g., pain, blood pressure change) after medication administration.

EQUIPMENT

- Disposable medication cups
- Glass of water, juice, or preferred liquid
- Drinking straw
- Pill-crushing device *(optional)*
- Paper towels
- Clean gloves (if handling medication)
- Medication administration record (MAR) (electronic or printed)

STEP	RATIONALE
ASSESSMENT	
1. Check accuracy and completeness of each medication administration record (MAR) with prescriber's original medication order. Check patient's name, drug name and dosage, route of administration, and time for administration. Clarify incomplete or unclear orders with health care provider before administration. Recopy or reprint any portion of printed MAR that is difficult to read.	The prescriber's order is the most reliable source and only legal record of drugs that patient is to receive. Ensures that patient receives the right medications. Illegible MARs are a source of medication errors (Jones and Treiber, 2010; Poon et al., 2010).
2. Assess for contraindications to patient receiving oral medication: Is patient able to swallow? Is patient able to have food and drink by mouth? Is patient experiencing nausea and vomiting? Was patient diagnosed as having bowel inflammation or reduced peristalsis? Has patient had recent gastrointestinal (GI) surgery? Does patient have gastric suction?	Alterations in GI function interfere with drug absorption, distribution, and excretion. Patients with GI suction do not receive benefit from the medication because it may be suctioned from the GI tract before it can be absorbed. Giving medications to patients who cannot swallow increases the risk for aspiration (Kaizer et al., 2012).
3. Review information related to medication, including action, purpose, desired effect, normal dose, route, side effects, time of onset and peak action, and nursing implications.	Allows you to determine if medication is appropriate for patient and anticipate effects of medication (Lehne, 2013).
4. Assess patient's medical history, history of allergies, medication history, and diet history. Make sure that patient's food and drug allergies are listed on each page of the MAR and prominently displayed on the patient's medical record per agency policy.	Identifies potential food and drug interaction. Reflects patient's need for medications. Effective communication of allergies is essential for all health care providers to provide safe, effective care.
5. Gather and review assessment and laboratory data that influence drug administration such as vital signs and renal and liver function laboratory findings.	Physical examination or laboratory data sometimes contraindicate drug administration. Alterations in liver and kidney function affect metabolism and excretion of medications (Lehne, 2013).

***Clinical Decision Point:* If patient has any contraindications to receiving oral medications or if in doubt about patient's ability to swallow oral medications, withhold medication and notify prescriber.**

STEP	RATIONALE
6. Assess patient's knowledge regarding health and medication usage.	Determines patient's need for medication education and helps to identify patient's adherence to drug therapy at home. Assessments can reveal drug use problems such as nonadherence, abuse, or addiction.
7. Assess risk for aspiration using a dysphagia screening tool if available (see Box 17-13 and Skill 33-1). Protect patient from aspiration by assessing swallowing ability.	Aspiration occurs when food, fluid, or medication intended for GI administration is inadvertently administered into the respiratory tract. Patients with altered ability to swallow are at higher risk for aspiration (Edmiaston et al., 2010; Kelly et al., 2011).
8. Assess patient's preferences for fluids. Maintain ordered fluid restriction (when applicable). Can medication be given with preferred fluid?	Fluids ease swallowing and facilitate absorption from the GI tract. It is necessary to maintain fluid restrictions. Some fluids (e.g., grapefruit juice) may interfere with drug absorption.

SKILL 17-1 ADMINISTERING ORAL MEDICATIONS—cont'd

STEP	RATIONALE
PLANNING	
1. Collect appropriate equipment (e.g., disposable medication cup) and MAR.	Enhances time management and efficiency.
2. Plan preparation to avoid interruptions. Do not take phone calls or talk with others. Follow agency "No Interruption Zone" policy.	Interruptions contribute to medication errors (Popescu et al., 2011).
IMPLEMENTATION	
1. Prepare medications:	
a. Perform hand hygiene.	Reduces transfer of microorganisms.
b. Arrange medication tray and cups in medication preparation area or move medication cart to position outside patient's room.	Organization of equipment saves time and reduces errors.
c. Log into automated dispensing system (ADS) or unlock medicine drawer or cart.	Medications are safeguarded when locked in cabinet, cart, or computerized medication dispensing system.
d. Prepare medications for *one patient at a time*. Follow the six rights of medication administration. Keep all pages of MARs or computer printouts for one patient together or look at only one patient's electronic MAR at a time.	A systematic approach prevents errors. Preventing distractions reduces medication preparation errors (Brady et al., 2009).
e. Select correct drug from stock supply or ADS. Compare label of medication with MAR computer printout (see illustration) or computer screen.	Reading label and comparing it with transcribed order reduce errors. *This is the first check for accuracy.*
f. Check expiration date on each medication one at a time. Exit ADS after removing drug(s).	Medications used past their expiration date are sometimes inactive, less effective, or harmful to patient. Exiting ADS ensures that no one else can remove medications using your identity.
g. Calculate drug dose as necessary. Double-check calculation. Ask another nurse to check calculations if needed.	Double-checking reduces risk for error (Dickinson et al., 2010).
h. If preparing controlled substance, check record for previous drug count and compare with supply available.	Controlled substance laws require careful monitoring of dispensed opioids.
i. Prepare solid forms of oral medications:	
(1) To prepare tablets or capsules from a floor stock bottle, pour required number into bottle cap and transfer medication to medication cup. Do not touch medication with fingers. Return extra tablets or capsules to bottle.	Maintains clean technique required of medication administration.
(2) To prepare unit-dose tablets or capsules, place packaged tablet or capsule directly into medicine cup. Do not remove wrapper (see illustration.)	Wrapper maintains cleanliness of medications and identifies drug name and dosage.
(3) If medication is in a blister pack, "pop" it through foil or paper backing into a medication cup.	Packs provide a 1-month supply; each "blister" usually contains a single dose.

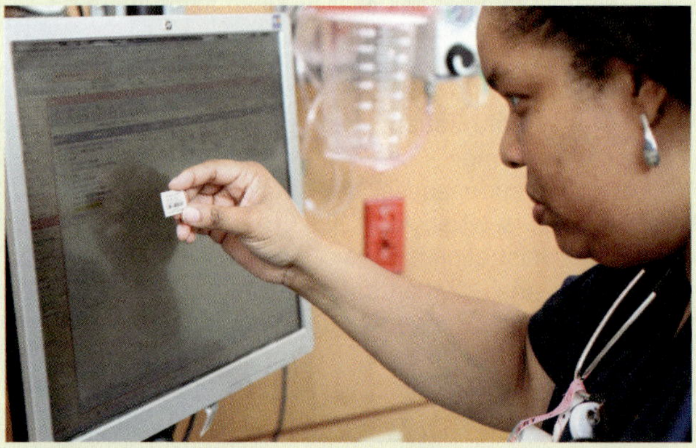

STEP 1e Check label of medication with patient's MAR.

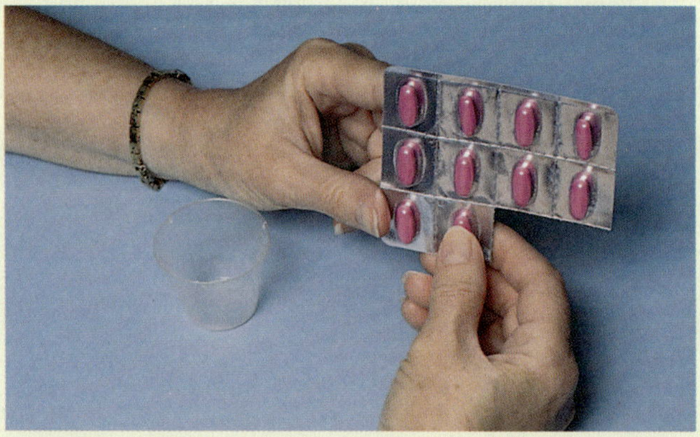

STEP 1i(2) Place tablet into medicine cup without removing wrapper.

STEP	RATIONALE
(4) If it is necessary to give half a tablet or pill for a proper dose of medication, pharmacy should split, label, package, and send medication to unit. If you must split medication, use clean, gloved hand to cut with clean pill-cutting device. Only cut tablets that are prescored by the manufacturer (line transverses the center of the tablet).	The ISMP (2006) recommends for inpatient settings if a pill *must* be split, that the pharmacist splits the pill, repackages and labels it, and sends it to the nurse for administration. Nurses *should not* split pills (ISMP, 2006).
(5) Place all tablets or capsules to be given to patient at same time in one medicine cup. Place medications requiring preadministration assessments (e.g., pulse rate, blood pressure) in separate cups.	Keeping medications that require preadministration assessments separate from others makes it easier for you to remember to make special assessments and withhold drugs as necessary.
(6) If patient has difficulty swallowing and liquid medications are not an option, use a pill-crushing device (see illustration) to grind pills. Clean device before and after use. If a pill-crushing device is not available, place tablet between two medication cups and grind with a blunt instrument. Mix ground tablet in small amount of soft food (e.g., custard, applesauce).	Large tablets are difficult to swallow. Ground tablet mixed with palatable soft food is usually easier to swallow. Cleaning pill-crushing device decreases risk for contaminating medications.

Clinical Decision Point: **Not all drugs can be crushed (e.g., capsules, enteric-coated drugs). Consult pharmacist and/or "Do Not Crush List" when in doubt (ISMP, 2013a).**

STEP	RATIONALE
j. Prepare liquids:	
(1) Gently shake container. Remove bottle cap from container and place cap upside down. If liquid is in a unit-dose container and has correct amount to administer, open it; no further preparation is necessary.	Shaking container ensures that medication is mixed before administration. Placing cap of bottle upside down prevents contamination of inside of cap.
(2) Hold bottle with label against palm of hand while pouring.	Spilled liquid does not soil or fade label.
(3) Place medication cup on hard surface (e.g., countertop), bend over if needed so you are at eye level with the medication cup, and fill to desired level (see illustration *A*). Make sure that scale is even with fluid level at its surface or base of meniscus, not edges. For small doses of liquid medications, draw liquid into a calibrated 10-mL syringe designed for enteral administration (see illustration *B*).	Ensures accuracy of measurement. Use of special syringe for oral medications is more accurate for measuring small doses of liquid medications and prevents accidental parenteral administration (ISMP, 2010).
(4) Discard any excess liquid into sink. Wipe lip and neck of bottle with paper towel.	Prevents contamination of contents of bottle and prevents bottle cap from sticking.
(5) Administer liquid medications packaged in single-dose cups directly from the single-dose cup. Do not pour them into medicine cups.	Avoids unnecessary manipulation of dose.
k. Return unused multiple-dose medications to shelf, drawer, or refrigerator. Label medication cups and poured medications with patient's name before leaving medication preparation area. Do not leave drugs unattended.	Ensures that correct medications are prepared for correct patient.

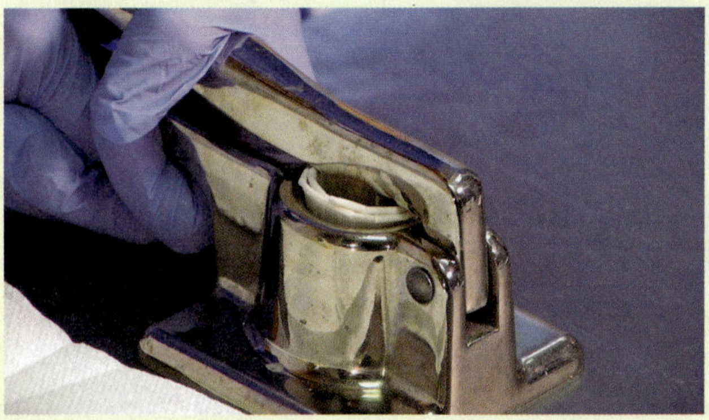

STEP 1i(6) Pill-crushing device used to crush pills when necessary.

SKILL 17-1 ADMINISTERING ORAL MEDICATIONS—cont'd

STEP	RATIONALE
l. Compare patient's name and name of medication on label of prepared medications with MAR before going to patient's room.	*This is the second check for accuracy to reduce medication error.*
2. Administer medications:	
a. Take medications to patient at correct time (see agency policy). Give STAT, first-time or loading doses, and single-order medications at time ordered. Give time-critical medications no later than 30 minutes before or after scheduled dose. Give non–time-critical scheduled medications within a range of either 1 or 2 hours of scheduled dose (ISMP, 2011b). Perform hand hygiene.	Ensures that intended therapeutic effect complies with professional standards. Hospitals need to adopt a medication administration policy and procedure for the timing of medication administration that considers patient needs, the prescribed medication, and the specific clinical indications (CMS, 2011; ISMP, 2011b). Hand hygiene decreases transfer of microorganisms.
b. Identify patient using two identifiers (e.g., name and birthday or name and account number) according to agency policy. Compare identifiers with information on patient's MAR or medical record.	Ensures correct patient. Complies with The Joint Commission requirements for patient safety (TJC, 2014).

Clinical Decision Point: **Replace patient identification bracelets that are missing, illegible, or faded.**

STEP	RATIONALE
c. Compare label of medications with MAR at patient's bedside.	Final check of medication label against MAR at patient's bedside reduces medication administration errors. *This is the third check for accuracy.*
d. Explain purpose of each medication and its action to patient. Allow patient to ask any questions about drugs.	Patient has right to be informed about medication therapy. Questions often indicate need for teaching, nonadherence to therapy, or potential medication error. Makes patient a participant in care, which minimizes anxiety.
e. Perform necessary assessments required before giving medications (e.g., blood pressure, pulse).	Helps you determine if you need to temporarily withhold any medications at this time.
f. Help patient to sitting or Fowler's position. Use side-lying position if sitting is contraindicated. Have patient stay in this position for 30 minutes.	Sitting position prevents aspiration during swallowing (Metheny et al., 2010). Remaining seated for 30 minutes helps medications move through the stomach.
g. Administer medication:	
(1) **For tablets:** Patients sometimes wish to hold solid medications in hand or cup before placing in mouth. Offer water or juice to help patient swallow medications. Give a full glass of water if not contraindicated.	Patient becomes familiar with medications by seeing each drug. Choice of fluid improves fluid intake and provides patient-centered care. Taking tablets and capsules with a full glass of water or other liquid helps medications enter stomach.

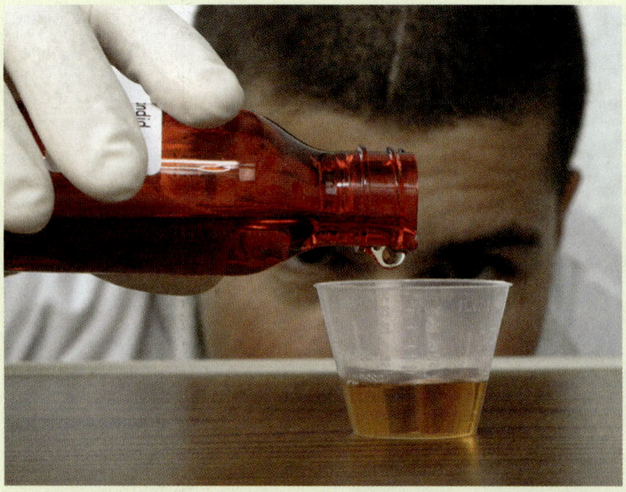

STEP 1j(3)A Pour desired volume of liquid so base of meniscus is level with line on scale.

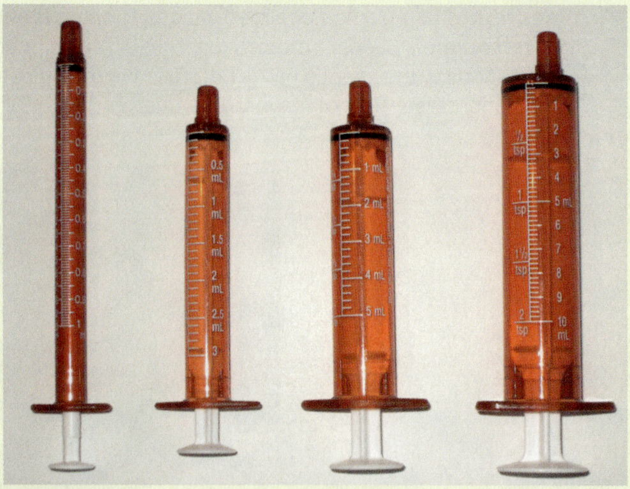

STEP 1j(3)B Use special enteric syringe to draw up liquid medications.

STEP	RATIONALE
(2) **For sublingual medications:** Help or have patient place medication under tongue in sublingual pocket and allow it to dissolve completely. Caution patient against swallowing tablet whole (see Figure 17-3).	Drug is absorbed through blood vessels of undersurface of tongue. If it is swallowed, gastric juices destroy the drug, or the liver rapidly detoxifies it so patient does not attain therapeutic blood levels.
(3) **For buccal medications:** Help or have patient place medication in mouth against mucous membranes of cheek until it dissolves (see Figure 17-4). Avoid administering liquids until buccal medication has dissolved.	Buccal medications act locally on mucosa or systemically as patient swallows them in saliva.
(4) **For powdered medications:** Mix with liquids at bedside and give to patient to drink.	When prepared in advance, powdered drugs thicken and even harden, making swallowing difficult.
(5) **For crushed medications mixed in food:** Give each medication separately in teaspoon of food.	Ensures that patient takes all medicine.
(6) Caution patient against chewing or swallowing lozenges.	Drug acts through slow absorption through oral mucosa, not gastric mucosa.
(7) Give effervescent powders and tablets immediately after dissolving.	Effervescence improves unpleasant taste of drug and often relieves GI problems.
h. If patient is unable to hold medications, place medication cup to lips and gently introduce each drug into mouth or place in proper location one at a time. Do not rush.	Administering single tablet or capsule eases swallowing and decreases risk for aspiration.

Clinical Decision Point: **If tablet or capsule falls to the floor, discard it and repeat preparation.**

STEP	RATIONALE
i. Stay until patient has completely swallowed each medication. Ask patient to open mouth if uncertain whether he or she has swallowed medication.	You are responsible for ensuring that patient receives ordered dosage. If left unattended, patient may not take dose or may save drugs, causing risk to health.
j. For highly acidic medications (e.g., aspirin), offer patient nonfat snack (e.g., crackers) if not contraindicated by patient's condition.	Reduces gastric irritation.
k. Help patient return to comfortable position.	Maintains patient's comfort.
l. Dispose of soiled supplies and perform hand hygiene.	Reduces transmission of microorganisms.
m. Replenish stock such as cups and straws, return cart to medicine room if used, and clean work area.	Clean working space helps other staff complete duties efficiently.
EVALUATION	
1. Evaluate patient's response to medications at times that correlate with onset, peak, and duration of medication. Evaluate patient for both desired and adverse effects.	Evaluates therapeutic benefit of drug and detects onset of side effects or allergic reactions.
2. Use Teach Back—State to the patient, "I want to be sure I explained your medications correctly. Can you tell me the name of each of your medications, why you are taking them, how much to take, when to take them, and which side effects you may experience?" Revise your instruction now or develop plan for revised patient teaching to be implemented at an appropriate time if patient is not able to teach back correctly.	Evaluates what the patient is able to explain or demonstrate.

RECORDING AND REPORTING

- Record administration of oral medications on MAR immediately after administering medication. If using paper copy of MAR, include your initials or signature.
- If you withheld any medication, record the reason and follow agency policy to record withheld medication on MAR.
- Report and record evaluation of medication effect to prescriber if required (e.g., report urine output following diuretic administration if ordered by prescriber).
- Document your evaluation of patient learning.

UNEXPECTED OUTCOMES AND RELATED INTERVENTIONS

- Patient exhibits adverse effects (e.g., side effect, toxic effect, allergic reaction).
  - Assess for symptoms such as urticaria, rash, pruritus, rhinitis, and wheezing that indicate allergic reaction.
  - Always notify prescriber and pharmacy when patient exhibits adverse effects.
  - Withhold further doses and add allergy information to patient's chart.

SKILL 17-1 ADMINISTERING ORAL MEDICATIONS—cont'd

- Patient refuses medication.
  - Explore reasons why patient does not want medication.
  - Educate if misunderstandings of medication therapy are apparent.
  - Do not force patient to take medication; patients have the right to refuse treatment.
  - If patient continues to refuse medication despite education, record why drug was withheld on patient's chart and notify prescriber.

SKILL 17-2 ADMINISTERING EYE MEDICATIONS

View Video!

DELEGATION CONSIDERATIONS

The skill of administering eye medications cannot be delegated to nursing assistive personnel (NAP). The nurse instructs NAP to:

- Report potential side effects of medications, including the potential for visual changes, to the nurse.

EQUIPMENT

- Medication bottle with sterile eyedropper or ointment tube or medicated intraocular disk
- Cotton ball or tissue
- Wash basin filled with warm water and washcloth if eyes have crust or drainage
- Eye patch and tape *(optional)*
- Clean gloves
- Medication administration record (MAR) (electronic or printed)

STEP	RATIONALE
ASSESSMENT	
1. Check accuracy and completeness of each MAR with prescriber's original medication order. Check patient's name, drug name and dosage (e.g., number of drops [if a liquid] and which eye), route of administration, and time for administration. Clarify incomplete or unclear orders with health care provider before administration. Recopy or reprint any portion of the MAR that is difficult to read.	The prescriber's order is the most reliable source and only legal record of drugs that patient is to receive. Ensures that patient receives the right medications. Illegible MARs are a source of medication errors (Jones and Treiber, 2010; Poon et al., 2010).
2. Review information related to medication, including action, purpose, desired effect, normal dose, route, side effects, time of onset and peak action, and nursing implications.	Allows you to determine if medication is appropriate for patient and anticipate its effects (Lehne, 2013).
3. Assess condition of external eye structures (see Chapter 16). (You may do this just before drug instillation.)	Provides baseline to later determine if local response to medications occurs. Also indicates need to clean eye before drug application.
4. Assess patient's medical history, allergies (including latex), and medication history. If patient has latex allergy, use nonlatex gloves.	Knowledge of medical history influences how some medications act. Protects patient from risk for allergic drug response.
5. Determine whether patient has any symptoms of visual alterations.	Certain eye medications act to either lessen or increase these symptoms. Provides baseline data to allow you to recognize change in patient's condition.
6. Assess patient's level of consciousness and ability to follow directions.	If patient becomes restless or combative during procedure, greater risk for accidental eye injury exists.
7. Assess patient's knowledge regarding drug therapy and desire to self-administer medication.	Patient's level of understanding indicates need for health teaching. Motivation influences teaching approach.
8. Assess patient's ability to manipulate and hold equipment necessary for eye medication (e.g., dropper, tube of ointment, intraocular disk).	Reflects patient's ability to self-administer drug.
PLANNING	
1. Collect appropriate equipment and MAR.	Enhances time management and efficiency.
2. Plan preparation to avoid interruptions. Do not take phone calls or talk with others. Follow agency "No Interruption Zone" policy.	Interruptions contribute to medication errors (Popescu et al., 2011).

STEP	RATIONALE
IMPLEMENTATION	
1. Perform hand hygiene and prepare medication (see Skill 17-1, Implementation Steps 1a-g, k, and l). Preparation usually involves taking eyedrops out of refrigerator and rewarming to room temperature before administering to patient. Check expiration date on container. Be sure to check label 2 times while preparing medication.	Following the same routine when preparing medications, eliminating distractions, and checking the label of the medication with MAR reduces errors. *This is the first and second accuracy check.* Warming eyedrops reduces irritation to eye.
2. Take medications to patient at correct time (see agency policy). Give STAT, first-time or loading doses, and single-order medications at time ordered. Give time-critical medications no later than 30 minutes before or after scheduled dose. Give non–time-critical scheduled medications within a range of either 1 or 2 hours of scheduled dose (ISMP, 2011b). Perform hand hygiene.	Ensures that intended therapeutic effect complies with professional standards. Hospitals need to adopt a medication administration policy and procedure for the timing of medication administration that considers patient needs, prescribed medication, and specific clinical indications (CMS, 2011; ISMP, 2011b). Hand hygiene decreases transfer of microorganisms.
3. Identify patient using two identifiers (e.g., name and birthday or name and account number) according to agency policy. Compare identifiers with information on patient's MAR or medical record.	Ensures correct patient. Complies with The Joint Commission requirements for patient safety (TJC, 2014).
4. Compare label of medication against MAR for third time at patient's bedside.	*Third check for accuracy ensures that right medication is administered.*
5. Explain procedure to patient regarding positioning and sensations to expect such as burning or stinging of eye.	Relieves anxiety about medication being instilled into eye.
6. Arrange supplies at bedside; apply clean gloves.	Reduces transmission of microorganisms.
7. Gently roll eyedrop container between your hands.	Ensures that medication is mixed before administration. Shaking container creates bubbles, which affects size of drops.
8. Ask patient to lie supine or sit back in chair with head slightly hyperextended.	Position provides easy access to eye for medication instillation and minimizes drainage of medication through tear duct.

Clinical Decision Point: **If patient has a cervical spine injury, do not hyperextend the neck.**

STEP	RATIONALE
9. If crusts or drainage are present along eyelid margins or inner canthus, gently wash away. Apply damp washcloth or cotton ball over eyelid for a few minutes to soak crusts that are dried and difficult to remove. Always wipe clean from inner to outer canthus.	Crusts or drainage harbors microorganisms. Soaking allows easy removal and prevents pressure from being applied directly over eye. Cleansing from inner to outer canthus avoids entrance of microorganisms into lacrimal duct.
10. Hold cotton ball or clean tissue in nondominant hand on patient's cheekbone just below lower eyelid.	Cotton or tissue absorbs medication that escapes eye.
11. With tissue or cotton resting below lower lid, gently press downward with thumb or forefinger against bony orbit.	Technique exposes lower conjunctival sac. Retraction against bony orbit prevents pressure and trauma to eyeball and fingers from touching eye.
12. Ask patient to look at ceiling.	Action retracts sensitive cornea up and away from conjunctival sac and reduces stimulation of blink reflex.
13. Administer ophthalmic drops:	
a. With dominant hand resting on patient's forehead, hold filled medication eyedropper or ophthalmic solution approximately 1 to 2 cm (½ to ¾ inch) above conjunctival sac (see illustration).	Helps prevent accidental contact of eyedropper with eye structures, thus reducing risk for injury to eye and transfer of infection to dropper. Ophthalmic medications are sterile.

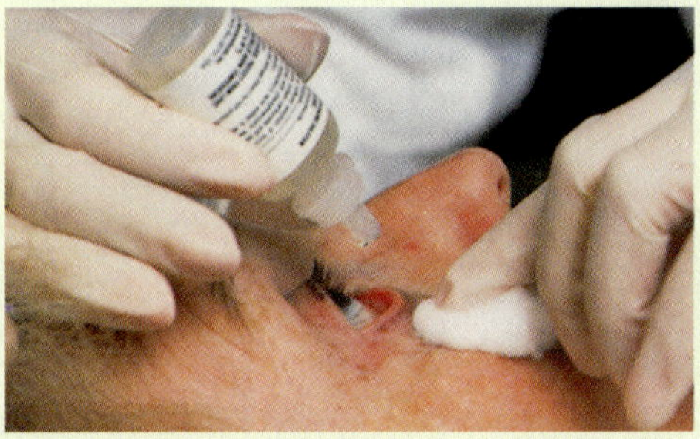

STEP 13a Hold eyedropper above conjunctival sac.

SKILL 17-2 ADMINISTERING EYE MEDICATIONS—cont'd

STEP	RATIONALE
b. Drop prescribed number of medication drops into conjunctival sac.	Conjunctival sac normally holds 1 or 2 drops. Provides even distribution of medication across eye.
c. If patient blinks or closes eye or if drops land on outer lid margins, repeat procedure.	Therapeutic effect of drug is obtained only when drops enter conjunctival sac.
d. After instilling drops, ask patient to close eye gently.	Helps to distribute medication. Squinting or squeezing the eyelids forces medication out of conjunctival sac (ASHP, 2013).
e. When administering drugs that cause systemic effects, apply gentle pressure with your finger and clean tissue on patient's nasolacrimal duct for 30 to 60 seconds.	Prevents overflow of medication into nasal and pharyngeal passages. Prevents absorption into systemic circulation (ASHP, 2013).
f. If patient receives more than one eye medication to the same eye at the same time, wait at least 5 minutes before administering the next medication and use a different cotton ball or tissue with each medication.	Avoids interactions between medications (ASHP, 2013).
14. Instill ophthalmic ointment:	
a. Holding ointment applicator above lower lid margin, apply thin stream of ointment evenly along inner edge of lower eyelid on conjunctiva (see illustration) from inner canthus to outer canthus.	Distributes medication evenly across eye and lid margin.
b. Have patient close eye and rub lid lightly in circular motion with cotton ball if rubbing is not contraindicated.	Further distributes medication without traumatizing eye.
15. Administer intraocular disk:	
a. Open package containing disk. Apply gloves. Gently press finger of dominant hand against disk so it adheres to your finger. Position convex side of disk on your fingertip (see illustration).	Allows you to inspect disk for damage or deformity.
b. With your other hand gently pull the patient's lower eyelid away from eye. Ask patient to look up.	Prepares conjunctival sac for receiving medicated disk.
c. Place disk in conjunctival sac so it floats on the sclera between the iris and lower eyelid (see illustration).	Ensures delivery of medication (Alvarez-Lorenzo, Hiratani, and Concheiro, 2006).
d. Pull patient's lower eyelid out and over disk (see illustration).	Ensures accurate medication delivery.

Clinical Decision Point: **You should not be able to see the disk at this time. Repeat Step 15d if you can see the disk.**

STEP	RATIONALE
16. Removal of intraocular disk:	
a. Perform hand hygiene and put on gloves.	Reduces transmission of microorganisms.
b. Explain procedure to patient.	Relieves anxiety about manipulation of disk in eye.
c. Gently pull down on patient's lower eyelid with nondominant hand.	Exposes intraocular disk.
d. Using the forefinger and thumb of your opposite hand, pinch disk and lift it out of patient's eye (see illustration).	

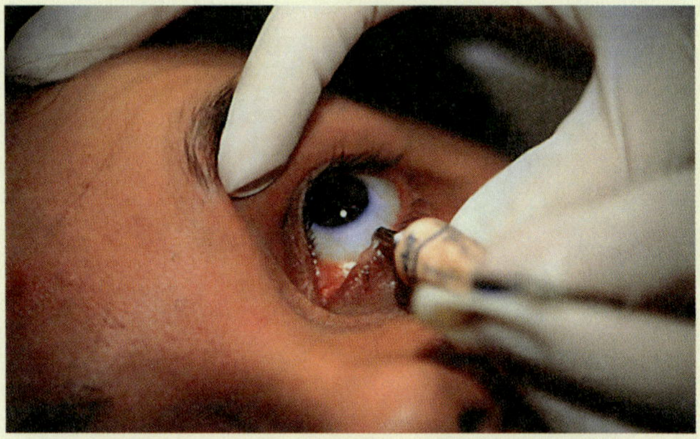

STEP 14a Apply ointment along lower eyelid.

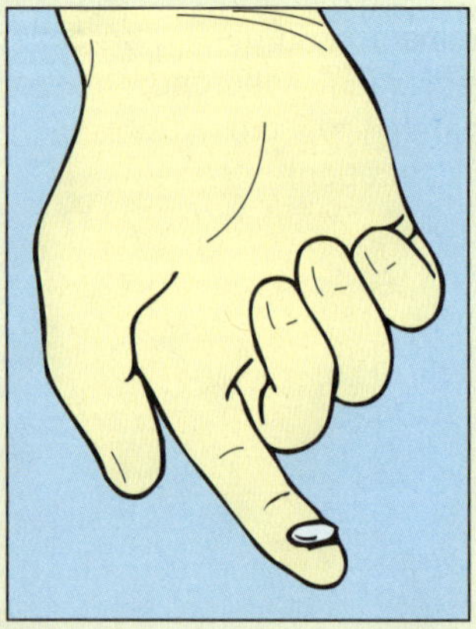

STEP 15a Gently position convex side of disk against your fingertip.

STEP	RATIONALE
17. If excess medication is on eyelid, gently wipe it from inner to outer canthus.	Promotes comfort and prevents trauma to eye (ASHP, 2013).
18. If patient had eye patch, apply clean one by placing it over affected eye so entire eye is covered. Tape securely without applying pressure to eye.	Clean eye patch reduces chance of infection.
19. Remove gloves, dispose of soiled supplies in proper receptacle, and perform hand hygiene.	Maintains neat environment at bedside and reduces transmission of microorganisms.
EVALUATION	
1. Note patient's response to instillation; ask if he or she felt any discomfort.	Determines if you performed procedure correctly and safely and if patient is experiencing adverse effects of medication.
2. Observe response to medication by assessing visual changes and noting any side effects.	Evaluates effects of medication.
3. Use Teach Back—State to the patient, "I want to be sure I explained your eye drops correctly. Can you tell me the name of your eye drops, why you are taking them, how much to take, when to take them, and which side effects you may experience?" Also state, "Show me how you will administer your eye drops at home." Revise your instruction now or develop plan for revised patient teaching to be implemented at an appropriate time if patient is not able to teach back correctly.	Evaluates what the patient is able to explain and demonstrate.

RECORDING AND REPORTING

- Record drug, concentration, number of drops, time of administration, and eye (left, right, or both) that received medication on electronic or printed MAR.
- Record appearance of eye in nurses' notes.
- Document your evaluation of patient learning.

UNEXPECTED OUTCOMES AND RELATED INTERVENTIONS

- Patient cannot instill drops without supervision.
    - Reinforce teaching and allow patient to self-administer drops as much as possible to enhance confidence.
    - If patient cannot self-administer drops, teach others such as family members to instill them into patient's eye.
- Patient displays signs of allergic reaction (e.g., tearing, reddened sclera) or systemic response (e.g., bradycardia) to medication.
    - Hold medication and speak with prescriber.
    - Follow institutional policy or guidelines for reporting adverse or allergic reaction to medications.
    - Add information about allergy to medical record per agency policy.

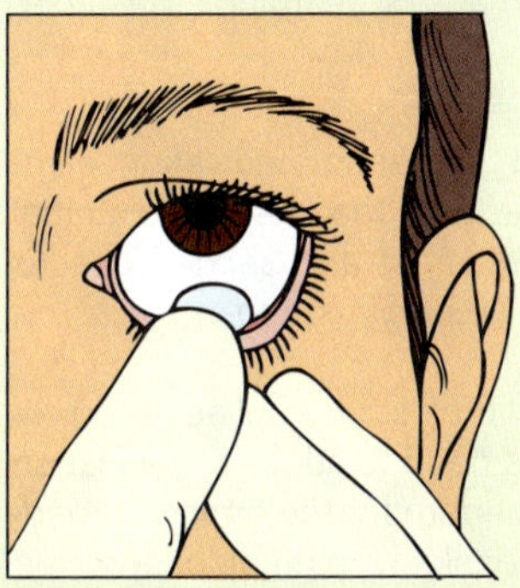

STEP 15c Place disk in conjunctival sac between iris and lower eyelid.

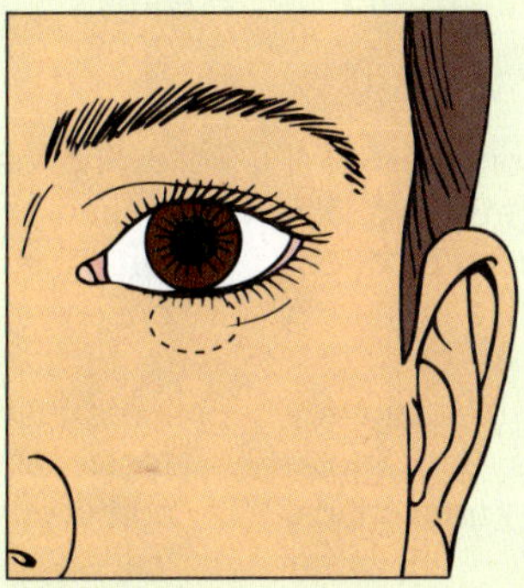

STEP 15d Gently pull lower eyelid over disk.

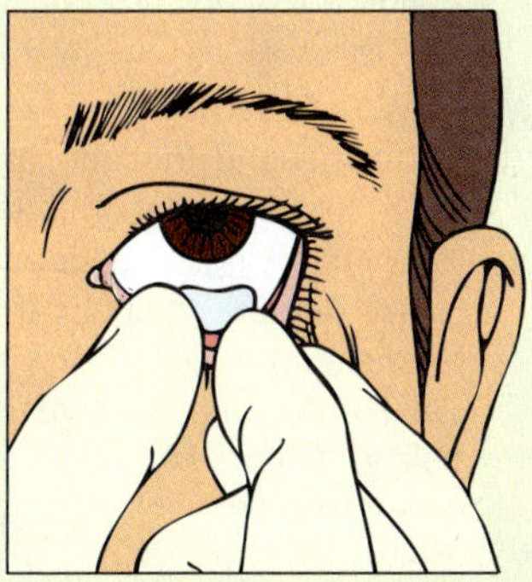

STEP 16d Carefully pinch disk to remove it from patient's eye.

SKILL 17-3 USING METERED-DOSE OR DRY POWDER INHALERS

DELEGATION CONSIDERATIONS

The skill of administering inhaled medications cannot be delegated to nursing assistive personnel (NAP). The nurse informs NAP about:

- Potential side effects of medications (e.g., increased coughing, breathing difficulties) and to report their occurrence.

EQUIPMENT

- Metered-dose inhaler or dry powder inhaler (MDI or DPI)
- Spacer (optional with MDI)
- Facial tissues *(optional)*
- Wash basin or sink with warm water
- Paper towel
- Medication administration record (MAR) (electronic or printed)

STEP	RATIONALE
ASSESSMENT	
1. Check accuracy and completeness of each MAR with prescriber's original medication order. Check patient's name, drug name and dosage, route of administration, and time for administration. Clarify incomplete or unclear orders with health care provider before administration. Recopy or reprint any portion of printed MAR that is difficult to read.	The prescriber's order is the most reliable source and only legal record of drugs that patient is to receive. Ensures that patient receives the right medications. Illegible MARs are a source of medication errors (Jones and Treiber, 2010; Poon et al, 2010).
2. Review information related to medication, including purpose, action, desired effect, normal dose, route, side effects, time of onset and peak action, and nursing implications.	Allows you to determine if medication is appropriate for patient and anticipate its effects (Lehne, 2013).
3. Assess patient's medical history, allergies, and medication history.	Knowledge of medical history influences how some medications act. Protects patient from risk for allergic drug response.
4. Assess respiratory pattern and auscultate breath sounds (Chapter 16).	Establishes baseline for airway status for comparison during and after treatment.
5. If patient was previously instructed in self-administration of inhaled medicine, assess technique in using an inhaler. Also assess patient's ability to hold, manipulate, and depress canister and inhaler.	Nurse's instruction sometimes requires only simple reinforcement, depending on patient's level of dexterity. Any impairment of grasp or coordination impairs patient's ability to use MDI or DPI correctly.
6. Assess patient's readiness and ability to learn: patient asks questions about medication, disease, or complications; requests education in use of inhaler; is mentally alert; not fatigued, in pain, or in respiratory distress; participates in own care.	Influences patient's motivation to understand explanations and actively participate in teaching process. Mental or physical limitations affect patient's ability to learn and methods nurse uses for instruction (Bastable, 2008).
7. Assess patient's knowledge and understanding of disease and purpose and action of prescribed medications.	Knowledge of disease and medications is essential for patient to realistically understand use of inhaler.
8. Determine drug schedule and number of inhalations prescribed for each dose.	Influences explanations that nurse provides for use of inhaler.
PLANNING	
1. Collect appropriate equipment and MAR.	Enhances time management and efficiency.
2. Plan preparation to avoid interruptions. Do not take phone calls or talk with others. Follow agency "No Interruption Zone" policy.	Interruptions contribute to medication errors (Popescu et al, 2011).
3. Provide adequate time for teaching session.	Prevents interruptions and enhances learning (Bastable, 2008).
IMPLEMENTATION	
1. Perform hand hygiene and prepare medication: See Skill 17-1, Implementation Steps 1a-f, k, l. Preparation usually involves taking inhaler device out of storage and into patient room. Be sure to check the label two times while preparing medication.	Following the same routine when preparing medication, eliminating distractions, and checking the medication label with the MAR reduces errors. *First and second checks ensure that right medication is administered.*
2. Take medications to patient at correct time (see agency policy). Give STAT, first-time or loading doses, and single-order medications at time ordered. Give time-critical medications no later than 30 minutes before or after scheduled dose. Give non–time-critical scheduled medications within a range of either 1 or 2 hours of scheduled dose (ISMP, 2011b). Perform hand hygiene.	Ensures that intended therapeutic effect complies with professional standards. Hospitals need to adopt a medication administration policy and procedure for the timing of medication administration that considers patient needs, the prescribed medication, and the specific clinical indications (CMS, 2011; ISMP, 2011b). Hand hygiene decreases transfer of microorganisms.

STEP	RATIONALE
3. Identify patient using two identifiers (e.g., name and birthday or name and account number) according to agency policy. Compare identifiers with information on patient's MAR or medical record.	Ensures correct patient. Complies with The Joint Commission requirements for patient safety (TJC, 2014).
4. Compare the label of the medication with the MAR one more time at the patient's bedside.	*Third check for accuracy ensures that right medication is administered.*
5. Help patient get into a comfortable position such as sitting in chair in hospital room or at kitchen table in home.	Patient is more likely to remain receptive to nurse's explanations in comfortable environment (Bastable, 2008).
6. Have patient manipulate inhaler, canister, and spacer device. Explain and demonstrate how canister fits into inhaler.	Patient needs to be familiar with how to use equipment.

Clinical Decision Point: **If patient is using an MDI and the inhaler is new or has not been used for several days, push a "test spray" into the air. You do not need to do this for a DPI.**

STEP	RATIONALE
7. Explain what metered dose is and warn patient about overuse of inhaler and medication side effects.	Makes sure that patient does not administer excessive inhalations because of risk for serious side effects. Side effects are minimized if patients take medication as ordered.
8. Explain steps for administering squeeze-and-breathe MDI (demonstrate steps when possible): **a.** Insert MDI canister into the holder. **b.** Remove mouthpiece cover from inhaler.	Use of simple, step-by-step explanations allows patient to ask questions during procedure (Bastable, 2008).

Clinical Decision Point: **If dirt or foreign objects are in mouthpiece, clean before using inhaler to avoid inhalation of unwanted material.**

STEP	RATIONALE
c. Shake inhaler strongly 5 or 6 times.	Aerosolizes fine particles.
d. Tell patient to sit up straight or stand and take a deep breath and exhale.	Empties lungs and prepares patient's airway to receive medication.
e. Have patient position inhaler in one of two ways: **(1)** Close mouth around mouthpiece with opening toward back of throat with lips held tight around it (see illustration). This is the most common method. **(2)** Position mouthpiece 2 to 4 cm (1 to 2 inches) in front of mouth (see illustration).	Proper positioning of inhaler is essential to administering medication correctly.
f. With inhaler positioned correctly, have patient hold inhaler with thumb at mouthpiece and index finger and middle finger at the top. This is called a *three-point or lateral hand position.*	MDIs work best when patients use a three-point or lateral hand position to activate canisters.
g. Instruct patient to tilt head back slightly and inhale slowly and deeply through mouth for 3 to 5 seconds while fully pressing down on canister.	Medication is distributed to airways during inhalation. Inhalation through mouth rather than nose draws medication into airways better.
h. Have patient hold breath for as long as comfortable, up to 10 seconds.	Allows medication to settle into patient's airway (MayoClinic.com, 2011b).

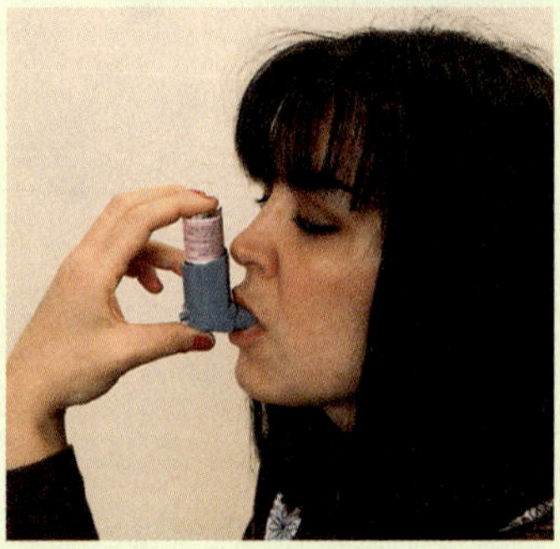

STEP 8e(1) One technique for use of inhaler. Patient opens lips and places inhaler in mouth with opening toward back of throat.

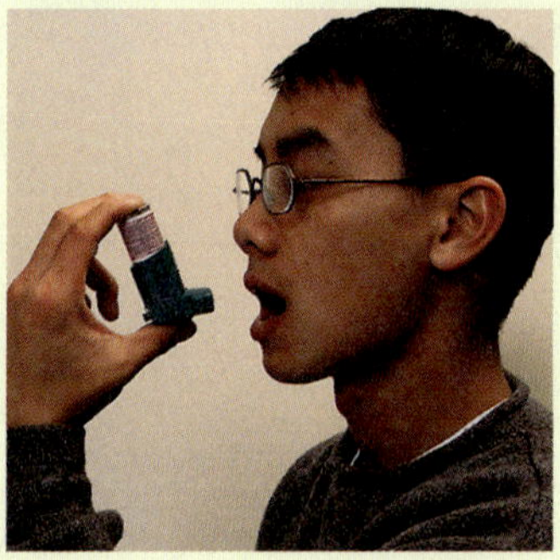

STEP 8e(2) One technique for use of inhaler. Patient positions mouthpiece 1 to 2 inches from mouth. This is considered the best way to deliver medication.

SKILL 17-3 USING METERED-DOSE OR DRY POWDER INHALERS—cont'd

STEP	RATIONALE
i. Remove MDI from mouth and exhale slowly through pursed lips.	Keeps small airways open during exhalation.
9. Explain steps to administer MDI using a spacer such as an Aerochamber (demonstrate steps when possible):	Use of simple, step-by-step explanations allows patient to ask questions at any point during procedure (Bastable, 2008).
a. Insert canister into holder. Remove mouthpiece covers from inhaler and spacer. Inspect spacer for foreign objects; if the spacer has a valve, make sure that it is intact.	Inhaler fits into end of spacer.
b. Shake inhaler strongly 5 or 6 times.	Ensures that fine particles are aerosolized.
c. Insert MDI holder mouthpiece into end of spacer.	Spacer traps medication released from MDI; patient then inhales the medication from the device. Spacers break up and slow down the medication particles, increasing the absorption of medication into the airway (MayoClinic.com, 2011a).
d. Instruct patient to place spacer mouthpiece into mouth and close lips. Avoid inserting beyond raised lip on mouthpiece and covering small exhalation slots with lips (see illustration).	Prevents medication from escaping through mouth.
e. Have patient take a deep breath, exhale, and breathe normally through spacer mouthpiece.	Empties lungs and prepares patient's airway to receive the medication.
f. Have patient press medication canister one time, spraying one puff into spacer.	MDI releases spray that allows finer particles to be inhaled. Large droplets are kept in spacer.
g. Instruct patient to inhale slowly and deeply through mouth for 3 to 5 seconds.	Maximizes amount of medication that enters lungs.
h. Instruct patient to hold breath for approximately 10 seconds.	Allows distribution of all medication.
i. Remove MDI and spacer before exhaling.	Allows patient to exhale normally.
10. Explain steps to administer DPI or breath-activated MDI (demonstrate when possible):	Use of simple step-by-step explanations allows patient to ask questions at any point during the procedure (Bastable, 2008).
a. Remove mouthpiece cover. *Do not shake* inhaler.	
b. Prepare medication as directed by manufacturer (e.g., hold inhaler upright and turn wheel to the right and then to the left until a click is heard; load medication pellet).	Primes inhaler, ensuring that medication is delivered to patient (Mayoclinic.com, 2011b).
c. Exhale away from inhaler.	Prevents loss of powder.
d. Position mouthpiece between lips (see illustration).	Keeps medication from escaping through mouth.
e. Inhale deeply and forcefully through mouth.	Creates aerosol.
f. Hold full breath for 5 to 10 seconds.	Allows distribution of medication.

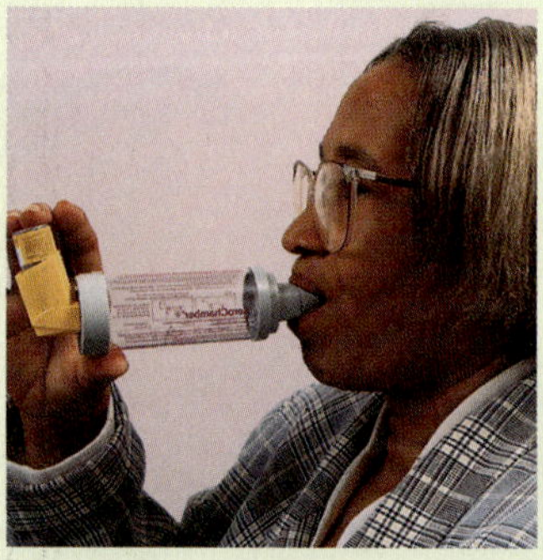

STEP 9d Have patient place mouthpiece in mouth and close lips, being careful to keep exhalation slots exposed.

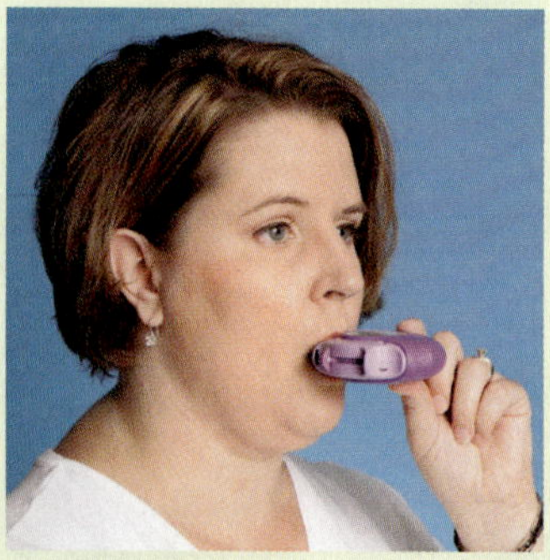

STEP 10d Have patient place mouthpiece of DPI between lips.

STEP	RATIONALE
11. Instruct patient to wait at least 20 to 30 seconds between inhalations of the same medication and 2 to 5 minutes between inhalations of different medications or as ordered by prescriber. Administer bronchodilators to open airways before steroids (Lilley at al., 2011).	Patients need to inhale medications slowly. First inhalation opens airways and reduces inflammation. Second or third inhalation penetrates deeper airways.

Clinical Decision Point: **If patient uses a corticosteroid, have him or her rinse mouth with water or salt water or brush teeth after inhalation to reduce risk for fungal infection. Also teach patient to inspect oral cavity daily for redness, sores, or white patches. Report abnormal assessment findings to the patient's health care provider (MayoClinic.com, 2011b).**

STEP	RATIONALE
12. Tell patient not to repeat inhaler doses until next scheduled dose.	Health care providers prescribe medications at intervals during the day to provide constant drug levels and minimize side effects.
13. Explain that patient may feel gagging sensation in throat caused by droplets of medication on pharynx or tongue. Have patient rinse mouth out with warm water approximately 2 minutes after using inhaler.	Results when inhalant is sprayed and inhaled incorrectly.
14. Instruct patient in how to clean inhaler:	
a. Once a day remove canister from inhaler. Rinse inhaler and cap in warm running water. Make sure that inhaler is completely dry before using.	Accumulation of spray around mouthpiece interferes with proper distribution during use.
b. Twice a week wash the L-shaped plastic mouthpiece with antibacterial soap and warm water. Rinse and air-dry well before putting canister back into mouthpiece.	Removes residual medication and decreases transfer of microorganisms. Do not place inhalers holding cromolyn, nedocromil, or hydrofluoroalkane (HFA) in water.
EVALUATION	
1. Ask if patient has any questions.	Clarifies information.
2. After medication has been taken, assess patient's respiratory status, including ease of respirations. Auscultate lungs and use a peak flowmeter if ordered (see Chapter 16).	Determines status of breathing pattern and adequacy of ventilation and confirms desired effect of medication. A peak flowmeter measures the peak expiratory flow (PEF) or how fast air is exhaled when a person breathes out forcefully. Patients often self-monitor PEF to monitor airway status.
3. Ask patient to calculate how many days the inhaler will last.	Helps patient determine when to reorder prescription.
4. Use Teach Back—State to the patient, "We covered a lot today about your inhaler, and I want to make sure that I explained things clearly. So let's review what we discussed. Can you tell me the name of your inhaler, why you are using it, when to take it, which side effects you may experience, and when you need to call your health care provider? Also, please show me how you will use your inhaler at home." Revise your instruction now or develop plan for revised patient teaching to be implemented at an appropriate time if patient is not able to teach back correctly.	Evaluates what the patient is able to explain or demonstrate.

RECORDING AND REPORTING

- Document your evaluation of patient learning.
- Record medication, time of administration, and amount of puffs on the MAR.
- Record patient's response to medication in nurses' notes.
- Report any undesirable effects from medication.

UNEXPECTED OUTCOMES AND RELATED INTERVENTIONS

- Patient needs bronchodilator more than every 4 hours.
  - Indicates respiratory problems; reassess type of medication and delivery methods needed.
  - Notify health care provider.
- Patient experiences cardiac dysrhythmias, light-headedness, and/or syncope, especially if receiving beta-adrenergics.
  - Withhold all further doses of medication.
  - Consult with prescriber.
- Patient is not able to self-administer medication properly.
  - Explore alternative delivery routes or methods.
- Patient experiences paroxysms of coughing.
  - Aerosolized particles irritate posterior pharynx. Notify prescriber; need to reassess type of medication or delivery method.

SKILL 17-4 PREPARING INJECTIONS FROM VIALS AND AMPULES

DELEGATION CONSIDERATIONS

The skill of preparing injections cannot be delegated to nursing assistive personnel (NAP).

EQUIPMENT

Medication in an Ampule

- Safety syringe, needle, and filter needle
- Small gauze pad or unopened alcohol swab

Medication in a Vial

- Safety syringe
- Needles:
  - Blunt tip vial access cannula (if needleless system used)
  - Filter needle if indicated
  - Needle for drawing up medication (if needed)
  - Safety needle for injection
- Small gauze pad or antiseptic swab
- Diluent (e.g., normal saline or sterile water) (if indicated)

Both

- Medication in vial or ampule
- Medication administration record (MAR) (electronic or printed)
- Puncture-proof container for disposal of syringes, needles, and glass

STEP	RATIONALE
ASSESSMENT	
1. Check accuracy and completeness of each MAR with prescriber's original medication order. Check patient's name, drug name and dosage, route of administration, and time for administration. Clarify incomplete or unclear orders with health care provider before administration Recopy or reprint any portion of the MAR that is difficult to read.	The prescriber's order is the most reliable source and only legal record of drugs that patient is to receive. Ensures that patient receives the right medications. Illegible MARs are a source of medication errors (Jones and Treiber, 2010; Poon et al., 2010).
2. Review information related to medication, including purpose, action, desired effect, normal dose, route, side effects, time of onset and peak action, and nursing implications.	Allows you to determine if medication is appropriate for patient and anticipate effects of medication (Lehne, 2013).
3. Assess patient's medical history, allergies, and medication history.	Knowledge of medical history influences how some medications act. Protects patient from risk for allergic drug response.
4. Assess patient's body build, muscle size, and weight if giving subcutaneous or intramuscular (IM) medication.	Determines type and size of syringe and needles for injection.
PLANNING	
1. Collect appropriate equipment and MAR.	Enhances time management and efficiency.
2. Plan preparation to avoid interruptions. Do not take phone calls or talk with others. Follow agency "No Interruption Zone" policy.	Interruptions contribute to medication errors (Popescu et al., 2011).
IMPLEMENTATION	
1. Perform hand hygiene and assemble supplies.	Reduces transmission of microorganisms and saves nursing time.
2. Prepare medication: See Skill 17-1, Implementation Steps 1a-h. Be sure to check the label two times while preparing medication.	Following the same routine when preparing medications, eliminating distractions, and checking the label of the medication with the MAR reduces errors. *First and second checks ensure that right medication is administered.*
A. **Ampule Preparation:**	
(1) Tap top of ampule lightly and quickly with finger until fluid moves from neck of ampule (see illustration).	Dislodges any fluid that collects above neck of ampule. All solution moves into lower chamber.
(2) Place small gauze pad or unopened alcohol pad around neck of ampule (see illustration).	Placing pad around neck of ampule protects fingers from trauma as glass tip is broken off.
(3) Snap neck of ampule quickly and firmly away from hands (see illustration).	Protects nurse's fingers and face from shattering glass.
(4) Draw up medication quickly using a filter needle long enough to reach bottom of ampule.	System is open to airborne contaminants. Makes sure that needle is long enough to access medication for preparation. Filter needles filter out any fragments of glass (Nicoll and Hesby, 2002).
(5) Hold ampule upside down or set it on a flat surface. Insert filter needle into center of ampule opening. Do not allow needle tip or shaft to touch rim of ampule.	Broken rim of ampule is considered contaminated. When ampule is inverted, solution dribbles out if needle tip or shaft touches rim of ampule.

STEP	RATIONALE
(6) Aspirate medication into syringe by gently pulling back on plunger (see illustrations).	Withdrawal of plunger creates negative pressure within syringe barrel, which pulls fluid into syringe.
(7) Keep needle tip under surface of liquid. Tip ampule to bring all fluid within reach of needle.	Prevents aspiration of air bubbles.
(8) If you aspirate air bubbles, do not expel air into ampule.	Air pressure forces fluid out of ampule, and medication is lost.
(9) To expel excess air bubbles, remove needle from ampule. Hold syringe with needle pointing up. Tap side of syringe to cause bubbles to rise toward needle. Draw back slightly on plunger and push plunger upward to eject air. Do not eject fluid.	Withdrawing plunger too far removes it from barrel. Holding syringe vertically allows fluid to settle in bottom of barrel. Pulling back on plunger allows fluid within needle to enter barrel so you do not expel fluid. You then expel air at top of barrel and within needle.
(10) If syringe contains excess fluid, use sink or other specially designed area for disposal of extra medication. Hold syringe vertically with needle tip up and slanted slightly toward sink. Slowly eject excess fluid into sink. Recheck fluid level in syringe by holding it vertically.	Safely disperses medication into sink. Position of needle allows you to expel medication without having it flow down needle shaft. Rechecking fluid level ensures proper dose.
(11) Cover needle with its safety sheath. Replace filter needle with regular safety needle or needleless access device for injection.	Prevents contamination of needle. Do not use filter needles for injection.
B. Vial Containing a Solution:	
(1) Remove cap covering top of unused vial to expose sterile rubber seal. If a multidose vial has been used before, cap is already removed. Firmly and briskly wipe surface of rubber seal with antiseptic swab and allow it to dry.	Vial comes packaged with cap that cannot be replaced after seal removal. Not all drug manufacturers guarantee that caps of unused vials are sterile; you need to swab all seals with alcohol before preparing medication. Swabbing reduces transmission of microorganisms. Allowing alcohol to dry prevents it from coating needle and mixing with medication.
(2) Pick up syringe and remove needle cap or cap covering needleless vial access device (see illustration). Pull back on plunger to draw amount of air into syringe equivalent to volume of medication to be aspirated from vial.	Injecting air into vial prevents buildup of negative pressure in vial when aspirating medication.

***Clinical Decision Point:* Some medications and agencies require use of filter needle when preparing medications from vials. Check agency policy or medication reference to determine if filter needle is required. If you use a filter needle to aspirate medication, you need to change it to a regular needle of the appropriate size to administer the medication (Nicoll and Hesby, 2002).**

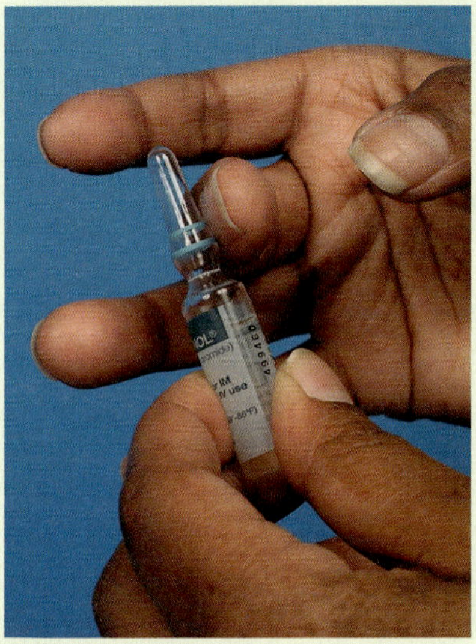

STEP 2A(1) Tapping ampule moves fluid down neck.

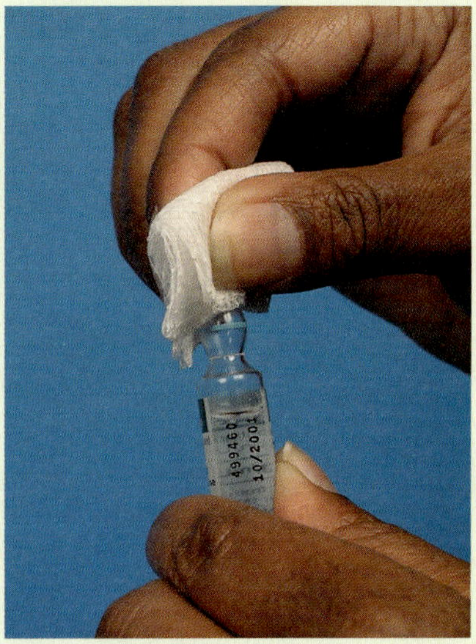

STEP 2A(2) Gauze pad placed around neck of ampule.

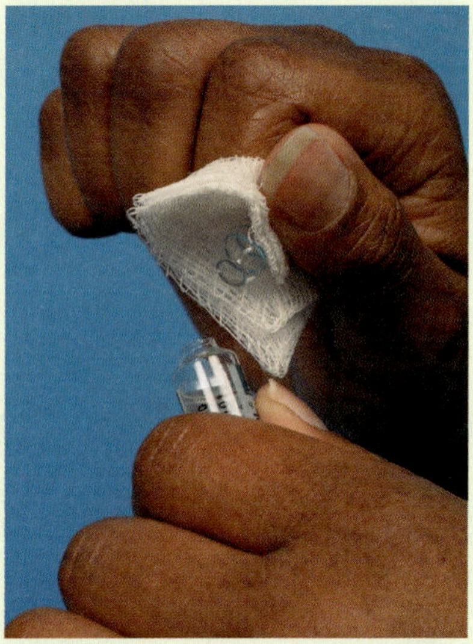

STEP 2A(3) Snapping neck away from hands.

SKILL 17-4 PREPARING INJECTIONS FROM VIALS AND AMPULES—cont'd

STEP	RATIONALE
(3) With vial on flat surface, insert tip of needle or needleless vial access device through center of rubber seal (see illustration). Apply pressure to tip of needle during insertion.	Center of seal is thinner and easier to penetrate. Using firm pressure prevents coring of rubber seal, which could enter vial or needle.
(4) Inject air into air space of vial, holding on to plunger. Hold plunger with firm pressure; plunger sometimes is forced backward by air pressure within the vial.	You need to inject air before aspirating fluid to create vacuum needed to get medication to flow into syringe. Injecting into air space of vial prevents formation of bubbles and inaccuracy in dosage.
(5) Invert vial while keeping firm hold on syringe and plunger (see illustration). Hold vial between thumb and middle fingers of nondominant hand. Grasp end of syringe barrel and plunger with thumb and forefinger of dominant hand to counteract pressure in vial.	Inverting vial allows fluid to settle in lower half of container. Position of hands prevents forceful movement of plunger and permits easy manipulation of syringe.
(6) Keep tip of needle below fluid level.	Prevents aspiration of air.

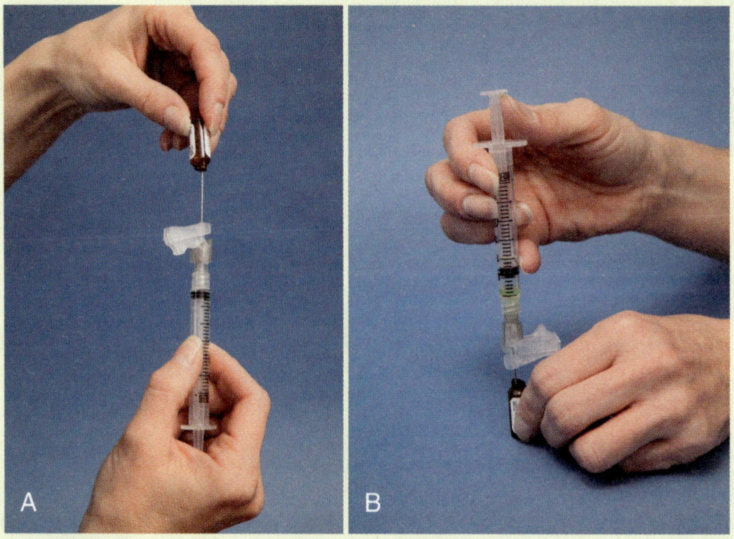

STEP 2A(6) **A,** Medication aspirated with ampule inverted. **B,** Medication aspirated with ampule on flat surface.

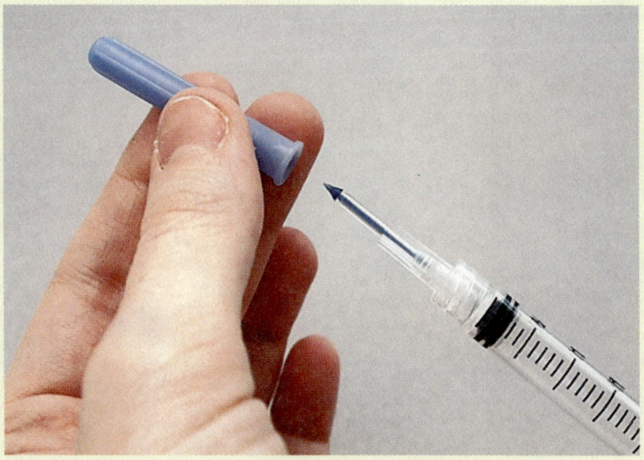

STEP 2B(2) Syringe with needleless adapter.

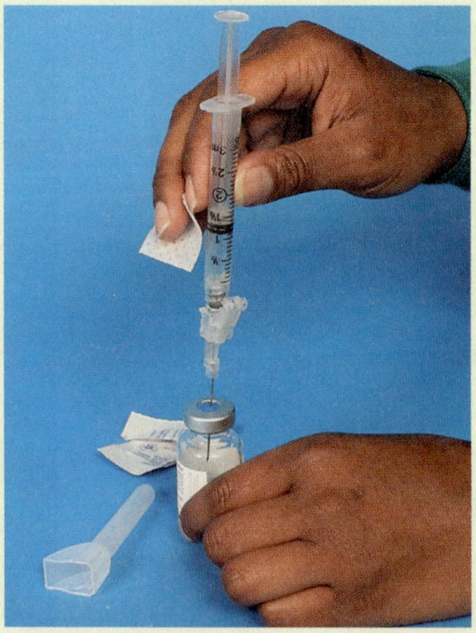

STEP 2B(3) Insert safety needle through center of vial diaphragm (with vial flat on table).

STEP	RATIONALE
(7) Allow air pressure from vial to fill syringe gradually with medication. If necessary, pull back slightly on plunger to obtain correct amount of solution.	Positive pressure within vial forces fluid into syringe.
(8) When you obtain desired volume, position needle into air space of vial; tap side of syringe barrel carefully to dislodge any air bubbles. Eject any air remaining at top of syringe into vial.	Forcefully striking barrel while needle is inserted in vial may bend needle. Accumulation of air displaces medication and causes dosage errors.
(9) Remove needle or needleless vial access device from vial by pulling back on barrel of syringe.	Pulling plunger rather than barrel causes plunger to separate from barrel, resulting in loss of medication.
(10) Hold syringe at eye level, at 90-degree angle, to ensure correct volume and absence of air bubbles. Remove any remaining air by tapping barrel to dislodge any air bubbles (see illustration). Draw back slightly on plunger; then push plunger upward to eject air. Do not eject fluid. Check volume of medication one more time.	Holding syringe vertically allows fluid to settle in bottom of barrel. Pulling back on plunger allows fluid within needle to enter barrel so you do not expel fluid. You then expel air at top of barrel and within needle.
(11) If you need to inject medication into patient's tissue, change needle to appropriate gauge and length according to route of medication administration.	Inserting needle through a rubber stopper dulls beveled tip. New needle is sharper. Because no fluid is along shaft, needle will not track medication through tissues. You cannot inject needleless access device into the body.
(12) For multidose vial, make label that includes date of opening vial and your initials.	Ensures that nurses will prepare future doses correctly. You discard some drugs after certain number of days after opening a vial.
C. Vial Containing a Powder (Reconstituting Medications):	
(13) Remove cap covering vial of powdered medication and cap covering vial of proper diluents. Firmly swab both caps with antiseptic swab and allow to dry.	Vial comes packaged with cap that cannot be replaced after seal removal. Not all drug manufacturers guarantee that caps of unused vials are sterile; you need to swab all seals with alcohol before preparing medication. Swabbing reduces transmission of microorganisms. Allowing alcohol to dry prevents it from coating needle and mixing with medication.
(14) Draw up diluents into syringe following Steps 2B(2) through 2B(10).	Prepares diluents for injection into vial containing powdered medication.
(15) Insert tip of needle or needleless access device through center of rubber seal of vial of powdered medication. Inject diluents into vial. Remove needle.	Diluent begins to dissolve and reconstitute medication.
(16) Mix medication thoroughly. Roll in palms. *Do not shake.*	Ensures proper dispersal of medication throughout solution.

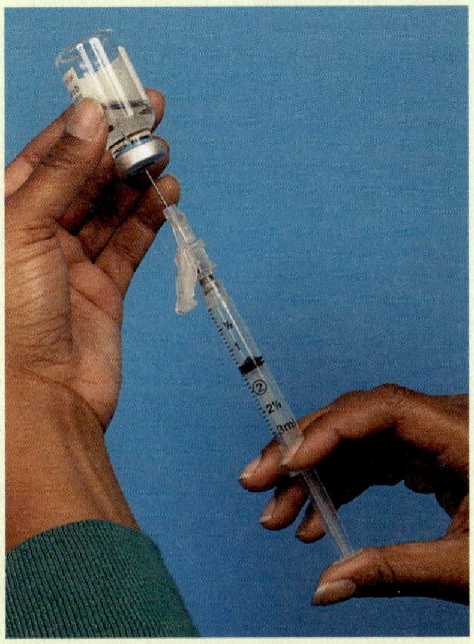

STEP 2B(5) Withdraw fluid with vial inverted.

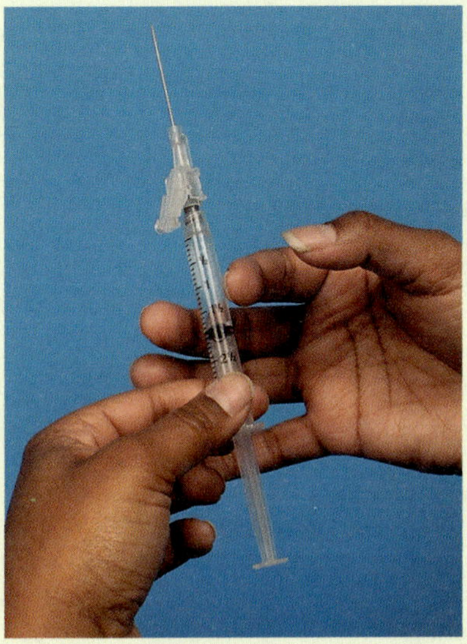

STEP 2B(10) Hold syringe upright; tap barrel to dislodge air bubbles.

SKILL 17-4 PREPARING INJECTIONS FROM VIALS AND AMPULES—cont'd

STEP	RATIONALE
(17) Reconstituted medication in vial is ready for you to draw into new syringe. Read label. Carefully determine dose after reconstitution.	Once you add diluent, concentration of medication (milligrams per milliliter) determines dose you give. Reading medication label carefully decreases administration errors.
(18) Draw up reconstituted medication in syringe following Steps 2B(2) through 2B(12).	Prepares medication for administration.

Clinical Decision Point: **Some agencies require that you verify medications prepared for parenteral administration for accuracy by another nurse. Check guidelines before administering medication.**

STEP	RATIONALE
3. Compare label of medication with MAR for final time at patient's bedside before administering medication.	*Third check for accuracy ensures that right medication is administered.*
4. Return unused multiple-dose medications to shelf, drawer, or refrigerator.	
5. Dispose of soiled supplies. Place broken ampule and/or used vials and used needle or needleless access device in puncture-proof and leak-proof container. Clean work area and perform hand hygiene.	Proper disposal of glass and needle prevents accidental injury to staff. Controls transmission of infection.
EVALUATION	
1. Compare dose in syringe with desired dose.	Determines that dose is accurate.

UNEXPECTED OUTCOMES AND RELATED INTERVENTIONS

- Air bubbles remain in syringe.
  - Expel air from syringe and add medication to syringe until you prepare the correct dose.
- You prepared incorrect dose.
  - Discard prepared dose and prepare corrected new dose.

SKILL 17-5 ADMINISTERING INJECTIONS

DELEGATION CONSIDERATIONS

The skill of administering injections cannot be delegated to nursing assistive personnel (NAP). The nurse informs NAP about:

- Potential side effects of medications and to report their occurrence along with any changes in vital signs or level of consciousness (e.g., sedation) to the nurse.

EQUIPMENT

- Proper-size syringe and safety needle:
  - *Subcutaneous:* Syringe (1 to 3 mL) and needle (25 to 27 gauge, $\frac{3}{8}$ to $\frac{5}{8}$ inch)
  - *Subcutaneous U-100 insulin:* Insulin syringe with preattached needle (28 to 31 gauge, $\frac{5}{16}$ to $\frac{1}{2}$ inch)
  - *Subcutaneous U-500 insulin:* 1-mL Tuberculin syringe with needle (25 to 27 gauge, $\frac{1}{2}$ to $\frac{5}{8}$ inch)
  - *Intramuscular (IM):* Syringe (2 to 3 mL for adult, 0.5 to 1 mL for infants and small children)
    - Needle length corresponds to site and type of injection and age and size of patient. Refer to following guidelines; length needed may vary outside these guidelines in patients who are smaller or larger than average. Needle gauge often depends on length of needle. Administer most biologicals and medications in aqueous solutions with 20- to 25-gauge needle. Use 18- to 25-gauge needles for medications in oil-based solutions (Nicoll and Hesby, 2002).
    - Children (Hockenberry and Wilson, 2011):
      - Preterm and small infants: 16-25 mm ($\frac{5}{8}$-1 inch)
      - Infants: 25 mm (1 inch)
      - Toddlers: 25-32 mm (1-$1\frac{1}{4}$ inch)
      - Older children: 38-51 mm ($1\frac{1}{2}$-2 inch)
    - Adults (Nicoll and Hesby, 2002):
      - Vastus lateralis: 16-25 mm ($\frac{5}{8}$-1 inch)
      - Ventrogluteal: 38 mm ($1\frac{1}{2}$ inch)
      - Deltoid: 25-38 mm (1-$1\frac{1}{2}$ inch)
  - Immunizations: Based on weight and body mass index (CDC, 2012)
    - Subcutaneous: 23-25 gauge, 16 mm ($\frac{5}{8}$ inch)
    - Intramuscular: 22-25 gauge
      - Male or female less than 59 kg (less than 130 pounds): 16-25 mm ($\frac{5}{8}$-1 inch)
      - Female 59-91 kg (130-200 pounds), Male 59-118 kg (130-260 pounds): 25-38 mm (1-$1\frac{1}{2}$ inch)
      - Female more than 91 kg (200 pounds), Male more than 118 kg (260 pounds): 38 mm ($1\frac{1}{2}$ inch)
- *Intradermal (ID):* 1-mL tuberculin syringe with needle (25 to 27 gauge, $\frac{1}{2}$ to $\frac{5}{8}$ inch)

- Small gauze pad
- Antiseptic swab
- Vial or ampule of medication or skin test solution
- Clean gloves
- Medication administration record (MAR) (electronic or printed)
- Puncture-proof container

STEP	RATIONALE
ASSESSMENT	
1. Check accuracy and completeness of each MAR with prescriber's original medication order. Check patient's name, drug name and dosage, route of administration, and time for administration. Clarify incomplete or unclear orders with health care provider before administration. Recopy or reprint any portion of the MAR that is difficult to read.	The prescriber's order is the most reliable source and only legal record of drugs that patient is to receive. Ensures that patient receives the right medications. Illegible MARs are a source of medication errors (Jones and Treiber, 2010; Poon et al., 2010).
2. Review information related to medication, including desired effect, normal dose, route, side effects, time of onset and peak action, and nursing implications.	Allows you to determine if medication is appropriate for patient and anticipate its effects (Lehne, 2013).
3. Assess patient's medical history, allergies (including latex), and medication history. **NOTE:** If patient has latex allergy, use nonlatex gloves.	Knowledge of medical history influences how some medications act. Protects patient from risk for allergic drug response.
4. Observe verbal and nonverbal responses toward receiving injection.	Injections are sometimes painful. Patients often have anxiety, which increases pain.
5. Assess for contraindications:	
a. For subcutaneous injections: Assess for factors such as circulatory shock or reduced local tissue perfusion. Assess adequacy of patient's adipose tissue.	Reduced tissue perfusion interferes with drug absorption and distribution. Physiological changes of aging or patient illness influences the amount of subcutaneous tissue that a patient has. This influences methods for administering injections.
b. For IM injections: Assess for factors such as muscle atrophy, reduced blood flow, or circulatory shock.	Atrophied muscle absorbs medication poorly. Factors interfering with blood flow to muscles impair drug absorption.
c. For ID injections: Assess for history of severe adverse reactions or necrosis that happened after a previous ID injection.	Medications are potent and can cause severe anaphylaxis.
6. Assess patient's knowledge regarding medication to be received.	Determines need for patient education.

Clinical Decision Point: **Because of documented adverse effects of IM injections, other routes of medication injection are safer. Consider calling prescriber for alternate route of medication administration (Nicoll and Hesby, 2002; WHO, 2006).**

STEP	RATIONALE
PLANNING	
1. Collect appropriate equipment and MAR	Enhances time management and efficiency.
2. Plan preparation to avoid interruptions. Do not take phone calls or talk with others. Follow agency "No Interruption Zone" policy.	Interruptions contribute to medication errors (Popescu et al., 2011).
IMPLEMENTATION	
1. Perform hand hygiene and prepare medication using aseptic technique (see Skill 17-4). Check label of medication carefully with the MAR two times while preparing medication.	Following the same routine when preparing medications, eliminating distractions, and checking the label of the medication with MAR reduces errors and ensures that medication is sterile. Preparation techniques vary for ampule and vial. *This is the first and second accuracy check.*
2. Take medications to patient at correct time (see agency policy). Give STAT, first-time or loading doses, and single-order medications at time ordered. Give time-critical medications no later than 30 minutes before or after scheduled dose. Give non–time-critical scheduled medications within a range of either 1 or 2 hours of scheduled dose (ISMP, 2011b). Perform hand hygiene.	Ensures that intended therapeutic effect complies with professional standards. Hospitals need to adopt a medication administration policy and procedure for the timing of medication administration that considers patient needs, the prescribed medication, and the specific clinical indications (CMS, 2011; ISMP, 2011b). Hand hygiene decreases transfer of microorganisms.
3. Close room curtain or door.	Provides privacy.

SKILL 17-5 ADMINISTERING INJECTIONS—cont'd

STEP	RATIONALE
4. Identify patient using two identifiers (e.g., name and birthday or name and account number) according to agency policy. Compare identifiers with information on patient's MAR or medical record.	Ensures correct patient. Complies with The Joint Commission requirements for patient safety (TJC, 2014).
5. Compare label of medication against MAR for third time at patient's bedside.	*Third check for accuracy ensures that right medication is administered.*
6. Explain steps of procedure and tell patient that injection will cause a slight burning or stinging.	Helps minimize patient's anxiety.
7. Apply clean gloves. **NOTE:** If patient has latex allergy, use latex-free gloves.	Reduces transmission of microorganisms.
8. Keep sheet or gown draped over body parts not requiring exposure.	Respects dignity of patient while exposing injection area.
9. Select appropriate injection site. Inspect skin surface over sites for bruises, inflammation, or edema.	Injection sites are free of abnormalities that interfere with drug absorption. Sites used repeatedly become hardened from lipohypertrophy (increased growth in fatty tissue). Do not use an area that is bruised or has signs associated with infection.
a. *Subcutaneous:* Palpate sites and avoid those with masses or tenderness. Rotate insulin sites within an anatomic area. Be sure that needle is correct size by grasping skinfold at site with thumb and forefinger. Measure fold from top to bottom. Make sure that needle is one-half length of fold. For immunizations in children less than 12 months use site in thigh; for patients greater than 12 months use site in upper arm (CDC, 2012).	You can mistakenly give subcutaneous injections in the muscle, especially in the abdomen and thigh sites. Appropriate size of needle ensures that you inject the medication in the subcutaneous tissue (Birkebaek et al., 2008). Sites for immunizations are based on age (CDC, 2012).
b. *IM:* Note integrity and size of muscle and palpate for tenderness or hardness. Avoid these areas. If you give injections frequently, rotate sites. Use ventrogluteal site in all patients if possible. May use vastus lateralis in children less than 12 months and deltoid in patients older than 12 months. For immunizations use vastus lateralis in children less than 3 years and deltoid in patients older than 3 years (CDC, 2012).	The ventrogluteal site is the preferred injection site for adults. This site is also preferred for children who are receiving irritating or viscous solutions (Hockenberry and Wilson, 2011; Nicoll and Hesby, 2002). Sites for immunizations are based on age (CDC, 2012).
c. *ID:* Note lesions or discolorations of skin. If possible select site three to four finger widths below antecubital space and one hand width above wrist. If you cannot use the forearm, inspect the upper back. If necessary use sites appropriate for subcutaneous injections.	An ID injection site is free of discolorations or hair so you can see the results of skin test and interpret them correctly (CDC, 2013).
10. Help patient to comfortable position:	
a. *Subcutaneous:* Have patient relax arm, leg, or abdomen, depending on site chosen for injection.	Relaxation of site minimizes discomfort.
b. *IM:* Position patient depending on site chosen (e.g., sitting, supine, on side).	Reduces strain on muscle and minimizes discomfort of injections.
c. *ID:* Have patient extend elbow and support it and forearm on flat surface.	Stabilizes injection site for easiest accessibility.
d. Talk with patient about subject of interest.	Distraction reduces anxiety.

Clinical Decision Point: **Ensure that patient's position is not contraindicated by medical condition.**

STEP	RATIONALE
11. Relocate site using anatomical landmarks.	Injection into correct anatomical site prevents injury to nerves, bones, and blood vessels (Nicoll and Hesby, 2002).
12. Clean site with an antiseptic swab. Apply swab at center of site and rotate outward in a circular direction for about 5 cm (2 inches) (see illustration).	Mechanical action of swab removes secretions containing microorganisms.
13. Hold swab or gauze between third and fourth fingers of nondominant hand.	Gauze or swab remains readily accessible when withdrawing needle.

STEP	RATIONALE
14. Remove needle cap from needle by pulling it straight off.	Preventing needle from touching sides of cap prevents contamination.
15. Hold syringe between thumb and forefinger of dominant hand:	
a. *Subcutaneous:* Hold as dart, palm down (see illustration).	Quick, smooth injection requires proper manipulation of syringe parts.
b. *IM:* Hold as dart, palm down.	
c. *ID:* Hold bevel of needle pointing up.	With bevel up you are less likely to deposit medication into tissues below dermis.
16. Administer injection:	
A. Subcutaneous:	
(1) For average-size patient pinch skin with nondominant hand.	Pinching skin elevates subcutaneous tissue and desensitizes area.
(2) Inject needle quickly and firmly at 45- to 90-degree angle. Release skin if pinched. *Option:* Continue to pinch skin and release after injecting medications.	Quick, firm insertion minimizes discomfort. (Injecting medication into compressed tissue irritates nerve fibers.) Correct angle prevents accidental injection into muscle.
(3) For obese patient pinch skin at site and inject needle at 90-degree angle below tissue fold.	Obese patients have fatty layer of tissue above subcutaneous layer.

Clinical Decision Point: **Aspiration after injecting a subcutaneous medication is not necessary (Lilley et al., 2011). Piercing a blood vessel in a subcutaneous injection is very rare.**

STEP	RATIONALE
(4) Inject medication slowly (see illustration).	Minimizes discomfort.
B. Intramuscular:	
(1) Position ulnar aspect of nondominant hand just below site and pull skin approximately 2.5 to 3.5 cm down or laterally to administer in a Z-track. Hold position until medication is injected. With dominant hand inject needle quickly at 90-degree angle into muscle.	Z-track creates zigzag path through tissues that seals needle track to avoid tracking of medication (Nicoll and Hesby, 2002). A quick, dartlike injection reduces discomfort.
(2) *Option:* If patient's muscle mass is small, grasp body of muscle between thumb and fingers.	Ensures that medication reaches muscle mass (Hockenberry and Wilson, 2011).

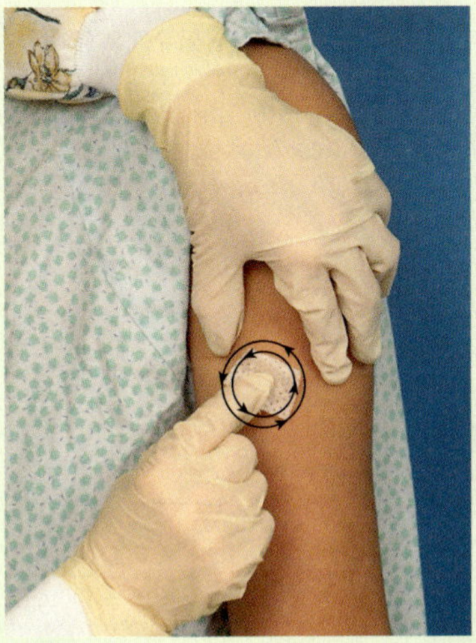

STEP 12 Clean site with circular motion.

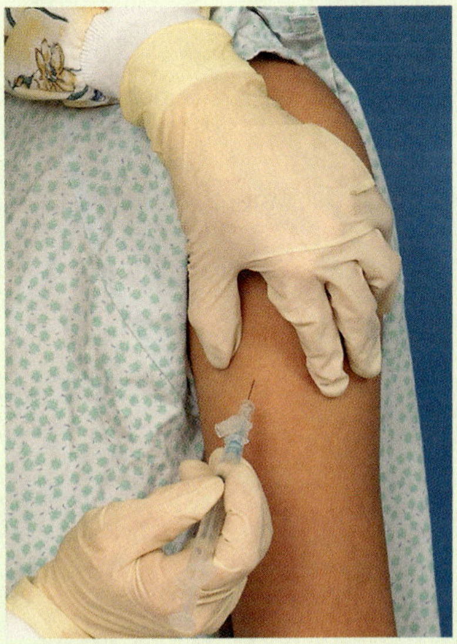

STEP 15a Hold syringe as if grasping a dart.

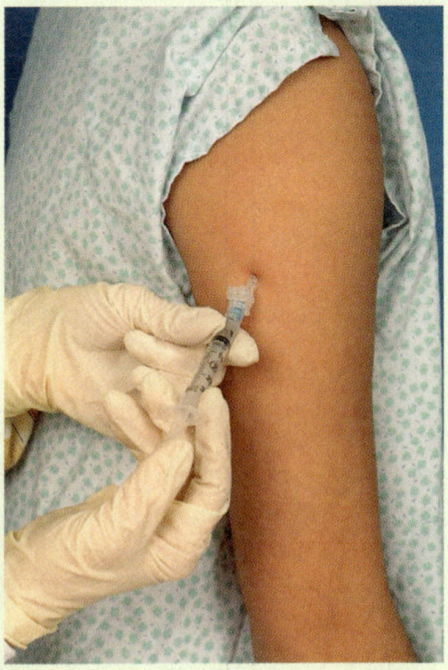

STEP 16A(4) Inject medication slowly.

SKILL 17-5 ADMINISTERING INJECTIONS—cont'd

STEP	RATIONALE
(3) Insert needle into the muscle using a smooth and steady motion. Grasp syringe barrel with thumb and forefinger of nondominant hand to stabilize syringe. Continue to pull skin tightly with nondominant hand. Move dominant hand to end of plunger. Do not move syringe.	Smooth manipulation of syringe reduces discomfort from needle movement (Nicoll and Hesby, 2002). Skin remains pulled until after you inject drug to ensure Z-track administration.
(4) Pull back on plunger 5 to 10 seconds. If no blood appears, inject medication slowly at a rate of 1 mL/10 sec.	Pulling back on syringe for 5 to 10 seconds ensures that needle is not in a low-flow vessel (Nicoll and Hesby, 2002). Aspiration of blood into syringe indicates intravenous (IV) placement of needle. Slow injection reduces pain and tissue trauma (Hockenberry and Wilson, 2011; Nicoll and Hesby, 2002). The CDC (2012) states that there is no need to aspirate *when administering vaccines* to reduce injection site discomfort. Follow agency policies for aspiration of IM injections.

Clinical Decision Point: **If blood appears in syringe, remove needle, dispose of medication and syringe properly, and prepare another dose of medication for injection.**

STEP	RATIONALE
(5) Wait 10 seconds and smoothly and steadily withdraw needle; then release skin.	Allows time for medication to absorb into muscle before removing syringe (Nicoll and Hesby, 2002).
C. **Intradermal:**	
(1) With nondominant hand stretch skin over site with forefinger or thumb.	Needle pierces tight skin more easily.
(2) With needle almost against patient's skin, insert it slowly at a 5- to 15-degree angle until resistance is felt. Then advance it through epidermis to approximately 3 mm (1/8 inch) below skin surface. You see needle tip through skin.	Ensures that needle tip is in dermis. You obtain inaccurate results if you do not inject needle at correct angle and depth (CDC, 2013).
(3) Inject medication slowly. Normally you feel resistance. If not, needle is too deep; remove and begin again.	Slow injection minimizes discomfort at site. Dermal layer is tight and does not expand easily when you inject solution.
(4) While injecting medication, note that small bleb (approximately 6 mm [1/4 inch]) resembling mosquito bite appears on skin surface (see illustration).	Bleb indicates that you deposited medication in dermis.
17. After withdrawing needle, apply alcohol swab or gauze gently over site.	Support of tissue around injection site minimizes discomfort during needle withdrawal. Dry gauze minimizes discomfort associated with alcohol on nonintact skin.
18. Apply gentle pressure. *Do not massage site.* Apply bandage if needed.	Massage damages underlying tissue. Massage of ID site disperses medication into underlying tissue layers and alters test results.
19. Help patient to comfortable position.	Gives patient sense of well-being.

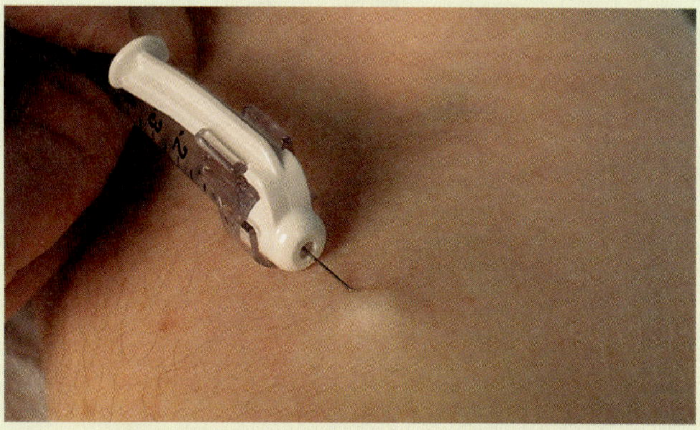

STEP 16C(4) Injection creates small bleb.

STEP	RATIONALE
20. Discard uncapped needle or needle enclosed in safety shield and attached syringe into puncture-proof and leakproof receptacle.	Prevents injury to patient and health care personnel. Recapping needles increases risk for needlestick injury (OSHA, n.d.b).
21. Remove gloves and perform hand hygiene.	Reduces transmission of microorganisms.
22. Stay with patient and observe for any allergic reactions.	Dyspnea, wheezing, and circulatory collapse are signs of severe anaphylactic reaction.
EVALUATION	
1. Return to room and ask if patient feels any acute pain, burning, numbness, or tingling at injection site.	Continued discomfort indicates injury to underlying bones or nerves.
2. Inspect site, noting any bruising or induration. Document findings and notify health care provider. Provide warm compress to site.	Bruising or induration indicates complication associated with injection.
3. Observe patient's response to medication at times that correlate with its onset, peak, and duration.	The body rapidly absorbs IM medications. Adverse effects of parenteral medications develop rapidly. Evaluation determines effectiveness of medication.
4. Use Teach Back—State to the patient, "I want to be sure I explained your medications correctly. Can you tell me the name of each of your medications, why you are taking them, how much to take, when to take them, and which side effects you may experience?" Revise your instruction now or develop plan for revised patient teaching to be implemented at an appropriate time if patient is not able to teach back correctly.	Evaluates what the patient is able to explain or demonstrate.
5. *For ID injections:* Use skin pencil to draw circle around perimeter of injection site. Read site within appropriate amount of time, designated by type of medication or skin test you give.	Pencil mark makes site easy to find. You determine the results of skin testing at various times, based on the type of medication used or the type of skin testing completed. Refer to manufacturer directions to determine when to read the test results.

Clinical Decision Point: **Read tuberculin test at 48 to 72 hours. Induration (hard, dense, raised area) of skin around injection site indicates positive tuberculin reaction of:**
- **15 mm or more in patients with no known risk factors for tuberculosis (TB).**
- **10 mm or more in patients who are recent immigrants; injection drug users; residents and employees of high-risk settings; patients with certain chronic illnesses; children less than 4 years of age; and infants, children, and adolescents exposed to high-risk adults.**
- **5 mm or more in patients who are human immunodeficiency virus (HIV) positive, immunocompromised patients, or patients recently exposed to TB (CDC, 2013)**

RECORDING AND REPORTING

- Document medication, dose, route, site, time, and date given on MAR.
- Document your evaluation of patient learning.
- Record patient's response to medications in nurses' notes.
- Report any undesirable effects from medication to prescriber.
- Document if medication is withheld or refused per agency policy.

UNEXPECTED OUTCOMES AND RELATED INTERVENTIONS

- Raised, reddened, or hard zone (induration) forms around ID test site.
  - Notify patient's health care provider.
  - Document sensitivity to injected allergen or positive test if tuberculin skin testing was completed.
- Hypertrophy of skin develops from repeated subcutaneous injections.
  - Do not use this site for future injections.
  - Instruct patient not to use site for 6 months.
- Patient develops signs and symptoms of allergy or side effects.
  - Follow agency policy or guidelines for appropriate response to adverse drug reactions.
  - Notify patient's health care provider immediately.
  - Document allergy information in patient's medical record.
- Patient states that he or she has localized pain, numbness, tingling, or burning at injection site.
  - Assess injection site and document findings.
  - Notify patient's health care provider.

SKILL 17-6 ADMINISTERING MEDICATIONS BY INTRAVENOUS BOLUS

DELEGATION CONSIDERATIONS

The skill of administering medications by intravenous (IV) bolus cannot be delegated to nursing assistive personnel (NAP). The nurse informs NAP about:

- Potential side effects of medications and the need to report their occurrence.
- The need to report discomfort at infusion site as soon as possible.
- Obtaining any required vital signs and reporting these findings.

EQUIPMENT

- Watch with second hand
- Medication administration record (MAR) (electronic or printed)
- Clean gloves
- Antiseptic swab
- Medication in vial or ampule
- Safety syringe for medication preparation
- Needleless device or sterile safety needle (21 to 25 gauge)
- Intravenous lock: Vial of appropriate flush solution (saline most common, but heparin flush may also be used; if heparin flush is used, most common concentration is 10 to 100 units per milliliter; check agency policy).

STEP	RATIONALE
ASSESSMENT	
1. Check accuracy and completeness of each MAR with prescriber's original medication order. Check patient's name, drug name and dose, route of administration, and time for administration. Clarify incomplete or unclear orders with health care provider before administration Recopy or reprint any portion of the MAR that is difficult to read.	The prescriber's order is the most reliable source and only legal record of drugs that patient is to receive. Ensures that patient receives the right medications. Illegible MARs are a source of medication errors (Jones and Treiber, 2010; Poon et al., 2010).

Clinical Decision Point: **Some IV medications can be pushed safely only when the patient is monitored continuously for dysrhythmias, blood pressure changes, or other adverse effects. Therefore you can push some medications only in specific areas within a health care agency. Confirm agency guidelines regarding requirements for special monitoring and the recommended rate of injection before giving these medications (Lehne, 2013).**

STEP	RATIONALE
2. Review drug reference information necessary to administer drug safely, including action, purpose, side effects, normal dose, time of peak onset, how slowly to give the medication, and nursing implications such as the need to dilute the medication or administer it through a filter.	Allows you to determine if medication is appropriate for patient, anticipate effects of medication, and prevent incompatible drug reaction (Lehne, 2013).
3. If you give drug through existing IV line, determine compatibility of medication with IV fluids and any additives within IV solution.	IV medication is sometimes not compatible with IV solution and/or additives.
4. Perform hand hygiene. Assess condition of IV needle insertion site for signs of infiltration or phlebitis (see Chapter 18).	Do not administer medication if site is edematous or inflamed.
5. Assess patient's medical history, allergies (including latex), and medication history. If patient has latex allergy, use nonlatex gloves.	Knowledge of medical history influences how some medications act. Protects patient from risk for allergic drug response. IV bolus delivers drug rapidly. Allergic reaction could prove fatal.
6. Assess patient's understanding of purpose of drug therapy.	Reveals need for education.
PLANNING	
1. Collect appropriate equipment and MAR.	Enhances time management and efficiency.
2. Plan preparation to avoid interruptions. Do not take phone calls or talk with others. Follow agency "No Interruption Zone" policy.	Interruptions contribute to medication errors (Popescu et al., 2011).

Clinical Decision Point: **Some IV medications require dilution before administration. Verify with agency policy. If a small amount of medication is given (e.g., less than 1 mL), dilute medication in small amount (e.g., 5 mL) of normal saline or sterile water so the medication does not collect in the "dead spaces" (e.g., Y-site injection port, IV cap) of the IV delivery system. Verify that medication can be diluted by consulting medication reference or checking with pharmacist first.**

STEP	RATIONALE
IMPLEMENTATION	
1. Perform hand hygiene and prepare medication from ampule or vial using aseptic technique (see Skill 17-4). Check label of medication carefully with MAR 2 times.	Ensures that medication is sterile. Preparation techniques differ for ampule and vial. Following the same routine when preparing medications, eliminating distractions, and checking the label of the medication with MAR reduces errors. *This is the first and second accuracy check.*
2. Take medications to patient at correct time (see agency policy). Give STAT, first-time or loading doses, and single-order medications at time ordered. Give time-critical medications no later than 30 minutes before or after scheduled dose. Give non–time-critical scheduled medications within a range of either 1 or 2 hours of scheduled dose (ISMP, 2011b). Perform hand hygiene.	Ensures that intended therapeutic effect complies with professional standards. Hospitals need to adopt a medication administration policy and procedure for the timing of medication administration that considers the patient needs, the prescribed medication, and the specific clinical indications (CMS, 2011; ISMP, 2011b). Hand hygiene decreases transfer of microorganisms.
3. Identify patient using two identifiers (e.g., name and birthday or name and account number) according to agency policy. Compare identifiers with information on patient's MAR or medical record.	Ensures correct patient. Complies with The Joint Commission requirements for patient safety (TJC, 2014).
4. Compare label of medication against MAR for third time at patient's bedside.	*Third check for accuracy ensures that right medication is administered.*
5. Explain procedure to patient. Encourage patient to report symptoms of discomfort at IV site.	Keeps patient informed and involved in care; helps identify possible infiltration early.
6. Put on clean gloves. **NOTE:** If patient has a latex allergy, use latex-free gloves.	Reduces transmission of microorganisms. There is risk of blood exposure during medication administration.
7. Intravenous push (existing line):	
a. Select injection port of IV tubing closest to patient. Whenever possible use needleless injection port. Use IV filter if required by medication reference or agency policy.	Follows provisions of The Needle Safety and Prevention Act of 2001 (OSHA, n.d.a).

Clinical Decision Point: **Never administer IV medications through tubing that is infusing blood, blood products, or parenteral nutrition solutions.**

STEP	RATIONALE
b. Clean port with antiseptic swab and allow to dry.	Prevents transfer of microorganisms during needle insertion.
c. Connect syringe to IV line: Insert needleless tip of syringe or small-gauge safety needle containing drug through center of port (see illustration).	Prevents damage to port diaphragm.
d. Occlude IV line by pinching tubing just above injection port (see illustration). Pull back gently on syringe plunger to aspirate for blood return.	Final check ensures that medication is delivered into bloodstream.

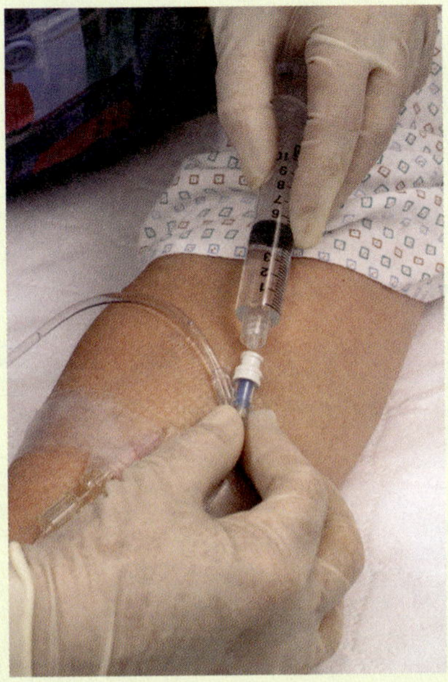

STEP 7c Connecting syringe to IV line with blunt needleless cannula tip.

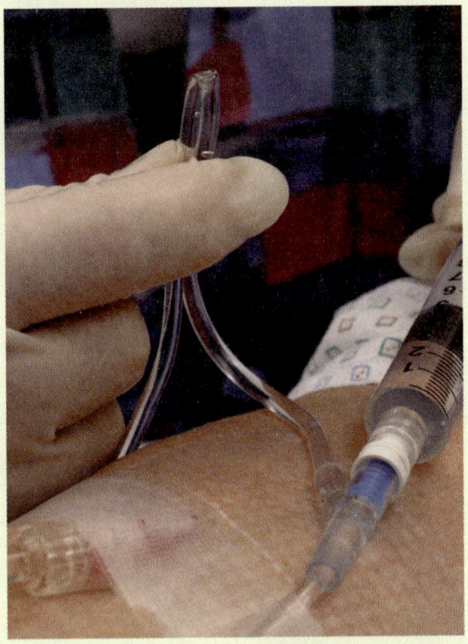

STEP 7d IV line pinched above injection port to aspirate for blood return.

SKILL 17-6 ADMINISTERING MEDICATIONS BY INTRAVENOUS BOLUS—cont'd

STEP	RATIONALE
Clinical Decision Point: **In some cases, especially with a smaller-gauge IV needle, blood return is not aspirated, even if IV line is patent. If IV site does not show signs of infiltration and IV fluid is infusing without difficulty, proceed with IV push.**	
e. Release tubing and inject medication within amount of time recommended by institutional policy, pharmacist, or medication reference manual. Use a watch to time administrations (see illustration). You can pinch the IV line while pushing medication and release it when not pushing medication. Allow IV fluids to infuse when not pushing medication.	Ensures safe drug infusion. Rapid injection of IV drug can be fatal. Allowing IV fluids to infuse while pushing IV drug enables medication to be delivered to patient at prescribed rate.
Clinical Decision Point: **If IV medication is incompatible with IV fluids, stop the IV fluids, clamp the IV line, flush with 10 mL of normal saline or sterile water, give the IV bolus over the appropriate amount of time, flush with another 10 mL of normal saline or sterile water at the same rate as the medication was administered, and restart the IV fluids at the prescribed rate. This allows you to give IV push medication through the existing line without creating potential risks associated with IV incompatibilities. If IV infusion that is currently hanging is a medication (e.g., ranitidine), disconnect IV line and administer IV push medication as outlined in Step 8 to avoid giving a sudden bolus of the medication in the existing IV line to the patient. Verify institutional policy regarding stopping IV fluids or continuous IV medications. If unable to stop IV infusion, start a new IV site (see Chapter 18) and administer medication using the IV push (IV lock) method.**	
f. After injecting medication, withdraw syringe and recheck fluid infusion rate.	Injection of bolus often alters rate of fluid infusion. Rapid fluid infusion causes circulatory fluid overload.
8. IV push (IV lock):	
a. Prepare two syringes filled with 2 to 3 mL of normal saline (0.9%).	Normal saline is effective in keeping IV locks patent and do not carry risk of thrombocytopenia associated with heparin flushes.
b. Administer medication:	
(1) Clean lock injection port with antiseptic swab and allow to dry.	Prevents transfer of microorganisms during needle insertion.
(2) Insert syringe with normal saline (0.9%) through injection port of IV lock (see illustrations).	

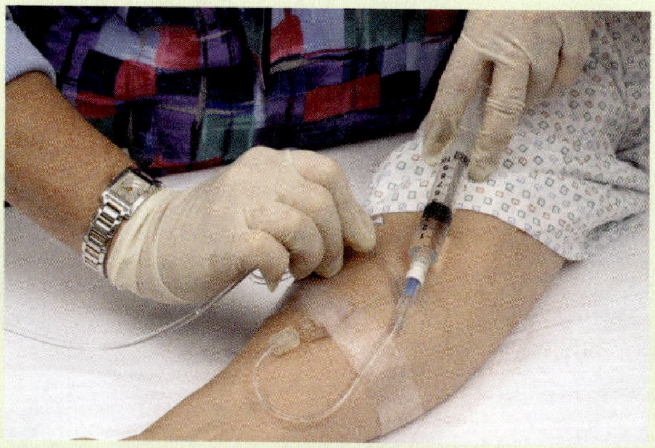

STEP 7e Using watch to time an IV push medication.

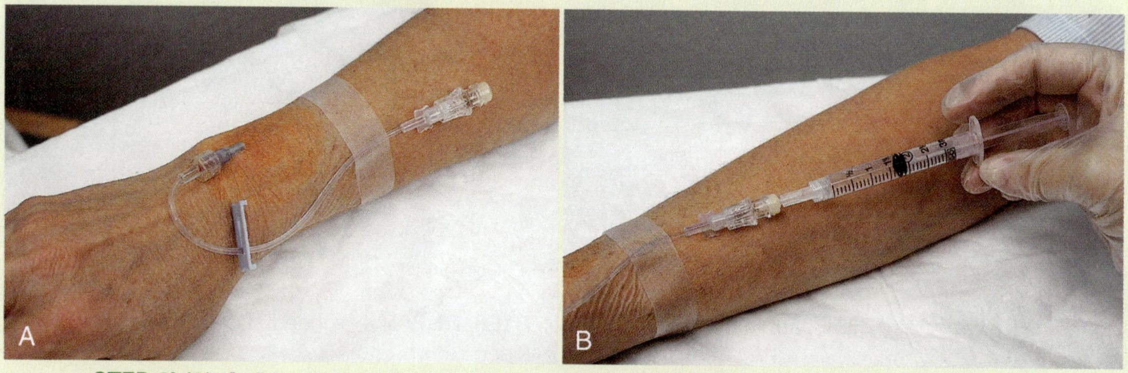

STEP 8b(2) A, IV catheter with saline lock adapter. **B,** Syringe inserted into injection port.

STEP	RATIONALE
(3) Pull back gently on syringe plunger, and check for blood return.	Indicates if needle or catheter is in vein.

Clinical Decision Point: In some cases, especially with a smaller-gauge IV needle, blood return is usually not aspirated, even if IV line is patent. If IV site does not show signs of infiltration and IV flushes without difficulty, proceed with IV push.

STEP	RATIONALE
(4) Flush IV site with normal saline by pushing slowly on plunger.	Cleans needle and reservoir of blood. Flushing without difficulty indicates patent IV line.

Clinical Decision Point: Carefully observe the area of skin above the IV catheter. Note any puffiness or swelling as you flush the IV line. Swelling indicates infiltration into the vein and requires removal of catheter.

STEP	RATIONALE
(5) Remove saline-filled syringe.	
(6) Clean lock injection port with antiseptic swab.	Prevents transmission of infection.
(7) Insert syringe containing prepared medication through injection port of IV lock.	Allows administration of medication.
(8) Inject medication within amount of time recommended by agency policy, pharmacist, or medication reference manual. Use watch to time administration.	Many medication errors are associated with IV pushes being administered too quickly. Following guidelines for IV push rates promotes patient safety (Lehne, 2013).
(9) After administering bolus, withdraw syringe.	
(10) Clean lock injection site with antiseptic swab.	Prevents transmission of infection.
(11) Flush injection port by attaching syringe with normal saline and inject normal saline flush at same rate that medication was delivered. Remove syringe.	Flushing IV line with saline prevents occlusion of IV access device and ensures that all medication is delivered. Flushing IV site at same rate as medication ensures that any medication remaining within IV needle is delivered at the correct rate.
9. Dispose of uncapped needles and syringes in puncture-proof and leakproof container.	Prevents accidental needlestick injuries and follows CDC guidelines for disposal of sharps (OSHA, n.d.a).
10. Remove gloves and perform hand hygiene.	Reduces transfer of microorganisms.
EVALUATION	
1. Observe patient closely for adverse reactions during administration and for several minutes thereafter.	IV medications act rapidly.
2. Observe IV site during injection for sudden swelling.	Swelling indicates infiltration into tissues surrounding vein.
3. Assess patient's status after giving medication to evaluate its effectiveness.	Some IV bolus medications cause rapid changes in the patient's physiological status. Some drugs require careful monitoring and assessment and possibly future laboratory testing (e.g., vasopressors and antiarrhythmics require blood pressure and heart rate monitoring, whereas heparin requires laboratory studies after administration to determine if it is in a therapeutic level).
4. Use Teach Back—State to the patient, "I want to be sure I explained your medications correctly. Can you tell me the name of each of your medications, why you are taking them, how much to take, when to take them, and which side effects you may experience?" Revise your instruction now or develop plan for revised patient teaching to be implemented at an appropriate time if patient is not able to teach back correctly.	Evaluates what the patient is able to explain or demonstrate.

RECORDING AND REPORTING

- Record medication administration, including drug name, dose, route, and time of administration.
- Document your evaluation of patient learning.
- Record patient's response to medication in nurses' notes.
- Report any adverse reactions to patient's health care provider. Patient's response may indicate need for additional medical therapy.

UNEXPECTED OUTCOMES AND RELATED INTERVENTIONS

- Patient develops adverse reaction to medication.
  - Stop delivering medication immediately and follow agency policy or guidelines for appropriate response and reporting of adverse drug reactions.
  - Add allergy information to patient's medical record per agency policy.

SKILL 17-6 ADMINISTERING MEDICATIONS BY INTRAVENOUS BOLUS—cont'd

- IV site shows symptoms of infiltration or phlebitis (see Chapter 18).
  - Stop infusing medication.
  - Treat IV site as indicated by agency policy.
  - Insert new IV site if continuing IV therapy.
- Patient is unable to explain medication information.
  - Patient requires reinstruction or is unable to learn at this time.

SKILL 17-7 ADMINISTERING INTRAVENOUS MEDICATIONS BY PIGGYBACK, INTERMITTENT INTRAVENOUS INFUSION SETS, AND MINI-INFUSION PUMPS

DELEGATION CONSIDERATIONS

The skill of administering intravenous (IV) medications cannot be delegated to nursing assistive personnel (NAP). The nurse informs NAP about:

- Potential side effects of medications and to report their occurrence.
- Reporting patient's report of any discomfort at infusion site to nurse.
- Reporting any change in the patient's condition or vital signs to nurse.

EQUIPMENT

- Adhesive tape *(optional)*
- Antiseptic swab
- IV pole
- Medication administration record (MAR) (electronic or printed)
- Clean gloves

Piggyback or Mini-infusion Pump

- Medication prepared in 5- to 250-mL labeled infusion bag or syringe
- Short microdrip, macrodrip, or mini-infusion IV tubing set, preferably with needleless system attachment
- Needleless access device (**Note:** Stopcocks are not recommended [INS, 2011])
- Mini-infusion pump if indicated

Volume-Control Administration Set

- Volutrol or Buretrol
- Infusion tubing (may have needleless device system attachment)
- Safety syringe (1 to 20 mL)
- Vial or ampule of ordered medication

STEP	RATIONALE
ASSESSMENT	
1. Check accuracy and completeness of each MAR with prescriber's original medication order. Check patient's name, drug name and dosage, route of administration, and time for administration. Clarify incomplete or unclear orders with health care provider before administration. Recopy or reprint any portion of MAR that is difficult to read.	The prescriber's order is the most reliable source and only legal record of drugs that patient is to receive. Ensures that patient receives the right medications. Illegible MARs are a source of medication errors (Jones and Treiber, 2010; Poon et al., 2010).
2. Assess patient's medical history, allergies (including latex), and medication history. **Note:** If patient has latex allergy, use nonlatex gloves.	Helps you anticipate therapeutic effect of medication. IV medications act rapidly. Allergic reactions can be fatal.
3. Review drug reference information necessary to administer drug safely, including action, purpose, side effects, normal dose, time of peak onset, how slowly to give the medication, and nursing implications such as the need to dilute the medication or administer it through a filter.	Allows you to determine if medication is appropriate for patient, anticipate effects of medication, and prevent incompatible drug reaction (Lehne, 2013).
4. Assess compatibility of drug with existing IV solution.	Drugs that are incompatible with IV solutions result in clouding or crystallization solution in IV tubing, which harms the patient.
5. Assess patency of patient's existing IV infusion line (see Chapter 18).	For medication to reach venous circulation effectively, IV line needs to be patent, and fluids should infuse easily.

Clinical Decision Point: **If the patient's IV site is saline locked, cleanse the port with alcohol and assess the patency of the IV line by flushing it with 2 to 3 mL of sterile normal saline. Attach appropriate IV tubing to the saline lock and administer the medication via piggyback, mini-infusion, or volume-control administration set. When the infusion is completed, disconnect the tubing, cleanse the port with alcohol, and flush the IV line with 2 to 3 mL of sterile normal saline. Maintain sterility of IV tubing between intermittent infusions.**

STEP	RATIONALE
6. Perform hand hygiene. Assess IV insertion site for signs of infiltration or phlebitis: redness, pallor, swelling, or tenderness on palpation.	Confirmation of placement of IV needle or catheter and integrity of surrounding tissues ensures that you administer medication safely.
7. Assess patient's understanding of purpose of drug therapy.	Reveals need for education.

STEP	RATIONALE
PLANNING	
1. Collect appropriate equipment and MAR.	Enhances time management and efficiency.
2. Plan preparation to avoid interruptions. Do not take phone calls or talk with others. Follow agency "No Interruption Zone" policy.	Interruptions contribute to medication errors (Popescu et al, 2011).
IMPLEMENTATION	
1. Perform hand hygiene and prepare medication from ampule or vial using aseptic technique (see Skill 17-4). Check label of medication carefully with MAR two times.	Ensures that medication is sterile. Preparation techniques differ for ampule and vial. Following the same routine when preparing medications, eliminating distractions, and checking the label of the medication with MAR reduces errors. *This is the first and second accuracy check.*
2. Take medications to patient at correct time (see agency policy). Give STAT, first-time or loading doses, and single-order medications at time ordered. Give time-critical medications no later than 30 minutes before or after scheduled dose. Give non–time-critical scheduled medications within a range of either 1 or 2 hours of scheduled dose (ISMP, 2011b). Perform hand hygiene.	Ensures that intended therapeutic effect complies with professional standards. Hospitals need to adopt a medication administration policy and procedure for the timing of medication administration that considers the patient needs, the prescribed medication, and the specific clinical indications (CMS, 2011; ISMP, 2011b). Hand hygiene decreases transfer of microorganisms.
3. Identify patient using two identifiers (e.g., name and birthday or name and account number) according to agency policy. Compare identifiers with information on patient's MAR or medical record.	Ensures correct patient. Complies with The Joint Commission requirements for patient safety (TJC, 2014).
4. Explain purpose of medication and side effects to patient and that you will give medication through existing IV line. Encourage patient to report symptoms of discomfort at site.	Keeps patient informed of planned therapies, minimizing anxiety. Patients who verbalize pain at IV site help detect IV infiltrations early, lessening damage to surrounding tissues.
5. Compare label of medication against MAR for third time at patient's bedside.	*Third check for accuracy ensures that right medication is administered.*
6. Put on clean gloves. **NOTE:** If patient has a latex allergy, use latex-free gloves.	Reduces transmission of microorganisms. There is risk of blood exposure during medication administration.
7. Administer infusion:	

Clinical Decision Point: **Never administer IV medications through tubing that is infusing blood, blood products, or parenteral nutrition solutions.**

STEP	RATIONALE
A. **Piggyback Infusion:**	
(1) Connect infusion tubing to medication bag (see Chapter 18). Allow solution to fill tubing by opening regulator flow clamp. Once tubing is full, close clamp and cap end of tubing.	Filling infusion tubing with solution and freeing air bubbles prevent air embolus.
(2) Hang piggyback medication bag above level of primary fluid bag (see Figure 17-24). (Use hook to lower main bag.)	Height of fluid bag affects rate of flow to patient.
(3) Wipe off needleless port of main IV line with antiseptic swab and allow to air dry. Connect tubing of piggyback infusion to appropriate connector on upper Y-port of primary infusion line and insert tip of piggyback infusion tubing (see illustration).	Connection allows IV medication to enter main IV line.

Clinical Decision Point: **Any add-on device such as a stopcock or extension set increases the chances for contamination. Number of manipulations and accidental disconnections or misconnections should be limited. The use of stopcocks is not recommended because of increased infection risk. When a stopcock is attached, always attach a sterile cap to the port of the stopcock to provide a closed system when not in use (INS, 2011).**

STEP	RATIONALE
(4) Regulate flow rate of medication solution by adjusting regulator clamp or IV pump infusion rate (see Chapter 18). Infusion times vary. Refer to medication reference or agency policy for safe flow rate.	Provides slow, safe infusion of medication and maintains therapeutic blood levels.

SKILL 17-7 ADMINISTERING INTRAVENOUS MEDICATIONS BY PIGGYBACK, INTERMITTENT INTRAVENOUS INFUSION SETS, AND MINI-INFUSION PUMPS—cont'd

STEP	RATIONALE
(5) After medication has infused, check flow rate on primary infusion. The primary infusion automatically begins to flow after piggyback solution is empty. If stopcock is used, turn it to off position.	Back-check valve on piggyback stops flow of primary infusion until medication infuses. Checking flow rate ensures proper administration of IV fluids.
(6) Regulate main infusion line to ordered rate if necessary.	Infusion of piggyback sometimes interferes with main line infusion rate.
(7) Leave IV piggyback bag and tubing in place for future drug administration or discard in appropriate containers.	Establishing secondary line produces route for microorganisms to enter main line. Repeated changes in tubing increase risk for infection transmission (check agency policy).
B. Mini-infusion Administration:	
(1) Connect prefilled syringe to mini-infusion tubing.	Special tubing designed to fit syringe delivers medication to main IV line.
(2) Carefully apply pressure to syringe plunger, allowing tubing to fill with medication.	Ensures that tubing is free of air bubbles to prevent air embolus.
(3) Place syringe into mini-infusion pump (follow product directions). Be sure that syringe is secured (see illustration).	Correct placement is necessary for proper infusion.
(4) Wipe off needleless port of IV tubing with disinfectant swab and allow to dry. Connect mini-infusion tubing to main IV line.	OSHA (n.d.a) recommends needleless system to reduce risk for needlestick injuries.
(5) Hang infusion pump with syringe on IV pole alongside main IV bag. Set pump to deliver medication within time recommended by agency policy, a pharmacist, or a medication reference manual. Set alarm if infusing medication through saline lock. Press button on pump to begin infusion.	Pump automatically delivers medication at safe, constant rate based on volume in syringe.
(6) After medication has infused, check flow rate on primary infusion. Infusion automatically begins to flow once pump stops. Regulate main infusion line to desired rate as needed.	Maintains patency of primary IV line.

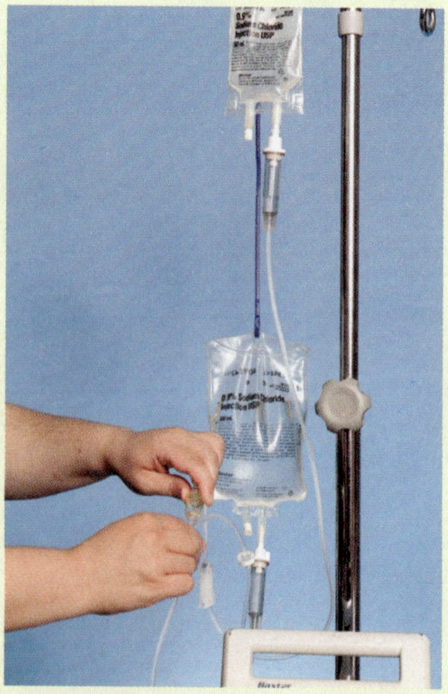

STEP 7A(3) For needleless system, insert tip of piggyback infusion tubing into port.

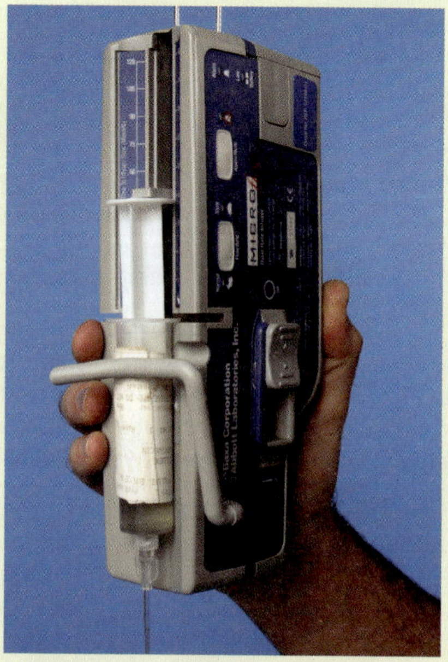

STEP 7B(3) Ensure that syringe is secure after placing it into mini-infusion pump.

STEP	RATIONALE
C. Volume-Control Administration Set (e.g., Buretrol):	
(1) Fill Buretrol with desired amount of fluid (50 to 100 mL) by opening clamp between Buretrol and main IV bag (see illustration).	Small volume of fluid dilutes IV medication and reduces risk for fluid infusing too rapidly.
(2) Close clamp and check to be sure that clamp on air vent of Buretrol chamber is open.	Prevents additional leakage of fluid into Buretrol. Air vent allows fluid in Buretrol to exit at regulated rate.
(3) Clean injection port on top of Buretrol with antiseptic swab and allow to dry.	Prevents introduction of microorganisms during needle insertion.
(4) Remove needle cap or sheath and insert syringe needle through port; inject medication (see illustrations). Gently rotate Buretrol between hands.	Rotating mixes medication with solution in Buretrol to ensure equal distribution.
(5) Regulate IV infusion rate to allow medication to infuse in time recommended by agency policy, a pharmacist, or a medication reference manual.	For optimal therapeutic effect, drug needs to infuse in prescribed time interval.
(6) Label Buretrol with name of drug; dosage; total volume, including diluent; and time of administration following ISMP (2013b) safe IV medication label format (see Figure 17-25).	Alerts nurses to drug being infused. Prevents other medications from being added to Buretrol.
(7) If patient is receiving a continuous IV infusion, check continuous infusion after Buretrol infusion is complete to ensure the appropriate rate of IV fluid administration.	Ensures appropriate fluid balance.
(8) Dispose of uncapped needle or needle enclosed in safety shield and syringe in proper container.	Prevents accidental needlesticks (OSHA, n.d.a).
(9) Discard supplies in appropriate container. Perform hand hygiene.	Reduces transmission of microorganisms.
EVALUATION	
1. Assess patient's status after giving medication.	Evaluates effect of medication.
2. Observe patient for signs of adverse reactions.	IV medications act rapidly.
3. During infusion periodically check infusion rate and condition of IV site.	IV system needs to remain patent for proper drug administration. Development of infiltration requires discontinuing infusion.
4. Use Teach Back—State to the patient, "I want to be sure I explained your medications correctly. Can you tell me the name of each of your medications, why you are taking them, how much to take, when to take them, and which side effects you may experience?" Revise your instruction now or develop plan for revised patient teaching to be implemented at an appropriate time if patient is not able to teach back correctly.	Evaluates what the patient is able to explain or demonstrate.

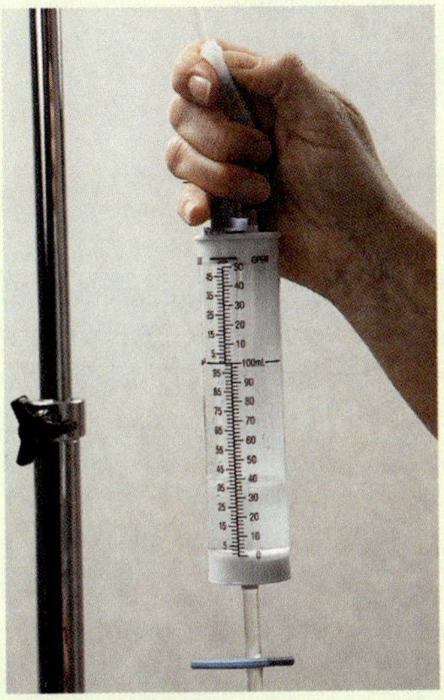

STEP 7C(1) Filling volume-control administration device.

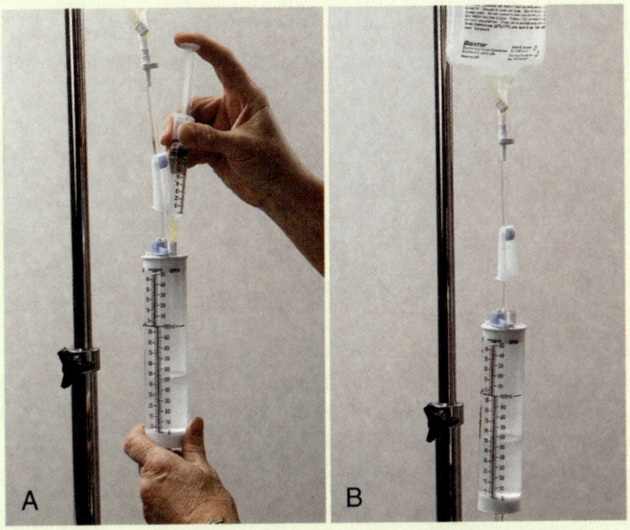

STEP 7C(4) **A,** Inject medication into device. **B,** Prepared dose.

SKILL 17-7 ADMINISTERING INTRAVENOUS MEDICATIONS BY PIGGYBACK, INTERMITTENT INTRAVENOUS INFUSION SETS, AND MINI-INFUSION PUMPS—cont'd

RECORDING AND REPORTING

- Record drug, dose, route, and time administered on MAR.
- Record volume of fluid in medication bag or Buretrol as fluid intake.
- Document your evaluation of patient learning.
- Report any adverse reactions to patient's health care provider.

UNEXPECTED OUTCOMES AND RELATED INTERVENTIONS

- Patient develops adverse drug reaction.
  - Stop medication infusion immediately.
  - Follow agency policy or guidelines for appropriate response and reporting of adverse drug reactions.
  - Add allergy information to patient's medical record.
- Medication does not infuse over desired period.
  - Determine reason (e.g., improper calculation of flow rate, poor positioning of IV needle at insertion site, infiltration).
  - Take corrective action as indicated.
- IV site shows symptoms of infiltration or phlebitis (see Chapter 18).
  - See related interventions in Skill 17-6.

KEY POINTS

- Learning medication classifications helps you better understand nursing implications for administering medications with similar characteristics.
- Handle all controlled substances according to strict procedures that account for each medication.
- Apply understanding of the physiology of medication action when timing administration, selecting routes, initiating interventions to promote the potency of a medication, and observing responses to medications.
- The older adult's body undergoes structural and functional changes that alter medication actions and influence the manner in which nurses provide medication therapy.
- Always prepare and calculate medication doses in a location without distractions and use the calculation method that works best for you. Have another nurse double-check your calculations, especially if the calculation is complex or if you are giving a high-alert medication that has a potential to cause great harm if given in the wrong amount.
- The body absorbs medications given parenterally more quickly than medications administered by other routes.
- Each medication order includes the patient's name; the time and date the order was written; the medication name; dosage, route, time and frequency of administration; and the prescriber's signature.
- Always clarify medication orders that are not clear to you (e.g., written illegibly, contain dangerous abbreviations).
- When you take a patient's medication history, include allergies, medications, including prescription medications, OTC medications, vitamins, and herbal supplements; and the patient's adherence to therapy.
- The six rights of medication administration enhance safe medication preparation and administration.
- Only administer medications that you prepare and never leave medications unattended.
- Document medications immediately after administration.
- Use clinical nursing judgment when determining the best time to administer prn medications.
- Report any actual and potential medication errors immediately.
- When preparing medications, check the medication container label against the MAR or computer printout 3 times before administration.
- When administering medication to patients, verify your patients' identity by using at least two patient identifiers.
- The Z-track method for IM injections protects subcutaneous tissues from irritating parenteral fluids.
- Failure to select injection sites by anatomical landmarks leads to tissue, bone, or nerve damage.

CLINICAL DECISION-MAKING EXERCISES

While Emilio is caring for Esther, her nurse practitioner (NP) comes to assess Esther and evaluate her progress. Emilio tells the NP that Esther's blood pressure has been a little higher than usual the past few days and that she has 2+ edema in her ankles bilaterally. The NP orders 60 mg furosemide intravenous push (IVP) now and q8h.

1. What information does Emilio need to know before he gives the furosemide?
2. Three 8-mL vials of furosemide arrive from the pharmacy. The label on each vial says, "80 mg furosemide in 8 mL." Using dimensional analysis, calculate how much medication Emilio will prepare in the syringe.

3. While Emilio flushes Esther's saline lock with saline before administering the intravenous (IV) furosemide, he assesses swelling, warmth, redness, and tenderness at the IV site. Which interventions does Emilio need to implement at this time?

evolve

Answers to Clinical Decision-Making Exercises can be found on the Evolve website.

QSEN ACTIVITY: SAFETY

Emilio is sitting with Esther's primary nurse at the nurses' station. Esther's physician walks by the nurse's station and gives the nurse several orders to change Esther's medications. When the nurse checks Esther's electronic health record, she and Emilio notice that the physician did not enter the medication changes into the computerized ordering system. The nurse asks Emilio, "What should I do? Should I go ahead and enter the orders into the computer for the physician?"

How should Emilio respond?

evolve

Answers to QSEN Activities can be found on the Evolve website.

REVIEW QUESTIONS

1. The nurse notices that the skin of a patient receiving a second dose of intravenous (IV) penicillin is beginning to have raised, reddened, and edematous patches of skin that the patient describes as "itchy." Which of the following statements best explains why the nurse stops the IV infusion?
   1. The patient is experiencing a side effect.
   2. The patient is experiencing an allergic reaction.
   3. The patient is experiencing a medication toxic effect.
   4. The patient is experiencing an idiosyncratic reaction.
2. A mother calls the nurse at the clinic because her 3-year-old child who is taking diphenhydramine (Benadryl) is having difficulty sleeping. How does the nurse document a description of this symptom?
   1. An expected side effect
   2. Tolerance to the medication
   3. An idiosyncratic medication reaction
   4. A desired response to the medication
3. You receive a telephone order to mix 800 mg of dopamine in an intravenous (IV) bag of 250 mL D_5W and administer it to your patient STAT. What must you do first?
   1. Contact the pharmacist
   2. Make sure that the patient wants to take the medication
   3. Prepare 800 mg of dopamine in a syringe using aseptic technique
   4. Gather all the supplies you need to mix the medication in the medication room
4. A female patient who weighs 59 kg is to receive a vaccine. The nurse needs to give the medication using the intramuscular (IM) route. Which size needle does the nurse plan to use to give the immunization?
   1. 18 gauge, 1¼ inch
   2. 20 gauge, 1 inch
   3. 24 gauge, ½ inch
   4. 25 gauge, 1 inch
5. A patient has an order for 3 tablespoons (tbsp) of magnesium hydroxide for constipation. How many milliliters (mL) does the nurse prepare?
   1. 15 mL
   2. 30 mL
   3. 45 mL
   4. 60 mL
6. A physician's order for a medication states: "digoxin 125 mcg QOD." The physician is very busy, does not like to be bothered, and is known for being difficult to work with. What is the nurse's priority action?
   1. Call the physician and verify the order
   2. Consult a pharmacist to interpret the order
   3. Administer 125 mcg of digoxin every other day
   4. Talk to the unit secretary on the floor who is good at reading the physician's handwriting
7. A patient is to receive 30 mg aripiprazole (Abilify) PO. The drawer of the automated medication dispensing system opens. There are five tablets, each labeled 10 mg, in the drawer. The nurse should give:
   1. ½ tablet
   2. 1 tablet
   3. 2 tablets
   4. 3 tablets
8. A nurse is going to give a patient an intramuscular (IM) injection in the ventrogluteal site using the Z-track method. The nurse uses the following steps to give the injection. In which order does the nurse implement the steps?
   1. Pull back on plunger for 5 to 10 seconds.
   2. Wait 10 seconds and pull out the needle in a smooth motion.
   3. Administer medication slowly (1 mL/10 seconds).
   4. Using the ulnar side of the nondominant hand, pull the skin just below the site down or laterally 2.5 to 3.5 cm and prepare site with an antiseptic swab.
   5. Move dominant hand to end of plunger without moving syringe.
   6. Inject needle at 90-degree angle into the muscle with the dominant hand using a smooth and steady motion.
   7. While continuing to pull skin tightly, grasp syringe barrel with thumb and forefinger of nondominant hand to stabilize syringe.
9. A nursing professor is with a nursing student while the student is giving medications to a patient. Which of the following actions requires the nursing professor to intervene?
   1. The student checks the patient's medications in a medication manual before preparing the medications.

2. The patient has an order for 6.25 mg of captopril; the student splits a prescored 12.5 mg tablet in half during preparation.
3. After the student pours a liquid medication into a medicine cup, the student wipes the medication bottle with a paper towel.
4. The nursing student pauses at the patient's bedside to verify the patient's identity and compare the labels of the medications with the medication administration record (MAR).

10. You give 500 mg of a medication to a patient at 1200. The biological half-life of the medication is 3 hours. How much of the total medication will the patient excrete by 1800?
    1. 125 mg
    2. 250 mg
    3. 375 mg
    4. 500 mg

evolve

Rationales for Review Questions can be found on the Evolve website.

1. 2; **2.** 3; **3.** 1; **4.** 4; **5.** 3; **6.** 1; **7.** 4; **8.** 4, 6, 7, 5, 1, 3, 2; **9.** 2;
10. 3

REFERENCES

Alexander AJ, et al: Medication reconciliation campaign in a clinic for homeless patients, *Am J Health Syst Pharm AJHP* 69(7):558, 2012.

Alvarez-Lorenzo C, Hiratani H, Concheiro A: Contact lenses for drug delivery: achieving sustained release with novel systems, *Am J Drug Deliv* 4(3):131, 2006.

American Diabetes Association (ADA): Insulin administration: position statement, *Diabetes Care* 27(1S):S106, 2004.

American Diabetes Association (ADA): Standards of medical care in diabetes—2012: position statement, *Diabetes Care* 35(1):S11, 2012.

American Hospital Association (AHA): *The patient care partnership*, 2003, http://www.aha.org/advocacy-issues/communicatingpts/pt-care-partnership.shtml. Accessed September 11, 2011.

American Nurses Association (ANA): *Nursing: scope & standards of practice*, ed 2, Silver Spring, MD, 2010, The Association.

American Society of Health-System Pharmacists (ASHP): *Healthcare leaders vow to stop intravenous medication errors*, 2008, http://www.ashp.org/menu/AboutUs/ForPress/PressReleases/PressRelease.aspx?id=511. Accessed November 11, 2012.

American Society of Health-System Pharmacists (ASHP): *How to use eye drops properly*, 2013, http://www.safemedication.com/safemed/MedicationTipsTools/HowtoAdminister/HowtoUseEyeDropsProperly.aspx. Accessed September 15, 2013.

American Society of Health-System Pharmacists [ASHP]: The ASHP discussion guide for compounding sterile preparations: summary and implementation of USP chapter <797>, http://www.ashp.org/s_ashp/docs/files/HACC_797guide.pdf, n.d. Accessed September 15, 2013.

Annersten M, Willman A: Performing subcutaneous injections: a literature review, *Worldviews Evid Based Nurs* 2(3):122, 2005.

Bae JP, et al: Adherence and dosing frequency of common medications for cardiovascular patients, *Am J Manage Care* 18(3):139, 2012.

Balon J, Thomas S: Comparison of hospital admission medication lists with primary care physician and outpatient pharmacy lists, *J Nurs Scholarsh* 43(3):292, 2011.

Bankhead R, et al: Enteral nutrition practice recommendations, *JPEN J Parenter Enteral Nutr* 33(2):122, 2009.

Barnason S, et al: Pilot testing of a medication self-management transition intervention for heart failure patients, *West J Nurs Res* 32(7):849, 2010.

Bastable SB: *Nurse as educator: principles of teaching and learning for nursing practice*, ed 3, Sudbury, MA, 2008, Jones & Bartlett.

Birkebaek NH, et al: A 4-mm needle reduces the risk of intramuscular injections without increasing backflow to skin surface in lean diabetic children and adults, *Diabetes Care* 31(9):e65, 2008.

Boullata J: Drug administration through an enteral feeding tube, *Am J Nurs* 109(10):34, 2009.

Brady A, et al: A literature review of the individual and systems factors that contribute to medication errors in nursing practice, *J Nurs Manage* 17(6):679, 2009.

Camden SG: Obesity: an emerging concern for patients and nurses, *OJIN Online J Issues Nurs* 14(1):1, 2009. Accessed November 10, 2012.

Centers for Disease Control and Prevention (CDC): *Epidemiology and prevention of vaccine-preventable diseases*, ed 12, second printing, Washington, DC, 2012, Public Health Foundation, http://www.cdc.gov/vaccines/pubs/pinkbook/index.html#chapters. Accessed September 15, 2013.

Centers for Disease Control and Prevention (CDC): *Tuberculosis*, 2013, http://www.cdc.gov/tb/. Accessed September 15, 2013.

Centers for Medicare & Medicaid Services (CMS): Updated guidance on medication administration, hospital appendix A of the State Operations Manual *(SOM)*, 2011, https://www.cms.gov/Medicare/Provider-Enrollment-and-Certification/SurveyCertificationGenInfo/downloads/SCLetter12_05.pdf. Accessed September 4, 2013.

Cocoman A, Murray J: Intramuscular injections: a review of best practice for mental health nurses, *J Psych Mental Health Nurs* 15(5):424, 2008.

Cornett S: Assessing and addressing health literacy, *Online J Issues Nurs* 14(3):1, 2009.

Cramer JA, et al.: Medication compliance and persistence: terminology and definitions. *Value Health* 11:44, 2008.

Dickinson A, et al: Paediatric nurses' understanding of the process and procedure of double-checking medications, *J Clin Nurs* 19(5-6):728, 2010.

Edelman CL, Mandle CL: *Health promotion throughout the life span*, ed 7, St Louis, 2010, Mosby.

Edmiaston J, et al: Validation of a dysphagia screening tool in acute stroke patients, *Am J Crit Care* 19(4):357, 2010.

Foulon V, et al: Patient adherence to oral anti-cancer drugs: an emerging issue in modern oncology, *Acta Clinical Belgium* 66(2):85, 2011.

Frankel SW, Leonard MW, Denham CR: Fair and just culture, team behavior, and leadership engagement: the tools to achieve high reliability, *Health Serv Res* 41(4 Pt 2):1690, 2006.

Giger JN: *Transcultural nursing: assessment and intervention*, ed 6, St Louis, 2013, Mosby.

Gray Morris D: *Calculate with confidence*, ed 5, St Louis, 2010, Mosby.

Haw C, Cahill C: A computerized system for reporting medication events in psychiatry: the first two years of operation, *J Psychiatr Ment Health Nurs* 18(4):308, 2011.

Hewitt P: Nurses' perceptions of the causes of medication errors: an integrative literature review, *Medsurg Nurs* 19(3):159, 2010.

Hockenberry MJ, Wilson D: *Wong's nursing care of infants and children*, ed 9, St Louis, 2011, Mosby.

Hong I, et al: Safety concerns involving transdermal patches and magnetic resonance imaging (MRI), *Hosp Pharm* 45(10):771, 2010.

Hook J, et al: *Using barcode medication administration to improve quality and safety: findings from the AHRQ health IT portfolio*, Prepared by the AHRQ National Resource Center for Health IT under Contract No. 290-04-0016, AHRQ Publication No. 09-0023-EF, Rockville, MD, December 2008, Agency for Healthcare Research and Quality, http://healthit.ahrq.gov/sites/default/files/docs/page/09-0023-EF_bcma_0.pdf. Accessed September 4, 2013.

Infusion Nurses Society (INS): Infusion Nursing Standards of Practice, *J Infusion Nurs* 34(1S):S31, 2011.

Institute of Medicine (IOM): *Report brief: to err is human: building a safer health system*, 1999, http://www.iom.edu/~/media/Files/Report%20Files/1999/To-Err-is-Human/To%20Err%20is%20Human%201999%20%20report%20brief.pdf. Accessed October 21, 2013.

Institute of Safe Medication Practices (ISMP): *Tablet splitting: do it only if you "half" to, and then do it safely*, 2006, http://www.ismp.org/Newsletters/acutecare/articles/20060518.asp. Accessed September 4, 2013.

Institute for Safe Medication Practices (ISMP): Patches: what you can't see can harm patients, *Nurse Advise-ERR* 5(4):1, 2007a.

Institute of Safe Medication Practices (ISMP): *Humulin R concentrate U-500*, 2007b, http://www.ismp.org/Newsletters/ambulatory/archives/200708_2.asp. Accessed September 15, 2013.

Institute for Safe Medication Practices (ISMP): *Never use parenteral syringes for oral medications*, 2010, http://www.accessdata.fda.gov/psn/transcript.cfm?show=94#9. Accessed September 15, 2013.

Institute of Safe Medication Practices (ISMP): *ISMP's list of error-prone abbreviations, symbols, and dose designations*, 2011a, http://www.ismp.org/Tools/confuseddrugnames.pdf. Accessed September 4, 2013.

Institute for Safe Medication Practices (ISMP): *ISMP acute care guidelines for timely administration of scheduled medications*, 2011b, http://www.ismp.org/Tools/guidelines/acutecare/tasm.pdf. Accessed September 11, 2013.

Institute of Safe Medication Practices (ISMP): *Read this important information before using fentanyl patches*, 2011c, http://www.ismp.org/download/files/ismp-Brochure-fentanyl–Dec_2010.pdf. Accessed September 11, 2013.

Institute of Safe Medication Practices (ISMP): *Avoiding inadvertent IV injection of oral liquids*, 2012, http://www.ismp.org/Newsletters/acutecare/showarticle.asp?id=29. Accessed September 15, 2013.

Institute of Safe Medication Practices (ISMP): *Oral dosage forms that should not be crushed*, 2013a, http://www.ismp.org/tools/donotcrush.pdf. Accessed September 15, 2013.

Institute of Safe Medication Practices (ISMP): *ISMP guidelines*, 2013b, http://www.ismp.org/Tools/guidelines/default.asp. Accessed September 15, 2013.

Jones J, Treiber L: When 5 rights go wrong: medication errors from the nursing perspective. *J Nurs Care Qual* 25(3):240, 2010.

Kaizer F, et al: Promoting shared decision-making in rehabilitation: development of a framework for situations when patients with dysphagia refuse diet modification recommended by the treating team, *Dysphagia* 27(1):81, 2012.

Kelly J, et al: An analysis of two incidents of medicine administration to a patient with dysphagia, *J Clin Nurs* 20(1-2):146, 2011.

Koohestani H, Baghcheghi N: Comparing the effects of two educational methods of intravenous drug rate calculations on rapid and sustained learning of nursing students: formula method and dimensional analysis method, *Nurse Educ Pract* 10(4):233, 2010.

Kripalani S, Yao X, Haynes RB: Interventions to enhance medication adherence in chronic medical conditions: a systematic review, *Arch Intern Med* 167(6):540, 2007.

Kuitunen T, et al: Medication errors made by health care professionals: analysis of the Finnish Poison Information Centre data between 2000 and 2007, *Eur J Clin Pharmacol* 64(8):769, 2008.

Lam P, et al: Impact of a self-administration of medications programme on elderly inpatients' competence to manage medications: a pilot study, *J Clin Pharm Ther* 36:80, 2011.

Lavik E, et al: Novel drug delivery systems for glaucoma, *Eye* 25(5):578, 2011.

Lehne RA: *Pharmacology for nursing care*, ed 8, St Louis, 2013, Elsevier.

Lenz TL, Gillespie N: Transdermal patch drug delivery interactions with exercise, *Sports Med* 41(3):177, 2011.

Lilley LL, et al: *Pharmacology and the nursing process*, ed 6, St Louis, 2011, Mosby.

Mandrack M, et al: Nursing best practices using automatic dispensing cabinets: nurses' key role in improving medication safety, *Medsurg Nurs* 21(3):134, 2012.

MayoClinic.com: *Asthma inhalers: Which one's right for you?* 2011a, http://www.mayoclinic.com/health/asthma-inhalers/HQ01081. Accessed September 15, 2013.

MayoClinic.com: *Using a metered dose asthma inhaler and spacer*, 2011b, http://www.mayoclinic.com/health/asthma/MM00608. Accessed September 15, 2013.

Metheny NA, et al: Effectiveness of an aspiration risk-reduction protocol, *Nurs Res* 59(1):18, 2010.

National Coordinating Council for Medication Error Reporting and Prevention (NCCMERP): *Recommendations to reduce medication errors associated with verbal medication orders and prescriptions*, 2006, http://www.nccmerp.org/council/council2001-02-20.html. Accessed September 4, 2013.

National Coordinating Council for Medication Error Reporting and Prevention (NCCMERP): *Statement opposing the criminalization of errors In healthcare*, 2012, http://

www.nccmerp.org/council/council2012-01-19.html. Accessed September 4, 2013.

National Institutes of Health, National Institute on Drug Abuse (NIH NIDA): *Drug facts: prescription and over-the-counter medications*, 2013, http://www.drugabuse.gov/publications/drugfacts/prescription-over-counter-medications. Accessed September 4, 2013.

National Quality Forum (NQF): *Serious reportable events*, 2013, http://www.qualityforum.org/Topics/SREs/Serious_Reportable_Events.aspx. Accessed September 4, 2013.

Nicoll LH, Hesby A: Intramuscular injection: an integrative research review and guideline for evidence-based practice, *Appl Nurs Res* 16(2):149, 2002.

Novo Nordisk: *Welcome to Levemir*, 2013, http://www.levemir.com/Default.aspx. Accessed September 15, 2013.

Occupational Safety and Health Administration (OSHA): *Bloodborne pathogens and needlestick prevention*, n.d.a, http://www.osha.gov/SLTC/bloodbornepathogens/index.html. Accessed September 15, 2013.

Occupational Safety and Health Administration (OSHA): *Bloodborne pathogens and needlestick prevention: OSHA standards*, n.d.b, http://www.osha.gov/SLTC/bloodbornepathogens/standards.html. Accessed September 15, 2013.

Ownby RL, et al: Tailored information and automated reminding to improve medication adherence in Spanish- and English-speaking elders treated for memory impairment, *Clin Gerontol* 35(3):221, 2012.

Poon EG, et al: Effect of bar-code technology on the safety of medication administration, *N Engl J Med* 362(18):1698, 2010.

Popescu A, et al: Multifactorial influences on and deviations from medication administration safety and quality in the acute medical/surgical context, *Worldviews Evid Based Nurs* 8(1):15, 2011.

Prettyman J: Subcutaneous or intramuscular? Confronting a parenteral administration dilemma, *Medsurg Nurs* 14(2):93, 2005.

Restrepo RD, Gardner DD: Selecting the best inhaler device not always an easy task, *J Respir Care Pract* 23(6):8, 2010.

Ruppar TM, et al: Medication adherence interventions for older adults: literature review, *Res Theory Nurs Pract Int J* 22(2):114, 2008.

Saini SD, et al: Effect of medication dosing frequently on adherence in chronic diseases, *Am J Manage Care* 15(6):e22, 2009.

Samann KH, et al: Addressing safety concerns about U-500 insulin in a hospital setting, *Am J Health Syst Pharm* 68(1):63, 2011.

Sanofi-Aventis: *Dosing and administration of Lovenox*, 2012, http://www.lovenox.com/hcp/dosing/lovenox-administration.aspx. Accessed September 15, 2013.

Skidmore-Roth L: *Mosby's 2013 nursing drug reference*, ed 26, St Louis, 2013, Mosby.

Teunissen R, et al: Clinical relevance of and risk factors associated with medication administration time errors, *Am J Health Syst Pharm* 70(12):1052, 2013.

The Joint Commission (TJC): *Joint Commission alert: preventing pediatric medication errors*, 2008a, http://www.jointcommission.org/assets/1/18/SEA_39.PDF. Accessed September 4, 2013.

The Joint Commission (TJC): *Standards FAQ details*, 2008b, http://www.jointcommission.org/standards_information/jcfaqdetails.aspx?StandardsFaqId=145&ProgramId=1. Accessed September 4, 2013.

The Joint Commission (TJC): *2013* Hospital accreditation standards, Oak Brook IL, 2013a, The Commission.

The Joint Commission (TJC): *Facts about the official "do not use" list*, 2013b, http://www.jointcommission.org/assets/1/18/Do_Not_Use_List.pdf. Accessed September 4, 2013.

The Joint Commission (TJC): *National Patient Safety Goals*, Oakbrook Terrace, IL, 2014, The Commission. Available at http://www.jointcommission.org/standards_information/npsgs.aspx.

Touhy TT, Jett K: *Ebersole and Hess' toward healthy aging*, ed 8, St Louis, 2012, Mosby.

Twin Cities Health Professionals (TCHP) Education Consortium: *Management of the obese patient*, 2005, http://tchpeducation.com/homestudies/generalinterest/obesity/obesitybook_2011_final.pdf. Accessed September 15, 2013.

US Food and Drug Administration (USFDA): *MedWatch: The FDA safety information and adverse event reporting program*, 2013, http://www.fda.gov/Safety/MedWatch/default.htm. Accessed September 4, 2013.

Walsh K: The relationship among mathematics anxiety, beliefs about mathematics, mathematics self-efficacy, and mathematics performance in associate degree nursing students, *Nurs Educ Perspect* 29(4):226, 2008.

Williams NT: Medication administration through enteral feeding tubes, *Am J Health System Pharm* 65(24):2347, 2008.

World Health Organization(WHO): *Injection safety: misuse and overuse of injection worldwide*, 2006, http://www.who.int/mediacentre/factsheets/fs231/en/. Accessed September 15, 2013.

Wright K: Do calculation errors cause medication errors in clinical practice? A literature review, *Nurse Educ Today* 30(1):85, 2010.

Zwicker D, Fulmer T: *Medication: nursing standard of practice protocol: reducing adverse drug events*, 2012, Hartford Institute for Geriatric Nursing, http://consultgerirn.org/topics/medication/want_to_know_more#item_5. Accessed September 11, 2013.

CHAPTER

18

Fluid, Electrolyte, and Acid-Base Balances

evolve WEBSITE

http://evolve.elsevier.com/Potter/essentials

- Video Clips
- Crossword Puzzle
- Butterfield's Fluids and Electrolytes Tutorial
- Audio Glossary

OBJECTIVES

- Describe basic physiological mechanisms responsible for maintaining fluid, electrolyte, and acid-base balances.
- Discuss risk factors for fluid, electrolyte, and acid-base imbalances.
- Describe fluid, electrolyte, and acid-base imbalances.
- Identify appropriate clinical assessments for specific fluid, electrolyte, and acid-base imbalances.
- Discuss appropriate nursing interventions for patients with fluid, electroiyte, and acid-base imbalances.
- Describe purpose and procedures for initiation and maintenance of intravenous therapy.
- Calculate an intravenous flow rate.
- Discuss complications of intravenous therapy and what to do if they occur.
- Describe how to change intravenous solutions, tubing, and dressings.
- Describe the procedure for initiating a blood transfusion and complications of blood therapy.

KEY TERMS

acidosis, p. 471
active transport, p. 465
ADH, p. 466
aldosterone, p. 466
allogeneic transfusion, p. 490
alkalosis, p. 471
angiotensin, p. 466
anion gap, p. 471
anions, p. 464
arterial blood gas (ABG), p. 471
autologous transfusion, p. 489
buffers, p. 467
cations, p. 464
clinical dehydration, p. 468
colloid osmotic pressure, p. 465
colloids, p. 482
concentration, p. 468
crystalloids, p. 482
diffusion, p. 465
electrolyte, p. 464
electronic infusion device (EID), p. 483
extracellular fluid volume (ECV) deficit, p. 473
extracellular fluid volume (ECV) excess, p. 468
filtration, p. 465
fluid, p. 464
fluid homeostasis, p. 466
hemolysis, p. 489
hydrostatic pressure, p. 465
hypercalcemia, p. 468
hyperchloremia, p. 468
hyperkalemia, p. 468
hypermagnesemia, p. 468
hypernatremia, p. 468
hypertonic, p. 465
hypocalcemia, p. 468
hypochloremia, p. 468
hypokalemia, p. 468
hypomagnesemia, p. 468
hyponatremia, p. 468
hypotonic, p. 465
hypovolemia, p. 468
infiltration, p. 487
insensible water loss, p. 466
ions, p. 464
isotonic, p. 465
metabolic acidosis, p. 471
metabolic alkalosis, p. 471
oncotic pressure, p. 465
osmolality, p. 465
osmoreceptors, p. 466

KEY TERMS—cont'd

osmosis, p. 465
osmotic pressure, p. 465
parenteral nutrition (PN), p. 482
phlebitis, p. 487
respiratory acidosis, p. 471
respiratory alkalosis, p. 471
transfusion reaction, p. 490
vascular access device (VAD), p. 482
venipuncture, p. 484

CASE STUDY *Mrs. Reynolds*

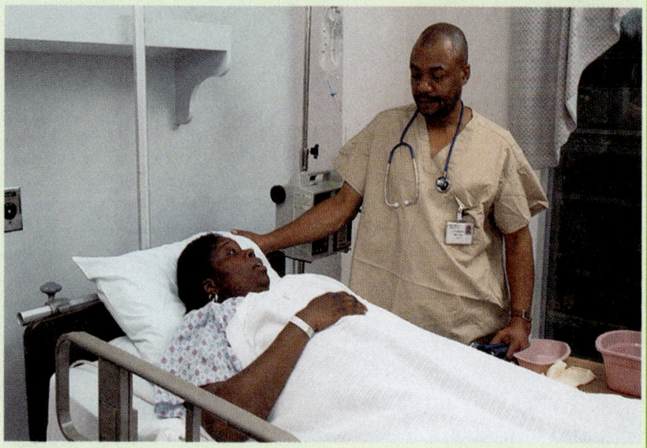

Susan Reynolds, a 42-year-old married accountant, was admitted yesterday to an acute care unit with a history of nausea, loss of appetite, and diarrhea for 7 days. She believes that her symptoms are related to "bad food" that she had on her recent business trip. Past medical history includes hypertension controlled by hydrochlorothiazide 25 mg by mouth once a day and a no added–salt diet.

Robert is a nursing student assigned to Mrs. Reynolds. He has cared for other patients with gastrointestinal (GI) disorders but none with fluid and electrolyte imbalances. Robert plans his care by reviewing Mrs. Reynolds' medical record and health care provider's orders.

Fluid, electrolyte, and acid-base balances within the body maintain health and function of all body cells, organs, and systems. The body maintains fluid and electrolyte balance by adjusting the intake and output (I&O) of water and electrolytes and their distribution in the body. Because cellular metabolism creates acid, the body maintains acid-base balance by buffering and excreting acid. Factors that alter these normal processes can cause fluid, electrolyte, and/or acid-base imbalances. In this chapter you learn how the body maintains balance; how imbalances develop and affect patients; and nursing interventions that help your patients maintain or restore fluid, electrolyte, and acid-base balance.

SCIENTIFIC KNOWLEDGE BASE

Water is the largest single component of the body; 60% of the average adult male's weight is fluid. The proportion of water is lower in women and older adults but higher in infants (Hall, 2011). The term **fluid** means water that contains

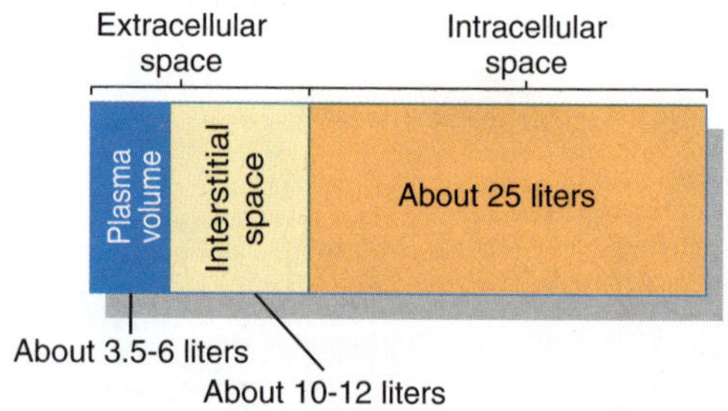

FIGURE 18-1 Normal distribution of total body water. (From Ignatavicius DD, Workman ML: *Medical-surgical nursing: patient-centered collaborative care,* ed 7, St Louis, 2013, Saunders.)

dissolved or suspended substances such as glucose, mineral salts, and proteins.

Distribution of Body Fluids

Body fluids are distributed in two major compartments, one containing intracellular fluid (ICF), and the other extracellular fluid (ECF) (Figure 18-1). ICF is inside cells. In adults the ICF is approximately two thirds of total body water (Hall, 2011).

ECF is all fluid outside the cells, approximately one third of total body water. The ECF is divided into two important compartments plus a minor one: intravascular (within blood vessels), interstitial (within tissues), and transcellular (minor). Intravascular fluid is the liquid portion of the blood, the plasma. Interstitial fluid is located between cells and outside the blood vessels. Transcellular fluid is secreted by epithelial cells and includes cerebrospinal, GI, peritoneal, and synovial fluids (Hall, 2011).

Composition of Body Fluids

Body fluid contains mineral salts known technically as electrolytes. An **electrolyte** is a compound that separates into **ions** (charged particles) when dissolved in water. Positively charged ions are **cations.** Major cations within body fluids include sodium (Na^+), potassium (K^+), calcium (Ca^{2+}), and magnesium (Mg^{2+}). Negatively charged ions are **anions.** The three major body fluid anions are chloride (Cl^-), bicarbonate (HCO_3^-), and phosphate (PO_4^{3-} and other forms). Electrolyte concentration is measured in milliequivalents per liter (mEq/L), millimoles per liter (mmol/L), or milligrams per deciliter (mg/dL).

Movement of Water and Electrolytes

Cell membranes and capillary walls separate the body compartments. Water and electrolytes move between body compartments by processes that allow the compartments to have

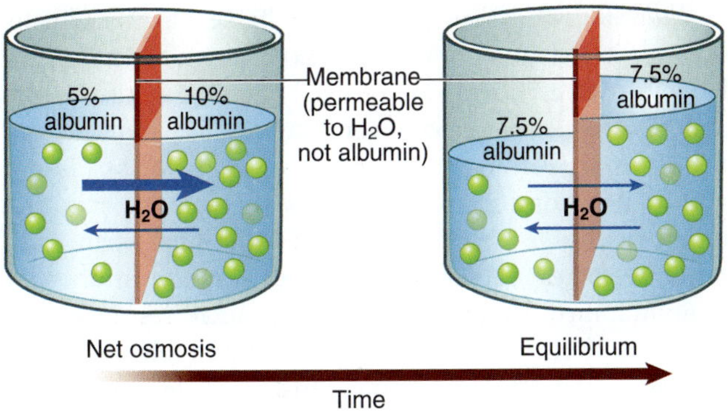

FIGURE 18-2 Osmosis moves water through a semipermeable membrane. (From Patton KT, Thibodeau GA: *Anatomy and physiology*, ed 7, St Louis, 2010, Mosby.)

different electrolyte concentrations while maintaining the overall particle concentration (osmolality) equal in all compartments. They move across cell membranes by four processes: active transport, diffusion, osmosis, and filtration.

Active transport is the energy-requiring movement of electrolytes or other substances across cell membranes against a concentration gradient (from an area of low concentration to one of higher concentration). This process requires energy, usually in the form of adenosine triphosphate (ATP). An example of active transport is the sodium-potassium pump that moves sodium ions out of a cell and potassium ions into it, thus keeping ICF lower in sodium and higher in potassium than the ECF.

Diffusion is passive movement of electrolytes or other particles from an area of higher concentration to one of lower concentration. In other words, the electrolytes move down their concentration gradient until the electrolyte concentration is equal in all areas. Electrolytes cannot diffuse across cell membranes unless the membranes have proteins that serve as ion channels. When ion channels are open, an electrolyte can diffuse across a membrane; when they are closed, no electrolytes pass. Opening and closing of ion channels play an important role in nerve and muscle function.

Osmosis is movement of water across a semipermeable membrane from a compartment of lower particle concentration to one that has a higher particle concentration (Figure 18-2). Osmosis equalizes the concentration of particles on each side of a membrane. Cell membranes are known as semipermeable membranes because water crosses them easily but electrolytes do not. The particles in any fluid compartment exert an inward-pulling force called **osmotic pressure.** If a semipermeable membrane separates two fluid compartments with different particle concentrations, water is drawn through the membrane to the more concentrated side because it has higher osmotic pressure (inward-pulling force). Osmosis continues until the particle concentration is equal in both fluid compartments. This process controls movement of water between interstitial fluid and the intracellular compartment. The **osmolality** of a fluid is a measure of the number of particles per kilogram of water, reported in milliosmoles per kilogram (mOsm/kg). Changes in extracellular

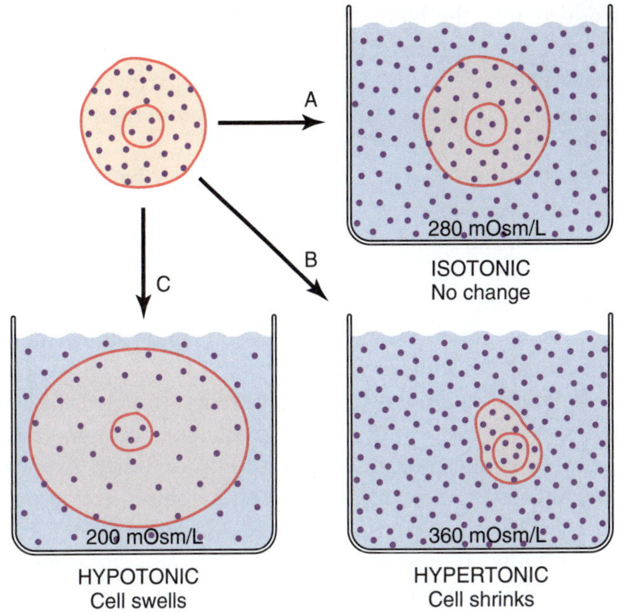

FIGURE 18-3 Effects of isotonic, hypotonic, and hypertonic solutions. (From Hall JE: *Guyton and Hall textbook of medical physiology*, ed 12, Philadelphia, 2011, Saunders.)

osmolality cause rapid shifts of water into or out of cells to equalize the osmolality. Osmosis is a passive process that does not require energy from the cells.

Intravenous (IV) solutions are hypertonic, isotonic, or hypotonic (Figure 18-3). Infusion of **hypotonic** IV solutions (more concentrated than normal blood) such as 3% sodium chloride, pulls fluid from cells by osmosis, causing them to shrink. **Isotonic** solutions such as 0.9% sodium chloride (same osmolality as normal blood) expand the extracellular fluid volume (ECV) of the body without causing water to shift in or out of cells. Physiologically **hypotonic** solutions (less concentrated than normal blood after they are infused) such as dextrose 5% in water (D_5W), move water from the extracellular compartment into the cells by osmosis, causing them to swell. When health care providers write fluid orders for an IV, they prescribe the type of IV fluid that will distribute to specific fluid compartments as needed by each patient's condition.

Filtration is the net effect of several forces that tend to move fluid across a membrane. Fluid moves into and out of capillaries (between the vascular and interstitial spaces) by filtration. **Hydrostatic pressure** is the force of a fluid pressing outward against the walls of its container. Thus capillary hydrostatic pressure is an outward-pushing force. Capillary hydrostatic pressure is greater at the arterial end of a capillary. **Colloid osmotic pressure (oncotic pressure)** is an inward-pulling force caused by the presence of protein molecules. Blood colloid osmotic pressure is greater at the venous end of a capillary. Normally fluid leaves a capillary at the arterial end (high outward-pushing capillary hydrostatic pressure), carrying oxygen and nutrients to cells; fluid enters the capillary at the venous end (high inward-pulling colloid osmotic pressure) carrying carbon dioxide and other waste products into the blood for disposal. The lymph channels return excess fluid and a few small proteins that entered the interstitial space to the intravascular compartment. Edema occurs when alterations in these forces cause fluid to accumulate in the interstitial space.

Fluid Balance. Fluid homeostasis is the dynamic interplay of three processes: fluid intake and absorption, fluid distribution, and fluid output (Felver, 2013b). Our daily fluid output consists of hypotonic sodium-containing fluid. To maintain fluid balance we must have an intake of an equivalent amount of hypotonic sodium-containing fluid (water plus foods with some salt).

Fluid Intake. Fluid intake occurs orally, through drinking, and also through eating because most foods contain some water. Food metabolism creates additional water. Average fluid intake by these routes for healthy adults is approximately 2200 to 2700 mL (Table 18-1), although it varies widely. Other routes of fluid intake that nurses encounter include IV, gastrointestinal (tube feedings), rectal (e.g., enemas), and irrigation of body cavities that results in fluid absorption.

Although you might think that the major regulator of oral fluid intake is thirst, habit and social reasons actually account for the majority of fluid intake. Thirst, a conscious desire for water, regulates fluid intake when plasma osmolality increases (osmoreceptor-mediated thirst) or the blood volume decreases (baroreceptor-mediated thirst and angiotensin II-mediated thirst) (Thornton, 2010). The thirst-control mechanism is in the hypothalamus of the brain. Osmoreceptors continually monitor plasma osmolality; when osmolality increases, the hypothalamus stimulates thirst. This thirst mechanism becomes less active in older adults. Dryness of oral mucous membranes also causes thirst. Thirsty people who can obtain fluid or communicate their thirst to others increase their fluid intake to restore fluid balance.

Fluid Distribution. Fluid distribution is movement of fluid between its various compartments. Fluid moves between the vascular and interstitial portions of the ECF (in and out of capillaries) by filtration. It distributes between the extracellular and intracellular compartments by osmosis.

TABLE 18-1 HEALTHY ADULT AVERAGE DAILY FLUID INTAKE AND OUTPUT

FLUID INTAKE	(ML)	FLUID OUTPUT	(ML)
Oral fluid	1100-1400	Kidneys	1200-1500
Solid foods	800-1000	Skin	500-600
Oxidative metabolism	300	Lungs	400
		Gastrointestinal	100-200
Total gains	**2200-2700**	**Total losses**	**2200-2700**

From Hall JE: *Guyton and Hall textbook of medical physiology,* ed 12, Philadelphia, 2011, Saunders.

Fluid Output. Fluid output (see Table 18-1) normally occurs through four organs: the skin, lungs, GI tract, and kidneys. When patients are seriously ill, output also occurs abnormally such as through vomiting, wound drainage, and hemorrhage (Felver, 2013b). Insensible water loss is not visible; it is continuous and occurs through the skin and lungs. Insensible water output from the lungs changes in response to respiratory rate and depth. Administration of nonhumidified supplemental oxygen increases insensible water loss from the lungs. Output of insensible water also increases with fever (Metheny, 2012). Visible perspiration (sweat) is secreted by the sweat glands. Sweat contains sodium chloride and water.

The GI tract plays a vital role in fluid balance. Approximately 3 to 6 L of fluid moves into the GI tract daily and returns again to the ECF. An average healthy adult excretes only 100 to 200 mL of fluid each day through feces. However, diarrhea causes a large fluid output from the GI tract.

The kidneys are the major regulator of fluid output because they respond to hormones that influence urine production. When healthy people drink more water, they make a larger urine volume to maintain fluid balance. If they drink less water, sweat a lot, or lose fluid by vomiting, their urine volume decreases to maintain fluid balance. These adjustments primarily are the result of the actions of antidiuretic hormone (ADH), aldosterone, and atrial natriuretic peptides (Halperin et al., 2010).

Antidiuretic Hormone. ADH regulates osmolality of body fluids by influencing how much water is excreted in urine. The hypothalamus controls release of ADH from the posterior pituitary gland. It circulates to the kidneys where it acts on the collecting ducts, causing them to resorb water (Hall, 2011). This antidiuretic effect removes water from the renal tubules and puts it back into the blood, diluting the blood. More ADH is released when plasma osmolality increases; increased ADH causes more water resorption and dilutes the plasma back to normal. Conversely less ADH is released when plasma osmolality decreases; less water is resorbed so it leaves the body in the urine and plasma osmolality returns to normal. Pain, nausea, stressors, some medications, and severely decreased blood volume increase the secretion of ADH and thus can cause plasma to become more dilute than normal. Ethyl alcohol decreases ADH release, which is why people urinate frequently when they drink alcoholic beverages.

Aldosterone. Aldosterone regulates ECV by influencing how much sodium and water are excreted in urine. The adrenal cortex releases aldosterone in response to increased plasma potassium concentration or as the end product of the renin-angiotensin-aldosterone system (RAAS). Renin released by the kidneys acts on the inactive protein angiotensinogen to produce angiotensin I, which other enzymes in the lung capillaries convert to angiotensin II. Angiotensin II causes vasoconstriction of many blood vessels, which helps regulate blood pressure; and it stimulates the release of aldosterone, which assists fluid homeostasis. Aldosterone circulates to the kidneys where it acts on the distal tubules, causing them to resorb sodium and water in isotonic proportions. Removing sodium and water from the renal tubules and returning it to the blood increases ECV. If ECV decreases such as through vomiting and diarrhea, the kidneys release more renin, and the RAAS produces more aldosterone to increase sodium and water resorption and restore the ECV. Aldosterone also contributes to electrolyte and acid-base balance by increasing urinary excretion of K^+ and H^+.

Atrial Natriuretic Peptide. Atrial natriuretic peptide (ANP) is a hormone that opposes the action of aldosterone and promotes vasodilation. It is secreted from the cells of the heart in response to atrial stretching and an increased circulating blood volume. ANP causes sodium and water to be excreted in the urine, thus decreasing ECV slightly (Hall, 2011).

Electrolyte Balance. Electrolyte homeostasis is the dynamic interplay among electrolyte intake and absorption, electrolyte distribution, and electrolyte output (Felver, 2013b). To maintain electrolyte balance, electrolyte intake must equal electrolyte output, and the electrolyte distribution must be normal.

Sodium Regulation. Normal serum Na^+ concentration ranges from 135 to 145 mEq/L. Sodium is the most abundant cation in ECF but has a smaller concentration inside cells. This unequal distribution is maintained by the Na^+-K^+ pump in cell membranes, which also maintains an unequal K^+ distribution. The concentration of Na^+ in ECF is greatly influenced by the relative amount of water and reflects the osmolality (concentration) of the ECF. Sodium concentration imbalances really are water imbalances and are discussed under the Fluid Imbalances heading.

Potassium Balance. The normal range for serum K^+ concentration is 3.5 to 5 mEq/L. In contrast to this small concentration of K^+ in the ECF, K^+ has a high intracellular concentration (Hall, 2011). This unequal distribution of K^+ maintains the resting membrane potential of cardiac, skeletal, and smooth muscle contraction, allowing for normal muscle function (Halperin et al., 2010). K^+ absorbs easily with dietary intake of food sources such as bananas, spinach, and apricots. Insulin, epinephrine, and alkalosis shift K^+ into cells. Acute and chronic diarrhea increase output of K^+ from the GI tract. Aldosterone facilitates K^+ renal excretion, as does polyuria.

Calcium Balance. Ca^{2+} in blood has two major forms: bound and free. Ca^{2+} bound to albumin and other blood components is inactive. Free (ionized) Ca^{2+} is available for physiological actions. Normal serum total Ca^{2+} levels (bound plus free) are 8.4 to 10.5 mg/dL. Normal serum ionized Ca^{2+} levels range from 4.5 to 5.3 mg/dL. Most of the calcium in the body is in bone, although intracellular Ca^{2+} has important functions. Ca^{2+} influences the excitability of nerve and muscle cells and is necessary for muscle contraction and blood clotting. Plasma Ca^{2+} concentration is regulated primarily by the actions of parathyroid hormone (shifts Ca^{2+} out of cells) and calcitonin (shifts Ca^{2+} into cells). Vitamin D is necessary to make proteins responsible for dietary Ca^{2+} absorption in the duodenum. Chronic diarrhea and undigested fat increase output of Ca^{2+} in the feces.

Magnesium Balance. Normal plasma concentration of Mg^{2+} ranges from 1.5 to 2.5 mEq/L. Similar to Ca^{2+}, some Mg^{2+} in the blood is bound and inactive. Most of the Mg^{2+} in the body is in bones and inside cells. Mg^{2+} is essential for action of many enzymes and for normal action at neuromuscular junctions. Absorption of dietary Mg^{2+} occurs primarily in the terminal ileum. Chronic diarrhea and undigested fat increase output of Mg^{2+} in the feces. Renal Mg^{2+} excretion increases with a rising blood alcohol.

Chloride Regulation. Normal serum Cl^- concentration ranges from 95 to 105 mEq/L. Cl^- is the major anion in ECF, and it is an important part of gastric hydrochloric acid.

Bicarbonate Regulation. Normal arterial bicarbonate levels range between 22 and 26 mEq/L; normal venous bicarbonate is 24 to 30 mEq/L. Bicarbonate is a base and serves as a key component of the bicarbonate buffering system essential to acid-base balance. The kidneys assist with regulating bicarbonate levels.

Phosphate Balance. Normal serum phosphate level ranges from 2.7 to 4.5 mg/dL. Phosphate exists in three forms ($H_2PO_4^-$, HPO_4^{2-}, and PO_4^{3-}), which are added together in the laboratory measurement. Most phosphate in the body is in bone and inside cells. Insulin and epinephrine shift phosphate into cells. Phosphate is necessary for production of ATP, the energy source for cellular metabolism. Ca^{2+} and phosphate blood levels are inversely proportional; if one rises, the other falls, except during end-stage renal disease. The GI tract absorbs dietary phosphate easily, except in the presence of aluminum or magnesium antacids. Renal excretion is the largest route of phosphate output and decreases greatly with oliguria.

Acid-Base Balance. Optimal cell function requires a balance between acids and bases. Acids release H^+; bases (alkaline substances) take up H^+. Acid-base homeostasis is the dynamic interplay of acid production, acid buffering, and acid excretion (Felver, 2013a). Acid-base balance requires acid excretion to be equal to acid production, with acid buffering in blood and renal tubular fluid.

The pH is a measure of fluid acidity or alkalinity. A pH value of 7.0 is neutral; below 7.0 is acid, and above 7.0 is alkaline. The greater the concentration of H^+, the more acidic the solution, and the lower the pH; the lower the concentration of H^+ ions, the more alkaline the solution, and the higher the pH. Normal pH range of arterial blood is 7.35 to 7.45.

Acid Production. Cellular metabolism constantly produces two kinds of acid: carbonic and metabolic. Carbonic acid (H_2CO_3) arises from the carbon dioxide (CO_2) that cells produce. Metabolic acids are all other acids produced by cells that are not carbonic acid such as lactic acid and citric acid.

Acid Buffering. **Buffers** are pairs of chemicals that work together to maintain normal pH of body fluids. If there are too many free H^+ ions, a buffer can take them up so they no longer are free and cannot decrease the pH. If there are not enough free H^+ ions, a buffer can release H^+ to restore a normal pH. All body fluids contain buffers. The major buffer in ECF is the bicarbonate buffer system, which buffers metabolic acids. Other buffers include hemoglobin, protein buffers, and phosphate buffers. Buffers normally keep the blood from becoming too acidic when acids produced by cells are circulating to lungs and kidneys for excretion.

Acid Excretion. The body has two acid excretion mechanisms: lungs (excrete carbonic acid) and kidneys (excrete metabolic acids). The lungs excrete carbonic acid in the form of CO_2 and water. The chemoreceptors regulate this excretion by altering respiratory rate and depth. If more carbonic acid should be excreted, respirations increase; if less should be excreted, respirations decrease (within limits). The kidneys excrete all acids except carbonic acid, using several mechanisms to adjust the amount of H^+ excreted in the urine to maintain acid-base homeostasis (Rose, 2013).

Disturbances in Fluid, Electrolyte, and Acid-Base Balances

Disturbances in fluid, electrolyte, and acid-base balances disrupt normal body processes and often occur together. As a nurse you need to be familiar with these imbalances and their effects on body functioning.

Fluid Imbalances. Fluid imbalances are isotonic (volume) and/or osmolality (concentration) imbalances (Table 18-2 and Figure 18-4). An isotonic deficit or excess exists when water and sodium are lost or gained in equal proportions, thus affecting the volume of the ECF. In contrast, an osmolality imbalance is a loss or excess of only water, which affects the **concentration** (osmolality) of the body fluids.

Extracellular Fluid Volume Imbalances. **ECV excess** is too much isotonic fluid in the extracellular compartment (see Table 18-2). Signs and symptoms come from too much vascular volume and interstitial volume. ECV deficit, as the name indicates, is too small a volume of isotonic fluid in the vascular and interstitial areas. The term **hypovolemia** refers to the decreased vascular volume in ECV deficit (Metheny, 2012).

Osmolality Imbalances. **Hypernatremia** is abnormally high Na^+ concentration in ECF caused by loss of relatively more water than salt or gain of relatively more salt than water (see Table 18-2) (Felver, 2013c). Water leaves cells by osmosis, and they shrivel. Signs of cerebral dysfunction occur when brain cells shrivel. Hypernatremia often occurs in combination with ECV deficit; the two together are **clinical dehydration.**

Hyponatremia is abnormally low Na^+ concentration in the ECF, which occurs from gaining relatively more water than salt or losing relatively more salt than water (see Table 18-2) (Felver, 2013c). Water enters cells by osmosis, causing them to swell. Signs of cerebral dysfunction occur when brain cells swell.

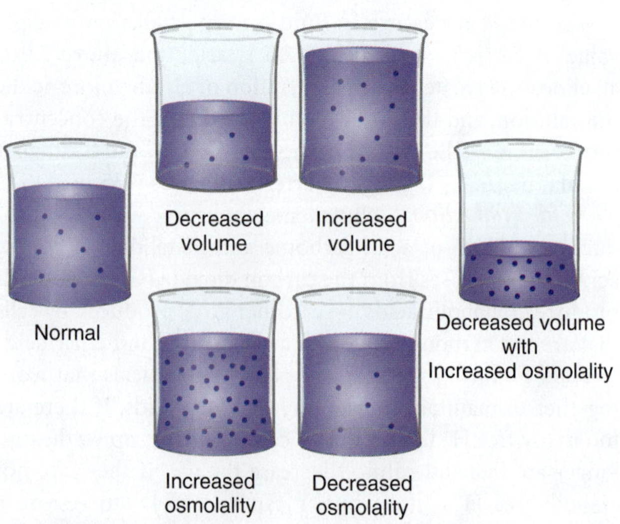

FIGURE 18-4 Fluid volume and osmolality imbalances. (From Copstead LC, Banasik JL: *Pathophysiology online for pathophysiology*, ed 4, St Louis, 2010, Saunders.)

Electrolyte Imbalances

Potassium Imbalances. **Hypokalemia,** a common electrolyte imbalance, is an inadequate level of K^+ in the blood. Common causes of hypokalemia involve increased K^+ output not balanced by K^+ intake: diarrhea and use of K^+-wasting diuretics (Table 18-3) (Felver, 2013b). Hypokalemia causes muscle weakness and, if severe, cardiac dysrhythmias.

Hyperkalemia is abnormally high blood K^+ concentration. Its causes are increased K^+ intake, shift of K^+ out of cells, and decreased K^+ output. Hyperkalemia produces muscle weakness and dangerous dysrhythmias.

Calcium Imbalances. **Hypocalcemia** is abnormally low blood concentration of total Ca^{2+} or ionized Ca^{2+}. It usually results from decreased Ca^{2+} intake and absorption or shift of Ca^{2+} into bones or unavailable forms (see Table 18-3) (Felver, 2013c). Signs and symptoms are caused by increased neuromuscular excitability.

Hypercalcemia is abnormally high Ca^{2+} concentration in the blood. Hypercalcemia often occurs from an underlying disease such as cancer or hyperparathyroidism that causes bone resorption, shifting Ca^{2+} from bones into the ECF. The person may develop pathological fractures from the weak bones that result.

Magnesium Imbalances. **Hypomagnesemia,** abnormally low blood Mg^{2+} level, often occurs with chronic alcoholism and causes increased neuromuscular excitability (see Table 18-3). **Hypermagnesemia,** abnormally high blood Mg^{2+} level, is the result of excess Mg^{2+} intake or decreased Mg^{2+} excretion with oliguric renal disease. It causes decreased neuromuscular excitability.

Chloride Imbalances. **Hypochloremia** is abnormally low blood chloride level. It frequently is associated with alkalosis and conditions that cause loss of hydrochloric acid (vomiting, nasogastric suction, and gastric fistula drainage). It always occurs with other imbalances and has no unique signs and symptoms.

Hyperchloremia is abnormally high blood chloride level, which occurs with some types of acidosis, some renal conditions, and other electrolyte imbalances. It also has no unique signs and symptoms.

TABLE 18-2 FLUID IMBALANCES

IMBALANCE AND RELATED CAUSES	SIGNS AND SYMPTOMS
Isotonic Imbalances—Water and Sodium Lost or Gained in Equal or Isotonic Proportions	
Extracellular Fluid Volume Deficit—Body Fluids Have Decreased Volume but Normal Osmolality	
Sodium and Water Intake Less Than Output, Causing Isotonic Loss: Severely decreased oral intake of water and salt Increased GI output: Vomiting, diarrhea, laxative overuse, drainage from fistulas or tubes Increased renal output: Use of diuretics, adrenal insufficiency Loss of blood or plasma: Hemorrhage, burns Massive sweating without water and salt intake	*Physical examination:* Sudden weight loss (overnight), postural hypotension, tachycardia, thready pulse, dry mucous membranes, poor skin turgor, slow vein filling, flat neck veins when supine, dark yellow urine If severe: Thirst; restlessness; confusion; hypotension; oliguria (urine output **below** 30 mL/hr); cold, clammy skin; hypovolemic shock *Laboratory findings:* Increased hematocrit, increased BUN **above** 25 mg/dL (hemoconcentration); urine specific gravity usually **above** 1.030, unless renal cause
Extracellular Fluid Volume Excess—Body Fluids Have Increased Volume but Normal Osmolality	
Sodium and Water Intake Greater Than Output, Causing Isotonic Gain: Excessive intake of Na^+-containing isotonic IV fluids or oral intake of salty foods and water Renal retention of Na^+ and water: Heart failure, cirrhosis, aldosterone or glucocorticoid excess, acute or chronic oliguric renal disease	*Physical examination:* Sudden weight gain (overnight), edema (especially in dependent areas), full neck veins when upright or semi-upright, crackles in lungs If severe: Confusion, pulmonary edema *Laboratory findings:* Decreased hematocrit, decreased BUN **below** 10 mg/dL (hemodilution)
Osmolality Imbalances	
Hypernatremia (Water Deficit; Hyperosmolar Imbalance)—Body Fluids Too Concentrated	
Loss of Relatively More Water Than Salt: ADH deficiency (diabetes insipidus) Osmotic diuresis Large insensible perspiration and respiratory water output without increased water intake **Gain of Relatively More Salt Than Water:** Administration of salt tablets, tube feedings or hypertonic parenteral fluids Lack of access to water, deliberate water deprivation, inability to respond to thirst (e.g., immobility, aphasia) Dysfunction of osmoreceptor driven thirst drive	*Physical examination:* Decreased level of consciousness (confusion, lethargy, coma), perhaps thirst; seizures if develops rapidly or is very severe *Laboratory findings:* Serum sodium level **above** 145 mEq/L, serum osmolality **above** 300 mOsm/kg
Hyponatremia (Water Excess; Hypoosmolar Imbalance)—Body Fluids Too Dilute	
Gain of Relatively More Water Than Salt: Excessive ADH (SIADH) Psychogenic polydipsia or forced excessive water intake Excessive IV administration of D_5W Use of hypotonic irrigating solutions Tap water enemas **Loss of Relatively More Salt Than Water:** Replacement of large body fluid output (diarrhea, vomiting) with water but no salt	*Physical examination:* Decreased level of consciousness (confusion, lethargy, coma); seizures if develops rapidly or is very severe *Laboratory findings:* Serum sodium level **below** 135 mEq/L, serum osmolality **below** 280 mOsm/kg
Combined Isotonic and Osmolity Imbalance	
Clinical Dehydration (ECV Deficit plus Hypernatremia)—Body Fluids Have Decreased Volume and Are Too Concentrated	
Sodium and Water Intake Less Than Output, with Loss of Relatively More Water Than Salt: Most of the causes of ECV deficit (see previous causes) plus poor or no water intake; often with fever causing increased insensible water output	*Physical examination and laboratory findings:* Combination of those for ECV deficit plus those for hypernatremia (see previous signs)

ADH, Antidiuretic hormone; *BUN,* Blood urea nitrogen; *ECV,* extracellular fluid volume; *GI,* gastrointestinal; *D_5W,* dextrose 5% in water; *SIADH,* syndrome of inappropriate ADH.

TABLE 18-3 ELECTROLYTE IMBALANCES

IMBALANCE AND RELATED CAUSES	SIGNS AND SYMPTOMS
Hypokalemia—Low Serum Potassium (K^+) Concentration	
Decreased K^+ Intake: Excessive use of K^+-free IV solutions **Shift of K^+ into Cells:** Alkalosis; treatment of diabetic ketoacidosis with insulin **Increased K^+ Output:** Acute or chronic diarrhea, vomiting, or other GI losses; use of potassium-wasting diuretics; aldosterone excess; polyuria; glucocorticoid therapy	*Physical examination:* Bilateral muscle weakness, abdominal distention, decreased bowel sounds, constipation, dysrhythmias *Laboratory findings:* Serum K^+ level **below** 3.5 mEq/L; ECG abnormalities: U waves, flattened or inverted T waves; ST segment depression
Hyperkalemia—High Serum Potassium (K^+) Concentration	
Increased K^+ Intake: Iatrogenic administration of large amounts of IV K^+; rapid infusion of stored blood; excess ingestion of K^+ salt substitutes **Shift of K^+ out of Cells:** Massive cellular damage (e.g., crushing trauma, cytotoxic chemotherapy); insufficient insulin (e.g., diabetic ketoacidosis); some types of acidosis **Decreased K^+ Output:** Acute or chronic oliguria (e.g., severe ECV deficit, end-stage renal disease); use of potassium-sparing diuretics; adrenal insufficiency	*Physical examination:* Bilateral muscle weakness, transient abdominal cramps, diarrhea, dysrhythmias; cardiac arrest if severe *Laboratory findings:* Serum potassium level **above** 5 mEq/L; ECG abnormalities: peaked T waves; widened QRS complex; PR prolongation; terminal sine-wave pattern
Hypocalcemia—Low Serum Calcium (Ca^{2+}) Concentration	
Decreased Ca^{2+} Intake and Absorption: Calcium-deficient diet; vitamin D deficiency (includes end-stage renal disease); chronic diarrhea, laxative misuse; steatorrhea **Shift of Ca^{2+} Into Bone or Inactive Form:** Hypoparathyroidism; rapid administration of citrated blood; hypoalbuminemia; alkalosis; pancreatitis **Increased Ca^{2+} Output:** Chronic diarrhea; steatorrhea	*Physical examination:* Numbness and tingling of fingers and circumoral (around mouth) region, positive Chvostek's sign (contraction of facial muscles when facial nerve is tapped), hyperactive reflexes, muscle twitching and cramping, tetany, seizures, laryngospasm, dysrhythmias *Laboratory findings:* Total serum calcium **below** 8.4 mg/ dL or serum ionized calcium level **below** 4.5 mEq/L; ECG abnormalities: prolonged ST segments
Hypercalcemia—High Serum Calcium (Ca^{2+}) Concentration	
Increased Ca^{2+} Intake and Absorption: Milk-alkali syndrome **Shift of Ca^{2+} out of Bone:** Prolonged immobilization; hyperparathyroidism; bone tumors; nonosseous cancers that secrete bone-resorbing factors **Decreased Ca^{2+} Output:** Use of thiazide diuretics	*Physical examination:* Anorexia, nausea and vomiting, constipation, diminished reflexes, lethargy, decreased level of consciousness, personality change; cardiac arrest if severe *Laboratory findings:* Total serum calcium level **above** 10.5 mg/dL or serum ionized calcium level **above** 5.3 mEq/L; ECG abnormalities: heart block, shortened ST segments
Hypomagnesemia—Low Serum Magnesium (Mg^{2+}) Concentration	
Decreased Mg^{2+} Intake and Absorption: Malnutrition; chronic alcoholism; chronic diarrhea, laxative misuse; steatorrhea **Shift of Mg^{2+} into Inactive Form:** Rapid administration of citrated blood **Increased Mg^{2+} Output:** Chronic diarrhea; steatorrhea; other GI losses (e.g., vomiting, nasogastric or fistula drainage); use of thiazide or loop diuretics; aldosterone excess	*Physical examination:* Positive Chvostek's sign, hyperactive deep tendon reflexes, muscle twitching and cramping, grimacing, dysphagia, tetany, seizures, insomnia, tachycardia, hypertension, dysrhythmias *Laboratory findings:* Serum magnesium level **below** 1.5 mEq/L; ECG abnormalities: prolonged QT interval
Hypermagnesemia—High Serum Magnesium (Mg^{2+}) Concentration	
Increased Mg^{2+} Intake and Absorption: Excessive use of Mg^{2+}-containing laxatives and antacids; parenteral overload of Mg^{2+} **Decreased Mg^{2+} Output:** Oliguric end-stage renal disease; adrenal insufficiency	*Physical examination:* Lethargy, hypoactive deep tendon reflexes, bradycardia, hypotension Acute elevation in Mg^{2+} levels: Flushing, sensation of warmth Severe acute hypermagnesemia: Decreased rate and depth of respirations, dysrhythmias, cardiac arrest *Laboratory findings:* Serum magnesium level **above** 2.5 mEq/L; ECG abnormalities: prolonged PR interval

ADH, Antidiuretic hormone; *AV,* atrioventricular; *BUN,* blood urea nitrogen; *ECG,* electrocardiogram; *ECV,* extracellular fluid volume; *GI,* gastrointestinal; *NG,* nasogastric.

Acid-Base Imbalances. Acid-base imbalances disrupt cell function and therefore can be fatal if untreated. Arterial blood gas (ABG) analysis is an effective method of evaluating acid-base balance and oxygenation. Measurement of ABG levels involves understanding the physiology of six components: pH, $PaCO_2$, PaO_2, SaO_2, base excess, and HCO_3^-. Deviation from normal values indicates that a patient has an acid-base imbalance.

pH. The pH measures H^+ concentration in body fluids. Even a slight change is potentially life threatening. An increase in concentration of H^+ makes a solution more acidic; a decrease makes the solution more alkaline. Normal arterial blood pH value is 7.35 to 7.45 (acidic is less than 7.35, and alkalotic is greater than 7.45).

$PaCO_2$. $PaCO_2$ is the partial pressure of carbon dioxide in arterial blood and reflects the amount of H_2CO_3 in the blood. Normal range is 35 to 45 mm Hg. Hyperventilation produces a $PaCO_2$ below 35 mm Hg. As rate and depth of respiration increase, more CO_2 is exhaled, decreasing the $PaCO_2$. Conversely, hypoventilation produces a $PaCO_2$ above 45 mm Hg. As rate and depth of respiration decrease, less CO_2 is exhaled while cells continue to produce it, which increases the $PaCO_2$.

PaO_2. PaO_2 is the partial pressure of oxygen in arterial blood. Normal range is 80 to 100 mm Hg. When PaO_2 is within normal range, it has no primary role in acid-base regulation. A PaO_2 less than 60 mm Hg leads to anaerobic metabolism, causing lactic acid production and metabolic acidosis. Hypoxemia can cause hyperventilation leading to respiratory alkalosis.

SaO_2 (Oxygen Saturation). Oxygen saturation (SaO_2) is the percentage of hemoglobin molecules that are carrying as much oxygen as is possible (saturated). Normal range is 95% to 100%. Changes in temperature, pH, and $PaCO_2$ affect SaO_2 levels.

Base Excess. Base excess (or deficit) is the amount of blood buffer (hemoglobin and bicarbonate) present in the blood. The normal range is ±2 mmol/L. A higher positive value indicates alkalosis, and a lower negative value indicates acidosis.

Bicarbonate. Normal range of bicarbonate (HCO_3^-) is 22 to 26 mEq/L. HCO_3^- is the principal buffer in the ECF. Bicarbonate levels reflect the action of the kidneys in managing metabolic acid. Levels below 22 mEq/L usually indicate metabolic acidosis; a level above 26 mEq/L indicates metabolic alkalosis.

Types of Acid-Base Imbalances. Acid-base imbalances are either respiratory or metabolic. The four primary types of acid-base imbalance are respiratory acidosis, respiratory alkalosis, metabolic acidosis, and metabolic alkalosis (Table 18-4). It is possible to have two primary (mixed) acid-base imbalances.

Respiratory acidosis is an increased $PaCO_2$ and an increased hydrogen ion concentration (pH below 7.35) that reflect the excess carbonic acid (H_2CO_3) in the blood. Hypoventilation produces respiratory acidosis, which causes cerebrospinal fluid and brain cells to become acidic, thus decreasing the level of consciousness (see Table 18-4).

Respiratory alkalosis is a decreased $PaCO_2$ and increased pH (above 7.45) that reflect the deficit of carbonic acid (H_2CO_3) in the blood. Hyperventilation produces respiratory alkalosis, which causes cerebrospinal fluid and brain cells to become alkalotic, decreasing the level of consciousness (see Table 18-4).

Metabolic acidosis results from conditions that increase metabolic acids in the body or decrease the amount of base (bicarbonate) (Felver, 2013a). The bicarbonate level always is low because the bicarbonate system buffers metabolic acids. Diabetic ketoacidosis is a common cause of metabolic acidosis (see Table 18-4). Calculation of the anion gap is useful for identifying the cause of metabolic acidosis. An anion gap reflects unmeasurable anions present in plasma. One way of calculating anion gap is by summing the Cl^- and bicarbonate levels and subtracting this number from the Na^+ concentration (Rose, 2013).

Metabolic alkalosis results from a gain of bicarbonate or from excessive excretion of metabolic acid (Felver, 2013a). The most common causes are vomiting and gastric suction (see Table 18-4).

NURSING KNOWLEDGE BASE

Fluid and electrolyte imbalances occur in all patients, regardless of age, gender, race, or culture. Your nursing knowledge base regarding these variables helps you understand how fluid and electrolyte imbalances affect patients. For example, you apply knowledge of growth and development when managing patients with fluid and electrolyte imbalances. Infants are at significant risk because of their limited ability to respond independently to early warnings of a problem (Hockenberry and Wilson, 2011). Your knowledge of normal growth and development is helpful in recognizing behavioral changes from fluid and electrolyte alterations. Similarly, adults who are severely ill, disoriented, and immobile have difficulty expressing symptoms when fluid and electrolyte imbalances develop. A nursing knowledge base regarding communication and health assessment techniques is invaluable in detecting problems early.

CRITICAL THINKING

Synthesis

You will apply elements of critical thinking whenever you perform the nursing process with patients. Consider the scientific knowledge you have learned, your experience, critical thinking attitudes, and standards to ensure an individualized approach to patient care (Box 18-1). Patients' conditions often change quickly in the presence of a fluid and electrolyte imbalance. Clinical decision making and judgment are necessary to analyze clinical data and make decisions regarding patient care. Use professional standards as guidelines for comprehensive assessment.

Knowledge. To provide care for patients with alterations in fluid and electrolyte or acid-base imbalance, use previously learned nursing knowledge and related knowledge acquired

TABLE 18-4 ACID-BASE IMBALANCES

IMBALANCE AND RELATED CAUSES	SIGNS AND SYMPTOMS
Respiratory Acidosis—Excessive Carbonic Acid Resulting From Alveolar Hypoventilation	
Impaired Gas Exchange: Type B COPD (chronic bronchitis) or end-stage type A COPD (emphysema) Bacterial pneumonia Airway obstruction Extensive atelectasis (obstruction of small airways often caused by retained mucus) Severe acute asthma episode **Impaired Neuromuscular Function:** Respiratory muscle weakness or paralysis from hypokalemia or neurological dysfunction Respiratory muscle fatigue, respiratory failure Chest wall injury or surgery causing pain with respiration **Dysfunction of Brainstem Respiratory Control:** Drug overdose with a respiratory depressant Some types of head injury	*Physical examination:* Headache, light-headedness, decreased level of consciousness (confusion, lethargy, coma), dysrhythmias *Laboratory findings:* Arterial blood gas alterations: pH **below** 7.35, $PaCO_2$ **above** 45 mm Hg, bicarbonate level normal (if uncompensated) or **above** 26 mEq/L (if compensated)
Respiratory Alkalosis—Deficient Carbonic Acid Resulting From Alveolar Hyperventilation	
Hypoxemia from any cause (e.g., initial portion of asthma episode, pneumonia) Acute pain Anxiety, psychological distress, sobbing Inappropriate mechanical ventilator settings Stimulation of brainstem respiratory control (meningitis, gram-negative sepsis, head injury, salicylate overdose)	*Physical examination:* Light-headedness; numbness and tingling of fingers, toes, and circumoral region; tachypnea; excitement and confusion possibly followed by decreased level of consciousness; dysrhythmias *Laboratory findings:* Arterial blood gas alterations: pH **above** 7.45, $PaCO_2$ **below** 35 mm Hg, bicarbonate level normal (if short lived or uncompensated) or **below** 22 mEq/L (if compensated)
Metabolic Acidosis—Excessive Metabolic Acids	
Increase of Metabolic Acids (High Anion Gap): Ketoacidosis (diabetes, starvation, alcoholism) Hypermetabolic state (severe hyperthyroidism, burns, severe infection) Oliguric renal disease (acute kidney injury, end-stage renal disease) Circulatory shock (lactic acidosis) Ingestion of acid or acid precursors (e.g., methanol, ethylene glycol, boric acid, aspirin overdose) **Loss of Bicarbonate (Normal Anion Gap):** Diarrhea Pancreatic fistula or intestinal decompression Renal tubular acidosis	*Physical examination:* Decreased level of consciousness (confusion, lethargy, coma), abdominal pain, dysrhythmias, increased rate and depth of respirations (compensatory hyperventilation) *Laboratory findings:* Arterial blood gas alterations: pH **below** 7.35, $PaCO_2$ normal (if uncompensated) or **below** 35 mm Hg (if compensated), bicarbonate level **below** 22 mEq/L
Metabolic Alkalosis—Deficient Metabolic Acids	
Increase of Bicarbonate: Excessive administration of sodium bicarbonate Massive blood transfusion (liver converts citrate to bicarbonate) Mild or moderate ECV deficit **Loss of Metabolic Acid:** Excessive vomiting or gastric suctioning Hypokalemia Excess aldosterone	*Physical examination:* Light-headedness; numbness and tingling of fingers, toes, and circumoral region; muscle cramps; possible excitement and confusion followed by decreased level of consciousness; dysrhythmias (may be caused by concurrent hypokalemia) *Laboratory findings:* Arterial blood gas alterations: pH **above** 7.45, $PaCO_2$ normal (if uncompensated) or **above** 45 mm Hg (if compensated), bicarbonate level **above** 26 mEq/L; K^+ level often decreased (below 3.5 mEq/L)

COPD, Chronic obstructive pulmonary disease; *ECV,* extracellular fluid volume.

BOX 18-1 SYNTHESIS IN PRACTICE

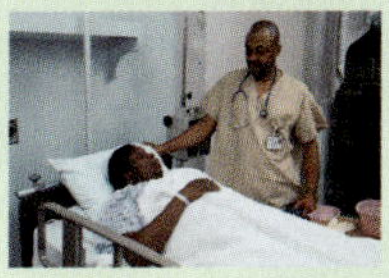

Robert reviews Mrs. Reynolds' clinical condition. Her history reveals that Mrs. Reynolds has loss of appetite, episodes of diarrhea, and continued use of hydrochlorothiazide (a potassium-wasting diuretic) for hypertension. She is at risk for fluid and electrolyte imbalances from gastrointestinal (GI) disturbance and continued use of a diuretic. The cause of her GI symptoms is unclear; therefore her health care provider plans further diagnostic tests. Robert reviews the physiology of fluid and potassium balance and studies the signs and symptoms of extracellular fluid volume (ECV) deficit and hypokalemia. He also reads recommendations in a pharmacology text on how to minimize the risk for hypokalemia when taking diuretics. Robert anticipates the need to perform a focused physical assessment and manage and monitor Mrs. Reynolds' intravenous (IV) therapy. He knows that patient education will eventually be important for this patient because her therapy for hypertension will continue after discharge.

Just a few weeks ago Robert cared for a patient with ulcerative colitis. Although Mrs. Reynolds' condition is different, both patients had diarrhea. Robert knows that Mrs. Reynolds will require careful monitoring of intake and output and stabilization of GI function. The lessons learned from his previous patient will help Robert to be more alert if Mrs. Reynolds' clinical condition changes during his care.

Robert applies the critical thinking attitude of discipline by completing a thorough examination and assessment. The attitude of curiosity is important when a clinical sign or symptom may be unclear and further information is needed.

When Robert checks the policy and procedures at his institution for an IV therapy protocol, he applies professional standards in practice. He reviews the standards for initiating and maintaining IV sites to be familiar with the procedures.

in anatomy, physiology, pharmacology, and/or chemistry courses. Consider all factors contributing to a patient's health problem. *For example, Mrs. Reynolds is at high risk for ECV deficit from her diarrhea, diuretic use, and decreased fluid intake. Her nurse, Robert, knows that she is at risk for becoming light-headed when she gets out of bed because of orthostatic hypotension. In the case study synthesizing previously learned knowledge about ECV deficit and orthostatic hypotension helps Robert plan and provide appropriate patient care.*

Experience. Professional experience helps you when caring for patients with fluid, electrolyte, or acid-base imbalances. Understanding patients' clinical signs and symptoms helps you identify and make appropriate clinical decisions when presented with a similar assessment. Prior patient care experiences make you more adept at future problem solving and decision making.

Attitudes. Accountability and discipline are two of the critical thinking attitudes to use when caring for patients with fluid, electrolyte, and acid-base imbalances. Be accountable by reporting changes in patient behavior or physical assessment findings immediately and follow standards of practice. Patients with fluid and electrolyte imbalances often present with a group of signs and symptoms; therefore use discipline in conducting a thorough and comprehensive assessment.

Standards. Apply intellectual standards of accuracy, relevancy, and significance in obtaining a health history for a patient with fluid and electrolyte imbalances. Apply Infusion Nurses Society (INS) standards of care for establishing, maintaining, monitoring, and discontinuing IV therapy (INS, 2011). Also apply the standards of infection control for invasive procedures such as IV therapy (O'Grady et al., 2011). Laboratory standards provide normal electrolyte ranges.

NURSING PROCESS

ASSESSMENT

It is important to use knowledge of fluid, electrolyte, and acid-base balance to guide assessment. By gathering assessment data and using critical thinking skills, nurses identify patients at risk and those with imbalances. Thorough assessment enables identification of appropriate nursing diagnoses.

Nursing History. Assessment begins with a patient history, which reveals risk factors or preexisting conditions that cause or contribute to fluid, electrolyte, and acid-base imbalances. Explore these factors with the patient and integrate the information with knowledge of regulation of fluid, electrolyte, and acid-base balances.

Age is an important assessment consideration. Infants and very young children have relatively more body water than older children and adults. They have greater water needs and immature kidneys (Hockenberry and Wilson, 2011). They are at greater risk for ECV deficit and hypernatremia because their body water loss is proportionately greater per kilogram of weight. Children ages 2 through 12 have less stable regulatory responses to imbalances; therefore they have a narrow range of tolerance for severe fluid or electrolyte imbalances. Adolescent girls have greater ECV fluctuations because of hormonal changes associated with the menstrual cycle.

Older Adult Considerations. Older adults experience a number of age-related changes that can affect fluid, electrolyte, and acid-base balances. These changes include a reduction in body water, diminished thirst sensation, and decreased ability to concentrate urine, which increase the risk of ECV deficit and hypernatremia (Felver, 2013c). Kidney changes of normal aging make it more difficult to excrete a large metabolic acid load, increasing the risk for metabolic acidosis. Normal aging changes, chronic diseases, and multiple medications often make maintaining fluid and electrolyte balance a challenge.

Medical History. A patient's prior medical history provides valuable data about fluid, electrolyte, and acid-base imbalances. When patients have chronic diseases (e.g., cancer, heart failure, oliguric renal disease), review these conditions to understand how they affect fluid, electrolyte, and acid-base balance. Assess duration of the disease and treatment regimens. In addition to chronic health problems, determine if a patient has a history of recent GI alterations (e.g., diarrhea or vomiting), nasogastric suctioning, or intestinal drainage.

Loss of GI fluids predisposes patients to ECV deficit, hypokalemia, and other electrolyte imbalances.

Recent surgery, head injury, respiratory disorders, and burns place patients at high risk for fluid and electrolyte imbalances. The physiological stress response to surgery causes increased secretion of aldosterone, cortisol, and ADH in the first few postoperative days. These changes cause increased ECV, decreased osmolality, and increased K^+ excretion. In otherwise healthy patients these imbalances resolve without difficulty, but patients with preexisting imbalances or additional risk factors may need treatment.

Environment. Hot environments increase fluid output through sweating. Sweat is a hypotonic Na^+-containing fluid. Ask patients whether they engage in vigorous physical work or exercise in hot environments. If so, are Na^+-containing fluid replacements available during activity?

Dietary Intake. Assess dietary intake of fluids, salt, and foods rich in K^+, Ca^{2+}, and Mg^{2+}. Assess recent changes in appetite and ability to chew and swallow, which affect nutritional status and fluid hydration. Starvation diets or high-fat, no-carbohydrate diets can cause metabolic acidosis.

Lifestyle. Take an alcohol intake history. Chronic alcohol abuse commonly causes hypomagnesemia, in part because it increases renal Mg^{2+} excretion.

Medications. Obtain a complete list of current medications, including over-the-counter (OTC) and herbal preparations, to assess risk for fluid, electrolyte, and acid-base imbalances. Box 18-2 lists commonly used medications that can cause these imbalances. If assessment reveals a medication that causes an electrolyte or acid-base imbalance, assess pertinent laboratory values.

BOX 18-2 COMMONLY USED MEDICATIONS THAT CAUSE FLUID, ELECTROLYTE, AND ACID-BASE IMBALANCES

- **ACE inhibitors** (e.g., captopril) and **angiotensin II receptor antagonists** (e.g., losartan): Hyperkalemia
- **Antidepressants**, SSRI (e.g., fluoxetine): Hyponatremia
- **Calcium carbonate antacids:** Hypercalcemia, mild metabolic alkalosis
- **Corticosteroids** (e.g., prednisone): Hypokalemia, metabolic alkalosis
- **Diuretics, potassium-wasting** (e.g., furosemide, thiazides): ECV deficit, hypokalemia, hypomagnesemia, mild metabolic alkalosis
- **Diuretics, potassium-sparing** (e.g., spironolactone): Hyperkalemia, mild metabolic acidosis
- **Effervescent (fizzy) antacids and cold medications** (high Na^+ content): ECV excess
- **Laxatives** (overuse): ECV deficit, hypokalemia, hypocalcemia, hypomagnesemia, metabolic acidosis
- **Magnesium hydroxide** (e.g., Milk of Magnesia): Hypermagnesemia
- **Nonsteroidal antiinflammatory drugs** (NSAIDs [e.g., ibuprofen]): Mild ECV excess, hyponatremia
- **Opioid analgesics, overdose** (e.g., morphine): Respiratory acidosis
- **Penicillin G, IV** medication (contains K^+): Hyperkalemia

Data from Lehne RA: *Pharmacology for nursing care*, ed 8, St Louis, 2013, Saunders Elsevier.
ECV, Extracellular fluid volume; *IV,* intravenous; *NSAID,* nonsteroidal antiinflammatory drugs; *SSRI,* selective serotonin reuptake inhibitor.

Focused Physical Assessment. Data gathered through a focused physical assessment validates and extends information gathered in the patient history. Table 18-5 summarizes assessments for patients with fluid, electrolyte, and acid-base imbalances. Focus your assessment on the areas pertinent to each patient situation. For example, for patients at risk for ECV imbalances, focus your assessment on body weight changes and clinical markers of vascular and interstitial volume. Assessments for patients at high risk of electrolyte and acid-base imbalances include specific cardiac, respiratory, neuromuscular, and GI markers. Grouping your assessments under these categories helps you know which assessments to prioritize and enables you to assess effectively. Table 18-6 provides a focused assessment of fluid status for Mrs. Reynolds.

Daily Weights and Fluid Intake and Output Measurement. Daily weights are an important indicator of fluid status (Metheny, 2012). Each kilogram (2.2 lbs) of weight gained or lost overnight is equal to 1 L of fluid gained or lost. Weigh patients with heart failure or those who are at high risk for or actually have ECV excess daily. Obtain the weight at the same time each day with the same calibrated scale after a patient voids. Have patients wear clothes that weigh the same each time they weigh. If you are using a bed scale, always use the same number of linens. Teach patients with heart failure to take and record daily weights at home and to contact their health care provider if weight increases suddenly according to parameters their providers set. Recognizing trends in daily weights is important. Classic research shows that patients who are hospitalized for decompensated heart failure often experience steady increases in daily weights during the week before hospitalization (Chaudry et al., 2007).

Measuring and recording all liquid I&O during a 24-hour period is an important aspect of fluid balance assessment. Compare 24-hour intake with 24-hour output. The two measures should be approximately equal if the person has normal fluid balance. Recognizing I&O trends is important (e.g., a gradually decreasing fluid output with increased intake may indicate a developing ECV excess).

In most health care settings I&O measurement is a nursing assessment. Some agencies require a health care provider's order for I&O. Check your agency policies if you want to measure I&O for a patient with compromised fluid status. Fluid intake includes all liquids that a person eats (e.g., gelatin, ice cream, broth), drinks (e.g., juice, coffee, tea, water), or receives through nasogastric or jejunostomy feeding tubes (see Chapter 16). IV fluids (continuous and intermittent) and blood components also count as intake. A patient receiving tube feedings may receive numerous liquid medications;

TABLE 18-5 PHYSICAL AND BEHAVIORAL NURSING ASSESSMENT FOR FLUID, ELECTROLYTE, AND ACID-BASE IMBALANCES

ASSESSMENT	IMBALANCES
Body Weight Changes from Previous Day	
Loss of 2.2 lbs (1 kg) or more in 24 hours for adults	ECV deficit
Gain of 2.2 lbs (1 kg) or more in 24 hours for adults	ECV excess
Clinical Markers of Vascular Volume	
Blood Pressure	
Hypotension or orthostatic hypotension	ECV deficit
Light-headedness on sitting upright or standing	ECV deficit
Pulse Rate and Character	
Rapid, thready	ECV excess
Bounding	ECV excess
Fullness of Neck Veins	
Flat or collapsing with inspiration when supine	ECV deficit
Full or distended when upright or semi-upright	ECV excess
Other Assessments of Vascular Volume	
Capillary refill: Sluggish	ECV deficit
Lung auscultation, dependent portions: Crackles or rhonchi with progressive dyspnea	ECV excess
Urine output: Small volume of dark yellow urine	ECV deficit
Clinical Markers of Interstitial Volume	
Edema: Present in dependent areas (ankles or sacrum) and possibly fingers or around eyes	ECV excess
Mucous membranes: Dry between cheek and gum, tears decreased or absent	ECV deficit
Skin turgor: Pinched skin fails to return to normal position within 3 seconds	ECV deficit
Thirst	
Thirst present	Hypernatremia, severe ECV deficit
Behavior and Level of Consciousness	
Restlessness and mild confusion	Severe ECV deficit
Decreased level of consciousness (confusion, lethargy, coma)	Hyponatremia, hypernatremia, hypercalcemia, acid-base imbalances
Cardiac and Respiratory Signs of Electrolyte or Acid-Base Imbalances	
Pulse rhythm and ECG abnormalities	K^+, Ca^{2+}, Mg^{2+}, and/or acid-base imbalances
Rate and Depth of Respirations	
Increased rate and depth	Metabolic acidosis (compensatory mechanism); respiratory alkalosis (cause)
Decreased rate and depth	Metabolic alkalosis (compensatory mechanism); respiratory acidosis (cause)
Neuromuscular Markers of Electrolyte or Acid-Base Imbalances	
Muscle Strength	
Muscle weakness, bilateral, especially quadriceps	Hypokalemia, hyperkalemia

Continued

TABLE 18-5 PHYSICAL AND BEHAVIORAL NURSING ASSESSMENT FOR FLUID, ELECTROLYTE, AND ACID-BASE IMBALANCES—cont'd

ASSESSMENT	IMBALANCES
Reflexes and Sensations	
Decreased deep tendon reflexes	Hypercalcemia, hypermagnesemia
Hyperactive reflexes, positive Chvostek's sign	Hypocalcemia, hypomagnesemia
Muscle twitching and cramping	Hypocalcemia, hypomagnesemia, respiratory alkalosis
Numbness; tingling in fingertips, around mouth	Hypocalcemia, hypomagnesemia, respiratory alkalosis
Tremor	Hypomagnesemia
Gastrointestinal Signs of Electrolyte Imbalances	
Inspection and Auscultation	
Abdominal distention	Hypokalemia
Decreased bowel sounds	Hypokalemia
Motility	
Constipation	Hypokalemia, hypercalcemia

ECG, Electrocardiogram; *ECV,* extracellular fluid volume.

TABLE 18-6 FOCUSED PATIENT ASSESSMENT

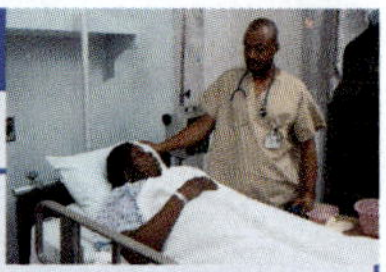

FACTORS TO ASSESS	QUESTIONS	PHYSICAL ASSESSMENT
Vital signs and neck veins	Do you get light-headed when you stand up?	Palpate patient's pulse and auscultate heart rate. Monitor patient's blood pressure and pulse when supine and then at 1 minute after sitting with legs dependent or at 1 minute after standing. Observe patient for light-headedness (unsteady gait). Inspect neck veins when patient is supine to see if they are flat or collapsing with inspiration.
Intake and output (I&O)	Are you thirsty? How often do you usually urinate?	Monitor patient's 24-hour I&O; note if having diarrhea fluid. Inspect urine (expect dark yellow color).
Skin, mucous membranes, and daily weight	Is your mouth dry? Is your skin more dry than usual?	Check dryness of mucous membranes between cheek and gum. Inspect patient's skin; test for turgor over sternum. Obtain a baseline weight and monitor daily.

ECV, Extracellular fluid volume.

water is used to flush the tube before and/or after the medications. During a 24-hour period these liquids can amount to significant intake and always should be recorded on the I&O record. Patient and family cooperation is essential for maintaining accurate I&O measurements. Ask alert patients to help measure their oral intake and explain to families why they should not eat or drink from the patient's meal tray or water pitcher.

Liquid output includes urine, diarrhea, vomitus, gastric suction, and blood and drainage from postsurgical wounds, burns, or other tubes (see Chapter 16). Record urinary output after each voiding. Instruct alert ambulatory patients to save their urine in a calibrated (graduated) insert that attaches to the rim of a toilet bowl (Figure 18-5). Teach patients and families the purpose of I&O; tell them to notify a nurse or nursing assistive personnel (NAP) to empty the container

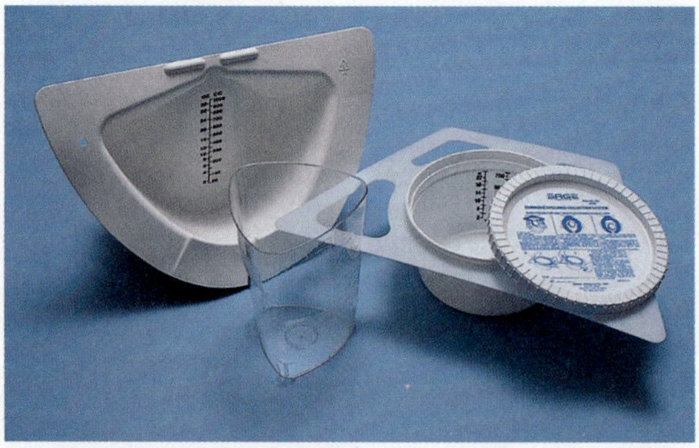

FIGURE 18-5 Graduated measuring containers. *Clockwise from top left:* "hat" receptacle, specimen, and measurement container.

TABLE 18-7 ARTERIAL BLOOD GAS ASSESSMENT

TEST	NORMAL RANGE FOR ADULTS	SIGNIFICANCE OF ABNORMAL FINDINGS
pH	7.35-7.45	Increased: Metabolic or respiratory alkalosis Decreased: Metabolic or respiratory acidosis (Small changes in pH indicate large changes in H^+ concentration and are clinically important.)
PaO_2 (mm Hg)	80-100	Decreased: Poor oxygenation of the blood
SaO_2 (%)	95-100	Decreased: Poor oxygenation of the blood
$PaCO_2$ (mm Hg)	35-45	Increased: Respiratory acidosis or compensation for metabolic alkalosis (differentiate with the pH) Decreased: Respiratory alkalosis or compensation for metabolic acidosis (differentiate with the pH)
Bicarbonate (mEq/L or mmol/L)	22-26	Increased: Metabolic alkalosis or compensation for respiratory acidosis (differentiate with the pH) Decreased: Metabolic acidosis or compensation for respiratory alkalosis (differentiate with the pH)

with voided fluid or teach them how to measure and record the result themselves. Patients need good vision and motor skills to perform these assessments. When a patient has an indwelling urinary catheter, drainage tube, or suction, record that output (e.g., at the end of each nursing shift or every hour) as the patient's condition requires.

You can delegate portions of I&O measurement to NAP. Classic research shows that visual estimates of fluid volumes often are unreliable; actual measurement is preferable (McConnell et al., 2007). In many agencies NAP can record oral intake but not intake through tubes or IV lines; they can record urine, diarrhea, and vomitus output but not drainage through tubes. Work as a team with the NAP to record measurements in the designated location in the electronic health record (EHR) or appropriate paper forms. Accurate I&O facilitates ongoing evaluation of a patient's hydration status.

Laboratory Studies. Review the patient's laboratory test results and compare them with normal ranges to obtain additional data about fluid, electrolyte, and acid-base balances. Box 18-3 and Table 18-7 summarize laboratory data useful for this purpose. The frequency of electrolyte level measurement depends on the severity of a patient's illness. Serum electrolyte tests are performed routinely on patients entering a hospital to screen for imbalances and serve as a baseline for future comparisons.

Patient Expectations. Fluid, electrolyte, and acid-base imbalances often accompany serious illness that prevents a review of patient expectations. With an alert patient a review of expectations may reveal short-term (e.g., provision of comfort from nausea) or long-term (e.g., understanding how to prevent imbalances in the future) needs. Strengthen a patient's trust through competent responses to sudden changes in condition and by keeping patients and/or family members informed so they become active participants in their care.

BOX 18-3 LABORATORY DATA REFLECTING FLUID, ELECTROLYTE, AND ACID-BASE IMBALANCES

FLUID AND ELECTROLYTES
- Alterations in serum sodium, osmolality, potassium, magnesium, calcium, phosphate, and chloride
- Alterations in hematocrit and blood urea nitrogen (BUN)
- Alterations in urine specific gravity

METABOLIC ALKALOSIS
- pH >7.45
- $PaCO_2$ normal or >45 mm Hg if lungs are compensating
- HCO_3^- >26 mEq/L
- Ionized calcium <4.5 mg/dL
- K^+ <3.5 mEq/L

METABOLIC ACIDOSIS
- pH <7.35
- $PaCO_2$ normal or <35 mm Hg if lungs are compensating
- HCO_3^- <22 mEq/L
- K^+ >5 mEq/L

RESPIRATORY ALKALOSIS
- pH >7.45
- $PaCO_2$ <35 mm Hg
- HCO_3^- <22 mEq/L if kidneys are compensating
- Ionized calcium <4.5 mg/dL
- K^+ <3.5 mEq/L

RESPIRATORY ACIDOSIS
- pH <7.35
- $PaCO_2$ >45 mm Hg
- HCO_3^- normal if early respiratory acidosis or >26 mEq/L if kidneys are compensating
- K^+ >5 mEq/L

NURSING DIAGNOSIS

When caring for patients with potential fluid, electrolyte, or acid-base imbalances, use critical thinking to formulate nursing diagnoses. The assessment data that establish the risk for or the actual presence of a nursing diagnosis may be subtle, but patterns and trends emerge after astute assessment. Multiple body systems may be involved, so carefully analyze the defining characteristics in clusters. For example, relevant assessment data for the nursing diagnosis *Deficient Fluid Volume* include defining characteristics such as insufficient oral intake, sudden weight loss, dry oral mucous membranes, decreased skin turgor, decreased blood pressure, and increased heart rate.

In addition to accurate clustering of assessment data, another part of developing nursing diagnoses is identifying the relevant causes or related factor. For example, *Deficient Fluid Volume related to loss of GI fluids from vomiting* requires interventions to manage the patient's vomiting and restore fluid volume (e.g., administer antiemetics, remove sights and odors that induce nausea, and provide IV fluid replacement). The same nursing diagnosis with a different related factor, such as *Deficient Fluid Volume related to elevated body temperature,* requires different interventions (e.g., administer antipyretics and provide oral fluids).

Possible nursing diagnoses for patients with fluid, electrolyte, and acid-base alterations include:

- *Decreased Cardiac Output*
- *Acute Confusion*
- *Risk for Electrolyte Imbalance*
- *Deficient Fluid Volume*
- *Excess Fluid Volume*
- *Risk for Imbalanced Fluid Volume*
- *Impaired Gas Exchange*
- *Risk for Injury*
- *Deficient Knowledge (regarding disease management)*
- *Impaired Oral Mucous Membrane*
- *Ineffective Peripheral Tissue Perfusion*

PLANNING

Goals and Outcomes. During the planning phase collaborate with each patient to establish goals and expected outcomes for each nursing diagnosis (see Care Plan). Make sure that goals are individualized and realistic with measurable outcomes. *In the nursing care plan Robert sets goals for improving Mrs. Reynolds' fluid status. Later Robert determines if these goals are met (e.g., by monitoring the outcome of focused assessments and I&O). Each goal and outcome needs a time frame for achievement. For Mrs. Reynolds this time frame is for her goals to be met before hospital discharge.*

In the acute care setting a long-term goal is to anticipate the needs of a patient and family to ease the transition to home or long-term care. *For example, Mrs. Reynolds likely will be discharged home with new medications or recommendations for a diet that causes less GI upset.* When creating a patient care plan, remember to take into consideration the patient's personal preferences, knowledge and skills of the patient and any family caregiver, and available resources.

Setting Priorities. A patient's clinical condition determines which diagnosis takes the greatest priority. Many nursing diagnoses in the area of fluid, electrolyte, and acid-base balance are of highest priority because the consequences for the patient can be serious or even life threatening. *For example, in the concept map* (Figure 18-6) *Mrs. Reynolds has diarrhea, which has created ECV deficit. The nursing diagnosis Deficient Fluid Volume ranks highest priority, requiring intervention to stabilize her status and prevent further complications.* As a patient's status changes, the priority nursing diagnoses also change. For example, the priority nursing diagnosis changes to *Deficient Knowledge* once a patient is well enough to be discharged home. The priority at this time is to ensure that the patient returns safely to the home, which often requires extensive patient and family education (see Chapter 12).

Collaborative Care. Consult with a patient's health care provider to identify realistic time frames for the goals of care, particularly when a patient's physiological status is unstable. Planning care for a patient requires collaboration with other members of the health care team such as the dietitian or pharmacist. You cannot delegate administration of IV medications and/or oxygen therapy to the NAP. When a patient is stable, you can delegate daily weights, I&O measurement, and direct physical patient care. Establish a rapport of open communication and teamwork with NAP, as with any member of the interdisciplinary team, to ensure timely and effective administration of care.

Continuity of care is essential as a patient moves from one health care setting to another or to home. Therapeutic regimens established in one setting continue until completed in the next setting. For example, a patient who will continue to monitor I&O at home needs to know how to measure and document fluid I&O. When the patient's discharge has been ordered, it is important to identify which resources are available for him or her to promote positive outcomes. Dietitians are a valuable resource for recommending food sources to increase or reduce intake of specific electrolytes. Chapter 33 describes various therapeutic diets (e.g., low Na^+). Pharmacists can provide information about a patient's prescription and OTC medications that may cause electrolyte or acid-base imbalances. The health care provider directs the treatment of any fluid, electrolyte, or acid-base imbalance. Be sure that a patient who will be discharged has the resources for continuing therapeutic regimens to return to a state of optimal functioning. A case manager or social worker might be able to connect patients with those resources.

IMPLEMENTATION

Health Promotion. Health promotion activities focus primarily on patient education. Teach patients and their family caregivers how to recognize risk factors for development of imbalances and implement appropriate preventive measures. For example, parents of infants need to understand

CARE PLAN

Extracellular Fluid Volume Deficit

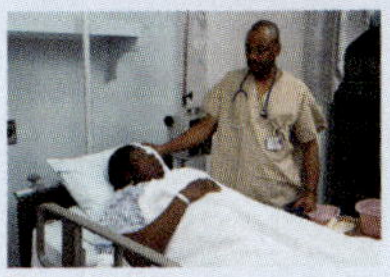

ASSESSMENT

Mrs. Susan Reynolds, a 42-year-old married accountant, was admitted yesterday to an acute care unit with a history of nausea, loss of appetite, and diarrhea for 7 days. After obtaining a blood sample for electrolyte levels, complete blood count, and an electrocardiogram (ECG), her health care provider admitted her for observation. Orders include intravenous (IV) infusion of 0.9% saline at 125 mL/hr, intake and output (I&O) recordings, vital signs every 4 hours, and daily weights.

ASSESSMENT ACTIVITIES	FINDINGS/DEFINING CHARACTERISTICS*
Ask Mrs. Reynolds to describe when her nausea began and which accompanying signs and symptoms she is experiencing.	Mrs. Reynolds states that she became nauseous after a business trip; has no appetite; is nauseous; and has had diarrhea for 7 days. She still is taking her furosemide (Lasix).
Assess vital signs.	Vital signs: temperature 99.6° F (37.6° C); **pulse, 100 beats/min** and regular; supine **blood pressure (BP), 105/60 mm Hg** with no changes when standing; respirations 18/min and nonlabored; lung sounds clear to auscultation bilaterally.
Assess abdomen and I&O.	Bowel sounds present and hyperactive in all four quadrants. Abdomen soft to palpation. Mrs. Reynolds reports less nausea since yesterday and only two loose stools since midnight. Twenty-four–hour intake was 1850 mL, with output of 2200 mL **(urine output accounted for only 1000 mL).** She voids without difficulty, with **dark yellow urine.**
Assess skin, mucous membranes, and daily weight for indicators of extracellular fluid volume (ECV) deficit.	Skin is **dry,** without discoloration, but **turgor is decreased.** Neck veins barely visible when supine. **Dry mucous membranes** between cheek and gum. Her **weight** of 143 lbs (65 kg) is **decreased 1 lb** (0.45 kg) since her admission yesterday.
Evaluate laboratory values and ECG results.	Laboratory result: hematocrit 44% (suggesting hypovolemia); serum K^+ 3.5 mEq/L (low normal because of diarrhea) and Na^+ 140 mEq/L. Electrocardiogram (ECG) showed normal sinus rhythm.

*__Defining characteristics__ are shown in **bold** type.

NURSING DIAGNOSIS: Deficient Fluid Volume related to increased fluid output from diarrhea and diuretic.

PLANNING

GOAL	EXPECTED OUTCOMES (NOC)†
	Fluid Balance
• Mrs. Reynolds' fluid volume will return to normal by time of discharge.	• Urine output equals intake of at least 1500 mL in 2 days. • Urine color becomes light yellow within 24 hours. • Heart rate and BP return to normal in 24 hours. • Mucous membranes are moist in 24 hours. • Skin turgor returns to normal within 24 hours. • Daily weights do not vary ± 2 lbs over next 2 days.
• Mrs. Reynolds will describe how to manage fluid balance at home before hospital discharge.	• Mrs. Reynolds describes how to replace diarrhea fluid loss with fluids that contain sodium. • She describes signs and symptoms that indicate the need to increase fluid and sodium intake.
	Electrolyte and Acid-Base Balance
• Mrs. Reynolds will achieve normal electrolyte balance by discharge.	• Serum electrolyte levels are within normal limits within 48 hours.
• Mrs. Reynolds will indicate plans to maintain a high dietary intake of potassium-rich foods at home.	• Mrs. Reynolds identifies potassium-rich foods that she enjoys and can access at home.

†Outcomes classification labels from Moorhead S, et al, editors: *Nursing outcomes classification (NOC),* ed 5, St Louis, 2013, Mosby.

Continued

CARE PLAN—cont'd

Extracellular Fluid Volume Deficit

INTERVENTIONS (NIC)[‡]	RATIONALE
Fluid and Electrolyte Management	
• Administer IV fluids (0.9% sodium chloride) at 125 mL/hr as prescribed.	Replacement of isotonic fluid restores blood volume; isotonic solutions expand ECV without causing fluid shift into cells.
• Provide patient with an additional 480 mL of her favorite noncaffeinated oral fluids at her preferred temperature during every 8 hours.	Patient-centered care takes individual preferences into account. Cultural preferences regarding temperature of oral fluid when ill influence fluid intake (Giger, 2013).
• Administer bismuth subsalicylate (Pepto-Bismol) as ordered for diarrhea.	Pepto-Bismol is an antidiarrheal that inhibits gastrointestinal secretions, stimulates absorption of fluid and electrolytes, and inhibits intestinal inflammation (Lehne, 2013).
• Maintain accurate intake and output (I&O) measurements.	Documents hydration and fluid balance for directing therapy.
• Weigh Mrs. Reynolds daily and monitor trends.	Daily weights provide an indication of fluid balance (Metheny, 2012).
• Teach Mrs. Reynolds and family about specific dietary modification (K^+-rich foods). Begin patient teaching regarding types of foods that are sources of K^+.	Hydrochlorothiazide is a K^+-wasting diuretic (Lehne, 2013). The body does not store K^+, thus requiring dietary intake rich in K^+.

[‡]Interventions classification label from Bulechek GM, et al, editors: *Nursing interventions classification (NIC),* ed 6, St Louis, 2013, Mosby.

EVALUATION

NURSING ACTIONS	PATIENT RESPONSE/FINDING	ACHIEVEMENT OF OUTCOME
Monitor electrolyte levels, daily weights, and I&O trends.	Serum electrolyte levels: K^+ 3.7 mEq/L and Na^+ 140 mEq/L; weight, 143 lbs (65 kg). Mrs. Reynolds' 24-hour intake is 2800 mL, and output is 2200 mL with 1800 mL urine. Urine is light yellow.	Electrolyte levels within normal range. Daily weight stable. Mrs. Reynolds' fluid balance is improving with urine output exceeding stool output.
Assess oral mucous membranes, neck vein fullness, skin turgor, heart rate, and blood pressure.	Mucous membranes remain dry. Neck veins full when supine. Skin turgor normal. Heart rate 80 beats/min, BP 126/78.	ECV is returning to normal.
Listen to lungs and inspect for edema during IV therapy with isotonic saline to detect overload.	Lungs are clear; no edema present.	No signs of ECV excess are present.
Evaluate effectiveness of teaching regarding maintaining fluid and electrolyte balance at home.	Mrs. Reynolds identifies Na^+-containing broth for replacing diarrhea fluid and K^+-rich foods she will eat to maintain electrolyte balance.	Mrs. Reynolds describes effective home management of fluid and electrolyte balance.

that GI losses lead quickly to serious fluid imbalances; therefore, when vomiting or diarrhea occurs, they should promptly begin rehydrating with Na^+-containing fluid. People of all ages need to learn to replace body fluid losses with Na^+-containing fluid and water (Box 18-4).

Patients with chronic health alterations need to understand their own risk factors and measures to take to avoid imbalances. For example, patients with end-stage renal disease often need to restrict intake of fluid, Na^+, K^+, Mg^{2+}, and phosphate. Patients with heart failure must limit their intake of liquids and high-sodium foods to prevent fluid retention. Through diet education these patients learn the types of foods to avoid and the daily volume of fluid they are permitted. Teach patients with chronic diseases and their family caregivers the early signs and symptoms of fluid, electrolyte, and acid-base imbalances for which they are at risk and what to do about them. For example, teach patients with heart failure to measure body weight each day at the same time and inform their health care provider of significant changes in weight from one day to another.

Acute Care. Although patients with fluid, electrolyte, and acid-base imbalances can be found in all health care settings, it is common to manage them in acute care settings. Acute care nurses conduct frequent and often complex monitoring (e.g., arterial blood gas measurement) and administer oral and IV fluids and medications to replace fluid and electrolyte deficits or maintain normal balance. They also manage parenteral nutrition (see Chapter 33) and patients' oxygenation needs (see Chapter 30).

Enteral Replacement of Fluids. Oral replacement of fluids and electrolytes is appropriate when a patient is physiologically stable enough for oral fluids to be replaced rapidly. Oral

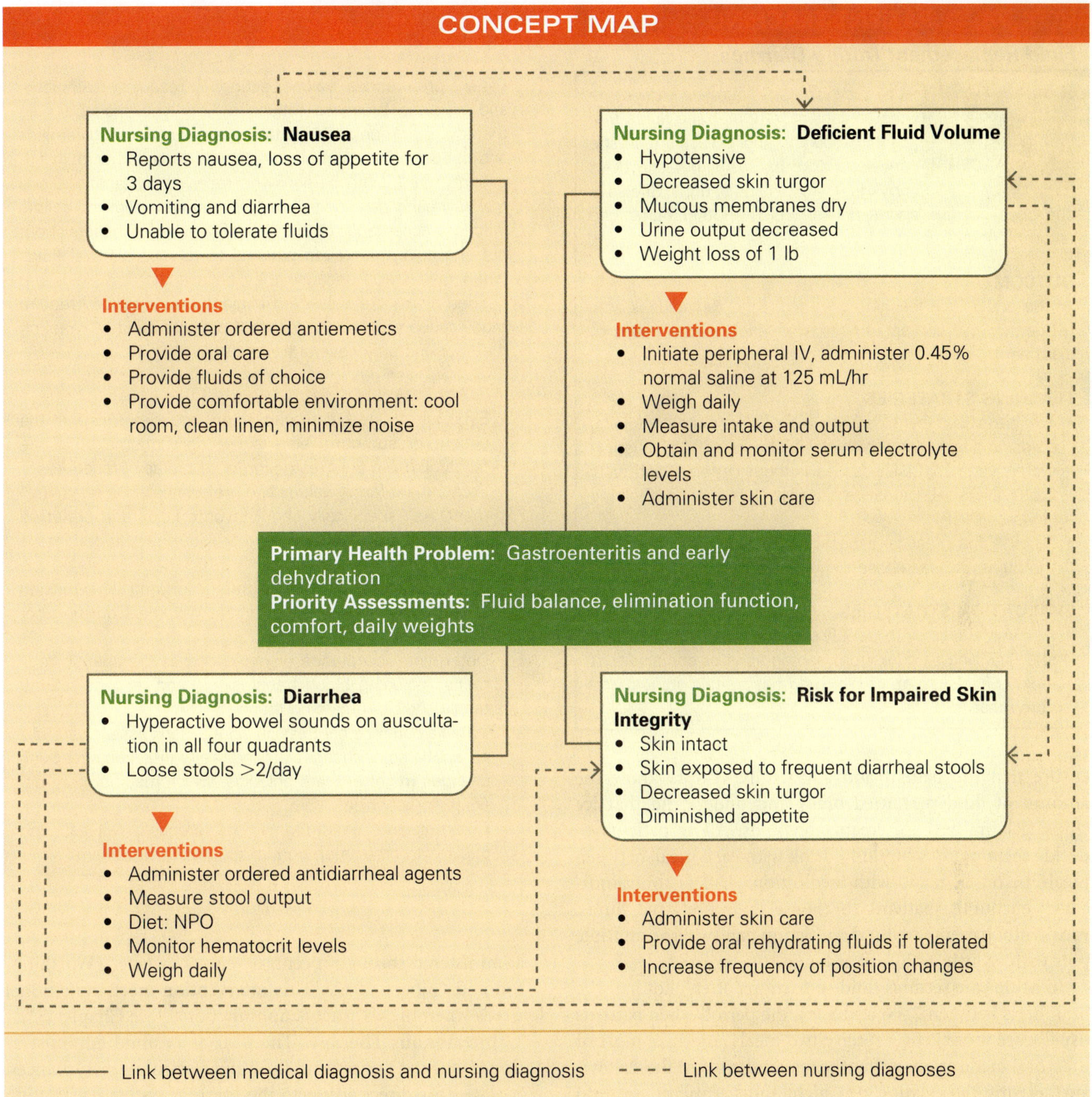

FIGURE 18-6 Concept map.

replacement is contraindicated when a patient has a mechanical obstruction of the GI tract, is at high risk for aspiration, or has impaired swallowing. Patients unable to tolerate solid foods may still be able to ingest fluids. Strategies to encourage fluid intake include offering small sips of fluid frequently, popsicles, and ice chips. If possible, provide each patient's preferred fluids at the preferred temperature (Box 18-5). Cultural beliefs regarding appropriate fluid temperature can interfere with fluid intake unless the preferred-temperature fluid is available (Giger, 2013).

When replacing fluids by mouth in a patient with ECV deficit, choose fluids that contain Na^+ (e.g., Pedialyte and Gastrolyte). Liquids containing lactose, caffeine, or low-Na^+ content are not appropriate when a patient has diarrhea. A feeding tube is used for fluid replacement when a patient's GI tract is healthy but the patient cannot ingest fluids (e.g., after oral surgery or with impaired swallowing) (see Chapter 33).

Restriction of Fluids. Patients who have hyponatremia usually require restricted water intake so their kidneys can resolve the imbalance. Patients who have very severe ECV excess may have both sodium and fluid restrictions. Fluid restriction is difficult for patients, particularly if they take medications that dry the oral mucous membranes or if they are mouth breathers. Explain why fluids are restricted and

BOX 18-4 PATIENT TEACHING

Fluid Replacement During Diarrhea

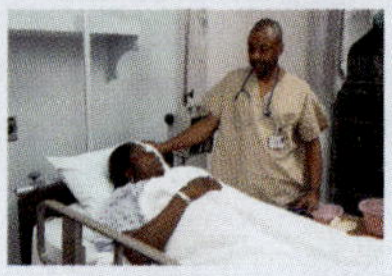

Mrs. Reynolds says that she knows she should drink more water and fluids that contain sodium and potassium if she develops diarrhea again, but she does not know which fluids to drink. She says she does not like sports drinks, which another nurse had recommended to her.

OUTCOME

At the end of the teaching sessions, Mrs. Reynolds is able to identify the appropriate fluids to drink in the event of diarrhea

TEACHING STRATEGIES

- Provide Mrs. Reynolds with a list of sodium-containing fluids and ask her which ones she is willing to drink: water, vegetable juice, sodas without caffeine, and salty broth (National Digestive Disease Information Clearing House, 2012)
- Discuss the practical aspects of obtaining and preparing the fluids she has chosen.

EVALUATION STRATEGIES

- Ask Mrs. Reynolds to identify sodium-containing fluids that she is willing to drink from photographs or containers of various fluids, some of which do not contain sodium and some that do.

ensure that the patient and any family visitors know the amount of fluid permitted orally and understand that ice chips, gelatin, and ice cream are fluids. Allow patients to decide the amount of fluid to drink with each meal, between meals, before bed, and with medications. Unless contraindicated, encourage patients to choose their preferred fluids. Frequently patients on fluid restriction can swallow multiple pills with as little as 30 mL of liquid.

In acute care settings fluid restrictions often allot half the oral fluids between 7 AM and 3 PM, the period when patients usually are more active, receive two meals, and take most of their oral medications. Offer the remainder of the fluid allowance during the evening and night shifts. Patients on fluid restriction need frequent mouth care to moisten mucous membranes, decrease mucosal drying and cracking, and maintain comfort (see Chapter 29).

Parenteral Replacement of Fluids and Electrolytes. Fluid and electrolytes may be replaced through infusion of fluids intravenously, meaning directly into veins. Parenteral replacement includes parenteral nutrition (PN), IV fluid and electrolyte therapy (crystalloids), and blood product (colloids) administration. Practice standard body fluid precautions (see Chapter 14) when administering parenteral fluids to minimize your own risk for exposure to bloodborne pathogens. Understand and follow the policy and procedures for parenteral infusions at each agency for which you work.

Parenteral Nutrition. PN is a nutritionally adequate solution consisting of glucose, other nutrients, and electrolytes

BOX 18-5 PATIENT-CENTERED CARE

FLUID THERAPY

Patient preferences, values, economic resources, ethnicity, and religious practices influence how you manage fluid therapy. Communication patterns may vary among families and cultures. For example, the family elder rather than the patient may be the person who receives explanations and makes health care decisions. Cultural and religious beliefs influence acceptance of therapies. For example, beliefs about hot and cold may cause patients to refuse cold oral fluids when they are ill because they believe that hot fluids are needed to restore balance. Religious practices may require modification of IV tubing length if patients need to kneel on the floor and pray several times daily.

IMPLICATIONS FOR PRACTICE

- Establish trusted communication and determine if the patient or someone else is the decision maker in the family. Explain fluid restriction or IV therapy procedures.
- Elicit patient/family values and preferences in your assessment. Ask specifically about favorite fluids and preferred temperature of oral fluids and provide them (if oral intake is allowed) (Giger, 2013).
- Incorporate one or more segments of long IV extension tubing into the IV setup if patient will kneel on the floor to pray.
- Determine acceptance or avoidance of therapeutic regimens, including blood transfusions, and respect patient/family choices regarding therapy.
- When a patient's natural skin color is dark, assess carefully for subtle color changes around the IV insertion site. Such changes might indicate phlebitis, which may be more difficult to recognize.
- Communicate patient/family preferences, values, and choices to other members of the health care team.

IV, Intravenous.

administered through a central venous catheter (Worthington and Gilbert, 2012). This intervention meets nutritional needs when the GI tract is nonfunctional (see Chapter 33).

Intravenous Therapy. The goal of IV fluid administration is to correct or prevent fluid and electrolyte disturbances. It allows for direct access to the vascular system, permitting continuous or intermittent infusion of fluids and medications. IV fluid therapy requires frequent monitoring to detect ongoing changes in a patient's fluid and electrolyte balance. To provide safe care to patients who require IV fluid administration, you need knowledge of the correct solution ordered, the reason it was ordered, the equipment needed, evidence-based procedures required to initiate an infusion, how to regulate the infusion rate and maintain the system, how to identify and correct problems, and how to discontinue the infusion. Whenever you care for a patient who requires IV therapy, it is imperative that you follow specific standards to decrease the incidence of infection related to the therapy (Box 18-6).

Vascular Access Devices. Vascular access devices (VADs) are catheters or infusion ports designed for repeated access

BOX 18-6 INS STANDARDS TO DECREASE INTRAVASCULAR INFECTION RELATED TO INTRAVENOUS THERAPY

- Palpate catheter insertion site for tenderness daily through the intact dressing.
- Directly inspect a catheter site if patient develops tenderness at site, fever without obvious source, or symptoms of local or bloodstream infection.
- Perform hand hygiene before and after palpating, inserting, replacing, or dressing any intravascular device.
- Clean skin site vigorously before venipuncture with an appropriate single-use antiseptic solution.
- Allow site to air-dry before proceeding with procedure: 2% chlorhexidine for 30 seconds, povidone-iodine for at least 2 minutes.
- Do not palpate insertion site after skin has been cleaned with single-use antiseptic solution.
- Use a catheter stabilization device that allows visual inspection of access site.
- Change gauze dressings that cover a catheter site every 48 hours.
- Leave transparent dressings in place until the IV tubing is replaced (INS, 2011).
- IV tubing administration sets can remain sterile for 96 hours.
- Replace dressing over peripheral venous catheters when replacing catheter or when dressing becomes damp, loosened, or soiled.
- Clean injection ports with single-use antiseptic solution before accessing system.
- Replace short peripheral catheters and rotate sites based on clinical assessment indicating signs or symptoms of IV-related complications.

Modified from Infusion Nurses Society: Infusion nursing standards of practice, *J Infus Nurs* 34(Suppl 1):S1, 2011.
INS, Infusion Nurses Society; *IV,* intravenous.

to the vascular system. Peripheral catheters are for short-term use (e.g., to restore fluid volume). Devices for long-term use include central lines, peripherally inserted central catheters (PICCs), and implanted ports. These devices are more effective than peripheral catheters for administering PN and medications and solutions that are irritating to veins. Nurses need specialized education in the care of these central devices to provide safe care (Segreti et al., 2011).

Types of Solutions. Many prepared IV solutions are available for use. An IV solution is isotonic, hypotonic, or hypertonic. Solutions that contain glucose have a greater tonicity in the IV container than their effective concentration in the body because the glucose enters cells rapidly; thus the rest of the infused fluid determines the effective physiological concentration (Table 18-8). Sodium-containing isotonic solutions are used for ECV replacement (e.g., ECV deficit after prolonged vomiting). A health care provider bases the decision to use a physiologically hypotonic or hypertonic solution on a patient's specific fluid and electrolyte imbalance. For example, a patient with hypernatremia that cannot be treated with oral water generally receives a hypotonic solution to dilute the ECF and rehydrate the cells. Administer all IV fluids carefully because too-rapid or excessive infusion of any IV fluid can cause serious patient problems.

Additives such as potassium chloride (KCl) are common in IV solutions. An IV therapy order includes the IV solution and any additives plus the volume and prescribed infusion time or rate. Usually a pharmacist prepares the solution. An example of an order follows:

> Infusion No. 1: 1000 mL D_5½ NS with 20 mEq KCl and 1 ampule of multivitamins at 125 mL/hr

Patients with normal renal function who do not have oral intake need to have potassium added to IV solutions. The body does not store potassium; and, even when plasma levels fall, the kidneys continue to excrete potassium. Hypokalemia develops quickly without potassium intake. Remember that failure to verify that a patient has adequate renal function and urine output before administering an IV solution containing potassium could cause hyperkalemia. *Under no circumstances should you give KCl by IV push (directly through a port in IV tubing). A direct IV infusion of KCl is fatal. IV administration of KCl requires dilution in solution and infusion over a period of time.*

Equipment. Correct selection and preparation of IV equipment ensures safe and quick placement of an IV line. Because fluids infuse directly into the bloodstream, sterile technique is necessary. Organize all equipment at the bedside for efficient insertion. IV equipment includes VADs, tourniquet, clean gloves, dressings, IV fluid containers, various types of tubing, and **electronic infusion devices (EIDs),** also called *IV pumps.* Peripheral IV catheters are available in a variety of gauges (e.g., 20 gauge, 22 gauge). A larger gauge indicates a smaller-diameter catheter.

You use different types of infusion tubing to administer medications or IV fluids. EIDs are commonly used in acute and critical care settings and in some care settings outside of hospitals to ensure a constant, regulated rate. Use the tubing that is designated for the particular EID that you are using, typically a macrodrip tubing. Macrodrip tubing delivers large drops (standard drop size is 10 or 15 gtt/mL depending on the manufacturer). In contrast, microdrip tubing provides a standard drop size of 60 gtt/mL, which facilitates precise regulation of IV fluids at slow rates. Add IV extension tubing to increase patient mobility and decrease manipulation and potential contamination of the insertion site.

Initiating Peripheral Intravenous Access. After organizing collected equipment at the bedside, prepare to insert the IV catheter by assessing the patient for a venipuncture site. The most common IV sites are on the inner arm (Figure 18-7). You may insert an IV in a foot vein in children, but avoid this site in adults because of the danger of thrombophlebitis (INS, 2011). When assessing patients for potential venipuncture sites, consider conditions that exclude certain sites. For example, because older adults and patients receiving corticosteroids have fragile veins, avoid sites that are easily

TABLE 18-8 INTRAVENOUS SOLUTIONS

SOLUTION	CONCENTRATION IN THE IV CONTAINER AND AT TIP OF VAD	EFFECTIVE CONCENTRATION IN THE BODY	COMMENTS
Dextrose (Glucose) in Water Solutions			
Dextrose 5% in water (D_5W)	Isotonic	Hypotonic	Isotonic when first enters vein; dextrose enters cells rapidly, leaving free water, which dilutes ECF; most of the water then enters cells by osmosis.
Dextrose 10% in water ($D_{10}W$)	Hypertonic	Hypotonic	Hypertonic when first enters vein; dextrose enters cells rapidly, leaving free water, which dilutes ECF; most of the water then enters cells by osmosis.
Saline (NaCl in Water) Solutions			
0.45% Sodium chloride (half NS; ½NS)	Hypotonic	Hypotonic	Expands ECV (vascular and interstitial) and rehydrates cells.
0.9% Sodium chloride (NS; 0.9% NaCl)	Isotonic	Isotonic	Expands ECV (vascular and interstitial); does not enter cells.
3% or 5% Sodium chloride (hypertonic saline; 3% or 5% NaCl)	Hypertonic	Hypertonic	Draws water from cells into ECF by osmosis.
Dextrose in Saline Solutions			
Dextrose 5% in 0.45% sodium chloride (D_5½NS; $D_5$0.45% NaCl)	Hypertonic	Hypotonic	Dextrose enters cells rapidly, leaving 0.45% NaCl.
Dextrose 5% in 0.9% sodium chloride (D_5NS; $D_5$0.9% NaCl)	Hypertonic	Isotonic	Dextrose enters cells rapidly, leaving 0.9% NaCl.
Multiple Electrolyte Solutions			
Lactated Ringer's (LR) solution	Isotonic	Isotonic	LR contains Na^+, K^+, Ca^{2+}, Cl^-, and lactate, which the liver metabolizes to HCO_3^-; expands ECV (vascular and interstitial); does not enter cells.
Dextrose 5% in LR (D_5LR)	Hypertonic	Isotonic	Dextrose enters cells rapidly, leaving LR.

ECF, Extracellular fluid; *ECV,* extracellular fluid volume; *IV,* intravenous; *NS,* normal saline; *VAD,* vascular access device.

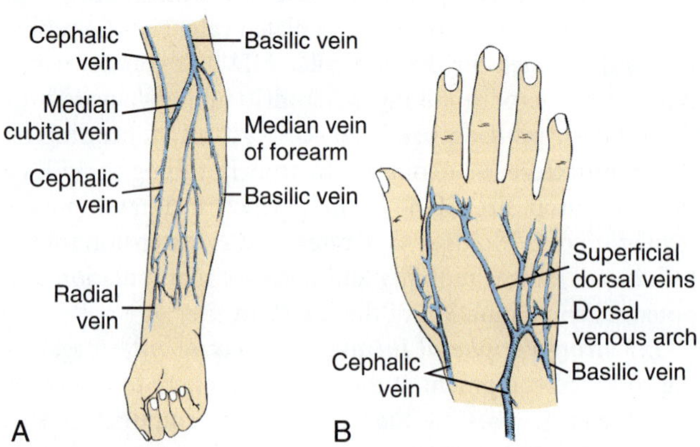

FIGURE 18-7 Common IV sites. **A,** Inner arm. **B,** Dorsal surface of hand.

bumped or moved such as the dorsal surface of the hand (Box 18-7).

Venipuncture is contraindicated in a site that has signs of inflammation, infiltration, or thrombosis. An infected site is red, tender, swollen, and possibly warm to the touch. Avoid using an extremity with a vascular (dialysis) graft or fistula or on the same side as a mastectomy (breast surgery). Initially place IV catheters at the most distal point, which allows for the use of proximal sites later if the patient needs a venipuncture site change (INS, 2011).

Venipuncture is the technique for accessing a vein by puncture through the skin using a sharp rigid stylet (e.g., metal needle). To collect a blood specimen, the needle has an attached syringe or collection tube. To start an IV infusion you use a stylet partially covered with a plastic catheter (over-the-needle catheter [ONC]). You use aseptic technique to prepare the skin. Only experienced practitioners perform venipuncture on patients with fragile veins (e.g., infants or older persons).

BOX 18-7 CARE OF THE OLDER ADULT

Protection of Skin and Veins During Intravenous Therapy

- Avoid using a tourniquet when selecting a vein. Position the arm in a dependent position to fill the veins sufficiently for a venipuncture or use a blood pressure cuff for better protection of older-adult skin. If using a tourniquet, place it over the patient's sleeve (Miller, 2012).
- Use the smallest-gauge IV catheter or needle possible such as 22 or 24 gauge to protect fragile veins. A smaller gauge allows better blood flow to provide increased hemodilution of the IV fluids or medications (Fabian, 2010).
- Avoid placing IV in veins that are easily bumped because older adults have less subcutaneous support tissue.
- Avoid the back of the hand, which may compromise a patient's need for independence and mobility.
- Use strict aseptic technique because an older adult patient is more likely to be immunocompromised.
- Do not slap the arm to visualize the patient's veins or use vigorous friction while cleansing the site to prevent tearing fragile skin.
- Decrease venipuncture insertion angle to 10 to 15 degrees after penetrating skin because of decreased supportive tissue (Fabian, 2010).
- Veins roll away from the needle easily as a result of loss of subcutaneous tissue. To stabilize the vein, apply traction to the skin below the projected insertion site (Fabian, 2010).
- Secure IV site with a catheter stabilization device and a mesh dressing for protection, avoiding excessive use of tape on fragile skin (Fabian, 2010).
- Use electronic infusion devices or controllers to titrate infusion volume and rate.

IV, Intravenous.

BOX 18-8 EVIDENCE-BASED PRACTICE

PICO Question: Does the use of nurses trained using a standard protocol for IV insertion reduce the number of ineffective peripheral IV insertion attempts for adult hospitalized patients compared with nurses trained in absence of a protocol in IV competencies?

SUMMARY OF EVIDENCE

Nurses who start IV lines need the knowledge and skills to apply the *Infusion Nursing Standards of Practice* (INS, 2011). Ineffective IV insertion attempts cause patient distress and increase the risk of infection. Many practicing nurses indicate lack of confidence in their IV insertion skills (Lyons and Kasker, 2012). Experts recommend using an education needs survey for infusion therapy to match nurses' perceived needs with continuing education to meet infusion competencies (Czaplewski, 2010). Hospital nurses who have specific continuing nursing education in IV insertions using simulation models make fewer ineffective IV insertion attempts than nurses who have continuing education using a "see one, do one, teach one" approach (Wilfong et al., 2011). Creating an IV team of skilled nurses on four admission units and implementing a standard procedure for IV insertion reduced the number of ineffective IV insertion attempts and also the occurrence of phlebitis (da Silva, Priebe, and Dias, 2010).

APPLICATION TO NURSING PRACTICE

- Request continuing nursing education in IV insertion competency.
- Follow a standard protocol for IV insertion to reduce ineffective IV insertion attempts (Czaplewski, 2010; da Silva et al., 2010).
- Use an education needs survey for infusion therapy to plan continuing education for staff nurses (Czaplewski, 2010).
- Provide competency-based continuing education using simulation models for staff nurses (Wilfong et al., 2011).

IV, Intravenous.

General purposes of venipuncture are to collect a blood specimen, start an IV fluid infusion, instill a medication, or inject a tracer for diagnostic examinations. Use intermittent infusion when a patient requires medications only at certain times, in an emergency situation, and to avoid the discomfort of repeated injections. An intermittent infusion involves the same techniques as a continuous IV drip, but after you give the complete dose of medication, you disconnect the tubing from the IV access device. A continuous infusion of fluids, with or without medications, is achieved over a 24-hour period through use of a VAD. Skill 18-1 describes the technique for initiating peripheral IV fluid infusion and incorporates INS standards of practice (INS, 2011) (Box 18-8).

Regulating the Infusion Flow Rate. After initiating an IV infusion and checking it for patency, regulate the rate of infusion according to the health care provider's orders (see Skill 18-2). An infusion rate that is too slow fails to reverse cardiovascular and circulatory collapse in a critically ill patient who is in shock or dehydrated. An infusion rate that is too rapid can cause fluid and electrolyte overload.

Calculate IV infusion rates to maintain a consistent flow at the ordered rate (e.g., 125 mL/hr). EIDs deliver an accurate hourly IV infusion rate. Familiarize yourself with the brand of EID in use at your institution so you can set the flow rate accurately. Safeguards are in place for EIDs to prevent free flow of infusion and sudden volume infusion when regulators are removed from the tubing housing. However, if you open a clamp on an infusion tubing that is not yet properly inserted in an EID or gravity-flow IV system, the IV fluid may infuse very rapidly. Nonelectronic volume-control devices are used occasionally above an EID to prevent accidental infusion of a large fluid volume, especially in pediatrics. These devices hold small amounts of fluid and hang between the IV fluid container and the EID. They also may be used with gravity-flow infusions. The rate of infusion with an IV gravity controller depends on the height of the IV fluid container, IV tubing size, and fluid viscosity. Regardless of the device in use, monitor the patient regularly to verify correct infusion of IV fluid and detect complications.

Patency of an IV catheter means that fluid flows easily through it. To be patent, the catheter tip needs to be free from clots and be away from the vein wall. A blocked catheter slows

TABLE 18-9 INFUSION NURSES SOCIETY PHLEBITIS SCALE

GRADE	CLINICAL CRITERIA
0	No symptoms
1	Erythema at access site with or without pain
2	Pain at access site with erythema and/or edema
3	Pain at access site with erythema, streak formation, palpable venous cord
4	Pain at access site with erythema, streak formation, palpable venous cord >2.5 cm (1 inch) in length, purulent drainage

From Infusion Nurses Society: Infusion nursing standards of practice, *J Infus Nurs* 34(Suppl 1):S1, 2011.

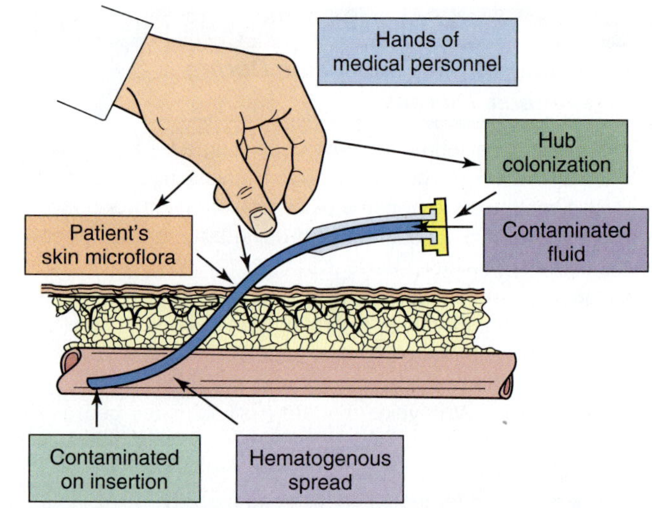

FIGURE 18-8 Potential sites for contamination of an intravascular device.

or stops the infusion of IV fluids. Infiltration (fluid leaking into tissues), a knot or kink in the tubing, external pressure on the tubing, and patient position changes decrease IV flow rates. If the IV flow decreases or stops, perform an assessment of the system until you locate the problem. Start the assessment at the catheter insertion site for signs and symptoms of infiltration and phlebitis (Table 18-9). The clinical presentation of infiltration is easily confused with phlebitis or irritant reactions (INS, 2011). Systematically continue your assessment by inspecting the area around the insertion site and the tubing for anything blocking the flow of IV fluids, such as a patient lying or sitting on the tubing. Frequently the flow rate resumes after you remove the tubing obstruction. Check for proper function of the EID. For gravity-flow systems the height of an IV container affects flow rates. Raising the container usually increases the rate because of increased driving pressure.

Flexion of an extremity, particularly at the wrist or elbow, often decreases the IV flow rate by pushing the tip of the catheter against the vein wall or compressing the vein. Although VAD placement in areas of flexion is discouraged, occasionally it becomes necessary. In that case INS standards specify use of an arm board or other joint stabilization device to protect the IV site by keeping the joint extended (INS, 2011). Use padding with arm boards because of the increased risk for skin or nerve damage from pressure. Sometimes it is more comfortable for a patient to have an infusion started in a new location rather than relying on a site that causes problems. Before discontinuing the current infusion, choose another site and start the infusion to verify that the patient has other accessible veins.

Maintaining the System. You must maintain an IV system once a catheter is in place and the flow rate is regulated. Agency policies regulate the maintenance of IV lines. IV line maintenance includes (1) keeping the system sterile and intact; (2) changing IV fluid containers, tubing, and contaminated site dressings; (3) assisting a patient with self-care activities (e.g., bathing) so the IV system is not disrupted; and (4) monitoring for complications of IV therapy.

Patient safety requires maintaining the integrity of an IV line to prevent infection (Hadaway, 2012). Figure 18-8 shows potential sites for contamination of a VAD. The procedure for IV insertion minimizes contamination during catheter insertion. After insertion prevent infection through conscientious use of infection control principles, including thorough hand hygiene before and after handling any part of the IV system and maintaining sterility of the system during tubing and fluid container changes.

Always maintain the integrity of an IV system. Never disconnect tubing because it becomes tangled or because it is more convenient to position or move a patient or apply a gown. If a patient needs more room to maneuver, add extension tubing to an IV line using aseptic technique. *Never let IV tubing touch the floor.* Avoid stopcocks for connecting multiple solutions to a single IV site because they are sources of contamination (INS, 2011). IV tubing contains injection ports through which you can insert syringes or other adapters for medication administration. Clean an injection port thoroughly with 2% chlorhexidine (preferred), 70% alcohol, or povidone-iodine and let it dry before accessing the system (INS, 2011).

Changing IV Fluid Containers, Tubing, and Dressings. Patients receiving IV therapy over several days require periodic changing of IV fluid containers. Organize your tasks so you can change solutions before a clot forms in the catheter. Recommended frequency of IV tubing change depends on whether it is used for continuous or intermittent infusion. INS standards (INS, 2011) specify that *continuous* infusion tubing changes should occur *no more frequently than every 96 hours* unless the tubing has been compromised or contaminated, which requires immediate tubing change. In contrast, you should change tubing for *intermittent* infusion every 24 hours because of the increased risk of contamination from opening the IV system (INS, 2011). Blood products and lipids easily promote bacterial growth in tubing. Thus you change tubing containing blood products every 4 hours, and tubing for continuous IV lipids every 24 hours (INS, 2011). Whenever possible, schedule tubing changes when it is time to hang a new IV container to decrease risk of infection (INS, 2011) (see Skill 18-3). To prevent entry of microorganisms into the bloodstream, maintain sterility during tubing and IV fluid container changes (INS, 2011).

A sterile dressing over an IV site reduces the entrance of bacteria into the insertion site. Transparent dressings, the most common type, help secure the VAD, allow continuous visual inspection of the IV site, and stay cleaner and drier than gauze dressings. Leave transparent dressings in place until the IV tubing is replaced (INS, 2011). If a gauze dressing is used, change it every 48 hours (INS, 2011). You change either form of dressing when the IV device is removed or when the dressing becomes damp, loosened, or soiled (INS, 2011) (see Skill 18-4). Agency policy may require routine dressing changes in different time frames.

Helping Patients Protect IV Integrity. To prevent accidental disruption of an IV system, patients often need assistance with hygiene, comfort measures, meals, and ambulation. Bathing and changing gowns are difficult for a patient with an IV line in the arm. Teach NAP and patients that they must not break the integrity of an IV line because this leads to contamination. If available, use a gown with snaps along the top sleeve seam to facilitate gown changes without disturbing the venipuncture site. Change regular gowns by following these steps:

1. To remove a gown, remove the sleeve of the gown from the arm without the IV line, maintaining the patient's privacy.
2. Remove the sleeve of the gown from the arm with the IV line.
3. Remove the IV solution container from its stand and pass it and the tubing through the sleeve. If this involves removing the tubing from an EID, use the roller clamp to slow the infusion to prevent accidental infusion of a large volume of fluid.
4. To apply a gown, place the IV solution container and tubing through the sleeve of the clean gown and hang it back on the stand. If the IV infusion is controlled by an EID, reassemble, turn on the pump, and open the roller clamp.
5. Place the arm with the IV line through the new gown sleeve.
6. Place the arm without the IV line through the new gown sleeve.

Mechanical catheter securement devices extend the time that a VAD can be used. Commercial protective devices also prevent accidental dislodgment of an IV catheter (Figure 18-9).

A patient with an arm or a hand infusion is able to walk unless contraindicated. Offer a rolling IV pole on wheels. See that the patient has help to get out of bed, if needed, and place the pole next to the involved arm. Teach the patient to hold on to the pole with the involved hand and push it while walking. Check that the IV container is at the proper height, there is no tension on the tubing, and the flow rate is correct.

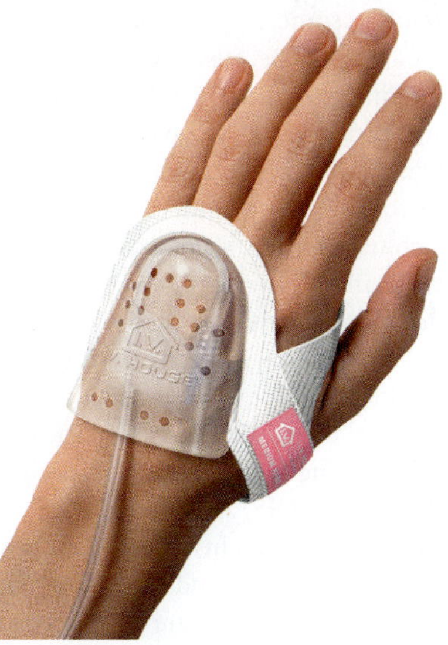

FIGURE 18-9 I.V. House protective device. (Courtesy I.V. House, St Louis, MO.)

Instruct the patient to report any blood in the tubing, stoppage in flow, an EID alarm, or increased discomfort.

Complications of Intravenous Therapy. An **infiltration** occurs when IV fluids leak into the subcutaneous tissue around the venipuncture site because the catheter tip no longer is in the vein. Infiltration causes swelling (from increased interstitial fluid), paleness, and coolness (from decreased circulation) around the venipuncture site. The IV infusion may slow or stop. Pain may occur, increasing as the infiltration progresses. The INS recommends using an infiltration scale for assessment (INS, 2011).

If infiltration occurs, discontinue the infusion and remove the VAD unless the solution contained a tissue-damaging solution that needs an antidote. If IV therapy still is necessary, insert a new VAD in a vein at a new location. To reduce discomfort elevate the extremity to promote venous drainage and decrease edema. Apply a warm, moist compress to the site for 20 minutes 3 to 4 times during the day to promote venous return and reduce pain and edema.

Certain IV medications, especially potassium and some antibiotics, cause discomfort and burning sensations at the IV site. Evaluate the source of discomfort, decrease the infusion rate if allowed, or start a new IV line in a larger vein if needed.

Phlebitis is inflammation of a vein. Risk factors include acidic or hypertonic IV solutions; rapid IV rate; irritating IV drugs such as KCl and vancomycin; VAD in area of flexion; poorly secured catheter; poor hand hygiene; and lack of aseptic technique (Roszell and Jones, 2010). Signs and symptoms include redness, tenderness, and warmth along the course of the vein starting at the access site, with possibly a red streak and/or palpable cord along the vein (INS, 2011). The INS Phlebitis Scale (see Table 18-9) is easy to use, valid, and reliable (Groll et al., 2010).

If phlebitis develops, discontinue the IV line and insert a new line in another vein. Warm, moist compresses on the site of phlebitis offer some relief to patients (see Chapter 36). Phlebitis is dangerous because blood clots (thrombophlebitis) can form, increasing the risk for an embolus (i.e., a clot that becomes dislodged and travels to the lungs). Phlebitis sometimes damages veins permanently. Although some agencies require routine removal of VADs and site rotation to prevent phlebitis, the INS Standards of Practice (2011) recommend replacing a peripheral VAD only if clinically indicated in adults (Webster et al., 2010). Assess the VAD site at least every 4 hours and more frequently with critically ill patients, children, and patients receiving IV solutions containing irritating drugs or vasoconstrictors (Gorski et al., 2012). Avoid routine replacement of peripheral VADs in infants and children (INS, 2011).

Local infection at a VAD insertion site is possible, showing redness and/or edema and exudate. Before removing a VAD, immediately notify the health care provider to find out if you need to send the exudate of the catheter tip for a culture. After you take the culture sample, remove the VAD and insert a new one in another site if continued IV therapy is necessary. If the health care provider orders antibiotics, do not start them until a blood culture is taken if ordered.

Another complication of IV therapy is overload of the IV fluid from a too-rapid infusion. Assessment findings depend on the type of solution. Overinfusion of a sodium-containing isotonic solution causes ECV excess, with shortness of breath and crackles in the lungs. If these clinical signs are present, slow the rate of IV infusion, notify the health care provider, raise the head of the bed, provide supplemental oxygen and diuretics as ordered, and monitor the patient's vital signs. Overinfusion of D_5W causes hyponatremia with confusion, lethargy, and possibly seizures. Whenever your patient has an IV running, monitor for the effects of overload of that particular IV fluid.

Discontinuing Peripheral Intravenous Access. Discontinuing a VAD is necessary after the prescribed amount of fluid is infused, when infiltration occurs, if phlebitis is present, or if a clot develops in the catheter. Review the health care provider's order before discontinuing a VAD. Explain to patients the reason for discontinuing the IV infusion and that they might feel a burning sensation when the catheter is removed. Perform hand hygiene and apply clean gloves. Prevent spillage of fluid by turning off the EID and closing the roller clamp or, if no EID, close the IV tubing roller clamp that controls the rate. Remove the IV site dressing and any manufactured catheter stabilization device. Then remove any tape securing the catheter without using scissors (INS, 2011). Remove secretions around the skin puncture site by holding the catheter hub and using antiseptic swab. Allow skin to dry completely. Place sterile gauze over the venipuncture site and apply light pressure while withdrawing the catheter by pulling away from the insertion site in a slow, steady motion (Figure 18-10). Keep the catheter hub parallel to the skin during withdrawal. Inspect the catheter end for intactness after removal. Keep gauze in place and apply continuous pressure to the site for 2 to 3 minutes to control bleeding and minimize hematoma formation (INS, 2011). If a patient receives anticoagulants or platelet inhibitors, apply steady pressure for 5 to 10 minutes and assess bleeding. Apply a sterile folded gauze dressing over the removal site and secure it with tape. Record the amount of fluid infused and the time the IV infusion was discontinued. Routinely inspect the site for redness, edema, and tenderness for 48 hours. In some settings LPNs discontinue peripheral IV infusions (consult agency policy or state Nurse Practice Act).

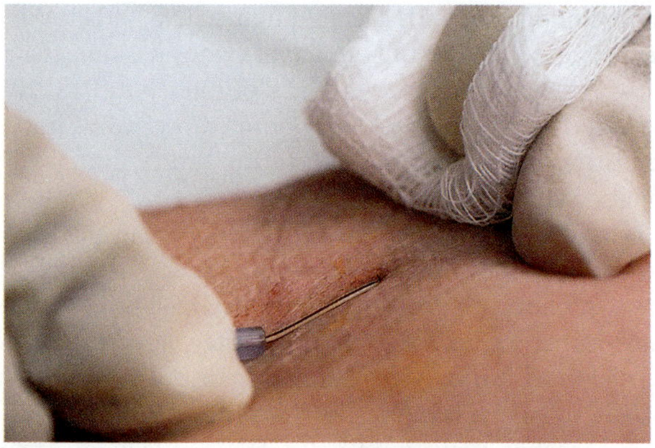

FIGURE 18-10 Withdraw IV catheter slowly, keeping catheter parallel to vein.

Blood Replacement. Blood replacement or transfusion is the IV administration of whole blood or a blood component such as plasma, packed red blood cells (RBCs), or platelets. Objectives for blood transfusions include (1) increasing circulating blood volume after surgery, trauma, or hemorrhage; (2) increasing the number of RBCs to maintain hemoglobin levels in patients with severe anemia; and (3) providing selected cellular components as replacement therapy (e.g., clotting factors, platelets, albumin).

Transfusing blood or blood components is a nursing procedure requiring an order from a health care provider. Perform thorough patient assessment before, during, and after a transfusion. Adverse blood transfusion events are National Quality Forum patient safety measures that are included in the public reporting of safety events of a health care institution (NQF, 2010). Before a transfusion assess the patient to determine if he or she knows the reason for the blood transfusion and whether he or she has had a previous transfusion or transfusion reaction. Patients who have had a transfusion reaction usually are not at greater risk for a reaction with a subsequent transfusion. However, they usually are anxious about the transfusion, requiring nursing intervention. Before starting a transfusion explain the procedure and instruct the patient to report any side effects (e.g., chills, lightheadedness, or fever) once transfusion begins. Ensure that the patient or representative has signed an informed consent. People from certain cultural backgrounds may refuse blood transfusions or seek alternatives to it (Tolich, 2008; Whyte, 2008). Be sensitive to patient preferences.

Because of the danger of transfusion reactions, your pretransfusion assessment includes baseline vital signs. These data allow you to determine when changes in vital signs occur

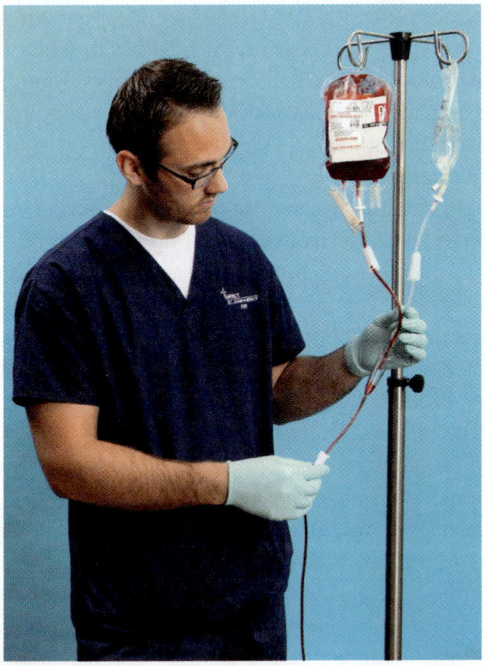

FIGURE 18-11 Filling tubing for blood administration.

as a result of a transfusion reaction. ABO incompatibility is a serious error with transfusions. It commonly involves misidentification of the patient, unit of blood, or label on the pretransfusion blood sample. For patient safety follow agency procedure to verify three things: that blood components delivered are the ones that were ordered; that blood delivered is compatible with the patient's blood type listed in the medical record; and that the right patient receives the blood. Many hospitals use bar-code technology to identify patients and verify compatible blood before beginning transfusions. Nurses are responsible for determining that the blood delivered to a patient corresponds to the patient's blood type documented in the medical record. Together two registered nurses (RNs) or one RN and a licensed practical nurse (LPN) (check agency policy and procedures) must check the label on the blood product against the medical record and the patient's identification number, blood group, and complete name (Clark, 2011). *If even a minor discrepancy exists, do not give the blood. Notify the blood bank immediately.*

When administering a transfusion, you need an appropriately sized IV catheter and special tubing with a 20-μm in-line filter (Figure 18-11). Adults require a large catheter such as 18 or 20 gauge because blood is more viscous than crystalloid IV fluids. Prime the tubing with 0.9% sodium chloride to reduce **hemolysis** (breakdown of RBCs). Initiate a transfusion slowly to allow for early detection of a transfusion reaction. Maintain the ordered infusion rate, monitor for side effects, assess vital signs, and promptly record all findings. Stay with the patient during the first 15 minutes, the time when a reaction is most likely to occur. After that time period continue to monitor the patient and obtain vital signs periodically during the transfusion as directed by agency policy.

BOX 18-9 NURSING INTERVENTIONS FOR BLOOD TRANSFUSION REACTION

1. *STOP the transfusion immediately,* even when you just suspect a reaction.
2. Remove blood component and tubing containing blood product. Replace them with new primed tubing with a container of 0.9% sodium chloride (normal saline). Connect tubing to hub of IV catheter.
3. **Caution:** Do not turn off the blood and simply turn on the 0.9% sodium chloride (normal saline) that is connected to the Y-tubing infusion set. This would cause blood remaining in the Y-tubing to infuse into the patient. Even a small amount of mismatched blood can cause a major reaction.
4. Maintain patent IV line using 0.9% normal saline.
5. Remain with the patient, observing signs and symptoms and monitoring vital signs as often as every 5 minutes.
6. Immediately notify the health care provider or emergency response team.
7. Notify blood bank.
8. Prepare to perform CPR and administer emergency drugs such as antihistamines, vasopressors, fluids, and corticosteroids per health care provider's order or protocol.
9. Save the blood container, tubing, attached labels, and transfusion record for return to the blood bank.
10. Obtain blood and first voided urine specimens per health care provider's order or protocol. **Note:** If patient is unable to void, insert a catheter to obtain this urine specimen.
11. Document the transfusion reaction, description, treatment, and outcome.

CPR, Cardiopulmonary resuscitation; *IV,* intravenous.

If you suspect a transfusion reaction, *STOP* the transfusion immediately and follow the guidelines in Box 18-9.

The transfusion rate usually is specified in the health care provider's orders. Ideally a unit of whole blood or packed RBCs is transfused in 2 hours. You lengthen the time to 4 hours if a patient is at risk for ECV excess. Beyond 4 hours there is an increased risk for bacterial contamination of the blood.

When patients have a severe blood loss such as with hemorrhage, they often receive rapid transfusions through a central venous catheter. A blood-warming device is necessary because the tip of the central venous catheter lies in the superior vena cava, above the right atrium. Rapid administration of cold blood can cause cardiac dysrhythmias. Patients who receive large-volume transfusion of citrated blood have high risk of hyperkalemia, hypocalcemia, hypomagnesemia, and metabolic alkalosis.

Autologous Transfusion. **Autologous transfusion** (autotransfusion) is the collection and reinfusion of a patient's own blood. Blood for an autologous transfusion usually is obtained by preoperative donation up to 6 weeks before the scheduled surgery, depending on the type of surgery and ability of the patient to maintain an acceptable hematocrit. Blood for autologous transfusion also can be obtained at the time of surgery by normovolemic hemodilution or through blood salvage. After surgery blood can be salvaged from drainage from chest tubes or joint cavities. Autologous transfusions are safer for patients because they decrease the risk of mismatched blood and exposure to bloodborne infectious agents (Trick, 2010).

Allogeneic Transfusion. Infusion of a donor's blood into a patient is **allogeneic transfusion.** In the United States the blood is collected in a donation center and goes through numerous tests to ensure that it is free from infectious agents such as human immunodeficiency virus (HIV) and hepatitis B (HBV) and C (HCV) viruses before it is infused. Blood testing positive for infectious agents is discarded; the donor is notified and placed on a list (deferral registry) that prohibits the donor from donating blood again (AABB, 2013).

ABO System. A blood transfusion must be matched to each patient to avoid dangerous incompatibility. Blood-typing systems are used to ensure a close match between transfused products and a patient's blood. The presence or absence of specific antigens on the surface of RBCs determines blood type in the ABO system. When the type A antigen is present, the blood group is type A. When the type B antigen is present, the blood group is type B. When both A and B antigens are present, the blood group is type AB; and, when neither A nor B antigens are present, the blood group is type O (Trick, 2010).

Antibodies that react against the A and B antigens naturally are present in the plasma of people whose RBCs do not carry the antigen. These antibodies react against the foreign antigens from mismatched transfusions. For example, if a person who is type A accidentally receives type B blood, antibodies in the person's blood attack the type B antigens. Incompatible RBCs agglutinate (clump together), causing a potentially life-threatening immune response known as a hemolytic **transfusion reaction.** People with type A blood have anti-B antibodies; people with type B blood have anti-A antibodies. People with type AB blood have neither antibody and can receive all blood types. People with type O blood have both A and B antibodies and can receive only type O blood.

Rh System. Another consideration for matching blood for transfusion is presence of Rh factor, an antigenic substance on most people's RBCs. A person with Rh factor is Rh positive, whereas a person without it is Rh negative. Unlike ABO antigens, there are no naturally occurring antibodies to the Rh antigen. A person with Rh-negative blood must first be exposed to Rh-positive blood before developing antibodies. People who are Rh negative should receive only Rh-negative blood components.

Transfusion Reactions and Other Adverse Effects. A transfusion reaction is an immune system response to a transfusion that ranges from a mild response to severe anaphylactic shock or acute intravascular hemolysis, both of which are life threatening. Prompt nursing intervention is essential to maintain a patient's physiological stability (see Box 18-9).

Circulatory overload is a risk when a patient receives massive transfusions for hemorrhagic shock or when a patient with normal intravascular volume receives blood. Older adults and those with cardiopulmonary diseases have high risk for circulatory overload and need careful monitoring during transfusion.

Another category of adverse transfusion effects is diseases transmitted by blood from infected donors who are asymptomatic. Symptoms of these diseases often arise long after the transfusion. Diseases transmitted through transfusions include malaria, HBV and HCV, HIV infection and acquired immunodeficiency syndrome (AIDS), and cytomegalovirus infection. Blood collected for blood banks in developed countries undergoes screening for HIV, HBV, HCV, and syphilis, which reduces the risk for acquiring these bloodborne infections (Trick, 2010).

Interventions for Acid-Base Imbalances. Nursing interventions to promote acid-base balance support prescribed medical therapies and aim at reversing the underlying disorder causing the acid-base imbalance while providing for patient safety. Imbalances are often life threatening and require a rapid nursing response to deliver treatment. Maintain a patent IV line and check for changes in prescribed therapies. Give fluid and electrolyte replacements and prescribed drugs promptly. In addition, monitor patients closely for changes in their status. Use protective measures such as bedrails for patients with decreased level of consciousness.

Arterial Blood Gas Measurement. Patients with serious fluid and electrolyte imbalance often require frequent ABG monitoring. ABG analysis reveals a patient's acid-base status and the adequacy of ventilation and oxygenation. The analysis involves removing a blood sample from an artery. A qualified RN or other personnel draws arterial blood from a peripheral artery (usually the radial) or from an arterial line (see agency policy and procedures). Before an arterial blood draw, ensure that the patient has an ulnar pulse to prevent loss of blood flow to the hand in the event of radial artery damage. After the arterial puncture, apply pressure to the puncture site for at least 5 minutes to reduce risk of hematoma formation. Apply pressure for a longer period if the patient takes anticoagulant medications or has a clotting disorder. Reassess the radial pulse after removing pressure. After obtaining the specimen, prevent air from entering the syringe because this alters the blood gas results. To reduce oxygen use by RBCs, submerge the syringe in crushed ice and transport it immediately to the laboratory.

Restorative and Continuing Care. After experiencing acute fluid, electrolyte, or acid-base imbalances, patients often require ongoing maintenance to prevent recurrence. Older adults require special considerations to prevent complications from developing.

Home Intravenous Therapy. Intravenous therapy often continues at home for patients requiring long-term hydration, parenteral nutrition, or long-term medication administration. A home IV therapy nurse works closely with a patient and/or family caregivers to ensure that they know how to maintain a sterile IV system; how to dispose of sharps and materials exposed to blood safely; techniques for ambulation, hygiene, and other activities of daily living without dislodging the IV catheter or disconnecting the system; and how to avoid complications or recognize and report them promptly.

Nutritional Support. Most patients who have electrolyte or acid-base imbalances require ongoing nutritional support. Depending on the type of disorder, you encourage or restrict certain fluids or food. Teach patients or family caregivers who are responsible for meal preparation the nutritional content of foods and how to read the labels of commercially prepared foods.

Medication Safety. Numerous prescription and OTC drugs and supplements contain components or create side effects that alter fluid and electrolyte balance. Patients with chronic disease who receive multiple medications and those with renal disorders have high risk for fluid and electrolyte imbalances. Teach patients and families regarding potential side effects and drug interactions that alter fluid, electrolyte, or acid-base balance. Review all medications with patients and family caregivers and encourage them to consult their local pharmacist before trying a new OTC drug or supplement.

EVALUATION

Patient Care. Evaluation of a patient's clinical status is important if an acute fluid, electrolyte, or acid-base imbalance exists. You need to recognize the signs and symptoms of impending problems by considering a patient's presenting risk factors and clinical status, effects of the present treatment regimen, and the potential causative agent. Perform an evaluation to determine if changes have occurred from the previous patient assessment. For example, if a patient's hypokalemia is improving, you expect the signs and symptoms of hypokalemia to diminish. The patient's heart rhythm becomes more regular, muscle strength improves, and bowel function returns. The serum potassium level returns to normal levels.

For patients with less acute alterations, evaluation occurs over a longer period of time. In these situations you focus evaluation more on behavioral changes (e.g., the patient's adherence to dietary restrictions and medication schedules). Also evaluate the family's ability to anticipate alterations and prevent problems from recurring.

A patient's level of progress determines whether you continue or revise the current plan of care. If goals are not met, consult with other members of the health care team to discuss additional methods such as increasing the frequency of an intervention (e.g., provide more fluids to a dehydrated patient), introducing a new therapy (e.g., initiate insertion of an IV), or discontinuing a particular therapy. Once a patient meets the outcomes of care, the nursing diagnosis is resolved and you can focus on other priorities, including maintaining normal fluid, electrolyte, and acid-base balance.

Patient Expectations. Review with patients how well their major concerns regarding fluid, electrolyte, or acid-base situations were alleviated or addressed. For example, if a person's concern was feeling uncomfortable with very dry mouth, you ask, "How does your mouth feel now?" (Box 18-10). If a patient's concerns involve having a better understanding of a newly diagnosed problem, evaluate patient satisfaction with the education provided. Often a patient's level of satisfaction with care also depends on success in involving family and friends. If patients have concerns about returning home or to a different care setting, it is important to evaluate how well prepared they feel for the transition from acute care.

BOX 18-10 EVALUATION

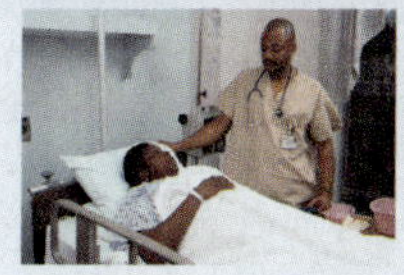

Robert continues to care for Mrs. Reynolds 2 days after her admission. He asks her how she feels and prepares to conduct a brief physical assessment. Mrs. Reynolds remarks, "I feel much better. I have had no nausea since early yesterday and no diarrhea since late yesterday afternoon." The IV infusion of 0.9% sodium chloride (normal saline) still is in place, infusing now at 100 mL/hr. However, the patient's physician just ordered to reduce the rate to 40 mL/hr. She has been tolerating oral fluids. During examination Robert notices that her oral mucosa is still slightly dry; skin turgor has returned to normal. Mrs. Reynolds' vital signs are blood pressure, 126/78 mm Hg; pulse, 80 beats/min; and respirations, 18 breaths/min. She is afebrile. The serum potassium level drawn at 7 AM was 4 mEq/L.

Robert is encouraged by Mrs. Reynolds' progress. He brings her breakfast meal tray, which includes the first soft food that she has had since being hospitalized. Robert sits down and discusses with Mrs. Reynolds what she has learned from their discussion about food sources for potassium. Robert asks, "Now that we've discussed the importance of potassium in your diet, tell me which foods you would select that are high in potassium." Mrs. Reynolds identifies five different sources of potassium among foods that she enjoys and can routinely include in her diet.

DOCUMENTATION NOTE

"Denies nausea and reports feeling better. No diarrheal stool since yesterday afternoon around 4 PM. On inspection oral mucosa remains dry without lesions or inflammation. Skin turgor is normal. Bowel sounds are normal in all four quadrants, abdomen soft to palpation. IV of 0.9% sodium chloride is infusing in left cephalic vein in forearm at 40 mL/hr per MD order. No tenderness or inflammation at IV site. Is able to identify five food sources for potassium to include in diet. Is resting comfortably, out of bed in a chair, and ate all of breakfast. Will continue to monitor."

IV, Intravenous.

SAFETY GUIDELINES FOR NURSING SKILLS

Ensuring patient safety is an essential role of a professional nurse. To ensure patient safety, communicate clearly with members of the health care team, assess and incorporate the patient's priorities of care and preferences, and use the best evidence when making decisions about your patient's care. When performing the skills in this chapter, remember the following points to ensure safe, individualized care.

- Check that you have the necessary information, an order if required, and equipment available for the procedure before beginning.
- Determine if patient has latex allergy and use nonlatex items if allergy is present (INS, 2011).
- Use special designated tubing for the brand of EID and for blood transfusions and some medications.
- Review the steps of the procedure mentally before entering a patient's room, considering modifications that you may need to make for each specific patient and verifying that the type of IV solution is appropriate for the patient.
- Maintain strict aseptic and sterile techniques when required and sterility and integrity of the IV system to prevent development of bloodstream infections (INS, 2011).
- If you contaminate a sterile object during the procedure, do not use it. Use a new sterile one.
- Use standard body fluid precautions during procedures and place all disposable blood-contaminated and sharp items in designated puncture-resistant biohazard containers (INS, 2011).

SKILL 18-1 INITIATING INTRAVENOUS THERAPY

View Video!

DELEGATION CONSIDERATIONS

The skill of initiating peripheral intravenous (IV) therapy cannot be delegated to nursing assistive personnel (NAP). Delegation to licensed practical nurses (LPNs) varies by state Nurse Practice Act. The nurse instructs NAP to inform the nurse if:

- Patient indicates burning, bleeding, swelling, or coolness at the catheter insertion site.
- An IV dressing becomes wet or loose.
- The IV fluid container is almost empty or the electronic infusion device (EID) alarm is signaling.

EQUIPMENT

- Facility-approved, proper safety mechanism–equipped vascular access device (VAD) (Figure 18-12) (varies with patient's vein size and reason for IV fluid administration). For continuous fluid infusion: peripheral 20-gauge catheter for an adult, 22-gauge for older adults and children are recommended (Perucca, 2010). Use a steel winged device only for short-term therapy or a single dose (INS, 2011).

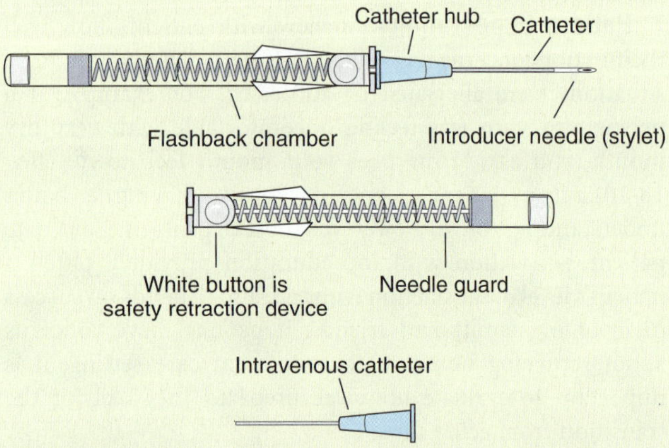

FIGURE 18-12 Intravenous access device options.

- IV start kit (available in some agencies): Contains a sterile drape, tourniquet, cleansing and antiseptic preparations, sterile dressing, and small roll of sterile tape
- If IV start kit not available:
  - Disposable drape or towel
  - Tourniquet (Determine type based on patient assessment [e.g., blood pressure (BP) cuff (older adult), rubber band (infant)]). Use a single-use tourniquet to prevent transfer of microorganisms between patients (Perucca, 2010)
  - Antiseptic swabs (chlorhexidine preferred)
  - Transparent dressing or, less commonly, 2 × 2 or 4 × 4 gauze sponge
  - Nonallergenic tape and sterile tape
- Short extension tubing with fused needleless connector or separate needleless connector (also called *injection cap,* IV plug, saline lock, heparin lock, PRN adapter, buff cap, or buffalo cap)
- Prefilled 5-mL syringe with flush agent (preservative-free sterile 0.9% sodium chloride (normal saline) solution for adults (INS, 2011).
- Local anesthetic (e.g., intradermal lidocaine, topical transdermal anesthetic, vapocoolant) *(optional).*
- Manufactured catheter stabilization device if available (INS, 2011)
- IV site protection device *(optional)*
- Clean gloves
- Protective equipment: Goggles, mask (*optional*; check agency policy)
- Patient gown with snaps at shoulder seam if available
- Needle disposal container (sharps container)

For Continuous IV Fluid Infusion, in Addition to Preceding List

- Correct IV solution in correct container size
- Electronic infusion device (EID)
- IV tubing with spike (primary administration set) appropriate for the EID
- If gravity-flow IV drip is infusing, use microdrip tubing when infusing small or very precise volumes; use macrodrip tubing to infuse more rapidly

- In-line filter if particulate matter is likely, long-term or high-volume IV therapy is expected, or if required by agency policy; size appropriate to type of solution (e.g., 0.22 micron for nonlipid solution, 1.2 μm for lipid solution)
- Long extension tubing if desired for patient mobility (see Box 18-5)
- IV pole: Rolling, ceiling mounted, or attached to bed
- Bar-code scanner, if using bar-code system

STEP	RATIONALE
ASSESSMENT	
1. Review accuracy and completeness of health care provider's order for patient name, type and amount of IV fluid, medication additives, infusion rate, and length of therapy. Follow six rights of medication administration (see Chapter 17).	Before administering solutions or medications, an order from a licensed independent practitioner (LIP) is needed (INS, 2011).
a. Check approved online data base, drug reference book, or pharmacist about IV fluid composition, purpose, potential incompatibilities, and side effects.	Ensures safe and correct administration of IV therapy and appropriate selection of VAD.
2. Assess patient's knowledge of procedure, reason for prescribed therapy, and arm placement preference.	Provides patient-centered care by determining level of emotional support and instruction needed (INS, 2011).
3. Assess for clinical variables that will respond to or be affected by IV fluid administration:	Provides baseline to determine effect that IV fluids have on patient's fluid and electrolyte balance.
a. Body weight	Daily weights reflect fluid retention or loss. One liter of fluid weighs 2.2 lbs (1 kg). Gain or loss of 1 kg in 24 hours indicates gain or loss of 1 L of fluid. Body fat gain or loss takes longer (Felver, 2013c).
b. Clinical markers of vascular volume:	Assess signs and symptoms as a group to interpret them accurately. Infusion of Na^+-containing fluid expands extracellular fluid volume (ECV) (vascular and interstitial).
(1) Blood pressure (BP) (orthostatic hypotension or hypotension with ECV deficit)	Decreased BP may indicate ECV deficit caused by decreased stroke volume.
(2) Pulse (rapid, thready with ECV deficit; bounding with ECV excess)	Baroreceptor response causes tachycardia with ECV deficit.
(3) Condition of neck veins (flat or collapsing with inhalation when supine with ECV deficit; full or distended when upright or semiupright with ECV excess)	With normal ECV neck veins are full when person is supine and flat when person is upright or semiupright.
(4) Capillary refill (sluggish with ECV deficit)	Indicates poor tissue perfusion.
(5) Auscultation of lungs	Crackles or ronchi in dependent portions of lungs may signal fluid buildup in the lungs because of ECV excess.
(6) Urine output (decreased; dark yellow with ECV deficit)	Kidneys respond to ECV deficit by reducing urine production and concentrating the urine. Average adult urine output is 1500 mL/24 hr; oliguria is less than 400 mL/24 hr. Kidney disease also can cause oliguria. Dark yellow indicates concentrated urine.
c. Clinical markers of interstitial volume:	Assess signs and symptoms as a group to interpret them accurately. Infusion of Na^+-containing fluid expands ECV (vascular and interstitial).
(1) Dependent edema—pitting or nonpitting; +1 for barely detectable edema to +4 for deep, persistent pitting (see Chapter 16)	Edema, indicating expanded interstitial volume, is most evident in dependent areas (i.e., feet and ankles if sitting or sacrum if bedfast).
(2) Oral mucous membranes (dry between cheek and gum with ECV deficit)	Dryness of opposing mucous membranes is more reliable indicator than dry lips or skin.
(3) Skin turgor (pinch skin over sternum or inside of forearm).	Pinched skin that stays elevated for several seconds is called *poor skin turgor* or *tenting.* It may occur from ECV deficit, rapid weight loss, or normal aging.
d. Thirst	Occurs with hypernatremia and severe ECV deficit. Not a reliable indicator for older adults because thirst sensation decreases with age.

***Clinical Decision Point:* Choose appropriate assessments for each patient. Skin turgor and thirst are less reliable indicators for older adults because of physiological changes of aging.**

SKILL 18-1 INITIATING INTRAVENOUS THERAPY—cont'd

STEP	RATIONALE
e. Behavior and level of consciousness:	
(1) Restlessness and mild confusion	Occurs with severe ECV deficit caused by lack of blood flow to brain.
(2) Decreased level of consciousness (lethargy, confusion, coma)	May occur with osmolality imbalances (hyponatremia; hypernatremia) and acid base imbalances.
f. Cardiac signs of electrolyte or acid-base imbalances: Irregular pulse and electrocardiogram (ECG) changes	Rhythm and ECG changes may occur with K^+, Ca^{2+}, Mg^{2+}, and/or acid-base imbalances.
4. Assess patient's previous experience with and perceptions of IV therapy, need for local anesthetic agent before venipuncture, understanding of purpose of IV therapy, and arm placement preference.	Provides patient-centered care by determining level of emotional support and instruction necessary. If patient is apprehensive about venipuncture, use a local anesthetic (Anderson et al., 2010).
5. Determine if patient is to undergo any planned surgeries or procedures.	Allows anticipation and placement of appropriate VAD (larger gauge) for fluid infusion and avoids placement in area that will interfere with medical procedures.
6. Assess for the following risk factors: child or older adult, presence of heart failure or oliguric renal disease, skin lesions or infection near potential venipuncture sites, low platelet count or receiving anticoagulants.	Older adults have proportionately less body water; people with heart failure cannot adapt to sudden increases in vascular volume; people with oliguria cannot eliminate excess extracellular fluid, K^+, or Mg^{2+}. Skin lesion or infection influences choice of access site. Low platelet count or anticoagulant use increases patient's risk for bleeding from VAD site and seepage of blood from puncture site during venipuncture.
7. Assess laboratory data.	Helps determine priority assessments; establishes baseline for determining if therapy is effective; may allow detection of an inadvisable fluid order.

***Clinical Decision Point:* If current K^+, Ca^{2+}, or Mg^{2+} serum values are high, clarify order with health care provider before administering an IV solution containing the elevated electrolyte to avoid worsening the electrolyte excess.**

STEP	RATIONALE
8. Assess patient's history of allergies, especially to iodine, adhesive, or latex.	Equipment used during insertion of VAD may contain substances to which patient is allergic. Use alternatives if patient has allergy.
PLANNING	
1. Identify patient using two identifiers (e.g., name and birthday or name and account number) according to agency policy. Compare identifiers with information on patient's MAR or medical record.	Ensures correct patient. Complies with The Joint Commission requirements for patient safety (TJC, 2014).
2. Collect and organize equipment. Be sure that you have the correct infusion set for the EID that will be used. If the IV container is rigid rather than collapsible, you need IV tubing with a vented spike.	Promotes comfort and relaxation for patient. Provides proper body mechanics for nurse. Aids in successful vein location.
IMPLEMENTATION	
1. Perform hand hygiene. Organize equipment on clean, clutter-free bedside stand or over-bed table.	Reduces transmission of infection and contamination of equipment (INS, 2011).
2. Change patient's gown to a more easily removed gown with snaps at shoulder if available. Position patient comfortably so that he or she is able to remain still during procedure. Caution against touching sterile work area.	Use of special IV gown makes gown removal easier and protects VAD site from trauma during gown changes. Prevents patient from touching sterile work area.
3. Open sterile packages using sterile aseptic technique (see Chapter 14).	Maintains sterility of equipment and reduces spread of microorganisms.
4. *Option:* Prepare short extension tubing with needleless connector or the stand-alone saline lock (check agency policy and procedures) to attach to VAD catheter hub.	Short extension tubing prevents traction on VAD. Many facilities use short extension tubing for continuous infusions and stand-alone saline locks (capped catheters). Continuous infusion attaches to the needleless connector on short extension tubing. Saline locks provide IV access when continuous IV infusions are not needed.

***Clinical Decision Point:* Consider using a short extension set with a short peripheral catheter and Luer-Lok connections to decrease potential contact with hub and reduce blood contact (INS, 2011).**

STEP	RATIONALE
a. Remove protective cap from needleless connector and attach syringe with 1-3 mL 0.9% sodium chloride, maintaining sterility. Slowly inject enough saline to prime the short extension tubing (if used) and connector, removing all the air. Leave syringe attached to tubing (see illustration).	Replaces air with normal saline, preventing air from entering patient's vein.
b. Maintain sterility and set aside for attaching to catheter hub after successful venipuncture.	Prevents touch contamination that allows microorganisms to enter infusion equipment and bloodstream.
5. *For continuous infusion:* Prepare IV infusion tubing and solution.	
a. Check IV solution, using six rights of medication administration (see Chapter 17). If using bar-code system, scan bar code on patient's wristband and then bar code on the IV fluid container. Be sure that prescribed additives such as potassium and vitamins are included and noted on bag label. Check solution for color, clarity, and expiration date. Check bag for leaks.	IV solutions are medications and need to be checked carefully to reduce risk for error. Bar-code systems reduce medication errors by verifying right patient, medication, dose, and time with the electronic medical record (Poon et al., 2010). Do not use solutions that are discolored, contain particles, or are expired. Do not use leaky bags because they present an opportunity for infection (INS, 2011).
b. Open infusion set, maintaining sterility of both ends of tubing. EIDs sometimes have a special dedicated administration set.	Prevents touch contamination, which allows microorganisms to enter infusion equipment and bloodstream.
c. Removing appropriate end caps, attach extension tubing with injection port to distal end of infusion set, maintaining sterility of the connection. Do not touch point of entry of connection. Leave end cap on the distal end of extension tubing.	Distal end of extension tubing with injection port attaches to IV catheter hub after venipuncture. Extra tubing provides greater ease of access and ability to change easily between continuous and intermittent IV infusion. Prevents touch contamination, which allows microorganisms to enter infusion equipment and bloodstream.
d. Place roller clamp of IV tubing about 2 to 5 cm (1 to 2 inches) below drip chamber and close roller clamp (see illustrations).	Close proximity of roller clamp to drip chamber allows more accurate regulation of flow rate. Closing clamp prevents accidental spillage of IV fluid on patient, nurse, bed, or floor.
e. Remove protective sheath from IV tubing port on plastic IV solution bag (see illustration) or top of bottle while maintaining sterility.	Provides access for insertion of infusion tubing into the solution while preventing touch contamination.
f. Insert infusion set into fluid bag or bottle: Remove protector cap from tubing insertion spike (not touching spike) and insert it into port of IV bag (see illustration). Cleanse rubber stopper on glass-bottled solution with single-use antiseptic and insert spike into black rubber stopper of IV bottle.	Prevents contamination of IV solution during insertion of spike. Flat surface on top of bottled solution may contain contaminants, whereas opening to plastic bag is recessed.

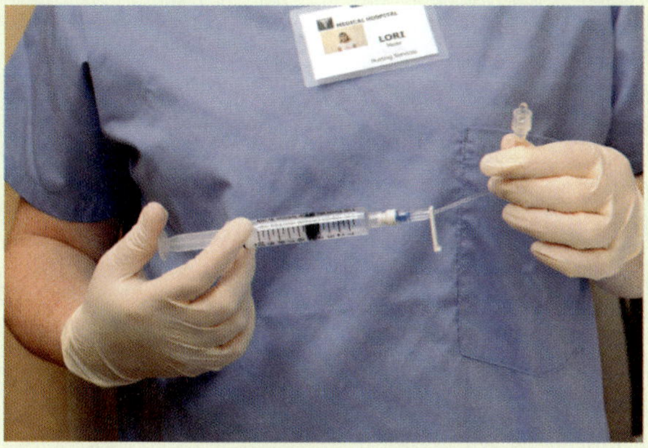

STEP 4a Prime short extension tubing, leaving syringe attached.

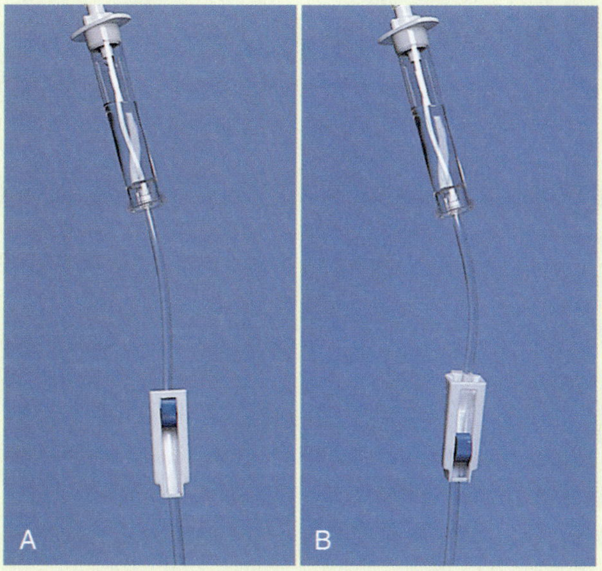

STEP 5d A, Roller clamp in open position. **B,** Roller clamp in closed or off position.

SKILL 18-1 INITIATING INTRAVENOUS THERAPY—cont'd

STEP	RATIONALE
***Clinical Decision Point:* Do not touch spike because it is sterile. If contamination occurs (e.g., you accidentally touch outside of bag with the spike or drop spike), discard that IV tubing and obtain a new one).**	
g. Compress drip chamber and release, allowing it to fill one-third to one-half full (see illustration).	Creates suction effect; fluid enters drip chamber, which prevents air from entering tubing.
h. Prime infusion and extension tubing by filling with IV solution: Remove protective cap on end of tubing (you can prime some tubing without removal) and slowly open roller clamp to allow fluid to travel from drip chamber through tubing to needle adapter. Invert Y-connector to displace air. Return roller clamp to "off" position after priming tubing. Replace protective cap on end of tubing if you removed it.	Priming ensures that tubing is clear of air before connecting with VAD. Slow fill of tubing decreases turbulence and chance of bubble formation. Closing clamp prevents continued flow of fluid. Cap on end of tubing maintains system sterility.
i. Be certain that tubing is clear of air and air bubbles. To remove small air bubbles, firmly tap tubing where air bubbles are located (see illustration). Check entire length of tubing to ensure that all air bubbles are removed. If using multiple port tubing, turn ports upside down and tap to fill and remove air.	Tapping causes air bubbles to rise up to drip chamber. Large air bubbles may act as emboli.
***Clinical Decision Point:* Consider adding long extension tubing to IV tubing to allow for more length, which enables patient to move more freely while still keeping IV line stable.**	
j. If using optional long extension tubing (not short extension tubing in Step 4), remove protective cap and attach it to the distal end of the IV tubing, maintaining sterility. Prime long extension tubing.	Priming replaces the air in tubing with IV solution so air does not enter patient's vein.
k. Insert primed tubing into EID with power off.	Facilitates starting infusion as soon as IV site is ready.
***Clinical Decision Point:* You apply gloves before or after assessing veins. You always apply gloves before VAD insertion.**	
6. Perform hand hygiene and apply clean gloves. Wear eye protection and mask (check agency policy) if splash or spray of blood is possible.	Reduces transmission of microorganisms. Prevents spraying of blood on your mucous membranes.

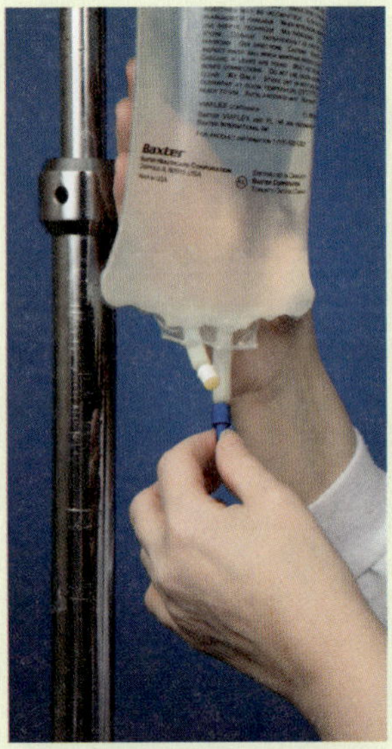

STEP 5e Remove protective covering from IV solution tubing port.

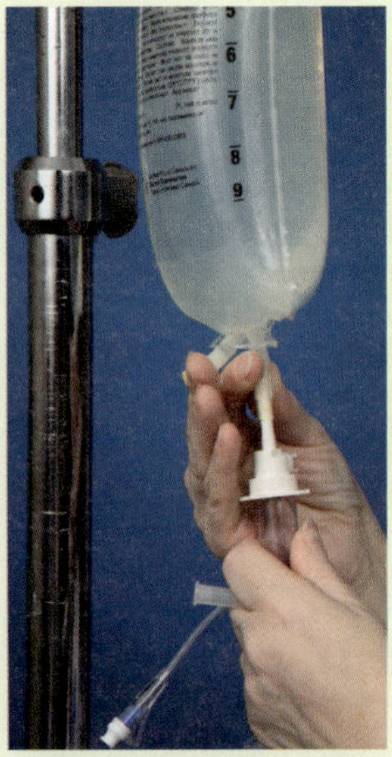

STEP 5f Insert tubing spike into IV container.

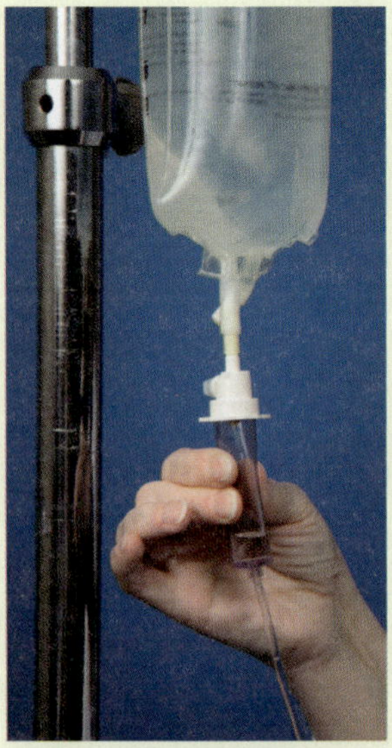

STEP 5g Squeeze the drip chamber to fill with fluid.

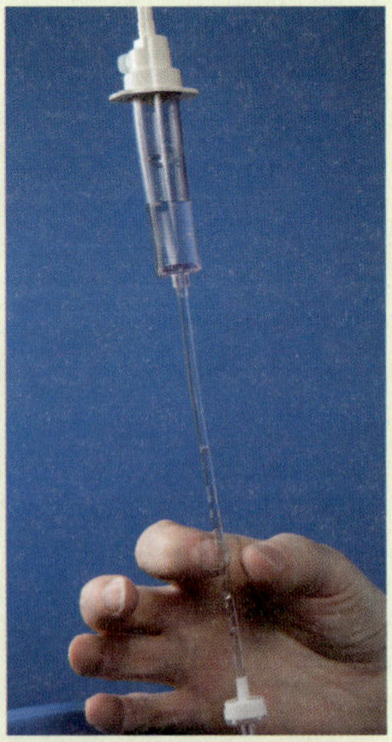

STEP 5i Remove air bubbles from tubing.

STEP	RATIONALE
7. Apply tourniquet to begin vein selection: Apply tourniquet around arm above antecubital fossa or 10-15 cm (4-6 inches) above proposed insertion site (see illustration). Do not apply it too tightly to avoid injury or bruising to skin or occluding arterial flow. Check for presence of radial pulse. *Option a:* Apply tourniquet on top of a thin layer of clothing such as a gown sleeve to protect fragile or hairy skin. *Option b:* Use BP cuff instead of tourniquet. Inflate it to a level just below the patient's normal diastolic pressure (less than 50 mm Hg).	Tourniquet needs to be tight enough to decrease venous return but not too tight to occlude arterial flow (INS, 2011). If patient has fragile veins, apply tourniquet loosely or not at all to prevent damage to veins or bruising. Avoid using antecubital fossa for IV insertion because a VAD at this site limits mobility; instead use this site for blood draws. Use of BP cuff reduces trauma to skin and underlying tissue.
8. Select vein for VAD insertion. Veins on dorsal and ventral surfaces of upper extremities (e.g., cephalic, basilic, and median veins) are preferred in adults (see Figure 18-7).	Ensures adequate vein that is easy to puncture and less likely to rupture. Do not routinely use veins in lower extremities for IV therapy in adults because of risk of tissue damage and thrombophlebitis (INS, 2011).
a. Use the most distal site in the nondominant arm, if possible.	VAD placement in dominant arm interferes with activities of daily living (ADLs). Perform venipuncture distal to proximal, which increases the availability of other sites for future IV therapy (INS, 2011).
b. Select a well-dilated vein. Methods to foster venous distention include:	Increased volume of blood in the vein at the venipuncture site makes vein more visible.
(1) Placing extremity in dependent position if possible and stroke from distal to proximal below proposed venipuncture site.	Promotes venous filling.
(2) Applying warmth to extremity for several minutes (e.g., with a warm washcloth).	Increases blood in vein by dilating it.

***Clinical Decision Point:* Choose appropriate dilation method. Vigorous friction and multiple tapping of a vein, especially in older adults, can cause hematoma and/or venous constriction.**

STEP	RATIONALE
9. Select a vein large enough for a VAD (sometimes you will remove gloves in order to palpably feel vein).	Prevents interruption of venous flow while allowing adequate blood flow around the catheter.
a. With your index finger, palpate vein by pressing downward. Note resilient, soft, bouncy feeling while releasing the pressure (see illustration).	Fingertip is sensitive for assessing vein location and condition.
b. Avoid vein selection in these areas:	
(1) Areas with tenderness, pain, infection, or wound	May indicate inflamed vein or increased risk of infection.
(2) Extremity affected by previous stroke (cerebrovascular accident [CVA]), paralysis, mastectomy, or dialysis graft	Increased risk for complications such as lymphedema or vessel damage.
(3) Site distal to previous venipuncture site, sclerosed or thrombotic veins, infiltrate site, bruised areas, and areas of venous valves	Such sites cause infiltration around newly placed VAD and excessive vessel damage.
(4) Fragile dorsal veins in older adult patients and vessels in an extremity with compromised circulation	Small fragile veins have increased risk of infiltration, hematoma from vessel rupture, and phlebitis from vessel damage.

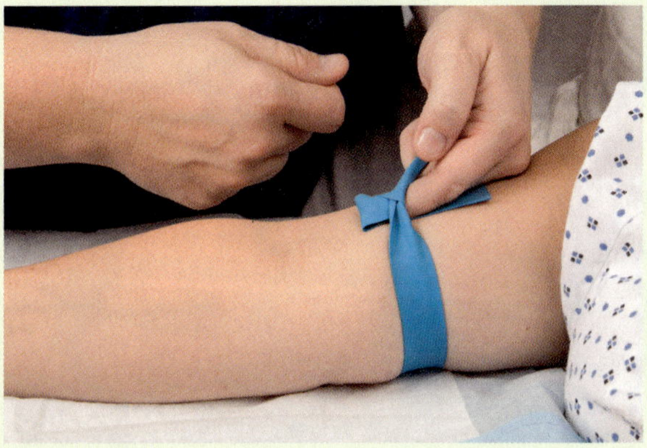

STEP 7 Tourniquet placed on arm for initial vein selection.

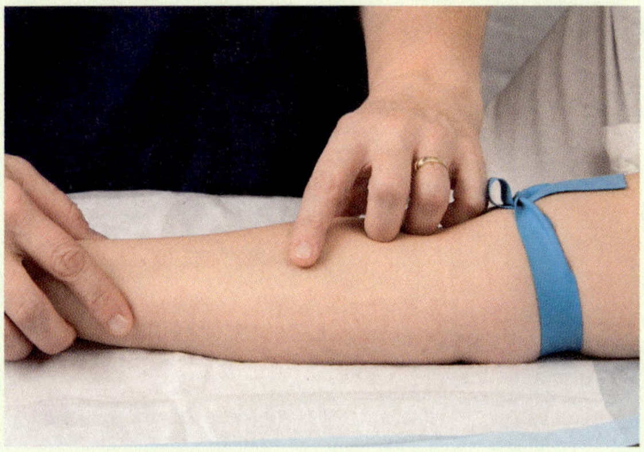

STEP 9a Palpate vein for resilience.

SKILL 18-1 INITIATING INTRAVENOUS THERAPY—cont'd

STEP	RATIONALE
c. Choose a site that will not interfere with patient's ADLs, use of mobility aids such as a cane, or planned procedure.	Keeps patient as mobile and independent as possible.
10. Release tourniquet temporarily and carefully. Clip arm hair with scissors if necessary (explain to patient). *Option:* At this point in the procedure there is the option of applying a local anesthetic to site. Monitor patient for allergic reaction.	Restores blood flow and prevents venospasm when preparing for venipuncture. Hair impedes venipuncture or adherence of dressing. Local anesthetic reduces procedural pain (Anderson et al., 2010).

Clinical Decision Point: **If hair removal is needed, do not shave area with a razor. Shaving causes microabrasions that increase risk of infection (INS, 2011).**

STEP	RATIONALE
11. Apply clean gloves if not done.	Reduces transmission of microorganisms.
12. Place adapter end of short infusion tubing/saline lock from Step 4 or adapter end of long infusion tubing from Step 5 nearby on sterile gauze or sterile towel, avoiding touch contamination.	Permits smooth, quick connection of infusion to VAD after accessing vein. Prevents microorganisms from entering infusion equipment and bloodstream.
13. If area of insertion appears to need cleansing, use soap and water first, then dry. Use chlorhexidine antiseptic swab to cleanse insertion site applying friction in a horizontal plane with first swab, vertical plane with second swab, and circular motion, moving outward with third swab (see illustration). Allow to dry completely. Refrain from touching cleansed site unless using sterile technique. Allow drying time between agents if agents are used in combination (alcohol and Betadine).	Mechanical friction allows penetration of antiseptic solution to epidermal layers of the skin. Allowing antiseptic solutions to air-dry completely reduces microbial counts and risk of phlebitis. Chlorhexidine 2% preparation is preferred (INS, 2011). Touching cleansed area introduces microorganisms from glove to site. If this happens, prepare site again.
14. Reapply tourniquet or BP cuff 10 to 12.5 cm (4 to 6 inches) above anticipated insertion site. Keep BP cuff inflated <50 mm Hg until venipuncture is completed. Verify presence of distal pulse.	Diminished arterial flow prevents venous filling. Pressure of tourniquet causes vein to fill and dilate.
15. Perform venipuncture. Anchor vein by placing thumb over vein and stretching skin against direction of insertion 4 to 5 cm (1½ to 2 inches) distal to site (see illustration).	Stabilizes vein for needle insertion. Places VAD parallel to vein.
a. Warn patient of a sharp, quick stick.	Prepares patient to avoid movement of extremity during venipuncture.
b. Insert with bevel up at 10- to 30-degree angle slightly distal to actual site of venipuncture in direction of vein (see illustration).	Places needle at optimal angle to vein to reduce risk of puncturing posterior vein wall. Superficial veins require a smaller angle. Deeper veins require a greater angle.

Clinical Decision Point: **Use each VAD only once for each insertion attempt.**

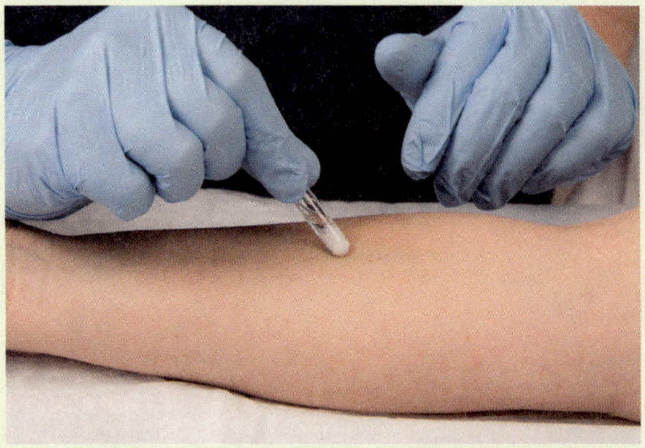

STEP 13 Cleanse site with chlorhexidine.

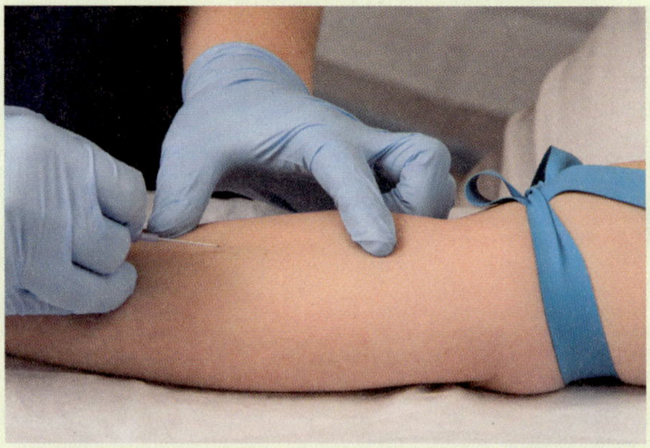

STEP 15 Stabilize vein below insertion site.

STEP	RATIONALE
16. Observe for blood return in flashback chamber of catheter, indicating that needle has entered vein (see illustration A). Lower catheter until almost flush with skin. Advance catheter approximately 0.6 cm (¼ inch) into vein and loosen stylet. Continue to hold skin taut and advance catheter into vein until hub is near venipuncture site. *Do not reinsert stylet once it is loosened.* Advance catheter while safety device automatically retracts stylet (see illustration B). (Techniques for retracting stylet vary with different VADs.) Follow manufacturer guidelines for specific safety catheter use. Place stylet directly into sharps container.	Increased venous pressure from tourniquet increases backflow of blood into catheter or tubing. Allows full penetration of the vein wall, placement of catheter in vein lumen, and advancement of catheter off stylet. Reduces risk of introducing microorganisms along catheter. Advancing entire stylet into vein may penetrate posterior vein wall, causing a hematoma. Reinsertion of stylet can cause catheter shearing and potential catheter embolization (INS, 2011).

***Clinical Decision Point:* Do not make more than two attempts at initiating the IV access (INS, 2011). After two attempts have another nurse attempt the insertion.**

STEP	RATIONALE
17. Stabilize catheter with one hand and release tourniquet or BP cuff with other. Apply gentle but firm pressure with middle finger of nondominant hand 3 cm (1¼ inches) above insertion site. Keep catheter stable with index finger.	Permits venous flow, reduces backflow of blood, and allows connection with administration set with minimal blood loss (INS, 2011).
18. Quickly connect Luer-Lok end of the primed short extension tubing or the prepared saline lock (prepared in Step 4) to the catheter. Do not touch point of entry of connection. Secure connection.	Prompt connection of infusion set maintains patency of vein and prevents risk for exposure to blood. Maintains sterility.

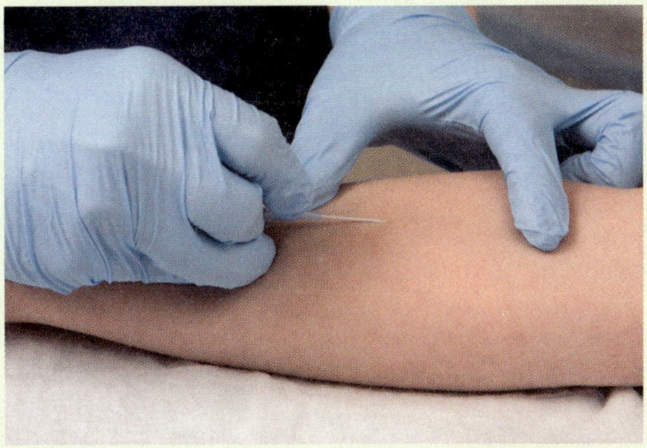

STEP 15b Puncture vein with catheter at a 10- to 30-degree angle. Catheter enters vein.

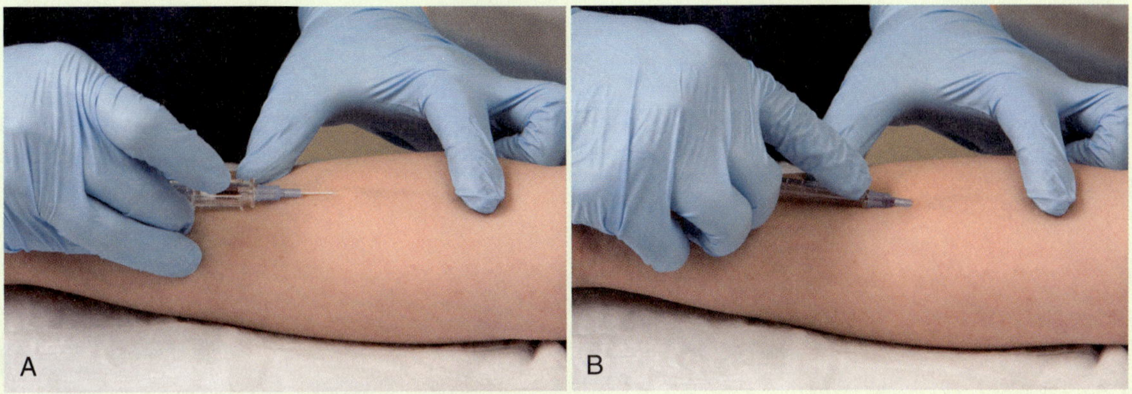

STEP 16 A, Look for blood return in flashback chamber. **B,** Advance catheter into vein until hub is near insertion site.

SKILL 18-1 INITIATING INTRAVENOUS THERAPY—cont'd

STEP	RATIONALE
19. Flush VAD. Slowly flush the primed extension set with remaining saline from the attached prefilled syringe (see illustration) or connect end of primary infusion tubing to short extension set. Then slowly open slide clamp or adjust roller clamp of IV tubing and allow fluid to infuse. Observe for swelling.	Positive-pressure flushing creates positive pressure in catheter and prevents reflux of blood into catheter lumen (INS, 2011). Initiates flow of fluid through IV catheter, preventing clotting of device. Swelling during flush indicates that infiltration and site must be discontinued.
20. Remove the syringe. For continuous infusion attach distal end of IV tubing to needleless connector on short extension tubing that is attached to catheter (see illustration). Insert tubing of IV administration set into EID. Check ordered rate of infusion, turn on EID, program it, and begin infusion at correct rate (see Skill 18-2). If using gravity flow instead of EID, begin infusion by slowly opening roller clamp to regulate rate.	Initiates flow of fluid through IV catheter, preventing clotting of device.

Clinical Decision Point: **Be sure to calculate rate (see Skill 18-2) and set EID correctly to infuse IV solution at prescribed rate.**

STEP	RATIONALE
21. Secure catheter and apply sterile dressing over site (procedures differ; check agency policy):	Prevents accidental dislodgement of catheter and protects site from infection.
a. *Manufactured catheter stabilization device* (see illustration): Wipe selected area with single-use skin protectant and allow to dry completely (10-15 seconds). Apply sterile adhesive strip over catheter hub. Place retainer over tubing end just behind spin nut. Peel off half of liner; press to adhere to skin. Repeat on other side. Apply transparent dressing.	A manufactured catheter stabilization device holds catheter in place, improving patient outcomes by reducing risk of catheter dislodgement, phlebitis, and other complications (INS, 2011).
b. *Transparent dressing:* Continue to secure catheter with nondominant hand.	Prevents accidental dislodgement of catheter.
(1) Remove adherent backing. Apply one edge of dressing and gently smooth remaining dressing over IV site, leaving connection between IV tubing and catheter hub uncovered. Remove outer covering and smooth dressing gently over site (see illustration).	Occlusive dressing protects site from bacterial contamination. Connection between administration set and hub needs to be uncovered to facilitate changing tubing if necessary.
(2) If manufactured catheter stabilization device is not used, secure catheter by placing a 1-inch piece of transparent tape over extension tubing or administration set (see illustration). Do not apply tape on top of transparent dressing.	Removal of tape from a transparent dressing might accidentally dislodge catheter. Tape on top of a transparent dressing prevents moisture from being carried away from the skin.

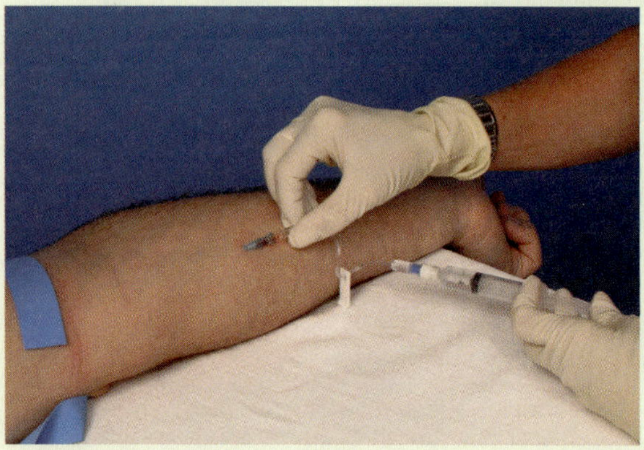

STEP 19 Flush catheter gently to ensure patency.

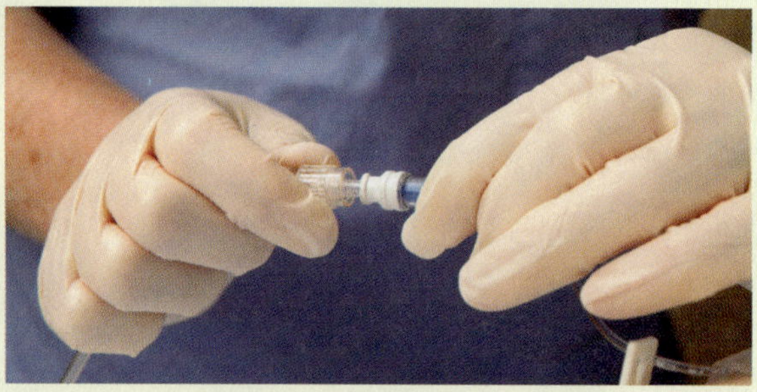

STEP 20 Connect IV tubing to the short extension set that is attached to catheter.

STEP	RATIONALE
c. *Sterile gauze dressing:* If manufactured catheter stabilization device is not used, secure catheter by placing a narrow piece (½ inch) of sterile tape over catheter hub. Place sterile tape only on hub, *never* over the insertion site. Secure site for easy visualization. Avoid applying tape or gauze around arm.	Use of sterile tape prevents site contamination. Regular adhesive tape is potential source of pathogenic bacteria (INS, 2011). Secure taping prevents back-and-forth motion of catheter. Wrapping anything around arm may compress veins or prevent visualization of the site.
(1) Place sterile 2 × 2 gauze pad over insertion site and catheter hub. Secure all edges with tape. Do not cover connection between IV tubing and catheter hub (see illustration).	A secure dressing is less likely to allow entrance of microorganisms.
(2) Fold 2 × 2 gauze in half and cover with a 1-inch-wide tape extending about an inch from each side. Place under tubing/catheter hub junction.	Tape on top of gauze makes it easier to access hub/tubing junction. Gauze pad elevates hub off skin to prevent pressure area.

***Clinical Decision Point:* Think carefully about where you place tape. Do not apply it over catheter insertion site, over connection between tubing or port and IV catheter hub, or on top of transparent dressing.**

STEP	RATIONALE
22. Curl loop of tubing along the arm and place second piece of tape directly over tubing to secure it (see illustration).	Securing loop of tubing reduces risk of dislodging catheter if IV tubing is pulled (i.e., loop comes apart before catheter dislodges).
23. For continuous infusion, check ordered rate of infusion programmed into EID and be sure it is functioning properly. If using gravity-flow IV infusion, recheck flow rate to correct drops per minute (see Skill 18-2).	Manipulation of catheter during dressing application may alter flow rate. Maintains correct rate of flow for IV solution.

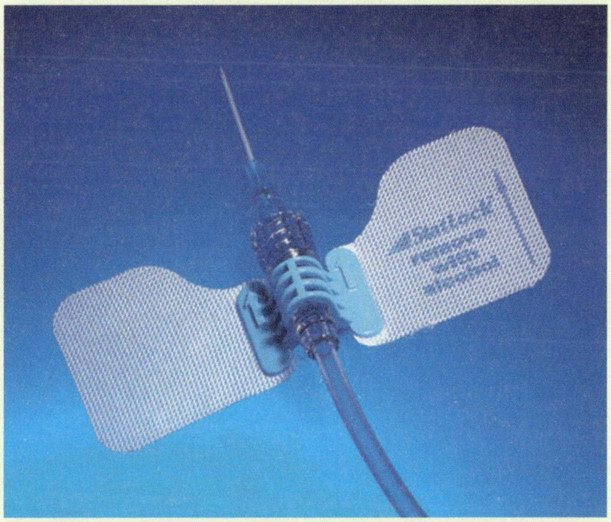

STEP 21a Catheter stabilization device. (Copyright C.R. Bard, Inc. Used with permission.)

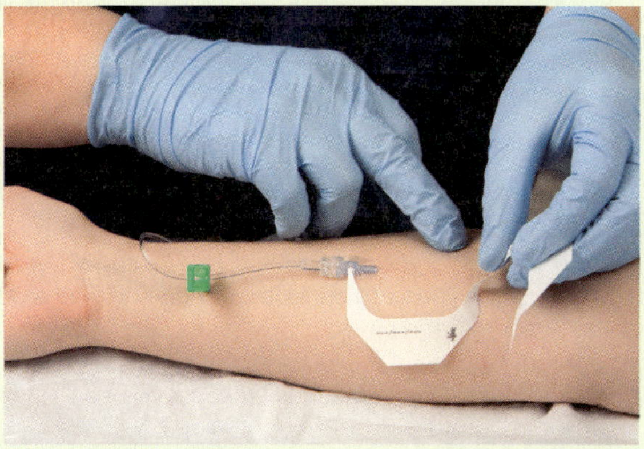

STEP 21b(1) Apply transparent dressing.

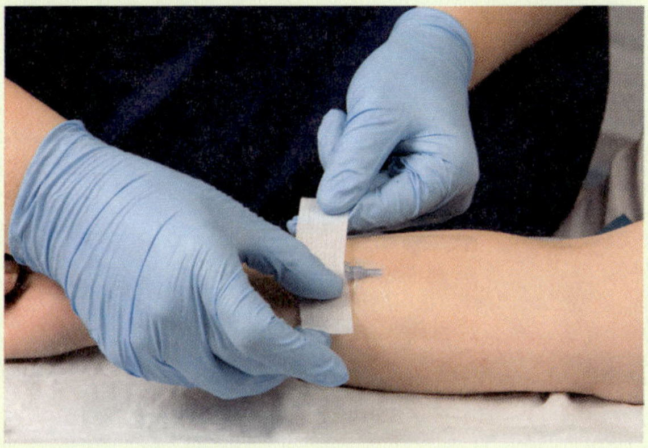

STEP 21b(2) Place tape over extension tubing.

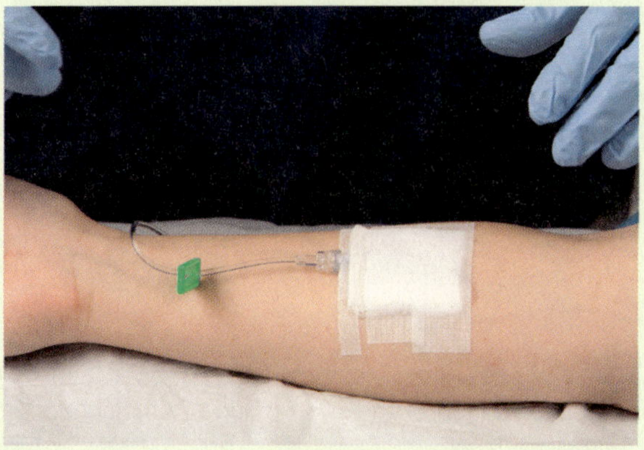

STEP 21c(1) Place 2 × 2 gauze over insertion site and catheter hub.

SKILL 18-1 INITIATING INTRAVENOUS THERAPY—cont'd

STEP	RATIONALE
24. Label dressing per agency policy. Include date and time of IV insertion, date and time of dressing change, VAD gauge size and length, and your initials (see illustration).	Provides immediate access to data as to when IV was inserted and when to rotate site.
25. Dispose of used stylet or other sharps in appropriate sharps container. Discard supplies. Remove gloves and perform hand hygiene.	Reduces transmission of microorganisms, prevents accidental needlestick injuries, and follows Centers for Disease Control and Prevention guidelines for disposal of sharps.
26. Instruct patient how to position arm or move or turn without dislodging VAD.	Prevents accidental dislodgement of catheter.

Clinical Decision Point: **Change peripheral IV access per agency policy, per health care provider's orders, or immediately on suspected contamination or complication. Change dressing only if it is soiled or no longer intact (INS, 2011).**

EVALUATION

STEP	RATIONALE
1. Observe patient every 1 to 2 hours or at established intervals per agency policy and procedures:	Frequency of site assessment should be determined by characteristics of patient and IV solution (Gorski et al., 2012).
a. Check that correct amount of IV solution has infused by observing fluid level in IV container.	Administration of prescribed fluid amount maintains or restores fluid balance.
b. Check rate on EID or count drip rate (if gravity drip).	Accurate monitoring of rate further ensures administration of correct amount of fluid.
c. Check patency of VAD.	Flow rate slows or stops if catheter becomes partially occluded.
d. Observe patient during palpation of vessel for signs of discomfort.	Tenderness can be an early sign of phlebitis.
e. Inspect insertion site, note skin color (e.g., redness, pallor). Inspect for presence of swelling, infiltration, and phlebitis (see Table 18-9). Palpate temperature of skin above dressing.	Redness, inflammation, tenderness, and warmth indicate phlebitis. Swelling above insertion site and cool temperature may indicate infiltration of fluid into tissues.
2. Observe patient to determine response to therapy (e.g., intake and output, weights, vital signs).	Purpose of IV fluids and additives is to maintain or restore fluid and electrolyte balance. Early recognition of problems leads to prompt treatment.
3. Use Teach Back—State to patient, "I want to be sure that I explained how you should position your arm and move about while this IV line is in place. Can you show me now how to position your arm correctly and turn on your side?" Revise your instruction now or develop plan for revised patient teaching to be implemented at an appropriate time if patient is not able to teach back correctly.	Evaluates what the patient is able to explain or demonstrate.

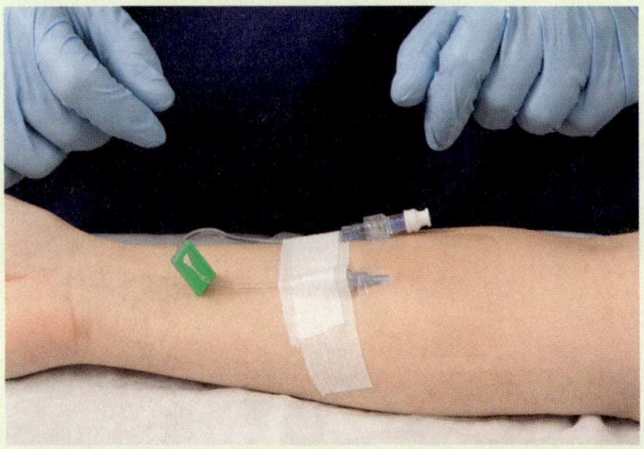

STEP 22 Curl a loop of the short or long IV tubing along the arm. Secure tubing.

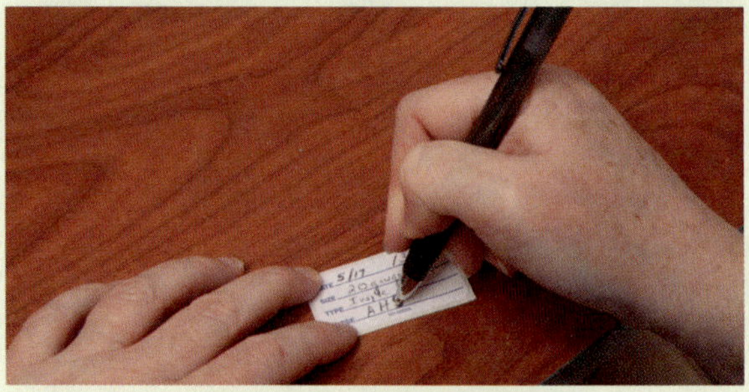

STEP 24 Label IV dressing.

RECORDING AND REPORTING

- Document in nurses' notes or other designated location in an electronic health record the date and time of insertion; number and sites of attempts; precise description of insertion site (e.g., cephalic vein on dorsal surface of right lower arm, 2.5 cm above wrist); any arm positioning restrictions; length and brand of catheter; type of dressing and catheter stabilization; flow rate; type of infusion; EID use; and your identity (INS, 2011). If using a bar-code system, fluid type and time records automatically.
- Document your evaluation of patient learning.
- Record patient's status, IV fluid, amount infused, and integrity and patency of system according to agency policy.
- Report to oncoming nursing staff: type of fluid, flow rate, status of VAD, amount of fluid remaining in present solution, expected time to hang subsequent IV container, and patient condition.
- Report to health care provider any adverse reactions.

UNEXPECTED OUTCOMES AND RELATED INTERVENTIONS

- Sudden infusion of large volume of solution, with patient having dyspnea, crackles in lungs, and bounding pulse, indicating ECV excess.
  - Slow infusion to keep vein open (KVO) rate.
  - Notify health care provider immediately.
  - Raise head of bed; administer oxygen and diuretics if ordered.
  - Monitor vital signs and laboratory reports.
  - Health care provider may adjust additives in IV solution or type of IV fluid; watch for and implement order.
- Infiltration or phlebitis (see Table 18-9)
  - Stop infusion and remove VAD.
  - Start new VAD in other extremity or proximal to previous insertion site if continued therapy is necessary.
  - Elevate affected extremity (infiltration) and apply warm moist compress to affected site.
  - Document degree of infiltration or phlebitis and nursing intervention.
- Local infection at insertion site
  - Notify health care provider before removing VAD. Anticipate order to culture catheter tip and/or the exudate around site.
  - Remove VAD after cultures are obtained (if ordered).
  - If antibiotic therapy is ordered, do not begin until blood cultures are obtained (if ordered).
- Bleeding at venipuncture site.
  - Verify that VAD is patent and place a pressure dressing over site or change dressing.
  - Start new VAD if VAD is dislodged or bleeding from site does not stop and if continued therapy is necessary.

SKILL 18-2 REGULATING INTRAVENOUS FLOW RATE

View Video!

DELEGATION CONSIDERATIONS

The skill of regulating intravenous (IV) flow rate cannot be delegated to nursing assistive personnel (NAP). Delegation to licensed practical nurses (LPNs) varies by state Nurse Practice Act. The nurse instructs NAP to inform the nurse if:

- Patient indicates burning, bleeding, swelling, or coolness at the catheter insertion site.
- The electronic infusion device (EID) alarm signals.
- The fluid container is almost empty.

EQUIPMENT

- For an EID: IV pump
- For gravity infusion: Volume-control device, watch with second hand
- Calculator or paper and pen/pencil
- Tape
- Label

STEP	RATIONALE
ASSESSMENT	
1. Review accuracy and completeness of health care provider's order for patient name, type and amount of IV fluid, medication additives, infusion rate, and length of therapy. Follow six rights of medication administration (see Chapter 17).	Before administering solutions or medications, an order from a licensed independent practitioner (LIP) is needed (INS, 2011).
2. Assess patient's knowledge of how positioning of IV site affects flow rate.	Fosters patient participation in maintaining most effective position of arm with IV equipment.
3. Perform hand hygiene.	Reduces transmission of microorganisms.
4. Observe for patency of vascular access device (VAD) and IV tubing.	For fluid to infuse at proper rate, IV tubing and VAD must be free of kinks, knots, and clots.

SKILL 18-2 REGULATING INTRAVENOUS FLOW RATE—cont'd

STEP	RATIONALE
5. Inspect IV site and verify with patient how venipuncture site feels (e.g., determine if any tenderness, pain, or burning exists).	Tenderness, pain, or burning may be early indication of phlebitis. Includes patient in own care.
6. Assess patient risk for fluid and electrolyte imbalance, given type of IV fluid (e.g., neonate, cardiac, or kidney disorder).	Helps prioritize nursing assessments.
PLANNING	
1. Identify patient using two identifiers (e.g., name and birthday or name and account number) according to agency policy. Compare identifiers with information on patient's MAR or medical record.	Ensures correct patient. Complies with The Joint Commission requirements for patient safety (TJC, 2014).
2. Gather paper and pen/pencil or calculator to calculate flow rate.	Use accurate mathematical calculations to obtain correct rate for patient safety.
3. Perform hand hygiene. Inspect IV site for signs and symptoms of IV-related complications such as pain, swelling, or redness.	Observation or report of an IV-related complication indicates need to reestablish patient IV access.
4. Check order to see how long to infuse each liter of fluid. If hourly rate (mL/hr) is not provided in the order, calculate milliliters per hour by dividing volume by hours. For example: Milliliters per hour = Total infusion volume (mL)/Hours of infusion 1000 mL/8 hr = 125 mL/hr *or* If 3 L is ordered for 24 hours, 3000 mL/24 hr = 125 mL/hr	Provides even infusion of fluid over prescribed hourly rate. A volume of 1 L = 1000 mL.

Clinical Decision Point: **Health care providers commonly write abbreviated IV orders such as "D_5W with 20 mEq KCl 125 mL/hr continuous." This order implies that you maintain the IV infusion at this rate until an order has been written to change the rate or for IV infusion to be discontinued. Occasionally an IV order calls for 1 L "TKO" or "KVO," either of which means at a slow rate to keep vein open. Clarify with the provider if any part of the order is not clear.**

STEP	RATIONALE
5. If KVO (or TKO) rate is ordered, check order or agency policy regarding the flow rate. KVO often falls in the range of 10-25 mL/hr.	KVO rate prevents catheter clotting, thus preserving IV access, while infusing a minimal amount of fluid. INS standards (2011) indicate that KVO orders contain a specific infusion rate.
6. Use hourly rate to program EID (see Implementation) or, if gravity-flow infusion, to calculate flow rate (drops/min).	
7. *For gravity-flow infusion:*	Use microdrip tubing when infusing small or very precise volumes. Use macrodrip tubing to infuse fluid more rapidly.
a. Determine drop factor (calibration) in drops per milliliter (gtt/mL) of infusion set currently available: *Microdrip:* 60 gtt/mL *Macrodrip:* 10 or 15 gtt/mL; see label on administration set packaging.	Drop factor for macrodrop tubing varies with the manufacturer.
b. Select one of the following formulas to calculate minute flow rate (drops/min) based on drop factor of infusion set: (1) Milliliters per hour/60 min = Milliliters per minute and Drop factor × Milliliters per minute = Drops per minute Or (2) Milliliters per hour × Drop factor/60 min = Drops per minute Example: Using formula (2) above, calculate minute flow rate for an IV infusion that is ordered to infuse at 125 mL/hr:	Formulas compute correct flow rate per minute.

STEP	RATIONALE
Microdrip: 125 mL/hr × 60 gtt/min/60 min = 125 gtt/min *Macrodrip with drop factor of 15 gtt/min:* 125 mL/hr × 15 gtt/min/60 min = 31-32 gtt/min	When using microdrip, milliliters per hour always equals drops per minute.
IMPLEMENTATION	
1. *Using an EID (infusion pump or smart pump):*	Smart pumps with medication software are designed for administration of IV fluid that contains medications.
a. Consult manufacturer directions for setup of the infusion. Use tubing compatible with the EID.	Special infusion tubing is required for most EIDs. It is designed to prevent free flow of fluid when tubing is removed from the device. Check agency equipment and associated policy and procedures.
b. Close roller clamp on primed IV tubing and insert tubing into chamber of EID control mechanism or pump module per manufacturer directions (see illustration). Roller clamp on IV tubing goes between EID and patient.	Most electronic infusion pumps use positive pressure to infuse. They move fluid through the IV tubing by compressing and milking the tubing.
c. Turn on EID power, test the alarm, select required volume per hour, volume to be infused (VTBI), and any other information required. Close control chamber door if not already done and press run/start button. If a smart pump alarms immediately and shuts down, your settings were outside the unit parameters. Recalculate the infusion rate and set the EID again.	Program EID per manufacturer instructions for patient safety. Smart pumps require additional information such as patient unit and medication. Smart pumps contain a computer that matches the pump setting against a drug dose database. If your setting does not match the database, the pump will alarm and automatically shut down for patient safety.
d. Open roller clamp completely while EID is in use.	Ensures that EID regulates infusion rate.
e. Monitor infusion rate and IV site for complications according to agency policy. Use watch to verify rate of infusion even when using EID.	EIDs do not replace frequent, accurate nursing evaluation. They may continue to infuse IV fluids even after an infiltration or other complication (INS, 2011).
f. Assess patency of system and resolve the problem if EID alarm sounds.	Alarm indicates a problem in the system. Empty solution container, kinked tubing, air in tubing, closed clamp, infiltration, clotted catheter, or low battery trigger the EID alarm.
2. *Using gravity flow:* Confirm hourly rate and minute rate based on drop factor of infusion set. Microdrip infusion set has a drop factor of 60 gtt/mL. Regular drip or macrodrip infusion set, used in this example, has a drop factor of 15 gtt/mL. Using formula (see Planning Step 7), calculate minute flow rate.	
a. Ensure that IV fluid container is 36 inches above IV site for adults.	Pressure caused by gravity is necessary to overcome venous pressure and resistance from tubing and catheter.

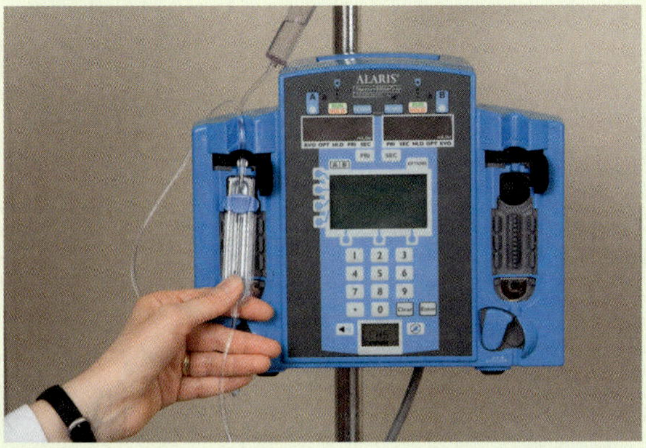

STEP 1b Insert IV tubing into chamber of EID control mechanism.

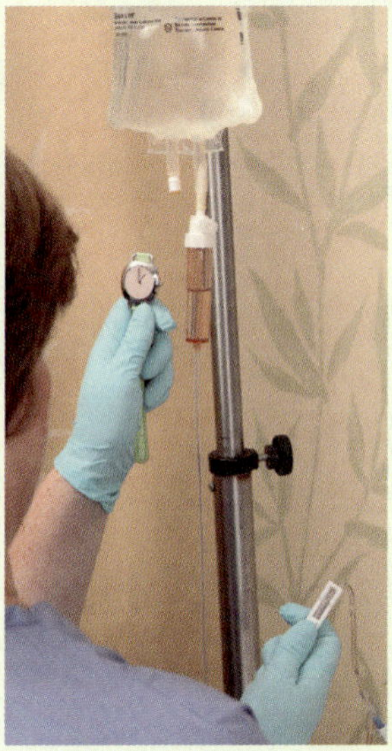

STEP 2b Nurse counting drip rate on gravity-flow infusion.

SKILL 18-2 REGULATING INTRAVENOUS FLOW RATE—cont'd

STEP	RATIONALE
b. Slowly open roller clamp on tubing until you see drops in drip chamber. Hold a watch with a second hand at same level as drip chamber and count drip rate for 1 minute (see illustration). Adjust roller clamp to increase or decrease drip rate until you obtain the desired number of drops per minute.	Regulates flow to prescribed rate.
c. Monitor drip rate at least hourly.	Many factors influence drip rate; frequent monitoring ensures IV fluid administration as prescribed.
3. *Using volume-control device with gravity flow:*	The device is a graduated chamber with tubing inserted in an IV line just below the IV fluid container. It is used in pediatric units if an EID is not used.
a. Insert volume-control device spike into IV container and insert spike of infusion set into bottom end of volume-controller tubing, using aseptic technique.	Delivers small volume of fluid to prevent bolus administration in case of equipment malfunction; especially important in pediatric units. You need to refill it when fluid volume becomes low.
b. Place no more than 2 hours' allotment of fluid into device by opening clamp between IV fluid container and device (see illustration).	Allows for continuous infusion of fluid if you do not return in exactly 60 minutes to refill volume controller. If infusion rate accidentally increases, patient receives only a 2-hour portion of fluid.
c. Regulate flow rate manually with roller clamp by counting drops in drip chamber for 1 minute by watch and adjusting roller clamp to increase or decrease infusion rate.	Regulate to prescribed rate of fluid infusion.
d. Assess system at least hourly; add fluid to volume control device. Regulate flow rate.	Maintains patency of system and provides patient monitoring.
4. Attach label to IV fluid container with date and time of container change (check agency policy). If using polyvinylchloride (PVC) container, mark only on label and not on container.	Provides data to determine next time for container change, especially with KVO rate. Ink may leach into IV fluid through PVC container.
5. Instruct patient to avoid raising hand or arm with IV line because that can affect flow rate, to avoid touching control clamp or other equipment, and about the purpose of EID alarms.	Provides information so patient does not alter infusion rate. Ask patient to instruct family if appropriate.
EVALUATION	
1. Monitor IV infusion at least every hour, noting volume of IV fluid infused and rate.	Ensures that correct volume infuses over prescribed time period.
2. Observe patient for signs of overhydration or dehydration to determine response to therapy.	Signs and symptoms of new overhydration or continued dehydration warrant changing rate of fluid infused. Contact health care provider for new infusion rate order.
3. Evaluate for signs of complications with IV flow rate: infiltration, inflammation at site, occluded VAD, or kink or obstruction in infusion tubing.	Prevents or identifies complications that decrease or stop flow rate.

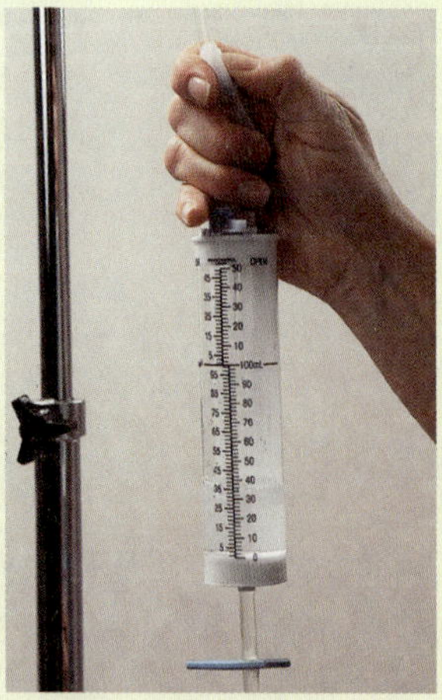

STEP 3b Open regulator clamp to fill volume-control device.

RECORDING AND REPORTING

- Record rate of infusion in milliliters per hour (or drops per minute with gravity flow) and use of EID or volume control device in IV flow sheet or other appropriate form.
- Immediately record any new IV fluid rate.
- At change of shift or when leaving on break, report rate of and volume left in infusion to nurse in charge or next nurse assigned to care for patient.

UNEXPECTED OUTCOMES AND RELATED INTERVENTIONS

- Sudden infusion of large volume of solution, with patient having dyspnea, crackles in lungs, and bounding pulse, indicating extracellular fluid volume excess
  - Slow infusion to KVO rate.
  - Notify health care provider immediately.
  - Raise head of bed; administer diuretics if ordered.
  - Monitor vital signs and laboratory reports.
  - Health care provider may adjust additives in IV solution or type of IV fluid; watch for and implement order.
- IV fluid container empties with subsequent loss of VAD patency
  - Discontinue present IV infusion and start new IV line in other extremity or proximal to previous insertion site.
- IV drip infuses more slowly than ordered.
  - Check for positional change that might affect rate, EID malfunction (or insufficient height of gravity-flow IV fluid container), tubing kink or obstruction, infiltration or other complication at VAD site.
  - Consult health care provider for new order to provide necessary fluid volume.

SKILL 18-3 CHANGING INTRAVENOUS SOLUTION AND TUBING

DELEGATION CONSIDERATIONS

The skill of changing intravenous (IV) solutions and tubing cannot be delegated to nursing assistive personnel (NAP). Delegation to licensed practical nurses (LPNs) varies by state Nurse Practice Act. The nurse instructs NAP to inform the nurse if:

- Any leakage occurs from or around the IV tubing.
- IV solution has any cloudiness or visible particles.
- IV container is near completion.

EQUIPMENT

- Correct volume and type of IV solution as ordered by the health care provider
- Infusion tubing
- Tape or label
- Filter (size appropriate to solution) and extension tubing (if necessary)
- Clean gloves
- Handheld bar-code scanner if using bar-code system

In Addition for Continuous Intravenous Infusion

- Infusion tubing
- 0.22-µm filter and extension tubing (if necessary)
- Tubing label
- Antiseptic swab (2% chlorhexidine)

In Addition for Intermittent Saline Lock

- Syringe containing 1 to 3 mL of preservative-free 0.9% sodium chloride (INS, 2011)
- 2 × 2 gauze pads (optional)
- Loop or short extension tubing (if necessary), injection cap or PRN adapter
- Antiseptic swab (2% chlorhexidine)

STEP	RATIONALE
ASSESSMENT	
1. *Changing IV fluid container:*	
a. Review accuracy and completeness of health care provider's order for patient name, type and amount of IV fluid, medication additives, infusion rate, and length of therapy. Follow six rights of medication administration (see Chapter 17). If order is written for keep vein open (KVO or TKO) rate, note date and time of last fluid container change and refer to agency policy to determine need for IV fluid container change.	Before administering solutions or medications, an order from a licensed independent practitioner (LIP) is needed (INS, 2011). Agency policy determines how often IV fluid container change is required for KVO infusion rate.
b. Check IV solution for integrity, including but not limited to discoloration, cloudiness, leakage, expiration date. Determine compatibility of all IV fluids and additives by consulting approved online database, drug reference book, or pharmacist.	If there has been a break in integrity of solution container, a new bag is needed. Incompatibilities can cause physical and chemical changes with adverse patient outcomes (INS, 2011).

SKILL 18-3 CHANGING INTRAVENOUS SOLUTION AND TUBING—cont'd

STEP	RATIONALE
2. *Changing IV tubing:*	
a. Assess current tubing for puncture, contamination, or occlusion, which requires immediate tubing change.	Compromised tubing allows fluid leakage, bacterial contamination, and entry of pathogens into patient's bloodstream. Blood, blood components, or incompatible mixtures can occlude or partially occlude tubing because viscous solutions adhere to walls of tubing, decreasing size of lumen.
b. Note date and time of last tubing change. Agency policy indicates frequency of routine change for IV administration sets and tubing used intermittently with saline locks.	INS (2011) recommends changing continuous IV tubing no more often than 96-hour intervals unless tubing becomes compromised. Change primary intermittent tubing set every 24 hours (INS, 2011).
3. Determine patient's/family's understanding of need for IV therapy.	Reveals need for patient teaching.
PLANNING	
1. Collect appropriate equipment. *For changing IV fluid container:* Have next solution prepared at least 1 hour before needed. If prepared in pharmacy, ensure that it has been delivered to patient care unit. Check that solution is correct and properly labeled. Allow it to warm to room temperature if refrigerated. Check solution expiration date. Observe for particles, discoloration, and leakage.	Adequate planning for changing solution reduces risk of clot formation at catheter tip resulting from lack of flow from empty IV container. Checking that solution is correct prevents medication error.
2. Coordinate tubing changes with IV fluid container changes if possible.	Promotes patient safety by reducing number of times IV system is open.
3. Identify patient using two identifiers (e.g., name and birthday or name and account number) according to agency policy. Compare identifiers with information on patient's MAR or medical record. If using bar-code system, scan bar-code on patient's wristband and then bar-code on the IV fluid container.	Ensures correct patient. Complies with The Joint Commission requirements for patient safety (TJC, 2014). Bar-code systems reduce medication errors by verifying right patient, medication, dose, and time with electronic medical record (Poon et al., 2010).
4. Explain to patient/family the procedure, its purpose, and what is expected of patient.	Promotes patient cooperation and decreases anxiety.
IMPLEMENTATION	
1. Perform hand hygiene.	Reduces transmission of microorganisms.
2. Determine patency of current vascular access device (VAD) site: Look for swelling, coolness to touch, or tenderness around VAD site. With electronic infusion device (EID) use, VAD should be patent if site is not infiltrated and EID functions without alarm signals. If not using EID, carefully adjust roller clamp to see an increase in flow rate and then regulate back to prescribed rate. With saline lock, cleanse port with alcohol and allow to dry; insert syringe and then aspirate for blood return to confirm VAD patency.	New IV access site needed if infiltration or phlebitis is present, IV tubing is compromised, or VAD site is not patent. EID alarm signals when system is occluded. In absence of EID, adjusting roller clamp increases flow rate when there is no obstruction.

Clinical Decision Point: **Choose appropriate method to determine patency of VAD site. Lowering IV fluid container below level of IV site for presence of blood return is an unreliable indicator of patency.**

STEP	RATIONALE
3. *Changing IV fluid container with existing tubing of continuous IV infusion:*	
a. Begin to change container when about 50 mL of fluid remains in old container. Be sure that drip chamber is at least half full.	Prevents air from entering tubing and vein from clotting from lack of flow.
b. Prepare new IV fluid container. If using plastic bag, remove protective cover from IV tubing port. If using glass bottle, remove metal cap and disks.	Permits quick, smooth, and organized change from old to new solution.
c. Close roller clamp to stop flow of existing solution. Remove tubing from EID. Then remove old IV fluid container from IV pole and hold it with tubing port pointing upward.	Prevents solution remaining in drip chamber from emptying while changing IV fluid container. Port held upward prevents IV fluid from spilling.

STEP	RATIONALE
d. Quickly remove spike from old solution container and, without touching tip, insert spike into new container (see illustrations).	Reduces risk of drip chamber becoming empty and maintains sterility.
***Clinical Decision Point:* If you contaminate the spike, discard that IV tubing and use a new one.**	
e. Hang new fluid container on IV pole.	Gravity assists delivery of fluid into drip chamber.
f. Check for air in tubing. If bubbles form, remove them by closing roller clamp below bubbles, stretching tubing downward, and tapping tubing with fingers (bubbles rise in fluid to drip chamber). For larger amount of air, swab port below air with alcohol and allow to dry; insert needleless syringe into port and aspirate air into syringe.	Reduces risk for air entering the tubing. Use of an air-eliminating filter also reduces this risk.
g. Make sure that drip chamber is one-third to one-half full. If it is too full, pinch off tubing below drip chamber, invert container, squeeze drip chamber to push fluid into container, release tubing, and hang container.	Reduces risk of air entering tubing. If chamber is completely filled, you cannot observe drips.
h. Insert tubing into EID and restart pump at prescribed rate. If no EID, regulate flow to prescribed rate with roller clamp.	Delivers IV fluid as ordered.
i. Attach piece of tape or label to IV fluid container with date and time of container change (check agency policy). If using polyvinylchloride (PVC) container, mark only on label and not on container.	Provides reference to determine next time for container change, especially with deep vein open (KVO) rate. Ink may leach into fluid through PVC container.
4. *Changing IV tubing:*	
a. Open new infusion set and connect add-on pieces (e.g., filters, extension tubing). Keep protective coverings over infusion spike and distal connector for VAD. Secure all connections.	Protective covers maintain sterility. Securing connections reduces risk of contamination, infection, and hemorrhage.
b. Apply clean gloves.	Reduces transmission of microorganisms.
c. If catheter hub is not accessible, remove IV dressing (see Skill 18-4). Do not remove tape that secures catheter to skin. Leave old tubing connected to catheter hub until tubing is prepared.	Catheter hub must be accessible to provide smooth transition when removing old and inserting new tubing.
d. *Change IV fluid container and tubing of existing continuous IV infusion:*	
(1) Close roller clamp on new IV tubing.	Prevents fluid spillage after spiking container.
(2) Slow rate of infusion to existing IV by regulating roller clamp on old tubing to KVO rate.	Prevents complete infusion of fluid remaining in tubing, thus decreasing risk of VAD clotting.
(3) Compress and fill drip chamber of old tubing.	Ensures that drip chamber contains enough fluid to maintain IV patency while changing tubing.
(4) Invert old IV fluid container and remove old tubing. Keep spike sterile and upright. *Optional:* Tape old drip chamber to IV pole without contaminating spike.	Allows fluid to continue to flow through VAD while new tubing is prepared.

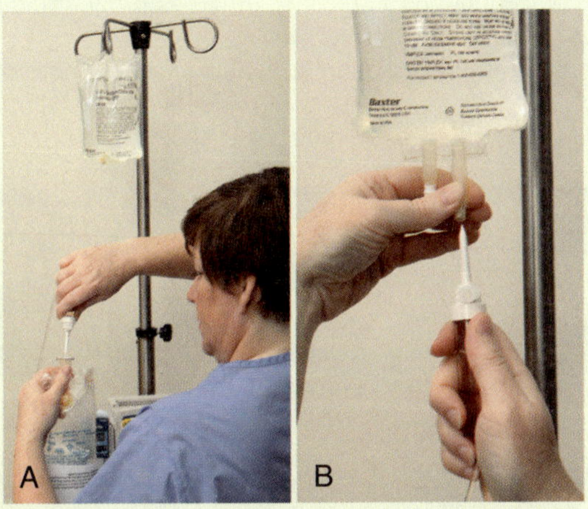

STEP 3d **A,** Quickly remove spike from old solution container. **B,** Without touching tip, insert spike into new container.

SKILL 18-3 CHANGING INTRAVENOUS SOLUTION AND TUBING—cont'd

STEP	RATIONALE
(5) Place insertion spike of new tubing into new IV fluid container. Hang container on IV pole, compress and release drip chamber on new tubing, and fill drip chamber one-third to one-half full. If you contaminate spike before inserting it into container, discard that IV tubing and use new one.	Permits flow of fluid from fluid container into new infusion tubing. Maintains sterility to prevent infection.
(6) Slowly open roller clamp, remove protective cap from adapter (if necessary), and flush new tubing with solution. Close roller clamp when tubing is full. Replace cap. Place capped end of adapter near patient's IV site.	Removes air from tubing, replacing it with fluid. Priming slowly reduces formation of air bubbles in tubing. Positions equipment for quick smooth connection of new tubing.
(7) Stop EID if used and close roller clamp on old tubing.	Prevents fluid spillage when tubing is removed from VAD.
(8) Remove manufactured catheter stabilization device from tubing if present. Gently disconnect old tubing from catheter hub and quickly insert adapter of new tubing into catheter hub, maintaining sterility of point of entry of connections.	Allows smooth transition from old to new tubing, minimizing time system is open to contamination. Careful technique prevents VAD dislodgement or vein trauma during tubing change and prevents transmission of microorganisms.
(9) Open roller clamp on new tubing, allowing solution to run rapidly for 30-60 seconds. Then regulate drip rate using EID or roller clamp if no EID.	Brief rapid flow ensures catheter patency and prevents occlusion. Regulation restores infusion rate to deliver IV fluid as prescribed.
e. *Change existing saline lock:*	
(1) If a loop or short extension tubing is needed, use sterile technique to connect new injection cap to new loop or tubing.	Sterile technique prevents infection.
(2) Swab injection cap with antiseptic swab and let dry. Insert syringe with 1 to 3 mL saline solution and inject through injection cap into loop of extension tubing. Place capped end of tubing near patient's IV site.	Removes air from tubing, preventing it from entering vein. Maintains patency of VAD.
(3) Gently disconnect old tubing from extension tubing and quickly insert adapter of new tubing connection, maintaining sterility of point of entry of connections (see illustrations).	Allows smooth transition from old to new tubing, minimizing time that system is open to contamination.
f. Apply new manufactured catheter stabilization device if used. Form loop of tubing and secure it to patient's arm with a strip of tape.	Avoids accidental pulling against IV site and stabilizes the catheter.
g. Attach label with date and time of solution change onto tubing, below drip chamber if a continuous infusion.	Provides reference to determine next time for tubing change.
h. Remove and discard used supplies. If necessary apply new dressing (see Skill 18-4). Remove and dispose of gloves. Perform hand hygiene.	Reduces transmission of microorganisms.
EVALUATION	
1. Observe connections for leakage. For continuous infusion: Evaluate IV flow rate and patency of system hourly.	Ensures proper fluid administration.
2. Observe patient for signs of overhydration or dehydration to determine response to IV therapy.	Signs and symptoms of new overhydration or continued dehydration warrant changing rate of fluid infused. Contact health care provider for new infusion rate order.

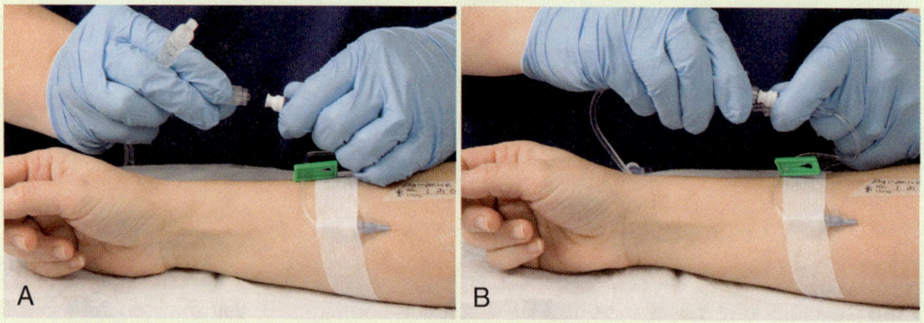

STEP 4e(3) **A,** Disconnect old tubing. **B,** Insert adapter of new tubing.

RECORDING AND REPORTING

- Record amount and type of fluid infused, amount and type of fluid started, and tubing change on appropriate IV flow sheet and intake and output record according to agency policy.

UNEXPECTED OUTCOMES AND RELATED INTERVENTIONS

- Flow rate is incorrect or absent; patient receives too little or too much fluid.
  - Readjust infusion rate to ordered rate.
  - Evaluate patient for adverse effects; notify health care provider if apparent.
  - Determine and correct cause of incorrect or absent flow rate (e.g., positional change that might affect rate, EID malfunction or incorrect programming of EID (or insufficient height of gravity-flow IV fluid container), tubing kink or obstruction, infiltration or other complication at VAD site).
  - Notify health care provider if patient's anticipated infusion is 100-200 mL less than or greater than expected (check agency policy).

SKILL 18-4 CHANGING A PERIPHERAL INTRAVENOUS DRESSING

DELEGATION CONSIDERATIONS

The skill of changing a peripheral intravenous (IV) dressing cannot be delegated to nursing assistive personnel (NAP). The nurse instructs NAP to:

- Report to the nurse if a patient mentions moistness or loosening of IV dressing.
- Protect the IV dressing during hygiene and activities of daily living.

EQUIPMENT

- Antiseptic swabs (2% chlorhexidine)
- Skin protectant swab *(optional)*
- Adhesive remover *(optional)*
- Clean gloves
- Strips of nonallergenic tape
- Manufactured catheter stabilization device if available
- Commercially available IV site protection device *(optional)*
- Sterile transparent dressing

or

- Sterile 2 × 2– or 4 × 4–inch gauze pad

STEP	RATIONALE
ASSESSMENT	
1. Determine when dressing was last changed. Dressing label includes date and time applied; size, and type of venous access device (VAD); and date VAD was inserted.	Provides information regarding length of time that present dressing has been in place. In addition, you are able to plan for dressing change (INS, 2011).
2. Perform hand hygiene. Observe present dressing for moisture and intactness. Determine whether moisture is from site leakage or external source.	Moisture is medium for bacterial growth and renders dressing contaminated. Loose dressing increases risk for bacterial contamination of venipuncture site or displacement of VAD.
3. Observe IV system for proper functioning or complications. Apply clean gloves if dressing is moist. Palpate VAD site through the intact dressing, assessing for pain or burning.	Unexplained decrease in flow rate requires investigating VAD placement and patency. Pain is associated with both phlebitis and infiltration.
4. Monitor body temperature.	Elevated body temperature sometimes is related to infection at the VAD site or systemic complication. (There are many other causes of elevated body temperature.)
5. Assess patient's understanding of the need for continued IV infusion.	Determines need for patient teaching.
PLANNING	
1. Identify patient using two identifiers (e.g., name and birthday or name and account number) according to agency policy. Compare identifiers with information on patient's MAR or medical record.	Ensures correct patient. Complies with The Joint Commission requirements for patient safety (TJC, 2014).
2. Explain procedure and purpose to patient and family. Explain that patient needs to hold affected extremity still and how long procedure will take.	Decreases anxiety, promotes cooperation, and gives patient time frame around which to plan personal activities.

SKILL 18-4 CHANGING A PERIPHERAL INTRAVENOUS DRESSING—cont'd

STEP	RATIONALE
3. Following procedure explain to patient the importance of alerting nurse to burning sensations at venipuncture site or leakage of IV solution on dressing.	Indicates an occlusion of IV catheter or dislodgement of catheter itself.
IMPLEMENTATION	
1. Perform hand hygiene. Collect equipment. Apply clean gloves.	Reduces transmission of microorganisms.
2. Remove transparent dressing by pulling up one corner and pulling dressing laterally while holding catheter hub and tubing with nondominant hand (see illustration). Leave tape that secures IV catheter in place. *For gauze dressing,* stabilize catheter hub while removing old dressing one layer at a time. Be cautious if catheter tubing becomes tangled between two layers of dressing.	Prevents accidental displacement of VAD.
3. Observe insertion site for signs and symptoms of infiltration, phlebitis (see Table 18-9), and local infection (inflammation and exudate). Discontinue infusion if complication exists.	Presence of infiltration, phlebitis, or local infection requires removal of VAD and new IV start in other extremity or proximal to previous insertion site if continued therapy is necessary.
4. Prepare new strips of sterile adhesive. If IV infusion is infusing properly, gently remove tape that secures VAD. Stabilize VAD with one hand. Use adhesive remover to cleanse skin and remove adhesive residue if needed.	Exposes venipuncture site. Stabilization prevents accidental displacement of VAD. Adhesive residue decreases ability of new tape to adhere tightly to skin.

Clinical Decision Point: **Keep one finger stabilizing VAD at all times until tape or dressing is applied. If patient is restless or uncooperative, ask another nurse to assist.**

STEP	RATIONALE
5. While stabilizing VAD, cleanse insertion site. Use an antiseptic swab, applying friction in a horizontal plane. Then discard and take a new swab, applying friction in a vertical plane. Use a third swab to clean in a circular pattern moving from the insertion site outward (see illustration). Allow antiseptic to dry completely.	Mechanical friction in this pattern allows penetration of antiseptic solution into epidermal layer of the skin.
6. *Optional:* Apply skin protectant solution to area where you will apply the tape or transparent dressing. Allow to dry.	Coats skin with protective solution to maintain skin integrity, prevents irritation from adhesive, and promotes adhesion of dressing.
7. While securing catheter, apply sterile dressing over site (procedures differ; follow agency policy).	
a. *Manufactured catheter stabilization device:* Apply as directed in Skill 18-1, Implementation Step 21a.	A manufactured catheter stabilization device is a sterile, adhesive pad that holds the catheter in place, improving patient outcomes by reducing risk of catheter dislodgement, phlebitis, and other complications (INS, 2011).
b. *Transparent dressing:* Apply as directed in Skill 18-1, Implementation Step 21b.	Occlusive dressing protects site from bacterial contamination.

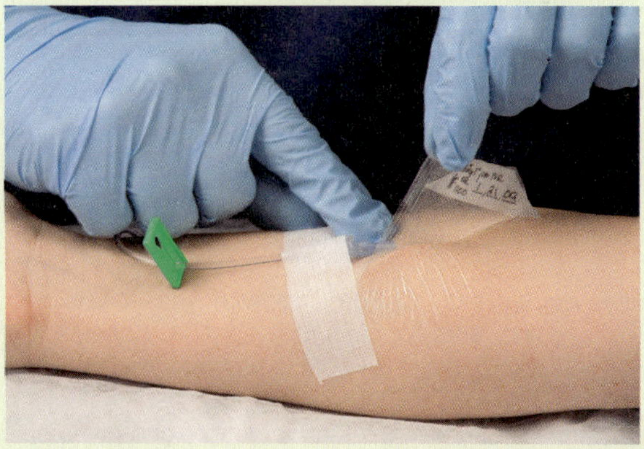

STEP 2 Remove transparent dressing by pulling it laterally.

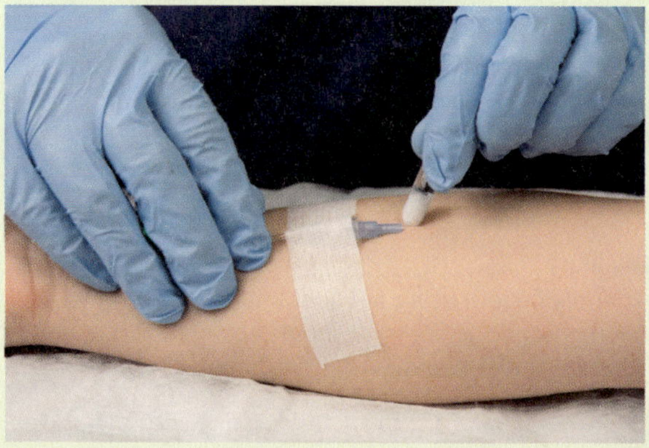

STEP 5 Cleanse peripheral insertion site with antiseptic swab.

STEP	RATIONALE
c. *Gauze dressing:* Apply as directed in Skill 18-1, Implementation Step 21c.	Less frequently used than transparent dressing.

***Clinical Decision Point:* Think carefully about where you place tape. Do not apply it over catheter insertion site, over connection between tubing or port and catheter hub, or on top of transparent dressing.**

STEP	RATIONALE
8. Remove and discard gloves.	Reduces transmission of microorganisms.
9. *Optional:* Apply a protective device (see Figure 18-9) over area if patient may pick at or bump dressing.	Site protection devices include vented plastic or stretch netting coverings and mitts for hands. Reduces risk for phlebitis, infiltration, or catheter displacement from mechanical motion.
10. Anchor IV tubing with additional pieces of tape if necessary.	Prevents accidental displacement of VAD.
11. Label dressing per agency policy. Label information includes date and time of original IV insertion, VAD gauge and length.	Labeling with IV insertion date and VAD length facilitates appropriate site rotation and safe discontinuation of IV access.
12. Discard equipment and perform hand hygiene.	Reduces transmission of microorganisms.
EVALUATION	
1. Observe function, patency of IV system, and flow rate after changing dressing.	Validates that IV is patent and functioning correctly. Manipulation of catheter and tubing may affect rate of infusion.
2. Inspect dressing after some time elapses to ensure that it has not become loose or moist again.	Validates that dressing replacement has been effective, maintaining patient safety.
3. Use Teach Back—State to patient, "I want to be sure that I explained why you need to alert the nurse if the IV loosens or begins to leak. Can you tell me why this is important?" Revise your instruction now or develop plan for revised patient teaching to be implemented at an appropriate time if patient is not able to teach back correctly.	Evaluates what patient is able to explain or demonstrate.

RECORDING AND REPORTING

- Record time that peripheral IV dressing was changed, reason for change, type of dressing material used, patency of system, and description of venipuncture site on IV flow sheet or appropriate form.
- Record any patient education regarding integrity of venipuncture site in nurses' notes.
- Document your evaluation of patient learning.
- Report any complications to health care provider and document that you did so.
- Report to nurse in charge or oncoming nursing shift that dressing was changed and any significant information about integrity of system.

UNEXPECTED OUTCOMES AND RELATED INTERVENTIONS

- Accidental VAD dislodgement or removal
  - Start new VAD in other extremity or proximal to previous insertion site if continued therapy is needed.
  - Reinforce to patient need to inform nurse if is dislodged.
- Infiltration or phlebitis (see Table 18-9)
  - Stop infusion and remove VAD.
  - Start new VAD in other extremity or proximal to previous insertion site if continued therapy is necessary.
  - Elevate affected extremity (infiltration) and apply warm moist compress to affected site.
  - Document degree of infiltration or phlebitis and nursing intervention.
- Local infection at insertion site
  - Notify health care provider before removing VAD. Culture of catheter tip and/or exudate probably will be ordered.
  - Remove VAD after cultures are obtained if ordered.
  - If antibiotic therapy is ordered, do not begin until blood cultures are obtained if ordered.

KEY POINTS

- Body fluids, consisting of water and the substances dissolved or suspended in it, are distributed in ECF (vascular plus interstitial) and ICF compartments.
- To maintain normal fluid and electrolyte balance, daily intake must equal the output and the fluid, and electrolytes must be distributed normally between body fluid compartments.
- Fluid output normally occurs through skin, lungs, GI tract, and kidneys and may also occur through abnormal routes in patient populations.
- Patients who are very young or very old; whose I&O of fluid and/or electrolytes are not equal; or who have various hormone imbalances, chronic diseases, or trauma are at greatest risk for fluid, electrolyte, and acid-base imbalances.
- ECV excess and deficit are abnormal volumes of isotonic sodium-containing fluid, manifested as sudden changes in body weight and changes in markers of vascular and interstitial volume.
- Osmolality imbalances are abnormal concentration of body fluids, manifested as altered serum sodium concentration and altered level of consciousness.
- Treatment for ECV excess is sodium restriction plus fluid restriction if severe; treatment for hyponatremia usually is water restriction.
- Enteral or parenteral administration of appropriate fluids prevents or treats ECV deficit, hypernatremia, and electrolyte deficits.
- Cellular metabolism constantly produces carbonic and metabolic acids; to maintain normal acid-base balance, carbonic acid must be excreted through the lungs, and metabolic acid must be buffered and then excreted through the kidneys.
- Acid-base imbalances are respiratory (excess or deficit of carbonic acid) or metabolic (excess or deficit of metabolic acids), manifested as changes in pH, $PaCO_2$, HCO_3^-, and level of consciousness.
- Initiation and maintenance of IV therapy require clinical decision making, skill, and organized procedures to maintain sterility and patency of the system.
- Nurses monitor for complications of IV therapy that include infiltration, phlebitis, infection, and overload of the specific IV fluid (see QSEN Activity: Quality Improvement).
- Administration of blood products entails a specific procedure for identification of the patient and the blood product and frequent monitoring during the transfusion for patient safety.
- Risks of blood transfusion include transfusion reactions, circulatory overload, infection, hyperkalemia, hypocalcemia, and hypomagnesemia from rapid administration of blood.
- Nursing interventions for acid-base imbalances support prescribed medical therapies and aim at treating the underlying disorder while providing for patient safety.

CLINICAL DECISION-MAKING EXERCISES

During Robert's assessment he finds that Mrs. Reynolds has decreased skin turgor and dry mucous membranes. The health care provider ordered assessing vital signs every 4 hours, nothing by mouth, I&O measurement, blood chemistry analysis, an IV infusion of 0.9% normal saline (NS) with 20 mEq KCl at 125 mL/hr, and an abdominal radiograph. Initial nursing diagnoses for Mrs. Reynolds are: Deficient Fluid Volume: Risk for Electrolyte Imbalance; and Deficient Knowledge of disease management related to fluid replacement for diarrhea.

1. What is the priority nursing diagnosis for Mrs. Reynolds now? Why?
2. Review Mrs. Reynolds' earlier case study. Which factors contributed to Mrs. Reynolds' fluid imbalance?
3. Additional assessment reveals that Mrs. Reynolds has a temperature of 38.2° C (100.9° F). How does this affect her condition?
4. When should *Deficient Knowledge of disease management related to fluid replacement for diarrhea* become the priority nursing diagnosis?

evolve

Answers to Clinical Decision-Making Exercises can be found on the Evolve website.

QSEN ACTIVITY: QUALITY IMPROVEMENT

Mrs. Reynolds is receiving IV 0.9% sodium chloride with 20 mEq KCl at 125 mL/hr. Nurses on the unit where Mrs. Reynolds is a patient are performing a quality improvement project to decrease the complications of IV therapy on their unit. They formed a day-shift IV team that performs all IV starts and coaches nurses on IV maintenance and monitoring on day shift. Evening and night shifts do not yet have IV teams.

List at least four outcomes that should be measured to determine effectiveness of this quality improvement project. Which comparisons of these items should be incorporated to determine effectiveness?

evolve

Answers to QSEN Activities can be found on the Evolve website.

REVIEW QUESTIONS

1. Which patient should you assess using Chvostek's sign?
   1. A 78-year-old with a metastatic cancer
   2. A 62-year-old with chronic diarrhea
   3. A 35-year-old with oliguric renal disease
   4. A 42-year-old with bacterial pneumonia

2. You have four patients with new signs and symptoms of ECV excess. Which assessment should you report most urgently to a health care provider?
   1. Daily weight increase of 1 kg
   2. Full neck veins when semiupright
   3. Crackles in the lung bases
   4. Bilateral swollen ankles
3. Your patient has diabetic ketoacidosis. Which of these arterial blood gas values is consistent with that diagnosis?
   1. pH, 7.52; PaO_2, 90 mm Hg; $PaCO_2$, 42 mm Hg; HCO_3^-, 36 mEq/L
   2. pH, 7.52; PaO_2, 80 mm Hg; $PaCO_2$, 28 mm Hg; HCO_3^-, 24 mEq/L
   3. pH, 7.22; PaO_2, 90 mm Hg; $PaCO_2$, 30 mm Hg; HCO_3^-, 12 mEq/L
   4. pH, 7.26; PaO_2, 80 mm Hg; $PaCO_2$, 55 mm Hg; HCO_3^-, 24 mEq/L
4. You need to prepare an IV solution and tubing before placing a VAD. Place the following steps in the correct order:
   1. Turn off the roller clamp on the IV tubing.
   2. Verify the correct solution and six rights of medication administration.
   3. Remove protective covering and insert spike into IV solution container, maintaining sterility.
   4. Check the health care provider's fluid order.
   5. Check the solution for color, abnormal particles, and expiration date and the bag for leaks.
   6. Prime the infusion tubing and clear air bubbles; replace protective cap on end if removed.
   7. Remove protective covering from IV tubing port on solution container, maintaining sterility.
   8. Maintaining sterility, open infusion set.
5. Your patient who is receiving a blood transfusion develops chills, flushing, tachycardia, and hypotension. You stop the infusion. What should you do next?
   1. Keep the IV line open by turning on the 0.9% NaCl that currently is connected to the Y tubing of the infusion set.
   2. Keep the IV line open by replacing the blood tubing at the VAD hub with primed new tubing attached to 0.9% NaCl.
   3. Notify the health care provider after checking the patient's vital signs.
   4. Notify the health care provider and then check the patient's vital signs.
6. To prevent ECV deficit, you should teach patients to replace diarrhea fluid output with fluid that contains __________.
7. Your patient has an aldosterone-secreting tumor. Which assessments do you use to detect the fluid and electrolyte imbalances for which this patient has high risk?
   1. Neck veins when upright and quadriceps muscle strength
   2. Urine output, blood pressure, and cardiac rate and rhythm
   3. Daily weights and Chvostek's sign
   4. Level of consciousness and arterial blood gases
8. Your patient was hospitalized with heart failure and is receiving a diuretic. His daily weights for 3 days show a downward trend. How should you interpret this assessment, and what should you do?
   1. Therapy is not effective; report that to the health care provider.
   2. Therapy is not effective; assess for signs of worsening heart failure.
   3. Therapy is effective; tell the patient that he will go home soon.
   4. Therapy is effective; assess for signs and symptoms of ECV deficit.
9. While changing an IV solution container using the existing tubing, you accidentally drop the tubing, and the spike hits the IV pole before you catch it. It does not touch the floor. What should you do?
   1. Insert the spike in the new solution container and check for air in the tubing
   2. Chart that tubing replacement should be scheduled within the next 24 hours
   3. Insert new tubing into the new solution container, prime it, and replace the old tubing
   4. Start a new VAD site, attach new tubing to the new container, and connect it to the VAD.
10. The health care provider has ordered IV potassium chloride (KCl) 20 mEq/L in 0.9% NaCl to be infused at 150 mL/hr. What should you assess before hanging this solution?
   1. Respiratory rate
   2. Liver enzymes
   3. Arterial blood gases
   4. Urine output

evolve
Rationales for Review Questions can be found on the Evolve website.

1. 2; 2. 3; 3. 3; 4. 4, 2, 5, 8, 1, 7, 3, 6; 5. 2; 6. Sodium; 7. 1;
8. 4; 9. 3; 10. 4

REFERENCES

AABB: *Blood donation FAQs*, 2013, http://www.aabb.org/resources/donation/pages/donatefaqs.aspx. Accessed April 2013.

Anderson S, et al: Administration of local anesthetic agents to decrease pain associated with peripheral vascular access, *J Infus Nurs* 33(6):353, 2010.

Chaudry SI, et al: Patterns of weight change preceding hospitalization for heart failure, *Circulation* 116(14):1549, 2007.

Clark CT: Recent efforts and available technologies for safety in delivery of blood products, *J Infus Nurs* 34(1):23, 2011.

Czaplewski L: Clinician and patient education. In Alexander M, et al, editors: *Infusion nursing: an evidence-based approach*, ed 3, St Louis, 2010, Saunders.

da Silva G, Priebe S, Dias FN: Benefits of establishing an intravenous team and the standardization of peripheral intravenous catheters, *J Infus Nurs* 33(3):156, 2010.

Fabian B: Infusion therapy in the older adult. In Alexander M, et al, editors: *Infusion nursing: an evidence-based approach*, ed 3, St Louis, 2010, Saunders.

Felver L: Acid-base balance. In Giddens JF, editor: *Concepts for nursing practice*, St Louis, 2013a, Mosby.

Felver L: Fluid and electrolyte balance. In Giddens JF, editor: *Concepts for nursing practice*, St Louis, 2013b, Mosby.

Felver L: Fluid and electrolyte homeostasis and imbalances. In Copstead LC, Banasik JL, editors: *Pathophysiology*, ed 5, St Louis, 2013c, Saunders.

Giger JN: *Transcultural nursing: assessment and intervention*, ed 6, St Louis, 2013, Mosby.

Gorski L, et al: Recommendations for frequency of assessment of the short peripheral catheter site, *J Infus Nurs* 35(5):290, 2012.

Groll D, et al: Evaluation of the psychometric properties of the phlebitis and infiltration scales for the assessment of complications of peripheral vascular devices, *J Infus Nurs* 33(6):385, 2010.

Hadaway L: Short peripheral intravenous catheters and infections, *J Infus Nurs* 35(4):230, 2012.

Hall JE: *Guyton and Hall textbook of medical physiology*, ed 12, Philadelphia, 2011, Saunders.

Halperin ML, et al: *Fluid, electrolyte, and acid-base physiology: a problem-based approach*, ed 4, St Louis, 2010, Saunders.

Hockenberry MJ, Wilson D: *Wong's nursing care of infants and children*, ed 9, St Louis, 2011, Mosby.

Infusion Nurses Society (INS): Infusion nursing standards of practice, *J Infus Nurs* 34(Suppl 1):S1, 2011.

Lehne RA: *Pharmacology for nursing care*, ed 8, St Louis, 2013, Saunders.

Lyons MG, Kasker J: Outcomes of a continuing education course on intravenous catheter insertion for experienced registered nurses, *J Contin Ed Nurs* 43(4):177, 2012.

McConnell JS, et al: "About a cupful"—a prospective study into accuracy of volume estimation by medical and nursing staff, *Accident Emerg Nurs* 15(2):101, 2007.

Metheny NM: *Fluid and electrolyte balance: nursing considerations*, ed 5, Sudbury, MA, 2012, Jones and Bartlett Learning.

Miller SL: Vascular access challenges: small fragile veins and tissue-paper skin, *Nursing* 42(2):62, 2012.

National Digestive Disease Information Clearing House: *What I need to know about diarrhea*, 2012, http://digestive.niddk.nih.gov/DDISEASES/pubs/diarrhea_ez/. Accessed November 18, 2013.

National Quality Forum (NQF): *National voluntary consensus standards for public reporting of patient safety event information: a consensus report*, Washington, DC, 2010, NQF.

O'Grady NP, et al: *Guidelines for the prevention of intravascular catheter-related infections*, 2011, http://www.cdc.gov/hicpac/pdf/guidelines/bsi-guidelines-2011.pdf. Accessed November 17, 2013.

Perucca R: Peripheral venous access devices. In Alexander M, et al, editors: *Infusion nursing: an evidence-based approach*, ed 3, St Louis, 2010, Saunders.

Poon EG, et al: Effect of bar-code technology on the safety of medication administration, *N Engl J Med* 362(18):1698, 2010.

Rose BD: *Clinical physiology of acid-base disorders*, ed 6, New York, 2013, McGraw-Hill.

Roszell S, Jones C: Intravenous administration issues: a comparison of intravenous insertions and complications in vancomycin versus other antibiotics, *J Infus Nurs* 33(2):112, 2010.

Segreti J, et al: Consensus conference on prevention of central line–associated bloodstream infections, 2011, *J Infus Nurs* 34(2):126, 2011.

The Joint Commission (TJC): *National Patient Safety Goals*, Oakbrook Terrace, IL, 2014, The Commission. Available at http://www.jointcommission.org/standards_information/npsgs.aspx.

Thornton SN: Thirst and hydration: physiology and consequences of dysfunction, *Physiol Behav* 100(1):15, 2010.

Tolich D: Alternatives to blood transfusion, *J Infus Nurs* 31(1):46, 2008.

Trick NL: Blood component therapy. In Alexander M, et al, editors: *Infusion nursing: an evidence-based approach*, ed 3, St Louis, 2010, Saunders.

Webster J, et al: Clinically indicated replacement versus routine replacement of peripheral venous catheters, *Cochrane Database Syst Rev* (3):CD007798, 2010.

Whyte A: A serious ethical dilemma, *Nurs Stand* 22(30):18, 2008.

Wilfong DN, et al: The effects of virtual intravenous and patient simulator training compared to the traditional approach of teaching nurses, *J Infus Nurs* 34(1):55, 2011.

Worthington PH, Gilbert KA: Parenteral nutrition, *J Infus Nurs* 35(1):35, 2012.

CHAPTER

19

Caring in Nursing Practice

evolve WEBSITE

http://evolve.elsevier.com/Potter/essentials

- Crossword Puzzle
- Audio Glossary

OBJECTIVES

- Discuss the role that caring plays in building nurse-patient relationships.
- Describe the commonalities among theories of caring.
- Discuss the evidence that exists about patients' perceptions of caring.
- Explain how the ethic of care influences nurses' decision making.
- Describe ways to express caring in practice.
- Describe the therapeutic benefit of listening to patients.
- Describe how health care institutions stress the importance of caring practices in achieving patient satisfaction.
- Explain the relationship between knowing a patient and clinical decision making.

KEY TERMS

caring, p. 518 **presence, p. 523** **transcultural, p. 519**

In the case study (see next page) Sue displays caring through her words and actions. Her calm presence, eye contact, and attention to the patient's concerns all convey a relationship-centered, comforting approach to care (Winsett and Hauck, 2011). Caring is central to nursing practice, but perhaps it has never been more important because of today's fast-paced health care environment. Financial pressures and fewer resources place demands on nurses that make it difficult to establish interpersonal connections that are an important part of caring practice (Potter et al., 2010). Despite these challenges, more professional organizations are stressing the importance of nurse caring in health care. The American Nurses Association (ANA) states in *Nursing's Agenda for the Future*, "Nursing is *the* pivotal health care profession highly valued for its specialized knowledge, skill, and *caring* in improving the health status of the public …." (ANA, 2002). In addition, the American Organization of Nurse Executives (AONE) (2005) describes caring and knowledge as the core of nursing, with caring being a key component of what a nurse brings to a patient experience (Figure 19-1). Now more than ever it is time to value and embrace the caring practices and expert knowledge that are the heart of competent nursing practice (Benner et al., 2010). When you engage patients in a caring and compassionate way, you learn that the therapeutic gain in caring contributes to the health and well-being of your patients. In addition, when you display caring practices when you administer nursing interventions (e.g., personal hygiene, initiate an intravenous (IV) line, or change a patient's dressing), you also engage the patient in the care practices, thus providing an opportunity for a patient to state his or her care preferences; as a result, the patient is usually more satisfied with care.

CASE STUDY *Mrs. Levine*

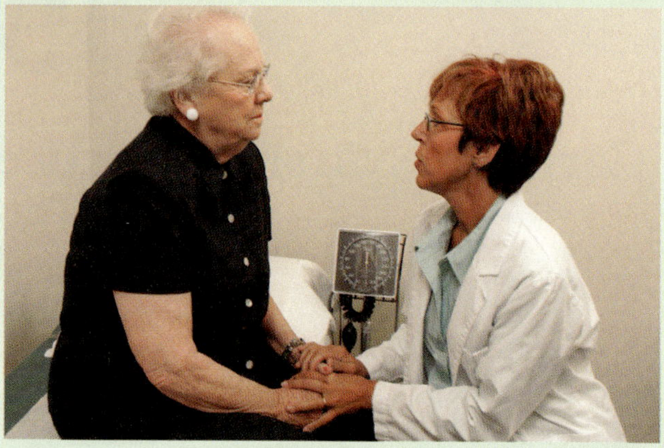

Mrs. Levine is an 82-year-old patient diagnosed 2 months ago with lymphoma, a cancer of the lymph tissue. She is experiencing weakness and fatigue. Over the last 4 weeks she has lost 8 lbs. She has been relatively independent before her diagnosis, playing bridge each week with friends and going to lunch with fellow church members. But now she has much less energy to do the things she enjoys. Her son, Jim, lives only a few miles away and is a consistent resource when she needs transportation to the health care provider or trips to the grocery. She will begin a research protocol for chemotherapy treatments this week at the oncology clinic.

Sue is an oncology nurse. She enters the examination room where Mrs. Levine is waiting, introduces herself, and sits down next to her patient. Sue states, "Mrs. Levine, I am here to understand your story. I want to listen and learn how I can best help you." She uses eye contact while talking and leans toward Mrs. Levine to establish a physical presence. Mrs. Levine nods, smiles, and begins her story. "I've had a good life. I just don't know what's going to happen." Sue replies, "Go on." Mrs. Levine explains, "The doctor tells me the cancer is serious. I worry about what's going to happen to me and how it will affect my son, Jim. I don't want to become a burden to him." Sue responds in a calm, soothing tone, "Mrs. Levine, your concerns are very normal. It is important for you to remain as independent as possible; let's talk about ways to help you retain your independence."

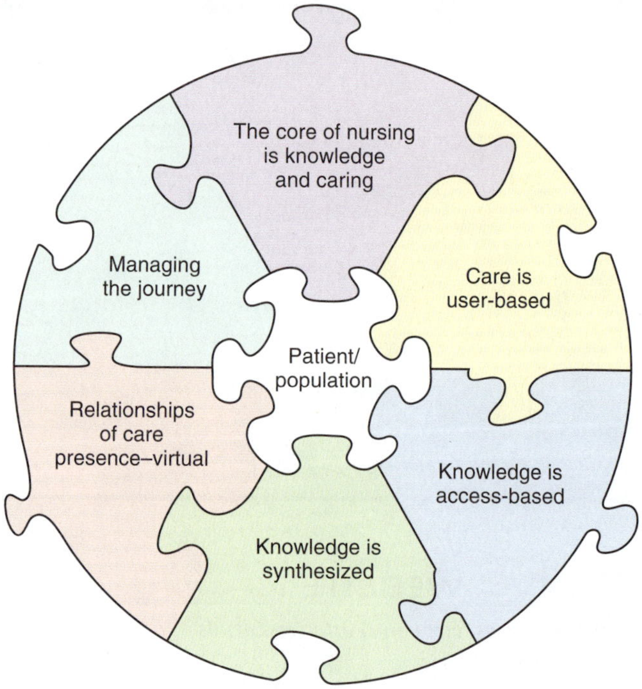

FIGURE 19-1 AONE guiding principles for future care delivery. (From American Organization of Nurse Executives (AONE): *Guiding principles for patient care delivery toolkit,* 2005, http://www.aone.org/aone/resource/toolkit.html. Accessed May 9, 2006.)

THEORETICAL VIEWS ON CARING

Caring is a universal phenomenon influencing the ways we think, feel, and behave in relation to one another. Since Florence Nightingale, nurses have studied caring from a variety of philosophical and ethical perspectives. A number of nursing scholars developed theories on caring because of its importance to nursing practice. This chapter does not detail all of the theories of caring, but it helps you understand how caring is at the heart of a nurse's ability to work with all patients in a respectful and therapeutic way.

Caring Is Primary

After spending time studying and analyzing the clinical stories of expert nurses, Patricia Benner (1984) describes caring as the essence of excellent nursing practice. The stories revealed the many behaviors and decisions that express nurses' caring. Caring means that people, events, projects, and things matter to people; it is a word for being connected (Benner and Wrubel, 1989). Because caring determines what matters to a person, it describes a range of involvements, from parental love to friendship, from caring about one's work to caring for one's pet to caring for and about one's patients (Burtson and Stichler, 2010). Understanding how to provide humanistic caring, and compassion begins early in nursing education and continues to mature through experiential practice (Gallagher-Lepak and Kubsch, 2009). In other words, "caring creates possibility" (Benner and Wrubel, 1989). *In the case study, Sue's concern for Mrs. Levine provides motivation and direction for Sue to better understand the meaning that cancer has for Mrs. Levine and the impact on her life and to provide the best approach in helping the patient cope with her cancer.*

Patients are not all the same. Each person brings a unique background of experiences, values, and cultural perspectives to a health care encounter. Caring is always specific and relational for each nurse-patient encounter. As nurses acquire more experience, they learn that caring helps them focus on the patients for whom they care. Caring facilitates a nurse's ability to know a patient, allowing the nurse to recognize a patient's problems and find and implement individualized solutions.

Because illness is the human experience of loss or dysfunction, any treatment or intervention given without consideration of its meaning to an individual is likely to be much less effective. Expert nurses understand the differences between health, illness, and disease. Through caring relationships nurses listen to patients' stories to understand the meaning of their illness. With this understanding, they provide therapeutic, patient-centered care. *When Mrs. Levine first began to feel fatigued, she thought it was just a part of being older. However, once the fatigue became serious enough to threaten her ability to manage her home and care for herself, she sought medical care. Through listening to Mrs. Levine's story, Sue is able to begin to understand her illness within the context of her life.*

Leininger's Transcultural Caring

Madeleine Leininger (1991) offers a **transcultural** view of caring. She describes the concept of care as the essence and unifying domain that sets nursing apart from other health care disciplines. Care is an essential human need, necessary for the health and survival of all individuals. Care, unlike cure, helps an individual or group improve a human condition. Acts of caring refer to nurturing and skillful activities, processes, and decisions that help people in ways that are empathetic, compassionate, and supportive. A caring act depends on the needs, problems, and values of a patient. Leininger's studies of numerous cultures around the world found that care protects, develops, nurtures, and provides survival to people. It is universal and vital to recovery from illness and the maintenance of healthy life practices in all cultures.

Caring is also very personal. One challenge is to find ways to communicate with patients so as to learn the culturally specific behaviors and words that reflect human caring (Box 19-1) (see Chapter 20).

BOX 19-1 PATIENT-CENTERED CARE

As a nurse you show caring through connecting with a patient and explaining your role in providing care. This includes asking about patient preferences; respecting privacy, diversity, and individual needs; interacting and listening to the patient and his or her family; providing a healing environment; and going the extra mile and asking your patient if there is anything else you can do (Winsett and Hauck, 2011). Communication helps a nurse understand a specific patient's cultural values and beliefs and provide patient-centered care (Suliman et al., 2009). In many ways caring communication is culturally universal.

When a nurse cares for patients from diverse backgrounds, it is not possible to become familiar with all of the patients' attitudes, values, practices, and beliefs that may conflict with his or her own. Often clinicians believe that "knowing" a patient's culture involves familiarizing oneself with a list of beliefs, but this tendency is the clinician's way to systematize or "tidy up" culture. In fact, people often have overlapping membership in several cultural communities (e.g., being an older adult, a member of an ethnic minority, a disabled person). A barrier to effective communication is the languages that a patient and nurse speak, both verbally and nonverbally. When communicating with patients of diverse backgrounds, it helps to acknowledge one another's difficulty in talking to put all involved at ease (Chambers, 2008).

IMPLICATIONS FOR PRACTICE

- Explore with patients your difficulty in understanding their cultural frame for communication. For example, say, "In my culture we believe that ..." or "As a nurse, I tend to value. ..."
- Ask patients to describe and explain the history of some of their beliefs and practices (e.g., seeking and accepting medical care).
- Allow your patients to share the impact of their own perspective on their health care plan.
- In some cultures discussion of a patient's common customs and popular culture create a common ground for communication.
- Understand how patients choose to communicate their feelings. For example, in some cultures it is considered unwise or even dangerous to express one's opinion.

Watson's Transpersonal Theory of Caring

Patients and their family members expect a high quality of human interaction from nurses, and caring is viewed as the central focus of nursing (Papastavrou et al., 2011). Unfortunately many conversations between patients and their nurses are very brief and disconnected. Workload demands create situations in which the development of a "close" relationship with a patient is limited (Henderson et al., 2007). Watson's transpersonal theory of caring (2005, 2010) is a holistic model that describes a conscious recognition that caring for a person involves sensitivity, respect, and a high moral and ethical commitment. The theory integrates human caring processes with healing environments, incorporating the life-generating and life-receiving processes of caring and healing for nurses and their patients (Watson, 2006b). The theory describes a consciousness that allows nurses to raise new questions about nursing, illness, and caring. The transpersonal caring theory rejects the disease orientation of health care and places care before cure (Watson, 2010). A nurse looks beyond a patient's disease and its treatment. Instead transpersonal caring looks for deeper sources of inner healing to protect, enhance, and preserve a person's dignity and inner harmony.

Caring becomes almost spiritual because it preserves human dignity in a cure-dominated health care system (Watson, 2006b). Nurses connect with patients at a deep spiritual level, sometimes only for a moment, and that "connectedness" allows both a nurse and patient to heal. The theory emphasizes the care of the whole patient rather than the pathologic condition and treatment of the patient's disease.

Watson's theory supports a holistic approach that allows a caring nurse to gain a unique level of understanding. Consider the example of performing a nursing assessment. A nurse who applies Watson's theory during an assessment is able to plan care in a way that goes beyond the physical aspect of a disease. *For example, Sue wants to assess Mrs. Levine's nutritional status to ensure a holistic approach to her patient's nutritional needs. Her assessment would go beyond what Mrs. Levine eats, her weight, and her sense of an appetite. Sue would also consider Mrs. Levine's desire for food, her food preferences, hunger, availability of food, social environment, and emotional attachment to food to determine a deeper understanding of the patient's nutritional status.* When applying the transpersonal theory of caring, the nurse accurately assesses a patient's physical needs and combines them with the patient's preferences, social environment, and emotional needs.

The emphasis in Watson's theory is on the nurse-patient relationship. How a nurse chooses to be with a patient and family in any given moment influences the caring-healing relationship. Watson (2005, 2008) identified 10 carative factors that offer a framework for nursing care (Table 19-1). The carative factors are tools for providing caring and humane nursing therapies.

Swanson's Theory of Caring

Kristen Swanson's study of patients and professional caregivers (1991) led to the development of a theory of caring for nursing practice. She interviewed three different groups: women who miscarried, parents and health care professionals in a newborn intensive care unit, and socially at-risk mothers who received long-term public health care. The researchers asked each group questions about how they experienced or expressed caring in their situation. After analyzing the stories, Swanson developed a theory of caring that consists of five categories or processes (Table 19-2). She defines caring as a nurturing way of relating to a valued other, toward whom one feels a personal sense of commitment and responsibility (Swanson, 1991). The theory supports that caring is a central nursing phenomenon but not necessarily unique to nursing practice.

Swanson's theory provides direction for how to develop useful and effective caring strategies. Each of the caring processes has definitions and subdimensions that serve as the basis for nursing interventions. For example, if a nurse provides an intervention by "doing for" patients, he or she will anticipate the risks associated with the procedure, administer the intervention skillfully, and explain aspects of the procedure to minimize a patient's anxiety.

An example is the way Sue administers chemotherapy. Knowing that chemotherapy is toxic and can cause adverse reactions, Sue begins the administration slowly as ordered, has the necessary equipment available if a reaction develops, and explains the reasons for each step of the administration. Nursing care and caring are crucial in making positive differences in patient's health and well-being (Palese et al., 2011).

Summary of Theoretical Views

Many theoretical views of caring have commonalities. Duffy, Hoskins, and Siefert (2007) identify these commonalities as human interaction or communication, mutuality, appreciating the uniqueness of individuals, and improving the welfare of patients and families. Caring is highly relational. A nurse

TABLE 19-1 WATSON'S 10 CARATIVE FACTORS

CARATIVE FACTOR	EXAMPLE IN PRACTICE
Forming a human-altruistic value system	Use loving kindness to extend yourself. Use self-disclosure appropriately to promote a therapeutic alliance with your patient.
Instilling faith-hope	Provide a connectedness with the patient that offers purpose and direction when trying to find the meaning of an illness.
Cultivating a sensitivity to one's self and others	Learn to accept yourself and others for their full potential. A caring nurse matures into becoming a self-actualized nurse.
Developing a helping-trusting, human, caring relationship	Learn to develop and sustain helping-trusting, authentic caring relationships through effective communication with your patients.
Promoting and accepting the expression of positive and negative feelings	Support and accept your patients' feelings. In connecting with your patients, show a willingness to take risks in what you share with one another.
Using creative problem-solving, caring processes	Apply the nursing process in a systematic way to provide patient-centered care.
Promoting transpersonal teaching-learning	Learn together while educating the patient to acquire self-care skills. The patient assumes responsibility for learning.
Providing for a supportive, protective, and/or corrective mental, physical, societal, and spiritual environment	Create a healing environment at all levels, physical and nonphysical. This promotes wholeness, beauty, comfort, dignity, and peace.
Meeting human needs	Assist patients with basic needs with an intentional care and caring consciousness.
Allowing for existential-phenomenological-spiritual forces	Allow spiritual forces to provide a better understanding of oneself and your patient.

Data from Watson J: *Caring science as a sacred science*, Philadelphia, 2005, FA Davis; and Watson J: *The philosophy and science of caring*, Boulder, 2008, University Press of Colorado.

TABLE 19-2 SWANSON'S THEORY OF CARING

CARING PROCESS	DEFINITIONS	SUBDIMENSIONS
Knowing	Striving to understand an event as it has meaning in the life of the other	Avoiding assumptions Centering on the one cared for Assessing thoroughly Seeking cues Engaging the self or both
Being with	Being emotionally present to the other	Being there Conveying ability Sharing feelings Not burdening
Doing for	Doing for the other as he or she would do for self if it were at all possible	Comforting Anticipating Performing skillfully Protecting Preserving dignity
Enabling	Facilitating the other's passage through life transitions (e.g., birth, death) and unfamiliar events	Informing/explaining Supporting/allowing Focusing Generating alternatives Validating/giving feedback
Maintaining belief	Sustaining faith in the other's capacity to get through an event or transition and face a future with meaning	Believing in/holding in esteem Maintaining a hope-filled attitude Offering realistic optimism "Going the distance"

Data from Swanson KM: Empirical development of a middle-range theory of caring, *Nurs Res* 40(3):161, 1991.

and patient enter into a relationship that is much more than one person simply doing tasks for another. There is a mutual give-and-take that develops as nurse and patient begin to know and care for one another (Sumner, 2010).

Caring seems invisible at times when a nurse and patient enter a relationship of respect, concern, and support. A nurse's empathy and compassion become a natural part of each patient encounter. However, when caring is absent, it becomes very obvious. For example, if a nurse is disinterested or avoids a patient's request for help, the nurse's inaction quickly conveys an uncaring attitude. Henderson et al. (2007) observed nurse-patient interactions on medical-surgical nursing units in Australia and then interviewed patients' perceptions of those interactions. Their study found that negative nurse-patient interactions were best described as "forgetfulness" (i.e., incidences in which nurses did not remember or follow up with patient requests). Patients are perceptive of nurses' behaviors and capable of recognizing when nurses show an uncaring approach. They quickly know when nurses fail to relate to them.

As you practice caring, your patients sense your commitment and willingness to enter into a relationship, allowing you to gain an understanding of their experience of illness (Winsett and Hauck, 2011). Patients particularly sense caring when nurses are accessible and optimistically able to look forward to the future, whatever it holds (Duffy et al., 2007). As a nurse-patient relationship forms, a nurse becomes a coach and partner rather than a detached provider of care.

In the case study Sue works with Mrs. Levine to help her remain independent. By considering Mrs. Levine's relationship with her son, the effects of her cancer, and upcoming treatment, Sue's caring behavior becomes enabling. When a nurse practices enabling, a patient and nurse work together to identify alternatives and resources. For example, are there ways for Mrs. Levine to organize her day so that she can take frequent rest periods and still complete her daily tasks? As Sue enables Mrs. Levine, she explains the effects of cancer and chemotherapy and supports the patient in identifying ways to complete self-care activities. By understanding Mrs. Levine's unique needs, Sue improves her patient's sense of well-being.

PATIENT SATISFACTION

Caring is a moral imperative, not a commodity to be bought and sold. Caring for other human beings protects, enhances, and preserves human dignity. It is a professional, ethical covenant that nursing has with its patients (Watson, 2010). Current evidence shows a connection between patient satisfaction and nurse caring (Box 19-2). Put simply, when the nurses within an organization successfully demonstrate caring, nursing care improves, and more patients are satisfied and more likely to return to the health care setting. Nurses also benefit when there are interventions that link nursing actions, caring processes, and expectations (Tonges and Ray, 2011). When patients sense that health care providers are sensitive, sympathetic, compassionate, and interested in them as people, they usually become active partners in the plan of care (Palese, et al., 2011; Papastavrou et al., 2011). More health care settings are adopting patient-centered care models that incorporate relationship-centered caring approaches. An organization needs to measure caring from a patient's point of view to show the value of nursing. Duffy et al. (2007) developed the Caring Assessment Tool (CAT) for that purpose. The tool was tested among hospitalized patients representing diverse ethnic groups. It is useful to you as a beginning nurse to appreciate the type of behaviors that hospitalized patients identify as caring. The CAT includes eight major factors, with three-to-six items that describe nursing behaviors for each (Box 19-3). Each major factor is consistent with caring theories (Duffy et al., 2007).

Mutual Problem Solving

A caring nurse helps hospitalized patients understand how to think about their health and illness and figure out questions

BOX 19-2 EVIDENCE-BASED PRACTICE

PICO Question: Do patient satisfaction rates among hospitalized adults improve when carative nursing practices are used?

SUMMARY OF EVIDENCE

Researchers identify a strong, positive correlation between nurse caring behaviors and patient satisfaction. Caring facilitates healing and improves patient satisfaction with nursing care (Osterman et al., 2010). There is evidence to show that patient satisfaction is more likely to improve if nurses adapt their work to accommodate patients' specific requests or communicate why these requests cannot be addressed immediately (Palese et al., 2011). The higher the patient satisfaction with nursing care, the higher their overall satisfaction with their health care experience (Winsett and Hauck, 2011). Caring nursing practices improve patient's functional status, coping, or self-care (Muller-Staub et al., 2006; Papastavrou et al., 2011). In addition, nursing caring is the most influential dimension of patient advocacy and is predictive of patient satisfaction (Burtson and Stichler, 2010).

APPLICATION TO NURSING PRACTICE

- Respond promptly to a patient request, either personally or by directing unlicensed nursing assistive personnel to respond (Palese et al., 2011).
- Discuss limitations that possibly lead to a delay in responding to requests (e.g., having to help another patient first or choosing to wait until a pain medication takes effect) (Palese, et al., 2011).
- Advocate for your patient such as initiating a change in pain-control measures or changing the timing of physical therapy (Burtson and Stichler, 2010).
- Connect with your patient, discuss all aspects of care, and include personal preferences. Explain how you will include or adapt personal preferences with your patient.

BOX 19-3 FACTORS AND ITEMS CONSTITUTING THE CARING ASSESSMENT TOOL (CAT)

Each item begins with the stem: Since I have been a patient here, the nurse(s):

MUTUAL PROBLEM SOLVING
- Help me understand how I am thinking.
- Ask me how I think treatment is going.
- Help me explore alternative ways of dealing.
- Ask me what I know.
- Help me figure out questions to ask.

ATTENTIVE REASSURANCE
- Are available.
- Seem interested.
- Support sense of hope.
- Help me believe in self.
- Anticipate my needs.

HUMAN RESPECT
- Listen to me.
- Accept me.
- Treat me kindly.
- Respect me.
- Pay attention to me.

ENCOURAGING MANNER
- Support my beliefs.
- Encourage me to ask questions.
- Help me to see some good.
- Encourage me to go on.
- Help me deal with bad feelings.

APPRECIATION OF UNIQUE MEANINGS
- Are concerned with how I view things.
- Know what is important to me.
- Acknowledge my inner feelings.
- Show respect for things having meaning.

HEALING ENVIRONMENT
- Check up on me.
- Pay attention to me when I am talking.
- Make me feel comfortable.
- Respect my privacy.
- Treat my body carefully.

AFFILIATION NEEDS
- Are responsive to my family.
- Talk openly with my family.
- Allow my family to be involved.

BASIC HUMAN NEEDS
- Make sure I get food.
- Help me with routine needs for sleep.
- Help me feel less worried.

Modified from Duffy JR, Hoskins L, Seifert RF: Dimensions of caring: psychometric evaluation of the Caring Assessment Tool, *Adv Nurs Sci* 30(3):235, 2007.

to ask their health care providers (Duffy et al., 2007). In addition, a caring nurse helps patients explore options for resolving health problems and provides information and instruction. Using evidence in practice is an aspect of mutual problem solving, with a nurse continuously learning and engaging patients and families in discussions about their health issues (Winsett and Hauck, 2011).

Attentive Reassurance

Patients perceive nurses to be caring when they are accessible and show interest in their well-being. Being able to foresee the future and confidently express possibilities often gives patients hope (Duffy et al., 2007; Palese et al., 2011). Attentive reassurance is consistent with Watson's faith-hope, sensitivity, and helping-trust relationship factors. It is also consistent with Swanson's maintaining belief.

Human Respect

Respect for patients is integral to providing care. Human respect refers to nurses being able to appreciate the value of human beings and displaying behaviors that demonstrate value such as accepting or paying attention to a patient (Duffy et al., 2007). By showing respect a nurse honors the worth of individuals (Watson, 2010).

Encouraging Manner

Hospitalized patients face very difficult situations: numerous diagnostic tests, anxiety and fear of not knowing what the future holds, family role changes, and many physical ailments. Patients perceive nurses as caring when nurses display professional behaviors, such as staying calm, being cheerful, and pointing out the good in difficult situations (Duffy et al.,

2007). Displaying an encouraging manner also involves helping patients deal with negative feelings. Patients perceive how nurses' attitudes and behaviors reflect an encouraging manner (Palese et al., 2011).

Appreciation of Unique Meanings

In Swanson's theory of caring (1991), knowing involves nurses' attempts at understanding the lived experiences of patients. Duffy et al. (2007) identified that hospitalized patients recognize when nurses know what is important to them and their families. This is especially important because nurses care for patients from different cultural environments (see Chapter 20). This aspect of caring is challenging because it takes time for nurses to develop a relationship with patients that allows for an appreciation of their inner feelings (Winsett and Hauck, 2011).

Healing Environment

Florence Nightingale was the first nurse to understand how changing patients' environments (e.g., providing nutrition, hygiene, and comfort) promote healing. A healing environment is one in which nurses check patients frequently, respect patient privacy, reduce noise, and treat the patient carefully. Such an environment leads patients to a sense of security and protection from harm (Winsett and Hauck, 2011).

Affiliation Needs

Including family members in a patient's care is basic nursing practice. It is a key element in discharge planning (see Chapter 2). Hospitalized patients perceive nurses as caring when they are responsive to patients' families and allow them to be involved in the patient's care (Duffy et al., 2007). This means you actively engage families in conversation and explain (when appropriate) the care that a patient is receiving. Family members influence decisions regarding how a patient will manage health care needs in the home. A caring nurse involves the family in such decisions.

Basic Human Needs

All humans have basic needs (Maslow, 1987) (see Chapter 1). Unfortunately these needs are not readily met when nurses instead become focused on managing technological demands and complex therapies. Often registered nurses delegate basic human need care measures to unlicensed nursing assistive personnel (see Chapter 12). However, patients perceive nurses as caring when they take patients' basic needs into account (Duffy et al., 2007).

As you begin clinical practice, consider how patients perceive caring and determine the best way to provide individualized care. Always focus on building a relationship that allows you to learn what is important to your patients.

CARING IN NURSING PRACTICE

There are no known ways that ensure that you will become a caring professional. For those who find caring a normal part of their life, it is a product of their culture, values, experiences, and relationships with others. People who do not experience care in their lives often find it difficult to act in caring ways. As nurses deal with health and illness in their practice, most grow in the ability to care. Caring nurses use a caring approach in each patient encounter.

Providing Presence

The concept of **presence** is an interpersonal process that is characterized by sensitivity, holism, intimacy, vulnerability, and adaptation to unique circumstances (Finfgeld-Connett, 2006). Put more simply, providing presence is a person-to-person encounter conveying closeness and a sense of caring. Presence occurs within an atmosphere of intimacy and sensitivity and is characterized by open and honest interactions (Finfgeld-Connett, 2008a). The process of presence is mutual. Patients demonstrate openness to presence while nurses create an environment and display professional behaviors to promote presence (Finfgeld-Connett, 2006).

Presence involves "being there" and "being with." Being there is more than a physical presence; it also includes communication and understanding. The interpersonal relationship of being there depends on a nurse being attentive and receptive to a patient. *For example, in the case study Sue decides that it is important to be with Mrs. Levine during her first chemotherapy treatment. Sue tells her patient, "You know, I want to be the one who gives you the first chemotherapy treatment. I know this has been an anxious moment for you." Sue sits down next to Mrs. Levine and prepares the infusion supplies carefully while continuing their conversation. When Sue sees Mrs. Levine's son at the doorway, she invites him in to sit with his mother.*

Nursing requires being present with patients at a moment of crisis or need. Eye contact, body language, expressions, listening, and a positive and encouraging manner act together to create openness and understanding (Figure 19-2). Presence conveys a message that the other's experience matters to the

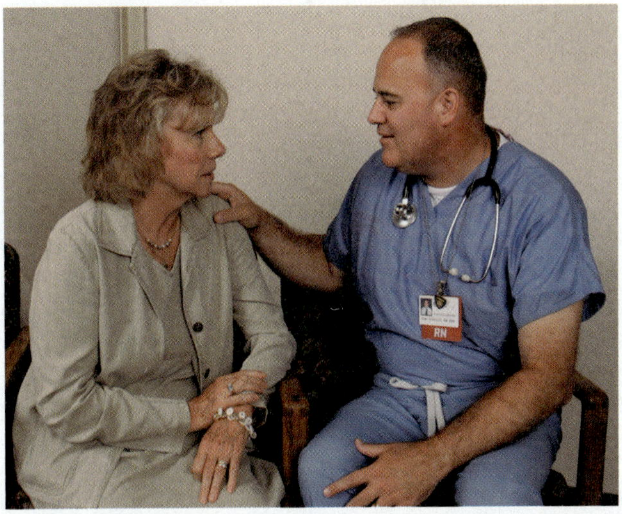

FIGURE 19-2 Nurse conveying presence to a patient.

one caring (Swanson, 1991). Establishing presence enhances your ability to learn from each patient. This strengthens your ability to provide effective patient-centered care. Nurses offer their presence to help patients achieve positive outcomes, diminish the intensity of unwanted feelings, or promote reassurance (Finfgeld-Connett, 2008b; Palese et al., 2011).

Being with a patient is interpersonal. A nurse and patient share personal insights in verbal and nonverbal ways (Finfgeld-Connett, 2008a). A nurse gives himself or herself, which means being available and open to a patient. If patients accept their nurse, they invite him or her to see, share, and touch their vulnerability and suffering. Through presence a nurse enters a patient's world. A patient is able to put words to feelings and understand himself or herself in a way that leads to identifying solutions, seeing new directions, and making choices.

Establishing presence when patients are experiencing stressful events or situations is very important. Awaiting a doctor's report of test results, preparing for an unfamiliar procedure, and planning for a return home after serious illness are just a few examples that create unpredictability and dependency on nurses. A nurse's presence calms anxiety and fear related to stressful situations. Giving reassurance and thorough explanations about a procedure, remaining at a patient's side, and coaching a patient through the experience convey a presence that promotes a patient's well-being.

Touch

Patients face situations that are embarrassing, frightening, and painful. Whatever the feeling or symptom, patients look to nurses for comfort. The use of touch is one comforting approach that reaches out to patients to communicate concern and support. However, you need to remember a simple gesture of touching a patient on the arm can be either consoling and sympathetic or invasive and offensive according to different cultures (Winsett and Hauck, 2011).

Touch is relational and often leads to a connection between nurse and patient. Fredriksson (1999) describes three categories of touch: task-oriented, caring, and protective. Nurses use task-oriented touch when performing a task or procedure. The skillful and gentle performance of a nursing procedure conveys security and competence. Expert nurses learn that any procedure is more effective when they administer it carefully and in consideration of any patient concern. For example, if a patient is anxious about the insertion of a nasogastric tube, offer comfort through a full explanation of the procedure and what the patient will feel. Then you convey that you will perform the procedure safely, skillfully, and successfully in the way you prepare supplies, position the patient, and gently manipulate and insert the nasogastric tube. Throughout any procedure talk quietly with a patient to provide reassurance and support.

Caring touch is a form of nonverbal communication, which successfully influences a patient's comfort and security, enhances self-esteem, increases confidence of caregivers, and improves mental well-being (Osterman et al., 2010). You express this in the way you hold a patient's hand, give a back massage, gently position a patient, or participate in a conversation. When using caring touch, you make a connection with a patient and show acceptance of the individual.

Protective touch is a form of touch that protects a nurse and/or patient (Fredriksson, 1999). A patient views it either positively or negatively. The most obvious form of protective touch is preventing an accident (e.g., holding and bracing a patient to avoid a fall). It is also a kind of touch that protects a nurse emotionally. A nurse withdraws from a patient when he or she is unable to tolerate suffering or needs to escape from a situation that is causing tension. When used in this way, protective touch elicits negative feelings in a patient (Fredriksson, 1999).

Because touch conveys many messages, use it with discretion. Touch itself is a concern when crossing cultural boundaries of either a patient or a nurse (Benner, 2004; Benner et al., 2010). However, do not assume that touch is only a cultural issue. In a recent study, researchers found that some patients who experienced trauma did not like to be touched a lot because touching increased their pain. In the case of trauma caused by physical violence, patients did not want to be touched because touching evoked fear. In these cases touching is not a caring intervention (Hayes and Tyler-Ball, 2007). Most patients allow task-oriented touch because most individuals give nurses and physicians an unwritten license to enter their personal space to provide care. Know and understand if patients are accepting of touch and how they interpret your intentions before providing hands-on care.

Listening

Caring is an interpersonal interaction that is much more than two people simply talking back and forth (Bunkers, 2010). In a caring relationship a nurse establishes trust, opens lines of communication, and listens to what a patient has to say. Listening is critical because it conveys a nurse's full attention and interest. Listening includes "taking in" what a patient says, interpreting and understanding it, and giving back that understanding to the patient (Shipley, 2010). Listening to the meaning of what a patient says creates a mutual relationship. True listening leads to knowing and responding to what really matters to a patient and family.

When an individual becomes ill, he or she usually has a story to tell about the meaning of their illness. Any critical or chronic illness affects all of a patient's life choices and decisions, sometimes even his or her identity. Being able to tell that story helps a patient break the distress of illness. A story needs a listener. Frank (1998) described his own feelings during his experience with cancer: "I needed a [health care professional's] gift of listening in order to make my suffering a relationship between *us,* instead of an iron cage around *me.*" He needed to be able to express what he needed when he was ill. The personal concerns that are part of a patient's illness story determine what is at stake for the patient. Caring through listening enables you to participate in a patient's life.

Through active listening you begin to know your patients and what is important to them. Learning to listen to a patient is sometimes difficult. It is easy to become distracted by tasks at hand, colleagues shouting instructions, or other patients waiting to have their needs met. However, the time taken to listen effectively is worthwhile both in the information gained and the strengthening of the nurse-patient relationship. Listening allows you to help patients find meaning, release fears, and answer their own questions.

Knowing the Patient

One of the five caring processes described by Swanson (1991) is knowing the patient. The concept comprises both a nurse's understanding of a specific patient and subsequent selection of interventions (Radwin, 2000). Knowing develops over time as a nurse learns the clinical conditions within a specialty and the behaviors and physiological responses of patients. Knowing helps a nurse respond to what really matters to a patient. To know a patient means that you avoid assumptions, focus on the patient, and engage in a caring relationship that reveals information and cues that facilitate critical thinking and clinical judgments (see Chapter 8). Knowing the patient is at the core of clinical decision making. Through caring you develop an understanding that helps you to better know the patient as a unique individual and choose the most appropriate and efficacious nursing therapies.

The caring relationships that a nurse develops over time, coupled with the nurse's growing knowledge and experience, provide a rich source of meaning that allows a nurse to recognize changes in a patient's clinical status. Expert nurses develop the ability to detect changes in patients' conditions almost effortlessly. Clinical decision making involves various aspects of knowing the patient, including responses to therapies, routines and habits, coping resources, physical capacities and endurance, and body typology and characteristics. The experienced nurse knows additional facts about his or her patients such as their experiences, behaviors, feelings, and perceptions. When you make clinical decisions accurately in the context of knowing a patient well, improved patient outcomes result. Swanson (1991) notes that when nurses base care on knowing the patient, the patients perceive care as personalized, comforting, supportive, and healing.

How can you develop your skill in knowing patients early in your practice?

- Routinely round on patients at the beginning of a work shift and ongoing as appropriate.
- Do not depend on other's observations; be thorough and make your own assessment.
- Always go back and observe how a patient responded to your interventions.
- Reflect about what you have learned each time you either assess or evaluate a patient.

Knowing the patient is at the core of clinical decision making. Success in knowing a patient lies in the relationship that you form together. To know a patient is to enter into a caring, social process, which results in a nurse-patient relationship; and the patient comes to feel known by the nurse (MacDonald, 2008). When patient care is fragmented, knowledge of the patient declines, and patient-centered care is compromised (Crocker and Scholes, 2009).

Spiritual Caring

Spiritual caring is about developing caring relationships with patients through fostering connections to promote spiritual comfort and well-being (Chapter 21). Research shows a link between mind, body, and spirit. An individual's beliefs and expectations have effects on a person's physical well-being.

Establishing a caring relationship with a patient involves interconnectedness between a nurse and a patient. This interconnectedness is why Watson (2006a, 2008, 2009, 2010) describes the caring relationship in a spiritual sense. Spirituality offers intrapersonal (connected with oneself), interpersonal (connected with others and the environment), and transpersonal (connected with the unseen, God, or a higher power) connectedness. In a caring relationship a patient and a nurse come to know one another so both move toward a healing relationship by doing the following (Watson, 2008):

- Mobilizing hope for the patient and the nurse
- Finding an understanding of illness, symptoms, or emotions that is acceptable to the patient
- Helping the patient use social, emotional, or spiritual resources
- Recognizing that caring relationships connect us human to human

Relieving Pain and Suffering

Relieving pain and suffering is more than giving pain medications, repositioning the patient, or cleaning a wound. The relief of pain and suffering are caring nursing actions that give a patient comfort, dignity, respect, and peace. By ensuring that a patient care environment is clean, reasonably quiet, pleasant, and inclusive of personal items, you make the physical environment a place that soothes and heals the mind, body, and spirit (Gallagher-Lepak and Kubsch, 2009).

Skillful and accurate assessment helps you identify the type and frequency of a patient's pain and the impact of the pain on his or her lifestyle. This accurate assessment is foundational to design a patient-centered plan of care to improve a patient's level of comfort. The skills previously discussed of presence, touching, listening, and knowing your patients help you and your patient develop goals for pain relief.

Human suffering is multifaceted and affects patients physically, emotionally, socially, and spiritually. In addition, it affects the patient's family and friends. *Mrs. Levine has multiple pain-control challenges. In addition, she is trying to maintain independence as long as her illness allows. Her son wants to help but also respects his mother's needs and concerns. Both Mrs. Levine and her son experience emotional suffering.* Their emotional suffering encompasses anger, guilt, fear, or grief. Although you cannot fix their suffering, you can provide comfort through a listening, nonjudgmental caring presence. Patients and their families are comforted by a caring listener (Hudacek, 2008).

BOX 19-4 NURSE CARING BEHAVIORS AS PERCEIVED BY FAMILIES

- Being honest
- Advocating for patient's care preferences
- Giving clear explanations
- Keeping family members informed
- Asking permission before doing something to a patient
- Providing comfort: Offering a warm blanket, finding food a patient can swallow, rubbing a patient's back
- Reading patients passages from religious texts, a favorite book, cards or mail
- Providing for and maintaining patient privacy
- Ensuring the patient that nursing services will be available
- Helping patients to do as much for themselves as possible
- Teaching the family how to keep the patient physically comfortable

Family Care

Each individual experiences life through relationships with others. Thus caring for a patient cannot occur in isolation from that person's family. As a nurse it is important for you to know a patient's family almost as thoroughly as you know a patient. The family is an important resource (see Chapter 24). Success with nursing interventions often depends on their willingness to share information about the patient, their acceptance and understanding of therapies, whether the interventions fit with the family's daily practices, and whether the family is willing to provide the therapies recommended. It is critically important to know who the primary family caregiver is. In some cases it may be more than one individual.

Families perceive many nurse caring behaviors to be important to patients' well-being. Ensuring a patient's well-being and being able to be active participants in care are critical for family members. *In the case study Sue spends time discussing with Mrs. Levine's son how he can help his mother manage her side effects from the chemotherapy. Sue prepares him to deal with any nausea or loss of appetite his mother experiences.* The behaviors listed in Box 19-4 offer useful guidelines for developing a caring relationship with all families. Begin a relationship by learning who makes up the patient's family and what their roles are in the patient's life. Showing the family care and concern for the patient creates an openness that then enables you to form a relationship with them. Caring for the family considers the context of the patient's illness and the stress it imposes on all members (see Chapter 24).

THE CHALLENGE OF CARING

Assisting individuals during a time of need is the reason many enter nursing. When nurses affirm themselves as caring individuals, they achieve a meaning and purpose to their lives (Benner, 2004; Benner et al., 2010). Caring motivates people to become nurses, and it is a source of satisfaction when nurses know they have made a difference in their patients' lives.

In today's health care system there are many challenges to provide caring to those who need help the most: the patient. Being a part of the helping professions is difficult and demanding. Nurses are torn between the human caring model and the task-oriented biomedical model and institutional demands that consume their practice (Tonges and Ray, 2011; Winsett and Hauck, 2011). They have increasingly less time to spend with patients, making it much harder to know who they are. A reliance on technology and cost-effective health care strategies and efforts to standardize and refine work processes all undermine the nature of caring. Too often patients become just a number, with their real needs either overlooked or ignored. In addition, nurses, especially those practicing in inpatient settings, deal with multiple stressors (e.g., interdepartmental, technology, paperwork stressors). As a result they are at risk for burn out and compassion fatigue (Potter et al., 2010).

The ANA, National League for Nursing, AONE, and American Association of Colleges of Nursing recommend strategies to reverse the current nursing shortage. A number of the strategies have potential for creating work environments that enable nurses to demonstrate more caring behaviors. Environmental factors promote artful nursing, presence, and caring (Finfgeld-Connett, 2006). A healthy work environment is one that is geographically designed to facilitate care activities, offers a way for staff to discuss problems and concerns about being able to provide care, and has adequate resources. To create environments conducive to caring, health care organizations must introduce greater flexibility into the work environment structure, reward experienced nurse mentors, offer programs for compassion fatigue, improve nurse staffing, and provide nurses with autonomy over their practice (Burtson and Stichler, 2010).

If health care is to make a positive difference, human beings cannot be treated like machines or robots. Instead health care has to become more humanizing. Nurses play an important role in making caring an integral part of health care delivery. This begins by their making caring a part of the philosophy and environment in the workplace and incorporating care concepts into standards of nursing care and guidelines for professional conduct. Consistent with the wisdom and vision of Nightingale, nursing is a lifetime journey of caring and healing, seeking to understand and preserve the wholeness of human existence and to offer compassionate, informed knowledgeable human caring (Watson, 2009).

KEY POINTS

- Caring is the essence of clinical nursing practice.
- Human caring is universal; the expressions, processes, and patterns of caring vary among cultures.

- When the nurses within an organization successfully demonstrate caring, patient satisfaction increases.
- An understanding of the behaviors that patients associate with caring offers you an excellent starting point to establish a caring practice.
- When a nurse establishes presence, eye contact, body language, voice tone, listening, and having a positive attitude, these factors act together to create an openness and understanding.
- Because touch conveys many messages, use it with discretion.
- Listening includes "taking in" what a patient says, interpreting and understanding what the patient is saying, and giving back that understanding to the person talking.
- Through caring you develop an understanding that helps you to better know the patient as a unique individual and choose the most appropriate and efficacious nursing therapies.
- Most patients and families seek spiritual care from nurses, not as a conscious or planned process but simply as a way of being human.
- Showing the family care and concern for the patient creates an openness that then enables you to form a relationship with the family.

CLINICAL DECISION-MAKING EXERCISES

Mrs. Levine has consistently relied on her son, Jim, to provide caregiving support through transportation and being a day-to-day resource. Jim brings his mother to the outpatient oncology clinic for her first chemotherapy infusion. The total treatment will last for approximately 5 hours. Sue invites Jim to sit in the treatment area with his mother.

1. As Sue prepares to administer the chemotherapy, identify three ways that she can demonstrate to Jim her caring for Mrs. Levine.
2. Jim asks Sue outside of the treatment room, "How will my mother respond to this chemotherapy? What should we expect?" Based on Swanson's theory of caring, what is an appropriate response on Sue's part in "maintaining belief?"
3. Three hours into the infusion Mrs. Levine asks Sue for a glass of water and begins talking about her pet cat and her desire to return home and be able to visit with one of her bridge partners tomorrow. Sue has another patient down the hall who has an infusion that has been under way for about an hour. What should Sue do to show her caring for Mrs. Levine?

evolve

Answers to Clinical Decision-Making Exercises can be found on the Evolve website.

QSEN ACTIVITY: PATIENT-CENTERED CARE

Mrs. Levine and her son, Jim, want to "look down the road" as her treatments continue and her disease progresses and ask Sue to help guide them in this journey. Mrs. Levine is happy with her life and wants to remain independent. When she and her son talked, they identified other challenges such as pain control, fatigue management, and nutritional needs. Jim is clear in his desire to partner with his mother during her illness. He shared with her that it is just as important to him to be with her and to give any assistance as it is for her to be independent. What they want from Sue is strategies that both can practice to "care" for one another. Mrs. Levine tells her son that as a mother it is important for her to worry and care for him and help him through this process. Jim also wants to care for his mom but not make her an invalid.

Which caring strategies can Sue teach each of them as Mrs. Levine transitions back to her home?

evolve

Answers to QSEN Activities can be found on the Evolve website.

REVIEW QUESTIONS

1. A nurse hears a colleague tell a nursing student that she never touches patients unless she is performing a procedure or doing an assessment. The nurse tells the colleague that from a caring perspective:
   1. She does not touch the patients either.
   2. Touch is a type of verbal communication.
   3. Touch forms a connection between nurse and patient.
   4. There is never a problem with using touch.
2. A young Mexican-American woman comes to a clinic for the first time for a gynecological examination. Which nursing behavior applies Swanson's caring process of "knowing" the patient?
   1. Sharing feelings about the importance of having regular gynecological examinations
   2. Explaining risk factors for cervical cancer
   3. Recognizing that the patient is modest, keeping her covered as much as possible during the examination
   4. Asking the patient what it means to have a vaginal examination
3. Helping a surgical patient adapt his learning style to discharge teaching demonstrates which of Swanson's five caring behaviors?
   1. Being with
   2. Doing for
   3. Enabling
   4. Knowing
4. When a nurse helps a patient find the meaning of cancer by supporting his beliefs about life, this is an example of:
   1. Instilling faith and hope.
   2. Forming a human-altruistic value system.

3. Cultural caring.
4. Being with.

5. Which of the following is a strategy for creating work environments that enable nurses to demonstrate more caring behaviors?
   1. Increasing technological support
   2. Increasing staff working hours
   3. Creating a setting that allows flexibility, autonomy, and the ability to discuss care
   4. Encouraging increased input concerning nursing functions from health care providers
6. Which of the following is an example of a nurse caring behavior that families perceive to be important to a patient's well-being?
   1. Making health care decisions for the patient
   2. Having family members provide a patient's total personal hygiene
   3. Injecting the nurse's personal views about death into a patient's story
   4. Asking permission before performing a procedure on a patient
7. A nurse is caring for an older adult male who is going to an assisted-living facility following discharge. Which of the following descriptions is an example of listening that displays caring?
   1. The nurse encourages the patient to talk about his concerns while reviewing a computer screen at the patient's bedside.
   2. The nurse sits at the patient's bedside, listens as he relays his fear of never seeing his home again, and then asks if he needs anything for pain.
   3. The nurse listens to the patient's story while sitting on the side of the bed and summarizes an interpretation of the patient's story.
   4. The nurse enters the patient's room, listens as he talks about his fears of not returning home, and tells the patient to think positively.
8. Listening is not only "taking in" what a patient says; it also includes:
   1. Incorporating the views of the health care provider.
   2. Correcting any errors in the patient's understanding.
   3. Injecting the nurses' personal views and statements.
   4. Interpreting and understanding what the patient means.
9. Presence involves a person-to-person encounter that:
   1. Enables a patient to care for self.
   2. Provides personal care to a patient.
   3. Conveys a closeness and a sense of caring.
   4. Incorporates own personal beliefs and values.
10. Match the following caring behaviors with their definitions:

1. ____Knowing	a. Sustaining faith in one's capacity to get through a situation
2. ____Being with	b. Striving to understand the meaning of an event for another person
3. ____Doing for	c. Being emotionally there for another person
4. ____Maintaining belief	d. Providing for another as he or she would do for themselves

evolve

Rationales for Review Questions can be found on the Evolve website.

1. 3; 2. 4; 3. 2; 4. 1; 5. 3; 6. 4; 7. 3; 8. 4; 9. 3; 10. 1=b, 2=c, 3=d, 4=a.

REFERENCES

American Nurses Association (ANA): *Nursing's agenda for the future: a call to the nation*, 2002, http://www.nursingworld.org/naf. Accessed May 9, 2008.

American Organization of Nurse Executives (AONE): *Guiding principles for patient care delivery toolkit*, 2005, http://www.aone.org/aone/resource/toolkit.html. Accessed May 9, 2006.

Benner P: *From novice to expert*, Menlo Park, CA, 1984, Addison-Wesley.

Benner P: Relational ethics of comfort, touch, solace-endangered arts, *Am J Crit Care* 13(4):346, 2004.

Benner P, Wrubel J: *The primacy of caring: stress and coping in health and illness*, Menlo Park, CA, 1989, Addison Wesley.

Benner P, et al: *Educating nurses: a call for radical transformation*, Stanford, CA, 2010, Carnegie Foundation for the Advancement of Teaching.

Bunkers SS: The power and possibility in listening, *Nurs Sci Q* 23(1):22, 2010.

Burtson L, Stichler JF: Nursing work environment and nurse caring: relationship among motivational factors, *J Adv Nurs* 66(8):1819, 2010.

Chambers T: Cross-cultural issues in caring for patients with cancer, *Cancer Treat Res* 140:45, 2008.

Crocker C, Scholes J: The importance of knowing the patient in weaning from mechanical ventilation, *Nurs Crit Care* 14(6):289, 2009.

Duffy JR, Hoskins L, Siefert RF: Dimensions of caring: psychometric evaluation of the caring assessment tool, *Adv Nurs Sci* 30(3):235, 2007.

Finfgeld-Connett D: Meta-synthesis of presence in nursing, *J Adv Nurs* 55:708, 2006.

Finfgeld-Connett D: Qualitative convergence of three nursing concepts: art of nursing, presence, and caring, *J Adv Nurs* 63(5):527, 2008a.

Finfgeld-Connett D: Qualitative comparison and synthesis of nursing presence and caring, *Intl J Nurs Terminol Classifications* 19(3):111, 2008b.

Frank AW: Just listening: narrative and deep illness, *Fam Syst Health* 16(3):197, 1998.

Fredriksson L: Modes of relating in a caring conversation: a research synthesis on presence, touch, and listening, *J Adv Nurs* 30(5):1167, 1999.

Gallagher-Lepak S, Kubsch S: Transpersonal caring: a nursing practice guideline, *Holistic Nurs Pract* 23(3):171, 2009.

Hayes JS, Tyler-Ball S: Perceptions of nurses' caring behaviors by trauma patients, *J Trauma Nurs* 14(4):187, 2007.

Henderson A, et al: "Caring for" behaviours that indicate to patients that nurses "care about" them, *J Adv Nurs* 60(2): 146, 2007.

Hudacek SS: Dimensions of caring: a qualitative analysis of nurses' stories, *J Nurs Educ* 47(3):124, 2008.

Leininger M: *Culture and care diversity and universality: a theory of nursing*, Pub No 15-2402, New York, 1991, New York.

MacDonald M: Technology and its effect on knowing the patient: a clinical analysis, *Clin Nurse Spec* 22(3):149, 2008.

Maslow AH: *Motivation and personality*, ed 3, Upper Saddle River, NY, 1987, Prentice Hall.

Muller-Staub M, et al: Nursing diagnoses, interventions and outcomes-application and impact on nursing practice: systematic review, *J Adv Nurs* 56:514, 2006.

Osterman PLC, et al: An exploratory study of nurses' presence in daily care on an oncology unit, *Nurs Forum* 45(3):197, 2010.

Palese A, et al: Surgical patient satisfaction as an outcome of nurses' caring behaviours: a descriptive correlational study in six European countries, *J Nurs Scholarship* 43(4):341, 2011.

Papastavrou E, et al: Nurses' and patients' perceptions of caring behaviours: quantitative systematic review of comparative studies, *J Adv Nurs* 67(6):1191, 2011.

Potter PA, et al: Compassion fatigue and burnout: prevalence among oncology nurses, *Clin J Oncol Nurs* 14(5):E56, 2010.

Radwin L: Oncology patients' perceptions of quality nursing care, *Res Nurs Health* 23(3):179, 2000.

Shipley SD: Listening: a concept analysis, *Nurs Forum* 45(2):125, 2010.

Suliman WA, et al: Applying Watson's nursing theory to assess patient perceptions of being cared for in a multicultural environment, *J Nurs Res* 17(4):293, 2009.

Sumner J: A critical lens on the instrumentation of caring in nursing theory, *Adv Nurs Sci* 33(1):E17, 2010.

Swanson KM: Empirical development of a middle-range theory of caring, *Nurs Res* 40(3):161, 1991.

Tonges M, Ray J: Translating caring theory into practice-the Carolina model, *J Nurs Admin* 41(9):374, 2011.

Watson J: *Caring science as a sacred science*, Philadelphia, 2005, FA Davis.

Watson J: Can an ethic of caring be maintained? *J Adv Nurs* 15:125, 2006a.

Watson J: Caring theory as an ethical guide to administrative and clinical practices, *Nurs Adm Q* 30(1):8, 2006b.

Watson J: *The philosophy and science of caring*, Boulder, 2008, University Press of Colorado.

Watson J: Caring science and human caring theory: transforming personal and professional practices of nursing and health care, *J Health Human Serv Admin* 31(4):466, 2009.

Watson J: Caring science and the next decade of holistic healing: transforming self and system from the inside out, *Am Holistic Nurses Assoc* 30(2):14, 2010.

Winsett RP, Hauck S: Implementing relationship-based care, *J Nurs Admin* 41(6):285, 2011.

CHAPTER 20

Cultural Awareness

evolve WEBSITE

http://evolve.elsevier.com/Potter/essentials

- Crossword Puzzle
- Audio Glossary

OBJECTIVES

- Describe social and cultural influences in health, illness, and caring patterns.
- Analyze the impact of culture on health, illness, and caring patterns.
- Describe health disparities.
- Describe steps toward developing cultural competence.
- Use cultural assessment to plan culturally competent care.
- Discuss research findings applicable to culturally competent care.

KEY TERMS

core measures, p. 534
cultural assessment, p. 536
cultural competence, p. 535
culturally congruent care, p. 533
culture, p. 532
explanatory model, p. 537
health disparity, p. 531
intersectionality, p. 532
ladder of cultural competence, p. 535
linguistic competence, p. 536
marginalized groups, p. 531
oppression, p. 532
social determinants of health, p. 534
transcultural nursing, p. 533
world view, p. 533

The United States is a complex multicultural society. The changing demographics of the U.S. population create challenges for the health care system. By the year 2050 the percentage of racial and ethnic minority groups in the United States is expected to climb to 50%. According to the Administration on Aging (2013), the population of people ages 65 and older is projected to double from 41.4 million in 2011 to 92 million in 2060. In 2010 15.1% (46.2 million) people officially lived in poverty. The American Community Survey 2007-2011 indicated that 42.7 million people or 14.3% of the U.S. population had income below the poverty level with African-Americans, Hispanics, and Native Americans having the highest national poverty rates (U.S. Census Bureau, 2013). According to the 2003 *National Adult Assessment of Literacy* (NAAL), only 12% of U.S. adults are proficient in obtaining, processing, and understanding basic health information and services needed to make appropriate health decisions (NCES, 2006). Additionally, more than ever before, individuals are openly expressing their religious views, sexual orientation, and gender identities. All of these factors contribute to the complexities of delivering health care in the United States. Thus, nurses and other health care providers need to consider what skills, knowledge, attitude and policies can help them deliver the best care to all patients.

The Joint Commission (TJC), the National Quality Forum (NFQ), and the National Commission on Quality Assurance (NCQA) are a few of the influential organizations that have responded to these complexities by implementing new standards focused on cultural competency, health literacy, and patient- and family-centered care. These standards recognize

CASE STUDY *Ms. Tatum*

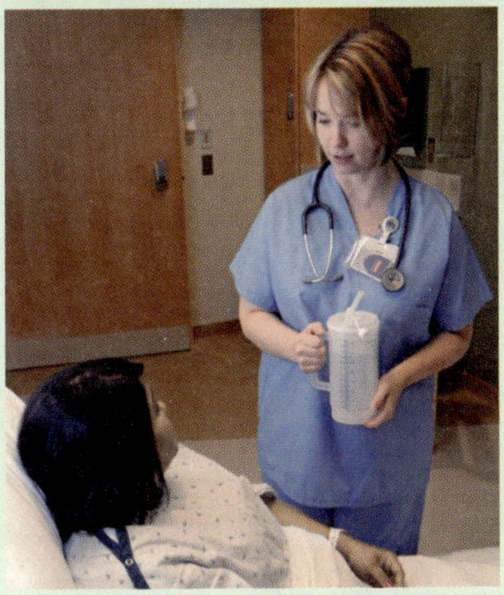

Ms. Tatum is a 27 year-old woman who is overweight, was diagnosed with diabetes 2 years ago, and now requires insulin to control her blood sugars. A major storm in 2011 destroyed her home. When she became homeless, she also lost her job and health insurance. She was admitted to the hospital with a blood sugar of 322 (the normal range is 80 to 120) and a hemoglobin A1C of 11% (normal is approximately 5%). Marina, a 23-year-old nursing student, is assigned to care for Ms. Tatum. After reading the patient's medical record, Marina notices that Ms. Tatum has come to the emergency department (ED) three times during the past 6 months for the same reason. Ms. Tatum's previous health care providers documented that she verbalized an understanding of how to manage her diabetes but has difficulty following her treatment plan. Marina teaches Ms. Tatum that it is important to take her insulin as prescribed. She also explains how to make healthy food choices. As Marina provides patient education, Ms. Tatum nods. Marina gives Ms. Tatum her insulin and ensures that she eats her scheduled meals and snacks as ordered. Before discharge, Marina gives Ms. Tatum a chance to ask questions, but Ms. Tatum says she has none.

that valuing each patient's unique needs improves the overall safety and quality of care.

HEALTH DISPARITIES

What is quality of care? More than a decade ago, a report by the Institute of Medicine (IOM, 2001) defined it as health care that is safe, effective, patient centered, timely, efficient, and equitable, or fair. Although the U.S. health care system has improved in most of those areas since the IOM report was published, the system still does not emphasize equality of care (Mutha et al., 2012). As a result, many health disparities remain.

Healthy People 2020 defines a **health disparity** as "a particular type of health difference that is closely linked with social, economic, and/or environmental disadvantage" (USDHHS, 2010). The word *parity* means "equality," so a health *dis*parity is literally an inequality or difference—a gap—between the health status of a disadvantaged group, such as people with low incomes, and an advantaged group, such as people in the upper class. Members of the disadvantaged group bear a burden of disease, injury, and violence that is out of proportion to the size of the group. They also have fewer opportunities to achieve optimal health by preventing illness and injury (CDC, 2008).

Disadvantaged groups face greater obstacles to health based on one or more of the following factors: racial or ethnic group; religion; socioeconomic status; gender; age; mental health; cognitive, sensory, or physical disability; sexual orientation or gender identity; geographic location; or other characteristics historically linked to discrimination or exclusion (USDHHS, 2010). For example, African-American children are hospitalized for asthma 4 to 5 times more often than Caucasian children. Such racial/ethnic disparities in health care are found even when comparing groups of similar socioeconomic status. For example, the infant mortality rate among children born to college-educated African-American women is significantly higher than among babies born to Caucasian women who are similarly educated (Kaiser Family Foundation, 2008).

Furthermore, although Americans' health overall has improved during the past few decades, the health of members of **marginalized groups** has actually declined (CDC, 2011). People in marginalized groups are more likely to have poor health outcomes and die at an earlier age because of a complex interaction between individual behaviors, public and health policy, community and environmental factors, and quality of health care (United Health Foundation, 2013). Poor access to health care is one social determinant of health that contributes to health disparities. Access to primary care is an important indicator of broader access to health care services. A patient who regularly visits a primary care provider is more likely to receive adequate preventive care than a patient who lacks such access. The 2011 National Healthcare Disparities Report (AHRQ, 2013b) revealed that African-Americans, Asians, and Hispanics are less likely than non-Hispanic Caucasians to see a primary care provider regularly.

A similar disparity in access to care exists in other disadvantaged groups. Less care is available or accessible to people in low- and middle-income groups compared with people in high-income groups. People who are lesbian, gay, and bisexual are less likely to have a regular source of basic health care than people who are heterosexual (Krehely, 2009). Uninsured people ages 0 to 64 are less likely to have a regular primary care provider than those with private or public insurance (AHRQ, 2013b).

A large body of research shows that health care systems and health care providers sometimes contribute significantly to the problem of health disparities. Inadequate resources, poor patient-provider communication, a lack of culturally competent care, fragmented delivery of care, and inadequate access to language services all compromise patient outcomes (NQF, 2012; National Research Council, 2003).

Studies also link poor health outcomes to limited health literacy. According to the National Research Council (2004), when compared with those who have adequate health literacy, individuals with limited health literacy report poorer health status and are less likely to use preventive services. They experience more serious medication errors, higher rates of emergency room visits and hospitalizations, increased mortality, and worse health care for their children (Brach et al., 2012). About nine out of ten people in the United States experiences challenges in using health care information (NCES, 2006). Patients who are especially vulnerable are elderly (age 65+), from immigrant populations, have low-incomes, do not have a high-school diploma or GED, and have chronic mental and/or physical health conditions (AMA, 2007).

ADDRESSING HEALTH CARE DISPARITIES

Developing health care providers' cross-cultural communication skills can help eliminate health care disparities. **Culture** was historically associated with norms, values, and traditions passed down through generations. It also has been perceived to be the same as ethnicity, race, nationality, and language (Kleinman and Benson, 2006). A more modern view of culture acknowledges its many other facets such as gender, sexual orientation, class, and immigration status (Kleinman and Benson, 2006). This more dynamic perspective recognizes that we all belong to multiple social groups at the same time, which affect our identity and experience of the world around us.

Culture develops as people share their experiences within a changing social and political landscape (Warrier, 2005). Members from the same culture share similar experiences, such as that of being an immigrant, Caucasian, and able-bodied. At the same time, significant differences exist among group members based on their individual perspectives and experiences. For example, two people share the experience of being poor, but one has a physical disability whereas the other does not.

Intersectionality

The model of **intersectionality** suggests that each of us stands at the intersection of two categories: privilege and oppression. Privilege and oppression are organizing principles formed from the building blocks of identity and culture, which include race, class, gender, age, sexual orientation, and religion (Box 20-1). **Oppression** is a formal and informal system of advantages and disadvantages tied to our membership in a social group (Adams, Bell, and Griffin, 2007). Oppression occurs on many levels—individual, cultural, and institutional. Including oppression in our definition of culture helps us recognize the profound effect it has on the individual and group experiences of those living in oppression. For example, a patient experiencing oppression has limited access to resources such as health care, housing, education, employment, and legal services. Those who support the theory of intersectionality believe that we must each determine how privileged and how oppressed we are in order to understand ourselves and the choices we make (Murphy et al., 2009). Social groups affect our daily lives, shape our world view, control our access to resources, and ultimately determine our health outcomes. Whether we live in a disadvantaged community or in a community with access to social power and resources, we are all affected by the system of oppression. Understanding the different levels of oppression and where you stand helps you develop cultural competence (Figure 20-1).

To apply the intersectionality model to daily nursing practice, think about Ms. Tatum, a 27-year-old homeless woman with diabetes; an 85-year-old African-American retired nurse from rural Alabama; a 32-year-old Latina lesbian executive in San Francisco who is Catholic; and a woman who is an undocumented immigrant from Eastern Europe and has a 3-year-old child with a developmental disability. How might the experiences of each of these women compare with the experiences of other Americans? How do their experiences with the health care system differ? How does age affect their perspective? How would these answers change if you looked at their lives 15 years ago or 35 years ago? How would the experiences change if these individuals were men or transgender? These scenarios are likely to draw a wide range of responses. The idea of intersectionality supports a broad view

BOX 20-1 KEY CONCEPTS OF INTERSECTIONALITY

- Social inequality: Groups have unequal access to resources, services, and positions.
- Over inclusion and under inclusion: Many groups have been overlooked in research and the design of interventions. For example, much of what is currently known about racial and ethnic disparities is drawn from national information sources and combines both sexes despite the large body of evidence of sex and gender differences in the prevalence of health conditions and the use of health services (James et al., 2009).
- Marginalization: Groups are left out (e.g., limited access or exclusion from facets of the society such as political system, labor market, positions of power).
- Social location: One's place in society is based on membership in a social group (e.g., gender, race, class, sexual orientation) that determines access to resources. Social location is not based on biology but on the meaning that society constructs and gives to one's social group. For example, evidence shows that race is not a biological category. Nevertheless, race in the United States has a profound effect on people's lives partly because of centuries of discrimination.
- Matrix of domination: Instead of thinking about race, gender, immigration status, and class as descriptive categories only, it is important to understand them within the context of the larger system of power and privilege that permeates society.

Adapted from Murphy Y, et al: *Incorporating intersectionality in social work practice, research, policy, and education,* Washington, DC, 2009, NASW Press.

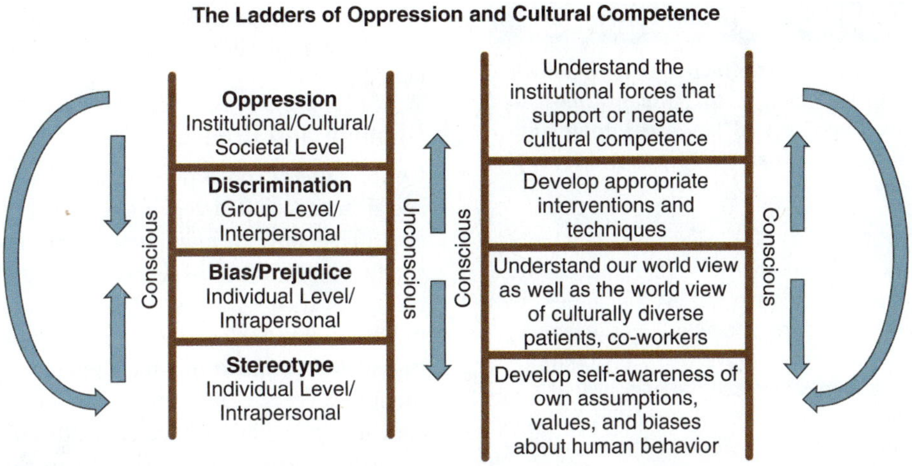

FIGURE 20-1 Ladders of oppression and cultural competence. Each level of the ladder of cultural competence offers a response to the ladder of oppression. Because of the extensiveness and complexity of the systems of oppression, individuals and organizations move up and down both ladders simultaneously. (©2011 BJH Center for Diversity and Cultural Competence.)

of culture by allowing consideration of a multitude of experiences within the context of power, privilege, and oppression. Use the intersectionality model to provide effective, evidence-based patient education (Box 20-2).

World View

Historical and social realities shape an individual's or group's **world view,** which determines how people perceive others, how they interact and relate to reality, and how they process information (Walker et al., 2010). World view refers to "the way people tend to look out upon the world or their universe to form a picture or value stance about life or the world around them" (Leininger, 2006). The cycle of socialization is the lifetime process of interacting with family, peers, communities, organizations, media, and institutions through which we develop our world view (Figure 20-2).

As a nurse, it is important that you advocate for a patient based on his or her world view. Plan and provide nursing care in partnership with each patient to ensure that it is safe, effective, and culturally sensitive (McFarland and Eipperle, 2008).

In any intercultural encounter there is an insider perspective (emic world view) and an outsider perspective (etic world view). For example, a Korean woman requests seaweed soup for her first meal after giving birth. This request puzzles her nurse. The nurse has an insider's view of professional postpartum care but is an outsider to the Korean culture. As such, the nurse is not aware of the meal's significance to the patient. Conversely, the Korean patient has an outsider's view of American professional postpartum care and assumes that seaweed soup is available in the hospital because according to her cultural beliefs, the soup cleanses the blood and promotes healing and lactation (Edelstein, 2011).

It is easy for nurses to stereotype various cultural groups after reading general information about ethnic practices and beliefs (Dein, 2006). Avoid stereotypes or unwarranted generalizations about any particular group that prevents an accurate assessment of an individual's unique characteristics and world view. Instead approach each person individually and ask questions to gain a better understanding of a patient's perspective and needs.

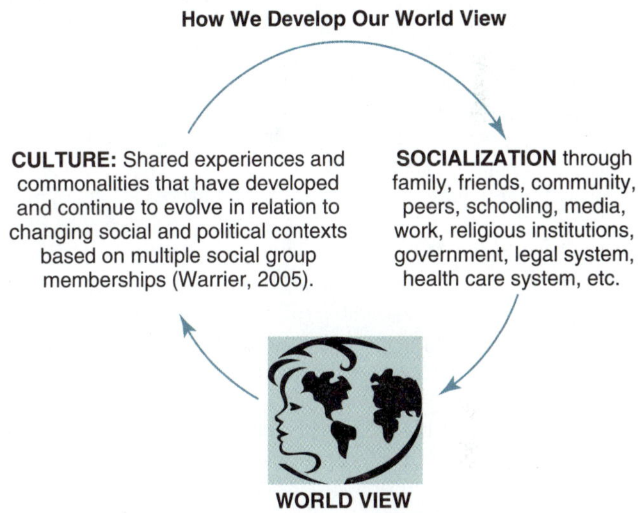

FIGURE 20-2 How we develop our world view. (©2011 BJH Center for Diversity and Cultural Competence.)

Culturally Congruent Care

Leininger (2002) defines **transcultural nursing** as a comparative study of cultures in order to understand their similarities (culture that is universal) and the differences among them (culture that is specific to particular groups). The goal of transcultural nursing is to provide **culturally congruent care,** or care that fits a person's life patterns, values, and system of meaning. Patterns and meaning are generated by people themselves, rather than from predetermined criteria. Culturally congruent care is sometimes different from the values and meanings of the professional health care system. Discovering patients' cultural values, beliefs, and practices as

BOX 20-2 EVIDENCE-BASED PRACTICE

PICO Question: What is the most effective way to deliver information about breast cancer to African-American women who are low income and have less than high school education to increase their participation in mammography screening?

SUMMARY OF EVIDENCE

Some research studies show that culturally appropriate interventions are more likely to have positive outcomes for populations affected by health disparities. For example, Kreuter et al. (2010) found that narrative forms of communication such as storytelling may increase the effectiveness of interventions to reduce cancer health disparities among some low income African-American women. The women in this study who watched a narrative video that included stories better remembered information and had more discussions with family members about breast cancer than the women who watched a video with the same content but with a more straightforward teaching approach that did not include stories. Women who watched the narrative video also reported fewer barriers to mammography and more confidence that mammograms work. They were also more likely to view cancer as an important problem affecting African-Americans. The narrative videos were especially helpful among the women who had less than a high school education, who had no close friends or family with breast cancer, and who were less trusting of traditional cancer information sources. Hall et al. (2012) evaluated the effectiveness of stories told by African-American breast cancer survivors through a mass media campaign. The stories aired on radio stations with a large number of female African-American listeners. The campaign also provided homes in predominantly African-American neighborhoods with culturally sensitive print materials to promote breast cancer awareness and the importance of breast cancer screening and early detection. Evaluation of this program found that it effectively reached African-American women and increased their awareness of breast cancer screenings available to them. Both studies suggest that narratives and culturally appropriate information is effective with certain population subgroups. Identifying these groups and matching them to specific communication approaches may increase the effectiveness of interventions.

APPLICATION TO NURSING PRACTICE

- Develop nursing interventions that take the patient's cultural experiences into consideration.
- Consider each patient individually instead of making broad generalizations.
- Modify educational approaches based on a patient's preferences to ensure the effectiveness of patient education.

they relate to nursing and health care requires you to assume the role of learner and to partner with your patients and their families to determine what is needed to provide meaningful and beneficial nursing care (Leininger and McFarland, 2002). Effective nursing care integrates the cultural values and beliefs of individuals, families, and communities with the perspectives of a multidisciplinary team of health care providers (Webber, 2008).

Disease and Illness

Culture affects social determinants of health, which are the social factors that determine health (WHO, 2013). Culture also affects how an individual defines the meaning of illness (see Chapter 2). **Social determinants of health** include resources such as access to health care, job opportunities, nutritious food, clean air, and transportation. Culture also provides the context in which a person interacts with family members, peers, community members, and institutions (e.g., educational, religious, media, health care, legal). Culture and life experiences shape a person's world view about health, illness, and health care.

To provide culturally congruent care, you need to understand the difference between disease and illness. Illness is the way that individuals and families react to disease, whereas disease is a malfunctioning of biological or psychological processes. People tend to react differently to disease based on their unique cultural perspective. Most health care providers in the United States are primarily educated to treat disease, whereas most individuals seek health care because of their experience with illness. In addition, there is a lack of cultural diversity among health care providers (OMH, 2013). This often frustrates patients and providers, fostering a lack of trust, lack of adherence, and poor health outcomes. Providing safe, quality care to all patients means taking into consideration both disease and illness.

Core Measures

The Joint Commission (TJC) and the Centers for Medicare and Medicaid Services (CMS) are two of the many regulatory bodies that hold health care providers accountable for considering patients' unique cultural perspectives in order to provide safe and quality care.

To improve health outcomes, TJC and the CMS developed a set of evidence-based, scientifically researched standards of care called *core measures* (TJC, 2013). The **core measures** are key quality indicators that help health care institutions improve performance, increase accountability, and reduce costs. All of the core measures, such as screening for depression and controlling high blood pressure, are consistent with national health priorities. They represent clinical conditions like heart failure, acute myocardial infarction, pneumonia, and surgical-site infections. Following these standards of care on a nationwide scale is expected to reduce mortality, complications, and inpatient readmissions (VanSuch et al., 2006; Chassin et al., 2010).

In addition, the core measures are intended to reduce health disparities. According to the 2011 National Health Care Disparities Report, African-Americans, American Indians, and Alaska Natives received worse care than Caucasians for 40% of core measures; Asians received worse care than Caucasians for 20% of core measures; Hispanics received worse care than Caucasians for 60% of core measures; and people who were poor received worse care than those with high incomes for 80% of core measures (AHRQ, 2013b).

CULTURAL COMPETENCE

Cultural competence is the ongoing process in which a health care professional strives to work effectively within the cultural context of a patient (individual, family, and community). A variety of models for acquiring cultural competence have been proposed. One model suggests that nurses see themselves as *becoming* rather than *being* culturally competent (Campinha-Bacote, 2007), since cultural competence is a developmental process that evolves over a lifetime. Campinha-Bacote's (2002) model of cultural competency has five interrelated components:

1. *Cultural awareness*: An in-depth self-examination of one's own background, recognizing biases, prejudices, and assumptions about other people
2. *Cultural knowledge*: Sufficient comparative knowledge of diverse groups, including the values, health beliefs, care practices, world view, and bicultural ecology commonly found within each group
3. *Cultural skills*: Ability to assess social, cultural, and biophysical factors that influence patient treatment and care
4. *Cultural encounters*: Cross-cultural interactions that provide opportunities to learn about other cultures and develop effective intercultural communication
5. *Cultural desire*: The motivation and commitment to caring that moves an individual to learn from others, accept the role as learner, be open to and accepting of cultural differences, and build on cultural similarities

You need to have specific knowledge, skills, and attitudes to deliver culturally congruent care to individuals, families, and communities. When you provide culturally competent care, you bridge cultural gaps to provide meaningful and supportive care for all patients. For example, during nursing school you are assigned to care for a female patient who observes Muslim beliefs. You notice the woman's discomfort with several of the male health care providers. You wonder if this discomfort is related to your patient's religious beliefs. While preparing for clinicals, you learn that Muslims differ in their adherence to tradition but that modesty is the "overarching Islamic ethic" pertaining to interaction between the sexes (Rabin, 2010). Thus you say to the patient, "I know that for many of our Muslim patients, modesty is very important. Is there some way I can make you more comfortable?" You do not assume that the information will automatically apply to this patient. Instead you combine your knowledge about a cultural group with an attitude of helpfulness and flexibility in order to provide quality, patient-centered, culturally congruent care.

Another model of cultural competence is the framework developed in the field of social work by Sue (2006). It includes four components:

- Developing self-awareness
- Understanding the worldview of others
- Developing appropriate strategies, skills and interventions
- Understanding organizational and institutional forces that either enable or inhibit cultural competence.

The ladder of cultural competence (see Figure 20-1) integrates Sue's model with the ladder of oppression to emphasize how culturally competent organizations and individuals can work to eliminate health care disparities. The integrated model implies that systems of oppression produce health inequities and operate at individual, group, and institutional levels. Culturally competent providers and institutions consider *all* of these levels in their efforts to deliver safe and quality care to all patients.

Self-Awareness

Curiosity about other ways of being in the world is an important attitude for cultural competence; however, it is also important for you to understand the forces that influence your own world view. Everyone holds biases about human behavior. A bias is a predisposition to see people or things in a certain light, either positive or negative (Aguilar, 2006). Becoming more aware of your biases and attitudes about human behavior is the first step on the ladder of cultural competence, which leads to positive change.

World View of Providers and Patients

Research supports the idea that group membership, such as membership in a professional group, shapes one's world view (Sue, 2006). Health care has its own culture of hierarchies, power dynamics, values, beliefs, and practices. Most health care providers educated in Western traditions are immersed in the culture of science and biomedicine through their coursework and professional experience. Consequently they often have a world view that differs from that of their patients. As a nurse, you need to assume that every patient encounter will be a cross-cultural one.

Even when a patient and health care provider are similar in age or have the same gender or ethnicity, two different perspectives are present each time they interact. When patients access the health care system they want to: (1) see their health care provider and (2) feel better. In return the health care providers expect patients to: (1) make and keep appointments; (2) give a medication history; (3) give informed consent; (4) follow (discharge) instructions; (5) read, understand, and use health education materials; (6) correctly complete insurance forms; (7) pay their bills; and (8) go home and manage their care by taking their medication the right way, eating the right foods, and stopping/starting/changing a variety of behaviors (AMA, 2007, p. 11). This list shows how complex each patient interaction is even before the interaction begins. The complexity increases as you consider the interactive effect between a health care provider's and patient's multiple social group identities and unique life experiences.

You, the patient, and all other health care providers bring each of your world views into the care process. The Iceberg Analogy (Figure 20-3) is a tool that helps you visualize the

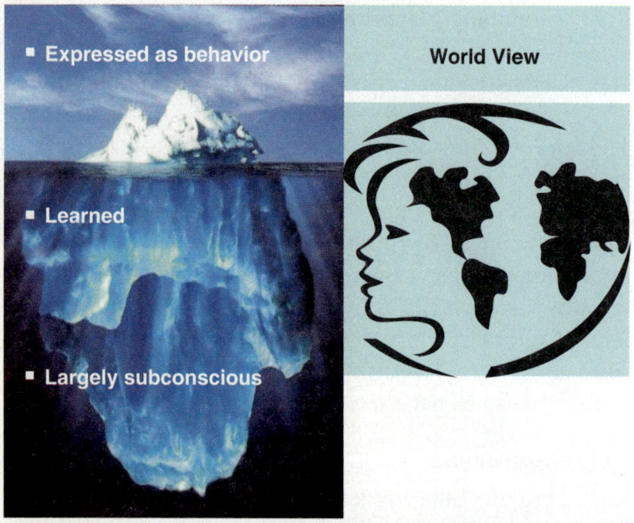

FIGURE 20-3 This model has been adapted from Campinha-Bacote et al. (2005) Iceberg Analogy. It incorporates the Kleinman (1980) explanatory model to emphasize that both nurse and patient act in accordance with their own world views. (©2011 BJH Center for Diversity and Cultural Competence.)

visible and invisible aspects of your world view. Just as most of an iceberg lies beneath the surface of the water, most aspects of a person's world view lie outside of his or her awareness and are invisible to those around the person. For example, a patient who has willingly agreed to be admitted to the hospital for a serious medical condition requiring surgery may refuse the surgery for religious reasons. In the patient's view, she came to the hospital for help to eliminate the pain and infection from her illness. At the same time she believes that she needs to seek God for a decision that entails removing a body part. The patient's health care provider assumes the patient is in the hospital to receive care for a serious illness and is willing to accept any and all treatments to cure the illness. The patient's deeply held religious beliefs about removing a body part are not obvious by assessing for a religious preference. Thus the nurse needs to conduct a comprehensive **cultural assessment** to understand how the patient's religious values will affect her willingness to receive care. These deeply held values reside underneath the iceberg. The observed behavior (in this case, coming to the hospital) is a visible sign of a person's world view, but the beliefs, attitudes, knowledge, and experiences that guide the behavior are not visible to others. Conflict arises when health care providers interpret the behaviors of patients through their own world view lens instead of trying to uncover the world view that guides the behavior of their patients.

Because of differences in age, gender, political association, class, religion, or other variables, cultural values frequently differ within a single social group, such as a family or a group of nurses. For patients, family members, and members of the health care team alike, culture is a process through which ordinary activities, such as greeting another person or selecting a doctor, take on an emotional tone and moral meaning beyond that which appears on the surface (Kleinman and Benson, 2006). Think about the complexity of cultural competence. Realize the need to develop your assessment skills and cultural interventions that will allow you to successfully negotiate the various world views present in all patient encounters.

Skills and Interventions

You need to develop skills and interventions to become culturally competent (Sue, 2006). Cultural skill is defined as the ability to collect relevant cultural data about a patient's presenting health problem(s) and use the collected data to ensure quality and safe care (Campinha-Bacote, 2011). Critical to success is your ability to conduct a systematic cultural assessment, communicate effectively, and have the skills to successfully manage world view differences with others.

Institutional Forces

In the past, health care agencies promoted a culturally competent health care environment by focusing on health care providers' efforts to become self-aware and learn about other cultures. Currently, the focus is on approaches that integrate cultural competence skills into everyday administrative processes and the provision of care. Health care regulatory agencies, national think-tanks, and government agencies expect health care organizations to incorporate cultural competence into policies and practices to ensure effective communication, patient safety and quality, and patient-centered care. Some examples of such organizational policies and practices include:

- Instituting a requirement for all staff to be trained in cultural competence.
- Embedding a broad description of family in written policies.
- Expanding visitation policies and practices to include a patient's preferences.
- Requiring nursing staff to conduct and document a cultural assessment on all patients within the clinical documentation system.
- Ensuring that persons who are deaf or speak limited English have access to an interpreter.
- Embedding health literacy principles in written and verbal communication.

Nurses and other health care providers need to be familiar with how policies and institutional forces enable or inhibit their ability to provide culturally competent, patient-centered, high-quality, safe care to all of their patients. When policies impede the delivery of effective care, you and your colleagues must advocate for policy change.

LINGUISTIC COMPETENCE

The National Center for Cultural Competence (2006) distinguishes linguistic competence from cultural competence. **Linguistic competence** is the ability of an organization and its staff to communicate effectively and convey information in a manner that is easily understood by diverse audiences. These audiences include people of limited English proficiency, those who have low literacy skills or are not literate, individuals with disabilities, and those who are deaf or hard of hearing. Linguistic competency requires organizational resources (e.g., interpreters) and providers who are able to respond effectively to the health and mental health literacy needs of the populations served. Nurses and other health care providers need organizational policies, procedures, structures, practices, and dedicated resources to understand and communicate effectively with all patients (Goode and Jones, 2009).

EVOLUTION OF CULTURAL COMPETENCE IN HEALTH CARE

Since 2000 the field of cultural competence has grown exponentially. According to Saha, Beach, and Cooper (2008), more than 1000 published health care journal articles contain the terms "cultural competence" or "cultural competency." A broad range of national and international efforts now address health care inequities through cultural competence education, interventions, and policies. In 2000 the Office of Minority Health developed Culturally and Linguistically Appropriate Standards (CLAS). In 2013, after 10 years of successful implementation, the OMH updated the standards to reflect the tremendous growth in the field and the increasing diversity of the nation. The enhanced National CLAS Standards are intended to advance health equity, improve quality, and help eliminate health care disparities by establishing a blueprint to help individuals and health care organizations implement culturally and linguistically appropriate services (OMH, 2013).

In its early stages the field of cultural competence primarily focused on the cultural barriers between health care providers educated in Western health care practices and immigrants arriving from non-Western parts of the world. Berlin and Fowkes (1982), Kleinman (1980), and Leininger (2002) were early pioneers in cross-cultural medicine who in the late 1970s and early 1980s outlined a set of universal skills to help health care providers work effectively with patients from any culture. These skills include: (1) respecting a patient's health beliefs as valid and understanding the effect of a patient's beliefs on health care delivery; (2) shifting a model of understanding a patient's experience from a disease happening in his or her organ systems to that of an illness occurring in the context of culture (biopsychosocial) context; (3) ability to elicit a patient's explanation of an illness and its causes (patient's **explanatory model**); (4) ability to explain to a patient in understandable terms the health care provider's perspective on the illness and perceived causes; and (5) being able to negotiate a mutually agreeable safe and effective treatment plan (Saha et al., 2008).

Expanding their original focus on interpersonal skills, many of the current approaches to cultural competence now also focus on: (1) all marginalized groups and not just immigrants; (2) prejudice, stereotyping, and social determinants of health; and (3) the health system, communities, and institutions (Saha et al, 2008).

You broaden your understanding of the world by learning about other people's world views, customs, values and experiences through reading, watching movies, taking courses, and traveling. However, this learning process can be tricky. Focusing too narrowly on learning about "others" potentially turns dynamic cultures into little more than encyclopedia entries. Unique, lively individuals become static objects of study. In trying to understand those who differ from the majority in some respect—appearance, language, national origin, religion, or sexual orientation, for example—you may be tempted to categorize people according to simplistic differences (Kumagai and Lypson, 2009). By describing people only in terms of how they differ from the majority, you unintentionally reinforce the dominant culture and lose the details of each individual's character and behavior. As a nurse, you are responsible for investigating whether a patient's health issue is associated with underlying societal conditions. You need to either find or develop theoretical frameworks to structure nursing interventions (Grace and Willis, 2012). As a member of the nursing profession, you need to understand principles of health and well-being and be able to discover and address injustice (Grace and Willis, 2012).

CULTURAL ASSESSMENT AND PATIENT-CENTERED CARE

Although cultural competence and patient-centered care both aim to improve health care quality, their focus is slightly different. Patient-centered care provides individualized care and restores an emphasis on personal relationships. It aims to elevate quality for all patients. Alternatively, cultural competence reduces health disparities and increases health equity and fairness by concentrating on people of color and other marginalized groups (Beach, Saha, and Cooper, 2006). Both patient-centered care and cultural competence recognize each patient as a unique person. You need to have cultural competence to provide effective patient-centered care to all patients (Campinha-Bacote, 2011).

Cultural Assessment

Cultural skill involves performing a systematic cultural assessment of individuals, groups, and communities as to their cultural beliefs, values and practices. When done correctly and appropriately you are able to form a mutually acceptable and culturally relevant treatment plan for each patient (Campinha-Bacote, 2011).

Numerous models facilitate cultural assessment, including Leininger's Sunrise Model (2002), Giger and Davidhizar's Transcultural Assessment Model (2002), and the Purnell Model for Cultural Competence (Purnell, 2002). Regardless of which one you select, using a cultural assessment model will help you focus on the information that is most relevant to your patient's problems. It will also help you better understand the complex factors that influence your patient's cultural world view. You need to assess and interpret a patient's

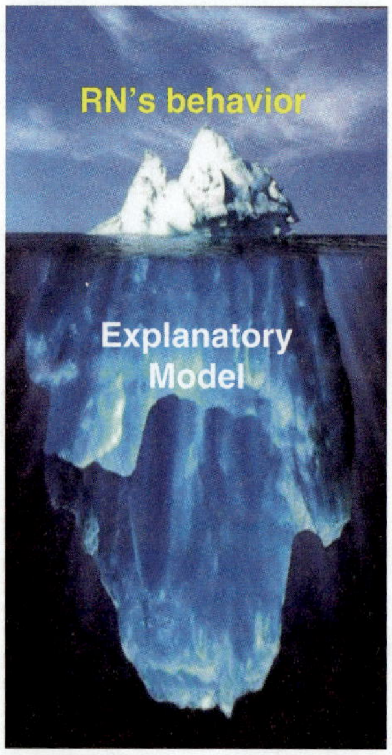

1. What do you call the problem? What name does it have?
2. What do you think has caused the problem?
3. Why do you think it started when it did?
4. What does your sickness do to you? How does it work?
5. How severe is it? Will it last a long or short time?
6. What do you fear most about this sickness?
7. What are the chief problems your sickness has caused for you?
8. What type of treatment do you think you should receive? What are the most important results you hope to receive from the treatment?

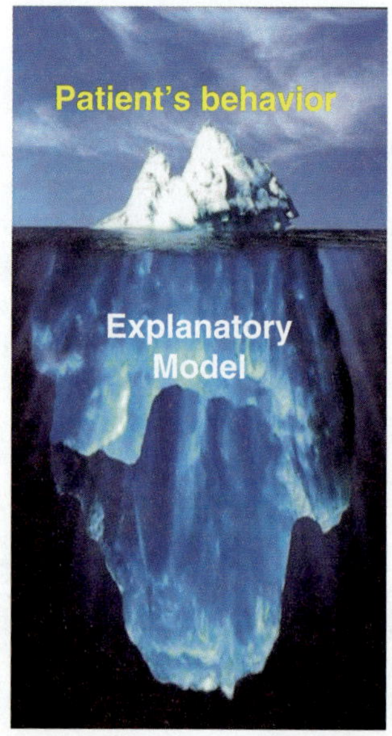

FIGURE 20-4 Cultural model that integrates Kleinman's explanatory model with the Iceberg Analogy. (©2011 BJH Center for Diversity and Cultural Competence.)

perspective during your assessment. Use open-ended, focused, and contrast questions. Encourage your patients to describe the values, beliefs, and practices that are significant to their care. Culturally oriented questions are by nature broad and require many descriptions (Box 20-3).

One effective approach to assessment is to ask questions that will help you understand a patient's definitions of health, wellness, and illness. Understanding a patient's perceptions of these concepts and the relationships between them helps you provide patient-centered care that combines a patient's values and beliefs with your perspectives. Using a cultural model during your assessment (such as the one in Figure 20-4 that integrates Kleinman's explanatory model with the previously discussed Iceberg Analogy) will help you develop open-ended questions that effectively reveal your patient's views on illness (Kleinman and Benson, 2006).

Table 20-1 summarizes and contrasts a patient's explanatory model of illness with the biomedical explanatory model of illness (Lynch and Medin, 2006). *In Ms. Tatum's case, she responds to Marina's biomedical assessment, indicating that she understands how to take her medications. Yet Ms. Tatum has come to the ED several times for the same problem. If Marina uses Kleinman's explanatory model to assess Ms. Tatum's perception of her problem, she will discover Ms. Tatum's beliefs and fears about her illness as well as her willingness to change or adopt behaviors to prevent future ED visits.*

Establishing Relationships

In contrast to other types of interviews, cultural assessment is intrusive and time consuming and requires a trusting relationship between participants. Miscommunication commonly occurs in intercultural transactions. This is because of language communication differences between and among

BOX 20-3 NURSING ASSESSMENT QUESTIONS

OPEN-ENDED
- What do you think caused you to become sick?
- How do you want us to help you with your problem?

FOCUSED
- Did you have this problem before?
- Is there someone you want us to talk to about your care?

CONTRAST
- How different is this problem from the one you had a month ago?
- What is the difference between what we are doing and what you think we should be doing for you?

ETHNOHISTORY
- How long have you/your parents lived in this country?
- What is your ethnic background or ancestry?
- Tell me how you left your homeland.

SOCIAL ORGANIZATION
- Who lives with you?
- What is your significant other/partner's name?
- Who are your family members?
- Where do other members of your family live?
- Who makes the decisions for you or your family?

CARING BELIEFS AND PRACTICES
- What do you do to keep yourself well?
- What do you do to show someone you care?
- How do you take care of sick family members?
- Which caregivers do you seek help from when you are sick?

TABLE 20-1 EXPLANATORY MODEL COMPARISON

PATIENT'S EXPLANATORY MODEL	BIOMEDICAL EXPLANATORY MODEL
What do you call your problem? What name does it have?	Etiology
What do you think has caused your problem? Why do you think it started when it did?	Time and mode of onset
What do you think your sickness does to you? How does this illness work inside your body?	Pathophysiology
What will happen to you? What do you fear most about your sickness? What are the chief problems your sickness has caused for you?	Course of illness (including symptom severity & trajectory: acute, chronic, impaired)
How should your sickness be treated?	Recommended treatment

Adapted from Lynch E, Medin D: Explanatory models of illness: study of within-culture variation, *Cogn Psychol* 53(4):285, 2006. Epub April 18, 2006.

participants and differences in interpreting one another's behaviors. You use transcultural communication skills to interpret a patient's behavior and to behave in a culturally congruent way. Effective communication is a critical skill in culturally competent care and helps you engage a patient/family in respectful, patient-centered dialogue. Transcultural communication manages the impression you make on a patient to achieve desired outcomes of communication (Purnell and Paulanka, 2008).

Mnemonics, or memory aids, make it easier to perform assessments and communicate effectively with patients (Table 20-2). They help you remember the steps of each communication technique. Cultural assessment requires a level of negotiation. Leininger (2006) describes cultural care negotiation as assistive, accommodating, facilitative, or enabling creative provider care actions or decisions that help people with different backgrounds adapt to or negotiate with others for culturally congruent care.

Heath Literacy and Teach Back

The concept of linguistic competence encompasses both health literacy and limited English proficiency. The dual challenges of limited health literacy and cultural differences are likely to increase with an expanding, increasingly diverse, and older population. Evidence suggests that health care providers who attend to both issues help reduce medical errors and improve adherence, patient-provider-family communication, and outcomes of care at both individual and population levels (Lie et al., 2012). Clear communication is essential for

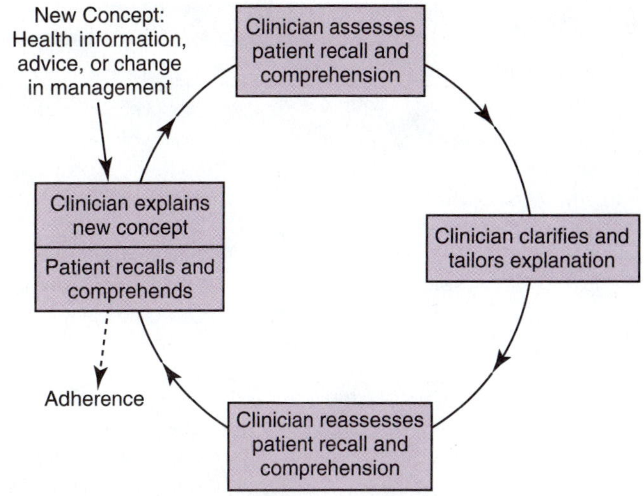

FIGURE 20-5 Using Teach Back technique to close the loop. (From the U.S. Health Resources and Services Administration.)

effective delivery of quality and safe health care, but most patients experience significant challenges when communicating with their health care providers. Use the Teach Back method to confirm that you have explained what a patient needs to know in a manner that the patient understands. The Teach Back technique is an ongoing process of asking patients for feedback through explanation or demonstration and of presenting information in a new way until you feel confident that you communicated clearly and that your patient has a full understanding of the information presented (Figure 20-5). You also use Teach Back to help you identify explanations and communication strategies your patients most commonly understand (AHRQ, 2013a).

When using the Teach Back technique do not ask a patient, "Do you understand?" or "Do you have any questions?" Instead ask open-ended questions to verify a patient's understanding. You can ask the question in the following ways.

- "I've given you a lot of information to remember. Please explain it back to me so I can be sure that I gave you the information you want and need to take good care of yourself."
- "What will you tell your wife [or husband/partner/child] about the changes we made to your medications today?"
- "We've gone over a lot of information today about how you might change your diet, and I want to make sure I explained everything clearly. In your own words, please review what we talked about. How will you make it work at home?"

It is important to understand that Teach Back is not intended to test a patient but rather to confirm the clarity of your communication (AHRQ, 2013a). Many patients are embarrassed by their inability to sort out health information or instructions. By regarding Teach Back as a test of your communication skills, you take responsibility for the success or failure of the interaction and create a shame-free environment for your patients.

TABLE 20-2 COMMUNICATION TECHNIQUES USING MNEMONICS

COMMUNICATION TECHNIQUE	PROCESS
Learn Berlin EA, Fowkes WC Jr: A teaching framework for cross-cultural health care, *West J Med* 139(6):934, 1982.	*L*isten with sympathy and understanding to patient's perception of problem. *E*xplain your perceptions of the problem (physiological, psychological, spiritual and/or cultural). *A*cknowledge and discuss cultural differences and similarities between you and your patient. *R*ecommend treatment (involving patient). *N*egotiate agreement (incorporate selected aspects of patient's culture into patient-centered plan).
Respect Bigby JA, editor: *Cross-cultural medicine,* Philadelphia, 2003, American College of Physicians p 20.	*R*apport Connect on a social level. Seek the patient's point of view. Consciously attempt to suspend judgment. Recognize and avoid making assumptions. *E*mpathy Remember that the patient has come to you for help. Seek out and understand the patient's rationale for his or her behaviors or illness. Verbally acknowledge and legitimize the patient's feelings. *S*upport Ask about and try to understand barriers to care and compliance. Help the patient overcome barriers. Involve family members if appropriate. Reassure the patient that you are and will be available to help. *P*artnership Be flexible with regard to issues of control. Negotiate roles when necessary. Stress that you will be working together to address medical problems. *E*xplanations Check often for understanding. Use verbal clarification techniques. *C*ultural *C*ompetence Respect the patient and his or her culture and beliefs. Understand that the patient's view of you may be influenced by stereotypes. Be aware of your own biases and preconceptions. Know your limitations in addressing medical issues across cultures. Understand your personal style and recognize when it may not be working with a given patient. *T*rust Self-disclosure may be difficult for some patients. Do not assume trust; instead take necessary time and consciously work to earn trust.
Ethnic Levin S, Like RC, Gottlieb JE: ETHNIC: A framework for culturally competent clinical practice, Patient Care 9(special issue):188, 2000.	*E*xplanation—Patient explains his or her perception of problem, or you ask what most concerns the patient. *T*reatment—What types of treatments has the patient tried for the problem? *H*ealers—Has the patient sought advice from alternative health practitioners (Table 20-3)? *N*egotiate—Try to find an option that is mutually acceptable. *I*ntervention—Agree on an appropriate intervention, which may incorporate alternate treatments. *C*ollaboration—Include patient, family members, and other health care professionals, healers, and community resources.
C-LARA *LARA* was developed by the organization Love Makes a Family; *C* (check your pulse) addition has been contributed by the organization Nonviolent Peaceforce.	*C*alm yourself down. Take a deep breath. Check your pulse. *L*isten to the patient's and family's perspective. *A*ffirm: Express connection with something that was shared: a feeling, perspective, principle. *R*espond: To what was said. Answer the question. *A*dd: Share additional information for the patient and family to consider. In this step you can educate.

TABLE 20-3 HEALERS THAT A PATIENT MAY MENTION WHEN ASSESSING EXPLANATORY MODELS

HEALER	NATURE OF PRACTICE
Herbalist	Person who combines plant, animal, and mineral products to prevent and treat illness
Acupuncturist	Practitioner who treats patients by using needles to restore balance and flow of *qi*
Shaman	Spiritual healer who combines prayers, chanting, and herbs to treat illnesses
Ayurvedic provider	Therapist who combines dietary, herbal, and other naturalistic therapies to prevent and treat illness
Homeopath	Practitioner who uses natural remedies in titrated doses
Chaplain	Spiritual adviser who offers counseling and prayer to treat illness or cope with personal and psychosocial problems related to illness
Curandero/a	Traditional healer who combines herbs, prayer, and other rituals to treat illness, especially in children
Partera Lay midwife	Person who assists women in childbirth and with newborn care
Yerbero Herbalist	Consultant for traditional herbal treatment of illnesses
Sabador Bonesetter	Healer who massages and manipulates bones and joints and treats a variety of ailments
Priest/Pastor	Person with the authority to lead or perform ceremonies in some religions, especially in some Christian religions
Rabbi	Person trained to make decisions about what is lawful in Judaism, perform Jewish ceremonies, or lead a Jewish congregation
Imam	Muslim religious leader; the prayer leader of a mosque
Doula	Woman experienced in childbirth who provides advice, information, emotional support, and physical comfort to a mother before, during, and just after childbirth
Chiropractor	Licensed practitioner whose system of therapy is based on the belief that disease results from a lack of normal nerve function and who manipulates and adjusts specific body structures (such as the spinal column)
Massage therapist	Practitioner who manipulates tissues (as by rubbing, kneading, or tapping) with the hand or with an instrument for therapeutic purposes

Below are helpful hints to consider when trying the Teach Back method:

- *Plan your approach.* Think about how you will ask your patient to teach back in a shame-free way. Keep in mind that some situations are not appropriate for Teach Back (AHRQ, 2013a).
- *Use handouts, pictures, and models* to reinforce your teaching (AHRQ, 2013a).
- *Clarify.* If a patient cannot remember or accurately repeat your instructions, clarify your information and allow him or her to teach it back again. Do this until the patient is able to teach back in his or her own words without parroting back what you said (AHRQ, 2013a). Understand Teach Back as a process of "closing the loop." (Schillinger et al., 2003) (see Figure 20-5).
- *Practice.* Although it takes time to get used to Teach Back, studies show that it does not take longer to perform once it becomes a part of your routine (AHRQ, 2013a). Box 20-4 provides an example of how Marina

BOX 20-4 PATIENT TEACHING

Taking Insulin As Prescribed and Nutritional Education

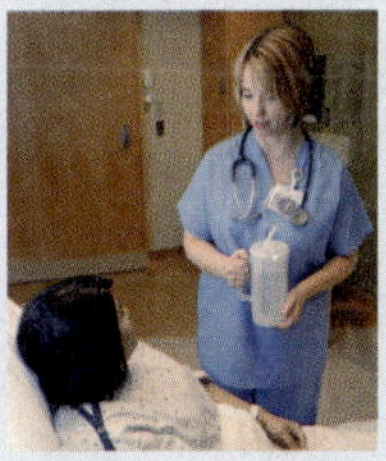

Marina knows it is important for Ms. Tatum to understand her health problems and prescribed treatments. Thus Marina plans to use Teach Back to ensure Ms. Tatum understands how to effectively manage her diabetes.

OUTCOME

At the end of the teaching session, Ms. Tatum will be able to:

- Verbalize in her own words how she will take her insulin
- Describe how she plans to make healthy food choices

TEACHING STRATEGIES

- Create a shame-free environment by demonstrating a general attitude of helpfulness.
- Assess Ms. Tatum's base line understanding of her diabetes and management strategies. This allows Marina to tailor education to Ms. Tatum's specific needs.
- Use nonmedical language and define in plain language all the medical terms.
- Sit instead of stand, and speak slowly.
- Use pictures, models, and written handouts to help Ms. Tatum better remember relevant information.
- Give Ms. Tatum the opportunity to prepare her own insulin whenever possible, and provide encouragement and feedback when needed.

EVALUATION STRATEGIES

- Have Ms. Tatum prepare her insulin in a syringe, evaluating each step and providing feedback as needed.
- State, "We've gone over a lot of information today about changes you plan to make to your diet. In your own words, please review what we talked about. How will you make it work at the shelter?"

used some of these strategies to educate Ms. Tatum on how to take insulin and manage her diet.

WORKING WITH INTERPRETERS

Most health care providers and virtually all health care organizations nationwide are subject to federal civil rights laws. These laws outline requirements for provision of language access services. They also help ensure meaningful access to health care for people with limited English proficiency (LEP) and offer effective communication services for those who are deaf or hard-of-hearing (TJC, 2013). As a nurse, it is critical for you to know that these laws require health care organizations to do the following:

- Provide language assistance services at all points of contact free of charge to all patients who speak limited English or are deaf.
- Notify patients, both verbally and in writing, of their right to receive language-assistance services.
- Take steps to provide auxiliary aids and services, including qualified interpreters, note takers, computer-aided transcription services, and written materials.
- Ensure that interpreters are competent in medical terminology and understand issues of confidentiality and impartiality.

Do not use a patient's family members to interpret for you or other health care providers. Cultural dynamics, lack of interpreting skills, low health literacy, and bias could lead to inaccurate interpretation. Box 20-5 provides guidelines for effectively working with an interpreter.

BOX 20-5 WORKING WITH INTERPRETERS

If a patient needs an interpreter:

- Introduce yourself to the interpreter and briefly describe the purpose of the meeting.
- Determine the interpreter's qualifications.
- Make sure the interpreter can speak the patient's dialect.
- Watch for differences in educational and socioeconomic status between the patient and the interpreter.
- Make sure that both the patient and interpreter are compatible and that both understand the expectations of the interpreter role.
- Introduce the interpreter to the patient.
- Do not expect the interpreter to interpret your statements word for word. Although the interpreter must ensure that everything that was said is interpreted, he or she may need to use more or fewer words to convey the meaning of your conversation with a patient.
- If you sense that the interpretation is not going well, stop and address the situation directly with the interpreter.
- Pace your speech by using short sentences, but do not break your sentences. Allow time for the patient's response to be interpreted.
- Direct your questions to the patient. Look at the patient, instead of looking at the interpreter.
- Ask the patient for feedback and clarification at regular intervals.
- Observe the patient's nonverbal and verbal behaviors.
- Thank both patient and interpreter.

Data from Pacquiao DF: Impression management: an alternative to assertiveness in intercultural communication, *J Transcult Nurs* 11(1):5, 2000.

KEY POINTS

- A health disparity that involves differences in the burden of disease, injury, violence, or opportunities to achieve optimal health experienced by socially disadvantaged groups is preventable.
- Members of marginalized groups are more likely to have poor health outcomes and to die at an earlier age.
- Health care systems and providers contribute to the problem of health disparities as a result of inadequate resources, poor patient-provider communication, a lack of culturally competent care, system fragmentation and inadequate access to language services.
- Culture is complex and dynamic. It includes race, ethnicity, nationality, gender, sexual orientation, class, immigration status, and other forms of identification. All of us are members of multiple social groups at the same time.
- Intersectionality is a model that helps you understand a person's location at the intersection of privilege and oppression. These socially constructed categories are influenced by race, class, gender, age, sexual orientation, and other characteristics.
- Culturally congruent care is sometimes different from the values and meanings of the professional health care system.
- A person's culture and life experiences shape his or her world view about health, illness, and health care.
- Nurses who provide culturally competent care bridge cultural gaps to provide meaningful and supportive care for all patients.
- For the patient, his or her family members, and members of the health care team, culture is a process through which ordinary activities such as greeting a person or selecting a health care provider take on an emotional tone and moral meaning.
- Cultural competency requires you to conduct systematic cultural assessments, communicate effectively, and have the skills to negotiate world view differences with others.
- One effective approach to cultural assessment is to ask patients questions that reveal their explanatory model of health, wellness, and illness.
- Current evidence shows that attending to limited health literacy and cultural differences often reduces medical errors and improves adherence, patient-provider-family communication, and outcomes of care.
- Use the Teach Back method to confirm that you have explained to a patient what he or she needs to know in a way that the patient understands.

CLINICAL DECISION-MAKING EXERCISES

After Marina conducts a cultural assessment using an explanatory model with questions similar to those in Table 20-1, she learns that Ms. Tatum fears she will eventually die because her mother died of diabetes. She also learns that Ms. Tatum has no way of getting her medications filled because she does not have health insurance. After obtaining this information, Marina consults with a social worker, who tells Marina about a community health center within five blocks of the homeless shelter where Ms. Tatum is living. This health center has a diabetes management program and can offer ongoing support to Ms. Tatum. Marina spends time with Ms. Tatum explaining that people do not die from diabetes if they manage it effectively. She discusses with Ms. Tatum some realistic ways to manage her diabetes given her challenging circumstances. Marina realizes that there is an opportunity for her to learn more about the social determinants of health that affect Ms. Tatum's ability to manage his or her care. She also realizes that by gaining skills in cultural competence she will be more confident in providing culturally competent care to her patients.

1. List some of the social determinants of health that Marina most likely discovered while conducting a cultural assessment with Ms. Tatum.
2. Based on a cultural assessment Marina discovers that Ms. Tatum believes that she may die. Select one of the communication mnemonics listed in this chapter and plot a discussion that might help Ms. Tatum understand that diabetes is a manageable chronic illness that does not have to result in death.
3. Ms. Tatum is discharged and returns to the ED several months later because she is having difficulty managing her diabetes again. You are assigned to care for Ms. Tatum. How will Ms. Tatum's weight, history of noncompliance, and past visits to the ED possibly affect your treatment of Ms. Tatum? How could these factors trigger biases and assumptions that will get in the way of providing quality care? How could self-awareness help you reduce the effect of bias on the quality of care you provide?

evolve

Answers to Clinical Decision-Making Exercises can be found on the Evolve website.

QSEN ACTIVITY: SAFETY

After teaching Ms. Tatum about diabetes management, Marina finishes the conversation by asking, "Do you have any questions?" Ms. Tatum states that she does not.

What is a more effective way to end this conversation and ensure safe care? How could thinking about the impact of health literacy on patient safety allow Marina to provide the highest quality of care to Ms. Tatum?

evolve

Answers to QSEN Activities can be found on the Evolve website.

REVIEW QUESTIONS

1. A nurse enters the examination room of the emergency clinic and meets a 56-year-old patient who has gained 6 lbs in 2 weeks and reports having a difficult time breathing because he did not take his medications as ordered at home. The patient is morbidly obese, and the nurse notes from the medical record that he has heart failure. He just had a discussion with a physician who was frustrated and impatient because the patient did not take his medications as prescribed. The patient confronts the nurse, saying, "I'm tired of being treated this way; no one cares. What are you going to do to help me?" Using the C-LARA mnemonic, match the nurse's response to the correct letter of the mnemonic.
   1. C ____
   2. L ____
   3. A ____
   4. R ____
   5. A ____

   a. The nurse affirms the patient by acknowledging that it is absolutely reasonable for patients to expect that their health care providers care about their situations and that it is disappointing when they have experiences that make them feel like they do not.
   b. The nurse uses a relaxation technique before responding to the patient's concerns. Calm yourself down. Take a deep breath. Check your pulse.
   c. The nurse says, "I want to help you. I can do that better if you tell me what's making it difficult for you to take your medicine each day."
   d. The nurse maintains eye contact and actively listens to the patient's perspective.
   e. The nurse explains, "One thing I want you to understand is that your heart medicine will only work if you take the same amount each day."
2. Which of the following is considered a social determinant of health? (Select all that apply.)
   1. A car maker closing one of the production plants causing a significant shortage of jobs in a community
   2. Lack of affordable health insurance
   3. Poor quality public school education that prevents a person from gaining college admission
   4. Absence of grocery stores selling fresh vegetables in the neighborhood
   5. The difference in infant mortality rate between two countries

3. Which of the following population groups are likely to have access to a primary health care provider?
   1. Hispanics
   2. Low-income families
   3. A lesbian couple
   4. A male with a high income
4. Which of the following are examples of problems with the health care system that contribute to health disparities? (Select all that apply.)
   1. The discharge nurse at a hospital uses Teach Back with a patient to ensure that she has communicated the discharge instructions clearly.
   2. A community hospital lacks an adequate staff of social workers who are able to ensure patients' access to resources they need to take care of their health.
   3. A hospital discharges a patient without ensuring that the patient has a primary care provider and has made a follow-up appointment.
   4. A nurse uses a family member as an interpreter instead of a medically trained interpreter.
5. Using the LEARN mnemonic to communicate with a patient, place the following steps in the correct order.

1. ______	a. Openly acknowledge the differences and commonalities between the perspectives.
2. ______	b. Involve the patient when recommending treatment.
3. ______	c. Listen to a patient's description of a problem with an open mind.
4. ______	d. Describe your perceptions of the patient's problem.
5. ______	e. Negotiate agreement.

6. A 32-year-old woman in labor is admitted through the ED. The nurse assesses the patient and quickly learns from her husband that she speaks little English. Spanish is her primary language. The nurse calls for an interpreter. What are appropriate nursing interventions the nurse needs to implement at this time? (Select all that apply.)
   1. Ask the husband to confirm the interpreter's ability to speak the patient's dialect.
   2. Once the interpreter arrives at the ED, tell him or her where to find the patient.
   3. Determine the interpreter's qualifications.
   4. Observe for obvious differences in the educational level of interpreter and patient.
7. A nursing professor is teaching nursing students about the components of Campinha-Bacote's (2002) model of cultural competency and asks the students to provide examples of the use of this model. Which of the following examples provided by a nursing student indicates that he or she needs further education about the model?
   1. A nurse regularly attends continuing education workshops that provide an in-depth understanding of diverse groups, including their health beliefs and world views.
   2. A preceptor ensures that a new graduate nurse is able to assess social, cultural, and biophysical factors influencing the treatment and care of their patients.
   3. A nurse understands how institutional forces support or inhibit cultural competence.
   4. A nurse is motivated to learn from others, accept the role as learner, be open and accepting of cultural differences, and build on cultural similarities because of a personal commitment to caring.
8. Which statement made by a new graduate nurse about the Teach Back technique requires intervention and further instruction by the nurse's preceptor?
   1. "After teaching a patient how to use an inhaler, I need to use the Teach Back technique to test my patient technique."
   2. "The Teach Back technique is an ongoing process of asking patients for feedback."
   3. "Using Teach Back will help me identify explanations and communication strategies that my patients will most commonly understand."
   4. "Using pictures, drawings, and models can enhance the effectiveness of the Teach Back technique."
9. Which of the following reasons support why nurses need to become culturally competent? (Select all that apply.)
   1. Improve quality and safety of care for all patients, regardless of their background
   2. Reduce health disparities
   3. Regulatory expectations
   4. Patients usually understand the information health care providers give them
   5. Ethics
10. Which of the following are ways to ensure effective cross-cultural communication in health care settings? (Select all that apply.)
    1. Use family members as interpreters because they have a good understanding of the patient's situation.
    2. Ask open-ended questions to gain an understanding of the patient's explanatory model.
    3. After you go over discharge instructions ask the patient: "Do you understand?" "or "Do you have any questions?"
    4. Check your pulse and practice relaxation techniques when working with others, especially when a patient's or co-worker's statement annoys you or causes you to feel judgmental.

evolve

Rationales for Review Questions can be found on the Evolve website.

1. 1b, 2d, 3a, 4c, 5e; **2.** 1, 2, 3, 4; **3.** 4; **4.** 2, 3, 4; **5.** 1c, 2d, 3a, 4b, 5e; **6.** 3, 4; **7.** 3; **8.** 1; **9.** 1, 2, 3, 5; **10.** 2, 4

REFERENCES

Adams M, Bell LA, Griffin P: *Teaching for diversity and social justice*, ed 2, New York, 2007, Routledge.

Administration on Aging: *Aging statistics*, 2013, http://www.aoa.gov/Aging_Statistics/. Accessed December 29, 2013.

Agency for Healthcare Research and Quality (AHRQ): *Health literacy universal precautions toolkit*, 2013a, http://www.ahrq.gov/professionals/quality-patient-safety/quality-resources/tools/literacy-toolkit/index.html. Accessed December 29, 2013.

Agency for Healthcare Research and Quality (AHRQ): *2012 National Healthcare Disparities Report*, 2013b, http://www.ahrq.gov/research/findings/nhqrdr/nhdr12/index.html. Accessed April 5, 2013.

Aguilar L: *Ouch! This stereotype hurts*, Flower Mound, TX, 2006, The Walk the Talk Co.

American Medical Association (AMA): *Health literacy and patient safety: help patients understand*, Chicago, 2007, American Medical Association Foundation.

Beach MC, Saha S, Cooper LA: The role and relationship of cultural competence and patient-centeredness in health care quality, Commonwealth Fund Publication No. 960, *Medicine* 82(2):193, 2006.

Berlin EA, Fowkes WC Jr: A teaching framework for cross-cultural health care, *West J Med* 139(6):934, 1982.

Bigby JA, editor: *Cross-cultural medicine*, Philadelphia, 2003, American College of Physicians, p 20.

Brach C, et al: *Ten attributes of health literate health care organizations*, 2012, Institute of Medicine, http://www.iom.edu/global/perspectives/2012/healthlitattributes.aspx. Accessed December 29, 2013.

Campinha-Bacote J: The process of cultural competence in the delivery of healthcare services: a model of care, *J Transcult Nurs* 13(3):181, 2002.

Campinha-Bacote J, et al: *Transforming the face of health professions through cultural and linguistic competence education: the role of the HRSA centers of excellence*, Washington, DC, 2005, US Department of Health and Human Services (USDHHS).

Campinha-Bacote J: *The process of cultural competence in the delivery of healthcare services: the journey continues*, ed 5, Cincinnati, OH, 2007, Transcultural C.A.R.E. Associates.

Campinha-Bacote J: Delivering patient-centered care in the midst of a cultural conflict: the role of cultural competence, *Online J Issues Nurs* 16(2):5, 2011.

Centers for Disease Control and Prevention (CDC): *Community health and program services (chaps): health disparities among racial/ethnic populations*, Atlanta, 2008, US Department of Health and Human Services.

Centers for Disease Control and Prevention (CDC): Health disparities and inequalities report—United States, 2011, *MMWR* 60(suppl):1, 2011.

Chassin MR, et al: Accountability measures—using measurement to promote quality improvement, *N Engl J Med* 363(7):6838, 2010.

Dein S: Race, culture and ethnicity in minority research: a critical discussion, *J Cult Diversity* 13(2):68, 2006.

Edelstein S: *Food, cuisine and cultural competency for culinary, hospitality and healthcare professionals*, Sudbury, MA, 2011, Jones & Bartlett.

Giger JN, Davidhizar RD: The Giger and Davidhizar transcultural assessment model, *J Transcult Nurs* 13(3):185, 2002.

Goode T, Jones W: *Linguistic competence*, modified 2009, National Center for Cultural Competence, Georgetown University Center for Child & Human Development, http://nccc.georgetown.edu/documents/Definition%20of%20Linguistic%20Competence.pdf. Accessed October 2, 2013.

Grace P, Willis D: Nursing responsibilities and social justice: an analysis in support of disciplinary goals, *Nurs Outlook* 60(4):198, 2012.

Hall IJ, et al: The African American women and mass media campaign: a CDC breast cancer screening project, *J Womens Health* 21(11):1107, 2012.

Institute of Medicine (IOM): *Crossing the quality chasm: a new health system for the 21st century*, Washington DC, 2001, National Academy of Sciences, National Academies Press.

James C, et al: *Putting women's health care disparities on the map: examining racial and ethnic disparities at the state level*, Menlo Park, CA, 2009, Kaiser Family Foundation, http://kff.org/disparities-policy/report/putting-womens-health-care-disparities-on-the/. Accessed December 29, 2013.

Kaiser Family Foundation (KFF): *Eliminating racial/ethnic disparities in health care: what are the options?* 2008, http://kff.org/disparities-policy/issue-brief/eliminating-racialethnic-disparities-in-health-care-what/. Accessed December 29, 2013.

Kleinman A: *Patients and healers in the context of culture*, Berkeley, 1980, University of California Press.

Kleinman A, Benson P: Anthropology in the clinic: the problem of cultural competency and how to fix it, *PLoS Med* 3(10):e294, 2006. DOI:10.1371/journal.pmed.0030294.

Krehely J: *How to close the LGBT health disparities gap*, 2009, The Center for American progress, http://www.americanprogress.org/issues/lgbt/report/2009/12/21/7048/how-to-close-the-lgbt-health-disparities-gap/. Accessed December 29, 2013.

Kreuter MW, et al: Comparing narrative and informational videos to increase mammography in low-income African American women, *Patient Educ Counsel* 81(suppl 1):S6, 2010.

Kumagai A, Lypson M: Beyond cultural competence: critical consciousness, social justice, and multicultural education, *Acad Med* 84(6):782, 2009.

Leininger MM: Culture care theory: a major contribution to advance transcultural nursing knowledge and practices, *J Transcult Nurs* 13(3):189, 2002.

Leininger MM: Cultural care diversity and universality theory and evolution of the ethnonursing method. In Leininger MM, McFarland MR, editors: *Culture care diversity and universality: worldwide nursing theory*, ed 2, Sudbury, MA, 2006, Jones and Bartlett Learning, p 1.

Leininger MM, McFarland MR: *Transcultural nursing: concepts, theories, research and practice*, ed 3, New York, 2002, McGraw-Hill.

Lie D, et al: What do health literacy and cultural competence have in common? Calling for a collaborative health professional pedagogy, *J Health Communication* 17:13, 2012.

Lynch E, Medin D: Explanatory models of illness: a study of within-culture variation, *Cogn Psychol* 53(4):285, 2006. Epub April 18, 2006.

McFarland MR, Eipperle MK: Culture care theory: a proposed practice theory guide for nurse practitioners in primary care settings, *Contemp Nurse* 28(1-2):48, 2008.

Murphy Y, et al: *Incorporating intersectionality in social work practice, research, policy, and education*, Washington, DC, 2009, NASW Press.

Mutha S, et al: *Bringing equity into quality improvement: an overview and opportunities ahead*, San Francisco, 2012, Center for the Health Professions at the University of California, http://futurehealth.ucsf.edu/Public/Publications-and-Resources/Content.aspx?topic=Bringing_Equity_Into_QI_1. Accessed December 29, 2013.

National Center for Cultural Competence (NCCC): *The cultural competence and linguistic competence policy assessment (CLCPA)*, Washington, DC, 2006, Georgetown University Center for Child and Human Development, http://www.clcpa.info/. Accessed December 29, 2013.

National Center for Education Statistics (NCES): *The health literacy of America's adults: results from the 2003 National Assessment of Adult Literacy*, Washington, DC, 2006, US Department of Education, http://nces.ed.gov/pubsearch/pubsinfo.asp?pubid=2006483. Accessed December 29, 2013.

National Quality Forum (NQF): *Healthcare disparities and cultural competence consensus standards: technical report*, 2012, http://www.qualityforum.org/Publications/2012/09/Healthcare_Disparities_and_Cultural_Competency_Consensus_Standards_Technical_Report.aspx. Accessed December 29, 2013.

National Research Council (NRC): *Unequal treatment: confronting racial and health disparities in health care* (full printed version), Washington DC, 2003, National Academies Press.

National Research Council (NRC): *Health literacy: a prescription to end confusion*, Washington, DC, 2004, National Academies Press.

Office of Minority Health (OMH), US Department of Health and Human Services (USDHHH): *Think cultural health: CLAS and continuing education*, 2013, https://www.thinkculturalhealth.hhs.gov/index.asp. Accessed December 29, 2013.

Purnell L: The Purnell model for cultural competence, *J Transcult Nurs* 13(3):193, 2002.

Purnell LD, Paulanka BJ: *Transcultural healthcare: a culturally competent approach*, ed 3, Philadelphia, 2008, FA Davis.

Rabin RC: *Respecting Muslim patient's needs*, 2010, New York Times, http://www.nytimes.com/2010/11/01/health/01patients.html?_r=0. Accessed December 29, 2013.

Saha S, Beach M, Cooper L: Patient centeredness, cultural competence, and healthcare quality, *J Natl Med Assoc* 100(11):1275, 2008.

Schillinger D, et al: Closing the loop physician communication with diabetic patients who have low health literacy, *Arch Intern Med* 163(1):83, 2003.

Sue DW: *Multicultural social work practice*, Ken, NJ, 2006, John Wiley & Sons.

The Joint Commission (TJC): *Core measure sets*, Chicago, 2013, TJC, http://www.jointcommission.org/core_measure_sets.aspx. Accessed December 29, 2013.

United Health Foundation: *America's health rankings: United States overview: 2012 edition results*, 2013, http://www.americashealthrankings.org/Rankings. Accessed December 29, 2013.

US Census Bureau: *The American community survey, 2008-2012*, 2013, http://www.census.gov/acs/www/. Accessed December 29, 2013.

US Department of Health and Human Services (USDHHS): *Healthy people 2020*, 2010, http://www.healthypeople.gov/2020/default.aspx. Accessed December 29, 2013.

VanSuch M, et al: Effect of discharge instructions on readmission of hospitalized patients with heart failure: do all of the Joint Commission on Accreditation of Healthcare Organization's heart failure core measures reflect better care? *Qual Saf Health Care* 15(6):414, 2006.

Walker RL, et al: Ethnic group differences in reasons for living and the moderating role of cultural worldview, *Cult Diversity Ethnic Minority Psychol* 16(3):372, 2010. DOI:10.1037/a0019720.

Warrier S: *Culture handbook. family violence prevention fund*, 2005, http://www.futureswithoutviolence.org/userfiles/file/ImmigrantWomen/Culture%20Handbook.pdf. Accessed December 29, 2013.

Webber P: Yes, Virginia, nursing does have laws, *Nurs Sci Q* 21(1):68, 2008.

World Health Organization (WHO): *Social determinants of health*, Commission on Social Determinants of Health, 2005-2008, 2013, http://www.who.int/social_determinants/thecommission/finalreport/key_concepts/en/index.html. Accessed December 29, 2013.

CHAPTER

21

Spiritual Health

evolve WEBSITE

http://evolve.elsevier.com/Potter/essentials

- Crossword Puzzle
- Audio Glossary

OBJECTIVES

- Describe the relationship among faith, hope, and spiritual well-being.
- Compare and contrast the concepts of religion and spirituality.
- Discuss the relationship of spirituality to an individual's total being.
- Assess a patient's spirituality and spiritual health.
- Discuss nursing interventions designed to promote spiritual health.
- Establish presence with patients.
- Evaluate how patients attain spiritual health.

KEY TERMS

agnostic, p. 549
atheist, p. 549
connectedness, p. 556
faith, p. 549
holistic, p. 547
hope, p. 550
self-transcendence, p. 548
spiritual distress, p. 550
spiritual well-being, p. 549
spirituality, p. 547
transcendence, p.548

The word *spirituality* comes from the Latin word *spiritus,* which refers to breath or wind. The spirit gives life to a person. It signifies whatever is at the center of all aspects of a person's life. **Spirituality** is an awareness of one's inner self and a sense of connection to a higher being, nature, or some purpose greater than oneself (Gall, Malette, and Guirguis-Younger, 2011). A person's health depends on a balance of physical, psychological, sociological, cultural, emotional, developmental, and spiritual variables. This **holistic** view of health is the focus and heart of nursing practice. Spiritual care is often an overlooked part of nursing; however, the spiritual dimension does not exist in isolation from our physical and psychological being (Cobb, 2012). Spirituality is an important factor that helps people achieve the balance needed to maintain health and well-being and to cope with illness. Current evidence shows that spirituality positively affects health, quality of life, health promotion behaviors, and disease prevention activities (Hurlbut, Robbins, and Hoke, 2011; Visser, Garssen, and Vingerhoets, 2010).

Too often nurses and other health care providers fail to recognize the spiritual dimension of human nature. In addition some health care providers do not believe in God or an ultimate being or believe that they do not have time to address spiritual needs. Frequently people use the concepts of spirituality and religion interchangeably, but spirituality is a much broader and more unifying concept than religion (Boswell and Boswell-Ford, 2010; Cohen et al., 2012). Florence Nightingale believed that spirituality is a force that provides energy needed in a healthy hospital environment. She also believed that caring for a person's spiritual needs is just as important as caring for his or her physical needs (Dolamo, 2010). The human spirit is powerful, and spirituality has

CASE STUDY *Victoria Timms*

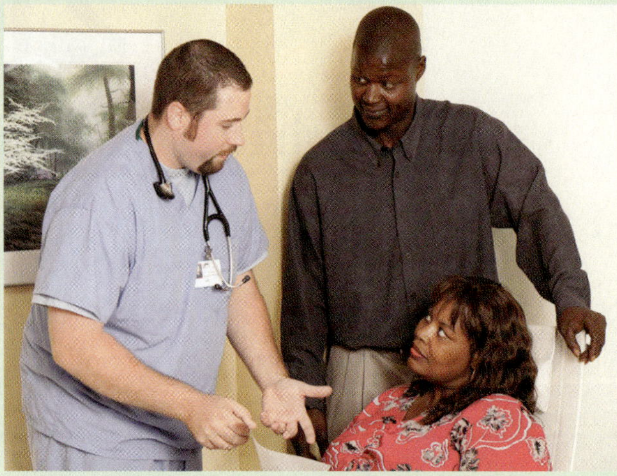

Victoria Timms is a 48-year-old African-American college professor, diagnosed 3 months ago with breast cancer. She is married to Joe, an insurance salesman, and is the mother of two children: Valerie, who is 16 years old, and Peter, who is 12. Victoria describes her family as being very close and supportive. Surgeons removed Victoria's cancerous tumor and two involved lymph nodes. Because of the lymphatic involvement, Victoria is at increased risk for the cancer to spread. Victoria has completed a course of radiation and now visits the local cancer clinic with her husband 3 times a week for chemotherapy treatments. Both Victoria and Joe discuss their concern for their children. Valerie and Peter attend Sunday school weekly after going to church with their parents. Their Sunday school teacher informed Victoria and Joe that Valerie and Peter are very angry about their mother's illness.

Jeff is a 36-year-old, married student nurse assigned to the oncology clinic. Jeff's preceptor, a nursing case manager, assigns Jeff to follow Victoria during her clinic visits. Jeff is in his last semester at school and hopes to get a position in the clinic after graduation. Victoria's experience is significant for Jeff because he has children who are the same age as Victoria's and he wonders how his children would react if his spouse became ill.

During one of their clinic visits Victoria and Joe appear very calm and relaxed when discussing cancer therapy. Joe explains, "We both have a lot of faith in God." Victoria responds, "Even though I know I have cancer, I hope to be able to continue to go to church with my family and my children. My family is very supportive, and together I know that we'll make it through this experience. But I'm worried about my children. With God's help I can help them cope with my illness better."

different meanings for different people. Therefore you need to understand your own spirituality to integrate spirituality into your patients' care. Nursing care involves helping patients use their spiritual resources as they identify and explore what is meaningful in their lives and find ways to cope with illness and stressors of life (Nixon and Narayanasamy, 2010).

SCIENTIFIC KNOWLEDGE BASE

The relationship between spirituality and health is not fully understood. However, people often are healthier when they believe in a higher power. For example, religious and spiritual beliefs protect college students from experiencing depression (Berry and York, 2011), and prayer is frequently associated with positive health outcomes (French and Narayanasamy, 2011). Current evidence shows a link connecting the mind, body, and spirit. An individual's beliefs and expectations often have effects on his or her physical and psychological well-being (Burris et al., 2009). Many of these effects are tied to hormonal and neurological function. For example, talking about concerns, relaxation exercises, and guided imagery can improve individuals' immune function (Cohen et al., 2011) and reduce perceptions of pain and anxiety (Mizrahi et al., 2012). Laughter raises pain thresholds, boosts antibody production, reduces stress hormones, relieves tension, and elevates mood (Harkins, 2009; Lebowitz et al., 2011). A person's inner beliefs and convictions are powerful resources for healing. As a nurse you will be more successful in helping patients achieve desirable health outcomes after learning to support patients and their families spiritually.

NURSING KNOWLEDGE BASE

Concepts in Spiritual Health

Current research supports the link between spirituality and health. Thus it is important for you to understand spiritual health and the concepts of spirituality, spiritual well-being, faith, religion, and hope to provide supportive spiritual care.

Spirituality. Definitions of spirituality differ. However, experts agree that it is complex and diverse (Cohen et al., 2012; Pike, 2011). It is unique for each individual and exists in everyone, regardless of religious beliefs (Nixon and Narayanasamy, 2010). Our culture, development, life experiences, beliefs, and ideas about life influence our definition of spirituality (McSherry, 2007). Spirituality exists in all people, regardless of their religious beliefs; and it gives people the *energy* needed to maintain health and cope with difficult situations. Current definitions of spirituality include five distinct but overlapping constructs (Figure 21-1).

Self-transcendence refers to connecting to your inner self, which allows one to go beyond oneself to understand the meanings of experiences (Wiggs, 2010), whereas **transcendence** is the belief that there is a positive force outside of and greater than oneself that allows one to develop new perspectives that are beyond physical boundaries (McCarthy, 2011). Examples of transcendent moments include the feelings of awe when holding a new baby or watching the sun rise over the mountains. Spirituality offers a sense of *connectedness* intrapersonally (connected with oneself), interpersonally (connected with others and the environment), and transpersonally (connected with God, the unseen, or a higher power). Through connectedness patients are able to move beyond the stressors of everyday life and find comfort, faith, hope, peace,

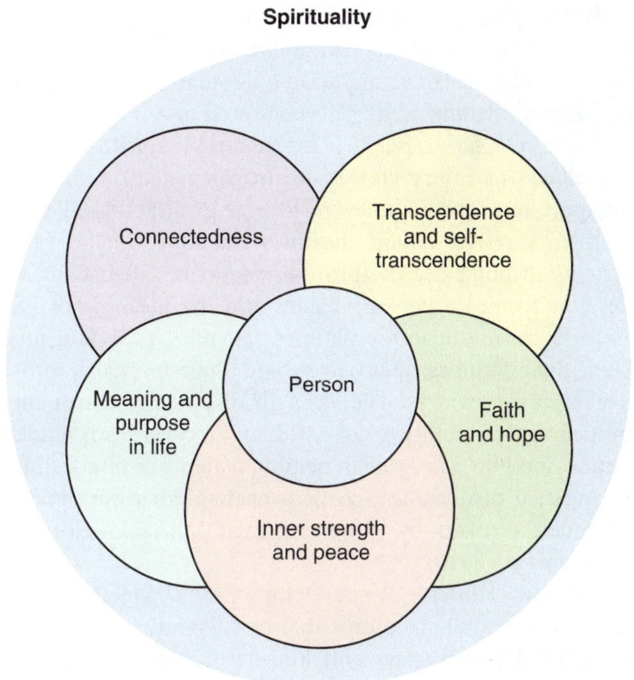

FIGURE 21-1 The concept of spirituality has five distinct but overlapping constructs.

and empowerment (Nelson-Becker, Nakashima, and Canda, 2007). *Faith* allows a person to have firm beliefs about something despite the lack of physical evidence. Although many associate faith with religious beliefs, faith can exist without them (Dyess, 2011). *Hope* has several meanings. It usually refers to a source of energy that helps a person plan and achieve goals (Redlich et al., 2010). *Inner strength* is an energy source that instills hope, provides motivation, and promotes a positive outlook on life, even during difficult times (Lundman et al., 2010). *Inner peace* fosters calm and positive feelings despite life experiences of chaos, fear, and uncertainty. These feelings help people feel comforted and find peace even in times of great distress (Haswell et al., 2010). Finally spirituality helps people find *meaning and purpose in life* in both negative and positive life events (Vachon, Fillion, and Achille, 2009).

Spirituality is an important concept for individuals who either do not believe in the existence of God (atheist) or who believe that any ultimate reality is unknown or unknowable (agnostic) (O'Connell and Skevington, 2010). Atheists search for meaning in life through their work and relationships with others. It is important for agnostics to discover meaning in what they do or how they live because they find no ultimate meaning for the way things are. They believe that we, as people, bring meaning to what we do.

Spirituality is an integrating theme in life. A person's concept of spirituality begins in childhood and continues to grow throughout adulthood (Mueller, 2010). Spirituality represents the totality of one's being, serving as the overriding perspective that unifies the various aspects of an individual. It spreads throughout the physiological, psychological, and sociocultural dimensions of a person's life, whether or not the individual acknowledges or develops it.

Spiritual Well-Being. There are four dimensions of spiritual well-being (Rowold, 2011). The personal dimension refers to how you relate with yourself in finding meaning and purpose in life. The communal dimension relates to the quality of your interpersonal relationships. The environmental dimension describes how you interact in the world, including your sense of awe with the environment. The transcendental dimension refers to the relationship between you and some higher power (e.g., God, Buddha). Spiritual well-being has a positive effect on health and leads to spiritual health. If you are spiritually healthy, you experience joy, forgive yourself and others, accept hardship and mortality, experience enhanced quality of life, and have a positive sense of physical and emotional well-being (Holt-Lunstad et al., 2011; Rowold, 2011).

Faith. In addition to being a part of the definition of spirituality, the concept of faith has other common definitions. Faith is a cultural or institutional religion such as Buddhism, Christianity, or Islam. It also is a relationship with a divinity, higher power, authority, or spirit that incorporates a reasoning faith (belief) and a trusting faith (action). Reasoning faith is a person's belief and confidence in something for which there is no proof. It is an acceptance of what our reasoning cannot explain. Sometimes it involves a belief in a higher power, spirit guide, God, or Allah. Faith also is how a person chooses to live life. In this sense it enables action. Patients who are ill frequently have a positive outlook on life and continue to participate in daily activities rather than resigning themselves to the symptoms of their disease. In these cases a patient's faith often becomes stronger because illness is viewed as an opportunity for personal growth (Ford et al., 2010). *For example, Victoria is living with breast cancer. She has faith; thus she has a positive outlook on life and continues to complete daily activities rather than giving into the symptoms caused by her breast cancer. Her faith becomes stronger because she views her cancer as an opportunity for growth.*

Religion. Religion is associated with the "state of doing" or a specific system of practices associated with a particular denomination, sect, or form of worship. Religion refers to the system of organized beliefs and worship that a person practices to outwardly express spirituality. Many people practice a faith or belief in the doctrines of a specific religion or sect such as the Lutheran church within Christianity or Orthodox Judaism. People from different religions view spirituality differently. For example, a Buddhist believes in Four Noble Truths: life is suffering; suffering is caused by clinging; suffering can be eliminated by eliminating clinging; and to eliminate clinging and suffering one follows an eightfold path. The path includes the right understanding, intention, speech, action, livelihood, effort, mindfulness, and concentration. This path promotes wisdom, moral behavior, and meditation. A Buddhist turns inward, valuing self-control, whereas a Christian looks to the love of God to provide enlightenment and direction in life.

When providing spiritual care to patients, you need to know the differences between religion and spirituality. Although closely related, these terms are not synonymous (Pike, 2011). Religious care helps patients follow their belief systems and worship practices. Spiritual care helps people maintain personal relationships and a relationship with a higher being or life force to identify meaning and purpose in life.

Hope. Spirituality and faith bring hope. When a person has the attitude of living for and looking forward to something, hope is present. **Hope** is multidimensional and gives comfort while a person endures hardship and personal challenges. It is closely associated with faith. It is energizing, giving individuals a motivation to achieve and the resources to use toward that achievement. People express hope in all aspects of their lives as a force that helps them deal with life stressors. It is a valuable personal resource and brings comfort when people face a loss (see Chapter 25) or a challenge that seems difficult to achieve (Kelsey et al., 2011).

Spiritual Health

People gain spiritual health by finding a balance between their life values, goals, and belief systems and their relationships within themselves and with others. Throughout life a person sometimes grows more spiritual, becoming increasingly aware of the meaning, purpose, and values of life. In times of stress, illness, loss, or recovery, a person often turns to previous ways of responding or adjusting to a situation. Often these coping styles lie within the person's spiritual beliefs.

Spiritual beliefs change as patients grow and develop (Table 21-1). Spirituality begins as children learn about themselves and their relationships with others. When you understand a child's spiritual beliefs, it is easier to care for and comfort the child (Bryant-Davis et al., 2012; Mueller, 2010). As children mature into adulthood, they experience spiritual growth by entering into lifelong relationships. An ability to care meaningfully for others and self is evidence of a healthy spirituality. Older adults often turn to important relationships and give themselves to others (Edelman and Mandle, 2010).

The Effect of Illness on Spirituality

When illness, loss, grief, or a major life change affects a person, spiritual resources help the person move to recovery. Without spiritual resources, concerns and doubts develop within an individual. **Spiritual distress** is "the impaired ability to experience and integrate meaning and purpose in life through connectedness with self, others, art, music, literature, nature, and/or a power greater than oneself" (NANDA International, 2012). Spiritual distress causes doubt, a loss of faith, and a sense of feeling alone or even abandoned. Individuals question their spiritual values, raising questions about their way of life and purpose for living. Spiritual distress also occurs when there is conflict between a person's beliefs and a prescribed health treatment plan or the inability to practice usual rituals.

Acute Illness. Sudden, unexpected illness that threatens a patient's life, health, and/or well-being creates significant spiritual distress. For example, an older man who has a heart attack and a young adult who is injured in a motor vehicle accident both face crises that threaten their spiritual health. The illness or injury creates an unanticipated scramble to integrate and cope with new realities (e.g., disability). People look for ways to remain faithful to their beliefs and value systems through use of spiritual resources. Often conflicts develop around a person's beliefs and the meaning of life. Anger is common; and sometimes patients express it against God, their families, themselves, and their nurses or other health care providers. The strength of patients' spirituality influences their ability to cope with and recover from sudden illness. You play a key role in helping patients resolve feelings of spiritual distress. You create a healing environment and maximize recovery by enhancing their spiritual well-being (Yeager et al., 2010).

Chronic Illness. People with chronic illnesses often suffer debilitating symptoms that permanently change their lifestyles. The uncertain and long-term nature of chronic illness and the potential for outcomes such as pain, changes in body image, and the need to confront death all lead to spiritual distress. Patients struggle with questions about the meaning and purpose of their lives because their independence is threatened, which often causes fear, anxiety, and powerlessness. The nursing diagnosis *Spiritual Distress* is appropriate to use for patients who experience these symptoms. A person's spirituality is a significant factor in how he or she adapts to the changes resulting from chronic illness. Successfully adapting to these changes strengthens a person spiritually, but it sometimes takes a long-term plan to help a patient with a chronic illness achieve spiritual well-being. As a nurse you are in a unique position to help patients reevaluate their lives and achieve spiritual health (Box 21-1). Patients who have a sense of spiritual well-being are often better able to cope with their illnesses and experience enhanced quality of life (Dalmida et al., 2012; Tan, Wutthilert, and O'Connor, 2011).

Terminal Illness. Terminal illness commonly causes fears of physical pain, isolation, the unknown, and dying. When patients feel uncertain about what death means, they are susceptible to spiritual distress. On the other hand, spirituality helps patients and families find resolution and peace by helping them prepare for and accept death (Vachon et al., 2009). Individuals experiencing a terminal illness often find themselves reviewing their life and questioning its meaning. Common questions asked include, "Why is this happening to me?" or "What have I done?" Terminal illness affects family and friends just as much as the patient. It causes members of the family to ask important questions about the meaning of life and how the illness will affect their relationship with the patient (see Chapter 26).

When caring for dying patients, help them gain a greater sense of control over their illness, whether they are in a health care setting (e.g., the hospital) or at home. Dying is a holistic process encompassing the patient's physical, social,

TABLE 21-1 RELATIONSHIP BETWEEN DEVELOPMENTAL STAGE AND SPIRITUAL BELIEFS

ERICKSON'S DEVELOPMENTAL STAGE	SPIRITUAL BELIEFS
Trust vs. mistrust Birth to 18 months	Spiritual well-being provided by parents Trust provides basis for hope Love, affection, security, and a stimulating environment promote spirituality
Autonomy vs. shame and doubt 20-36 months	Fascination with magic and mystery Often believes that illness is related to bad behavior Begins to learn the difference between right and wrong Imitates parents' spiritual or religious actions; recites prayers and sings simple religious songs, but does not understand their meanings Interprets meanings literally
Initiative vs. guilt 3-6 years	Feels guilty when not acting responsibly Influenced by spiritual and religious stories, examples, moods, and actions Models moral behaviors of parents Begins to ask about God or supreme beings
Industry vs. inferiority 6-12 years	Wants to learn about spirituality Has a clear picture of God or supreme being, morality, and the difference between right and wrong Sorts fantasy from fact Demands proof of reality and believes literal meanings of spiritual stories
Identity vs. identity confusion Adolescence	Reflects on inconsistencies in stories Begins to question spiritual practices, forms own opinions, and occasionally discards parents' beliefs Abstract reasoning leads to exploration of moral issues Spirituality comes from connectedness with family, nature, and God or a supreme being
Intimacy vs. isolation and loneliness Young adulthood	Establishes self-identity and world view Forms independent beliefs, attitudes, and lifestyles Uses principles to solve problems when individual's and society's rules conflict
Generativity vs. stagnation Middle-age adulthood	Develops appreciation of past spiritual experiences Embraces people from different faiths and religions Reviews value system during crisis Values others
Ego identity vs. despair and disgust Older adulthood	Values love and interactions with others Focuses on overcoming oppression and violence Beliefs vary based on many factors such as gender, past experiences, religion, economic status, and ethnic background

Data from Edelman CL, Mandle CL: *Health promotion throughout the life span,* ed 7, St Louis, 2010, Mosby; and Mueller CR: Spirituality in children: understanding and developing interventions, *Pediatr Nurs* 36(4):197, 2010.

psychological, and spiritual health (Hayden, 2011; Phelps et al., 2012).

Near-Death Experience. You may care for a patient or have a family member who has had a near-death experience (NDE). NDE is a psychological phenomenon in which people have either been close to clinical death or recovered after being declared dead. It is not associated with a mental disorder. Instead experts agree that NDE describes a powerfully close brush with physical, emotional, and spiritual death. For example, people who have an NDE after cardiopulmonary arrest often tell the same story of feeling themselves rising above their bodies and watching caregivers initiate lifesaving measures. Commonly patients who experience an NDE describe feeling totally at peace, having an out-of-body experience, being pulled into a dark tunnel, seeing bright lights and a tunnel, and encountering people who preceded them in death. Instead of moving toward the light, they learn that it is not time for them to die, and they return to life (Agrillo, 2011; Cant et al., 2012).

Patients who have an NDE are often reluctant to discuss it, thinking family or caregivers will not understand. Isolation and depression often occur. Furthermore, not all NDEs are positive experiences (Rominger, 2010). However, individuals experiencing an NDE who discuss it openly with family or caregivers find acceptance and meaning from this powerful experience. They are often no longer afraid of death, and they have a decreased desire to achieve material wealth. They also report increased sensitivity to different chemicals such as

BOX 21-1 EVIDENCE-BASED PRACTICE

PICO Question: How do perceptions of spirituality affect well-being and quality of life in patients with chronic illnesses?

SUMMARY OF EVIDENCE

All aspects of a patient's life are affected by a chronic illness. Current research supports that spirituality helps patients cope with the effects of their chronic illnesses, leading to enhanced well-being and quality of life (QOL). For example, existential well-being (having a purpose in life and being satisfied with life) significantly contributes to the health status of patients living with human immunodeficiency virus (HIV) (Cobb, 2012; Dalmida et al., 2012) and cancer (Visser et al., 2010). High levels of spirituality are associated with positive QOL in older adults who have at least one chronic illness (Tan et al., 2011); whereas religiosity and closeness to God help patients accept death (Daaleman and Dobbs, 2010). Nursing interventions, including prayer, establishing presence, establishing a caring relationship, having patients discuss spirituality in groups, and supporting patients within a faith community help patients with chronic illnesses thrive even at the end of life (Dyess and Chase, 2010; Tuck, 2012).

APPLICATION TO NURSING PRACTICE

- Provide spiritual care as an essential component of holistic care to your patients (Tan et al., 2011).
- Pray with your patients if they desire; prayer enhances connectedness to God or another higher being and often provides a source of strength, enhancing well-being and quality of life (Daaleman and Dobbs, 2010; Dyess and Chase, 2010).
- Help patients with chronic illnesses find meaning and hope, even if they are facing a hopeless situation (Cobb, 2012).
- Encourage patients with chronic illnesses to maintain connections with others and their faith community (Dyess and Chase, 2010; Tuck, 2012).

BOX 21-2 SYNTHESIS IN PRACTICE

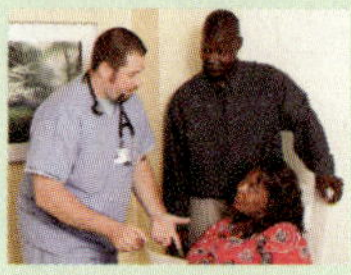

Jeff plans for Victoria and Joe's return to the oncology clinic. He spends time learning more about Victoria's disease and treatment plan so he is able to explain what to expect as chemotherapy progresses. Jeff knows that Joe usually comes to the clinic, and Victoria describes him as a strong source of support. However, Jeff does not know enough about the couple's relationship and wants to explore this further. The role of family members in providing support, particularly with regard to decision making, is important for Jeff to understand before he develops a plan of care. In reviewing information about loss and grieving, Jeff recognizes that Victoria shows acceptance of her disease because she is able to discuss cancer and the plan for treatment. Jeff knows that, as patients begin to accept the diagnosis of a life-threatening disease, it is important to offer opportunities to share feelings and discuss future plans.

Jeff's previous experiences with patients who have cancer taught him that, when patients express hope, they move forward and cope better with the challenges of their disease. During the last clinic visit Victoria stated that she hoped she would be able to continue to attend religious services at her church. Jeff reflected on that experience and thinks that Victoria and Joe have a strong sense of spiritual well-being that will help them cope with cancer. However, further assessment is necessary.

Jeff wants to completely assess Victoria and Joe's level of spiritual health. He is Lutheran and does not know very much about the Baptist faith, the couple's religion. However, he knows that the Baptist sense of community is very strong and that it is important to learn more about how members of the Timms' church play a role in offering support to the family. Jeff recognizes that spiritual well-being is more complex than religion. He spends time reflecting on his own value and belief systems so he remains open and receptive to understanding Victoria and Joe's spiritual belief systems. By understanding his own beliefs, Jeff is also better able to help Victoria and Joe cope with Victoria's diagnosis of cancer.

alcohol and medications. After patients have survived an NDE, promote spiritual well-being by remaining open, giving patients a chance to explore what happened, and supporting them as they share the experience with significant others (Cant et al., 2012).

CRITICAL THINKING

Synthesis

You apply elements of critical thinking whenever you perform the nursing process with patients. Consider the scientific knowledge you have learned, your experience, critical thinking attitudes, and standards to ensure an individualized approach to patient care (Box 21-2).

Knowledge. The helping role is an important domain of nursing practice (Benner, 1984). Patients look to nurses for help that is different from the help they seek from other health care professionals. To effectively care for your patients' spiritual needs, you first need to be comfortable with your own spirituality (Ronaldson et al., 2012). By fostering your own personal, emotional, and spiritual health, you become a resource for your patient. Use your awareness of your own spirituality as a tool when caring for yourself and your patients. Differentiate your personal spirituality from that of the patient. This becomes important during the delivery of care, when you need to be able to engage a patient spiritually rather than try to exercise personal spiritual convictions. Your role is not to solve the spiritual problems of patients but to provide an environment for them to express their spirituality (Hayden, 2011).

After becoming comfortable with your own spirituality, use your nursing expertise to anticipate your patients'

BOX 21-3 PATIENT-CENTERED CARE

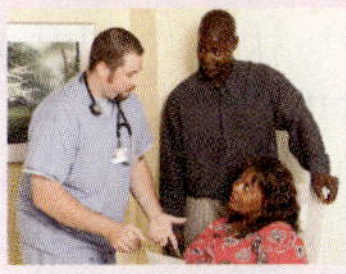

Through studying Jeff found that African-American women have the second-highest breast cancer incidence rate and the highest mortality rate (U.S. Cancer Statistics Working Group, 2012). Jeff also knows that patients' spiritual needs are often associated with their cultural, social, and ethnic background. African-American women generally express a deep relationship with God and strong moral and ethical values. Spirituality for African-Americans often provides a source of healing, coping, and peace. Furthermore, being connected with a caring community environment such as a neighborhood or church is particularly important for African-American women who have breast cancer because caring communities provide great emotional and social support (Heiney et al., 2011). Jeff applies this information when he assesses Victoria's spiritual needs, validates that this perspective is shared by Victoria, and uses this understanding of breast cancer and spirituality among African-American women to provide patient-centered care for Victoria and her family.

IMPLICATIONS FOR PRACTICE

- Jeff encourages Victoria and her family to strengthen their spiritual health as they continue to cope with Victoria's breast cancer diagnosis and cancer treatment.
- After asking Victoria if there are any communities with whom she feels connected, Jeff discovers that she is close to the members of her church and her work group.
- Jeff determines that Victoria's church has a parish nurse. With Victoria's permission he shares her health problems and concerns with the parish nurse who agrees to contact Victoria and arrange a time for them to meet.
- Jeff determines that Victoria and Joe have used prayer in the past to cope with different stressors. Thus Jeff prays with Victoria and Joe during their visits to the oncology clinic, encourages them to continue to read the Bible together at home, and encourages Joe to attend church even if Victoria is too ill to attend.
- Because breast cancer and its treatment often interfere with employment, Jeff explores ways that Victoria can remain connected with her peers at work to help her maintain this important source of support (Lewis et al., 2012).

personal issues and the resulting effect on spiritual well-being. Your knowledge about the concept of spirituality and a patient's faith and belief systems helps to provide appropriate spiritual care. Knowledge of a patient's values, beliefs, preferences, and needs provides additional insight into a person's spiritual practices. Application of therapeutic communication principles (see Chapter 11) and caring (see Chapter 19) helps you establish therapeutic trust with patients. An individual's spiritual beliefs are very personal. When you integrate patient preferences into spiritual care, you provide patient-centered care, respecting the diversity of your patient's experience (QSEN Institute, n.d.) (Box 21-3).

When caring for patients who have a terminal illness or are experiencing some other type of loss, knowledge of loss and grief dynamics is important (see Chapter 26). Spirituality influences personal reactions to loss and response to grief. Also consider family dynamics while providing spiritual care (see Chapter 24). For many individuals their spiritual health is often integrated with the relationships among family members. Therefore consider the family's beliefs when planning spiritual care for your patient.

Finally a sound understanding of ethics and values (see Chapter 6) is essential when providing spiritual care. A person's values or beliefs about the worth of a given idea, attitude, or custom are linked to the individual's spiritual well-being. Application of ethical principles ensures respect for a patient's spiritual and religious convictions.

Experience. You often care for patients who are in spiritual distress. Use these experiences when helping others select coping options. Because spirituality is more than religion, you need to consider personal views and philosophies about life and reflect on whether your own spirituality is beneficial in helping patients. If you sense a personal faith and hope regarding life, it is likely that you will be better able to help patients. Previous personal and professional experiences with dying patients, patients with chronic disease, or patients who have experienced significant losses provide lessons in how to help them face difficult challenges and how to offer support to family and friends.

Attitudes. Do not take a patient's reaction to illness or loss for granted. Humility becomes very important, particularly when caring for patients from diverse cultural and/or religious backgrounds. Recognize any limitations in your own knowledge about a patient's spiritual beliefs and religious practices and be willing to pursue the knowledge needed to provide appropriate, individualized care. Show genuine concern for patients as you ask them about their beliefs and how spirituality influences their health. Also exhibit integrity; realize the importance of refraining from expressing your opinions about religion or spirituality when they conflict with that of a patient. Finally show confidence in dealing with spiritual issues as you build a caring relationship with a patient. Confidence works to build trust.

Standards. A nurse who thinks critically is thorough and ensures that information about a patient is significant and relevant when making decisions about his or her spiritual needs. The nature of a person's spirituality is complex and highly individualized. Therefore avoid making assumptions about his or her religion and beliefs. Significance and relevance are standards of critical thinking that ensure that you explore the issues that are most meaningful to patients and most likely to affect their spiritual well-being. Apply ethical standards of care when providing spiritual care.

The Joint Commission sets standards for quality health care. It requires health care organizations to acknowledge patients' rights to spiritual care and provide for patients' spiritual needs through pastoral care or others who are certified, ordained, or lay individuals. The standards also require that you assess and provide for your patients' denomination, beliefs, and spiritual practices (TJC, 2014).

The American Nurses Association's Code of Ethics for Nurses (Fowler, 2010) sets standards for quality nursing care. The Code requires you to practice nursing with compassion by accepting the dignity and worth of all of your patients despite their socioeconomic status, personal characteristics, or type of health problems. You promote an environment that respects your patients' values, customs, and spiritual beliefs.

NURSING PROCESS

Understanding a patient's spirituality and then appropriately identifying the level of support and resources needed require a broad perspective and an open mind. As a nurse you make a commitment to care. To care for and meet the spiritual needs of your patients, it is essential to respect each patient's personal beliefs. People experience the world and find meaning in life in different ways. Application of the nursing process from the perspective of a patient's spiritual needs is not simple. It goes beyond assessing his or her religious practices. Caring for your patients' spiritual needs requires you to be compassionate and remove any personal biases or misconceptions. Be willing to share and discover their meaning and purpose in life, illness, and health. Identify common values and respect unique commitments and values with your patients by having quiet conversations, listening effectively, and communicating using presence and touch (Daaleman, 2012).

You need to recognize that not all patients have spiritual problems. Patients bring certain spiritual resources that help them assume healthier lives, recover from illness, or face impending death. Supporting and recognizing the positive side of a patient's spirituality allows you to deliver safe, effective, patient-centered nursing care.

ASSESSMENT

Before you complete a spiritual assessment on your patient, be aware of your own spiritual beliefs, values, and biases. Understanding your own spirit is essential when you provide spiritual care to your patients. Remember that spirituality is very subjective and has different meanings for different people. You are able to gather an accurate assessment of your patients' spirituality when you take time to build therapeutic relationships with them. Once you establish a trusting relationship with a patient, you and the patient reach a point of learning together, and spiritual caring occurs (Bailey, Moran, and Graham, 2009). Conduct an ongoing spiritual assessment the entire time you care for a patient (McSherry, 2007). Focus your assessment on aspects of spirituality most likely to be influenced by life experiences, events, and questions in the case of illness and hospitalization (Table 21-2). Conducting an assessment is therapeutic for you and your patient because it conveys a level of caring and support.

Assess your patient's spiritual health in several different ways. One way is to ask the patient direct questions. This approach requires you to feel comfortable asking others about their spirituality. Some health care agencies and researchers have created assessment tools to clarify values and assess spirituality. For example, the spiritual well-being scale (SWB) has 20 questions that assess a patient's relationship with God and his or her sense of life purpose and life satisfaction (Life Advance, 2009). The FICA assessment tool (Borneman, Ferrell, and Puchalski, 2010) evaluates spirituality and is closely correlated to quality of life. FICA stands for the following:

F—**Faith** or belief
I—**Importance** of spirituality
C—Individual's spiritual **Community**
A—Interventions to **Address** spiritual needs

Effective assessment tools such as the SWB and FICA help you remember important areas to assess. Patient responses to the assessment items on the tools indicate areas that you need to investigate further. For example, if, after using the FICA tool with a patient who is having difficulty accepting a new diagnosis of prostate cancer, you find out that he does not want you or his pastor to help him address this issue, you need to spend time understanding how the patient plans to manage this new illness. Remember, when using any spiritual assessment tool, do not impose your personal values on your patient. This is sometimes difficult, especially when a patient's values and beliefs are similar to yours, because it is very easy for you to make false assumptions. When you understand the overall approach to spiritual assessment, you are able to enter into thoughtful discussions with patients, gain a greater awareness of the personal resources they bring to a situation, and incorporate the resources into an effective plan of care.

TABLE 21-2 FOCUSED PATIENT ASSESSMENT

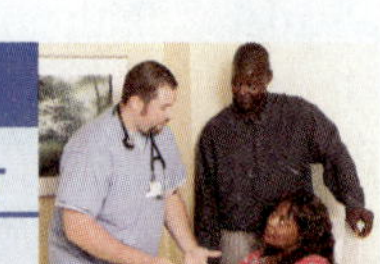

FACTORS TO ASSESS	QUESTIONS	PHYSICAL ASSESSMENT
Past experiences with loss	How would you describe the ways you cope spiritually when faced with difficult times?	Observe patient's facial expressions and mannerisms during the discussion.
Fear of the unknown resulting from a terminal illness	Describe the people who mean the most to you. In what way do you look to them for support? Do you consider yourself a spiritual person? If so, what gives you comfort? If not, what provides you a sense of peace?	Fear is associated with anxiety. Be alert for changes in vital signs. Observe the patient's mood, willingness to initiate conversation, and interest in surroundings.

Faith. Although individual definitions vary, faith helps people find meaning in their life experiences (Dyess, 2011). When assessing a patient's faith, first determine his or her beliefs, especially those that influence hope. For example, ask how a patient believes that a treatment will affect a newly diagnosed serious illness. Determine which of your patient's beliefs serve as a guide and help the patient find meaning in life events. Ask your patient if he or she is able to live according to his or her beliefs. Finally assess to what extent your patient interrelates with self, others, and/or a source of authority. A patient's source of authority is usually God or some other supreme being (Dyess, 2011). Faith in an authority provides a sense of confidence that guides a person in exercising beliefs and experiencing growth. Assess a person's faith in an authority by asking, "To whom do you look to for guidance in life?" The patient's response will likely open the door for a meaningful discussion. Listen carefully and explore what is meaningful to the patient.

Determine if patients have a religious source of guidance that conflicts with their medical treatment plans. This seriously affects the treatment options that nurses and other health care providers are able to offer patients. For example, if a patient is a Jehovah's Witness, blood products are not an acceptable form of treatment. Christian Scientists often refuse any medical intervention, believing that their faith will heal them.

It is also important to understand a patient's philosophy of life. Asking a patient, "Describe for me what is most important in your life," or "Tell me what gives your life meaning or purpose," helps to assess the basis of his or her spiritual belief system. This information often reveals how illness, loss, or disability affects a person's life. A patient's religious practices, views about health, and response to illness influence how you will provide support (Table 21-3).

Life and Self-Responsibility. Assessing spiritual well-being includes looking at your patient's life and

TABLE 21-3 RELIGIOUS BELIEFS ABOUT HEALTH

RELIGIOUS OR CULTURAL GROUP	HEALTH CARE BELIEFS	RESPONSE TO ILLNESS	IMPLICATIONS FOR HEALTH AND NURSING
Hinduism	Accept modern medical science.	Past sins cause illness. Prolonging life is discouraged.	Allow time for prayer and purity rituals. Allow use of amulets, rituals, and symbols.
Sikhism	Accept modern medical science.	Females to be examined by females. Removing undergarments causes great distress.	Provide time for devotional prayer. Allow use of religious symbols.
Buddhism	Accept modern medical science.	Sometimes refuse treatment on holy days. Nonhuman spirits invading the body cause illness. Sometimes want a Buddhist priest. Usually permit withdrawal of life support. Do not practice euthanasia. Often do not take time off from work or family responsibilities when sick.	Health is an important part of life. Good health is maintained by caring for yourself and others. Do not always accept medications because of belief that chemical substances in the body are harmful.
Islam	Must be able to practice the Five Pillars of Islam. Sometimes have a fatalistic view of health.	Use faith healing. Family members are a comfort. Group prayer is strengthening. Sometimes permit withdrawal of life support. Do not practice euthanasia. Believe that time of death is predetermined and cannot be changed. Maintain a sense of hope and often avoid discussions of death.	Women prefer female health care providers. During month of Ramadan Muslims do not eat anything from dawn until sunset. Health and spirituality are connected. Family and friends visit during times of illness. Organ transplantation or donation and postmortem examinations are usually not considered.

Continued

TABLE 21-3 RELIGIOUS BELIEFS ABOUT HEALTH—cont'd

RELIGIOUS OR CULTURAL GROUP	HEALTH CARE BELIEFS	RESPONSE TO ILLNESS	IMPLICATIONS FOR HEALTH AND NURSING
Judaism	Believe in the sanctity of life. God and medicine have a balance. Observance of the Sabbath is important. Some refuse treatments on the Sabbath.	Visiting the sick is an obligation. Obligation to seek care, exercise, sleep, eat well, and avoid drug and alcohol abuse. Euthanasia is forbidden. Life support is discouraged.	Believe it is important to keep yourself healthy. Expect nurses to provide competent health care. Allow patients to express their feelings. Allow family to stay with the dying patient.
Christianity	Accept modern medical science. Complementary or alternative medicine often used.	Use prayer, faith healing. Appreciate visits from clergy. Some use "laying on" of hands. Some take holy communion. Anointing of the sick is given when individual is ill, in acute setting, or near death (Catholic).	Are in favor of organ donation. Health is important to maintain. Allow time for patients to pray by themselves, with family or friends.
Navajos	Concepts of health have a fundamental place in their concept of humans and their place in the universe.	Blessingway is a practice that attempts to remove ill health by means of stories, songs, rituals, prayers, symbols, and sand paintings.	Prefer holistic approach to health care. Often are not on time for appointments. Promote physical, mental, spiritual, and social health of people, families, and communities. Allow family members to visit. Provide teaching about wellness, not disease prevention, when possible.
Appalachians	External locus of control. Nature controls life and health. Accept folk healers. Good Christian members of community are called as servants to minister to disabled.	Dislike hospitals. Tend to not follow medical regimens but expect help when seeking episodic treatment.	Become anxious in unfamiliar settings. Encourage communication with family and friends when ill.

self-responsibility. People who accept change, make decisions about their lives, and are able to forgive themselves and others in times of difficulty have a higher level of spiritual well-being. During illness patients often are unable to accept limitations or know what to do to regain a functional and meaningful life. Their sense of helplessness reflects spiritual distress. However, if a patient is able to adapt to changes and seek solutions for how to deal with any limitations, spiritual well-being reflects an important coping resource. Assess the extent to which a patient understands any limitations or threats posed by an illness and the manner in which the patient chooses to adjust to them. Ask, "Tell me how you feel about the changes caused by your illness," and "How do these changes affect what you now need to do?"

Connectedness. Connectedness is a dimension of spirituality. Patients who are connected to themselves, others, nature, God, or another supreme being usually report higher levels of physical and emotional health (Register, Herman, and Tavakoli, 2011). Patients remain connected with God by praying (Figure 21-2). Prayer is personal communication with one's god. It provides a sense of hope, strength, and security and is woven into one's faith. Patients often use prayer when other treatments are ineffective (Dezutter, Wachholtz, and Corveleyn, 2011). You help patients become or remain connected by respecting each patient's unique sense of spirituality. Assess whether a patient loses the ability to express a sense of relatedness to something greater than self. You assess a patient's connectedness by asking, "What feelings do you have after you pray?" or "Who do you believe is the most important person in your life?"

Life Satisfaction. Spiritual well-being is tied to a person's satisfaction with life and what he or she has accomplished (Chlan, Zebracki, and Vogel, 2011). When people are satisfied with life and how they are using their abilities, more energy is available to deal with new difficulties and resolve problems. You assess a patient's satisfaction with life by

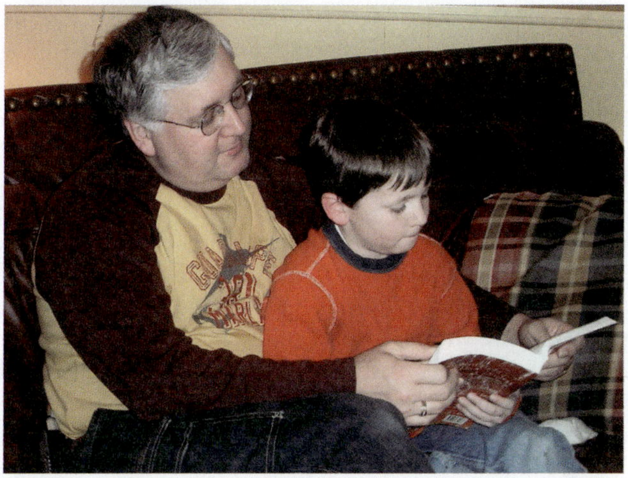

FIGURE 21-2 Praying together enhances connectedness between parents and their children.

asking, "How happy or satisfied are you with your life?" or "Tell me to what extent you feel satisfied with what you have accomplished in life."

Fellowship and Community. Fellowship is one kind of relationship that an individual has with other people, including immediate family, close friends, associates at work or school, fellow members of a church, and neighbors. More specifically this includes the extent of the community of shared faith between people and their support networks. Many times social support from faith-based groups helps patients cope with illness (Heiney et al., 2011) and participate in health promotion behaviors (Newlin et al., 2012). To assess a patient's supportive community, ask questions such as, "With whom do you bond?" "Who do you find to be the greatest source of support in times of difficulty?" or "When you've faced difficult times in the past, who has been your greatest resource?"

Explore the extent and nature of a person's support networks and their relationship with the patient. It is unwise to assume that a given network offers the kind of support that a patient desires. For example, calling a patient's pastor to request a visit is inappropriate if the patient finds little fellowship with the pastor or the pastor's faith community. Does the patient have one significant fellowship or several? What level of support does the community give? Do they visit, say prayers, or support the patient's immediate family? Learn whether openness exists between a patient and the people with whom a fellowship has formed.

Ritual and Practice. The use of rituals and practice is easy to assess and helps you understand a patient's spirituality. Rituals include participation in a religious group or private worship, prayer, sacraments such as baptism or communion, fasting, singing, meditating, scripture reading, and making offerings or sacrifices. Different religions have different rituals for life events. For example, Buddhists practice baptism later in life and find burial or cremation acceptable at death. Muslims wash the body of a dead family member and wrap it in white cloth with the head turned toward the right shoulder. Orthodox and Conservative Jews have their newborn sons circumcised 8 days after birth. Determine whether illness or hospitalization has interrupted a patient's usual rituals or practices. A ritual provides a patient with structure and support during difficult times. If rituals are important to a patient, use them as part of your nursing intervention (Sreevani and Reddemma, 2012).

Vocation. Individuals express their spirituality daily in their work, play, and relationships. Spirituality is often a part of a person's identity and vocation in life. Determine if illness or hospitalization has altered the ability to express some aspect of spirituality as it relates to a person's work or daily activities. Expression of spirituality is highly individual and includes showing an appreciation for life in the variety of things people do, living in the moment and not worrying about tomorrow, appreciating nature, expressing love toward others, and being productive. Assess how patients routinely express spirituality. Questions to ask include, "Has your illness affected the way you live your life spiritually at home or where you work?" or "Has your illness affected your ability to express what's important in life for you?"

Older Adult Considerations. Spirituality often plays a more pronounced and important role in the lives of older adults (Hodge et al., 2012). Older adults often experience many losses, including the loss of a home, spouse, friends, and siblings. Although spirituality varies among older adults, it is strongly related to their ability to cope and manage stress (Edelman and Mandle, 2010). Older adults frequently participate in spiritual practices such as praying, reading the Bible, and enjoying nature. They also often have a strong relationship with God or another higher being, strive to find meaning and purpose in difficult situations, and need to connect with others (Hodge et al., 2012). When caring for older adults, ask open-ended questions to assess their spiritual needs (Edelman and Mandle, 2010). Questions such as, "Which spiritual practices do you use most frequently?" and "What brings you hope?" help you identify spiritual needs and show that you care about and value the older adult.

Patient Expectations. Patients often need to make difficult health-related decisions, and many use spirituality to achieve a sense of well-being (Yuen, 2011). Thus it is essential to take the time to establish a trusting and therapeutic relationship with your patients to accurately assess their expectations in their spiritual care. Active listening and maintaining presence leads to an accurate assessment of a patient's spiritual needs. To determine a patient's expectations about spiritual care and needs, consider asking the following questions: "What are your spiritual goals?", "How does your faith help you cope?", and "Would you like me to contact your minister, pastor, or rabbi to visit you?" Questions such as these indicate respect for your patient and allow you to include his or her expectations in the plan of care.

NURSING DIAGNOSIS

When you review your patient's spiritual assessment, you know a great deal about the patient's spirituality. Exploring a patient's spirituality sometimes reveals responses to health problems that require nursing intervention, or it reveals a strong set of resources for the patient to use in coping. Use your critical thinking skills to analyze data and discover patterns of defining characteristics. Potential nursing diagnoses affected by spiritual health include the following:

- *Anxiety*
- *Ineffective Coping*
- *Fear*
- *Hopelessness*
- *Powerlessness*
- *Spiritual Distress*
- *Risk for Spiritual Distress*
- *Readiness for Enhanced Spiritual Well-being*

As you identify nursing diagnoses for a patient, it is important to recognize the significance that spirituality has for all types of health problems. You may need to apply spiritual care principles if your patient has nursing diagnoses such as *Acute Pain, Chronic Pain, Fear, Anxiety,* and *Compromised Family Coping.*

Three nursing diagnoses accepted by NANDA International (2012) pertain specifically to spirituality. *Readiness for Enhanced Spiritual Well-Being* is based on defining characteristics that show a pattern of inner strength and interconnectedness that comes from inner faith and hope. Patients with this nursing diagnosis have a strong faith; are in harmony with self, others, and a higher power; and have a good sense of life purpose and meaning. A patient with enhanced spiritual well-being has resources on which to draw when faced with other nursing diagnoses. You help the patient explore how to use these resources when facing health problems.

The nursing diagnoses of *Spiritual Distress* and *Risk for Spiritual Distress* create different clinical pictures. Defining characteristics from your assessment show patterns that reflect a person's actual or potential dispiritedness (e.g., expressing concern with the meaning of life and beliefs, anger toward God, and verbalizing conflicts about personal beliefs). Patients likely to be at risk for spiritual distress include those who have poor relationships, have experienced a recent loss, or are suffering some form of mental or physical illness.

Validate defining characteristics and clarify them with the patient before you make a diagnosis and develop a plan of care. With spiritual care the importance of your own spiritual well-being and perceptions cannot be overemphasized. Do not impose your personal beliefs. Be sure that any diagnosis has an accurate related factor (e.g., a situational loss or relationship conflict) so your interventions are purposeful and goal directed.

PLANNING

During planning integrate the knowledge gathered from assessment and knowledge relating to resources and therapies available for spiritual care to develop an individualized plan of care (see Care Plan). Match a patient's needs with evidence-based interventions that are supported and recommended in the clinical and research literature. Use a concept map (Figure 21-3) to organize your patient's care and show how his or her medical diagnosis, assessment data, and nursing diagnoses are interrelated. Focus on building a caring relationship with the patient so you enter into a healing relationship together.

CARE PLAN

Readiness for Enhanced Spiritual Well-Being

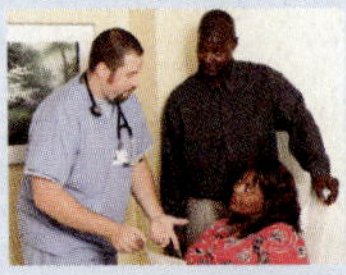

ASSESSMENT

Jeff learns that doctors told Victoria that her prognosis is promising, although she will need treatment to prevent spread of her disease. Joe has been helping Victoria more at home and has been trying to arrange work so he is able to take her to the clinic. This means that he has less time in the evening to spend with the children. In the past Joe and Victoria have always had discussions with the children during mealtime, but recently this has been difficult. Jeff knows that current evidence shows many African-American women use spirituality to cope with breast cancer; therefore he decides to assess Victoria's spirituality.

ASSESSMENT ACTIVITIES	FINDINGS/DEFINING CHARACTERISTICS*
Assess Victoria's connections with herself.	Victoria used to feel good about herself. However, since her cancer treatments, she is more tired and feels less positive at times. She states, **"I wish I had more hope about my prognosis."**
Assess Victoria's connections with her family and significant others.	Before Victoria's illness the **children were very close to their parents and shared their faith in God.** However, **now they are not coping well with Victoria's illness.** Victoria and Joe **attend their church regularly and hope to continue** doing so even during the chemotherapy. **Members of their church have offered support** by taking Victoria to the clinic if Joe is unable.
Determine Victoria's connections with a power greater than herself.	Victoria **expresses a connectedness with her God,** "I don't feel alone; God is with me. I have a better appreciation of each day God gives me, and I believe God's strength will help me continue to be active in my church."

***Defining characteristics** are shown in **bold** type.

CARE PLAN—cont'd

Readiness for Enhanced Spiritual Well-Being

NURSING DIAGNOSIS: Readiness for Enhanced Spiritual Well-Being related to desire to be more connected with self, family, and God

PLANNING

GOAL	EXPECTED OUTCOMES (NOC)[†] *Spiritual Health*
• Victoria will restore connectedness with children within 2 months.	• In 2 weeks Victoria, Joe, and children discuss patient's beliefs about the future and her hope of having the cancer cured. • In 6 weeks Victoria reports son and daughter's ability to discuss fears with mother.
• Victoria will remain connected with herself, her husband, and God within 1 month.	• By the end of this week, Victoria makes a formal time in her day to pray with family members. • In 3 weeks Victoria reports that she and Joe are able to discuss their feelings and fears on a daily basis.

[†]Outcomes classification label from Moorhead S et al, editors: *Nursing outcomes classification (NOC),* ed 5, St Louis, 2013, Mosby.

INTERVENTIONS (NIC)[‡]	RATIONALE
Spiritual Support	
• Use therapeutic communication (see Chapter 11) to establish presence and trust and demonstrate empathy with Victoria and Joe.	Establishing rapport, active listening, and trust is necessary to connect with patients who have spiritual needs (Stovall and Baker, 2010).
• Pray with Victoria and her family.	When people pray, they often experience enhanced health outcomes and connectedness (French and Narayanasamy, 2011).
• Encourage Victoria and her family to continue to attend church and participate in religious practices.	African-Americans who attend church and actively participate in religious activities experience improved spiritual, mental, and physical health (Samuels, 2011).
Family Integrity Promotion	
• Identify typical family coping mechanisms during a conference scheduled late in afternoon at the cancer clinic when the children are able to attend. Provide discussion of their mother's progress. Establish a presence and express a realistic hope of mother's prognosis.	Diagnosis of cancer causes entire family to grieve. Discussing coping mechanisms used in the past helps children cope with illness. Discussion of illness ensures that children will have accurate perception of mother's clinical condition and treatment. Religious and spiritual coping helps children make sense of traumatic experiences (Bryant-Davis et al., 2012).
• Encourage Joe to communicate frequently and openly with Victoria so he can better understand her feelings and to create special times every day to talk about feelings and fears and connect with one another.	Couples who are facing breast cancer and receive and provide daily support for one another have an enhanced sense of connectedness, which allows them to maintain intimacy during the breast cancer experience (Belcher et al., 2011).

[‡]Intervention classification labels from Bulechek GM et al, editors: *Nursing interventions classification (NIC),* ed 6, St Louis, 2013, Mosby.

EVALUATION

NURSING ACTIONS	PATIENT RESPONSE/FINDING	ACHIEVEMENT OF OUTCOME
Ask Victoria about her daily routine. Determine if it includes time for prayer with the family.	Victoria reports that she spends at least 10 minutes every morning in prayer while sitting in her garden. Husband has joined her at times. She meditates for 10 to 15 minutes every day and reports that she is going to church regularly.	Victoria is attending to her spiritual health daily and is maintaining connections with herself and with God.
Ask Victoria and Joe about their relationship with themselves and their children.	Victoria and Joe set time aside every day to talk about what is happening that day, but they are having difficulty finding time to spend with their children because of their hectic school schedule.	Victoria is spending time with her husband regularly; she needs some help working out a schedule that will allow her to spend time with her children. Suggest that Victoria plan a family game night or some other fun family activity to allow time for enhanced interaction with children.

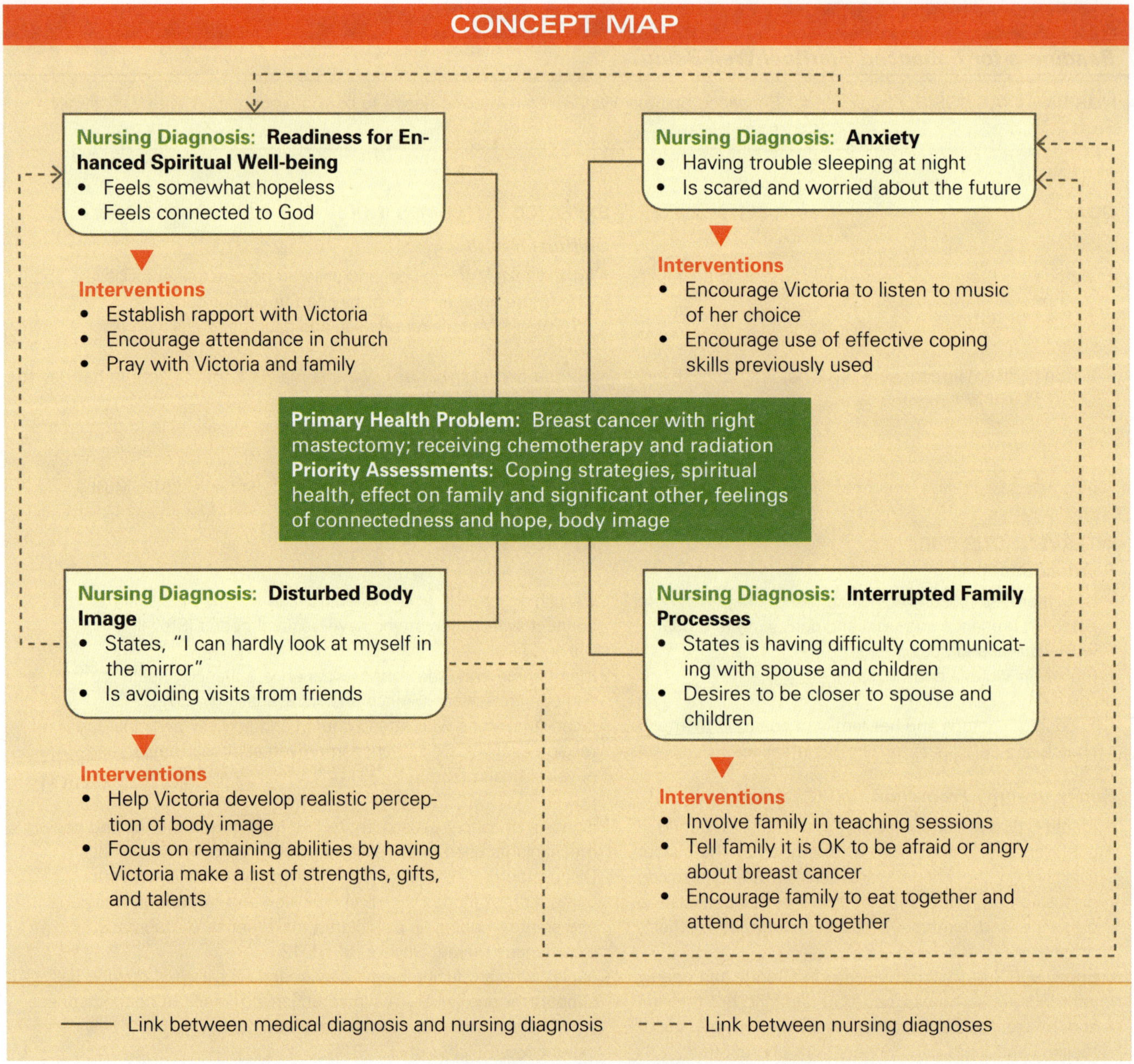

FIGURE 21-3 Concept map.

Goals and Outcomes. A spiritual plan of care includes realistic and patient-centered goals along with relevant outcomes. This requires you to work closely with each patient in setting goals and outcomes and ultimately choosing nursing interventions. In cases in which spiritual care requires helping patients adjust to loss or stressful situations, some goals are long term (e.g., regaining spiritual comfort or affirming a purpose in life). Short-term goals such as renewing participation in religious practices are helpful to allow patients to move toward a more spiritually healthy situation. Outcomes need to relate to what you have learned about a patient. For example, if you know that a patient once practiced regular prayer and meditation, you state an outcome for the goal of regaining spiritual comfort as "Patient prays and meditates daily."

Setting Priorities. Spiritual care is very personalized. Your relationship with a patient allows you to understand your patient's priorities. If you have developed a mutually agreed–on plan with a patient, he or she is able to relate what is most important. Do not sacrifice spiritual priorities for physical care priorities. For example, if your patient is in acute distress, focus your care to help the patient gain a sense of control. In the case of a terminally ill patient, spiritual care is possibly the most important intervention that you provide (Cowey, 2012).

Collaborative Care. To ensure ongoing spiritual care, it sometimes becomes necessary to involve family members, significant others, and clergy to lend support. This means that you learned from the assessment that individuals or groups have a fellowship with the patient. These individuals become involved in all levels of your care plan. The patient's support network help in sharing quiet moments of prayer, reading scripture to the patient, and even giving physical care. In a hospital setting the pastoral care department is a valuable resource. These professionals provide insight about how and when to best support patients and families. When caring for patients with spiritual needs in the community setting, make a referral to a parish nurse if possible. Parish nurses work in a variety of churches and other faith communities. They help bring people closer to God during times of illness and crisis (Van Dover and Pfeiffer, 2012). Their practice emphasizes health and healing within the faith community; and they provide a variety of holistic nursing interventions to their patients, respecting their diverse needs (King, 2011).

IMPLEMENTATION

If a patient is in spiritual distress or has a health problem that requires the use of spiritual resources, a caring relationship between you and the patient is necessary (see Chapter 19). Both you and the patient must feel free to let go and discover together the meaning that illness or loss poses for the patient and the effect it has on the meaning and purpose of life. When you achieve this level of understanding with a patient, it enables you to deliver care in a sensitive, creative, and appropriate manner.

Health Promotion. Spiritual care needs to be a central theme in promoting an individual's overall well-being because of its importance in health promotion (Kemppainen et al., 2011). Spirituality is one personal resource that influences the balance between health and illness. You are able to use the interventions described here at any level of health care.

Establishing Presence. You contribute to a sense of well-being and provide hope for recovery when you spend quality time with your patients. Behaviors that establish your presence include giving attention, answering questions, listening, and having a positive and encouraging (but realistic) attitude. Presence is part of the art of nursing (Milligan, 2011). Benner (1984) explains that presence involves "being with" a patient versus "doing for" a patient. Presence is being able to offer closeness with a patient physically, psychologically, and spiritually. It helps to prevent emotional and environmental isolation (see Chapter 19).

When health promotion is the focus of care, your presence becomes important in instilling confidence in patients' abilities to take the steps necessary to remain healthy. You convey a caring presence by listening to patients' concerns, willingly involving family in discussions about a patient's health, showing self-confidence when providing health instruction, and supporting your patients when they make decisions about their health.

Trust is fundamental to any relationship. The attitude you convey when first interacting with a patient sets the tone for all conversations (see Chapter 11). Actively listening to the meaning of what a patient says is most important. It involves paying attention to the person's words and tone of voice and entering his or her frame of reference. By observing the patient's expressions and body language, you find cues to help him or her explore ways to achieve inner peace, take action, or manage pain. Your role as a nurse is not to solve patients' spiritual problems but to provide an environment in which they can express spirituality.

Supporting a Healing Relationship. When giving spiritual care, look beyond isolated patient problems and recognize the broader picture of a patient's holistic needs. For example, do not look at a patient's back pain as just a problem to solve with quick remedies but rather look at how the pain influences his or her ability to function and achieve goals established in life. A holistic view enables you to assume a helping role. When you develop a helping role with your patients, you establish healing relationships (Benner, 1984). Three steps are evident when you establish healing relationships with your patients:

1. Mobilizing hope for you and for your patients
2. Finding an interpretation or understanding of the illness, pain, anxiety, or other stressful emotion that is acceptable to patients
3. Helping patients use social, emotional, or spiritual resources (Benner, 1984)

Mobilizing a patient's hope is central to a healing relationship. Hope motivates people to face challenges in life (Yeager et al., 2010). You help patients find realistic things for which to hope. For example, a patient newly diagnosed with diabetes becomes hopeful when you help him learn how to manage the disease so as to continue a productive and satisfying way of life. Your focus on controlling a terminally ill patient's pain and other symptoms raises hope that she will be able to attend her daughter's graduation and live each day to the fullest.

Hope has both short- and long-term implications. From a long-term perspective, it gives individuals a determination to endure and carry on with life responsibilities. In the short term hope provides an incentive for constructive coping with obstacles and finding ways to realize the object of hope. Hope is future oriented and helps a patient work toward goals (Kelsey et al., 2011). You help patients achieve hope by working with them to find explanations for their situations that are mutually acceptable. Then help each patient realistically exercise hope. This includes supporting a patient's positive attitude toward life or a desire to be informed and make decisions.

To further support a healing relationship, remain aware of a patient's spiritual resources and needs. It is always important for patients to be able to express and exercise their beliefs and find spiritual comfort. When illness or treatment creates confusion or uncertainty for a patient, recognize the possible effect that this can have on his or her well-being. How can spiritual resources be used and strengthened? Having a clear sense of what illness will be like helps a person apply all resources toward recovery.

Acute Care. Within an acute care setting, support and enhancement of a patient's spiritual well-being are challenging when the focus of health care is on treatment and cure rather than care. Lack of time and patient privacy are other barriers to spiritual care in acute care settings (Ronaldson et al., 2012; Tuck, 2012). Patients often experience multiple stressors and feel like they are losing control. To overcome these challenges, display a soothing presence and supportive touch as you implement nursing interventions. Some patients are fearful of experiencing an illness that threatens their loss of control, and they look for someone to offer competent direction. Your artful use of hands, encouraging words of support, promotion of connectedness, and calm and decisive approach establish a presence that builds trust. Work closely with patients to maximize resources that support their spirituality. For example, you build trust with your patients when you perform procedures competently. You promote connectedness and build trust by listening to a dying patient's concerns, providing reassurance and comfort, and helping a patient complete unfinished business.

Support Systems. Use of support systems is important in any health care setting. They serve as a human link connecting the patient, the nurse, and the patient's lifestyle before an illness. In today's society support comes from many areas, including the family, friends, and support groups. Families often influence how patients perceive their illness. You enhance a patient's support network when you include a patient's family and friends in planning care. A patient's support system often is a source of coping, faith, and hope.

When a patient depends on family, friends, spiritual advisors, and members of the clergy for support, encourage them to visit the patient regularly. Make all the patient's visitors welcome on nursing units and ensure privacy during visits to provide spiritual comfort. If the patient desires, ask the pastoral care department to notify his or her clergy of the patient's admission. Often illness and the hospital environment produce uncertainty that frightens family members and friends. Help the family feel welcome and use their support and presence to promote the patient's healing. For example, including family members in prayer is a thoughtful gesture if it is appropriate to the patient's religion and if family members are comfortable participating. Encouraging the family to bring meaningful religious symbols to the patient's bedside and facilitating the administration of sacraments, rites, and rituals offers significant spiritual support. Do not forget to support the family as well. When you support the family's spirituality and faith practices, you decrease their anxiety and feelings of uncertainty (Kim et al., 2011).

Diet Therapies. Food and nutrition are important aspects of nursing care. Food is also an important component of some religious observances. For example, people in some Hindu and Islamic sects are vegetarian. Muslims are not allowed to eat pork, and they fast during the month of Ramadan. Orthodox Jewish patients observe kosher dietary restrictions. Native Americans have food practices influenced by individual tribal beliefs. Like many aspects of a particular culture or religion, food and the rituals surrounding the preparation and serving of food are important to a patient's spirituality. Integrate a patient's dietary preferences into daily care when possible and consult with the dietitian in the health care institution. If a hospital or other health care agency cannot prepare food in the preferred way, ask the family to bring meals that are appropriate for dietary restrictions posed by the patient's condition.

BOX 21-4 CARE OF THE OLDER ADULT

Supporting Older Adults' Spirituality

- Religious activities, attitudes, and spiritual experiences are very common among older adults. Those who experience spiritual well-being have strong social support, better emotional health, and to some extent improved physical health (Wang, 2011).
- Respecting privacy and dignity is an essential part of nursing care, especially when meeting spiritual needs of the older adult (Ellis and Narayanasamy, 2009).
- Older adults use a variety of strategies such as exercise, relaxation, and biofeedback to cope with pain and chronic illness. Including religious activities positively enhances coping (Prommer and Ficek, 2012; Unsanit et al., 2012).
- Feelings of connectedness are important for the older adult. Enhance connectedness by helping the older patient find meaning and purpose in life, listening actively to concerns, and being present (The Joanna Briggs Institute, 2010).
- Beliefs in the afterlife increase as adults grow older. Make visits from clergy, social workers, lawyers, and even financial advisors available so patients feel as though they have completed all unfinished business. Leaving a legacy to loved ones prepares the older adult to leave the world with a sense of meaning (Touhy and Jett, 2014). Legacies include oral histories, works of art, publications, photographs, or other objects of significance.

Supporting Rituals. You become active in your patients' spiritual care by supporting their participation in spiritual rituals and activities. This is especially important for older adults (Box 21-4). Plan care to allow time for religious readings, spiritual visitations, or even attendance at religious services. Some churches and synagogues offer audiotapes of religious services. Allow family members to plan a prayer session or an organized reading when appropriate. Taped meditations, religious music, televised religious services, and some Internet sites provide other effective options. Be respectful of icons, medals, prayer rugs, or crosses that patients bring to a health care setting and make sure that they are not accidentally lost or misplaced.

Restorative and Continuing Care

Prayer and Meditation. The act of prayer gives an individual the opportunity to renew personal faith and belief in a higher being in a specific, focused way that is either highly ritualized and formal or quite spontaneous and informal. Prayer is an effective coping resource for physical and psychological symptoms (Oliver and Dutney, 2012). Patients pray in private or pursue opportunities for group prayer with family, friends, or clergy. Some patients pray while listening to music. Be supportive of prayer by giving the patient privacy if desired, learning if the patient wishes to have you participate,

BOX 21-5 PATIENT TEACHING

Meditation

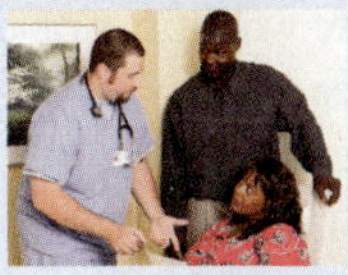

At one of her clinic visits, Victoria tells Jeff, "My friend told me yesterday that, when she had cancer, she used meditation to help her cope with the side effects of her chemotherapy. I was thinking that I might try meditating to see if it would help me, but I don't know how to meditate. Can you help me?" Jeff develops the following teaching plan for Victoria:

OUTCOME

Victoria verbalizes feelings of relaxation and self-transcendence after meditation.

TEACHING STRATEGIES

- Provide a brief description of what will be taught.
- Give Victoria a patient-teaching sheet that describes how to meditate.
- Help Victoria identify at least one quiet place in her home that has minimal interruptions.
- Encourage her to use soft background noise such as a fan or soft music during meditation to block out distractions.
- Teach Victoria the steps of meditation—sit in a comfortable position with the back straight; breathe slowly; and focus on a sound, a prayer, or an image.
- Encourage Victoria to meditate for 10 to 20 minutes 2 times a day.
- Answer any questions.
- Reinforce information as needed.

EVALUATION STRATEGIES

- Ask Victoria to identify what she learned about herself and how she feels after meditating.

BOX 21-6 EVALUATION

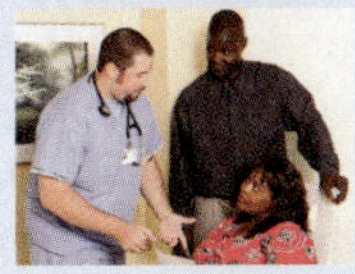

Victoria returns to the clinic 1 week after making a plan to enhance her spiritual health with Jeff. A member of her church accompanies Victoria because Joe is out of town on a business trip. Jeff wants to evaluate whether Victoria continues to feel connected with herself, Joe, her children, and God. Jeff asks, "Tell me, Mrs. Timms, have you had a chance yet to try any of the approaches we talked about last week to give yourself, Joe, and the kids a chance to talk about their feelings? If so, what were the results?" Victoria reports, "Yes, I spend at least 10 minutes every morning in prayer while I sit in my garden, and I've been meditating for 10 to 15 minutes every day. Joe and I set aside at least 15 minutes a day to talk in private after the kids go to bed. If he's not in town, we talk on the phone. Joe and I planned a family game night last Saturday evening with the kids. We shared lots of funny family stories and began to talk with them about my cancer treatment. The kids really seemed to enjoy being together as a family. They asked many questions, and we talked about chores they could do to help me. They are looking forward to coming to the clinic Thursday. I hope this will help them feel less frightened." Jeff also determines that Victoria has spoken with close friends from her church and they plan to visit her this week. Victoria states that she is going to see the physical therapist today.

In an effort to evaluate whether the clinic has met Victoria's expectations, Jeff asks, "Your faith is strong, and it is my hope you have felt comfortable in talking about your worries. Do you believe that we have helped you so far with your concerns about your family?" Victoria replies, "The best thing you've done is listen and recognize how important my family is to me. Your suggestions have helped so far; I am truly blessed to have met all of you nice people at the clinic."

DOCUMENTATION NOTE

"Visited the clinic for the third week of chemotherapy. Denies nausea but is complaining of some soreness in the mouth and a loss of hair. Asks questions readily and made an appointment with the physical therapist as recommended. States has enhanced her connectedness with herself and her family by taking time to pray and meditate, talking and listening with her family, and having fun with her children. Expresses hope that her children will feel less frightened over the diagnosis and states that they will be coming to the next clinic visit."

and suggesting prayer when you know that it is a coping resource for the patient. If prayer is not suitable for a patient, alternatives include listening to calming music or reading a book, poetry, or inspirational texts selected by the patient.

Meditation is effective in creating a relaxation response that reduces daily stress. Patients who meditate often state that they have an increased awareness of their spirituality and of the presence of God or a supreme being (Box 21-5). Meditation exercises give patients relief from pain, insomnia, anxiety, and depression and increase coping and the ability to relax (Cole et al., 2012; Williams-Orlando, 2012). Meditation involves sitting quietly in a comfortable position with eyes closed and repeating a sound, phrase, or sacred word in rhythm with breathing while disregarding intrusive thoughts. Individuals who meditate regularly (twice a day for 10 or 20 minutes) experience decreased metabolism and heart rate, easier breathing, and slower brain waves. Chapter 32 addresses relaxation approaches.

EVALUATION

Patient Care. Attainment of spiritual health is a lifelong goal. Patients experience the need to clarify values (see Chapter 6), reshape philosophies, and live the experiences that help to shape purpose in life. As you provide spiritual care, always evaluate whether the patient achieved planned outcomes and goals (Box 21-6). Compare the patient's level of spiritual health with the behaviors and perceptions noted in the nursing assessment. For example, if your assessment found a patient losing hope, the follow-up evaluation involves a discussion to determine if the patient has regained an attitude that life is worth living. Family and friends are a useful source of evaluative information. Successful outcomes reveal a patient developing an increased or restored sense of connectedness with family; maintaining, reviewing, or reforming a sense of purpose in life; and for some a confidence and trust in a Supreme Being or higher power.

For patients with a serious or terminal illness, evaluation focuses on the goal of helping them retain faith and hope or express openly the uncertainties life poses. Evaluate how well a patient accepts an illness and whether hope has enabled him or her to recognize individual mortality and focus on living for each day. You cannot assume that all patients have faith in a higher power. However, your support helps patients find meaning in life and death, accept their destiny, and be at peace (Ronaldson et al., 2012).

Patient Expectations. You use critical thinking to evaluate whether your spiritual care met your patient's expectations and contributed to your patient's health. When you evaluate spiritual care, include your patient in the evaluation of outcomes. Ask patients if you and the health care team met their expectations and if there is anything you can do to enhance their spiritual well-being. With respect to the nurse-patient relationship, does your patient express trust and confidence in you? Taking time to ask a patient to reflect on the quality of the nurse-patient relationship is time well spent. Asking a patient, "Have you felt comfortable in saying what you feel is important to you spiritually?" determines whether you developed an effective healing relationship.

KEY POINTS

- Attending to a patient's spirituality ensures a holistic focus to nursing practice.
- Frequently the concepts of spirituality and religion are interchanged, but spirituality is a much broader and more unifying concept than religion.
- An individual's beliefs and spiritual well-being influence physical health status.
- Faith and hope are closely linked to a person's spiritual well-being, providing an inner strength for dealing with illness and disability.
- Research suggests that there is a link between a patient's spirituality and potential for healing.
- Acute and chronic illness, terminal illness, and NDEs pose spiritual problems for individuals.
- Providing appropriate spiritual care requires you to critically apply knowledge from principles related to caring, cultural care, loss and grief, and therapeutic communication.
- Avoid biases when assessing and planning spiritual care.
- Learning to practice caring and compassion helps you discover a patient's life values and meaning.
- Connectedness and fellowship with other people are a source of hope for a patient.
- Patients often have spiritual strengths that you use as resources to help them assume healthier lives.
- Interruptions in or changes to customary religious practices affect the support that religion contributes to a person's well-being.
- Common religious rituals include private worship, prayer, singing, use of a rosary, and scripture reading.
- The personal nature of spirituality requires open communication and the establishment of trust between you and a patient.
- Establishing presence involves giving attention, answering questions, having an encouraging attitude, and conveying a sense of trust.
- Part of a patient's caregiving environment is the regular presence of family, friends, and spiritual advisors.

CLINICAL DECISION-MAKING EXERCISES

Victoria and Joe return to the oncology clinic with their children for Victoria's first chemotherapy treatment. Jeff continues his spiritual assessment of the family unit and determines how well they are coping with Victoria's diagnosis.

1. During his assessment, Jeff wants to establish presence with Victoria and her family. Describe at least three ways that he can accomplish this.
2. While Victoria is receiving her chemotherapy, Jeff takes her children to the family waiting room to have a snack. While they are sitting in the family room, the children tell Jeff that they are angry about their mother's breast cancer and they are really upset that she is going to lose her hair because of her treatments. They both ask Jeff why God has done this to their family and say they are no longer inviting friends over to their house. Which nursing diagnosis does Jeff add to his care plan to address the children's needs?
3. After the children finish their snack, Jeff walks with them back to Victoria. He begins to speak with Joe. Joe says, "I'm having trouble sleeping at night because I'm so worried about Victoria. I'm also having trouble focusing at work because I can't get her off my mind." Based on this information, Jeff determines that *Anxiety related to change in health status of wife* is an appropriate nursing diagnosis for Joe at this time. List two nursing interventions that will enhance Joe's spiritual health and decrease his anxiety.

evolve

Answers to Clinical Decision-Making Exercises can be found on the Evolve website.

QSEN ACTIVITY: EVIDENCE-BASED PRACTICE

To provide evidence-based, patient-centered care to Victoria, Jeff wonders what effects prayer has on the severity of side effects of breast cancer treatment. He also wonders if the clinic nurses should routinely start praying with their patients. The manager of the clinic, who believes that Jeff's question may lead to an evidence-based practice change at the clinic, informs Jeff that the first step of the evidence-based practice process is to ask a clinical question.

Using the PICO format, develop an appropriate and clinically relevant question that Jeff could use to guide his search of the current evidence (see Chapter 7).

evolve

Answers to QSEN Activities can be found on the Evolve website.

REVIEW QUESTIONS

1. You are caring for a patient who has just had a heart attack. When you walk into the waiting room, your patient's spouse is wringing her hands, and she is tearful when she speaks. You ask the spouse, "Is there someone I can call who can sit with you while you are in the waiting room?" What are you demonstrating in this example?
   1. Presence
   2. Connecting
   3. Establishing hope
   4. Offering support systems
2. You are completing a spiritual assessment on a 27-year-old male patient admitted to the hospital following a spinal cord injury. When you ask him if he prays to God, he replies, "I don't pray. I don't believe that God exists." Based on his reply, this man most likely is an:
   1. Agenic.
   2. Atheist.
   3. Agnostic.
   4. Anarchist.
3. You are caring for a 16-year-old male patient who is paralyzed as a result of a recent all-terrain vehicle (ATV) accident. The patient states, "I can't believe that God did this to me. My girlfriend hates me now, and I can't stand it when my parents come to visit me; they're worthless." Which nursing diagnosis is this patient likely experiencing?
   1. *Spiritual Distress*
   2. *Ineffective Coping*
   3. *Risk for Spiritual Distress*
   4. *Readiness for Enhanced Spiritual Well-being*
4. You are working in an emergency department when a patient comes in because of severe abdominal pain. During your assessment you discover that the patient has human immunodeficiency virus (HIV) and recently lost his job. You can smell alcohol on his breath. You can tell that something is really bothering him. You pull up a chair next to the patient's bed, sit in the chair, and ask him, "Tell me what concerns you have." Which intellectual standard for critical thinking are you demonstrating?
   1. Risk taking
   2. Significance
   3. Compassion
   4. Completeness
5. You are caring for an elderly patient who has chronic dementia and her 55-year-old daughter who is the patient's caregiver on a daily basis. The daughter is very anxious because she is making some difficult decisions about the long-term care of her mother and is experiencing spiritual distress. While talking with the daughter, you discover that she enjoys spending time at the beach with her grandchildren. Based on this information, which of the following interventions do you implement to reduce the daughter's anxiety and enhance her spiritual health? (Select all that apply.)
   1. Giving the patient an antianxiety medication
   2. Asking the daughter if she would like to pray with you
   3. Suggesting that the daughter continue participating in spiritual rituals that bring her comfort.
   4. Asking the daughter to tell you about a time when she was at the beach with her grandchildren
6. A patient who is recovering after recently experiencing third-degree burns shows transcendence when she states:
   1. "My pain medicine helps me feel better."
   2. "I know I will get better if I just keep trying."
   3. "I see God's grace and become relaxed when I watch the sun set at night."
   4. "I have had a great life and a good marriage. My husband has been so helpful in my healing."
7. You are caring for a male patient who is very angry and depressed and decide to complete a spiritual assessment using the FICA tool. Which of the following assessment questions addresses the F in FICA?
   1. How have your beliefs influenced how you take care of yourself?
   2. What gives meaning to your life?
   3. Who is most important to you?
   4. What can I do to help you with your spiritual needs?
8. You are caring for a hospitalized patient who is Muslim and has diabetes. Which of the following items do you need to remove from the meal tray when it is delivered to the patient?
   1. Small container of vanilla ice cream
   2. 15 red grapes
   3. Bacon, lettuce, and tomato sandwich
   4. Garden salad with ranch dressing
9. A nursing student is providing a presentation to fellow students about spiritual well-being. Which of the following statements made by the student requires clarification by the nursing professor?
   1. "The personal dimension of spiritual well-being shows how you find purpose in your life."
   2. "People who are spiritually healthy have difficulty forgiving other people."
   3. "One part of spiritual well-being relates to how you interact with and encounter nature."
   4. "A person's relationship with a higher power such as Buddha is called the *transcendental dimension.*"

10. A group of oncology nurses is talking about the recent death of a patient. One of the nurses states, "I am so blessed to be able to be an oncology nurse. My patients give me more than I give them." What best describes this belief?
    1. Fellowship and community
    2. Connectedness
    3. Life satisfaction
    4. Vocation

evolve

Rationales for Review Questions can be found on the Evolve website.

1. 4; 2. 2; 3. 1; 4. 3; 5. 2, 3, 4; 6. 3; 7. 2; 8. 3; 9. 2; 10. 4

REFERENCES

Agrillo C: Near-death experience: out-of-body and out-of brain? *Rev Gen Psychol* 15(1):1, 2011.

Bailey ME, Moran S, Graham MM: Creating a spiritual tapestry: nurses' experiences of delivering spiritual care to patients in an Irish hospice, *Int J Palliat Nurs* 15(1):42, 2009.

Belcher AJ, et al: Daily support in couples coping with early-stage breast cancer: maintaining intimacy during adversity, *Health Psychol* 30(6):665, 2011.

Benner P: *From novice to expert*, Menlo Park, CA, 1984, Addison-Wesley.

Berry DM, York K: Depression and religiosity and/or spirituality in college: a longitudinal survey of students in the USA, *Nurs Health Sci* 13(1):76, 2011.

Borneman T, Ferrell B, Puchalski CM: Evaluation of the FICA tool for spiritual assessment, *J Pain Symptom Manage* 40(2):163, 2010.

Boswell GEH, Boswell-Ford KC: Testing a SEM model of two religious concepts and experiential spirituality, *J Religion Health* 49(2):200, 2010.

Bryant-Davis T, et al: Religiosity, spirituality, and trauma recovery in the lives of children and adolescents, *Prof Psychol Res Pract* 43(4):306, 2012.

Burris JL, et al: Factors associated with the psychological well-being and distress of university students, *J Am Coll Health* 57(5):536, 2009.

Cant R, et al: The divided self: near death experiences of resuscitated patients—a review of literature, *Int Emerg Nurs* 20(2):88, 2012.

Chlan KM, Zebracki K, Vogel LC: Spirituality and life satisfaction with pediatric-onset spinal cord injury, *Spinal Cord* 49(3):371, 2011.

Cobb R: How well does spirituality predict health status in adults living with HIV disease: a Neuman Systems Model study, *Nurs Sc Q* 25(4):347, 2012.

Cohen L, et al: Presurgical stress management improves postoperative immune function in men with prostate cancer undergoing radical prostatectomy, *Psychosom Med* 73(3):218, 2011.

Cohen MZ, et al: A platform for nursing research on spirituality and religiosity: definitions and measures, *West J Nurs Res* 34(6):795, 2012.

Cole BS, et al: A randomised clinical trial of the effects of spirituality-focused meditation for people with metastic melanoma, *Ment Health Religion Cult* 15(2):161, 2012.

Cowey E: End-of-life care for patients following acute stroke, *Nurs Stand* 26(27):42, 2012.

Daaleman TP: A health services framework of spiritual care, *J Nurs Manage* 20(8):1021, 2012.

Daaleman TP, Dobbs D: Religiosity, spirituality, and death attitudes in chronically ill older adults, *Res Aging* 32(2):224, 2010.

Dalmida SG, et al: The meaning and use of spirituality among African American women living with HIV/AIDS, *Wes J Nurs Res* 34(6):736, 2012.

Dezutter J, Wachholtz A, Corveleyn J: Prayer and pain: the mediating role of positive re-appraisal, *J Behav Med* 34(6):542, 2011.

Dolamo BL: Spiritual nursing, *Nurs Update* 34(4):22, 2010.

Dyess SM: Faith: a concept analysis, *J Adv Nurs* 67(12):2723, 2011.

Dyess S, Chase SK: Caring for adults living with a chronic illness through communities of faith, *Int J Human Caring* 14(4):38, 2010.

Edelman CL, Mandle CL: *Health promotion throughout the life span*, ed 7, St Louis, 2010, Mosby.

Ellis HK, Narayanasamy A: An investigation into the role of spirituality in nursing, *Br J Nurs* 18(14):886, 2009.

Ford D, et al: Factors associated with illness perception among critically ill patients and surrogates, *Chest* 138(1):59, 2010.

Fowler MDM: *Guide to the code of ethics for nurses: interpretation and application.* Silver Springs, MD, 2010, American Nurses Association.

French C, Narayanasamy A: To pray or not to pray: a question of ethics, *Br J Nurs* 20(18):1198, 2011.

Gall TL, Malette J, Guirguis-Younger M: Spirituality and religiousness: a diversity of definitions, *J Spirituality Ment Health* 13(3):158, 2011.

Harkins LE: Literature analysis of humor therapy research, *Am J Recreation Ther* 8(4):35, 2009.

Haswell MR, et al: Psychometric validation of the growth and empowerment measure (GEM) applied with indigenous Australians, *Aust NZ J Psychiatry* 44(9):791, 2010.

Hayden D: Spirituality in end-of-life care: attending the person on their journey, *Br J Community Nurs* 16(11):546, 2011.

Heiney SP, et al: Antecedents and mediators of community connection in African Women with breast cancer, *Res Theory Nurs Pract* 25(4):252, 2011.

Hodge DR, et al: Older adults' spiritual needs in health care settings: a qualitative meta-synthesis, *Res Aging* 34(2):131, 2012.

Holt-Lunstad J, et al: Understanding the connection between spiritual well-being and physical health: an examination of ambulatory blood pressure, inflammation, blood lipids and fasting glucose, *J Behav Med* 34(6):477, 2011.

Hurlbut JM, Robbins LK, Hoke MM: Correlations between spirituality and health-promoting behaviors among sheltered homeless women, *J Community Health Nurs* 28(2):81, 2011.

Kelsey K, et al: Obesity, hope and health: findings from the HOPE works community survey, *J Community Health* 36(6):919, 2011.

Kemppainen J, et al: Health promotion behaviors of residents with hypertension in Iwate, Japan and North Carolina, USA, *Jpn J Nurs Sci* 8(1):20, 2011.

Kim S, et al: Spirituality and psychological well-being: testing a theory of family interdependence among family caregivers and their elders, *Res Nurs Health* 34(2):103, 2011.

King MA: Parish nursing: holistic nursing care in faith communities, *Holistic Nurs Pract* 25(6):309, 2011.

Lebowitz KR, et al: Effects of humor and laughter on psychological functioning, quality of life, health status, and pulmonary functioning among patients with chronic obstructive pulmonary disease: a preliminary investigation, *Heart Lung* 40(4):310, 2011.

Lewis PE, et al: Psychosocial concerns of young African American breast cancer survivors, *J Psychosoc Oncol* 30(2):168, 2012.

Life Advance: *The spiritual well-being scale*, http://www.lifeadvance.com/spiritual-well-being-scale.html, 2009. Accessed November 30, 2013.

Lundman B, et al: Inner strength: a theoretical analysis of salutogenic concepts, *Int J Nurs Stud* 47(2):251, 2010.

McCarthy VL: A new look at successful aging: exploring a mid-range nursing theory among older adults in a low-income retirement community, *J Theory Construct Test* 15(1):17, 2011.

McSherry W: *The meaning of spirituality and spiritual care within nursing and health care practice*, London, 2007, Quay Books.

Milligan S: Addressing the spiritual care needs of people near the end of life, *Nurs Stand* 26(4):47, 2011.

Mizrahi MC, et al: Effects of guided imagery with relaxation training on anxiety and quality of life among patients with inflammatory bowel disease, *Psychol Health* 27(12):1463, 2012.

Mueller CR: Spirituality in children: understanding and developing interventions, *Pediatr Nurs* 36(4):197, 2010.

NANDA International: *Nursing diagnoses: definitions and classification, 2012-2014*, Oxford, 2012, Wiley-Blackwell.

Nelson-Becker H, Nakashima M, Canda ER: Spiritual assessment in aging: a framework for clinicians, *J Gerontol Soc Work* 48(3/4):331, 2007.

Newlin K, et al: A methodological review of faith-based health promotion literature: advancing the science to expand delivery of diabetes education to black Americans, *J Religion Health* 51(4):1075, 2012.

Nixon A, Narayanasamy A: The spiritual needs of neuro-oncology patients from patients' perspectives, *J Clin Nurs* 19(15-16):2259, 2010.

O'Connell KA, Skevington SM: Spiritual, religious, and personal beliefs are important and distinctive to assessing quality of life in health: a comparison of theoretical models, *Br J Health Psychol* 15(Pt 4):729, 2010.

Oliver IN, Dutney A: A randomized, blinded study of the impact of intercessory prayer on spiritual well-being in patients with cancer, *Altern Ther Health Med* 18(5):18, 2012.

Phelps AC, et al: Addressing spirituality within the care of patients at the end of life: perspectives of patients with advanced cancer, oncologists, and oncology nurses, *J Clin Oncol* 30(20):2538, 2012.

Pike J: Spirituality in nursing: a systematic review of the literature from 2006-10, *Br J Nurs* 20(12):743, 2011.

Prommer E, Ficek B: Management of pain in the elderly at the end of life, *Drugs Aging* 29(4):285, 2012.

QSEN Institute: *Pre-licensure KSAs*, http://qsen.org/competencies/pre-licensure-ksas/, n.d. Accessed November 30, 2013.

Redlich D, et al: Mediated learning experience intervention increases hope of family members coping with a relative with severe mental illness, *Community Ment Health J* 46(4):409, 2010.

Register ME, Herman J, Tavakoli AS: Development and psychometric testing of the register connectedness scale for older adults, *Res Nurs Health* 34(1):60, 2011.

Rominger R: Postcards from heaven and hell: understanding the near-death experience through art, *Art Ther: J Am Art Ther Assoc* 27(1):18, 2010.

Ronaldson S, et al: Spirituality and spiritual caring: nurses' perspectives and practice in palliative and acute care environments, *J Clin Nurs* 21(15/16):2126, 2012.

Rowold J: Effects of spiritual well-being on subsequent happiness, psychological well-being, and stress, *J Religion Health* 50(4):950, 2011.

Samuels AD: The underserved aged and the role of the African American church, *J Cult Diversity* 18(4):129, 2011.

Sreevani R, Reddemma K: Depression and spirituality—a qualitative approach, *Int J Nurs Educ* 4(1):90, 2012.

Stovall S, Baker JD: A concept analysis of connection relative to aging adults, *J Theory Construct Test* 14(2):52, 2010.

Tan H, Wutthilert C, O'Connor M: Spirituality and quality of life in older people with chronic illness in Thailand, *Prog Palliat Care* 19(4):177, 2011.

The Joanna Briggs Institute: The Joanna Briggs Institute best practice information sheet: the psychosocial and spiritual experiences of elderly individuals recovering from a stroke, *Nurs Health Sci* 12(4):515, 2010.

The Joint Commission (TJC): *2014 Hospital Accreditation Standards*, 2014, The Commission.

Touhy TA, Jett KF: *Ebersole and Hess' gerontological nursing & healthy aging*, ed 4, St Louis, 2014, Mosby.

Tuck I: A critical review of a spirituality intervention, *West J Nurs Res* 34(6):712, 2012.

Unsanit P, et al: Development and evaluation of the Thai spiritual well-being assessment tool for elders with a chronic illness, *Pac Rim Int J Nurs Res* 16(1):13, 2012.

US Cancer Statistics Working Group: *United States Cancer Statistics: 1999-2010 Incidence and mortality web-based report*, Atlanta, 2012, Department of Health and Human Services, Centers for Disease Control and Prevention, and National Cancer Institute, http://www.cdc.gov/uscs. Accessed November 30, 2013.

Vachon M, Fillion L, Achille M: A conceptual analysis of spirituality at the end of life, *J Palliat Med* 21(1):53, 2009.

Van Dover L, Pfeiffer J: Patients of parish nurses experience renewed spiritual identity: a grounded theory study, *J Adv Nurs* 68(8):1824, 2012.

Visser A, Garssen B, Vingerhoets A: Spirituality and well-being in cancer patients: a review, *Psycho-Oncology* 19(6):565, 2010.

Wang J: A structural model of the bio-psycho-socio-spiritual factors influencing the development toward gerotranscendence in a sample of institutionalized elders, *J Adv Nurs* 67(12):2628, 2011.

Wiggs CM: Creating the self: exploring the life journey of late-midlife women, *J Women Aging* 22(3):218, 2010.

Williams-Orlando C: Spirituality in integrative medicine, *Integrative Med: Clinician's J* 11(4):34, 2012.

Yeager S, et al: Embrace hope: an end-of-life intervention to support neurological critical care patients and their families, *Crit Care Nurs* 30(1):47, 2010.

Yuen E: Spirituality and the clinical encounter, *Int J Hum Caring* 15(2):42, 2011.

CHAPTER

22

Growth and Development

evolve WEBSITE

http://evolve.elsevier.com/Potter/essentials

- Crossword Puzzle
- Audio Glossary

OBJECTIVES

- Compare the frameworks for growth and development as described by major developmental theorists.
- Describe the growth and development changes that occur in individuals from conception through old age.
- Identify factors that promote or interfere with normal growth and development of individuals at each stage of life.
- Specify the physical and psychosocial health concerns of infants, children, adolescents, and adults.
- Use knowledge of growth and development to enhance use of the nursing process for individuals across the life span.
- Identify specific nursing interventions for the health promotion of patients across the life span.
- Use critical judgment to determine appropriate teaching topics for individual patients across the life span.

KEY TERMS

adolescence, p. 577
Alzheimer's disease, p. 584
climacteric, p. 580
delirium, p. 584
dementia, p. 584
depression, p. 584
development, p. 568
geriatrics, p. 582
growth, p. 568
ischemic vascular dementia (IVD), p. 584
maturation, p. 569
menarche, p. 577
menopause, p. 580
neonate, p. 571
polypharmacy, p. 586
puberty, p. 577
reality orientation, p. 586
reminiscence, p. 585
teratogens, p. 571

As a nurse, you care for individuals of all ages. Human growth and development are orderly, predictable processes beginning with conception and continuing until death. Knowledge of these patterns helps you provide anticipatory guidance to help the families for whom you care.

SCIENTIFIC KNOWLEDGE BASE

Concept of Growth and Development

When the terms *growth* and *development* are used together, they refer to all of the many changes that take place throughout an individual's lifetime (Hockenberry and Wilson, 2013). **Growth** is the measurable aspect of a person's increase in physical dimensions. Measurable growth indicators include changes in height, weight, teeth and bone, and sexual characteristics. **Development** is an interaction of biological, sociological, and psychological forces. It occurs gradually and refers to changes in skill and capacity to function. These changes are qualitative in nature and difficult to measure in exact units. However, there are certain predictable characteristics that are measurable such as development proceeds from simple to complex.

CASE STUDY *Crystal Taylor*

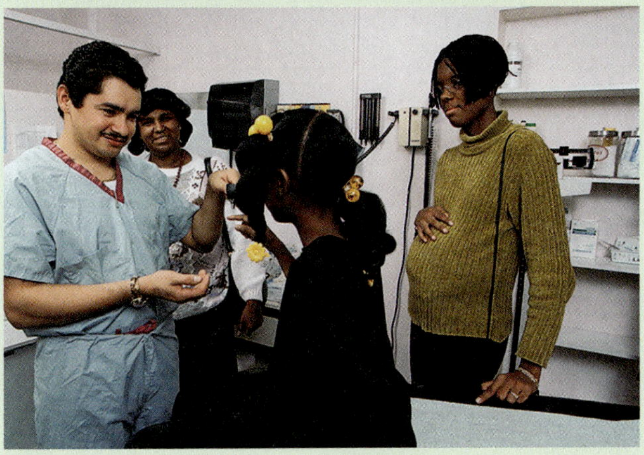

Crystal Taylor, a 25-year-old African-American woman, is a single parent of 2½-year-old Zachary and 6-year-old Monica, who has recently learned to ride a bicycle. Crystal is a smoker and is currently 6 months pregnant. She lives with her 44-year-old mother and 15-year-old brother. Crystal's 68-year-old maternal grandmother and aunt live next door and often help care for Zachary and Monica. Crystal has a strong family history for breast cancer. Her grandmother and aunt are both breast cancer survivors. Crystal mentioned that her mother had a mammogram 6 years ago but has not had any other routine screenings. Crystal's family has used the health care center for years, and she now brings her children to the neighborhood clinic for their health care. Today she has brought Monica to the clinic for her checkup before beginning school.

Louis Ruiz is a 28-year-old nursing student assigned to the clinic. He has to select a family to follow throughout the semester. Louis, who is married and has a 4-year-old son who attends day care, was a medical technician in the army for 4 years. The clinic is Louis' first clinical experience as a nursing student, and he is eager to become involved in health promotion activities but is also anxious about his new role as a professional nurse.

An example of this is learning to crawl before learning to walk.

Maturation is the biological plan for the predictable milestones for growth and development. Physical growth and motor development are a function of maturation. Examples of age-related behaviors that follow a specific sequence are sitting, walking, and running, which are a result of maturation.

A critical period of development refers to a specific phase or period when the presence of a function or reasoning has its greatest effect on a specific aspect of development. For example, if a child does not walk by 20 months, there is delayed gross-motor ability, which slows exploration and manipulation of the environment. The success or failure experienced within a phase affects the child's ability to complete the next phases.

Theories of Human Development

Developmental theories provide a framework for examining, describing, and appreciating human development. It is helpful to look at multiple theories to understand the person as a whole (Burns, 2009). Useful theories explain behavior and predict behavior that is measurable and observable (Table 22-1). Some theories view development as a continuous process involving gradual, cumulative changes slowly over a period of time. Others consider it as discontinuous, with distinct stages. An example of a continuous change is a seedling that grows into an apple tree, whereas the child learning words is discontinuous and the result of weeks and months of practice and development.

Sigmund Freud. Sigmund Freud (1856-1939) provided the first formal structured theory of personality development. Freud's psychoanalytic model of personality development is grounded in the belief that two internal biological forces drive the psychological change in a child: sexual (libido) and instinctive forces. The theory describes a series of five stages, each associated with a pleasurable zone, serving as the focus of gratification. In the first stage, the oral stage, sucking and oral satisfaction are vital to life and also very pleasurable. During the anal stage the focus of pleasure changes to the anal zone. In Stage 3, phallic stage, the genital organs become the focus of pleasure. In the latency stage Freud believed that the sexual urges from the earlier phallic stage are repressed and channeled into productive activities that are socially acceptable. The genital stage occurs during adolescence and is a turbulent time for the child and family. The child's sexual urges reawaken, and social activities begin to occur outside the family circle.

Erik Erikson's Eight Stages of Development. Erik Erikson (1902-1994) expanded Freud's psychoanalytic stages into a psychosocial model that covered the whole life span (Erikson, 1963). In this theory Erikson divided life into eight stages, known as Erikson's eight stages of development (Erikson, 1963, 1997). According to this theory, individuals need to accomplish a particular task before successfully completing the stage. Each task is framed with opposing conflicts such as trust versus mistrust. Each stage builds on the successful attainment of the previous developmental conflict. Unlike Freud, Erikson described three additional stages, including young adulthood, middle adulthood, and old adulthood. The task for stage 6, young adulthood, is intimacy versus isolation. This occurs as young adults develop a sense of identity and deepen their capacity to love others and care for them. Generativity versus self-absorption and stagnation (stage 7) occurs during the middle adult years. Erikson believed that the task at this stage was for adults to accept themselves and be accepting of others. Middle-age adults should strive to give of themselves, be creative, and develop ways to improve society. The last stage, ego integrity versus despair, occurs through the aging process. As the adult ages, he or she begins to struggle with losses such as the loss of loved ones, changes in family, or losses in functional status. These changes challenge the person to adjust while continuing to live a full and rich life.

TABLE 22-1 **COMPARISON OF MAJOR DEVELOPMENT THEORIES OF CHILDHOOD**

DEVELOPMENTAL STAGE (APPROXIMATE AGE)	FREUD (PSYCHOSEXUAL DEVELOPMENT)	ERIKSON (PSYCHOSOCIAL DEVELOPMENT)	PIAGET (LOGICAL, COGNITIVE, AND MORAL DEVELOPMENT)	KOHLBERG (DEVELOPMENT OF MORAL REASONING)
Infancy (birth to 18 months)	Oral stage	Trust vs. mistrust Ability to trust others	Sensorimotor period Progress from reflex activity to simple repetitive actions	
Early childhood/toddler (18 months to 3 years)	Anal stage	Autonomy vs. shame and doubt Self-control and independence	Preoperational period—thinking using symbols; egocentric	Preconventional level Punishment-obedience orientation
Preschool (3-5 years)	Phallic stage	Initiative vs. guilt Highly imaginative	Use of symbols; egocentric	Preconventional level Premoral Instrumental orientation
Childhood (6-12 years)	Latent stage	Industry vs. inferiority Engaged in tasks and activities	Concrete operations period Logical thinking	Conventional level Good-boy, nice-girl orientation
Adolescence (12-19 years)	Genital stage	Identity vs. role confusion Sexual maturity, "Who am I?"	Formal operations period Abstract thinking	Postconventional level Social contract orientation
Young Adulthood		Intimacy vs. isolation Affiliation and love		
Adulthood		Generativity vs. stagnation Production and care		
Maturity		Ego integrity vs. despair Renunciation and wisdom		

Piaget's Theory of Cognitive Development. Jean Piaget (1896-1980) developed the theory of cognitive development, which describes children's intellectual organization and how they think, reason, and perceive the world. The theory includes four periods: sensorimotor, preoperational, concrete operations, and formal operations (see Table 22-1). As a child grows from infancy into adolescence, the intellectual development progresses, starting with reflex and repetitive motion responses, to the use of symbols and objects from the child's point of view, to logical thinking, and finally to abstract thinking (Burns, 2009).

Kohlberg's Moral Developmental Theory. Lawrence Kohlberg (1927-1987) expanded on Piaget's work. According to Kohlberg (1964), moral development is one component of psychosocial development. It involves the reasons that an individual makes a decision about right and wrong behaviors within a culture. Moral development depends on a child's ability to accept social responsibility and integrate personal principles of justice and fairness. In addition, a child's knowledge of right and wrong and behavioral expression of this knowledge must be founded on respect and regard for the integrity and rights of others (Burns, 2009). Cognitive development aids the progression of a person's morality from level to level.

Maslow's Theory of Human Needs. Abraham Maslow (1908-1970) developed a theory of human needs from his study of healthy individuals without physical or mental illness (Figure 22-1). He described an ordering (hierarchy) of needs that motivate human behavior. This ordering is often depicted as a pyramid composed of five levels (Maslow, 1970). When the most basic needs such as hunger and oxygen are met, a person strives to satisfy the needs for safety and security on the next highest level. Disturbances at lower levels interfere with the highest level, self-actualization or the realization of one's potential. This theory has made a valuable contribution to understanding human development through its positive viewpoint and recognition of needs that motivate all humans. However, critics have noted that it does not differentiate according to age-groups.

NURSING KNOWLEDGE BASE

A strong body of knowledge about growth and development gives you good insight regarding how individuals perceive an

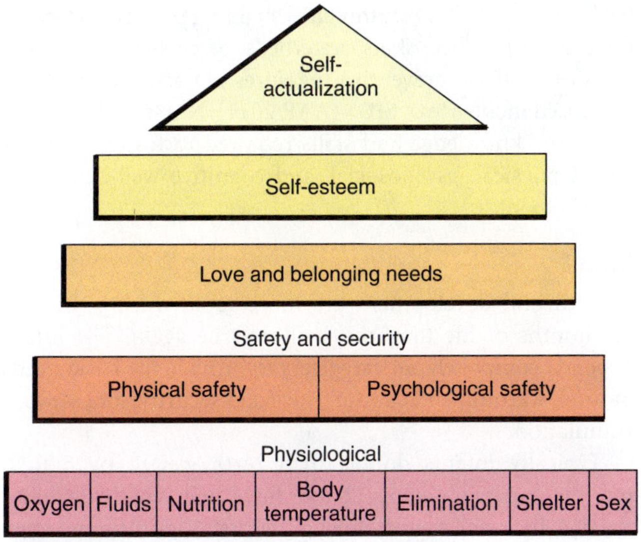

FIGURE 22-1 Maslow's hierarchy of needs. (Redrawn from Maslow AH: *Motivation and personality,* ed 3, Upper Saddle River, NJ, 1970, Prentice Hall.)

event or behave in response to a given situation at a particular age or stage of life. The following is an overview of the stages of life and related health concerns.

Conception and Fetal Development

From the moment of conception, human development proceeds rapidly. The ovum and sperm each carry half the genetic material that guides biochemical processes essential to the developing organism. Intrauterine life generally lasts approximately 9 calendar or 10 lunar months or 266 days, beginning with fertilization and ending with the birth of a baby. Pregnancy may be divided into three periods: germinal, embryonic, and fetal. The germinal period occurs from the time of fertilization until implantation about 2 weeks. The embryonic period extends from the second week until the eighth week after conception. During this time cells differentiate, and organs appear. The fetal period extends from 2 months after conception until birth. Another way is to divide the pregnancy into three trimesters.

The first trimester is the first 3 calendar months. During this time several organ systems are developing at the same time; the disruption of one system can affect the development of other systems.

The second trimester is the period from the third to the sixth prenatal months of life. Some organ systems continue basic development during this time, and the functional capabilities of others are refined. By the end of the second trimester most organ systems are complete and able to function. The fetus weighs about 0.7 kg (1½ lbs) and is approximately 30 cm (12 inches) long.

During the last 3 months of intrauterine life the fetus grows to approximately 50 cm (20 inches) in length. Weight increases to approximately 3.2 to 3.4 kg (7 to 7½ lbs). The skin thickens, lanugo (soft, downy hair) begins to disappear, and the fetal body becomes rounder and fuller. A tremendous spurt in brain growth begins during this trimester and lasts well into the first few years of life. The central nervous system has established its total number of neurons and connections between neurons, and myelination of nerve fibers progresses rapidly. Damage to the central nervous system during the third trimester can potentially alter higher-level cognitive functions.

Health Promotion. Abnormalities in the genes or chromosomes alter health. Other health problems such as fetal alcohol syndrome result from environmental factors (e.g., the mother's diet or tobacco use). **Teratogens** are chemical or physiological agents capable of having adverse effects on a fetus. Exposure to potential teratogens can affect fetal development during any of the trimesters; however, vulnerability is increased during the first trimester when fetal cells are differentiating and organs are forming. Because the placenta is extremely porous, teratogens pass easily from mother to fetus. Some examples of teratogens are viruses, drugs (prescribed, over-the-counter, and street drugs), alcohol, and environmental pollutants such as lead. The fetal effect of these harmful agents depends on the developmental stage in which exposure takes place. Some teratogens produce defects only if the fetus is exposed to the agent at a critical time when the vulnerable organ is developing. For example, the rubella or measles virus is primarily dangerous if a fetus is exposed to it in the first trimester. This virus can cause spontaneous abortion; stillbirth; or defects of the eyes, ears, and heart.

Many drugs are teratogenic during the period of rapid organ growth in the first trimester. Barbiturates, alcohol, anticonvulsants, antibiotics, anticoagulants, and over-the-counter medications can cause fetal abnormalities. Health care providers weigh the benefits of prescribed medications against potentially harmful fetal effects. In addition, there is evidence that mothers who smoke deliver infants with lower birth weights than nonsmoking mothers.

You explore lifestyle changes that can help women abstain from tobacco, alcohol, and drugs not only during pregnancy but also while planning for pregnancy. Preconception counseling is a growing trend in health care. The goal is to secure the best outcome for mother, fetus, and significant others through good prenatal care.

Neonate

The neonatal period is the first 28 days of life. The newborn's physical functioning is primarily reflexive, and stabilization of major organ systems is the primary task of the body. The average full-term **neonate** weighs 3.4 kg (about 7½ lbs), is 50 cm (20 inches) in length, and has a head circumference of 35 cm (14 inches). Neonates lose up to 10% of their birth weight in the first few days of life, primarily through fluid losses by respirations, urination, defecation, and low fluid intake. They usually regain the weight by the end of the second week of life.

Physically the neonate may have lanugo on the skin of the back; cyanosis of the hands and feet (acrocyanosis), especially during activity; and a soft, protuberant abdomen.

Behaviorally the newborn has periods of sucking, crying, sleeping, and activity. The newborn's movements are generally sporadic, but they are symmetrical and involve all extremities. Newborns respond to sensory stimuli, particularly the caregiver's face, voice, and touch.

Early cognitive development begins with innate behaviors, reflexes, and sensory functions. For example, the rooting reflex permits neonates to turn to the nipple instinctively when their cheek is stroked. Other automatic and involuntary reflexes help an infant respond to its environment. Newborns are able to focus on objects 20 to 25 cm (8 to 10 inches) from their faces and respond to auditory stimuli. Therefore you need to teach parents the importance of talking to their babies and providing appropriate visual stimulation.

Health Promotion. Parental concerns during the neonatal period most frequently center on the baby's crying, feeding, eliminating, and sleeping behaviors (Box 22-1). New parents are not always aware of the newborn's immature immune system and need information about how to protect the baby from infection (e.g., avoiding exposure to crowds of people such as at church or the grocery store).

The American Academy of Pediatrics (AAP) recommends placing healthy infants on their backs while they sleep to decrease the risk for sudden infant death syndrome (SIDS). Side sleeping is not advised because it is not as safe as back sleeping. Help new parents by teaching the phrase "face up to wake up" as a reminder to always place children on their backs. The AAP also recommends avoiding placing infants on thick bedding, sheepskins, waterbeds, or cushions. Research shows that these preventive measures are associated with a decreased incidence of SIDS (AAP, 2011). Nurses help parents attain the knowledge and skills required to foster the newborn's physical, psychosocial, and cognitive well-being and development.

BOX 22-1 HEALTH PROMOTION GUIDELINES FOR PARENTS OF NEWBORNS

- Selection of a crib with slats less than approximately 6 cm (2⅜ inches) apart (Hockenberry and Wilson, 2013)
- Mattress fitting snugly against the slats
- No pillows or bumper pads in baby's crib
- Positioning infants on their backs in the crib, "face up to wake up" (AAP, 2011)
- Know expected physiological newborn behaviors and variability of behavioral cycles (sleep-awake states)
- Principles and techniques for feeding method chosen; the American Academy of Pediatrics (2012) recommends breastfeeding, and breastfeeding moms need support and interventions for some minor problems such as sore nipples and temporary decline in milk production
- Appropriate stimulation techniques and support for parents' attempts to provide sensory stimulation to the newborn
- Know feeding patterns and behaviors
- Schedule of well-baby visits and immunization schedule
- Care measures, including hygiene, dressing, comfort
- Protective measures, including asepsis, safety, cardiopulmonary resuscitation (CPR), thermoregulation
- Cleansing of umbilical cord stump with alcohol until it falls off
- Circumcision care
- Signs and symptoms of newborn requiring evaluation by a health care professional

Infant

Growth and development are more rapid during the first 12 months of life than they will ever be again. The infant depends completely on caregivers to provide for basic needs of food, warmth, and comfort; love and security; and sensory stimulation.

Typically infants double their birth weight by 5 to 6 months and triple it by 12 months. Their length increases about 1 inch per month during the first 6 months and then ½ inch per month to the end of their first year. Play is solitary, and it provides opportunities for the infant to develop many motor skills. Rattles, plastic stacking rings, and wooden blocks are just a few examples of toys that promote fine-motor development of the hands and fingers (Figure 22-2).

Health Promotion. In addition to health promotion activities regarding feeding, crying, eliminating, and sleeping for the newborn, new health promotion activities for the 1- to 12-month-old infant are often related to dentition, immunizations, and safety.

The first tooth to erupt is usually one of the lower central incisors at the average age of 7 months. Most babies have six teeth by their first birthday (Hockenberry and Wilson, 2013). The use of a chilled teething ring may soothe swollen, sore gums. Tooth decay is preventable by providing adequate fluoride through formula or otherwise, cleaning inside the baby's

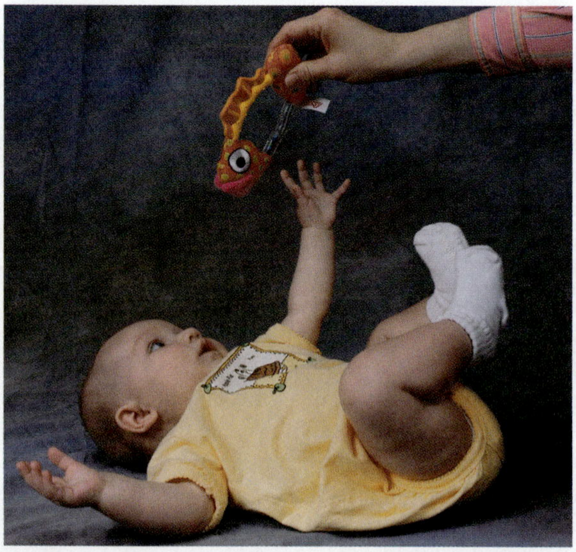

FIGURE 22-2 Three-month-old infant focuses on visual subject and reaches toward it. (Courtesy Paul Vincent Kuntz, Texas Children's Hospital, Houston, TX. From Hockenberry ML, Wilson D: *Wong's nursing care of infants and children*, ed 8, St Louis, 2009, Mosby.)

mouth at least once a day with a wet washcloth, and not allowing the baby to take the bottle to bed (Hockenberry and Wilson, 2013).

Sleep varies from infant to infant. Most neonates sleep 10 to 20 hours a day. After this sleep patterns vary; however, by 4 months of age most infants are sleeping at night with 1 to 2 naps during the day.

The quality and quantity of nutrition influence an infant's growth and development. Breastfeeding is recommended for infants. It is associated with a decreased frequency of gastroenteritis, otitis media, food allergies, diabetes, childhood leukemia, obesity, and pneumonia (Hockenberry and Wilson, 2013). However, when the parent cannot or does not want to breastfeed, an acceptable alternative is iron-fortified commercially prepared formula. Infants should not have any type of cow's milk during the first year because the high protein content may increase the chance of food allergies (Hockenberry and Wilson, 2013).

The use of immunizations has resulted in a dramatic decline of infectious diseases over the past 50 years. Some parents have chosen not to vaccinate their children, citing fears regarding side effects of the vaccines. Although there are small risks from the vaccines, the risks of not receiving the vaccines are far more serious (CDC, 2011). Nurses play a major role in helping community organizations promote immunizations and eliminate preventable childhood disease.

Infants' quickly developing motor skills increase their mobility and their ability to place all types of objects in their mouths. They need constant supervision when not sleeping. You can help parents raise their level of awareness regarding potential hazards in their homes. Common accidents during infancy include automobile accidents, aspiration, burns, drowning, falls, poisoning, and suffocation (Box 22-2). The AAP recommends that infants not sleep with a blanket until they are 1 year old. Some day care facilities recommend blanket sleepers and do not allow blankets in the cribs.

Erikson (1963) described the task for the infant stage as trust. Basic trust is established by having the caregivers meet the infant's needs in a timely manner. Infants who are neglected develop mistrust.

Acute Care. When an infant becomes ill, it is important that you maintain his or her routine daily care. When this is impossible, limit the number of caregivers who have contact with the infant and follow the parents' directions for care. If hospitalization is necessary, infants sometimes have difficulty establishing physical boundaries because of repeated bodily intrusions and painful sensations. Limiting these negative experiences and providing pleasurable sensations support early psychosocial development.

Toddler

The toddler period ranges from 12 to 36 months of age. The rapid development of fine- and gross-motor skills allows a child to participate in feeding, dressing, and toileting. Toddlers walk in an upright position with a broad-stance gait, bowed legs, protuberant abdomen, and arms flung out to the sides for balance. Soon the child begins to navigate stairs, run, jump, stand on one foot for several seconds, and kick a ball.

Because moral development is closely associated with cognitive ability, the moral development of toddlers is just beginning. Toddlers are also egocentric. They do not fully understand concepts of right and wrong. However, they do grasp that some behaviors bring pleasant results and others bring unpleasant results.

Toddlers are generally able to speak in short sentences. Common questions they ask are, "Who's that?" and "What's that?" By 3 years of age toddlers have a beginning mastery of speech; are possessive of their toys; and are often heard to say, "That's mine!" They begin to learn that sharing is a desirable behavior when they offer parents toys to hold and the parents express pleasure. Play is frequently solitary in nature. However, toddlers often participate in parallel play, playing beside another child with a similar toy or object but not actively interacting through their play. Gradually play begins to include the exchanging or sharing of objects when playing beside another toddler engaged in a similar activity.

Health Promotion. Slower growth rates often occur with a decrease in caloric needs and a smaller food intake. Confirming a child's pattern of growth with standard growth charts is reassuring to parents concerned about his or her decreased, fussy appetite known as physiological anorexia. Encourage parents to offer a variety of nutritious foods, in reasonable servings, for mealtime and snacks. Special dietary considerations are necessary for the toddler who is ill, going to have surgery, or on a vegetarian diet. Finger foods allow the toddler to be independent.

BOX 22-2 HEALTH PROMOTION GUIDELINES FOR PARENTS OF INFANTS

- Keeping crib away from radiators, the blast of air ducts, and cords from drapes or blinds
- Expected growth and developmental norms
- Play activities to stimulate gross- and fine-motor development
- Techniques to encourage development of language
- Readiness for weaning from breast or bottle to cup
- Addition of solid foods (usually at 6 months) and other fluids by introducing only one new food at a time to assess for food allergies
- Need for immunizations and immunization schedule
- Safety measures related to use of approved car seats, falls, drowning, and use of mouth to explore everything in environment
- Avoiding exposure to secondhand smoke
- Development of attachment, stranger awareness, and separation anxiety
- Use of voice, eyes, and facial gestures as disciplinary measures
- Signs of illness, measures for assessment (temperature taking), and appropriate action
- Criteria to use when choosing day care

Toilet training is a major task of toddlerhood. The success of toilet training is based on three primary factors: physical ability to control anal and urethral sphincters (after the child learns to walk), the child's ability to recognize urge and communicate it to the parent, and the desire to please the parent by holding on and letting go at appropriate times. The average age for achieving control is 2 years for daytime and 3 years for nighttime control. Girls usually toilet train earlier than boys (Hockenberry and Wilson, 2013).

According to Erikson's theory of psychosocial development, toddlers are developing autonomy and want to do things for themselves (Erikson, 1963). The natural curiosity and mobility of toddlers without good reasoning abilities make them an accident waiting to happen. Toddlers want to put everything into their mouths (e.g., bugs, bleach, or electrical cords) or place their hands, feet, or entire bodies into dangerous places (e.g., electrical outlets, clothes dryers, tubs with very hot water). They need constant supervision unless they are in a totally childproofed area such as their crib or playpen. Toddlers have little awareness of physical safety, and accidents continue to be the leading cause of death and injury. The most common accidents are burns, drowning, falls, motor vehicle accidents, and poisoning (CDC, 2012). You can help parents anticipate the safety needs of their toddlers and make appropriate suggestions (Box 22-3).

Acute Care. When toddlers are ill, it is important to provide care consistent with a child's developmental needs. Use the responses of children and their parents to determine children's specific care. For a young child, being separated from one's family in an unfamiliar environment during an illness is a stressful experience. Parents are more likely to remain with their young child when the nurse and members of the health care team create a comfortable environment for them. Whenever possible encourage the family to bring in the child's favorite toy, blanket, or familiar object. If a significant caregiver cannot remain with the toddler, it is especially important that one nurse assume responsibility for providing the toddler with consistent and appropriate care. Limiting the number of strange caregivers helps establish trust and reduces separation anxiety for the toddler. During times of stress or illness children often regress to behaviors of an earlier time that provide them comfort and security. This regression of behavior is often disturbing to parents, and they need reassurance that the behavior is normal and the child will return to more mature behavior patterns when the stressful situation is resolved.

Toddlers cannot clearly identify where they feel pain and often find anything that causes pressure intrusive or extremely painful. Reduce physical discomfort by keeping periods of restraint or immobility to a minimum. A soft voice, physical contact, and a security item also comfort a child.

BOX 22-3 HEALTH PROMOTION GUIDELINES FOR PARENTS OF TODDLERS

- Play activities to stimulate gross- and fine-motor development (e.g., push/pull, nesting toys)
- Reading to the child
- Good nutritional habits and feeding of self
- Techniques to encourage development of language
- Readiness and appropriate methods for toilet training
- Need for independence and setting limits on behavior
- Need to set limits and provide firm, gentle discipline to resolve negativism and temper tantrums
- Continued separation anxiety and development of ritualism
- Safety measures, including childproofing the home environment (e.g., storage of cleaning products and medication, use of car seats, selection of appropriate safe toys, pool and water precautions, outdoor play, placing plants out of reach and getting rid of poisonous ones)
  - Keeping electrical cords out of reach and covering unused electrical outlets
  - Blocking stairways and balconies and not leaving infant unsupervised near water
  - Reducing the risk for injuries: not leaving iron on ironing board, turning handles of saucepans and frying pans to inside of stove when cooking
- Continued need for immunization and developmental assessments

Preschool Child

Early childhood is a period between the ages of 3 and 5 years when children refine the mastery of their bodies and eagerly await the beginning of formal education. Many parents find this age-group more enjoyable than toddlerhood because children are more cooperative, share thoughts with greater accuracy, and interact and communicate more effectively. Physical development continues at a slow pace, whereas cognitive and psychosocial development accelerates. According to Erikson, this is the time when children develop a sense of moral responsibility (Erikson, 1963).

Three-year-olds are able to recognize people, objects, and events by their outward appearance. For example, they prefer having two nickels over a dime because it appears to be more. The continued egocentricity of early thinking makes it difficult to suggest acceptable alternatives to a preschooler. When they are hungry, they expect others also to be hungry, and they think they must eat now!

In addition, preschoolers are increasingly able to solve problems intuitively on the basis of one aspect of a situation. For example, they can classify objects according to either size or color but not both. They ask many questions. Erikson described the task for this stage as initiative versus guilt. Initiative is described as the point in which children see themselves as separate individuals. They also have a great sense of imagination. Adults often misinterpret preschoolers' "tall tales" as lying; however, they are actually presenting their own reality. Their imagination also contributes to the development of fears, the greatest of which in this age-group is the fear of bodily harm. For example, this manifests as fear of various animals, the dark, or procedures such as having their blood pressure measured.

If two events are related in time or space, children link them causally. For example, the hospitalized child reasons, "I cried last night, and that's why the nurse gave me the shot." As children near age 5, they begin to use rules to understand cause and effect. They then begin to reason from the general to the particular.

Health Promotion. Ingestion of large amounts of carbohydrates and fats from junk foods results in overweight and undernourishment. Encourage parents to be role models for good eating habits and to offer their children a varied diet that prevents deficiencies and excesses. Children enjoy helping prepare healthy snacks such as fruit slices, carrot sticks, celery stuffed with peanut butter, and popcorn. Family meals also help improve the quality of food eaten.

Preschoolers require role models and instruction to develop good hygiene measures such as brushing their teeth after meals and sugary snacks, covering their mouths and noses when coughing or sneezing, keeping their fingers out of their noses and eyes, and washing their hands before eating and after using the toilet.

Accidents are the major cause of mortality for this age-group, and motor vehicle accidents (usually as a pedestrian) are the major cause of death. Parents need education to help meet the health promotion needs of their child (Box 22-4). This is a good time for you to teach children what to do in case of fire, safety regulations for crossing the street, and the necessity of riding in the back seat of the car buckled in an approved car seat. Preschool children can be taught how to get help when someone is hurt.

BOX 22-4 HEALTH PROMOTION GUIDELINES FOR PARENTS OF PRESCHOOL CHILDREN

- Encouraging parents to support their child's sense of initiative and recognizing that the child will be unable to complete all activities begun
- Nutritional requirements for optimal growth
- Methods to stimulate continued progress in the development of motor skills, language, cognitive skills, and social skills: reading to the child, using play groups, encouraging the child to do small chores and activities for the family
- Knowing signs of common childhood communicable diseases and measures to reduce their risk and spread
- Beginning instruction for children for personal safety (e.g., do not talk to strangers; tell an adult about inappropriate touching, strangers in the area)
- Criteria to use when evaluating preschool education programs:
  - Teaching methods used to help preschoolers learn about their health, including nutrition, exercise, and rest
  - Safety measures and education related to motor vehicles, tricycles, and fire
- Increased sexual curiosity and need for use of correct anatomical terminology
- Child abuse, including how to protect children, identifying signs of abuse, and knowing community agencies available for assistance

Acute Care. When preschoolers become ill, their beginning abilities to reason and understand make illness less stressful. Although they have developed object permanence and recognize that their parents still exist when out of sight, most tolerate only short absences without becoming distressed. Encourage parents to tell the child when they are leaving and when they will return in terms the child can understand (e.g., "I am leaving and will be back after lunch."). Be present when parents leave to provide distraction and support for the child. Reduce children's fear by allowing the child to sit up for assessments and procedures when possible and demonstrating procedures on another person or doll. Also allow the child to see and handle equipment and help with a procedure as appropriate. Encouraging parents to be present during procedures and leaving the room door open at night if the child requests it reduce fear as well. Simple and factual information is especially important to this age-group because of their great sense of imagination (Hockenberry and Wilson, 2013).

School-Age Child

The foundation for adult roles in work, recreation, and social interaction occurs during the "middle years" of childhood (ages 6 to 12). Great developmental strides are made in physical, cognitive, and psychosocial skills. Children become "better" at things. For example, they run faster and farther as proficiency and endurance develop.

Educational experience in school expands a child's world and transitions him or her from a life of relatively free play to one of structured play, learning, and work. The school and home influence growth and development. For optimal development to occur, a child has to learn to cope with the rules and expectations of school and peers. School-age children have some reasoning and logical thoughts. Children at this stage adopt their parents' moral standards to seek their approval.

School-age children become more graceful as they gain increasing control over their bodies (Figure 22-3). Strength doubles, and large-muscle coordination improves. Participation in the basic gross-motor skills of running, jumping, balancing, throwing, and catching refines neuromuscular function and skills. Holding a pencil and printing letters and words are evidence of fine-motor coordination improvement in 6-year-olds. By age 12, a child makes detailed drawings and writes sentences. Assessment of neurological development is often based on fine-motor coordination. Teachers often ask school nurses to conduct fine-motor assessment of children if they observe a lack of these motor skills.

The middle childhood years are often referred to as the "age of the loose tooth," because children often lose all of their primary teeth during this period. The secondary teeth are much larger in proportion and are often referred to as "tombstone teeth." Regular dental visits confirm that children are brushing their teeth with regularity and proper technique.

As children begin to move into the school world, there are many opportunities for them to gain a sense of competence

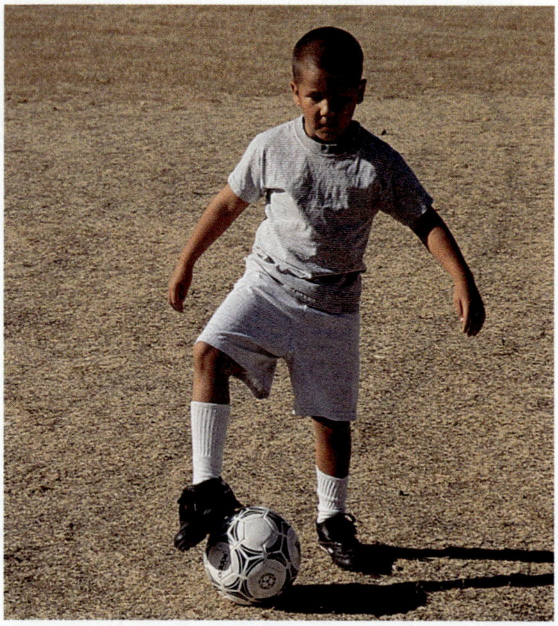

FIGURE 22-3 Coordination improves in school-age children as they gain control over their bodies.

as they learn reading, writing, and other academic skills. They also have the ability to follow the rules of a new authority person and to compete and cooperate with peers in play and work. The recognition that a child receives at home for achievements also improves the child's developing self-esteem and provides reason to put forth further good efforts. Children's success in work and play leads to an increasing sense of independence and a need to participate in any decisions that involve them. As children move through these middle years of childhood, they confront a number of stressors in the school, in their home, and from peers.

The school-age child prefers same-sex peers to opposite-sex peers. In general girls and boys view the opposite sex negatively. Peer influence becomes diverse during this stage.

Health Promotion. Accidents and injuries are major health problems affecting school-age children and are the causative factor in a large number of deaths in this age-group. Motor vehicle accidents, followed by drowning, fires, burns, and firearms are the most frequent fatal accidents. Other major causes of accidents involve recreational activity, most frequently involving bicycles, swings, skateboards, and contact sports. Encourage parents of school-agers to have their children assume some responsibility for their own safety by establishing rules and acting as good role models (Box 22-5).

Blood pressure elevation in childhood is the single best predictor of adult hypertension. This recognition has reinforced the significance of making blood pressure measurement a part of every annual assessment of a school-age child (Hockenberry and Wilson, 2013; NHBPEP, 2012). Measure on at least three separate occasions with the appropriate-size cuff and in a relaxed situation before concluding that the child's blood pressure is elevated and needs further medical attention.

BOX 22-5 HEALTH PROMOTION GUIDELINES FOR SCHOOL-AGERS AND THEIR PARENTS

- Expected growth parameters and developmental tasks, including the middle childhood growth spurt and puberty
- Measures to enhance adjustment to school and reduce school-related stressors
- Influence and importance of peers as they learn to follow rules and be competitive
- Development and expression of sexuality, including sex play (e.g., masturbation)
- Parental modeling of safety practices
- Instruction for children for personal safety (e.g., do not talk to strangers, tell an adult about inappropriate touching, strangers in the area, bullying)
- Monitoring of and limiting recreational screen time (computer, video games, television) to 1 to 2 hours a day
- Educating parent to read violence and sexual language ratings on video and computer games and media
- Reinforcing Internet safety (e.g., placing the computer in an interactive family area rather than in the child's room, blocking inappropriate e-mail messages and pop-up messages, emphasizing the need to tell an adult when there is "something funny" on the screen or in the e-mail)
- Recreational safety, including helmets for sports, bicycling, and skateboarding
- Substance abuse (tobacco, alcohol, drugs), including dangers, signs of use, and available community agency support
- Responsibility for health promotion activities, including nutrition, exercise, and safety

Childhood obesity is a prominent health problem, which increases a child's risk for hypertension, diabetes, coronary artery disease, and other chronic health problems. In addition, overweight children are frequently the targets of teasing and bullying, and these children are less likely to be chosen for team or peer activities. Daily exercise and maintaining normal body weight are important as both interventions and prevention (Hockenberry and Wilson, 2013).

Acute Care. During illness school-agers usually tolerate the absence of their parents better than the younger child because of their reasoning abilities. Although they understand that their parents often need to be elsewhere, they want and expect daily visits and phone calls and texts. The items that school-agers often bring from home such as their own pillows and favorite books give them a sense of security and independence. During times of illness and hospitalization, honesty, factual information, and interest in their concerns are helpful in establishing a trusting relationship with school-age children.

School-agers are usually able to pinpoint their pain, describe it with moderate assistance, and sometimes attempt to explain its cause. They often use play to cope with their pain or withdraw in an attempt to deal with their discomfort. They are usually aware that they receive medication for pain but sometimes do not ask for it until the pain is intense. They are quick to learn to use a scale to assess their discomfort. Most school-agers are eager learners who enjoy learning to find their various pulses, read a thermometer, or operate the blood pressure machine during hospitalization. Many are able to help check their urine for sugar or protein or learn to do their own fingersticks for blood samples. School-agers who become ill are often threatened by a loss of their recently developed independence by needing to use a bedpan, having help with bathing, bed rest, or having someone else select their menus.

Preadolescent

At present children experience more emotional and social pressures than did youngsters 30 years ago. As a result, children 10 to 12 years of age are now having experiences that were once unique to 14- and 15-year-old youths. This transitional period between childhood and adolescence is preadolescence. Others refer to this period as *late childhood, early adolescence, pubescence,* and *transescence*. Physically it refers to the beginning of the second skeletal growth spurt, when the physical changes such as the development of pubic hair and female breasts begin. Children also become more social, and their behavioral patterns become much less predictable.

Puberty. A wide variation exists between the sexes and within the same sex as to when the physical changes of puberty begin. Use the ranges of normal growth to assess the progress of growth for an adolescent patient. As with increases in height and weight, the pattern of sexual changes is more significant than their time of onset. Large deviations from normal time frames require attention. Visible and invisible changes take place during puberty as a result of hormonal changes.

The physical changes of puberty enhance achievement of sexual identity. These changes encourage the development of masculine and feminine behaviors. If these physical changes involve deviations, the person has more difficulty developing a comfortable sexual identity.

Girls attain 90% to 95% of their adult height by **menarche,** the onset of menstruation, and reach their full height by 1 to 2 years after menarche. Boys continue to grow taller until 18 to 20 years of age. Adolescents are sensitive about physical changes that make them different from peers. Thus they are generally interested in the normal pattern of growth and their personal growth curves.

Adolescent

Adolescence is the transition from childhood to adulthood, usually between 13 and 18 years of age but sometimes extending until graduation from college. The term *adolescence* refers to the psychological maturation of an individual, whereas **puberty** refers to the point when reproduction is possible. A steady progression of physical, social, cognitive, psychological, and moral changes all characterize this period. According to Erikson's theory of psychosocial development, this is a period when adolescents search for a sense of identity (Erikson, 1963). The adaptations required by these changes push them to develop individualized coping mechanisms and styles of behaviors, which they will continue to use or adapt throughout life.

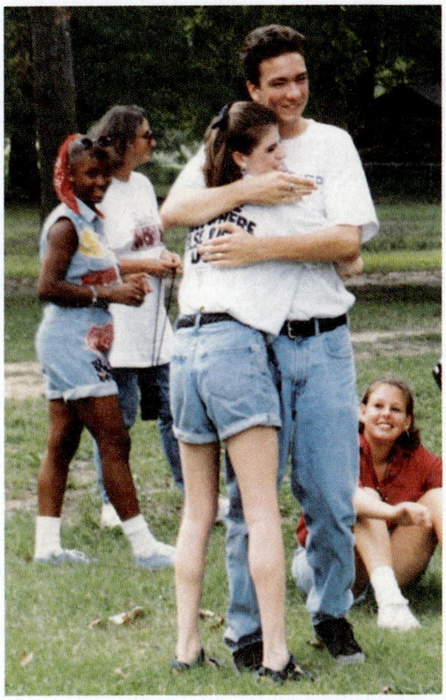

FIGURE 22-4 Heterosexual relationships are an important part of adolescence. (From Hockenberry ML, Wilson D: *Wong's nursing care of infants and children,* ed 8, St Louis, 2009, Mosby.)

Physical Development. Although timing varies greatly, physical changes occur rapidly during adolescence. Sexual maturation follows the development of primary and secondary sexual characteristics. Primary characteristics are physical and hormonal changes necessary for reproduction. Secondary characteristics differentiate males from females externally.

Adolescents depend on the development of the secondary sex characteristics to define their maleness or femaleness. In addition, this helps them feel secure and similar to their peers. Cultural attitudes, expectations of sex role behavior, and available role models also influence sexual identity. The masculine and feminine behaviors that teenagers see and the expectations they perceive for behaving as a man or woman affect how they express sexuality. Adolescents master age-appropriate sexuality when they feel comfortable with sexual behaviors, choices, and relationships (Figure 22-4).

Language development is fairly complete by adolescence, although vocabulary continues to expand. The primary focus becomes developing diverse communication skills to use effectively in many situations, which the person will refine later in life. Adolescents need to communicate thoughts, feelings, and facts to peers, parents, teachers, and other people of authority.

Developing moral judgment depends on cognitive and communication skills and peer interaction. Moral development, begun in early childhood, matures. Adolescents learn to understand that rules are cooperative agreements that can be changed to fit the situation rather than absolutes. They learn to apply rules by using their own judgment rather than simply to avoid punishment as in the earlier years. They judge themselves by internalized ideals, which often lead to conflict between personal and group values.

Adolescents are more likely to engage in risk-taking behaviors that often jeopardize their safety. The prefrontal area of the brain, which is responsible for impulse control, is not fully developed until 25 years of age. Adolescents have a sense of invulnerability, which also increases risk-taking behavior. It is during adolescence that the incidence of motor vehicle accidents, STIs, and substance experimentation and addiction increases.

The search for personal identity is the major task of adolescent psychosocial development. Teenagers establish close peer relationships or remain socially isolated. Erikson (1963) sees identity (or role) confusion as the prime task of this stage. Teenagers have to become emotionally independent from their parents and yet retain family ties. They also need to develop their own ethical systems based on personal values.

Health Promotion. A component of personal identity is perception of health. Healthy adolescents evaluate their own health according to feelings of well-being, ability to function normally, and absence of symptoms. Health problems causing severe or long-term alteration of these factors permanently alter self-identity. Along with parents, you help adolescents take responsibility for their own health status and practices (Box 22-6).

The major causes of mortality in the adolescent age period are injuries, homicide, and suicide (Hockenberry and Wilson, 2013). Motor and other vehicular accidents, pregnancy, STIs, and substance abuse are major causes of morbidity. Mental disorders, chronic illness, and eating disorders are other causes.

Health services for adolescents need to be readily available, affordable, and approachable if parents and communities expect teens to use them. Adolescents also tend to use school-based programs. Health care workers need skills in interviewing adolescents and identifying those more at risk. Successful health promotion activities actively involve teenagers at all times. The involvement of teens in organizations that promote responsible behaviors such as Students Against Destructive Decisions (SADD) is a key element. Through your efforts in the school and community you can make many contributions to help meet the *Healthy People 2020* objectives (USDHHS, 2013). The use of seat belts when in a motor vehicle and refraining from texting while driving are important topics to emphasize with adolescents.

Substance abuse is a major concern to those who work with teenagers. All adolescents are at risk for experimental or recreational substance use. You assess those at risk, educate them to prevent accidents related to substance abuse, and counsel those in rehabilitation.

Suicide is the third leading cause of death in people between 15 and 24 years of age and the second leading cause of death for Caucasian males in this age-group (National Institute of Mental Health, 2010). Depression and social isolation commonly precede a suicide attempt, but suicide most likely results from a combination of several factors. Be alert to the following warning signs, which often occur for at least 1 month before a suicide attempt (Hockenberry and Wilson, 2013):

1. Decrease in school performance
2. Withdrawal
3. Loss of initiative
4. Loneliness, sadness, or crying
5. Appetite and sleep disturbances
6. Verbalization of suicidal thoughts

Make immediate referrals to mental health professionals when your assessment suggests that an adolescent is considering suicide. Guidance helps focus on the positive aspects of life and strengthens coping abilities.

Sexual experimentation is common among adolescents. Peer pressure, physiological and emotional changes, and

BOX 22-6 HEALTH PROMOTION GUIDELINES FOR ADOLESCENTS AND THEIR PARENTS

- Setting clear, reasonable limits for acceptable behavior and consequences for breaking the rules
- Automobile safety, including driver's education course; use of seat belts; risks to self and others associated with drinking, drugs, and driving; use of helmets by bicyclists and motorcyclists
- Developing a mutual plan so the adolescent never gets into a car when the driver has been drinking or the adolescent never drives if he or she has been drinking; plan to include who to call to pick up the child
- Awareness of warning signs of depression and suicide, alternatives to suicide, and methods to deal with a suicidal peer
- Potential of social isolation and the excessive use of computer for recreational activities (e.g., searching the Internet, solitary computer games)
- Discussing threats to safety from the Internet (e.g., identity theft, sexual predators)
- Dealing with peer pressure, school-related stressors, anger, and violent feelings through decision-making skills, conflict resolution, and positive coping strategies
- Prevention of unintentional injuries (e.g., classes on use of firearms, danger of swimming alone or under the influence of alcohol or drugs)
- Sexual experimentation and measures to prevent STIs and pregnancy, including abstinence, transmission of infection, symptoms of disease, prophylactic measures, and community organizations that provide assistance
- Supporting development of sexual identity (i.e., homosexual, heterosexual, and bisexual)
- Importance of routine HIV testing for at-risk adolescents
- Allowing increasing independence within limits of safety and well-being
- Breast and testicular self-examination

HIV, Human immunodeficiency virus; *STIs,* sexually transmitted infections.

societal expectations contribute to heterosexual and homosexual relations. About 50% of adolescent students have had sexual intercourse during their lifetime. Two thirds of these sexually active teenagers are inconsistent in their use of safe sex, including condom use. The risk-taking behaviors of adolescent sexual activity and drug use make adolescents vulnerable to the threat of human immunodeficiency virus (HIV) infection and acquired immunodeficiency syndrome (AIDS).

The United States has one of the highest rates of teenage pregnancy in the world. Adolescent pregnancy occurs across socioeconomic classes, in public and private schools, among all ethnic and religious backgrounds, and in all parts of the country.

Acute Care. Hospitalization imposes rules and separates adolescents from their usual support system, restricts their independence, and threatens their personal identity. Adolescents who are forced into dependency or have their need for privacy ignored respond with frustration, anger, or self-assertion. Although most hospitals allow peers to visit, some adolescents isolate themselves until they are able to compete on an equal basis with peers. The telephone is often the lifeline between adolescents and their friends and helps them maintain their place in their social group. Many adolescents welcome peer visitors, and hospitals often allow patients to go to a lounge or cafeteria with them.

Adolescents who are more independent from their parents usually do well with intermittent visiting but expect some type of daily contact. Some request that their parent remain with them throughout the hospitalization, demonstrating that they also experience regression with the stress of illness. It is important that you address the patient rather than the parents during the assessment process.

Adolescents usually describe their pain with minimal assistance, pinpoint its location, and often explain its cause. They are usually aware of the medication they receive for pain and like to be in control of when you give it to them. Many of them are able to use distraction and relaxation techniques to decrease their discomfort.

Young Adult

Adult developmental changes are based on earlier characteristics that help shape subsequent behaviors. Each person's development is a unique process. Young adulthood is defined as the ages between 20 and 40 (Linton et al., 2012). During this phase the individual moves away from the family and marries or remains single. Young adults are active and adapt to new experiences and newly acquired independence.

Young adults have reached physical maturity, have achieved the highest level of cognitive ability according to Piaget, and are expected to exhibit a high degree of psychosocial maturity. Many young adults recognize that they are continuously in the process of becoming more mature in their behavior.

Physical Development. Young adults usually complete their physical growth by the age of 20. They are usually at their peak of health and less commonly experience severe illnesses compared with other adults. Although physical changes associated with aging have begun, the effects are not great enough to be noticed or require attention.

Cognitive Development. Rational thinking habits and flexibility of thought increase steadily through the adult years. Formal and informal educational experiences, general life experiences, and occupational opportunities dramatically increase conceptual, problem-solving, and motor skills. A rich, stimulating environment for the growing and maturing adult encourages the development of full creative potential. An understanding of how adults learn helps you develop teaching plans for them (see Chapter 12).

Psychosocial Development. The emotional health of young adults is related to their ability to effectively address personal and social tasks. According to developmental theorists, certain patterns or trends are relatively predictable. Once young adults have begun to work in their chosen area, they have more time and energy to select a mate (if they have not already done so) and develop a greater sense of intimacy. Many choose to marry, but an increasing number of young adults are choosing to remain single.

Identifying a preferred occupational area is a major task of young adults. When individuals know their skills, talents, and personality characteristics, occupational choices are easier, and they are generally more satisfied with their choices. In the young and middle adult years job satisfaction is a major factor in achievement and responsibility.

The developmental tasks of young adults are potentially filled with stressful situations. Most young adults have the physical and emotional resources and support systems to meet the many challenges, tasks, and responsibilities they face. You often help them develop time-management skills or mobilize their resources and support systems, especially when one of their immediate family members is ill or hospitalized.

Health Promotion. Health teaching and counseling are often directed at helping patients improve their health habits. Understanding the dynamics of behavior and habits assists you in designing interventions that help patients develop or reinforce health-promoting behaviors. To help patients form positive health habits, you become a teacher and facilitator. You need to remember that you do not always change patients' habits but you are able to raise their level of knowledge regarding the potential impact of behavior on health. Patients have control of and are responsible for their own behaviors. When working with a patient, explain psychological principles of changing habits, offer information about health risks, and provide positive reinforcement of health-directed behaviors and decisions. Minimize or eliminate barriers to change such as lack of knowledge or motivation to bring about change.

Young adults are generally active and have no major health problems. However, their fast-paced lifestyles put them at risk for illnesses or disabilities during their middle or older adult years. Motor vehicle accidents and violence are the greatest cause of mortality and morbidity among young adults. Poor adherence to routine screening schedules puts patients at risk for severe illnesses because of failed early detection.

Encourage your patients to follow cancer screening guidelines for breast self-examination (BSE), testicular self-examination (TSE), and genital self-examination (see Chapter 16).

Family stressors occur at any time. Family life has peaks, when everyone in the family works together, and valleys, when everyone appears to pull apart. Situational stressors occur during events such as births, deaths, illnesses, marriages, divorces, and job losses. The psychosocial assessment allows you to identify areas of particular stress for the young adult (see Chapter 25). After identifying these stressors, work with the patient to modify the stress response.

Acute Care. Many young adults do not experience hospitalization; but when they do, it is often threatening because it interferes with their employment and fulfillment of family responsibilities. Scheduled hospitalizations allow adults to effectively plan to meet the needs of their families and expectations of their employment. Unanticipated hospitalizations often cause chaos for adults and all those directly involved in their lives. If they do not have a strong support system, they usually welcome your help to establish priorities and mobilize their resources. Adults are often impatient with the time and energy requirements that a chronic health problem requires for good management. Support groups often help patients deal with these challenges.

Middle-Age Adult

Middle adulthood usually refers to the years between 40 and 65. For many it is a period when one has both grown children and older-adult parents. Most have experienced personal and career achievements, along with socioeconomic stability. Using leisure time in satisfying and creative ways is a challenge that, if met satisfactorily, enables middle-age adults to prepare for retirement.

Physical Changes. Accepting and adjusting to the physiological changes of middle age is one of the major developmental tasks of this age period. Because middle adulthood spans 25 years, many of the physical changes described usually do not occur until later in the developmental period. Middle-age adults use much energy to adapt self-concept and body image to physiological realities and changes in physical appearance. Table 22-2 summarizes these expected physical assessment findings.

Climacteric. Climacteric is a term that describes the decline of reproductive capacity and accompanying changes brought about by the decrease in sexual hormones. It affects men and women differently. Men begin to experience decreased fertility, but they are able to continue to father children. Menopause, when a woman stops ovulating and menstruating, occurs only when 12 months have passed since the last menstrual flow.

Cognitive Development. Changes in the cognitive function of middle-age adults are few except during illness or trauma. Performance on intelligence tests indicates increases in some areas, particularly verbal abilities and tasks involving stored knowledge. Although middle-age adults sometimes perform more slowly and are not as adept at solving new or unusual problems, the ability to solve practical problems based on experience peaks at midlife because of the ability for integrative thinking.

Psychosocial Development. According to Erikson (1963), the primary developmental task of the middle-age adult years is to achieve generativity, which is the willingness to establish and guide the next generation and care for others. Many find particular joy in helping their children and other young people become productive and responsible adults.

Expected changes in the middle-age adult involve expected events such as children moving away from home (the empty-nest syndrome) or unexpected events such as a marital separation or the death of a spouse or parent. Another increasingly common situation is that many middle adults find themselves caring for both their own children still living at home and at the same time having to care for an elderly parent. For this reason middle adults are frequently referred to as the "sandwich generation." These changes result in stress that affects the middle-age adult's overall level of health.

Career changes occur by choice or as a result of changes in the workplace or society as a whole. In recent decades middle-age adults more often change occupations because they find themselves less satisfied with their present employment. In some cases technological advances or changes in the direction of industry force them to change work situations. Such changes, especially when unanticipated, result in stress that affects family relationships, self-concept, and financial security for the later years.

Marital changes that occur during middle age include death of a spouse, separation, divorce, and the choice of remarrying or remaining single. A widowed, separated, or divorced patient goes through a period of loss and grief during which it is necessary to adapt to the change in marital status. If the single middle-age adult decides to marry, the stressors of marriage are similar to those for the young adult. In addition, the couple sometimes has to cope with the social expectations and pressures related to middle-age marriage.

The increasing life span in the United States and Canada has led to increased numbers of older adults in the population. Therefore greater numbers of middle-age adults address the personal and social issues confronting their aging parents. Adult children frequently assume partial or total caregiving responsibilities for their older parents. This means that adult children help with personal care, decision making, housekeeping, financial matters, transportation, and medical care management tasks. The burden placed on adult family caregivers increases if they are also employed and continuing to raise children. Twenty percent of female caregivers over age 50 who also work full time suffered symptoms of depression compared to 8% of noncaregiving peers (MetLife, 2011). The middle-age adult and the older-adult parent have conflicting relationship priorities. The older adult often desires to remain independent, whereas the adult child strives to protect the parent. Negotiations and compromises are useful in defining and resolving such problems.

Health Promotion. Because middle-agers experience physiological changes and face certain health realities, their perceptions of health and health behaviors are often

TABLE 22-2 PHYSICAL ASSESSMENT FINDINGS IN THE MIDDLE-AGE ADULT

BODY SYSTEM	NORMAL OR EXPECTED FINDINGS
Integument	Intact Appropriate distribution of pigmentation Slow, progressive decrease in skin turgor Graying and loss of hair
Head and neck	Symmetry of scalp, skull, and face
Eyes	Visual acuity by Snellen chart that is less than 20/50 Loss of accommodation of lens to focus light on near objects Pupillary reaction to light and accommodation Normal visual fields and extraocular movements Normal retinal structures
Ears	Normal auditory structures; acuity of high-pitched sounds declines
Nose, sinuses, and throat	Patent nares and intact sinuses, mouth, and pharynx Location of trachea at midline Nonpalpable lateral thyroid lobes
Thorax and lungs	Increased anteroposterior diameter Respiratory rate 10-20 breaths/min and regular Normal tactile fremitus, resonance, and breath sounds
Heart and vascular system	Normal heart sounds Systole: S_1 less than S_2 at base Diastole: S_1 less than S_2 at apex Point of maximal impulse: at fifth intercostal space in midclavicular line and 2 cm or less in diameter Vital signs Temperature: 36.0°-37.6° C (96.8°-99.6° F) Pulse: 60-100 beats/min (conditioned athlete, 50 beats/min) Blood pressure: <120 mm Hg systolic <80 mm Hg diastolic All pulses palpable
Breasts	Decreased size resulting from decreased muscle mass Normal nipples and areola
Abdomen	No tenderness or organomegaly Decreased strength of abdominal muscles
Female reproductive system	Change in menstrual cycle and duration and quality of menstrual flow "Hot flashes" Change in cervical mucosa
Male reproductive system	Normal penis and scrotum Prostatic enlargement in some individuals
Musculoskeletal system	Decreased muscle mass Decreased range of joint motion
Neurological system	Appropriate affect, appearance, and behavior Lucidity and appropriate level of cognitive ability Intact cranial nerves Adequate motor responses Responsive sensory system

important factors in maintaining health. Middle-age adults are more prone to stress-related illnesses such as heart attacks, hypertension, migraine headaches, backache, arthritis, cancer, and autoimmune diseases.

The leading causes of death in people between the ages of 45 and 64 years are heart disease, cancer (primarily lung, breast, and colorectal), stroke, accidental injuries, and chronic obstructive pulmonary diseases. Middle-age adults need to continue the same recommended health practices outlined in the discussion on the young adult. It is important that you understand cultural implications when providing health screening to your patients (Box 22-7). It is also important for middle-age patients to follow cancer screening guidelines (see Chapter 16).

BOX 22-7 PATIENT-CENTERED CARE

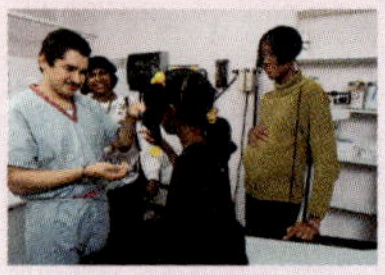

As Louis prepared to help develop health promotion activities for Crystal and her family, he read about the impact of a patient's culture on health care practices. Louis knows that it is important to respect his patient's cultural beliefs and practices, but he also understands the value of routine health screenings (Phillips and Cohen, 2011). Because there is a strong family history for breast cancer, Louis wants to help Crystal and her mother develop breast health practices. He knows that breast cancer survival rates are increasing, but he also recognizes that cultural beliefs and practices influence adherence to breast cancer screening. Although the 5-year survival rate for breast cancer is steadily improving, the survival rate for African-American women remains lower. African-American women are not as diligent in having routine clinical breast examinations (CBEs) or mammograms as are Caucasian women. Louis learns that Crystal's mother, at age 44, has not yet had a mammogram. Her risk for cancer makes her a candidate for screening. More African-American women delay breast cancer screening and at time of diagnosis are often diagnosed with late-stage breast cancer (Conway-Phillips and Millon-Underwood, 2009). Louis wants to learn if the mother has talked with her doctor about screening.

IMPLICATIONS FOR PRACTICE

- Assess Crystal and her mother to determine their family's beliefs and practices about breast self-examination, CBE, and mammography.
- Ask Crystal about the role of their family's spirituality and spiritual practices in coping with illness, symptoms, and other life stressors.
- Contact the breast health center at the city clinic. Determine if Crystal and her mother desire to be introduced to culturally specific breast health practices from a female health care provider.

When middle-age adults seek health care, you need to develop goals for positive health behaviors. For example, women need to increase the calcium in their diets to decrease the risk for osteoporosis. Simple things such as increasing dietary calcium and vitamin D supplements are effective. In addition, organizations such as exercise and fitness clubs give men and women the opportunity to participate in many physical activities. These activities help improve balance, coordination, and activity tolerance.

Acute Care. Middle-agers hold the same family and occupational concerns regarding hospitalization as do young adults. There is sometimes less stress because of the security of employment or because the children who are still at home are usually old enough to care for themselves. However, underinsured middle-agers face serious financial threats. Middle-age adults are at risk for a decline in their physical health. Chronic health problems such as sickle cell anemia, arthritis, asthma, diabetes, and lung disease require ongoing medical care and often brief hospitalizations. The middle-age adult is usually interested in his or her health and wants to be informed.

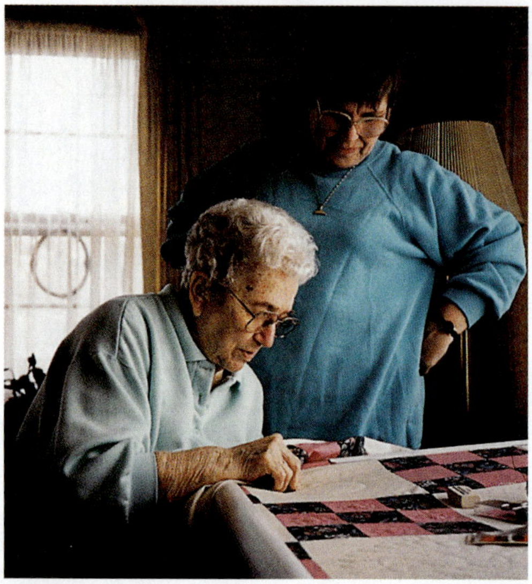

FIGURE 22-5 Quilting keeps this older adult active.

Older Adult

Most older adults are physically active, intelligent, and socially engaged (Figure 22-5). Extended life spans allow many older adults to enjoy their retirement by pursuing interests for which they previously had little time. The number of older adults in the United States continues to grow. In addition, statistics project that the diversity of this population will increase. By 2050 it is expected that the older adults from minority groups (e.g., African-American, American Indians, Asian/Pacific Islanders, Hispanics, and Islamic) will account for 33% of the total over the age of 65 (U.S. Census Bureau, 2010).

Older adulthood traditionally begins after retirement, but the time when people retire varies greatly. Some people retire at age 50, and others work into their 80s and 90s. It is not unusual for those who write about older adults to divide them into the "young old," who are vital, vigorous, and active, and the "old old," who are frail and infirm. The fastest growing subset is people over the age of 90, whose growth rate tripled between 1980 and 2010 and is expected to quadruple between 2010 and 2050 (He and Muenchrath, 2011). **Geriatrics** is the branch of health care dealing with the physiology and psychology of aging and with the diagnosis and treatment of diseases affecting older adults. Gerontology is the study of all aspects of the aging process and its consequences.

Nursing care of older adults poses special challenges because of diversity in patients' physical, cognitive, and psychosocial health. Older adults vary in level of function and productivity. Before making a health assessment, be aware of the normal expected findings on physical and psychosocial assessment for an older adult and consider the normal changes of aging.

TABLE 22-3 COMMON PHYSICAL CHANGES OF AGING

SYSTEM	NORMAL OR EXPECTED FINDINGS
Integument	
Skin color	Brown age spots and spotty pigmentation in areas exposed to sun; pallor even in absence of anemia
Moisture	Dry, scaly
Temperature	Extremities cooler; perspiration decreased
Texture	Decreased elasticity; wrinkles; folding, sagging
Fat distribution	Decreased on extremities; increased on abdomen
Hair	Thinning and graying on scalp; axillary and pubic hair and hair on extremities sometimes decreased; facial hair in men decreased; chin and upper lip hair present in women
Nails	Decreased growth rate
Head and neck	
Head	Nasal and facial bones sharp and angular; loss of eyebrow hair in women; men's eyebrows become bushier
Eyes	Decreased visual acuity; decreased accommodation; reduced adaptation to darkness; sensitivity to glare; diminished light reflex
Ears	Decreased pitch discrimination; diminished hearing acuity
Nose and sinuses	Increased nasal hair; decreased sense of smell
Mouth and pharynx	Use of bridges or dentures; decreased sense of taste; atrophy of papillae of lateral edges of tongue; occasionally change in voice pitch
Neck	Thyroid gland nodular; slight tracheal deviation resulting from muscle atrophy
Thorax and lungs	Increased anteroposterior diameter; increased chest rigidity; increased respiratory rate with decreased lung expansion
Heart and vascular system	Blood pressure (BP) remains within normal limits, <120/80 mm Hg (NHBPEP, 2012); BP between 120/80 and 139/89 mm Hg is considered prehypertension; elevations in BP are not a normal aspect of aging, and older adults need minor elevations monitored (NHBPEP, 2012); peripheral pulses easily palpated; pedal pulses weaker, and lower extremities colder, especially at night; orthostatic hypertension common
Breasts	Diminished breast tissue; pendulous
Gastrointestinal system	Decreased salivary secretions, which make swallowing more difficult; decreased peristalsis; decreased production of digestive enzymes, hydrochloric acid, pepsin, and pancreatic enzymes, leading to indigestion and constipation
Reproductive system	
Female	Decreased estrogen; decreased uterine size; decreased secretions; atrophy of epithelial lining of the vagina; vaginal dryness
Male	Decreased testosterone; decreased sperm count; erections less firm and slower to develop; decreased testicular size
Urinary system	Decreased renal filtration and renal efficiency; subsequent loss of protein from kidney; nocturia
Female	Urgency and stress incontinence from decrease in perineal muscle tone
Male	Frequent urination resulting from prostatic enlargement
Musculoskeletal system	Decreased muscle mass and strength; bone demineralization (more pronounced in women); shortening of trunk from intervertebral space narrowing; decreased joint mobility; decreased range of joint motion; kyphosis (usually in women); slowed reaction time
Neurological system	Decreased rate of voluntary or automatic reflexes; decreased ability to respond to multiple stimuli; insomnia; shorter sleeping periods

Modified from Ebersole P et al.: *Toward healthy aging: human needs and nursing response*, ed 8, St Louis, 2012, Mosby.
NHBPEP, National High Blood Pressure Education Program.

Physical Development. An older adult must adjust to the physical changes of aging. These changes are not associated with a disease state but are the normal changes anticipated with aging. The physiological changes that occur with advancing age vary with each patient. Table 22-3 describes the common types of physiological changes. They occur in all people but take place at different rates and depend on accompanying circumstances in an individual's life.

Cognitive Development. Older adults often remain alert and highly perceptive until the time of their death. Nevertheless the misconception that they always have cognitive impairments and suffer from memory loss and confusion persists. Because cognitive impairment occurs in this age-group, be aware of the nature and type of these impairments.

Certain aspects of short-term memory (e.g., numbers) decrease with age; but visual memory, which allows a person to remember how to read, remains strong. Long-term memory for newly learned information decreases significantly with age, but recall for distant experiences and procedural experiences (e.g., driving) do not seem to be affected in the later years of life. Both intelligence and memory vary greatly among individuals. Most older people who want and need to learn new skills and information do so when they are presented more slowly over a long period. Continuing mental activity is essential to keeping older adults alert, and older people benefit from memory training (Linton et al., 2007).

Three common conditions affect cognition in older adults: delirium, dementia, and depression (Box 22-8). It is important that you learn how to distinguish among these three conditions to select appropriate interventions for your patients. Use a valid assessment tool to accurately assess for patient's cognitive changes. In addition, take time to learn how to correctly use these cognitive assessment tools (Linton, et al., 2007).

Delirium is an acute confusional state and requires prompt assessment. It is a potentially reversible cognitive impairment that often has physiological causes such as electrolyte imbalance, hypoglycemia, infection, and medications. In addition, very slight body temperature alterations cause delirium in older adults. This condition often accompanies infections such as pneumonia. The characteristics of delirium usually include fluctuations in cognition that develop over a short time such as a reduced ability to focus, sustain, or shift attention; and there are acute changes in mood, arousal, and self-awareness. Other signs are hallucinations, transient incoherent speech, disturbed sleep pattern, and disorientation.

Dementia is a broad category of disorders that refers to a generalized impairment of intellectual functioning that interferes with social and occupational functioning. Dementia differs from delirium in that it is a gradual, progressive, irreversible dysfunction. The many causes of dementia include neurological disorders, vascular disorders, inherited disorders, and infections (National Institutes of Health, 2013). Thus early recognition is important, requiring you to make thorough observations of patient behavior, neurological function (see Chapter 16), and laboratory diagnostic studies. Family and friends are valuable resources in detecting behavioral changes since this disorder may go unnoticed in those who see the person infrequently.

Alzheimer's disease is the most common form of dementia. It is a progressive loss of memory (amnesia), loss of ability to recognize objects (agnosia), loss of the ability to perform familiar tasks (apraxia), and loss of language skills (aphasia). As the disease progresses some patients also experience changes in personality and behavior such as anxiety, suspiciousness, agitation, and delusions or hallucinations (Alzheimer's Association, 2012).

Ischemic vascular dementia (IVD) is the second most common form of dementia. It can be characterized by either an abrupt loss of function, usually from a stroke, or general slowing of cognitive abilities. The person may have difficulty with cognitive tasks such as planning. For some people the condition develops slowly with a gradual loss of function and/or thinking (Ebersole et al., 2012).

Depression among older adults is increasing. This diagnosis was once overlooked and assumed to be a normal response to aging, physical losses, or other life events. Depression is treatable and often reversible. Health care workers must look at the possible underlying or contributing factors in an attempt to find the proper treatment methods.

Psychosocial Development. The older adult has to adapt to many psychosocial changes that occur with aging. Among the more common transitions that occur with aging are retirement, volunteerism, and loss of spousal roles (Ebersole et al., 2012). Despite the changes that occur, the older adult has the potential for developing new and fulfilling life patterns.

BOX 22-8 EVIDENCE-BASED PRACTICE

PICO Question: How does an anticipatory preparation educational program for adult-children caregivers impact role strain and depressive symptoms related to caring for parents with dementia?

SUMMARY OF EVIDENCE

Older adults in the United States who require assistance because of chronic illnesses or disabilities frequently receive help from their family to live independently. According to the U.S. Census Bureau (2010), over 22 million American families report providing care for someone over the age of 50. Typically caregivers are middle-age females who are employed full time and spend an average of 21 hours per week providing care for their elderly family member. Research has shown that the way in which a woman has come into the caregiver role influences how much emotional stress and strain she feels. Women who felt they had a choice in caring for their family member had lower levels of emotional stress than those who didn't believe they had a choice (Pope et al., 2012). The demands of working can also affect the adult child caregiver's role strain (Wang et al, 2010).

APPLICATION TO NURSING PRACTICE

- Encourage adult children to discuss caregiving plans with their parents to give them a sense of control in assuming the caregiving role.
- Encourage adult children who are going to be assuming a caregiving role to discuss resources with their siblings (Wang et al., 2010).
- Help adult children who are caregivers locate community support groups and respite resources.
- Encourage caregivers to reconcile their work schedules, when possible, with family caregiving responsibilities.
- Assess caregivers for work flexibility to identify high-risk groups.

Most older adults want to work as long as they are physically able (Ebersole et al., 2012). The time a person chooses to retire is often based on type of work, status achieved, and length of time employed. When a patient describes retirement, it is important to know whether the individual is fully retired, partially retired, or retired from one position to assume another.

Retirement represents a developmental stage that may occupy 30 years of one's life. It also represents a highly productive and fulfilling period of life. Help patients and their families prepare for retirement by gathering information as to why the patient is considering it. Retirement also affects more individuals than the retired person; it affects spouses, adult children, and grandchildren. In addition, the retired person may be spending more time alone for the first time in his or her life.

Reminiscence, or life review, is a technique that facilitates an individual's preparation for the end of life. It is an adaptive function of older adults that allows them to recall the past to assign new meaning to past experiences. Reminiscence is the natural way that older adults revive their past in an attempt to establish order and meaning and reconcile conflicts and disappointments as they prepare for death (Alea et al., 2010).

Death. Most older adults experience death of spouses, friends, and in some cases children. These losses require individuals to go through a process of grieving (see Chapter 26). Some older adults experience loss when they lose a partner after many years in a satisfying relationship (Ebersole et al., 2012). For many older adults the grief associated with loss of a spouse lasts for many years. Experiencing the grieving process requires support from family, nurses, and other health professionals. You lend support by showing warmth and caring to help patients feel they are not alone.

A common misconception is that the death of an older adult is always a blessing and the culmination of a full and rich life. Many dying older adults still have life goals and are not emotionally prepared to die.

Aloneness and Loneliness. With advancing age more people live alone. This is particularly common for older Caucasian women. However, living alone is not equivalent to the feeling of loneliness. A person can be surrounded by others yet still feel lonely. Ebersole et al. (2012) define loneliness as an affective state of longing and emptiness; whereas being alone is to be solitary, apart from others, and undisturbed. Many patients choose to be alone or isolated simply because of the desire for privacy or an opportunity for self-reflection and creativity. Loneliness, on the other hand, is sometimes a passive and painful emotion, influenced by psychological, economic, sociological, and physiological factors.

Housing and Environment. Changes in social roles, family responsibilities, and health status influence an older patient's choice of living arrangements. An older adult sometimes needs to change living arrangements because of the death of a spouse or a change in health status. A change in an older patient's living arrangements requires an extended period of adjustment during which assistance and support will be needed from family and friends and health care professionals.

Health Promotion. The possibility of an individual being reasonably healthy and fit in later life often depends on his or her lifestyle. Older adults need to continue the same recommended health practices introduced in the young-adult section. Some older adults need encouragement to maintain a pattern of physical exercise and activity. It is not too late for an older person to begin an exercise program; however, older adults need to have a complete physical examination, which usually includes a stress cardiogram or stress test. Assessment of activity tolerance helps you and the patient plan a program that meets physical needs while allowing for physical impairments (Box 22-9).

Most older adults are in good health; however, chronic medical conditions increase dramatically with age. The effect of a particular chronic health problem on mobility and independence depends greatly on the individual. Most older adults are capable of taking charge of their lives and assume responsibility for preventing disability.

Sensory impairments are common in the older adult (see Chapter 38). These changes are frequently the result of the normal aging process. Help the older adult identify resources to help correct visual and auditory problems. The sense of touch usually remains strong. Older adults who become

BOX 22-9 CARE OF THE OLDER ADULT

Health Promotion and Independence

- Provide information from the American Association of Retired Persons (http://www.aarp.org) regarding supplemental health insurance, group discounts for older adults, and medical and legal information.
- Discuss housing alternatives to help the older adult make a decision regarding the sale of the home, relocation to another area of the country, or retirement communities.
- Instruct patient in health maintenance programs such as exercise activities that are designed to increase exercise tolerance, flexibility, and socialization.
- Teach patient that the need for annual influenza and routine pneumonia vaccines increases, especially when chronic illness is present.
- Teach patient about safe and appropriate administration of prescribed drugs: purpose; effect; possible other prescription, over-the-counter, or dietary interactions; and reportable side effects.
- Encourage patient to use one pharmacy for prescription and over-the-counter preparations.
- Instruct patient about importance of making sure to tell health care providers about all prescription, over-the-counter preparations, and supplements that they take.
- Instruct patient regarding environmental safety issues (e.g., home lighting, floor coverings, stairs, shoes, electrical cords) to reduce the risk for falling.
- Instruct patient in nutritional aspects related to disease (e.g., a low-fat diet with hypertension, the need for a balanced diet with reduced total calories because of aging changes, and lower energy expenditures).

victims of social isolation are often deprived of touching and holding, which convey affection and friendliness. The touch of nurses and all caregivers who work with older adults serves to provide sensory stimulation; reduce anxiety; relieve physiological and emotional pain; orient older adults to reality; and provide comfort, particularly during the dying process.

As a group, adults over 65 years of age are the greatest users of prescription drugs. Many drugs interact with one another, potentiating or negating the effect of another drug. Some drugs cause confusion; affect balance; cause dizziness, nausea, or vomiting; or promote constipation or urinary frequency. **Polypharmacy,** the prescription, use, or administration of more medications than are indicated clinically, is a common problem of older adults. The combined use of multiple drugs causes serious problematic effects.

Acute Care. Hospitalization of older adults is often disturbing to them because they are not accustomed to the environment and routines. Even those who are able to live independently with some assistance from their families become temporarily disoriented by the strange surroundings of a hospital. Monitor the patient for confusion and encourage frequent visitation by family members. In addition, use reality orientation techniques to help reorient the older adult who has been disoriented by a change in environment, surgery, illness, or emotional stress.

Reality orientation is a communication modality used for making a patient aware of time, place, and person. The major purposes of reality orientation include the following:

- Restoring patients' sense of reality
- Improving their level of awareness
- Promoting socialization
- Elevating patients to a maximal level of independent functioning
- Minimizing confusion, disorientation, and physical regression

Environmental changes within a hospital such as the bright lights and lack of windows in intensive care and the noise from nearby roommates often lead to disorientation and confusion. A patient's environment and the nursing personnel are constantly changing in the hospital; and the immediate environment is unstable, making coping and adaptation difficult. Anticipate disorientation and confusion as a consequence when older adults are hospitalized and incorporate reality orientation interventions into their care.

When an older adult is hospitalized or has an acute or chronic illness, the related physical dependence makes it difficult for the person to maintain a positive body image. You are able to have an influence on the older-adult patient's appearance. Help him or her maintain a pleasant appearance and present a socially acceptable image.

CRITICAL THINKING

Synthesis

You apply elements of critical thinking whenever you perform the nursing process with a patient. Consider the scientific knowledge you have learned, your experience, critical thinking attitudes, and standards to ensure an individualized approach to patient care. When caring for an individual patient or family, a variety of factors influence your care. In addition to your knowledge, you and your patients bring unique backgrounds and personal experiences to each care setting. Although you do not always discuss these individual perspectives openly, they do influence your care. Both you and your patients have preexisting ideas as to how to best meet their developmental needs.

Knowledge. Before assessing your patient, review the developmental theories that relate to him or her. In addition, as you work with your patients in attaining an optimal level of health, it is essential that you know the expected physical developmental milestones, psychosocial developmental crises, cognitive development, and health concerns for each age-group.

Another important area of knowledge to consider when caring for a patient's developmental needs is that of cultural awareness (see Chapter 20). Together with the patient, explore the cultural variations in family roles and relationships as they influence an individual's development to have a clear understanding of patient needs.

Experience. If you are a parent or have been involved in teaching children, you are aware that the thinking abilities of individuals of different ages differ, and it is necessary to change your approach to gain their cooperation. In addition, your family, social, and educational experiences with individuals of various ages make it easier for you to determine age-specific appropriate or inappropriate behaviors and health concerns.

Attitudes. Humility is an important attitude for you to apply when collecting data about a patient's developmental history. It is easy to form opinions about patients' developmental needs on the basis of developmental theory and related psychosocial principles. However, as is the case in any nursing situation, do not assume that you know what a patient's needs are without gathering a clear picture of his or her physical and psychosocial health concerns. Often information about a patient's health practices reflects his or her cultural background, which is sometimes very different from yours. Creativity is a valuable critical thinking attitude when you conduct an assessment of an infant or child. Often you incorporate play or other activities into the assessment to better visualize the child's physical developmental capacities.

Standards. Critical thinking standards help to ensure that you are making the right decisions. When developing a plan of care that incorporates growth and development principles and approaches, strive to apply the intellectual standards of relevance and completeness. It is important that you use a developmental approach that fits with the patient's level of maturation. *Referring to the case study, for example, asking Zachary to attempt a motor skill such as coloring a detailed picture or successfully using eating utensils is not within his ability, is irrelevant, and is inappropriate for promoting developmental enrichment.* When selecting a plan of care, you need to be sure that the plan uses psychosocial, cognitive, and physical approaches that complement and strengthen the patient's developmental abilities.

Also use professional standards when providing care to patients of various age-groups. For example, when supporting parents' health promotion practices, it is important to refer to the Centers for Disease Control and Prevention or the AAP standards for adult and childhood immunizations (Box 22-10). These standards help to determine the required immunizations for certain age-groups. Similarly, the American Cancer Society lists a variety of health screenings for adults. Refer to these standards when providing patient education.

BOX 22-10 SYNTHESIS IN PRACTICE

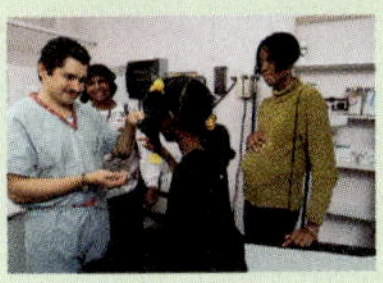

Louis selected Crystal Taylor and her family to follow throughout this semester of his nursing program. As he prepares to begin an assessment, he focuses on 6-year-old Monica, whom Crystal has brought to the clinic for a checkup before beginning school. Louis recalls the physical, psychosocial, and cognitive developmental characteristics that are typical of the older preschool child and prepares to use this information as a basis for his observations. He plans to engage Monica in play activities with dolls to ensure that observations of her physical abilities are relevant and complete. He is also interested in any concerns that Crystal has regarding Monica's health. In preparation for doing anticipatory guidance with Monica and her mother, he reviews types of accidents common among her age-group and appropriate health promotion activities. He is also interested in observing the quality of the interaction between Monica and her mother and assessing how Crystal copes with being a single parent.

As the parent of a 4-year-old, Louis knows the importance of immunizations in keeping children free of many contagious diseases with serious consequences, and he is aware that children are not admitted to school without the completion of certain immunizations. His own child has made him very conscious of the great fear that young children have for bodily harm and the fact that Monica may have difficulty cooperating with an injection. He recalls the approach he has used to help his own son cooperate with and recover from the discomfort of an injection. Louis refers to the standards for immunizations that the American Academy of Pediatrics, the American Academy of Family Physicians, and the Centers for Disease Control and Prevention update twice a year to determine Monica's immunization needs. Louis knows that the key to having a positive effect on the practice of health promotion activities by Crystal Taylor's family members is the development of trust through positive interactions.

Louis' nursing instructors have informed him that he is responsible for encouraging health promotion activities among his patients. He recognizes that *Healthy People 2020: National Objectives for Improving Health* is a guide for choosing health promotion activities for Crystal's family (see Chapter 2). He knows he cannot be judgmental of Ms. Taylor as a single parent and that he needs to assess the resources she has to support health promotion in her family. Understanding that Crystal probably has some definite ideas about parenting and health promotion ensures that Louis is complete in assessing patient needs and offering appropriate suggestions to support Crystal and her family.

NURSING PROCESS

ASSESSMENT

Nursing assessment of individuals across the life span requires you to be familiar with the physiological, cognitive, and psychosocial changes that occur during each stage of development and the health concerns for each age-group. Table 22-4 is an example of a focused assessment for a school-age child such as Crystal's daughter, Monica. A number of assessment tools facilitate concise but comprehensive data collection for individuals of various ages. Observe the interactions between the patient and any family member present during the health history, physical assessment, and developmental assessment. Data gathered provides information regarding the patient's lifestyle, level of functioning, family relationships, health concerns, and health promotion activities.

Throughout life illness and hospitalization are stressful experiences. Many factors affect the ability of individuals to cope such as their level of development, their coping skills, their previous experiences with illness and hospitalization, and the seriousness of the diagnosis. The degree to which the illness interferes with activities of daily living and lifestyle and the availability of a support system also have an impact on how individuals cope. Be sure your assessment demonstrates an awareness of specific patient concerns at various stages of life.

Patient Expectations. During your assessment it is important to determine what patients and/or their families expect from caregivers. At the beginning of a home visit ask, "What do you think is most important for us to accomplish today?" or when preparing to leave, ask, "Have I met your expectations for this visit?" In the outpatient setting ask what expectation(s) the patient and/or family have for the visit. In the hospital setting it is wise to determine if family members want to participate in the care of the patient and how members of the health team can help. As the patient's primary nurse you begin each day with a brief assessment to determine any change in condition and the patient's perceptions of the care received.

NURSING DIAGNOSIS

Your nursing assessment of the patient and, when appropriate, the family reveals clusters of data from the nursing history, physical examination, and developmental assessment. These data include defining characteristics, which you analyze through critical thinking to select the nursing diagnoses that apply. Accuracy is important because the defining characteristics differentiate the nursing diagnosis that applies to the clinical situation. For example, *Parental Role Conflict* and *Impaired Parenting* are two distinctly different nursing diagnoses. Carefully review all information before selecting the

TABLE 22-4 FOCUSED PATIENT ASSESSMENT

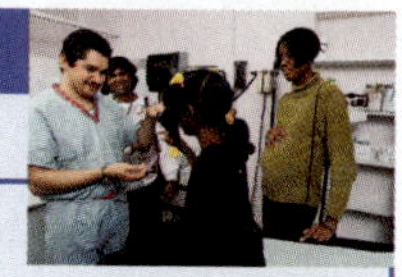

FACTORS TO ASSESS	QUESTIONS	PHYSICAL ASSESSMENT
Home safety	Where do you keep household cleaners, medications?	Observe patient's home environment. Observe child's play area.
	Has your child had any accidents playing at home or other home-based accidents during the last year? If so, please tell me about them.	
	Does your family have a home evacuation plan and a meeting place?	Along with parent, play out a situation when the home needs to be evacuated (e.g., fire) and observe evacuation drill and congregation of family at meeting place.
	Where do you keep your computer? Does your child have unsupervised use of the Internet? Do you have any parental controls that block unsafe sites?	If able, observe child's use of home computer if home visit is made.
Health promotion activities	Does your child have all the immunizations? How current are your immunizations? Where do you keep this information?	Conduct an immunization history.
	Tell me about your child's usual food intake.	Measure height and weight and compare with standards.
Sibling interaction	How do your children get along? Do they play together? Are there any changes in your child's behavior, independence?	Observe child playing and interacting with sibling.

nursing diagnosis that applies to the patient's and family's needs. Defining characteristics for the nursing diagnosis of *Ineffective Sexuality Pattern* include factors such as difficulties or limitations in sexual functioning, expressions of concern about sexuality, and inappropriate verbal and nonverbal sexual behavior. The following are more examples of nursing diagnoses for patients with developmental problems throughout the life span:

- *Risk for Delayed Development*
- *Caregiver Role Strain*
- *Compromised Family Coping*
- *Delayed Growth And Development*
- *Readiness for Enhanced Self-Health Management*
- *Risk for Injury*
- *Impaired Social Interaction*

The second part of the nursing diagnostic statement states suspected causes or related factors for the patient's response to the health problem. Revealed in the assessment data, the related factors allow you to target specific interventions toward the patient's diagnosis. For example, the nursing diagnosis of *Ineffective Sexuality Pattern* might be related to the stress of an impaired relationship with a significant other, fear of pregnancy, or lack of a significant other. The related factors are different, and each requires different nursing strategies.

PLANNING

Goals and Outcomes. The plan addresses each identified nursing diagnosis and appropriate goals, patient outcomes, and interventions for the alleviation or resolution of the diagnosis. The goal for each nursing diagnosis identifies a specific and measurable patient outcome that is realistic and reflects the patient's highest level of wellness and independence in function. An example of a goal is "Patient will acquire healthy physical and mental health behaviors within 3 months." An example of an outcome is "Patient participates in scheduled exercise activities within 6 weeks." See the Care Plan for detailed examples of goals and outcomes.

Collaboration with patients and their families is essential when determining goals and outcomes. Patients' degree of participation in planning depends on their developmental status and physiological and psychological condition. For example, because young children are often unable to articulate feelings and needs, their parents need to become involved in establishing goals. The participation of patients and their families in this process increases their motivation for achievement of identified goals and outcomes (see Care Plan).

Setting Priorities. During the planning phase of the nursing process, formulate a plan of care directed toward the identified nursing diagnoses. Patients and their families often have multiple nursing diagnoses, and these diagnoses often interact with one another (Figure 22-6). Address the nursing diagnoses in order of priority, giving the most pressing problems immediate attention. Base your priorities of nursing diagnoses on such factors as the nature of the problem (e.g., whether it is life threatening, interferes with activities of daily living, or affects level of comfort) and the degree of importance attributed to it by the patient or family.

CARE PLAN

Ineffective Health Maintenance

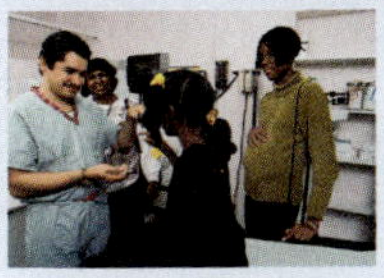

ASSESSMENT

Louis knows that this family has multiple health promotion needs. He wants to ensure that the children are on target with their growth and development and developmental tasks, especially Monica, who is entering school. In addition, he wants to determine any of Crystal's concerns as she enters the last trimester of her pregnancy.

ASSESSMENT ACTIVITIES	FINDINGS/DEFINING CHARACTERISTICS*
Complete height and weight examination on Monica.	Monica is in the 60th percentile for weight and the 75th percentile for height of a 6-year-old.
Using the Denver II (Denver Developmental Screening Test), observe Monica as she completes developmental tasks.	Monica balances on each foot for 6 seconds. Monica defines words such as *house* and *banana.* She can copy a square. Crystal says that she independently brushes her teeth and dresses, prepares her own cereal, and plays board games. Monica enjoyed showing and telling Louis about the pictures she is coloring and often giggles.
Ask Crystal about how the children interact with one another.	Crystal explains that **Monica is very protective of and bossy with her brother** and she always **wants to sit on Crystal's lap when she is holding Zachary.**
Ask about immunizations and safety concerns.	Crystal is **unsure of the status of the children's immunizations and states, "I'm not sure they help."** Crystal states that all medications and cleaning agents are locked in a cabinet in the garage and she has the only key. Crystal states that she is **concerned about Monica riding her bike without the training wheels.** Monica **tries to play with a cigarette lighter.**
Ask Crystal about preparation for the new baby.	Crystal states that she has **done nothing in particular.** Monica **asks how the baby will get out.** Crystal **asks about suggestions to prepare her children for the arrival of the new baby.**
Ask Crystal about her tobacco use.	Crystal states that she **smokes a half-pack of cigarettes daily and would like to quit.**

*__Defining characteristics__ are shown in **bold** type.

NURSING DIAGNOSIS: Ineffective Health Maintenance related to a lack of knowledge regarding age-related health promotion activities.

PLANNING

GOAL	EXPECTED OUTCOMES (NOC)†
	Knowledge: Health Promotion
• Crystal will become more knowledgeable about health concerns related to her children's ages within the next 3 months.	• Crystal will begin to discuss the safety needs of her children with all other family members who participate in their care before her next clinic visit. • Crystal will talk to other family caregivers and Monica about protecting Monica from the danger of playing with fire before the next clinic visit. • Crystal will talk to other family members about the importance of making sure that Monica always wears a safety helmet when riding her bicycle. • Crystal will begin to prepare Monica and Zachary for the birth of a sibling within the next month.
• Crystal will become more knowledgeable about smoking cessation strategies within the next month.	• Crystal will implement smoking cessation activities within the next month. • Crystal will begin to remove/clean smoke residue from residence.

Continued

CARE PLAN—cont'd

Ineffective Health Maintenance

Health Promoting Behavior

- Crystal will keep her children's appointments for well-baby or well-child checkups and have the children receive appropriate immunizations during the next clinic visit.
- Crystal will insist that Monica always wear her bicycle helmet when riding her bicycle.
- Crystal will stop smoking within 1 month.

†Outcomes classification labels from Moorhead S et al., editors: *Nursing outcomes classification (NOC)*, ed 5, St Louis, 2013, Mosby.

INTERVENTIONS (NIC)‡	RATIONALE
Health Education	
• Provide Crystal with literacy-appropriate handouts that describe safety measures according to age of child.	Written information provides both initial information and allows for a quick review of information whenever needed (Kääriäinen et al., 2011).
• Discuss with Crystal measures to decrease Monica's risk for playing with fire.	Adults need to keep potentially hazardous items out of reach of children; a lighter such as a match is an adult tool (Hockenberry and Wilson, 2013).
• Provide Crystal with a list of books about preparing children for a new sibling.	The list helps Crystal find these books in a bookstore or at the local library.
• Enroll Crystal in a child health class.	Class provides alternative learning approach.
• Help Crystal develop a smoking cessation plan.	Feelings of personal control are increased when assistance is available. Research has demonstrated that advice from health care professionals can significantly increase the quit rates of patients and with follow-up the effect is even greater (Zhu et al., 2012).
• Discuss the removal of secondhand smoke residue from the residence.	Secondhand smoke residue contains toxins that build up on surfaces where smoking has occurred. Children coming into contact with items such as carpeting and furniture are exposed to highly toxic particles.
Decision-Making Support	
• Provide Crystal with a pocket schedule for required childhood immunizations. • Provide a copy of her children's actual immunization records.	Immunization education that includes immunization schedules, appointment reminder methods, and the importance for routine immunizations is essential.

‡Intervention classification labels from Bulechek GM et al., editors: *Nursing interventions classification (NIC)*, ed 6, St Louis, 2013, Mosby.

EVALUATION

NURSING ACTIONS	PATIENT RESPONSE/FINDING	ACHIEVEMENT OF OUTCOME
Provide Crystal with handouts describing safety measures.	Crystal continues to lock up medicines and cleaning agents but also locks up any lighters and matches in her own home.	Crystal's home is improved for safety.
	Crystal was able to get grandmother to move medicines and cleaning agents to a locked cabinet.	Crystal is modifying her grandmother's home for safety risks.
	Crystal requested that all family members insist that Monica wear a helmet when riding her bicycle.	Crystal is making sure that there is consistency among caregivers in providing safe care.
Ensure that Crystal receives appointment card for next visit and an up-to-date immunization schedule.	Crystal kept next appointment. Crystal provided child's school with an up-to-date record of immunizations.	This is ongoing, and Crystal needs to maintain appointments for checkups and immunizations.
Ask Crystal if she received list of books and tapes to prepare children for arrival of new sibling.	Children were able to talk about the "almost new baby." "Baby is coming for Halloween."	Preparation for new sibling is progressing but remains ongoing.
Ask Crystal how she is doing in regard to her smoking cessation plan.	Crystal quit smoking 2 weeks after her last clinic visit, although at times she still has strong cravings for a cigarette.	Crystal continues to follow her smoking cessation plan by using resources to help her cope with the tobacco cravings.
Ask Crystal about her progress in remediating her residence from smoke residue.	Crystal has had window treatments, carpets, and upholstery cleaned.	Home environment is remediated from smoke residue.

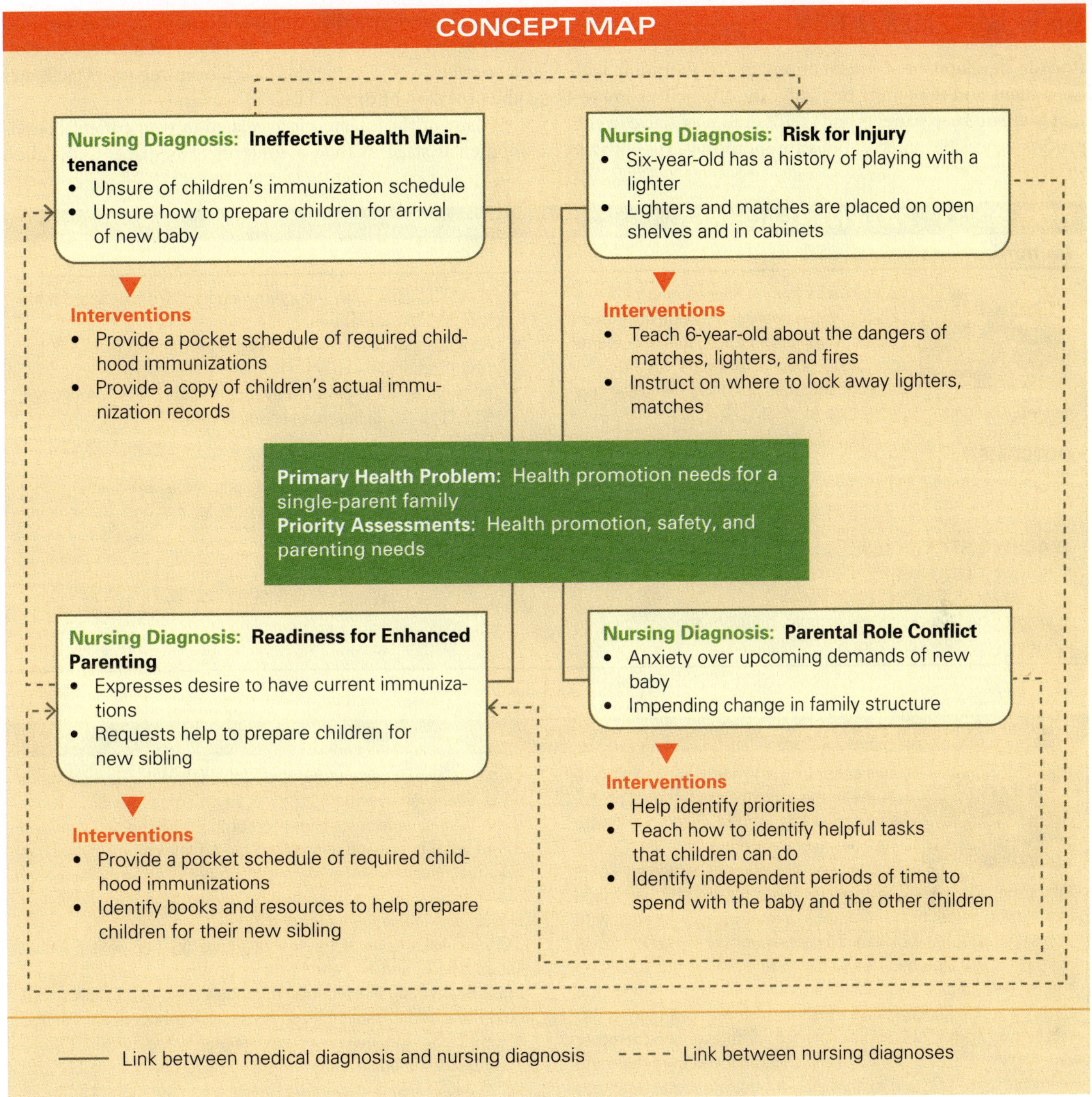

FIGURE 22-6 Concept map.

Maslow's theory of human needs is helpful as a guide when arranging nursing diagnoses in order of priority. A high-priority nursing diagnosis is not always a physiological problem. *For example, Louis has concerns over the fact that Crystal is unsure about the children's immunization schedule; thus he views fear as a priority for care in the initial clinic visit, especially when immunizations are necessary.*

Collaborative Care. Collaboration and consultation with other members of the health care team provide valuable resources for care for patients. Such collaboration identifies community resources to help parents of a child with developmental disabilities or help a family find adult day care activities for an older adult. In addition, these resources often help to provide continuity in discharge planning.

Begin discharge planning at the time of admission to the hospital because the length of stay is usually very brief. Effective planning involves the health care team, the patient, and the patient's support system. Make sure that you individualize nursing interventions for the patient and modify them accordingly for home- or hospital-based nursing care. Make needed referrals to community agencies coincide with the patient's arrival home.

IMPLEMENTATION

Provide developmental interventions in collaboration with the patient and the family or significant others. It is important that you keep patients and their families as active in this process as possible. Interventions are appropriate for both the patient's developmental level and his or her unique needs to support and promote normal developmental processes. Collaboration with a variety of health team members facilitates the provision of optimal care for patients.

Many of the interventions related to your patients' developmental stage include a component of patient education

BOX 22-11 PATIENT TEACHING

Immunizations

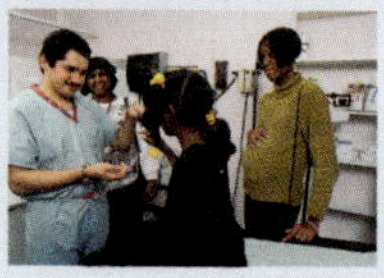

Louis knows that he is developing a therapeutic nurse-patient relationship with Crystal. Crystal told Louis that she wants to provide good health care for her children but she does not understand the suggested immunization schedule for them.

OUTCOME

At the end of the teaching session, Crystal is able to state the routine immunization schedule for her children.

TEACHING STRATEGIES

- Provide Crystal with the American Academy of Pediatrics schedule for routine immunizations.
- Using Crystal's personal calendar, highlight the dates when the immunizations are due.
- Provide Crystal with the phone contact for the appropriate clinic for immunizations.
- Show Crystal how to safely keep a permanent record of the immunizations.
- Tell Crystal to provide only copies of the immunization records to the children's school.

EVALUATION STRATEGIES

- Ask Crystal when the next immunizations are due.
- Review Crystal's personal calendar for a scheduled appointment for immunizations.
- Ask Crystal where she keeps the children's immunization records.

BOX 22-12 EVALUATION

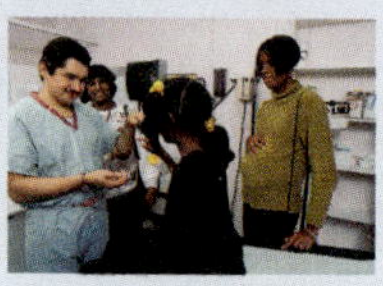

Louis sees Crystal 1 month later when she returns to the clinic for a scheduled prenatal visit. She has left the children at home with their grandmother. While Crystal waits to see her primary caregiver, Louis takes the opportunity to evaluate the progress she has made in meeting expected outcomes. Crystal proudly shares with Louis that she has not had a cigarette in over 2 weeks. Louis asks Crystal if she has been able to find any of the books on the list he had given her about preparing young children for the birth of a sibling. Crystal reports that the librarian helped her locate two books, one appropriate for her toddler and the other one for Monica. She adds that the children loved the books and want her to read them every night at bedtime. Louis asks her if she thinks the content of the books was the kind of information she wanted to share with her children, and she replies that they explained childbirth so simply that it really made it easy for her to talk about the new baby with both children.

During the previous clinic visit Louis had also given Crystal pamphlets that described important safety measures for infants and young children. He asks her if she has discussed any of this information with any family members. Crystal tells him that her mother and grandmother have looked at the pamphlets and told her that it is a big responsibility to watch grandchildren and it is very hard to keep up with them. She also reports that they have all talked to Monica about not playing with candles, matches, or lighters; and Crystal locks up these items as well. She tells Louis about the evening news on television talking about a child who hid in her bedroom playing with a lighter and caught herself and the mattress on fire and almost died. The story seemed to scare Monica, and they talked about what young children should do if anything caught fire around them. She says Monica has often brought up the situation and asked what happened to the little girl on television. Crystal has also discussed with her family members the importance of Monica wearing a safety helmet every time she rides her bicycle.

Crystal asks Louis if he will be there for her next prenatal appointment, and he tells her that he plans to be. He asks if there is anything in particular that she would like to talk about next time, and Crystal replies, "Just tell me how I can manage a new baby and my other two at the same time!" Before leaving Crystal again tells Louis she likes having him be with her at each clinic visit and that he has given her helpful information. Louis is satisfied that they are developing a therapeutic relationship and that he has helped her develop her knowledge base for managing health promotion activities for her children.

DOCUMENTATION NOTE

After the primary caregiver has documented Crystal's prenatal visit, Louis adds the following documentation in Crystal's clinic chart:

"While waiting for primary caregiver, reports she has not smoked in over 2 weeks and has begun to prepare her two children for the birth of a new sibling through reading books and talking about the event. States she has shared safety measures for children, particularly in regard to fire and bicycle safety, with family caregivers. Has requested additional information pertaining to child rearing; will assess further during next visit."

(see Chapter 12). Patient education is an effective tool to teach your patients about health promotion practices, desired behavioral changes, and the need for age-appropriate screening practices. However, patients from different cultures or countries have different languages and beliefs that affect their ability to understand or talk to a health care provider (Singleton and Krause, 2010). Effective patient education considers your patient's health literacy, and it is planned according to the patient's needs (Box 22-11).

Earlier in this chapter nursing strategies for health promotion and acute care were discussed for each age-group. Restorative care measures for older adults were also outlined. Refer to each of the developmental age-groups for specific interventions regarding age-related health concerns. It is important to remember to incorporate a patient's developmental needs into any plan of care, regardless of the nature of the patient's health problem. Whether the patient has serious physiological alterations or merely is seeking health promotion information, developmental care considerations ensure a more individualized and thorough nursing approach.

EVALUATION

Patient Care. During evaluation measure the patient's progress and the degree to which the planned interventions were effective in meeting the expected outcomes and goals of care (see Case Study). Evaluate the patient's behavioral response to the interventions and determine the success or failure of the nursing action. This includes observing family members interact, having the patient describe health promotion habits, or visiting the home to see if the recommendations for making the home safe have been followed. You and the patient and/or family evaluate if the expected outcomes were met in the manner anticipated. When outcomes are not met, a review determines if they were realistic and appropriate or if there is a need to modify an approach. Ongoing evaluation is necessary to ensure that progress toward defined goals is achieved (Box 22-12).

Patient Expectations. Nurse-patient relationships are often long term when you start a developmental plan of care. Always remember to determine if the patient's expectations of care are continuing to be met. Over time the patient's expectations sometimes change. To add to the complexity of evaluation, expectations sometimes vary when family members are involved. Basic to understanding the patient's and family members' expectations is trust. When you and the patient have established trust, it becomes easier to evaluate on a frequent basis how your relationship with the patient is proceeding and whether the patient senses that his or her health care needs are being adequately and professionally addressed.

KEY POINTS

- Growth and development are orderly, predictable, interdependent processes that continue throughout the life span.
- Growth is most rapid during the prenatal and infancy stages and continues to slow until the second skeletal growth spurt announces that puberty is approaching.
- People progress through similar stages of growth and development but at an individual pace and with individual behaviors.
- Theories of growth and development such as those of Freud, Erikson, and Piaget provide nurses with a framework for understanding individual behaviors.
- Physiological, cognitive, and psychosocial development continue across the life span. You must be familiar with normal expectations to determine potential problems and promote normal development.
- Patients need specific immunizations throughout life, not just in childhood. These immunizations help to protect individuals against illness and infections.
- Young adults have few health problems but need to develop positive health habits to avoid problems in middle and late adulthood.
- The health concerns of the middle adult commonly involve hormonal changes, stress-related illnesses, situational stressors, screening for health problems, and adoption of positive health habits.
- The health concerns of older adults are related to chronic illnesses, lifestyle changes, functional ability changes, accidents, and infectious diseases such as the flu.

CLINICAL DECISION-MAKING EXERCISES

As indicated in the case study, Monica, 6 years old, is having a checkup in preparation for beginning school. Louis needs to perform a number of procedures, which Monica may perceive as threatening because of their intrusive or invasive nature (e.g., measure her blood pressure, check her throat, and look in her ears). Louis needs to address a number of other health-related teaching opportunities with Crystal.

1. During the checkup Monica was able to help with the examination by answering questions and reading the eye chart. She also had the chance to play with the equipment and has had her blood pressure and other vital signs taken. During the review of immunizations Louis notes that up to now Monica's vaccinations have been up-to-date, but she needs two shots and is fearful of injections. How should Louis approach this?
2. Crystal is worried about secondhand smoke in her home environment. What information can Louis give her?
3. Crystal is also concerned that her 15-year-old brother may soon become sexually active and wants to be sure that he knows the risks involved and how to protect himself from STIs (including AIDS) and from becoming a father before he is ready for the responsibility. How should Louis advise her?
4. As noted in the case study, Crystal is pregnant with her third child; she is a single parent as well. After Louis does the well-child examination on the children, he is able to

turn his attention to Crystal. What information should he obtain from her?

evolve

Answers to Clinical Decision-Making Exercises can be found on the Evolve website.

QSEN ACTIVITY: TEAMWORK AND COLLABORATION

As indicated in the case study, Crystal needs help from a variety of health care team members. It is important that Louis be able to collaborate and communicate effectively with other members of the health care team to achieve the best possible outcome for Crystal and her family.

How can Louis best communicate, collaborate, and integrate the skills of the other health care team members to help Crystal and her family achieve her health goals?

evolve

Answers to QSEN Activities can be found on the Evolve website.

REVIEW QUESTIONS

1. The nurse discusses a child's weight gain with the mother at a well-child checkup. Which of the following terms most appropriately describes this specific measurement?
   1. Growth
   2. Development
   3. Maturation
   4. Health promotion
2. While assessing a preschooler's growth and developmental status, it is important to remember that: (Select all that apply.)
   1. It is difficult to suggest acceptable alternative behaviors because of the preschooler's egocentricity.
   2. Each preschooler progresses at the same rate of development.
   3. The preschooler is afraid of being harmed and may be fearful of a clinical procedure.
   4. The preschooler does not have sufficient motor skills to assist in self-care activities.
3. During the hospitalization of a toddler, the mother indicates that she is concerned because her child suddenly started sucking her thumb again. Which of the following is the nurse's best response?
   1. Toddlers often suck their thumbs.
   2. Your child may have seen another patient suck her thumb and is imitating the behavior.
   3. It is not unusual for children to regress to earlier behaviors when they are ill.
   4. Your child probably is hungry.
4. You are caring for a 16-year-old boy whose mother brought him to the clinic because he has not been eating or sleeping well for the past 2 weeks. Which of the following safety issues should you be most concerned about with this patient?
   1. A motor vehicle accident caused by the patient falling asleep at the wheel
   2. Susceptibility to a communicable disease because of increased physiological stress
   3. Depression leading to a suicide attempt
   4. An underlying gastrointestinal problem
5. A newly diagnosed 36-year-old patient with type 1 diabetes shares with you that he is frustrated with the time it takes to prepare meals, monitor his exercise and blood sugar, and worry about his insulin coverage. Given his age, which of the following suggestions would be most appropriate?
   1. Provide patient education materials that are easy to read
   2. Refer this patient to a diabetes support group
   3. Suggest that the patient make an appointment with a registered dietitian
   4. Refer the patient to his endocrinologist
6. An 82-year-old patient becomes very confused and combative after receiving soap-suds enemas before a procedure. Which of the following is the most likely diagnosis based on the information available?
   1. Delirium
   2. Dementia
   3. Depression
   4. Alzheimer's disease
7. Which of the following are forms of dementia? (Select all that apply.)
   1. Alzheimer's disease
   2. Ischemic vascular dementia (IVD)
   3. Deep vein thrombosis
   4. Depression
8. (Fill in the blank.) You are caring for an 84-year-old patient who was admitted to the hospital with an acute urinary tract infection. This patient is confused and disoriented. You explain to him or her where he or she is and what day it is. This communication modality is known as ____________________.
9. You are visiting a patient with diabetes for follow-up wound care in his or her home. What is the best opening statement for you to use as you prepare to give care?
   1. "How long has it been since your last dressing change?"
   2. "What do you think is the most important thing for us to accomplish?"
   3. "Do you have your blood sugar under control?"
   4. "Do you need additional supplies to monitor your blood sugar?"
10. The mother of your 14-year old patient is concerned because she believes her daughter spends too much time worrying about what her friends think. You can help this mother by explaining that this is normal

behavior and her daughter is which stage of psychosocial development?
1. Autonomy vs. Shame and Doubt
2. Initiative vs. Guilt
3. Industry vs. Inferiority
4. Identity vs. Role Confusion

evolve

Rationales for Review Questions can be found on the Evolve website.

1. 1; **2.** 1, 3; **3.** 3; **4.** 3; **5.** 2; **6.** 1; **7.** 1, 2; **8.** Reality orientation; **9.** 2; **10.** 4.

REFERENCES

Alea N, et al: The content of older adults' autobiographical memories predicts the beneficial outcomes of reminiscence group participation, *J Adult Dev* 17(3):135, 2010.

Alzheimer's Association: *Alzheimer's disease symptoms*, Chicago, 2012, The Association, http://www.alz.org/alzheimers_disease_symptoms_of_alzheimers.asp. Accessed May 2013.

American Academy of Pediatrics (AAP): *SIDS and other sleep-related infant deaths: expansion of recommendations for a safe infant sleeping environment*, 2011, www.pediatrics.org/cgi/doi/10.1542/peds.2011-2284. Accessed May 2013.

American Academy of Pediatrics (AAP): Policy statement: breastfeeding and the use of human milk, *Pediatrics* 129(3):e827–e841, 2012. DOI:10.1542/peds.2011-3552. Accessed May 2013.

Burns CE, et al: Pediatric primary care [4] (VitalSource Bookshelf), 2009, http://pageburstls.elsevier.com/books/978-1-4160-4087-3/id/B9781416040873500119_para123. Accessed May 2013.

CDC Vital Signs: *Unintentional injury deaths among persons aged 0-19 years—United States, 2000-2009*, 2012, http://www.cdc.gov/mmwr/preview/mmwrhtml/mm61e0416a1.htm?s_cid=mm61e0416a1_w#tab1. Accessed May 2013.

CDC Vaccine Safety: *Vaccine safety information for parents*, 2011, http://www.cdc.gov/vaccinesafety/populations/parents.html. Accessed May 2013.

Conway-Phillips R, Millon-Underwood S: Breast screening behaviors of African-American women: a comprehensive review, analysis, and critique of nursing research, *Assoc Black Nurs Faculty J* 20(4):97, 2009.

Ebersole P, et al: *Toward healthy aging: human needs and nursing response*, ed 8, St Louis, 2012, Mosby.

Erikson E: *Childhood and society*, New York, 1963, WW Norton.

Erikson E: *The lifecycle completed*, New York, 1997, WW Norton.

He W, Muenchrath MN, US Census Bureau: *American Community Survey Reports, ACS-17, 90+ in the United States: 2006-2008*, Washington, DC, 2011, US Government Printing Office.

Hockenberry M, Wilson D: *Wong's essentials of pediatric nursing*, ed 9, St Louis, 2013, Mosby.

Kääriäinen M, et al: Improving the quality of rheumatoid arthritis patients' education using written information, *Musculoskeletal Care* 9(1):19, 2011.

Kohlberg L: Development of moral character and moral ideology. In Hoffman ML, Hoffman LNW, editors: *Review of child development research* (vol 1), New York, 1964, Russell Sage Foundation.

Linton AD, et al: *Matteson & McConnell's gerontological nursing: concepts and practice*, ed 3, Philadelphia, 2007, Saunders.

Linton AD, et al: *Introduction to medical-surgical nursing*, ed 5, St Louis, 2012, Saunders.

Maslow AH: *Motivation and personality*, ed 3, Upper Saddle River, NJ, 1970, Prentice Hall.

MetLife Mature Market Institute: *The MetLife study of caregiving costs to working caregivers: double jeopardy to baby boomers caring for their parents*, 2011, http://www.caregiving.org/wp-content/uploads/2011/06/mmi-caregiving-costs-working-caregivers.pdf. Accessed May 2013.

National High Blood Pressure Education Program; National Heart, Lung, and Blood Institute; National Institutes of Health: *The seventh report of the Joint National Commission on detection, evaluation, and treatment of high blood pressure*, 2012, http://www.nhlbi.nih.gov/about/nhbpep/, Accessed May 2013.

National Institutes of Health (NIH): *Senior health: depression*, http://nihseniorhealth.gov/depression/aboutdepression/01.html, 2013. Accessed September 2013.

National Institutes of Mental Health: *Suicide in the US: statistics and prevention*, http://www.nimh.nih.gov/health/publications/suicide-in-the-us-statistics-and-prevention/index.shtml#children, 2010. Accessed May 2013.

Phillips J, Cohen MZ: The meaning of breast cancer risk for African-American women, *J Nurs Scholarship* 43(3):239, 2011. DOI 10.1111/j.1547-5069.2011.01399.x.

Pope ND, et al: How women in late midlife become caregivers, *J Women Aging* 24:242–261, 2012. DOI:10.1080/08952841.2012.639676.

Singleton K, Krause EMS: Understanding cultural and linguistic barriers to health literacy, *KY Nurse* 58(4):4, 2010.

US Census Bureau: *The next four decades: the older population in the United States: 2010 to 2050*, 2010, http://www.aoa.gov/AoARoot/Aging_Statistics/future_growth/DOCS/p25-1138.pdf. Accessed May 2013.

US Department of Health and Human Services (USDHHS): *Healthy People 2020*, 2013, http://www.healthypeople.gov/2020/topicsobjectives2020/default.aspx. Accessed December 7, 2013.

Wang Y, et al: Reconciling work and family caregiving among members of adult-child family caregivers of older people with dementia: effects on role strain and depressive symptoms, *J Adv Nurs* 67(4):829, 2010. DOI:10.1111/j.1365-2648.2010.05505.x.

Zhu S-H, et al: Interventions to increase smoking cessation at the population level: how much progress has been made in the last two decades? *Tobacco Control* 21:110–118, 2012. DOI:10.1136/tobaccocontrol-2011-050371.

CHAPTER

23

Self-Concept and Sexuality

evolve WEBSITE

http://evolve.elsevier.com/Potter/essentials

- Crossword Puzzle
- Audio Glossary

OBJECTIVES

- Discuss factors that influence the following components of self-concept: identity, body image, and role performance.
- Identify stressors that affect self-concept, self-esteem, and sexuality.
- Describe the components of self-concept as each relates to Erikson's developmental stages.
- Discuss ways in which your self-concept and nursing actions affect your patient's self-concept and self-esteem.
- Discuss your role in maintaining or enhancing a patient's sexual health.
- Apply the nursing process to promote a patient's self-concept and sexual health.

KEY TERMS

body image, p. 598
identity, p. 598
role performance, p. 599
self-concept, p. 596
self-esteem, p. 599
sexual dysfunction, p. 601
sexual orientation, p. 601
sexuality, p. 596
sexually transmitted infection, p. 602

Self-concept and sexuality include a complex mixture of unconscious and conscious thoughts, attitudes, and perceptions. As a nurse you care for patients who face a variety of health problems that threaten their self-esteem and sexuality. For example, patients who experience a loss of body function or a change in their physical appearance are at risk for experiencing a change in self-concept and sexuality. Help your patients adjust to alterations in self-concept and sexuality to promote successful coping.

SCIENTIFIC KNOWLEDGE BASE

Self-concept is your view of who you are. It directly affects your self-esteem and how you feel about yourself. What you think and how you feel about yourself affect the way in which you care for yourself physically and emotionally. Self-concept also influences the way in which you care for others. You need to have knowledge of factors that affect self-concept and self-esteem. Be aware of differences in self-concept and self-esteem across age, gender, ethnicity, socioeconomic status, and other cultural variables to individualize your approach to patient care (see Chapter 20).

Sexuality is a broad term that refers to all aspects of being sexual. It is a part of who a person is and is important for overall health. It is possible for people to be sexually healthy in numerous ways. Sex is considered a basic physiological need, and sexual intimacy throughout the life span is equally important for sexual health. Healthy sexuality enables a person to develop and maintain their fullest potential. Sexuality includes a person's thoughts and feelings about the body, a sense of femaleness or maleness, romantic and erotic attachments toward others, and attitudes toward sexual

CASE STUDY *Paul Taylor*

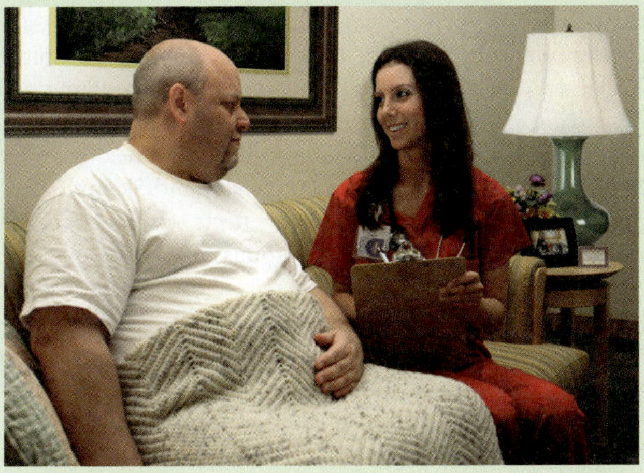

Paul Taylor, a 58-year-old man, suffered a stroke. He experienced the stroke suddenly and unexpectedly while working at his job as a construction manager. The stroke was unexpected and sudden. He did not know that he had hypertension because he had not been getting annual checkups. Mr. Taylor woke up in the hospital bed to find that he could not move his right hand. He was not able to care for himself or to turn himself for days. With daily rehabilitation activities, he is finally able to transfer from his bed into a chair. Mr. Taylor wonders what lies ahead. His body image has dramatically changed from that of a man of strength to that of a helpless individual. Mr. Taylor worries about his family and what will happen. He and his wife, Meredith, are terrified. Although Mrs. Taylor works, their savings are minimal. The family is worried they will not have enough money for their children's education without both incomes. Mr. Taylor's role as primary breadwinner for the family will be drastically changed if his condition does not improve.

Mr. Taylor's self-esteem lessens as his recovery and rehabilitation move slowly. His self-concept has changed from that of a strong laborer, one who did his own plumbing and car repairs, to a man who must rely on others. Although he is now at home in the rehabilitation process, Mr. Taylor is not able to perform tasks for the family and waits until his wife and son get home to help him with things that require strength. Moreover, because of the sexual side effects of the antihypertensive medication he is taking, there is a lack of intimacy with his wife, and this is affecting their relationship. Mr. Taylor's adaptation capabilities are stretched to the maximum. His identity is not clear to him anymore. He has no clear role within the family, his body image has been drastically altered, his sexual health has suffered, and his self-esteem has never been lower.

Maria Kendal is a 27-year-old nursing student assigned to care for Mr. Taylor. She recognizes that changes in health status often result in stressors that affect a person's self-concept and sexuality. Such stressors influence a person's ability to interact with others and function effectively. Maria's knowledge of self-concept and sexuality helps to identify stressors that affect Mr. Taylor and promote effective planning to support his growth and adaptation to change.

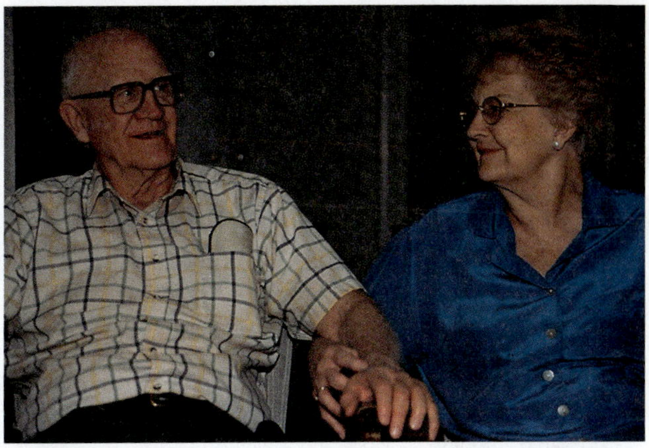

FIGURE 23-1 Sexuality is important across the life span.

functioning. Our sexual health is based on our ability to form healthy relationships with others (Figure 23-1).

NURSING KNOWLEDGE BASE

To provide evidence-based care to patients, incorporate professional nursing knowledge developed from the humanities and sciences, nursing research, and clinical practice. A broad knowledge base allows you to have a holistic view of patients, thus promoting quality patient care that best meets the self-concept and sexual health needs of each patient and family.

Development of Self-Concept

The development of self-concept is a complex process that begins at birth and continues throughout life and involves many factors. Erikson's psychosocial theory of development (1963) is helpful in understanding key tasks that individuals face at various stages of development. Each stage builds on the tasks of the previous stage. Completing each developmental stage successfully leads to a solid sense of self.

You use Erikson's theory to identify the stage of psychosocial development of a patient based first on his or her biological age and then adjusted based on any significant life events. You also assess the patient's psychosocial development stage by determining how the patient is handling the developmental tasks of that stage. For example, an adolescent with a strong sense of identity demonstrates more self-assurance and confidence than an adolescent who lacks a sense of identity (Rhee and Johnson, 2011). Awareness of lifelong developmental tasks (Box 23-1) allows you to select individualized nursing actions tailored to your patient's needs.

Components and Interrelated Terms of Self-Concept

A positive self-concept gives a sense of meaning and wholeness to a person. Nurses care for patients who experience threats to the various components of self-concept, including identity, body image, role performance, and self-esteem. Sexuality also has an effect on self-concept. Likewise, identity,

BOX 23-1 ERIKSON'S DEVELOPMENTAL TASKS AND IMPACT ON SELF-CONCEPT AND SEXUALITY

TRUST VS. MISTRUST (BIRTH TO 1 YEAR)
- Develops trust from consistency in caregiving and nurturing interactions with caregivers
- Distinguishes self from environment

AUTONOMY VS. SHAME AND DOUBT (1 TO 3 YEARS)
- Begins to communicate likes and dislikes
- Increasingly independent in thoughts and actions
- Appreciates body appearance and function (including dressing, feeding, talking, and walking)

INITIATIVE VS. GUILT (3 TO 6 YEARS)
- Takes initiative
- Identifies with a gender
- Enhances self-awareness
- Increases language skills, including identification of feelings

INDUSTRY VS. INFERIORITY (6 TO 12 YEARS)
- Incorporates feedback from peers and teachers
- Increases self-esteem with new skill mastery (e.g., reading, math, sports, music)
- Sexual identity strengthens
- Aware of strengths and limitations

IDENTITY VS. ROLE CONFUSION (12 TO 20 YEARS)
- Accepts body changes/maturation
- Examines attitudes, values, and beliefs; establishes goals for the future
- Feels positive about expanded sense of self

INTIMACY VS. ISOLATION (MID-20s TO MID-40s)
- Has intimate relationships with family and significant others
- Has stable, positive feelings about self
- Experiences successful role transitions and increased responsibilities

GENERATIVITY VS. SELF-ABSORPTION (MID-40s TO MID-60s)
- Able to accept changes in appearance and physical endurance
- Reassesses life goals
- Shows contentment with aging

EGO INTEGRITY VS. DESPAIR (LATE 60s TO DEATH)
- Feels positive about one's life and its meaning
- Interested in providing a legacy for the next generation

body image, role performance, and self-esteem affect sexual health. Although overlap exists among concepts, this chapter presents each one separately.

Identity involves the sense of individuality and being distinct and separate from others. Being "oneself" or living a life that is genuine and authentic is the basis of true identity. The achievement of identity is necessary for intimate relationships because identity is expressed in relationships with others. Sexuality is a part of your identity. Gender identity is a person's private view of maleness or femaleness, and gender role is the feminine or masculine behavior exhibited. Racial or cultural identity develops from identifying and socializing within an established group and through incorporating the responses of individuals who do not belong to that group into one's self-concept (Anderson and Skemp, 2012). The opinion or approval of others affects self-esteem differently among racial and cultural groups.

Body image involves attitudes related to the perception of the body, including physical appearance, femininity and masculinity, youthfulness, health, and strength. These views are not always the same as the person's actual physical structure or appearance and are ever changing. When a change in health status occurs, as in the case of Mr. Taylor, an individual sometimes has exaggerated disturbances in body image. The way others view a person's body and the feedback offered are also influential. For example, a controlling, violent husband tells his wife that she is ugly and that no one else would want her. Over the years of marriage she incorporates this criticism into her self-concept.

Cultural and societal attitudes and values influence body image and sexuality. For example, when compared with European American youths, one study showed that some Hispanic/Latino youths are more accepting of individuals who are slightly overweight because this body type represents being healthy and prosperous in this culture (Ceballos and Czyzewska, 2010). Race, gender, and the social environment (family, peers, media) also affect an adolescent's body image (Holmqvist and Frisen, 2010; Martin et al., 2009). Studies suggest that body dissatisfaction is more common in wealthier countries where people have adapted a western lifestyle, which embraces a thin body as ideal (Holmqvist and Frisen, 2010).

Body art such as tattoos and piercings is increasingly common among all ages of individuals and has become a popular way to express individuality, which is part of one's body image. No federal regulation of piercing and tattoo practices exists in the United States, and regulations vary by state (CDC, 2010; Nelius et al., 2011). Complications from piercings occur more frequently than from tattoos; the most common complication of both is localized site infection (Holbrook et al., 2012; Urdang et al., 2011). Using sterile technique during the initial procedure and basic hygienic practices following the procedure minimizes infection.

Tattoos and body piercings may interfere with diagnostic imaging, and jewelry may have to be removed to safely perform some procedures such as those involving electrocautery (Durkin, 2012; Holbrook et al., 2012). Nurses should be familiar with the mechanics of basic types of jewelry in case a patient is unable to help with removal. A plastic piercing retainer can be inserted to keep the piercing tract open because some sites may occlude quickly. A 14- or 16-gauge intravenous catheter without the needle can be used as a spacer if a piercing removal kit is not available (Nelius et al., 2011). Acknowledging the importance of the piercing shows acceptance and caring by the nurse and may enhance the therapeutic relationship (Young et al., 2010). Whenever possible, collaborative decision making about jewelry removal and education about site care should occur.

Body image depends only partly on the reality of the body. When physical changes occur, individuals may or may not incorporate these changes into their body image. For example, a patient who experiences significant weight loss does not perceive herself as thin and tells you that there is still a "fat person" inside. Body image issues are often associated with negative self-concept and self-esteem. Most men and women experience some degree of body dissatisfaction, which often affects body image and overall self-concept. As a nurse you are in an ideal position to influence a patient's body image.

Normal developmental changes such as puberty and aging have a more obvious effect on body image than on other aspects of self-concept. Hormonal changes during puberty and menopause in later adulthood influence body image. The development of secondary sex characteristics and changes in body fat distribution have a tremendous impact on the self-concept of an adolescent. Female adolescents struggle more with body-image issues than do their male counterparts (Anderson and Skemp, 2012; Ceballos and Czyzewska, 2010). Changes associated with aging (e.g., wrinkles; graying hair; and decrease in visual acuity, hearing, and mobility) affect body image in older adults.

As a person grows and develops, so does his or her sexuality. Each stage of development brings changes in sexual functioning, sexual focus, and sexual relationships. Knowledge of sexual development and changes throughout the life span is essential for a nurse. The adult has achieved physical maturation but is continuing to explore and define emotional maturation in relationships. Even into adulthood people continue to struggle with questions about who they are, how they want to present ourselves, and what type of partners they find most attractive. As a nurse, it helps to have a clear sense of your own sexual orientation because it influences your ability to form open relationships, which is needed to support patients' sexual health. You provide care to individuals whose sexual orientation is heterosexual (attracted to different-sex partners), lesbian or gay (same-sex partners), bisexual (both male and female partners), or transgender (people whose gender identity or expression is different from their sex at birth). You also care for patients who are involved in intimate relationships with several partners and for patients whose sexual relationships occur outside of marriage. You may not learn a great deal about a patient's sexual preferences. However, as a caregiver you learn to accept a person's sexual orientation and help the individual understand the implications that his or her health condition has on maintaining healthy sexual relationships.

Role performance is the way in which a person views his or her ability to carry out significant roles. Common roles include mother or father, wife or husband, daughter or son, sister or brother, employee or employer, and nurse or patient. For example, stating, "I am a good father" or "I am a caring and competent nurse" reflects a positive self-concept and self-esteem. Each role involves meeting certain expectations. In the case of Mr. Taylor, his role as a father and employee requires him to earn a salary as a construction manager and to support his wife and children. Fulfillment of these expectations leads to an enhanced sense of self. Difficulty or failure to meet role expectations leads to decreased self-esteem or altered self-concept.

Self-esteem is an individual's overall sense of personal worth or value. It is positive when one feels capable, worthwhile, and competent (Erol and Orth, 2011). Once established, basic feelings about the self tend to be constant, even though sometimes a little fluctuation exits. A situational crisis such as a hospitalization often temporarily affects one's self-esteem.

Self-evaluation is an ongoing mental process. A positive sense of self-worth, or self-esteem, is an important factor in determining how an individual functions in the world. A person's ability to contribute in a meaningful way to society often affects self-concept and self-esteem. Some individuals who are chronically ill feel a sense of worthlessness. Your acceptance of a patient as an individual with worth and dignity helps to maintain and improve the patient's self-esteem.

Stressors Affecting Self-Concept and Sexuality

A self-concept stressor is any real or perceived change that threatens identity, body image, or role performance (Figure 23-2). An individual's perception of the stressor is the most important factor in determining his or her response. For example, Mr. Taylor's stroke caused a deficit that makes him believe he will no longer be able to be the active construction site manager he has prided himself as being. This perception of what the stroke will mean to his lifestyle can lead to depression. However, another man may view his stroke as a message to slow down and enjoy his life.

Any change in health is a stressor that potentially affects self-concept. A physical change in the body leads to an altered body image, affecting identity and self-esteem. Chronic illnesses often alter role performance, which frequently alters a person's identity and self-esteem. Living with a chronic illness requires a person to cope with a lost sense of self while a new self emerges. After adjustment to the loss, the person has to develop a new self-concept. For example, the loss of a partner sometimes leads to a loss of identity and a lower self-esteem.

A crisis occurs when a person cannot cope with stressors with usual methods of problem solving and adaptation. Any crisis potentially threatens self-concept and self-esteem. Some crises such as Paul Taylor's in the case study, directly affect all components of self-concept. If people are unable to adapt to such stressors, their health is at risk, and illness often results.

Identity Stressors. Stressors throughout life affect an individual's identity; but identity is particularly vulnerable during adolescence, which is a time of great change. Adolescents are trying to adjust to the physical, emotional, and

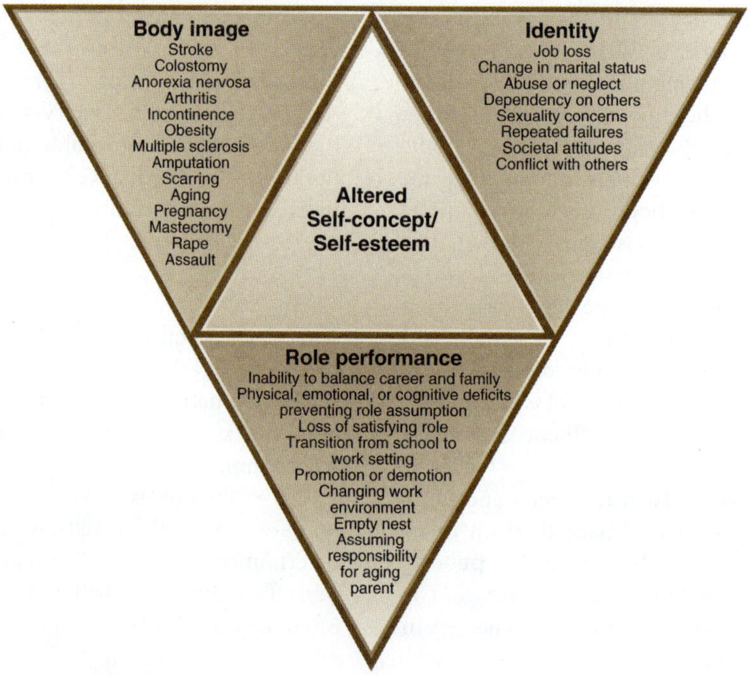

FIGURE 23-2 Common stressors that influence self-concept.

mental changes of increasing maturity, which results in insecurity and anxiety. For example, an adolescent who wants to be identified as part of the popular crowd at school develops a poor self-concept if not included in that group. Family and cultural factors sometimes influence negative health practices such as cigarette smoking. Promoting a change in a patient's self-concept demands an evidence-based practice approach supported by the entire health care team.

An adult generally has a stable identity and thus a more developed self-concept than an adolescent. Once a person has established his or her identity, the adult is better able to handle stressors such as marriage, divorce, menopause, aging, and retirement. Retirement for some means the loss of an important means of achievement. Some people at retirement begin to reevaluate their identities and accomplishments. More and more older people are working past the traditional retirement age or change careers following retirement. Some do so because of a financial need, whereas others have a desire to remain involved and productive (Quell, 2012). Sometimes loss of a significant other leads a person to reexamine aspects of his or her identity.

Body Image Stressors. Changes in the appearance or function of a body part require an adjustment in body image. An individual's perception of the change and the relative importance placed on body image in the individual's self-concept affect the significance of the loss or change. For example, if a woman considers her breasts key to her femininity, a mastectomy negatively affects her body image. Changes in the appearance of the body such as an amputation, facial disfigurement, or burns are obvious stressors affecting body image. Surgical procedures, potentially undetected by others, have a significant impact on the individual. Elective changes such as breast augmentation or reduction also affect body image. Chronic illnesses such as heart and lung disease involve a change in function (less tolerant of exercise), in which the body no longer performs at an optimal level. Physical changes associated with aging or treatment for medical conditions negatively affect body image as well. In addition, the effects of pregnancy, significant weight gain or loss, medication management of an illness, and radiation therapy all change body image. Negative body image sometimes leads to adverse health outcomes.

Many people associate success with a specific body part or function. For example, some athletes consider their bodies and physical activities to be the focus of personal success. Their adaptation and rehabilitation is often affected if an injury prevents future participation in athletics. Body image changes require reevaluation of long-accepted self-perceptions and alterations in lifestyle.

Role Performance Stressors. Throughout life a person undergoes many role changes. Normal changes associated with maturation result in changes in role performance. For example, when a couple has a child, both the male and female need to adjust to new parenting roles and changes in their personal relationship. When a middle-age woman with young children assumes responsibility for the care of her older parents, she adapts to the increased demands of this new role. Acute and chronic illnesses alter a person's ability to carry out various roles, which affects self-esteem and identity.

All people must adapt to changes that occur with aging. Role performance changes associated with retirement differ for men and women. Many women have adjusted to several different roles throughout their lifetime and are more likely than men to have developed friendships that are not work related. Adjusting to changes in role performance has an impact on the marital relationship. Changes in role performance following the loss of a spouse or partner also affect self-concept. A widow who has never paid bills or one who needs to learn to cook needs help to change roles.

Self-Esteem Stressors. Individuals with high self-esteem are generally better able to cope with demands and stressors than those with low self-esteem. Low self-worth contributes to feeling unfulfilled and misunderstood and results in depression and anxiety. Illness, surgery, or accidents that change life patterns also influence feelings of self-worth. The more that chronic illness such as diabetes, arthritis, and heart disease interferes with the ability to engage in activities contributing to feelings of worth or success, the more they affect self-esteem.

Self-esteem stressors vary with developmental stages. A child's self-worth lessens if the child believes that he is unable to meet his parents' expectations or if his parents harshly criticize or inconsistently discipline him. The self-esteem of an adolescent is also vulnerable because he or she directs so much energy to worrying about appearance, searching for identity, and being overly concerned about what others think. A 14-year study examining the development of self-esteem in individuals ages 14 to 30 years found that self-esteem increases steadily during adolescence and into young adulthood (Erol and Orth, 2011). No differences were found between male and female adolescents, but by age 30 blacks and Hispanics had higher self-esteem than whites. Stressors affecting the self-esteem of an adult include failures at work and in relationships. Box 23-2 discusses ways to promote self-esteem in older adults.

Sexuality Stressors. As a nurse you work with patients who are making decisions or dealing with issues related to sexuality on a regular basis. For example, people of all ages face reproductive health issues, including contraception, infertility, sexual dysfunction, and sexual satisfaction. Understanding some of the decisions and issues that patients face increases your effectiveness in helping them reach their maximum level of sexual health.

Lesbian, gay, bisexual, or transgender (LGBT) individuals have unique stressors related to their sexual orientation (Doty et al., 2010; Williamson, 2010). Peer, family, and social support is often lacking. This places individuals in this population at high risk for health issues such as sexually transmitted infections, human immunodeficiency virus (HIV), depression, and victimization (Williamson, 2010). Nurses are in a unique position to support a patient and provide education and resources based on his or her individual needs.

Alterations in sexual health occur from a variety of situations such as illness, infertility, trauma, and abuse. Sexual dysfunction involves problems with desire, arousal, or orgasm. Erectile dysfunction is a common problem among older men. It is generally related to chronic diseases such as diabetes, kidney disease, alcohol dependence, depression, neurological disorders, vascular insufficiency, and diseases of the prostate (Touhy and Jett, 2010). In addition, side effects of medications or medical conditions also contribute to sexual dysfunction. Examples of common medications that can cause sexual dysfunction include statins, antihypertensives, antidepressants, antipsychotics, and benzodiazepenes. The causes of sexual dysfunction are physiological or psychological. Sometimes the cause of a dysfunction cannot be identified or is a result of a combination of several factors.

Because sexual dysfunction sometimes results from the use of medications, it is important to include a discussion of sexual side effects in patient teaching. Your patient is more likely to adhere to a treatment plan if you discuss side effects of medications that alter sexual function with both partners and the patient is able to make an informed decision. Our current state of health greatly influences sexual response (from desire to arousal to orgasm). The availability of sexual performance–enhancing medication such as sildenafil (Viagra) and tadalafil (Cialis) has changed the lives of many couples. These medications treat erectile dysfunction but are contraindicated in men with coronary artery disease or those taking common cardiac drugs.

Changing physical appearance and concerns about physical attractiveness affects sexual functioning. The loss of sexual

BOX 23-2 CARE OF THE OLDER ADULT

Promoting Self-Concept and Self-Esteem

Gender and ethnicity affect self-esteem across the lifespan (Orth et al., 2010). Self-esteem rises steadily across the life span, peaks at around age 60, and then begins to decline. Women demonstrate lower self-esteem than men as young adults, but the two equalize by old age. Whites and blacks also have higher self-esteem in young and middle adulthood, but self-esteem in blacks declined more sharply than whites in older age. In some individuals aging promotes improved coping strategies that protect against the declining feelings of self-esteem, despite all the physical and emotional changes associated with aging. Nursing interventions aimed at promoting resiliency and enhancing self-concept and self-esteem in older adults are essential.

- Clarify what the life changes mean and the impact on self-concept for the older adult (Resnick, 2011; Troutman, 2012).
- Be alert to preoccupation with physical complaints. Assess complaints thoroughly; if no physical explanation exists, encourage the older adult to verbalize needs (fear, insecurity, loneliness) in a nonphysical way (Meiner, 2011; Troutman, 2012).
- Identify positive and negative coping mechanisms. Support and teach effective strategies (Troutman, 2012).
- Encourage reminiscence through the use of storytelling and review of old photographs (Touhy and Jett, 2010).
- Communicate that the older adult is worthwhile by actively listening to and accepting the person's feelings, being respectful, and praising healthy behaviors (Touhy and Jett, 2010).
- Allow additional time to complete tasks. Reinforce the older adult's efforts at independence (Touhy and Jett, 2010).

activity and the absence of a self-concept that includes being a sexual person are not inevitable aspects of aging. Some older people face health concerns and societal attitudes that make it difficult for them to continue sexual activity. Although declining physical abilities sometimes make sex as they knew it painful or impossible, with intervention older adults are able to experiment with and learn alternative ways of sexual expression.

Hormonally stimulated changes brought on by developmental maturation are also stressors that affect sexuality across the life span. Menarche, the onset of menstrual cycle in girls, is occurring at an earlier age in the United States; and some adolescent girls are unaware that it is normal to grow pubic, underarm, and body hair and deposit more fat on their hips and breasts, all of which also affect body image (Deardorff et al., 2012). Early maturation in females is linked to negative health outcomes throughout the life span such as obesity and cardiovascular disease.

As boys approach puberty, physical changes include nocturnal emissions and ejaculation, increasing sexual desire, and increased hygiene needs. Patient teaching needs to include instruction on breast and testicular self-examinations and prevention of **sexually transmitted infections (STIs),** which are spread through oral, anal, or vaginal activity. The use of latex condoms reduces the risk of STIs (Box 23-3).

Older women experiencing menopause (i.e., the cessation of menstrual periods) experience changes in vaginal lubrication and sexual interest. Most menopausal woman recognize the importance of maintaining an active sex life; but many report reduced sex drive, decreased sexual interest, and mood changes that may require intervention by a health care provider (Sobecki et al., 2012).

Approximately 20 million people in the United States are infected with genital human papillomavirus (HPV), and 50% of these infections occur in adolescents and young adults ages 15 to 24 (CDC, 2013b). The Gardasil vaccine is recommended for males and females in early adolescence to decrease the risk for cancers associated with HPV, including genital warts and cancers of the cervix, vagina, vulva, and anus (CDC, 2013c). Cervarix is prescribed only for females. The greatest benefit occurs when individuals receive the vaccines before sexual activity or exposure to the virus.

Sexual abuse, assault, and rape are also stressors that affect self-concept. Be alert to clues that suggest abuse (Box 23-4). In addition, observe the interaction between the patient and partner for additional clues. Controlling behaviors such as speaking for the person or refusing to leave him or her alone with a caregiver are suggestive of emotional and perhaps physical or sexual abuse. If you suspect abuse, interview the patient privately. A patient will probably not admit to problems of abuse with the abuser present. Some of the following questions are useful: "Are you in a relationship in which someone is hurting you?" or "Have you ever been forced to have sex when you didn't want to?" When you recognize or report abuse, mobilize treatment immediately for the victim and the family. The most important factor to consider is the safety of the suspected victim. Often all family members require therapy to promote healthy interactions and relationships.

BOX 23-3 EVIDENCE-BASED PRACTICE

PICO Question: Do youths in monogamous sexual relationships use condoms more consistently than youths involved with multiple sex partners?

SUMMARY OF EVIDENCE

Adolescents have one of the highest rates of sexually transmitted infections (STIs) and unplanned pregnancy in the United States; using latex condoms reduces the risk for both of these occurrences (CDC, 2013a). Condom use by sexually active youths increased between 1990 and 2003, but there has been no significant increase in this practice during the last decade (CDC, 2012).

The stability of the relationship between partners affects consistency of condom use in youths (Manning et al., 2012). Youths involved in relationships with less commitment, lower levels of communication and disclosure about sexual habits, and more conflict exhibit more consistent condom use than those in more stable, sexually exclusive relationships. Condom use also occurs less consistently in monogamous relationships of longer duration, when partners are together for 6 months or longer (Bearinger et al., 2011).

APPLICATION TO NURSING PRACTICE

- Help the adolescent see how risky sexual behavior could interfere with his or her personal goals in relation to education, sports, or careers (Manning et al., 2012).
- When completing a sexual history, explore the duration and quality of the relationship(s) of the adolescent and his or her partner(s) (Bearinger et al., 2011).
- Use strategies such as role play or scenarios to enhance communication skills in adolescents (Scott et al., 2011).
- Provide community resources for STI screenings, birth control, and counseling (Scott et al., 2011).
- Educate adolescents about effective birth control methods and concurrent use of a condom to decrease the risk of unplanned pregnancy and protect from STIs (Scott et al., 2011).

The Nurse's Influence on the Patient's Self-Concept and Sexuality

As a nurse you have the ability to positively influence a patient's self-concept. Your acceptance of a patient with an altered self-concept helps promote positive change. Your words and actions convey sincere interest and acceptance and have a profound effect on patients. When a patient's physical appearance has changed, both the patient and the family watch your verbal and nonverbal responses and reactions to the changed appearance. A positive and matter-of-fact approach to care provides a model for the patient and family to follow. It is important that health care providers understand the degree to which self-esteem and sexuality affect patient outcomes.

How you respond to patients who have experienced changes in body appearance sets the stage for how they come

BOX 23-4 SIGNS AND SYMPTOMS THAT MAY INDICATE CURRENT SEXUAL ABUSE OR A HISTORY OF SEXUAL ABUSE

- Unexplained bruises, lacerations, or abrasions, especially around breasts, genital or anal areas
- Unexplained vaginal or anal soreness or bleeding
- Unexplained genital or sexually transmitted infection
- Frequent visits to health care providers
- Headaches
- Gastrointestinal problems
- Abdominal pain
- Dysmenorrhea
- Premenstrual syndrome
- Sleep pattern disturbances
- Nightmares
- Repetitive dreams
- Depression
- Social withdrawal
- Anxiety
- Eating disorders
- Substance abuse
- Decreased self-esteem
- Difficulty developing trust
- Difficulties with intimate relationships
- Impaired school or work performance
- Reports of being sexually assaulted or raped

Note: No physical symptoms may be present.

Modified from Stuart GW: *Principles and practice of psychiatric nursing,* ed 10, St Louis, 2013, Mosby.

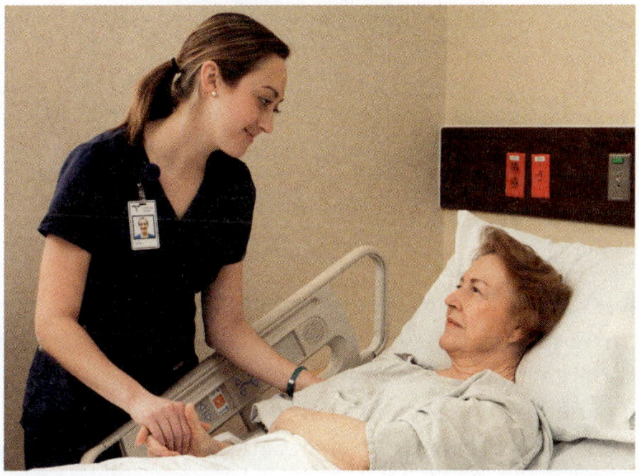

FIGURE 23-3 Nurses use touch and eye contact to enhance a patient's self-esteem.

to see themselves. The patient with a change in body functioning or appearance is often extremely sensitive to your verbal and nonverbal responses (Figure 23-3). Building a trusting nurse-patient relationship and appropriately including a patient in decision making will support most patients' self-concepts. Sometimes individualized approaches, including supporting the use of alternative healing techniques or methods of spiritual expression, help a patient adapt to changes in self-concept.

As a nurse you affect your patient's body image. For example, you have a positive influence on the body image of a patient who has had disfiguring surgery by showing acceptance of the surgical scar. On the other hand a shocked or disgusted facial expression causes a patient to develop a negative body image. It is very important to monitor your responses toward each patient. Matter-of-fact statements such as "This wound is healing nicely" or "This looks healthy" enhance the body image of a patient.

Inadvertently nonverbal communication such as frowning or grimacing when performing procedures has a profound effect on patients. Your nonverbal behavior conveys the level of caring that exists for your patient and affects his or her self-esteem. For example, when a patient who is incontinent perceives that you find the situation unpleasant, it threatens the patient's self-concept. Anticipate your own reactions, acknowledge them, and focus on the patient instead of the unpleasant task or situation. Put yourself in the patient's position to lessen his or her embarrassment, frustration, and anger.

When you consider the sexuality of patients, think about your own knowledge regarding sexual development, sexual orientation, sexual response, STIs, contraception, and alterations in sexual health. Also consider your knowledge base about communication (see Chapter 11). Your own sexuality, sexual experiences, and communication style are valuable when trying to understand your patient's experiences. Be sure not to convey your feelings to patients. Attempts at self-exploration teach us about our bodies and the potential for providing pleasure. Your attitude about masturbation may have stemmed from personal experience or from values or beliefs communicated by other people. Games such as "doctor" and "nurse" may have provided other early sex play and exploration. In addition, your own sexual experiences add to understanding about what a first sexual encounter may have been like or what it is like to introduce the topic of STIs or intercourse. In addition to personal experiences related to sexuality, use what you have learned through working with other patients as you assess and develop trust with current patients.

CRITICAL THINKING

Synthesis

You apply elements of critical thinking whenever you perform the nursing process with a patient. Consider the scientific knowledge you have learned, your experience, critical thinking attitudes, and standards to ensure an individualized approach to patient care. Your nursing expertise allows you to anticipate and respond to stressors that affect your patient's

BOX 23-5 SYNTHESIS IN PRACTICE

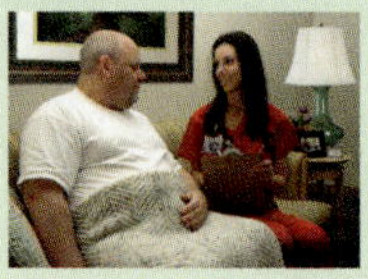

As Maria prepares to care for Mr. Taylor, she thinks about what she knows about self-concept and sexuality. She realizes that Mr. Taylor's stroke and resulting neurological deficits along with the sexual side effects of his antihypertensive medications are significant stressors in regard to his self-concept and sexuality. Mr. Taylor's independence is threatened because he is in the hospital and dependent on the nurses for most of his care. He may never be able to go back to work again, and he does not consider himself a strong man anymore. Therefore his family role as provider is threatened. Maria recognizes the significance of these changes and their potential influence on his self-concept and sexuality.

Maria's father had a stroke 2 years ago. Although his neurological symptoms finally improved enough to allow him to go back to work, Maria remembers the struggle her father went through as he coped with the physical and emotional changes that the stroke created. Maria's experience as a single mother also provides insight into what it is like to assume a new role within a family. She uses these two different experiences to guide her assessment of Mr. Taylor's concerns.

Maria needs to learn as much as she can about Mr. Taylor's thoughts and feelings about his self-concept and sexuality. To do this she realizes that she must first establish a trusting relationship with him and his wife, Meredith. Because Maria feels uncomfortable discussing sexuality with her patients, she reviews the PLISSIT assessment of sexuality (see Box 23-8) the night before she cares for Mr. Taylor and writes out some questions that she wants to ask him. Maria also plans to talk with both Mr. and Mrs. Taylor about their relationship before and after the stroke.

self-concept and sexual health. Consider changes in your patient's identity, body image, role performance, and self-esteem as important aspects of care (Box 23-5).

Knowledge. In addition to considering the various aspects of a patient's self-concept, use knowledge of how various medications, certain medical conditions, and chronic pain or fatigue influence your patient's ability to perform self-care and function at an optimal level. When you care for patients who have alterations in self-concept, be particularly alert to the patient who is experiencing chronic pain or fatigue. Chronic pain predisposes a person to a decreased ability to function sexually, irritability, and decreased sleep. Patients with chronic fatigue often feel exhausted and lack the energy for sexual interaction. These types of changes negatively affect self-concept. Another area of knowledge to consider is the patient's cultural background. Culture influences the importance that people place on such things as appearance, role performance, and acceptance by others (see Chapter 20).

Experience. Throughout life all individuals, including nurses, have experience with self-concept issues. Personal memories of changes in appearance or times when you were unable to carry out usual roles because of a temporary illness help you be empathetic with patients who are experiencing stressors to their self-concept or sexuality. Past experiences with patients who have undergone changes in self-concept or experienced self-concept stressors also provide useful insight into how to work effectively with a current patient.

BOX 23-6 PATIENT-CENTERED CARE

Body art (i.e., piercings and tattoos) are increasingly common in the U.S. population, especially among younger adults. Clinical facilities are concerned that visible body art in nurses may negatively influence patient satisfaction and care outcomes (Wittmann-Price et al., 2012). Patients respond to male and female health care providers with non-earlobe piercings and visible tattoos less positively than those without such modifications (Westerfield et al., 2012). Female providers with tattoos are considered less professional than males with similar tattoos. In addition, nurses with the most body art are perceived to be the least caring, skilled, and knowledgeable by patients (Thomas et al., 2010).

IMPLICATIONS FOR PRACTICE

- The patient's perception of competence and caring is often based on the appearance of the nurse.
- The patient's view of the nurse influences the ability to achieve positive interactions and health outcomes.
- Older adults have more negative views of tattoos and tend to be more influenced by appearances than younger patients.
- Dress code polices need to include guidelines about acceptable body art and consider both freedom of expression and professional image issues.

Attitudes. Attitudes to adopt when caring for patients with threats to self-concept and sexuality are acceptance, respect, and compassion. Some patients have values, attitudes, or behaviors that differ from your own. A patient-centered approach to care is important in order to support patients with alterations in self-concept and sexuality (Box 23-6). Developing a therapeutic nurse-patient relationship based on mutual respect, professional compassion, and unconditional acceptance promotes positive patient outcomes.

Standards. There are several codes of professional conduct for nurses; each reflects a commitment to the principle of respect for patient autonomy. Autonomy means that individuals have the freedom to choose their own life plan. Supporting your patients' autonomy to make choices and live in an authentic way consistent with personal values and beliefs supports the development and maintenance of a strong and positive self-concept.

NURSING PROCESS

ASSESSMENT

When assessing self-concept and self-esteem, focus on all components (identity, body image, and role performance)

BOX 23-7 BEHAVIORS SUGGESTIVE OF ALTERED SELF-CONCEPT AND SEXUALITY

- Avoidance of eye contact
- Slumped posture
- Unkempt appearance
- Overly apologetic
- Hesitant speech/withdrawn
- Overly critical or angry
- Frequent or inappropriate crying
- Negative self-evaluation
- Excessively dependent
- Hesitant to express views or opinions
- Lack of interest in what is happening
- Passive attitude
- Difficulty making decisions

and on behaviors suggestive of altered self-concept, self-esteem, or sexuality (Box 23-7). Also assess actual and potential self-concept stressors (see Figure 23-2). Determining a patient's current and past coping patterns is also important. If a patient shows mood changes such as depression, a mental status examination may also be helpful. In addition to direct questioning, you effectively gather much of the data regarding self-concept by observing a patient's nonverbal behavior and paying attention to what he or she says. Take note of the manner in which patients talk about the people in their lives because this provides clues to both stressful and supportive relationships. It also suggests key patient roles and obligations.

Apply your knowledge of developmental stages (see Box 23-1) to determine what aspects of self-concept are likely to be important to the patient, and inquire about these aspects of the person's life. For example, ask a 65-year-old male patient about his life now that retirement is approaching and what is now most important to him. Spend time asking a school-age patient how he or she has adjusted to transferring to a new school and whether he or she has been able to make friends. The individuals' conversations will likely provide data relating to role performance, identity, self-esteem, stressors, and coping patterns. At appropriate times specific questions are useful (Table 23-1).

Every complete nursing history needs to include a few questions related to a person's sexual health. Start with a general open-ended questions such as "Sex is an important part of life and can be affected by health status. Tell me how you would describe your sexual health" or "Share with me any questions or concerns you have about how your health will affect your sex life." Once you approach the topic, the patient is able to talk about concerns and explore possible ways to resolve the problem. When you address sexuality in a sensitive, relaxed, matter-of-fact manner, patients feel safe to bring up areas of concern. Use gender-neutral terms and questions when completing a sexual history. For example, say "chest" versus "breast." The intimacy of a nurse-patient relationship, whether it is involved in providing physical care or discussing the impact of a recent diagnosis, provides a unique opportunity for discussing a person's sexual concerns. The acronym PLISSIT is a helpful format for discussing sexuality with patients (Box 23-8).

BOX 23-8 PLISSIT MODEL FOR ASSESSING AND APPROACHING SEXUALITY

Permission for health care provider to discuss sexuality issues and for patient to discuss sexuality concerns.

Limited **I**nformation—Assess and clarify misinformation, dispel myths, provide simple factual information.

Specific **S**uggestions—Provide specific suggestions directly related to particular problem (only when the nurse is clear about the problem).

Intensive **T**herapy—Provide individualized therapy by referring to a professional with advanced training if necessary.

Modified from Annon J: The PLISSIT model: a proposed conceptual scheme for the behavioral treatment of sexual problems, *J Sex Educ Ther* 2(2):1, 1976.

Assessment of sexuality involves physical, psychological, social, and cultural variables. It is sometimes unnerving to inquire about another person's sexual functioning. You may worry that the patient does not appreciate being asked about sexuality and sexual practices. However, patients want to know how medications, treatments, and surgical procedures influence their sexual relationships. With experience you come to recognize that many patients welcome the opportunity to talk about their sexuality, especially when they are experiencing difficulty in sexual functioning.

It is important to first understand the reasons for changes in a patient's perceived sexual health. How a person responds to any physical or functional change in sexuality and intimacy following an illness depends on their self-concept, support of sexual partner, and attitudes regarding sexuality. Many health professionals fail to address the sexual needs of their patients. To promote sexual health, assess the effect of a diagnosis and its treatment and medications on your patient's perception of sexuality or sexual performance as you develop a treatment plan. For example, when caring for a man who has had a heart attack, you might ask, "Following a heart attack, men have questions about sexuality such as when they are able to resume sexual intercourse. Do you have questions like this that I can answer?" Or in the case of a patient with spinal cord injury resulting in paralysis, "It is natural for you to have concerns about being able to perform sexually. Would you like to discuss any concerns that you have?" A variety of physical factors positively or negatively influence sexual desire and function. For example, sexual intercourse sometimes results in pain or discomfort from arthritis, angina, endometriosis, or lack of vaginal lubrication. Even anticipation that sex may hurt such as during the postpartum period or after surgery lessens sexual desire. Learn to what extent these physical factors affect a patient's sexual performance.

Body image can also be affected by adherence to medical and treatment regimens. For example, many chemotherapy agents used in the treatment of cancer often result in infertility. You ask a patient, "Tell me if you have any concerns about whether your chemo medicine will affect your ability to have

TABLE 23-1 FOCUSED PATIENT ASSESSMENT

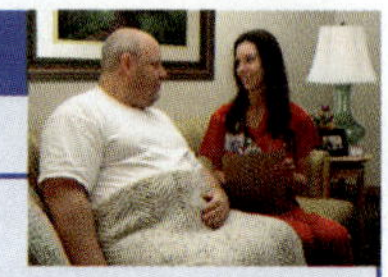

FACTORS TO ASSESS	QUESTIONS	PHYSICAL ASSESSMENT
Identity	How would you describe yourself?	Note verbal and nonverbal responses. Watch for hesitant speech, poor eye contact, and slumped posture. Derogatory answers (e.g., "I don't know; there's not too much worth mentioning") raise concern.
Body image	Which aspects of your appearance do you like? Are there any aspects of your appearance that you would like to change? If yes, describe the changes you would make.	Determine ability to identify something positive about appearance or body functions (e.g., "People have always told me I have nice eyes" or "I'm strong"). People who do not identify positive characteristics often have negative body image and poor self-esteem.
Self-esteem	Tell me about the things you do that make you feel good about yourself. How do you feel about yourself? If you were to describe yourself to someone else, which characteristics would you use?	Observe verbal and nonverbal responses. With prompting, most patients can identify something favorable. Statements about not having any strengths or not being able to do anything well raise concern and require additional assessment.
Role performance	Tell me about your primary roles (e.g., partner, parent, friend, sister, professional role, and volunteer). How effective are you at carrying out each of these roles? Do you have any barriers to fulfilling your roles?	Listen for the number of primary roles identified. A large number of primary roles will put the patient at risk for role conflicts and role overload. Patients who do not think that these roles are met adequately may be experiencing alterations in self-concept.
Sexuality	How has your illness, medication, or surgery affected your sex life? Are your needs for intimacy being met? Do you have any concerns about your sexual functioning?	Identify concerns about sexual functioning (e.g., erectile dysfunction in men, changes in vaginal lubrication in women) or overall change in sex drive. Determine if patient is hesitant to bring up issues of sexuality.

children." Such risks seriously lessen the likelihood of patients remaining adherent to their medications. Some medications affect sexual desire or cause physical changes that affect performance. Drinking alcohol or using drugs clouds judgment and results in sexual intercourse or other activities that lead to STIs or pregnancy. Gather a complete history of any medications or illicit drugs that the patient is taking or has taken in the past. You also need to obtain the same information for the patient's partner.

Another important area to assess is sexual decision making, including patients' use of contraception and safe sex practices. Adolescents' best respond to a question such as "Many people your age have questions about sexually transmitted infections or whether their bodies are developing at the right rate. What questions about sex can I answer?"

Older Adult Considerations. Reviewing sexuality changes associated with aging is also important. Approximately 50% of older women experience some type of sexual problem such as low desire or vaginal dryness (Sobecki et al., 2012). In men the penis does not become firm as quickly and is not as firm as it is at a younger age. Ejaculation takes longer to achieve and is shorter in duration, and the erection often diminishes more quickly. When assessing sexual changes, you need to ask about a patient's past sexual experiences, perceptions, and difficulties.

Your nursing assessment includes consideration of previous coping behaviors; the nature, number, and intensity of stressors; and a patient's internal and external resources. Knowing how a patient has dealt with self-concept stressors in the past provides insight into his or her style of coping. Not all patients address issues in the same way, but often a person uses a familiar coping pattern for newly encountered stressors. As you identify previous coping patterns, it is useful to determine whether these patterns contributed to healthy functioning or created more problems. For example, the use of drugs or alcohol during times of stress often creates additional stressors.

Exploring resources and strengths such as availability of significant others or prior use of community resources is important when formulating a realistic and effective plan. For example, midlife women who are recently single as a result of separation, divorce, or widowhood may be unaware that they are at risk for unintended pregnancies and STIs (Taylor and James, 2012). These women need screening for infections and education about safe sex and contraception. In addition, the physiological changes associated with aging such as changes in vaginal mucosa can make the middle- or older-adult woman at higher risk for infection than an adolescent. All mature adults need education about safe sex and STI screenings since they may not be aware of the health risks of unprotected sex (*Older People and AIDs*, 2012; USDHHS, 2009). Adults in the United States over the age of 50 are one of the fastest growing populations for HIV and acquired immunodeficiency syndrome (AIDS).

Valuable assessment data often evolve from conversations with family and significant others. Sometimes significant others have insights into a person's way of dealing with stressors and knowledge about what is important to the person's self-concept. The way in which a loved one talks about a patient, including his or her nonverbal behaviors, provides information about what kind of support is available for the patient. Ask patients' if they feel comfortable when they are relating to their partner and whether there is openness in the interaction.

Patient Expectations. The patient's expectations are also important to assess. Asking a patient how he or she believes medical and nursing interventions will make a difference provides useful information regarding the patient's expectations. This provides an opportunity to discuss the patient's goals. For example, when working with a patient who is experiencing anxiety related to an upcoming diagnostic study, ask the patient about his or her expectations of the relaxation exercise that you have been practicing together. The patient's response provides valuable information about his or her beliefs and attitudes regarding the effectiveness of the interventions and the potential need to modify the nursing approach. When nursing care involves consideration of a patient's sexuality, you need to be sensitive and understanding and always maintain the patient's confidentiality.

NURSING DIAGNOSIS

Carefully consider assessment data to identify a patient's actual or potential problem areas. You rely on knowledge and experience, apply appropriate critical thinking attitudes and professional standards, and look for clusters of defining characteristics that indicate a nursing diagnosis. Possible nursing diagnoses (NANDA International, 2012) related to self-concept and sexual functioning include the following:

- *Disturbed Body Image*
- *Disturbed Personal Identity*
- *Ineffective Role Performance*
- *Readiness for Enhanced Self-Concept*
- *Chronic Low Self-Esteem*
- *Situational Low Self-Esteem*
- *Sexual Dysfunction*
- *Ineffective Sexuality Pattern*

Forming nursing diagnoses about self-concept or sexuality is complex. Often isolated data are defining characteristics for more than one nursing diagnosis. If a person who has recently been laid off from work expresses a predominantly negative self-appraisal, including inability to handle situations or events and difficulty making decisions, these characteristics suggest a nursing diagnosis of *Situational Low Self-Esteem related to inability to fulfill previous roles*. Assessing information regarding recent events in the patient's life and how he or she has viewed himself or herself in the past is important. Likewise, identifying a nursing diagnosis regarding sexuality often requires you to clarify that defining characteristics exist and the patient perceives difficulty with regard to sexuality. Clues to help you identify defining characteristics of a possible nursing diagnosis include surgery of reproductive organs or changes in appearance, chronic fatigue or pain, past or current physical abuse, chronic illness, and developmental milestones such as puberty or menopause. Determining the contributing factors is important. Interventions depend on selecting the correct related factors. When you include all relevant contributing factors, you plan effectively. For example, the nursing diagnosis *Ineffective Sexuality Pattern related to difficulty with acceptance of recent loss and fear of pain* is appropriate for a woman who recently had a mastectomy. Further expanding the "related to" section to include more about how the mastectomy is affecting sexuality is helpful. For example, altered sexuality is possibly related to postoperative pain or fear of pain, fear of diminished attractiveness, and/or difficulty in moving.

PLANNING

Goals and Outcomes. Develop an individualized plan of care for each nursing diagnosis and help the patient set realistic expectations for care. Individualize goals and set realistic and measurable outcomes. While establishing goals, consult with the patient about whether the goals are perceived as realistic (see Care Plan). Consult with significant others to develop a more comprehensive and workable plan. Once you formulate a goal, consider how the data that illustrated the problem would change if the problem were diminished. Reflect these changes in the outcome criteria. For example, Mr. Taylor was diagnosed with *Situational Low Self-Esteem related to negative view of self and uncertainty about future roles.* He described feeling "less than a man" and lost interest in self-care activities. These are the defining characteristics. Formulate the goal that Mr. Taylor will experience fewer alterations in self-concept and the outcome that he will discuss his concerns before discharge. Additional expected outcomes include that Mr. Taylor performs self-care within 2 days and verbalizes feelings of self-acceptance in 4 days. As you develop your patient's plan of care, remember that patients have more than one interrelated problem (Figure 23-4).

Setting Priorities. The care plan presents the goals, expected outcomes, and interventions for a patient with an alteration in self-concept or sexuality. Your interventions focus on helping the patient adapt to the stressors that led to the disturbance and supporting and reinforcing the development of coping methods. The patient often needs time to adapt to physical changes. Self-concept priorities include maximizing his or her ability to address physical and psychological needs. Priorities for sexual health typically

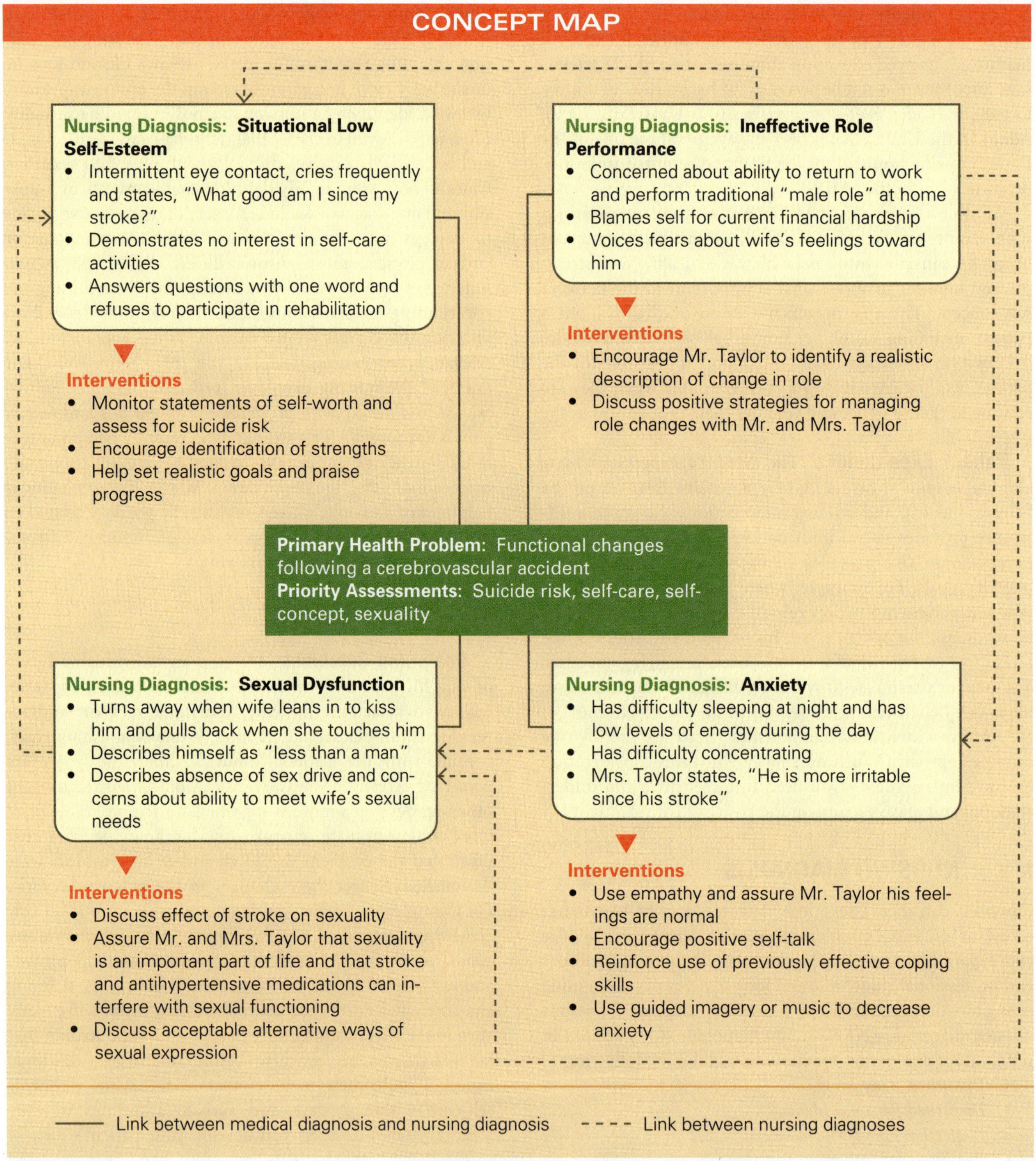

FIGURE 23-4 Concept map.

include resuming sexual activities. Look for strengths in both the individual and the family and provide resources and education to turn limitations into strengths. Patient teaching communicates the normalcy of certain situations (e.g., nature of a chronic disease, change in relationships, effect of a loss). It is important to determine your patients' needs and plan accordingly. For example, when caring for a patient whose sexual health is altered, include private time for your patient and partner to quietly sit in the room and have dinner and watch a movie without any interruptions.

Collaborative Care. The perceptions of significant others are important to incorporate into the plan of care. Sometimes individuals who experienced deficits in self-concept before the current episode of treatment have established a system of support, including mental health clinicians, clergy, and other community resources. Before involving

CARE PLAN

Situational Low Self-Esteem

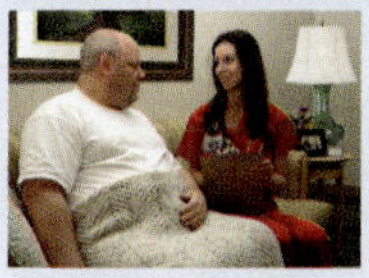

ASSESSMENT

After Maria completes Mr. Taylor's physical assessment and helps him with his self-care activities, she sits down with Mr. and Mrs. Taylor to discuss how the stroke has affected Mr. Taylor's self-concept and sexual health.

ASSESSMENT ACTIVITIES	FINDINGS/DEFINING CHARACTERISTICS*
Assess identity concerns (e.g., sexual role, masculinity, and breadwinner). Ask how the stroke has affected Mr. Taylor's sense of self.	Mr. Taylor **looks away, shakes his head,** and states, "**I feel less of a man.** My wife says she's just thankful I'm alive, but that's not enough for me." Is not able to perform physical activities by self or fulfill role within family.
Observe Mr. Taylor's mood, affect, nonverbal communication, and interactions with others; interview family as appropriate.	Mrs. Taylor reports that Mr. Taylor demonstrates **intermittent eye contact, frequent crying when alone, blank staring** at his flaccid hand, and **superficial conversations** with family members.
Determine Mr. Taylor's interest and involvement in self-care activities.	Mr. Taylor **refuses to bathe or comb his hair.** He **eats less** than 50% of meals and **demonstrates avoidance** of the prescribed rehabilitation activities.

*__Defining characteristics__ are shown in **bold** type.

NURSING DIAGNOSIS: Situational Low Self-Esteem related to negative view of self as less than whole following stroke and uncertainty of future personal, family, and professional roles.

PLANNING

GOAL	EXPECTED OUTCOMES (NOC)†
• Mr. Taylor will experience fewer alterations in self-concept, including low self-esteem, disturbed body image, altered role performance, and impaired sexuality by discharge.	***Self-Esteem*** • Mr. Taylor will verbalize feelings of self-acceptance and self-worth within 4 days. ***Role Performance*** • Mr. Taylor will describe role changes associated with his stroke in 2 days. ***Body Image*** • Mr. Taylor will demonstrate adjustment to changes in body function in performing self-care activities within 1 week.

†Outcomes classification labels from Moorhead S, et al, editors: *Nursing outcomes classification (NOC)*, ed 5, St Louis, 2013, Mosby.

INTERVENTIONS (NIC)‡	RATIONALE
Self-Esteem Enhancement	
• Facilitate an environment and activities (e.g., writing in a journal, reflection, praying, talking with a nurse) that increase self-esteem.	A therapeutic nurse-patient relationship promotes positive patient outcome, including behavior change (Stuart, 2013).
• Reinforce Mr. Taylor's statements of self-worth during care activities.	Positive self-esteem can improve quality of life and adaptive functioning (Choi et al., 2011).
• Encourage increased responsibility for self and help patient accept dependence on others as appropriate.	Self-management allows patients and families to be active participants in care and promotes empowerment (Leuven, 2012).

Continued

CARE PLAN—cont'd

Situational Low Self-Esteem

Role Enhancement

• Help Mr. Taylor identify specific role changes brought on by the stroke and seek ways in which to make adaptations.	Role strain occurs when one feels unable to fulfill certain roles and can be brought on by changes in health. Alternative choices can be proposed only after the problem is accurately defined (Stuart, 2013).

Body Image Enhancement

• Discuss changes in function and physical appearance caused by change in medical condition.	People who have a positive body image are more likely to report high self-esteem (Stuart, 2013).

Sexual Counseling

• Include Mrs. Taylor while teaching Mr. Taylor about the effects of his paralysis and medications on sexual function. Explain that sexuality is an important part of life and how Mr. Taylor can make adaptations in order to perform sexually.	Sexuality is a basic need and concern for both men and women yet is one of the most difficult discussions for patients to initiate. Many nurses believe that patients do not expect the nurse to address sexuality concerns and lack comfort and confidence in addressing concerns (Ivarsson et al., 2010).

‡Intervention classification labels from Bulechek GM, et al, editors: *Nursing interventions classification (NIC),* ed 6, St Louis, 2013, Mosby.

EVALUATION

NURSING ACTIONS	PATIENT RESPONSE/FINDING	ACHIEVEMENT OF OUTCOME
Ask Mr. Taylor how effective he feels in his ability to identify and express feelings verbally and nonverbally.	Mr. Taylor reports, "I've been able to talk with my wife, even about my concerns that she won't find me attractive anymore."	Improved verbal and nonverbal communication noted
Monitor changes in Mr. Taylor's statements about himself.	Mr. Taylor is making fewer negative comments and is evaluating body image more realistically but remains dissatisfied with appearance and strength of hand.	Small improvement in self-esteem; body image more realistic but remains negative Discusses body image with wife and primary nurse
Ask Mr. Taylor to describe how his roles have changed since his stroke and which adaptations have been made.	Mr. Taylor states, "Although I can't work right now, Meredith is going to pick up some extra hours at her job to help make ends meet. I may not be able to bring home any money right now, but I can do other things around the house to help."	Relationship with wife strengthened; beginning to accept change in family role
Observe Mr. Taylor's participation in self-care related to stroke.	Mr. Taylor assumes responsibility for basic hygiene; he is able to do most of his bath independently; and, although his gait remains unsteady, he is able to walk short distances with a walker.	Meeting self-care need; seeks assistance as needed
Encourage Mr. Taylor to identify resources outside the hospital.	Mr. Taylor expresses interest in attending local stroke recovery support group and connecting with friends.	Scheduled to attend stroke recovery support group 2 days after discharge and plans to invite a close friend over within 1 week of discharge, which indicate adjustment to changes in body function and appearance.

the family, consider a patient's desires for significant others to be involved and cultural norms regarding who most frequently makes decisions in the family. Sexual conflict in marriage, intimacy issues stemming from past sexual assault, or incest often require intensive treatment with mental health professionals. Resolving self-concept issues is a long-term goal and includes referrals to a clinical psychologist, advanced practice psychiatric nurse, social worker, or professional counselor.

IMPLEMENTATION

As with all of the steps of the nursing process, a therapeutic nurse-patient relationship is central to the implementation phase. Once you have developed goals and outcomes, consider nursing interventions that help move your patient toward his or her goals. To develop effective nursing interventions, consider the nursing diagnosis and related interventions that address the diagnosis. Individualize standard interventions to your patient. You develop nursing interventions based on the "related to" component of the nursing diagnosis. Developing interventions that affect the "related to" factors often decreases the problem reflected in the nursing diagnosis. In the case of Mr. Taylor (see Care Plan), the "related to" component of the nursing diagnosis focuses on the areas to explore when talking with the patient and family.

Nursing interventions are designed to promote a patient's healthy self-concept and sexuality. Strategies help patients regain or restore the elements that contribute to a strong and secure sense of self. The approaches that you choose vary according to the level of care required. Effective nursing care includes promoting sexual health in acute and restorative settings by helping patients understand their problems and exploring methods to deal with them effectively.

Health Promotion. Work with patients to help them develop healthy lifestyle behaviors that contribute to a positive self-concept. Measures that support adaptation to stress such as proper nutrition, regular exercise within a patient's capabilities, adequate sleep and rest, and stress-reducing practices contribute to a healthy self-concept. As a nurse you are in a unique position to identify lifestyle practices that place patients' self-concepts at risk or are suggestive of altered self-concepts. For example, a college student visits an outpatient clinic with complaints of being unable to sleep and anxiety attacks. In gathering the patient history, you learn of lifestyle practices such as too little rest, a large number of life changes occurring simultaneously, irregular menstrual cycles, and excessive use of alcohol. These data suggest actual or potential self-concept disturbances. You then talk with the patient to determine how she views the various lifestyle elements, to facilitate her insight into behaviors, and to make appropriate referrals or provide needed health teaching.

Exploring a person's sexuality and providing useful sex education require good communication skills. Make sure that the environment and timing provide privacy, uninterrupted time, and patient comfort. For example, discuss contraception methods with a woman in an office rather than in the examination room when she is only partially clothed. Plan the discussion so there are no interruptions and sit down while showing your interest and readiness to support her needs.

Teaching topics on sexuality vary based on the age of the patient. Education offers explanation of normal developmental changes. For example, you talk to a school-age child about the appearance of breast buds or pubic hair. When discussing sexual health with patients of childbearing age, always consider your patient's cultural and religious beliefs regarding contraception. The discussion includes their desire for children, usual sexual practices, and acceptable methods of contraception. Review all methods of contraception to provide necessary information for an informed patient choice. Reinforce that the best method is the one the patient will use consistently. Teaching needs for an adult include details of physiological changes resulting from illness or treatment effects. Box 23-9 summarizes a teaching plan for educating adults about their sexual health.

Individuals need to learn more about safe sex practices when they have more than one sex partner or when their partner had other sexual experiences. Provide information on STIs, including their symptoms, use of condoms, and high-risk sexual activities. Safe sex also means considering a patient's emotional risks within a relationship. Role play is a useful teaching tool to help a patient learn to say "no" or to negotiate with a partner to use a condom.

Acute Care. In the acute care setting you are likely to encounter patients who are experiencing potential threats to their self-concept because of the nature of the treatment and diagnostic procedures. Threats to a patient's self-concept result in anxiety and/or fear. Numerous stressors, including unknown diagnoses, the need to make changes in lifestyle, and change in functioning, are present; and you need to address them. In the acute care setting there is often more than one stressor, thus increasing the overall stress level for patients and their families.

You also care for patients who are faced with the need to adapt to an altered body image as a result of surgery or other physical change. Often a visit by someone who has experienced similar changes and adapted to them is helpful. The timing of such a visit is important. Because addressing these needs is often difficult to do while in an acute care setting, appropriate follow-up and referrals, including home care, are essential. Be sensitive to a patient's level of acceptance of the change. Forcing confrontation with the change before a patient is ready delays the patient's acceptance. Signs that a person is receptive to such a visit include the patient's asking questions related to how to manage a particular aspect of what has happened or looking at the changed area. As the patient expresses readiness to integrate the body change into his or her self-concept, you either let him or her know about groups that are available or ask if he or she wants you to make the initial contact. In addition, you facilitate adjustment to a change in physical appearance through your own response to the wound or change. As you

BOX 23-9 PATIENT TEACHING

Promoting Sexual Function

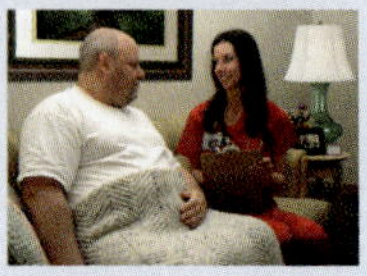

After talking with Mr. and Mrs. Taylor, Maria decides to develop a teaching plan that will help the couple adapt to the changes in sexuality that resulted from Mr. Taylor's stroke.

OUTCOME

Mr. and Mrs. Taylor state at least three ways to attain a satisfactory level of sexual activity.

TEACHING STRATEGIES

- Provide teaching on normal sexual changes that occur with aging and following a stroke.
- Encourage Mr. and Mrs. Taylor to discuss which types of intimate behavior provide the most sexual stimulation and satisfaction.
- Discuss side effects of medications that commonly alter sexual function and response.
- Encourage selection of a time of day when Mr. Taylor feels most rested and a comfortable/nonthreatening setting.
- Instruct Mrs. Taylor to use a water-based lubricant during intercourse to promote comfort.
- Encourage alternative positions for intercourse (e.g., side-lying, lying on a bed with legs over the side) that decrease discomfort during intercourse.
- Inform Mr. and Mrs. Taylor that a longer period of foreplay helps to achieve penile firmness.
- Instruct Mr. and Mrs. Taylor to conserve strength by not working hard at the beginning of intercourse to avoid tiring before climax.

EVALUATION STRATEGIES

- Ask Mr. and Mrs. Taylor to verbalize plan for improved sexual health.
- Ask Mr. and Mrs. Taylor to evaluate their satisfaction with their sexual relationship.

Modified from Meiner SE: *Gerontologic nursing*, ed 4, St Louis, 2011, Mosby.

respond with acceptance, you model acceptance for both the patient and the family.

Both physical and psychological aspects of illness have the potential to affect sexuality. Never assume that sexual functioning is not a concern merely because of an individual's age or severity of prognosis. After identifying concerns, address them in the context of the patient's value system. When a patient experiences physical limitations to sexual performance, provide the following suggestions: planning sexual activity when the patient is rested, experimenting with positions that are more comfortable, encouraging partners to give one another more time, and encouraging the use of foreplay to achieve arousal.

Restorative and Continuing Care. If you work in a home care or restorative care environment, you will have the opportunity to work with a patient to attain a more positive self-concept. Interventions designed to help a patient reach the goal of adapting to changes in self-concept or attaining a positive self-concept are based on the premise that the patient first develops insight and self-awareness concerning problems and stressors and then acts to solve the problems and cope with the stressors. You incorporate this approach into patient teaching for alterations in self-concept, including situational low-self-esteem, which is sometimes present in the home care setting. Increase a patient's self-awareness by establishing a trusting relationship that allows him or her to openly explore thoughts and feelings. A priority nursing intervention continues to be the expert use of communication skills to clarify the expectations of the patient and family. Open exploration makes the situation less threatening for the patient and encourages behaviors that expand self-awareness. Encourage the patient's self-exploration by accepting his or her thoughts and feelings, helping him or her to clarify interactions with others, and being empathetic. Also encourage self-expression and stress the patient's self-responsibility.

Promoting a patient's self-evaluation involves helping him or her define problems clearly and identify positive and negative coping mechanisms. Work closely with each patient to help analyze adaptive and maladaptive responses, consider alternatives, and discuss outcomes. Collaborating with a patient in establishing realistic goals involves helping him or her identify alternative solutions and develop realistic goals based on them. This facilitates real change and encourages further goal-setting behaviors. You design opportunities that result in success, reinforce the patient's skills and strengths, and help the patient get needed assistance.

Teach patients to move away from ineffective coping mechanisms and develop successful coping strategies. Supporting attempts that are health promoting is essential because with each success a patient is more motivated to make another attempt at promoting health. Supporting adaptive, flexible coping is critical to intervening in self-concept alterations. Patients who are experiencing threats to or alterations in self-concept often benefit from collaboration with mental health and community resources to promote increased awareness. Knowledge of available community resources allows you to make appropriate referrals.

Use a nonjudgmental, respectful approach to encourage honest and open discussions about sexual health. Management of sexuality concerns is important as you promote sexual intimacy and provide closeness and closure between partners at the end of life. Give priority to patients in middle and older adulthood when you address sexuality concerns resulting from illness, medications, or physical changes. Provide information on how the specific illness will limit sexual activity and ideas for adapting or facilitating sexual activity. Interventions range from giving permission for a partner to lie in bed and hold a patient to coordinating nursing care and medications in a way that provides opportunity for privacy and intimacy. In the home environment it is important to help patients create an environment comfortable for sexual activity. For example, this sometimes involves making recommendations for ways to rearrange a patient's bedroom to accommodate any limitations. Patients and partners need to know how to accommodate barriers such as Foley catheters or drainage tubes that make sexual positioning difficult.

Research shows that middle- and older-age adults who are sexually active have greater independence, better overall health, and longer life expectancy (Lindau and Gavrilova, 2010; Tenenbaum, 2009). As the U.S. population ages, it is estimated that approximately 12 million adults over the age of 65 will need long-term care by the year 2030 (Bentrott and Margrett, 2011). In the long-term care setting, facilities need to make proper arrangements for privacy during a patient's sexual experience (Brown, 2012; Tarzia et al., 2012). Staff at such facilities need to be educated about the importance of sexuality and ways to support intimacy and sexual expression among consenting adults. In addition, do not assume that all older patients are heterosexuals.

Establishing a therapeutic relationship is critical to successfully intervening with patients who have alterations in self-concept, whether care is focused on health promotion, dealing with an acute process, or addressing restorative care. To support the development of a positive self-concept in a patient, convey genuine caring for the patient (see Chapter 19). Then and only then do you establish a partnership with the patient to address underlying problems.

EVALUATION

Patient Care. Expected outcomes for a patient with a self-concept disturbance include nonverbal behaviors indicating a positive self-concept, statements of self-acceptance, and acceptance of change in appearance or function (see Care Plan; Box 23-10). For example, a patient who has difficulty making eye contact demonstrates a more positive self-concept by making more frequent eye contact and smiling during conversation. Adequate self-care and acceptance of the use of prosthetic devices indicate progress. A positive attitude toward rehabilitation and increased movement toward independence facilitate a return to preexisting roles at work or at home. Patterns of interacting often reflect changes in self-concept. For example, a patient who was hesitant to express his or her views more readily offers opinions and ideas as self-esteem increases.

Sometimes initial goals are unrealistic or require modification as the patient's condition changes. You and the patient need to revise the plan in these cases. Patient adaptation to major changes sometimes takes a year or longer, but the fact that this period is long does not suggest problems with adaptation. Look for signs that the patient has reduced some stressors and that some behaviors have become more adaptive. This requires a follow-up discussion with the patient to determine if the level of satisfaction with sexual performance or sexual function has improved. Sometimes the patient achieved the goal and outcome criteria, but sexual functioning is still not ideal. Consider which other steps are appropriate. Changes in self-concept and sexuality take time. Although change is slow, care of the patient with a self-concept disturbance is rewarding.

BOX 23-10 EVALUATION

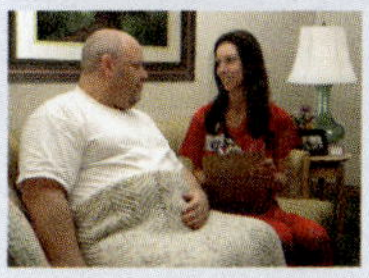

Because Mr. Taylor was in the hospital for 2 weeks, Maria was able to care for him and watch him adapt to the changes he experienced as a result of his stroke. On the last day that Maria cared for Mr. Taylor, he reported that he was going to a rehabilitation center that specializes in helping people who have had strokes. Mr. Taylor is able to complete most of his bath independently. Although his gait is a little unsteady, he is able to walk short distances with a walker. During his bath he jokes, "I think my new haircut makes me look a lot younger!" This improvement in function and acceptance of self has helped Mr. Taylor become more satisfied with himself and his progress in therapy. He is hopeful that he will be able to return to work after he leaves the rehabilitation center. Both Mr. and Mrs. Taylor have worked with a therapist who specializes in helping couples who have sexual problems. Mr. Taylor states that the therapy sessions have helped him grow closer to his wife and have strengthened their relationship. Several of his bowling friends visited him last night. Mr. Taylor states, "I can't wait to get better. I have a lot of things to do and a lot to live for."

DOCUMENTATION NOTE

"Ability to perform ADLs improving. Only needs help to wash back during bath. Improvements in function have led to reports of enhanced self-esteem and acceptance of body image. Actively participates in sexual therapy with spouse and is maintaining relationships with friends. States is highly motivated to get better and return to work soon. Plans to continue to work on improving neurological deficits at the stroke rehabilitation center."

ADLs, Activities of daily living.

Patient Expectations. In evaluating care provided to patients with alterations in self-concept and sexual health, determine if their expectations are met. After determining the achievement of targeted outcomes, ask if the patient thinks that nursing care was effective and supportive. Remain aware of any personal limitations in being able to counsel the patient. In some cases referrals to other health care providers is still necessary.

KEY POINTS

- Self-concept is an integrated set of conscious and unconscious attitudes and perceptions about the self.
- Components of self-concept are identity, body image, and role performance. Self-esteem and sexuality are closely related terms.
- Each developmental stage involves factors that are important to the development of a healthy, positive self-concept.

- Identity is particularly vulnerable during adolescence.
- Body image is the mental picture of one's body and is not necessarily consistent with a person's actual body structure or appearance.
- Body image stressors include changes in physical appearance, structure, or functioning caused by normal developmental changes or illness.
- Self-esteem is the emotional appraisal of self-concept and reflects the overall sense of being capable, worthwhile, and competent.
- Self-esteem stressors include developmental and relationship changes, illness (particularly chronic illness involving changes in what were normal activities), surgery, accidents, and the responses of other individuals to changes resulting from these events.
- The nurse's self-concept and nursing actions often have an effect on a patient's self-concept.
- Planning and implementing nursing interventions for self-concept disturbance involve expanding the patient's self-awareness, encouraging self-exploration, aiding in self-evaluation, helping formulate goals in regard to adaptation, and helping the patient achieve these goals.
- Sexuality is related to all dimensions of health. Therefore address sexual concerns or problems as part of nursing care.
- Sexual health involves physical and psychosocial aspects and contributes to an individual's sense of self-worth and positive interpersonal relationships.
- Development and life changes, ethical decisional issues, fertility, personal and emotional conflicts, illness, and hospitalization all affect a patient's sexuality.

CLINICAL DECISION-MAKING EXERCISES

Mr. Taylor comes to the stroke rehab unit. He states he is having a bad day. He is feeling depressed and less interested in his rehabilitation. During the morning he shared with Maria some of his concerns about when he will be able to return to work. He says, "I just want to get back to my normal self."

1. Describe how Maria should respond to Mr. Taylor's comment regarding "getting back to normal."
2. Mrs. Taylor reports that Mr. Taylor has no interest in being intimate and he rejects her when she attempts to initiate sexual contact. How should Maria approach issues of sexuality with the Taylors?
3. Maria suspects that Mr. Taylor's depressed mood and loss of interest in usual activities is now a higher priority than the previous diagnosis of *Situational Low Self-Esteem.* Describe which assessment data are needed to modify his plan of care. Identify priority nursing interventions.

evolve

Answers to Clinical Decision-Making Exercises can be found on the Evolve website.

QSEN ACTIVITY: QUALITY IMPROVEMENT

Maria notices that discharge instructions given to patients who had myocardial infarctions (MIs) do not always include counseling regarding resumption of sexual activity. She realizes that some patients may be hesitant to bring up this subject but knows that sexually active adults report higher quality of life than adults who are not sexually active. When she asked some of the nurses about this omission, some said that it was because of time constraints, and others said they didn't feel knowledgeable enough to be discussing this with a patient.

How could this information be used to create an approach for improving the quality of care for post MI patients?

How should the nurses measure if any changes in their approach have beneficial effects?

evolve

Answers to QSEN Activities can be found on the Evolve website.

REVIEW QUESTIONS

1. A 57-year-old divorced woman tells the nurse that she has just started dating again. Based on this information, the nurse realizes that the patient needs information about:
   1. Breast self-examination and mammograms.
   2. The HPV vaccine.
   3. Safe sex practices and screenings for STIs.
   4. Birth-control options.
2. A 64-year-old patient says that she has not been intimate with her partner since her mastectomy 2 months ago. The nurse realizes that the woman is having difficulty adjusting to changes in which of the following aspects of self-concept? (Select all that apply.)
   1. Self-esteem
   2. Sexuality
   3. Gender identity
   4. Body image
3. When assessing a patient's adjustment to the role changes brought about by a medical condition such as a stroke, the nurse asks about which of the following? (Select all that apply.)
   1. What are your thoughts about returning to work?
   2. What questions do you have about your medications?
   3. How has your health affected your relationship with your partner?
   4. What level of physical activity is the patient able to perform?
4. The nurse is educating a group of adolescents about the HPV vaccines. The nurse knows that further instruction is needed when several of the youths state:
   1. "The vaccines can decrease the occurrence of genital warts."

2. "Both vaccines can only be administered to females."
3. "The vaccines can protect against the cancers of the anus."
4. "The vaccines are most effective when given before exposure to the virus."

5. Mr. Alvarez is being discharged after recovery from a myocardial infarction (MI). The nurse plans to include information about resumption of sexual activity in the discharge instructions. He says that his wife will be in to take him home later in the day after work. Why should the nurse wait until Mrs. Alvarez is present before giving discharge instructions? (Select all that apply.)
   1. The nurse will feel more comfortable discussing intimate issues with a female present.
   2. The nurse needs to determine Mrs. Alvarez's sexual identity.
   3. Health issues can alter a couple's relationship.
   4. The nurse can encourage open communication between the couple.
6. A nurse is taking a sexual history during the admission process and wants to establish a relaxed and matter-of-fact approach to help the patient feel safe. Which of the following questions is the best example of this practice?
   1. Have you ever had a homosexual experience?
   2. Are you a heterosexual?
   3. Tell me how you would describe your sexual health.
   4. How often do you have sexual intercourse with your wife since your illness?
7. A healthy 68-year-old man tells the nurse that he is having difficulty sustaining an erection. He is not currently on any medications. What is the most appropriate response for the nurse to make?
   1. "It is not unusual for men your age to have this issue."
   2. "You should consider performance-enhancing medications."
   3. "I'll arrange for you talk to a sex therapist about this issue."
   4. "This is probably a temporary issue, and I wouldn't be too concerned unless it continues."
8. A nurse is questioning the policy at a clinical facility about the need for nursing staff to cover tattoos or remove multiple piercings when delivering care. The nurse says that this policy infringes on the right to self-expression and individuality. What is the best response by the unit manager?
   1. Disregard the comments to minimize conflict with staff
   2. Inform the nurse to abide by the policy or he or she could lose her job
   3. Explain to the nurse recent research findings about patient perceptions of professionals with visible piercings and tattoos
   4. Consider making an exception to the policy since the nurse is well qualified
9. A nurse is working with an older black adult who has recently moved to an assisted-living facility because of declining physical capabilities associated with the normal aging process. Which nursing interventions are directed at promoting self-esteem in this patient?
   1. Commending the patient's efforts at completing self-care tasks
   2. Assuming that the patient's physical complaints are attention-seeking measures
   3. Minimizing time discussing memories and past achievements spent with the patient
   4. Limiting decision-making opportunities for the patient to reduce stress
10. Match the following assessment questions listed below to the appropriate category in the PLISSIT model.

1. P_____	a. What do you know about ways to adjust positioning for intimacy? Let me explain.
2. LI_____	b. You have described a number of sexual problems, I would like you to talk to our psychologist, if that is OK.
3. SS_____	c. Are you comfortable in talking about how your surgery may affect your sexual health?
4. IT_____	d. You know it is not unusual for older adults to want sexual intimacy, how do you feel about that?

evolve

Rationales for Review Questions can be found on the Evolve website.

1. 3; 2. 1, 2, 4; 3. 1, 3; 4. 2; 5. 3, 4; 6. 3; 7. 1; 8. 3; 9. 1; 10. 1c, 2d, 3a, 4b.

REFERENCES

Anderson DM, Skemp KM: Self-image differences as related to body image of students in a middle school, *Am J Health Behav* 36(4):533, 2012.

Bearinger LH, et al: Adolescent condom use consistency over time: global versus partner-specific measures, *Nurs Res* 60:3(suppl):568, 2011.

Bentrott MD, Margrett JA: Taking a person-centered approach to understanding the sexual expression among longer-term care residents: theoretical perspectives and research challenge, *Ageing Int* 36:401, 2011.

Brown PS: Intimacy, sexuality, and aging. In Lange JW, editor: *The nurse's role in promoting optimal health of older adults*, Philadelphia, 2012, FA Davis.

Ceballos N, Czyzewska M: Body image in Hispanic/Latino vs. European American adolescents: implications for treatment and prevention of obesity in underserved populations, *J Health Care Poor Underserved* 21:823, 2010.

Centers for Disease Control and Prevention (CDC): *Workplace and safety health topics, follow regulations*, 2010, http://www.cdc.gov/niosh/topics/body_art/stateRegs.html. Accessed May 7, 2013.

Centers for Disease Control and Prevention (CDC): Trends in HIV-related risk behaviors among high school students—United States, 1991–2011, *MMWR* 61(29):556–560, 2012, http://www.cdc.gov/mmwr/preview/mmwrhtml/mm6129a4.htm?s_cid=mm6129a4_w. Accessed May 7, 2013.

Centers for Disease Control and Prevention (CDC): *Adolescent and school health: sexual risk behavior: HIV, STD, & teen pregnancy prevention*, 2013a, http://www.cdc.gov/HealthyYouth/sexualbehaviors/index.html. Accessed May 7, 2013.

Centers for Disease Control and Prevention (CDC): *Genital infection fact sheet*, 2013b, http://www.cdc.gov/std/HPV/STDFact-HPV.html. Accessed May 7, 2013.

Centers for Disease Control and Prevention (CDC): *HPV, HPV vaccines*, 2013c, http://www.cdc.gov/hpv/vaccine.html. Accessed May 7, 2013.

Choi KB, et al: Sexual life and self-esteem in married elderly, *Arch Gerontol Geriatr* 53:17, 2011.

Deardorff J, et al: Does neighborhood environment influence girls' pubertal onset? Findings from a cohort study, *BMC Pediatrics* 12:27, 2012, http://www.biomedcentral.com/1471-2431/12/27. Accessed May 7, 2013.

Doty ND, et al: Sexuality related social support among lesbian, gay, and bisexual youth, *J Youth Adolescence* 39:1134, 2010.

Durkin SE: Tattoos, body piercing, and healthcare concerns, *J Radiology Nurs* 31(1):20, 2012.

Erikson E: *Childhood and society*, ed 2, New York, 1963, WW Norton.

Erol RY, Orth U: Self-esteem development from age 14 to 30 years: a longitudinal study, *J Personality Social Psychol* 101:3, 2011.

Holbrook J, et al: Body piercing complications and prevention of health risks, *Am J Clin Dermatol* 13(1):1, 2012.

Holmqvist K, Frisen A: Body dissatisfaction across cultures: findings and research problems, *Eur Eat Disorders Rev* 18:133, 2010.

Ivarsson B, et al: Health professionals' views on sexual information following MI, *BJN* 19(16):1052, 2010.

Leuven KA: Population aging: implications for nurse practitioners, *J Nurse Pract* 8(7):554, 2012.

Lindau ST, Gavrilova B: Sex, health, and years of sexually active life gained due to good health: evidence from two US population-based cross-sectional surveys of ageing, *BMJ* 340:c810, 2010.

Manning WD, et al: Young adult dating relationships and the management of sexual risk, *Population Res Policy Rev* 31:165, 2012.

Martin MA, et al: Gender and race/ethnic differences in inaccurate weight perceptions among US adolescents, *Womens Health Issues* 19:292, 2009.

Meiner SE: Gerontologic assessment. In Meiner SE, editor: *Gerontologic nursing*, ed 4, St Louis, 2011, Mosby.

NANDA International: *Nursing diagnoses: Definitions and classifications 2012-2014*, ed 9, Hoboken, NJ, 2012, Wiley-Blackwell.

Nelius T, et al: Genital piercings: diagnostic therapeutic implications for urologists, *Urology* 78:(5):998, 2011.

Older People and AIDS, Fact sheet 616, 2012, http://www.aidsinfonet.org/fact_sheets/view/616. Accessed May 7, 2013.

Orth U, et al: Self-esteem development from young adulthood to old age: a cohort-sequential longitudinal study, *J Personality Social Psychol* 98(4), 2010.

Quell TT: Opportunities and challenges of growing old. In Lange JW, editor: *The nurse's role in promoting optimal health of older adults*, Philadelphia, 2012, FA Davis.

Resnick B: Health promotion in illness/disability prevention. In Meiner SE, editor: *Gerontologic nursing*, ed 4, St Louis, 2011, Mosby.

Rhee J, Johnson KP: Investigating relationships between adolescents' liking for an apparel brand and brand self-congruency, *Young Consum* 13(1):74, 2011.

Scott ME, et al: Exploration of the effect unsafe sex has on reproduction, *Perspect Sex Reprod Health* 43(2):110, 2011.

Sobecki JN, et al: What we don't talk about when we don't talk about sex: results of a national survey of US obstetricians/gynecologists, *J Sex Med* 9:1285, 2012.

Stuart GW: *Principles and practice of psychiatric nursing*, ed 10, St Louis, 2013, Mosby.

Tarzia L, et al: Dementia, sexuality and consent in residential aged care facilities, *J Med Ethics* 2012.

Taylor D, James EA: Risks of being sexual in midlife: what we don't know can hurt us, *Female Patient* 37:17, 2012.

Tenenbaum EM: To be or to exist: standards for deciding whether dementia patients in nursing homes should engage in intimacy, sex, and adultery, *Indiana Law Rev* 42(3):675, 2009.

Thomas CM, et al: Perception of nurse caring, skills, and knowledge based on appearance, *JONA* 40(11):489, 2010.

Touhy TT, Jett KF: *Ebersole and Hess' Gerontological nursing healthy aging*, ed 3, St Louis, 2010, Mosby.

Troutman M: Mid-range theory of successful aging. In Lange JW, editor: *The nurse's role in promoting optimal health of older adults*, Philadelphia, PA, 2012, FA Davis.

US Department of Health and Human Services (USDHHS), National Institute of Health, National Institute on Aging: *HIV, AIDS, and older people*, 2009, http://www.nia.nih.gov/health/publication/hiv-aids-and-older-people, Accessed May 7, 2013.

Urdang M, et al: Tattoos and piercings: a review for the emergency physician, *West J Emerg Med* 12(4):393, 2011.

Westerfield HV, et al: Patients' perceptions of patient care providers with tattoos and/or body piercings, *J Nurs Admin* 42(3):160, 2012.

Williamson C: Providing care to transgender persons: a clinical approach to primary care, hormones, and HIV management, *J Nurses AIDS Care* 21(3):221, 2010.

Wittmann-Price RA, et al: Nurses and body art what's your perception? *Nursing2012* 42(6):62, 2012.

Young C, et al: A triad of evidence for care of women with genital piercings, *J Am Acad Nurse Pract* 22(2):70, 2010.

CHAPTER

24

Family Context in Nursing

evolve WEBSITE

http://evolve.elsevier.com/Potter/essentials

- Crossword Puzzle
- Audio Glossary

OBJECTIVES

- Examine current trends in the American family.
- Discuss how the term *family* is defined to reflect family diversity.
- Discuss common family forms and their health implications.
- Explain how the relationship between family structure and patterns of functioning affects the health of individuals within a family and the family as a whole.
- Discuss the role of families and family members as caregivers.
- Compare and contrast nursing care that views family as context with family as patient and with family as system and explain how these different perspectives influence nursing practice.
- Use the nursing process to provide for the health care needs of a family.

KEY TERMS

family, p. 618
family as context, p. 622
family as patient, p. 622
family as system, p. 622
family forms, p. 619
hardiness, p. 621
resiliency, p. 621

The family remains a strong part of American society. However, the concept, structure, and functioning of a family unit changes over time. Families face many challenges, including the effects of health and illness, changing economics, childbearing and childrearing, changes in family structure and dynamics, and caring for older parents. Family characteristics or attributes such as durability, resiliency, and diversity help families adapt to these challenges.

Family durability is a system of support and structure within a family that extends beyond the walls of the household. Through divorce, remarriages, or cohabitation new members are added to a family. In addition, an extended family also includes contact with former spouses or partners. For example, in the case study on the next page, Patrick and Michelle are part of an extended family because of their relationship with Lois. Michelle keeps her husband connected with her grandmother. The players may change, the parents may remarry, the children may or may not leave home as adults, but the "family" transcends long periods and inevitable lifestyle changes.

Family resiliency is the ability of a family to cope with expected and unexpected stressors. One stressor on the O'Connell family is Patrick's potential job loss. Not only does Patrick's job provide income and insurance benefits, it defines part of Patrick's role in his family. Patrick's and Michelle's resiliency will affect how they adjust to this stressor. For example, if Michelle needs to resume full-time work with benefits, will Patrick be able and willing to take over household tasks and care for Lois? The family's ability to adapt to role changes, developmental milestones, and crises shows

CASE STUDY ***The O'Connell Family***

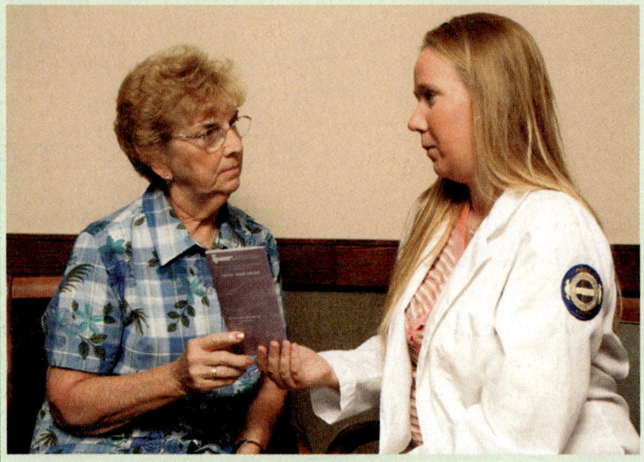

Patrick and Michelle O'Connell have been married for 10 years. Patrick is 44 years old and works in the Department of Public Safety. Recently he learned that he is in danger of being laid off in the next round of cuts. He has borderline hypertension and admits that his stress level is an 8 on a scale of 0 to 10. He enjoys watching television, playing war games on the computer, and playing with the family's pet dogs and cats. The family has health insurance through Patrick's job. Michelle is 42 years old, is employed part-time as a receptionist at a building supply company, and attends nursing school. They are a childfree couple by choice. Michelle was diagnosed with cervical cancer 3 months after their wedding and had a hysterectomy. Michelle is very worried about their financial problems and the health problems of her grandmother, Lois. She describes herself as spiritual and attends church occasionally.

Michelle is the oldest daughter in her family and the only one of the siblings to maintain routine contact with her 80-year-old grandmother. Her parents live out-of-state and are unable to travel to visit often. Her two sisters live approximately 4 to 6 hours away by car. Michelle has learned that Lois has become more forgetful and less tolerant of physical activity related to severe heart disease. She needs support, and it is probable that this needed support will increase over time. Michelle worries that the only alternative is for Lois to move in with the O'Connells. If so, Michelle would have to rid the house of pets to which Lois is allergic, and her home would require major renovations.

Bethany, age 28, is the nursing student assigned to care for Lois in her community health rotation. She sees Lois living alone in a clean mobile home in a nice park. Although Lois receives Social Security and has Medicare, she cannot afford supplemental insurance.

resilience (see Chapter 25). The goal of the family is not only to survive "the challenge" but also to thrive and grow as a result of newly gained knowledge.

Family diversity is the uniqueness of each family unit. As a nurse, you work with many different kinds of families. Some families are experiencing marriage for the first time and having children in later life, whereas others of the same age are grandparents. You also work with families that are headed by a single parent and those with two parents. Every person within a familial unit has specific needs, strengths, and important developmental considerations.

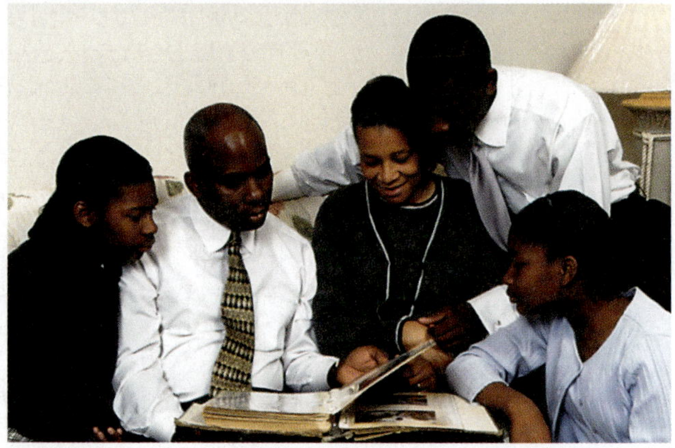

FIGURE 24-1 Family celebrations and traditions strengthen the family.

When you care for patients and their families you are responsible for first understanding the makeup (configuration), structure, function, and coping capacity of the family and then building on the family's relative strengths and resources (Duhamel, 2010). The goal of family-centered nursing care is to advocate for, promote, and provide for the well-being of the patient, family, and individual family members (Brazil et al., 2012; Popejoy, 2011).

SCIENTIFIC KNOWLEDGE BASE

Concept of Family

For some the term *family* evokes a visual image of adults and children living together in a satisfying, harmonious manner. For others this term has the exact opposite image. Families represent more than a set of individuals, and a family is more than a sum of its individual members (Kaakinen et al., 2010). Families are as diverse as the individuals who compose them. Patients have deeply ingrained values about their families that deserve respect. It is important that you understand how your patient defines a family. In other words, think of a family as a set of relationships that a patient identifies as family or as a network of individuals who influence one another's lives, whether there are actual biological or legal ties (Figure 24-1).

Definition: What Is Family?

Defining family seems simple at first. However, different definitions cause debates among social scientists and legislators. The definition of family is significant and affects who is included on health insurance policies, who has access to children's school records, who files joint tax returns, and who has eligibility for sick-leave benefits or public assistance programs. A **family** is a set of interacting individuals related by blood, marriage, or adoption who usually live together and fulfill functions of socialization, division of labor, and economic provisions and cooperatively meet affective and

BOX 24-1 FAMILY FORMS

NUCLEAR FAMILY
A nuclear family consists of husband and wife (and perhaps one or more children).

EXTENDED FAMILY
An extended family includes relatives (aunts, uncles, grandparents, and cousins) in addition to the nuclear family.

SINGLE-PARENT FAMILY
A single-parent family is formed when one parent leaves the nuclear family because of death, divorce, or desertion or when a single person decides to have or adopt a child.

BLENDED FAMILY
A blended family is formed when parents bring unrelated children from prior or foster parenting relationships into a new, joint living situation.

ALTERNATIVE PATTERNS OF RELATIONSHIPS
These relationships include multiadult households, "skip-generation" families (grandparents caring for grandchildren, which commonly results from legal interventions such as when the parent is convicted of a crime or dies and there is no other parent available), communal groups with children, "nonfamilies" (adults living alone), and cohabitating partners.

emotional needs of the individuals within the family unit. In addition, individuals living together, regardless of their relationship or whether they fulfill common social functions, constitute a household. When you provide individualized family care, understand that families take many forms and have diverse cultural and ethnic orientations. In addition, no two families are alike. Each has its own strengths, weaknesses, resources, and challenges.

Current Trends and New Family Forms

Family forms are patterns of people who are identified as family members. These family members are included in the family (Box 24-1). Although all families have some things in common, each family form has unique strengths and challenges. Maintain an open mind about who makes up a family so you do not overlook potential resources and concerns.

Families are constantly changing. People may marry later or delay childbirth; couples may choose to have fewer children or none at all. The number of people living alone is expanding and accounts for approximately 26% of households. Divorce rates have tripled since the 1950s; and, although the rate appears to have stabilized, it is estimated that 54% of all marriages will end in divorce (U.S. Census Bureau, 2010).

The number of single-parent families appears to be stabilizing at about 26% of all families with children. Although mothers head 83% of single-parent families, father-only families are on the rise. Forty-one percent of children are living with mothers who have never married; many of these children result from an adolescent pregnancy (U.S. Census Bureau, 2010).

Adolescent pregnancy is an ever-increasing concern. The majority of adolescent mothers continue to live with their families. A teenage pregnancy tends to have long-term consequences for the mother and often severely stresses family relationships and resources. In addition, there is an increased risk for continued poverty for the family (Harper et al., 2010). Teenage fathers also experience stressors when their partner becomes pregnant. These young men have poorer support systems and fewer resources to teach them how to parent (Biello et al., 2010). As a result, both adolescent parents often struggle with the normal tasks of development and identity and are also forced to accept a responsibility for which they are not ready physically, emotionally, socially, and/or financially.

Although unable to marry by law in all states, homosexual couples define their relationship in family terms. Approximately half of all gay male couples live together, compared with three fourths of lesbian couples. Individuals in same-sex relationships have become more open about their sexual preferences and more vocal about their legal rights.

Factors Influencing Family Forms

Families face many challenges, including changing structures and roles related to the changing economic status of society. There are family challenges related to divorce and the aging of its older members. Social scientists identify six additional trends as threats or concerns facing the family: (1) changing economic status (e.g., declining family income, need for dual incomes, decreased health insurance, or lack of access to health care); (2) homelessness; (3) domestic violence, (4) the presence of acute or chronic illness, (5) trauma, or (6) end-of-life care.

Economic Factors. Making ends meet is a daily concern for many people because of the declining economic status of families. Economics have particularly affected families at the lower end of the income scale, and single-parent families are especially vulnerable. As a result, many families have inadequate or no health insurance, and they have difficulty accessing health care. There are 16.4 million children living below the poverty level, and 7.9 million children are uninsured (CDF, 2012). The Affordable Care Act aims to address this issue by making health insurance for families more affordable, but challenges in accessing health care in the U.S. persist (USDHHS, 2014). *As you read in the case study, the O'Connell family is faced with a potential decline in economic resources. Not only will this loss affect the family finances, but there is a potential loss of health insurance benefit if Patrick loses his job.*

Homelessness. Another factor influencing family forms is homelessness. The fastest growing segment of the homeless population is families with children. This includes complete nuclear families and single-parent families. More than 794,000 homeless are enrolled in the public school systems (National Coalition for the Homeless, 2012).

Homelessness severely affects the functioning, health, and well-being of the family and its members. Children of homeless families are often in fair or poor health and have higher rates of asthma, ear infections, stomach problems, mental illness, and poor immunization documentation. Usually the only access to health care for these children is through the emergency department.

Children who are homeless face barriers such as meeting residency requirements for public schools and inability to obtain previous enrollment records when enrolling and attending school. They frequently lack adult supervision to help them with homework and other school-related projects and issues. As a result, they are more likely to drop out of school, develop risky behaviors, and become unemployable. Homelessness greatly increases the risk for developing long-term health, psychological, and socioeconomic problems in families and children, thus posing a major challenge for our entire society.

Adults who are homeless face health risks as well. They are more likely to suffer from mental health issues and chronic health problems. They are exposed to the elements and have poor nutrition and limited access to health care. When a shelter is present, it is usually an evening/night shelter only. Because adults who are homeless usually live "on the street," they are vulnerable to physical and emotional violence, injury, and trauma.

Domestic Violence. Domestic violence includes not only intimate partner relationships of spousal, live-in partners, and dating relationships but also familial, elder, and child abuse. Abuse generally falls into one or more of the following categories: physical battering, sexual assault, and emotional or psychological abuse; and it generally escalates over a period of time (Futures Without Violence, 2014).

The cause of family violence is complex and multidimensional. Stress, poverty, social isolation, psychopathology, and learned family behavior are all factors associated with violence. In addition, other factors such as alcohol and drug abuse, pregnancy, sexual orientation, and mental illness increase the incidence of abuse within a family. Although abuse sometimes ends when a person leaves a specific family environment, there are often negative long-term physical and emotional consequences. One of these consequences includes moving from one abusive situation to another. For example, a child sees marriage as a way to leave an abusive home and in turn marries a person who continues the abuse within the marriage.

Acute or Chronic Illness. Any acute or chronic illness influences a family economically, socially, and functionally and affects the family's decision-making and coping resources. Hospitalization of a family member is stressful for the whole family. Hospital environments are foreign, physicians and nurses are strangers, the medical language is difficult to understand or interpret, and family members are separated from one another.

During an acute illness such as a trauma, myocardial infarction, or surgery, family members are often left in waiting rooms anticipating information about their loved one. Communication and support among family members may be misdirected from fear and worry. In some families previous family conflicts rise to the surface, whereas others are suppressed. In addition, a shortened length of stay often leads to fragmented care, which in turn increases family and patient anxieties and fears (Laitinen et al., 2011). When implementing a patient-centered care model, patients' family members and surrogate decision makers must become active partners in decision making, care, advocacy, and quality-of-life issues (Brazil et al., 2012).

Chronic illnesses are a global health problem. They are common, and adaptations to them pose unique challenges for families (Weinert et al., 2008). Often a family needs to reorganize family patterns, interactions, social activities, work and household schedules, economic resources, and other family needs and functions to adapt to the chronic illness or disability. Families must also learn how to manage many aspects of their loved one's illness or disability (Tamayo, 2010). Astute nursing care helps a family prevent and/or manage medical crises, control symptoms, learn how to provide specific therapies, adjust to changes over the course of an illness, avoid isolation, obtain community resources, and resolve conflict. Families and the health care team need to develop partnerships to identify available health care and community resources for disease management (Weinert et al., 2008). As with all serious illnesses, caring for a family member whose chronic illness worsens is socially, emotionally, and financially devastating; and it affects the entire family.

Trauma. Trauma is a sudden unplanned event. Family members need to cope with the challenges of a severe, life-threatening event, which can include the stressors associated with an intensive care environment, anxiety and depression, and economic burden, not to mention the impact on a family's functioning and decision making (McDaniel and Allen, 2012). When caring for family members, answer their questions honestly. When you do not know the answer, find someone who does. Provide realistic assurance; giving false hope breaks the nurse-patient trust and also affects how the family can adjust to "bad news." Take time to be sure that the family is comfortable. You can bring them something to eat or drink, give them a blanket, or encourage them to get a meal. Sometimes telling the family that you will stay with their loved one while they are gone is all they need to feel comfortable in leaving.

End-of-Life Care. At times, a family member becomes terminally ill. Although people equate terminal illness with cancer, there are other diseases with terminal aspects (e.g., heart failure and neuromuscular diseases). Even if family members are prepared for their loved one's death, their need for information, support, assurance, and presence are great (see Chapter 26). The more you know about your patient's family, how they interact with one another, their strengths, and their weaknesses, the better. Each family approaches and copes with end-of-life decisions differently. Give the family information about the dying process. Help set up home care and obtain hospice and other appropriate resources, including grief support. Be sure that the family knows what to do at the time of death. If you are present at the time of death, be sensitive to the family's needs (e.g., provide for privacy and allow sufficient time for saying good-byes).

Structure

Structure is based on the ongoing membership of the family and the pattern of relationships, which are often numerous and complex. Each family has a unique structure and way of functioning. For example, in the case study you see that Michelle has relationships with her husband, grandmother, employer, and colleagues in school. Each of these relationships has different demands, roles, and expectations. The multiple relationships and their expectations are often sources for personal and family stress (see Chapter 25).

Although the definitions of structure vary, you can assess family structure by asking the following questions: "Who is included in the family?" "Who performs which tasks?" and "Who makes which decisions?" Structure either enhances or detracts from the family's ability to respond to the expected and unexpected stressors of daily life. Structures that are too rigid or flexible often threaten family functioning. Rigid structures specifically dictate who accomplishes different tasks and also limits the number of people outside the immediate family allowed to assume these tasks. For example, in a rigid family the mother is the only acceptable person to provide emotional support for the children and/or to perform all of the household chores. The husband is the only acceptable person to provide financial support, maintain the vehicles, do the yard work, and/or do all of the home repairs. A change in the health status of the person responsible for a task places a burden on a rigid family because no other person is available, willing, or considered acceptable to assume that task. An extremely flexible structure also presents problems for the family. An absence of stability often impairs the ability to take action during a crisis or rapid change.

Function

Family functioning is what a family does. Specific functional aspects include how a family reproduces, interacts to socialize its young, cooperates to meet economic needs, and relates to the community or larger society. Family functioning also focuses on the processes used by a family to achieve its goals. These processes include communication among family members, goal setting, conflict resolution, nurturing, and use of internal and external resources. Although many families pursue these goals at various times during their development, the provision of psychological support remains an important goal throughout the life span.

Developmental Stages

Families, like individuals, change and grow over time. Although families are far from identical to one another, they have a basic pattern and similarity in experiences resulting in predictable stages. Each of these developmental stages has its own challenges, needs, and resources and includes tasks that need to be completed before the family is able to successfully move on to the next stage (Table 24-1).

Family and Health

Multiple factors influence the health of a family (e.g., its social resources, economic resources, geographical location, and genetic factors). The family is the primary social context in which health promotion and disease prevention take place. A family's beliefs, values, culture, and practices strongly influence health-promoting behaviors of its members. When a family satisfactorily meets its goals through adequate functioning, its members tend to feel positive about themselves and their family. Conversely, when they do not meet goals, families view themselves as ineffective.

Good health is not always highly valued; in fact, harmful practices are acceptable in some families; some of these practices might include poor dietary habits such as high-caloric, high-fat diets. A long-term illness in one of the family members affects the well-being and health of the entire family. In addition, long-term habits such as smoking also influence the health of members in the family unit. Although illness strains relationships, research indicates that family members have the potential to be a primary force for coping.

Hardiness and **resiliency** are factors that moderate a family's stress. Family hardiness is the internal strengths and durability of the family unit. A sense of control over the outcome of life, a view of change as beneficial and growth producing, and an active rather than passive orientation in adapting to stressful events characterize family hardiness (McCubbin, McCubbin, and Thompson, 1996). Resiliency helps to evaluate healthy responses when individuals and families are experiencing stressful events. Resources and techniques that a family or individuals within the family use to maintain a balance or level of health enhance a family's resiliency. *Hardiness and resiliency are important for the O'Connell family. The strong marital bond between Patrick and Michelle helps them balance the new demands as Lois's health declines.*

Genetic factors reflect a family's heredity or genetic susceptibility to a disease that may or may not result in actual development of the disease (U.S. Department of Energy, Genomic Science Program, 2012). Sometimes genetic factors and genetic counseling information help family members decide whether or not to test for the presence of the disease and/or have children. Some families choose not to have children; other families choose not to know genetic risks and have children; and other families choose to know the risk and then determine whether or not to have children. Some of these diseases such as heart or kidney disease are manageable. With genetic risks for certain cancers such as breast cancer, a family member may choose to have prophylactic mastectomies to reduce the risk for developing the disease. Families with genetic neurological diseases such as Huntington's disease may choose not to have children. When families know of these risks, they have the opportunity to make informed decisions about their lifestyle and health behaviors, are more

TABLE 24-1 STAGES OF THE FAMILY LIFE CYCLE

FAMILY LIFE CYCLE STAGE	EMOTIONAL PROCESS OF TRANSITION: KEY PRINCIPLES	CHANGES IN FAMILY STATUS REQUIRED TO PROCEED DEVELOPMENTALLY
Unattached young adults	Accepting parent-offspring separation	Differentiating self in relation to family of origin Developing intimate peer relationships Establishing self in work
Joining of families through marriage: newly married couple	Committing to new family system	Forming marital system Realigning relationships with extended families and friends to include spouse
Family with young children	Accepting new generation of members into system	Adjusting marital system to make space for children Taking on parenting roles Realigning relationships with extended family to include parenting and grandparenting roles
Family with adolescents	Increasing flexibility of family boundaries to include children's independence	Shifting parent-child relationships to permit adolescents to move into and out of system Refocusing on midlife marital and career issues Beginning shift toward concerns for older generation
Family with young adults	Accepting multitude of exits from and entries into family system	Renegotiating marital system as couple or unit of only two Developing adult-to-adult relationships between grown children and their parents Realigning relationships to include in-laws and grandchildren Dealing with disabilities and death of parents (grandparents)
Family without children		Refocusing on new career opportunities Refocusing on marital and career issues Renegotiating recreational activities
Family in later life	Accepting shifting of generational roles	Maintaining own or couple functioning and interests in face of physiological decline; exploring new familial and social role options Supporting more central role for middle generation Making room in system for wisdom and experience of older adults; supporting older generation without overfunctioning for them Retiring; change in role Dealing with loss of spouse, siblings, and other peers and preparing for own death; reviewing life and integrating

Data from Duvall EM, Miller BC: *Marriage and family development,* ed 6, Boston, 2005, Allyn and Bacon.

vigilant about changes in their health, and in some cases seek medical intervention earlier.

NURSING KNOWLEDGE BASE

To begin work with families you need a scientific knowledge base in family theory and family nursing. The two concepts interact to affect the care that you deliver to the family. All practice settings and health care environments emphasize family nursing.

Family Nursing: Family as Context, as Patient, and as System

In caring for a family, your goal is to help a family and its individual members reach and maintain maximum health in any given situation throughout and beyond the illness experience. Family nursing is based on the assumption that all people, regardless of age, are a member of some type of family form (see Box 24-1). *In the case study Bethany either telephones or meets with Michelle every 2 weeks and strives to offer Michelle strategies that allow her to help Lois adapt to the physical limits of her heart disease. In addition, Bethany also offers Patrick and Michelle preparation strategies to adjust to the impending changes in their family life resulting from Lois's illness and the change in the family's finances.*

There are different approaches for family nursing practice. This chapter presents three levels of approaches: (1) **family as context,** (2) **family as patient,** and (3) **family as system.** Family as system is a newer model and includes both relational and transactional concepts. All approaches recognize that a nursing intervention for one member influences all members and affects family functioning. Families are continually changing. As a result, the need for family support changes over time, and it is important for you to understand that the family is more complex than simply a combination of individual members.

Family as Context. When you view the family as context, your primary focus is on the health and development of an individual member existing within a specific environment (i.e., the patient's family). Although you focus the nursing process on the individual's health status, you also assess the extent to which the family provides the individual's basic needs. These needs vary, depending on the individual's developmental level and situation. Because families provide more than just material essentials, you also need to consider their ability to help the patient meet psychological needs.

Family as Patient. When you view the family as patient, the family processes and relationships (e.g., parenting or family caregiving) are your primary focus of care. Focus your nursing assessment on the family patterns versus individual member characteristics. Concentrate on patterns and processes that are consistent with reaching and maintaining family and individual health. In the case study Bethany focuses on the O'Connell family as the patient. Care is planned to meet not only the patient's needs but also the changing needs of the family. Use an interdisciplinary approach when a family's needs are complex. Know the limits of nursing practice and make referrals when appropriate.

Family as System. It is important to understand that, although you make theoretical and practical distinctions between the family as context and the family as patient, they are not necessarily mutually exclusive. When you care for the family as a system, you are caring for each family member (family as context) and the family unit (family as patient), using all community, social, and psychosocial resources.

CRITICAL THINKING

You apply elements of critical thinking whenever you perform the nursing process with patients. Consider the scientific knowledge you have learned, your experience, critical thinking attitudes, and standards to ensure an individualized approach to patient care. Critical thinking is crucial in the care of patients and their families. As a nurse you synthesize all aspects of critical thinking to give individualized, compassionate family care. The care of a family is an ongoing mutually acceptable relationship. As you begin to provide family-centered care, you continually assess, analyze, and reflect on the changing needs and health care goals of your patients and their families.

Synthesis

Scientific and family nursing knowledge, experience, critical thinking attitudes, and standards enable you to identify the needs of both patients and their families. Synthesis of these elements enables you to assess the family as context, as patient, or as a system and to gain information about the family life cycle perspective, family structure and functioning, and family health (Box 24-2).

BOX 24-2 SYNTHESIS IN PRACTICE

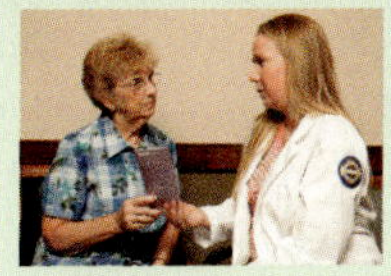

Bethany assesses Lois's health care demands and basic physiological needs. She analyzes the role strain on Michelle and how this affects her relationship with Patrick. She also is aware of the impact of stress on Patrick's health status and control of his hypertension. She knows that Lois wants to stay in her home and Michelle wants to help that happen. Bethany asks about any extended-family members. Michelle says that she has two sisters who live 4 and 6 hours away. They are willing to come and help care for Lois. Michelle's two sisters plan on alternating visits every month to help Patrick and Michelle.

If Bethany views the family as the context, she focuses on each member of the family. Lois's changes in health affect the family greatly, and Bethany's care helps Lois improve her ability to tolerate exercise and maximize her independence. In addition, Bethany helps Michelle reduce stress by teaching her relaxation and meditation techniques, helping her to plan "down time," and giving her some time-management techniques. Bethany assesses Patrick's knowledge of ways to manage his blood pressure (e.g., reducing the number of high-sodium foods and using stress-reduction techniques) and helps him plan "down time" as well.

When she views the family as a patient, Bethany assesses the family's goals for Lois's care and independence. She assesses their caregiving strengths, needs, and weaknesses, as well as the resources available to the family as they assume the role of caregiver. She observes the impact that caregiving has on Michelle and Patrick and also asks about Michelle's siblings who are helping with the care.

As Bethany views the family as a system, she needs to work with the entire family to help Lois transition from her own home. One possible solution to this problem is to help the family select an assisted-living community located halfway between the O'Connell home and the homes of Michelle's two sisters.

Knowledge. The health and functioning of each family member to some degree depends on the health of the family system as a whole. Family care draws on knowledge from growth and development, psychology, communication, family theories, sociology, and the family life cycle. When a family is in a transitional phase of the life cycle perspective (e.g., birth of a first child) or there is an additional stressor to the family unit (e.g., chronic illness), it creates considerable anxiety and stress within the family system. Your knowledge of stress and coping helps in family care.

Experience. Your past experiences in related situations help you solve problems. We all draw on life experiences even if we are not able to draw on nursing knowledge. Experiences in your own family help you design family-centered care. Carefully appraise past experiences and your use of experience-related information because no two families are alike.

It is possible for illness to bring family members closer together because they all share duties, roles, and responsibilities. Conversely, illnesses, especially critical or life-threatening illnesses, have the potential to pull families apart. *In the case study as Lois's health declines, Patrick and Michelle look for ways to help her. As the case study progresses you see that Michelle begins to reach out to her siblings for help.*

Attitudes. Keep an open mind to identify a patient's needs and begin to solve problems and apply critical thinking attitudes such as creativity, perseverance, and risk taking. Partner with a patient and family to use the strengths from a patient's family structure and function, beliefs, values, and expectations to develop a comprehensive, multidisciplinary plan of care.

Standards. As a nurse you apply nursing standards (e.g., critical care, obstetrical, or gerontological) that pertain to a family. In the case study Bethany applies gerontological nursing standards when offering guidelines for Lois's care. In addition, it is important to apply ethical principles when supporting family decisions such as helping family members accept the advance directives of their loved ones. You need to keep all information about a family confidential in all health care settings. In family-centered care there may be many health care providers; therefore be sure to document pertinent information accurately and consistently.

NURSING PROCESS

The nursing process is the same whether the focus is family as patient, context, or system. It is also the same as that used with individuals and incorporates the needs of the family and those of the patient.

ASSESSMENT

Family assessment is a priority for providing adequate family care and support. You have an essential role in helping families adjust to acute and chronic illnesses; however, you must first understand the family unit, what the patient's illness means to the family members and family functioning, and the support the family needs (Kaakinen et al., 2010). It is essential to assess a patient and family thoroughly (Table 24-2). The family as a whole differs from individual members. The measure of family health is more than a summation of the health of all members. Areas included in family assessment are the form, structure, and function of the family; its developmental stage; and its progress toward or accomplishment of developmental tasks. Begin assessment by considering the views of a patient toward the family. To determine the family form and membership, ask the patient to tell you about the family: "Who do you consider your family?" or "With whom do you share your concerns?" If the patient is unable to express a concept of family, ask with whom the patient lives, spends time, and shares confidences. Then ask the patient to confirm that people mentioned are his or her family: "Do you consider this person to be family or like family to you?"

Structure and Function. It is important to assess family structure and function and determine the effects of illness and the support the family requires (Anderson and Friedemann, 2010). Family structure provides information about composition of the family (e.g., whether it is a nuclear

TABLE 24-2 **FOCUSED PATIENT ASSESSMENT**

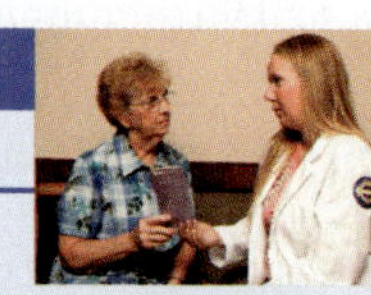

FACTORS TO ASSESS	QUESTIONS	PHYSICAL ASSESSMENT
Family resources	Are there significant relatives and friends not occupying immediate residence? How does your family cope? What do you see as your family's coping strengths/coping challenges or needs? How does your family obtain health services?	When possible, observe family member interaction. Review past medical experiences of the family. Observe for physical signs of stress or coping difficulties (e.g., rapid speech, difficulty focusing, weight gain/loss, increased blood pressure, heart rate) (see Chapter 25).
Family patterns	Who works outside the home, type of work, and hours worked? How does your family divide the work of the family such as household chores (e.g., housekeeping, shopping, repairs), childrearing responsibilities, and care of older parents? How are decisions made (e.g., day-to-day decisions, financial decisions, health care decisions)?	Observe communication patterns with individual family members. Observe family members as they make decisions (e.g., regarding health care, discharge planning) to help obtain this information.
Family function	Does your family have any short- and long-term goals regarding a variety of subjects (e.g., childrearing, retirement, health care)? Do these goals change because of an illness of a family member?	Observe communication and interaction patterns within the family.

or extended family). To assess family structure it is helpful to determine the following: who is the head of the household, who is the wage earner, how are decisions made, and who maintains the household. To assess family functioning, ask questions to determine the power structure and patterning of roles and tasks. For example, "How are financial decisions made?" "Who makes decisions for the family?" "How are the tasks divided in your family (e.g., who does the laundry and who mows the lawn)?" and "Who decides where to go on vacation?"

Cultural Aspects. Conduct a comprehensive, culturally sensitive family assessment to form an understanding of family life, current changes in family life, and overall goals and expectations, as well as to plan family-centered care. A family's cultural background (see Chapter 20) is an important variable when assessing the family. Education, geographic location of home, race, and ethnicity affect structure, function, health beliefs, values, and the way a family perceives events. The United States is increasingly more diverse. A large number of immigrants enter the country daily, adding to both the number and the variety of ethnic groups that make up the population. American health care institutions tend to operate from a white, middle-class perspective; and immigrant populations often have difficulty understanding and "fitting into" the system.

Forming conclusions about families' needs based on cultural backgrounds requires critical thinking. It is imperative to remember that categorical generalizations are often misleading (e.g., Asian Americans consume low-fat diets, impoverished patients are unmotivated.) Overgeneralizations do not lead to greater understanding of the culturally diverse family. Culturally different families vary in meaningful and significant ways; however, neglecting to examine similarities leads to inaccurate assumptions and stereotyping.

Knowing about a family's culture and the meaning of that culture to a family's structure and functioning, health practices, and family celebrations helps you design family-centered care (Box 24-3). To determine the influence of culture on a family, you ask a patient about his or her cultural background. Then ask questions concerning cultural practices. For example, "What type of foods do you eat?" "Who cares for sick family members?" "Have you or anyone in your family been hospitalized?" "Did family members remain at the hospital?" "Do you use some of the health practices of your culture such as acupuncture or meditation?" "What role do grandparents play in raising your children?"

Family-Focused Care. Use a family-focused approach to enhance your nursing care. When you establish a relationship with a family, it is important to identify potential and external resources. A complete patient and family assessment provides this information. Together with your patient and his or her family, develop a plan of care that all members clearly understand and on which they mutually agree. Goals you establish need to be concrete and realistic, compatible with the family's developmental stage, and acceptable to family members.

BOX 24-3 FAMILY-CENTERED CARE

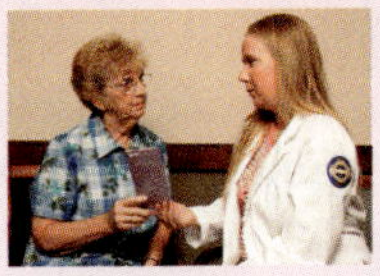

Bethany knows that families have their unique perspectives and characteristics. They have differences in values, beliefs, and philosophies. The cultural heritage of the family often affects religious, child-rearing, and nutritional practices; recreational activities; and health promotion behaviors. As she studies and reviews the literature, Bethany learns that nurses need to have cultural competence and sensitivity when caring for families. Incorporating cultural preferences helps provide family- and patient-centered care, which increases a patient's adherence to therapy, helps the family transition from hospital to home, and provides a unique aspect for care.

IMPLICATIONS FOR PRACTICE

- Focus on the needs of the family and understand the family's beliefs, values, customs, and roles when designing care (Brazil et al., 2012). Perception of certain events varies across cultural groups and has particular impact on families. For example, the care of a grandmother has great significance to the extended family.
- Family caregiving values, practices, and roles vary across cultures (Plank et al., 2012). Bethany knows that in some cultures it is a sign of disrespect to your elders to place them in nursing homes. She knows that Lois's family wants to help her live as independently as possible.
- Intergenerational support and patterns of living arrangements are related to cultural background (Giger, 2013). For example, traditional Chinese, African-American, Japanese, and Hispanic people are more likely to live in extended family households than their Caucasian counterparts.
- Health beliefs differ among various family forms and cultures. These beliefs affect the family's health care decisions about when and where to seek help. Trust in the health care system is a cross-cultural influence. When family members and caregivers have a sense of trust in the health care system, they are more likely to use the system as a resource for decision making (Funk et al., 2010).

Collaboration with family members is essential, whether the family is the patient or the context of care. Collaborate closely with all appropriate family members when determining what they hope to achieve with regard to the family's health. You base a positive collaborative relationship on mutual respect and trust. The family needs to feel "in control" as much as possible. By offering alternative actions and asking family members for their own ideas and suggestions, you help reduce the family's feelings of powerlessness. For example, offering options for how to prepare a low-fat diet or how to rearrange the furnishings of a room to accommodate a family member's disability gives the family an opportunity to express their preferences, make choices, and ultimately feel as though they have contributed.

When you view a family as the patient, you need to support communication among all family members. This ensures that the family remains informed about the goals and interventions for health care. Often you participate in conflict resolution between family members so each member is able to confront and resolve problems in a healthy way. Help the family identify and use external and internal resources as necessary. Ultimately your aim is to help the family reach a point of optimal function, given the family's resources, capacities, and desire to become healthier.

Assessment of family functions includes determining their ability to cope with their current health problem or situation, the need for social and emotional support for members, the appropriateness of their goal setting, and progress toward achievement of developmental tasks (see Table 24-1). Because families' goals vary, make sure that measures of family health are flexible. During assessment assess whether a family is able to provide and distribute sufficient economic resources and if a family's social network is extensive enough to provide support.

Community Assessment. Assess a family's home environment and community. When assessing a patient's home, determine the size of the home, provision for privacy, and safety factors such as presence of smoke detectors and safe bathrooms and stairwells (see Chapter 28). When assessing a community, determine the presence of health care resources, proximity of emergency services, and municipal services (see Chapter 4). If there is a strong extended family, how far away does the extended family live from the patient? Do they live together, in the same neighborhood, or the same city? If the family lives together, how large is their living space?

Patient Expectations. Families, like individual patients, have certain expectations for care. Some families expect to be consulted as a whole unit when discussing care of their loved one. Others wish to have a designated decision maker. The family sometimes expects the health care system to meet all of their needs, not only those related to health issues. When assessing a family's expectations, be clear whether the family or the family member is the patient and receiver of care. Determining these expectations early in the assessment helps to avoid problems resulting from misunderstandings in the future.

NURSING DIAGNOSIS

Nursing assessment results in clustering relevant data and seeing patterns that support nursing diagnoses. The nursing diagnoses selected often include a family's health needs, current and potential health problems, level of wellness, or a combination of these areas. Examples of nursing diagnoses for family-focused care include the following:

- *Risk for Caregiver Role Strain*
- *Compromised Family Coping*
- *Disabled Family Coping*
- *Interrupted Family Processes*
- *Impaired Parenting*
- *Ineffective Role Performance*
- *Risk for Other-Directed Violence*

The nursing diagnosis often focuses on a family's ability to cope with its current situation, whether it is an acute illness, an anticipated developmental transition, or negative behaviors that threaten short- or long-term health. Appropriate use of internal and external resources allows a family to cope with day-to-day challenges and unexpected occurrences that threaten health and equilibrium. A nursing diagnosis often focuses on changes in family processes or roles of members. During times of acute illness, a family becomes extremely distressed and focuses solely on the ill member, neglecting the needs of the other family members. For example, consider the diagnosis of *Risk for Caregiver Role Strain* a possibility when extended care of a family member is necessary.

The diagnostic statement indicates related factors contributing to the health problem. For example, *unrealistic expectations* is a possible related factor. *In the case study Michelle initially wanted to assume responsibility for Lois. However, after making repeated trips to Lois's home and trying to support Patrick, Michelle becomes more stressed when trying to handle all the demands of care. In this case the nursing diagnosis* Risk for Caregiver Role Strain *is appropriate. Another potential nursing diagnosis,* Interrupted Family Processes related to caregiving demands, *is the result of a change in the relationship between Michelle and Patrick. Because of the caregiving demands, Michelle and Patrick are not able to relax and spend time together as a couple.*

PLANNING

Goals and Outcomes. After you develop nursing diagnoses, the next step is to plan care with the family. Goal setting is mutual. The goals need to be concrete, realistic, compatible with a family's developmental stage and expectations, and acceptable to the family. The plan of care for the O'Connell family is represented in a concept map (Figure 24-2) and Care Plan.

A family-focused approach enhances nursing practice. Goals for a plan of care incorporating a family approach include those that view the family as context, the family as patient, the family as system, or a combination. The patient situation and availability of family members define the types of goals that are feasible, thus helping family members to confront and resolve conflict in a healthy way. An example of a goal is "The family will gain improved understanding of family caregiving," with the expected outcome being "Communication clearly describes the role and expectation for each caregiver."

Setting Priorities. Setting priorities focuses on a patient, a patient/family unit, or a family alone. It is imperative that the family and patient clearly understand and agree on the plan of care and priorities. The priorities for a patient and family are sometimes different. For example, the priorities for your patient are to obtain physiological or emotional stability, self-care, or progress to a rehabilitation facility. However, the

CARE PLAN

Caregiver Role Strain

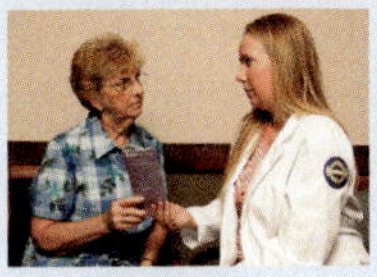

ASSESSMENT

Patrick and Michelle are caregivers to Michelle's grandmother, Lois, who has heart disease and is still living in her own home. Lois suffers fatigue and forgetfulness and poses numerous caregiving demands. She frequently complains about how Michelle helps with household chores. Michelle and Patrick have frequent arguments over how to best help Lois. They both believe that, although they are committed to caring for Lois and maintaining her independence, the caregiving responsibilities take time away from their marital, social, and professional relationships.

ASSESSMENT ACTIVITIES	FINDINGS/DEFINING CHARACTERISTICS*
Ask Michelle if she notices any changes in her sleeping or eating.	**Difficulty sleeping**—includes both **falling asleep** and **remaining asleep** **Poor eating habits**—Michelle notes that she does not eat regularly; and when she eats it is frequently a high-fat, high-carbohydrate fast-food meal.
Ask Patrick to describe changes in lifestyle since Michelle increased her caregiving activities.	Time spent together is decreased. They have **increased arguments.** He **complains about the time Michelle spends with her grandmother and the amount of time she spends worrying about her grandmother.** **He admits to doing less around the home to help Michelle.**
Ask Patrick about any changes in his health status.	Patrick's health care provider said that his blood **pressure is higher.**
Use a scale of 0 to 10 to ask Patrick and Michelle to rate their stress level.	**Patrick rates his stress as an 8.** **Michelle rates her stress as a 7.**
Ask Michelle to describe how she feels about taking care of her grandmother.	**She describes being fearful of "not doing things well for her grandmother."** She **feels anxious** when actually helping with tasks and when at home with Patrick.

*__Defining characteristics__ are shown in **bold** type.

NURSING DIAGNOSIS: Caregiver Role Strain related to Lois's increasing health care needs and unrealistic expectations

PLANNING

GOAL	EXPECTED OUTCOMES (NOC)†
	Caregiver Well-Being
• Michelle and Patrick will gain improved understanding of stress and adaptive management techniques within 1 month.	• Michelle and Patrick are able to identify and share four caregiving activities within 1 week. • Michelle and Patrick demonstrate correct meditation techniques within 1 month. • Michelle and Patrick meditate together 4 nights a week within 6 weeks.
• Patrick and Michelle will use community-based resources within 1 month.	• Michelle and Patrick contact the local council on aging within 3 weeks.

†Outcomes classification label from Moorhead S, et al, editors: *Nursing outcomes classification (NOC),* ed 5, St Louis, 2013, Mosby.

INTERVENTIONS (NIC)‡	RATIONALE
Caregiver Support	
• Discuss with Patrick and Michelle the effects of stress on themselves and the family. • Listen to their individual concerns.	For stress-reduction techniques to be effective, caregivers need guidance to identify specific stressors and their potential effects (Funk et al., 2010).
• Teach relaxation exercises and meditation techniques to reduce their stress response.	Teaching specific problem-solving and coping skills improves family caregiver's abilities to adjust to expectations and changes as patient's disease worsens (Mattila et al., 2010).

Continued

CARE PLAN—cont'd

Caregiver Role Strain

Intervention	Rationale
• Provide a list of support services such as volunteers from faith-based groups or the local council on aging who provide respite care for Patrick and Michelle.	Interprofessional care such as physical therapy (PT), occupational therapy (OT), speech therapy, and meals on wheels are now foundational to transition from hospital to home (Funk et al., 2010). Promoting health maintenance and/or restoration assistance is complex and at times requires community-based groups to help families and reduce strain on caregiver (Marsh and Brown, 2011).
• Call Patrick and Michelle weekly to coach them in use of the caregiving and stress-reduction activities.	Helps satisfy caregivers' needs for hope, confidence, reinforcement, and safety (Plank et al., 2012).
• Consult with Patrick and Michelle to establish a list of community resources, assisted-living facilities, and family support to help with caregiver tasks.	Provides family with organized system of providing supportive, safe care for an older adult who is living in the community (Mattila et al., 2013).

‡Intervention classification labels from Bulechek GM, et al, editors: *Nursing interventions classification (NIC)*, ed 6, St Louis, 2013, Mosby.

EVALUATION

NURSING ACTIONS	PATIENT RESPONSE/FINDING	ACHIEVEMENT OF OUTCOME
Ask Patrick and Michelle to describe how they will divide caregiving activities.	Patrick and Michelle describe new activities for which they assumed responsibility and activities that remained shared.	Patrick is sharing more caregiving activities.
Ask Patrick and Michelle how often they meditate each week and how they feel after they meditate.	Patrick and Michelle state that they meditate 3 times per week together. Michelle states, "It is difficult to find the time to meditate, but we are much more relaxed after we do it."	Meditation is effective. Need to work with couple to reinforce need to schedule meditation 4 times per week.
Ask Patrick, Michelle, and Lois to identify resources found through the local agency on aging.	Patrick and Michelle state they were able to locate resources through their church. The ladies from church come once a week to stay with Lois. Lois is happy with meals on wheels.	Michelle and Patrick have located community resources to help meet caregiving demands.

family priorities include obtaining temporary housing so they are near their ill family member, spiritual support, assistance with decision making, and understanding the complexities of the health care delivery system. In some instances the priorities of the family and patient are different but require simultaneous interventions.

Collaborative Care. In today's health care environment more family members are becoming caregivers, and the transition from hospital to home is at times overwhelming. The family caregiver feels "responsible for everything" and needs to feel "in control" as much as possible (Plank et al., 2012). Collaboration with all appropriate family members when planning care is essential. Base your collaborative relationship on mutual respect and trust. By offering alternative actions and asking family members for their own ideas and suggestions, you help to reduce the family's feelings of powerlessness. For example, offering options for how to rearrange a kitchen and plan meals to accommodate a family member's disability gives the family an opportunity to express their preferences, make choices, and ultimately feel as though they have contributed. Collaborating with other disciplines such as physical therapy and social services increases the likelihood of a comprehensive approach to the family's health care needs, and it ensures better continuity of care. Making referrals to other disciplines is particularly important when discharge planning from a health care facility to home or an extended care facility or from home to an extended care facility (McDaniel and Allen, 2012).

IMPLEMENTATION

Family nursing is used in a variety of health care settings, whether the nurse is providing health promotion, acute care, or restorative and continuing care. Regardless of the setting, some general facts about family nursing are applied across all health care settings. Knowing about challenges for family nursing and principles for implementing family-centered nursing is important to help you develop individualized care for your patients and their families.

Challenges for Family Nursing. Family caregivers are crucial to health care systems and provide the majority of physical and emotional care to patients wishing to remain in their home (Funk et al., 2010). Demographic and social factors contribute to the increased need of family caregivers. Factors such as the increasing percentage of older adults and increased chronic illnesses all contribute to the growing need for family caregiving (Plank et al., 2012).

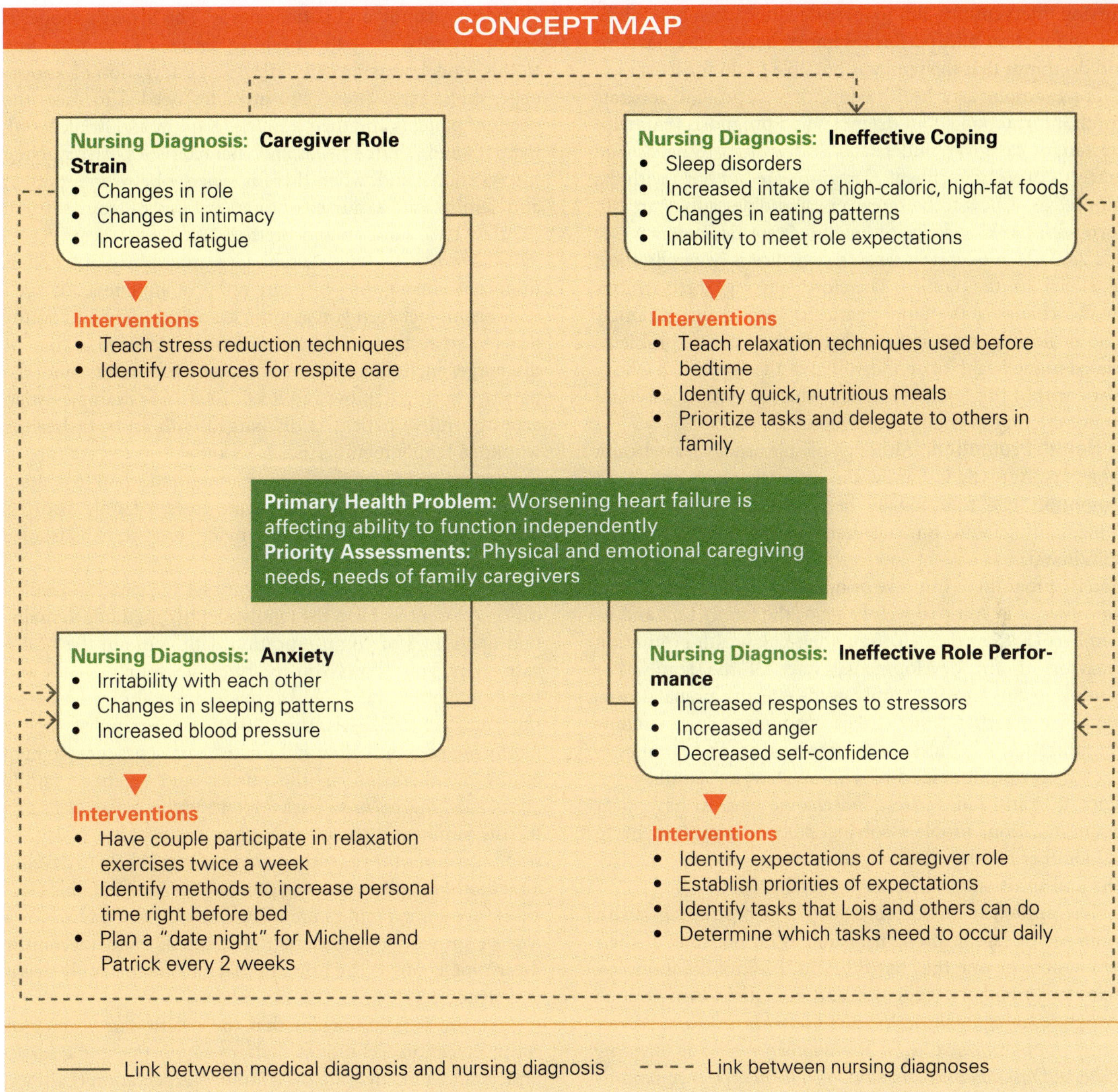

FIGURE 24-2 Concept map.

Delegation in the management of nursing care activities is a challenge in family nursing. Incorporating day-to-day learning outcomes for family caregivers better prepares them for their role and often reduces the stress following the transition home (Frank-Bader et al., 2011). Often nurses try to affect family health by delegating duties to family members or other members of the health care team. For example, you help family members learn how to provide certain types of procedures to care for an ill family member. With earlier discharge and more complex family needs at the time of discharge, planning for discharge begins with the initiation of care.

Using family caregivers is an important resource and challenge for family nursing. Family caregivers need to learn aspects of physical and emotional care for the patient. For example, many family caregivers are now faced with having to perform complex nursing procedures at home such as wound care, enteral nutrition, and intravenous therapy. However, they have physical and emotional health care needs as well. Teach them how to meet their needs. Family caregivers are often used in restorative and continuing care areas; this is discussed in a later section of this chapter.

Implementing Family-Centered Care. Whether you provide care for the family as context, patient, or system, nursing interventions aim to increase family members' abilities to function and perform, remove health care barriers, and do things that the family is not able to do for itself.

For example, as a health educator you provide accurate health information about diagnosis and prognosis that helps the family caregiver understand and anticipate needs and concerns of a care recipient. Caregivers are not born with the knowledge of how to be caregivers, and older adults are not born with the knowledge of how to accept dependency (see Box 24-3). A moderately flexible structure is generally most beneficial to the family. Therefore nursing interventions involve changing the family patterns away from extremely rigid or flexible structures if either extreme causes problems related to the health of an individual or the family as a whole. Work within the family structure when providing care and do not attempt to change the structure.

Health Promotion. Although people usually learn health behaviors from their family, the primary focus on health promotion has traditionally been on individuals. When implementing family nursing, design health promotion interventions such as low-fat, low-carbohydrate meals or a family exercise program to improve or maintain the physical, social, emotional, and spiritual well-being of the family unit and its members (Duhamel, 2010). You often link health promotion behaviors to the developmental stage of the family. For example, a childbearing family needs effective prenatal care, and a childrearing family needs encouragement to follow immunization schedules. Encourage patients and families to reach their optimum level of wellness. "Strong" families that adapt to transitions, crises, and change tend to have clear communication, problem-solving skills, a commitment to one another and to the family unit, and a sense of cohesiveness and spirituality (Schumacher et al., 2006).

One approach for meeting goals and promoting health is the use of family strengths. Families do not look at their own system as one that has inherent, positive components. Help the members recognize and use their own unique strengths. *For example, in the case study Michelle and Patrick clearly communicated with one another regarding dividing household tasks. Family strengths often include clear communication, adaptability, healthy childrearing practices, support and nurturing among family members, and the use of crisis for growth.*

Help family members focus on their strengths instead of their problems and weaknesses. *For example, Bethany points out to Patrick and Michelle that their 10-year marriage probably endured a variety of crises and transitions. As a result they are likely to have the capabilities to adapt to this latest challenge.* Prevention programs aimed at enhancing or developing these attributes are available for families and children in many communities. You need to be aware of family-oriented offerings so you are able to refer patients as needed.

Acute Care. The family is becoming more of the focus within the context of health care delivery in a managed care environment. Acute care settings discharge patients very quickly, and the complexities of today's acute health care settings require you to be astute in assessing, understanding, and supporting family and patient needs. The Synergy Model is useful in providing patient-family centered care. According to this model, nursing care reflects an integration of knowledge, skills, experiences, and attitudes needed to meet the needs of patients and their families (Kaplow and Reed, 2008). Patient's and family's needs and characteristics drive nursing interventions; and, when there is synergy between a patient and family and a nurse, optimal patient outcomes result (Curley, 2007; Gralton and Brett, 2012).

Discharge Planning. Discharge planning with a family is important during the acute care phase of an illness. An open relationship between you as a nurse and a patient and family leads to an accurate assessment of what is needed at time of discharge, including resources in the community and the patient's home (Kaplow and Reed, 2008). For example, when a postoperative patient is discharged with an open healing wound, a family member needs to know how to take care of the wound and recognize complications and when to contact a health care professional. In some cases a family also has home care services, which can provide short-term assistance with wound care.

Communication. In an acute care setting clear communication is essential. Help the family identify methods to maintain open lines of communication with you and the health care team. This allows you to anticipate your patient's and family members' needs and provide optimal care based on these unique needs (Arashin, 2010). For example, when a family member is ill, how will you use caring practices to help family members inform the nuclear and extended family about any progress or setbacks? Identify who makes decisions for the family and consistently go to the decision maker. In some situations the decision maker also needs help to develop a method to clearly communicate any decisions. In this electronic age some families are using blogs on the Internet as a way of providing consistent information. Help the family determine if this is the best approach for their family needs and structure.

Likewise it is important that the health care team uses communication techniques that are supportive and clear to understand and advocate for a family's expectation (Laitinen et al., 2011). In addition, clear communication from the health care team untangles medical terminology and enables the family to understand their health care issues, types of decisions to be made, and possible health care outcomes.

Restorative and Continuing Care. Family nursing emphasizes maintenance of a patient's functional abilities. This means working closely with a family to provide well-timed, individually targeted information; practical guidance; and instructions to help the family understand the specific care taking place in the home (Plank et al., 2012). For example, when family caregivers help with medication administration, it is important for them to understand the importance and aspects of safe medication practices (Box 24-4).

When there are changes in a person's functional abilities, make sure that the home environment is adaptive to the patient's strengths and limitations. Referral to home care nursing is essential. Clear, concise, and accurate communication

BOX 24-4 PATIENT TEACHING

Medication Administration

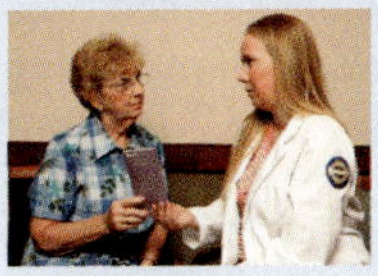

Michelle tells Bethany that Lois's medications were changed. Some of these medications may need to be "held" if Lois's pulse changes. Michelle is fearful of giving her grandmother the wrong medication or giving the medication incorrectly.

OUTCOMES

At the end of the teaching sessions, Michelle and Patrick are able to do the following:

- Correctly place all of Lois's medications in the weekly medication dispenser
- Correctly obtain an apical pulse
- State that, if Lois's pulse rate is 60 beats/min or less or 100 beats/min or greater, she should not be given the digoxin 0.25 mg, and they should notify the home care nurse

TEACHING STRATEGIES

- Provide Michelle and Patrick with a laminated card that lists all medications: include action, side effects, precautions, and premedication assessments (e.g., need for pulse measurement).
- Demonstrate to both Michelle and Patrick how to fill the weekly medication dispenser.
- Demonstrate how to take an apical pulse.
- Discuss with Michelle and Patrick situations in which digoxin is not given.

EVALUATION STRATEGIES

- Ask Michelle and Patrick to identify which medication requires a preadministration apical pulse.
- Observe weekly medication dispenser to determine accurate medication administration.
- Observe and validate Michelle and Patrick obtaining an apical pulse.
- Ask Michelle and Patrick about situation in which digoxin should not be given.

BOX 24-5 SANDWICH GENERATION

- Usually a daughter or daughter-in-law is the caregiver
- Conflicting responsibilities for aging parents, children, spouse, and job (McDaniel and Allen, 2012)
- Feels responsible for everything (McDaniel and Allen, 2012)
- Usually does not recognize need for or request help
- Potential interventions
  - Help families identify additional caregivers in the family or community
  - Help families set realistic priorities
  - Assess for application of "flex time" with caregiver's employer
  - Identify available resources (e.g., respite care, meal delivery, housekeepers)

BOX 24-6 CARE OF THE OLDER ADULT

Caregiver Concerns

- Assess for caregiver stress such as tension in relationships with family and care recipient, changes in level of health, changes in mood, and anxiety and depression (Wang et al., 2010).
- Value and appreciate caregivers' presence to help them feel more positive about their caregiving roles (Plank et al., 2012).
- Later-life families have a different social network than younger families because friends and same-generation family members often have died or been ill themselves. Look for social support within the community and church affiliation (Tamayo et al., 2010).
- Caregivers often feel "trapped" in the care environment. Identify family members, friends, and neighbors who will take the time to socialize with caregiver (Funk et al., 2010).
- Abuse of older adults in families occurs across all social classes. Spouses are the most frequent abusers. Report unexplained bruises and skin trauma to state protective agencies.

with a home care nurse helps to provide continuity of care and facilitate the transition from hospital to home. Educate family members about providing ongoing care and making changes in the home so the patient becomes self-sufficient whenever possible.

Family Caregiving. Family caregiving is a social issue that is becoming more and more prevalent because of the aging population and the increase in chronic illnesses (Marsh and Brown, 2011). It involves the routine provision of services and personal care activities for a family member by spouses, siblings, or parents. Family caregiving is more than activities that include personal care, monitoring for complications or side effects of medications, and performing instrumental activities of daily living (shopping or housekeeping); it also includes ongoing emotional support, decision making, advocating for their loved one, and maintaining the integrity of the family unit (Brazil et al., 2012; Corcoran, 2011).

The fastest-growing age-group is 65 years and older. This "graying" of America affects the family life cycle; it is perhaps most significant for the middle generation. These caregivers are part of the "sandwich generation" (Box 24-5). They find that they need to balance their own needs with those of their offspring and the needs of their aging parents. This balance often occurs at the expense of their well-being and resources. In addition, many of these caregivers report that support received from professional health professionals is often lacking (McDaniel and Allen, 2012; Wang et al., 2010).

The majority of family caregivers provide an average of 20 hours of care per week (Schumaker et al., 2006). Caring for a frail or chronically ill relative is a primary concern for a growing number of families. It is not uncommon for people in their 60s and 70s to be the major caregivers for one another; as a result there are major caregiver concerns for this age-group (Box 24-6).

When family members assume the role of caregiver, their relationship with their significant other often changes (Mattila et al., 2009). One way to best provide family care is through support of family caregivers. Whenever an individual becomes dependent on another family member for care and assistance, significant stress affects both the caregiver and the care recipient. In addition, the caregiver needs to continue to meet the demands of his or her usual lifestyle (e.g., raising children, working full time, or dealing with personal problems or illness). In many instances adult children are trying to take care of their parents while meeting the needs of their own family (Wang et al., 2010). You can support the caregiver in many ways; for example, simply listening to the caregiver's stories and offering suggestions on how to deliver care or find community resources are often beneficial. Also connect the caregiver with other caregivers in the community and, when appropriate, online resources. Finally help the caregiver develop ways to effectively communicate with the extended family.

Caregiving is more than simply a series of tasks, and it occurs within the context of a family. Whether it is a wife caring for a husband or a daughter caring for a mother, caregiving is an interactional process. The interpersonal dynamics among family members influence the ultimate quality of caregiving. Thus you have a key role in helping family members develop better communication and problem-solving skills to build the relationships needed for caregiving to be successful. Caregiving occurs in all aspects of care. As health care costs continue to increase, families are important caregivers. One expanding area for family caregivers is end-of-life care (Box 24-7). You can help family members in their role as caregiver by showing them how to perform specific aspects of physical care (e.g., dressing changes), helping them find home care equipment (e.g., oxygen therapy), and helping them identify community resources. Preparing members of the family for care activities and responsibilities helps caregiving become a meaningful experience for both caregiver and patient.

BOX 24-7 EVIDENCE-BASED PRACTICE

PICO Question: Does an end-of-life caregiving education program compared with standard disease-based discharge planning improve caregiver satisfaction during end-of-life family caregiving?

SUMMARY OF EVIDENCE

Meeting the education and support needs of the family and family caregivers is essential during end-of-life care, whether the patient is in a family home, critical care area, hospital, or extended care setting. Although these settings are different, each family makes the decision based on its own needs and physical, fiscal, and emotional resources (Cohen et al., 2010). Regardless of the setting, family caregivers' priorities are learning about maintaining a quality of life and managing end-of-life symptoms such as breathlessness, anorexia, and fatigue. In addition caregivers want guidance about pain control, comfort measures, and hygiene and nutrition needs (Funk et al., 2010). Families appreciate communication strategies that provide information to detangle medical language and compassion and caring from the professional caregiver (Brazil et al., 2012). For the most part families do not fear having their loved one die in their home or in the family caregivers' presence. What they do fear is an inability to meet the end-of-life needs of the patient such as not knowing how to provide physical and emotional comfort to the patient.

APPLICATION TO NURSING PRACTICE

- Assess family understanding and expectations for end-of-life care. This helps to develop patient-centered care for the dying family member (Brazil et al., 2012).
- Avoid medical jargon and terminology. Help family caregivers become comfortable using the words "dying" or "death" (Brazil et al., 2012).
- Identify patient's priority symptoms and provide specific tips for managing patient-specific symptoms (Plank et al., 2012).
- Avoid the temptation to give too much information about pharmacology or disease process (Brazil et al., 2012).
- Provide opportunities for caregivers to express the burdens of caregiving (e.g., emotional, physical, and economic burdens) (Funk et al., 2010).
- Help caregivers understand that their silent presence next to their loved one's bedside is beneficial; they do not need to be "doing something" all the time (Funk et al., 2010; Cohen et al., 2010).
- Help family caregivers develop an action plan when death is imminent or has occurred. Family caregivers need and want to know the signs and symptoms of impending death.
- Be sure that family members have bereavement resources.

EVALUATION

Patient Care. When a patient's family functions as the context, the evaluation focuses on attainment of patient needs. Thus evaluation is patient centered, although nursing measures have involved helping the patient adapt to the family environment. You compare the response of a patient with predetermined outcomes (see Care Plan).

When the family is the patient, the measure of family health is more than an evaluation of the health of all family members. For example, a family's attainment of family developmental tasks is a useful criterion. You evaluate a family's change in functioning and its satisfaction with the new level of functioning.

When you care for a family as a system, evaluation focuses on the effects that interventions have on the entire family, including extended family. For example, if you are caring for an older adult who has begun chemotherapy for a new cancer diagnosis, you evaluate how the frequent trips to the oncology clinic and the cancer diagnosis affect the patient, the spouse, the children, and the grandchildren.

Evaluation is an ongoing process. Use critical thinking skills and clinical decision making to evaluate your patient's

BOX 24-8 EVALUATION

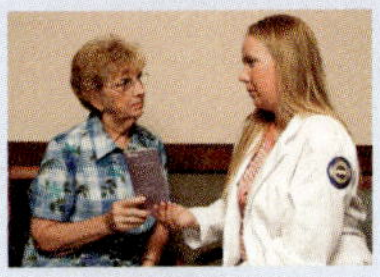

Recently Lois's health status declined, and she needed more supervision with medication administration and her activities. As a result, she needed to move in with Michelle and Patrick. Michelle's two sisters continue to alternate monthly visits to give Patrick and Michelle a 3-day weekend.

Bethany visits Lois periodically throughout the semester and checks to see how the family's short-term goals are progressing for caregiving and maintaining their own family life. She checks to see how Lois's goals are being fulfilled regarding her care in her granddaughter's home, activity tolerance, and forgetfulness. Bethany assesses Michelle's and Patrick's stress levels at school, at home, and when meeting Lois's health care needs. To assess Michelle and Patrick, she requests that the family arrange a meeting once a month. This ongoing evaluation requires a multidisciplinary effort from the home care nurse who knows the family best, the family members themselves, their health care provider, the chaplain, the social worker, and the nutritionist. The nurse is the true coordinator and evaluator of care provided, and Bethany knows this.

Michelle has more free time to concentrate on her studies every other night so she is able to "hurry through school to get a better job to help their financial future plans," as she and Patrick have wanted. One evening a week another family member comes to Michelle and Patrick's home to stay with Lois so the couple can have an evening out.

Bethany discussed the long-term goals of including the community in Lois's care. A registered nurse visits for 1 hour per week, which allows Michelle time to run errands. A volunteer from their church takes Lois to the Senior Enrichment Program on Mondays, and a clergyman visits once per week. Lois sees the nurse practitioner once a month and her physician every 4 months. Michelle's sisters are great resources, and the plan is working well. However, they are also in the process of investigating assisted-living/nursing home facilities for Lois as her health declines.

DOCUMENTATION NOTE

"Patrick and Michelle both report that sitting down together helps them deal with the stress of their jobs, school, and Lois's care. Michelle feels that she and Patrick are partners in the work of the family. Both Patrick and Michelle know that Lois will eventually need an assisted-living setting or nursing home care and have begun looking at placements together along with other family members."

responses to interventions (Box 24-8). Often a patient and/or family does not know the best way to deliver care. For example, a family thinks that a pain medication does not work at all. You make an adjustment in scheduling, and the medication is more effective. Each patient and family is unique. Family nursing requires the use of therapeutic communication skills, scientific and family nursing knowledge, critical thinking skills, knowledge of oneself, and extensive learning about the patients and their families.

Patient Expectations. It is important to obtain a family's perspective of nursing care: how you planned and delivered the care with them; whether it was satisfactory; whether it met the family's goals; and, if not, what they think was lacking. This evaluation is continuous to modify or adjust care delivery techniques (e.g., how soon the home care nurse was able to make a visit, adequacy of comfort measures, or timeliness of care) or even to adjust care delivery personnel.

KEY POINTS

- Because the concept of family is highly individualized, base care on a patient's views toward his or her family.
- Families are as diverse as the individuals who compose them, and patients have deeply ingrained values about their families that deserve respect.
- Family functioning involves the processes used by a family to achieve its goals.
- The goal of family nursing is to help a family and its individual members reach and maintain maximum health throughout and beyond the illness experience.
- The nurse views a family as an important context for an individual family member or views a family unit as the patient or as a system. The approach for any family depends in part on the situation.
- Families face many challenges, including changing structures and roles, especially as the economic status of society changes.
- The family is the primary social context in which health promotion and disease prevention take place.
- As you begin to provide family-centered care, you continually assess, analyze, and reflect on the changing needs and health care goals of patients and their families.
- Goals for a care plan that incorporate a family approach include those that view the family as patient, context, system, or a combination of the three.
- Whether you are caring for a patient with the family as context, family as patient, or family as system, you direct your nursing interventions to increasing family members' abilities to function and perform, remove barriers to health care, and do things that the family cannot do for itself.

CLINICAL DECISION-MAKING EXERCISES

Patrick and Michelle are caring for Michelle's grandmother, Lois, who is in the last stages of heart failure. They are married without children. At present they have health insurance and are facing potential reduction in income because Patrick may lose his job. Lois is easily fatigued, and she needs more help in her activities of daily living. The following are the nursing diagnoses for this family:

- *Risk for Caregiver Role Strain*
- *Compromised Family Coping*
- *Ineffective Coping*

- *Interrupted Family Processes*
- *Ineffective Role Performance*

1. Which stressors are placed on this family?
2. As Lois's health status changes, the physician warns the family her disease will progress. Which additional stressors do you anticipate?
3. Identify priority nursing interventions for caregiver role strain and state why they are priority.
4. What family experiences do you bring to this situation?

evolve

Answers to Clinical Decision-Making Exercises can be found on the Evolve website.

QSEN ACTIVITY: EVIDENCE-BASED PRACTICE

Bethany knows that Patrick and Michelle are committed to their role as family caregivers. However, this commitment has potential stressors that impact that role and also their personal and professional roles. Bethany learns that many of the nurses in the agency are also concerned about family caregiver stress. Bethany works with the medical librarian at the university to conduct a literature search on family caregiving stress. She wants collaboration with the librarian to help her refine the literature search so it is relevant for family caregivers caring for older adults who wish to remain independent as long as possible. She locates six articles: three are studies that surveyed the caregiver stressors, two studies surveyed both caregiver and patient stressors, and one study was a pilot test using meditation as a stress-reduction intervention for family caregivers of community-dwelling older adults.

How would you describe the strength of the evidence? How can this evidence be used to intervene with caregiver stress?

evolve

Answers to QSEN Activities can be found on the Evolve website.

REVIEW QUESTIONS

1. The Collins family includes a mother, Jean; stepfather, Adam; two teenage biological daughters of the mother, Lisa and Laura; and a biological daughter of the father, 25-year-old Stacey. Stacey just moved home following the loss of her job in another city. The family is converting a study into Stacey's bedroom and is in the process of distributing household chores. When you talk to members of the family, they all believe that their family can adjust to lifestyle changes. This is an example of family:
   1. Diversity.
   2. Durability.
   3. Resiliency
   4. Configuration.
2. The most common reason that grandparents are called on to raise their grandchildren is because of:
   1. Single parenthood.
   2. Legal interventions.
   3. Dual-income families.
   4. Increased divorce rate.
3. David Singer is a single parent of a 3-year-old boy, Kevin. Kevin has well-managed asthma and misses day care infrequently. David is in school studying to be an information technology professional. His income and time are limited, and he admits to frequent fast-food restaurants for dinner. He and his son spend a lot of time together. David receives state-supported health care for his son, but he does not have health insurance or a personal physician. David has his son enrolled in a government-assisted day care program. Which of the following are risks to this family's level of health? (Select all that apply.)
   1. Economic status
   2. Asthma
   3. Underinsurance
   4. Government-assisted day care
4. The Cleric family, which includes a mother, Jean; father, Adam; and two teenage biological daughters, is an example of a(n):
   1. Nuclear family.
   2. Blended family.
   3. Extended family.
   4. Alternative family.
5. The Carson family is composed of John, 52 years old; his wife, Sandy, 54 years old; and Sandy's two daughters from a previous marriage: Kera, who is 21 years old and Kathy, who is 23 years old. John's mother, Agnes, who is 78 years old, lives with them. Everyone is healthy. The two girls are teachers, Sandy is a head nurse, John is an aerospace engineer, and Agnes occasionally cooks for the family. For the last 6 years on New Year's Day the family has had a brunch, and the five of them sit down and discuss their personal and family goals for the year, vacations, and activities. This family brunch is an example of:
   1. Family functioning.
   2. Family forms.
   3. Family structure.
   4. Family support.
6. The Carson family structure (in question 5) includes blended family members and intergenerational family members. Which of the following statements best describes family structure?
   1. The process used by the family to achieve its goals
   2. The patterns of people who are considered to be family members
   3. The ongoing membership of the family and the pattern of relationships
   4. The intrafamilial system of support and structure extending beyond the walls of the household

7. Communication is important in family dynamics. Which of the following are possible outcomes for a family with clear communication? (Select all that apply.)
   1. Personal goals
   2. Decision making
   3. Clear methods of discipline
   4. Coping
8. Diane is a hospice nurse who is caring for the Robinson family. This family is providing end-of-life care for the grandmother who has terminal breast cancer. When Diane visits the home 3 times a week she focuses on symptom management for the grandmother, helps the daughter with coping skills, works with the family to identify care resources, and discusses with the son-in-law how he can help the children understand what is happening. Of which of the following is this an example?
   1. Family as context
   2. Family as patient
   3. Family as system
   4. Family as structure
9. Which of the following are included in a family assessment? (Select all that apply.)
   1. Cultural practices
   2. Decision making
   3. Rituals and celebrations
   4. Residential history
10. A college freshman and his mother go to a clinic. The nurse teaches the new freshman and his mother about immunization updates, including the vaccination for bacterial meningitis; stress-relief measures; and the need for regular exercise. Which type of nursing interventions are these?
   1. Health promotion activities
   2. Acute care activities
   3. Restorative care activities
   4. Growth and development care activities

evolve

Rationales for Review Questions can be found on the Evolve website.

1. 3; 2. 2; 3. 1, 3; 4. 1; 5. 1; 6. 3; 7. 2, 3, 4; 8. 2; 9. 1, 2, 3; 10. 1

REFERENCES

Anderson KH, Friedemann ML: Strategies to teach family assessment and intervention through an online international curriculum, *J Fam Nurs* 16(2):213, 2010.

Arashin KA: Using the synergy model to guide the practice of rapid response teams, *Dimens Crit Care Nurs* 29:120, 2010.

Biello KB, et al: Effect of teenage parenthood on mental health trajectories: does sex matter? *Am J Epidemiol* 162(3):279, 2010.

Brazil K, et al: Family caregiver views on patient-centered care at the end of life, *Scand Caring Sci* 26:513, 2012.

Children's Defense Fund (CDF): *CDF statement on uninsured children and children in poverty in 2010*, 2012, http://www.childrensdefense.org/. Accessed January 19, 2014.

Cohen CJ, et al: Family caregiving to hospitalized end-of-life and acutely ill geriatric patients, *J Gerontol Nurs* 36(8):42, 2010.

Corcoran MA: Caregiving styles: a cognitive and behavioral typology associated with dementia, *The Gerontologist* 51(4):463, 2011.

Curley MA: *Synergy: The unique relationship between nurses and patients*, Sigma Theta Tau International, 2007, Indianapolis.

Duhamel F: Implementing family nursing: how do we translate knowledge into clinical practice? Part 2, *J Fam Nurs* 16(1):8, 2010.

Frank-Bader M, et al: Improving transplant discharge education using a structured teaching approach, *Progress Transplant* 21:332, 2011.

Funk L, et al: Part 2: Home-based family caregiving at the end of life: a comprehensive review of published qualitative research (1998-2008), *Palliat Med* 24:594, 2010.

Futures Without Violence: *National health resource center on domestic violence*, 2014, http://www.futureswithoutviolence.org/content/features/detail/790/. Accessed January 19, 2014.

Giger J: *Transcultural nursing: assessment and intervention*, ed 6, St Louis, 2013, Mosby.

Gralton LS, Brett SA: Integrating the Synergy Model for patient care at children's hospital of Wisconsin, *J Pediatr Nurs* 27:74, 2012.

Harper CC, et al: Abstinence and teenagers: prevention counseling practices of health care providers serving high-risk patients in the United States, *Perspect Sexual Reprod Health* 42(2):125, 2010.

Kaakinen JR, et al: *Family health care nursing: theory, practice, and research*, ed 4, Philadelphia, 2010, FA Davis.

Kaplow R, Reed KD: The AACN Synergy Model for patient care: a nursing model as a force of magnetism, *Nurs Econ* 26(1):17, 2008.

Laitinen H, et al: When time matters: the reality of patient care in acute care settings, *Int J Nurs Pract* 17:388, 2011.

Marsh AG, Brown S: Family caregiving: the issue of our time, *Caring* 30(5):22. 2011.

Mattila E, et al: Nursing interventions studies on patients and family members: a systematic literature review, *Scand J Caring Science* 23:611, 2009.

Mattila E, et al: Support for hospital patients and associate factors, *J Caring* 24(4):734, 2010.

Mattila E, et al: The method of nursing support in hospital and patients' and family members' experiences of the effectiveness of the support, *Scand J Caring Sciences* 27:112, 2013.

McCubbin MA, McCubbin HI, Thompson AI: Family Hardiness Index (FHI). In McCubbin HI, Thompson AI, McCubbin MS, editors: *Family assessment: resiliency, coping, and adaptation, inventories for research and practice*, Madison, 1996, University of Wisconsin Press.

McDaniel KR, Allen DG: Working and care-giving: the impact on caregiver stress, family-work conflict, and burnout, *J Life Care Plan* 10(4):21, 2012.

National Coalition for the Homeless: *Who is homeless?* Washington, DC, 2012, The Coalition, http://www.nationalhomeless.org/factsheets/education.html. Accessed January 19, 2014.

Plank A, et al: Becoming a caregiver: new family careers experience during the transition from hospital to home, *J Clin Nurs* 21:2072, 2012.

Popejoy LL: Complexity of family caregiving and discharge planning, *J Fam Nurs* 17:61, 2011.

Schumacher K, et al: Family caregivers, *Am J Nurs* 106(8):40, 2006.

Tamayo GJ, et al: Caring for the caregiver, *Oncol Nurs Forum* 37(1):E50, 2010.

US Census Bureau: *Population profile of the United States: households and families* 2010 (Internet release, April 2012 update), Washington, DC, 2010, The Bureau, http://www.census.gov/prod/cen2010/briefs/c2010br-14.pdf. Accessed January 19, 2014.

US Department of Energy, Genomic Science Program: *Genome Program's biological and environmental research information system (BERIS)*, 2012, http://genomicscience.energy.gov/berismission.shtml#page=news. Accessed January 19, 2014.

U.S. Department of Health and Human Services (USDHHS): *Read the law*, 2014, http://www.hhs.gov/healthcare/rights/law/index.html. Accessed January 19, 2014.

Wang YN, et al: Reconciling work and family caregiving among adult-child family caregivers of older people with dementia: effects on role strain and depressive symptoms, *J Adv Nurs* 67(4):829, 2010.

Weinert C, et al: Evolution of a conceptual model for adaptation to chronic illness, *J Nurs Scholarship* 40(4):364, 2008.

CHAPTER

25

Stress and Coping

evolve WEBSITE

http://evolve.elsevier.com/Potter/essentials

- Crossword Puzzle
- Audio Glossary

OBJECTIVES

- Define stress and coping.
- Describe the three stages of the general adaptation syndrome.
- Identify how stress and coping relate to health.
- Discuss the integration of stress theory with nursing theories.
- Formulate nursing diagnoses based on assessment data.
- Identify stress-management techniques used in coping with stress.
- Develop a care plan for a patient experiencing stress.
- Discuss the relevance of compassion fatigue for health care.

KEY TERMS

compassion fatigue, p. 642
coping, p. 637
crisis, p. 650
crisis intervention, p. 650
endorphins, p. 639
general adaptation syndrome (GAS), p. 638
primary appraisal, p. 640
secondary appraisal, p. 640
stress, p. 637
stress management, p. 640
stressor, p. 637

Responding to environmental stimuli involves both physiological and psychological processes and may manifest in such a way as to adversely affect health. When an event is viewed as a threat, exceeding our ability to immediately deal with it, **stress** results. A **stressor** is any perceived event that can evoke stress. An important part of determining whether an event leads to stress lies in the meaning that we attach to it. How we react to stress depends on how we perceive and value the event, our social and other supports, and usual coping mechanisms. **Coping** refers to strategies or practices that help people deal with stress (Box 25-1). Depending on the degree of stress and the presence of other factors such as social support, coping may or may not be effective. When ineffective, a degree of crisis may result. An important part of nursing is helping to promote positive adaptation in both patients and families. This requires the ability to recognize stress in others and an awareness of how people respond to stress. To intervene effectively you first need to be able to successfully assess for the presence of stress and patterns of coping. In addition, stressful events will occur in the course of your clinical practice that can affect your performance as a nurse. Thus an understanding of stress and coping is an important part of nursing.

SCIENTIFIC KNOWLEDGE BASE

In the early part of the twentieth century the fight-or-flight response was described. This arousal of the sympathetic nervous system prepares a person for action by increasing heart rate; diverting blood from the intestines to the brain and striated muscles; and increasing blood pressure, heart rate, respiratory rate, and blood glucose levels. In an

CASE STUDY ***Rachael Bennett, RN***

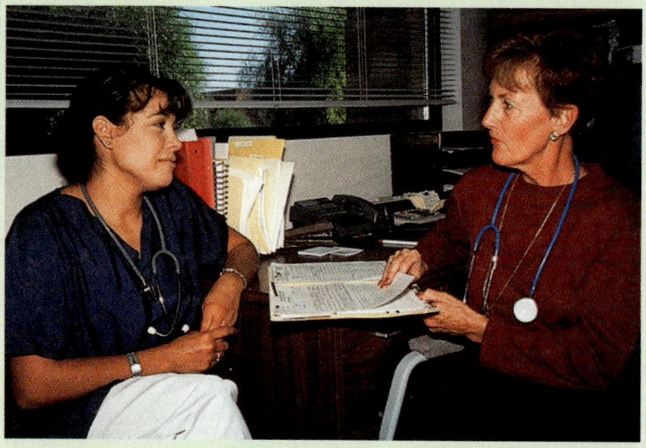

Rachael Bennett, a 32-year-old married mother of three children, works as the nurse manager in a medical intensive care unit. Until recently she has felt very happy with her job. However, patient and staff satisfaction have been declining, and Rachael feels pressured to improve the unit satisfaction scores. In addition, within the past year Rachael's husband has had several hospitalizations related to heart disease, and he is unable to work. For the past 6 weeks she has been feeling defeated and hopeless, has no energy, and has difficulty organizing her thoughts. When her supervisor noticed Rachael's frequent severe headaches, reported lack of sleep, and use of wine at night to relax, her supervisor referred her to the hospital employee health office. One of the duties of this department is to help employees cope with their stress. Becky Howard, a nurse practitioner in the office, does preliminary screening and crisis intervention with staff members experiencing stress and potential substance-abuse problems. The behavioral health care resources are included in Rachael's employee health-benefit package.

expansion of this concept, a three-stage response to stress, the **general adaptation syndrome (GAS),** was described. The GAS was viewed as a reaction to stress consisting of three distinct stages. A pattern of alarm is followed by a stage of resistance as a person attempts to compensate for changes induced by the alarm stage. A state of exhaustion follows if the person cannot adapt during the stage of resistance successfully (Selye, 1993) or if stress remains unrelieved. When stress reaches chronic, harmful levels, deleterious consequences follow, from compromised immune function to weight gain to developmental impairment.

BOX 25-1 FACTORS INFLUENCING THE RESPONSE TO STRESSORS

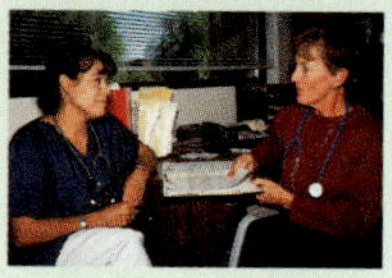

ASPECTS OF A STRESSOR THAT INFLUENCE THE STRESS RESPONSE

As Becky interviews Rachael, she learns more about Rachael's stressors and how she perceives them.

Intensity

Rachael experiences pressures at work and home. This combination of stressors creates continuous intensity.

Scope

Rachael's stress pervades her life, both at work and at home, day and night.

Duration

Rachael has been feeling the effects of stress for about 6 weeks, having problems sleeping and feelings of hopelessness.

Number and Nature of Other Stressors Present

Rachael has multiple stressors. She has stress at home from her husband's hospitalizations and at work with low staff and patient satisfaction scores.

Predictability

Rachael is unable to anticipate or control the stressor of her husband's illness or the poor satisfaction scores.

CHARACTERISTICS OF THE INDIVIDUAL THAT INFLUENCE THE STRESS RESPONSE

Level of Personal Control

Rachael feels no control over patient and staff satisfaction at work or her husband's disability.

Feelings of Competence

Rachael questions her competence at work with the lower satisfaction scores.

Cognitive Appraisal

Rachael is telling herself that she is a failure, and she is afraid of losing her job. Her identity as a nurse and her image of nursing conflict with the events in her life.

Availability of Social Supports

Rachael does not report having the support of other people who could help reduce her stress.

General Adaptation Syndrome

The GAS is a pattern of physiological responses to stress. It involves the autonomic nervous system and the endocrine system, resulting in numerous symptoms (Table 25-1). When an environmental stressor such as an injury or some physical or emotional demand occurs, the hypothalamic-pituitary-adrenal (HPA) axis of the endocrine system is stimulated. Neurons in the hypothalamus release corticotropin-releasing hormone (CRH) and arginine-vasopressin (AVP). CRH is transported to the anterior pituitary, where it stimulates the secretion of corticotropin. Consequently corticotropin stimulates the adrenal gland to increase the production of corticosteroids, including cortisol, the primary hormone impacting the stress response. Cortisol increases blood glucose, enhances the use of glucose by the brain, and increases the availability of substances for tissue repair. Vasopressin increases resorption of water by the kidneys and induces vasoconstriction, thereby raising blood pressure. The adrenal gland also releases the catecholamines adrenaline and noradrenaline into the bloodstream. The pituitary gland secretes endorphins in

TABLE 25-1 INDICATORS OF STRESS

SYSTEM	ASSESSMENT FINDINGS	SYSTEM	ASSESSMENT FINDINGS
Physical		**Psychological**	
Cardiovascular	Tightness of chest Increased heart rate Elevated blood pressure	Cognitive	Forgetfulness/preoccupation Denial Poor concentration Inattention to detail Orientation to past instead of present Decreased creativity Slower thinking, problem solving, reactions Learning difficulties Apathy Confusion Decreased attention span Calculation difficulties Memory problems
Respiratory	Breathing shallow Tachypnea	Emotional	Disruption of logical thinking Blaming others Lack of motivation to get up in the morning Crying tendencies Lack of interest Irritability Isolation Diminished initiative
Neuroendocrine	Headaches, migraines Fatigue, exhaustion Insomnia, sleep disturbances Feeling uncoordinated Restlessness, hyperactivity Tremors (lips, hands) Profuse sweating (palms) Dry mouth Cold hands and feet	Behavior/lifestyle	Worrying Decreased involvement with others Withdrawal Change in interactions with others Increased or decreased food intake Increased smoking or alcohol intake Overvigilance to environment Excessive humor or silence No exercise
Gastrointestinal/ genitourinary	Urinary frequency Nausea, diarrhea, vomiting Weight gain or loss of more than 10 lbs Change in appetite Gastrointestinal bleeding		
Diagnostic	Blood in stools/vomitus Elevated blood glucose level Elevated cortisol levels		
Musculoskeletal	Backaches, muscle aches Bruxism (clenched jaw) Slumped posture		
Reproductive	Amenorrhea Failure to ovulate Impotency in men Loss of libido		
Immunological	Frequent or prolonged colds/flu		

response to stress. **Endorphins** are hormones that interact with the opiate receptors in the brain to reduce our perception of pain and produce a sense of well-being (Chrousos, 2009).

In response to stress the sympathetic system is activated and influences most bodily organs (e.g., the heart and lungs). This response is mediated by the parasympathetic system, a set of nerves that inhibit the sympathetic responses and attempt to bring the body back to a state of homeostasis. Homeostasis is a state of physiological balance in which the body has a chance to recover or recuperate from the physiological activation experienced during stress. Over time the body may experience an excessive state of activation that cannot be inhibited by the parasympathetic system. Alternatively the ability of the parasympathetic system to respond to stress may be reduced. This pattern of response reflects the stages of resistance and exhaustion.

During the alarm reaction rising hormone levels result in increased blood volume, blood glucose levels, heart rate, blood flow to muscles, oxygen intake, and mental alertness. In addition, the pupils of the eyes dilate to produce a greater visual field. This change in body systems prepares an individual for fight or flight and lasts from 1 minute to many hours. If the stressor poses an extreme threat to life or remains for a long time, the person progresses to the second stage, resistance (Selye, 1993).

During the resistance stage the body stabilizes and responds in an opposite manner to the alarm reaction. Antiinflammatory adrenocortical hormones are released, and healing occurs. Hormone levels, heart rate, blood pressure, and cardiac output return to normal; and the body repairs any damage that occurred. However, if the stressor remains and adaptation does not happen, the person enters the third stage, exhaustion. The exhaustion stage occurs when the body is no longer able to resist the effects of the stressor and the struggle to maintain adaptation drains all available energy. The physiological response intensifies, but the person has so little energy left that adaptation to the stressor diminishes. The body can no longer defend itself against the impact of the event; and, if the stress continues, it damages the heart along with other bodily organs and lowers resistance to illness. Persistent elevated cortisol levels are associated with chronic health conditions such as obesity, heart disease, depression and anxiety, diabetes, and osteoporosis (Schoorlemmer et al., 2009). Unhealthy coping choices such as the use of alcohol or tobacco negatively affect a person's health and increase the perception of stress (McEwen, 2004; Selye, 1993).

Reaction to Psychological Stress

The transactional model of stress refers to a process of interaction between the person and the environment. When a person encounters an event, there is an immediate process of **primary appraisal** or rating of the event. If this appraisal results in the event being identified as either a potential harm, loss, threat, or challenge, the person has stress. Therefore you need to determine how the patient perceives the event. Following the recognition of stress, **secondary appraisal** focuses on the resources or coping strategies that can meet the stress (Lazarus and Folkman, 1984).

No single coping strategy works for everyone or for every stressor. The same person copes differently from one time to another. In stressful situations people use both problem-focused and emotion-focused coping. In other words, when they are under stress and believe they can do something about the problem, they use problem-focused coping. They obtain information and take action to change the situation. On the other hand, if a problem or challenge seems to be beyond their control, they are more likely to rely on emotion-focused coping and regulate their emotions tied to the stress. In some cases they avoid thinking about the situation or change the way they think about it without changing the actual situation itself (Lazarus and Folkman, 1984).

Psychological adaptive behaviors, or ego-defense mechanisms, regulate emotional distress and thus protect a person from anxiety and stress (Box 25-2). When you recognize that a patient is using an ego-defense mechanism such as denial or displacement, do not point this out to the patient or suggest that the defense mechanism is unhealthy. Denial often helps a patient reduce stress to a manageable level until he or she can cope with it. Displacement means transferring emotions from a stressful situation to a less anxiety–producing substitute. For example, this can happen if a patient acts angrily toward a nurse when the patient is worried about his or her illness, pain, or trauma.

Stress management techniques used to cope with generalized stress and arousal aim to relax and soothe the body and mind. For example, physical exercise, relaxation strategies, and letting go of excess anger reduce physical and psychological tension. Exercise improves circulation and triggers the release of endorphins. The relaxation response, elicited by meditation or progressive muscle relaxation, lowers blood pressure, pulse rate, and respiratory rate.

As a person becomes stressed, the state of sympathetic dominance becomes longer, which compromises the functioning of the higher-order brain systems such as language, motor activity, filtering, and compassion (Ohlensehlen, 2011). Self-regulation skills are effective in relaxing the muscles in the pelvic region to affect systemic muscle relaxation. The relaxation of the pelvic muscles during a time of perceived threat facilitates a shift from the sympathetic system (i.e., fight-or-flight reflex used during periods of perceived threat) to the parasympathetic system (i.e., relaxation and optimal functioning used during periods of safety). This return to parasympathetic dominance allows an individual to regain optimal functioning of speech, language, motor coordination, filtering, and compassion (Ohlensehlen, 2011).

Meditation and other emotive strategies can also alleviate stress. The practice of mindfulness-based stress reduction has been shown to reduce levels of stress (Chiesa and Serretti, 2009; Marchand, 2012). Forgiveness, or letting go of excess anger, also reduces stress-provoking hormone levels. Other well-known stress-management techniques include massage, yoga, cognitive therapy, and nutrition (Seaward, 2012; Varvogli and Darviri, 2011).

BOX 25-2 EXAMPLES OF EGO-DEFENSE MECHANISMS

Compensation: Making up for a deficiency in one aspect of self-image by strongly emphasizing a feature considered an asset *(Example:* A person who is a poor communicator relies on organizational skills.)

Conversion: Unconsciously repressing an anxiety-producing emotional conflict and transforming it into nonorganic symptoms (e.g., difficulty sleeping, loss of appetite).

Denial: Avoiding emotional conflicts by refusing to consciously acknowledge anything that causes intolerable emotional pain *(Example:* A person refuses to discuss or acknowledge a personal loss.)

Displacement: Transferring emotions, ideas, or wishes from a stressful situation to a less anxiety–producing substitute *(Example:* A person transfers anger over a job conflict to a malfunctioning computer.)

Identification: Patterning behavior after that of another person and assuming that person's qualities, characteristics, and actions

Dissociation: Experiencing a subjective sense of numbing and a reduced awareness of one's surroundings

Regression: Coping with a stressor through actions and behaviors associated with an earlier developmental period

NURSING KNOWLEDGE BASE

Nursing Theory and the Role of Stress

Many nursing theories explain and describe stress. For example, explanation of the concepts of stress and reaction to stress constitute Betty Neuman's Neuman Systems Model. Because the Neuman Systems Model uses a systems approach, it helps you understand your patients' individual responses to stressors and also families' and communities' responses. A systems approach explains that a stressor at one place in a system affects other parts of the system; a system is a person, family, or community. Events are multidimensional and not caused or affected by only one thing. Every person develops a set of responses to stress that constitute the "normal line of defense" (Neuman and Fawcett, 2010). This line of defense helps to maintain health and wellness. Physiological, psychological, sociocultural, developmental, or spiritual influences buffer stress. When a patient cannot buffer stress, the normal line of defense is broken, resulting in disease. The Neuman Systems Model of nursing views a patient, family, or community as constantly changing in response to the environment and stressors.

On the other hand, Pender's Health Promotion Model focuses on promoting health and managing stress. She contends that people want to live in ways that enable them to be as healthy as possible and capable of assessing their own abilities and assets. Pender, Mudaugh, and Parsons (2010) advocate increasing physical activity, improving diet and nutrition, and using stress-management strategies to become healthy and remain healthy.

Situational, Maturational, and Sociocultural Factors

Potential stressors and coping mechanisms vary across the life span. For example, adolescence, adulthood, and old age bring different stressors related to separating from family, establishing oneself as an adult, and making a contribution to society. Likewise, coping strategies fluctuate from an emphasis on primarily emotional coping to problem solving as our minds grow and thinking develops.

Situational Factors. Work stress for nurses happens with work overload (patient load, distractions, conflicting priorities), heavy physical work, long work shifts, patient concerns (dealing with death and medical treatment), and interpersonal problems with other health care professionals and staff (Moustaka and Constantinidis, 2010; Sabo, 2011). Coping strategies vary with the individual and the situation. Some nurses often ease coping with shift work by knowing their own circadian rhythms. People who function best in the morning have the greatest difficulty with night work and changing shifts. As people age they tend to become more morning oriented. Morning people need to be counseled about the potentially negative effects of night work for them. In general, people doing shift work need to maintain as consistent a sleep and mealtime schedule as possible (Sabo, 2011).

Adjusting to chronic illness can result in situational stress. The physical limitations posed by a disease state, the uncertainty regarding the future, and other stressors associated with chronic illness provoke stress in not only patients but also their families (Stanton and Revenson, 2011). Furthermore the stress experienced while caring for someone with a chronic illness (e.g., Alzheimer's disease) can lead to adverse health consequences. Family members caring for those with Alzheimer's disease have been found to be at increased risk for the development of cardiovascular complications (Roepke et al., 2012). In addition, family members caring for cancer patients have been shown to display immunological changes that can contribute to the development of inflammatory disease (Rohleder et al., 2009).

Maturational Factors. Stressors and coping strategies vary with life stage. Babies use the emotion-focused coping mechanisms of thumb sucking, rocking, and crying. Children learn to manage the reactions of their caregivers with problem-focused coping strategies. In general problem-focused coping strategies aim to alter the situation and behavior of others, change the person's own attitudes, and develop new skills and responses. Emotion-focused coping strategies aim to manage emotional distress. Examples of emotion-focused coping among adults include physical exercise, meditation, expressing feelings, and seeking support (Kleinke, 2007). Older adults may use a pattern of coping that relies on the interaction between two people (partners, friends, or family members) working together to adapt to stress (Box 25-3) (Aldwin, 2007).

People who cope successfully take responsibility for finding a solution to their problems. They assess the situation, get advice and support, and make a plan. They view challenges as growth-producing opportunities; and they use hope, patience, and a sense of humor. On the other hand, people who do not cope successfully meet challenges with denial and avoidance. They may become angry and aggressive or depressed and passive; they blame themselves or others for their problems (Kleinke, 2007).

BOX 25-3 CARE OF THE OLDER ADULT

Coping Strategies Used by Older Adults

Some older adults report better mental health than younger adults because older adults appraise and cope with stress differently. For example, for older adults healthy coping includes the following:

- Organizing objects in their environment such as using canes, walkers, handrails, hearing aids, amplifiers on telephones, and magnifying glasses to enhance their daily functioning
- Making their daily activities routine and predictable
- Deemphasizing their health problems by using positive comparisons with their peers and finding others who are more disabled with whom they can compare themselves
- Dissociating their body from an illness by attributing the illness episode to external factors such as food poisoning or a hazardous environment
- Making a fatalistic appraisal by attributing control of their health to inevitability, fate, or luck
- Using dyadic coping (two people), or joint coping, to compensate for memory problems and other physical deficits; happens when one spouse or partner anticipates the other's needs and helps as needed, often without being asked
- Arranging one's schedule or actions to help the spouse or partner to facilitate the other person's coping

Data from Aldwin C: *Stress, coping, and development: an integrative perspective,* ed 2, New York, 2007, Guilford.

Sociocultural Factors. Potential stressors affect any age-group, but they are especially stressful for young people. These include prolonged poverty, physical handicap, and chronic illness. The vulnerability of children escalates when they lose relationships with parents and caregivers through divorce, imprisonment, or death or when parents have mental illness or substance-abuse disorders. Furthermore, living under conditions of continuing violence, disintegrated neighborhoods, or homelessness affects people of any age; but these factors are especially stressful to young people (Pender et al., 2010).

Cultural variations produce stress, particularly if a person's values differ from the dominant culture in aspects of gender roles, family relationships, and religious beliefs (Box 25-4). Other aspects of cultural variations begin with language difference, geographical location, family relationships, time orientation, access to health care programs, and disparities in health care (Pender et al., 2010). Uncertainty about immigration status and citizenship can contribute to increased stress.

The culture of being a nurse carries many expectations for people who are nurses. For example, nurses expect themselves to be altruistic and a role model of adaptive and growth-producing behavior. They expect themselves to approach life with a sense of growing, hopefulness, and adapting (Stuart, 2013). When a nurse's home and/or professional life becomes chaotic or overwhelming, the nurse might feel unsuccessful and subsequently stressed.

Cultural differences exist in both problem-focused and emotion-focused coping. Because problem-focused coping attempts to control or manage a situation, culture heavily influences these coping strategies. For example, Americans or Israelis might confront a problem directly. On the other hand, people from Asian cultures might use indirect methods that nevertheless confront a problem situation such as asking an older relative to address a difficult interpersonal situation. However, indirect action does not necessarily indicate passive behavior (Aldwin, 2007). Remember that each individual is unique; thus do not bias your assessment of patients' coping strategies simply on the basis of their ethnic background.

In the realm of emotion-focused coping strategies, various ethnic groups use social support differently. European Americans might go outside the family to social support groups, whereas Africans and Hispanics might rely more heavily on family members rather than on friends. Culture strongly influences expression or control of feelings. Generally people from northern European cultures prefer emotional control, yet Italian and Jewish ethnic groups are more expressive. Many cultures view mental illness as temporary reactions to stress, not necessarily pathological as long as they are time limited (Aldwin, 2007).

BOX 25-4 PATIENT-CENTERED CARE

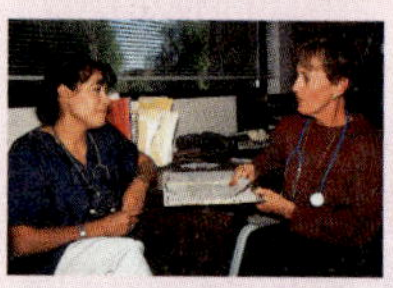

Stress and anxiety may lead to insomnia, as it did for Rachael. Cultural factors are also related to poor sleeping. There are significant differences in rates of insomnia among ethnic groups. Seventy-one percent of the African-American women in one study experienced trouble getting to sleep, waking up during the night, or awakening too early in the morning. European American, Eastern European, and Dominican women had similar high rates. On the other hand, only about a third of Caribbean and Haitian women reported insomnia-related symptoms.

IMPLICATIONS FOR PRACTICE

- Ethnic differences in sleep and insomnia influence interventions for insomnia. Interventions for anxiety-related sleep problems need to be culturally appropriate.
- Suggesting daytime naps may be more culturally acceptable for some cultures such as African-American and Spanish women.
- Ask patients what their family members, especially their parents, do when they cannot sleep to learn about their cultural values associated with insomnia.
- Help patients connect their insomnia with the stress that they are experiencing by asking them what they think about while they are lying in bed awake.
- Ask women with insomnia which coping strategies they have tried.
- When assessing women with insomnia, determine if their coping measures include sleep medication.

Data from Jean-Louis G, et al: Insomnia symptoms in a multiethnic sample of American women, *J Womens Health* 17(1):15, 2008.

Compassion Fatigue

Compassion fatigue is a term used to describe a state of burnout and secondary traumatic stress (Potter et al., 2013). Secondary traumatic stress is the trauma that health care providers experience when witnessing and caring for others suffering trauma. Examples include an oncology nurse who cares for patients undergoing surgery and chemotherapy over the long term for their cancer or a spouse who witnesses his wife deteriorating over the years from Alzheimer's disease. Burnout is the condition that occurs when perceived demands outweigh perceived resources (Potter et al., 2013). It is a state of physical and mental exhaustion that often affects health care providers because of the nature of their work environment. Over time, giving of oneself in often intense caring environments can result in emotional exhaustion, leaving a nurse feeling irritable, restless, and unable to focus and engage with patients. This condition may be viewed as a failure of coping because it often occurs in situations in which there is a lack of social support, organizational pressures influencing staffing, and the inability of the nurse to practice self-care. Compassion fatigue can result in feelings of hopelessness, a decrease in the ability to take pleasure from previously enjoyable activities, a state of hypervigilance, and anxiety (Coetzee and Klopper, 2010).

The feelings of hopelessness and anxiety from compassion fatigue can result in feelings of inadequacy and lower self-esteem. These factors can then lead to the sufferer lashing out in an attempt to cope with these feelings and the attendant stress. This can manifest in what is referred to as *lateral violence,* which refers to health care providers engaging in bullying and potentially assaultive behaviors toward co-workers (Embree and White, 2010).

CRITICAL THINKING

Synthesis

You apply elements of critical thinking whenever you perform the nursing process with a patient. Consider the scientific knowledge you have learned, your experience, critical thinking attitudes, and standards to ensure an individualized approach to patient care. This approach helps you identify specific health care needs and design individualized interventions (Box 25-5).

Knowledge. Physiological changes occur in a patient experiencing the alarm reaction, resistance stage, and exhaustion stage of the GAS. Apply knowledge of these physiological changes. Your knowledge of communication principles helps you assess the patient's behaviors. Consider your patient's perception of the stress. Determine his or her ability to cope with it. If the patient does not succeed with his or her usual coping skills, you need to refer him or her to crisis intervention counseling.

Experience. Your experience teaches you to understand a patient's unique perception of stressors and responses to stress. View every person as an individual, recognizing that no two people are exactly alike. Experience with patients also helps you recognize responses to stress. In addition, your own personal experiences with stress and coping increase your ability to empathize with a patient temporarily immobilized by stress. Understanding a patient's position enables you to intervene more effectively.

BOX 25-5 SYNTHESIS IN PRACTICE

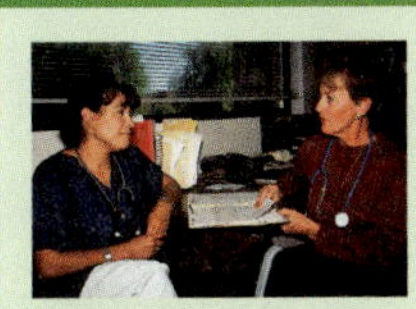

When Becky talks with Rachael, she learns that Rachael worries about losing her job because of the declining quality of patient care on her unit. Rachael provides sole support for her family at this time. She also learns about Mr. Bennett's recent illness and the effect it has on Rachael's overall well-being. Becky has also talked with Rachael's supervisor and knows that Rachael has been having headaches and difficulty concentrating when making decisions.

Becky takes time to reflect on other employees that she sees in the employee health office. Many of the registered nurses have had physical complaints of stress, including headaches, sleep problems, changes in eating habits, and flare-ups of existing medical problems. Becky knows that she wants to be thorough in assessing the responses and symptoms that Rachael has been experiencing. Previous experience with other employees has taught Becky the importance of learning about the employee's family, the type of support they offer, and the person's appraisal of the situation.

Attitudes. Use confidence and believe that you and a patient are able to manage stress effectively. Patients respect your advice and counsel and gain confidence from your belief in their ability to move past stressful events or illnesses. Patients experiencing a crisis often lack the ability, at least initially, to act on their own behalf. They require either direct intervention or guidance. You need to have an attitude of integrity through which you respect a patient's perception of or perspective about a stressor. Make the effort to have patients explain their unique viewpoints and situations.

Standards. Accurately assess a patient's stress, coping mechanisms, and support system before intervening. Clearly and precisely understand a patient's perception of the stress and focus on factors significant to his or her well-being. In addition, select interventions that respect the individuality of the patient. Be especially aware of your ethical responsibility in caring for someone who has less independence because of being in a crisis state.

NURSING PROCESS

ASSESSMENT

Assessment of a patient's stress level and coping resources requires that you first establish a trusting nurse-patient relationship. You ask the patient and family to share personal and sensitive information (see Chapter 9). Learn from the patient by asking questions and making observations of nonverbal behavior, interactions with the family, and the patient's environment. Synthesize the information you obtain and adopta critical thinking attitude while observing and analyzing patient behaviors. Often a patient has difficulty describing the most bothersome aspects of a situation until someone else has time to listen and encourage the patient to explore it.

Subjective Findings. When you assess a patient's stress level and coping resources, sit with the patient in comfortable chairs in a private setting facing one another. Assume a listening posture, establish eye contact, and allow time for the patient to talk. Gather information about the health status of the patient from his or her perspective and begin the process of developing a trusting relationship.

Use the interview to determine a patient's view of the situation that provoked stress; assess safety issues, coping resources, any possible maladaptive coping, and adherence to prescribed medical recommendations such as medication or diet (Table 25-2) (Stuart, 2013). If the patient uses denial as a coping mechanism, be alert to whether the person overlooks necessary information. Listen for any recurrent themes in the patient's conversation. As in all interactions with a patient, respect the confidentiality and sensitivity of the information shared.

If your patient is experiencing a crisis, assess safety concerns such as potential for suicide or homicide and ability to care for one's own activities of daily living. Assessment includes determining the patient's emotions, behaviors, cognitive state, and precrisis level of functioning. In addition, assess for prior trauma, symptoms of mental illness, and use of legal and illegal drugs. Assess whether this crisis is a one-time situation or part of a pattern of a crisis-oriented life history. Finally assess alternatives, coping mechanisms, and support systems (Kanel, 2012).

Objective Findings. Obtain objective findings related to stress and coping through your observation of a patient's appearance and nonverbal behavior. Observe grooming and hygiene, gait, characteristics of the patient's handshake, actions of the patient while sitting, quality of speech, eye contact, and the attitude of the patient toward you during the interview (see Chapter 16). During this part of the interview you need to keep in mind cultural norms that may influence a patient's responses. Before the interview begins or at the end of the interview, depending on the anxiety level of the patient, take basic vital signs to assess for physiological signs of stress such as elevated blood pressure, heart rate, or respiratory rate.

Patient Expectations. Recognize the importance of the meaning of the precipitating event to the patient and the ways in which stress affects the patient's life. Allow time for the patient to express priorities for coping with stress. For example, you are caring for a woman who has just found out about a breast mass identified on a routine mammogram. It is important for you to know what the patient wants and needs most from you. Ask her what she wants to know about the next steps (e.g., surgical or diagnostic procedure). Although some people in this situation identify their need for information about biopsy or mastectomy as their personal priority, other women need guidance and support in discussing how to share the news with family members. Remember that in some cases nothing will change or improve the situation. Allowing a patient to use denial as a coping mechanism is helpful. Gaining an understanding of patient expectations does not mean that you exclude certain types of care that are important simply because a patient does not identify them as needs. However, by inquiring about patient expectations and priorities, you are better able to ensure that his or her needs are addressed in some way.

NURSING DIAGNOSIS

When selecting a nursing diagnosis be sure that there are defining characteristics from your assessment that confirm the diagnosis. For example, major defining characteristics of *Ineffective Coping* include verbalization of an inability to cope and an inability to ask for help. You identify defining characteristics during the assessment (e.g., by asking the patient what concerns him or her most at the time of the interview) and, importantly, allow the patient sufficient time to answer (see Table 25-2). Observe for psychological indicators of

TABLE 25-2 FOCUSED PATIENT ASSESSMENT

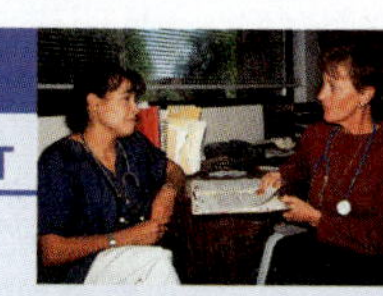

FACTORS TO ASSESS	QUESTIONS	PHYSICAL ASSESSMENT
Patient safety	Do you have thoughts of harming yourself? How are you sleeping? Do you have problems going to sleep or awakening during the night? How has your appetite changed? How does stress affect your work? Are you having problems concentrating? Have you had accidents at home, in the car, or on the job?	Observe for indicators of anxiety, anger, or tension. For example, you may observe such nonverbal behaviors as irritability, crying, and inappropriate laughing.
Perception of stressor	What do you believe is stressing you? What do you think about when you can't sleep? What does this situation or stressor mean in your opinion?	Observe for nonverbal indicators of stress such as rapid talking, crying, changes in posture (e.g., folding arms over chest). Listen for recurrent themes.
Available coping resources	Are you keeping in touch with your friends? How often do you see your family members? What have you done before to cope with similar problems or stress? What do you do for fun? How do you spend your leisure time?	Observe whether the person is alone or with others. Observe the person's communication skills. Observe if the person is able to ask for help. Observe developmental level and sociocultural circumstances.
Maladaptive coping used	How much do you smoke? How much do you drink? Do you use any over-the-counter or herbal medications for your stress? How much coffee or soda do you drink in a day?	Observe for effects of smoking, alcohol, drugs, and caffeine (e.g., difficulty sleeping, nervousness, or difficulty concentrating).
Adherence to healthy practices	How long has it been since you saw a health care provider? Do you get regular check-ups? What type of a diet do you follow? Do you eat regular meals at home? What type of exercise do you get?	Obtain vital signs and palpate for any tender areas. Obtain weight.

stress and nonverbal signs of anxiety, fear, anger, and irritability. After selecting the diagnosis, identify the related factor so you can select appropriate interventions that are relevant and likely to resolve the diagnosis once they are implemented.

The nursing diagnoses that are most applicable to stress and coping focus on ineffective coping responses and the consequences of stress. Other appropriate diagnoses target a patient or family member who is ready for additional education regarding coping strategies. Examples of stress-related nursing diagnoses include the following:

Coping-Specific Diagnoses

- *Compromised Family Coping*
- *Ineffective Denial*
- *Defensive Coping*
- *Ineffective Coping*
- *Readiness for Enhanced Coping*

Stress-Specific Diagnoses

- *Relocation Stress Syndrome*
- *Stress Overload*

Potential Consequences of Ineffective Coping or Overwhelming Stress

- *Anxiety*
- *Fear*
- *Hopelessness*
- *Moral Distress*
- *Post-Trauma Syndrome*

PLANNING

Goals and Outcomes. Desirable goals for people experiencing stress are (1) coping with the stressor(s), (2) family coping, and (3) psychosocial adjustment: life change. Expected outcomes are behavioral markers that show progress toward goal achievement. For example, if a patient is to cope with stress, outcomes may include increasing interaction with others and improved sleep. After setting goals and outcomes, select interventions for managing the specific stressor and improving coping (Stuart, 2013).

Plan care using nursing interventions designed within the framework of primary, secondary, and tertiary prevention. At the primary level of prevention, nursing interventions include preparing patients for turning points in life such as the birth of a baby or the death of a parent. Nursing interventions at the secondary level include actions directed at symptoms such as protecting the patient from self-harm. Tertiary-level interventions help your patient readapt and often include relaxation and time-management training.

Patients' perceptions of stress and coping depend on recognition of the problem and use of coping resources. Similarly, selecting appropriate interventions requires a partnership with a patient and support system, usually the family. In the case of a family or community stressor and impaired family or community coping, your view of the situation and resources would be broader (see Care Plan).

CARE PLAN

Stress and Individual Coping

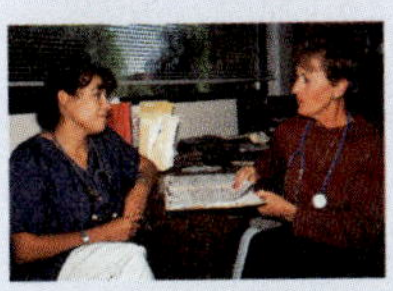

ASSESSMENT

During her initial contact with Rachael, Becky detects a great deal of anxiety but also some anger. Becky knows that it is important to build trust with Rachael as quickly as possible. She knows that Rachael's anger is not directed at her but reflects Rachael's frustration. As a single parent herself, Becky identifies with Rachael's crisis of being the sole financial support for the family. Yet Becky decides not to tell her life history to Rachael because she recognizes that no two persons have exactly the same experience or use the same coping strategies to get through difficult times. Becky wants to be able to work closely with Rachael and establish priorities that are realistic for her to achieve.

ASSESSMENT ACTIVITIES	FINDINGS/DEFINING CHARACTERISTICS*
Observe for signs of stress.	She observes Rachael frequently licking her lips, picking at her fingernails, and being easily startled. Rachael uses poor eye contact and then bursts into tears and expresses feelings of being overwhelmed.
Measure vital signs.	Rachael's **vital signs show changes in response to stress:** pulse, 120 beats/min; respirations, 24 breaths/min; blood pressure, 168/84 mm Hg.
Ask Rachael about recent weight loss.	Rachael appears thin and pale and reports that she has **lost 20 lb in the last 3 months.**
Ask Rachael about changes in sleep.	She also reports difficulty in falling and remaining asleep at night.
Assess Rachael's perception of the stress.	Rachael expresses fear of both losing her job and being unable to support her family. She also expresses **feelings of shame and embarrassment.** She **thinks of herself as a failure for not coping better.**
Ask Rachael about current coping methods.	Rachael admits to having started drinking at night to help herself "unwind."

*__Defining characteristics__ are shown in **bold** type.

Continued

CARE PLAN—cont'd

Stress and Individual Coping

NURSING DIAGNOSIS: Ineffective Coping related to increased pressure at work and multiple family stresses and responsibilities

PLANNING

GOAL	EXPECTED OUTCOMES (NOC)[†] *Coping*
• Rachael will manage stressors that have been taxing her individual resources.	• Rachael differentiates effective and ineffective coping patterns. • Rachael verbalizes a decrease in stress. • Rachael modifies her lifestyle to reduce stress. • Rachael uses her personal support system. • Rachael verbalizes need for assistance.

[†]Outcomes classification label from Moorhead S, et al, editors: *Nursing outcomes classification (NOC)*, ed 5, St Louis, 2013, Mosby.

INTERVENTIONS (NIC)[‡] *Coping Enhancement*	RATIONALE
• Encourage Rachael to identify a realistic description of her changing roles.	A cognitive reappraisal helps Rachael reframe the poor patient satisfaction scores so she does not take all the responsibility for them. How she defines the reality and the personal meaning it has for her directly affects her stress level (Stuart, 2013).
• Use a calm, reassuring approach.	For treatment goals to be accomplished in a short time, Rachael sees the nurse as being nonthreatening, reliable, and understanding (Varcarolis and Halter, 2009).
• Help Rachael develop an objective appraisal of her situation.	Rachael's primary appraisal of the stressor and her secondary appraisal of her coping strategies define the stressful situation (Kleinke, 2007).
• Explore with Rachael previous methods of dealing with life problems.	A problem-solving approach empowers Rachael and improves her self-confidence (Kleinke, 2007).
• Explore Rachael's previous achievements.	Emphasizing the positive helps a person feel more optimistic, which leads to positive actions and results (Stuart, 2013).
• Encourage Rachael to identify own strengths and abilities.	To manage stress and cope with change, people need to know their strengths and abilities and what is important to them (Stuart, 2013).
• Help Rachael break down complex goals into small, manageable steps.	Changing her cognitive view of her situation reduces her stress. Small successes accumulate for her and reduce the magnitude of her stress (Stuart, 2013).
• Help Rachael identify available support systems such as family members and support groups.	Talking with others relieves tension for a person, and helping others as in a support group reduces self-absorption and stress (Stuart, 2013).
• Teach Rachael strategies to increase her resistance to stress.	Increasing resistance to stress is one of the primary modes for intervention for stress management (Pender et al., 2010).

[‡]Intervention classification labels from Bulechek GM, et al, editors: *Nursing interventions classification (NIC)*, ed 6, St Louis, 2013, Mosby.

EVALUATION

NURSING ACTIONS	PATIENT RESPONSE/FINDING	ACHIEVEMENT OF OUTCOME
Ask Rachael about her perception of stress on her life and changes she has made.	Rachael appears less anxious. She exercises by walking with her husband 3 times a week. Her blood pressure is 140/82 mm Hg, and pulse is 88 beats/min. She has a 3-lb weight gain and is eating healthy foods. She is not drinking wine to reduce her stress. During the past week she began sleeping through the night.	Rachael is decreasing the effect of stress by using healthy lifestyle habits.
Ask Rachael about the use of new and former support systems.	Rachael resumed a friendship with a neighbor. She now asks her husband for help at home and her co-workers for help at work.	Rachael is increasing her use of personal support systems at home and work. Consider helping Rachael locate a support group to provide further support.

Setting Priorities. People experiencing stress often have multiple nursing diagnoses that interact with one another. Prioritizing their diagnoses is important in planning care (Figure 25-1). One way to prioritize is to first ask, "What has happened that caused you to come for help today?" or "What happened in your life that is *different?*" This requires some focusing by the patient. Next learn about the patient's perception of the event, available situational supports, and what the patient usually does about a problem that he or she is not able to solve (Kanel, 2012). As in all areas of nursing, make the safety of the patient and others in the patient's environment the highest priority. For example, if a patient is suicidal, determine if he or she is at risk for harming himself or herself. Ask, "Are you thinking of hurting yourself?" If the answer is yes, ask for more information such as whether or not the person has attempted suicide previously, has a plan for committing suicide, and has the means to carry out the specific plan. These questions are sometimes difficult to ask, but a patient who is highly stressed and has thought about suicide at some point is usually relieved when someone else brings up the subject.

Prioritize diagnoses by determining the degree of disruption in the person's life with work, school, home, and family. If your assessment has been thorough, you are able to prioritize problems, ensure the patient's safety, and begin the problem-solving process (Stuart, 2013).

Collaborative Care. An effective plan requires you to collaborate appropriately with health care providers. There are times when nursing practice alone does not meet all of a patient's needs. Patients experiencing stress from medical

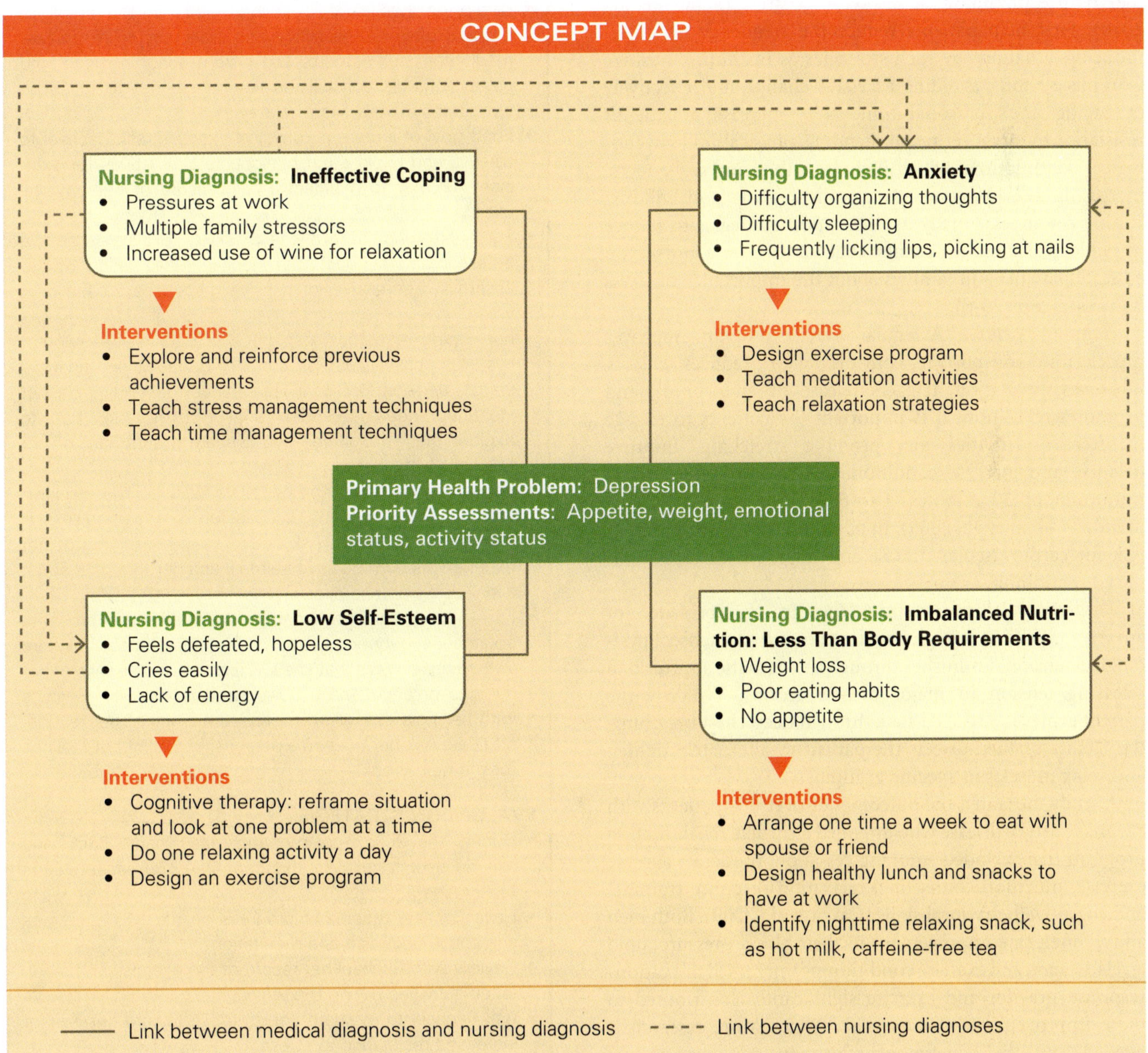

FIGURE 25-1 Concept map.

conditions or psychiatric disorders present needs that make it necessary for you to consult with advanced practice mental health nurses, psychiatrists, psychologists, pastoral care professionals, or psychiatric social workers. Such a multidisciplinary approach to care addresses the holistic needs of your patients. Make the patient and family partners in care. Recognize the need for collaboration and consultation; inform the patient about potential resources; and make arrangements for consultations, group sessions, or therapy as needed.

IMPLEMENTATION

Health Promotion. Intervention for relieving stress has a three-pronged approach: (1) decrease stress-producing situations, (2) increase resistance to stress, and (3) learn skills that reduce physiological response to stress (Pender et al., 2010). First help patients reduce the frequency of stress-inducing situations by such strategies as instituting positive workplace habits, avoiding excessive change, and effectively managing one's personal time. Next increase a patient's resistance to stress by recommending physical and psychological conditioning, which includes enhancing self-esteem, increasing assertiveness, setting realistic goals, and building coping resources. Finally use relaxation strategies to reduce physiological arousal (Pender et al., 2010). As a nurse you educate patients and families about the importance of stress reduction (Box 25-6).

Regular Exercise. A regular exercise program improves muscle tone and posture, controls weight, reduces tension, improves circulation, triggers release of endorphins, and promotes relaxation. It is important for patients to engage in exercise activities that promote stretching, improve balance, and increase conditioning. Aerobic exercise for a minimum of 30 minutes, 4-to-6 times a week is recommended (Khan et al., 2009). In addition, exercise reduces the risk for cardiovascular disease and improves cardiopulmonary functioning.

Progressive Muscle Relaxation. In the presence of anxiety-provoking thoughts and events, muscles tense. Physiological tension diminishes through a systematic approach to releasing tension in major muscle groups. Typically the patient achieves a relaxed state through deep chest breathing; the facilitator then directs the patient to alternately tighten and relax muscles in specific groupings.

A study measured the outcomes of over 600 patients with coronary artery disease who attended a cardiac rehabilitation program that included smoking cessation, moderate aerobic exercise, nutrition counseling, relaxation-response training, and cognitive/behavioral skills (Casey et al., 2009). Both men and women saw improvement in their blood pressure, lipid levels, weight, and exercise conditioning. Increased relaxation-response practice and exercise significantly contributed to these improvements (Casey et al., 2009). More research is needed, but the benefits of relaxation and exercise are promising.

BOX 25-6 PATIENT TEACHING

Stress Reduction

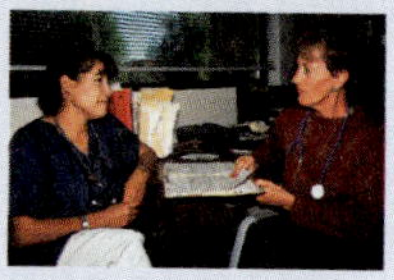

Becky recognizes that Rachael wants to learn how to increase her resistance to stress. Becky develops the following teaching plan for Rachael.

OUTCOME

At the end of the teaching session, Rachael verbally identifies two methods to reduce her stress.

TEACHING STRATEGIES

- Meet with Rachael in a quiet and private setting at a time when Rachael has about 1 hour to talk without interruptions.
- Schedule a follow-up hour about a week after the first session.
- Based on Rachael's identified needs in the areas of physical exercise, assertiveness skills, coping resources, meditation, self-esteem, and insight about personal and professional responsibilities, encourage her to focus on two stress-management strategies.
- For a goal of increasing physical exercise, ask Rachael to discuss and explore her reasonable alternatives for exercise. Ask her to maintain a daily record of her physical exercise.
- For increasing assertiveness skills, explain assertive behavior and suggest that Rachael keep a log of her assertive, aggressive, or passive responses for the next week.
- For coping resources, explore with Rachael her support system, possibilities for continuing education, financial status, and her personal appearance, depending on her identified needs (Pender et al., 2010). Ask her to explore these resources and prepare a summary of her findings.
- For self-esteem describe cognitive skills such as positive self-talk and becoming successful in a particular skill (Pender et al., 2010). Ask her to keep a daily log of her experiences with positive self-talk and her thoughts about a skill at which she excels.
- For developing insight about maintaining appropriate boundaries between work and personal space, explore with Rachael ways that she will increase awareness of her feelings of anger, pain, hurt, sadness, and joy. Discuss with her how she will recognize the limits of her responsibilities. Ask her to keep a personal journal of her feelings for the next week.

EVALUATION STRATEGIES

- During the follow-up meeting use Teach Back and ask Rachael to explain the benefits of stress-reduction techniques.
- Have Rachael report her progress on the two strategies she chose: exercise and meditation.
- Review with Rachael her record of the exercise and meditation activities during the week.
- Ask Rachael to evaluate her progress toward her goal of increased resistance to stress.

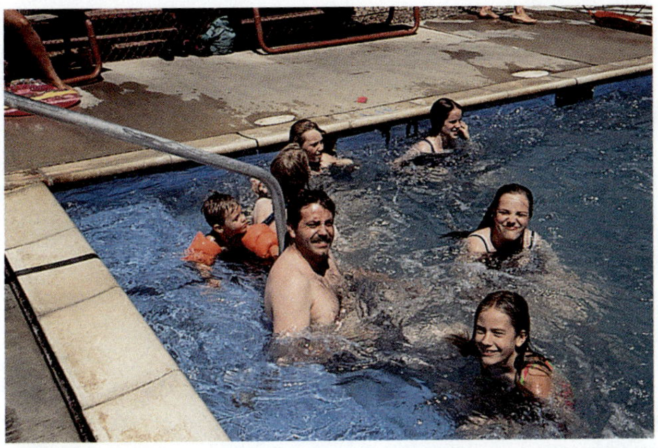

FIGURE 25-2 Sharing recreation with family and friends promotes relaxation. (Courtesy Michael S. Clement, MD, Mesa, Ariz.)

Support Systems. A support system of family and friends who listen, offer advice, share recreation time, and provide emotional support benefits a patient experiencing stress (Figure 25-2). People with strong networks of friends, neighbors, and family tend to be healthier than those without support systems (Box 25-7). Many organizations such as the American Heart Association, the American Cancer Society, local hospitals and churches, and mental health organizations offer support group services to individuals. Acceptable support systems vary by cultural group. For example, one cultural group relies heavily on church members for support. Another cultural group values individual privacy and prefers to avoid a self-help group with "strangers."

Cognitive Therapy. Cognitive therapy teaches patients how certain thinking patterns cause symptoms of stress or depression. For example, all-or-none thinking leads people to believe that consequences of a situation are catastrophic. Cognitive therapy focuses on changing ways of thinking so a patient feels empowered and in control of his or her own life. People using cognitive therapy examine whether or not they are overestimating the catastrophic nature of a situation by asking, "What is the worst thing that can happen?" or "Would it be so terrible if that really took place?" (Stuart, 2013).

Cognitive therapy uses reframing of perceptions, a strategy that involves focusing on other aspects of a problem and encouraging a person to see the issue from a different perspective. Reframing helps a person see an adversity as a potentially positive event. For example, a job loss may be perceived as a stressor, but by reframing the situation a person could see the job loss as an opportunity to pursue a new job or career (Stuart, 2013). However, in the process be cautious about minimizing a patient's view of a stressor. Suggest that the patient reframe the perception rather than offering your own reframing.

Assertiveness Training. Assertiveness training teaches individuals to communicate effectively regarding their needs and desires. The ability to resolve conflict with others through assertiveness training reduces stress. When a group leader teaches assertiveness, the effects of interacting with other people increase the benefits of the experience.

Stress Management in the Workplace. The interventions described previously address activities and responses that you can make in your personal life or teach your patients to use. Dealing with stress in the workplace requires a different approach. Rapid changes in health care technology, diversity in the workforce, organizational restructuring, and changing work systems place stress on nurses. It is also difficult to care for the acutely ill day after day, especially if you have formed relationships with patients over time. Additional causes of job stress include particular job assignments, difficult schedules,

BOX 25-7 EVIDENCE-BASED PRACTICE

PICO Question: Do nurses who show resistance to stress vs. those who experience traumatic stress have greater work satisfaction?

SUMMARY OF EVIDENCE

A study of 464 nurses across five acute care hospitals examined factors that predicted job satisfaction among nursing staff. Several potential factors thought to influence job satisfaction and the likelihood of staying in a nursing position were examined. Among other factors, control, job stress, leadership structure, and empowerment were evaluated. The presence of a degree of stress resistance, or resiliency, was found to be the strongest predictor of likelihood of staying in a nursing position. Stress resiliency contributed to a sense of empowerment and job satisfaction (Larrabee et al., 2010). In a separate study telephone interviews were conducted with nurses randomly selected across the United States. Thirteen nurses were thought to be highly resistant to stress and were compared with 14 nurses who were displaying signs of traumatic stress. Several themes were found in the nurses seen as highly resistant to stress; they had good social networks, were more optimistic, and had good role models. These findings were not seen in the nurses experiencing adverse levels of stress (Mealer, Jones, and Moss, 2012).

These studies are attempts to identify the characteristics of nurses who are better prepared to deal with work stress. The findings indicate that nurses who had friends and loved ones with whom they could talk, had a sense of spiritual connection, and were more optimistic appeared to be more resistant to workplace stress and were more likely to continue working as nurses.

APPLICATION TO NURSING PRACTICE

- Identify your social supports.
- Seek out a positive role model for nursing.
- Advocate for shared decision making and nurse participation on your work unit.
- Assess your coping mechanisms and strategies to identify positive means of dealing with stress.
- Consider establishing a support group of other nurses to help discuss strategies for dealing with workplace stress.
- Have someone with whom you can talk and share your difficult patient care experiences.

shift work, fear of failure, and inadequate support services. Compassion fatigue occurs as a result of chronic stress and is often associated with the human service professions (Potter et al., 2013).

If you recognize feelings of compassion fatigue, learn how to identify perceived threats that are sources of stress (e.g., angry co-worker, added patient assignment, sense of not getting work done) and practice relaxation when you perceive them. In addition, identify the limits and scope of your responsibilities at work. Recognize the areas over which you have control and the ability to change and those for which you do not have responsibility. Make a clear separation between work and home life as well. Strengthening friendships outside of the workplace, socially isolating oneself for personal "recharging" of emotional energy, and spending off-duty hours in interesting activities all help reduce burnout (Showalter, 2010).

Acute Care

Crisis Intervention. When stress overwhelms a person's usual coping mechanisms and demands mobilization of all available resources, the stress becomes a **crisis. Crisis intervention** is different from counseling and focuses on how intensely a patient views his or her problems as intolerable or how emotionally unstable the patient is. Crisis intervention provides more direction than brief psychotherapy or counseling. Any member of the interdisciplinary health care team who has been trained in its techniques is able to initiate crisis intervention (Kanel, 2012). It requires excellent nurse-patient communication skills (see Chapter 11).

Crisis intervention begins with defining the problem, ensuring patient safety, and providing support. First determine that a patient is safe and not at risk for injury to self or others. Then use crisis intervention to examine alternatives, make plans, and obtain a commitment to positive action from the patient. Ideally these last three steps are completed collaboratively with a patient, but a patient in crisis may be unable to participate actively and may need a very directive approach or a crisis interventionist (Kanel, 2012).

When using crisis intervention, help a person become aware of present feelings such as anger, grief, guilt, or tension. Using open-ended questions elicits feelings and responses with deeper meaning. Closed-ended questions provide important information early in the crisis intervention process. Emphasize focusing on the specific problem and help a patient avoid all-encompassing, catastrophic interpretations. You may need to provide guidance and direction for obtaining resources and assistance. Provide an atmosphere of calm acceptance, yet be aware of situations that require a direct approach to ensure the safety of the patient. Capitalize on a patient's strengths when identifying coping strategies with him or her; these might include previous hobbies, an interest in music or sports, or religious faith (Kanel, 2012; Whitehead and Bergeman, 2012).

Restorative and Continuing Care. A person under stress recovers when the stress disappears or coping strategies succeed. However, a person who experienced a crisis has changed, and the effects sometimes last for years or for the rest of the person's life. In the final stage of adapting to a crisis, a patient acknowledges the long-term implications of the crisis. If a person successfully copes with a crisis and its consequences, he or she becomes more mature and healthy. When a person has recovered from a stressful situation, teach him or her stress-management skills to reduce the number and intensity of the stress response in future situations.

EVALUATION

Patient Care. By evaluating the goals and expected outcomes of care, you know if your nursing interventions were effective and if the patient copes with the identified stress. Assess the patient's perception of the effectiveness of the plan. Review the behaviorally stated, measurable goals and evaluate whether or not the patient has met the criteria for success as stated in the outcomes. If the nursing interventions have not been effective in helping the patient achieve targeted goals, reevaluate the strategies implemented and revise the plan of care in consideration of the patient's current health status.

Observe patient behaviors and talk with the patient and family, if appropriate, to evaluate a patient experiencing stress (Box 25-8). Remember that coping with stress takes time. If you are in a setting in which contact with a patient ends before achieving goals or resolution, refer your patient to appropriate resources so as not to delay or interrupt progress.

Patient Expectations. Maintain ongoing communication with patients regarding the plan of care. Patients under severe stress often experience feelings of powerlessness, vulnerability, and loss of control. Actively involve patients

BOX 25-8 EVALUATION

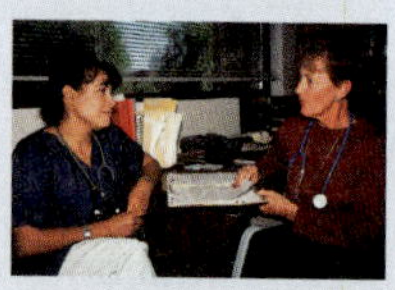

Three weeks after their initial discussion, Rachael makes her routine appointment at the employee health office to see Becky. Becky is relieved to see that Rachael is less anxious and looking better. The nervous behaviors previously assessed are no longer present. Feeling less drained, Rachael is making progress on developing professional and personal boundaries. Her neighbors and friends know about her situation and provide casseroles for the family to eat. Rachael accepts this help by reminding herself that it is only temporary. She is encouraged by the insight she gets from individual and group counseling sessions. Although the Bennett family has not yet found full resolution for their stress, they are making progress toward achievable, short-term goals.

DOCUMENTATION NOTE

"Reports that she feels 'more hopeful.' Blood pressure is 140/82 mm Hg, and pulse is 88 beats/min. Weight increased by 3 lbs since her last visit, and this week began sleeping through the night. States is going with husband to a family support group meeting held every week at the rehabilitation facility."

and families in problem identification (assessment), prioritizing, and goal setting and evaluation. Involving patients in these processes gives them an opportunity to direct their energy in a positive way and moves them toward taking greater responsibility for health maintenance and promotion.

Engaging a patient as a partner in his or her health care sets the stage for open communication. This gives the patient a sense of control and begins to promote independence, which are both crucial to the patient's successful resolution of the situation. In such an environment the patient feels more freedom to give important feedback to you about interventions that are successful. This helps you better understand why some interventions fail to meet the established goals.

KEY POINTS

- The general adaptation syndrome (GAS), an immediate physiological response to stress, involves the autonomic nervous system and the endocrine system.
- Physiological responses to stress also include immunological changes.
- Stress makes people ill as a result of both increased levels of powerful hormones such as cortisol that change bodily processes and coping choices that are unhealthy such as not getting enough rest or a proper diet or use of tobacco, alcohol, or caffeine.
- A person experiences psychological stress only if he or she evaluates the event or circumstance as personally significant; this is called *primary appraisal.*
- Stress includes work stress, family stress, chronic stress, acute stress, daily hassles, trauma, and crisis.
- Potential stressors and coping mechanisms vary across the life span, from childhood through adolescence, adulthood, and old age and from one culture to another.
- Coping, a process that constantly changes to manage demands on a person's resources, means making an effort to manage psychological stress.
- A patient who has such severe stress that he or she is unable to cope in ways that worked before is experiencing a crisis.

CLINICAL DECISION-MAKING EXERCISES

Case Recap: Rachael Bennett, a 32-year-old married mother of three children, works as the nurse manager in a medical intensive care unit. Work pressures in combination with significant family events engendered a state of stress that adversely affected her health. She was evaluated by a nurse practitioner working within employee health. During the assessment interview Rachael reported uncertainty related to her husband's medical status and a lack of control in the work and home settings. This perceived uncontrollability of life and work events contributed to stress and decreased feelings of self-worth. Reported coping attempts include an increase in the use of alcohol. The nurse practitioner began to work with Rachael on developing increased social supports and cognitive reframing. Use this information and the information from the initial case study in the chapter to answer the following questions.

1. At this point in Rachael's care there are three relevant nursing diagnostic labels: *Caregiver Role Strain, Compromised Family Coping,* and *Ineffective Coping.* Prioritize these potential nursing diagnoses for Rachael Bennett. Provide the rationale for your priority selection.
2. List three cultural factors to assess when meeting with Rachael.
3. Identify four long-term strategies that Rachael can use to better deal with work stress.

evolve

Answers to Clinical Decision-Making Questions can be found on the Evolve website.

QSEN ACTIVITY: SAFETY

During Rachael's assessment Becky collects a great deal of information regarding the stressors that she is experiencing. Through a process of systematic assessment she also identifies the coping strategies and mechanisms that Rachael uses most frequently. Becky then needs to identify ineffective coping patterns and evaluate for adverse consequences of stress.

How could the use of prepared checklists and assessment measures help Becky perform that task? What are some objective signs of ineffective coping? For which subjective statements should Becky assess?

evolve

Answers to QSEN Activities can be found on the Evolve website.

REVIEW QUESTIONS

1. Your 63-year-old male patient reports feeling a high level of stress. He identifies that he works out when feeling stressed. This would be an example of:
   1. Primary appraisal.
   2. Secondary appraisal.
   3. Denial.
   4. The alarm stage.
2. Your 52-year-old co-worker tells you that she "no longer cares about her patients." You conclude that she is experiencing compassion fatigue. Which other signs and symptoms would you expect to find?
   1. Hopelessness, depression, and social isolation
   2. Hopelessness, loss of pleasure in previously enjoyable activities, and anxiety
   3. Hopelessness, flashbacks, and resilience
   4. Hypervigilance, increased risk taking, and flashbacks

3. What would you expect a patient experiencing the alarm stage of the general adaptation syndrome to display?
   1. Increased heart rate and pupillary dilation.
   2. Decreased heart rate and pupillary constriction.
   3. Rapid fluctuating heart rate along with slowing of respirations.
   4. An irregular pulse and atrial fibrillation.
4. A family has three children. Over the last year the husband lost his job, and the wife had a serious illness. The husband reports that he thinks that being there for his wife is more important at this point in time and is no longer stressed by being out of work. This would be referred to as:
   1. Primary appraisal.
   2. Secondary appraisal.
   3. Problem-focused coping.
   4. Emotion-focused coping.
5. During the case study Rachael shared several feelings with Becky. During her initial contact with Rachael, Becky detected a high level of anxiety and stress. Which of the following interventions would be most effective to encourage Rachael to use as a coping strategy?
   1. Begin drawing and painting in her free time
   2. Walking
   3. Imagining herself in a relaxing place
   4. Meditating
6. You are working with a 50-year-old male who experienced a complete spinal cord injury of the cervical spine 5 years ago. He reports that he will walk again and is participating actively in therapy and social activities. Which of the following nursing diagnoses would be most appropriate for this patient?
   1. *Denial*
   2. *Ineffective Denial*
   3. *Stress Overload*
   4. *Ineffective Coping*
7. You are talking with a patient recently admitted for angina. He reports that his chest pain is of recent onset and is accompanied by increased anger and frustration. These feelings are tied to his recently assuming care for his elderly mother who had a stroke. Which of the following nursing diagnoses would be most appropriate?
   1. *Anxiety*
   2. *Caregiver Role Strain*
   3. *Fear*
   4. *Ineffective Coping*
8. An elderly female patient has care responsibilities for her older uncle. He has significant physical limitations, and one of her children just lost her job and may need to move back home. How would these events be termed?
   1. Family pressures
   2. Family demands
   3. Stress
   4. Stressors
9. You are caring for a 75-year-old female with a history of diabetes who had elective knee-replacement surgery yesterday. She had a poor appetite before the surgery and has only taken in clear liquids since the operation. You checked her blood glucose this morning and found it elevated. What possible explanation is there for this elevation?
   1. The surgery adversely affected the release of insulin from her system.
   2. The surgery is a physical stressor that resulted in a release of cortisol.
   3. The psychological trauma from the surgery is related to the increase in glucose.
   4. She has not been taking her insulin since the surgery.
10. A nurse experiencing work-related stress should take which of the following actions first?
    1. Determine the particular cause of the workplace stress for him or her
    2. Begin a walking-based exercise program
    3. Use relaxation strategies
    4. Increase assertiveness and set realistic goals

evolve

Rationales for Review Questions can be found on the Evolve website.

1. 2; 2. 2; 3. 1; 4. 4; 5. 4; 6. 1; 7. 2; 8. 4; 9. 2; 10. 3

REFERENCES

Aldwin C: *Stress, coping, and development: an integrative perspective*, ed 2, New York, 2007, Guilford.

Casey A, et al: A model for integrating a mind body approach to cardiac rehabilitation: outcomes and correlators, *J Cardiopulm Rehabil Prev* 29(4):230, 2009.

Chiesa A, Serretti A: Mindfulness-based stress reduction for stress management in healthy people: a review and meta-analysis, *J Altern Complement Med* 15(5):593, 2009.

Chrousos G: Stress and disorders of the stress system, *Nature Rev Endocrinol* 5:374, 2009.

Coetzee SK, Klopper HC: Compassion fatigue within nursing practice: a concept analysis, *Nurs Health Sci* 12(2):235, 2010.

Embree JL, White AH: Concept analysis: nurse-to-nurse lateral violence, *Nurs Forum* 45(3):166, 2010.

Kanel K: *A guide to crisis intervention*, ed 4, Belmont, CA, 2012, Cengage.

Khan NA, et al: The 2009 Canadian Hypertension Education Program recommendations for the management of hypertension. Part 2: Therapy, *Can J Cardiol* 25(5):287, 2009.

Kleinke CL: What does it mean to cope? In Monat A, Lazarus RS, Reevy G, editors: *The Praeger handbook on stress and coping*, Westport CN, 2007, Praeger, p 289.

Larrabee JH, et al: Influence of stress resiliency on RN job satisfaction and intent to stay, *West J Nurs Res* 32:81, 2010.

Lazarus RS, Folkman S: *Stress, appraisal, and coping*, New York, 1984, Springer.

Marchand WR: Mindfulness-based stress reduction, mindfulness-based cognitive therapy, and Zen meditation for depression, anxiety, pain, and psychological distress, *J Psychiatr Pract* 18(4):233, 2012.

McEwen BS: *The end of stress as we know it*, Washington, DC, 2004, Joseph Henry Press.

Mealer M, Jones J, Moss M: A qualitative study of resilience and posttraumatic stress disorder in United States ICU nurses, *Intensive Care Med* 38:1445, 2012.

Moustaka E, Constantinidis TC: Sources and effects of work-related stress in nursing, *Health Sci J* 4(4):210, 2010.

Neuman B, Fawcett J: *The Neuman systems model*, ed 5, Upper Saddle River, NJ, 2010, Pearson.

Ohlensehlen L: *Secondary trauma and self-care*, Naswida-ho.files.wordpress.com/2011/04/professional.self care1.doc, 2011. Accessed March 17, 2013.

Pender N, Mudaugh CL, Parsons MA: *Health promotion in nursing practice*, ed 6, Upper Saddle River, NJ, 2010, Pearson.

Potter P, et al: Evaluation of a compassion fatigue resiliency program for oncology nurses, *Oncol Nurs Forum* 40(2):180, 2013.

Roepke SK, et al: Relationship between chronic stress and carotid intima-media thickening in elderly Alzheimer's disease caregivers, *Stress* 15(2):121, 2012.

Rohleder N, et al: Biologic cost of caring for a cancer patient: dysregulation or pro- and anti-inflammatory pathways, *J Clin Oncol* 31:2909, 2009.

Sabo B: Reflecting on the concept of compassion fatigue, *Online J Issues Nurs* 16(1):1, 2011.

Schoorlemmer RM, et al: Relationships between cortisol level, mortality, and chronic diseases in older persons, *Clin Endocrinol (Oxford)* 71(6):779, 2009.

Seaward BL: *Managing stress: principles and strategies for health and well-being*, ed 7, Burlington, MA, 2012, Jones and Bartlett.

Selye H: History of the stress concept. In Goldberger L, Breznitz S, editors: *Handbook of stress: theoretical and clinical aspects*, ed 2, New York, 1993, Free Press, p 7.

Showalter SE: Compassion fatigue: what is it? Why does it matter? Recognizing the symptoms, acknowledging the impact, developing the tools to prevent compassion fatigue, and strengthening the professional already suffering from the effects, *Am J Hosp Palliat Med* 27(4):239, 2010.

Stanton AL, Revenson TA: Adjustment to chronic disease: progress and promise in research. In Friedman HS: *The Oxford handbook of health psychology*, New York, 2011, Oxford, p 241.

Stuart GW: *Principles and practice of psychiatric nursing*, ed 10, St Louis, 2013, Elsevier.

Varcarolis EM, Halter MJ: *Foundations of psychiatric mental health nursing: a clinical approach*, ed 6, St Louis, 2009, Saunders.

Varvogli L, Darviri C: Stress management techniques: evidence-based procedures that reduce stress and promote health, *Health Sci J* 5(2):74, 2011.

Whitehead BR, Bergeman CS: Coping with daily stress: differential role of spiritual experience on daily positive and negative affect, *J Gerontol B Psychol Sci Soc Sci* 67(4):456, 2012.

CHAPTER

26

Loss and Grief

evolve WEBSITE

http://evolve.elsevier.com/Potter/essentials

- Crossword Puzzle
- Audio Glossary

OBJECTIVES

- Discuss five categories of loss.
- Review grief and loss theories.
- Describe types of grief.
- Discuss variables that influence a person's response to grief.
- Identify assessment parameters in a patient experiencing loss and grief.
- Identify nursing interventions for helping patients cope with loss, death, and grief.
- Develop a care plan for a patient and family members experiencing loss and grief.
- Discuss principles of palliative and hospice care.
- Identify ways to educate and involve family members in providing palliative care.
- List the steps in caring for a body after death.
- Discuss nurses' experiences of loss when caring for dying patients.

KEY TERMS

acceptance, p. 656
actual loss, p. 655
anger, p. 656
anticipatory grief, p. 657
autopsy, p. 671
bargaining, p. 656
bereavement, p. 656
complicated grief, p. 657
denial, p. 654
depression, p. 656
disenfranchised grief, p. 657
disorganization and despair, p. 656
grief, p. 656
hope, p. 667
hospice, p. 666
maturational loss, p. 655
mourning, p. 656
necessary losses, p. 655
normal or uncomplicated grief, p. 657
numbing, p. 656
palliative care, p. 666
perceived loss, p. 655
postmortem care, p. 670
reorganization, p. 656
reminiscence, p. 657
situational loss, p. 656
yearning and searching, p. 656

People need nursing care for many reasons. They want to learn how to stay healthy, prevent illness, or cope with chronic illness. People also need nurses to help them recover from an acute illness or injury. At some point most people will need nursing care at the end of life. Nurses have a long and proud history of caring for patients who face loss, grief, and death. Situations that involve loss and grief often bring out stress, fear, and uncertainty in caregivers (Showalter, 2010). Fortunately nursing knowledge regarding the care of people who are dying and grieving has expanded greatly in the last decade (American Association of Colleges of Nursing [AACN], 2013; Keegan and Drick, 2011). Grief and loss affect a person's health physically, psychologically, socially, and spiritually. Care at the end of life is enhanced when nurses

CASE STUDY ***The Kelly Family***

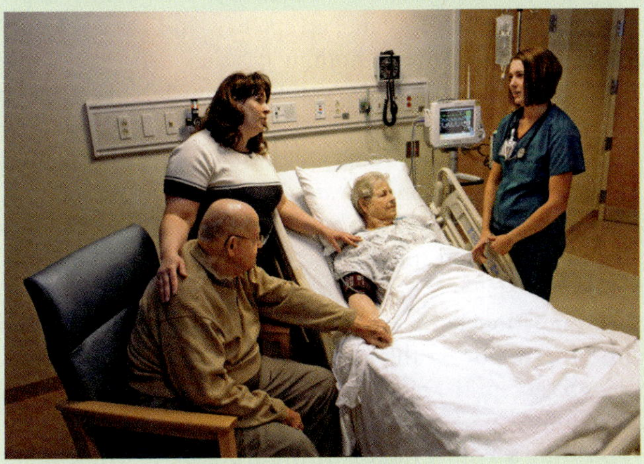

Mrs. Kelly is a 79-year-old woman who has end-stage heart disease secondary to diabetes mellitus. Her quality of life has declined greatly because of shortness of breath, anorexia, fatigue, lack of sleep, decreased strength, and poor oxygenation. She takes pain medication for severe back pain and frequently has constipation. She was admitted to the hospital 4 times in the past year for heart failure or for care of her venous stasis ulcers. She is now in the intensive care unit for chest pain and heart failure. Tests indicate that her heart function is worsening. Mrs. Kelly no longer wants to be hospitalized every time her medical condition deteriorates, and she wants to go home to die. Mrs. Kelly is being evaluated for home hospice care and will temporarily receive home care.

Mrs. Kelly lives with her husband of 54 years. Her daughter, Lilly, visits her parents every day. Lilly does not agree with the plan to begin hospice care. She believes that her mother is "giving up" too soon. Mr. Kelly does not understand hospice and is not sure if he will be a good caregiver.

Nursing student Jennifer Brown will be caring for the Kelly family as she learns how to give care in the home. She has never taken care of a person at the end of life in a home setting and feels anxious about her abilities to care for Mrs. Kelly. She will be taking care of Mrs. Kelly's symptoms, physical needs, and the family's grief issues.

provide holistic patient care (Thornton, 2012). Patients at the end of life need knowledge, compassion, and expert nursing care as they live with illnesses that cannot be cured and come to the end of their lives.

SCIENTIFIC KNOWLEDGE BASE

Loss

Throughout our lives from birth to death we form attachments and suffer losses. We become independent from our parents, leave home to attend school, begin careers, and form new lifelong relationships. Growing up is natural and positive, yet throughout life we experience **necessary losses.** Often losses are replaced by something different or better. For example, a person leaves behind family members to begin college but makes new friends and begins a meaningful career. Other necessary losses such as death of a loved one challenge a person's sense of security and coping skills.

How we perceive loss depends on what we value. Our family, friends, society, culture, and faith traditions shape our priorities and help us determine what matters most in life. A person experiences loss when a meaningful object, person, body part or function, emotion, or idea is no longer present. There are several types of loss (Table 26-1). People experience an **actual loss** when they can no longer touch, hear, see, or have near them valued people or objects. Examples include the loss of a body part, pet, friend, life partner, or job. People feel grief when a valued object becomes worn out, lost, stolen, or ruined by disaster. A child often grieves after losing a favorite toy. **Perceived losses** are uniquely experienced by a grieving person and are often less obvious to others. A perceived loss is very real to the person who has had the loss. For example, a person perceives that she is less loved by her parents and experiences a loss of self-esteem. Other people often misunderstand perceived losses.

People experience **maturational losses** as they go through a lifetime of normal developmental processes. For example, when a child goes to school for the first time he or she spends less time with his or her parents, leading to a change in the

TABLE 26-1 TYPES OF LOSS

DEFINITION	IMPLICATIONS OF LOSS
Loss of external objects (e.g., loss, misplacement, theft, destruction by nature)	Extent of grieving depends on object's value, sentiment attached to it, and its usefulness.
Loss of a known environment (e.g., moving from a neighborhood, hospitalization, a new job, moving to a long-term care facility)	Loss occurs through maturational or situational events and with injury or illness. Loneliness in unfamiliar setting threatens self-esteem and makes grieving difficult.
Loss of a significant other (e.g., divorce; loss of a family member, friend, trusted nurse, or pet; family rifts)	Significant others meet a person's need for psychological safety, love and belonging, and self-esteem.
Loss of an aspect of self (e.g., body part, psychological or physiological function, job; financial uncertainty)	Illness, injury, or developmental changes result in a loss that causes changes in body image, self-concept, and level of independence.
Loss of life (e.g., death of family member, friend, or acquaintance; own death)	Loss of a life creates grief for those left behind. Persons facing death often fear pain and loss of control or independence.

parent-child relationship. Grieving maturational losses help a person cope with the change. **Situational loss** occurs as a result of an unpredictable life event. A situational loss often involves multiple losses. For example, a divorce begins with the loss of a life companion but often leads to financial strain, changes in living arrangements, less contact with one's children, and loss of friends who were part of the couple's married life.

How an individual interprets the meaning of any loss and the type of loss affects how that person grieves. People respond to loss differently. For some people the loss of a possession, pet, or social status causes the same level of grief as the loss of a person. The value that people place on an absent object or changed social status (e.g., loss of job and income) influences their emotional response to the loss.

People experience multiple losses when they become ill or need to be hospitalized. They often lose their privacy, modesty, sense of safety, and control over body functions and daily routines. Chronic, debilitating illness often adds financial concerns, requires job changes, threatens independence, forces changes in lifestyle, and challenges family relationships.

Death is the ultimate loss. Although death is a part of life and is experienced by all living things, its mysterious, uncertain character often produces anxiety and fear (Matzo and Sherman, 2010). Death ends relationships with family and friends and separates people from the physical presence of those important to them. Persons at the end of life and their caregivers often experience sorrow; uncertainty; fear; or physical, emotional, and spiritual challenges throughout the dying process. Loss experiences can also lead to personal growth and a meaningful reprioritization of life. Close friends and caregivers of a dying person are reminded of their own mortality. Most people do not want to become dependent on others at the end of life, yet they do not want to die alone.

Facing death often brings out emotions such as guilt, anger, sadness, and fear. Some family members and caregivers, fearful of the intensity of the experience, withdraw at a time when the dying person most needs their love and support. A person's basic beliefs and values, culture, and spirituality and the quality of emotional support influence the way a person and family approach dying. They need individually designed, compassionate end-of-life care.

Grief

Grief is the emotional response to a loss. People respond to grief in different ways, based on their experiences, cultural expectations, and spiritual beliefs (Hooyman and Kramer, 2008; see Chapters 20 and 21). Grief involves **mourning,** the conscious and unconscious behaviors associated with loss. **Bereavement** includes grief and mourning, the inner feelings and outward behaviors of a survivor. Many theorists describe the grief process that occurs with any loss, including death, chronic illness, or sudden loss of body function. The following classic grief theories describe commonly experienced psychological and behavioral characteristics (Corless, 2010).

Kübler-Ross' Five Stages of Grief. Kübler-Ross' classic theory (1969) identifies five responses to loss: denial, anger, bargaining, depression, and acceptance. Individuals in the **denial** stage act as though nothing has changed. They cannot believe or understand that a loss has occurred. In the **anger** stage a person resists the loss, is angry about the situation, and sometimes becomes angry with God. During **bargaining** the individual postpones awareness of the loss and tries to prevent it from happening by making deals or promises. A person realizes the full significance of the loss during the **depression** stage. When depressed, the person feels overwhelmingly lonely or sad and withdraws from interactions with others. During the stage of **acceptance** the individual begins to accept the reality and inevitability of loss and looks to the future.

Bowlby's Four Phases of Mourning. Attachment, the foundation of Bowlby's four phases of mourning (1980), is an instinctive behavior, which leads to the development of lifelong bonds of affection between children and their primary caregivers. In the **numbing** phase a person has periods of extremely intense emotion and reports feeling "stunned" or "unreal." The numbing phase lasts from several hours to a week. The **yearning and searching** phase evokes emotional outbursts, tearful sobbing, and acute distress. To move forward people need to experience this painful phase of grief. Common physical symptoms include tightness in the chest and throat, shortness of breath, a feeling of weakness and lethargy, insomnia, and loss of appetite. This phase lasts for months or intermittently for years. During the phase of **disorganization and despair** an individual spends much time thinking about how and why the loss occurred. The person often expresses anger at anyone he or she believes to be responsible. Gradually this phase gives way to an acceptance that the loss is permanent. During the final phase of **reorganization,** which usually requires a year or more, the person accepts unaccustomed roles, acquires new skills, and builds new relationships.

Worden's Four Tasks of Mourning. The four tasks of mourning theory (Worden, 1982) describe how individuals help themselves through mourning and ask others for help. Although the time needed varies from person to person, moving through Worden's tasks typically takes at least 1 year.

- Task I: *Accept the reality of the loss.* People experience a period of disbelief and surprise that a loss has happened, even when a death is expected. In this phase people realize that a person or object is gone and will not return.
- Task II: *Work through the pain of grief.* It is impossible to experience a loss without some degree of emotional pain. Individuals who deny or suppress the pain often prolong their grief.
- Task III: *Adjust to the environment in which the deceased is missing.* A person does not realize the full impact of a loss for at least 3 months. After the first few weeks after a death, visitors and friends become less attentive, and a person experiences the full impact of the loss. Adjustment happens as a person takes on roles

formerly filled by the deceased and participates in new activities.

- Task IV: *Emotionally relocate the deceased and move on with life.* People who move on with life do not forget the deceased or devalue the relationship but begin the difficult task of giving the deceased a less central place in their emotional life. Eventually a person is able to love other people without loving the deceased person less.

Rando's R Process Model. Rando's model of mourning (1993) is specific to western society. Mourning is an action-oriented process involving recognizing the loss, reacting to the pain of separation, reminiscence, relinquishing old attachments, and readjusting to life after loss. Reminiscence is an important activity in grief and mourning. In reminiscence a person recollects and reexperiences the deceased and the relationship by mentally or verbally reliving and remembering the person and past experiences.

Postmodern Grief Theories. The phase and task theories described in the previous paragraphs often lack empirical evidence and do not consider cultural differences (Buglass, 2010; Walter and McCoyd, 2009). Recent studies about grief focus on the multiple ways that people react to loss based on their personal, cultural, and social circumstances. Research suggests that people do not grieve in predictable, linear stages nor do they necessarily complete the grieving tasks. Instead they move back and forth between stages, experience phases in an overlapping manner, or do not exhibit typical emotions (e.g., depression or anger) or grief behaviors. People rarely "get over" a significant loss but instead learn to live with loss. They experience distress associated with the loss for a lifetime. Denial and repressed coping help some people demonstrate resilience (Holman et al., 2010). Because people experience grief differently, you need to listen as people tell their stories and engage them as their story unfolds (Wittenberg-Lyles, Goldsmith, and Ragan, 2010). Theories of loss, death, grief, or mourning help you understand common shared feelings and behaviors. Use these theories to develop individualized interventions based on a patient's experiences.

Types of Grief

Normal Grief. Normal or uncomplicated grief consists of commonly expected emotional and behavioral reactions to a loss (e.g., resentment, sorrow, anger, crying, loneliness, and temporary withdrawal from activities). When patients feel supported and valued as they grieve, they often come to view the experience later as growth producing and positive.

Anticipatory Grief. The process of "letting go" before an actual loss or death has occurred is called anticipatory grief. For example, after a person and family members accept the reality of a terminal diagnosis, they begin saying good-bye and complete life affairs before death occurs. After a prolonged dying process a patient's family members often do not respond with shock and disbelief at the time of death, and feelings of sadness mingle with some relief that the suffering is over. There are risks associated with anticipatory grieving. Some family members begin withdrawing emotionally from the patient as a self-protective mechanism, leaving the patient with less support as death approaches. On the other hand, if a person thought to be near death survives longer than anticipated, others can have difficulty reconnecting or feel resentful that the stressors associated with anticipating a death continue.

Complicated Grief. Complicated grief happens when a person has difficulty progressing through the loss experience. The person does not accept the reality of the loss, and the intense feelings associated with acute grief do not go away (Field and Filanosky, 2009). A person experiencing complicated grief feels strain in relationships and finds it hard to go forward in life. The following are four types of complicated grief:

- *Chronic grief:* When the active acute mourning experienced in normal grief reactions does not decrease and continues over long periods of time, a person experiences chronic grief. The person verbalizes an inability to "get past" the grief.
- *Delayed grief:* When people consciously or unconsciously avoid the pain of loss and do not experience common grief reactions at the time of the loss, they have a delayed grief reaction. The grief arises later, often in response to a different, seemingly lesser loss. For example, a wife suppresses the pain of loss after the death of her husband and quickly resumes her busy career life. A year later she becomes severely depressed and withdraws from her children when one of them moves out of town. The extreme reaction to the relocation is a delayed response to the death of her husband.
- *Exaggerated grief:* People having an exaggerated grief response are overwhelmed by their loss, have difficulties functioning, and display significant behavioral dysfunction. Evidence of exaggerated grief includes severe phobias; deep depression; or self-destructive behaviors such as alcoholism, substance abuse, or suicide.
- *Masked grief:* After a significant loss some people are unable to recognize that the behaviors making normal functioning difficult are a result of their loss. For example, a person who loses a pet develops changes in sleeping patterns but does not see the connection between the two events. "Unmasking" the connections between grief and unwanted behaviors helps the healing process.

Disenfranchised Grief. Individuals experience disenfranchised grief when they cannot openly acknowledge a loss or receive full social support from others. This type of grieving is difficult for others to understand. Disenfranchised grief occurs in situations in which others view a person's loss as insignificant or invalid. For example, a grieving woman does not experience support from her parents when experiencing the loss of her ex-husband. People often experience disenfranchised grief when a loss is deeply private or secretly experienced (e.g., early miscarriage or death of a family member as a result of alcoholism).

NURSING KNOWLEDGE BASE

Nurses care for people who have experienced all types of losses and who express their grief in different ways. You use interventions supported by research and evidence-based practice to help patients during difficult life transitions. Nurses need knowledge of the multiple factors that influence a person's response to loss and grief.

Factors Influencing Loss and Grief

Human Development. A person's age and stage of development affect the ability to understand loss (see Chapter 22). Expressions of grief evolve as individuals mature. For example, toddlers cannot understand the permanence of death but feel anxiety over loss of objects and separation from parents. Although school-age children are able to understand the significance of loss more completely, they see their loss as a challenge to their emerging identity or self-concept. Middle-age adults often use grief experiences to reexamine or reprioritize their lives. Older adults anticipate grief as they encounter declining physical function or life opportunities, give up employment or social status, or lose loved ones.

Psychological Perspectives of Grief and Loss. Individuals respond to loss by using their usual coping strategies. Sometimes when people experience multiple losses or lose something of great significance, their usual coping strategies are inadequate. At the end of life people often find new coping mechanisms and new resources to maintain control and stability (McSherry, 2011; Chapter 25).

Socioeconomic Status. Socioeconomic status influences access to resources and support for coping with loss. Generally people feel greater burden from a loss when they lack financial, educational, or occupational resources. For example, a person with limited financial resources is unable to replace a home lost in a fire or afford the medical care needed to manage a newly diagnosed disease.

Nature of Personal Relationships. If you gain information about the quality and meaning of a relationship that a person had with the deceased, you will better understand a person's grief. If the two people were close and well-connected, the surviving person often finds it very difficult to cope with the loss. If there was conflict or abuse in the relationship, the survivor often feels guilt, remorse, regret, or relief.

Nature of the Loss. The visibility of a loss influences the amount of support a person receives. For example, a family who loses a home in a tornado gets strong support from the community, whereas a family in the same community who loses an early-term pregnancy experiences less support. Many people empathize with the first very public loss. In the case of a private loss, fewer people know about it or appreciate its significance. People respond differently to sudden, unexpected, or stigmatized deaths (e.g., suicide) than to anticipated or seemingly inevitable losses.

Culture and Ethnicity. Patient-centered, culturally competent care focuses on respecting individual differences, including cultural, ethnic, and religious responses to grief and loss (Box 26-1). Cultural belief systems provide the structures and interpretations that people need to cope with change, loss, illness, or death. For example, in western societies many people grieve privately and restrain their emotions. In other cultures survivors wail loudly and publically display their sorrow to communicate the significance of their loss to others. Although members of a cultural or religious group often share similar beliefs, each person still responds in his or

BOX 26-1 PATIENT-CENTERED CARE

People across the world rely on culturally specific rituals and mourning practices to achieve a sense of acceptance and inner peace and participate in socially accepted expressions of grief. One's culture greatly influences behaviors and rituals expected at the time of death. Institutional guidelines and end-of-life care procedures should provide standards based on compassion, maintaining privacy and dignity, and respect for all patients' and family members' cultural beliefs and practices. Expert end-of-life care allows time for patients and their families to make private and public preparations and complete unfinished communication. Understanding the uniqueness of cultural expectations at the end of life helps you know what questions to ask. You need to understand patients' culture-specific practices surrounding end-of-life care. The cultural or religious practices described in the following list are not necessarily exclusive to the culture named but are offered to give you ideas of some culturally specific concerns that you may encounter in end-of-life care.

- European Americans affirm the life of the whole person and seek closure and a sense of completion at the end of life.
- Orthodox Jews stay with a person who is dying throughout the entire process and have community members (minyan) praying at the bedside.
- Members of religious faiths that believe in reincarnation (e.g., Hindu religion) support refusal of nourishment and pain medications because of the implications for the dying person's next life.
- Religious leaders in devout Muslim and Jewish communities play a key role in resolving conflicts between medical practices and religious beliefs.
- Some religious groups or cultures object to a person being told that he or she has a terminal condition.
- Members of the Catholic Church often receive an anointing by a priest and Holy Communion. Christians usually believe in heaven or an afterlife.

IMPLICATIONS FOR PRACTICE

- Assess patient and family preferences for care of the end of life.
- Ensure that end-of-life and postmortem care is culturally sensitive by communicating patient and family preferences to the health care team.
- Include religious or spiritual leaders in patient care when appropriate.

Data from Anderson, et al: Culturally based health and illness beliefs and practices across the life span, *J Transcult Nurs* 21(4):152S, 2010; Fiorelli R, Jenkins W: Cultural competency in grief and loss, *Beginnings* 32(3):11, 2012.

her own unique way. Gain knowledge and appreciation of values and beliefs as they apply to each individual's culture (Fiorelli and Jenkins, 2012).

Spiritual Beliefs. People use their faith in a higher power, a community of friends, their sources of hope and meaning in life, and religious rituals and practices to cope with life challenges and grief (Hayden, 2011; Milligan, 2011; see Chapters 21 and 25). Regardless of their beliefs, all people have a need for love, meaning, and purpose. A loss often provokes questions related to spiritual values and the meaning of life. Spirituality helps patients buffer the stress of chronic illness and other life challenges (Bephage, 2009).

CRITICAL THINKING

Synthesis

You apply elements of critical thinking whenever you perform the nursing process with patients. Consider the scientific knowledge you have learned, your experience, critical thinking attitudes, and standards to ensure an individualized approach to patient care. Each patient for whom you care has different developmental, spiritual, and cultural backgrounds. Consider all of these dimensions of critical thinking when you develop a comprehensive, holistic plan of care (Box 26-2). You use all of your critical thinking skills to review data; recognize patterns; interpret the meaning of the data; make nursing diagnoses; and plan, implement, and evaluate a plan of care.

Knowledge. Knowledge of loss and grief theories helps you understand a patient's unique responses to grief, loss, and death. Applying knowledge of therapeutic communication principles (see Chapter 11) allows you to have helpful discussions with patients and family members to better understand their experience and perspectives. When loss is related to a particular disease or illness, knowledge about the disease process helps you design educational interventions and offer patients a realistic description of what to expect. Understanding cultural and religious diversity allows you to individualize your approach. Finally principles of caring (see Chapter 19) and family dynamics (see Chapter 24) enable you to provide inclusive, compassionate care.

Experience. Most of us have experienced some type of loss. Personal experience with loss prepares you to understand and empathize with others going through difficult times. You need to reflect on your own mortality as well. Each time you care for a patient or family member who is coping with grief, loss, or death, you gain valuable life wisdom and experience. Reflect on these experiences and apply what you have learned when caring for other patients.

Attitudes. Critical thinking attitudes of risk taking, self-confidence, and humility help you make accurate assessments and decisions about your patients (see Chapter 8). Many nurses become anxious when caring for dying patients or people coping with grief and loss. Confidence helps you understand that, even if there is nothing you can do or say to change the situation, patients need your compassionate presence and a personal connection. Confidence helps you accept the responsibility to remain present even in difficult situations. By silently sharing a moment of sadness with a patient or family member, you communicate caring and send the message that you respect and accept their feelings in the moment. You cannot know everything there is to know about a patient's loss. Humility helps you put aside personal assumptions about how the patient interprets loss to better hear his or her concerns and remain present with the patient in his or her grief or loss (Newman, 2008).

Standards. The use of appropriate standards guides you during the assessment phase of the nursing process so you gather the data most pertinent to the patient's situation. Professional standards, including bioethical principles (see Chapter 6), the *Dying Person's Bill of Rights* (2004) (Box 26-3), the End-of-Life Nursing Consortium basic and advanced curricula for end-of-life care (AACN, 2013), and the Hospice and Palliative Nurses Association [HPNA] and American Nurses Association's [ANA] *Scope and Standards of Hospice and Palliative Practice* (2007), are available. Guidelines for the care of the elderly at the end of life are offered by the National Institutes of Health [NIH] Institute on Aging (2010).

BOX 26-2 SYNTHESIS IN PRACTICE

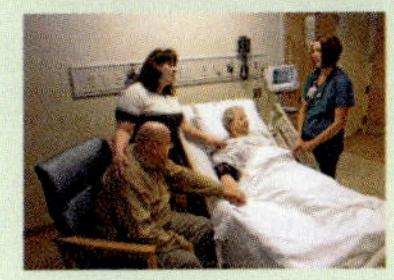

Before Jennifer meets the Kelly family for the first time, she reviews the information needed to complete a thorough assessment. She identifies the key symptoms to look for in a person with end-stage heart disease with chronic pain and will be sensitive to any embarrassment that Mrs. Kelly feels about her constipation and decreased functional abilities. Jennifer understands that people experience grief differently, and she understands that not all members of the Kelly family agree on the plan of care.

Jennifer worries that she will be asked questions for which she has no answer. She feels more comfortable talking about heart disease than about end-of-life decisions and care. She knows that attitudes of humility and willingness to take risks will help her form helping, trusting relationships. If the family members' ask her difficult questions about death or to predict what will happen, Jennifer plans to use open-ended questions to explore their concerns. She knows that she cannot "fix things" for the Kelly family, but she can assure them that they will have help. If family members share intense emotions, Jennifer will listen carefully and validate their feelings.

Jennifer will ensure that Mrs. Kelly's pain is well managed before asking about her other priorities for care. She knows that Mr. Kelly and Lilly have never given end-of-life care; therefore she plans to provide teaching for their priority concerns. She anticipates that they will want to learn how to help Mrs. Kelly conserve her energy, give medications, help with ambulation, and position her for comfort. Jennifer knows that above all she will honor patient and family preferences, culture, and religious traditions during this meaningful event in the Kelly's family history.

BOX 26-3 THE DYING PERSON'S BILL OF RIGHTS

- I have the right to be treated as a living human being until I die.
- I have the right to be in control.
- I have the right to maintain a sense of hopefulness, however changing its focus may be.
- I have the right to be cared for by those who can maintain a sense of hopefulness, however changing this might be.
- I have the right to have a sense of purpose.
- I have the right to express my feelings and emotions about my approaching death in my own way.
- I have the right to participate in decisions concerning my care.
- I have the right to expect continuing medical and nursing attention even though "cure" goals must be changed to "comfort" goals.
- I have the right not to die alone.
- I have the right to be free from pain.
- I have the right to have a respected spirituality.
- I have the right to have my questions answered honestly.
- I have the right not to be deceived.
- I have the right to have help from and for my family in accepting my death.
- I have the right to die in peace and dignity.
- I have the right to retain my individuality and not be judged for my decisions that may be contrary to beliefs of others.
- I have the right to discuss and enlarge my religious and/or spiritual experiences, whatever these may mean to others.
- I have the right to expect that the sanctity of the human body will be respected after death.
- I have the right to be cared for by caring, sensitive, knowledgeable people who will attempt to understand my needs and be able to gain some satisfaction in helping me face my death.

Modified from Barbus AJ: The dying person's bill of rights, *Am J Nurs* 75:99, 1975; *Dying person's bill of rights,* 2004.

NURSING PROCESS

ASSESSMENT

Begin with an open heart and mind and an accepting, humble attitude as you assess a patient or family experiencing a loss (Galvin and Todres, 2009). The assessment process continues throughout all patient interactions. Be aware that any assumptions you make can interfere with the accuracy of your assessment. Do not assume that other people react to loss or grief as you do or that a particular behavior necessarily indicates grief. For example, crying expresses different feelings—grief, relief, sorrow, happiness, or gratitude. Encouraging patients to tell stories about their loved one gives them an opportunity to provide information in a natural, unstructured, and meaningful way. Remain aware of verbal and nonverbal communication as you ask questions and gather information about the way patients and family members experience their grief (Table 26-2).

Provide opportunities in a therapeutically safe environment for patients and family members to talk about their feelings with others. To maintain confidentiality and encourage conversation, talk to patient and family members separately unless they want to speak together. Listen carefully while observing responses and behaviors. Assume a neutral but interested perspective and remain alert for nonverbal cues such as facial expressions, voice tones, and avoidance of certain topics. Collaborate with other members of the health care team to complete your assessment.

Type and Stages of Grief. Most people exhibit some signs and symptoms of grief in situations of serious illness, loss, or impending death (Box 26-4). Your assessment becomes more specific as you begin to observe behaviors, listen to patients' conversations, and identify their type and/or stage of grief. Application of a grief theory helps you assess a situation accurately. For example, a patient who complains of loneliness and difficulty falling asleep may be in a yearning

TABLE 26-2 FOCUSED PATIENT ASSESSMENT

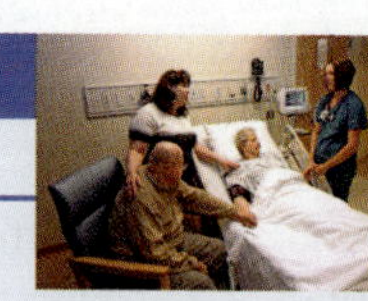

FACTORS TO ASSESS	QUESTIONS	PHYSICAL ASSESSMENT
Phase of grief	Tell me how you're feeling now. Validate patient's feelings: • You seem (angry/sad); tell me more about that. • This can be a confusing time.	Observe patient's behaviors: • Frequent sighing or crying • Withdrawn behaviors (e.g., decreased communication, silence, does not want visits) • Poor eye contact • Unwilling to talk about feelings and disagreements
Family member's response to loss	It is so difficult to deal with these kinds of decisions. What do you think your wife is going through right now? What are *you* feeling right now? You feel guilt/sadness/regret because . . . ? Do you believe you could have changed what is happening?	Observe nonverbal behaviors as members of family interact: • Tone of conversation • Frequency of interaction • Detachment behaviors (e.g., changing topic, walking away) • Seeks physical closeness

or searching phase. To gather more data, ask questions such as, "When did the loss occur?" or "How long have you been feeling this way?" Ask patients to describe their losses and how their lives have changed. You understand the patient's grief better by assessing in detail the factors that influence grieving (Table 26-3).

Coping Resources. Determine which coping patterns and resources a patient typically uses to get through difficult challenges. Use open-ended questions when you want to learn more about coping patterns: "Tell me how you usually adjust to change or loss." Use direct questioning to find out if certain activities (e.g., relaxation exercises, massage, meditation, reading, or exercise) help a patient cope with stress (see Chapter 25). Include some of those interventions in your care plan. Assess family members' coping patterns and methods too. If they are coping well, their care for the patient is enriched.

End-of-Life Decisions. Patients who have the capacity to make their own decisions should be encouraged to express their wishes for end-of-life care. Look for information about a patient's advance directives or medical durable power of attorney (a person who will make decisions for a patient if the patient cannot make health care decisions) in the patient's medical record (see Chapter 5). If there is no information in the record, ask if a patient has either of these legal documents and place a copy in the chart. If a person does not have an advance directive, ask the patient and/or family about their preferences, including their wishes for the use of life-sustaining measures, where the patient prefers to die, and their expectations about pain control and symptom management (Mahon, 2010). If you feel uncomfortable assessing a patient's wishes, find a health care team member (e.g., social worker or spiritual care provider) who has experience with discussing sensitive, complex issues. Patients' cultural or religious beliefs often influence their wishes for end-of-life care (Bullock, 2011).

Older Adult Considerations. Thoroughly assess older adults who are experiencing grief and loss. Ask questions about recent relationships that have been lost, significant life events, and other stressful events that are happening at this time. Many times older adults experience several stressful events all at once. The risk for impaired grieving increases with the number of stressors being experienced simultaneously. Explore ways that an older adult has coped with loss previously, and assess the social and economic effect of the loss to help you develop appropriate, patient-centered nursing interventions (Touhy and Jett, 2012).

Patient Expectations. A patient's perceptions, preferences, and expectations for care influence how you prioritize nursing diagnoses. Use current evidence to guide your assessment of patient and family members' expectations for nursing care (Box 26-5). Attend to acute, distressing symptoms before attempting to discuss a patient's care expectations. If a patient is in severe pain, he or she is less able to identify other needs. Assess patient or family member expectations by asking questions such as, "What is the most important thing I could do to help you through this?" Ask family members if they understand health care team members' roles and offer clarification if necessary. Early communication about expectations and goals provides clarity and helps prevent misunderstandings.

BOX 26-4 SYMPTOMS OF NORMAL GRIEF

FEELINGS
- Sadness
- Anger
- Guilt or self-reproach
- Anxiety
- Loneliness
- Fatigue
- Helplessness
- Shock/numbness (lack of feeling)
- Yearning
- Relief

COGNITION (THOUGHT PATTERNS)
- Disbelief
- Confusion
- Preoccupation about the deceased
- Sense of the presence of the deceased
- Hallucinations
- Hopelessness ("I'll never be OK again.")

PHYSICAL SENSATIONS
- Hollowness in the stomach
- Tightness in the chest
- Tightness in the throat
- Oversensitivity to noise
- Sense of depersonalization ("Nothing seems real.")
- Feeling short of breath
- Muscle weakness
- Lack of energy
- Dry mouth

BEHAVIORS
- Sleep disturbances
- Appetite disturbances
- Dreams of the deceased
- Sighing
- Crying
- Carrying objects that belonged to the deceased

NURSING DIAGNOSIS

You review and interpret a patient's assessment data to cluster defining characteristics and identify relevant nursing diagnoses. Several nursing diagnoses apply to patients who experience loss, grief, or death. In addition to diagnoses specific to grieving, you likely diagnose problems related to a patient's physical or mental states. Clustering data concerning patient or family behaviors, actual or potential losses, observed coping mechanisms, and information about the nature and meaning of loss leads to individualized nursing diagnoses. You need three or four defining characteristics to make an accurate diagnosis. Examples of nursing diagnoses frequently identified in situations of grief, loss, and end of life include the following:

- *Death Anxiety*
- *Ineffective Denial*
- *Fear*
- *Grieving*
- *Hopelessness*
- *Risk for Loneliness*
- *Social Isolation*
- *Spiritual Distress*
- *Readiness for Enhanced Spiritual Well-Being*

TABLE 26-3 ASSESSMENT OF FACTORS INFLUENCING GRIEVING

FACTORS	AREAS/SUGGESTED QUESTIONS TO EXPLORE
Hope	Explore goals, worth, adaptations to future changes. *Examples*: Tell me what you think about your treatment plan. What do you expect will happen to you? What do you most want to accomplish?
Nature of relationships	Explore functions of family, community, society. *Examples*: How have you and your husband coped during other hospitalizations? Tell me about your relationship with ________. Will it change? I see that you have lots of cards from church friends. Tell me about your church activities.
Social support system	Explore availability of family caregivers, friends, timing, family needs. *Examples*: How do other people best give you help? Tell me about the family/friends who are available to help you. Tell me about the people you talk to about your ________.
Nature of loss	Explore actual vs. perceived losses; death issues; impact on roles. *Examples*: How is the loss affecting your daily life? What past experiences have you had with loss? Tell me how you usually cope with disappointment or loss.
Cultural and spiritual beliefs	Values, practices, beliefs, and attitudes are shaped by culture/religion. *Examples*: What do you believe about death? Who makes health care decisions in your family/culture? Tell me about your family's/culture's funeral practices.
Personal life goals	Actual or perceived losses affect future decisions and options. *Examples*: How will your life change as a result of your diagnosis/loss? How does this loss change your personal goals? Tell me what you know about advance directives.

BOX 26-5 EVIDENCE-BASED PRACTICE

PICO Question: Do patients' and family members' perceptions about nursing care interventions affect their satisfaction with end-of-life care?

SUMMARY OF EVIDENCE

Patients and families require special care at the end of life. Effective communication typically leads to patient and family satisfaction during this difficult time (Jackson et al., 2012). Communication needs to be open and honest and include patients, family members, and health care providers (Jackson et al., 2012; Payne et al., 2010). Professional caregivers need to be competent and caring and provide up-to-date information. They also need to include patients and family members in making decisions, even when difficult decisions need to be made (Payne et al., 2010). Patients prefer less aggressive, comfort-focused care. Those who do not have advance directives are at higher risk for receiving more medical interventions at the end of life than they would prefer (Kelley et al., 2010). Thus patients and families value receiving information about advance directives. Other essential patient education includes the impending signs of death (Jackson et al., 2012). Murray et al. (2009) found that, although most patients with terminal cancer prefer to die at home, the majority die in an institution. Therefore it is also important to ask questions about where patients wish to die and help patients and family caregivers make appropriate plans for the end of life.

APPLICATION TO NURSING PRACTICE

- Provide frequent updates and patient-family teaching to enhance satisfaction with care.
- Collaborate with other health care providers such as social workers to help patients develop advance directives.
- Engage in open conversations to help patients, family caregivers, and health care providers make place of death plans consistent with patient preferences.

Some patients have several nursing diagnoses. For example, if you are caring for a patient who cries often, displays anger, and reports nightmares, you have identified defining characteristics that are common with *Acute or Chronic Pain, Ineffective Coping,* and *Spiritual Distress.* Look for other behaviors and symptoms to validate your selection of an accurate nursing diagnosis. Also identify the appropriate related factor for each diagnosis. For example, *Complicated Grieving related to loss of the ability to walk due to lower limb paralysis* requires different interventions than *Complicated Grieving related to the loss of a pregnancy.* Clarification of the related factor helps you select appropriate interventions.

PLANNING

Plan your nursing care to meet a patient's and family members' physical, emotional, developmental, and spiritual needs and select interventions to alleviate symptoms as much as possible (Figure 26-1). Patient input, preferences, and priorities are of primary importance in planning end-of-life care (see Care Plan).

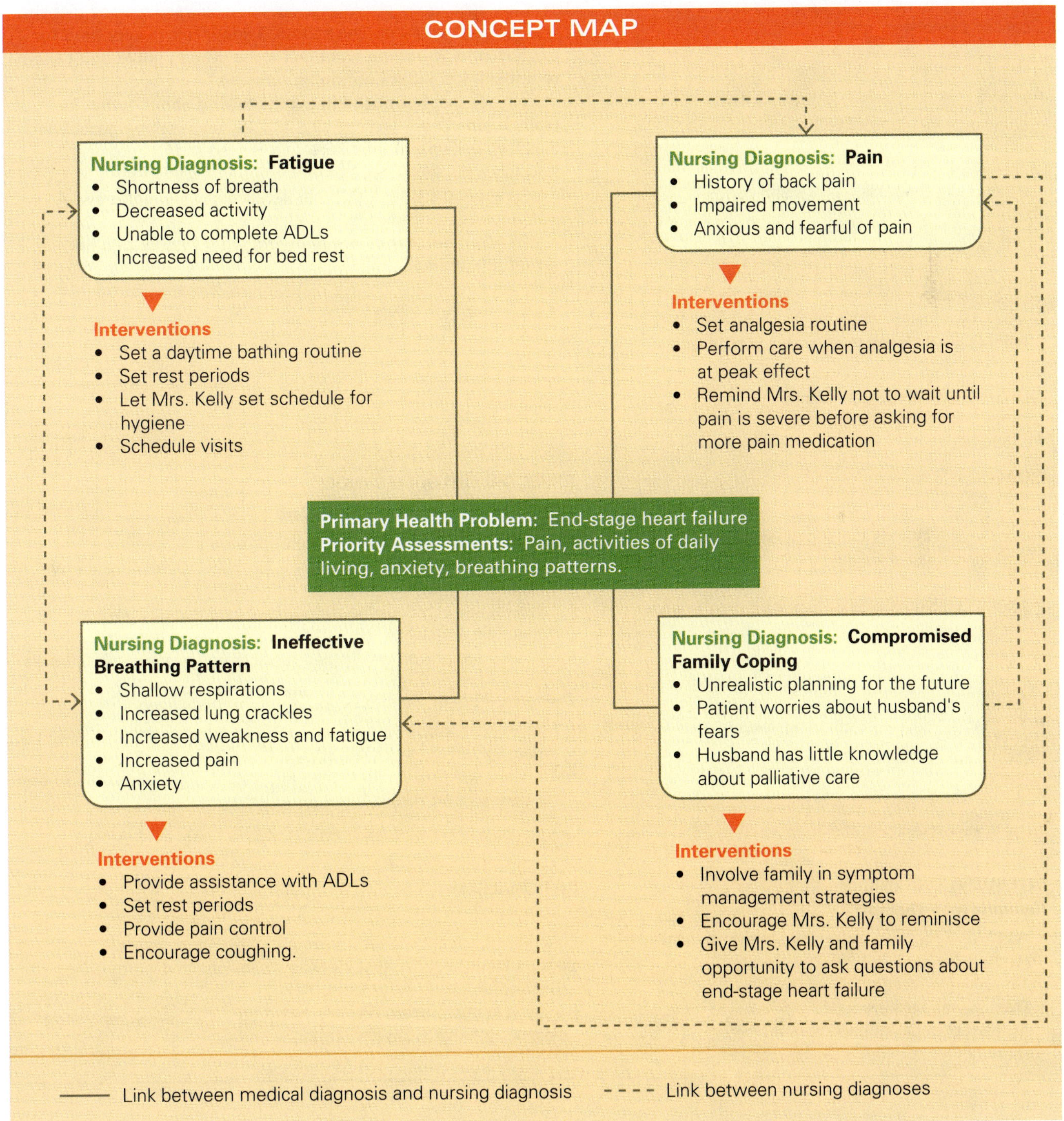

FIGURE 26-1 Concept map. *ADL,* Activities of daily living.

CARE PLAN

Loss and Grief

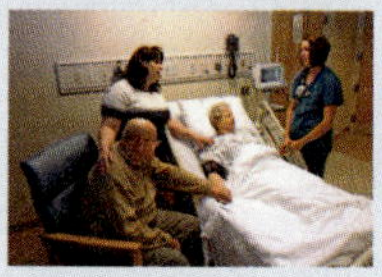

ASSESSMENT

At her first home visit 1 week after Mrs. Kelly's discharge from the hospital, Jennifer sees that Mrs. Kelly has a worried look on her face and she seems distressed. Mrs. Kelly cannot independently perform many activities of daily living because of shortness of breath. She is only able to eat small amounts of food and reports that she feels dizzy, weak, and "wobbly" when walking to the commode. Mrs. Kelly shares her feelings with Jennifer and asks many questions. While talking about her family, Mrs. Kelly states, "My daughter Lilly doesn't know what to do to help me."

ASSESSMENT ACTIVITIES	FINDINGS/DEFINING CHARACTERISTICS*
Arrange time to talk to Mrs. Kelly alone and observe patient's emotions.	Mrs. Kelly cries when she talks about her family and worries that she is a "burden" on them. She states, **"I know this is very hard for my husband to accept, but I feel alone when people don't seem to understand what I am going through."**
Ask Mrs. Kelly about how she thinks her family is doing.	She confides that **her husband avoids talking about "what is really happening,"** and she says that he keeps talking about the trips they will take in the future. Lilly is tired and has not been sleeping well.
Ask Mr. Kelly about his feelings and needs.	He talks about plans for a summer vacation, still 9 months away. He appears sad and anxious. He talks about **his fear of not knowing what to do when her symptoms worsen.** He states, "I still can't believe that she wants to die instead of staying here with Lilly and me."

*__Defining characteristics__ are shown in **bold** type.

NURSING DIAGNOSIS: Compromised Family Coping related to stress of impending death of wife/mother

PLANNING

GOAL	EXPECTED OUTCOMES (NOC)†
	Caregiver Performance: Direct Care
• Family understands the symptoms of end-stage heart condition within 2 weeks.	• Mr. Kelly describes end-stage heart disease in 1 week. • Mr. Kelly identifies the symptoms his wife may experience within 2 weeks.
• Family is able to provide palliative care interventions within 3 weeks.	• Mr. Kelly and Lilly describe the palliative care that Mrs. Kelly will need in the next 2 weeks. • Mr. Kelly and Lilly provide hygiene and comfort needs within 3 weeks.
	Caregiver-Patient Relationship
• The family develops affirming relationships within 1 month.	• Mrs. Kelly shares feelings about her life and relationship with husband and daughter within 2 weeks. • Mr. Kelly and Lilly verbalize their understanding of Mrs. Kelly's need for their support within 1 month.

†Outcomes classification label from Moorhead S et al, editors: *Nursing outcomes classification (NOC),* ed 5, St Louis, 2013, Mosby.

INTERVENTIONS (NIC)‡	RATIONALE
Reminiscence Therapy	
• Ask Mrs. Kelly to reminisce by sharing stories with her family.	Encouraging patients to tell stories about events and people allows them to sense that life was meaningful and worth living (Butler, 2009).
• Discuss with Mr. Kelly and Lilly the value of reminiscence as part of looking back and evaluating life and its meaning.	Engaging in this process helps to move the family along the process of anticipatory grieving (Butler, 2009).

CARE PLAN—cont'd

Loss and Grief

Caregiver Support

• Involve the Kelly family in a discussion about symptom recognition and management. • Offer the Kelly family a chance to ask questions about end-stage heart disease, the projected course of the condition, and Mrs. Kelly's wishes regarding the use of medications.	Even with a poor prognosis, social support and prompt symptom relief help maintain a higher quality of life for the patient and family. Clarifying expectations better prepares individuals to face changes that will happen as the disease progresses (Jeong et al., 2010).
• Explain that setting easily achievable goals helps give hope. Enlist family help to establish goals for the next week.	Restructuring goals to be short-term and achievable is a means of supporting and sustaining hope in terminally ill patients (McSherry, 2011).

‡Intervention classification labels from Bulechek GM et al, editors: *Nursing interventions classification (NIC)* ed 6, St Louis, 2013, Mosby.

EVALUATION

NURSING ACTIONS	PATIENT RESPONSE/FINDING	ACHIEVEMENT OF OUTCOME
Ask Mr. Kelly and Lilly about any changes they see in Mrs. Kelly.	Both note that Mrs. Kelly has less activity tolerance but she is able to rest with oxygen in place. They ask Mrs. Kelly if she is having pain more frequently instead of waiting until Mrs. Kelly states that she is in pain.	Mr. Kelly and Lilly are more skillful in recognizing subtle symptoms in Mrs. Kelly's status, and they are more proactive in controlling her symptoms.
Observe family members' caregiving activities and their level of comfort and involvement in care.	After 1 week Mr. Kelly and Lilly note that they were more at ease with their care activities.	Family continues to increase their knowledge of and ability to provide palliative care.
Ask Mrs. Kelly to describe her feelings after sharing stories and life review with family.	After 2 weeks the Kelly family notices that they look forward to sharing these stories and are becoming at ease with Mrs. Kelly's decision and their role in palliative care.	Developing and strengthening the relationship between her husband and daughter remain ongoing.

Goals and Outcomes. Establish realistic goals and expected outcomes. Consider the patient's available resources such as supportive family members, methods for coping, spiritual beliefs, and physical energy when establishing goals of care. For example, if a patient who is terminally ill has the diagnosis of *Powerlessness related to cancer diagnosis and treatment,* a goal of "Patient will discuss expected course of disease" is realistic if the patient has accepted his diagnosis enough that he can talk about the disease without excessive anxiety. An expected outcome of "Patient participates in series of short planned teaching discussions about disease" takes into account a patient's need for short, nonthreatening sessions to reduce uncertainty and anxiety.

Goals of care for a patient dealing with loss can be long- or short-term, depending on the nature of the loss, the patient's grief, and how long the patient has to live. Because a patient sometimes moves back and forth between phases of grief, be prepared to revise goals and outcomes with patient input. Some nursing care goals include accommodating grief, accepting the reality of a loss, and renewing relationships.

Setting Priorities. When a patient has multiple nursing diagnoses, it is not possible to address all of them at the same time. Address the patient's most urgent physical or psychological needs first and then gather information about his or her expectations and preferences for prioritizing care. If the patient meets a high-priority goal, address other unmet needs. *For example, Mrs. Kelly (see Care Plan) has been visited by physical therapy and is beginning to feel more secure using a walker, but she continues to have problems with constipation. Jennifer, the nursing student, needs to reassess Mrs. Kelly's bowel pattern and frequency and recommend dietary or medication changes. Base your goal setting and prioritization on the patient's expectations and preferences. If Mrs. Kelly wants comfort interventions and spiritual support more than help with her constipation, Jennifer needs to address Mrs. Kelly's spiritual needs first.*

Collaborative Care. End-of-life care draws on the resources of an interdisciplinary team. Social workers, spiritual care providers, and psychologists have skills to help patients and family members deal with grief, anger, or depression. A pain-management specialist offers an individualized plan to address chronic pain. A coordinated team approach ensures that a patient's plan of care will be managed well and thoroughly addressed. When patients choose to go home for end-of-life care, home care and hospice nurses collaborate closely with family members and other health care providers to ensure continuity of care.

IMPLEMENTATION

Health Promotion. A person experiencing grief needs support as he or she learns how to live with loss and move toward grief resolution. People facing significant disability, loss of body function, or even death want to achieve optimal physical and emotional well-being. Patients and family members feel sadness or emotional turmoil along the way but still want to cope with their life stressors. Nurses help patients learn how to deal with their loss; make effective decisions about their health care; and adjust to the disappointment, frustration, and anxiety created by their loss. Many times patients at the end of life wish to maintain as much self-care as possible (Johnston, 2010). With effective care and support, patients at the end of life often experience high levels of wellness.

Grief and Loss Support in Acute, Restorative, and Continuing Care Settings

Palliative Care. Interventions for patients with serious chronic illnesses or those near the end of life are based on a philosophy of total care called *palliative care.* **Palliative care** is practiced in any setting and focuses on the prevention, reduction, or relief of physical, emotional, social, and spiritual symptoms of disease or treatment at the end of life when cure is no longer possible. People of any age or diagnosis receive palliative care at any time and in any setting. Expert palliative care involves an interdisciplinary team composed of health care professionals (i.e., nurses, social workers, spiritual care professionals, nutritionists, physicians, psychologists, and pharmacists). Therapists who use complementary healing interventions (e.g., massage, music, healing touch, or aromatherapy) also work with palliative care teams (Keegan and Drick, 2011). The World Health Organization (2013) summarizes palliative care philosophy and practice as follows:

- Affirms life and regards dying as a normal process
- Neither hastens nor postpones death
- Provides relief from pain and other distressing symptoms
- Integrates psychological and spiritual aspects of patient care
- Offers a support system to help patients live as actively as possible until death
- Offers a support system to help families cope during the patient's illness and their own bereavement
- Enhances the quality of life
- Uses a team approach to meet the needs of patients and families

Above all palliative care ensures that patients with advanced chronic illness or those near death receive care that is as free of avoidable pain and suffering as possible; is consistent with patient and family wishes; and is consistent with clinical, cultural, and ethical standards.

Hospice Care. **Hospice** care provides services for patients who are at the end of life. Many people do not know about this option for care and depend on you to explain hospice services and care philosophy to them. Patients who meet the criteria for hospice care generally have less than 6 months to live. Hospice teams provide care in many settings (i.e., home, hospital, or extended care facilities) and physical, emotional, and spiritual care for patients and family members. Hospice care focuses exclusively on palliative care interventions to relieve the symptoms and burdens of illness or treatment and help patients live as fully as possible until death. Nurses base hospice care on a patient's goals and support patient and family preferences for maintaining comfort and a high quality of life. Hospice programs are built on the following core beliefs and services:

- Patient and family as the unit of care
- Coordinated home care with access to inpatient and nursing home beds when needed
- Symptom management
- Physician-directed services
- Provision of an interdisciplinary care team
- Medical and nursing services available at all times
- Bereavement follow-up after a patient's death
- Use of trained volunteers for visitation and respite support

For a patient to receive home hospice care, a family caregiver must be living in the home. The family caregiver receives support from professional and volunteer hospice team members who are available 24 hours a day. If a patient receiving home hospice care goes to the hospital for the management of acute symptoms, a hospice nurse coordinates care between the home and hospital settings (Hospice Foundation of America, n.d.). Figure 26-2 illustrates the relationship between palliative care and hospice.

Communicate Therapeutically. A trusting nurse-patient relationship enables you to support patients in grief and to provide palliative care. Trust develops as you relate to patients and family members with an open, nonassuming communication style (Lowey, 2008). Open-ended questions invite

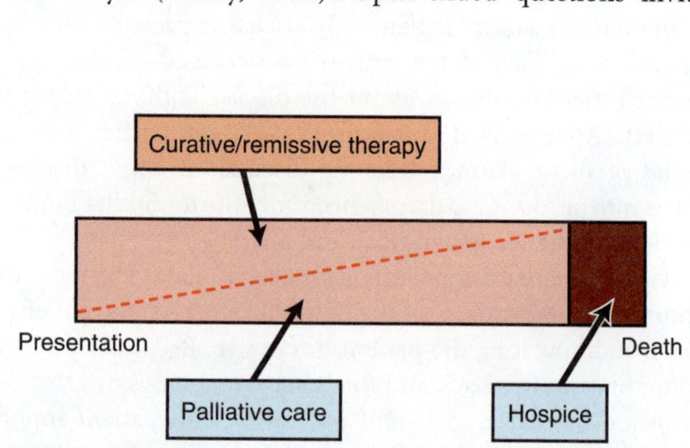

FIGURE 26-2 Continuum of palliative and hospice care. (From Emanuel L, VonGunten C, Ferris F: *Education in palliative and end of life care (EPEC) curriculum: the EPEC Project,* Chicago, 2003, Northwestern University Press.)

patients to expand on their thoughts and tell their stories. Closed-ended questions usually lead patients to give short answers (yes or no).

Use active listening, learn to be comfortable with silence, and use prompts (e.g., "go on" or "tell me more") to encourage continued conversation. Verbally empathize with the patient's grief and build a trusting relationship by offering your caring presence using intentional, meaningful touch (Kozlowska and Doboszynska, 2012; Thornton and Mariano, 2012).

Some people do not want to talk about their feelings of loss or grief with others. Do not take a person's inability or lack of desire to communicate with you personally. Some people cope with stress and loss by talking things out, whereas others need to process their loss privately before they can talk to others. Cultural or gender expectations also influence the degree to which people talk about their loss. If patients do not want to share feelings or concerns, convey a willingness to be available if they want to talk later. If you are respectful of patients' personal or cultural values and their need for dignity, respect, and privacy, a therapeutic relationship will develop.

Grief brings out intense feelings such as anger, denial, depression, or guilt. People often become demanding and accusing and take out their anger on family or caregivers. Recall that denial, anger, and depression are normal reactions to loss. Reflect on how you react to people who exhibit intense feelings or negative behaviors. If you show fear or disappointment when people express intense emotions, they do not find it easy to confide in you. Offer support by saying, "I can see this is very upsetting to you. I just want you to know I am available to talk if you want." Avoid creating barriers to communication such as denying a patient's grief, offering false reassurance, or offering unsolicited advice (see Chapter 11).

Do not avoid a topic that a patient who is dying wishes to discuss. When you sense that patients want to talk, find the time to listen. In a busy acute care setting you need to reprioritize your responsibilities so you can talk to your patients when they are ready. Respond to questions openly and honestly. Provide information to help patients understand their condition, consider the benefits and burdens of treatment choices, and clarify their personal values and goals.

Promote Hope and Spiritual Well-Being. **Hope,** a concept relevant to the human spirit, is the anticipation of a continued good or an improvement or lessening of something unpleasant. Hope energizes and comforts people and enhances their coping skills as they face personal challenges. To help patients feel more hopeful, remind them of their strengths and reinforce their expressions of courage, positive thinking, and realistic goal setting. Patients feel more hopeful when they have a sense of control. In a recent study, family members of dying persons identified the importance of maintaining connections, finding meaning in their situation, and coming to acceptance with hope-promoting activities (Revier et al., 2012). Offer information to patients about their illness, correct misinformation, and clarify patient's perceptions. Patients can behave in hopeful ways also. Help them practice healthy behaviors (e.g., enjoying meals, talking with friends, and getting rest) and suggest that they develop a workable schedule for each day. People give hope to one another. Encourage patients to nurture important relationships. When people have strong relationships and a sense of emotional connectedness to others, they know that help is available. Nurses connect with patients to foster hope (Yeager et al., 2010).

Facilitate Mourning. Nursing interventions help people acknowledge the reality of their loss. Discuss how and when the loss or illness occurred, under what circumstances, and other similar topics to help make the event more real and place it in perspective. Support efforts to live in the face of disability or in cases when the family must face being without the deceased person. Ask the people involved to identify and prioritize concerns and then facilitate the development of a plan to address their concerns. Encourage them to rely on their support network of family members, friends, professionals, and community resources. Suggest that they begin by reaching out to others in welcoming groups (e.g., religious communities or volunteer activities).

- Reinforce the understanding that people grieve differently and that feelings change or resolve over time. Some people have "anniversary reactions" (heightened or renewed feelings of loss or grief) months or years after a loss. They worry that they are losing ground when signs of grief reappear after a period of relative calm. Offer reassurance that anniversary reactions are common and encourage pleasant reminiscence.
- Provide continuing support. Patients and their families need to talk about their loved one and need support long after their loss. If you see the patient or family after an extended time, it is appropriate to ask them how they are doing after the loss. This gives them the opportunity to talk and lets them know that their loved one is remembered.

Manage Symptoms. Expert palliative care focuses primarily on managing the distress caused by unwanted symptoms of disease or side effects of treatments. Worry or fear concerning symptoms heightens a patient's perception of distress. Assess the character of a patient's symptoms carefully and individualize therapies. See Chapter 32 for a detailed discussion of both pharmacologic and nonpharmacologic pain management strategies, which are essential to achieve high-level palliative care. Patients at the end of life commonly experience other physical symptoms (e.g., dyspnea, fatigue, urinary incontinence, or nausea), psychological symptoms (e.g., anxiety, fear, or depression), social symptoms (e.g., loneliness, isolation, or loss of community), and spiritual symptoms (e.g., hopelessness, despair, or loss of meaning). A comprehensive care plan addresses symptoms identified by a patient as most distressing (Ferrell and Coyle, 2010; Matzo and Sherman, 2010). See Table 26-4 for a summary of nursing implications of commonly experienced symptoms.

Maintain Dignity and Self-Esteem. Help patients maintain dignity and self-esteem by providing spiritual care (see

TABLE 26-4 MANAGING SYMPTOMS IN THE TERMINALLY ILL PATIENT

SYMPTOMS	CHARACTERISTICS OR CAUSES	NURSING IMPLICATIONS
Pain	Pain can be related to the disease process, medical interventions, chronic conditions, prolonged bed rest, or pressure ulcers.	Address pain reports promptly; provide medication as ordered and multiple nonpharmacological measures such as massage, repositioning, relaxation, guided imagery, or music (Paice, 2010; see Chapter 32).
Discomfort	Discomfort can result from any source of physical irritation (e.g., dehydration, immobility) that causes pressure injuries and pain.	Provide thorough skin care, including daily baths; lubrication of skin; and dry, clean bed linens to reduce irritants (Chapter 29).
	As patients approach death, they breathe through the mouth, tongue becomes dry, and lips become dry and cracked.	Provide oral care at least every 2 to 4 hours. Use soft toothbrushes or foam swabs dipped in water for frequent mouth care. Apply a light film of petroleum jelly to lips and tongue (see Chapter 29).
	Blinking reflexes diminish near death; eyes often remain open, causing drying of cornea.	Gently remove crusts from eyelid margins. Artificial tears reduce corneal drying (see Chapter 29).
Fatigue	Increased metabolic demands, disease progression, pain, or declining heart function cause weakness and fatigue.	Help patient to identify valued or desired tasks; conserve energy for only those tasks. Help with activities of daily living.
	Exhaustion phase of the general adaptation syndrome causes energy depletion.	Plan frequent rest periods in a quiet environment and pace nursing care activities.
Nausea	Occurs as a side effect of medications, disease progression, or a result of severe pain.	Give antiemetics: provide oral care at least every 2 to 4 hours; offer clear liquids and ice chips; avoid liquids that cause stomach acidity, coffee, milk, and citrus juice (Acreman, 2009).
Constipation	Opioid medications and immobility slow peristalsis. Lack of bulk in diet or reduced fluid intake occurs as appetite decreases.	Increase fluid and fiber intake if possible. Give prophylactic stool softeners (Enck, 2009; Kyle, 2010).
Diarrhea	Diarrhea results from some disease processes and side effects of medications.	Assess for fecal impaction. Confer with health care provider to change medication if possible. Provide low-residue diet.
Urinary incontinence	Incontinence results from disease progression, decreased level of consciousness.	Protect skin from irritation or breakdown. Change linens frequently. Use indwelling urinary catheter or condom catheters if indicated (Kyle, 2010).
Decreased appetite	Decreased blood flow to the intestines at the end of life causes anorexia. Nausea and vomiting decrease appetite.	Give patients whatever food or fluids they enjoy. Offer frequent small meals and/or snacks rather than large meals. Do not force people to eat. Offer small portions of desired foods or home-cooked meals if patient prefers (Acreman, 2009; D'Arcy, 2012).
Dyspnea or shortness of breath	Disease progression involves lung tissue (e.g., pneumonia, pulmonary edema). Anemia reduces oxygen-carrying capacity. Anxiety increases oxygen demands. Fever increases oxygen demands.	Treat or control underlying cause. Maximize lung expansion and ease of breathing (e.g., position patient upright, provide supplemental oxygen if patient prefers; decrease anxiety or fever). Give medications (e.g., bronchodilators, anxiolytics, inhaled steroids, opioids) to suppress cough and ease breathing (Balkstra, 2010). Provide antipyretics as ordered.
Anxiety	Anxiety has physical causes such as shortness of breath, pain, fear of death, spiritual concerns, and relationship concerns.	Give anxiolytics as ordered (Pasacreta et al., 2010). Offer self as healing presence and provide information to decrease uncertainty (Sandor, 2012). Discuss spiritual or relational issues causing anxiety or fear (Edwards et al., 2010). Collaborate with spiritual care professionals. Discuss feelings/reasons associated with the anxiety.

Chapter 21). You enhance patients' self-esteem by helping them maintain a pleasing physical appearance. Cleanliness, absence of body odors, attractive clothing, and personal grooming often elevate a patient's mood. Demonstrate respect, patience, and willingness when helping patients with toileting and bathing, especially as they become increasingly dependent on caregivers. Patients experience added grief and embarrassment when they can no longer tend to their basic needs. Include patients in making care decisions (e.g., how to perform personal hygiene, diet preferences, and timing of activities). Inform patients in advance about activities and their anticipated effects. Provide privacy while giving care and give patients and family members quiet, uninterrupted time together.

Prevent Feelings of Abandonment and Isolation. Many people fear dying alone. In hospitals or extended care facilities, answer patients' call lights promptly and assure them that caregivers are available throughout the day and night. Be readily available to answer questions or interpret changes in a patient's condition. Offer your comforting presence and use gentle touch when providing care (Figure 26-3). Unless family members need privacy or are remaining with the patient around the clock, avoid placing patients in a private room. Patients who are dying often feel a sense of involvement and companionship when sharing a room and have more opportunities to interact with staff and visitors.

Family members who are having difficulty accepting a patient's impending death sometimes avoid visits. When family members visit, reassure them that their presence is important, encourage interaction, and offer information about what the patient was talking about or has recently experienced. Encourage family members to discuss normal family activities, reminisce about enjoyable times, and ask about the patient's concerns. Suggest simple and appropriate tasks for family members to perform (e.g., offering help with meals, simple hygiene or comfort activities, or filling out a menu).

Some people feel lonely or fearful at night and want a family member to stay with them. In acute care settings or extended care facilities, allow visitors to remain with a patient who is dying and relax other visiting restrictions (e.g., visits from children and number of visitors) to accommodate the patient's circumstances. Know how to contact family members so they can be notified at any time if a patient wants to see them or if the patient's condition changes. Older patients often have a smaller support group and age-related needs at the end of life (Box 26-6).

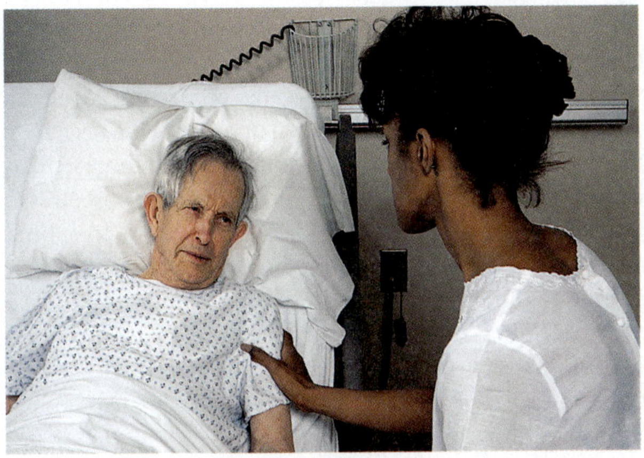

FIGURE 26-3 Offer your calm, comforting presence and use gentle touch when providing care.

Provide a Comfortable and Peaceful Environment. Promote patient comfort by repositioning, keeping bed linens dry, and controlling environmental noise. Keep the patient's immediate surroundings pleasant and clean. Open curtains so patients can experience the natural changes from day to night. Remove sources of unpleasant odors (e.g., stale food and used bedpans or emesis basins) promptly. Pictures, cherished objects, cards from friends and family, or plants create a comforting and familiar environment for patients and family members (Waller, 2011). Offer the patient frequent body massage if desired and provide opportunities for patients to hear their favorite music (Beck et al., 2009; Black and Penrose-Thompson, 2012; Osaka et al., 2009). A comfortable environment often helps patients relax, promotes sleep, and minimizes severity of symptoms.

Support Family Members. When a patient chooses to be at home at the end of life, family members become primary caregivers. Caring for a person dying at home is often rewarding yet physically exhausting and emotionally and spiritually

BOX 26-6 CARE OF THE OLDER ADULT

Caregiver Concerns

- There is little evidence that grief experiences differ due to age alone. Responses to loss are more likely related to the nature of the specific loss experience and individual differences.
- Older adults have likely faced multiple losses—loved ones, friends, valued objects, outliving a child, or declining health and a shrinking social network (Lee and Coakley, 2011).
- Older adults exhibit resilience. Others around them can learn from their courage and ability to respond to life challenges graciously, accepting life with integrity and wholeness (Walter and McCoyd, 2009).
- Older adults are at risk for complicated grieving due to multiple losses, potential for cognitive impairment, or decreased physical abilities. The risks include depression, loneliness, and accompanying functional decline.
- Pain is often reported and undertreated in older adults, particularly in people with dementia or cognitive impairments. Side effects of pain medications are often more pronounced in elderly (Matzo and Sherman, 2010).
- Older adults benefit from the same therapeutic techniques as persons in other age-groups and have opportunities for growth and development through their loss experiences (Hooyman and Kramer, 2008).
- Older adults are likely to be cared for across multiple health care settings, increasing the risk of fragmentation of care from one setting to another (Lee and Coakley, 2011).

BOX 26-7 PATIENT TEACHING

Preparing the Dying Patient's Family

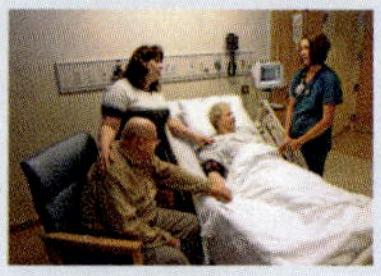

Jennifer establishes a teaching plan for Mr. Kelly and Lilly to help them learn how to perform palliative care interventions.

OUTCOME

At the end of the teaching session Mr. Kelly and Lilly demonstrate ways to help Mrs. Kelly with activities of daily living, pain management, and mobility safety.

TEACHING STRATEGIES

- Describe and demonstrate techniques for helping a person experiencing fatigue to eat safely and select easily chewed and swallowed foods.
- Demonstrate bathing, mouth care, and other hygiene interventions and allow family to perform a return demonstration.
- Show video on simple transfer techniques and use of walker to prevent injury to themselves and the patient. Observe family members practice the techniques.
- Describe ways the family can promote patient's comfort (e.g., frequent rest periods, giving massage, repositioning).
- Discuss medication purposes and side effects.
- Discuss ways to assess fatigue, bowel and bladder symptoms, and shortness of breath.
- Demonstrate how to assess pain, record pain intensity, and give medications.
- Teach family to recognize signs and symptoms of impending death and whom to call in an emergency and when death occurs.
- Invite questions from family and provide information as needed.

EVALUATION STRATEGIES

- Observe Mr. Kelly and Lilly as they provide supportive care to Mrs. Kelly.
- Ask Mr. Kelly and Lilly to describe the purpose and dosage of pain medications and how frequently they administer them to Mrs. Kelly.
- Ask Mr. Kelly and Lilly to describe hospice services and whom they will call when Mrs. Kelly dies.

BOX 26-8 SIGNS OF IMPENDING DEATH

- Minimal intake of food or water
- Increased sleeping and decreased consciousness
- Disorientation and restlessness
- Decreased urinary output and/or incontinence
- Cool hands and feet
- Noisy breathing
- Irregular breathing patterns with long pauses
- At the time of death, you will note:
  - Absence of breathing and heartbeat.
  - Bowel and bladder release.
  - Unresponsiveness.
  - Eyes fixed on a certain spot.
  - Dilated pupils.

stressful (Buck and McMillan, 2008). Family members benefit from education regarding the physical, emotional, and spiritual issues that often arise through each phase of the dying process (Box 26-7). They also need information about home care services, hospice, and community service resources. Hospice programs offer respite care for family caregivers to temporarily relieve them of their duties so they can get needed rest and rejuvenation. In some cases families need assistance and support in making the difficult decision about nursing home placement.

Provide family members with a description of common symptoms the patient will likely experience, the signs and symptoms of impending death, and the implications for care (Box 26-8). Encourage family members to talk openly with their loved one to give everyone a chance to discuss lingering concerns or requests. Family members often appreciate the opportunity to share their concerns with you in private. As death approaches encourage the use of silent vigil at the patient's bedside, touch, and verbal reassurances that the person is loved and not alone. After death help family members notify the funeral home, family members, and friends who were not present at the bedside; arrange for safe transportation of the body; and gather the patient's belongings.

Provide Care After Death. Provide a private area for the family to discuss organ donation if this is an option. Professionals educated in organ procurement and transplant procedures (e.g., transplant coordinators, social workers, or spiritual care providers) make the first contact with family members regarding requests for donation of organs or tissues. They consider the family's personal, religious, and cultural needs and discuss which tissues or organs are suitable for transplant; offer a description of the process, costs, and impact of donation on funeral plans; and answer family members' questions. For example, many people do not understand "brain death." For their loved one to donate major organs (e.g., heart, lungs, and liver), the body must be kept in good functional condition so the organs do not become damaged before donation. The patient remains on a ventilator until his or her organs are removed. Family members often believe that the person is still alive because his or her heart is still beating. Be available to reinforce explanations of the organ-retrieval process during this most stressful, tragic time. Nonvital tissues such as corneas, skin, long bones, and middle ear bones can be removed at the time of death without maintaining vital functions. If the patient left no communication regarding his or her preferences for organ donation, family members make that decision with support and conversation. Review your state laws regarding organ retrieval and the formal consent process.

A nurse assumes responsibility for **postmortem care** (i.e., care of the body after death) (Box 26-9). Give postmortem

BOX 26-9 CARE OF THE BODY AFTER DEATH

HEALTH CARE PROVIDER RESPONSIBILITIES

1. Confirm the time of death and take appropriate actions.
2. Determine the need for autopsy and order autopsy if indicated.
3. A staff member educated in making requests for organ and tissue donation discusses with family the donation options.

NURSE RESPONSIBILITIES

1. Perform hand hygiene and apply clean gloves.
2. Provide care with dignity and sensitivity to the patient and family members. Place the patient in a supine position and elevate the head of the bed 30 degrees or elevate with pillows to prevent discoloration of the face as you prepare for and complete postmortem care.
3. Check orders for any specimens to be collected or special postmortem instructions such as autopsy or retrieval of donated tissues.
4. Ask family members if and how they would like to help care for the body. Make arrangements for a member of the professional staff (e.g., spiritual care provider) to stay with family members if they do not wish to participate in body care. Ask family members if they have any special requests for body preparation (e.g., shaving, a special gown, Bible or rosary with the body).
5. Ask family about shaving male facial hair. Some cultures or religions prohibit shaving facial hair or cutting hair.
6. Remove all catheters, tubes, or indwelling devices from the patient's body, except in the case of autopsy. In that case leave medical devices in place. Remove medical equipment, supplies, and dirty linens from the room to create a clean, natural environment.
7. Bathe the body thoroughly, keeping the head of the bed elevated; apply clean sheets.
8. Brush and comb patient's hair. Apply patients' hairpieces, if possible, for natural appearance.
9. Position according to protocol. Close eyes gently by holding eyelids down briefly. Some cultural groups prefer that the eyes remain open. Dentures remain in the mouth to maintain facial alignment.
10. Cover the body with a clean sheet up to the chin with arms outside covers if possible.
11. Lower the lighting and reduce unpleasant odors as able.
12. Dispose of supplies, remove gloves, and perform hand hygiene.
13. Give family members an opportunity to view the body and accompany them to the bedside. Some will not want to view their dead loved one; assure them that either choice is acceptable.
14. Encourage the family to say good-bye with words and touch.
15. Do not rush the process of family visitation and body viewing. Once the family is more comfortable, *ask* if they would like to be left alone. Tell them how to find you easily.
16. Ask which personal belongings remain with or on the body. Give remaining personal items to a family member and document a description of the item and the date and time you transferred the belongings to the family's possession.
17. Do not throw away any personal belongings accidentally left behind by the family. Call a family member to describe the item(s) and arrange for someone to retrieve those they want to keep.
18. Apply name tags to the body according to agency protocol, usually on the right big toe and/or outside a shroud before transporting the body. Clearly mark the outside of the shroud if the body presents an isolation or contamination risk.
19. Document all care and any observations of injury to the skin in the nursing notes.
20. Remain sensitive to other hospitalized patients or visitors when transporting the body. Cover the body with a clean sheet and avoid moving it past groups of visitors when transporting it to the morgue or funeral home.
21. Follow all agency protocols and policies and comply with national or state laws regarding end-of-life issues.

care with dignity and sensitivity and in a manner consistent with a patient's religious or cultural beliefs. Because a body undergoes many physical changes after death, provide postmortem care as soon as possible to prevent tissue damage or disfigurement of body parts. For example, immediately after death, elevate the head of the bed to 30 degrees or place the patient's head on pillows to prevent pooling of blood, which can discolor the face.

Be aware that federal and state laws require that health care agencies formulate policies and procedures based on current laws to validate death, identify potential organ or tissue donors, request autopsy, and provide postmortem care. Following some deaths family members are asked to consent to an **autopsy,** the surgical dissection of a body after death to determine cause of death or how the person died or to contribute to knowledge of the disease. State legislation determines when an autopsy must be obtained, usually when death may have resulted from accident, homicide, or suicide. You alter your approach to care of the body after death if an autopsy is planned.

Nurses coordinate all aspects of care surrounding a patient's death. If a hospitalized patient dies while in a semi-private room, transfer the other patient temporarily to another room to provide privacy for the deceased patient and family and avoid exposing the roommate to the stressors related to postmortem care. Use postmortem care guidelines to make the body appear as natural and comfortable as possible.

After a patient's death shift your care to surviving family members. Make all appropriate resources available to them. They may want their family priest, minister, or rabbi to be with them; or they may appreciate the presence of the spiritual care staff at the health care agency. Social workers and counselors also offer valuable support. Remember that this is a very stressful but important event in this family's history. Do all you can to calmly and smoothly facilitate family members' requests, attend to their needs, and ask them about their preferences. Some family members prefer to be left alone and are unable to talk about the event until they have processed it privately.

Document all of the activities surrounding a death carefully to provide an accurate record of the final events of a patient's life. Sometimes your summary of activities is used for risk management or legal investigations. Include in your documentation the time and date of death, the name of the health care provider who pronounces the death, organ or tissue donation status (e.g., request made and donation decision), preparation of the body, medical devices left in or on the body, valuables or belongings left with the patient (e.g., dentures, glasses, or wedding ring) or given to the family (e.g., clothing, mail, or photographs), time of discharge, and destination of the body (e.g., morgue at the agency or funeral home). Become familiar with the policies and procedures for postmortem care used in your agency and be sure that your care and documentation reflect those guidelines.

EVALUATION

Patient Care. Nurses care for patients and families throughout a grief experience. Learn to recognize the behaviors and symptoms of a grief response and use your observations of behaviors and symptoms to evaluate how a patient or family is coping with loss and progressing through the grief process. Critical thinking ensures that the evaluation process is thorough and relevant to a patient's situation.

Refer to the goals and expected outcomes in your care plan and compare actual behaviors with expected outcomes to determine the patient's progress and make revisions to the care plan as needed. For example, if the goal is to have a patient share her feelings about death through reminiscing, you evaluate her verbal and nonverbal communication for cues that reflect normal grieving and healthy coping. Patient responses determine if the problem is resolving, if the patient needs new interventions, or if you need to revise existing strategies. Include patients and family members as active participants in the evaluation process (Box 26-10).

Patient Expectations. Maintain open lines of communication with patients so they feel free to evaluate their nursing care honestly. Patients who have a good relationship with you comfortably discuss their perceptions of care. Consider it a sign of a trusting relationship when a patient or family member offers feedback or suggestions to improve their care. When providing end-of-life care, ask often about patient and family satisfaction. Revise the care plan to include changing patient needs or requests for a different approach. Similarly be encouraged when patients or family members tell you that the care plan is helping them achieve their established goals.

Nurses' Self-Evaluation. Nurses who care for patients at the end of life and their family members often find their work to be very fulfilling and rewarding (Sinclair, 2011).

BOX 26-10 EVALUATION

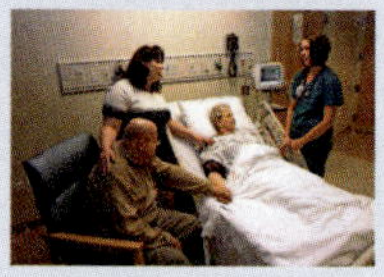

Two weeks after discussing her plan of care with the Kelly family, Jennifer observes Mr. Kelly helping his wife with her bath. He explains that Lilly is "taking a break to catch up on her school work." Mr. Kelly has obtained a walker, and Mrs. Kelly states that she feels less afraid of walking. Walking relieves the back pain that has become worse with bed rest. Mrs. Kelly explains that she and Lilly have enjoyed looking through old photo albums together and yesterday Mr. Kelly "wanted to join in the fun, too." Mr. Kelly tells Jennifer that his wife still reports some problems with constipation. He carefully records her pain medication schedule and frequency of bowel movements. He also tells Jennifer that he and his daughter received information about a support group for family caregivers sponsored by the hospital palliative care service.

DOCUMENTATION NOTE

"Uses walker to ambulate in the home. States she feels more secure. Husband involved in bathing. Husband and daughter working together in care activities. Bath in progress at time of visit. Skin has no redness, tenderness, or evidence of tissue breakdown. Continues to have problems with constipation. Assessed current bowel medication regimen and bowel movement frequency. States has some constant back pain, but current pain medication keeps in control. Sleeps well at night, waking once a night for pain meds. Family contacted palliative care team regarding support group."

However, experiencing repeated deaths of patients can feel overwhelming at times. Nurses grieve too. If you work in an area in which you experience multiple losses and fail to acknowledge your own feelings of loss, you may begin to feel overwhelmed by intense emotions (e.g., frustration, anger, guilt, sadness, or dissatisfaction with life) and become vulnerable to compassion fatigue (Showalter, 2010).

Frequently evaluate your own emotional well-being. We all have feelings and memories about previous illnesses and death. Use self-reflection or journaling to determine if your personal sadness is related to a patient or to an unresolved personal experience from your past. Knowing more about your own grief and past experiences helps you care for others more insightfully. Being a professional caregiver involves knowing when to get away from a stressful situation and how best to take care of one's self. Many nurses, especially those who routinely provide hospice care, attend a viewing at the mortuary or the funeral to show support for the family, honor the deceased's memory, and cope with their own grief. As a caregiver you were an important part of the patient's story at a very meaningful time of life. Develop your own support systems, take restful time away from your work, and find a person with whom you can safely share your feelings and concerns. Stress-management techniques (e.g., relaxation, meditation, yoga, or deep breathing) help to restore your energy and enjoyment in your work (Aycock and Boyle, 2009).

KEY POINTS

- The type and meaning of a loss influence how a person experiences and expresses grief.
- Theorists describe grief as a series of phases or tasks experienced by people as they adapt to loss and move on with life.
- Individuals move back and forth through the phases or tasks of grieving, experience them simultaneously over a period of time, or do not experience them at all.
- Knowing specific types of grief helps develop an effective plan of care.
- A person's age, developmental stage, beliefs, roles, culture, relationships, and socioeconomic status influence reactions to loss and expressions of grief.
- When assessing patients experiencing grief or loss, do not make assumptions about how you think they feel. Ask them to share their experience in their own words and tell their stories.
- Therapeutic communication fosters the development of trust and provides an opportunity for patients and family members to talk about their concerns.
- Nursing care of a patient who is grieving or dying focuses on enhancing a patient's sense of identity, dignity, and self-esteem and maintaining the highest possible quality of life.
- Patients of any age or diagnosis benefit from palliative care at any time in the course of their illness.
- Palliative and hospice care principles include involving patients and family caregivers in developing the plan of care; helping patients make informed choices; providing relief for physical, emotional, or spiritual symptoms; and offering support from an interdisciplinary team.
- Provide education and opportunities for family caregivers who want to be involved in end-of-life care.
- Provide care of a body after death and care for surviving family members with respect and sensitivity for their preferences, culture, and/or religion and based on evidence-based protocols and standards.
- Evaluate nursing care using identifiable grief behaviors and communication.
- Nurses benefit from acknowledging and attending to their own grief when caring for dying patients and their family members.

CLINICAL DECISION-MAKING EXERCISES

Two months have passed, and Mrs. Kelly is approaching death. She is having increased pain, weakness, and confusion and eats very little. She needs increased doses of pain medication. She becomes fatigued easily and speaks only in short sentences. Mrs. Kelly is receiving home hospice care, and Mr. Kelly and Lilly are the primary care providers. Mr. Kelly says to Jennifer, "This is happening so fast. I don't know what to expect next. I know that she really wants to celebrate our anniversary, so I think she'll get better again for a while. I can't imagine life without her."

1. Mr. Kelly is psychologically adjusting to his impending loss and grief. Which interventions help him mourn the loss of his life as he knows it and face the reality of his wife's impending death?
2. Mr. Kelly indicates that he does not know what to expect in the final phase of his care for his wife. What does Jennifer need to include in her teaching plan to help him?
3. Identify a goal of care and expected outcome for Mr. Kelly and Lilly as family caregivers.

evolve

Answers to Clinical Decision-Making Exercises can be found on the Evolve website.

QSEN ACTIVITY: TEAMWORK AND COLLABORATION

In making the transition from hospital care to home hospice care, the nurse needs to consider the multiple concerns that Mrs. Kelly and her family have about providing care at home. Although Mr. Kelly plans to be at home with his wife, he is not able to provide for all of her needs, and he will need respite care. Mrs. Kelly has lost strength as a result of decreased activity, shortness of breath, and back pain. She has a decreased appetite and no longer wants to help prepare meals. She feels anxious about the changes in her life and impending death and worries about how her family is coping.

How can the nurse in the hospital ensure a smooth discharge?

How will teamwork and interprofessional collaboration help Mrs. Kelly achieve her goal of receiving end-of-life care at home?

evolve

Answers to QSEN Activities can be found on the Evolve website.

REVIEW QUESTIONS

1. A woman experienced a very early loss of a pregnancy. None of her friends talk about her loss, and her sister tells her that this just was not the right time to have another child and to feel grateful for the two children she already has. The woman feels distressed that people don't understand her sadness, and she feels all alone. Which type of grief is this woman experiencing?
   1. Anticipatory
   2. Complicated
   3. Exaggerated
   4. Disenfranchised
2. Which of the following statements made by a patient with cancer best illustrates the acceptance stage of loss?
   1. "I have always taken such good care of my health. This isn't fair!"
   2. "If I get over this cancer, I'll never smoke again."
   3. "I plan to use the days I have left to enjoy my family as much as I can."

4. "I don't think my disease is really as serious as they say."

3. Place the following postmortem care activities in the correct order from the first intervention to be completed to the last.
   1. Bathe the body.
   2. Ask family members if they wish to participate in care.
   3. Elevate the head of the bed or place patient's head on pillows.
   4. Ask if an autopsy will be done on the body.
   5. Place identification tags on the body.
4. A patient recently diagnosed with a serious, life-limiting disease cries intermittently, no longer wants to interact with others, becomes angry with staff over small matters, and is unable to concentrate during conversations. Which of the following nursing diagnoses is the priority at this time?
   1. Grief related to diagnosis of terminal illness
   2. Pain related to tissue damage
   3. Readiness for Enhanced Comfort related to anger
   4. Ineffective Denial related to inability to concentrate
5. A patient's wife asks you to explain the difference between palliative care and hospice services. Which points do you include in your teaching? (Select all that apply.)
   1. The patient will continue to receive treatment for the disease while receiving palliative care.
   2. People must be considered as having less than 6 months to live to be eligible for palliative care.
   3. Hospice care is designed to meet the needs of patients nearing the end of life.
   4. Hospice care is only given in the home.
   5. Hospice and palliative care interventions focus on providing symptom relief and maintaining a high quality of life.
   6. A person eligible for palliative care and hospice receives care from an interdisciplinary team and volunteers.
6. A patient who is near the end of life tells you that she no longer wants to have visitors. Which of the following responses is most helpful at this time?
   1. "Can you share with me what you experience when you visit with others?"
   2. "You need to reconsider that decision. Social support helps people have a high quality of life."
   3. "It sounds like you're depressed. Sometimes talking to others helps."
   4. "Have you considered what not being able to see you will mean to your friends?"
7. A patient receiving end-of-life care in hospice is angry and withdrawn most of the time. He will not communicate with his family members and believes that it is unfair that he won't grow old with his wife. Which of the interventions best helps you respond to the patient's anger?
   1. Help the patient move past the anger to reach acceptance before he dies by involving spiritual care providers.
   2. Describe grief theories to the patient so he understands that his anger is just a phase that he's going through.
   3. Support the patient without judgment, recognizing that anger is a common emotional response to loss.
   4. Warn the family members that the patient's anger could hasten his death.
8. A patient diagnosed 1 year ago with a progressive neurological disease is no longer able to care for herself. She needs to make care decisions soon. Which of the following statements is appropriate to begin your assessment of the patient's care decisions?
   1. "Tell me what you already know about your options."
   2. "Have you thought about where you would like to die?"
   3. "Don't worry about it now. Things will work out."
   4. "I think it's time you consider getting a live-in caregiver."
9. You are performing postmortem care for a patient whose religious practices at the end of life require that family members cleanse the body as part of a purification ritual. They need a quiet, private place for this process. Which of the following nursing interventions is appropriate at this time? (Select all that apply.)
   1. Inform the family that a nurse needs to perform postmortem care in a hospital setting.
   2. Explain any legal requirements that apply to the situation (e.g., autopsy).
   3. Discuss with the family how you can include their religious practices in your care.
   4. Inform the family that it is impossible to provide quiet and privacy in a hospital setting.
   5. Offer to help the family manage any medical equipment or appliances that will complicate their bathing.
10. A patient's daughter is taking care of her mother at the end of life. The family used to eat together frequently before the mother became ill. The daughter asks, "How can I convince my mom to eat with me? I think if she ate with me she could keep up her strength." Which of the following responses is the most therapeutic?
    1. "Maybe you should look into high-protein, high-calorie milk shakes for your mother."
    2. "Your idea about more food would hurt your mother more than help her."
    3. "Let's start a food journal to see if there is a time of day when she is hungrier."
    4. "It sounds like you want to do what's best for your mother. What do you miss most about not being able to share meals with your mom?"

evolve

Rationales for Review Questions can be found on the Evolve website.

1. 4; **2.** 3; **3.** 3, 4, 2, 1, 5; **4.** 1; **5.** 1, 3, 5, 6; **6.** 1; **7.** 3; **8.** 1; **9.** 2, 3, 5; **10.** 4

REFERENCES

Acreman S: Nutrition in palliative care, *Br J Community Nurs* 14(10):127, 2009.

American Association of Colleges of Nursing [AACN]: *End-of-life nursing education consortium (ELNEC) fact sheet*, 2013, http://www.aacn.nche.edu/elnec/about/fact-sheet. Accessed November 13, 2013.

Aycock N, Boyle D: Interventions to manage compassion fatigue in oncology nursing, *Clin J Oncol Nurs* 13(2):183, 2009.

Balkstra C: Dyspnea. In Matzo M, Sherman D, editors: *Palliative care nursing: quality care at the end of life*, ed 3, New York, 2010, Springer.

Beck I, et al: To find inner peace: soft massage as an established and integrated part of palliative care, *Int J Palliat Nurs* 15(11):51, 2009.

Bephage G: Promoting spiritual comfort in palliative care settings, *Nurs Residential Care* 11(9):463, 2009.

Black B, Penrose-Thompson P: Music as a therapeutic resource in end-of-life care, *J Hosp Palliat Nurs* 14(2):118, 2012.

Bowlby J: *Attachment and loss, vol 3, Loss, sadness, and depression*, New York, 1980, Basic Books.

Buck H, McMillan S: The unmet spiritual needs of caregivers of patients with advanced cancer, *J Hosp Palliat Nurs* 10(2):91, 2008.

Buglass E: Grief and bereavement theories, *Nurs Stand* 24(41):44, 2010.

Bullock K: The influence of culture on end-of-life decision making, *J Soc Work End of Life Palliat Care* 7(1):83, 2011.

Butler F: Telling life stories, *J Psychosocial Nurs* 47(11):21, 2009.

Corless I: Bereavement. In Ferrell B, Coyle N, editors: *Textbook of palliative nursing*, ed 3, New York, 2010, Oxford University Press.

D'Arcy Y: Managing end-of-life symptoms, *Am Nurs Today* 7(7):22, 2012.

Dying person's bill of rights, 2004, http://learningplaceonline.com/stages/together/dying-rights.htm. Accessed November 6, 2013.

Edwards A, et al: Understanding of spirituality and the potential role of spiritual care in end-of-life and palliative care: a meta-study of qualitative research, *Palliat Med* 24(8):753, 2010.

Enck R: An overview of constipation and newer therapies, *Am J Hosp Palliat Med* 26(3):157, 2009.

Ferrell B, Coyle N: *Textbook of palliative nursing*, ed 3, New York, 2010, Oxford University Press.

Field NP, Filanosky C: Continuing bonds, risk factors for complicated grief and adjustment to bereavement, *Death Studies* 34:1, 2009, http://www.tandfonline.com/doi/full/10.1080/07481180903372269#.Unq1XBCQOM0. Accessed November 6, 2013.

Fiorelli R, Jenkins W: Cultural competency in grief and loss, *Beginnings* 32(3):11, 2012.

Galvin K, Todres L: Embodying nursing openheartedness, *J Holist Nurs* 27(2):141, 2009.

Hayden D: Spirituality in end-of-life care: attending the person on their journey, *Br J Community Nurs* 16(11):546, 2011.

Holman EA, et al: The myths of coping with loss in undergraduate psychiatric nursing books, *Res Nurs Health* 33(6): 486, 2010.

Hooyman N, Kramer B: *Living through loss: interventions across the lifespan*, New York, 2008, Columbia University Press.

Hospice Foundation of America: *Hospice services and expenses*, n.d., http://www.hospicefoundation.org/servicesandexpenses. Accessed November 6, 2013.

Hospice and Palliative Nurses Association [HPNA] and American Nurses Association [ANA]: *Scope and standards of hospice and palliative nursing practice*, Silver Spring MD, 2007, The Author.

Jackson J, et al: Family perspectives on end-of-life care, *J Hosp Palliat Nurs* 14(4):303, 2012.

Jeong S, et al: The essentials of advance care planning for end-of-life care for older people, *J Clin Nurs* 19(3-4):389, 2010.

Johnston B: Can self-care become an integrated part of end-of-life care? Implications for palliative nursing, *Int J Palliat Nurs* 16(5):212, 2010.

Keegan L, Drick C: *End of life: nursing solutions for death with dignity*, New York, 2011, Springer.

Kelley A, et al: Opiniones: end-of-life care preferences and planning of older Latinos, *J Am Geriatr Soc* 58(6):1109, 2010.

Kozlowska L, Doboszynska A: Nurses' nonverbal methods of communication with patients in the terminal phase, *Int J Palliat Nurs* 18(1):40, 2012.

Kübler-Ross E: *On death and dying*, New York, 1969, Macmillan.

Kyle B: Bowel and bladder care at the end of life, *Br J Nurs* 19(7):408, 2010.

Lee S, Coakley E: Geropalliative care: a concept synthesis, *J Hosp Palliat Nurs* 13(1):242, 2011.

Lowey S: Communication between the nurse and family caregiver in end-of-life care: a review of the literature, *J Hosp Palliat Nurs* 10(1):35, 2008.

Mahon M: Advanced care decision making: asking the right people the right questions, *J Psychosocial Nurs* 48(7):13, 2010.

Matzo M, Sherman D: *Palliative care nursing: quality care to the end of life*, ed 3, New York, 2010, Springer.

McSherry C: The inner life at the end of life, *J Hosp Palliat Nurs* 13(2):112, 2011.

Milligan S: Addressing the spiritual care needs of people near the end of life, *Nurs Stand* 26(4):47, 2011.

Murray M et al: Where the dying live: a systematic review of determinants of place of end-of-life cancer care, *Oncol Nurs Forum* 36(1):69, 2009.

National Institutes of Health (NIH) National Institute on Aging: *End of life: helping with comfort and care*, 2010, http://www.nia.nih.gov/health/publication/end-life-helping-comfort-and-care. Accessed November 6, 2013.

Newman M: *Transforming presence*, Philadelphia, 2008, FA Davis.

Osaka I, et al: Endocrinological evaluations of brief hand massage in palliative care, *J Altern Comp Med* 15(9):981, 2009.

Paice J: Pain at the end of life. In Ferrell B, Coyle N, editors: *Textbook of palliative nursing*, ed 3, New York, 2010, Oxford University Press.

Pasacreta JV, et al: Anxiety and depression. In Ferrell B, Coyle N, editors: *Textbook of palliative nursing*, ed 3, New York, 2010, Oxford University Press.

Payne S, et al: End-of-life issues in acute stroke care: a qualitative study of the experiences and preferences of patients and families, *Palliat Med* 24(2):146, 2010.

Rando T: *Treatment of complicated mourning*, Champaign, IL, 1993, Research Press.

Revier S, et al: The lived experience of hope in family caregivers caring for a terminally ill loved one, *J Hosp Palliat Nurs* 14(6):438, 2012.

Sandor MK: Holistic nursing: becoming a catalyst for conscious change at end of life, *Beginnings* 32(3):15, 2012.

Showalter S: Compassion fatigue: what is it? Why does it matter? Recognizing the symptoms, acknowledging the impact, developing the tools to prevent compassion fatigue and strengthen the professional already suffering from the effects, *Am J Hosp Palliat Med* 27(4):239, 2010.

Sinclair S: Impact of death and dying on the personal lives and practices of palliative and hospice care professionals, *Can Med Assoc J* 183(2):180, 2011.

Thornton L: The importance of holistic nursing in end-of-life care, *Beginnings* 32(3):2, 2012.

Thornton L, Mariano C: Evolving from therapeutic to holistic communication. In Dossey B, Keegan L, editors: *Holistic nursing: a handbook for practice*, Burlington MA, 2012, Jones and Bartlett.

Touhy TT, Jett K: *Ebersole and Hess' toward healthy aging: human needs and nursing response*, ed 8, St Louis, 2012, Elsevier.

Waller S: Giving end of life care environments a makeover, *Nurs Manage* 18(7):16, 2011.

Walter C, McCoyd J: *Grief and loss across the lifespan: a biopsychosocial perspective*, New York, 2009, Springer.

Wittenberg-Lyles EM, Goldsmith J, Ragan S: The COMFORT initiative: palliative nursing and the centrality of communication, *J Hospice Palliative Nurs* 12(5):293, 2010.

Worden JW: *Grief counseling and grief therapy*, New York, 1982, Springer.

World Health Organization (WHO): *Palliative care*, 2013, http://www.who.int/cancer/palliative/en/. Accessed November 6, 2013.

Yeager S, et al: Embrace hope: an end-of-life intervention to support neurological critical care patients and their families, *Crit Care Nurse* 30(1):47, 2010.

CHAPTER 27

Exercise and Activity

evolve WEBSITE

http://evolve.elsevier.com/Potter/essentials

- Video Clips
- Crossword Puzzle
- Audio Glossary

OBJECTIVES

- Describe the role of the skeleton, skeletal muscles, and nervous system in the regulation of movement.
- Discuss physiological and pathological influences on body alignment and joint mobility.
- Assess patients for impaired body alignment, exercise, and activity.
- Formulate nursing diagnoses for patients experiencing problems with exercise and activity.
- Develop a nursing care plan for a patient with impaired body alignment and activity.
- Describe the interventions for maintaining proper alignment, helping a patient move up in bed, repositioning a patient needing assistance, and transferring a patient from a bed to a chair.
- Evaluate the nursing care plan for maintaining body alignment and activity.

KEY TERMS

abduction, p. 690
active range-of-motion exercises, p. 692
activity tolerance, p. 684
adduction, p. 690
body mechanics, p. 680
center of gravity, p. 678
crutch gait, p. 695
dorsiflexion, p. 691
extension, p. 679
foot boot, p. 691
footdrop, p. 691
friction, p. 679
gait, p. 684
hand rolls, p. 689
hand-wrist splints, p. 690
hyperextension, p. 691
joint, p. 679
mechanical lift, p. 707
orthostatic hypotension, p. 692
passive range-of-motion exercises, p. 692
plantar flexion, p. 691
posture, p. 678
prone, p. 691
proprioception, p. 680
range of motion (ROM), p. 684
side rails, p. 690
supine, p. 689
trapeze bar, p. 690
trochanter rolls, p. 689

Walking, turning, lifting, or carrying are all common actions used to provide nursing care. Such activities require muscle exertion. You need to practice proper body mechanics and remain knowledgeable about current research, standards, and guidelines concerning safe transfer and positioning techniques to reduce the risk for injury (Box 27-1). This includes knowledge of the actions of various muscle groups; understanding of the factors involved in the coordination of body movement; and familiarity with the integrated functioning of the skeletal, muscular, and nervous systems.

CASE STUDY *Mr. Indelicato*

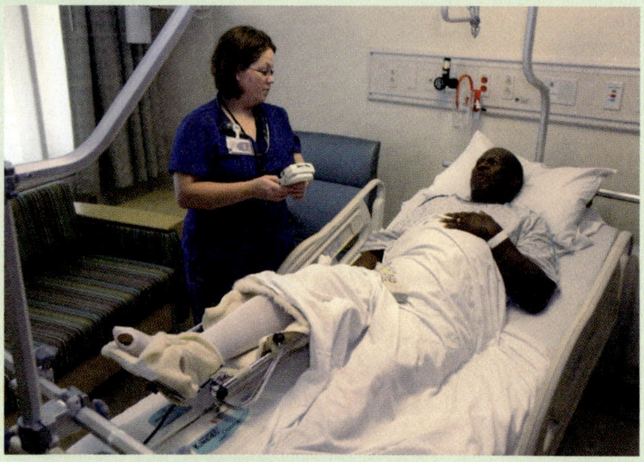

Mr. Indelicato, a 72-year-old African-American gentleman, is hospitalized for surgery on his right knee. His general level of health is good. He does not have underlying chronic illnesses and relates the problem with his knee to previous sports injuries. He "twisted my knee" at least 6 times over the last 30 years while playing racquetball. He first sought medical advice and treatment approximately 6 years ago. His last injury to his knee was approximately "5 or 6 years ago, and it hasn't worked the same since." He tried various treatments, including physical therapy, rest, and pain medication. His only preoperative medication is ibuprofen 600 mg every 6 to 8 hours. He has not taken his ibuprofen for the past few days because of the impending surgery. He wants the surgery so he can get back to being active. He and his wife enjoy golf, tennis, and bike riding. Mr. Indelicato's wife is also very healthy.

Marilyn Sweeney is a 30-year-old nursing student. She just finished a clinical rotation on a general surgical unit and is spending the remaining 6 weeks in the orthopedic/rehabilitation division of the agency. Her assignment is to follow Mr. Indelicato through his surgery and rehabilitation.

BOX 27-1 EVIDENCE-BASED PRACTICE

PICO Question: Does the use of lift devices compared to good body mechanics reduce injuries to nurses?

SUMMARY OF EVIDENCE

Musculoskeletal disorders are the most prevalent and debilitating occupational health hazard among nurses. There has been little improvement in the incidence of musculoskeletal injuries in health care workers. The total recordable injury incidence rate for hospitals is 7.1 per 100 full-time employees (Bureau of Labor Statistics, 2009). Back injuries among health care workers are estimated to cost $10,689 per case; thus back injuries are an economic burden and a major health concern (CDC, 2009; NIOSH, 2006). The National Institute of Occupational Safety and Health Administration recommends that manual lifting of patients be minimized in all cases and eliminated when feasible (NIOSH, 2006). In addition, many facilities have limited-lift policies (LLPs) that minimize patient handling by nurses and instead use lift devices to reduce on-the-job injuries (Nelson and Hughes, 2009; Tullar et al., 2010).

APPLICATION TO NURSING PRACTICE

- Use "lift teams" and patient-handling equipment such as mechanical lifts to prevent injury to yourself and patient. Lift devices reduce on-the-job injuries (Kutash et al., 2009; Sedlak et al., 2009; Zadvinskis and Salsbury, 2010).
- Minimize manual lifting of patients in all cases and eliminate lifting when possible (NIOSH, 2006).
- Use safe, efficient lifting techniques, including assistive equipment and devices to promote safe patient transfer and prevent injury to patients and health care workers (ANA, 2007; 2008; 2013).

SCIENTIFIC KNOWLEDGE BASE

The coordinated efforts of the musculoskeletal and nervous systems provide the foundation for body mechanics to maintain balance, posture, and body alignment during lifting, bending, moving, and performing activities of daily living (ADLs). Performing these activities correctly decreases the risk for musculoskeletal system injury, preventing muscle strain and excessive use of muscle energy.

Body Alignment

Body alignment refers to the relationship of one body part to another along a horizontal or vertical line. Correct alignment reduces strain on musculoskeletal structures, maintains adequate **muscle tone,** and contributes to balance.

Body Balance

You achieve body balance when you balance a relatively low **center of gravity** over a wide, stable base of support. A vertical line falls from the center of gravity through the base of support. The base of support is the foundation. When the vertical line from the center of gravity does not fall through the base of support, the body loses balance.

Posture also enhances body balance. The term **posture** means maintaining optimal body position. It means a position that most favors function; requires the least muscular work to maintain; and places the least strain on muscles, ligaments, and bones (Patton and Thibodeau, 2013).

Maintain proper body alignment and posture by using two simple techniques. First widen your base of support by separating your feet to a comfortable distance. Second, bring the center of gravity closer to your base of support to increase balance. You achieve this by bending the knees and flexing the hips until squatting and maintaining proper back alignment by keeping the trunk erect.

Coordinated Body Movement

Weight is the force exerted on a body by gravity. When you lift an object, you must overcome the weight of the object and be aware of its center of gravity. In symmetrical objects the center of gravity is located at the exact center of the object. The force of weight is always directed downward. An object that is unbalanced has its center of gravity away from the midline and falls without support. Like unbalanced objects, patients who fail to maintain a balance with their center of gravity are unsteady, placing them at risk for falling. Be able to identify patients with an unbalanced center of gravity and intervene to maintain safety.

Friction

Friction is the effect of rubbing or the resistance that a moving body meets from the surface on which it moves. As you turn, transfer, or move a patient up in bed, you need to overcome friction. Remember, the greater the surface area of the object you move, the greater the friction generated.

A patient who is passive or immobilized produces greater friction to movement. Thus when possible use some of a patient's strength and mobility when lifting, transferring, or moving a patient up in bed. You do this by explaining the procedure and telling the patient when to move. For instance, you decrease friction when patients are able to bend their knees and lift their hips while being moved up in bed. You also reduce friction by safe lifting techniques rather than pushing a patient. Lifting has an upward component and decreases the pressure between a patient and the bed or chair. The use of a drawsheet or transfer board reduces friction because you are able to move the patient more easily along the surface of the bed.

Regulation of Movement

Coordinated body movement involves the integrated functioning of the skeletal, muscular, and nervous systems. Because these three systems cooperate so closely in mechanical support of the body, they are often considered as a single functional unit.

Skeletal System. Bones perform five functions in the body: support, protection, movement, mineral storage, and hematopoiesis (blood cell formation). To provide support, bones serve as the framework and contribute to the shape, alignment, and positioning of body parts. Bones provide movement, using their joints as levers for muscle attachment (Patton and Thibodeau, 2013).

Joints. An articulation, or joint, is the connection between bones. Each joint is classified according to its structure and degree of mobility. Joints are classified as fibrous, cartilaginous, or synovial connective structures (Huether and McCance, 2012). Fibrous joints have a ligament or membrane that unites two bony surfaces such as the paired bones of the tibia and fibula. They are flexible and permit limited movement. The cartilaginous joint has little movement but is elastic. This type of joint allows for bone growth while providing stability such as the joint between the sternum and second rib. The synovial, or true joint, is a freely movable joint. Bony surfaces are covered by cartilage and connected by ligaments lined with a synovial membrane. An example is the hip joint.

Ligaments. Ligaments are white, shiny, flexible bands of fibrous tissue that bind joints and connect bones and cartilages. They are elastic and aid joint flexibility and support. In some areas of the body, they also have a protective function.

Tendons. Tendons are white, glistening, fibrous bands of tissue that connect muscle to bone. Tendons are strong, flexible, and inelastic and occur in various lengths and thicknesses.

Cartilage. Cartilage is nonvascular, supporting connective tissue with the flexibility of a firm, plastic material. The gristlelike nature of cartilage permits it to sustain weight and serve as a shock-absorber pad between articulating bones (Patton and Thibodeau, 2013).

Skeletal Muscle. In addition to facilitating movement, muscles determine body form and contour. Skeletal muscles span at least one joint and attach to both articulating bones. When contraction occurs, one bone is fixed while the other moves. The origin is the point of attachment that remains still; the insertion is the point that moves when the muscle contracts (Patton and Thibodeau, 2013).

Muscles Concerned with Movement. The muscles of movement are near the skeletal region, where a lever system causes movement (Patton and Thibodeau, 2013). The lever system makes the work of moving a weight or load easier. It occurs when specific bones such as the humerus, ulna, and radius and the associated joints such as the elbow act as a lever. Thus the force applied to one end of the bone to lift a weight at another point tends to rotate the bone in the opposite direction of the applied force. Muscles that attach to bones of leverage provide the necessary strength to move the object.

Muscles Concerned with Posture. Gravity pulls on parts of the body all the time; muscles exert pull on bones in the opposite direction to keep the body in position. Muscles accomplish this counterforce by maintaining a low level of sustained contraction. Poor posture places more work on muscles to counteract the force of gravity. This leads to fatigue and eventually interferes with bodily functions and causes deformities.

Muscle Groups. The nervous system coordinates the antagonistic, synergistic, and antigravity muscle groups that maintain posture and initiate movement. Antagonistic muscles bring about movement at the joint. During movement the active mover muscle contracts while its antagonist relaxes. For example, during extension of the arm, the active mover, the triceps brachii, contracts; and the antagonist, the biceps brachii, relaxes.

Synergistic muscles contract to accomplish the same movement. When you flex your arm, you increase the strength of the contraction of the biceps brachii by contracting the synergistic muscle, the brachialis.

Antigravity muscles help with joint stabilization. These muscles continuously oppose the effect of gravity on the body and permit a person to maintain an upright or sitting posture. In an adult the antigravity muscles are the extensors of the leg, the gluteus maximus, the quadriceps femoris, the soleus muscles, and the muscles of the back.

Skeletal muscles support posture and carry out voluntary movement. The muscles are attached to the skeleton by tendons, which provide strength and permit motion.

Nervous System. The nervous system regulates movement and posture. The motor strip, the major voluntary motor area, is located in the cerebral cortex (precentral gyrus). A majority of motor fibers descend from the motor strip and cross at the level of the medulla. The motor fibers from the right motor strip initiate voluntary movement for the left side of the body, and motor fibers from the left motor strip initiate voluntary movement for the right side of the body. Transmission of the impulse from the nervous system to the musculoskeletal system is an electrochemical event that requires a neurotransmitter (i.e., a chemical that transfers the electric impulse from the nerve to the muscle).

Proprioception. The nervous system also regulates posture. Posture requires coordination of proprioception and balance. **Proprioception** is the awareness of the position of the body and its parts and depends on impulses from the inner ear and receptors in joints and ligaments (Huether and McCance, 2012). Proprioceptors located on nerve endings in muscles, tendons, and joints monitor proprioception. While a person carries out ADLs, proprioceptors monitor muscle activity and body position. When a person walks, the proprioceptors on the bottom of the feet monitor pressure changes. Thus, when the bottom of the moving foot comes in contact with the walking surface, the individual automatically moves the stationary foot forward.

Balance. The cerebellum and the inner ear control **balance** through the nervous system. The major function of the cerebellum is to coordinate all voluntary movement. Within the inner ear are the fluid-filled semicircular canals. When you rotate your head suddenly in one direction, the fluid remains stationary for a moment while the canal turns with the head. This allows a person to change position suddenly without losing balance. When individuals have cerebellar or inner ear conditions, their balance is impaired and increases their risk for falling.

Body Mechanics

Using principles of **body mechanics** during routine activities helps prevent injury. However, body mechanics alone are not sufficient to prevent musculoskeletal injuries when positioning or transferring patients. Teaching the use of patient-handling equipment in combination with proper body mechanics is more effective than either one in isolation (Nelson and Hughes, 2009; Pelczarski, 2012; Waters et al., 2011a).

The U.S. National Institute of Occupational Safety and Health Administration released federal ergonomic guidelines to prevent musculoskeletal injuries in the workplace (NIOSH, 2006). Half of all back pain is associated with manual lifting tasks. The most common back injury is strain on the lumbar muscle group, which includes the muscles around the lumbar vertebrae. Injury to these areas affects the ability to bend forward, backward, and from side to side. The ability to rotate the hips and lower back is also decreased (Nelson and Hughes, 2009).

Manual lifting is the last resort. Do **not** use manual lifting when you need to lift most or all of a patient's weight (Pelczarski, 2012; Tullar et al., 2010; Waters et al., 2011a). Before lifting assess the weight to be lifted, the assistance needed, and the resources available. Use safe patient-handling equipment in conjunction with agency lift teams to reduce the risk of injury to a patient and members of the health care team (Table 27-1).

Pathological Influences on Body Alignment, Exercise, and Activity

Many pathological conditions (e.g., congenital defects; disorders of bones, joints, and muscles; central nervous system damage; and musculoskeletal trauma) affect body alignment, exercise, and activity.

Congenital Defects. Congenital abnormalities affect the musculoskeletal system in regard to alignment, balance, and appearance. Osteogenesis imperfecta is an inherited disorder that affects bone. Some characteristics of this disorder are fractures and bone deformity (Hockenberry et al., 2011). Bones are porous, short, bowed, and deformed; as a result, children experience curvature of the spine and shortness of stature. Scoliosis is a structural curvature of the spine associated with vertebral rotation. Muscles, ligaments, and other soft tissues become shortened. This affects balance and mobility in proportion to the severity of abnormal spinal curvatures (Huether and McCance, 2012).

Disorders of Bones, Joints, and Muscles. Osteoporosis is a well-known disorder of aging in which bone mass or density is reduced. The bone remains biochemically normal but has difficulty maintaining integrity and support. Many factors cause this, varying from hormonal imbalances to insufficient intake of nutrients (Huether and McCance, 2012).

Inflammatory and noninflammatory joint diseases and articular disruption all alter joint mobility. Some characteristics of inflammatory joint disease (e.g., arthritis) are inflammation or destruction of the synovial membrane and articular cartilage and systemic signs of inflammation. Noninflammatory diseases such as those caused from a traumatic injury have none of these characteristics, and the synovial fluid is normal (Huether and McCance, 2012).

Central Nervous System Damage. Damage to any component of the central nervous system that regulates voluntary movement results in impaired body alignment and mobility. For example, you are caring for a patient who experienced head trauma with damage to the motor strip in the cerebrum. The amount of voluntary motor impairment is directly related to the amount of destruction of the motor strip. A patient with a right-sided cerebral hemorrhage and damage to the right motor strip usually has left-sided hemiplegia.

Musculoskeletal Trauma. Trauma to the musculoskeletal system sometimes results in bruises, contusions, sprains, and fractures. A fracture is a disruption of bone tissue

TABLE 27-1 PREVENTING LIFT INJURIES IN HEALTH CARE WORKERS

ACTION	RATIONALE
When planning to move a patient, arrange for adequate help. If your institution has a lift team, use it as a resource.	A lift team is properly trained in techniques to prevent musculoskeletal injuries.
Use patient-handling equipment and devices such as height-adjustable beds, ceiling-mounted lifts, friction-reducing slide sheets, and air-assisted devices (Nelson and Hughes, 2009; Sedlak et al., 2009; Tullar et al., 2010).	These devices help to reduce the caregiver's muscular strain during patient handling.
Encourage patient to help as much as possible.	Promotes patient's independence and strength while minimizing workload.
Keep back, neck, pelvis, and feet aligned. Avoid twisting.	Reduces risk of injury to lumbar vertebrae and muscle groups. Twisting increases risk of injury.
Flex knees; keep feet wide apart.	A broad base of support increases stability.
Position self close to patient (or object being lifted).	Reduces horizontal reach and stress on caregiver's back.
Use arms and legs (not back).	Leg muscles are stronger, larger muscles capable of greater work without injury.
Slide patient toward yourself with a pull sheet or slide board. When transferring a patient onto a stretcher or bed, a slide board is more appropriate.	Sliding requires less effort than lifting. Pull sheet minimizes shearing forces, which can damage patient's skin.
Person with the heaviest load coordinates efforts of team involved by counting to three.	Simultaneous lifting minimizes the load for any one lifter.
Perform manual lifting as last resort and only if it does not involve lifting most or all of a patient's weight (Nelson and Hughes, 2009; Tullar et al., 2010).	Lifting is a high-risk activity that causes significant biochemical and postural stressors.

continuity. Fractures most commonly result from direct external trauma. They also occur because of some deformity of the bone, as with pathological fractures of osteoporosis.

NURSING KNOWLEDGE BASE

Knowledge from nursing practice enables you to meet activity and exercise needs of patients. Growth and development concepts, behavioral aspects, and cultural and ethnic origin are a few areas of nursing knowledge that you incorporate into the plan of care.

Growth and Development

Throughout the life span the appearance and functioning of the body undergo change. Knowledge of growth and development (see Chapter 22) helps you anticipate types of activities that patients are able to perform. A newborn infant's spine is flexed and lacks the anteroposterior curves of the adult. As growth and stability increase, the thoracic spine straightens; and the lumbar spinal curve appears, which allows sitting and standing. As an infant grows, musculoskeletal development permits support of weight for standing and walking. A toddler's posture is awkward because of the slight swayback and protruding abdomen (Hockenberry et al., 2011). From the third year through the beginning of adolescence, the musculoskeletal system continues to grow and develop. Greater coordination enables a child to perform tasks that require fine-motor skills. With aging changes in musculoskeletal function limit patient activity.

Behavioral Aspects

It is important to take into consideration a patient's knowledge of exercise and activity, barriers to a program of exercise and physical activity, and current exercise behavior or habits. Patients are more open to developing an exercise program if they are at the stage of readiness to change their behavior (Prochaska, Redding, and Evers, 2008). Patients' decisions to change behavior and include a daily exercise routine in their lives often occur gradually with repeated information individualized to their needs and lifestyle (Box 27-2).

Cultural and Ethnic Origin

Exercise and physical fitness are beneficial to all people. When developing a physical fitness program for culturally diverse populations, consider what motivates individuals to exercise and which activities are appropriate and enjoyable (Box 27-3).

CRITICAL THINKING

Synthesis

You will apply elements of critical thinking whenever you perform the nursing process with patients. Consider the scientific knowledge you have learned, your experience, critical

BOX 27-2 GENERAL GUIDELINES FOR INITIATING AN EXERCISE PROGRAM

STEP 1: ASSESS FITNESS LEVEL
- Seek approval from a health care provider to begin. Are there any limitations to consider before determining the exercises in the fitness program?
- Record baseline fitness scores such as pulse rate, how long it takes to walk 1 mile, waist circumference, and body mass index.

STEP 2: DESIGN THE FITNESS PROGRAM
- Consider fitness goals. Make goals attainable.
- Plan a logical progression of activities (e.g., walk a mile and gradually increase the pace).
- Build the program into a daily routine.
- Plan the fitness program with creativity and different activities.

STEP 3: ASSEMBLE EQUIPMENT
- Choose athletic shoes designed for the chosen exercise.
- Try equipment at a fitness center before purchasing to make sure that it fits into the fitness program.
- Buy used fitness equipment.
- Try homemade equipment (e.g., half-gallon milk jugs filled with sand for weights).

STEP 4: GET STARTED
- Start slowly, including a warm-up and cool-down period.
- Divide exercise time throughout day if time or fatigue is a barrier. Ten minutes of exercise 3 times a day instead of a single 30-minute workout may be better for some patients' schedules and medical conditions.

STEP 5: MONITOR PROGRESS
- Retake fitness assessment at 6 weeks and then every 3 to 6 months.
- If losing motivation: set new goals, exercise with a friend, or try new activities.

Modified from the American Academy of Orthopaedic Surgeons: *Starting an exercise program,* January, 2012, http://orthoinfo.aaos.org/topic.cfm?topic=A00416&return_link=0. Accessed May, 2013; and Mayo Clinic Tools for Healthier Lives: *Fitness programs: 5 steps to getting started,* 2010, http://www.mayoclinic.com/health/fitness/HQ00171/NSECTIONGROUP=2. Accessed May 2013.

BOX 27-3 PATIENT-CENTERED CARE

Studies of ethnic groups indicate that physical inactivity is one of the risk factors associated with type 2 diabetes. In the United States type 2 diabetes is more prevalent in blacks and the Native American population. Physical activity is identified as having an important role in the prevention and treatment of type 2 diabetes, yet blacks and Native Americans have a disproportionate number of individuals who are poor, unemployed, and disadvantaged and who lack access to the health care system (Huang et al., 2009; Maskarinec et al., 2009).

IMPLICATIONS FOR PRACTICE
- Physical inactivity is a modifiable risk factor for the development of type 2 diabetes. Prevention and treatment programs need to focus heavily on exercise and be tailored to the activity tolerance of the individual patient.
- Support promotion of physical activity through formal programs in schools, churches, and government agencies within black and Native American communities.
- Incorporate motivational factors into exercise programs such as providing a healthy snack or meal for participants and furnishing each patient with a log to monitor weight loss and blood glucose levels.
- Development of an exercise/prevention program needs to remove potential barriers such as transportation and cost to facilitate commitment to the program.

BOX 27-4 SYNTHESIS IN PRACTICE

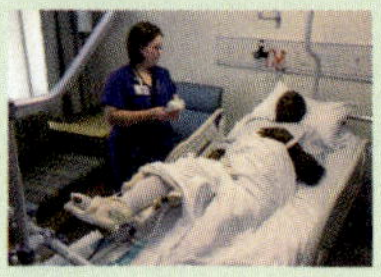

As Marilyn prepares to assess Mr. Indelicato, she reviews anatomy and physiology related to the musculoskeletal system and exercise physiology. She gathers information about the expected surgery, anticipated recovery, and physical therapy. During her previous rotation she cared for postoperative patients and knows relevant postoperative care measures to promote patient comfort and the implications of inactivity on postoperative recovery.

Marilyn knows that it is important to assist Mr. Indelicato in a prompt, immediate postoperative recovery and engage him in a steady, progressive physical therapy program. Although she has cared for patients who have required physical therapy, Marilyn has never cared for a patient requiring continuous passive motion equipment. She found and read literature about this equipment, and she consulted with the physical therapist who will be assigned to Mr. Indelicato.

Marilyn approaches this clinical experience with energy and creativity. She plans to collaborate and implement individualized care to promote Mr. Indelicato's comfort, increase activity, and improve range of motion.

thinking attitudes, and standards to ensure an individualized approach to patient care. This approach helps prevent complications, promotes rehabilitation, and promotes a timely return of patients to their homes (Box 27-4).

Knowledge. When you begin the process of problem solving for patient care, you need to consider a variety of concepts and weave them together to provide the best outcome for your patient. Knowledge of the musculoskeletal system, exercise physiology, and health alterations that create problems for a patient in the area of exercise and activity provides the foundation for decision making and planning care.

Experience. Past experiences with exercise or caring for patients with problems related to activity and exercise help you anticipate patients' needs such as pain control, positioning, transferring, and support of ADLs. Visits to a physical or occupational therapy unit in a hospital or community setting increase your experiential base.

TABLE 27-2 FOCUSED PATIENT ASSESSMENT

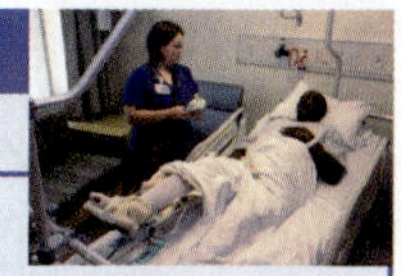

FACTORS TO ASSESS	QUESTIONS	PHYSICAL ASSESSMENT
Range of motion (ROM)	Do you have limited movement in your joints?	Observe patient's gait and ability to carry out activities of daily living (ADLs).
	Do you have a history of connective tissue disorders, fractures, and/or damage to ligaments or tendons?	Inspect joints for deformity. Measure range of motion of affected joints.
Pain	Do you experience pain or discomfort on movement? Do you need pain medication before ambulating (with assistance) or other exercise? Please rate your pain on a scale of 0 to 10 with 10 representing the worst pain.	Inspect joints for redness or swelling indicating potential inflammatory process. Observe for objective signs of pain such as grimacing, moaning, increasing respiratory rate, pulse, and blood pressure. (**NOTE:** These objective signs are not always present, and it is best to ask patient if pain is present.)
Activity tolerance	Do you feel fatigued? Do you have any difficulty with your daily activities because of muscle weakness? Do you feel short of breath, palpitations, light-headed, or dizzy?	Observe for signs of fatigue. Observe patient's performance of ADLs. Observe patient for paleness, obtain vital signs, and compare to baseline measures.

Attitudes. Attitudes of creativity and perseverance are essential because problems with activity and exercise are often prolonged. The more creative your approach for improving activity tolerance and mobility skills, the greater the chance for a patient's success. This is especially important with children. For example, creating a game that incorporates the goal of improving activity tolerance elicits better cooperation and participation from the child. In addition, providing colorful stickers to symbolize success is a creative approach to enhance cooperation (Hockenberry et al., 2011).

Standards. Professional standards and guidelines such as those from the American Nurses Association (ANA, 2007; 2008; 2013), U.S. Department of Health and Human Services (2010), National Institute of Occupational Safety and Health (NIOSH) (2006), and Quality and Safety Education for Nurses (Sherwood and Barnsteiner, 2012) concerning the use of assistive equipment and devices to safely transfer and position patients provide valuable safety guidelines for you and your patients. In addition, these standards help you promote a patient's independence while safely adhering to the prescribed rehabilitation plan.

NURSING PROCESS

ASSESSMENT

An assessment includes a patient's present activity tolerance and information about preillness functioning. Assess body alignment and posture with a patient standing, sitting, or lying down. Table 27-2 offers examples of factors to assess, related questions, and physical assessment techniques for assessing activity intolerance.

Through assessment you are able to determine patients' normal physiological changes in growth and development; deviations related to poor posture, trauma, muscle damage, or nerve dysfunction; and any learning needs. In addition, assessment provides opportunities for you to observe patients' posture and obtain important information about other factors that contribute to poor alignment such as fatigue, malnutrition, and psychological problems.

Body Alignment. The first step in assessing body alignment is to put a patient at ease so he or she does not assume unnatural or rigid positions. Remove pillows and positioning supports from the bed (if not contraindicated) and place the patient in the supine position.

Standing. Assessment of the patient includes the following:

- The head is erect and midline.
- Body parts are symmetrical.
- The spine is straight with normal curvatures (cervical concave, thoracic convex, and lumbar concave).
- The abdomen is comfortably tucked in.
- The knees are in a straight line between the hips and ankles and slightly flexed.
- The feet are flat on the floor and pointed directly forward and slightly apart to maintain a wide base of support.
- The arms hang comfortably at the sides (Figure 27-1).

A patient's center of gravity is in the midline, and the line of gravity is from the middle of the forehead to a midpoint between the feet. Laterally the line of gravity runs vertically from the middle of the skull to the posterior third of the foot (Seidel et al., 2011).

Sitting. Assess your patient for the following: the head is erect, and the neck and vertebral column are in straight alignment; the body weight is distributed on the buttocks and thighs; the thighs are parallel and in a horizontal plane (be careful to avoid pressure on the popliteal nerve and blood

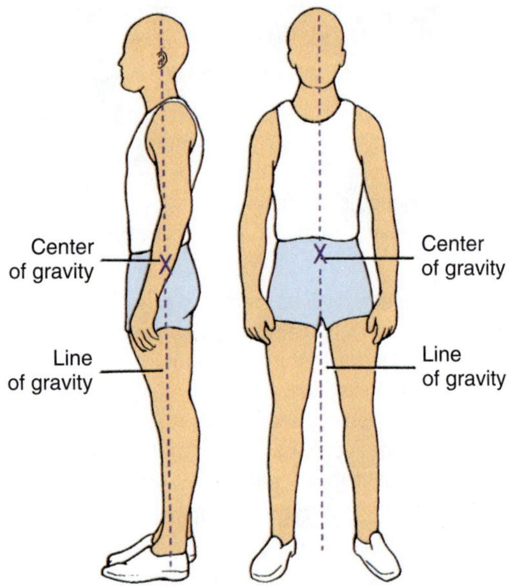

FIGURE 27-1 Correct body alignment with standing.

supply); the feet are supported on the floor; and the forearms are supported on the armrest, in the lap, or on a table in front of the chair.

Assessment of alignment in the sitting position is particularly important for the patient with neuromuscular disorders, muscle weakness, muscle paralysis, or nerve damage. A patient with these alterations has diminished sensation in affected areas and is unable to perceive pressure or decreased circulation. Proper sitting alignment reduces the risk for musculoskeletal system damage.

Recumbent. Position your patient in the lateral position with all but one pillow and all positioning supports removed from the bed. Make sure that the vertebrae are in straight alignment without observable curves. This assessment provides baseline data concerning a patient's body alignment.

Conditions that create a risk for damage to the musculoskeletal system when lying down include impaired mobility (e.g., spinal curvature), use of immobilization devices (e.g., traction), decreased sensation (e.g., hemiparesis from a stroke), impaired circulation (e.g., diabetes), and lack of voluntary muscle control (e.g., spinal cord injuries).

When a patient is unable to change position voluntarily, assess the position of body parts while he or she is lying down. Make sure that the vertebrae are in straight alignment without any observable curves. Normally the extremities are in alignment and do not cross over one another. The head and neck are aligned without excessive flexion or extension.

Mobility. The adequacy of your patient's mobility affects his or her coordination and balance while walking, the ability to carry out ADLs, and the ability to participate in an exercise program. The assessment of mobility has three components: range of motion, gait, and exercise.

Range of Motion. Observing **range of motion (ROM)** is one of the first assessment techniques used to determine the degree of limitation or injury to a joint. Assess ROM to further clarify the extent of joint stiffness, swelling, pain, limited movement, and unequal movement. Chapter 36 covers a thorough ROM assessment. Limited ROM indicates inflammation such as arthritis, fluid in the joint, altered nerve supply, or contractures. Increased mobility (beyond normal) of a joint indicates connective tissue disorders, ligament tears, and possible joint fractures.

Gait. **Gait** is the manner or style of walking, including rhythm, cadence, and speed. Assessing gait allows for conclusions about balance, posture, and the ability to walk without assistance (see Chapter 16). While a patient walks, look for conformity, a regular, smooth rhythm and symmetry in the length of leg swing; smooth swaying related to the gait phase; and a smooth, symmetrical arm swing (Seidel et al., 2011).

Exercise. Exercise is physical activity. It can be used for body conditioning, improving health, maintaining fitness, providing therapy for correcting a deformity, or restoring the body to a maximal state of health. During assessment determine a patient's level and frequency of exercise. This provides baseline information for both exercise and activity tolerance. In addition, baseline information is beneficial when establishing a patient's exercise and rehabilitation plan following an illness or injury. When a person exercises, physiological changes occur in body systems (Box 27-5).

During exercise you improve muscle tone, size, and strength and cardiopulmonary conditioning. As a result you are able to exercise longer with each strengthening of the muscles. Exercise also enhances joint mobility because the exercise itself requires movement of body parts.

Activity Tolerance. **Activity tolerance** is the type and amount of exercise or work that a person is able to perform without undue exertion or injury (Box 27-6). Observe patients after ambulation, self-bathing, or sitting in a chair for several hours and assess their verbal report of fatigue and weakness. Assess heart rate and blood pressure response to activity.

Patient Expectations. In assessing a patient's expectations concerning body alignment and joint mobility, determine your patient's perception of what is normal or acceptable in regard to mobility. For example, if exercising is painful or tiresome to patients, they may lack adherence and commitment to desired interventions. Some patients are content with their present range of motion or mobility and do not perceive a need for improvement. Unless there is a real threat to health maintenance, forcing patients to accept perspectives not in accordance with their own beliefs is a breach of standards of care.

Older Adult Considerations. The older adult often experiences a decline in physical activity and changes in joints that predispose to problems with mobility and limit joint flexibility. In addition, chronic conditions increase in older adults, and certain medications (e.g., cardiovascular medication, diuretics, or changes in dosages of these medications) affect a person's activity and exercise tolerance. It is important for older adults to exercise and remain active. A program of exercise promotes health, and improves illness, trauma, and rehabilitation outcomes (CDC, 2011). As people age they lose lifelong partners and friends, and opportunities for exercise

BOX 27-5 EFFECTS OF EXERCISE

CARDIOVASCULAR SYSTEM
- Increased cardiac output
- Improved myocardial contraction, thereby strengthening cardiac muscle
- Decreased resting heart rate
- Improved venous return

PULMONARY SYSTEM
- Increased respiratory rate and depth followed by a quicker return to resting state
- Improved alveolar ventilation
- Decreased work of breathing
- Improved diaphragmatic excursion

METABOLIC SYSTEM
- Increased basal metabolic rate
- Increased use of glucose and fatty acids
- Increased triglyceride breakdown
- Increased gastric motility
- Increased production of body heat

MUSCULOSKELETAL SYSTEM
- Improved muscle tone
- Increased joint mobility
- Improved muscle tolerance to physical exercise
- Possible increase in muscle mass
- Reduced bone loss

ACTIVITY TOLERANCE
- Improved tolerance
- Decreased fatigue

PSYCHOSOCIAL FACTORS
- Improved tolerance to stress
- Reports of "feeling better"
- Reports of decrease in illness (e.g., colds, influenza)

Data from Huether SE, McCance KL: *Understanding pathophysiology,* ed 5, St Louis, 2012, Mosby.

BOX 27-6 FACTORS INFLUENCING ACTIVITY TOLERANCE

PHYSIOLOGICAL FACTORS
- Skeletal abnormalities
- Muscular impairments
- Endocrine or metabolic illnesses (e.g., diabetes mellitus, thyroid disease)
- Hypoxemia
- Decreased cardiac function
- Decreased endurance
- Impaired physical stability
- Pain
- Sleep pattern disturbance
- Prior exercise patterns
- Infectious processes and fever

EMOTIONAL FACTORS
- Anxiety
- Depression
- Chemical addictions
- Motivation

DEVELOPMENTAL FACTORS
- Age
- Sex
- Pregnancy
- Physical growth and development of muscle and skeletal support

and activities lessen. Recommend approaches that help older adults increase exercise and activity, use proper body mechanics, and prevent injury (Box 27-7).

BOX 27-7 CARE OF THE OLDER ADULT

General Guidelines for Initiating an Exercise Program with the Older Adult

- Encourage older adults to avoid prolonged sitting and get up and stretch. Frequent stretching decreases joint contractures. Tai Chi exercise and meditative movements may be a suitable exercise alternative for the older adult (Piliae-Taylor et al., 2010; Rogers, Keller, and Larkey, 2010).
- Be sure that older adults maintain proper body alignment when sitting. Proper alignment minimizes joint and muscle stress.
- Teach patients how to use stronger joints or larger muscle groups to manipulate items such as spray cans and container lids. Efficient distribution of workload decreases joint stress and pain.
- Provide resources for planned exercise programs. Proper exercise activities slow further bone loss and prevent fractures in the older adult with osteoporosis (Blake and Hawley, 2012).
- It is never too late to begin an exercise program (Edelman and Mandle, 2010). Ensure older adults consult a health care provider before beginning an exercise program, particularly if they have heart or lung disease or other chronic illnesses (Neidrick et al., 2012).

NURSING DIAGNOSIS

A patient's assessment provides related clusters of data or defining characteristics that lead to the identification of nursing diagnoses, including these examples:

- *Activity Intolerance*
- *Risk for Activity Intolerance*
- *Disturbed Body Image*
- *Fatigue*
- *Risk for Injury*
- *Impaired Physical Mobility*
- *Acute Pain*
- *Chronic Pain*
- *Impaired Skin Integrity*
- *Risk for Impaired Skin Integrity*

Alterations in body alignment and joint mobility result from developmental changes, postural and bone formation abnormalities, impaired muscle development, damage to the central nervous system, or direct trauma to the musculoskeletal system. In some cases alterations in joint mobility or alignment are the defining characteristics to support a diagnosis. Nursing diagnoses often focus on an individual's ability to move. Make sure that the diagnostic label directs nursing interventions. For example, the diagnostic label *Impaired Physical Mobility related to pain and muscle weakness* directs you to initiate pain-relief and exercise measures.

PLANNING

Use data gathered during assessment and critical thinking to develop an individualized plan of care for your patients. You identify patient needs and, in collaboration with the patient and family, integrate these needs with the goals and outcomes of care, care priorities, and restorative and continuing care needs. This enables you to develop a plan of care to optimize the patient's exercise and activity levels (Figure 27-2).

Goals and Outcomes. Once you define appropriate nursing diagnoses, work with your patient to set goals and

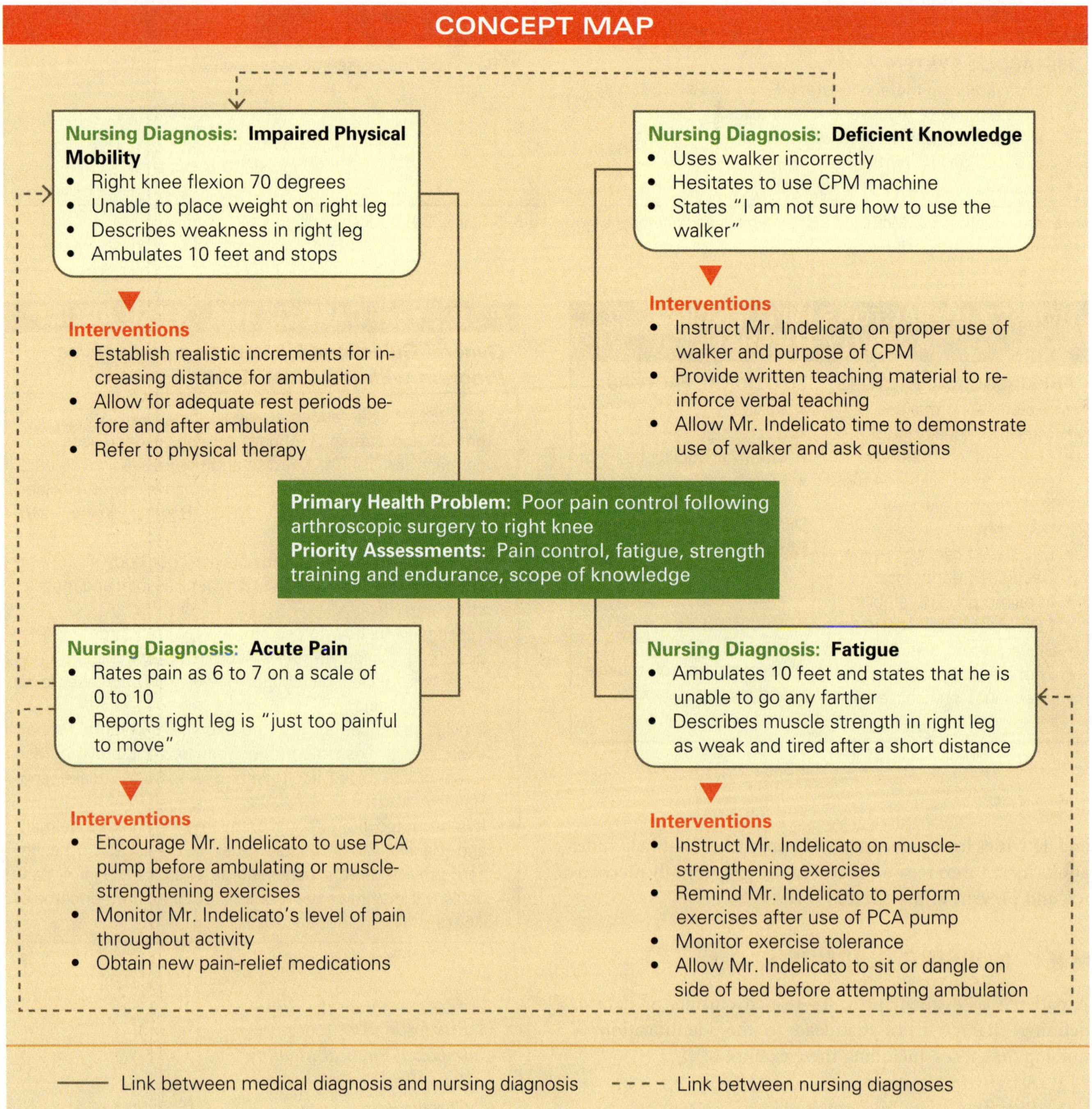

FIGURE 27-2 Concept map. *CPM,* Continuous passive motion; *PCA,* patient-controlled analgesia.

expected outcomes, which then direct nursing interventions. For example, the goal of achieving optimum ROM in the right knee has the outcome of achieving 90-degree flexion in the right knee by discharge. Nursing therapies include ROM and muscle strengthening. The plan considers risks for injury and preexisting health concerns. It is especially important to have knowledge of your patient's previous functional status and home environment.

Setting Priorities. Consider your patient's most immediate needs when individualizing a plan of care. Determine the immediacy of any problem by the effect the problem has on a patient's mental and physical health. For example, if a patient is in acute pain, relieving pain is a priority before you begin exercise therapy. Safety becomes a priority whenever you are assisting with the many skills associated with the care of patients with activity intolerance, improper body mechanics, and/or impaired mobility. For example, you must use caution to avoid a patient fall during transferring. Your priorities change from short term to long term when you plan for patients' return to their homes. For those who remain disabled or limited in mobility, be sure that family members are prepared to help with positioning and transfer techniques. When you perform skills that promote a patient's activity, always be vigilant in monitoring your patients and supervising nursing assistive personnel in carrying out activities to prevent complications and potential injury.

Collaborative Care. Planning also involves an understanding of a patient's need to maintain motor function and independence. Collaborate with other members of the health care team such as physical or occupational therapists. Long-term rehabilitation is sometimes necessary, and you begin discharge planning when a patient enters the health care system. In addition, always individualize a plan of care directed at meeting the actual or potential needs of your patient (see Care Plan).

IMPLEMENTATION

Health Promotion. Over the last few decades there has been an increase in exercise awareness; more community centers, shopping malls, and exercise facilities have indoor walking areas. Thus people are able to plan for walking as an exercise in climate-controlled and safe environments. Family and community gardens offer another method of exercise and help a person maintain and improve balance. Community centers, local adult education classes, and exercise facilities have exercise classes geared to a variety of age-groups and families. In addition, some facilities have exercise classes geared to individuals with chronic illnesses such as cardiac or pulmonary disease. All of these resources focus on improving exercise and activity.

Encourage patients to exercise daily; moderate 15- to 30-minute exercise is beneficial to maintain fitness, weight levels, and glycemic (blood sugar) control. Always encourage older adults or patients with underlying medical conditions to consult with their health care provider before beginning a vigorous exercise program. Direct patient-centered health promotion activities toward maintaining and/or improving exercise and activity that help return a patient to independence and a maximal state of health following trauma or

CARE PLAN

Impaired Physical Mobility

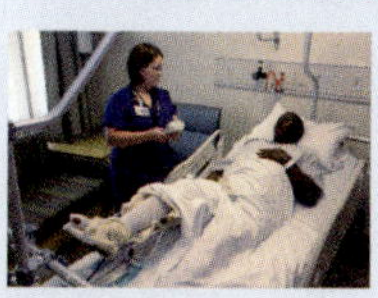

ASSESSMENT

Mr. Indelicato is a 72-year-old African-American hospitalized for surgery on his right knee. Over the past 5 years he has continued to experience pain and decreased mobility. He is now 2 days *postoperative* following total right knee replacement. His incision is healing, and there is no edema or redness.

ASSESSMENT ACTIVITIES	FINDINGS/DEFINING CHARACTERISTICS*
Assess Mr. Indelicato's pain level.	Mr. Indelicato is hesitant to ambulate or use his continuous passive motion (CPM) machine. He rates his **pain as 6 to 7 on a scale of 0 to 10** and is using a patient-controlled analgesia (PCA) pump. He states, **"I can't put all my weight on my right leg. It's just too painful."**
Assess Mr. Indelicato's baseline mobility and endurance.	His degree of **knee flexion is now 70 degrees.** He is able to **ambulate 10 feet with a walker but states, "I can't go any farther."** In addition, he further describes his muscle strength in his right leg as **feeling weak and tired after walking a short distance.**
Assess Mr. Indelicato's knowledge about proper use of his walker.	The nurse observes Mr. Indelicato using the walker incorrectly.

***Defining characteristics** are shown in **bold** type.

Continued

CARE PLAN—cont'd

Impaired Physical Mobility

NURSING DIAGNOSIS: Impaired Physical Mobility related to pain, muscle weakness, and limited joint motion.

PLANNING

GOALS	EXPECTED OUTCOMES (NOC)†
	Pain Control
• Mr. Indelicato will obtain a tolerable level of pain during ambulation.	• Mr. Indelicato's pain is 2 to 3 on a scale of 0 to 10 during ambulation.
	Endurance
• Mr. Indelicato will gain optimal functioning of the right knee with independent, purposeful movement.	• Mr. Indelicato ambulates 50 to 75 feet with aid of walker without reports of increasing fatigue. • Mr. Indelicato gains a minimum of 90-degree flexion in right knee by discharge.
	Knowledge: Prescribed Activity
• Mr. Indelicato will use walker properly while ambulating.	• Mr. Indelicato performs a return demonstration of proper use of walker.

†Outcomes classification labels from Moorhead S et al, editors: *Nursing outcomes classification (NOC),* ed 5, St Louis, 2013, Mosby.

INTERVENTIONS (NIC)‡	RATIONALE
Exercise Therapy: Ambulation	
• Encourage Mr. Indelicato to use patient-controlled analgesia (PCA) pump before ambulation.	Peak actions of analgesic occur as patient begins activity (Christo et al., 2011).
• Encourage Mr. Indelicato to sit in bed or on side of bed (dangle) before standing to ambulate.	Allowing patient to dangle before changing positions helps reduce or prevents orthostatic hypotension; maintains safety and prevents injury to patient.
• Establish realistic increments for Mr. Indelicato to increase walking distance during ambulation.	Gradually increasing physical activity and setting realistic goals for ambulation encourage activity in older adults (Chodzko-Zajko et al., 2009).
Exercise Promotion: Strength Training	
• Monitor exercise tolerance.	Presence of symptoms such as breathlessness, rapid pulse, pallor, or light-headedness indicates need for patient to stop activity (Lewis et al., 2011).
Teaching: Prescribed Exercise	
• Consult with physical therapist on proper use of walker.	Ensures safe use of assistive device.
• Instruct Mr. Indelicato and family caregivers on proper use of walker. Provide written material that reinforces verbal instructions.	Providing instructions in a quiet environment and giving written instructions in large, easy-to-read print enhance learning for the older adult (Touhy et al., 2014).

‡Intervention classification labels from Bulechek GM et al, editors: *Nursing interventions classification (NIC),* ed 6, St Louis, 2013, Mosby.

EVALUATION

NURSING ACTIONS	PATIENT RESPONSE/FINDING	ACHIEVEMENT OF OUTCOME
Ask Mr. Indelicato to rate the level of pain on a scale of 0 to 10.	Mr. Indelicato rates his pain at a 3 and states, "I am able to walk now that my knee doesn't hurt so badly anymore."	Mr. Indelicato's pain is under control, and he is able to ambulate with minimal discomfort.
Observe Mr. Indelicato's range of motion (ROM) or use of CPM machine.	Able to perform ROM and use CPM machine.	Outcome met. Mr. Indelicato expresses understanding of need for ROM and CPM machine.
Observe Mr. Indelicato's ambulation.	Steady gait with aid of walker.	Outcome met. Demonstrates correct use of walker.

illness. Although some patients require formal rehabilitation, many of these activities are implemented in a patient's home or neighborhood.

Acute Care

Lifting Techniques. In the clinical setting, patient care activities place health care providers at risk for injury during patient handling (see Chapter 36). In recent years the rate of injuries in occupational settings has increased dramatically. The most common back injury is strain on the lumbar muscle group, which includes the muscles around the lumbar vertebrae. Injury to these areas affects the ability to bend forward, backward, and side-to-side and to rotate the hips and lower back.

Lifting activities are necessary in acute care and restorative care settings. For example, you may care for an individual who is wheelchair dependent and healthy but needs assistance moving from bed to chair or chair to commode; or you may care for an individual who is unable to assist with any transfer and needs to be lifted from bed to chair or bed to stretcher. In any setting you need to know and use proper lifting techniques. Before lifting assess the weight that you will lift and what assistance, if any, you need. If you need help, assess if a second person is adequate or if you need mechanical assistance. Once you determine the amount of assistance you need, follow these steps:

1. Keep the weight you are lifting as close to your body as possible; this action places the object in the same plane as the lifter and close to the center of gravity for balance.
2. Bend at the knees; this maintains the center of gravity and uses the stronger leg muscles to do the lifting (Figure 27-3). Avoid twisting. Twisting overloads the spine and leads to serious injury.
3. Tighten abdominal muscles and tuck the pelvis; this provides balance and helps protect the back.
4. Keep your trunk erect and knees bent so multiple muscle groups work together in a coordinated manner.

However, note that injuries are not only related to lifting. You spend time in many activities involving bending and twisting that also cause injury (e.g., lifting and carrying supplies and equipment and pushing and pulling equipment (Waters et al., 2011b; 2011c).

Positioning Techniques. Patients with impaired nervous or musculoskeletal system functioning, patients with increased weakness, or those restricted to bed rest benefit from therapeutic positioning. During patient positioning determine areas of bony prominences where pressure, friction, and shear cause the most wear and tear. Through the use of proper positioning and pressure-relief methods, you are able to protect these areas (see Chapter 37).

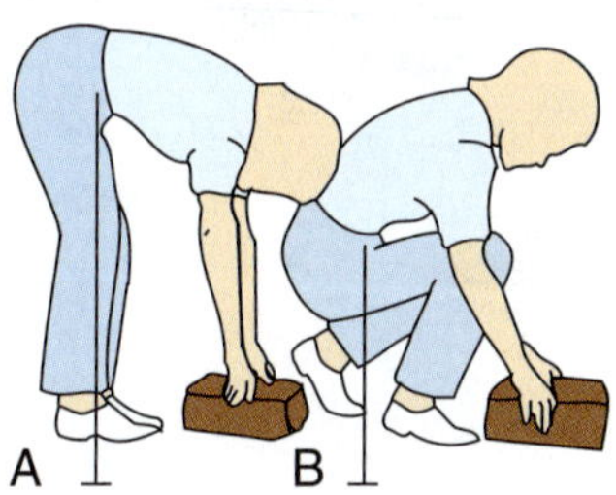

FIGURE 27-3 Incorrect **(A)** and correct **(B)** body position for lifting.

In general you reposition patients as needed and at least every 2 hours if they are in bed and 1 hour if they are sitting in a chair (Hartford Institute for Geriatric Nursing, 2008; WOCN, 2010). Improper positioning increases patients' risk for developing pressure ulcers or contractions, especially patients who have underlying condition such as diabetes mellitus or peripheral vascular diseases. You need to frequently reposition patients with contractures or patients who are at greater risk for skin breakdown over bony prominences. Positions that compromise peripheral blood flow also damage nerves. Every time you reposition a patient, make certain to check total body alignment, placement of extremities, skin breakdown, and joint contractures. The following also influence the frequency of position changes: level of comfort, amount of spontaneous movement, presence of edema, loss of sensation, and overall physical and mental status. Several devices are available to maintain a patient's body alignment after positioning (Table 27-3). Select the therapeutic position that maximizes your patient's comfort, safety, and ability to still use remaining function. Skill 27-1 describes the methods of positioning patients.

Fowler's and Semi-Fowler's Positions. Elevate the head of the patient's bed to the desired level and slightly elevate the patient's knees, avoiding pressure on the popliteal vessels. The head rests against the mattress or a small pillow for support. Use pillows to maintain natural alignment of the hands, wrists, and forearms. In semi-Fowler's position the head of the bed is at a 30- to 45-degree angle; you use this position for patients who cannot tolerate a supine position such as those with cardiac and respiratory problems. In supported Fowler's or high-Fowler's position the head of the bed is 60 to 90 degrees. Patients with severe respiratory distress breathe more easily in high-Fowler's position. Common trouble areas for patients in the Fowler's position include:

- Increased cervical flexion because the pillow at the head is too thick and head thrusts forward
- Extension of the knees, allowing the patient to slide to the foot of the bed
- Pressure on the posterior aspect of the knees, decreasing circulation to the feet
- External rotation of the hips
- Arms hanging unsupported at the patient's sides
- Unsupported feet or pressure on the heels
- Unprotected pressure points at the sacrum and heels
- Increased shearing force on the back and heels when you raise the head of the bed greater than 60 degrees

Supine Position. In the **supine** position the patient rests on the back. A small, flat pillow supports the head, neck, and upper shoulders (Pierson and Fairchild, 2013; Sorrentino et al., 2012). When a patient is immobile, use pillows, **trochanter rolls** (see Table 27-3), and **hand rolls** or arm splints

TABLE 27-3 DEVICES USED FOR PROPER POSITIONING

DEVICES	USES AND DESCRIPTIONS
Pillows	Make sure that pillows are appropriate size for the body part you will position. They provide support, elevate body parts, and splint incisional areas.
Foot boots	*Foot boots* maintain feet in *dorsiflexion.* Remove boots at least 2 to 3 times per day to assess skin integrity and joint mobility.
Trochanter rolls	*Trochanter rolls* prevent external rotation of legs when immobile patients are in the supine position. To form a trochanter roll, fold a cotton bath blanket or a sheet lengthwise to a width extending from the greater trochanter of the femur to the lower border of the popliteal space (Figure 27-4). Place the roll under the buttocks and roll it away from the patient until the thigh is in a neutral position or an inward position with the patella facing upward.
Hand rolls	*Hand rolls* maintain the thumb slightly adducted and in opposition to the fingers; they maintain fingers in a slightly flexed position (Figure 27-5). You make hand rolls by folding a washcloth in half, rolling it lengthwise, and securing the roll with tape. Place the roll against the palmar surface of the hand. Evaluate the position of the hand to make certain the hand is functional.
Hand-wrist splints	***Hand-wrist splints*** are individually molded for the patient to maintain proper alignment of the thumb in slight ***adduction*** and the wrist in slight dorsiflexion. Use these splints only for the patient for whom they were made.
Trapeze bar	The ***trapeze bar*** descends from a securely fastened overhead bar attached to the bed frame (Figure 27-6). The trapeze allows patient to use upper extremities to raise the trunk off the bed, to assist in transfer from bed to wheelchair, or to perform upper arm–strengthening exercises.
Side rails	***Side rails*** are bars positioned along the sides of the length of a hospital bed. They are designed to increase patient's ability to move and turn in bed (e.g., rolling from side to side or sitting up in bed).
Wedge pillow	A wedge or abductor pillow is a triangular-shaped pillow made of heavy foam. Use it to maintain the legs in ***abduction*** following total hip replacement surgery.

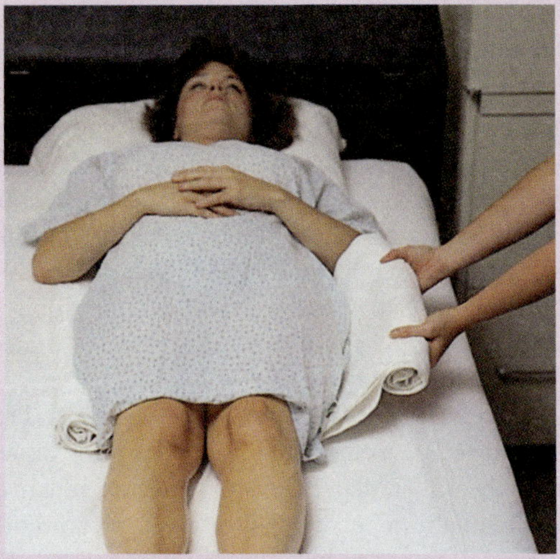

FIGURE 27-4 Trochanter roll.

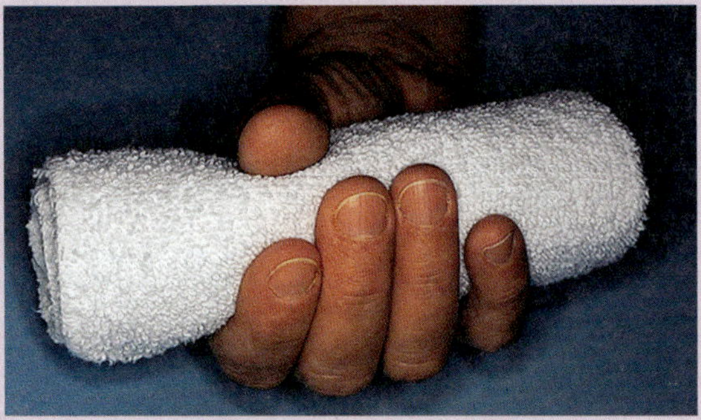

FIGURE 27-5 Hand roll.

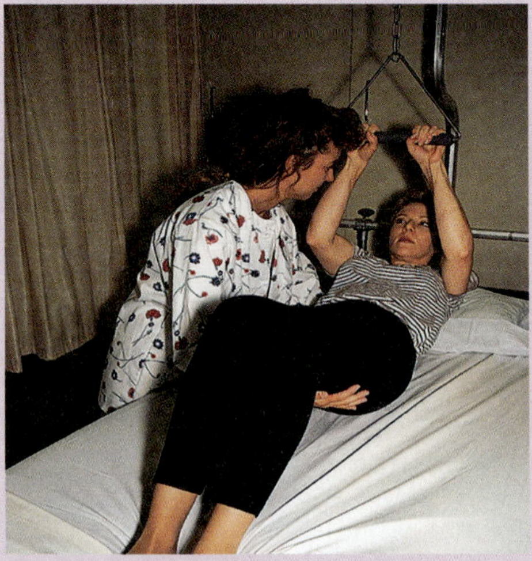

FIGURE 27-6 Patient using a trapeze bar.

to increase comfort and reduce injury to the skin or musculoskeletal system. The risk for aspiration is greater with this position; thus avoid the supine position when the patient is confused, agitated, experiencing a decreased level of consciousness, or at risk for aspiration.

Make sure that the mattress is firm enough to support the cervical, thoracic, and lumbar vertebrae. Avoid pressure on the back of the legs and heels. Use a **foot boot** to prevent **footdrop**, maintain proper alignment, and provide freedom of movement for the feet. The following are some common trouble areas for patients in the supine position:

- Pillow at the head that is too thick, increasing cervical flexion
- Head flat on the mattress
- Shoulders unsupported and internally rotated
- Elbows extended
- Thumb not in opposition to the fingers
- Hips externally rotated
- Unsupported feet
- Unprotected pressure points at the vertebrae, coccyx, elbows, heels, and the occipital region of the head

Prone Position. When **prone,** a patient is in the face-down position. Before placing a patient in the prone position, assess his or her medical record for any possible complications such as increasing intracranial pressure or cardiopulmonary disease.

Help the patient lie on the abdomen. Have him or her turn the head to the side. This facilitates respiration and drainage of oral secretions. Place a pillow under the head for comfort and relief from pressure. As an alternative place a wedge under the patient's chest or arms flexed over the head if it is more comfortable. Place a pillow under the lower leg; this promotes relaxation. If a pillow is unavailable, make sure that a patient's ankles are in **dorsiflexion** over the end of the mattress. Body alignment is poor when the ankles are continuously in **plantar flexion** and the lumbar spine remains in **hyperextension**. Sometimes lung expansion is compromised in this position, especially in people who are obese. Monitor your patient for signs of respiratory distress. You assess for and correct any of the following potential trouble points:

- Neck hyperextension
- Hyperextension of the lumbar spine
- Plantar flexion of the ankles
- Unprotected pressure points at the chin, elbows, hips, knees, and toes

Lateral Position. In the lateral (or side-lying) position a patient is supported on the right or left side with the opposite arm, thigh, and knee flexed and resting on the bed. Place a pillow under the patient's head to keep the head, neck, and spine in alignment. The upper arm is flexed and supported with a pillow. The upper leg is flexed at the hip and knee and positioned on a small pillow (Pierson and Fairchild, 2013; Sorrentino et al., 2012). Patients who are obese or older are often not able to tolerate this position for any length of time. The 30-degree lateral position is recommended as a position to avoid development of pressure ulcers (WOCN, 2010). The position differs from side-lying in that the dependent hip is brought forward so less pressure is directly on the bony prominence (Figure 27-7). The following trouble points are common in the side-lying position:

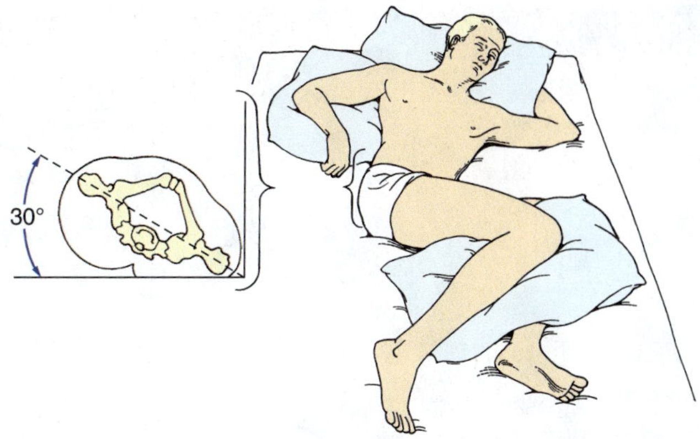

FIGURE 27-7 Thirty-degree lateral position at which pressure points are avoided. (Adapted from Bryant RA, Nix DP editors: *Acute and chronic wounds: current management concepts,* ed 4, St Louis, 2012, Mosby.)

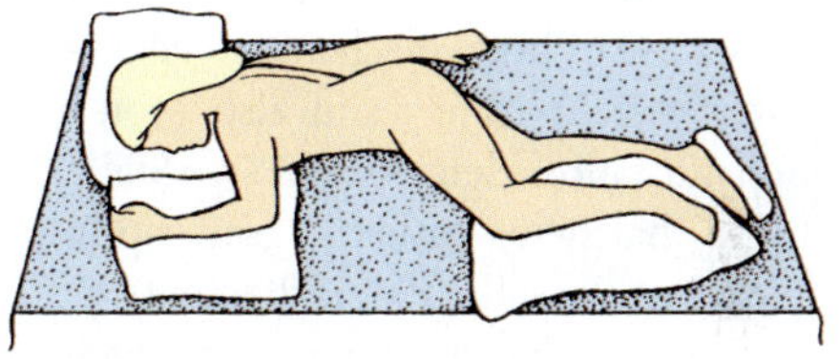

FIGURE 27-8 Patient in Sims' position.

- Lateral flexion of the neck
- Spinal curves out of normal alignment
- Shoulder and hip joints internally rotated, adducted, or unsupported
- Lack of support for the feet
- Lack of protection for pressure points at the ear, shoulder, anterior iliac spine, trochanter, and ankles
- Excessive lateral flexion of the spine if the patient has large hips and a pillow is not placed superior to the hips at the waist

Sims' Position. In the Sims' position a patient is semi-prone on the right or left side with the opposite arm, thigh, and knee flexed and resting on the bed (Figure 27-8). The Sims' position differs from the side-lying position in the distribution of the patient's weight. In this position you place the patient's weight on the anterior ilium, humerus, and clavicle. Trouble points common in Sims' position include the following:

- Lateral flexion of the neck
- Internal rotation, adduction, or lack of support to the shoulders and hips
- Lack of support for the feet
- Lack of protection for pressure points at the ilium, humerus, clavicle, knees, and ankles

Transfer Techniques. You often care for patients who are immobilized and need a position change, to be moved up in

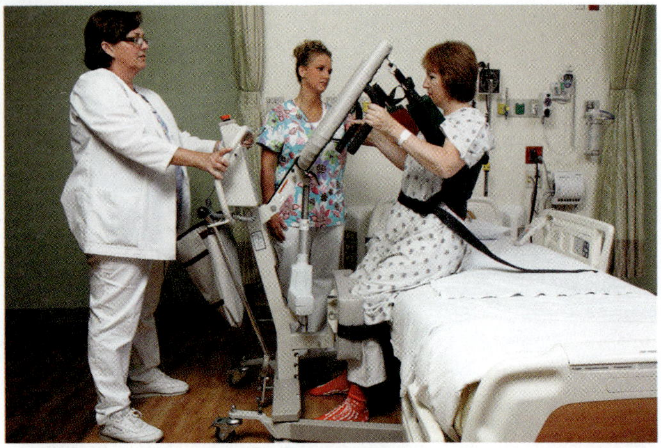

FIGURE 27-9 Patient grasps handles as nurse enables motorized lift.

bed, or to be transferred from a bed to a chair or a bed to a stretcher. Proper use of body mechanics enables you to move, lift, or transfer patients safely and also protects you from injury to your musculoskeletal system (see Skill 27-2). Transferring is a skill that helps patients regain optimal independence as quickly as possible. Physical activity maintains and improves joint motion, increases strength, promotes circulation, relieves pressure on skin, and improves urinary and respiratory functions. It also benefits the patient psychologically by increasing social activity and mental stimulation and providing a change in environment. Thus mobilization plays a crucial role in a patient's rehabilitation.

One of the major concerns during transfer is the safety of you and your patient. You prevent self-injury by using correct posture, minimal muscle strength, and effective body mechanics and lifting techniques. Always be aware of your patient's motor deficits, ability to aid in transfer, and body weight. As a rule of thumb, *GET HELP* to transfer a patient. If you or any other caregiver needs to lift more than 35 lbs (NIOSH 2006; Waters et al., 2011a), use assistive devices for the transfer (Figure 27-9). Explain the assistive device and procedure to the patient before the transfer.

When preparing to transfer patients, consider the type of problems that can develop. A patient who has been immobile for several days or longer is often weak or dizzy or sometimes develops **orthostatic hypotension** (a drop in blood pressure of 20 mm Hg or more systolic or 10 mm Hg or more diastolic when rising from a sitting position) when transferred (Freeman et al., 2011; Lagro, 2012; Lewis et al., 2011). A patient with neurological deficits sometimes has paresis (muscle weakness) or paralysis unilaterally or bilaterally, which complicates safe transfer. A flaccid arm sustains injury during transfer if unsupported. As a general rule use a transfer belt and obtain assistance for mobilization of patients with neurological deficits.

Joint Mobility and Ambulation

Range-of-Motion Exercises. The easiest intervention to maintain or improve joint mobility for patients and one that you are able to coordinate with other activities is the use of ROM exercises. In **active range-of-motion (ROM) exercises** a patient is able to move his or her joints. In contrast, you move the patient's joints in **passive range-of-motion (ROM) exercises.** The use of these exercises enables you to systematically assess and improve the patient's joint mobility (see Chapter 36).

Joints that are not moved periodically develop contractures, a permanent shortening of a muscle followed by the eventual shortening of associated ligaments and tendons. Over time the joint becomes fixed in one position, and a patient loses normal use of it. For a patient who does not have voluntary motor control, passive ROM exercises are the exercises of choice.

Mechanical devices are available for specific joints, which place these joints through continuous passive motion (CPM). Use these CPM machines after surgery to place joints through a selective repetitive ROM (see Chapter 36). A physician orders the machine to be set at certain degrees of joint mobility with increasing joint mobility or flexion as the goal. Patients who commonly use the CPM machine have had some form of total joint replacement surgery.

Unless contraindicated, the nursing care plan includes exercising each joint through as nearly a full ROM as possible. Initiate passive ROM exercises as soon as a patient loses the ability to move the extremity or joint (see Chapter 36).

Walking. Walking also increases joint mobility. In the normal walking posture the head is erect; the cervical, thoracic, and lumbar vertebrae are aligned; the hips and knees have appropriate flexion; and the arms swing freely in alternation with the legs. Illness or trauma reduces activity tolerance, requiring help with walking or the use of mechanical devices such as crutches, canes, or walkers.

Assisting a Patient to Walk. Helping a patient walk requires preparation. Assess a patient's activity tolerance, strength, coordination, and balance to determine the type of assistance needed. Also assess a patient's orientation and determine if there are any signs of distress. This precludes attempts at ambulation.

Assess the environment for safety before ambulation. Remove obstacles, be sure that the floor is clean and dry, and establish rest points in case the patient's activity tolerance decreases or the patient becomes dizzy. Also make sure that the patient wears supportive, nonslip shoes.

When preparing a patient for ambulation, dangling is an important technique. You help the patient to a sitting position with the legs dangling off the side of the bed and have him or her rest for 1 to 2 minutes before standing. The longer the period of immobility, the greater are the physiological changes. This is especially true with changes in circulation. When a patient has been flat for extended periods, blood pressure drops when he or she stands. Dangling helps to prevent this. After standing have the patient remain stationary for a minute or two before moving. If the patient becomes dizzy, the bed is still nearby, and you are able to quickly ease him or her back to bed.

You can use several methods to help a patient with ambulation. Use a gait belt to support him or her and maintain a

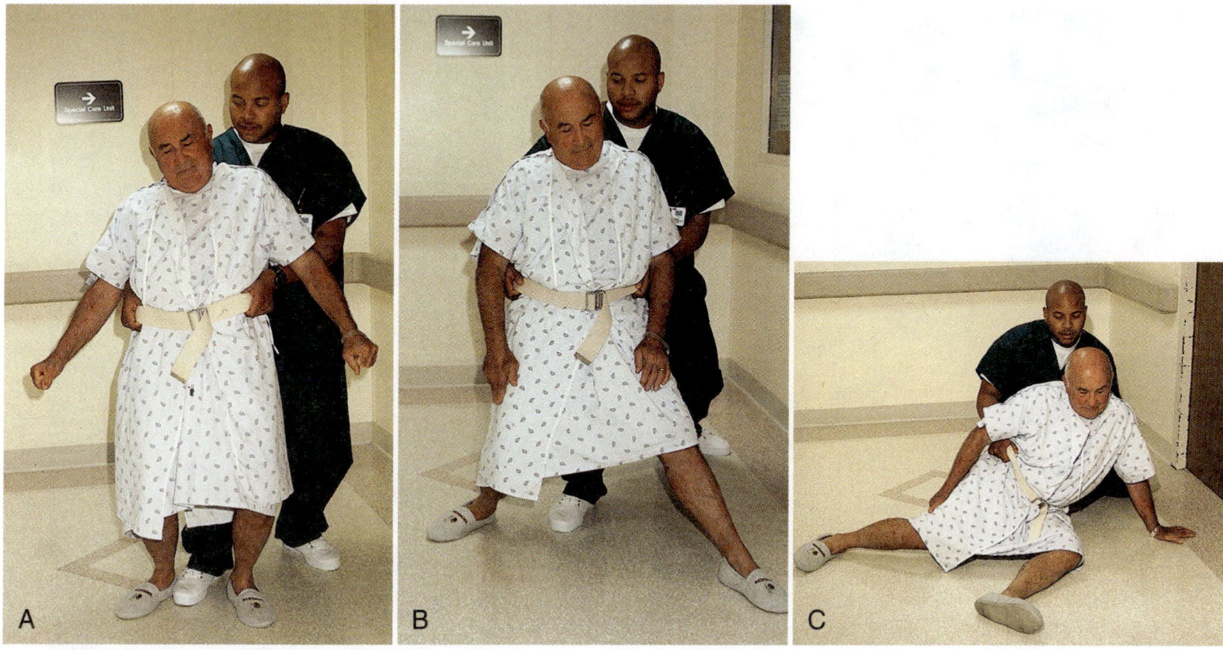

FIGURE 27-10 **A,** Stand with feet apart to provide broad base of support. **B,** Extend one leg and let patient slide against it to floor. **C,** Bend knees to lower body as patient slides to floor.

midline center of gravity. Make sure that he or she does not lean to one side because the center of gravity is no longer midline, which distorts balance and increases risk for falling.

Return a patient who appears unsteady or complains of dizziness to the closest bed or a chair. If the patient has a syncopal episode or begins to fall, assume a wide base of support with one foot in front of the other, thus supporting the patient's body weight. Gently lower the patient to the floor, protecting his or her head. Although lowering a patient to the floor is not difficult, practice this technique with a friend or classmate before attempting it in a clinical setting (Figure 27-10). Assess the patient for injuries at this time and notify his or her health care provider. Even if the patient is stable, obtain the assistance of a lift team to help you get the patient off the floor and back in bed or a chair.

Restorative and Continuing Care. Restorative and continuing care involving activity and exercise involves implementing strategies to assist the patient in ADLs after a patient no longer needs acute care. In collaboration with other health care professionals such as physical therapists, you promote activity and exercise by teaching the use of canes, walkers, or crutches, depending on the assistive device most appropriate for a patient's condition. Restorative and continuing care includes activities and exercises that restore and improve optimal functioning in a patient with chronic musculoskeletal illnesses such as arthritis, trauma, and other chronic illnesses such as coronary artery disease (CAD).

Assistive Devices for Walking

Walkers. Walkers are extremely light, movable devices, approximately waist high and made of metal tubing (Figure 27-11). They have four widely placed, sturdy legs. A walker is fitted correctly by having the patient step inside the walker.

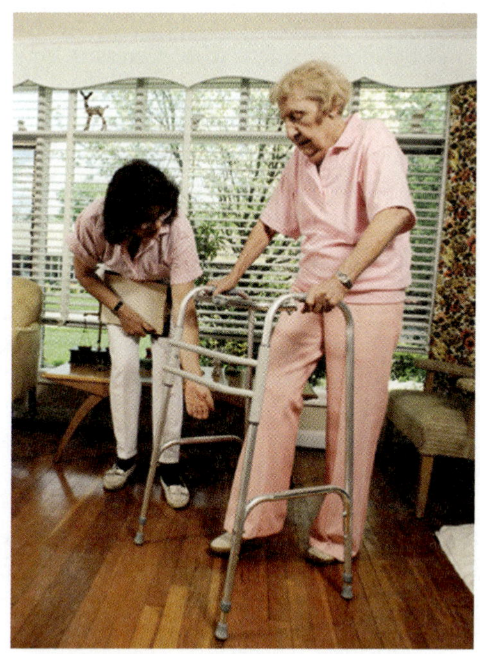

FIGURE 27-11 Patient using walker.

The person's elbow should bend comfortably, about 30 degrees, while holding onto the grips. When the person relaxes the arms at the side of the body, the top of the walker should line up with the crease on the inside of the wrist (Pierson and Fairchild, 2013). When walking, the patient holds the handgrips on the upper bars, takes a step, moves the walker forward, and takes another step. The patient should not lean over the walker or walk behind it; otherwise he or she might lose balance and fall.

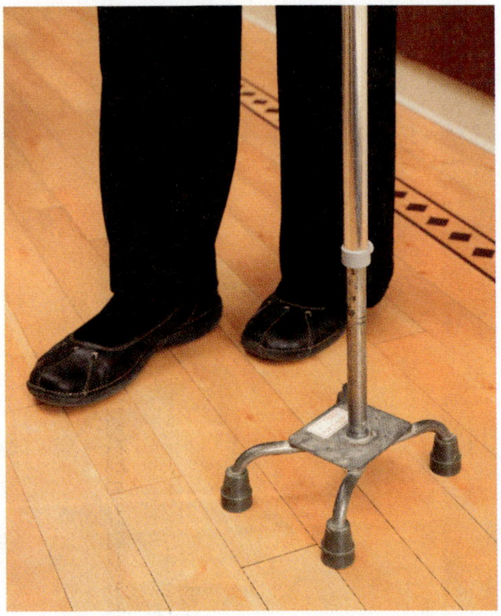

FIGURE 27-12 Base of quad cane.

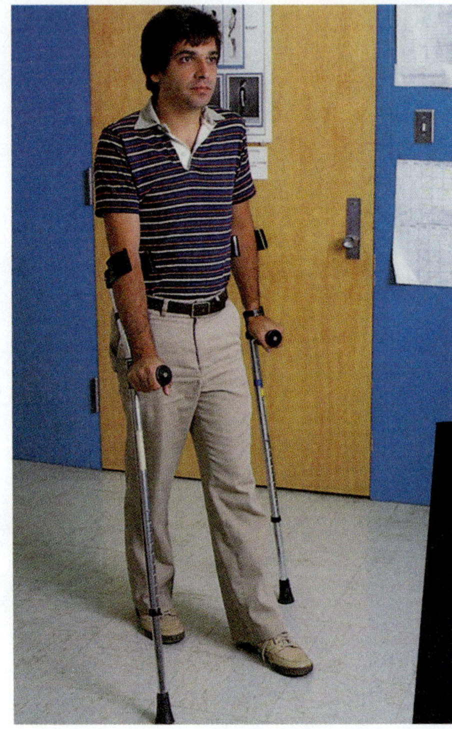

FIGURE 27-13 Double adjustable Lofstrand or forearm crutch.

Canes. Canes are lightweight, easily movable devices approximately waist high, made of wood or metal. Two common types of canes are the single straight-legged cane and the quad cane. The single straight-legged cane is used to support and balance a patient with decreased leg strength. Make sure that the patient keeps the cane on the stronger side of the body (Pierson and Fairchild, 2013). The nurse stands on the patient's weak side for support (Pierson and Fairchild, 2013). For maximum support when walking, the patient places the cane forward 15 to 25 cm (6 to 10 inches), keeping body weight on both legs. He or she moves the weaker leg to the cane, which divides body weight between the cane and the stronger leg. The patient then advances the stronger leg past the cane so the weaker leg and the body weight are supported by the cane and weaker leg. During walking the patient continually repeats these three steps. Teach the patient that two points of support such as both feet or one foot and the cane need to be touching the ground at all times.

The quad cane provides the most support and is used when there is partial or complete leg paralysis or some hemiplegia (Figure 27-12). You teach the same three steps used with the straight-legged cane to the patient.

Crutches. The use of crutches is usually temporary such as after ligament damage to the knee. However, some patients such as those with paralysis of the lower extremities need crutches permanently. A crutch is a wooden or metal staff. The two types of crutches are the double adjustable Lofstrand or forearm crutch (Figure 27-13) and the axillary wooden or metal crutch. The forearm crutch has a handgrip and a metal band that fits around the patient's forearm. The metal band and the handgrip are adjustable to fit the patient's height. The axillary crutch has a padded curved surface at the top, which fits under the axilla. The patient holds a handgrip in the form of a crossbar at the level of the palms to support the body. It is important to measure crutches for the appropriate length and teach patients to use their crutches safely. This includes teaching a patient to achieve a stable gait, ascend and descend stairs, and rise from a sitting position. You or a physical therapist teach the patient safety measures and guidelines associated with the use of crutches (Box 27-8).

Measuring for Crutches. The axillary crutch is the crutch more commonly used. There are three common methods to measure the length of the crutches. The first method multiplies the height of the patient by 77% (e.g., 70 inches × 77% = 53.90, or 54 inches) or subtracts 16 inches from the height (e.g., 70 inches – 16 inches = 54 inches) and uses the resulting value for the overall crutch length (i.e., axillary rest to tip). The second method is with the patient lying supine and measures the distance from the anterior axillary fold (i.e., the crease of the armpit) to a point approximately 6 to 8 inches lateral to the heel for the overall crutch length. The third method is used with the patient sitting and the upper extremities abducted at shoulder level. With one elbow extended and one elbow flexed to 90 degrees, measure from the olecranon process of the flexed elbow to the tip of the long finger of the hand of the opposite upper extremity. These methods often provide similar results, but sometimes you will find a difference in the measurements. Select the method that provides the best result consistently. These measurements are only estimates of the length of the crutch; confirm their fit with the patient standing (Pierson and Fairchild, 2013). When fitting crutches, the appropriate length of the crutch is from 3 to 4

BOX 27-8 PATIENT TEACHING

Crutch Safety

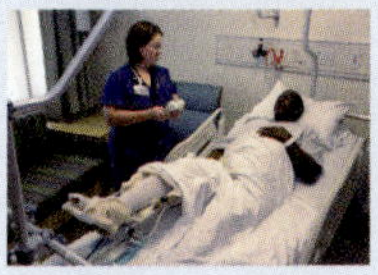

The physical therapist (PT) told Marilyn that Mr. Indelicato will need crutches for a short period of time because of limited weight bearing on the affected knee. It is important that Mr. Indelicato begins to use the crutches before discharge. Marilyn and the PT work together to develop the following teaching plan:

OUTCOME

Patient states the steps needed for safe crutch walking.

TEACHING STRATEGIES

- Demonstrate to patient how to inspect the crutch tips routinely. Make sure that the rubber tips are attached securely to the crutches. When the tips are worn, they need to be replaced immediately. Rubber crutch tips increase surface friction and prevent the crutches from slipping.
- Inform patient about the importance of keeping the crutch tips dry. If the tips become wet, the patient needs to dry them. Water decreases surface friction and increases the risk that the crutches will slip.
- Show patient how to inspect the structure of the crutches routinely. Cracks in a wooden crutch decrease the ability of the crutch to support weight. Bends in aluminum crutches alter body alignment, increasing the risk for further damage to the musculoskeletal system.
- Give patient a list of medical suppliers in the community. This allows the patient to obtain repairs and new rubber tips, handgrips, and crutch pads.
- Suggest that patient investigate the possibility of having a set of spare crutches and tips.

EVALUATION STRATEGIES

- Ask patient to describe how he will maintain crutch safety.
- Observe patient inspect his crutch tips and structure.
- Ask patient what he will do if his crutch breaks or he needs additional crutch tips.

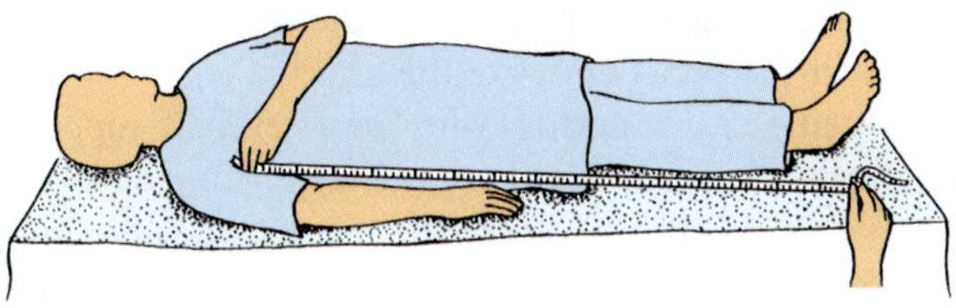

FIGURE 27-14 Measuring for crutch length.

finger widths from the axilla to a point 15 cm (6 inches) lateral to the patient's heel (Figure 27-14).

Make sure that you position the handgrips so the axillae do not support all of the patient's body weight. Pressure on the axillae increases pressure placed on underlying nerves, which sometimes results in partial paralysis of the arm. You determine the correct position of the handgrips with the patient upright, supporting weight by the handgrips with the elbows slightly flexed (20 to 25 degrees). You verify elbow flexion with a goniometer (Figure 27-15). When you have determined the height and placement of the handgrips, you again verify that the distance between the crutch pad and the patient's axilla is 3 to 4 finger widths (Figure 27-16).

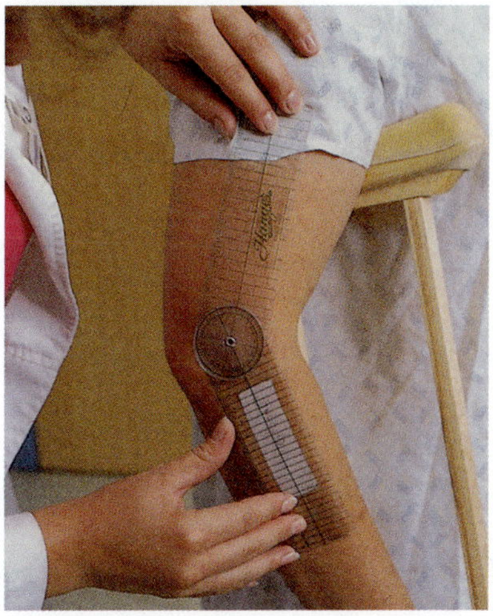

FIGURE 27-15 Using goniometer to verify correct degree of elbow flexion for crutch use.

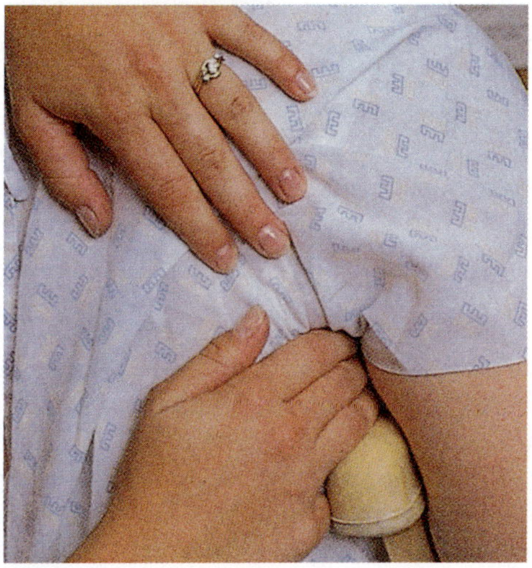

FIGURE 27-16 Verifying correct distance between crutch pad and axilla.

Crutch Gait. A patient assumes a **crutch gait** by alternately bearing weight on one or both legs and on the crutches. The health care provider determines the appropriate gait by assessing a patient's functional abilities, strength and weight-bearing ability, and the disease or injury that resulted in the need for crutches. This section summarizes the basic crutch stance and the four standard gaits: four-point alternating gait, three-point alternating gait, two-point gait, and swing-through gait.

The basic crutch stance is the tripod position, formed when the crutches are placed 15 cm (6 inches) in front of and

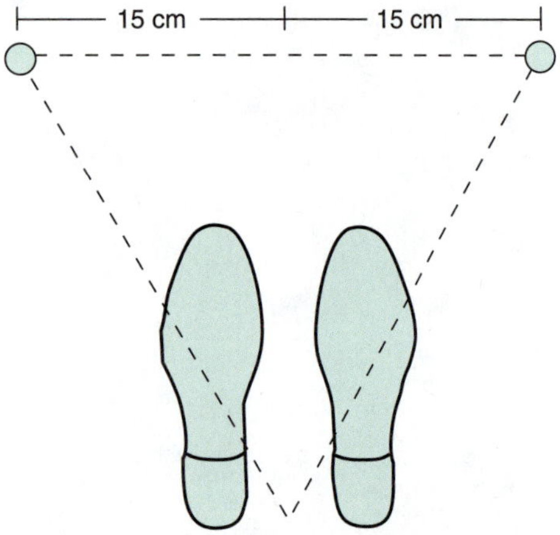

FIGURE 27-17 Tripod position, basic crutch stance.

15 cm to the side of each foot (Figure 27-17). This position improves the patient's balance by providing a wider base of support. The body alignment of the patient in the tripod position includes erect head and neck, straight vertebrae, and extended hips and knees. No weight should be borne by the axillae. The tripod position is used before crutch walking.

Four-point alternating or four-point gait gives stability to the patient but requires weight bearing on both legs. Each leg is moved alternately with each opposing crutch so that three points of support are on the floor at all times (Figure 27-18, *A*).

Three-point alternating or three-point gait requires a patient to bear all of the weight on one foot. In a three-point gait a patient puts weight on both crutches and then on the uninvolved leg and repeats the sequence (Figure 27-18, *B*). The affected leg does not touch the ground during the early phase of the three-point gait. Gradually the patient progresses to touchdown and full weight bearing on the affected leg.

The two-point gait requires at least partial weight bearing on each foot (Figure 27-18, *C*). The patient moves a crutch at the same time as the opposite leg so the crutch movements are similar to arm motion during normal walking.

People with paraplegia who wear weight-supporting braces on their legs frequently use the swing-through gait. With weight placed on the supported legs, the patient places the crutches one stride in front and then swings to or through the crutches while they support his or her weight.

Crutch Walking on Stairs. When ascending stairs on crutches, a patient usually uses a modified three-point gait (Figure 27-19). The patient stands at the bottom of the stairs and transfers body weight to the crutches. The patient advances the unaffected leg between the crutches to the stairs and shifts weight from the crutches to the unaffected leg. Finally, the patient aligns both crutches on the stairs. He or she repeats this sequence until the patient reaches the top of the stairs.

To descend the stairs (Figure 27-20), a patient also uses a three-phase sequence. The patient transfers body weight to the unaffected leg. The patient places crutches on the stair

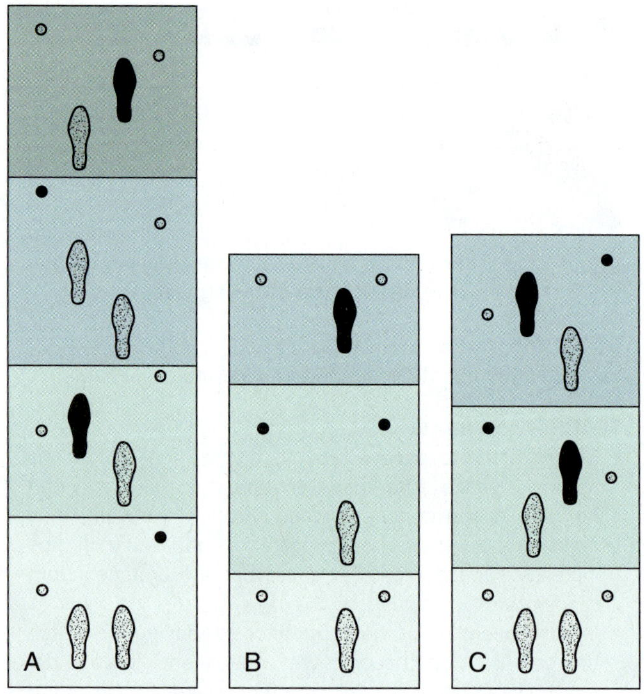

FIGURE 27-18 **A,** Four-point alternating gait. Solid feet and crutch tips show foot and crutch tip moved in each of the four phases. (Read from bottom to top.) **B,** Three-point gait with weight borne on unaffected leg. Solid foot and crutch tips show weight bearing in each phase. **C,** Two-point gait with weight borne partially on each foot and each crutch advancing with opposing leg. Solid areas indicate leg and crutch tips bearing weight.

and begins to transfer body weight to the crutches, moving the affected leg forward. Finally the patient moves the unaffected leg to the stairs with the crutches, repeating the sequence until reaching the bottom of the stairs.

Sitting in a Chair with Crutches. Sitting in a chair with crutches also involves phases and requires a patient to transfer weight (Figure 27-21). First the patient gets positioned at the center front of the chair with the posterior aspect of the legs touching the chair. Then the patient holds both crutches in the hand opposite the affected leg. If both legs are affected (e.g., a person who wears weight-supporting braces), the patient holds the crutches in the hand on the stronger side. With both crutches in one hand, the patient supports body weight on the unaffected leg and crutches. While still holding the crutches, the patient grasps the arm of the chair with the remaining hand and lowers the body into the chair. To stand the patient reverses the procedure and, when fully erect, assumes the tripod position before beginning to walk.

EVALUATION

Patient Care. You evaluate a patient's response to all nursing interventions by comparing a patient's actual response to the expected outcomes for each goal. You evaluate

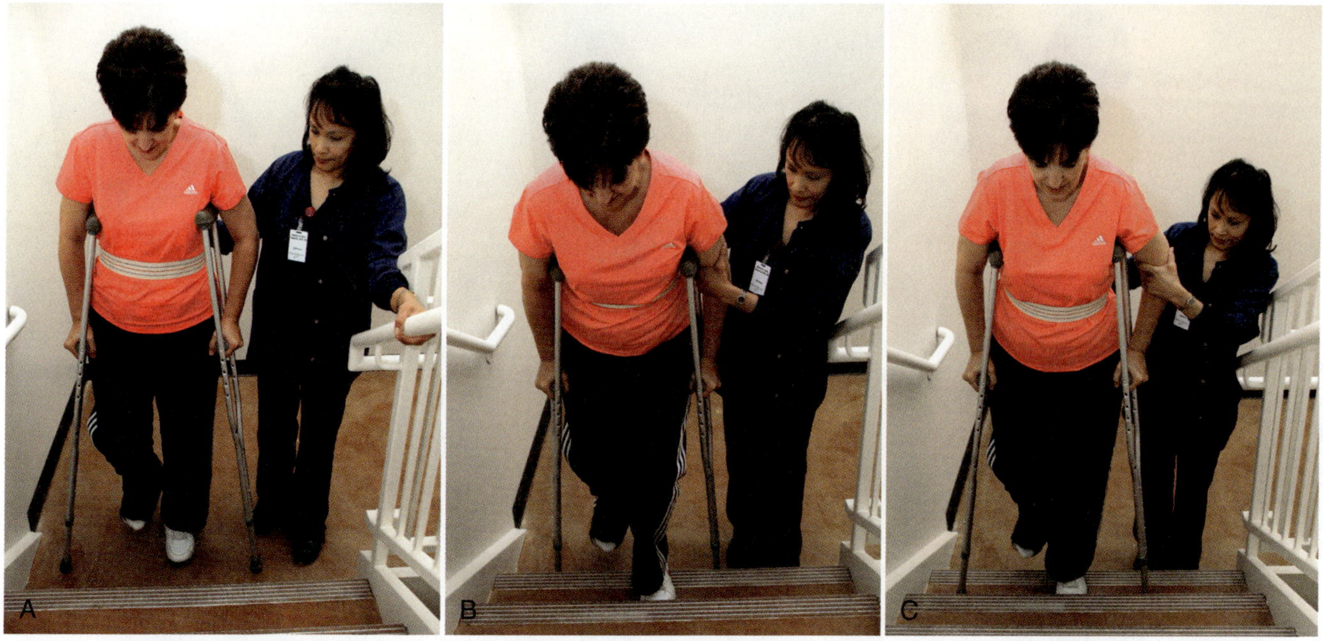

FIGURE 27-19 Ascending stairs. **A,** Weight is placed on crutches. **B,** Weight is transferred from crutches to unaffected leg on stairs. **C,** Crutches are aligned with unaffected leg on stairs.

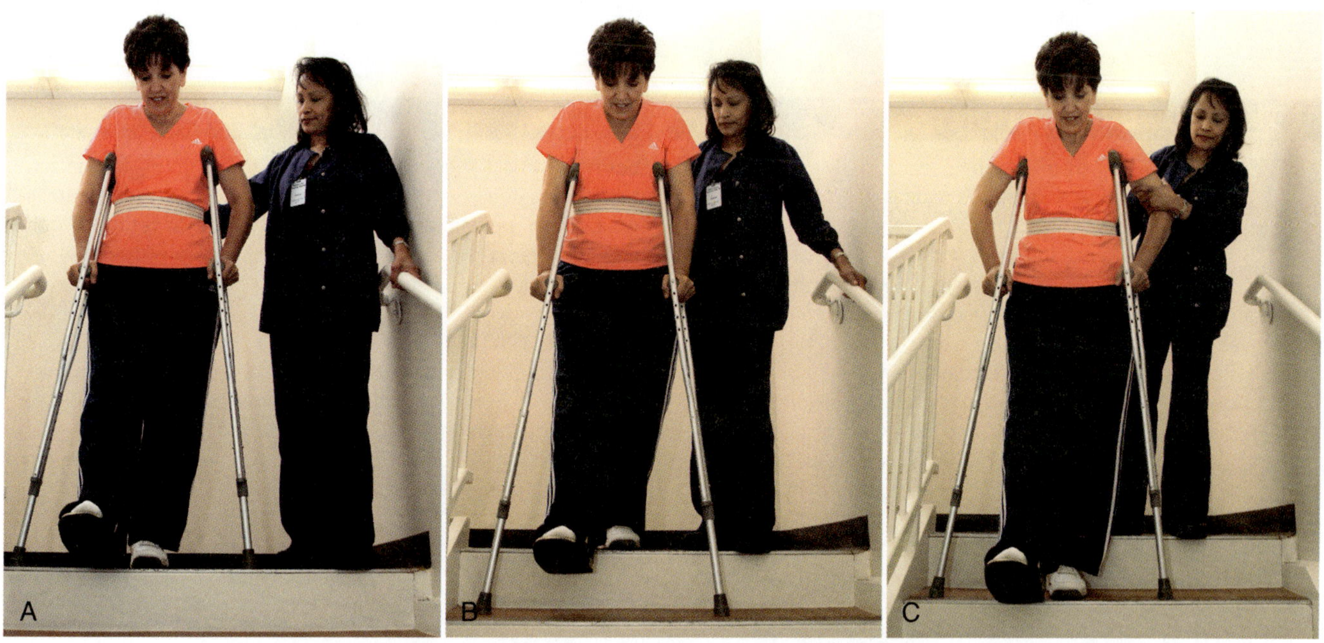

FIGURE 27-20 Descending stairs. **A,** Body weight on unaffected leg. **B,** Body weight transferred to crutches. **C,** Unaffected leg aligned on stairs with crutches.

specific outcomes designed to demonstrate improved activity and exercise tolerance. You need to revise the plan if the patient does not achieve the expected outcomes. For example, a patient may achieve improved joint range of motion, but if exercise tolerance is still poor, there may be a need to increase duration of exercise. The success in meeting each outcome is based on the use of evaluative measures such as ROM, ability to ambulate, distance of ambulation, and activity/exercise tolerance (Box 27-9). In many cases evaluation will occur in the long term (e.g., weeks or months) before patients regain full function.

Patient Expectations. For you to evaluate a patient's perception of interventions, first you need to know his or her expectations concerning joint mobility, posture, or body alignment. What is acceptable or anticipated on your part is sometimes vastly different from what a patient and family members anticipate or accept. Ask patients to describe their satisfaction with the plan of care.

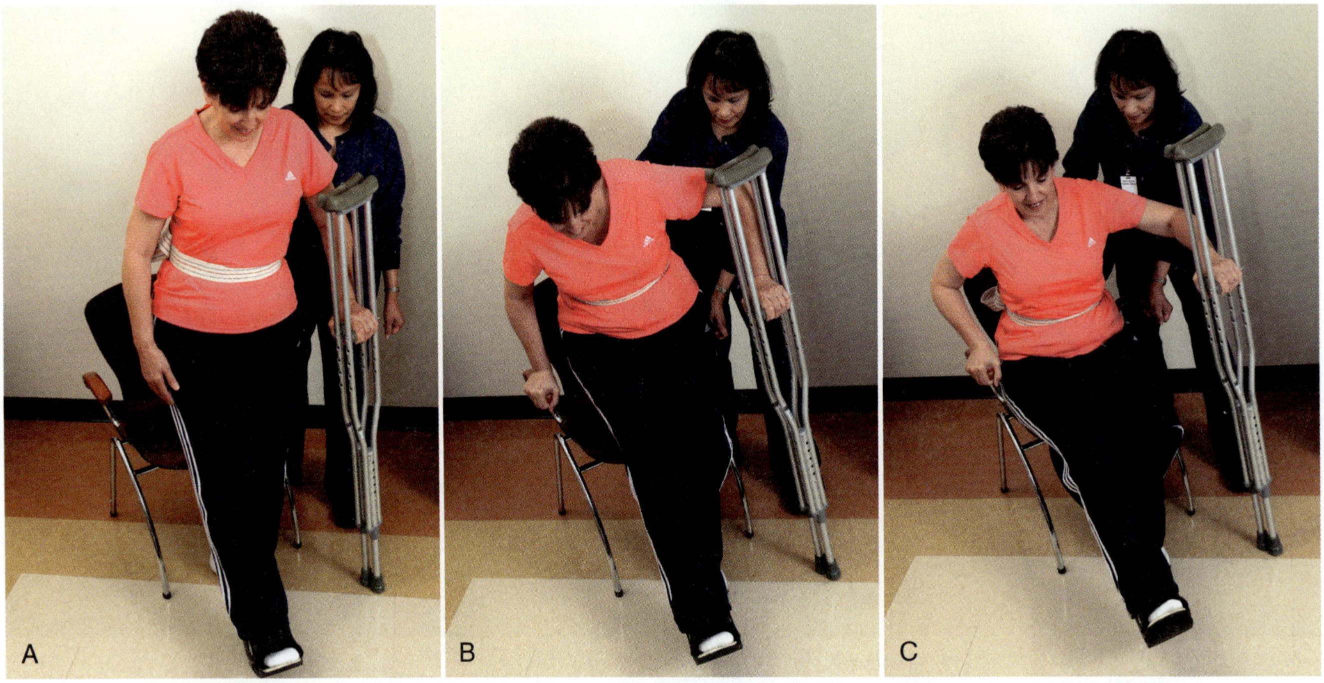

FIGURE 27-21 Sitting on chair. **A,** Both crutches are held by one hand. Patient transfers weight to crutches and unaffected leg. **B,** Patient grasps arm of chair with free hand and begins to lower herself into chair. **C,** Patient completely lowers herself into chair.

BOX 27-9 EVALUATION

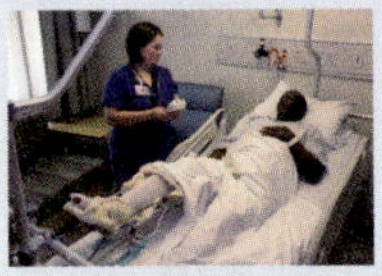

Marilyn began to care for Mr. Indelicato 5 weeks ago, and she has followed him in the outpatient rehabilitation setting over the past 4 weeks. He progressed steadily, increasing both weight bearing and range of joint motion of his affected knee. Mr. Indelicato's pain was difficult to manage. He expected pain to be completely resolved on hospital discharge and did not expect it to follow his physical therapy. Marilyn and the physical therapist worked with Mr. Indelicato and his orthopedic surgeon to identify pain-control measures following physical therapy. Currently Mr. Indelicato takes 600 mg of ibuprofen 45 minutes before physical therapy and every 8 to 12 hours thereafter. He reports that his pain is now almost totally gone. He is working on increasing strength so he is able to return to golf and bike riding. He says he will probably give up racquetball and tennis.

DOCUMENTATION NOTE

"Weight bearing and range of motion continue to improve. States takes 600 mg ibuprofen 45 minutes before coming to therapy and every 8 to 12 hours as needed for pain. Rates pain a 1 when exercising. States would like to begin riding bike and playing golf again in next 1 to 2 months."

SAFETY GUIDELINES FOR NURSING SKILLS

Ensuring patient safety is an essential role of the professional nurse. To ensure patient safety communicate clearly with members of the health care team, assess and incorporate the patient's priorities of care and preferences, and use the best evidence when making decisions about your patient's care. When performing the skills in this chapter, remember the following points to ensure safe, individualized patient care.

- Mentally review the transfer steps before beginning to ensure both the patient's and your safety.
- Assess the patient's mobility and strength to determine the assistance that he or she is able to offer during transfer.
- Determine the amount and type of assistance you require, including type of transfer equipment and the number of personnel it will take to safely transfer and prevent harm to a patient and yourself.
- Stand on a patient's strong side when he or she is not to place weight on the weak side (e.g., orthopedic surgery).

- Stand on a patient's weak side if he or she is supposed to increase weightbearing on the weak side.
- Raise the side rail on the side of the bed opposite of where you are standing to prevent the patient from falling out of bed on that side.
- Position the level of the bed to a comfortable and safe height.
- Arrange equipment (e.g., intravenous [IV] lines, feeding tube, Foley catheter) so it will not interfere with the transfer.
- Evaluate patient for correct body alignment and pressure areas on the skin after the transfer.

SKILL 27-1 MOVING AND POSITIONING PATIENTS IN BED

View Video!

DELEGATION CONSIDERATIONS

The skill of moving and positioning patients in bed can be delegated to nursing assistive personnel (NAP). The nurse informs the NAP about:

- Any limitations affecting movement and positioning of patient in bed.
- Scheduled times to reposition patient throughout the shift.
- When to request assistance (e.g., when patient is unable to assist nurse, has a lot of equipment, or is confused).

EQUIPMENT

- Pillows
- Therapeutic boots, splints, ankle support device, if needed
- Trochanter roll
- Hand rolls
- Side rails
- Appropriate safe patient-handling assistive device

STEP	RATIONALE
ASSESSMENT	
1. Assess patient's body alignment and comfort level while patient is lying down.	Provides baseline data for later comparisons. Determines ways to improve position and alignment.
2. Assess for risk factors that contribute to complications of immobility:	Increased risk factors require you to reposition patient more frequently (see Chapter 36).
a. Paralysis: Hemiparesis resulting from cerebrovascular accident (CVA); decreased sensation	Paralysis impairs movement; changes muscle tone; affects sensation. Because of difficulty moving and poor awareness of involved body part, patient is unable to protect and position body part for self.
b. Impaired mobility: Traction, arthritis, or other contributing disease processes	Traction or arthritic changes of affected extremity result in decreased range of motion (ROM).
c. Impaired circulation	Decreased circulation predisposes patient to pressure ulcers.
d. Age: Very young, older adult	Premature and young infants require frequent turning because their skin is fragile. Normal physiological changes associated with aging predispose older adults to greater risks for developing complications of immobility.
e. Level of consciousness and mental status	Patients who are comatose or semicomatose are unable to verbalize areas of skin pressure, increasing risk for skin breakdown.
3. Assess patient's physical ability to help with moving and positioning:	Enables nurse to use patient's mobility, coordination, and strength. Determines need for additional help. Ensures patient's and nurse's safety.
a. Age	Some older adult patients move more slowly with less strength.
b. Level of consciousness and mental status	Determines need for special aids or devices. Patients with altered levels of consciousness do not always understand instructions and are often unable to help.
c Disease process	Cardiopulmonary disease requires patient to have head of bed elevated.
d. Strength, coordination	Determines amount of assistance provided by patient during position change.
e. ROM	Limited ROM contraindicates certain positions.
4. Assess patient's height, weight, and body shape.	Devices for safe patient handling have different weight restrictions; bariatric patients require special beds, lifts, wheelchairs, and toileting and bathing equipment (Pelczarski, 2012).
5. Assess health care provider's orders. Clarify whether patient's condition contraindicates any positions (e.g., spinal cord injury; respiratory difficulties; certain neurological conditions; presence of incisions, drain, or tubing).	Placing patient in an inappropriate position causes injury.

SKILL 27-1 MOVING AND POSITIONING PATIENTS IN BED—cont'd

STEP	RATIONALE
6. Assess for presence of tubes, incisions, and equipment (e.g., traction).	They alter positioning procedure and affect patient's ability to independently change positions.
7. Assess condition of patient's skin.	Provides baseline to determine effects of positioning.
8. Assess ability and motivation of patient and family caregiver to participate in moving and positioning patient in bed in anticipation of discharge to home.	Determines ability of patient and family caregivers to help with positioning.
PLANNING	
1. Identify patient using two patient identifiers (e.g., name and birthday or name and account number) according to agency policy. Compare identifiers with information on patient's MAR or medical record.	Ensures patient safety. Complies with The Joint Commission requirements for patient safety (TJC, 2014).
2. Collect appropriate equipment. Get extra help as needed. Close door to room or close bedside curtains.	Having appropriate number of people to position patient prevents patient and nurse injury. Provides for patient privacy.
3. Perform hand hygiene.	Reduces transfer of microorganisms.
4. Explain procedure.	Decreases anxiety and increases patient cooperation.
5. Raise level of bed to comfortable working height. Remove all pillows and devices used for positioning.	Raises work toward nurse's center of gravity. Reduces any interference during positioning.
IMPLEMENTATION	
1. Position patient flat in bed on back if tolerated. Keep patient aligned.	Repositioning from flat position decreases friction and possible shear on patient's skin.

***Clinical Decision Point:* Before flattening bed, account for all tubing, drains, and equipment to prevent dislodgment or tipping if caught in mattress or bed frame as bed is lowered.**

STEP	RATIONALE
A. **Assist Patient in Moving Up in Bed (Two Nurses)**	This is not a one-person task. Helping a patient move up in bed without help from other co-workers or without the aid of an assistive device (i.e., friction-reducing pad) is no longer recommended or considered safe for the patient or nurse. If a patient is unable to assist fully, refer to Step 1B.
(1) Remove pillow from under head and shoulders and place it at head of bed.	Prevents striking patient's head against head of bed.
(2) Face head of bed.	Facing direction of movement prevents twisting your body while moving patient.
(3) Each nurse places one arm under patient's head and shoulders and one arm under patient's thighs.	Provides support across length of patient's body.
(4) *Alternative position if patient can assist:* Position one nurse at patient's upper body. Nurse's arm nearest head of bed is under patient's head and opposite shoulder; other arm is under patient's closest arm and shoulder. The second nurse's arms are under patient's lower back and torso.	Prevents trauma to patient's musculoskeletal system by supporting shoulder and hip joints and evenly distributing weight.
(5) Place feet apart with foot nearest head of bed in front of other foot (forward-backward stance).	Wide base of support increases balance. Stance enables you to shift body weight as you move patient up in bed, thereby reducing force needed to move load.
(6) Before moving patient, instruct him or her to flex knees with feet flat on bed.	Decreases friction and enables patient to use leg muscles during movement.
(7) Also instruct patient to flex neck, tilting chin toward chest.	Prevents hyperextension of neck when moving patient up in bed.
(8) Have patient assist moving by pushing with feet on bed surface.	Reduces friction. Increases patient mobility. Decreases workload.
(9) Flex your knees and hips, bringing forearms closer to level of bed.	Increases balance and strength by bringing your center of gravity closer to patient. Uses thighs instead of back muscles.

STEP	RATIONALE
(10) Instruct patient on count of 3 to push with heels and elevate trunk while breathing out, thus moving toward head of bed.	Prepares patient for move. Reinforces assistance in moving up in bed. Increases patient cooperation. Breathing out avoids Valsalva maneuver.
(11) On count of three, rock and shift weight from front to back leg. At the same time patient pushes with heels and elevates trunk.	Rocking enables you to improve balance and overcome inertia. Shifting weight counteracts patient's weight and reduces force needed to move load. Patient's assistance reduces friction and workload.
B. Move Immobile Patient Up in Bed With Drawsheet (Two or more nurses)	

Clinical Decision Point: **No caregiver should ever manually lift more than 35 lbs of a patient's weight (Waters et al., 2011a). Determine need for more caregivers to assist or consider assistive device to help move patient up in bed.**

STEP	RATIONALE
(1) Place drawsheet under patient by turning side to side. Extend sheet from shoulders to thighs. Return patient to supine position.	Supports patient's body weight and reduces friction during movement.
(2) Position one or more nurses at each side of patient's hips.	Distributes weight equally between nurses.
(3) Grasp drawsheet firmly near patient.	
(4) Place feet apart with forward-backward stance. Flex knees and hips. On count of 3 shift weight from front to back leg and move patient and drawsheet to desired position in bed (see illustration).	Facing direction of movement ensures proper balance. Shifting weight reduces force needed to move load. Flexing knees lowers center of gravity and thighs instead of back muscles.
(5) Realign patient in correct body alignment.	Prevents injury to musculoskeletal system.
C. Position Patient in Supported Fowler's Position (see illustration)	
(1) Elevate head of bed to 60 degrees if not contraindicated.	Increases comfort, improves ventilation, and increases patient's opportunity to socialize or relax.
(2) Rest head against mattress or on small pillow.	Prevents flexion contractures of cervical vertebrae.
(3) Use pillows to support arms and hands if patient does not have voluntary control or use of hands and arms.	Prevents shoulder dislocation from effect of downward pull of unsupported arms, promotes circulation by preventing venous pooling, and prevents flexion contractures of arms and wrists.
(4) Position pillow at lower back.	Supports lumbar vertebrae and decreases flexion of vertebrae.
(5) Place small pillow under thigh.	Prevents hyperextension of knee and occlusion of popliteal artery caused by pressure from body weight.
(6) Position patient's heels in heel boots or other heel pressure-relief device.	Heel pressure-relief devices are more effective than pillows for consistently reducing pressure from mattress on heels.

Clinical Decision Point: **To keep feet in proper alignment and prevent footdrop, use foot support devices such as ankle or foot boots (check agency policy).**

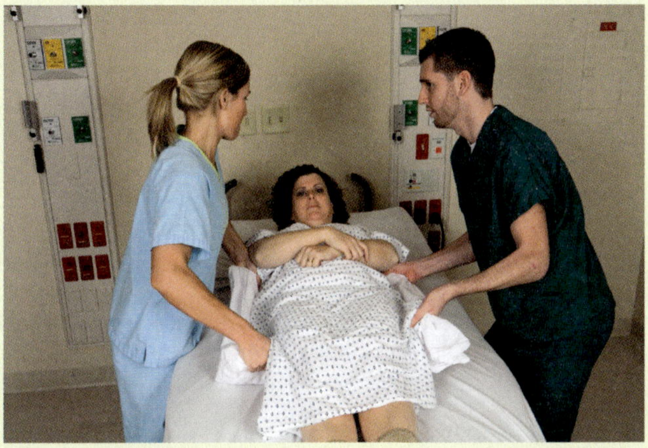

STEP 1B(4) Moving immobile patient up in bed with drawsheet.

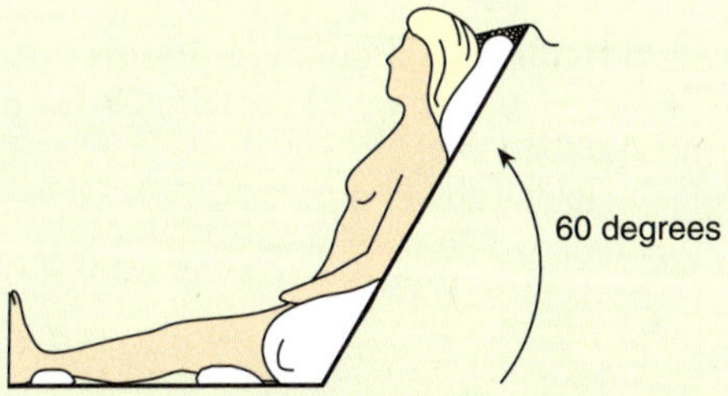

STEP 1C Supported Fowler's position.

SKILL 27-1 MOVING AND POSITIONING PATIENTS IN BED—cont'd

STEP	RATIONALE
D. Position Hemiplegic Patient in Supported Fowler's Position	
(1) Elevate head of bed to 60 degrees.	Increases comfort, improves ventilation, and increases patient's opportunity to relax.
(2) Position patient in sitting position as straight as possible.	Counteracts tendency to slump toward affected side. Improves ventilation and cardiac output and decreases intracranial pressure. Improves patient's ability to swallow and helps to prevent aspiration of food, liquids, and gastric secretions.
(3) Position head on small pillow with chin slightly forward. If patient is totally unable to control head movement, avoid hyperextension of neck.	Prevents hyperextension of neck. Too many pillows under head cause neck flexion contracture.

Clinical Decision Point: **If patient has a paralyzed extremity, provide support for involved arm and hand on over-bed table in front of patient. Place arm away from patient's side and support elbow with pillow. Position flaccid hand in normal resting position with wrist slightly extended, arches of hand maintained, and fingers partially flexed; use section of rubber ball cut in half; clasp patient's hands together. Position spastic hand with wrist in neutral position or slightly extended; extend fingers with palm down or leave fingers in relaxed position with palm up. At times it is difficult to position spastic hands without use of specially made splints for patient.**

STEP	RATIONALE
(4) Flex knees and hips by using pillow or folded blanket under knees.	Ensures proper alignment. Flexion prevents prolonged hyperextension, which impairs joint mobility.
(5) Place trochanter rolls along side of patient's legs.	Prevents external rotation of hips that often contributes to contractures.
(6) Support feet in dorsiflexion with foot support such as ankle or foot boots (check agency policy).	Prevents footdrop by placing ankle in neutral dorsiflexion. Stimulation of ball of foot by hard surface has tendency to increase muscle tone in patient with extensor spasticity of lower extremity.
E. Position Patient in Supine Position	
(1) Be sure that patient is comfortable on back with head of bed flat.	Some patients' physical conditions do not tolerate supine position.
(2) Place small rolled towel under lumbar area of back.	Provides support for lumbar spine.
(3) Place pillow under upper shoulders, neck, or head.	Maintains correct alignment and prevents flexion contractures of cervical vertebrae.
(4) Place trochanter rolls parallel to lateral surface of patient's thighs if patient is immobile.	Reduces external rotation of hip.
(5) Position patient's heels in heel boots or other heel pressure-relief device (check agency policy).	Heel pressure-relief devices are more effective than pillows for consistently reducing pressure from mattress on heels.
(6) If needed, support feet in dorsiflexion with foot support such as ankle or foot boots (check agency policy).	Prevents footdrop by placing ankle in neutral dorsiflexion. Stimulation of ball of foot by hard surface has tendency to increase muscle tone in patient with extensor spasticity of lower extremity.
(7) Place pillows under pronated forearms, keeping upper arms parallel to patient's body (see illustrations).	Reduces internal rotation of shoulder and prevents extension of elbows. Maintains correct body alignment.
(8) Place hand rolls in patient's hands. Consider physical therapy referral for use of hand splints.	Reduces extension of fingers and abduction of thumb. Maintains thumb slightly adducted and in opposition to fingers.
F. Position Hemiplegic Patient in Supine Position	
(1) Be sure that patient is comfortable on back with head of bed flat.	Some patients' physical conditions do not tolerate supine position.
(2) Place folded towel or small pillow under shoulder of affected side.	Decreases possibility of pain, joint contracture, and subluxation. Maintains mobility in muscles around shoulder to permit normal movement patterns.

STEP	RATIONALE
(3) Keep affected arm away from body with elbow extended and palm up. (*Alternative* is to place arm out to side, with elbow bent and hand toward head of bed.)	Maintains mobility in arm, joints, and shoulder to permit normal movement patterns. (*Alternative* position counteracts limitation of ability of arm to rotate outward at shoulder [external rotation]. Need external rotation to raise arm overhead without pain.)
(4) Place folded towel under hip of involved side.	Diminishes effect of spasticity in entire leg by controlling hip position.
(5) Flex affected knee 30 degrees by supporting it on pillow or folded blanket.	Slight flexion breaks up abnormal extension pattern of leg. Extensor spasticity is most severe when patient is supine.
(6) Position patient's heel in heel boots or other heel pressure-relief device (check agency policy).	Heel pressure-relief devices are more effective than pillows for consistently reducing pressure from mattress on heels. In addition, heel boot also maintains feet in dorsiflexion, which prevents footdrop.
(7) If needed, support feet in dorsiflexion with foot support such as ankle or foot boots (check agency policy).	Prevents footdrop by placing ankle in neutral dorsiflexion. Stimulation of ball of foot by hard surface has tendency to increase muscle tone in patient with extensor spasticity of lower extremity.
G. **Position Patient in Prone Position** (see illustration)	
(1) With patient supine, place arm on side to be turned, alongside body. Roll patient over arm positioned close to body, with elbow straight and hand under hip. Position on abdomen in center of bed.	Positions patient correctly to maintain alignment.
(2) Turn patient's head to one side and support head with small pillow.	Reduces flexion or hyperextension of cervical vertebrae.
(3) Place small pillow under patient's abdomen below level of diaphragm.	Reduces pressure on breasts of some female patients and decreases hyperextension of lumbar vertebrae and strain on lower back.

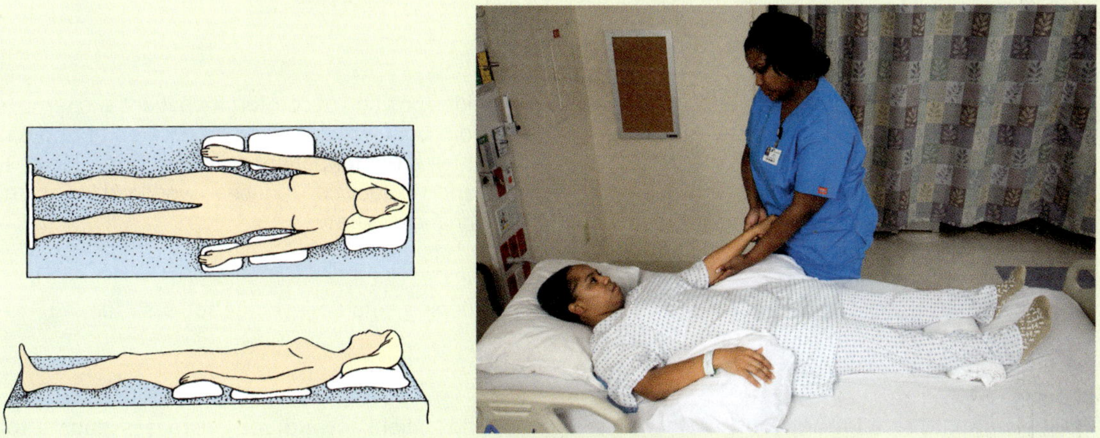

STEP 1E(7) Supine position with pillows in place.

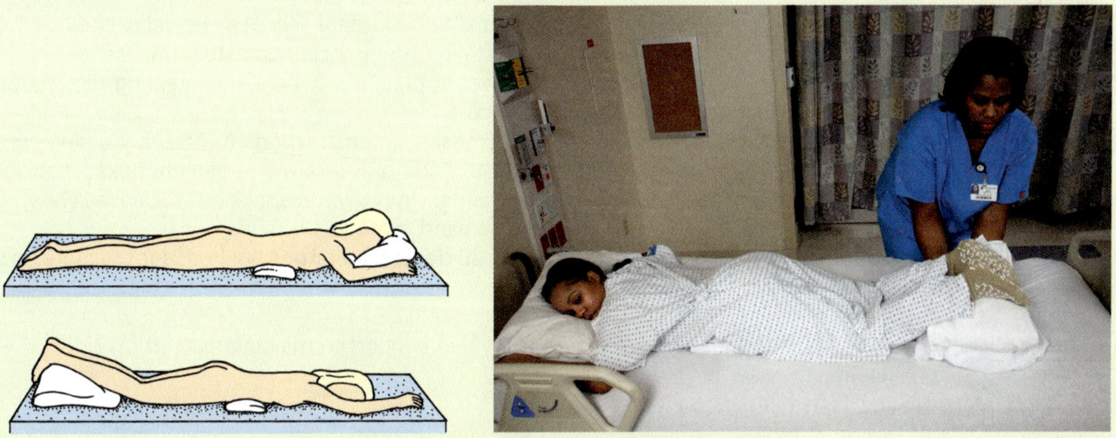

STEP 1G Prone position with pillows in place.

SKILL 27-1 MOVING AND POSITIONING PATIENTS IN BED—cont'd

STEP	RATIONALE
(4) Support arms in flexed position level at shoulders.	Maintains proper body alignment. Support reduces risk for joint dislocation.
(5) Support lower legs with pillow to elevate toes.	Prevents footdrop. Reduces external rotation of hips. Reduces mattress pressure on toes.
H. Position Hemiplegic Patient in Prone Position	

***Clinical Decision Point:* Increase frequency of positioning if pressure areas begin to appear, joint mobility becomes impaired or worsened, or patient demonstrates signs of discomfort. Consult with physical and occupational therapists as needed.**

STEP	RATIONALE
(1) Move patient toward unaffected side, with patient remaining supine.	Creates room for proper patient alignment in center of bed when patient is rolled onto abdomen.
(2) Place pillow on patient's abdomen.	Prevents sagging of abdomen when patient is rolled over; decreases hyperextension of lumbar vertebrae and strain on lower back.
(3) Roll patient onto affected side.	
(4) Roll patient onto abdomen by positioning involved arm close to patient's body, with elbow straight and hand under hip. Roll patient carefully over arm.	Prevents injury to affected side.
(5) Turn head toward involved side.	Promotes development of neck and trunk extension, which is necessary for standing and walking.
(6) Position involved arm out to side with elbow bent, hand toward head of bed, and fingers extended (if possible).	Counteracts limitation of ability of arm to rotate outward at shoulder (external rotation). Need external rotation to raise arm over head without pain.
(7) Flex knees slightly by placing pillow under legs from knees to ankles.	Flexion prevents prolonged hyperextension, which impairs joint mobility.
(8) Support feet with foot support devices such as ankle or foot boots (check agency policy).	Maintains feet in dorsiflexion.
I. Position Patient in 30-Degree Lateral (Side-Lying) Position	
(1) Patient lies supine with head of bed as low as patient tolerates.	Provides position of comfort for patient and removes pressure from bony prominences on back and buttocks.
(2) Position patient to one side of bed. Then move to opposite side of bed toward which patient is to be turned. Use friction-reducing device or mechanical lift per manufacturer guidelines if patient cannot help with moving.	Provides room for patient to turn to side. Use of safe patient-handling device reduces workload of caregivers and enhances safety.
(3) Prepare to turn patient onto side. Flex patient's knee that will not be next to mattress. Place one hand on patient's hip and one hand on patient's shoulder.	Positioning sets up leverage for easy turning.
(4) Roll patient onto side toward you.	Rolling patient toward you decreases trauma to tissues. In addition, positioning patient so leverage is on hip makes turning easy.
(5) Place pillow under patient's head and neck.	Maintains alignment. Reduces lateral neck flexion. Decreases strain on sternocleidomastoid muscle.
(6) Place hands under patient's dependent shoulder and bring shoulder blade forward.	Prevents patient's weight from resting directly on shoulder joint.
(7) Position both arms in slightly flexed position. Support upper arm with pillow level with shoulder, other arm by mattress.	Decreases internal rotation and adduction of shoulder. Supporting both arms in slightly flexed position protects joints. Improves ventilation because chest is able to expand more easily.
(8) Place hands under dependent hip and bring hip slightly forward so angle from hip to mattress is approximately 30 degrees (see Figure 27-7).	The 30-degree lateral position reduces pressure on trochanter.
(9) Place tuck-back pillow behind patient's back. (Make by folding pillow lengthwise. Smooth area is slightly tucked under patient's back.)	Provides support to maintain patient on side.

STEP	RATIONALE
(10) Place pillow under semiflexed upper leg level at hip from groin to foot.	Maintains leg in correct alignment. Prevents pressure on bony prominence.
(11) Support feet with foot support devices such as ankle or foot boots (check agency policy).	Maintains dorsiflexion of foot. Prevents footdrop.
J. **Position Patient in Sims' (Semiprone) Position**	
(1) Be sure that patient is comfortable in supine position.	Provides for proper body alignment while patient is lying down.
(2) Position patient in side-lying position, lying partially on abdomen, with dependent arm straight along patient's body.	Facilitates turning onto side. Avoids injury to arm; semiprone position places less pressure on abdomen.
(3) Carefully lift patient's dependent shoulder and bring arm back behind patient.	Patient is rolled only partially on abdomen.
(4) Place small pillow under patient's head.	Maintains proper alignment and prevents lateral neck flexion.
(5) Place pillow under flexed upper arm, supporting arm level with shoulder.	Prevents internal rotation of shoulder. Maintains alignment.
(6) Place pillow under flexed upper leg, supporting leg level with hip (see Figure 27-8).	Prevents internal rotation of hip and adduction of leg. Flexion prevents hyperextension of leg. Reduces mattress pressure on knees and ankles.
(7) Support feet with foot support devices such as ankle or foot boots (check agency policy).	Maintains foot in dorsiflexion. Prevents footdrop.
K. **Logrolling Patient (Three Nurses)**	

Clinical Decision Point: **Supervise and assist NAP when there is a health care provider's order to logroll patient. Patients who have suffered from a spinal cord injury or are recovering from neck, back, or spinal surgery often need to keep the spinal column in straight alignment to prevent further injury.**

STEP	RATIONALE
(1) Place small pillow between patient's knees.	Prevents tension on spinal column and adduction of hip.
(2) Cross patient's arms on chest.	Prevents injury to arms.
(3) Position two nurses on side of bed to which patient will be turned. Position third nurse on other side of bed (see illustration). If needed, use fourth caregiver who stands on same side as third person.	Distributes weight equally between nurses.
(4) Fanfold or roll drawsheet alongside of patient.	Provides strong handles to grip drawsheet without slipping.
(5) Move patient as one unit in smooth, continuous motion on count of 3 (see illustration).	This maintains proper alignment by moving all body parts at the same time, preventing tension or twisting of the spinal column.
(6) Nurse on opposite side of bed places pillows along length of patient (see illustration).	Pillows keep patient aligned.
(7) Gently lean patient as a unit back toward pillows for support (see illustration).	Ensures continued straight alignment of spinal column, preventing injury.
2. Perform hand hygiene.	Reduces transmission of microorganisms.

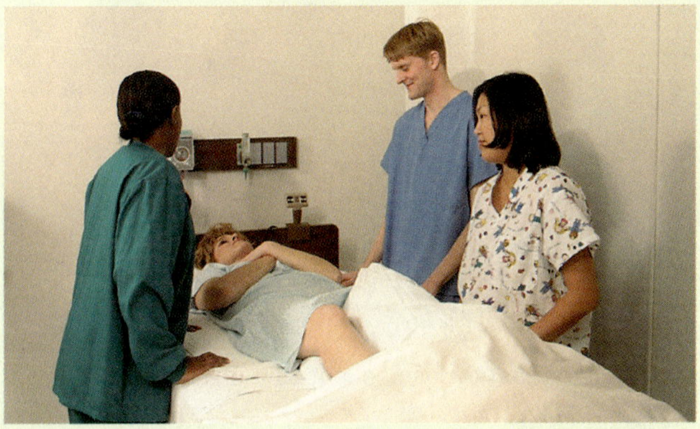
STEP 1K(3) Position nurses on each side of patient.

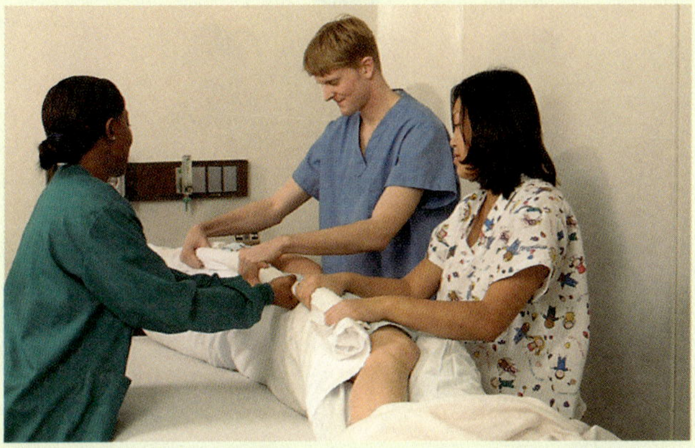
STEP 1K(5) Move patient as a unit, maintaining proper alignment.

SKILL 27-1 MOVING AND POSITIONING PATIENTS IN BED—cont'd

STEP	RATIONALE
EVALUATION	
1. Evaluate patient's body alignment, position, and level of comfort.	Determines effectiveness of positioning. Add or remove additional supports (e.g., pillows, bath blankets) to promote comfort and correct body alignment.
2. Measure ROM (see Chapter 36).	Determines if joint contracture is developing.
3 Observe for areas of erythema or breakdown involving skin.	Indicates complications of immobility or improper positioning of body part. Determines need for increasing frequency of repositioning patient.
4. Use Teach Back—State to patient, "I want to be sure I explained clearly why we change your position frequently and which types of positions are effective to reduce the risk for pressure ulcers or contractures. Can you tell me some of those reasons?" Revise your instruction now or develop plan for revised patient teaching to be implemented at an appropriate time if patient is not able to teach back correctly.	Evaluates what the patient is able to explain or demonstrate.

RECORDING AND REPORTING

- Record procedure and observations (e.g., condition of skin, joint movement, patient's ability to help with positioning and tolerance of position).
- Document your evaluation of patient learning.
- Report observations at change of shift and document in nurses' notes.
- Report turning schedule and frequency of repositioning patient at change of shift.

UNEXPECTED OUTCOMES AND RELATED INTERVENTIONS

- Joint contractures develop or worsen.
  - Ensure that patient is positioned properly.
  - Consider referral to physical or occupational therapy.
- Skin shows areas of erythema and breakdown.
  - Increase frequency of repositioning.
  - Place turning schedule above patient's bed.
  - Initiate skin care protocol (check agency policy) (Chapter 37).
- Patient avoids moving.
  - Medicate for pain as ordered by health care provider to ensure patient's comfort before moving.
  - Allow pain medication to take effect before proceeding.

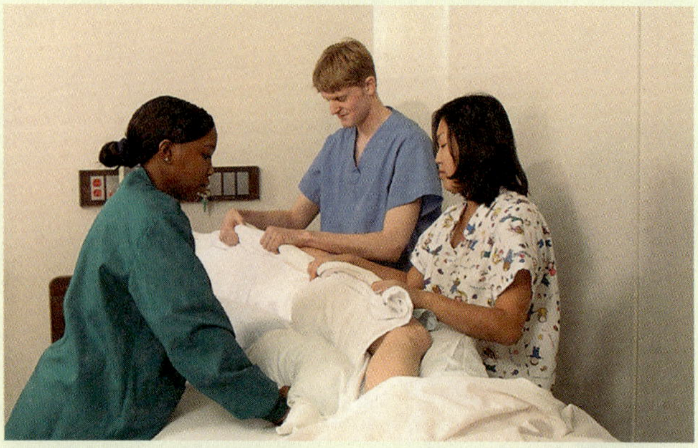

STEP 1K(6) Place pillows along patient's back for support.

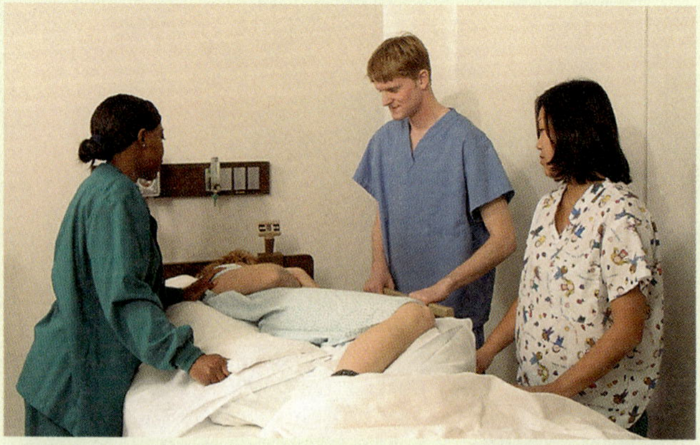

STEP 1K(7) Gently lean patient as a unit against pillows.

SKILL 27-2 USING SAFE AND EFFECTIVE TRANSFER TECHNIQUES

View Video!

DELEGATION CONSIDERATIONS

The skill of transfer techniques can be delegated to nursing assistive personnel (NAP). Patients whom you are transferring for the first time after prolonged bed rest, extensive surgery, critical illness, or spinal cord trauma require supervision by professional nurses. Before delegation, inform NAP about:

- Seeking assistance when moving or lifting a patient (e.g., when patient is overweight or confused).
- Patient limitations (e.g., changes in blood pressure, mobility restrictions) that affect safe transfer techniques.

EQUIPMENT

- Transfer belt, sling, or lapboard (as needed)
- Nonskid shoes, bath blankets, pillows
- Wheelchair
- Stretcher
- Mechanical lift: Use frame, canvas strips or chains, and hammock or canvas strips

STEP	RATIONALE
ASSESSMENT	
1. Assess physiological capacity to transfer:	Provides information relative to patient's abilities, physical status, ability to comprehend, and number of individuals needed to provide safe transferring.
a. Muscle strength (legs and upper arms)	Immobile patients have decreased muscle strength, tone, and mass. Affects ability to bear weight or raise body.
b. Joint mobility (range of motion [ROM]) and contracture formation	Immobility or inflammatory processes (e.g., arthritis) lead to contracture formation and impaired joint mobility.
c. Paralysis or paresis (spastic or flaccid)	Patient with central nervous system damage sometimes has bilateral paralysis (requiring transfer by swivel bar, sliding bar, or **mechanical lift**) or unilateral paralysis, which requires belt transfer to "best" side. Weakness (paresis) requires stabilization of knee while transferring. Flaccid arm needs support with sling during transfer.
d. Risk for orthostatic (postural) hypotension (e.g., previously on bed rest, first time arising from supine position following surgical procedure, history of dizziness when arising)	Determines risk for fainting or falling during transfer. Immobile patients have decreased ability for autonomic nervous system to equalize blood supply, resulting in drop of 20 mm Hg or more in blood pressure when rising from sitting position.
e. Activity tolerance (e.g., shortness of breath on walking)	Determines ability of patient to assist with transfer.
f. Level of comfort	Pain reduces patient's motivation and ability to be mobile. Pain relief before transfer enhances patient participation.
g. Vital signs	Vital sign changes such as increased pulse and respiration and change in blood pressure indicate activity intolerance (see Chapter 15).
2. Assess patient's sensory status: a. Adequacy of central and peripheral vision b. Adequacy of hearing c. Loss of peripheral sensation	Determines influence of sensory loss on ability to make transfer. Visual field loss decreases patient's ability to see in direction of transfer. Peripheral sensation loss decreases proprioception. Patients with visual and hearing losses need transfer techniques adapted to deficits. Patients with cerebrovascular accident (CVA) sometimes lose area of visual field, which profoundly affects vision and perception.

Clinical Decision Point: **Patients with hemiplegia also often "neglect" one side of the body (inattention to or unawareness of one side of body or environment), which distorts perception of visual field. If patient experiences neglect of one side, instruct him or her to scan all visual fields when transferring.**

STEP	RATIONALE
3. Assess patient's cognitive status.	Determines patient's ability to follow directions and learn transfer techniques.

Clinical Decision Point: **Patients with head trauma or CVA have perceptual cognitive deficits that create safety risks. If patient has difficulty comprehending, simplify instructions and maintain consistency.**

STEP	RATIONALE
4. Assess patient's level of motivation: a. Patient's eagerness versus unwillingness to be mobile b. Whether patient avoids activity and offers excuses	Altered psychological states reduce patient's desire to engage in activity.

SKILL 27-2 USING SAFE AND EFFECTIVE TRANSFER TECHNIQUES—cont'd

STEP	RATIONALE
5. Assess previous mode of transfer (if applicable).	Determines mode of transfer and assistance required to provide continuity. Use of transfer belts is necessary with all patients being transferred.
6. Assess patient's specific risk for falling or being injured when transferred (e.g., neuromuscular deficits, motor weakness, calcium loss from long bones, cognitive and visual dysfunction, altered balance).	Certain conditions increase patient's risk for falling or potential for injury.
7. Assess special transfer equipment needed for home setting. Assess home environment for hazards.	Prior teaching of family and support people, assessment of home for safety risks and functionality, and provision of applicable aids greatly enhance transfer ability at home.
PLANNING	
1. Gather appropriate equipment.	
2. Determine number of people needed to assist with transfer. Do not start procedure until all caregivers are available.	Ensures safe patient transfer.
3. Perform hand hygiene. Verify that bed brakes are locked.	Reduces transmission of microorganisms. Promotes patient and caregiver safety.
4 Explain procedure to patient.	Increases patient participation.
IMPLEMENTATION	
1. Transfer patient.	
A. **Assist Cooperative Patient to Sitting Position in Bed (when electrical bed is not available)**	
(1) Raise bed to waist level. Place patient in supine position.	Enables you to assess your patient's body alignment continually.
(2) Face head of bed at 45-degree angle and remove pillows.	Proper positioning reduces twisting of your body when moving the patient. Pillows cause interference when patient is sitting up in bed.
(3) Place feet in wide base of support, with foot closest to bed in front of other foot.	Improves balance and allows transfer of body weight as you move patient to sitting position.
(4) Place hand nearer head of bed under patient's shoulders, supporting patient's head and cervical vertebrae.	Maintains alignment of head and cervical vertebrae and allows for even lifting of patient's upper trunk.
(5) Place other hand on bed surface.	Provides support and balance.
(6) Raise patient to sitting position by shifting weight from front to back leg.	Improves balance, overcomes inertia, and transfers weight in direction in which you move patient.
(7) Push against bed with arm that is placed on bed surface.	Divides activity between arms and legs and protects back from strain. By bracing one hand against mattress and pushing against it as you lift patient, you transfer weight away from your back muscles through your arm onto the mattress.

Clinical Decision Point: **Careful assessment of your patient's ability to assist in the following positioning technique is extremely important. Consider the use of a mechanical lift. Your role in assisting your patient to a sitting position is to guide and instruct. If your patient can bear weight and move to a sitting position independently, allow him or her to do so and offer assistance.**

STEP	RATIONALE
B. **Assist Cooperative Patient Who Can Partially Bear Weight to Sitting Position on Side of Bed**	
(1) With bed flat and at waist level, turn patient to side, using assistance of another caregiver if necessary. Patient needs to face nurse on side of bed on which patient will be sitting (see illustration).	Decreases amount of work needed by you and your patient.
(2) Raise head of bed 30 degrees.	Facilitates raising patient to sitting position and protects patient from falling.
(3) Stand opposite patient's hips. Turn diagonally so you face patient and far corner of foot of bed.	Places your center of gravity nearer patient. Reduces twisting of your body because you are facing direction of movement.

STEP	RATIONALE
(4) Place feet apart with foot closest to bed in front of other foot (see illustration).	Improves balance and allows transfer of body weight as you move patient to sitting position.
(5) Place arm nearer head of bed under patient's shoulders, supporting patient's head and cervical vertebrae.	Maintains alignment of head and cervical vertebrae and allows for even lifting of patient's upper trunk.
(6) Place other arm over patient's thighs (see illustration).	Supports hip and prevents patient from falling backward during procedure.
(7) Move patient's legs and feet over side of bed. Pivot toward rear leg, allowing patient's upper legs to swing downward. At same time shift weight to back leg and elevate patient (see illustration).	Decreases friction and resistance. Weight of patient's legs when off bed allows gravity to lower legs, and weight of legs assists in pulling upper body to sitting position.
C. **Transferring Cooperative Patient Who Is Partially Weight Bearing From Bed to Chair**	

Clinical Decision Point: **If patient requires you to lift more than 35 lbs of patient's weight or is unpredictable in amount of assistance offered, obtain a motorized lift (see Figure 27-9) (Sedlak et al., 2009).**

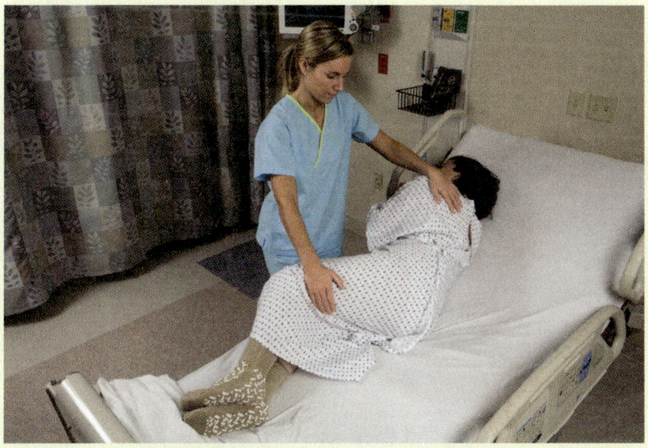

STEP 1B(1) Side-lying position.

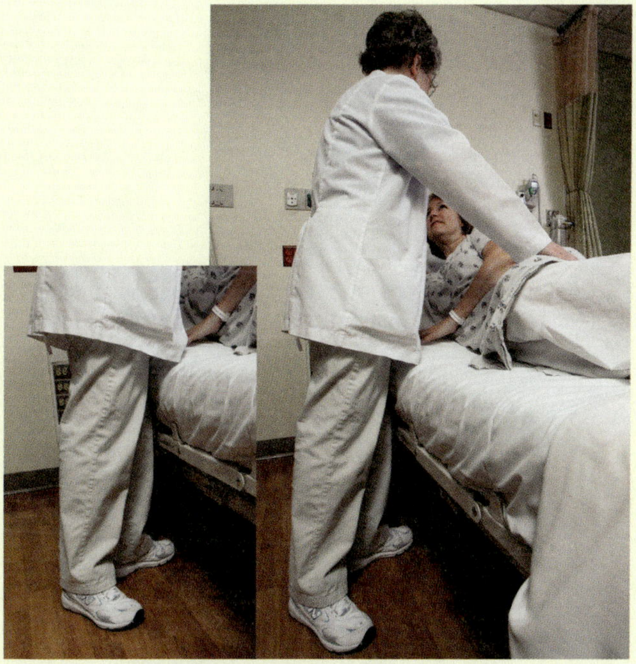

STEP 1B(4) Proper foot placement.

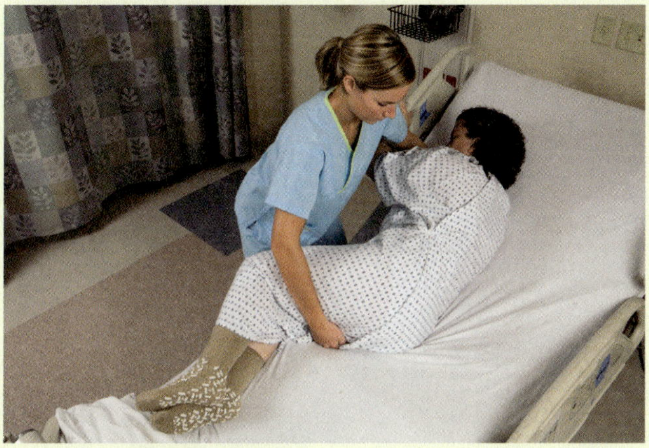

STEP 1B(6) Nurse places arm over patient's thighs.

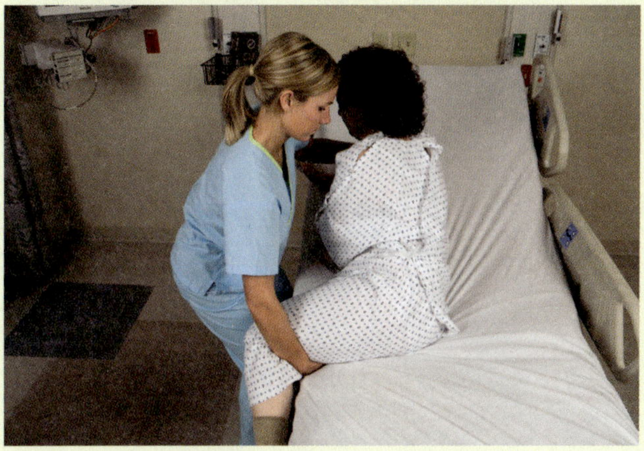

STEP 1B(7) Nurse shifts weight to rear leg and elevates patient.

SKILL 27-2 USING SAFE AND EFFECTIVE TRANSFER TECHNIQUES—cont'd

STEP	RATIONALE
(1) Assist patient to sitting position on side of bed (see Step 1B). Have chair in position at 45-degree angle to bed on patient's strong side. For wheelchair, lock brakes, remove footrests. Allow patient to sit on side of the bed (dangling) for a few minutes before transferring. Ask if patient feels dizzy. Do not leave unattended while dangling.	Positions chair within easy access for transfer. Placing chair on patient's stronger side allows patient to assist when transferring. Dangling helps equilibrate blood pressure, reducing risk for dizziness or fainting when standing.
(2) Apply transfer belt or other transfer aids.	Transfer belt maintains stability of patient during transfer and reduces risk for falling (Nelson et al., 2003a, 2003b; Pierson and Fairchild, 2013). Put patient's arm in sling if flaccid paralysis is present.
(3) Ensure that patient is wearing stable nonskid shoes. Place weight-bearing or strong leg forward, with weak foot back.	Nonskid soles decrease risk for slipping during transfer. Always have patient wear shoes during transfer; bare feet increase risk for falls. Patient stands on stronger, or weight-bearing, leg.
(4) Spread your feet apart.	Ensures balance with wide base of support.
(5) Flex your hips and knees, aligning knees with patient's knees (see illustration).	Flexion of knees and hips lowers center of gravity to object to be raised; aligning knees with patients allows for stabilization of knees when patient stands.
(6) Grasp transfer belt from underneath along patient's sides.	Grasping transfer belt at patient's side provides movement of patient at center of gravity. Never lift patients by arms or under arms (Nelson et al., 2003b; Owens et al., 1999; Pierson and Fairchild., 2013).

***Clinical Decision Point:* Use transfer belt or walking belt with handles in place of under-axilla technique. The under-axilla technique is physically stressful for nurses and uncomfortable for patients (Owens et al., 1999; Pierson and Fairchild., 2013).**

STEP	RATIONALE
(7) Rock patient up to standing position on count of 3 while straightening hips and legs and keeping knees slightly flexed (see illustration). Unless contraindicated, instruct patient to use hands to push up if applicable.	Rocking motion gives patient's body momentum and requires less muscular effort to lift patient.

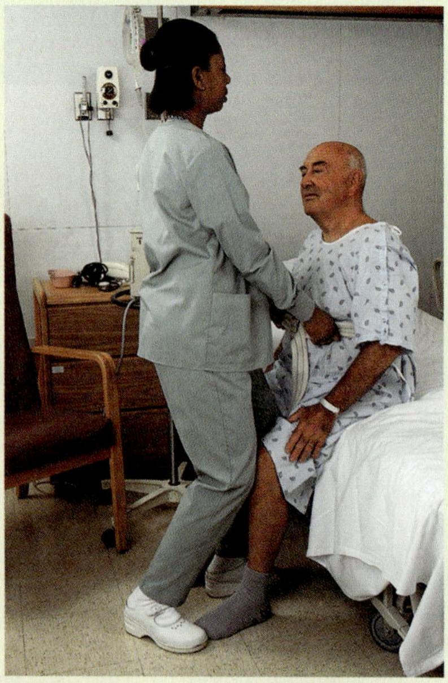

STEP 1C(5) Nurse flexes hips and knees, aligning knees with patient's knees.

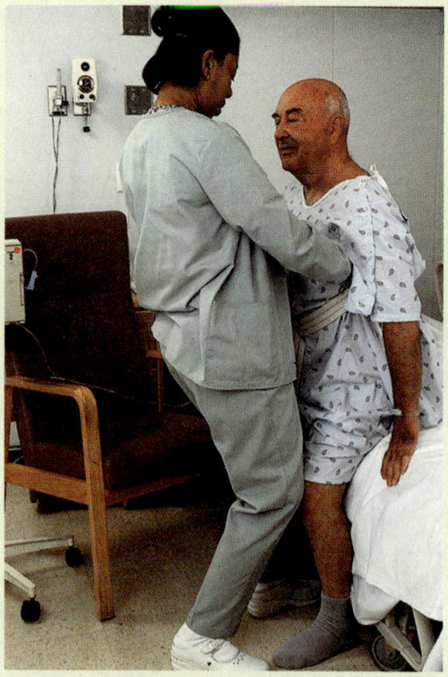

STEP 1C(7) Nurse rocks patient to standing position.

STEP	RATIONALE
(8) Maintain stability of patient's weak or paralyzed leg with knee.	Often patient maintains ability to stand on paralyzed or weak limb with support of knee to stabilize (Pierson and Fairchild, 2013).
(9) Pivot on foot farther from chair.	Maintains support of patient while allowing adequate space for patient to move.
(10) Instruct patient to use armrests on chair for support and ease into chair (see illustration).	Increases patient stability.
(11) Flex hips and knees while lowering patient into chair (see illustration).	Prevents injury from poor body mechanics.
(12) Assess patient for proper alignment for sitting position. Provide support for paralyzed extremities. Lapboard or sling supports flaccid arm. Stabilize leg with bath blanket or pillow.	Prevents injury to patient from poor body alignment.
(13) Praise patient's progress, effort, or performance.	Continued support and encouragement provide incentive for patient perseverance.
D. Use Mechanical Lift and Full-Body Sling to Transfer Uncooperative Patient Who Can Bear Partial Weight or Patient Who Cannot Bear Weight and Is Either Uncooperative or Does Not Have Upper Body Strength to Move From Bed to Chair	
(1) Position lift properly at bedside.	Ensures safe elevation of patient off bed. (Before using lift, be thoroughly familiar with its operation.)
(2) Position chair near bed and allow adequate space to maneuver lift.	Prepares environment for safe use of lift and subsequent transfer.
(3) Raise bed to high position with mattress flat. Lower side rail.	Maintains nurses' alignment during transfer.
(4) Keep bed side rail up on side opposite from you.	Maintains patient safety.
(5) Roll patient away from you.	Positions patient for use of lift sling.
(6) Place sling under patient. Place lower edge under patient's knees (wide edge) and upper edge under patient's shoulders (narrow piece).	Allows positioning of patient on mechanical/hydraulic lift. Places sling under patient's center of gravity and greatest portion of body weight.
(7) Roll patient to opposite side toward you and pull body sling through.	Completes positioning of patient on mechanical/hydraulic sling.
(8) Roll patient supine onto canvas seat.	Sling extends from shoulders to knees (hammock) to support patient's body weight equally.
(9) Remove patient's glasses if appropriate.	Swivel bar is close to patient's head and could break eyeglasses.

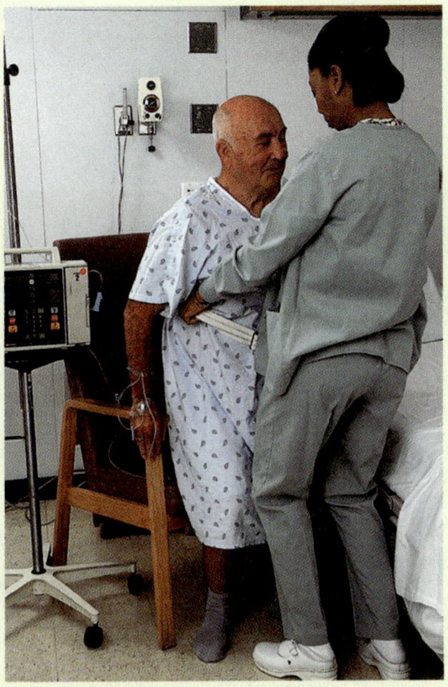

STEP 1C(10) Patient uses armrests for support.

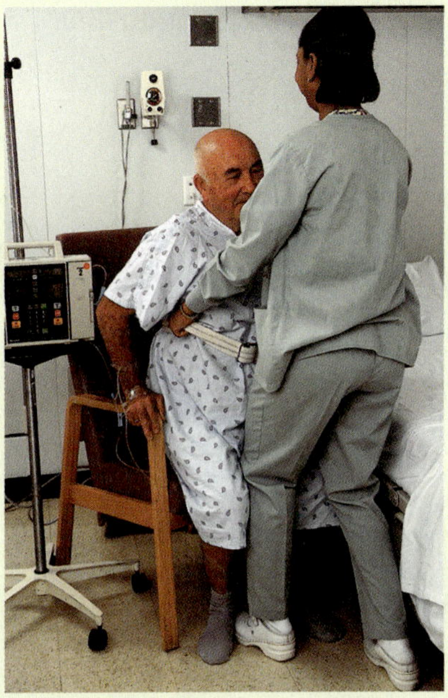

STEP 1C(11) Nurse eases patient into chair.

SKILL 27-2 USING SAFE AND EFFECTIVE TRANSFER TECHNIQUES—cont'd

STEP	RATIONALE
(10) If using a transportable Hoyer life, place horseshoe-shaped base of lift under side of bed (on side with chair).	Positions lift efficiently and promotes smooth transfer.
(11) Lower horizontal bar to sling level following manufacturer directions. Some lifts require valve to be locked.	Positions hydraulic lift close to patient. Locking valve prevents injury to patient.
(12) Attach hooks on strap to holes in sling. Short straps hook to top holes of sling; longer straps hook to bottom of sling.	Secures hydraulic lift to sling.
(13) Elevate head of bed.	Positions patient in sitting position.
(14) Fold patient's arms over chest.	Prevents injury to paralyzed arms.
(15) Use lift to raise patient off bed (see illustration).	Moves patient off bed.
(16) Use steering handle to pull lift from bed and maneuver to chair.	Moves patient from bed to chair.
(17) Move lift to chair.	Positions lift in front of the chair.
(18) Position patient and lower slowly into chair following manufacturer guidelines (see illustration).	Safely guides patient into back of chair as seat descends.
(19) Remove straps and mechanical/hydraulic lift.	Prevents damage to skin and underlying tissues from canvas or hooks.
(20) Check patient's sitting alignment and correct if necessary.	Prevents injury from poor posture.
E. Transfer Patient From Bed to Stretcher (Bed at Stretcher Level).	
(1) Raise bed to height of stretcher, which is aligned with bed. Lock stretcher brakes.	Bed and stretcher need to be at same level to allow patient to slide from bed to stretcher.
(2) Lower head of bed as much as patient can tolerate. Cross patient's arms on chest. Ensure that bed brakes are locked.	Prevents injury to arms during transfer.
(3) Lower side rails. Two caregivers stand on side where the stretcher will be while third caregiver stands on the other side.	Minimizes caregivers' stretching. Prevents patient from falling out of bed and promotes safety.
(4) Two caregivers help patient roll onto side toward them (use of drawsheet is *optional*) with smooth, continuous motion.	Positions patient for placing friction-reducing lateral transfer device.
(5) Place slide board under drawsheet or follow manufacturer guidelines (see illustrations). Gently roll patient back onto slide board.	Patient needs to be placed on transfer device properly to allow safe transfer.

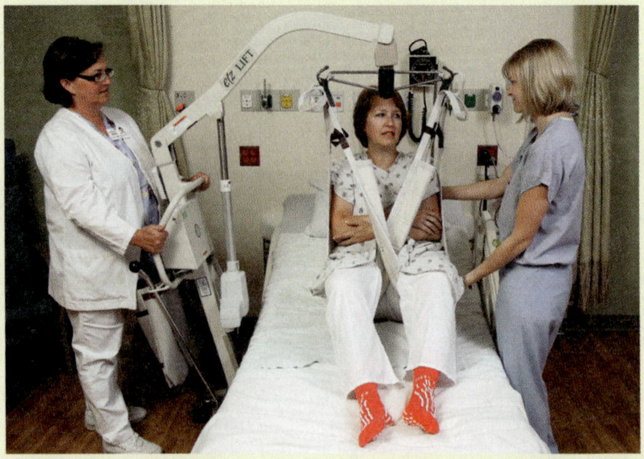

STEP 1D(15) Use mechanical lift to raise patient off bed.

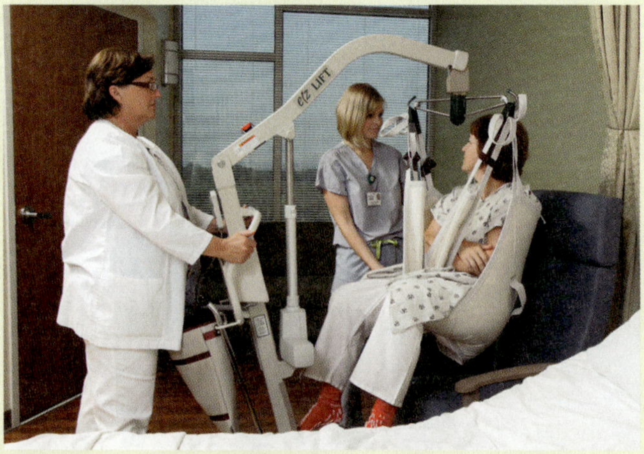

STEP 1D(18) Use mechanical lift to lower patient into chair.

STEP	RATIONALE
(6) Align stretcher alongside bed. Lock wheels of stretcher once it is in place. Instruct patient not to move.	Positions stretcher in correct position for transfer and prevents patient falling out of bed.
(7) All three caregivers place feet widely apart with one slightly in front of the other and grasp fiction-reducing device.	Prepares for transfer. Wide base of support allows nurse to shift weight and minimizes back strain.
(8) On count of three, two caregivers pull drawsheet or patient from bed onto stretcher while third person holds slide board in place. Using friction-reducing device, shift weight from front foot to back foot (see illustrations). Position patient in center of stretcher.	Transfers patient smoothly and efficiently to stretcher.
(9) Put up side rail of stretcher on side where caregivers are, unlock brakes, and roll stretcher away from bed. Put side rail up on that side.	Side rails prevent patient from falling off stretcher.
(10) Cover patient with sheet or blanket.	Promotes comfort and provides patient dignity.
2. Perform hand hygiene.	Reduces transmission of microorganisms.

EVALUATION

1. Evaluate vital signs. Ask if patient feels fatigued.	Evaluates patient's response to postural changes and activity. Minimizes risk for immobility complications.
2. Observe for correct body alignment and presence of pressure points on skin.	Prompt identification of poor alignment reduces risks to patient's skin and musculoskeletal systems.

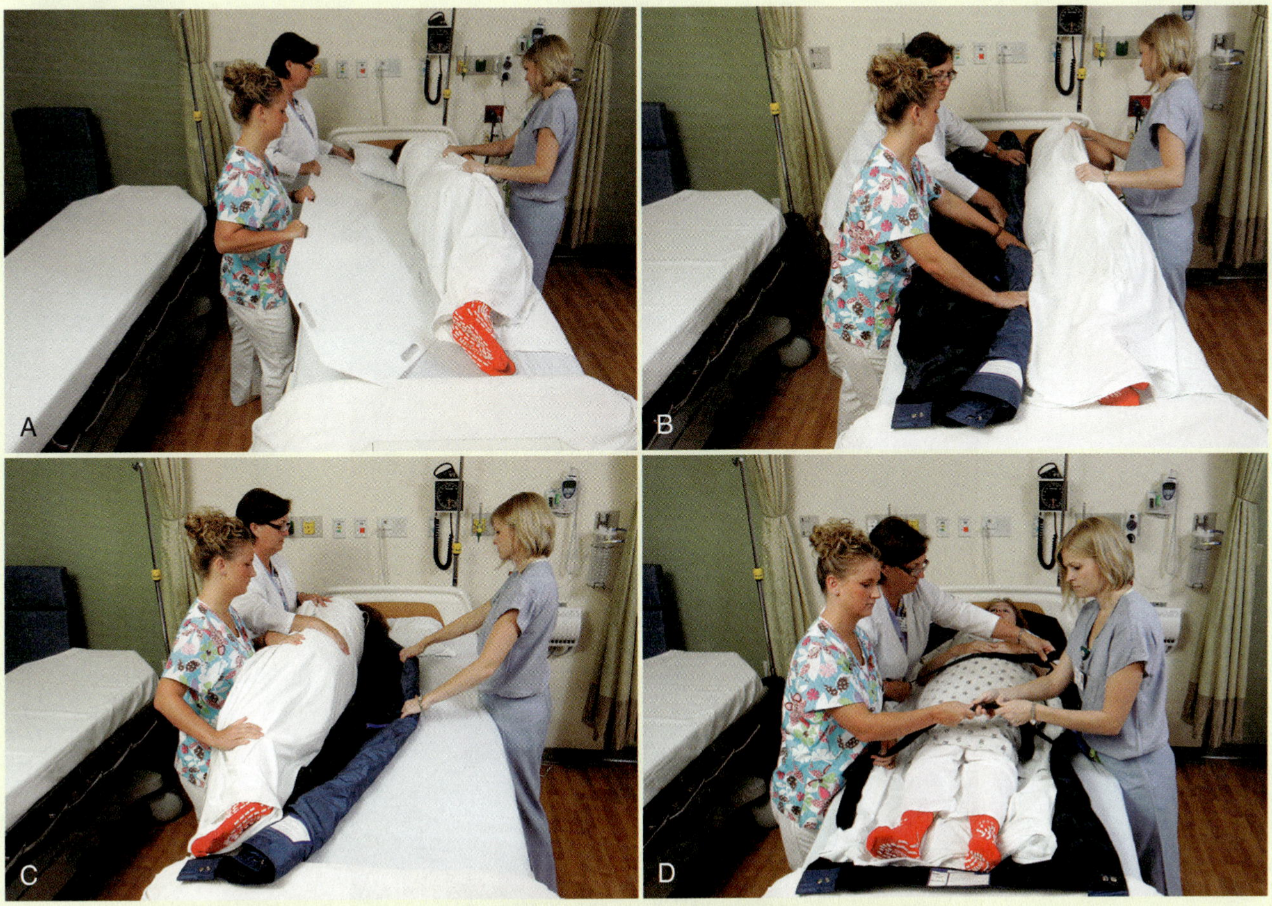

STEP 1E(5) **A,** Two caregivers position sliding board under patient. **B,** Two caregivers place air-assisted device under patient. **C,** Patient rolls to opposite side while other caregiver unrolls air-assisted device. **D,** Secure safety straps.

SKILL 27-2 USING SAFE AND EFFECTIVE TRANSFER TECHNIQUES—cont'd

STEP	RATIONALE
3. Ask if patient experienced pain during transfer.	Determines need for additional pain control or alteration of technique of transferring.
4. Use Teach Back—State to patient, "I want to be sure that I clearly explained why I need your assistance and cooperation when I transfer you from bed to chair. Can you tell me why I need them?" Revise your instruction now or develop plan for revised patient teaching to be implemented at an appropriate time if patient is not able to teach back correctly.	Evaluates what the patient is able to explain or demonstrate.

RECORDING AND REPORTING

- Record procedure, including pertinent observations: weakness, ability to follow directions, weight-bearing ability, balance, ability to pivot, number of personnel needed to assist, and amount of assistance (muscle strength) required.
- Document your evaluation of patient learning.
- Report any unusual occurrence to nurse in charge. Report transfer ability and assistance needed to next shift or other caregivers. Report progress or transfer difficulties to rehabilitation staff (physical therapist or occupational therapist).

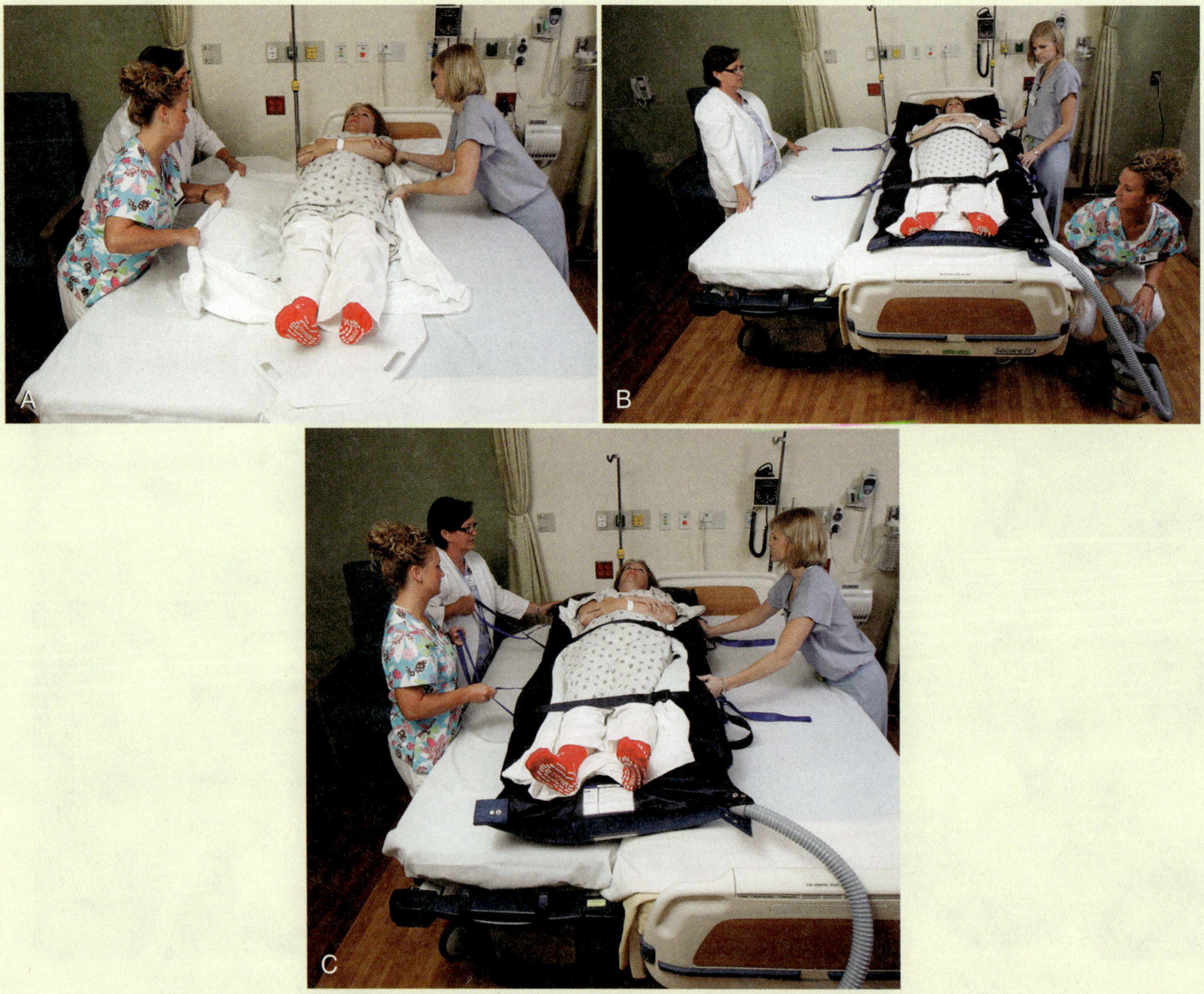

STEP 1E(8) **A,** Transfer of patient from bed to stretcher using sliding board. **B,** Inflating air-assisted transfer device. **C,** Transfer of patient using air-assisted device.

UNEXPECTED OUTCOMES AND RELATED INTERVENTIONS

- Patient unable to comprehend and follow directions for transfer.
  - Reassess continuity and simplicity of instructions.
- Patient sustains injury on transfer.
  - Evaluate incident that caused injury (e.g., assessment inadequate, change in patient status, improper use of equipment).
  - Complete occurrence report according to institution policy.
- Patient's level of weakness does not permit active transfer.
  - Obtain assistance from additional nursing personnel.
  - Increase bed activity and exercise to heighten tolerance.
- Patient continues to bear weight on non–weight-bearing limb.
  - Reinforce information about weight-bearing status.
- Patient transfers well on some occasions, poorly on others.
  - Assess patient for factors that affect ability to transfer (e.g., pain, fatigue, confusion) before transfer.
  - Allow for rest period before transferring, medicate for pain if indicated, or reorient patient.
  - Periodic confusion also alters performance.
- Patient is unable to stand for time required in transfer to chair.
  - Provide for adequate assistance during transfer.
  - Assess for orthostatic changes in blood pressure when transferring patient.
- Localized areas of erythema develop that do not disappear quickly (see Chapter 37).
  - Establish individualized skin care regimen.
  - Position patient in 30-degree lateral position.

KEY POINTS

- Muscles primarily associated with movement are located near the skeletal region, where movement results from leverage.
- Muscles primarily associated with posture are located in the lower extremities, trunk, neck, and back.
- Body alignment is the positioning of joints, tendons, ligaments, and muscles in various body positions.
- You achieve body balance when there is a wide base of support, the center of gravity falls within the base of support, and a vertical line falls from the center of gravity through the base of support.
- Conditions that affect body alignment and mobility include postural abnormalities, altered bone formation or joint mobility, impaired muscle development, central nervous system damage, and musculoskeletal system trauma.
- Assessment of a patient's mobility enables you to determine the patient's coordination, balance, and ability to complete ADLs and makes it possible to evaluate or plan an exercise program.
- Assessing gait allows you to draw some conclusions about the patient's balance, posture, and ability to walk without assistance.
- Patients with impaired body alignment require nursing interventions to maintain them in the supported Fowler's, supine, prone, side-lying, and Sims' positions.
- Transfer techniques require the use of correct body mechanics.
- Mechanical devices such as canes and walkers require specific nursing interventions to promote walking.

CLINICAL DECISION-MAKING EXERCISES

Mr. Indelicato is frustrated with his "lack of progress." Marilyn assesses his progress and asks him to demonstrate crutch walking. He refuses and tells Marilyn, "It's just too hard and painful." He is allowed partial weight bearing on his right leg.

1. During your assessment of Mr. Indelicato, which potential barriers is he experiencing that may be preventing him from participating in his treatment?
2. Which of the following statements from Mr. Indelicato do you address first? "My pain level is 8 out of 10. I just can't take it."; "I don't understand how to use those crutches."; or, "I've been so inactive for weeks, and I feel weak and tired."
3. Which is the most appropriate crutch gait for Mr. Indelicato? Explain your choice.

evolve

Answers to Clinical Decision-Making Exercises can be found on the Evolve website.

QSEN ACTIVITY: INFORMATICS

Marilyn meets with Mr. Indelicato at the outpatient rehabilitation setting 5 weeks after surgery on his right knee. He states, "I don't feel like I'm making progress or improvement; this is so frustrating. I can't keep track of when or if I did my exercises for the day." Marilyn notices that over the past several weeks Mr. Indelicato has entered his appointment times into his smartphone. She tells him that she will program his smartphone to help record his exercises each day.

What is the appropriate response to Mr. Indelicato's statements? Should Marilyn recommend the use of smartphone technology to address his concerns? Explain your answer.

evolve

Answers to QSEN Activities can be found on the Evolve website.

REVIEW QUESTIONS

1. A patient begins to fall during ambulation. Which of the following actions should you do first?
   1. Call for assistance.
   2. Slide the patient down your body to the floor.
   3. Instruct the patient to sit in the nearest chair.
   4. Contact the health care provider and document the fall.
2. A nursing assistive personnel asks for assistance in transferring a 160-lb patient from the bed to a wheelchair. The patient is unable to assist. What is the nurse's best response?
   1. "As long as we use proper body mechanics, no one will get hurt."
   2. "The patient only weighs 160 lbs. You don't need my assistance."
   3. "Call the lift team for additional assistance."
   4. "The two of us can easily lift the patient."
3. A patient has a head injury and has been in a coma for several days. The best intervention to include in the care plan to prevent complications of immobility such as footdrop would be:
   1. Active range of motion.
   2. Isometric exercises.
   3. Turn every 4 hours.
   4. Passive range of motion.
4. All of the following are necessary safety precautions when ambulating a patient except:
   1. Placing a transfer belt around patient's waist.
   2. Having patient wear well-fitting rubber-soled shoes or slippers.
   3. Having at least two people present to assist patient.
   4. Being sure that no pain medication was given for at least 3 hours before ambulation.
5. Mr. Rogers is able to walk but has a history of falls and reports feeling weak. He is 84 years old and lives alone. You are participating in his discharge planning. Which of the following pieces of equipment would be best to help Mr. Rogers in his home environment?
   1. A walker
   2. Crutches
   3. A wheelchair
   4. A mechanical lift device
6. Which statements apply to the proper use of a cane? (Select all that apply.)
   1. For maximum support when walking, the patient places the cane forward 15 to 25 cm (6 to 10 inches), keeping body weight on both legs. The weaker leg is moved forward to the cane so body weight is divided between the cane and the stronger leg.
   2. A person's cane length is equal to the distance between the elbow and the floor.
   3. Canes provide less support than a walker and are less stable.
   4. The patient needs to learn that two points of support such as both feet or one foot and the cane are present at all times.
7. Two nurses are standing on opposite sides of the bed to move a patient up in bed with a drawsheet. In relation to the patient, they stand even with the patient's:
   1. Hips.
   2. Chest.
   3. Knees.
   4. Shoulders.
8. A health care provider orders partial weight bearing on the left foot of a patient with a broken ankle and full weight bearing on the right foot. The crutch gait that the patient uses is the:
   1. Two-point.
   2. Four-point.
   3. Three-point.
   4. Swing-through.
9. Which of the following would best motivate a patient to participate in an exercise program?
   1. Given information on exercise
   2. Being at the stage of readiness to change behavior
   3. Diagnosed with a chronic disease such as diabetes
   4. Ordered by the health care provider to begin an exercise program
10. Which of the following methods of transfer from the bed to a chair is most appropriate for a patient who weighs 250 lbs and is able to minimally assist?
    1. Mechanical lift
    2. Sliding board
    3. Drawsheet with two caregivers
    4. Walker

evolve

Rationales for Review Questions can be found on the Evolve website.

1. 2; 2. 3; 3. 4; 4. 4; 5. 1; 6. 1, 3, 4; 7. 1; 8. 1; 9. 2; 10. 1

REFERENCES

American Nurses Association (ANA): *Nursing's legislative and regulatory initiatives for the 110th Congress: workplace health and safety*, 2007, http// www.anapoliticalpower.org.

American Nurses Association (ANA): *Handle with Care Position*, 2008, http:// www.safeliftingportal.com/documents/ safelifting-practices-for-nurses.pdf. Accessed May 2013.

American Nurses Association (ANA): ANA leads initiative to develop national safe patient handling standards, *Wyoming Nurse* 25(4):13, 2013.

Blake H, Hawley H: Effects of tai chi exercise on physical and psychological health of older people, *Curr Aging Sci* 5(1):19, 2012.

Bureau of Labor Statistics: *Occupational industries and illnesses: industry data*, 2009, http://stats.bls.gov/bls/ occupation.htm. Accessed June 17, 2013.

Centers for Disease Control and Prevention (CDC) and National Institute of Occupational Health and Safety (NIOSH): *State of the sector/healthcare and social assistance*, http://www.cdc.gov/ niosh/docs/2009-139/pdfs/2009-139.pdf, 2009. Accessed June 17, 2013.

Centers for Disease Control and Prevention (CDC): *How much physical activity do older adults Need?* http://www.cdc.gov/ physicalactivity/everyone/guidelines/ olderadults.htm, 2011. Accessed June 17, 2013.

Chodzko-Zajko WJ, et al: Exercise and physical activity for older adults, *Med Sci Sports Exercise* 41(7):1510, 2009.

Christo P, et al: Effective treatments for pain in the older patient, *Curr Pain Headache Rep* 15:22, 2011.

Edelman CL, Mandle CL: *Health promotion throughout the life span*, ed 7, St Louis, 2010, Mosby.

Freeman R, et al: Consensus statement on the definition of orthostatic hypotension, neutrally mediate syncope and the postural tachycardia syndrome, *Auton Neurosci* 161:46, 2011.

Hartford Institute for Geriatric Nursing (HIGN): Preventing pressure ulcers and skin tears. In Capezuti E, et al, editors: *Evidence-based geriatric nursing protocols for best practice*, ed 3, New York, 2008, Springer.

Hockenberry MJ, et al: *Wong's nursing care of infants and children*, ed 9, St Louis, 2011, Mosby.

Huang ES, et al: Racial/ethnic differences in concerns about current and future medications among patients with type 2 diabetes, *Diabetes Care* 32(2):311, 2009.

Huether SE, McCance KL: *Understanding pathophysiology*, ed 5, St Louis, 2012, Mosby.

Kutash M, et al: The lift team's importance to a successful safe patient handling program, *J Nurs Admin* 39(4):170, 2009.

Lagro J, et al: Diastolic blood pressure drop after standing as a clinical sign for increased mortality in older falls clinic patients, *J Hyperten* 30(6):1195, 2012.

Lewis S, et al: *Medical-surgical nursing: assessment and management of clinical problems*, ed 8, St Louis, 2011, Mosby.

Maskarinec G, et al: Diabetes prevalence and body mass index differ by ethnicity: the multiethnic cohort, *Ethnicity Dis* 19(1):49, 2009.

National Institute of Occupational Health and Safety (NIOSH): *Safe lifting and moving of nursing home patients*, 2006, http://www.cdc.gov/niosh/docs/2006-117/pdfs/2006-117.pdf. Accessed February 2, 2014.

Neidrick T, et al: Physical activity promotion in primary care targeting the older adult, *J Am Acad Nurs Pract* 24(7):405, 2012.

Nelson NA, Hughes RE: Quantifying relationships between selected work-related risk factors and back pain: a systematic review of object biomechanical measures and cost-related health outcomes, *Int J Industrial Ergonom* 39(1):202, 2009.

Nelson A, et al: Myths and facts about back injuries in nursing, *Am J Nurs* 103(2):32, 2003a.

Nelson A, et al: Safe patient handling and movement: preventing back injury among nurses requires careful selection of the safest equipment and techniques, *Am J Nurs* 103(3):32, 2003b.

Owens B, et al: What are we teaching about lifting and transferring patients? *Res Nurs Health* 22:3, 1999.

Patton KT, Thibodeau GA: *Anatomy and physiology*, ed 8, St Louis, 2013, Mosby.

Pelczarski KM: Back in action: design considerations for safe patient handling, *Health Facil Manage* 25(8):21, 2012.

Pierson F, Fairchild S: *Principles and techniques of patient care*, ed 5, St Louis, 2013, Saunders.

Piliae-Taylor RE, et al: Effects of Tai Chi and Western exercise on physical and cognitive functioning in healthy community-dwelling older adults, *J Aging Physical Activity* 18(3):261, 2010.

Prochaska JO, et al: The transtheoretical model and stages of change. In Glanz K, et al, editors: *Health behavior and health education*, ed 4, San Francisco, 2008, Jossey-Bass.

Rogers C, Keller C, Larkey L: Perceived benefits of meditative movement in older adults, *Geriatr Nurs* 31(1):37, 2010.

Sedlak C, et al: Development of the National Association of Orthopaedic nurses guidance statement on safe patient handling and movement in the orthopaedic setting, *Orthop Nurs* 28(2S):S2, 2009.

Seidel HM, et al: *Mosby's guide to physical examination*, ed 7, St Louis, 2011, Mosby.

Sherwood G, Barnsteiner J: *Quality and safety in nursing*, UK, 2012, Wiley-Blackwell.

Sorrentino SA, Remmert LN: *Mosby's textbook for nursing assistants*, ed 8, St Louis, 2012, Mosby.

The Joint Commission (TJC): *National Patient Safety Goals*, Oakbrook Terrace, IL, 2014, The Commission. Available at http://www.jointcommission.org/ standards_information/npsgs.aspx.

Touhy T, et al: *Ebersole and Hess's gerontological nursing and healthy aging*, ed 4, St Louis, 2014, Mosby.

Tullar JM, et al: Occupational safety and health interventions, *J Occup Rehabil* 20(2):199, 2010.

US Department of Health and Human Services (USDHHS): *Safe patient handling & lifting standards for a safer American workforce*, 2010, http://www .help.senate.gov/imo/media/doc/Collins4 .pdf. Accessed May 2013.

Waters T, et al: AORN Ergonomic tool 2: Positioning and repositioning the supine patient on the OR bed, *AORN J* 93(4), 2011a.

Waters T, et al: AORN Ergonomic tool 6: Lifting and carrying supplies and equipment in the perioperative setting, *AORN J* 94(2), 2011b.

Waters T, et al: AORN Ergonomic tool 7: Pushing, pulling, and moving equipment on wheels, *AORN J* 93(3), 2011c.

Wound, Ostomy, and Continence Nurses Society (WOCN): *Guideline for prevention and management of pressure ulcers*, Mount Laurel, NJ, 2010, WOCN.

Zadvinskis I, Salsbury SL: Effects of a multifaceted minimal-lift environment for nursing staff: Pilot results, *West J Nurs Res* 32:47, 2010.

CHAPTER

28

Safety

evolve WEBSITE

http://evolve.elsevier.com/Potter/essentials

- Video Clips
- Crossword Puzzle
- Audio Glossary

OBJECTIVES

- Describe environmental hazards that pose risks to patient safety.
- Discuss specific safety risks for patients at each developmental age.
- Discuss the importance of national patient safety resources and standards for promoting patient safety.
- Describe factors that create a culture of safety.
- Explain the concept of Never Events and a nurse's role in prevention.
- Assess risks to patients' safety within health care settings and the home.
- Identify relevant nursing diagnoses associated with risks to safety.
- Explain approaches for establishing a restraint-free environment.
- Identify factors to consider in the use of restraints.
- Develop a nursing care plan for patients whose safety is threatened.
- Describe nursing interventions specific to a patient's age for reducing risk for falls, fires, poisonings, and electrical hazards.
- Describe methods to evaluate interventions designed to maintain or promote safety.

KEY TERMS

carbon monoxide, p. 721
chemical restraints, p. 735
heat exhaustion, p. 722
hypothermia, p. 721
immunization, p. 723
Never Events, p. 719
pathogen, p. 723
restraint, p. 735
serious reportable events, p. 719

Patient safety is the most important initiative influencing how health care settings develop and implement programs for patient care. The Institute of Medicine (IOM) report (2000), *To Err is Human: Building a Safer Health System,* was a pivotal publication that brought patient safety to the forefront of health care in the United States. The report indicated that 44,000 to 98,000 people die each year as a result of preventable medical errors. Shortly thereafter the IOM published a second book, *Crossing the Quality Chasm: a New Healthcare System for the 21st Century* (IOM, 2001). This report recommended fundamental changes in the organization and delivery of health care in the United States. It also identified the need to focus on introducing processes and approaches for improving the quality of care delivered to patients, including forming new rules to redesign and improve health care, building organizational supports for change, applying evidence to health care delivery, and using information technology.

Much of the force behind the changes for improving safety in health care settings comes from regulatory and

CASE STUDY *Mr. Gonzales*

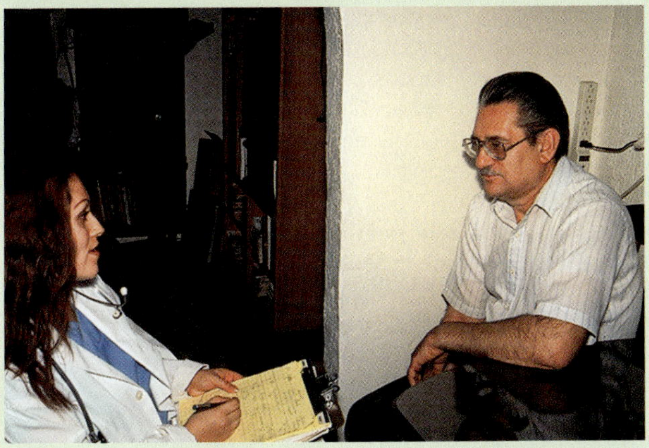

Mr. Gonzales is a 73-year-old man who has lived alone in a senior apartment building since his wife died 6 months ago. He and his wife were born in Mexico but came to live in the United States shortly after they were married. He is retired from a produce warehouse where he worked for 42 years. He and his wife raised three sons. The closest son, Carlos, is 30 minutes away by car. Carlos visits Mr. Gonzales every week to socialize and take him shopping. Mr. Gonzales is generally healthy but takes medication for high blood pressure. He also has decreased visual acuity, hearing loss from the noisy warehouse job, and some "arthritis" in his knees. He expects to live at least as long as his father, who lived to be 92 years old. Since his wife's death, Mr. Gonzales has attended Catholic mass every day at his parish church, where his wife had attended daily.

Joani Green, a 25-year-old married mother of two, is currently a nursing student at the local college. As part of the clinical requirements, she and her study partner are conducting health screenings and providing health promotion education for the residents of the apartment building where Mr. Gonzales lives. Part of her screening will include Mr. Gonzales' home environment.

accreditation agencies. The Joint Commission (TJC) and the Centers for Medicare and Medicaid Services (CMS) stress the importance of error prevention and patient safety. Their "Speak Up" campaign encourages patients to take a role in preventing health care errors by becoming active, involved, and informed participants in their health care (TJC, 2013a). For example, patients are encouraged to ask health care workers if they have washed their hands before providing care. The 2014 TJC National Patient Safety Goals (Box 28-1) are specifically directed at reducing the risk of medical errors.

The National Quality Forum (NQF) (2013a) has the mission of improving the quality of health care in America. It focuses on building consensus on national priorities and goals for performance improvement in health care. It also endorses national consensus standards for measuring and publicly reporting the performances of health care institutions. The NQF released its *National Voluntary Consensus Standards for Public Reporting of Patient Safety Events* (NQF, 2011). The report offers a framework for publicly reporting patient safety events, indicators, and measures about health care organizations to consumers. The NQF patient safety measures (e.g., falls with injury, incidence of pressure ulcers, and central-line bloodstream infection) are standards for judging health care quality. These measures are also used by organizations such as TJC and CMS. The NQF also endorses an updated list of 29 **serious reportable events** (SREs) (Box 28-2) that are a major focus for patient safety initiatives (NQF, 2013b). The CMS names select SREs as **Never Events** (adverse events that should never occur in a health care setting) (USDHHS, 2008). It now denies payment to hospitals for any hospital-acquired conditions resulting from or complicated by the occurrence of certain Never Events that were not present on admission (Box 28-3). Many of the hospital-acquired conditions are nurse-sensitive indicators, meaning that nursing interventions directly affect their development.

BOX 28-1 THE JOINT COMMISSION 2014 NATIONAL PATIENT SAFETY GOALS

HOSPITALS
- Identify patients correctly.
- Improve staff communication.
- Use medicines safely.
- Use alarms safely.
- Prevent infection.
- Identify patient safety risks (e.g., suicide).
- Prevent mistakes in surgery.

HOME CARE
- Identify patients correctly.
- Use medicines safely.
- Prevent infection.
- Prevent patients from falling.
- Identify patient safety risks (e.g., patients on oxygen, risk of fire).

Adapted from The Joint Commission (TJC): *National Patient Safety Goals*, Oakbrook Terrace, IL, 2014, The Commission. Available at http://www.jointcommission.org/standards_information/npsgs.aspx.

Health care organizations strive to create a culture of safety, one that consistently minimizes adverse events despite carrying out complex and hazardous work (USDHHS, 2012). A culture of safety requires a commitment that acknowledges the high-risk nature of the activities of an organization, the determination to achieve consistently safe operations, a blame-free environment in which individuals can report errors without fear or reprimand, and an organizational commitment of resources. These organizations foster a patient-centered safety culture by continually focusing on performance improvement efforts (see Chapter 7), risk-management findings, and safety reports to design a safe work environment. A safer work environment requires all staff to receive continuing education and have access to appropriate resources (Box 28-4).

As part of the health care team, you have the professional responsibility to engage in activities that support a patient-centered safety culture. The Quality and Safety Education for Nurses (QSEN) project was developed to meet the challenge of preparing future nurses to have the knowledge, skills, and attitudes needed to continuously improve the quality and

BOX 28-2 NATIONAL QUALITY FORUM LIST OF SERIOUS REPORTABLE EVENTS

SURGICAL OR INVASIVE PROCEDURE EVENTS

- Surgery or other invasive procedure performed on wrong site
- Surgery or other invasive procedure performed on wrong patient
- Wrong surgical or other invasive procedure performed on a patient
- Unintended retention of foreign object in patient after surgery or other invasive procedure
- Intraoperative or immediately postoperative/postprocedure death in an ASA class 1 patient

PRODUCT OR DEVICE EVENTS

- Patient death or serious injury associated with use of contaminated drugs, devices, or biologicals provided by health care setting
- Patient death or serious injury associated with use or function of a device in patient care in which device is used for functions other than as intended
- Patient death or serious injury associated with intravascular air embolism that occurs while being cared for in a health care setting

PATIENT PROTECTION EVENTS

- Discharge or release of patient/resident of any age who is unable to make decisions to other than an authorized person
- Patient death or serious injury associated with patient elopement (disappearance)
- Patient suicide, attempted suicide, or self-harm that results in serious injury while being cared for in a health care setting

CARE MANAGEMENT EVENTS

- Patient death or serious injury associated with medication error (e.g., errors involving wrong drug, wrong dose, wrong patient, wrong time, wrong rate, wrong preparation, or wrong route of administration)
- Patient death or serious injury associated with unsafe administration of blood products
- Maternal death or serious injury associated with labor or delivery in low-risk pregnancy while being cared for in a health care setting
- (NEW) Death or serious injury of a neonate associated with labor or delivery in a low-risk pregnancy
- Patient death or serious injury associated with a fall while being cared for in a health care setting
- Any stage 3, stage 4, and unstageable pressure ulcers acquired after admission/presentation to a health care setting
- Artificial insemination with wrong donor sperm or wrong egg
- (NEW) Patient death or serious injury resulting from irretrievable loss of an irreplaceable biological specimen
- (NEW) Patient death or serious injury resulting from failure to follow up or communicate laboratory, pathology, or radiology test results

ENVIRONMENTAL EVENTS

- Patient or staff death or serious injury associated with an electric shock in the course of a patient care process in a health care setting
- Any incident in which system that is designated for oxygen or other gas to be delivered to a patient contains no gas or wrong gas or is contaminated by toxic substances
- Patient or staff death or serious injury associated with a burn incurred from any source in the course of a patient care process in a health care setting
- Patient death or serious injury associated with use of physical restraints or bedrails while being cared for in a health care setting

RADIOLOGIC EVENTS

- (NEW) Death or serious injury of a patient or staff associated with introduction of a metallic object into magnetic resonance imaging (MRI) area

POTENTIAL CRIMINAL EVENTS

- Any instance of care ordered or provided by someone impersonating a physician, nurse, pharmacist, or other licensed health care provider
- Abduction of a patient/resident of any age
- Sexual abuse/assault on a patient or staff member within or on grounds of a health care setting
- Death or serious injury of a patient or staff member resulting from a physical assault (i.e., battery) that occurs within or on grounds of a health care setting

Adapted from NQF: *List of SREs*, 2013b, http://www.qualityforum.org/Topics/SREs/List_of_SREs.aspx#sre1. Accessed December 1, 2013.

safety of the health care systems where they work (QSEN Institute, 2013). The QSEN safety competency requires you to "minimize risk of harm to patients and providers through both system effectiveness and individual performance." Use of critical thinking skills (see Chapter 8) coupled with application of the nursing process (see Chapter 9) enables you to become a provider of safe patient care and an active participant in health promotion.

SCIENTIFIC KNOWLEDGE BASE

Safety (i.e., the freedom from psychological and physical injury) is a basic human need. Health care provided in a safe manner and a safe community environment is essential for patients' well-being. Vulnerable groups that require help in achieving a safe environment include infants, children, older adults, the ill or injured, the physically and mentally disabled, the illiterate, and the poor. To be effective, you need to understand factors that contribute to a safe environment in the home or health care agency and thoroughly assess the environment for threats to safety. You also need to understand how alterations in mobility, sensory function, and cognition affect patients' safety (see Chapters 36 and 38). A safe environment includes meeting basic human needs, reducing physical hazards, and reducing transmission of pathogens.

BOX 28-3 2013 CENTERS FOR MEDICARE AND MEDICAID SERVICES HOSPITAL-ACQUIRED CONDITIONS AND PRESENT-ON-ADMISSION INDICATORS

- Foreign object retained after surgery
- Air embolism
- Blood incompatibility
- Stages III and IV pressure ulcers
- Falls and trauma: fracture, dislocation, intracranial injury, crushing injury, burn, other injuries
- Catheter-associated urinary tract infections
- Vascular catheter-associated infections
- Manifestations of poor glycemic control: diabetic ketoacidosis, nonketotic hyperosmolar coma, hypoglycemic coma, secondary diabetes with ketoacidosis, secondary diabetes with hyperosmolarity
- Surgical site infections following:
    - Mediastinitis after coronary artery bypass graft (CABG)
    - Certain orthopedic procedures: spine, neck, shoulder, elbow
    - Bariatric surgery for obesity: laparoscopic gastric bypass, gastroenterostomy, laparoscopic gastric restrictive surgery
    - Cardiac implantable electronic device (CIED)
- Deep vein thrombosis and pulmonary embolism following certain orthopedic procedures: total knee replacement or hip replacement
- Iatrogenic pneumothorax with venous catheterization

From Centers for Medicare and Medicaid Services (CMS): *Hospital-acquired conditions,* 2012, http://www.cms.gov/Medicare/Medicare-Fee-for-Service-Payment/HospitalAcqCond/Hospital-Acquired_Conditions.html. Accessed December 1, 2013.

BOX 28-4 RESOURCES RELATED TO SAFETY AND SAFETY INITIATIVES

- The Joint Commission: http://www.jointcommission.org/topics/patient_safety.aspx
- Agency for Healthcare Research and Quality: http://www.psnet.ahrq.gov/
- Institute for Healthcare Improvement: http://www.ihi.org/ihi
- U.S. Department of Veterans Affairs: http://www.patientsafety.va.gov/
- Centers for Medicare and Medicaid Services: http://www.cms.gov
- Quality Improvement Organization Support Center: http://www.qualitynet.org
- National Quality Forum: http://www.qualityforum.org/Home.aspx
- ECRI Institute: http://www.ecri.org

Basic Human Needs

The physiological needs of adequate oxygen, nutrition, and favorable temperature and humidity are basic human needs often at risk from a variety of environmental hazards. These needs must be met before physical and psychological safety and security can be addressed.

Oxygen. Patients who require supplemental oxygen in health care settings can be at risk because of the potential for oxygen to support burning. A fire needs three things to remain burning: fuel, an adequate supply of oxygen, and a sufficient heat source. Strict codes regulate the use and storage of medical oxygen in health care facilities. This is not the case in the home environment. Smoking is by far the leading cause of burns, reported fires, deaths, and injuries involving home medical oxygen. Be sure to administer oxygen safely and provide patients and family caregivers the information needed to manage oxygen in the home (see Chapter 30).

Know factors in a patient's environment that decrease the amount of available oxygen. A hazard in the home is an improperly functioning heating system. A furnace, stove, or fireplace that is not properly vented introduces carbon monoxide into the environment. **Carbon monoxide** affects a person's oxygenation by binding strongly with hemoglobin; preventing the formation of oxyhemoglobin, and thus reducing the supply of oxygen delivered to the tissues (see Chapter 30). Low concentrations cause nausea, dizziness, headache, and fatigue. Higher concentrations are often fatal. Unintentional, non–fire-related (UNFR) carbon monoxide (CO) poisoning is one of the most common causes of poisoning in the United States and results in more than 20,000 emergency department visits annually (Iqbal et al., 2010).

Nutrition. Meeting nutritional needs requires knowledge about healthy food, food safety, and how to use environmental controls. Chapter 33 details the principles of balanced nutrition and therapeutic diets. Health care facilities are required to meet State Board of Health regulations for the storage, preparation, and provision of food. In the home some patients do not know how to properly refrigerate, store, and prepare food. A patient needs a refrigerator with a freezer compartment to keep perishable foods fresh. An adequate, clean water supply is necessary for drinking and to wash fresh produce and dishes. Provisions for garbage collection are necessary to maintain sanitary conditions. Foods need to be adequately cooked to kill any residing organisms. If a patient does not prepare or store foods properly, it increases his or her risk for infections and food poisoning from bacteria such as *Escherichia coli, Salmonella,* or *Listeria.* Groups at the highest risk for food poisoning are children, pregnant women, older adults, and people with compromised immune systems.

Temperature. A person's comfort zone is usually between 18.3° and 23.8° C (65° and 75° F). Temperature extremes, which often occur during the winter and summer, affect comfort, productivity, and safety. Exposure to severe cold for prolonged periods causes frostbite and accidental **hypothermia** (see Chapter 15). Older adults, the very young, patients with cardiovascular conditions, patients who have ingested drugs or excess alcohol, and the homeless are at high risk for hypothermia. Exposure to extreme heat changes body electrolyte balance and raises the core body temperature, resulting in heatstroke or heat exhaustion. People at risk from high environmental temperatures need to avoid extremely hot, humid environments; otherwise heat exhaustion results.

Physical Hazards

On average 33.5 million injuries take place each year, with most occurring inside or outside of the home (CDC, 2010). Physical hazards in the environment threaten a person's safety and often result in physical or psychological injury or death. Unintentional injuries are the fifth leading cause of death for Americans of all ages (National Center for Injury Prevention and Control, 2010). Motor vehicle accidents are the leading cause, followed by poisonings and falls. Additional hazards consist of fire and disasters. Your role as a nurse is to educate patients about common safety hazards and how to prevent injury while placing emphasis on hazards to which patients are more vulnerable.

Motor Vehicle Accidents. Vehicle design and equipment such as seat belts, air bags, and laminated windshields (remain in one piece when impacted) have improved vehicular safety. State laws relating to young drivers' licensing, safety belt use, child restraint use, and motorcycle helmets exist for protection of drivers. Child safety seats and booster seats appropriate for a child's age and weight and the type of car need to be used. The American Academy of Pediatrics (AAP) (2013) recommends the following:

1. All infants and toddlers should ride in a rear-facing car safety seat (CSS) until they are 2 years of age or until they reach the highest weight or height allowed by the manufacturer of their CSS.
2. All children 2 years or older, or those younger than 2 years who have outgrown the rear-facing weight or height limit for their CSS, should use a forward-facing CSS with a harness for as long as possible, up to the highest weight or height allowed by the manufacturer of their CSS.
3. All children whose weight or height is above the forward-facing limit for their CSS should use a belt-positioning booster seat until the vehicle lap-and-shoulder seat belt fits properly, typically when they have reached 4 feet 9 inches in height and are between 8 and 12 years of age.
4. When children are old enough and large enough to use the vehicle seat belt alone, they should always use lap-and-shoulder seat belts for optimal protection.
5. All children younger than 13 years should be restrained in the rear seats of vehicles for optimal protection.

Newer cars and trucks are equipped with a LATCH (Lower Anchors and Tethers for Children) system for installing child safety seats. However, if children and their car seats have a combined weight of 65 pounds, the strength of the anchors cannot be guaranteed. Child seats typically weigh 15 to 33 pounds. A new rule expected to be released in 2014 by the National Highway Transportation and Safety Administration warns that some children as light as 32 pounds might not be able to use a system designed to make child seats easier to install and, therefore, safer. Once children and their seats are past the weight limit for the lower anchors, parents can secure the child seat using the car's safety-belt system. The revision to the rule will apply only to the lower anchors. Use of the tether strap that is attached to the top anchor is not affected (Figure 28-1).

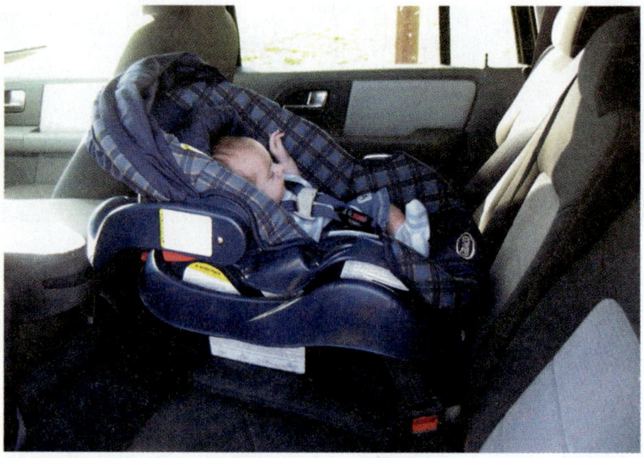

FIGURE 28-1 Rear-facing infant car seat. (Courtesy Brian and Mayannyn Sallee, Las Vegas, NV.)

According to the CDC the risk of motor vehicle accidents is higher among 16- to 19-year-old drivers than any other age-group (CDC, 2012a). Teens tend to underestimate dangerous situations or are not able to recognize hazardous situations (e.g., texting while driving). In addition, they tend to speed and allow shorter headways, ride with intoxicated drivers, and drive after using alcohol and drugs. Teens have the lowest rate of seat belt use. Older drivers are keeping their licenses longer and driving more miles than in the past. Age-related declines in vision and cognitive functioning (ability to reason and remember) and physical changes affect some older adults' driving abilities (CDC, 2013c). On the positive side older adults have a higher incidence of use of seat belts, they tend to drive when road conditions are the safest, and they are less likely to drink under the influence of alcohol.

Poison. A poison is any substance that impairs health or destroys life when ingested, inhaled, or absorbed by the body. Almost any substance is poisonous if too much is taken. Poisons impair the function of every major organ system. Health care providers are at risk from chemicals such as chemotherapy drugs and toxic cleaning agents. Sources of poison in people's homes include medicines, other solid and liquid substances, gases, and vapors. Toddlers, preschoolers, and young school-age children have a greater risk for accidental poisoning in the home because they often ingest household cleaning solutions, medications, or personal hygiene products. Emergency treatment is needed when a person ingests a poisonous substance or comes in contact with a chemical that is absorbed through the skin. A poison control center is the best resource for patients and parents needing information about the treatment of an accidental poisoning.

Fire. Home fires are a major cause of death and injury. In 2012 U.S. fire departments responded to 36,500 home structure fires, which caused 12,875 civilian injuries and 2,380 civilian deaths (National Fire Protection Association, 2013). Smoking materials such as cigarettes, cigars, and pipes are a primary source of home fires. Many fatal fires are the result of individuals smoking in bed and accidentally falling asleep. Another problem related to fatal fires is a failure to keep fresh batteries in home smoke detectors. The improper use of cooking equipment and appliances, particularly stoves, is another source for in-home fires. Smoke detectors and carbon monoxide detectors need to be placed strategically throughout a home. Multipurpose fire extinguishers need to be near the kitchen and any workshop areas.

Falls. Falls are a major public health problem. Among adults 64 years and older, falls in the home are the leading cause of unintentional death (CDC, 2010). Common physical hazards that lead to falls in the home include inadequate lighting, barriers along normal walking paths and stairs, and a lack of safety devices. Often a fall leads to serious injury such as fractures or internal bleeding. Injuries often result from accidental contact with objects on stairs, floors, and low-standing furniture. Forces from falls lead to injury with variable severity, depending on the height of the fall, body position on impact, and impact surface.

Disasters. When a disaster such as a flood, hurricane, tornado, or wildfire strikes, death and serious injury result. These types of disasters also leave many people homeless. Another type of disaster, bioterrorism, is a real threat to the safety of our general population. Threats of this type come in the form of biological, chemical, and radiological attacks. Bioterrorism, or the use of biological agents to create fear and threat, is the most likely form of a terrorist attack to occur. National preparedness for all forms of disaster has progressed during the last decade. Hospitals have plans and disaster drills for internal and external disasters (Veenema, 2011). Medical and public health professionals have joined the disaster preparedness community, the U.S. federal government increased investment in preparedness, and community partners and participants are involved in disaster preparedness (Inglesby, 2011).

Pathogen Transmission. Pathogens and parasites pose a threat to patient safety. A **pathogen** is any microorganism capable of producing an illness. The most common means of transmission of pathogens is by the hands. The most effective way to limit the transmission of pathogens is the medical aseptic practice of handwashing. Pathogens are also transmitted through human blood and body fluids and by insects (e.g., mosquitoes carrying malaria) and rodents. See details in Chapter 14 on how pathogens are transmitted and acquired and the means for controlling transmission of infectious microorganisms.

Health care agencies are concerned with the processing of biohazardous wastes, a source of pathogen transmission. It is important to properly dispose of needles, surgical dressings, sharps, and syringes to prevent the risk for exposure to the general population and employees. You also need to clean or dispose of bed linens and patient gowns contaminated by body fluids in proper containers to reduce threats to safety.

Immunization. **Immunization** is the process by which resistance to an infectious disease is produced or increased. The body acquires active immunity after a small amount of weakened or dead organisms and modified toxins from the organism (toxoids) is injected into the body. Passive immunity occurs when antibodies produced by other people or animals are introduced into a person's bloodstream for protection against a pathogen. Nurses must know immunization guidelines and inform members of the public about the importance of immunization in maintaining the health of their children.

Pollution. A healthy environment is free of pollutants (i.e., harmful chemical or waste materials discharged into the water, soil, or air). People often think of pollution only in terms of air, land, or water; but excessive noise is also a form of pollution that presents health risks. Air pollution is the contamination of the atmosphere with a harmful chemical. Prolonged exposure to it increases the risk of pulmonary disease. In urban areas industrial waste and vehicle exhaust are common contributors to air pollution. In the home, school, or workplace, cigarette smoke is the primary air pollutant. Improper disposal of radioactive and bioactive waste products can cause land pollution. Water pollution is the contamination of lakes, rivers, and streams, usually by industrial pollutants. If water becomes contaminated, the public needs to use bottled or boiled water for drinking and cooking. Flooding often damages water treatment stations and thus requires use of bottled or boiled water.

NURSING KNOWLEDGE BASE

Factors Influencing Patient Safety

A person's developmental stage, lifestyle habits, mobility status, sensory and cognitive function, and safety awareness all influence threats to safety. As a nurse be familiar with each patient's risks and the risks that are present within a health care setting.

Developmental Level

Infant, Toddler, and Preschooler. Injuries are a major cause of death during infancy, especially for children 6 to 12 months old (Hockenberry and Wilson, 2011). The leading causes of injury to infants are falls, ingestion injuries (poison, foreign body ingestion, and medication) and burns. Aspiration often occurs from the ingestion of foreign material such as small toys and food items. The nature of an injury is closely related to an infant's normal growth and development. Children at these early stages are curious; they explore their environment and, because of an increase in oral activity, put objects in their mouths. Accidents involving young children are largely preventable. Parents need to be aware of specific dangers. Accident prevention requires health education for parents and the removal of dangers whenever possible.

School-Age Child. When children enter school, their environment expands to include the school, the means of transportation to and from school, and after-school activities. School-age children learn how to perform more complicated motor activities and are often uncoordinated. Instruct parents and teachers about safe practices to follow at school and during play. Teach school-age children who are involved in team and contact sports rules for playing safely and how to use protective safety equipment. Head injuries resulting from falls, motor vehicle injuries, and bicycle injuries are a major cause of death (Hockenberry and Wilson, 2011). Precautions are needed to make a child's environment safe. Playground safety is especially important during the summer months.

Adolescent. As children enter adolescence, they develop greater independence and a sense of identity. The adolescent begins to separate emotionally from the family, and the peer group begins to have a stronger influence. Wide variations that swing from childlike to mature behavior are characteristic of adolescent behavior (Hockenberry and Wilson, 2011). To relieve the tensions associated with the physical and psychosocial changes and peer pressure, adolescents often engage in risk-taking behaviors such as smoking, drinking alcohol, and using drugs. This increases the risk for accidents such as drowning and motor vehicle accidents. According to the Insurance Institute for Highway Safety (2011), the fatal crash rate per mile driven for 16- to 19 year-olds in the United States is nearly 3 times the rate for drivers ages 20 and over. Fatal crash rates for teens are high largely because of their immaturity combined with driving inexperience. To assess for possible substance abuse, have parents look for environmental and psychosocial clues. Environmental clues include the presence of drug-oriented magazines, beer and liquor bottles, drug paraphernalia, blood spots on clothing, and the continual wearing of long-sleeved shirts in hot weather and dark glasses indoors. Psychosocial clues include failing grades, change in dress, increased absenteeism from school, isolation, increased aggressiveness, and changes in interpersonal relationships.

Adult. Threats to an adult's safety are often related to lifestyle habits. For example, a patient who uses alcohol or drugs excessively is at greater risk for motor vehicle accidents. Adults experiencing high levels of stress are at a greater risk for accidents and stress-related illnesses such as headaches, depression, gastrointestinal disorders, and infections.

Older Adult. The physiological changes associated with aging, effects of multiple medications, psychological factors, and acute or chronic disease increase an older adult's risk for falls and other types of accidents. One out of three adults age 65 and older falls each year, but fewer than half talk to their health care providers about it (CDC, 2013a). Among older adults (those 65 or older), falls are the leading cause of injury death. They are also the most common cause of nonfatal injuries and hospital admissions for trauma.

Most falls occur within or around the home, specifically in the bedroom, bathroom, and kitchen. Environmental factors such as broken stairs, icy sidewalks, inadequate lighting, throw rugs, and exposed electrical cords cause many accidents. Older adults typically fall while transferring from beds, chairs, and toilets; getting into or out of bathtubs; tripping over carpet edges or doorway thresholds; and slipping on wet surfaces or descending stairs. Fear of falling is common among community-dwelling older adults who both do and do not have a history of falling (Duckyoo, 2008). As a result of their fear, many older adults avoid activities or change the way in which they walk and position themselves, making them more at risk for falling. It is important to learn which conditions increase a person's fear of falling so steps can be taken to remove or change any hazards in the home.

Other Risk Factors

Lifestyle. Lifestyle choices increase safety risks. People who drive or operate machinery while under the influence of chemical substances or work at jobs that are dangerous are at greater risk for injury. People who are preoccupied by stress or anxiety are more accident prone because they fail to recognize the source of potential accidents such as a cluttered stair or stop sign.

Impaired Mobility. A patient with impaired mobility has many kinds of safety risks. Immobilization predisposes a patient to physiological and emotional hazards, which in turn further restrict mobility and independence (see Chapter 36). Patients with disabilities are at greater risk for injury when entering motor vehicles and buildings not equipped for the handicapped.

Sensory Impairments. Patients with visual, hearing, tactile, or communication impairments such as aphasia or language barrier are at greater risk for injury. Such patients are not always able to perceive a potential danger or express need for assistance (see Chapter 38).

Cognitive Impairments. Cognitive impairments associated with delirium, dementia, and depression place patients at greater risk for injury. These conditions contribute to altered concentration and attention span, impaired memory, and orientation changes. Patients with these alterations become easily confused about their surroundings and are more likely to have falls and burns.

Safety Awareness. Some patients are unaware of safety precautions such as keeping medicine, poisonous plants, or other poisons away from children or reading the expiration date on food products. This may be the result of their educational background, low health literacy, health beliefs, and access to informational resources. Your nursing assessment identifies a patient's level of knowledge regarding home safety so you are able to correct safety problems with an individualized care plan.

Risks in the Health Care Agency

Environmental safety pertains not only to a patient's home and community but also to a health care agency. However, there are risks in health care agencies that you also need to address.

Chemical Exposure. Various forms of chemicals used in patient care are a source of an environmental risk. Chemicals found in some medications such as chemotherapy agents, anesthetic gases, cleaning solutions, and disinfectants are potentially toxic if ingested or inhaled. Material safety data sheets (MSDSs) are a resource available in any health care agency. The sheets provide information on the chemical composition of a material, first aid measures for exposure, proper disposal methods, and technical information such as the physical and chemical properties of the material (U.S. Department of Labor, n.d.).

Falls. In addition to the home setting, the health care setting is a location where falls often occur. Up to 50% of hospitalized patients are at risk for falls, and almost half of those who fall suffer an injury (Fitzpatrick, 2011). Falls are a major contributor to a patient's functional decline and increased health care use. Even if a fall doesn't cause a serious injury, it may triple a patient's likelihood of requiring placement in a skilled nursing facility (Jorgensen, 2011). A fall can cause lasting pain and suffering and may limit physical, psychological, and social function, placing additional burdens on families and society. Falls also affect the cost per case that a health care organization incurs and the patient's length of stay. The average hospital stay for patients who fall is lengthened by 12.3 days, and injuries from falls lead to a 61% increase in patient-care costs (Fitzpatrick, 2011). Every health care institution has initiatives in place to reduce falls, including use of special fall risk assessment tools, fall prevention protocols, fall alert signs, and identification bands. To date no one intervention has demonstrated effectiveness in reducing falls in health care settings. Their cause is multifactorial. Common risk factors for falls in hospital settings are broken down into two categories: intrinsic and extrinsic (Kulik, 2011).

- *Intrinsic factors* are patient-related and include physiological conditions such as vision disturbances, urinary/stool frequency or incontinence, mental impairment, gait and balance disorders, polypharmacy, and older age.
- *Extrinsic factors* are environmentally related and include room clutter, loose electrical cords, and spills.

A number of evidence-based interventions, when used together, have been effective in reducing falls (Box 28-5).

Patient-Inherent Accidents. Patient-inherent accidents are those (other than falls) in which a patient is the primary reason for the accident. Examples are self-inflicted cuts, injuries, and burns; ingestion or injection of foreign substances; self-mutilation or setting fires; and pinching fingers in drawers or doors. One of the more common precipitating factors for a patient-inherent accident is a seizure. Place patients with seizure disorders on seizure precautions, which include protecting a patient from harm during a seizure, assisting with airway management if indicated, and administering antiseizure medications as ordered.

Procedure-Related Accidents. Health care providers cause procedure-related accidents. They include medication and fluid administration errors, not putting external devices on correctly, and improperly performing procedures such as dressing changes. Always follow the policies and procedure of an organization and standards of nursing practice to prevent procedure-related accidents. For example, correct use of body mechanics and transfer techniques reduces the risk for injuries when moving and lifting patients (see Chapter 27). All staff need to be aware that distractions and interruptions contribute to procedure-related accidents and need to be limited.

Equipment-Related Accidents. Equipment-related accidents result from an electrical hazard or the malfunction, disrepair, or misuse of equipment. To avoid rapid infusion of intravenous (IV) fluids, all general-use and patient-controlled analgesic pumps need to have free-flow protection devices. To avoid accidents, do not operate medical equipment without adequate instruction. If you discover a faulty piece of equipment, replace it with the proper working equipment, place a tag on the faulty one, take it out of service, and promptly report any malfunctions. Assess potential electrical hazards to reduce the risk of electrical fires, electrocution, or injury from faulty equipment. In health care settings the clinical engineering staff make regular safety checks of

BOX 28-5 EVIDENCE-BASED PRACTICE

PICO Question: Does a multifactorial fall-intervention program compared with single interventions reduce incidence of falls among hospitalized patients?

SUMMARY OF EVIDENCE

Research shows that fall prevention intervention programs in hospitals and other health care settings need to multifactorial (i.e., there needs to be a variety of interventions (Spoelstra, Given, and Given, 2012). Fall prevention interventions shown to have benefit in reducing hospital-related falls and fall-related injuries include fall-risk assessments, door/bed/ patient fall-risk alerts (e.g., bed alarms, signs, identification bands), environmental and equipment modifications, staff and patient safety education, improved medication management [reducing polypharmacy], and additional assistance with transfer and toileting. Hospitals need to use multiple evidence-based fall prevention interventions to reduce falls and injuries. Current research shows that having nurses make hourly rounds to check more frequently on patients helps to reduce fall incidence initially, but the intervention needs to be used consistently over time to have long term effects (Tucker et al., 2012).

APPLICATION TO NURSING PRACTICE

- Multiple interventions aimed at the patient's specific risk factors produce the best outcomes.
- Educate patient and family members about safe mobility practices (e.g., how to move safely with intravenous pole or indwelling urinary catheter).
- Provide patient and family with safety tips to prevent falls.
- Activate bed exit alarms at night or when patients are sleeping.
- Keep beds in proper position with wheels locked.
- Modify mobility signs posted on units. Post appropriate directions (e.g., "provide assistive device" or "assist to bathroom").
- Round on patients hourly.

equipment. Facilities must report all suspected medical device–related deaths to both the Food and Drug Administration (FDA) and the product manufacturer (FDA, 2013).

CRITICAL THINKING

Synthesis

You apply elements of critical thinking whenever you perform the nursing process with patients. Consider the scientific knowledge you have learned, your experience, critical thinking attitudes, and standards to ensure an individualized approach to patient care (Box 28-6).

Knowledge. When caring for a patient's safety needs, begin by reflecting on the knowledge you have about common safety risks and a patient's developmental stage. You need a complete picture of a patient's physical, cultural, physiological, psychosocial, and environmental information to protect him or her from injury. Consider information from pharmacology (e.g., medications being taken and possible interactions) and information about environmental hazards. Apply your assessment findings regarding a patient's environment and where most activities of daily living occur. Because all patients are different, prioritize factors that are threats to their safety and concentrate on probable threats. After you consider a patient's specific strengths, weaknesses, developmental stage, and environment, work with the patient and family to determine a patient-centered approach.

Experience. Use clinical and personal experience to recall safety incidents that occurred with other patients or your own family and the specific circumstances that led to a situation. For example, if your grandmother fell because her slipper became entangled in a throw rug at the top of the stairs, use the experience of your grandmother's fall and apply the knowledge gained when you assess a patient's home for safety hazards during a home visit.

Attitudes. Using critical thinking attitudes ensures that your plan of care for a patient's safety is comprehensive. For example, show perseverance in identifying all potential safety risks and threats. Be responsible for collecting unbiased, accurate data that are relevant to a patient's safety. It is important to show discipline to thoroughly assess a patient's home environment. View all situations as opportunities to protect a patient. Once they occur, injuries cause pain, immobility, loss of income, or even death.

Standards. The American Nurses Association's (ANA's) *Nursing: Scope and Standards of Practice* (2010) includes the concept of safety, stating that nurses will implement nursing interventions competently in a safe and appropriate manner. The ANA Code of Ethics (see Chapter 6) includes safety issues, describing a nurse's responsibility to promote, advocate for, and strive to protect the health, safety, and rights of patients. Regulatory agencies such as TJC and the Occupational Safety and Health Administration (OSHA) define standards and guidelines related to safety in health care settings (OSHA, 2013; TJC, 2014).

NURSING PROCESS

ASSESSMENT

To conduct a thorough patient assessment, consider possible threats to the patient's safety, including his or her immediate environment and any individual risk factors (Table 28-1). When you care for patients in the home, perform a home safety assessment to look for factors that are hazards within the home (Box 28-7). A thorough safety assessment covers topics such as adequacy of lighting, presence of safety devices, conditions (e.g., flooring, steps) that pose risks for falls, and safety of the kitchen and bathrooms. To assess a home, walk through the rooms with the patient and discuss how the patient normally conducts daily activities and whether the

BOX 28-6 SYNTHESIS IN PRACTICE

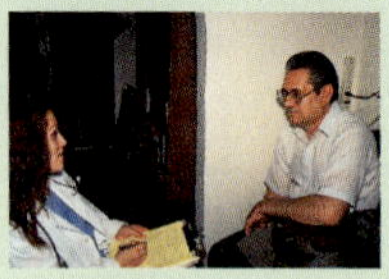

Joani completed a health screening on Mr. Gonzales. She knows that she needs to incorporate knowledge about fall and environmental risks as they relate to Mr. Gonzales' age, level of independence, health status, and expectations. Mr. Gonzales is the third patient Joani has cared for in the home; thus she is also able to draw on her past experiences. As Joani integrates knowledge with her previous experience, she remembers that Mr. Gonzales values his independence. As a result she considers ways to develop a plan of care to meet Mr. Gonzales' safety needs while helping him maintain his independence. She discovers that the lighting in his home is poor and that several throw rugs are near the chairs and bedside. The health screening revealed that Mr. Gonzales has decreased visual acuity and has not had a new pair of glasses for 3 years. He fell in his apartment about a month ago but did not have any injuries, nor did he tell his son.

BOX 28-7 HOME SAFETY ASSESSMENT

Look for these factors when assessing the safety of a home:

- Proper lighting inside and outside
- Storage areas within easy reach
- Appliances in good working order
- Extension cords placed along walls
- Presence of smoke detectors and a fire extinguisher
- Presence of carbon monoxide detector
- Flammable objects away from stove or heaters
- Gas pilot lights lit
- Hot water thermostat set to 120°F or less
- Handrails or grip bars installed
- Nonskid surfaces in bathroom and tub or shower
- Floor coverings secured and floors free of clutter
- Furniture and assistive devices promote ease of mobility
- Medications stored properly and not outdated
- Telephone accessible with readily available emergency phone numbers

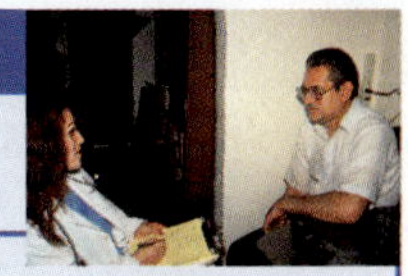

TABLE 28-1 FOCUSED PATIENT ASSESSMENT

FACTORS TO ASSESS	QUESTIONS	PHYSICAL ASSESSMENT
Environment	Describe times you have fallen in the past. Where do the falls commonly happen? Have you ever burned yourself?	Inspect the home environment both inside and outside for potential hazards: focus on the kitchen and bathroom.
Sensory	When do you wear your glasses? When was the last time you had your eyes checked? Can you hear your phone when it rings?	Observe patient's ability to read printed material accurately and ability to move about within the home. Assess ability to hear normal spoken word.
Physical mobility	How does your (arthritis, surgery, impaired gait) affect the way you walk and move around? Do you exercise? Describe how you exercise each day. Are you able to move around safely at home?	Observe patient's posture, gait, and balance during activities of daily living.

environment poses problems. For example, when assessing adequacy of lighting, inspect areas where a patient moves and works, particularly outside walkways, steps, interior halls, and doorways. Getting a sense of a patient's routines helps you recognize safety hazards.

Assessment of patients' risk factors for falling is a priority in health care settings. Many different fall assessment instruments are available such as the Morse Fall Scale (Morse, 2009); use the one chosen by your health care agency. Assess both intrinsic and extrinsic factors that increase a patient's risk. Intrinsic factors include a previous history of falling, being age 65 or over, reduced vision, orthostatic hypotension, gait instability, lower limb weakness, balance problems, urinary incontinence, frequency or need for assisted toileting, use of walking aids, agitation or confusion, and the effects of medications (e.g., sedatives, hypnotics, anticonvulsants, and certain analgesics) (Deandrea et al., 2010). Extrinsic factors include those within the hospital environment. Does the placement of equipment pose barriers when a patient attempts to ambulate? Does positioning of a patient's bed allow him or her to safely reach items on a bedside table? Does a patient need assistance with ambulation? Are self-care items at the bedside and is the call light arranged for accessibility? Another area of risk includes wheelchair-related falls involving older adults and people with disabilities. Patients are at risk for falls during transfer tasks and reaching while seated in a wheelchair (Opalek, Graymire, and Redd, 2009). Finally be sure that equipment is safe to use. Collaborate with the hospital clinical engineering staff if you have any questions about equipment functions.

Your nursing history includes data about a patient's level of wellness to determine if any underlying conditions pose a further threat to safety. Patients with conditions such as osteoporosis and bleeding disorders are more at risk for injury from falls. When you believe that a patient is a fall risk, assess for a fear of falling. Signs that a person is fearful of falling include concern or worry during walking, sweating or shaking while walking, clutching people or objects while walking, and reluctance to change position or walk. Other fall risk factors to assess include a patient's activity tolerance, level of cognition, presence of painful conditions, muscle strength in extremities, balance, and vision (see Chapter 16). Consider a patient's developmental level when you analyze your data. Review the type and number of medications that a patient is taking and if the patient is undergoing any procedures that pose risks.

Older Adult Considerations. When you assess older adults, recognize the types of physical changes that increase their risk for injury (Box 28-8). Research shows that even minor stride-to-stride variations in a person's gait increase the risk of falls. These gait changes are often too small to notice during normal walking alone but rather appear in combination with an additional task (e.g., walking a dog, carrying a bag of groceries) (Wolf et al., 2012). An assessment approach used within health care facilities is the Timed Get Up and Go Test (Mathias et al., 1986). Have the older adults wear regular footwear, sit back in a comfortable chair with an armrest, and use their normal assist device (if needed). Have a watch with a second hand or a digital second display ready. On the word "GO" time the person as he or she performs the following:

1. Stands up from the arm chair
2. Stands still momentarily
3. Walks 10 feet (3 meters) (in a line)
4. Turns around
5. Walks back to chair
6. Turns around
7. Sits down

Time the effort and observe the patient for postural stability, steppage, stride length, and sway. Normally a person completes the task in less than 10 seconds; an abnormal response is more than 20 seconds.

Patient Expectations. Patients expect to be safe in health care settings and in their homes. However, there are times when their view of what is safe does not agree with that of their health care providers and standards of care. For this

BOX 28-8 CARE OF THE OLDER ADULT

Physical Assessment Findings in Older Adults That Increase the Risk for Accidents

MUSCULOSKELETAL CHANGES
- Muscle strength decreased
- Joints becoming less mobile
- Brittle bones caused by osteoporosis
- Posture changes; some kyphosis common
- Limited range of motion (ROM)
- Change in walking gait

NERVOUS SYSTEM CHANGES
- Slower voluntary or autonomic reflexes
- Decreased ability to respond to multiple stimuli
- Decreased sensitivity of touch

SENSORY CHANGES
- Decreased peripheral vision and lens accommodation
- Decreased night vision and ability to adjust to changes in light
- Development of opacity (cataracts) in lens
- Increased stimuli threshold for light touch and pain
- Impaired hearing because high-frequency tones are less perceptible

GENITOURINARY CHANGES
- Increased nocturia
- Increased occurrence of incontinence

Modified from Touhy TA, Jett K: Ebersole and Hess P: *Toward healthy aging,* ed 8, St Louis, 2012, Mosby.

reason conduct a patient-centered assessment that includes a patient's own perceptions of his or her risk factors, knowledge of how to adapt to such risks, and previous experience with accidents. Ask what a patient expects from your care. For example, ask, "How can I provide care that will make you feel safe?" or "After we walk through your home, tell me what we need to do to help you feel safe." Patients usually do not purposefully put themselves in danger. When they are uninformed or inexperienced, threats to their safety occur. Always ask patients or family members about their ideas for ways to reduce hazards in their environment.

NURSING DIAGNOSIS

Gather data from your nursing assessment and analyze clusters of defining characteristics to identify relevant nursing diagnoses. Be thorough in analyzing defining characteristics. For example, the two nursing diagnoses of *Risk for Injury* and *Risk for Falls* have similar defining characteristics. In the case of *Risk for Falls* the defining characteristics are specific to conditions that increase fall risk, whereas defining characteristics for *Risk for Injury* are broader and cover areas such as infection and malnutrition risks. Nursing diagnoses for patients with safety risks include the following:

- *Risk for Falls*
- *Impaired Home Maintenance*
- *Risk for Injury*
- *Deficient Knowledge (regarding safety risks)*
- *Risk for Poisoning*
- *Risk for Suffocation*
- *Risk for Trauma*

Include specific related or contributing factors so the diagnosis allows you to individualize your nursing care. For example, the nursing diagnosis *Impaired Home Maintenance* could be related to injury or sensory alteration (e.g., visual). An injury that affects a person's mobility leads you to select such nursing interventions as placing handrails near toilets, showers, and bathtubs or teaching the proper use of safety devices such as side rails, canes, or crutches. Visual impairment as the related factor leads you to select different interventions such as keeping the area well lit or keeping eyeglasses clean, handy, and well protected. When you do not identify the correct related factor, the use of inappropriate interventions increases a patient's risk for injury.

PLANNING

Patients who have safety risks require a nursing care plan with interventions that prevent and minimize the intrinsic and extrinsic threats to safety. Design interventions to create a safe environment and help a patient actually feel safe to interact freely within that environment. The total plan of care needs to address all aspects of patient needs and use resources of the health care team and the community when appropriate.

Goals and Outcomes. Collaborate with a patient, family members, and other members of the health care team when you plan and set goals of care. Remember to keep goals realistic, within the resources available to a patient. When you involve a patient and family in planning, they become more alert to safety risks and potential hazards. For example, in the case of Mr. Gonzales, Joani identifies the goal "Reduce patient's fall risk." Expected outcomes include "Patient removes barriers to reaching the bathroom" and "Patient improves mobility in using lower extremities." Joani discusses the goal with Mr. Gonzales and his son, suggesting that they discuss ways the patient's bedroom and bath can be made safer and consider if there is a way to get Mr. Gonzales involved in an exercise program (see Care Plan).

Setting Priorities. Prioritize a patient's nursing diagnoses and interventions that are most important in terms of risk to safety and health promotion. In some situations you need to select more than one nursing diagnosis that best represents a patient's particular needs. For example, in the case study Joani has identified the nursing diagnoses *Risk for Falls, Impaired Physical Mobility, and Fear* (Figure 28-2). She establishes risk for falls as the first priority. She focuses nursing interventions on modifying the home after completing a comprehensive home safety assessment with Mr. Gonzales and his son. They discuss together the factors within the home that pose risk for injuries and falls. Once both the patient and son understand Mr. Gonzales' health risks, Joani can focus on specific interventions for reducing Mr. Gonzales'

CARE PLAN

Risk for Falls

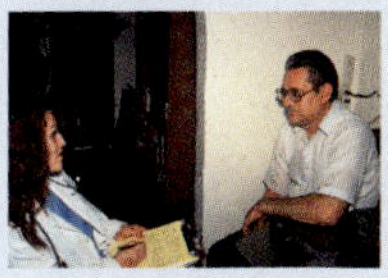

ASSESSMENT

Joani knows that people with impaired vision and mobility limitations are at increased risk for injury. She knows that she also needs to assess Mr. Gonzales' fall risks more thoroughly. When Joani meets with Mr. Gonzales, she learns that he fell in his home about 3 months ago. He expresses concern about his safety, "I'm afraid I might fall again. My knees make it harder to go upstairs." He wants to remain independent and live to a "ripe old age" but admits that his concern causes him to participate in fewer social activities. His son has talked with him about getting a cane to help him walk, but so far Mr. Gonzales has declined.

ASSESSMENT ACTIVITIES	FINDINGS/DEFINING CHARACTERISTICS*
Inspect Mr. Gonzales' home environment for safety hazards.	Joani discovers **throw rugs on the floors** near the chairs and at the bedside and **poor lighting** in the bedroom and bathroom.
Conduct a physical assessment to determine Mr. Gonzales' risk factors for falling.	Mr. Gonzales is unable to **read the labels on his medication bottles. His last visual examination was 3 years ago.** Gait assessment reveals that Mr. Gonzales **does not pick his feet up very high off the floor. He has reduced strength in his right leg. His movements are stiff and slow, especially when standing up from a chair.** Joani also learns that the patient exercises infrequently.
Joani asks Mr. Gonzales what he knows about fall risks and ways to prevent them.	Mr. Gonzales has **limited knowledge** about fall risks, except that he knows to use caution with stairs. He says that his doctor talked about things for which to watch after his fall, but **he can't recall the information.**

***Defining characteristics** are shown in **bold** type.

NURSING DIAGNOSIS: Risk for Falls

PLANNING

GOAL	EXPECTED OUTCOMES (NOC)†
	Safe Home Environment
• Mr. Gonzales' fall risk will be reduced within 2 months.	• Mr. Gonzales lists hazards in his apartment within 1 week. • Mr. Gonzales reduces modifiable hazards in his apartment by 100% within 1 month.
	Personal Safety Behavior
• Mr. Gonzales improves balance and mobility in using lower extremities.	• Mr. Gonzales will participate in a prescribed exercise program. • Mr. Gonzales will use assist device correctly.

†Outcomes classification label from Moorhead S et al, editors: *Nursing outcomes classification (NOC)*, ed 5, St Louis, 2013, Mosby.

INTERVENTIONS (NIC)‡	RATIONALE
Environmental Management: Safety	

• Review and discuss with Mr. Gonzales and his son the risks for accidents and falls. After completing a home safety checklist, recommend the following:
  • Removing throw rugs
  • Increasing lighting to a minimum of 75 watts per light
  • Installing nonslip surface in shower
  • Clearing pathways from bedroom to bathroom
	Identifying fall hazards in the home helps to prevent falls (CDC, 2012b).
	Home modification is one feature of a comprehensive program with multiple interventions that can reduce fear of falling and incidence of falls (Chase et al., 2012).

• Arrange for Mr. Gonzales to visit an ophthalmologist and get a new prescription for eyeglasses.	Reduced visual acuity is correctable. Routine eye examinations are recommended as part of a comprehensive program to reduce falls in older adults (Chase et al., 2012).
Exercise Promotion	
• Consult with Mr. Gonzales' health care provider about a physical therapy evaluation to recommend an exercise regimen for Mr. Gonzales and determine if an assist device is needed.	A progressive exercise program that focuses on moderate-to-high–intensity balance exercises appears to be effective in preventing falls (Shubert, 2011).

‡Intervention classification labels from Bulechek GM et al, editors: *Nursing interventions classification (NIC)*, ed 6, St Louis, 2013, Mosby.

Continued

CARE PLAN—cont'd

Risk for Falls

EVALUATION

NURSING ACTIONS	PATIENT RESPONSE/FINDING	ACHIEVEMENT OF OUTCOME
Visit and observe Mr. Gonzales' apartment for elimination of threats to safety.	Throw rugs have been removed or replaced with rubber-backed rugs. Lighting has been increased to 75 watts except in bedroom. Mr. Gonzales is able to identify most factors in home that increase his risk for falling.	Mr. Gonzales has reduced home hazards. Knowledge about barriers and risk factors within the apartment has improved but may need reinforcement.
Reassess motor, sensory, and cognitive status.	Mr. Gonzales has new glasses and is able to read medication bottle labels. Mr. Gonzales will start an exercise program established by physical therapist (PT) in 1 week. Mr. Gonzales is not in need of assist device as determined by PT.	Improved visual acuity. Still has reduced strength in right leg and problem with gait. Will reevaluate in 2 weeks after exercise program begins. Discontinue recommendation for assist device at this time.

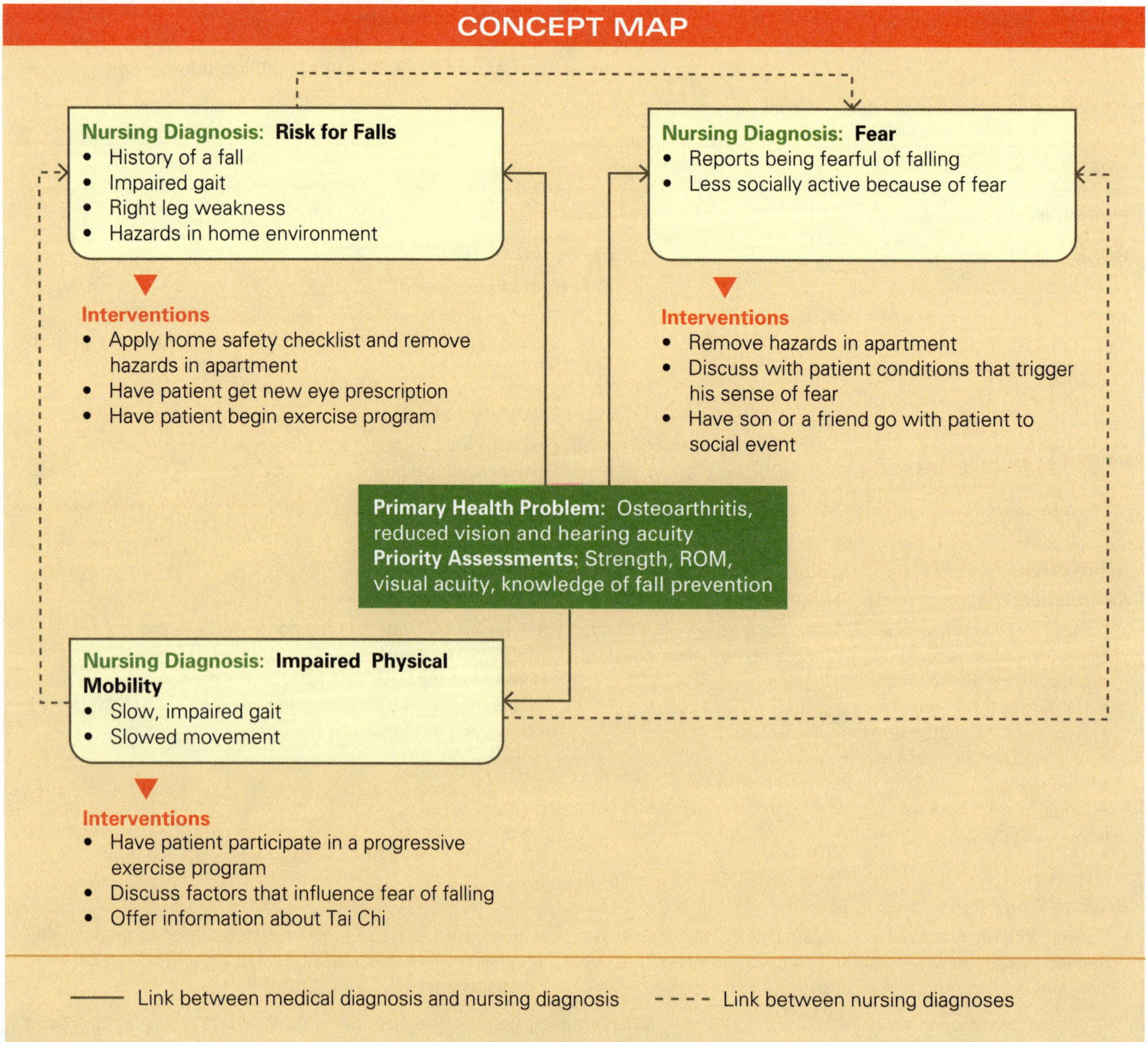

FIGURE 28-2 Concept map.

fear of falling and improving mobility to prevent falls and injuries.

Collaborative Care. It is important to collaborate with patients and other disciplines such as social work and occupational and physical therapy in planning a patient's care. Having appropriate resources within the home, being able to perform activities of daily living safely, and being able to move about with minimal risk are key factors in helping patients return to safe environments in their homes. Hospitalized patients also need to learn how to identify and select resources that are available within their community. For example, an older adult may need to go to an adult day care center during weekdays when family members are working and unable to provide regular assistance.

IMPLEMENTATION

The QSEN project outlines recommended skills to ensure nurse competency in patient safety (QSEN, 2013). These skills include those involving safe nursing practice during direct care:

- Demonstrate effective use of technology and standardized practices that support safety and quality.
- Demonstrate effective use of strategies to reduce risk of harm to self or others.
- Use appropriate strategies to reduce reliance on memory (such as forcing functions, checklists).

Direct nursing interventions toward maintaining a patient's safety in all settings. Always be safety conscious when you intervene to promote health, implement illness prevention measures, and prevent patient harm and injury.

Health Promotion. Health promotion requires a person to be in a safe environment and practice a lifestyle that minimizes risk of injury. Edelman and Mandle (2010) describe passive and active strategies aimed at health promotion. Passive strategies include public health measures and government legislative interventions (e.g., sanitation and clean water laws). Active strategies are those in which an individual is actively involved through changes in lifestyle (e.g., wearing seat belts or installing outdoor lighting along walking paths) and participation in wellness programs. As a nurse participate in health promotion activities by supporting legislation; acting as a positive role model; and recommending safety measures in the home, school, neighborhood, and workplace.

Developmental Interventions

Infant, Toddler, and Preschooler. Growing, curious children need adults to protect them from injury. Educate young parents or guardians about reducing risks of injuries to children and teach ways to promote safety in the home. Some examples are preventing access to poisonous substances; creating a safe sleeping environment; using car seats correctly; using safe, age-appropriate toys; and teaching young children safety rules (e.g., proper use of scissors, how to walk in parking lots with parents) (see Chapter 22). Children typically trust their environment and never perceive that they are in danger. Health promotion begins with well-informed parents or guardians. Educate parents about the importance of immunizations and how they protect a child from life-threatening diseases.

School-Age Child. School-age children increasingly explore their environment. They have friends outside their immediate neighborhood; and they become more active in school, church, and the community. Educate parents about the importance of children wearing seat belts whenever riding in a car; wearing helmets when riding a bicycle, skateboard, or scooter; and keeping adults informed of where they are. A child needs to know how to cross a street safely and to refrain from talking to or accepting rides or gifts from strangers. Teach children what to do if a stranger approaches and how to get help and to avoid unsafe and isolated areas.

Adolescent. Risks to an adolescent's safety involve many factors outside the home because they spend much of their time away from home and with their peer group. However, adults serve as role models for adolescents. Help them minimize safety risks by setting expectations and providing examples and education. Because adolescence is a time when sexual physical characteristics develop, adolescents often begin to have physical relationships with others. They need prompt, accurate instructions about abstinence and safe sexual practices. It is also important to educate them and their families about signs of school violence, including bullying, fighting, weapon use, gang violence, and electronic aggression (CDC, 2013b). Adolescents may benefit from developing better social skills and social problem solving with peers. When they learn to drive, they need education about complying with rules and regulations regarding safe driving and the use of a car (Box 28-9). Most schools have drivers' education programs.

Adult. Risks to young and middle-age adults frequently result from lifestyle factors such as child rearing, high-stress states, inadequate nutrition, use of firearms, and abuse of drugs or alcohol. In this fast-paced society there also appears to be more expression of anger. This anger can quickly precipitate motor vehicle collisions resulting from "road rage." Help adults understand their safety risks and guide them in making lifestyle modifications by referring them to resources such as classes to help quit smoking and for stress management and employee assistance programs. Encourage them to exercise regularly, maintain a healthy diet, practice relaxation techniques, and get adequate sleep (see Chapters 27 and 31 to 33).

Older Adult. Elimination of threats to the safety of the older adult focuses primarily on accident prevention. Advancing age and concurrent physiological changes predispose older adults to falls. Table 28-2 lists nursing interventions designed to prevent falls and compensate for the physiological changes of aging. Certain disease states common to older adults such as arthritis or strokes increase the chance of injury (Box 28-10). The effects of many medications such as sedatives, diuretics, and anticoagulants also increase the chance of injury.

BOX 28-9 PATIENT TEACHING

Safe Driving Habits

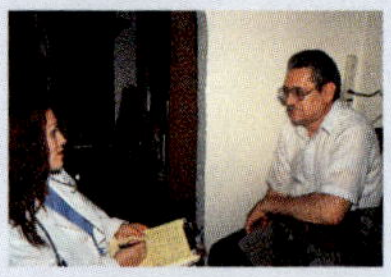

During a follow-up visit to Mr. Gonzales' apartment, Joani meets Carlos, Mr. Gonzales' son, and Carlos' son John. During the visit Carlos expresses concern to Joani about his 16-year-old son's safety while driving. Carlos wants John to learn how to drive safely, but the school has no driver's education program. He asks Joani for advice on how to keep his son safe. Joani develops the following teaching plan for Carlos and his son John.

OUTCOME

Carlos and John describe five ways to promote safe driving habits.

TEACHING STRATEGIES

- Recommend that Carlos and his son go to the CDC website "Parents are the Key" (http://www.cdc.gov/parentsarethekey) for information on teen driver safety.
- Explain the importance of using seat belts while driving and as a passenger. Include a discussion of injury rates when seat belts are not worn.
- Stress to Carlos the importance of being a role model by practicing safe driving habits.
- Encourage Carlos to provide frequent opportunities for John to practice driving in good and bad weather.
- Explain to John the safety risks associated with driving under the influence of drugs and alcohol.
- Explain the costs associated with traffic violations such as higher insurance premiums and possible loss of driver's license.
- Ask Carlos and John to form a contract regarding not driving and drinking. Instruct John never to enter an automobile when the driver has been using drugs or alcohol.

EVALUATION STRATEGIES

- Ask Carlos to identify when he will provide opportunities for John to practice driving.
- Ask John what he would do if he were drinking at a party and needed to get home.
- Ask John what will happen if he receives a traffic violation.
- Ask Carlos how he will demonstrate safe driving habits to John.
- Ask John to identify the risks of driving without a seat belt.

Provide information about neighborhood resources to help an older adult maintain an independent lifestyle. Older adults frequently relocate to new neighborhoods and must get acquainted with new resources such as modes of transportation, church schedules, and food resources (e.g., Meals on Wheels). Although retired from their jobs, older adults have a wealth of past experience to aid volunteer organizations. Some retirees even enjoy reentering the work force in a new capacity. Information about assistance resources such as daily "hello" programs, emergency services, and elder-abuse hot lines is also helpful.

BOX 28-10 CARE OF THE OLDER ADULT

Safety Education

- Because of visual impairments in older adults, teach patients to keep living areas well lighted and free of clutter, keep eyeglasses in good condition, and avoid night driving.
- Older adults have musculoskeletal changes that make movement difficult and increase the risk for falling. Teach patients to keep assistive devices in proper working order (canes, hand rails in tub and bathroom, and elevated seats) and to use nonskid strips in bathtubs.
- Advise older adults to avoid smoking in bed, lower thermostats on water heaters, avoid overloading electrical outlets, and install and maintain smoke and carbon monoxide detectors in the house.
- Driving helps older adults stay mobile and independent, yet they are more likely to have automobile accidents as a result of decreased hearing and visual acuity, altered depth perception, slowed reaction time, and poor peripheral vision. Advise them to drive only short distances and in the daylight; avoid driving in inclement weather; use side and rear view mirrors carefully; look behind them toward their blind spot before changing lanes; and keep a window rolled down to hear sirens and horns.
- Teach patients about the proper handling and storage of medications and safe methods of scheduling and taking them.
- Older adults have physiological changes that result in slower metabolism of drugs. Teach patients about drug interactions and signs and symptoms of drug toxicity to report to their health care provider.
- Some older adults suffer from irreversible dementia. Help family caregivers understand the nature of dementia. Teach them ways to match expectations with the patient's capabilities; how to incorporate earlier life skills and interests; and to provide a calm, caring, and structured environment.

Environmental Interventions. Nursing interventions directed at eliminating environmental threats include those associated with a person's basic needs and general preventive measures.

Basic Needs. Nurses contribute to a safer environment by helping patients meet their basic needs. When administering oxygen, follow the principles of medication administration and use precautions to prevent accidental fires. Contact with heat or a spark is needed to trigger combustion. When oxygen is in use, post "No Smoking" and "Oxygen in Use" signs in patients' hospital rooms and in their homes. Do not use oxygen around electrical equipment or flammable products. Store oxygen tanks upright in carts or stands to prevent tipping or falling over. Chapter 30 outlines guidelines for proper oxygen administration. If patients require oxygen in the home, a home medical provider and home health nurse educate them about safe oxygen use.

TABLE 28-2 MEASURES TO PREVENT FALLS IN OLDER ADULTS

MEASURE	RATIONALE
Home or Health Care Facility	
Stairs	
Install treads with uniform depth of 25.4-28 cm (10-11 inches) and 19-19.7 cm (7½-7¾ inches) risers (vertical face of steps).	When stairs are of uniform size, older adults do not have to continually look at the stairs and adjust their gait.
Install uniform-textured or plain-colored surfaces on each tread and mark edge of tread with contrasting color.	Uniform textures or color help to decrease vertigo. Marking edge of tread provides obvious visual clue to end of stair.
Ensure proper lighting of each tread. Block sun or light bulb glare with translucent shades or screen or use lower-wattage bulbs.	Older adults' vision is unable to adjust quickly to changes in lighting.
Ensure adequate head room so user does not have to duck to avoid hitting his or her head while going up or down the stairs.	Sudden changes in head position often result in dizziness, which increases the risk for falling.
Remove protruding objects from staircase walls.	Decreased peripheral vision prevents patient from seeing object. Moving to avoid protruding objects disrupts balance.
Maintain outdoor walkways and stairs in good condition and free of holes, cracks, and splinters.	Decreased visual acuity prevents patient from seeing any structural defect.
Handrails	
Install smooth but slip-resistant handrail at least 3.8 cm (1½ inches) from wall.	Ample distance needed to allow patient to grasp handrail firmly for support.
Secure handrail firmly to support user's weight, especially at bottom and top of stairway.	Older adults have greatest risk for falling at top and bottom of stairs because they shift their center of gravity, making balance unstable.
Install grab bars in bathroom near toilet and tub.	Enables patient to have support while rising from sitting to standing position.
Floors	
Ensure that patients wear properly fitting shoes or slippers with nonskid surface.	Reduces chances of slipping.
Secure all carpeting, mats, and tile; place nonskid backing under small rugs.	Sudden slip causes dizziness and inability to regain balance.
Place bath mats or nonskid strips on bathtub or shower stall floors.	Wet surfaces increase the risk for falling.
Secure electrical cords against baseboards.	Prevents tripping.
Health Care Facility	
Orientation	
Admit disoriented patients to a room near nurses' station.	Provides for more frequent observation by nursing staff.
Maintain close supervision of confused patients.	Confused patient often attempts to wander out of bed or room.
Show patient how to use call light at bedside and in bathroom and place within easy reach. Instruct patient to call for assistance with movement as needed.	Location and use of the call light are essential to patient safety.
Place bedside tables and over-bed tables close to the patient. Place articles within easy reach.	Prevents patient from searching or overreaching for items.
Keep bed in low position. Have patient rise from bed or chair slowly.	Prevents dizziness resulting from postural hypotension.
Leave one side rail up and one down on side where oriented and ambulatory patient gets out of bed.	Patient is able to use side rail for support when getting in and out of bed and to position self once in bed.
Transport	
Lock bed and wheelchair when transferring patient from bed to wheelchair or back to bed.	Provides stability and support during transfer.
Place side rails in up position and secure safety straps around patient on stretcher.	Prevents patient from rolling off stretcher.

Food safety requires a patient and family to understand principles of food preparation.

- Proper refrigeration, storage, and preparation of food decrease risk of foodborne illnesses. Store perishable foods in refrigerators to maintain freshness.
- Refrigerate foods at 4°C (40°F) within 2 hours of cooking.
- Thaw frozen foods in the refrigerator.
- Wash hands for at least 15 seconds before preparing food.
- Rinse fruits and vegetables thoroughly.
- Avoid cross-contamination of one food with another during preparation, especially with poultry.
- Use a separate cutting board for vegetables, meat, and poultry.
- Cook foods adequately to kill any residual organisms.
- Refrigerate leftovers promptly and label the date when leftovers are saved.

General Preventive Measures. Adequate lighting and security measures in and around a home, including the use of night-lights, exterior lighting, and locks on doors and windows, reduce a person's risk for injury from falls or crime. Local police departments and community organizations often hold safety classes on how not to become a victim of crime.

Help parents reduce the risk of accidental poisoning by teaching them to keep hazardous substances out of children's reach. Older adults are also at risk for poisoning because diminished eyesight may cause an accidental ingestion of toxic substances. When older adults have impaired memory, the accidental overdosage of prescription medications may occur. Educate patients or their family caregivers about keeping medications in original containers that are labeled in large print. Recommend the use of medication organizers that are filled once a week. Have patients keep poisonous substances out of the bathroom and properly discard old and unused medications.

To control pathogen transmission, teach patients how and when to wash hands (e.g., following toileting, before and after food preparation, before eating, and before wound care). Nurses use Standard Precautions when caring for all patients to protect themselves from contact with blood and body fluids (see Chapter 14). Patients also need to know how to dispose of infected material such as wound dressings and used needles in the home. The Environmental Protection Agency (EPA) encourages disposal of used needles by way of community drop-off programs, household hazardous waste facilities, or sharps mail-back programs or by using home needle destruction devices (Coalition for Safe Community Needle Disposal, 2010). Encourage patients to contact neighborhood community governments for guidelines on waste disposal methods.

Acute Care. Nurses implement specific interventions to ensure patient safety in acute care settings. You are responsible for making a patient's hospital room safe. Explain and demonstrate to patients how to use a call light or intercom system. Always place a call device close to a patient at the conclusion of any care activity. Respond quickly to call lights and bed/chair alarms so patients do not attempt to get up on their own. Many falls occur as patients try to get out of bed unassisted. Keep the environment around the bedside free from clutter. Also be prepared to conduct hourly rounds, a practice that many health care organizations have adopted. During rounding address toileting, turning, pain control, and hydration.

Falls. Patient-centered care is important, with nurses making patients their partners in recognizing fall risks and then taking preventive action. Fall prevention strategies must be targeted to specific patient risks. For example, if a patient has postural hypotension, a nurse chooses a low bed and has the patient dangle the legs for 5 minutes on the side of the bed before trying to ambulate. Or a nurse gives a patient with a history of urinary incontinence a bedside commode to use. Remember, patient situations change. Prevention of falls and fall-related injuries requires diligent ongoing nursing assessment and engagement of the entire health care team in the implementation of patient-specific interventions (Degelau et al., 2012). TJC has a "Speak up" campaign created for patients to follow in the home and hospital (TJC, 2013a). It offers tips and actions to help people reduce their risk of falling, whether at home or in a medical facility.

In health care settings color-coded wristbands are used to help communicate a patient's safety risk. In 2008 the American Hospital Association (AHA) issued a recommendation that hospitals standardize wristband colors: red for patient allergies, yellow for fall risk, and purple for do-not-resuscitate preferences. This recommendation came after a near-miss incident in which a nurse, working in two different hospitals, placed a wrong-colored band on a patient. Many state hospital associations and communities are now standardizing colors to reduce confusion both within and across health care organizations (AHA, 2008).

Modifying a patient's environment reduces fall risks. For example, a patient who is morbidly obese needs a bed, wheelchair, or commode specifically designed to support the additional weight. A patient with impaired mobility benefits from organizing the home so it becomes unnecessary to walk up or down stairs. In a health care facility use a gait belt for patients needing assistance to transfer or ambulate. Remove excess furniture and equipment and make sure that patients wear rubber-soled shoes or slippers to walk or during transfer. Use additional safety equipment and safe handling techniques when moving and positioning patients (see Chapter 36). Also provide a clear path to the bathroom and keep rooms well lit to promote safe ambulation. Inspect canes, walkers, and crutches to be sure that rubber tips are intact and connections are tight and that the assistive devices are at the appropriate height for the patient. Additional devices to use at a patient's bedside include a low bed, bedside commode, nonskid floor mat, and overhead trapeze (Figure 28-3).

Restraints. Patients who are confused or disoriented or who repeatedly fall or try to remove medical devices (e.g., IV lines or dressings) may require the temporary use of restraints

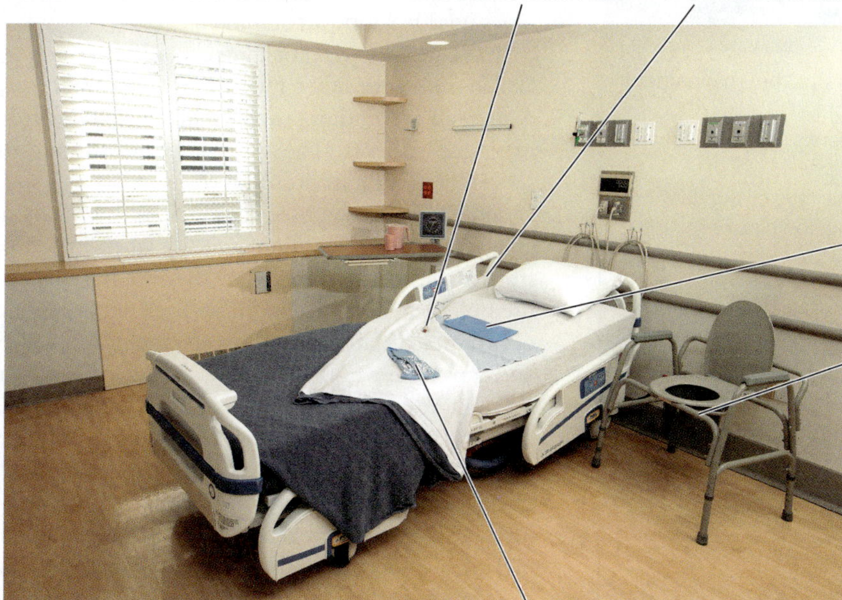

FIGURE 28-3 Safe patient room environment.

to keep them safe. Restraints are not a solution to a patient problem but rather a temporary means to maintain patient safety. All alternatives must be used before placing patients in restraints. Federal and state laws prohibit Medicare- and Medicaid-certified nursing homes from using restraints unless they are medically needed. **Chemical restraints** are medications such as anxiolytics and sedatives used to manage a patient's behavior and are not a standard treatment for a patient's condition. A physical **restraint** is any manual method, physical or mechanical device, material, or equipment that immobilizes or reduces the ability of a patient to move arms, legs, body, or head freely. A restraint does not include devices such as orthopedically prescribed devices, protective helmets, or methods that involve physically holding a patient to conduct an examination or test, protecting a patient from falling out of bed, or permitting a patient to participate in activities without the risk of physical harm (TJC, 2011).

The use of restraints is associated with serious complications resulting from immobilization such as pressure ulcers, pneumonia, constipation, and incontinence. In some cases death has resulted because of restricted breathing and circulation. Patients have been strangled while trying to get out of bed while restrained in a jacket or vest restraint. As a result, many health care facilities have eliminated the use of the jacket (vest) restraint (Capezuti et al., 2008). For this reason this text does not describe the use of the vest restraint. Loss of self-esteem, humiliation, and agitation are also serious concerns. Because of these risks, legislation emphasizes reducing the use of restraints. Regulatory agencies such as TJC and CMS enforce standards for the safe use of restraint devices. A restraint-free environment, either physical or chemical, is your first goal for all patients. Always try alternatives before using restraints (Box 28-11).

For patients who continue to try to ambulate without assistance, use low beds and electronic bed and chair alarm devices. Specially designed low beds reduce the distance from the edge of a mattress to the floor, making it easier for a person to get out of bed, and lower the distance to the floor. Use a low bed with an adjacent mat on the floor. Alarm devices warn nursing staff that a patient is attempting to leave a bed or chair unassisted. There are a variety of types, including a device with a knee band that sounds an alarm when the patient reaches a near-vertical position. An infrared type of alarm is affixed to a headboard or bed frame, allowing a patient to move freely within a bed. If a patient tries to leave the bed, the infrared beam detects motion and sends out an alarm tone. Other safety devices include pressure-sensitive strips placed beneath a patient under the buttocks or a tether alarm that is clipped to a patient's gown. Alarm devices help avoid physical restraints and, when responded to immediately, prevent a patient fall.

When restraints are required to protect a patient or others, involve the patient and family in the decision to use them. Help them adapt to this change by explaining the purpose of the restraint, expected care while the patient is in restraints, and that the restraint is temporary and protective. It is a requirement for nursing homes to obtain informed consent from family members before using restraints.

For legal purposes know agency-specific policies and procedures for appropriate use and monitoring of restraints. The use of a restraint must be clinically justified and part of a patient's prescribed medical treatment and plan of care. A physician's order is required, based on a face-to-face

BOX 28-11 ALTERNATIVES TO RESTRAINTS

- Orient patients and family members to the environment; explain all procedures and treatments.
- Provide companionship and supervision; use trained sitters; adjust staffing and involve family.
- Offer diversionary activities such as music, puzzles, crocheting, activity aprons, and folding towels. Enlist ideas and support from family.
- Assign confused or disoriented patients to rooms near nurses' stations and observe them frequently.
- Use calm, simple statements and physical cues as needed.
- Use de-escalation, time-out, and other verbal intervention techniques when managing aggressive behaviors.
- Provide appropriate visual and auditory stimuli (e.g., family pictures, clock, calendar).
- Remove cues that promote leaving the room (e.g., close doors to block view of stairs, do not wear street clothes).
- Promote relaxation techniques and normal sleep patterns.
- Institute exercise and ambulation schedules as allowed by patient's condition; consult physical therapy for mobility and exercise program.
- Attend frequently to needs for toileting, food and liquid, and pain management.
- Camouflage intravenous lines with clothing, stockinette, or Kling dressing.
- Evaluate all medications and ensure timely and effective pain management.
- Eliminate bothersome treatments as soon as possible. For example, discontinue tube feedings and begin oral feedings as quickly as a patient's condition allows.
- Use protective devices such as hip pads, helmet, skid-proof slippers, and nonskid strips near bed.

assessment of a patient. The order must be current, stating the type and location of the restraint, and specify the duration and circumstances under which it will be used. The orders need to be renewed within a specific time frame according to agency policy. In hospitals each original restraint order and renewal is limited to 4 hours for adults, 2 hours for ages 9 through 17, and 1 hour for children under 9 (CMS, 2013; TJC, 2011). Orders may be renewed to the time limits for a maximum of 24 consecutive hours. Restraints are not to be ordered PRN (as needed). Always make ongoing assessments of patients who are restrained. Properly document the behaviors that led to application of restraints, the procedure used in restraining, the condition of the body part restrained (e.g., color and pulse of extremity), and the evaluation of the patient response. Always remove a restraint periodically and assess if it continues to be necessary. Follow specific guidelines when using physical restraints (see Skill 28-1). The use of restraints must meet one of the following objectives:

1. Reduce the risk for patient injury from falls
2. Prevent interruption of therapy such as traction, IV infusions, nasogastric tube feeding, or Foley catheter
3. Prevent the confused or combative patient from removing life support equipment
4. Reduce the risk for injury to self or others

Collaborate with other members of the health care team to design fall prevention programs and a restraint-free environment for patients. The goal is to discontinue the use of restraints as soon as possible.

Side Rails. When used correctly, side rails help to increase a patient's mobility and/or stability when in bed or moving from a bed to chair. However, they are the most commonly used physical restraint and have been shown to increase the occurrence of falls when patients attempt to get out of bed and crawl over a rail. There are a variety of beds with different side-rail designs. Basically a patient needs to have a route to exit a bed safely and maneuver freely within the bed; in this case side rails are not considered a restraint. For example, raising only the two side rails at the top of the bed so the lower part of the bed is open gives a patient room to exit a bed safely. Side rails used to prevent a patient such as one who is sedated from falling out of bed are not considered a restraint. Always know agency policy about the use of side rails. Be sure that a bed is in the lowest position possible when side rails are raised. Always assess the risk of using side rails compared to not using them. Check their condition; bars between the bedrails need to be spaced close together to prevent entrapment. A potential exists for trapping a person's head and body in gaps and openings between the bed frame and mattress.

The use of side rails alone for a disoriented patient often causes more confusion and further injury. Frequently a confused patient or one determined to get out of bed because of pain, toileting needs, or anxiety tries to climb over a side rail or out at the foot of the bed. Either attempt often results in a fall. To reduce a patient's confusion, focus your interventions first on the cause such as a response to a new medication, dehydration, or pain. Frequently nurses mistake a patient's attempt to explore his or her environment or to self-toilet as confusion. Use of a low bed reduces the distance between the bed and floor, facilitating a roll rather than a fall from the bed. If all efforts to reduce confusion or restlessness fail and the patient is at risk for serious injury to self or others, a restraint is sometimes necessary. A less-restrictive restraint for the cognitively impaired is the Posey Bed Canopy. The canopy is a bed enclosure that allows a patient freedom of movement within a protected environment. However, remember that the goal is to remove the restraint at the earliest possible time.

Fires. Although smoking is usually not allowed in health care settings, smoking-related fires continue to pose a significant risk because of unauthorized smoking in beds or bathrooms. Institutional fires typically result from an electrical or anesthetic-related fire. The best intervention is to prevent fires. Nursing measures include complying with the smoking policies of an agency and keeping combustible materials away from heat sources. Box 28-12 highlights fire intervention guidelines in health care agencies. Regardless of where a fire occurs, always have an evacuation plan in place. Know where

BOX 28-12 FIRE INTERVENTION GUIDELINES IN HEALTH CARE AGENCIES

- Keep the phone number for reporting fires visible on the telephone at all times.
- Know the fire drill and evaluation plan of an agency.
- Know the location of all fire alarms, exits, extinguishers, and oxygen shut-off.
- Use the mnemonic RACE to set priorities in case of fire
  R—Rescue and remove all patients in immediate danger.
  A—Activate the alarm. Always do this before trying to extinguish even a minor fire.
  C—Confine a fire by closing doors and windows and turning off oxygen and electrical equipment.
  E—Extinguish a fire with an appropriate extinguisher.

fire extinguishers and gas shut-off valves are located and how to activate a fire alarm.

Some health care agencies have fire doors that are held open by magnets and close automatically when a fire alarm sounds. It is important to keep equipment away from blocking these doors. All personnel evacuate patients when appropriate. Patients who are close to the fire, regardless of its size, are at risk of injury and need to be moved to another area. If a patient requires oxygen but not life support, discontinue the oxygen, which is combustible and will fuel an existing fire. If the patient is on life support, maintain the patient's respiratory status manually with a bag-valve mask (e.g., Ambu-bag) (see Chapter 30) until you move the patient away from the fire. Direct ambulatory patients to walk by themselves to a safe area or have them help move patients in wheelchairs. Move bedridden patients from the scene by a stretcher, their bed, or a wheelchair or have one or two rescuers carry them. If you have to carry a patient, do so correctly (e.g., two-man carry). Another two-rescuer technique is the chair carry, in which the victim is seated in a chair and both rescuers carry the chair. If you must carry a patient, be careful not to overextend your physical limits for lifting because an injury to you results in further injury to the patient. If fire department personnel are on the scene, they help to evacuate patients.

After a fire has been reported and patients are out of danger, you and other personnel need to take measures to contain or put out the fire such as closing doors and windows, turning off oxygen and electrical equipment, and using a fire extinguisher. There are three types of extinguishers based on causes of fires: paper and rubbish (type A), grease and anesthetic gas (type B), and electrical (type C). There is also a multipurpose extinguisher (ABC) to use for all types of fires. To use an extinguisher correctly follow these steps: remember the word **PASS:**

- **P**ull the pin. Hold the extinguisher with the nozzle pointing away from you and release the locking mechanism.
- **A**im low. Point the extinguisher at the base of the fire.
- **S**queeze the lever slowly and evenly.
- **S**weep the nozzle from side to side.

Electrical Accidents. Electrical equipment used in health care settings is usually inspected and maintained regularly. The clinical engineering departments of hospitals inspect biomedical equipment such as beds, IV infusion pumps, and ventilators. You know that a piece of equipment is safe to use when you see a safety inspection sticker with an expiration date. Decrease the risk for electrical injury and fire by using properly grounded and functional equipment. The ground prong in an electrical outlet carries any stray electrical current back to the ground. Remove equipment that is not in proper working order or that sparks when plugged in or is out of service and notify appropriate hospital staff.

Radiation. Radiation is a health hazard in health care settings where radiation and radioactive materials are used in the diagnosis and treatment of patients. Hospitals have strict guidelines concerning the care of patients who are receiving radiation and radioactive materials. Know the agency established protocols. To reduce your exposure to radiation, limit the time spent near the source, make the distance from the source as great as possible, and use shielding devices such as lead aprons. Staff who work near radiation must wear devices that track the accumulative exposure to radiation.

Disasters. As a nurse be prepared to respond to and care for a sudden influx of patients during a disaster. TJC (2013b) requires hospitals to have an emergency-management plan that addresses identifying possible emergency situations and their probable impact, maintaining an adequate amount of supplies, and having a formal response plan. The plan must include actions to be taken by staff and steps to restore essential services and resume normal operations following an emergency. Infection control practices are critical in the event of a biological attack. You must manage all patients with suspected or confirmed bioterrorism-related illnesses with Standard Precautions (see Chapter 14). Additional precautions such as airborne or contact isolation precautions are needed for diseases such as smallpox and pneumonic plague. Most infections associated with biological agents are not transmissible from patient to patient. However, limit the transport and movement of patients only to movement that is essential for treatment.

EVALUATION

Patient Care. Evaluate your nursing interventions for reducing threats to safety by comparing the patient's response to the expected outcomes for each goal of care. This requires you to reassess a patient's condition to measure actual responses. When the expected outcomes are not achieved, revise your interventions. It is also possible that new nursing diagnoses have developed. Apply evaluative measures (reassessments) to determine a patient's progress toward outcomes and goals. An example of a goal, outcome, and evaluative measure includes the goal "Patient's environment will be adapted to his motor and sensory developmental needs." A possible outcome for this goal is "Modifiable hazards in the home are reduced by 100% within 2 weeks." Your evaluative measures would include "Observe environment for elimination of threats to safety" and "Reassess motor and sensory status for appropriate environmental modifications." Evaluate a patient's outcomes by comparing what you planned with what resulted and evaluate how well you implemented the plan (Box 28-13). Examine the planned interventions for appropriateness and effectiveness in each situation. By accomplishing goals and outcomes you validate effective care.

Patient Expectations. Patient-centered care requires a thorough evaluation of a patient's perspective related to safety and whether his or her expectations have been met. Expectations as a result of care include restoration of health, reduction in fall risks, a safer home environment, and improved recognition of safety risks. Patients are often unaware of the dangers in their homes and workplaces. Many make the needed adjustments to keep themselves and loved ones safe and injury free once you identify the dangers. Ask a patient questions such as, "Are you satisfied with the changes made to your home?" "Do you feel safer as a result of changes we made?" "Are you still afraid of falling?" Involve the family in the evaluation, especially if they live with the patient and provide assistance in the home.

BOX 28-13 EVALUATION

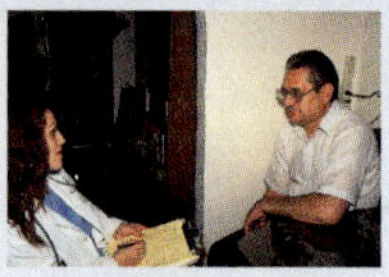

It has been 2 weeks since Joani implemented Mr. Gonzales' plan of care. She recommended modifications after conducting the home safety checklist. Mr. Gonzales' son helped to remove throw rugs in his father's home and adjust lighting. He plans to install a nonslip surface in the shower next week. With a new pair of glasses and after attending two sessions of a recommended exercise program, Mr. Gonzales is beginning to sense that his walking is improving. He tells Joani, "I feel a bit more relaxed moving around. I'm not as hesitant."

DOCUMENTATION NOTE

"Mr. Gonzales' home has improved lighting and fewer obstacles along walking path. He verbalizes benefit from his exercise program and is exercising on his own by walking twice a day. He states that he is less 'hesitant' to move about. No report of injury."

SAFETY GUIDELINES FOR NURSING SKILLS

Ensuring patient safety is an essential role of a professional nurse. To ensure patient safety, communicate clearly with members of the health care team, assess the patient's risks, incorporate priorities of care and preferences, and use the best evidence when making decisions about your patient's care. When performing the skill in this chapter, remember the following points to ensure safe, individualized patient care.

- Always attempt restraint alternatives (see Box 28-11) before using a restraint.
- If a restraint is needed, always use the least restrictive device.
- Because restraints limit a patient's ability to move freely, make clinical judgments appropriate to the patient's condition and agency policy.

SKILL 28-1 APPLYING PHYSICAL RESTRAINTS

View Video!

DELEGATION CONSIDERATIONS

The skill of applying a restraint can be delegated to trained nursing assistive personnel (NAP). However, the nurse is responsible for assessment of a patient's behavior, level of orientation, need for restraints, and appropriate type to use. The assessment while a restraint is in place cannot be delegated to NAP. The nurse directs the NAP by:

- Reviewing correct placement of the restraint.
- Reviewing when and how to change patient's position.
- Instructing NAP to notify nurse if there is a change in skin integrity, circulation of extremities, or patient breathing.
- Instructing to provide range of motion, nutrition and hydration, skin care, toileting, and opportunities for socialization.

EQUIPMENT

- Proper restraint
- Padding (if needed)

STEP	RATIONALE
ASSESSMENT	
1. Assess patient's behavior such as confusion, disorientation, agitation, restlessness, combativeness, repeated removal of therapies, creating a risk to other patients, and inability to follow directions.	If patient's behavior continues despite treatment or restraint alternatives, use of restraint is indicated. Use the least restrictive type of restraint.

STEP	RATIONALE
2. Determine if restraint alternatives fail. Review agency policies regarding restraints. Check health care provider's order for purpose and type of restraint, location, and duration of restraint. Consult attending physician as soon as possible if he or she did not write the original order. Determine if you need a signed consent for use of a restraint.	An authorized physician or licensed independent practitioner who is responsible for a patient's care must order the restraint. Unless state law is more restrictive, orders for the use of restraints for the management of violent or self-destructive behavior that jeopardize the immediate physical safety of a patient, staff, or others are renewed every 4 hours (for adults); 2 hours (for children ages 9 through 17); and 1 hour (for children under age 9). Orders are renewed to the time limits for a maximum of 24 consecutive hours (CMS, 2013; TJC, 2011).

Clinical Decision Point: **A physician or other licensed independent practitioner responsible for the care of a patient evaluates the patient in person within 1 hour of the initiation of restraint use for the management of violent or self-destructive behavior that jeopardizes the physical safety of the patient, staff, or others. A registered nurse or physician assistant may conduct the in-person evaluation if trained in accordance with the requirements and consultations with the primary health care provider after the evaluation as determined by hospital policy (TJC, 2011).**

STEP	RATIONALE
3. Review manufacturer instructions for restraint application before entering patient's room. Determine most appropriate size restraint.	Be familiar with all devices used for patient care and protection. Incorrect application of restraint device could result in patient injury or death.
PLANNING	
1. Perform hand hygiene and collect appropriate equipment.	Reduces transmission of microorganisms and promotes organization.
2. Approach patient in calm, confident manner and explain what you plan to do. Provide privacy.	Reduces patient anxiety and promotes cooperation.
3. Identify patient using two identifiers (e.g., name and birthday or name and account number) according to agency policy.	Ensures correct patient. Complies with The Joint Commission requirements for patient safety (TJC, 2014).
4. Introduce self to patient and family and assess their feelings about restraint use. Explain that restraint is temporary and designed to protect patient from injury.	Informs patient and family about use of restraint. In nursing homes informed consent is mandatory.
IMPLEMENTATION	
1. Adjust bed to proper height and lower side rail on side of patient contact.	Allows you to use proper body mechanics and prevents injury during application.
2. Be sure that patient is comfortable and in correct anatomical alignment. Inspect area where restraint will be placed. Assess condition of skin, sensation, adequacy of circulation, and range of motion.	Positioning prevents contractures and neurovascular impairment. Sometimes restraints compress and interfere with functioning of devices or tubes. Assessment provides baseline to monitor patient's condition.
3. Pad skin and bony prominences (if necessary) that will be under restraint.	Reduces friction and pressure from restraint to skin and underlying tissue.
4. Apply proper-size restraint. NOTE: Always refer to manufacturer directions.	
a. **Belt restraint:** Have patient in sitting position. Apply belt over clothes, gown, or pajamas. Make sure that you place restraint at waist, not chest or abdomen. Remove wrinkles or creases in clothing. Bring ties through slots in belt. Help patient lie down if in bed. Avoid applying belt too tightly (see illustrations).	Restrains center of gravity and prevents patient from rolling off stretcher, sitting up while on stretcher, or falling out of bed. Tight application interferes with breathing.
b. **Extremity (ankle or wrist) restraint:** Restraint designed to immobilize one or all extremities. Commercially available limb restraints are made of sheepskin with foam padding. Wrap limb restraint around wrist or ankle with soft part toward skin and secure snugly (not tightly) in place by Velcro straps or buckle.	Maintains immobilization of extremity to protect patient from injury from fall or accidental removal of therapeutic device (e.g., intravenous [IV] tube, urinary catheter). Tight application interferes with circulation.

Clinical Decision Point: **Patient with wrist and ankle restraints is at risk for aspiration if placed in flat, supine position. Place patient in lateral position rather than supine or keep head of bed elevated at least 30 degrees.**

SKILL 28-1 APPLYING PHYSICAL RESTRAINTS—cont'd

STEP	RATIONALE
c. **Mitten restraint:** Thumbless mitten device that restrains patient's hands (see illustration). Place hand in mitten, being sure that Velcro strap is around wrist and not forearm.	Prevents patients from dislodging invasive equipment, removing dressings, or scratching, yet allows greater movement than wrist restraint.
d. **Elbow restraint (freedom splint)**: Restraint consists of rigidly padded fabric that wraps around arm. It is closed with Velcro. Upper end has clamp that hooks to sleeve of patient's gown or shirt. Insert patient's arm so elbow joint rests against padded area, keeping joint rigid (see illustration).	Commonly used with infants and children to prevent elbow flexion (e.g., with IV lines). May also be used for adults. Keeps elbow joint rigid.
e. **For all splints:** Insert two fingers under secured restraint (see illustration) to be sure that it is not too tight.	Tight application interferes with circulation and potentially causes neurovascular injury.
5. Attach restraint straps to portion of bed frame that moves when raising or lowering head of bed (see illustrations). **Do not attach to side rails.** Attach restraint to chair frame for patient in chair or wheelchair, being sure that tie is out of reach.	Patient will be injured if you secure restraint to a side rail and it is lowered.
6. Secure restraint with quick-release buckle (see illustrations) or adjustable seat belt–like locking device. *Do not tie in knot.*	Allows for quick release in an emergency.

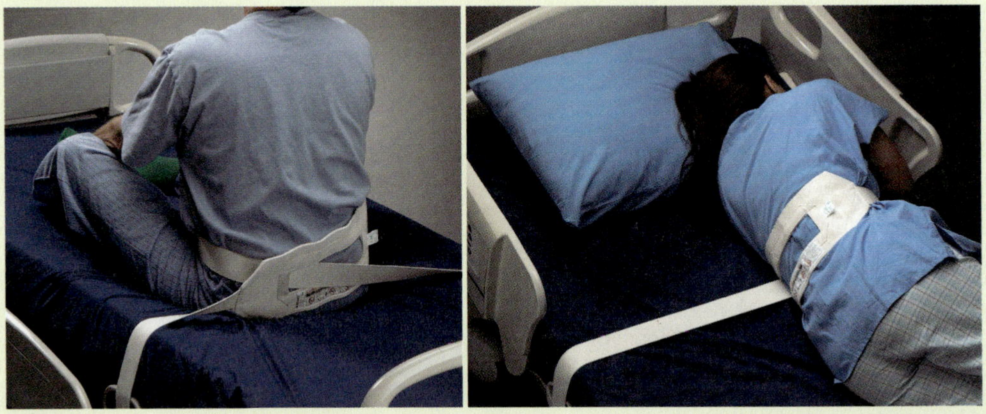

STEP 4a *Left,* Apply belt restraint with patient sitting. *Right,* Properly applied belt restraint allows patient to turn in bed. (Courtesy Posey Company, Arcadia, CA.)

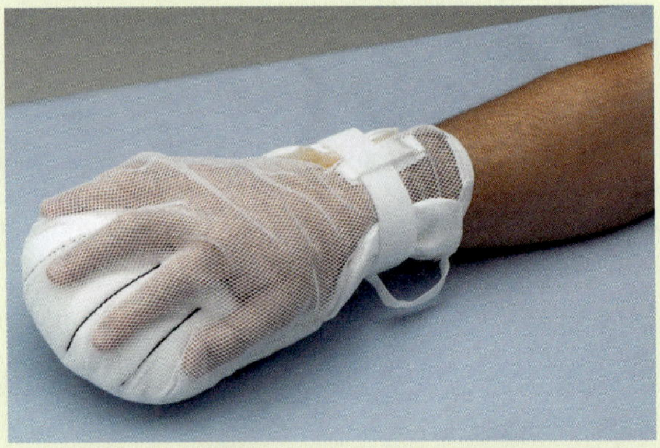

STEP 4c Mitten restraint. (Courtesy Posey Company, Arcadia, CA.)

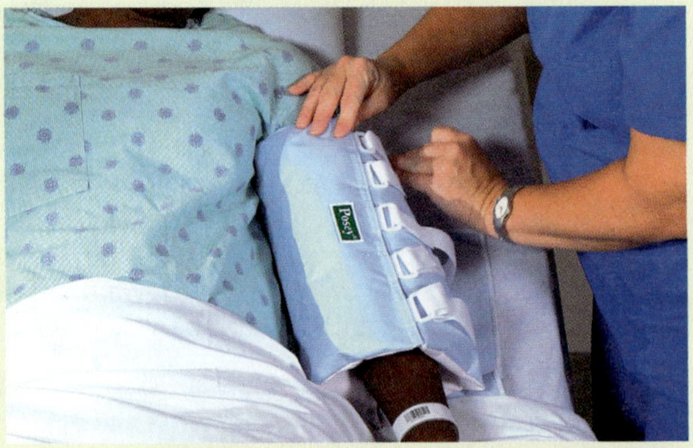

STEP 4d Freedom elbow restraint.

STEP	RATIONALE
7. Double check and insert two fingers under secured restraint. Assess proper placement of restraint, skin integrity, pulses, skin temperature and color, and sensation of restrained body part.	Provides baseline to later evaluate if injury develops from restraint placement.
8. Remove restraints **at least every 2 hours** (TJC, 2013b) or more frequently as determined by agency policy. If patient is violent or noncompliant, remove one restraint at a time and/or have staff assistance while removing restraints.	Removal provides opportunity to change patient's position, offer nutrients, perform full range of motion (ROM), assist with toileting and exercise, and assess condition of site and need for continuation.

Clinical Decision Point: **Do not leave violent or aggressive patients unattended while restraints are off.**

STEP	RATIONALE
9. Secure call light or intercom system within reach.	Allows patient, family, or caregiver to obtain assistance quickly.
10. Provide food and/or fluids and help with toileting and other activities as needed.	Ensures that basic needs are met when patient is unable to move about freely.
11. Leave bed with wheels locked. Make sure that bed is in the lowest position.	Locked wheels prevent bed from moving if patient attempts to get out. If patient falls when bed is in lowest position, this reduces chances of injury.
12. Perform hand hygiene.	Reduces transmission of microorganisms.

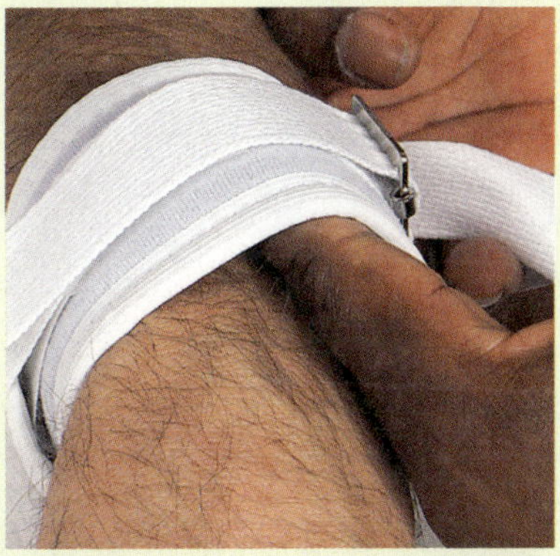

STEP 4e Insert two fingers under restraint to check for constriction.

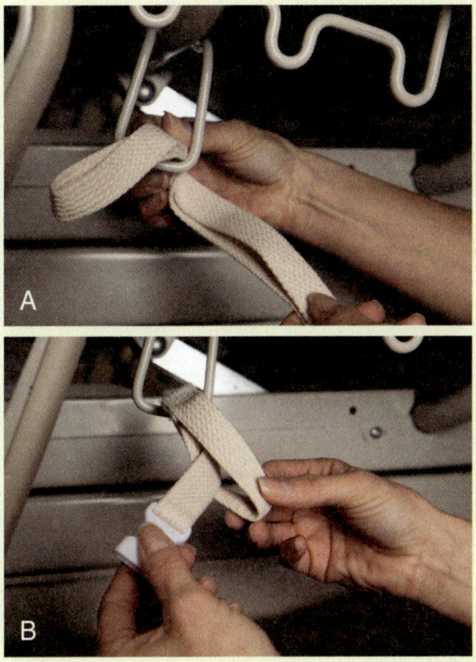

STEP 5 Attaching restraint to bed frame.

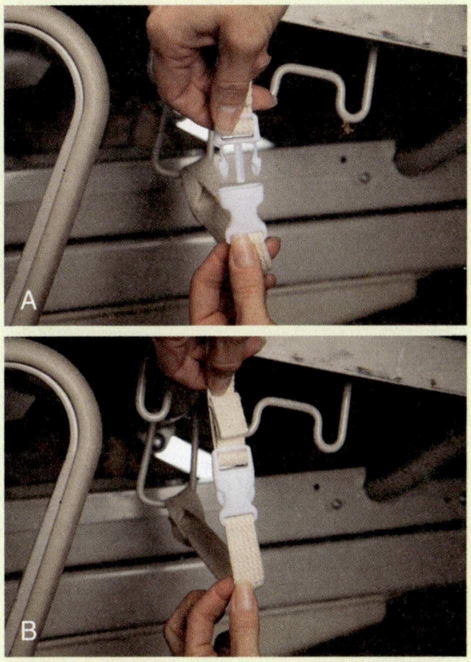

STEP 6 Connecting the quick-release buckle.

SKILL 28-1 APPLYING PHYSICAL RESTRAINTS—cont'd

STEP	RATIONALE
EVALUATION	
1. Monitor patient's condition according to facility policy. Use judgment and consider patient's condition and type of restraint when selecting physical assessment measures (e.g., circulation, nutrition and hydration, ROM in extremities, vital signs, hygiene and elimination, physical and psychological status, readiness for discontinuation). Perform visual checks if patient is too agitated to approach (TJC, 2013b).	Frequent evaluation prevents injury to patient and promotes removal of restraint at earliest possible time. Frequency of monitoring guides staff in determining appropriate intervals for evaluation based on patient's needs and condition, type of restraint used, and risks associated with use of chosen intervention.
2. Physician, licensed independent practitioner (LIP), or registered nurse trained according to CMS requirements (2007) needs to evaluate patient within either 1 or 4 hours after initiation of restraint, depending on hospital Medicare status (see agency policy).	Determines patient's immediate situation, reaction to restraints, medical and behavioral condition, and need to continue or terminate restraints (CMS, 2007).
3. After 24 hours, before writing a new order, a physician or LIP who is responsible for patient's care must see and evaluate patient.	Ensures that restraint application continues to be medically appropriate.
4. Observe IV catheters, urinary catheters, and drainage tubes to determine that you positioned them correctly.	Reinsertion is uncomfortable and increases risk for infection or interruption of therapy.
5. Use Teach Back—To determine patient's or family's understanding about restraints. State, "I want to be sure I explained how these restraints protect you from pulling out your urinary catheter. Can you explain to me why this restraint protects you?" Revise your instruction now or develop plan for revised patient teaching to be implemented at an appropriate time if patient is not able to teach back correctly.	Evaluates what the patient or family is able to explain.

RECORDING AND REPORTING

- Record patient behaviors before you applied restraints.
- Record restraint alternatives that you attempted and patient's response.
- Record patient's level of orientation and patient's or family's understanding of purpose of restraint and consent (when needed).
- Document your evaluation of patient's and family's learning.
- Record type and location of the restraint; time applied; times when assessments and releases are performed; and findings from the assessments concerning orientation, oxygenation, skin integrity, circulation, ROM, and positioning.
- Record patient's behavior and expected or unexpected outcomes after you applied the restraint.
- Record patient's response when you removed restraints (e.g., calm, cooperative).
- Report to charge nurse or health care provider if patient interrupts therapy or develops skin breakdown or other injury from restraint.

UNEXPECTED OUTCOMES AND RELATED INTERVENTIONS

- Patient experiences impaired skin integrity.
  - Reassess need for continued use of restraint and if alternatives can be used. If restraint is necessary, make sure that you apply it correctly and provide adequate padding.
  - Check skin under restraint for abrasions and remove restraints more frequently.
  - Provide appropriate skin/wound care (see Chapter 37).
  - Change wet or soiled restraints.
- Patient becomes more confused and agitated after you apply restraints.
  - Determine cause of the behavior and eliminate it if possible.
  - Determine need for more or less sensory stimulation.
  - Reorient as needed and/or attempt other restraint alternatives.
- Patient has altered neurovascular status of an extremity.
  - Remove restraint immediately, stay with patient, and notify health care provider.
  - Protect extremity from further injury.
- Patient releases restraint and suffers a fall or other injury.
  - Attend to patient's immediate physical needs.
  - Notify health care provider and reassess type of restraint and correct application.

KEY POINTS

- A culture of safety requires a commitment that acknowledges the high-risk nature of the activities of an organization, the determination to achieve consistently safe operations, a blame-free environment, and an organizational commitment to resources.
- Vulnerable groups that require help in achieving a safe environment include infants, children, older adults, the ill or injured, the physically and mentally disabled, the illiterate, and the poor.
- Your role as a nurse is to educate patients about common safety hazards and how to prevent injury while placing emphasis on hazards to which patients are more vulnerable.
- In the community a safe environment means that basic needs are achievable, physical hazards are reduced, transmission of pathogens and parasites is reduced, pollution is controlled, and sanitation is maintained.
- Caring for patients requires assessment of safety risks based on their developmental stage.
- Threats to an adult's safety are frequently associated with lifestyle habits.
- The physiological changes associated with aging, effects of multiple medications, psychological factors, and acute or chronic disease increase an older adult's risk for falls and other types of accidents.
- Risks to patient safety within a health care agency include falls and patient-inherent, procedure-related, and equipment-related accidents.
- Common risk factors for falls in hospital settings are broken down into two categories: intrinsic and extrinsic.
- Nurses are responsible for making patients' hospital rooms safe.
- Restraints are not a solution to a patient problem. All alternatives must be used before placing patients in restraints.
- A medical order for a restraint must be current, stating the type and location of restraint, and specify the duration and circumstances under which it will be used.
- Side rails are the most commonly used physical restraint and have been shown to increase the occurrence of falls when patients attempt to get out of bed and crawl over a rail.
- Continually evaluate the nursing care plan to promote safety to identify new or continued risks to a patient.

CLINICAL DECISION-MAKING EXERCISES

Mr. Gonzales' son makes arrangements to be at his father's home when Joani comes to visit 1 month later. Joani notices that there is clutter in Mr. Gonzales' living room, the area where he spends most of his time. The son tells Joani that he did not think it was a problem to let his dad decide how to arrange the room, especially since he now has new glasses.

1. How should Joani respond to the son's comments?
2. Mr. Gonzales tells Joani that he continues to feel more relaxed when he walks around the home since he started his new exercise program. Joani knows that it is important to reduce a patient's fear of falling. Why is reducing the fear of falling important, and which other steps can Joani take to reduce Mr. Gonzales' fear?
3. When Joani evaluates her plan of care for Mr. Gonzales, she finds that he is not able to identify all risk factors in his home environment. What approaches might she use to improve Mr. Gonzales ongoing knowledge?

evolve

Answers to Clinical Decision-Making Exercises can be found on the Evolve website.

QSEN ACTIVITY: INFORMATICS

Joani makes an appointment to visit with Mr. Gonzales and his son. As she completes her safety assessment of Mr. Gonzales' apartment, his son states, "I'm really worried that my dad will fall in his apartment. Since he lives alone, I'm afraid that, if he does fall, it could be hours or days before anyone finds him. We were thinking about getting some type of home safety device that my dad could use in his apartment to allow him to communicate to someone that he needs help. Do you know much about them?"

How should Joani respond? Conduct an Internet search to investigate home medical alert systems. What are the benefits of having a home medical alert system? How does this technology improve communication between a patient and a responder?

evolve

Answers to QSEN Activities can be found on the Evolve website.

REVIEW QUESTIONS

1. A nurse discovers an electrical fire in a patient's room. Which action should the nurse take first?
   1. Turn off the oxygen to the unit
   2. Evacuate any patients/visitors in immediate danger
   3. Close all doors and windows
   4. Use the nearest fire extinguisher to put the fire out
2. Which of the following activities reflect a culture of safety within a health care organization? (Select all that apply.)
   1. A hospital purchases a new bar-code system to check patient identification during medication administration.
   2. A hospital requires nurse managers to submit an annual safety plan for high-risk patients.
   3. A nurse commits an error while administering a high-risk medication and is released from her position.
   4. A hospital enforces routine monthly checks of electrical equipment.
3. Mr. Rosen is a 72-year-old patient who is scheduled for elective surgery. A review of his history shows that he

takes a total of six medicines daily. He is generally healthy but has an enlarged prostate that causes him to go to the bathroom frequently. He had a low-grade fever the night before surgery but is afebrile at 7 AM. Which factors place him at a fall risk? (Select all that apply.)
1. Low-grade fever
2. Multiple medications
3. Elective surgery
4. Urinary frequency

4. Place the steps for conducting a Get Up and Go test in the proper order.
1. Turn around.
2. Stand still and then walk 10 feet.
3. Stand up from chair.
4. Sit down.
5. Turn around and walk back to chair.

5. The nurse finds a 68-year-old woman wandering in the hallway and exhibiting confused behavior. The patient says that she is looking for the bathroom. Which interventions are appropriate to ensure the safety of the patient? (Select all that apply.)
1. Ask the physician or health care provider to order a restraint.
2. Insert a urinary catheter.
3. Provide scheduled toileting rounds every 2 to 3 hours.
4. Consult with the health care provider about ordering an antianxiety medication.
5. Keep the bed in low position with the side rails down.
6. Keep the pathway from the bed to the bathroom clear.

6. A home health nurse is visiting a patient and begins a discussion with the family caregiver about food safety. Which of the following statements made by the caregiver suggests that he or she requires further instruction?
1. "When I prepare a salad, I need to rinse the lettuce and mushrooms thoroughly."
2. "I always wash my hands before I start to make a meal."
3. "When I make meat loaf, I use the cutting board to cut up onion and then shape the hamburger loaf on the same board."
4. "I always cook my husband's pork chops well done."

7. Place the following steps for applying a wrist restraint in the correct order.
1. Pad the skin overlying the wrist.
2. Insert two fingers under secured restraint to be sure that it is not too tight.
3. Be sure that patient is comfortable and in correct anatomical alignment.
4. Secure restraint straps to bed frame with quick-release buckle.
5. Wrap limb restraint around wrist or ankle with soft part toward skin and secure snugly.

8. Which of the following patients are at risk for falls because of intrinsic factors? (Select all that apply.)
1. A patient with a tendency to have postural hypotension
2. A patient whose hospital room has a bedside commode and suction machine blocking the path to the bathroom
3. A patient who has bathroom floor mats that are thin and frayed
4. A patient who suffers dementia and has cataracts

9. A nursing team conference is being held to discuss a patient who wanders frequently. The 72-year-old gets lost on the nursing unit and goes into other patients' rooms. The nursing team selects a set of interventions. Which of the following is not an appropriate restraint alternative?
1. Arranging to have the patient work on a puzzle in her room
2. When the patient becomes aggressive with other patients, confronting her and immediately removing her from the room
3. Relocating the patient to a room near the nurses' station
4. Asking the patient's family to bring pictures of grandchildren to place in the patient's room

10. A young mother asks the nurse in the outpatient clinic what causes toddlers to often have accidents. Which of the following statements made by the nurse best answers the mother's question?
1. "Toddlers are curious about their surrounding environment."
2. "The toddler's environment expands."
3. "Toddlers take risks frequently."
4. "Many toddlers are exposed to stress in their daily activities."

evolve

Rationales for Review Questions can be found on the Evolve website.

1. 2; **2.** 1, 2, 4; **3.** 2, 4; **4.** 3, 2, 5, 1, 4; **5.** 3, 5, 6; **6.** 3; **7.** 3, 1, 5, 2, 4; **8.** 1, 4; **9.** 2; **10.** 1

REFERENCES

American Academy of Pediatrics (AAP): *Car safety seats: information for families for 2013*, Healthy Children.Org, 2013, http://www.healthychildren.org/English/safety-prevention/on-the-go/pages/Car-Safety-Seats-Information-for-Families.aspx. Accessed December 29, 2013.

American Hospital Association (AHA): *Quality advisory: implementing standardized colors for patient alert wristbands*, September 4, 2008, http://www.aha.org/advocacy-issues/tools-resources/advisory/2008/080904-quality-adv.pdf. Accessed December 3, 2013.

American Nurses Association (ANA): *Nursing: scope and standards of practice*, ed 2, Washington, DC, 2010, The Association.

Capezuti E, et al: Least restrictive or least understood? Waist restraints, provider practices, and risk of harm, *J Aging Soc Policy* 20(3):305, 2008.

Centers for Disease Control and Prevention (CDC): *Percentage distribution of injuries by place of occurrence among males and females—National health interview survey*, United States, 2004-2007, Morbidity and Mortality Weekly Report, Atlanta, GA, 2010, Office of Surveillance, Epidemiology and Laboratory Services, Centers for Disease Control and Prevention, United States, Department of Health and Human Services.

Centers for Disease Control and Prevention (CDC): *Injury prevention and control: motor vehicle safety*, 2012a, http://www.cdc.gov/Motorvehiclesafety/teen_drivers/teendrivers_factsheet.html. Accessed December 3, 2013.

Centers for Disease Control and Prevention (CDC): *Home and recreational safety: check for safety: a home fall prevention checklist for older adults*, 2012b, http://www.cdc.gov/HomeandRecreationalSafety/Falls/CheckListForSafety.html. Accessed December 3, 2013.

Centers for Disease Control and Prevention (CDC): *Falls among older adults: an overview*, 2013a, http://www.cdc.gov/HomeandRecreationalSafety/Falls/adultfalls.html/. Accessed December 3, 2013.

Centers for Disease Control and Prevention (CDC): *Injury center: violence prevention: school violence*, 2013b, http://www.cdc.gov/ViolencePrevention/youthviolence/schoolviolence/index.html. Accessed December 3, 2013.

Centers for Disease Control and Prevention (CDC): *Injury prevention and control, motor vehicle safety: older adult drivers: get the facts*, 2013c. http://www.cdc.gov/Motorvehiclesafety/Older_Adult_Drivers/adult-drivers_factsheet.html. Accessed December 3, 2013.

Centers for Medicare and Medicaid Services (CMS): *Revisions to Medicare conditions of participation*, 482.13, Bethesda, MD, 2007, US Department of Health and Human Services.

Centers for Medicare and Medicaid Services (CMS): *State operations manual.* Appendix A: *Survey protocol, regulations, and interpretive guidelines for hospitals*, 2013, http://www.cms.gov/manuals/downloads/som107ap_a_hospitals.pdf. Accessed December 3, 2013.

Chase CA, et al: Systematic review of the effect of home modification and fall prevention programs on falls and the performance of community-dwelling older adults, *Am J Occup Ther* 66(3):284, 2012.

Healthfinder.gov: *Coalition for safe community needle disposal*, 2010, http://www.healthfinder.gov/orgs/hr3706.htm. Accessed December 3, 2013.

Deandrea S, et al: Risk factors for falls in community dwelling older people: a systematic review and meta-analysis, *Epidemiology* 21(5):658, 2010.

Degelau J, et al: *Prevention of falls (acute care): health care protocol*, Bloomington, MN, 2012, Institute for Clinical Systems Improvement (ICSI).

Duckyoo J: Fear of falling in older adults: comprehensive review, *Asian Nurs Res* 2(4):214, 2008.

Edelman CL, Mandle CL: *Health promotion throughout the life span*, ed 7, St Louis, 2010, Mosby.

Fitzpatrick MA: Meeting the challenge of fall reduction, *Am Nurse Today* 2(suppl 6):1, 2011.

Food and Drug Administration (FDA): *Report a problem to the FDA*, 2013, http://www.fda.gov/safety/reportaproblem/. Accessed December 3, 2013.

Hockenberry M, Wilson D: *Wong's Nursing care of infants and children*, ed 9, St Louis, 2011, Mosby.

Inglesby TV: Progress in disaster planning and preparedness since 2011, *JAMA* 306(12):1372, 2011.

Insurance Institute for Highway Safety: *Fatality facts 2011 teenagers*, Arlington, VA, 2011, The Institute, http://www.iihs.org/iihs/topics/t/teenagers/fatalityfacts/teenagers. Accessed December 3, 2013.

Institute of Medicine (IOM) Committee on Quality of Health Care in America: *To err is human: building a safer health system*, Washington DC, 2000, National Academies Press.

Institute of Medicine (IOM) Committee on Quality of Health Care in America: *Crossing the quality chasm: a new health system for the 21st century*, Washington DC, 2001, National Academies Press.

Iqbal S, et al: Carbon monoxide–related hospitalizations in the US: evaluation of a web-based query system for public health surveillance, *Public Health Rep* 125(3):423, 2010.

Jorgensen J: Reducing patient falls: a call to action, *Am Nurse Today* 2(Suppl 6):2, 2011.

Kulik C: Components of a comprehensive fall risk assessment, *Am Nurse Today* 2(Suppl 6):6, 2011.

Mathias S, et al: The get up and go test, *Arch Phys Med Rehabil* 67:387, 1986.

Morse JM: *Preventing patient falls: establishing a fall intervention program*, ed 2, New York, 2009, Springer Publishing.

National Center for Injury Prevention and Control: *10 leading causes of death, United States 1999-2007*, 2010, http://webappa.cdc.gov/sasweb/ncipc/leadcaus10.html. Accessed December 3, 2013.

National Fire Protection Association: *The US fire problem*, 2013, http://www.nfpa.org/itemDetail.asp?categoryID=953&itemID=23071&URL=Research/Fire%20statistics/The%20U.S.%20fire%20problem. Accessed December 3, 2013.

National Quality Forum (NQF): *National voluntary consensus standards for public reporting of patient safety events*, Washington DC, 2011, NQF, http://www.qualityforum.org/Publications/2011/02/National_Voluntary_Consensus_Standards_for_Public_Reporting_of_Patient_Safety_Event_Information.aspx. Accessed December 29, 2013.

National Quality Forum (NQF): *Mission and vision*, Washington DC, 2013a, http://www.qualityforum.org/About_NQF/Mission_and_Vision.aspx. Accessed December 3, 2013.

National Quality Forum (NQF): *List of SREs*, 2013b, http://www.qualityforum.org/Topics/SREs/List_of_SREs.aspx#sre1. Accessed December 1, 2013.

Occupational Safety and Health Administration (OSHA): *Healthcare*, 2013, https://www.osha.gov/SLTC/healthcarefacilities/index.html. Accessed December 6, 2013.

Opalek JM, Graymire VL, Redd D: Wheelchair falls: 5 years of data from a level I trauma center, *J Trauma Nurs* 16(2):98, 2009.

QSEN Institute: *QSEN institute*, 2013, http://qsen.org/. Accessed December 1, 2013.

Shubert TE: Evidence-based exercise prescription for balance and falls prevention: a current review of the literature, *J Geriatr Phys Ther* 34(3):100, 2011.

Spoelstra SL, Given BA, Given CW: Fall prevention in hospitals: an integrative review, *Clin Nurs Res* 21(1):92, 2012.

The Joint Commission (TJC): *Comprehensive accreditation manual for hospitals*, Chicago, 2011, TJC.

The Joint Commission (TJC): *Speak up initiatives*, 2013a, http://www.jointcommission.org/speakup.aspx. Accessed December 3, 2013.

The Joint Commission (TJC): *Comprehensive accreditation manual for hospitals*, Chicago, 2013b, TJC.

The Joint Commission (TJC): *National Patient Safety Goals*, Oakbrook Terrace, IL, 20114, The Commission. Available at http://www.jointcommission.org/standards_information/npsgs.aspx.

Tucker SJ, et al: Outcomes and challenges in implementing hourly rounds to reduce falls in orthopedic units, *Worldviews Evid Based Nurs* 9(1):18, 2012.

US Department of Health and Human Services (USDHHS), Office of Inspector General: *Adverse events in hospitals: overview of key issues*, OEI-06-07-00470, Washington DC, 2008, USDHHS.

US Department of Health and Human Services (USDHHS): *Safety culture*, Washington, DC, 2012, Agency for Healthcare Research and Quality, http://psnet.ahrq.gov/primer.aspx?primerID=5. Accessed December 3, 2013.

US Department of Labor: *Occupational Safety and Health Administration:* Recommended format for material safety data sheets *(MSDSs)*, n.d., http://www.osha.gov/dsg/hazcom/msdsformat.html. Accessed December 3, 2013.

Veenema TG: Disaster preparedness 10 years after 911, *Am J Nurs* 111(9):7, 2011.

Wolf I, et al: Gait changes and fall risk, *Praxis* 101(3):175, 2012.

CHAPTER

29 Hygiene

evolve WEBSITE

http://evolve.elsevier.com/Potter/essentials

- Video Clips
- Crossword Puzzle
- Audio Glossary

OBJECTIVES

- Describe factors that influence personal hygiene practices.
- Perform a comprehensive assessment of a patient's hygiene needs.
- Discuss factors that influence the condition of the skin, mouth, hair, scalp, nails, and feet.
- Identify common problems involving the skin, feet, nails, hair, and scalp.
- Discuss appropriate interventions for hygiene problems.
- Correctly perform hygiene procedures for care of a patient's skin, perineum, feet, nails, mouth, eyes, ears, and nose.
- Explain the importance of foot care for a patient with diabetes.
- Discuss conditions that place patients at risk for impaired oral mucous membranes.
- Describe how hygiene for older adults differs from that for younger patients.
- Make an occupied and unoccupied hospital bed.
- Identify ways to foster patient-centered care when providing hygiene care.
- Incorporate safety measures into hygiene care activities.

KEY TERMS

alopecia, p. 757
dental caries, p. 749
denture stomatitis, p. 764
edentulous, p. 754
effleurage, p. 771
gingivitis, p. 749
maceration, p. 765
mucositis, p. 760
pediculosis capitis, p. 757
perineal care, p. 768
skin tears, p. 758
stomatitis, p. 759
xerosis, p. 757

Personal hygiene influences your patient's comfort, safety, and well-being. Hygiene care includes cleaning and grooming activities that maintain personal body cleanliness and appearance. A variety of personal, social, and cultural factors influence hygiene practices. Because hygiene care requires close contact with your patients, use communication skills (e.g., listening, reflecting, focusing) to promote caring therapeutic relationships (see Chapter 11). You can integrate other nursing activities during hygiene care, including patient assessment and interventions such as range-of-motion (ROM) exercises, application of dressings, or inspection and care of intravenous (IV) sites. During hygiene care try to preserve as much of a patient's independence as possible, assess each patient's ability to perform hygiene care, ensure privacy, convey respect, and foster a patient's safety and comfort.

CASE STUDY *Mrs. Winkler*

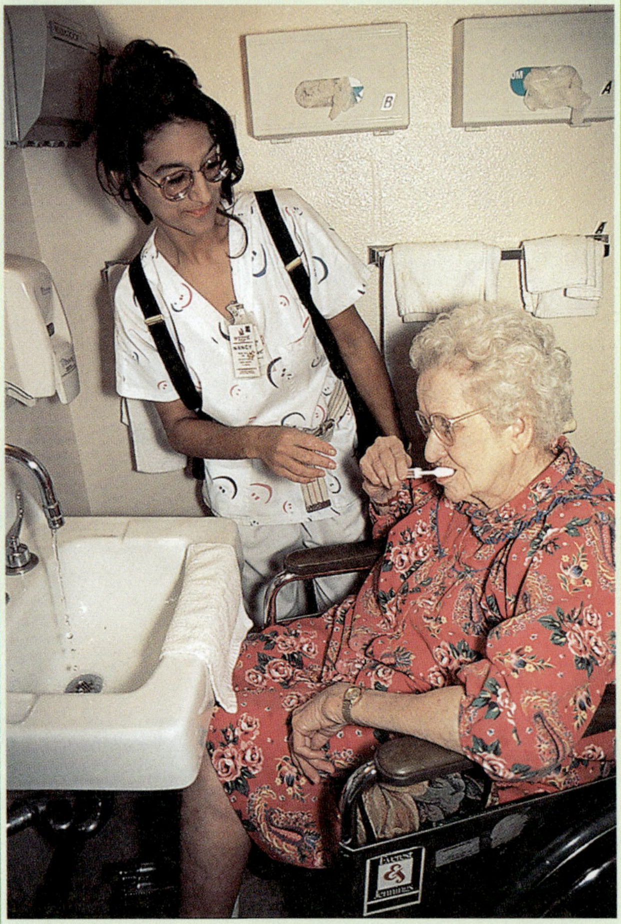

Mrs. Winkler is a 78-year-old woman with a medical history of rheumatoid arthritis and diabetes mellitus; she is a recently admitted resident of an extended care facility. The arthritis has resulted in chronic pain and deformity in her hands and knees. Mrs. Winkler has limited ability to use her hands as a result of the pain and joint deformity. Jamie Johnson is a nursing student assigned to care for Mrs. Winkler today, including helping Mrs. Winkler with her hygiene care.

To provide basic hygiene Jamie needs to learn about how to promote hygiene while giving attention to Mrs. Winkler's comfort level. When hygiene needs are not fulfilled, patients may experience complications, including skin or oral mucosa breakdown and infections. Jamie needs to review the effect of dependency on the patient's self-esteem and ways to provide opportunities to maintain self-care needs. At an optimal level of functioning with assistance, Mrs. Winkler is at risk for self-care deficits, impaired skin integrity, impaired oral mucosa, and risk for infection. During hygiene care Jamie interacts with Mrs. Winkler to assess her readiness to learn and teach health promotion practices. Jamie wants to preserve as much of Mrs. Winkler's independence as possible, ensure privacy, and foster physical well-being.

SCIENTIFIC KNOWLEDGE BASE

Providing hygiene for patients requires an understanding of the anatomy and physiology of the skin, nails, oral cavity, eyes, ears, and nose. Whether patients perform their own hygiene needs or you help provide them, effective hygiene techniques promote the normal structure and function of body tissues.

Skin

The skin serves several functions, including protection, secretion, excretion, body temperature regulation, and cutaneous sensation (Table 29-1). Two primary layers compose the skin: the epidermis and the dermis. Just beneath the skin lies the subcutaneous tissue (also known as the *hypodermis*), which shares some of the protective functions of the skin. The epidermis (outer layer) shields underlying tissues against water loss and injury, prevents entry of disease-producing microorganisms, and generates new cells to replace the dead cells that are continuously shed from the outer surface of the skin. Bacteria (normal flora) commonly reside on the outer epidermis; these normal flora inhibit disease-producing microorganisms. The dermis provides support for the epidermis and contains nerve fibers, blood vessels, sebaceous and sweat glands, and hair follicles. Sebaceous glands secret sebum, an oily fluid that softens and lubricates the skin, slows water loss from the skin, and also exerts bactericidal action. Subcutaneous tissue functions as a heat insulator, supports upper skin layers to withstand stresses and pressure, and anchors the skin loosely to underlying structures such as muscle.

The skin often reflects a change in a person's physical condition by alterations in color, thickness, texture, turgor, temperature, and moisture (see Chapter 16). Hygiene practices frequently influence skin status, having both beneficial and negative effects on the skin and its functions. For example, too-lengthy bathing and use of hot water can lead to dry, flaky skin and loss of protective oils.

Feet, Hands, and Nails

The feet, hands, and nails require special attention to prevent infection, odor, and injury. The condition of a patient's hands and feet influences the ability to perform hygiene care. Without the ability to bear weight, ambulate, or manipulate the hands a patient is at risk for losing self-care ability. Discomfort while standing or walking limits self-care abilities.

The nails grow from the root of the nail bed, which is located in the skin at the nail groove hidden by a fold of skin called the *cuticle*. A normal healthy nail appears transparent, smooth, and convex, with a pink nail bed and translucent white tip. The appearance of the nails reflects level of self-care. Inadequate nutrition and disease can cause changes in the shape, thickness, and curvature of the nail (see Chapter 16).

Oral Cavity and Teeth

The oral cavity consists of the lips, the cheeks, the tongue and its muscles, and the hard and soft palates. Mucous

TABLE 29-1 FUNCTIONS OF THE SKIN AND IMPLICATIONS FOR CARE

FUNCTION/DESCRIPTION	IMPLICATIONS FOR CARE
Protection	
The epidermis is the relatively impermeable skin layer that prevents entrance of microorganisms. Although microorganisms reside on skin surfaces and in hair follicles, relative dryness of the surface inhibits bacterial growth. Sebum removes bacteria from hair follicles. Acidic pH of skin further slows bacterial growth.	Weakening of epidermis occurs by scraping or stripping its surface as by use of dry razors, tape removal, or improper turning or positioning techniques. Excessive dryness causes cracks and breaks in skin and mucosa that allow bacteria to enter. Emollients soften and prevent moisture loss; soaking improves moisture retention; and hydration of mucosa prevents dryness. Constant exposure to moisture causes maceration or softening, which interrupts dermal integrity and promotes ulcers and bacterial growth. Keep bed linen and clothing dry. Misuse of soap, detergents, cosmetics, deodorant, and depilatories causes chemical irritation. Alkaline soaps neutralize the protective acid condition of the skin. Cleansing removes excess oil, sweat, dead skin cells, and dirt, which promote bacterial growth.
Sensation	
The skin contains sensory organs for touch, pain, heat, cold, and pressure.	Minimize friction to avoid loss of stratum corneum, which increases risk for pressure ulcers. Smoothing linen removes sources of mechanical irritation. Remove rings during bathing to prevent injuring a patient's skin. Make sure that bath water is not too hot or cold.
Temperature Regulation	
Radiation, evaporation, conduction, and convection control body temperature.	Factors that interfere with heat loss can alter temperature control. Wet bed linen or gowns increase heat loss. Excess blankets or bed coverings interfere with heat loss through radiation and conduction. Coverings conserve heat.
Excretion and Secretion	
Sweat promotes heat loss by evaporation. Sebum lubricates skin and hair.	Perspiration and oil sometimes harbor microorganism growth. Bathing removes excess body secretions, although excessive bathing causes dry skin.

membranes continuous with the skin line the oral cavity. Normal oral mucosa glistens and is pink, soft, moist, smooth, and without lesions. Healthy gums fit tightly around each tooth and are pink, moist, and smooth. Several glands secrete saliva into the oral cavity; saliva cleanses the mouth, dissolves food chemicals to promote taste, moistens food to facilitate bolus formation, and contains enzymes that start the breakdown of starchy foods. The effects of medications, exposure to radiation, dehydration, and mouth breathing may impair salivary secretion in the mouth.

A normal tooth consists of the crown, neck, and root. Healthy teeth appear white, smooth, shiny, and aligned. The condition of the oral cavity reflects overall health and also indicates oral hygiene needs (see Chapter 16).

Difficulty in chewing develops when the gums surrounding the teeth become inflamed or infected or when teeth are lost or become loosened. Regular oral hygiene helps to prevent **gingivitis** (i.e., inflammation of the gums) and **dental caries** (i.e., tooth decay produced by interaction of food with bacteria that form plaque).

Hair

Hair growth, distribution, and pattern indicate general health status (see Chapter 16). Hormonal changes, altered nutrition, emotional and physical stress, aging, infection, and certain illnesses can affect hair characteristics.

Eyes, Ears, and Nose

Chapters 16 and 38 describe the structure and function of the eyes, ears, and nose. When you provide hygiene care, a patient's eyes, ears, and nose also require careful attention. Clean the sensitive sensory tissues in a way that prevents injury and discomfort for a patient (e.g., use care not to get soap in the eyes). Specialized glands in the auditory canal secrete cerumen, which traps foreign bodies and repels insects. In some people cerumen can build up and become impacted. The eyes secrete tears, which contain substances that cleanse and lubricate the eye and protect it from bacteria. Patients with alterations in one or more of the senses often need help to meet their hygiene needs.

NURSING KNOWLEDGE BASE

A number of factors influence personal preferences for hygiene and the ability to maintain hygiene practices. Since no two individuals perform hygiene care in the same way, you individualize patient care based on assessing a patient's unique hygiene practices and preferences.

Hygiene care often involves intimate contact with a patient requiring use of communication skills to promote the therapeutic relationship. The time spent with a patient during hygiene care offers the opportunity to convey caring and more thoroughly assess the patient's needs. Personal hygiene activities such as taking a bath or shower, brushing and flossing the teeth, washing the hair, and performing nail care promote comfort, foster a positive self-image, and help prevent infection and disease.

Physical and Mental Status

Patients with limitations or disabilities associated with disease and injury often lack the physical energy and dexterity to perform hygiene self-care safely. A patient whose arm is in a cast or who has an IV line or other device connected to the body needs help with hygiene care. Inability to use the hands because of disease or injury can make using a toothbrush, washcloth, or hairbrush difficult or ineffective. Sensory deficits not only alter a patient's ability to perform care but also place him or her at risk for injury. Safety is a priority for a patient with a sensory deficit. For example, the inability to feel that the water is too hot can lead to burn injury.

Chronic illnesses (e.g., cardiac disease, chronic lung disease, cancer, or neurological disorders) often exhaust or incapacitate a patient. Patients who become fatigued need to have complete hygiene care provided. Include periods of rest during care to allow patients to participate in their care.

Pain that accompanies illness and injury limits a patient's ability to tolerate hygiene and grooming activities or perform self-care. Pain may limit ROM, resulting in impaired use of the arms or hands or limited ability to move about in the environment; any of these limitations impairs hygiene self-care ability. Sedation and drowsiness associated with analgesics used for pain management also limit a patient's ability to participate in care and could result in injury from a fall.

Limited mobility caused by a variety of factors (e.g., physical injury, weakness, surgery, pain, prolonged inactivity, medication effects, and presence of an indwelling catheter or IV line) decreases a patient's ability to perform hygiene self-care activities safely. Individualized care considers a patient's ability to perform care, the amount of assistance needed, and the need for assistive and safety devices to facilitate safe hygiene care.

Acute and chronic cognitive impairments such as stroke, brain injury, psychoses, and dementia often result in the inability to perform self-care independently. Patients with cognitive impairments may be unaware of their hygiene and grooming needs. Because of impaired ability to interpret stimuli, some patients with dementia become fearful and agitated during hygiene care, resulting in aggressive behavior (Hoeffer et al., 2006). Safe, effective patient care takes the impact of cognitive impairment into consideration and allows for appropriate modifications when providing hygiene care.

Socioeconomic Status

A person's economic resources influence the type and extent of hygiene practices used. Be sensitive in considering that a patient's economic status affects the ability to regularly maintain hygiene. A patient with limited funds may not be able to afford desired basic supplies such as deodorant, shampoo, and toothpaste or may find it difficult to make needed modifications in the home such as adding nonskid surfaces and grab bars in the bathroom for safety.

Developmental Stage

Apply knowledge of physical and psychosocial developmental changes as you assess your patients and plan, implement, and evaluate hygiene care. A patient's developmental stage not only influences the normal condition of body tissues and structures but also the person's ability to perform proper hygiene care. According to Erikson (1963), children in the early-childhood stage strive to develop a sense of autonomy and independence; caregivers can foster this development by supervising toddlers during hygiene care while allowing them to attempt the care. Erikson describes the preschool stage to include the development of "initiative" as a child exerts control over the environment and becomes more independent. During this stage caregivers should encourage children to explore hygiene care while helping them make appropriate care choices. When children enter school they have to cope with the social demands of that environment, including the influence of peers. Caregivers need to recognize that personal hygiene habits may change during this stage as the child struggles to fit in with his or her peer group (e.g., a young boy might rebel against a daily bath during this stage). During adolescence a teen tries to develop a sense of self and personal identity. He or she may experiment with a variety of hygiene and grooming choices; it is important for teens to be able to exert their personal style as they develop their individual identities in this stage.

Skin. A neonate's skin is relatively immature and thin, with the epidermis and dermis being loosely bound together. Friction against the skin layers may easily cause damage. Handle neonates carefully during bathing; any break in the skin may result in an infection. A toddler's skin layers become more tightly bound together, resulting in greater resistance to skin injury and infection. However, because a toddler is more active and does not have established independent hygiene habits, caregivers need to provide thorough hygiene and teach good hygiene habits. During adolescence growth and maturation of the skin increase. Sebaceous glands become more active, predisposing adolescents to acne. Sweat glands become fully functional during puberty. More frequent bathing and shampooing and use of antiperspirants become necessary to reduce body odors and eliminate oily skin and hair.

The condition of an adult's skin depends on hygiene practices and exposure to environmental irritants. Normally the skin is elastic, well hydrated, firm, and smooth. With aging the rate of epidermal cell replacement slows, and elastic collagen fibers shrink; the skin thins and loses resiliency, becoming fragile and subject to bruising and breaking. As the production of lubricating substances from skin glands decreases, the skin becomes dry and itchy (Meiner, 2011). These changes often lead to dry, cracked skin. Although bathing for too long and or with hot water or harsh soap causes the skin to become increasingly dry, a 5- to 10-minute bath or shower adds moisture to the skin (American Academy of Dermatology, 2012a).

Feet and Nails. With aging chronic foot problems are more likely to develop as a result of poor foot care, improper fit of footwear, and systemic disease. Older adults may not have the strength, flexibility, visual acuity, or manual dexterity to care for their feet and nails. Common problems of the feet affecting older adults include corns, calluses, bunions, hammertoe, and fungal infections. Painful feet result from a variety of deformities, weak structure, injuries, and diseases such as diabetes and rheumatoid arthritis.

Mouth. At approximately 6 to 10 months of age infants begin teething, with the first permanent teeth erupting at about 6 years of age (Hockenberry and Wilson, 2011). By age 13 years most children have 28 of their permanent teeth; the last of the permanent teeth to erupt are the third molars or "wisdom teeth," which usually begin to erupt between ages 17 and 21 years. From adolescence through middle adulthood the teeth and gums remain healthy if a person follows healthy eating patterns and oral care practices. As a person ages, numerous factors may contribute to poor oral health, including age-related changes of the mouth, chronic diseases such as diabetes mellitus, physical disabilities involving hand grasp or strength, lack of attention to oral care, and medications (e.g., chemotherapy) that have oral cavity side effects. With aging gums lose vascularity and tissue elasticity, which cause dentures to fit poorly if present.

Hair. Throughout life changes in the growth, distribution, and condition of the hair influence hair hygiene and grooming. As males reach adolescence, shaving becomes a part of routine grooming. Young girls who reach puberty often begin to shave their legs and axillae. With aging, as scalp hair becomes thinner and drier, shampooing is needed less frequently.

Eyes, Ears, and Nose. Chapter 38 describes changes in hearing, vision, and olfaction across the lifespan. Alterations in sensory function often require modifications in hygiene care. Use your knowledge of developmental changes when planning hygiene care.

Family customs play a major role during childhood in determining hygiene practices such as the frequency of bathing, the time of day bathing is performed, and even whether certain hygiene practices such as brushing teeth are performed or not.

Personal Preferences

Patients have individual desires and preferences about when to bathe, shave, and perform hair and oral care. Some patients prefer to shower, whereas others prefer to bathe in the bed. Patients select different hygiene products according to personal preference and needs. Knowing these desires and preferences helps you provide a patient-centered approach to hygiene. Safe and effective patient-centered nursing care elicits individual preferences, allows patients to make personal choices whenever possible, and promotes patient involvement and independence (Cronenwett et al., 2007).

Cultural Variables

A patient's cultural beliefs and practices influence hygiene care. People from diverse cultural backgrounds follow different self-care practices. Maintaining cleanliness may not hold the same importance for some ethnic or social groups as it does for others (Galanti, 2008). In North America it is common to bathe or shower daily and use deodorant. However, people from some cultures may not be sensitive to body odor and may prefer to bathe less frequently and not use deodorant. Avoid expressing disapproval when caring for a patient whose hygiene practices differ from yours. Do not force changes in hygiene practices unless the practices affect a patient's health. In these situations be tactful when speaking with the patient, provide information, and allow patient choices.

Be aware of the possible impact of a patient's cultural beliefs on hygiene care. For example, some East Indian Hindus believe that bathing before a meal can be injurious and that cold water should not be added to hot water when preparing a bath (Giger, 2013). When providing hygiene care for a Hindu patient, first determine if he or she holds such beliefs. You would need to schedule the bath at a time after mealtime and discard bath water that is too hot instead of merely adding cold water.

Religious beliefs associated with culture may influence hygiene practices. Females of the Muslim faith follow *hijab* or modesty in dress when in the presence of males and avoid touching or having close proximity to males (Giger, 2013). Clothing includes head covering, long sleeves, and long slacks or skirts covering legs. Because of these beliefs and practices, you need to ensure that care provided for these patients ensures enough privacy for bathing and toileting activities, appropriate bed clothing, and same-gender caregivers for hygiene care.

CRITICAL THINKING

Synthesis

You apply elements of critical thinking whenever you perform the nursing process with a patient. Consider the scientific knowledge you have learned, your experience, critical thinking attitudes, and standards to ensure an individualized approach to patient care (Box 29-1).

BOX 29-1 SYNTHESIS IN PRACTICE

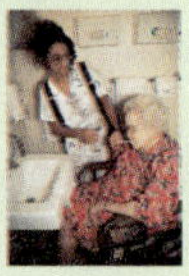

Before entering Mrs. Winkler's room, Jamie reviews and synthesizes knowledge about the effect of chronic illness on functional independence, reviews principles of therapeutic communication, and reviews the pathophysiologic effects of rheumatoid arthritis and diabetes mellitus. From previous clinical experience Jamie has learned that patients need to have input in how nurses implement nursing care. By applying the ethical standard of autonomy, Jamie encourages Mrs. Winkler to make decisions about how to proceed with her hygiene care by engaging her in a therapeutic conversation. Jamie learns that Mrs. Winkler wants to clean her face and hands and care for her dentures before breakfast. But then she tells Jamie that she can't do these things by herself and that she doesn't want to be "any trouble." At this time Jamie determines that reassuring Mrs. Winkler and helping her with prebreakfast hygiene are priorities.

Knowledge. Knowledge of the anatomy and physiology of the skin, oral cavity, nails, and sense organs helps you understand the implications of proper hygiene for a patient's total health status. As you develop a knowledge base about various pathological conditions, you more fully understand risk factors that increase the risk for hygiene problems. Apply this knowledge to guide the questions you ask patients about their hygiene care as you assess their care needs and their hygiene self-care status. Also use your knowledge to plan and implement patient care. For example, a patient with diabetes mellitus is at high risk for nail and foot problems because of the effects of the disease on circulation. Knowledge about the pathophysiology of diabetes and its potential effects on a patient's circulation and sensation provides you with the scientific knowledge base needed to implement safe and effective foot care.

You also apply knowledge of physical assessment skills (see Chapter 16) when providing hygiene. Performing an examination of the skin, oral and nasal cavities, eyes and ears, peripheral circulation, sensory-motor function, and degree of ROM while providing hygiene needs uses time efficiently and provides a database to identify hygiene problems and monitor a patient's progress over time.

Use knowledge of comfort measures and safety when planning and implementing hygiene care. For example, implement measures to limit pain before performing hygiene care. Provide for protection from injury by using aids to limit slipping or falling and checking water temperature to prevent burns.

Experience. Draw on your own experiences in meeting your personal hygiene needs as you help with your patients' hygiene care. You may have helped family members with their hygiene. Usually an early clinical experience involves providing hygiene for a patient. As your experience increases, your comfort and expertise in meeting the individualized hygiene needs of your patients increase as well.

Attitudes. Multiple critical thinking attitudes apply to hygiene care. Display curiosity; be thorough in your assessment of the condition of a patient's skin, nails, sensory organs, and oral cavity. Strive to know a patient's personal preferences and any cultural aspects that might influence hygiene care. Use creativity to collaborate with patients and determine the best way to meet individual hygiene needs. You need to be creative and supportive to help patients develop new hygiene practices or adapt existing ones when illness or loss of function impairs self-care abilities. For example, your patient may need to adapt to showering instead of a tub bath because of physical limitations. Because of variations in individual patients' physical strength and hygiene practices, it is important that you approach care with an attitude of flexibility. Encourage patient involvement while determining how and when care is provided. For example, you may need to include periods of rest to prevent exhaustion during hygiene care. Demonstrate responsibility and accountability when making a plan of care that promotes your patient's well-being.

Standards. The use of critical thinking standards ensures that assessment of hygiene needs is relevant and accurate. Be accurate and consistent when assessing for any skin alterations during hygiene care. Apply professional standards of care in your practice. For example, when caring for patients with diabetes, apply standards from the American Diabetes Association to ensure that you give proper foot care. Recommendations from the American Dental Association provide the basis for teaching oral care. Also apply standards of professional responsibility to advocate for a patient. For example, apply the ethical standard of autonomy by letting your patient choose the time and type of bath when possible. You adhere to the principle of beneficence when you use evidence-based, patient-centered bathing measures with a patient who is cognitively impaired and becomes agitated or aggressive when bathed (Hoeffer et al., 2006). Promote your patients' independence as much as possible while still maintaining their safety.

NURSING PROCESS

ASSESSMENT

Assessment of a patient's hygiene status and self-care abilities requires you to complete a nursing history and perform physical assessment. You do not routinely assess all body regions before providing hygiene. However, you need to conduct a brief history to determine priority areas and plan patient-centered hygiene care (Table 29-2). While helping a patient with personal hygiene, carefully assess the skin, nails, oral cavity, hair and scalp, and sensory organs (see Chapter 16). Visually inspect and palpate tissue, noting alterations in integrity. Pay particular attention to characteristics such as cleanliness of skin or hydration of oral mucosa, most influenced by hygiene measures. Assessment data help you determine any hygiene-related issues and identify the type and extent of hygiene care required.

Observe a patient as you are giving care to detect problems associated with inadequate hygiene practices. It is important

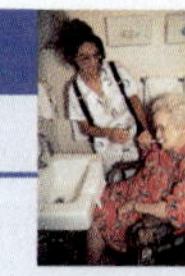

TABLE 29-2 FOCUSED PATIENT ASSESSMENT

FACTORS TO ASSESS	QUESTIONS	PHYSICAL ASSESSMENT
Skin care	Which skin care products do you use? Are any skin problems bothering you?	Inspect condition of skin and bony prominences. Observe skin surfaces and skinfolds for presence of dirt or debris.
Mouth care	Are you having any mouth pain, or have you noticed any sores in your mouth? Do you wear dentures or a partial plate?	Inspect condition of teeth, gums, and mouth. Observe patient during mouth care or eating to determine presence of oral pain or discomfort that impairs hygiene practices. Observe fit of dentures. Observe patient performing oral care.
Assistance with hygiene	Do you use any aids to help you with your bath such as grab bars in your tub or shower? Which parts of personal hygiene can you do for yourself? For which parts of hygiene care do you need help? How can I make helping you with your hygiene easier and more pleasant?	Observe patient's use of assistive devices, noting proper, safe use. Complete an environmental assessment to detect presence of safety devices or hazards related to hygiene care. Observe patient during hygiene activities, noting activities that are difficult for patient to perform.
Tolerance of hygiene	Do hygiene activities cause any symptoms such as shortness of breath, pain, or fatigue? What do you do to minimize these symptoms? What can I do to help you complete hygiene care most comfortably?	Observe patient before, during, and after hygiene. Palpate pulse, noting rate and rhythm changes. Observe breathing pattern, noting rate and ease of breathing. Observe patient for pallor and diaphoresis. Notice facial expressions that indicate pain.

to assess a patient's ability to tolerate hygiene procedures that are sometimes exhausting. During hygiene care you can assess for a variety of health care problems and thus better set health care priorities.

Self-Care Ability. Assess a patient's status as it relates to his or her ability to perform or help with hygiene care safely and efficiently. Assessing a patient's ability to provide self-care helps you make decisions about the kind and amount of hygiene care to provide and a patient's ability to participate in care while in a health care facility and after discharge. When a patient is unable to bathe or perform personal skin care, you need to provide assistance. To determine whether a patient requires a bed bath instead of a tub bath or shower, assess his or her balance, activity tolerance, and muscle strength and coordination and the presence of treatment-related tubs or equipment. When a patient is ordered to be on bed rest or to sit up in a chair for a limited time, your hygiene options are limited. Be alert for activity intolerance during hygiene care. Observe respirations, noting changes in rate and depth or any shortness of breath; observe for changes in skin color. Palpate the pulse to detect changes in rate and regularity and question the patient about dizziness, weakness, or fatigue. If a patient shows signs of intolerance and is up in a chair, return the patient to bed to lower the cardiovascular and respiratory demand and help prevent injury from a fall. To foster safety with bathing, assess a patient's ability to detect thermal and tactile stimuli.

The degree of assistance needed by a patient during bathing also depends on his or her vision, the ability to sit without support and perform hand grasps, and the degree of active ROM of extremities. Observe your patient's physical ability to perform eye, ear, and nose care and to care for any sensory aids. Patients who have limited upper-extremity mobility, have reduced vision, are seriously fatigued, or are unable to grasp small objects such as a hearing aid battery or contact lenses require assistance. Evidence shows that the degree of hand function plays a key role in the adequate removal of dental and denture plaque in institutionalized older people performing their own oral care (Padilha et al., 2007).

When patients have self-care limitations, family caregivers likely help with care in the home. In the hospital setting nurses begin discharge planning early in each hospitalization. It is a nurse's responsibility to assess if there is a need for hygiene care assistance and ensure that appropriate plans are made for care after discharge. For patients found to have postdischarge hygiene care needs, discharge planning should include arrangements for a home assessment/evaluation to promote an individualized plan of care.

Also assess your patient's cognitive status. A patient with impaired cognitive function may be unaware of hygiene care needs or less able to follow instructions and help with care. In the home setting patients with dementia may begin to no longer maintain their hygiene. An early warning sign of dementia is poor judgment. Patients may pay less attention to grooming or keeping themselves clean (Alzheimer's Association, 2009). In the hospital setting you may need to consult with therapists or specialists for patients with cognitive deficits. This usually requires an order from a health care provider.

Assessment of the Skin. Perform an assessment of the skin, noting color, texture, thickness, turgor, temperature, and hydration (see Chapter 16). Pay special attention to the presence and characteristics of any lesions. Note dryness of the skin indicated by flaking, redness, scaling, and cracking. Discovering manifestations of common skin problems influences how you administer hygiene care (Table 29-3). When caring for patients with dark skin pigmentation, be aware of assessment techniques and skin characteristics unique to highly pigmented skin.

Determine the degree of cleanliness by observing the appearance of the skin and detecting body odors that indicate previous inadequate cleansing or excessive perspiration caused by fever or pain. Inspect less obvious or difficult-to-reach skin surfaces such as under the breasts or scrotum, around a female patient's perineum, or in the groin for redness, excessive moisture, and soiling or debris. Separate skinfolds carefully for observation and palpation. Assess the condition and cleanliness of the perineal and anal areas during hygiene and with each toileting when patients require hygiene assistance. Most people consider these areas to be private. Your reluctance to expose the patient or your patient's reluctance may result in problems because of inadequate hygiene care. Use sensitivity in your approach.

Be attentive for characteristics of skin problems most influenced by hygiene measures. Is the skin dry from too much bathing or from use of hot water or irritating soap? Does the patient have a rash caused by an allergic reaction to a skin-care product? Certain conditions place patients at risk for impaired skin integrity (see Chapter 37). Because of increased risk be particularly alert when assessing patients with reduced sensation, vascular insufficiency, altered cognition, incontinence, nutrition or hydration alterations, body secretions, and decreased mobility. Carefully assess the skin in dark-skinned patients at risk for pressure ulcers (see Chapter 37). Patients may be unaware of skin problems because they are unable to feel pain or pressure or see their skin in some places (e.g., the back or the feet). Carefully assess the skin under orthopedic devices (braces, splints, casts) and beneath items such as tape.

Assessment of the Feet and Nails. A variety of common foot and nail problems can be caused by inadequate hygiene and are actually detected during hygiene care (Table 29-4). Problems sometimes result from abuse or poor care of the feet and hands such as nail biting or trimming nails improperly, exposure to harsh chemicals, and wearing poorly fitting shoes. Question patients to determine the type of footwear worn and usual foot and nail care practices.

Assess patients with diseases that affect peripheral circulation and sensation for the adequacy of circulation and sensation of the feet. Palpate the dorsalis pedis and posterior tibial pulses and assess for intact sensation to light touch, pinprick, and temperature (see Chapter 16). Observe a patient's gait. A variety of common foot problems contribute to pain and cause alterations in gait.

Inspect the condition of the fingernails and toenails, looking for lesions, dryness, inflammation, or cracking, which are often associated with a variety of common nail problems (see Table 29-4) or with nail-care practices. The cuticle that surrounds the nail can grow over the nail and become inflamed if nail care is not performed periodically. Ask patients whether they frequently polish their nails and use polish remover because chemicals in these products can cause excessive nail dryness. Some diseases change the condition, shape, and curvature of the nails (see Chapter 16). Inflammatory lesions and fungus of the nail bed cause thickened, horny nails that can separate from the nail bed.

Examine all skin surfaces of the feet, including areas between the toes and over the entire sole of the foot. Poorly fitting shoes may irritate the heels, soles, and sides of the feet. Inspect the feet for lesions, including noting areas of dryness, inflammation, or cracking.

Observe your patient's gait. Painful foot disorders or decreased sensation causes limping or an unnatural gait. Ask whether the patient has foot discomfort and determine factors that aggravate the pain. Foot problems sometimes result from bone or muscular alterations or poorly fitting footwear.

Assessment of the Oral Cavity. Inspect all areas of the mouth carefully for color, hydration, texture, and lesions (see Chapter 16). Patients may develop oral problems as a result of inadequate oral care or consequence of disease (e.g., oral malignancy) or as a side effect of medications, radiation, and chemotherapy. Localized pain or tenderness and infection accompany many common oral problems (Box 29-2).

Apply clean gloves to palpate any tender areas or lesions. If an older adult becomes **edentulous** (without teeth) and wears complete or partial dentures, assess underlying gums and palate. Observe for cleanliness and use olfaction to detect halitosis. If you identify any oral problems, notify the patient's health care provider. Early identification of poor oral hygiene

BOX 29-2 COMMON ORAL PROBLEMS

DENTAL CARIES (CAVITIES)

- Most common among young people
- Buildup of plaque causes acid destruction of tooth enamel; initially appears as chalky, white discoloration of the tooth

PERIODONTAL DISEASE (PYORRHEA)

- Most common after age 35
- Involves destruction of gingiva (gums) and other supporting structures with bleeding gums, inflammation, and receding gum lines, which may lead to tooth loss

OTHER PROBLEMS

- Oral mucositis (oral erythema, ulceration, and pain)
- Glossitis (inflammation of the tongue)
- Gingivitis (inflammation of the gums)
- Halitosis (bad breath)
- Cheilitis (cracked lips)
- Oral malignancy (mouth lumps or ulcers)

TABLE 29-3 COMMON SKIN PROBLEMS

PROBLEM	CHARACTERISTICS	IMPLICATIONS	INTERVENTIONS
Dry skin 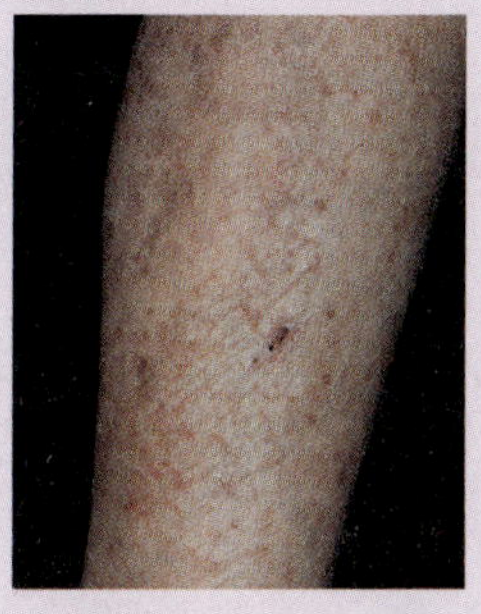	Flaky, rough texture on exposed areas such as hands, arms, legs, or face	Skin may become infected if epidermal layer cracks.	Effective treatment of dry skin does not require limiting frequency of bathing. Bathing daily for limited time (10 minutes or less) can help with hydration. To minimize drying use warm, not hot water and superfatted soap (e.g., Dove) for cleansing. Rinse body of all soap well because residue left can cause irritation and breakdown. Use a humidifier to add moisture to air. Increase fluid intake when skin is dry. Use moisturizing lotion to aid healing process; lotion forms protective barrier and helps maintain fluid within skin.
Acne 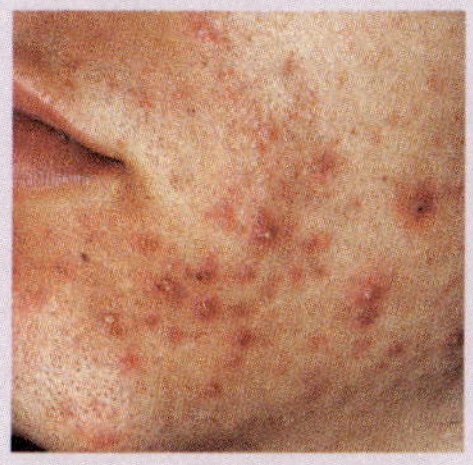	Inflammatory, papulopustular skin eruption, usually involving bacterial breakdown of sebum; appears on face, neck, shoulders, and back	Infected material within pustule spreads if area is squeezed or picked. Permanent scarring can result.	Wash hair and skin each day with soap and warm water to remove oil. Use oil-free cosmetics because oily cosmetics or creams accumulate in pores and make acne worse. Use prescribed topical antibiotics for severe acne. Implement necessary dietary restrictions by eliminating foods found to aggravate condition.
Skin rashes 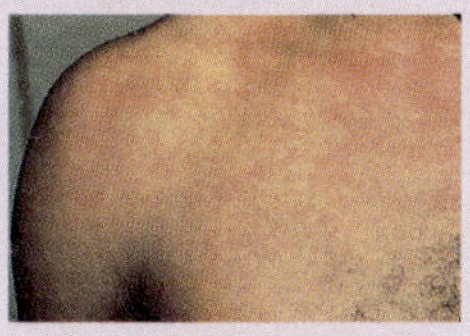	Skin eruption that may result from overexposure to sun or moisture or from allergic reaction; appears flat or raised, localized or systemic, pruritic or nonpruritic	If patient scratches skin, inflammation and infection occur. Rashes also cause discomfort.	Wash area thoroughly and apply antiseptic spray or lotion to prevent further itching and aid healing process. Warm or cold soaks may relieve inflammation and promote comfort.
Contact dermatitis 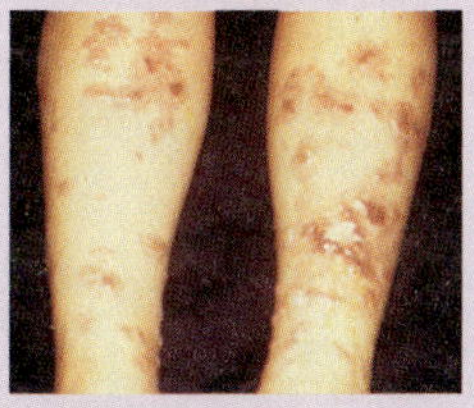	Inflammation of skin characterized by abrupt onset with erythema, pruritus, pain, and appearance of scaly, oozing lesions; seen on face, neck, hands, forearms, trunk, and genitalia	Dermatitis is often difficult to eliminate because person is usually in continual contact with substance causing skin reaction. Substance is sometimes hard to identify.	Identify and avoid contributing agents (e.g., cleansers, cosmetics, latex, poison ivy or oak). Treatment consists of removing the contributing agent and applying over-the-counter topical steroids or calamine lotion. In some cases prescription steroids may be ordered. Patients may find that tepid baths provide comfort.
Abrasion 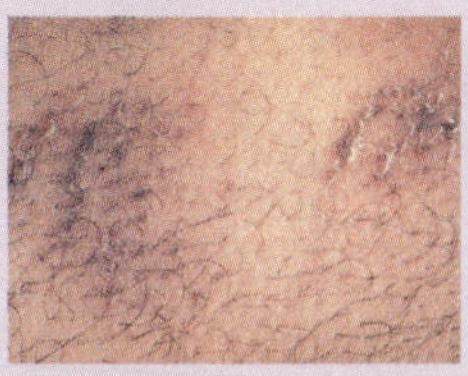 (From Cottran SR et al: From the Teaching Collection of the Department of Dermatology, University of Texas, Southwestern Medical School, Dallas.)	Scraping or rubbing away of epidermis; results in localized bleeding and later weeping of serous fluid	Infection occurs easily as result of loss of protective skin layer.	Be careful not to scratch patients with your jewelry or fingernails. Wash abrasions with mild soap and water. Dressing or bandage could increase risk for infection because of retained moisture.

TABLE 29-4 COMMON FOOT AND NAIL PROBLEMS

PROBLEM	CHARACTERISTICS	IMPLICATIONS	INTERVENTIONS
Callus 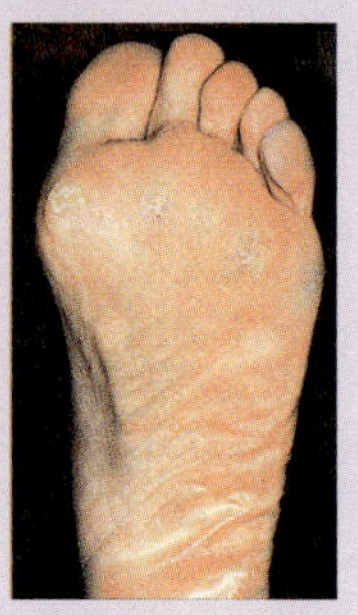	Thickened portion of epidermis, consisting of mass of horny, keratotic cells; usually flat and painless; found on undersurface of foot or on palm of hand; caused by local friction or pressure	Foot calluses often cause discomfort when wearing tight-fitting shoes.	Wear gloves when using tools or objects that create friction on palms. Wear comfortable shoes that fit. Soak callus in warm water and Epsom salts to soften cell layers (soaking feet is contraindicated in patients with diabetes and peripheral vascular disease). Use pumice stone to remove callus after it softens. Be careful not to use stone on noncallused skin. Applications of creams or lotions reduce recurrence. Use of orthotic devices (e.g., foam insoles, metatarsal pads, and various cushioning devices) redistributes weight and pressure away from callused area.
Corns 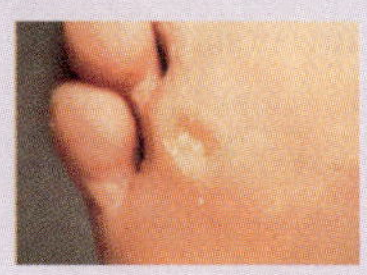	Keratosis caused by friction and pressure from shoes; mainly on toes, over bony prominence; usually cone shaped, round, and raised; calluses with painful core	Conical shape compresses underlying dermis, making it thin and tender. Tight shoes aggravate pain. Tissue attaches to bone if allowed to grow. Patient may suffer alteration in gait because of pain.	Surgical removal is sometimes necessary, depending on location and severity of pain and size of corn. Use oval corn pads carefully because they increase pressure on toes and reduce circulation. Do not use corn pads for patients with diabetes or impaired circulation.
Plantar warts 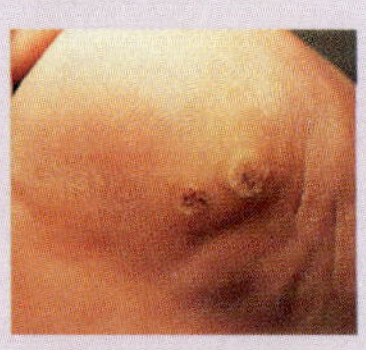	Fungating lesion that appears on sole of foot; caused by papillomavirus	Warts are sometimes contagious, are painful, and make walking difficult.	Treatment ordered by health care provider may include topical applications of acids, electrodessication (burning with electric spark), cryotherapy (freezing with carbon dioxide or liquid nitrogen), or laser therapy.
Athlete's foot (tinea pedis) 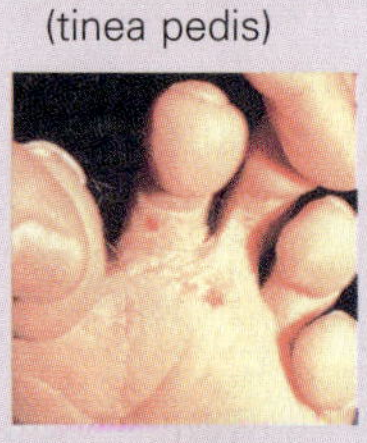	Fungal infection of foot; scaliness and cracking of skin between toes and on soles of feet; small blisters containing fluid appear, apparently induced by constricting footwear (e.g., sneakers)	Athlete's foot can spread to other body parts, especially hands. It is contagious and frequently recurs.	Make sure that feet are well ventilated. Drying feet well after bathing and applying powder help prevent infection. Wearing clean socks or stockings reduces incidence. Health care provider often orders application of griseofulvin, miconazole nitrate, or tolnaftate.
Ingrown nails 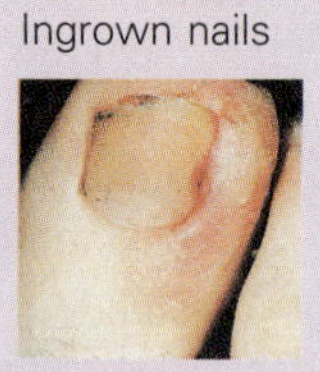	Toenail or fingernail growing inward into soft tissue around nail; results from improper nail trimming, poor shoe fit, or heredity	Ingrown nails cause localized pain in presence of pressure; some become infected.	Treatment is frequent warm soaks in antiseptic solution and removal of portion of nail that has grown into skin. Instruct patient in proper nail trimming techniques and to report purulent drainage. Recommend professional podiatry if needed.
Paronychia 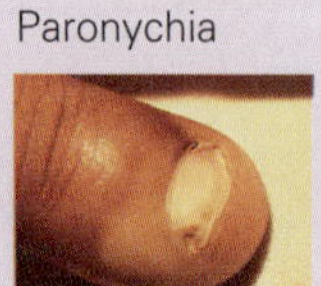	Inflammation of tissue surrounding nail after hangnail or other injury; occurs in people who frequently have their hands in water; common in patients with diabetes	Area sometimes becomes infected.	Treatment is warm compresses or soaks (*exception:* do not soak nail if patient has diabetes) and local application of antibiotic ointments. Careful manicuring prevents paronychia.
Foot odors	Result of excess perspiration promoting microorganism growth; faulty foot hygiene or improper footwear causes foot odor	Odor frequently embarrasses patient.	Frequent washing, use of foot deodorants and powders, and clean footwear prevent or reduce this problem.
Nail fungal infection	Results from excess moisture, use of artificial nails	Infection requires treatment with fungicide.	Wear clean, dry footwear (see athlete's foot).

practices and common oral problems reduces the risk for gum disease and dental caries or cavities.

Include specific questions and observations for a patient with dentures or a dental appliance. Observe under dentures and appliances for evidence of pressure areas or irritation. Note size and location of any lesions. Note how well the dentures or appliance fits. Question patients about any problems associated with dental devices, including tender areas and poor fit.

Assessment of the Hair and Hair Care. Before performing hygiene care, assess the condition of the hair and scalp (Box 29-3). Findings help you detect hair and scalp problems and determine the frequency and type of care needed (Table 29-5). During care observe your patient's ability to perform hair care. A person's appearance and feeling of well-being often are related to the way the hair looks and feels. Illness, disability, and conditions such as arthritis, fatigue, and the presence of physical barriers (e.g., cast or IV access) alter a patient's ability to maintain daily hair care. Assess an immobilized patient's hair for tangles and check hair around and beneath dressings for sticky blood residue or antiseptic solutions.

Ethnicity, culture, and personal preferences influence choice of hair style and hair-care practices. Assess a patient's practices and discuss any potential associated problems.

In community health and home care settings it is particularly important to inspect the hair and scalp for lice. If you suspect **pediculosis capitis** (head lice), protect yourself against self-infestation by handwashing and using gloves or tongue blades to inspect the hair and scalp. Notify the patient's health care provider if you assess presence of lice.

Alopecia (loss of hair) may result from effects of chemotherapy medications, hormonal changes, damaging hair-care practices, genetic predisposition, or psychological impairment. If noted be sure to question your patient about specific hair-care practices, especially the types of products used and heat application during hair care.

BOX 29-3 ASSESSMENT OF HAIR

PHYSICAL CHANGES

- Assess condition of hair and scalp (see Chapter 16). Consider age-appropriate changes.
- Consider racial or ethnic differences.
- Determine reasons for change in distribution or loss of hair.
- Check oiliness and texture of hair.
- Inspect scalp for lesions, inflammation, infection, or parasites.

SELF-CARE ABILITY

- Assess patient's ability to grasp comb or brush and raise arm for brushing or combing.
- Determine patient's ability to physically care for hair.
- Does patient become easily fatigued?

HAIR-CARE PRACTICES

- Assess patient's preferences in hair styling.
- Identify patient's preferences for hair care and shaving products.
- Assess adequacy of patient's hygiene practices.
- Determine patient's perceptions of own appearance.
- Assess patient's socioeconomic background.

Assessment of the Eyes, Ears, and Nose. Carefully inspect all external eye structures (see Chapter 16). The presence of redness indicates possible allergic or infectious conjunctivitis. The crusty drainage associated with infectious conjunctivitis easily spreads from one eye to the other. Wear gloves to examine the eyes and perform hand hygiene before and after the examination. Determine if a patient wears contact lenses, especially if he or she enters the health care agency in an unresponsive or confused state. An undetected contact lens may cause corneal injury when left in place too long.

Assessment of the external ear structures includes inspection of the auricle and external ear canal (see Chapter 16). Observe for the presence of accumulated cerumen (earwax) or drainage in the ear canal. Note evidence of local inflammation. Question patients about tenderness on palpation of the external ear or the presence of pain and ask how they usually clean their ears.

Inspect the nares for signs of inflammation, discharge, lesions, edema, and deformity (see Chapter 16). If your patient has any type of tubing in the nares (e.g., oxygen, nasogastric), observe for tissue damage (pressure ulcer), localized tenderness, inflammation, drainage, and bleeding.

For patients who wear eyeglasses, contact lenses, artificial eyes, or hearing aids, assess knowledge regarding methods used to care for the aids. Have your patient describe typical care for the aids and watch him or her perform care when possible.

Patients at Risk for Hygiene Problems. Some patients present risks that require more attentive and rigorous hygiene care (Table 29-6). These risks result from side effects of medications or other medical therapy; lack of knowledge; immobilization; an inability to perform hygiene; or a physical condition that potentially injures the skin, feet and nails, hair, or oral-cavity structures. Anticipate whether a patient is predisposed to any risks and follow through with a complete assessment. Timely identification of risks and preventive care reduces injury to skin, feet, nails, or oral mucosa. For example, patients who receive broad-spectrum antibiotics are at risk for the medication destroying normal flora in their mouths, allowing the overgrowth of opportunistic microbes. You need to more thoroughly and frequently observe their oral cavity for inflammation and lesions. Ask these patients if they have noticed sores or tenderness in the mouth.

Older Adult Considerations. Changes associated with aging affect the hygiene needs of older adults. Observe for **xerosis** (abnormal dryness of the skin), which is marked by cracking of the skin, especially on the extremities but also on the trunk and face (Touhy and Jett, 2010). Question older adults about itching, which accompanies xerosis; observe for evidence of skin trauma caused by scratching. Assess the usual frequency and time length of bathing, temperature of the water, and type of products used for skin care.

TABLE 29-5 HAIR AND SCALP PROBLEMS

PROBLEM	CHARACTERISTICS	IMPLICATIONS	INTERVENTIONS
Dandruff	Scaling of the scalp accompanied by itching; in severe cases dandruff on eyebrows	Dandruff may cause psychological distress or embarrassment; secondary bacterial or fungal infections may develop.	Shampoo regularly (preferably daily) with over-the-counter dandruff or medicated shampoo. Loosen scales by scrubbing vigorously with fingers for at least 5 minutes; rinse thoroughly. Make an appointment with health care provider if symptoms do not respond to over-the-counter treatments.
Ticks	Small gray-brown parasites that burrow into skin and suck blood	Ticks sometimes transmit Rocky Mountain spotted fever, Lyme disease, and tularemia.	Using fine-tipped tweezers, grasp tick as close to surface of skin as possible and pull upward with steady, even pressure. Hold until tick pulls out, usually for about 3-4 minutes. Avoid twisting or jerking because this can cause the mouth parts to break off. If this happens, remove the mouth parts with tweezers. After removing the tick, clean the area and perform hand hygiene. If you develop a rash or fever within the next several weeks see your health care provider, being sure to tell him or her about your recent tick bite (CDC, 2011).
Pediculosis capitis (head lice)	Tiny grayish-white parasitic insects that attach to hair strands; eggs look like oval particles, resemble dandruff; bites or pustules may be found behind ears and at hairline	Head lice are difficult to remove and if not treated spread to furniture and other people.	Wearing gloves, check entire scalp with tongue depressor or special lice comb. Caution against use of products containing lindane because the ingredient is a neurotoxin known to cause adverse reactions (CDC, 2010). Check hair for nits and comb with a nit comb for 2 to 3 days until all lice and nits have been removed. Vacuum infested areas of home and car upholstery.
Pediculosis corporis (body lice)	Tend to cling to clothing, making them difficult to see; body lice suck blood and lay eggs on clothing and furniture	Patient itches constantly; scratches on skin become infected; hemorrhagic spots appear on skin where lice are sucking blood.	Have patient bathe or shower thoroughly; after drying skin, apply lotion for eliminating lice; after 12 to 24 hours have patient take another bath or shower; bag infested clothing or linen until laundered.
Pediculosis pubis (crab lice)	Found in pubic hair; grayish-white with red legs	Lice spread through bed linen, clothing, furniture, or sexual contact.	Shave hair off affected areas; cleanse as for body lice; if lice were sexually transmitted, patient needs to notify partner.
Alopecia	Balding patches; hair becomes brittle and broken; caused by improper use of hair curlers and picks, tight braiding, hot styling tools, certain diseases	Patches of uneven hair growth and loss alter patient's appearance. Alopecia is very distressing for all patients, especially women.	Stop hair-care practices that damage hair (e.g., teasing hair, hair picks, tight braiding, excessive heat when blow-drying).

Too-lengthy bathing with hot water and harsh soaps can cause the skin of the older adult to become dry and easily damaged. Although dry skin may be a part of aging or the effect of environmental factors, overly dry skin may also indicate more serious systemic disease or dehydration. Include assessment of the older adult's fluid and nutrient intake because inadequacies can contribute to drying of an older adult's skin. Because the dermis loses about 20% of its thickness with aging (Saxon et al., 2010), carefully observe the skin for damage, especially in patients who have limited movement or those with impaired sensation. **Skin tears** (traumatic wounds in which the epidermis separates from the dermis)

TABLE 29-6 RISK FACTORS FOR HYGIENE PROBLEMS

RISKS	HYGIENE IMPLICATIONS
Oral Problems	
Patients who are unable to use upper extremities because of paralysis, weakness, or restriction (e.g., cast or dressing)	Patient lacks upper-extremity strength or hand dexterity needed to brush teeth.
Dehydration, inability to take fluids or food by mouth (NPO)	Causes excess drying and fragility of mucosa; increases accumulation of secretions on tongue and gums.
Presence of nasogastric or oxygen tubes; mouth breathers	Causes drying of mucosa, which increases risk for breakdown and infection.
Chemotherapeutic drugs	Drugs kill rapidly multiplying cells, including normal cells lining oral cavity. Ulcers and inflammation **(stomatitis)** develop with resulting discomfort.
Broad-spectrum antibiotics	Destroy normal oral flora, allowing overgrowth of opportunistic microbes.
Over-the-counter lozenges, cough drops, antacids, and chewable vitamins	Medications contain large amounts of sugar. Repeated use increases sugar or acid content in mouth, increasing risk for tooth and gum problems.
Altered blood clotting caused by medications or disease states	Predisposes to bleeding gums spontaneously or with oral care.
Endotracheal intubation with mechanical ventilation	Potential for ventilator-associated pneumonia (VAP) exists. Use of chlorhexidine gluconate 2% rinse reduces risk of VAP (Munro et al., 2009).
Radiation therapy to head and neck	Causes oral mucositis, which affects all mucosal folds within oral cavity, resulting in erythema, ulceration, and pain (NCI, 2013).
Oral surgery, trauma to mouth, placement of oral airway	Cause trauma to oral cavity with swelling, ulcerations, inflammation, and bleeding.
Immunosuppression; altered blood clotting	Predisposes to inflammation, infection, and bleeding gums.
Diabetes mellitus	Prone to dryness of mouth, gingivitis, periodontal disease, and loss of teeth.
Poorly fitting dentures	Food trapped under dentures causes mouth odor; increased risk for oral mucosa breakdown and stomatitis.
Inadequate brushing and flossing of teeth	Predisposes patients to periodontal disease.
Cardiovascular disease	Linked to periodontal disease.
Skin Problems	
Immobilization	Dependent body parts are exposed to pressure from underlying surfaces. The inability to turn or change position increases risk for pressure ulcers.
Reduced sensation caused by stroke, spinal cord injury, diabetes, local nerve damage	Patient does not receive normal transmission of nerve impulses when excessive heat or cold, pressure, friction, or chemical irritants are applied to skin.
Limited protein or caloric intake and reduced hydration (e.g., fever, burns, gastrointestinal alterations, poorly fitting dentures)	Limited caloric and protein intake predispose to impaired tissue synthesis. Skin becomes thinner, less elastic, and smoother with loss of subcutaneous tissue. Poor wound healing results. Reduced hydration impairs skin turgor.
Excessive secretions or excretions on skin from perspiration, urine, watery fecal material, and wound drainage	Moisture is medium for bacterial growth and causes local skin irritation, softening of epidermal cells, and skin maceration.
Presence of external devices (e.g., cast, restraint, bandage, dressing)	Device exerts pressure or friction against surface of skin.
Vascular insufficiency	Arterial blood supply to tissues is inadequate, or venous return is impaired, causing decreased circulation to extremities. Tissue ischemia and breakdown occur. Risk for infection is high.
Foot Problems	
Patient unable to bend over or has reduced visual acuity	Patient is unable to fully visualize entire surface of each foot, making it difficult to adequately assess condition of skin and nails.
Decreased sensation	Patient is unable to sense pressure, heat or cold, pain. Patient requires education on importance of regular foot inspection and potential for referral to podiatrist.
Eye Care Problems	
Reduced dexterity and hand coordination	Physical limitations create inability to safely insert or remove or cleanse contact lenses.

occur easily in thin skin as a result of minor trauma such as bumping an extremity or removing tape.

Decreasing circulation with advancing age can lead to yellowing, thickening, and brittleness of fingernails and toenails. Be aware that these changes may require more attention to nail care, which may not be possible for a patient because of loss of close vision acuity or limited manual dexterity (Touhy and Jett, 2012). Common foot problems of older adults include corns and calluses. Observe carefully for evidence of chemical burns or ulcerations that can occur when over-the-counter preparations are used or for evidence of damage from using razor blades or scissors to trim the corns or calluses (Touhy and Jett, 2010).

Patient Expectations. Hygiene is a very personal aspect of care for which patients have varying expectations. Personal preferences reflect a person's cultural or religious customs and beliefs. Assess your patient's usual practices and ask questions about cultural, personal, or religious practices that might affect hygiene care. When giving or helping with hygiene care, ask patients about preferred personal care items such as soap, lotion, toothpaste, and deodorant. Also ask the type of bath desired and preferred time to bathe. Ask about special grooming preferences such as hair styling, makeup, and shaving.

Each culture exhibits unique personal hygiene practices. When caring for patients from different cultures, learn as much as possible about and be sensitive to the customs, beliefs, and practices associated with the particular culture. Ask about preferred hygiene methods or any cultural restrictions. Recognize that patients from some cultures may express sensitivity to invasion of personal space and to gender of caregivers. When assessing patients ask, "How would you prefer that I bathe you?" "Are you comfortable with someone helping you? Would you feel more comfortable having a nurse of the same gender bathe you?" "Do you prefer that someone from your family helps you?"

NURSING DIAGNOSIS

Thorough assessment of a patient's hygiene status and self-care abilities identifies clusters of data or defining characteristics that support actual or at-risk hygiene-related diagnoses. Identification of the defining characteristics leads you to select the NANDA International diagnostic label that best communicates the individual patient's situation. For example, when caring for an older adult with degenerative arthritis, you observe a generally unkempt appearance. The patient states, "I can't do my own care anymore; I just can't do it." Your initial thinking is that this patient might have either *Bathing Self-Care Deficit* or *Activity Intolerance.* On closer, further assessment you observe swollen joints, weakness, and limited ROM in the dominant hand. Questioning of the patient indicates that he or she can't manipulate the basin or tub faucets. Your critical thinking and use of the NANDA–I diagnostic labels and defining characteristics help you accurately add the nursing diagnosis of *Bathing Self-Care Deficit* to the patient's care plan.

Determine whether a patient has an actual alteration (e.g., *Impaired Oral Mucous Membrane*) or is at risk (e.g., *Risk for Impaired Skin Integrity*) to appropriately focus nursing care. For example, a patient with open oral lesions requires more extensive hygienic oral care than usual, including cleansing and comfort measures and care to promote healing of the lesions. If the patient is at risk for a problem, take preventive measures. In the case of the patient at risk for impaired oral mucous membranes, keep the mucosa well hydrated, minimize foods irritating to oral tissues, and provide adequate cleansing.

Completing an actual nursing diagnosis requires identification of related factors that guide your selection of nursing interventions. A diagnosis of *Impaired Oral Mucous Membrane related to malnutrition* and a diagnosis of *Impaired Oral Mucous Membrane related to chemical trauma* require different interventions. When poor nutrition is a causal factor, consult with a dietitian for appropriate dietary supplements and incorporate patient education about diet into the plan. When chemotherapy injures the oral mucosa, follow cancer nursing guidelines regarding oral care for **mucositis** (i.e., painful inflammation of oral mucous membranes), including frequent gentle brushing with soft toothbrush, flossing, rinsing with bland rinse, limiting diet to soft foods, and applying water-based moisturizer to lips (Harris et al., 2008; ONS, 2007). Although many possible nursing diagnoses apply to patients in need of supported hygienic care, the following list offers examples of commonly associated nursing diagnoses:

- *Activity Intolerance*
- *Bathing Self-Care Deficit*
- *Dressing Self-Care Deficit*
- *Impaired Oral Mucous Membrane*
- *Risk for Activity Intolerance*
- *Risk for Infection*

PLANNING

During planning use collected data and critical thinking to develop an individualized plan of care. Identify patient goals and outcomes, set priorities for care, and plan for continuity of care. Use a concept map (Figure 29-1) to visualize how nursing diagnoses interrelate. Rely on knowledge, experience, and established standards of care, including evidence-based guidelines for care when developing a patient-centered plan for a patient's hygiene care. Consciously include the patient in this important step of the nursing process. Collaborate with other health care providers (e.g., occupational or physical therapists) in developing the plan whenever possible to promote a successful outcome.

Goals and Outcomes. Partner with a patient and family to identify goals and outcomes and develop an individualized plan of care based on the patient's nursing diagnoses (see Care Plan). Establish goals with the patient's self-care abilities, risks, preferences, and resources in mind. Focus on improving self-care abilities and the condition of the skin and oral cavity. State the patient outcomes in measurable and

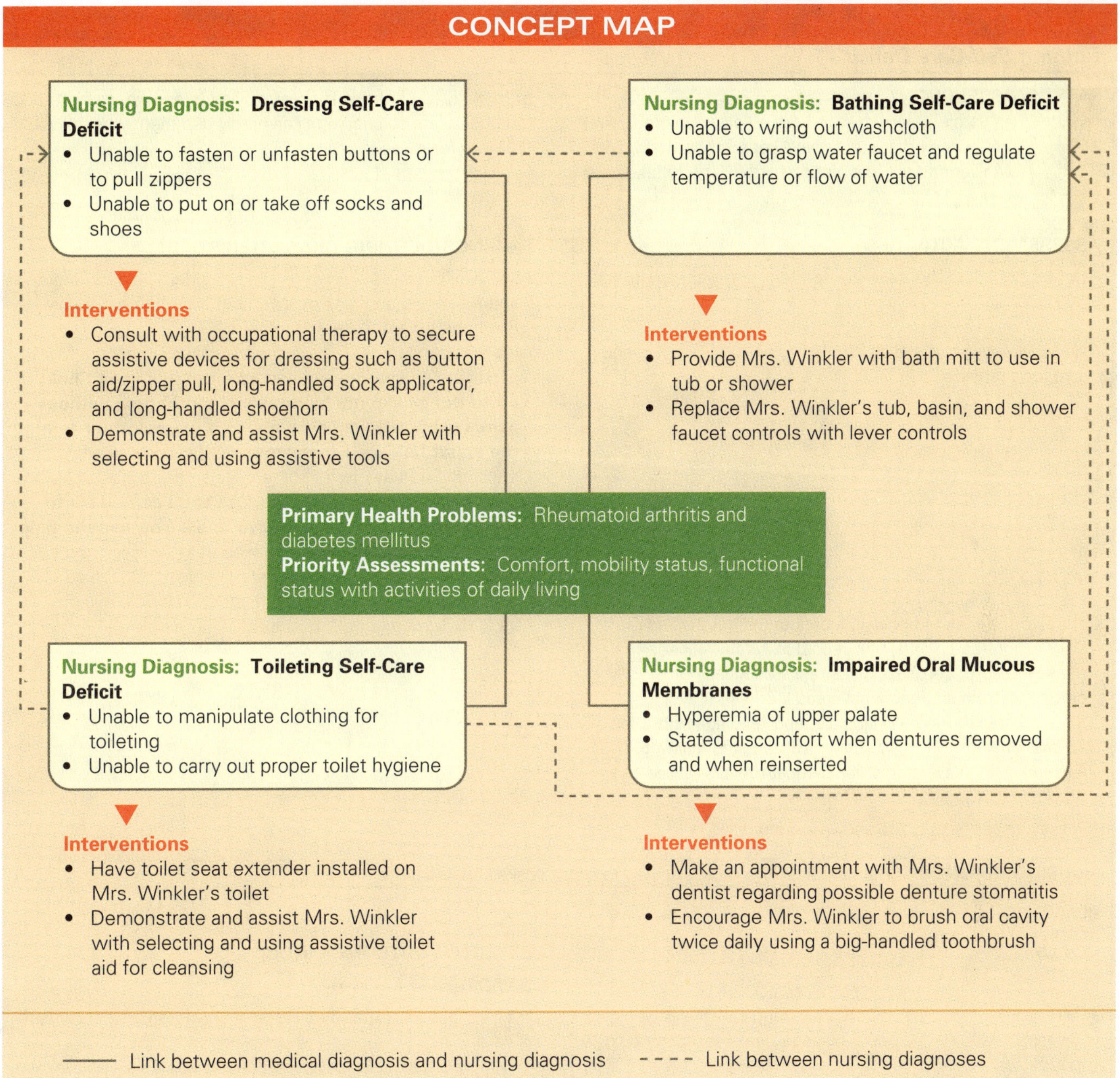

FIGURE 29-1 Concept map.

achievable terms within a patient's limitations. In addition, work with the patient to select individualized hygiene measures.

You care for a variety of patients with varying self-care abilities and hygienic needs. For example, you and the patient who has right-sided paralysis establish the following goal: "Patient's skin will remain free of breakdown." Then you create a series of realistic individualized expected outcomes. These outcomes would include the following:

- Patient's skin is clean, dry, and intact without signs of inflammation.
- Patient's skin remains elastic and well hydrated.
- Patient's skin is free from pressure areas.
- Patient tolerates bathing without excessive fatigue.

Setting Priorities. A patient's condition influences your priorities for hygiene care. Set priorities based on the necessary assistance required by patients, the extent of hygiene problems, and the patient's nursing diagnoses. For example, a patient who is seriously ill usually needs a daily bath because body secretions accumulate, but the patient is unable to independently maintain cleanliness. Some patients at home require a visit from a home care aide to help with a tub bath or shower. Patients who are normally inactive during the day and have skin that tends to be dry may need to bathe only twice a week, whereas a patient with urinary and bowel incontinence need perineal cleansing with each episode of soiling. A patient who has acute pain requires a bath, but it is necessary to administer pain medications before giving the

CARE PLAN

Bathing Self-Care Deficit

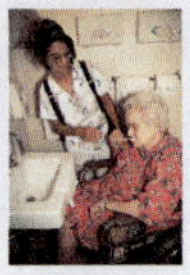

ASSESSMENT

As Jamie is talking with Mrs. Winkler before breakfast is served about helping her with her bath, Mrs. Winkler states, "It's just so hard for me to take care of myself. My arthritis makes my hands and knees hurt, and my fingers are so crippled I can hardly use them. I wish I could do more for myself."

ASSESSMENT ACTIVITIES	FINDINGS/DEFINING CHARACTERISTICS*
Ask Mrs. Winkler what care is important to her this morning.	Mrs. Winkler says, "I want to clean my dentures and mouth and feel clean and look nice without it hurting too much. But I don't want to be any trouble."
Assess Mrs. Winkler's ability to bathe, perform oral hygiene care, and dress.	Mrs. Winkler admits, "I have trouble using my hands. My hands are so crippled and hurt so much that I **can't hold on to things like my hairbrush or toothbrush without pain. I can't even squeeze my own washcloth or turn the water faucets.** I sometimes can't even button or zip my clothes. I have to let someone else dress me. Sometimes my knees hurt so much that **I can't walk to the bathroom by myself. I have to ask someone to help me."** Leaned heavily on nurse when transferring from bed to chair at bedside, did not bear full weight. Observed deformities of knee and hand (fingers and wrists) joints.
Complete the Katz Index of Independence in Activities of Daily Living (Katz ADLs) and record in Mrs. Winkler's medical record. The Katz ADLs ranks adequacy of performance in six functional areas (bathing, dressing, toileting, transferring, continence, and feeding) with total scores ranging from 6, which indicates full function, to 2 or less indicating severe functional impairment (Wallace and Shelkey, 2008).	Mrs. Katz's score is 3.

*Defining characteristics are shown in **bold** type.

NURSING DIAGNOSIS: Bathing Self-Care Deficit related to musculoskeletal impairment and pain

PLANNING

GOALS	EXPECTED OUTCOMES (NOC)†
	Self-Direction of Care
• Mrs. Winkler will be involved in directing caregivers who give or assist with her personal hygiene care within the next 2 days.	• Mrs. Winkler states two personal preferences for hygiene care today. • Mrs. Winkler selects which bathing assistive devices she wishes to use within 2 days.
	Self-Care: Bathing
• Mrs. Winkler will use assistive devices for bathing within the next week. • Mrs. Winkler will accept help from caregiver as needed and be satisfied with the bathing experience within the next week.	• Mrs. Winkler helps with bathing by using padded shower chair, bath mitt, and large-grip shower spray mounted in shower within the next week. • Mrs. Winkler regulates water flow and temperature in shower using lever handles within the next week. • Mrs. Winkler states satisfaction with use of assistive devices and help from caregiver when needed within the next week.

†Outcome classification labels from Moorhead S et al, editors: *Nursing outcomes classification (NOC)*, ed 5, St Louis, 2013, Mosby.

INTERVENTIONS (NIC)‡	RATIONALE
Self-Care Assistance: Bathing/Hygiene	
• Share results of the Katz ADLs Index with Mrs. Winkler and include her in selection of assistive devices for bathing.	Determining patient's preferences and expressed needs and including these in the plan of care fosters patient-centered care (Cronenwett et al., 2007).

CARE PLAN—cont'd

Bathing Self-Care Deficit

• Coordinate with social services and occupational therapy to obtain selected assistive devices for Mrs. Winkler.	The registered nurse coordinates care delivery.
• Teach Mrs. Winkler how to safely use the selected assistive devices by going over printed material and demonstrating and supervising her use of the devices. Allow adequate time for instruction and practice and encourage expression of concerns and questions.	Teaching plan addresses the three domains of learning (cognitive, affective, and psychomotor) and multiple teaching methods (Edelman and Mandle, 2010).

‡Intervention classification labels from Bulechek GM et al, editors: *Nursing interventions classification (NIC)*, ed 6, St Louis, 2013, Mosby.

EVALUATION

NURSING ACTIONS	PATIENT RESPONSE/FINDING	ACHIEVEMENT OF OUTCOME
Ask Mrs. Winkler to state two personal preferences for hygiene care.	Mrs. Winkler states that she prefers to have her care in the morning after breakfast and shower instead of taking a bath.	Able to be involved in direction of care and express personal preferences for type and timing of hygiene care.
Ask Mrs. Winkler to state which bathing assistive devices she has selected.	Mrs. Winkler states that she would like to try the padded shower chair, the bath mitt, the lever shower controls, and the large-grip shower spray.	Able to be involved in direction of care and express personal preferences by selecting bathing assistive devices.
Ask Mrs. Winkler if her hygiene needs were satisfactorily met by the caregiver, with consideration for her preferences.	Mrs. Winkler states, "You were so kind and gentle. I appreciate that. You helped me but let me do what I could. My joints feel better after the warm shower, and I feel clean. I am pleased with my care."	Verbally expresses satisfaction with hygiene care, including level of fulfillment and caregiver consideration of preferences and personal needs.
Observe patient during shower to note use of assistive devices.	Observed Mrs. Winkler safely maneuver the handheld spray and use the padded shower chair and bath mitt. Mrs. Winkler was not able to adequately grasp the lever shower controls and needed help to regulate flow and temperature of the shower.	Able to safely use all of the assistive devices except for the lever shower control. Need to search for another adaptation, perhaps increasing diameter of levers using foam overlays.
Caregiver asks patient to state level of satisfaction with use of assistive devices and help from caregiver.	Mrs. Winkler stated, "I feel so much happier since I can do more of my shower now. I love the bath mitt and the handheld shower spray. The lever handles are better than the old knobs, but I still have some trouble grasping them in my hands."	Verbally expresses satisfaction with all of the assistive devices except for the lever shower control.

bath. Plan to use assistive devices to ensure optimum level of independence and safety. For example, a patient with partial paralysis who has difficulty getting out of the tub needs to have a tub chair, handrails, or extra personnel available for help.

Timing is also important in planning hygiene care. Being interrupted in the middle of the bath for an x-ray film examination frustrates and embarrasses patients. If a patient is tired after extensive diagnostic tests, rest is an important patient priority. In this situation it is best to delay hygiene and allow the patient to rest.

Collaborative Care. Plan for care throughout a patient's hospital stay. Anticipate the need for postdischarge hygiene assistance when a patient is admitted. Consider the need to include other disciplines and services, including the social worker, occupational therapist, physical therapist, and home care agencies. Ensure continuity of care when patients are discharged to a rehabilitation facility or home. When your patient needs help because of a self-care deficit, family members often become caregivers and need to be included in the plan of care. Be mindful of the equipment and procedures needed so the patient and family caregiver are knowledgeable about the care, have the skill needed to provide it, and have access to necessary equipment on discharge.

Collaborate with other health care providers such as physical or occupational therapists and social workers. For example, physical therapists help patients with strengthening exercises needed for bathing, and occupational therapists fit patients with useful assistive devices that allow patients to pick up toileting items. Collaborate with the social worker to help gain access to community resources for hygiene activities.

IMPLEMENTATION

Although aspects of care differ, basic patient care frequently includes hygiene interventions. Regardless of patient characteristics or variations in setting, all patients require attention to hygiene. Include family caregivers in all educational interventions when appropriate.

Health Promotion. To promote healthy hygiene and self-care practices, educate and counsel patients and their family caregivers on proper hygiene techniques. Always stress ways to avoid injury and reinforce infection control practices. Incorporate adaptations for the patient's lifestyle, functional status, living arrangements, and preferences when teaching about hygiene care.

Skin Care. Teach patients ways to promote healthy skin. Demonstrate how to routinely inspect the skin for changes in color or texture and to report changes or abnormalities to their health care provider. Instruct patients to handle the skin gently, avoiding excessive or rough rubbing. Advise against use of hot water for bathing and too-lengthy bathing sessions to prevent loss of oils and excessive drying of skin. Also encourage patients to eat a balanced diet, including foods rich in antioxidants, vitamins, and minerals, and to drink adequate fluids. Stress safety concerns in the home such as failure to adjust the water temperature when bathing or showering or slipping on wet surfaces in the bathroom. Ensure that patients understand that healthy and intact skin protects them from infections.

Oral Care. Teach patients proper brushing and flossing techniques. The American Dental Association (2012) guidelines for effective oral hygiene include brushing the teeth at least twice a day with American Dental Association–accepted fluoride toothpaste. A soft-bristled toothbrush with a straight handle and a brush small enough to reach all areas of the mouth cleans best. Older-adult patients with reduced dexterity and grip may require an enlarged handle with an easier grip.

Demonstrate how to brush all tooth surfaces thoroughly. When teaching patients about mouth care, recommend that they not share toothbrushes with family members or drink directly from a bottle of mouthwash. Cross-contamination occurs easily. Instruct patients to rinse the toothbrush thoroughly after each use, store it upright between uses, and obtain a new toothbrush every 3 or 4 months (American Dental Association, 2012). Avoid using toothbrush covers, which can create a moist, enclosed environment that promotes bacterial growth.

Dental flossing removes plaque and tartar between teeth. Flossing involves inserting waxed or unwaxed dental floss between all tooth surfaces, one at a time. The seesaw motion used to pull floss between teeth removes plaque and tartar from tooth enamel. If you apply toothpaste to the teeth before flossing, fluoride comes in direct contact with tooth surfaces, aiding in cavity prevention. Instruct patients that flossing once a day is recommended (American Dental Association, 2012). Placing a mirror in front of a patient helps you demonstrate the proper methods for holding the floss and cleaning between the teeth.

Teach a patient that diet influences plaque formation and development of dental caries. Acidic fruits in a patient's diet help reduce plaque formation. A well-balanced diet contributes to the integrity of oral tissues. To prevent tooth decay, patients sometimes need to change eating habits (e.g., reduce intake of carbohydrates, especially sweet snacks, between meals). Encourage all patients to visit a dentist regularly for checkups. Teaching about common gum and tooth disorders (see Box 29-2) and methods to prevent these problems may motivate patients to follow recommended oral-hygiene practices. If finances limit options, check to see if a local dental hygiene clinic or dental school offers dental care at reduced cost.

Patients with dentures require instruction in proper care of their dentures and prevention of associated complications such as **denture stomatitis** (inflammation of the oral mucosa in contact with a denture surface) (Box 29-4). Teach a patient to remove and rinse dentures after eating by running water over them. Placing a towel in the sink helps reduce the chance of breaking the dentures if dropped. Instruct patient to clean the mouth after removing dentures with a soft-bristled toothbrush on any remaining natural teeth and on the tongue and palate. Dentures need to be brushed at least once daily with denture cleanser and a denture brush to remove food, plaque, and other deposits. Instruct a patient to avoid damaging the dentures by not using stiff-bristled brushes, strong cleansers, or regular toothpaste. Toothpastes with whitening agents are particularly abrasive and should not be used on dentures. Advise a patient to remove dentures, soak them overnight, and rinse well before replacing in the morning. Emphasize that taking the dentures out at night helps prevent denture stomatitis. Include in teaching that patients with dentures need to schedule regular dental checkups. Report any damage to dentures or any change in fit or development of tenderness or sore mouth.

Care of Eyes, Ears, and Nose. Teach patients how to safely clean the eyes, ears, and nose. Encourage them to clean the eyes by washing with a clean washcloth moistened in water. Explain or demonstrate how to clean from the inner to outer canthus and use a different section of the washcloth for each eye to limit transmission of infection.

Explain that routine ear care involves cleaning the ear with the end of a moistened washcloth rotated gently into the ear canal. Gentle, downward retraction at the entrance of the ear canal usually causes visible cerumen to loosen and slip out. Instruct your patient to never use objects such as bobby pins, toothpicks, paper clips, or cotton-tipped applicators to remove earwax. These objects can injure the ear canal and rupture the tympanic membrane. In addition, they may cause earwax to become impacted within the ear canal.

Teach patients to remove secretions from the nose by gently blowing into a soft tissue. Caution a patient against harsh blowing, which creates pressure capable of injuring the eardrum, nasal mucosa, and even sensitive eye structures. Bleeding from the nares is a key sign of harsh blowing.

Nail and Foot Care. Routine nail care involves soaking to soften cuticles and layers of horny cells, thorough cleansing, drying, and proper nail trimming. The one exception is a patient who has diabetes. *Never recommend soaking the nails if a person has diabetes or other peripheral vascular or*

BOX 29-4 PATIENT TEACHING

Preventing Denture Stomatitis

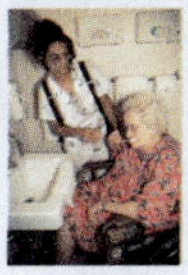

Mrs. Winkler wears full dentures. She does not usually remove her dentures at night. She finds it difficult to care for her dentures because of the deformity and pain in her hands. Usually her dentures are cleaned only once a day, and she does not rinse her mouth after eating because she is reluctant to ask others for help. To help Mrs. Winkler prevent denture stomatitis, Jamie develops the following teaching plan for her.

OUTCOME

At the end of the teaching session, Mrs. Winkler helps to perform preventive oral and denture care correctly.

TEACHING STRATEGIES

- Teach Mrs. Winkler the signs and symptoms of denture stomatitis such as redness and swelling under dentures, especially on upper palate, and small red sores on roof of mouth. Although mouth pain may not occur, patient may experience mouth discomfort with dentures in place or on inserting or removing dentures.
- Encourage Mrs. Winkler's involvement by encouraging her to report any symptoms to staff.
- Teach Mrs. Winkler that denture stomatitis commonly is caused by the following:
  - Poorly fitting dentures
  - Wearing dentures while sleeping
  - Inadequate cleansing and buildup of the yeast Candida albicans
- Teach Mrs. Winkler prevention strategies and encourage her involvement to prevent recurrence of stomatitis.
- Ask Mrs. Winkler to visit her dentist twice a year.
- Make sure that Mrs. Winkler's dentures fit properly. Encourage her to report any problems.
- Teach Mrs. Winkler what to do if her dentures become damaged (e.g., do not wear them, do not try to fix them, go to the dentist for needed repairs).
- Encourage Mrs. Winkler to rinse mouth and dentures after eating; assure her that it is appropriate to ask for staff help as needed.
- Encourage Mrs. Winkler to ask for help every night to take her dentures out and clean them with dental brush and paste. Leave teeth out overnight, soaking them in clean water. Mark calendar to clean once a week with an effervescent cleanser.
- Provide Mrs. Winkler with printed material about denture stomatitis so she can review the material after one-on-one instruction.

EVALUATION STRATEGIES

- Ask Mrs. Winkler to state the signs and symptoms of denture stomatitis and what to do if they occur.
- Ask Mrs. Winkler to state ways she can help prevent recurrence of denture stomatitis.
- Ask Mrs. Winkler to verbalize concerns about asking for help with care.

Data from Sciubba JJ, Elston, DM: *Denture stomatitis follow-up*, 2010, http://emedicine.medscape.com/article1075994-overview. Accessed August 24, 2012.

circulatory conditions. Teach patients to avoid use of harsh chemicals or long soaks in the tub. Prolonged soaking leads to softening or **maceration** of the tissue and can promote ulceration. Demonstrate proper trimming and filing techniques. For ongoing home care instruct patients or their family caregivers to use sharp manicure scissors or clippers to trim the nails straight across and round the tips by filing in a gentle curve. Explain that trimming is easiest when the nails are soft such as after the bath but to be sure that they have dried before filing to prevent splitting. Prevent drying of nails and cuticles by rubbing hand lotion into the fingernails and cuticles when applying hand lotion. Instruct to limit nail damage by not using fingernails as tools to pry things and not biting them or picking at the cuticles. If hangnails occur, carefully clip them instead of pulling them off.

People with diabetes develop many different foot complications associated with nerve damage and poor blood flow to the lower extremities. Foot injuries in the patient with diabetes can quickly turn into a serious problem with slow healing, infection, and the possibility of amputation. According to the American Diabetes Association (2012a) more than 60% of lower limb amputations for nontraumatic reasons are associated with diabetes. If a patient has diabetes or any other condition affecting peripheral circulation or sensation, recommend a podiatrist for regular examinations and trimming of nails (American Podiatric Medical Association, 2012). Also instruct these patients to report any of the following to their health care provider: abnormalities or changes in the nail, including changes in nail shape or color; bleeding around the nails; thinning or thickening of the nails; redness, swelling, or pain around the nails.

When teaching patients with diabetes about foot and nail care, advise them to use the following guidelines in a routine nail-care program (American Diabetes Association, 2012b):

- Receive a thorough foot examination at least once a year.
- Inspect the feet daily, including tops and soles of the feet, heels, and areas between the toes. Use a mirror to inspect all surfaces or ask a family member to check daily.
- Wash feet daily with lukewarm water. Gently but thoroughly pat the feet dry, especially between the toes.
- Keep skin soft and smooth by rubbing a thin coat of lotion over toes and bottoms of feet but not between toes where the increased and prolonged moisture can lead to maceration.
- Wear shoes and clean, dry socks at all times; never go barefoot. Check inside shoes before wearing them for rough areas or objects that may rub against the foot.
- If you can see and reach your toenails, trim them straight across and square; file the edges smooth.
- Keep the blood flowing to your feet by putting them up when sitting and wiggling your toes and moving your ankles up and down for 5 minutes 2 or 3 times a day. Do not cross your legs for long periods and don't smoke.

- Protect the feet from hot and cold. Do not use heating pads or electric blankets and always wear shoes at the beach or on hot pavement.

Hair Care. To best promote hair and scalp health, instruct patients to keep hair clean, combed, and brushed regularly.

Be sure to follow the practices unique to a patient's cultural or ethnic preferences (Box 29-5). Frequent brushing helps to keep hair clean and distributes oil evenly along hair shafts. Combing prevents hair from tangling.

Patients may also need to know how to check for and remove parasites (see Table 29-5). Tell patients to notify their primary health care provider of changes in the texture and distribution of hair, which may indicate a systemic problem.

Acute Care. The variety and timing of hygiene care vary across health care settings and according to individual patient needs. In the acute care setting factors such as more frequent diagnostic and treatment plans and the need for more extensive hygiene care resulting from acute illness or injury affect scheduling.

Bathing and Skin Care. Consider a patient's normal grooming routines, including type of hygiene products used and the time of day preferred for hygiene care. The extent, type, and timing or frequency of bathing and the methods used depend on a patient's physical abilities, health problems, and the degree of hygiene required. Use the tub bath or shower to give a more thorough bath than a bed bath (Skill 29-1). Clean the skin at the time of any soiling and at routine intervals. Problems such as incontinence, wound drainage, or excessive diaphoresis require more frequent cleansing to promote comfort and prevent skin breakdown and infection. A patient with overly dry skin is predisposed to skin impairment. Use soap and lotions that contain emollients to hydrate dry skin. Use the opportunity during a complete bath to reassess a patient's skin and help with joint ROM exercises.

Regardless of the type of bath (Box 29-6), use the following guidelines when bathing:

- *Provide privacy.* Close the door and/or pull room curtains around the bathing area. Expose only the areas being bathed by using proper draping.
- *Maintain safety.* Keep side rails up and the bed in low position when away from the bedside. Note: When side rails serve as a restraint, you need a health care provider's order (see agency-specific policy) for restraint usage (see Chapter 28). Place call light in patient's reach if leaving the bedside even temporarily. Protect patients from injury by assessing and controlling the bath water temperature. This is especially important for older adults and others with reduced sensation such as patients with diabetes, peripheral neuropathy, or spinal cord injuries. Use assistive devices such as bath chairs when indicated. Place a chair in the shower for a patient with weakness or poor balance. Both tubs and showers need grab bars for patients to hold during entry and exit and for maneuvering during the bath or shower.
- *Maintain warmth and comfort.* Keep room warm to prevent chilling. Control drafts and keep windows

BOX 29-5 PATIENT-CENTERED CARE

The structure of African-American hair makes it fragile and prone to breakage and damage. In addition, the hair tends to be naturally dry. According to the American Academy of Dermatology (2012b), hair loss is the fourth most common reason for African-Americans to visit a dermatologist. Ethnic hair styles often favored by African-Americans include styles that may excessively pull the hair (e.g., braids, cornrows, weaves); these styles are implicated in the development of traction alopecia, the most common form of permanent hair loss of African-American women.

Carefully observe the African-American patient for evidence of hair damage and developing hair loss. Ask for details about hair care practices and hair styles that might pull the hair. Include teaching about the risk of traction alopecia and ways to prevent or lessen this risk and promote healthy hair. Recognize that the choice of hair style and hair care practices is up to each patient; your role is to provide information and support for an informed decision. These key points should be part of your discussion (American Academy of Dermatology, 2012b).

IMPLICATIONS FOR PRACTICE

- Wash hair once a week or every other week; too-frequent washing dries the hair, but buildup of hair care products also dries.
- Use conditioner each time hair is washed, paying special attention to the ends.
- For those who work out regularly, rinse the hair to remove salty sweat buildup; apply conditioner after the water rinse.
- Use hair-care products with natural ingredients such as olive oil, Shea butter, aloe vera, or glycerin because these agents help hair retain moisture. Avoid lanolin-containing or greasy products; they may moisturize, but they also clog pores on the scalp.
- Avoid shampoos containing sulfates, which dry the hair.
- Hot oil treatments twice a month add moisture and elasticity to dry hair.
- Use heat protectant on hair after washing and before heat styling. Products with silicone provide heat shielding and hydration.
- Have hair relaxers applied only by a professional hair stylist to minimize hair damage.
- Avoid too-frequent use of relaxers, including touch-ups; allow 8 to 12 weeks between applications.
- Avoid overuse of thermal straightening devices; it is best to limit heat use to no more than once a week. Ceramic combs or irons with a dial temperature are safest.
- Protect the hair by wrapping it in a satin scarf or bonnet before bedtime.
- Braids, cornrows, and weaves can damage if too tight or in place too long. If these styles hurt, they are potentially damaging.
- Report even slight thinning of the hair or change in hair texture to your health care provider because this can be the start of hair loss.

BOX 29-6 TYPES OF BATHS

- **Complete bed bath:** Bath administered to totally dependent patient in bed (see Skill 29-1).
- **Partial bed bath:** Bed bath that consists of bathing only body parts that would cause discomfort if left unbathed such as the hands, face, axillae, and perineal area. Partial bath also includes washing back and providing a backrub. Give a partial bath to dependent patients in need of partial hygiene or self-sufficient bedridden patients who are unable to reach all body parts.
- **Sponge bath at the sink:** Involves bathing from a bath basin or sink with patient sitting in a chair. Patient is able to perform part of the bath independently. You help patient with hard-to-reach areas.
- **Tub bath:** Involves immersion in a tub of water that allows more thorough washing and rinsing than a bed bath. Patient may still require assistance. Some institutions have tubs equipped with lifting devices that facilitate positioning dependent patients in the tub.
- **Shower:** Patient sits or stands under a continuous stream of water. The shower provides more thorough cleansing than a bed bath but can be fatiguing.
- **Bag bath/travel bath:** Contains several soft, nonwoven cotton cloths that are premoistened in a solution of no-rinse surfactant cleanser and emollient. The bag bath offers an alternative because of the ease of use, reduced time bathing, and patient comfort.

closed. Cover your patient, exposing only the body part being washed.

- *Promote independence.* Encourage your patient to participate with bathing as much as he or she is able. Offer assistance as needed but assess carefully for activity intolerance.
- *Anticipate needs.* Implement actions to address a patient's pain or nausea relief before hygiene care.

A complete bed bath, tub bath, or shower (see Skill 29-1) may exhaust a patient. Be alert for a patient's activity intolerance during hygiene care. Observe respirations, noting changes in rate and depth or any shortness of breath; observe for changes in skin color. Palpate the pulse to detect changes in rate and regularity and question the patient about dizziness, weakness, or fatigue. If a patient experiences activity intolerance (e.g., rapid, irregular heart rate) during care, seek assistance, return him or her to bed, and observe carefully for improvement with rest. Provide a partial bed bath for a patient who is in need of only partial hygiene, who is too debilitated or unable to tolerate a complete bed bath, or who can perform self-care but needs help with completing the bath.

The question of whether to use bath basins with soap and water became an issue after a recent study conducted in intensive care units. Researchers found that, when using regular soap and water, bath basins provide a reservoir for bacteria and are a possible source of transmission of hospital-acquired infections (Johnson et al., 2009). There is a link between waterborne pathogens and the development of biofilm (multiple colonies of microorganisms attached to a surface such as a bath basin). The formation of a biofilm combined with transmission of organisms through contact with unwashed hands can create a reservoir of bacteria that can be transferred to and maintained in a patient's bath basin. Further study of this issue is needed on a wider variety of patient care areas. In contrast, the use of chlorhexidine gluconate (CHG) 4% solution in place of standard soap and water in wash basins has been shown to decrease bacterial growth in basins (Powers et al., 2012) Bathing with CHG 4% liquid solution using a bath basin and bath water does not increase the risk of exposing patients to bacterial contaminants from the basin itself. It is important to use a basin dedicated to bathing only and not for the storage of supplies. When using CHG be sure to dry basins completely after use, either with paper towels or by storing the basins upside down.

Currently health care–associated infections (HAIs) loom as one of the most common adverse events occurring during hospitalization, resulting in a large financial burden caused by prolonged hospitalization and in a high incidence of fatalities. Because of the high rate of central line–associated bloodstream infections with an associated mortality of up to 25% (Munoz-Price et al., 2012), several studies have been performed to test the effect of interventions to decrease these central line infections (Box 29-7). Among the interventions tested is daily bathing with impregnated chlorhexidine cloths or chlorhexidine liquid soap (e.g., Hibiclens). Findings consistently validate significant reductions in colonization and infection following use of chlorhexidine for bathing (Climo et al., 2013; Dixon and Carver, 2010; Evans et al., 2010; Kassakian et al., 2011; Munoz-Price et al., 2012; O'Horo et al., 2012). A recent study by Jury et al. (2011) investigated the effectiveness of patient bathing in decreasing the number of spores on the skin of patients with *Clostridium difficile* infections. This research provided evidence that, although neither bathing nor showering eliminated all spores, showering was more effective than bed bathing at reducing the spore load.

An alternative to the complete bed bath using soap and water or CHG and water is the use of 2% CHG no-rinse disposable cleansing cloths. There is some reported risk of skin irritation after repeated use; thus bathing a person with the cloths every other day may be an option. Another option is the bag bath. The bag bath contains a no-rinse surfactant, a humectant to trap moisture, and an emollient. Note that the bag bath does not contain CHG. When using cloths or the bag bath no bath basin is needed.

Patients with dementia require special considerations in bathing. These patients may become more confused and often combative as a result of pain, fatigue, weakness, anxiety from exposure during a bath, and discomfort from cold or drafty bathing areas (Rader et al., 2006). Bathing using the towel bath technique has been shown to be effective. This is a person-centered in-bed approach in which a nurse uses a large towel, one or two regular-size towels, washcloths, a bath blanket, and no-rinse soap and water. This technique has been shown to produce a marked reduction in behavioral

BOX 29-7 EVIDENCE-BASED PRACTICE

PICO Question: Does daily bathing with chlorhexidine compared with traditional soap-and-water bathing reduce the rate of central vascular catheter-associated bloodstream infections in hospitalized adults?

SUMMARY OF EVIDENCE

Health care–associated infections (HAIs) exist as one of the most common adverse events during hospitalization. Central line–associated bloodstream infections are one of the most frequent HAIs in the United States, with a staggering mortality of up to 25% (Munoz-Price et al., 2012). Multiple studies conducted in long-term acute care facilities and both medical and surgical intensive care units support that daily bathing with 2% chlorhexidine cloths substantially reduces colonization and bloodstream HAIs, including methicillin-resistant *Staphylococcus aureus* (MRSA) and vancomycin-resistant *Enterococcus* (VRE) infections (Dixon and Carver, 2010; Evans et al., 2010; Munoz-Price et al., 2009; Munoz-Price et al., 2012; Popovich et al., 2009). A recent study conducted on general medicine units showed a 64% decrease in the risk of acquiring an infection from methicillin-resistant MRSA and VCE infections when using chlorhexidine gluconate (CHG) (Climo et al., 2009; Kassakian et al., 2011). One of the studies (Munoz-Price et al., 2012) involved investigation of stepwise interventions, including not only the 2% chlorhexidine cloths but also use of chlorhexidine to "scrub-the hub" of central intravenous lines (see Chapter 18).

APPLICATION TO NURSING PRACTICE

- Provide educational programs to nursing staff on the effectiveness of chlorhexidine wipes for bathing in the reduction of HAIs.
- Instruct nursing staff on the correct use of chlorhexidine wipes.
- Effect changes in policy and procedure to adopt use of chlorhexidine wipes for bathing patients at high risk of developing HAIs (i.e., specifically central line–associated bloodstream infections).
- Adopt evidence-based care for central-line hubs, including use of chlorhexidine to cleanse the hubs (see Chapter 18).
- Expand study of the use of chlorhexidine for bathing other groups of patients at risk for HAIs.

symptoms when comparing the in-bed approach to showering (Rader et al., 2006).

Perineal Care. Cleansing patients' genital and anal areas is called **perineal care.** It occurs as part of a complete bed bath but also is performed at additional times as needed. Factors that result in the need for more frequent perineal care include urinary and bowel incontinence, presence of indwelling urinary catheters, menstruation, vaginal drainage or draining wounds, and obesity. Prolonged contact of urine on the skin can alter the normal protective skin flora by raising the pH of the skin; contact with moisture from incontinence weakens the skin, making it more prone to damage from friction (Chatham and Caris, 2013). Stool remaining on the skin contains active fecal enzymes that damage the skin; bacteria in the feces can also penetrate the skin and contribute to secondary infections (Chatham and Caris, 2012).

Encourage patients to perform their own perineal care if they are able. Sometimes you may feel embarrassed about providing perineal care, particularly to a patient of the opposite gender. Similarly a patient may feel embarrassed. Do not let these feelings cause you to overlook a patient's hygiene needs. When staffing permits, use a gender-congruent caregiver. A professional, dignified, and sensitive approach reduces embarrassment and helps put a patient at ease.

If a patient performs perineal care without assistance, various manifestations such as vaginal or urethral discharge, perineal irritation, and unpleasant odors may go undetected. Stress the importance of perineal care in preventing skin breakdown and infection. Be alert for complaints of burning during urination or localized soreness, excoriation, or pain in the perineum. Inspect vaginal and perineal areas and the bed linen for evidence of discharge and use your sense of smell to detect abnormal odors.

Oral Care. When patients become ill, many factors influence their need for oral hygiene. Base the frequency of care on the condition of the oral cavity and a patient's level of comfort (Box 29-8). Some patients require oral hygiene as often as every 1 to 2 hours.

Patients who are unconscious or have artificial airways (e.g., endotracheal or tracheal tubes) need special precautions with oral care because they often do not have a gag reflex (Box 29-9). While providing hygiene to an unconscious patient, you need to protect him or her from aspiration. The safest practice is to have two nurses provide the care. You can delegate nursing assistive personnel (NAP) to participate. One nurse does the actual cleaning, and the other removes secretions with oral suction equipment (see Chapter 30). While cleansing the oral cavity, use a small oral airway or a padded tongue blade to hold the mouth open. Never use your fingers. A human bite is highly contaminated. Explain the steps of mouth care and the sensations the patient will feel. Also tell the patient when the procedure is completed.

Proper oral hygiene requires keeping the mucosa moist and removing secretions that can lead to infection. Researchers have found that foam stick applicators stimulate the mucosal tissues but are ineffective in removing debris from the teeth (Grap et al., 2003). Limit the use of foam toothettes to situations in which gentle cleansing is required such as with patients who have bleeding tendencies or sustained trauma to the oral cavity. A pediatric-size toothbrush fits more easily around an endotracheal tube than an adult-size brush.

Current evidence-based practice guidelines include those for oral care in patients on mechanical ventilation. Colonization of microorganisms occurs in the oral pharynx of these patients. These microorganisms frequently move from the oral pharynx into the lungs, leading to ventilator-associated pneumonia (VAP). Dental plaque has also been implicated as a reservoir for microorganisms, leading to VAP. Current evidence supports the use of antiseptic chlorhexidine rinse as part of oral hygiene because it reduces the risk for VAP in

BOX 29-8 PROCEDURAL GUIDELINE

Performing Oral Hygiene

DELEGATION CONSIDERATIONS

The skill of performing oral hygiene can be delegated to nursing assistive personnel (NAP). However, the nurse is responsible for assessment of the patient's gag reflex to determine risk for aspiration. The nurse directs NAP to:

- Immediately report to the nurse excessive patient coughing or choking during or after oral hygiene.
- Report any bleeding of oral mucosa or gums, any patient report of pain, or any lesions.

EQUIPMENT

Tongue depressor; soft-bristled toothbrush; nonabrasive fluoride toothpaste; dental floss; water glass with cool water; normal saline or an essential oil-antiseptic mouth rinse *(optional: may follow patient preference)*; emesis basin; face towel; paper towels; clean gloves; linen bag or hamper

STEPS

1. Perform hand hygiene; apply clean gloves.
2. Identify patient using two identifiers (e.g., name and birthday or name and account number) according to agency policy.
3. Using tongue depressor, inspect integrity of lips, teeth, buccal mucosa, gums, palate, and tongue; also assess for presence of gag reflex and ability to swallow (see Chapter 16).
4. Identify presence of common oral problems (see Box 29-2).
5. Remove gloves and perform hand hygiene.
6. Explain procedure to patient, discussing preferences and willingness to help with oral care.
7. Assess patient's ability to grasp and manipulate toothbrush.
8. Place paper towels on over-bed table and arrange other equipment within easy reach.
9. Provide for privacy. Raise bed to comfortable working position. Raise head of bed (if allowed) and lower near side rail. Ask patient to move closer to side of bed or help patient move closer. Side-lying position can also be used.
10. Place towel over patient's chest.
11. Apply clean gloves.
12. Apply enough toothpaste to brush to cover length of bristles. Hold brush over emesis basin. Pour small amount of water over toothpaste.
13. Patient may help by brushing. Hold toothbrush bristles at 45-degree angle to gum line (see illustration). Be sure that tips of bristles rest against and penetrate under gum line. Brush inner and outer surfaces of upper and lower teeth by brushing from gum to crown of each tooth. Clean biting surfaces by holding top of bristles parallel with teeth and brushing gently back and forth (see illustration). Brush sides of teeth by moving bristles back and forth (see illustration).
14. Lightly brush over surface and sides of tongue. Avoid initiating gag reflex.
15. Allow patient to rinse mouth thoroughly by taking several sips of water, swishing water across all tooth surfaces, and spitting into emesis basin.
16. Have patient rinse mouth with antiseptic rinse for 30 seconds. Then have him or her spit-rinse into emesis basin.
17. Help wipe patient's mouth.
18. Floss or allow patient to floss between all teeth (see illustrations).

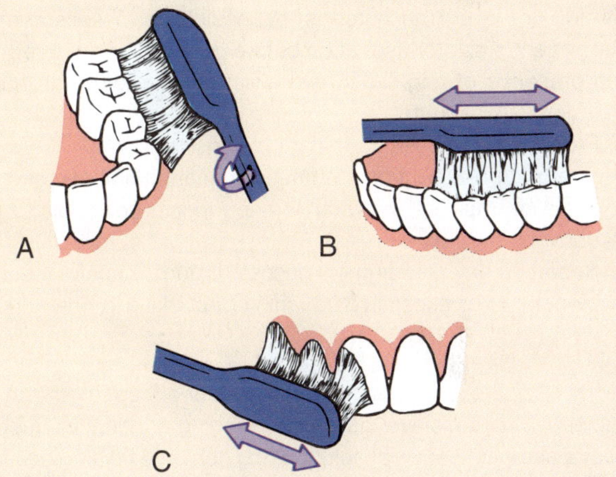

STEP 13 Direction for toothbrush placement. **A,** Forty-five–degree angle brushes gum line. **B,** Parallel position brushes biting surfaces. **C,** Lateral position brushes side of teeth.

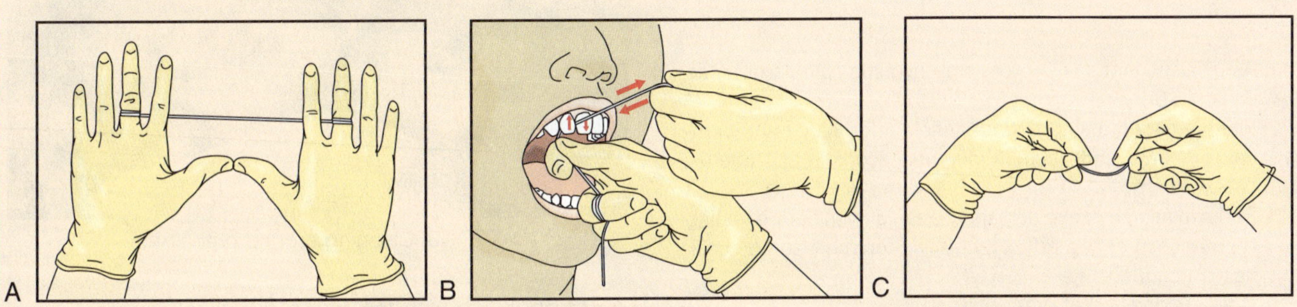

STEP 18 Flossing. **A,** Dental floss held between middle fingers to floss upper teeth. **B,** Floss moved in up-and-down motion between teeth. **C,** Floss held with index fingers to floss lower teeth.

Continued

BOX 29-8 PROCEDURAL GUIDELINE—cont'd

Performing Oral Hygiene

19. Allow patient to rinse mouth thoroughly with cool water and spit into emesis basin. Help wipe patient's mouth.
20. Inspect oral cavity to determine effectiveness of oral hygiene and rinsing. Ask patient if mouth feels clean or if there are any sore or tender areas. Remove towel and place in linen bag.
21. Use Teach Back—State to the patient, "We discussed how often you should brush your teeth each day. Tell me how often you should brush. Also explain what we discussed about the type of toothbrush to use." Revise your instruction now or develop plan for revised patient teaching to be implemented at an appropriate time if patient is not able to teach back correctly.
22. Remove gloves. Help patient to comfortable position, raise side rail, and lower bed to original position.
23. Perform hand hygiene. Apply clean gloves to clean and dry emesis basin before returning basin and nondisposable supplies.
24. Remove gloves and perform hand hygiene.
25. Record procedure, note condition of oral cavity and amount of care patient could perform and whether additional instruction is needed on oral care in nurse's notes.
26. Report bleeding, pain, or presence of lesions to nurse in charge or health care provider.

BOX 29-9 PROCEDURAL GUIDELINE

Performing Oral Hygiene for an Unconscious or Debilitated Patient

DELEGATION CONSIDERATIONS

The skill of performing oral care for an unconscious or debilitated patient can be delegated to nursing assistive personnel (NAP). However, the nurse is responsible for assessment of the patient's risk for aspiration before care, including determining presence of gag reflex and ability to swallow. The nurse instructs NAP about:

- Proper way to position patient for oral care.
- Use of an oral suction catheter for clearing oral secretions.
- Signs of impaired integrity of oral mucosa to report to the nurse.
- Reporting any bleeding of mucosa or gums, painful reaction by patient, or excessive coughing or choking to the nurse.

EQUIPMENT

Small pediatric, soft-bristled toothbrush or a foam toothette for patient with sensitive gums or bleeding tendency; fluoride toothpaste; antibacterial solution (e.g., chlorhexidine gluconate 2% rinse); tongue blade; small oral airway (optional for uncooperative patient or patient who shows bite reflex); face towel; paper towels; emesis basin; water glass with cool water; water-soluble lip lubricant; small-bulb syringe or suction catheter and machine (for patients with poor or absent gag reflex); clean gloves

STEPS

1. Assess patient's risk for oral hygiene problems (see Table 29-6).
2. Identify patient using two identifiers (e.g., name and birthday or name and account number) according to agency policy.
3. Perform hand hygiene and apply clean gloves before testing for presence of gag reflex by placing tongue blade on back half of tongue.
4. Inspect condition of oral cavity.
5. Remove gloves and perform hand hygiene.
6. Gather needed supplies.
7. Explain procedure to patient, even if patient is unconscious.
8. Pull curtain around bed and/or close room door.
9. Arrange equipment on over-bed table. If needed, turn on suction machine and connect tubing to suction catheter.
10. Unless contraindicated (e.g., head injury, neck trauma) raise bed, lower side rail, and position patient in Sims' position with head turned well toward dependent side and head of bed lowered. Raise side rail.
11. Perform hand hygiene and apply clean gloves.
12. Lower side rail. Place towel under patient's head and one across chest. Place an emesis basin under chin.
13. If patient is uncooperative or cannot keep mouth open, insert an oral airway. Insert airway upside down; turn sideways and then over tongue to keep teeth apart for cleaning. If possible, insert when patient is relaxed; do not force and do not insert your fingers into patient's mouth. Cleanse around airway (see illustration).

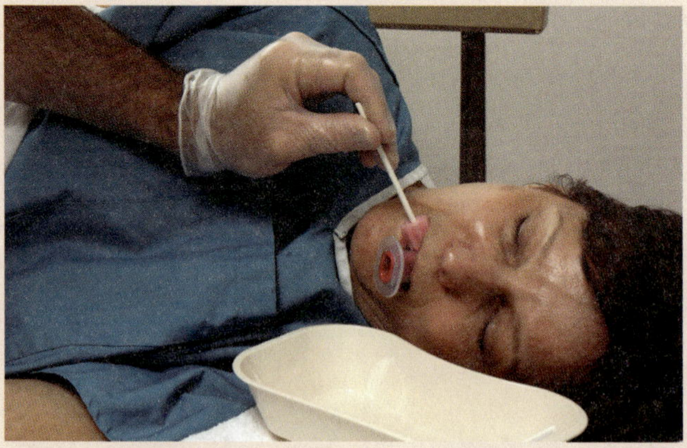

STEP 13 Cleaning around oral airway.

14. Clean mouth with toothbrush moistened in water. Apply toothpaste or use antiinfective solution first to loosen any crusts. Clean tooth surfaces with an up-and-down gentle motion. A toothette may be used for patients with sensitive gums or bleeding tendency. Clean chewing and inner tooth

BOX 29-9 **PROCEDURAL GUIDELINE—cont'd**

Performing Oral Hygiene for an Unconscious or Debilitated Patient

surfaces first. Clean outer tooth surfaces. Moisten brush with chlorhexidine solution to rinse. Use brush or toothette to clean roof of mouth, gums, and inside cheeks. Gently brush tongue but avoid stimulating gag reflex if present. Repeat rinsing several times. Use brush or toothette to apply water-based mouth moisturizer.

15. Suction secretions as they accumulate if necessary.
16. Apply thin layer of water-soluble jelly to lips (see illustration).
17. Inspect oral cavity to determine effectiveness of oral care. Ask patient who can respond if mouth feels clean.
18. Inform patient that procedure is completed.
19. Remove gloves and dispose of properly.
20. Raise side rail. Perform hand hygiene.
21. Raise bed and lower side rail. Reposition patient comfortably and return bed to low position with side rail up.
22. Apply clean gloves to gather used equipment. Clean equipment and return to proper place. Place soiled linen in proper receptacle and dispose of any trash.
23. Remove gloves and discard in trash. Perform hand hygiene.
24. Record procedure, including pertinent assessments (e.g., presence of bleeding gums, dry mucosa or lips, ulcerations, crusts on tongue, choking episode, tachypnea, or abnormal lung sounds).

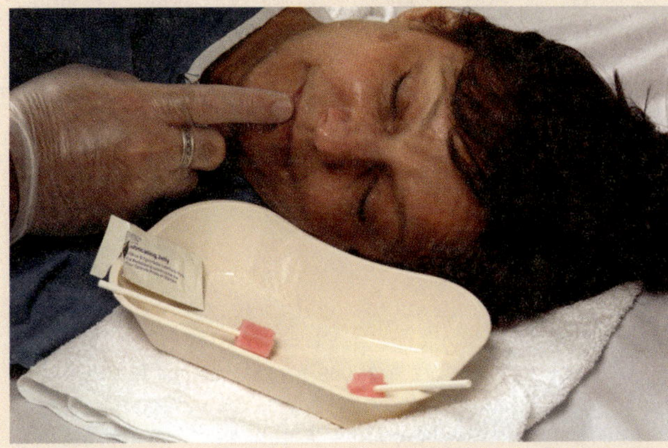

STEP 16 Application of water-soluble moisturizer to lips.

high-risk groups (Labeau et al., 2011; Munro et al., 2009; Snyders et al., 2011).

Patients receiving cancer chemotherapy, immunosuppressive agents, or head and neck radiation therapy or having nasogastric intubation or an infection of the mouth are susceptible to experiencing mucositis. Mucositis causes burning, pain, and a change in a person's food and fluid tolerance. For these patients brush with a soft toothbrush and floss gently to prevent bleeding of the gums. In some cases flossing needs to be omitted temporarily from oral care (e.g., excessive bleeding, use of anticoagulants, thrombocytopenia). Normal saline rinses on awakening in the morning, after each meal, and at bedtime help clean the oral cavity. Patients can increase the rinses to every 2 hours if needed. Instruct patients with mucositis to avoid alcohol and commercial mouthwash and to stop smoking. Consult with the health care provider to obtain topical or oral analgesics for pain control. Assess a patient's fluid and nutritional status regularly to detect inadequate food and fluid intake caused by oral discomfort (Harris et al., 2008; ONS, 2007).

Denture Care. When patients become disabled, someone must assume responsibility for denture care (Box 29-10). Dentures are the patient's personal property and need to be handled with care because they break easily. To prevent warping, keep them covered in water when they are not being worn and always store them in an enclosed, labeled cup with the cup placed in the patient's bedside stand. Discourage patients from removing their dentures and placing them on a napkin or tissue or in the bed or chair because they could easily be thrown away.

Backrub. A backrub usually follows the bath. It promotes relaxation, relieves muscular tension, and decreases pain perception. Evidence supports that **effleurage** (the long, light, gliding strokes used in a massage) may reduce anxiety, heart rate, and respiratory rate (Zullino et al., 2005). Research shows that slow-stroke back massages of 3 minutes' duration and hand massages of 10 minutes significantly improve both physiological and psychological indicators of relaxation in older people (Harris and Richards, 2010).

Always ask whether a patient would like a backrub or if he or she prefers gentle instead of deep massage because some patients dislike physical contact. In addition, consult a patient's record for any contraindications to a massage such as spinal cord injury, rib fractures, or other painful conditions.

Care of Eyes, Ears, and Nose. Give special attention to cleansing the eyes, ears, and nose during a patient's bath. Focus care on preventing infection and maintaining normal organ function.

Basic Eye Care. The unconscious patient requires more frequent eye care. Secretions collect along the lid margins and inner canthus when the blink reflex is absent or when the eye does not close totally. When an eye remains open, you may need to apply an eye patch over the involved eye to prevent corneal drying and irritation. Administer lubricating eyedrops according to the health care provider's orders.

Eyeglasses. Although eyeglasses are made of hardened glass or plastic that is impact resistant to prevent shattering,

BOX 29-10 PROCEDURAL GUIDELINE

View Video!

Cleaning Dentures

DELEGATION CONSIDERATIONS

The skill of cleaning dentures can be delegated to nursing assistive personnel (NAP). Instruct NAP to report:

- Cracked dentures or rough surfaces on dentures.
- Patient complaints of oral discomfort, sore mouth, or poorly fitting dentures.

EQUIPMENT

Soft-bristled toothbrush or denture toothbrush, emesis basin or sink, denture cleaning agent or toothpaste, denture adhesive *(optional)*, glass of water, 4 × 4–inch gauze, washcloth, denture cup, clean gloves

STEPS

1. Ask patient if dentures fit and if there is any gum or oral tenderness or irritation.
2. Ask patient about preferences for denture care and products used. You provide denture care for patients unable to care for their own dentures. Clean dentures for patient during routine oral care; dentures need to be cleaned as often as natural teeth.
3. Fill emesis basin with tepid water. If using sink, place washcloth in bottom and fill sink with approximately 1 inch of water.
4. Perform hand hygiene. Apply clean gloves.
5. Remove dentures. If patient is unable to do this independently, grasp upper plate at front with thumb and index finger wrapped in gauze and pull downward. Gently lift lower denture from jaw and tilt one side downward to remove from patient's mouth. Place dentures in emesis basin or sink.
6. Apply cleaning agent to brush and brush surfaces of dentures (see illustration). Hold dentures close to water. Hold brush horizontally and use back-and-forth motion to cleanse biting surfaces. Use short strokes from top of denture to biting surfaces of teeth to clean teeth surfaces. Hold brush vertically and use short strokes to clean inner tooth surfaces. Hold brush horizontally and use back-and-forth motion to clean undersurface of dentures.

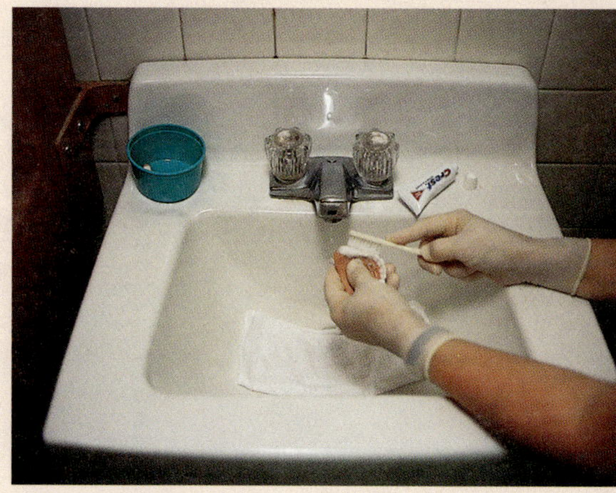

STEP 6 Brush surface of dentures.

7. Rinse thoroughly in tepid water.
8. For patient who uses an adhesive to seal dentures in place, apply thin layer to undersurface before inserting dentures.
9. If patient needs help to insert dentures, moisten upper denture and press firmly to seal in place. Then moisten and insert lower denture. Ask if dentures feel comfortable.
10. If patient does not want dentures to be inserted, place them in denture cup covered by tepid water. Label cup with patient's name and store it in safe location to prevent loss or breakage.
11. Dispose of supplies. Remove and discard gloves; perform hand hygiene.

you must use caution when handling or cleaning glasses. In addition, protect them from damage when they are not worn by placing them in a case and putting them in a drawer of the bedside table when not in use. You can cleanse the lenses with cool water and use a soft cloth for drying to prevent scratching them. Avoid use of paper towels for cleansing or drying glasses. Plastic lenses in particular scratch easily; special cleansing solutions and drying tissues are available.

Contact Lenses. Contact lenses are relatively easy to apply and remove. If patients are able, have them remove daily-wear lenses nightly for cleaning and disinfection, Extended-wear lenses may be worn overnight and are removed at least weekly for cleaning and disinfection.

Care of contact lenses includes proper cleaning, insertion and removal, and storage. When patients require help to clean their contact lenses, first perform hand hygiene and then clean and disinfect the lenses with the appropriate contact lens solution. Before reinsertion rinse the lenses with the appropriate solution such as sterile saline. Instruct the patient to never use saliva or homemade solutions when cleaning contacts to avoid potential eye infections and to clean the contact lens case frequently with warm water and allow to air dry.

When patients are admitted to hospitals or agencies in unresponsive or confused states, it is important to determine if they wear contact lenses and if the lenses are in place. If a seriously ill patient is wearing contact lenses and no one detects this, severe corneal injury results. If you determine that your patient has contact lenses in place and the patient cannot remove them, seek assistance in removing the lenses from the patient's eyes. Once you remove the lenses, be sure to document their removal, the condition of the patient's eyes following removal, and whether you gave the lenses to a relative or placed them with the patient's valuables.

Ear Care. To properly clean the outer ear, insert one end of a cotton swab along the pinna or outer shell of the ear at the top. Then swipe clean by moving the cotton swab down following the curve of the ear. Place the end of the cotton swab at the opening of the ear canal and gently wipe the entrance of the ear canal clean. Do not occlude the ear with the swab or try to clean the inside. This can damage the tympanic membrane and cause earwax to become impacted in the ear.

When earwax is impacted, you can usually remove it by irrigation, which requires a health care provider's order. Review the order for type of solution and ear(s) to receive the irrigation. Before irrigation question a patient for history of perforated eardrum and inspect his or her tympanic membrane to be sure that it is intact; a perforated tympanic membrane is a contraindication to irrigation. Visually inspect the pinna and external meatus for redness, swelling, drainage, and presence of foreign objects. If an object (e.g., dried bean) is in the ear canal, do not perform irrigation. Use an otoscope to inspect deeper portions of the auditory canal and the tympanic membrane (see Chapter 16). Determine the patient's ability to hear in the affected ear before irrigation.

To irrigate the ear, have a patient sit or lie on the side with the affected ear up. Place a curved emesis basin under the affected ear. For adults and children over 3 years of age, gently pull the pinna up and back. In children 3 years of age or younger, the pinna should be pulled down and back. Using a bulb irrigating syringe, gently wash the ear canal with warm solution (37° C [98.6° F]), being careful not to occlude the canal, which results in pressure on the tympanic membrane. Direct the fluid slowly and gently toward the superior aspect of the ear canal, maintaining the flow in a steady stream. Periodically during the irrigation ask if the patient is experiencing pain, nausea, or vertigo. These symptoms indicate that the solution is too hot or too cold or is being instilled with too much pressure. After the canal is clear, wipe off any moisture from the ear with cotton balls and inspect the canal for remaining earwax.

Nasal Care. If a patient is unable to remove nasal secretions, help by using a wet washcloth or a cotton-tipped applicator moistened in water or saline. Never insert the applicator beyond the length of the cotton tip. You can also remove excessive nasal secretions by gentle suctioning (see Chapter 30).

When patients have nasogastric, feeding, or endotracheal tubes inserted through the nares, change the tape anchoring the tube at least once a day. When the tape becomes moist from nasal secretions, the skin and mucosa can easily become macerated (softened by soaking). Friction from a tube causes a tissue injury. Anchor tubing correctly with tape or fixative devices to minimize tension or friction on the nares (Figure 29-2).

Nail and Foot Care. Routine care involves soaking to soften cuticles and layers of horny cells, thorough cleaning, drying, and proper nail trimming. In some settings or with specific patients such as a person with diabetes mellitus or peripheral vascular disease, you need a health care provider's order to trim toenails. You provide foot and nail care in bed for an immobilized patient or have the patient sit in a chair (Box 29-11).

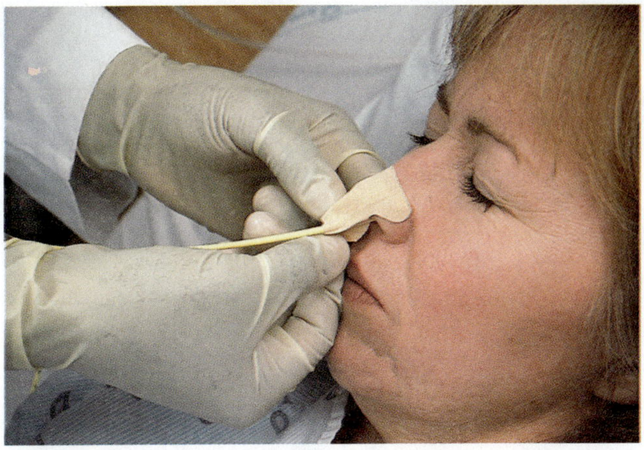

FIGURE 29-2 Apply new fixative device over feeding tube.

Recognize conditions that place a patient at increased risk for amputation such as uncontrolled diabetes, peripheral neuropathy, limited joint mobility, bony deformity, peripheral vascular disease, and a history of skin ulcers or previous amputation. Observe for changes that indicate peripheral neuropathy or vascular insufficiency (Box 29-12).

Hair Care. Patients appreciate the opportunity to have their hair brushed and combed before others visit them. Long hair easily becomes matted when a patient is confined to bed, even for a short period. Blood and topical medications also cause tangling when lacerations or incisions involve the scalp. Frequent brushing and combing keep long hair neatly groomed. Braiding helps to avoid repeated tangles. Ask permission before braiding a patient's hair.

To brush hair, part it into two sections and separate each into two more sections. It is easier to brush smaller sections of hair. Brushing from the scalp toward the hair ends minimizes pulling. Moistening the hair with water or an alcohol-free detangle product makes the hair easier to comb. Do not cut a patient's hair without consent.

Frequency of shampooing depends on a patient's preferences and the condition of the hair. Remind hospitalized patients that staying in bed, excess perspiration, or treatments that leave blood or solutions in the hair may require more frequent shampooing.

The patient who is able to take a shower or bath is usually able to shampoo the hair without difficulty. Use a shower chair for the ambulatory patient who becomes tired or faint. Handheld shower nozzles allow patients to wash the hair during a tub bath or shower. If the patient is allowed to sit in a chair, you usually shampoo the hair in front of a sink. If the patient sits at the bedside, shampoo the hair as the patient leans forward over a wash basin. However, bending is limited or contraindicated in certain conditions (e.g., after eye surgery or neck injury). In these situations teach the patient and family caregivers the degree of bending allowed.

Transfer patients who cannot sit but can be moved to a stretcher for transportation to a sink or shower equipped with a handheld nozzle. Place a towel or small pillow under the patient's head and neck, allowing the head to hang slightly

BOX 29-11 PROCEDURAL GUIDELINE

Performing Nail and Foot Care

DELEGATION CONSIDERATIONS

You can delegate nail and foot care of patients without sensory or circulatory compromise to nursing assistive personnel (NAP). Instruct NAP about:

- Not clipping patient's nails.
- Use of warm, not hot, water for soaking.
- Reporting any changes that may indicate inflammation or injury to tissue.
- Any special considerations for patient positioning.

EQUIPMENT

Wash basin, emesis basin, washcloth, towels, nail clippers (check agency policy), soft nail or cuticle brush, plastic applicator stick, emery board or nail file, lotion, bath mat, paper towels, linen bag or hamper, clean gloves if drainage or lesion present

STEPS

1. Obtain health care provider's order for cutting nails (required by most agencies).
2. Identify patient using two identifiers (e.g., name and birthday or name and account number) according to agency policy.
3. Explain procedure to patient, including fact that proper soaking requires several minutes. Determine what patient knows about nail and foot care. Provide explanation during procedure.
4. Perform hand hygiene. Arrange equipment on over-bed table.
5. Pull curtain around bed or close room door (if desired).
6. Help ambulatory patient sit in bedside chair. Help bed-bound patient to supine position with head of bed elevated. Place bath mat on floor under patient's feet or place towel on bed.
7. Fill wash basin with warm water. Test water temperature.
8. Place basin on bath mat or towel and help patient place feet in basin. Place call light within patient's reach.
9. With patient sitting in a chair or lying in bed, adjust over-bed table to low position and place it over patient's lap.
10. Fill emesis basin with warm water and place basin on paper towels on over-bed table.
11. Instruct patient to place fingers in emesis basin and arms in comfortable position.
12. Soak patient's feet and fingernails for 10 minutes. *Exception:* Patients with diabetes and peripheral vascular disease should not soak nails in advance.
13. Apply clean gloves if drainage or lesions present. Clean gently under fingernails with end of plastic applicator stick while fingers are immersed (see illustration). Remove emesis basin and dry fingers thoroughly.
14. Use nail clippers to clip fingernails straight across and even with tops of fingers (see illustration) or file fingernails straight across. Shape nails with emery board or file. If patient has circulatory or sensory deficits, do not cut nails. Only file them.
15. Use a soft cuticle brush or nailbrush to clean around cuticles. Remove hands from basin and dry thoroughly.
16. Move over-bed table away from patient.
17. Scrub callused areas of feet with washcloth.
18. Clean, file, and trim toenails following Steps 13 to 15. Do not file corners of toenails. Remove feet from basin and dry thoroughly.
19. Apply lotion to feet and hands, being sure that lotion is absorbed completely; help patient back to bed and into comfortable position.
20. Evaluate condition of nails and feet when completed. Look for any remaining areas of redness or breaks in skin.
21. Use Teach Back—State to the patient, "Remember that we discussed how often to look at your feet at home. Tell me how often you will check and when you should call the doctor." Revise your instruction now or develop plan for revised patient teaching to be implemented at an appropriate time if patient is not able to teach back correctly.
22. Clean and return supplies to appropriate location; place soiled linen in bag or hamper.
23. Perform hand hygiene.
24. Record appearance of nails and feet, condition of circulation, and care and instruction given.
25. Report any breaks in skin, any reddened or tender areas, and any discomfort.

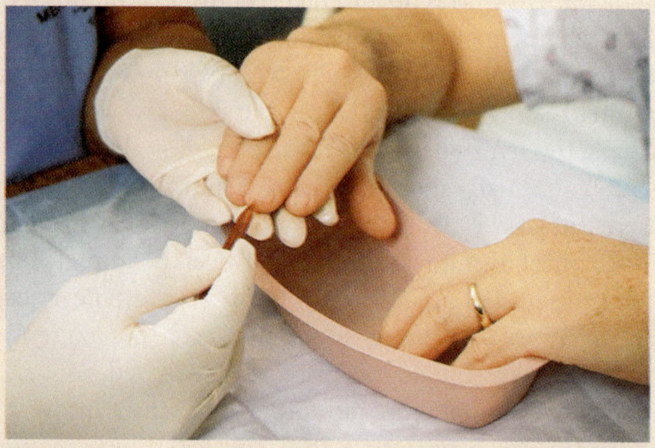

STEP 13 Clean under fingernails with end of plastic applicator stick.

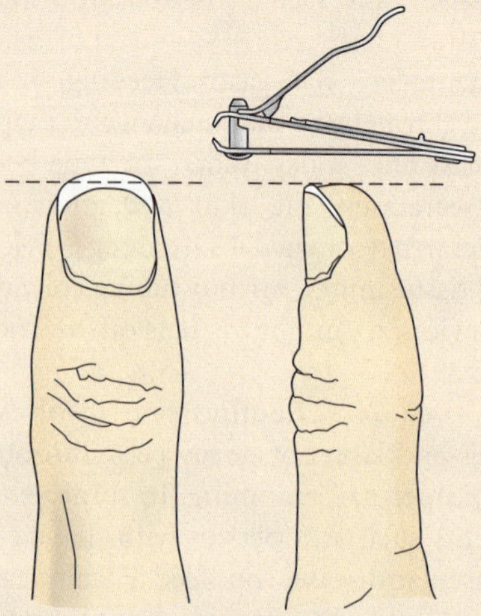

STEP 14 Clip fingernails straight across. Use nail clipper.

BOX 29-12 SIGNS OF PERIPHERAL NEUROPATHY OR VASCULAR INSUFFICIENCY

PERIPHERAL NEUROPATHY	VASCULAR INSUFFICIENCY
• Muscle wasting of lower extremities • Foot deformities • Soft tissue infection of lower extremities • Abnormal gait • Decreased or absent vibratory, touch, temperature, or painful stimuli	• Decreased hair growth on legs and feet • Absent or decreased pulses • Infection of the foot • Poor wound healing • Thickened nails • Shiny appearance of the skin • Blanching of the skin on elevation

over the edge of the stretcher. Use caution when shampooing patients with neck injuries because hyperextension of the neck can cause further injury. You need a health care provider's order to shampoo the hair of patients with neck injuries. Another option is to wash a patient's hair in the bed (Box 29-13).

When patients are unable to move, sit in a chair, be transferred to a stretcher, or tolerate a wet hair-washing procedure, various "dry" shampoo products are available. Read manufacturer guidelines carefully. In general you massage these products into the patient's hair and scalp. Some products require you to apply a towel to remove excess oil and dirt, whereas others require you to brush the product through the patient's hair.

Shaving. Shave facial hair after a bath or shampoo. Some women prefer to shave their legs or axillae while bathing. Use caution when helping a patient shave to avoid cutting the patient with the razor blade. Patients prone to bleeding (e.g., those receiving anticoagulants or high doses of aspirin or those with bleeding disorders such as thrombocytopenia and leukemia) need to use an electric razor. Before using an electric razor, check it for electrical hazards. Use electric razors on only one patient because of the risk for infection transmission.

When using a razor blade for shaving, the skin must be softened to prevent pulling, scraping, or cuts. Placing a warm washcloth over a male patient's face for a few seconds, followed by application of shaving cream or a lathering of mild soap, softens the skin. You need to shave patients when they are unable to shave themselves independently. To avoid causing discomfort or razor cuts, gently pull the skin taut and use short, firm razor strokes in the direction the hair grows. Short downward strokes work best to remove hair over the upper lip. A patient usually explains the best way to move the razor across the skin. Facial hair of African-Americans tends to be curly and becomes ingrown unless shaved close to the skin.

Mustache and Beard Care. Mustaches or beards require daily grooming. Grooming keeps food particles and mucus from collecting in the hair. You need to groom a patient's mustache and beard if the patient is unable to carry out self-care. Comb out beards gently and obtain a patient's permission before trimming or shaving off a mustache or beard.

Continuing and Restorative Care. In extended care facilities and nursing homes, hygiene care may be scheduled less frequently than in the acute care setting. Aging adults comprise the majority of patients cared for in extended care facilities. Both the normal effects of aging and abnormal changes such as urinary and bowel incontinence and increased incidence of dementia create special challenges for nurses when caring for patients in continuing and restorative care.

Bathing and Skin Care. Changes associated with aging include thinning, dryness, and roughness of the skin. These changes result in the need to adapt skin care when providing care for older adults (Box 29-14). The thinning of the skin and loss of elasticity associated with aging contribute to the increased frequency of skin tears among this population. These skin tears often occur where an age-related purpura has already formed. Ayello and Fulmer (2012) recommend the following interventions to decrease the risk of skin tears: Use a standardized assessment tool to determine skin tear risk; use a no-rinse, one-step bath product instead of the traditional washcloth, soap, and water bathing method; implement measures to limit trauma such as wearing long sleeves and pants; provide adequate light to decrease the chance of bumping into items, making the environment safe for patients who wander; and educate all staff and family caregivers on the risk for skin tears and ways to prevent them.

Bathing often creates discomfort for patients with dementia. Confusion causes these patients to feel vulnerable during bathing, resulting in screaming, crying, and even aggressively lashing out at caregivers. Research shows that using nontraditional bathing techniques and educating caregivers to provide person-centered care ease the conflict and reduce aggressive, negative behaviors associated with bathing activities (Hoeffer et al., 2006). Use person-centered techniques such as covering a person with towels as much as possible; avoiding rushing; using favorite soaps and no-rinse products; and padding the shower chair for comfort. Address factors that contribute to bathing difficulties such as noisy bathing areas, drafts, and overexposure of body during bathing; and support caregivers through education and provision of needed supplies (Rader et al., 2006).

Oral Care. Implement measures to prevent denture stomatitis when caring for patients who wear dentures. Also called *denture sore mouth,* denture stomatitis is a disease of the mouth and gums caused by ill-fitting dentures and poor dental hygiene habits (Sciubba and Elston, 2010). Measures to prevent denture stomatitis include rinsing the dentures after meals, cleaning them carefully, soaking them overnight, brushing and flossing remaining teeth, and teaching patients and family caregivers how to prevent this complication.

Hearing Aid Care. Hearing aids amplify sound in a controlled manner; the aid receives normal low-intensity sound

BOX 29-13 PROCEDURAL GUIDELINE

View Video!

Shampooing Hair of Bed-Bound Patient

DELEGATION CONSIDERATIONS

You can delegate shampooing hair of bed-bound patients to nursing assistive personnel (NAP). Instruct NAP:

- About the proper way to position patient with restrictions, especially those with head or neck mobility restriction.
- To inform the nurse if the patient reports neck pain.
- To inform the nurse of any skin or scalp lesions.

EQUIPMENT

Bath towels (two or more), washcloths, shampoo, hair conditioner *(optional)*, hydrogen peroxide *(optional)*, water pitcher and warm water supply, shampoo trough, wash basin, bath blanket, waterproof pad, clean gloves if open lesions on scalp, clean comb and brush, hair dryer *(optional)*, disposable gown *(optional)*, saline *(optional)*

STEPS

1. Before washing patient's hair, determine that there are no contraindications to this procedure. Certain medical conditions such as head and neck injuries, spinal cord injuries, and arthritis place patient at risk for injury during shampooing because of positioning and manipulation of patient's head and neck.
2. Perform hand hygiene. Apply clean gloves if needed.
3. Identify patient using two identifiers (e.g., name and birthday or name and account number) according to agency policy.
4. Inspect hair and scalp before initiating procedure to determine presence of any conditions that require use of special shampoos or treatments (e.g., dandruff, lice, dried blood). If lice are present, wear disposable gown and gloves during procedure.
5. Place waterproof pad under patient's shoulders, neck, and head. Position patient supine with head and shoulders at top edge of bed. Place trough under patient's head and wash basin at end of trough spout (see illustration). Be sure that trough spout or tubing extends beyond edge of mattress.
6. Place rolled towel under patient's neck and bath towel over patient's shoulders.
7. Brush and comb patient's hair.
8. Obtain warm water.
9. Ask patient to close eyes or hold face towel or washcloth over eyes.
10. Slowly pour water from water pitcher over hair until it is completely wet (see illustration). If hair contains matted blood, put on gloves, apply hydrogen peroxide to dissolve clots, and rinse hair with saline. Apply small amount of shampoo.
11. Work up lather with both hands. Start at hairline and work toward back of neck. Lift head slightly with one hand to wash back of head. Shampoo sides of head. Massage scalp by applying pressure with fingertips.
12. Rinse hair with water. Make sure that water drains into basin. Repeat rinsing until hair is free of soap.
13. Apply conditioner or crème rinse if requested and rinse hair thoroughly.
14. Wrap patient's head in bath towel. Dry patient's face with cloth used to protect eyes. Dry off any moisture along neck or shoulders.
15. Dry patient's hair and scalp. Use second towel if first becomes saturated.
16. Comb hair to remove tangles and dry with dryer if desired.
17. Apply oil preparation or conditioning product to hair if desired by patient.
18. Help patient to comfortable position and complete styling of hair.

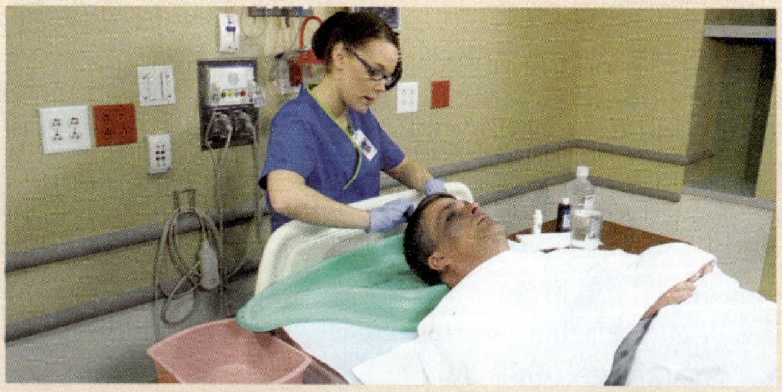

STEP 5 Patient positioned for shampoo.

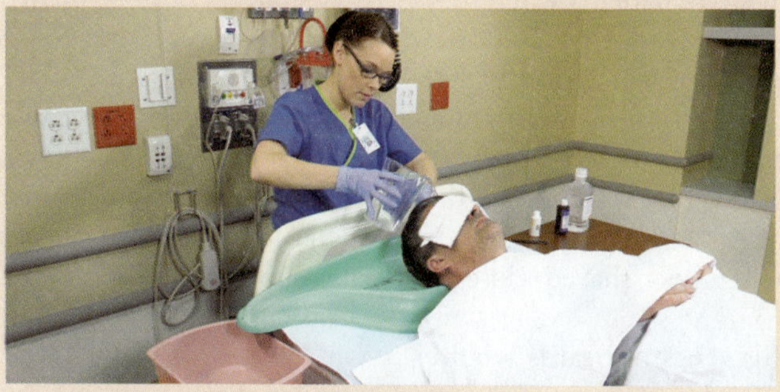

STEP 10 Wetting patient hair.

BOX 29-14 CARE OF THE OLDER ADULT

Skin Changes with Aging

- Skin changes associated with aging include thinning, dryness, and roughness. Epithelial renewal may take 30% to 50% longer in the older adult because keratinocytes become smaller and regeneration slows (Touhy and Jett, 2010).
- The dermis loses approximately 20% of its thickness with aging (Saxon et al., 2010).
- The American Academy of Dermatology (2010) recommendations for aging skin care include:
  - Bathing daily using warm (not hot) water, limiting bath or shower time to 5 to 10 minutes.
  - Closing bathroom door to maximize humidity.
  - Using only mild cleansers; avoiding deodorant bars, perfumed soaps, and any products with alcohol.
  - Gently patting skin dry.
  - Applying moisturizer within 3 minutes of getting out of bath or shower; this maximizes trapping of moisture in skin.
  - Moisturizing more frequently throughout the day as needed.
  - Selecting correct type of moisturizer. Ointments and creams are better suited for dry skin than lotions.
  - Checking ingredients in moisturizer. Those with lactic acid and urea alleviate severe dryness. Hyaluronic acid helps skin hold water, whereas dimethicone and glycerin can draw water to skin and keep it there. Mineral oil, lanolin, and petrolatum work well to trap moisture in skin.
  - Checking any antiaging products for presence of retinoids or an alpha-hydroxy acid, which can cause irritation and dry, itchy skin.
  - Considering using humidifier in dry environments.
  - Avoiding clothing that irritates such as wool or other rough, textured materials.
  - Protecting hands by wearing gloves when out in cold, dry air; applying hand cream after each handwashing; and wearing waterproof gloves if hands are frequently in water.
  - Wearing sunscreen daily, even in winter; using sunscreen with a Sun Protection Factor (SPF) of 30 or higher on all exposed skin.
  - Using lip balm with an SPF of at least 30.
  - Seeing a dermatologist if these measures do not relieve overly dry skin.

inputs and delivers them to the patient's ear as louder outputs. Hearing aids come in a variety of types (see Chapter 38). Box 29-15 outlines care for a patient with a hearing aid, including patient teaching.

BOX 29-15 CARE AND USE OF HEARING AIDS

Follow these guidelines when caring for a patient's hearing aids and when teaching patients about care of hearing aids:

- Perform hand hygiene before handling the aid.
- Check battery by holding hearing aid in your hand and turning up volume. If battery is working, you hear a "whistle." This is feedback noise.
- After inserting or applying the hearing aid, slowly turn up volume to one-third to one-half volume to obtain a comfortable hearing level for talking at a distance of 1 yard.
- A whistling sound while patient is wearing hearing aid indicates incorrect earmold insertion, improper fit of aid, or buildup of earwax or fluid.
- Do not wear aid under heat lamp or hair dryer or in very wet, cold weather.
- Do not store aid in warm place such as a windowsill or in a car. Heat can change the shape of the earmold, causing aid to not fit properly.
- Remove battery from hearing aid when it is not being used for a day or longer.
- Avoid dropping aid or twisting cord.
- Remove aid before radiological examination or radiation therapy to avoid damage.
- Protect aid from water, alcohol, aerosol sprays, perspiration, and cologne.
- Use manufacturer-recommended cleaning solution and soft, lint-free cotton cloth to clean earmold. Regularly remove cerumen from aid with a wax loop or device supplied with aid.

Data from National Institute on Deafness and Other Communication Disorders: Hearing aids, Pub. No. 08-4340, Bethesda, MD, 2008, National Institutes of Health, http://www.nidcd.nih.gov/staticresources/health/hearing/HearingAids07.pdf. Accessed August 22, 2012.

PATIENT'S ROOM ENVIRONMENT

Attempt to make a patient's room as comfortable as the home. The room needs to be safe and large enough to allow patients and their visitors to move about freely. Control room temperature, ventilation, noise, and odors.

Maintaining Comfort

Depending on age and physical condition, maintain the room temperature between 20° and 23° C (68° and 73.4° F). Infants, older adults, and the acutely ill often need a warmer room. However, certain ill patients benefit from cooler room temperatures to lower body metabolic demands. Protect the acutely ill, infants, and older adults from drafts by ensuring that they are adequately dressed and covered with a lightweight blanket.

An effective ventilation system keeps stale air and odors from lingering in a room. Good ventilation reduces lingering odors caused by draining wounds, emesis, bowel movements, and used bedpans and urinals. Always empty and cleanse bedpans or urinals promptly. Room deodorizers help remove many unpleasant odors. Before using room deodorizers, determine that your patient is not allergic or sensitive to the deodorizer itself.

Make every effort to control the noise level, especially when patients are trying to sleep. Explain the source of unfamiliar noises such as an IV pump or pulse oximeter alarm. Proper lighting provides for safety and comfort. A brightly lit room usually stimulates, whereas a darkened room promotes rest and sleep. Adjust room lighting by closing or opening drapes, regulating over-bed and floor lights, and closing or opening room doors. When entering a patient's room at night, avoid abruptly turning on the overhead light unless necessary.

Room Equipment

Although there are variations across health care settings, a typical room contains an over-bed table, bedside stand, chairs, and bed (Figure 29-3). An over-bed table rolls on wheels and adjusts to various heights over the bed or a chair. The table provides ideal working space for performing procedures. It also serves as a surface on which to place meal trays, toiletry items, and objects that a patient frequently uses. Clean the top of the over-bed table with an antiseptic cleaner before using it for meals. Do not place a bedpan or urinal on the over-bed table. Use the bedside stand to store a patient's personal possessions and hygiene equipment. Patients often use bedside stands for their telephone, water pitcher, and drinking cup.

Most patient rooms contain an armless straight-backed chair or an upholstered lounge chair with arms. Armless straight-backed chairs are convenient when temporarily transferring a patient from the bed such as during bed making. Upholstered lounge chairs or recliners tend to be more comfortable when patients are able to sit for an extended period.

Each room usually has an over-bed light and floor level night lighting. Patients often have access to lighting controls via their call light system. Additional portable or built-in special-examination lighting provides extra light during bedside procedures.

Other equipment usually found in a patient's room includes a call light, a television set, a wall-mounted blood pressure gauge, oxygen and vacuum wall outlets, and personal care items. Special equipment designed for promoting comfort or positioning patients includes footboards and foot boots, special mattresses, and bed boards.

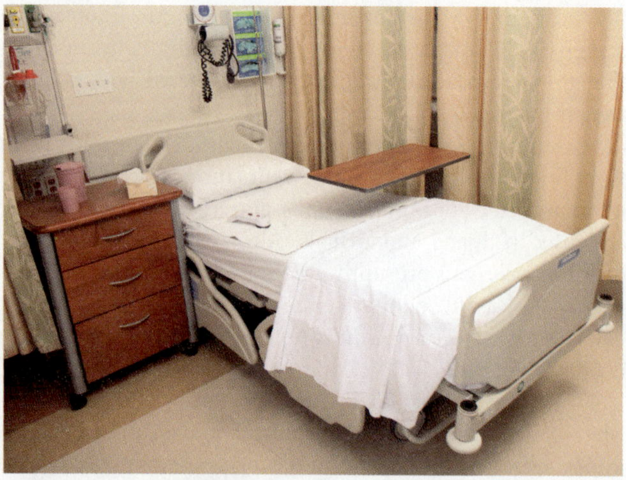

FIGURE 29-3 Room furniture.

Beds. Seriously ill patients may remain in bed for an extended time. The typical hospital bed has a firm mattress on a metal frame that you can raise and lower horizontally and that can be placed in various positions. You use different bed positions to promote patient comfort, minimize symptoms, promote lung expansion, and improve access during procedures (Table 29-7). You change the position of an electric bed by using electrical controls usually incorporated into the call light or in a panel on the side or foot of the bed. Become familiar with use of the bed controls. Instruct patients in the proper use of controls and caution them against raising the bed to a position that causes harm. Maintain the bed height at the lowest horizontal position when a patient is unattended.

Patients who are at risk for falling are often placed on low beds in the hospital (see Chapter 28). Special beds and mattress options are also available for patients who are at risk for pressure ulcers (see Chapter 37). Low-pressure mattresses, rotation beds, and special overlays are just examples.

All beds contain safety features such as locks on the wheels or casters. Lock wheels when a bed is stationary to prevent accidental movement. Side rails allow patients to move more efficiently in bed and prevent accidents. Do not use side rails to restrict a patient from moving in bed. When using side rails as a restraint, you need a health care provider's order (see Chapter 28). You can remove the headboard from most beds. This is important when the medical team needs to have easy access to the head such as during cardiopulmonary resuscitation.

Bed Making. Keep a patient's bed clean and comfortable. This requires frequent inspections to be sure that linen is clean, dry, and free of wrinkles. When patients are diaphoretic, have draining wounds, or experience incontinence, check more frequently for wet or soiled linen.

Usually you make a bed in the morning after a patient's bath or while a patient is bathing, in a shower, sitting in a chair eating, or out of the room for procedures or tests. Throughout the day straighten linen that becomes loose or wrinkled. In addition, check the bed linen for food particles after meals and for wetness or soiling. Change linen that becomes soiled or wet.

When changing bed linen, follow basic principles of medical asepsis by keeping soiled linen away from your uniform. Place soiled linen in linen bags before placing in the linen hamper. To avoid air currents that spread microorganisms, never shake linen. To avoid transmitting infection, do not place soiled linen or linen bags on the floor. Immediately place any clean linen that touches the floor or any unclean surface into a dirty linen container.

During bed making use safe patient-handling procedures and proper body mechanics (see Chapter 28). Always raise the bed to the appropriate height before changing linen so you do not have to bend or stretch over the mattress.

A patient's privacy, comfort, and safety are important when making a bed. If a patient is confined to bed, organize bed-making activities to conserve time and energy. Using side rails, keeping call lights within the patient's reach, and

TABLE 29-7 COMMON BED POSITIONS

POSITION	DESCRIPTION	USES
Fowler's 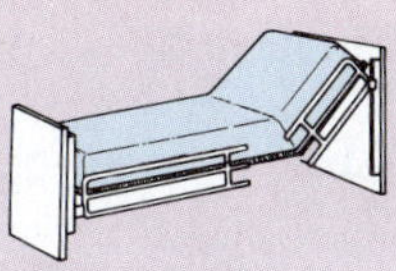	Head of bed raised to angle of 45 degrees or more; semi-sitting position; foot of bed may also be raised at knee	Used during meals and oral medication administration, nasogastric tube insertion, and nasotracheal suction Promotes lung expansion
Semi-Fowler's 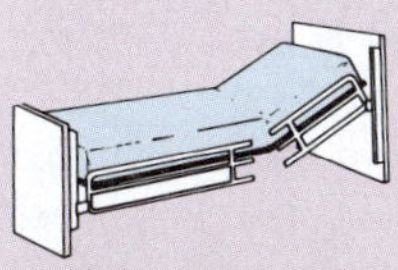	Head of bed raised approximately 30 degrees; incline less than Fowler's position; foot of bed may also be raised at knee	Promotes lung expansion Used when patients receive gastric feedings to reduce regurgitation and risk for aspiration
Trendelenburg's 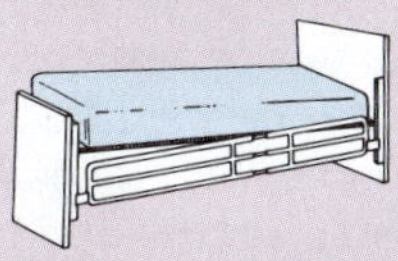	Entire bed tilted with head of bed down	Used for postural drainage Facilitates venous return in patients with poor peripheral venous perfusion
Reverse Trendelenburg's 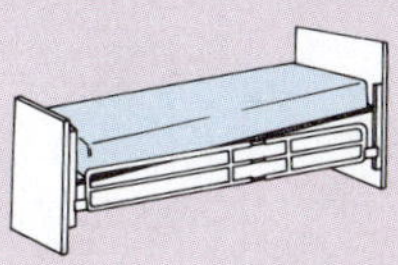	Entire bed frame tilted with foot of bed down	Used infrequently Promotes gastric emptying Prevents esophageal reflux
Flat 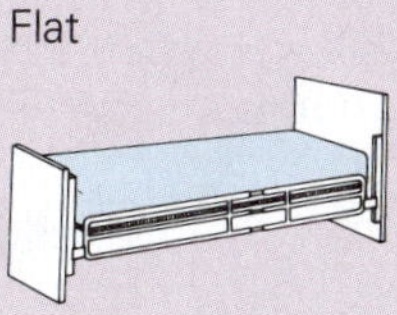	Entire bed frame horizontally parallel with floor	Used for patients with vertebral injuries and in cervical traction Used for patients who are hypotensive Generally preferred by patients for sleeping

maintaining the proper bed position help promote comfort and safety. After making a bed you always return it to the lowest horizontal position and verify that the wheels are locked to prevent accidental falls.

When possible, make a bed while it is unoccupied (Box 29-16). When making an unoccupied bed, follow the same basic principles used for making an occupied bed (Skill 29-2). The surgical, recovery, or postoperative bed is a modified version of the unoccupied bed. Fold the top covers of the surgical bed to one side or fanfold them to the bottom third of the bed to allow for easy transfer of a patient into the bed. After a patient is discharged, send all bed linen to the laundry. Housekeeping personnel usually clean and disinfect the mattress and bed and apply new bed linen following discharge.

Many agencies have "nurse servers" either within or just outside a patient's room where a daily supply of linen is stored. Because of the importance of cost control and prevention of infection transmission, avoid bringing excess linen into a patient's room. Once you bring linen into a patient's room, even if the linen is not used, it must be laundered before being used by another patient. Excess linen lying around a patient's room creates clutter and obstacles for patient care activities.

EVALUATION

Patient Care. Evaluation of hygiene measures occurs both while giving care and on completion of caregiving activities (Box 29-17). For example, while bathing a patient inspect the skin carefully to see if soiling or drainage is effectively removed. Once a bath is finished, evaluate the effectiveness of hygiene care by asking patients if they feel more comfortable and relaxed. Observe a patient's behavior during and after hygiene care to detect discomfort that might be caused by movement and activities associated with hygiene care. Is the patient restless or relaxed? Does his or her facial expression suggest a feeling of comfort? Is he or she free of body odor?

Conduct ongoing evaluation since it often takes time for hygiene care to result in an improvement in a patient's condition. For example, oral lesions and skin excoriation usually need repeated hygiene interventions. Evaluate by applying assessment measures to determine if the patient's condition and level of comfort improve over time. Throughout evaluation consider the goals of care and evaluate whether expected outcomes have been achieved. Use the established expected outcomes as the standards for evaluation.

Patient Expectations. During assessment you collect data about a patient's expectations of care. Both during and

BOX 29-16 PROCEDURAL GUIDELINE

Making an Unoccupied Bed

DELEGATION CONSIDERATIONS

You can delegate making an unoccupied bed to nursing assistive personnel (NAP). Instruct NAP:

- About any positioning or activity restrictions that apply to a patient's ability to get out of bed.

EQUIPMENT

Linen bag, mattress pad *(optional,* depending on facility practice; change only when soiled), bottom sheet (flat or fitted), drawsheet *(optional),* top sheet, blanket, bedspread, waterproof pads *(optional),* pillowcases, bedside chair or table, clean gloves (if linen is soiled), washcloth, and antiseptic cleanser

STEPS

1. Perform hand hygiene.
2. Determine if patient has been incontinent or if excess drainage is on linen. Gloves are necessary in these situations.
3. Assess activity orders or restrictions in mobility. Help to bedside chair or recliner.
4. Lower side rails on both sides of bed and raise bed to comfortable working position.
5. Remove soiled linen, holding it away from uniform, and place in linen bag. Avoid shaking or fanning linen.
6. Reposition mattress as needed and wipe off any moisture with a washcloth moistened in antiseptic solution (consult agency guidelines). Dry thoroughly.
7. Apply all bottom linen on one side of bed before moving to opposite side. Apply bottom sheet, flat or fitted.
   a. *For fitted bottom sheet:* Make sure that fitted sheet is placed smoothly over mattress from head to foot of bed and over mattress edges.
   b. *For flat bottom sheet:* Place sheet over mattress. Allow approximately 25 cm (10 inches) to hang over side mattress edge. Lower hem of sheet should lie seam down even with bottom edge of mattress. Pull remaining top portion of sheet over top edge of mattress. While standing at head of bed, miter top corner of bottom sheet (see Skill 29-2, Step 11). Tuck remaining portion of flat sheet under mattress.
8. *Optional:* Apply drawsheet, laying centerfold along middle of bed lengthwise. Smooth drawsheet over mattress and tuck excess edge under mattress, keeping palms down.
9. Move to opposite side of bed and spread bottom sheet smoothly over edge of mattress from head to foot of bed.
   a. *For fitted bottom sheet:* Make sure that fitted sheet is placed smoothly over mattress from head to foot of bed and over mattress edges.
   b. *For flat bottom sheet:* Miter top corner of bottom sheet, making sure that corner is taut. Grasp remaining edge of flat bottom sheet and tuck tightly under mattress, moving from head to foot of bed.
10. Smooth folded drawsheet over bottom sheet and tuck under mattress, first at middle of bed, then at top, and then at bottom.
11. If needed apply waterproof pad over bottom sheet or drawsheet.
12. Place top sheet over bed with vertical centerfold lengthwise down middle of bed. Open sheet out from head to foot, being sure that top edge of sheet is even with top edge of mattress.
13. Make horizontal toe pleat; stand at foot of bed and fanfold in sheet 5 to 10 cm (2 to 4 inches) across bed. Pull sheet up from bottom to make fold approximately 15 cm (6 inches) from bottom edge of mattress.
14. Tuck in remaining portion of sheet under foot of mattress. Then place blanket over bed with top edge parallel to top edge of sheet and 15 to 20 cm (6 to 8 inches) down from edge of sheet. *(Optional:* Apply additional spread over bed.)
15. Make cuff by turning edge of top sheet down over top edge of blanket and spread.
16. Standing on one side at foot of bed, lift mattress corner slightly with one hand; with other hand tuck top sheet, blanket, and spread under mattress. Be sure that toe pleats are not pulled out.
17. Make modified mitered corner with top sheet, blanket, and spread. After making triangular fold, do not tuck tip of triangle (see illustration).

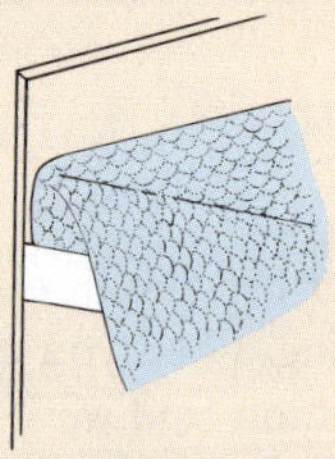

STEP 17 Modified mitered corner.

18. Go to other side of bed. Spread sheet, blanket, and spread out evenly. Make cuff with top sheet and blanket. Make modified corner at foot of bed. Alternatively fanfold sheet, blanket, and spread to foot of bed, with top layer ready to be pulled up (this leaves an open bed).
19. Apply clean pillowcase(s).
20. Place call light within patient's reach on bed rail or pillow and return bed to lowest position, allowing for patient transfer. Help patient to bed when desired.
21. Arrange patient's room. Remove supplies, returning them to proper locations. Perform hand hygiene.

after care determine from the patient that care is being provided in an acceptable manner. While giving care encourage the patient to verbalize any discomfort such as cool water temperature or discomfort with movement. To determine the patient's satisfaction with your care ask questions such as the following: "Do you think your bath helped you feel more comfortable?" "Are there ways that we can do a better job with your hygiene care?" Being aware of and addressing the patient's expectations and any concerns fosters a caring therapeutic relationship.

BOX 29-17 EVALUATION

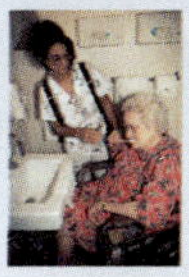

Jamie includes Mrs. Winkler in the plan to increase her self-care ability and feel more satisfied with her situation. She collaborates with occupational therapy and social services to obtain the assistive devices that Mrs. Winkler selects. After using the devices Mrs. Winkler verbally expresses satisfaction with both her involvement in hygiene care planning and with the caregivers' consideration of her preferences and needs. She states that she is much happier with her care using the assistive devices except for the shower lever handles. Jamie observes Mrs. Winkler performing care with the assistive devices, noting that she can use the devices easily and safely except for the shower levers. Jamie alters the plan to include seeking a way to make the levers larger to allow Mrs. Winkler to move them without needing to grasp them with her arthritic hands.

DOCUMENTATION NOTE

"Observed using assistive devices (bath mitt, padded shower chair, handheld shower spray, and shower levers); able to manipulate all devices without assistance except for shower levers; states 'the levers are better than the old knobs, but I still have some trouble grasping them in my hands; I feel so much happier since I can do more of my shower now'; will contact occupational therapy for ideas to improve lever grasp."

SAFETY GUIDELINES FOR NURSING SKILLS

SAFETY CONSIDERATIONS

To ensure patient safety communicate clearly with members of the health care team, assess and incorporate a patient's priorities of care and preferences, and use the best evidence when making decisions about your patient's care. When performing the skills in this chapter, remember the following points to ensure safe, individualized patient care:

- To reduce the risk of infection always perform hygiene measures moving from cleanest to less clean or dirty areas. This often requires you to change gloves and perform hand hygiene during care activities.
- Use clean gloves when you anticipate contact with nonintact skin or mucous membranes or when there is or may likely be contact with drainage, secretions, excretions, or blood during hygiene care.
- When using water or solutions for hygiene care, be sure to test the temperature to prevent burn injury.
- To avoid injury when performing hygiene care, use principles of body mechanics and safe patient handling.
- Remember that you are responsible and accountable for assessing and evaluating a patient both before and after care to detect unexpected outcomes and give proper direction to NAP when delegating hygiene care.

SKILL 29-1 BATHING AND PERINEAL CARE

View Video!

DELEGATION CONSIDERATIONS

The skill of bathing and perineal care can be delegated to nursing assistive personnel (NAP). The nurse directs NAP about:

- Not massaging reddened skin areas.
- Reporting early signs of impaired skin integrity, including redness or pallor.
- Reporting perineal drainage, discomfort, or tenderness.
- Proper ways to position male and female patients with musculoskeletal limitations and indwelling catheters.
- Reporting patient fatigue or report of pain during hygiene care.

EQUIPMENT

- Bar soap and soap dish or chlorhexidine 4% liquid soap (e.g., Hibiclens)
  - *Option:* chlorhexidine gluconate (CHG) cloths or disposable bag bath cloths
- 4 to 6 washcloths
- Bath towels
- Bath blanket
- Toiletry items (deodorant, powder)
- Body lotion (**Note:** if using CHG soap use a lotion that is hospital approved such as Aloe Vesta)
- Toilet tissue or hygiene wipes
- Warm water
- Clean hospital gown or patient's own pajamas or gown
- Laundry bag
- Clean gloves (when risk for contacting body fluids)
- Wash basin (used for bath water only)

STEP	RATIONALE
ASSESSMENT	
1. Assess patient's tolerance for bathing, activity tolerance, comfort level, cognitive ability, musculoskeletal function, and presence of shortness of breath.	Determines patient's ability to perform or tolerate bathing and type of bath to administer (e.g., tub bath, partial bed bath).

SKILL 29-1 BATHING AND PERINEAL CARE—cont'd

STEP	RATIONALE
***Clinical Decision Point:* Patients with dementia may become agitated during bathing activities. Observe for behaviors such as restlessness, yelling, and fighting with caregivers.**	
2. Assess patient's visual status, ability to sit without support, hand grasp, range of motion (ROM) of extremities.	Determines degree of assistance that patient needs for bathing.
3. Assess for presence of external medical device/equipment (e.g., intravenous [IV] line, oxygen tubing, urinary catheter).	Affects how you plan bathing activities and positioning.
4. Assess patient's bathing preferences: frequency and time of day preferred for bathing, type of hygiene products used, and other factors related to patient preferences and cultural awareness.	Promotes patient's comfort and willingness to cooperate. Includes cultural or personal hygiene preferences in care.
5. Ask if patient has noticed any problems related to condition of skin and genitalia.	Provides information to direct physical assessment of skin and genitalia during bathing. Also influences selection of skin-care products.
6. Before or during bath assess condition of patient's skin. Note presence of dryness (indicated by flaking, redness, scaling, and cracking), excessive moisture, areas of redness or inflammation, or pressure ulcers.	Provides a baseline for comparison over time in determining if bathing improves condition of skin.
7. Assess patient's knowledge of skin hygiene in terms of its importance, preventive measures to take, and common problems encountered. Include family caregivers in assessment if they ultimately will provide hygiene care after discharge.	Determines patient's learning needs.
PLANNING	
1. Review orders for specific precautions concerning patient's movement or positioning and check patient allergy history.	Prevents injury or allergic reactions from hygiene products during bathing activities. Determines level of assistance required by patient.
2. Check for health care provider's therapeutic bath order; if there is an order, note type of solution, length of time for bath, and body part to be treated.	Therapeutic baths are ordered for specific physical effect, which usually includes promotion of healing or soothing effects.
3. Explain procedure and ask patient for suggestions on how to prepare supplies. If partial bath, ask how much of bath patient wishes to complete.	Promotes patient's cooperation and participation.
4. Adjust room temperature and ventilation, close room doors and windows, and draw room divider curtain.	Warm room that is free of drafts prevents rapid loss of body heat during bathing. Privacy ensures patient's mental and physical comfort.
5. Prepare equipment and supplies. If it is necessary to leave room, be sure that call light is within patient's reach, bed is in low position, and wheels are locked.	Avoids interrupting procedure or leaving patient unattended to retrieve missing equipment. Provides for patient safety.
IMPLEMENTATION	
1. **Complete or Partial Bed Bath**	
***Clinical Decision Point:* Refer to hospital policy regarding bathing with bath basin and soap and water or use of CHG. Research suggests that bath basins holding soap and water can easily become contaminated with infectious microorganisms. CHG soap can be used successfully in bath basins without increasing infection risk.**	
a. Identify patient using two identifiers (e.g., name and birthday or name and account number) according to agency policy.	Ensures correct patient. Complies with The Joint Commission requirements for patient safety (TJC, 2014). Helps prevent injury from improper positioning or movement or from allergic reactions caused by misidentification of patient.
b. Offer patient bedpan or urinal. Apply clean gloves to help patient as needed. Provide toilet tissue. Discard gloves.	Patient feels more comfortable after voiding. Avoid raising side rail with soiled gloves.
c. Perform hand hygiene. If patient has nonintact skin or skin is soiled with drainage, excretions, or body secretions, apply clean gloves before beginning bath.	Reduces transmission of microorganisms.

STEP	RATIONALE
d. Raise bed to comfortable working height. Lower side rail closest to you and help patient assume comfortable supine position, maintaining body alignment. Bring patient toward side closest to you.	Prevents bed from moving. Helps you reach patient without stretching and reaching across bed, thus minimizing strain on back muscles.
e. Place bath blanket over patient. Have patient hold top of bath blanket and pull top sheet and bedspread down to foot of bed from under bath blanket without exposing patient.	Blanket provides warmth and privacy.
f. Remove patient's gown or pajamas.	Provides full exposure of body parts during bathing.
(1) If gown has snaps on sleeves, simply unsnap and remove gown without pulling IV tubing if present.	
(2) If an extremity is injured or has reduced mobility, remove gown from *unaffected* side first.	Undressing unaffected side first allows easier manipulation of gown over body part with reduced ROM.
(3) If patient has IV line and gown with no snaps, remove gown from arm *without IV line* first. Then remove gown from arm with IV line (see illustrations). Remove IV bag from pole and slide IV container and tubing through arm of patient's gown. Rehang IV container and check flow rate. Regulate if necessary.	Manipulation of IV tubing and container may disrupt flow rate.
(4) If IV pump is in use, turn pump off, clamp tubing, remove tubing from pump, and proceed as in Step (3). Reinsert tubing into pump, unclamp tubing, and turn pump on at correct rate. Observe flow rate and regulate if necessary. *Do not disconnect tubing.*	Regulation is necessary to prevent improper infusion of fluids. Disconnecting IV tubing places patient at risk for introduction of microorganisms into the IV line.
g. Raise side rail. Lower bed temporarily to lowest position and raise on return after filling wash basin two-thirds full with warm water. Place basin and supplies on over-bed table over bed. Check water temperature and also have patient place fingers in water to test temperature tolerance. Place plastic container of bath lotion in bath water to warm if desired.	Raising side rail and lowering bed position maintains patient's safety while you leave bedside. Warm water promotes comfort, relaxes muscles, and prevents unnecessary chilling. Testing temperature prevents accidental burns. Use of over-bed table allows you to move to opposite side of bed without having to move equipment

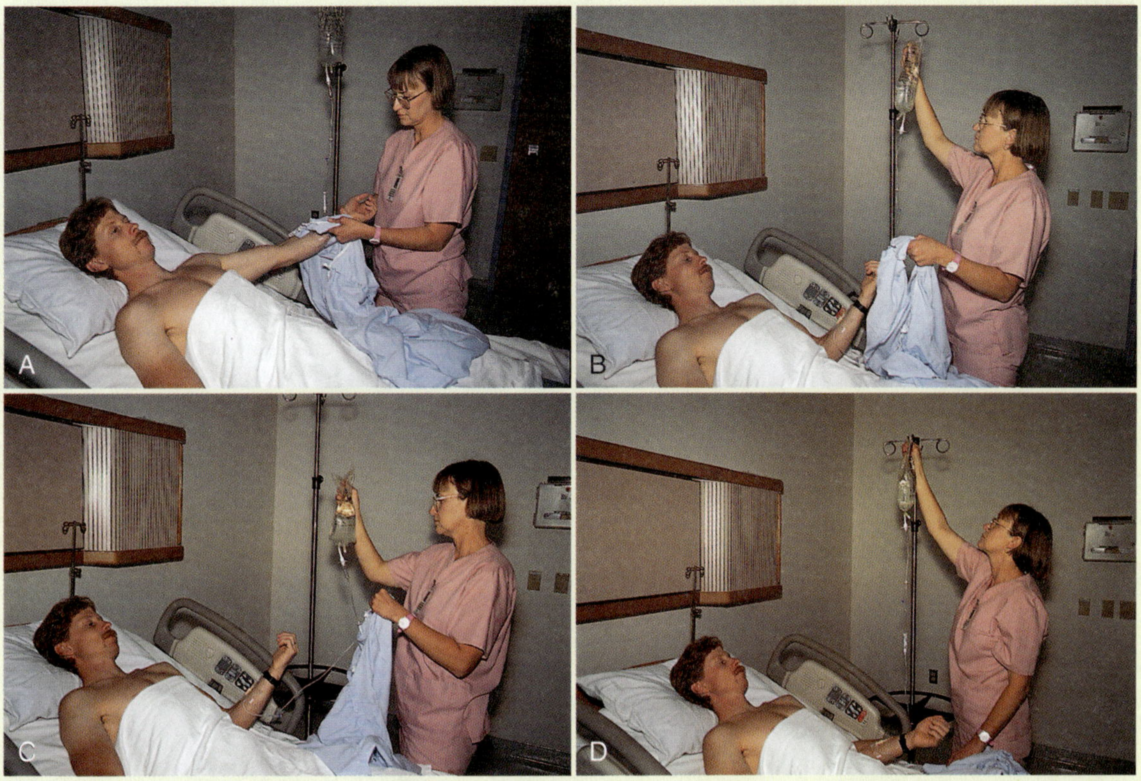

STEP1f(3) A, Remove patient's gown. **B,** Remove IV line from pole. **C,** Slide IV tubing and bag through arm of patient's gown. **D,** Rehang IV bag.

SKILL 29-1 BATHING AND PERINEAL CARE—cont'd

STEP	RATIONALE
h. Lower side rail, remove pillow if tolerated, and raise head of bed 30 to 45 degrees if allowed. Place bath towel under patient's head. Place second bath towel over patient's chest.	You do not have to reach across bed, thus minimizing strain on back muscles. Removal of pillow makes it easier to wash patient's ears and neck. Placement of towels prevents soiling of bed linen and bath blanket.
i. Wash face.	
(1) Ask if patient is wearing contact lenses. You may choose to remove at this time.	Prevents accidental injury to eyes.
(2) Immerse clean washcloth in plain water and wring out thoroughly. Form mitt with washcloth (see illustration).	Mitt retains water and heat better than loosely held washcloth; keeps cold edges from brushing against patient and prevents splashing.
(3) Wash patient's eyes with plain warm water while using clean area of mitt for each eye and bathing from inner to outer canthus (see illustration). Soak any crusts on eyelid for 2 to 3 minutes with damp cloth before washing and rinsing eyes. Dry eyes thoroughly but gently.	Soap irritates eyes. Use of separate sections of mitt reduces infection transmission. Bathing eye from inner to outer canthus prevents secretions from entering nasolacrimal duct.
(4) Ask if patient prefers to use soap on face. Otherwise wash, rinse, and dry forehead, cheeks, nose, neck, and ears without using soap. Ask men if they want to be shaved at this point or after bath.	Soap tends to dry face, which is exposed to air more than other body parts.

***Clinical Decision Point:* If using liquid soap containing 4% CHG, do not use on face. Use only plain water. CHG is irritating to mucous membranes.**

STEP	RATIONALE
j. Wash trunk and upper extremities.	
(1) Remove bath blanket from patient's arm that is closest to you. Place bath towel lengthwise under arm. Bathe arm with soap and water or add liquid soap (following package directions) to water. Use long, firm strokes from distal to proximal areas (fingers to axilla).	Towel prevents soiling bed. Soap lowers surface tension and facilitates removal of debris and bacteria. Long, firm strokes promote venous return.

***Clinical Decision Point:* When using CHG 4% liquid in a bath basin of water, use one washcloth for washing each major body part. Then dispose of cloth and use a new cloth for the next body part. Dipping cloth back into basin contaminates solution and makes CHG less effective. Also do not rinse after bathing. Allow CHG to simply dry on the skin.**

STEP	RATIONALE
(2) Raise and support arm above head (if possible) to wash, rinse, and dry axilla thoroughly (see illustration). Apply deodorant or powder to underarms if desired or needed.	Movement of arm exposes axilla and exercises normal ROM of joint. Respect patient's preference in use of hygiene products.
(3) Move to other side of bed, and repeat Steps (1) and (2) with other arm.	Provides for better access to patient and helps prevents back strain.
(4) Cover patient's chest with bath towel and fold bath blanket down to umbilicus. Bathe chest with long, firm strokes. Take special care with skinfolds under female and/or obese patient's breasts, lifting breast upward with back of hand, if necessary, while bathing underneath the breast. Keep patient's chest covered between wash and rinse periods. Rinse and dry well.	Draping prevents unnecessary exposure of body parts. Towel maintains warmth and privacy. Secretions and dirt collect easily in areas of tight skinfolds. Skin under breasts is vulnerable to excoriation if not kept clean and dry.

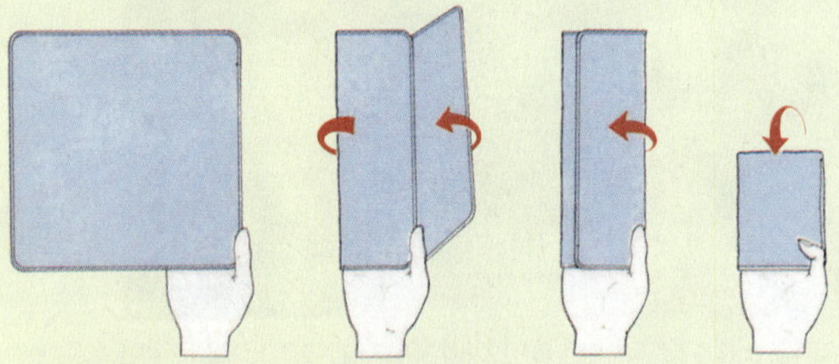

STEP1i(2) Steps for folding washcloth to form a mitt.

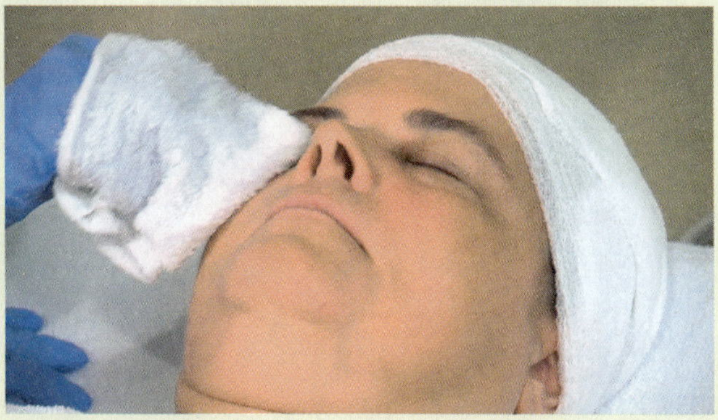

STEP1i(3) Wash eye from inner to outer canthus.

STEP	RATIONALE
k. Wash hands and nails.	
(1) Fold bath towel in half and lay it on bed beside patient. Place basin on towel. Immerse patient's hand in water. Allow hand to soak for 3 to 5 minutes before cleaning fingernails (see Box 29-11). Remove basin and dry hand well. Repeat for other hand.	Soaking softens cuticles and calluses of hand, loosens debris beneath nails, and enhances feeling of cleanliness. Thorough drying removes moisture from between fingers.
l. Check temperature of bath water and change water when cool or soapy.	Warm water maintains patient's comfort. Alkaline soap residue is irritating to skin and can decrease normal protectiveness of acid pH.

Clinical Decision Point: **When using CHG in water, do not discard water (unless in the original basin you filled one-half full with water and used one-half bottle of CHG). One bottle of CHG soap is sufficient for a complete bath.**

STEP	RATIONALE
m. Wash abdomen.	
(1) Place bath towel lengthwise over chest and abdomen. (You may need to use two towels.) Fold bath blanket down to just above pubic region. With unmitted hand lift bath towel. With mitted hand bathe and rinse abdomen, giving special attention to umbilicus and skinfolds of abdomen and groin. Stroke from side to side. Keep abdomen covered between washing and rinsing. Rinse and dry well.	Draping prevents unnecessary exposure of body parts and maintains warmth. Keeping skinfolds clean and dry helps prevent odor and skin irritation. Moisture and sediment that collect in skinfolds predispose skin to maceration (softening of tissue from prolonged contact with fluid).
(2) Apply clean gown or pajama top. If an extremity is injured or immobilized, dress affected side first. *Optional:* You may omit this step until completion of bath; make sure that gown does not become damp or soiled during remainder of bath.	Maintains patient's warmth and comfort. Dressing affected side first allows easier manipulation of gown over body part with reduced ROM.
n. Wash lower extremities.	
(1) Cover patient with bath blanket. Expose near leg only by folding blanket toward midline, being sure to keep perineum covered.	Prevents unnecessary exposure.
(2) Place bath towel under leg, supporting leg at knee and ankle.	Towel prevents soiling of bed linen. Support of joint and extremity during lifting prevents strain on musculoskeletal structures.
(3) Wash leg using long strokes from ankle to knee and from knee to thigh (see illustration). Rinse and dry well. Assess for areas of redness, warmth, swelling, or pain. Cleanse foot, making sure to bathe between toes. Rinse and dry toes and feet completely. Remove and discard towel.	Promotes circulation and venous return. Secretions and moisture may be present between toes, predisposing patient to maceration and breakdown. Warmth, redness, swelling, tenderness, and pain in lower extremities might be signs of deep vein thrombosis.
(4) Raise side rail, move to opposite side of bed, lower side rail, and repeat Steps (2) and (3) for other leg and foot. If skin is dry, apply moisturizer but be sure that it is massaged in and totally absorbed. When finished cover patient with bath blanket.	When applied within 3 minutes of bathing, moisturizers help prevent dryness and itching by trapping existing water in the skin (American Academy of Dermatology, 2010). Excess moisturizer can cause maceration.

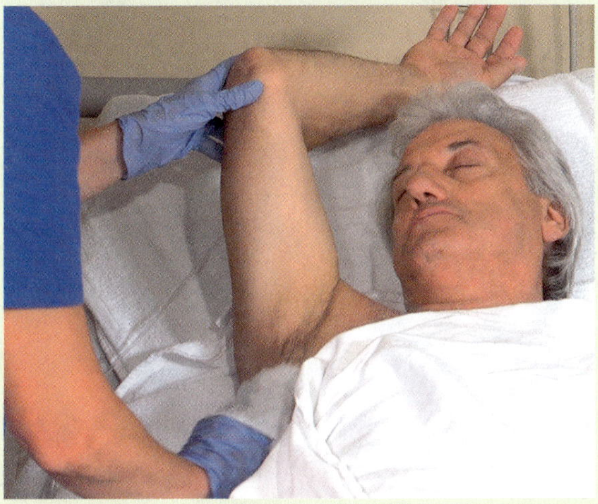

STEP1j(2) Positioning patient's arm to wash axilla.

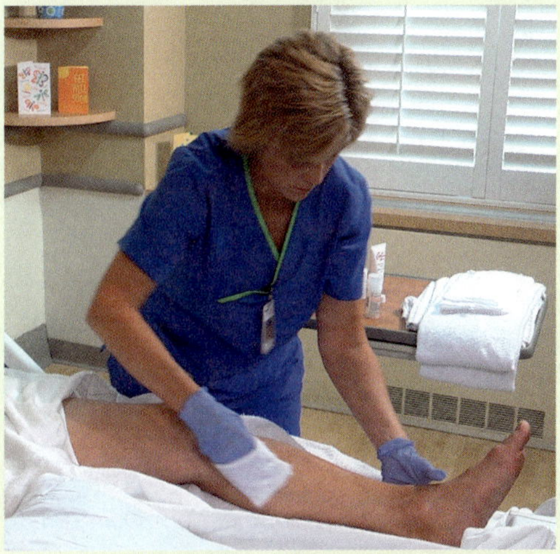

STEP1n(3) Wash patient's leg.

SKILL 29-1 BATHING AND PERINEAL CARE—cont'd

STEP	RATIONALE
***Clinical Decision Point:* Because of the risk of dislodging a deep vein thrombosis, do not use long, firm strokes to wash lower extremities of patients with history of deep vein thrombosis or blood-clotting disorder. Use short, light strokes instead. Avoid massaging legs.**	
o. Raise side rail, lower bed, provide call light before leaving bedside to change bath water.	Decreased bath water temperature causes chilling. Clean water reduces microorganism transmission.
p. Wash back.	
(1) Apply clean pair of gloves. Raise bed to working height. Lower side rail and help patient assume prone or side-lying position. Place towel lengthwise along patient's side.	Exposes back and buttocks for bathing. Protects bed from moisture and soiling.
(2) Keep patient draped by sliding bath blanket over shoulders and thighs during bathing. Wash, rinse, and dry back from neck to buttocks with long, firm strokes.	Maintains warmth and prevents unnecessary exposure.
(3) Cleanse buttocks and anus, washing from front to back (see illustration). Cleanse, rinse, and dry area thoroughly. Pay special attention to folds of buttocks and anus. If fecal material is present, enclose in a fold of underpad or toilet tissue and cleanse with disposable wipes. If needed place a clean pad under patient's buttocks.	Cleansing buttocks and anus prevents contamination of back. Skinfolds near buttocks and anus may contain fecal excretions and microorganisms.
(4) Remove gloves, perform hand hygiene, and give backrub if patient desires.	Promotes patient relaxation.
(5) Position patient supine; cover patient with bath blanket, raise side rail, lower bed, provide call light before leaving bedside to change bath water.	Provides for patient safety. Clean water reduces microorganism transmission to perineal structures.
q. Provide perineal care.	
(1) If patient is able to maneuver and handle washcloth, allow cleansing perineum on own.	Maintains patient's dignity and self-care ability.
(2) Female Patient	
(a) Perform hand hygiene and apply clean gloves. Raise bed to working height. Lower side rail. Help patient assume dorsal recumbent position with waterproof pad under buttocks. Drape patient with bath blanket placed in shape of diamond. Lift lower edge of bath blanket to expose perineum (see illustration).	Provides full exposure of female genitalia. Draping limits exposure and shows respect for patient's dignity. Gloves provide a barrier to prevent transmission of microorganisms.
(b) Fold lower corner of bath blanket up between patient's legs onto abdomen. If not already cleansed during bath, start perineal care by washing, rinsing, and drying patient's upper thighs.	Keeping patient draped until procedure begins minimizes anxiety. Buildup of perineal secretions soils surrounding skin surfaces. Removal of these secretions before perineal care prevents resoiling of area.

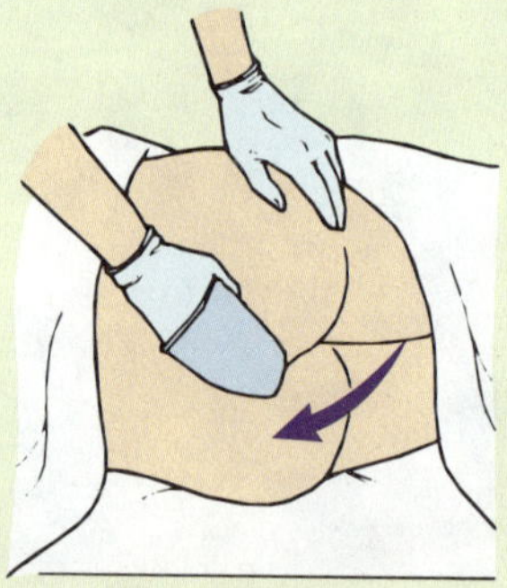

STEP1p(3) Cleanse buttocks from front to back.

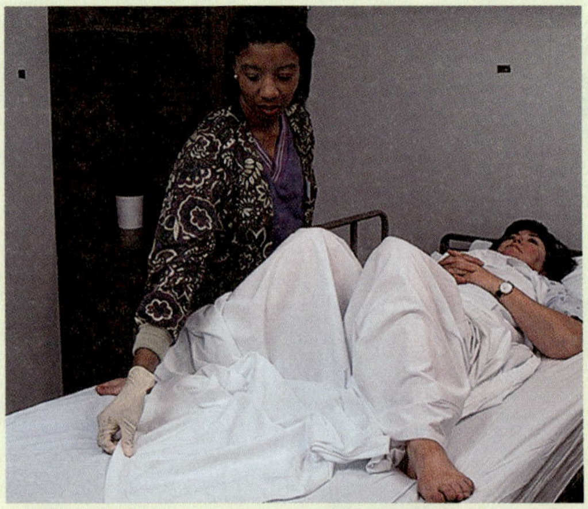

STEP1q(2)(a) Drape patient for perineal care.

STEP	RATIONALE
(c) Wash labia majora. Use nondominant hand to gently retract labia from thigh: with dominant hand, wash carefully in skinfolds. Wipe in direction from perineum to rectum (front to back). Repeat on opposite side with separate section of washcloth. Rinse and dry area thoroughly.	Perineal care involves thorough cleansing of patient's external genitalia and surrounding skin. Skinfolds may contain body secretions that harbor microorganisms. Wiping front to back reduces chance of transmitting fecal organisms to urinary meatus.

Clinical Decision Point: **Package directions for CHG products warn against use on mucous membranes. However, CHG solutions may be used to clean the external genitalia only.**

STEP	RATIONALE
(d) Gently separate labia with nondominant hand to expose urethral meatus and vaginal orifice. With dominant hand wash downward from pubic area toward rectum in one smooth stroke (see illustration). Use separate section of cloth for each stroke. Cleanse thoroughly over labia minora, clitoris, and vaginal orifice. Avoid placing tension on indwelling catheter if present and clean area around catheter thoroughly.	Cleansing method reduces transfer of microorganisms to urinary meatus.
(e) Provide catheter care as needed (see Chapter 34).	Cleansing along catheter from exit site reduces incidence of hospital-associated urinary tract infection.
(f) Rinse area thoroughly. May use bedpan and pour warm water over perineal area. Dry thoroughly from front to back.	Rinsing removes soap and microorganisms more effectively than wiping. Retained moisture harbors microorganisms.

Clinical Decision Point: **To aid in prevention of skin breakdown consider using cleanser with emollient (instead of soap and water) for perineal care following incontinence (Geraghty, 2011).**

STEP	RATIONALE
(g) Fold lower corner of bath blanket back between patient's legs and over perineum. Ask patient to lower legs and assume comfortable position.	
(3) Male Patient	
(a) Apply new pair of clean gloves. Raise bed to working height. Lower side rail. Help patient to supine position.	Provides full exposure of male genitalia. Gloves provide barrier to prevent transmission of microorganisms.
(b) Fold lower half of bath blanket up to expose upper thighs. If not already cleansed during bath, start perineal care by washing, rinsing, and drying patient's upper thighs.	Buildup of perineal secretions soils surrounding skin surfaces.
(c) Cover thighs with bath towels. Raise bath blanket to expose genitalia. Gently raise penis and place bath towel underneath. Gently grasp shaft of penis. If patient is uncircumcised retract foreskin. If patient has an erection defer procedure until later.	Draping minimizes patient anxiety. Towel prevents moisture from collecting in inguinal area. Gentle but firm handling of penis reduces chance of an erection. Secretions capable of harboring microorganisms collect underneath foreskin.
(d) Wash tip of penis at urethral meatus first. With circular motion cleanse from meatus outward (see illustration). Discard washcloth and repeat with clean cloth until penis is clean. Rinse and dry gently.	Direction of cleansing moves from area of least contamination to area of most contamination, preventing microorganisms from entering urethra.

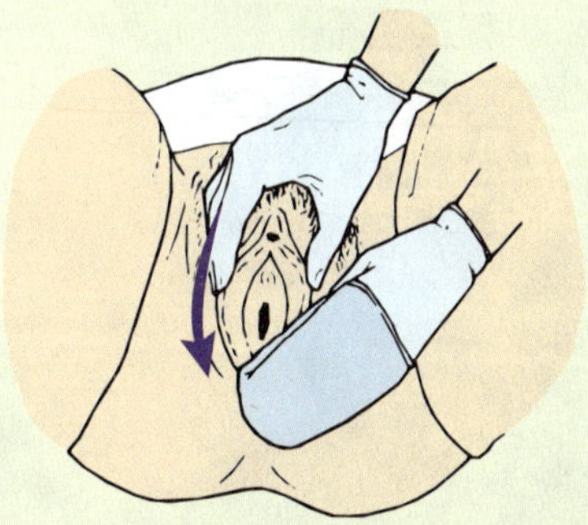

STEP1q(2)(d) Cleanse from perineum to rectum (front to back).

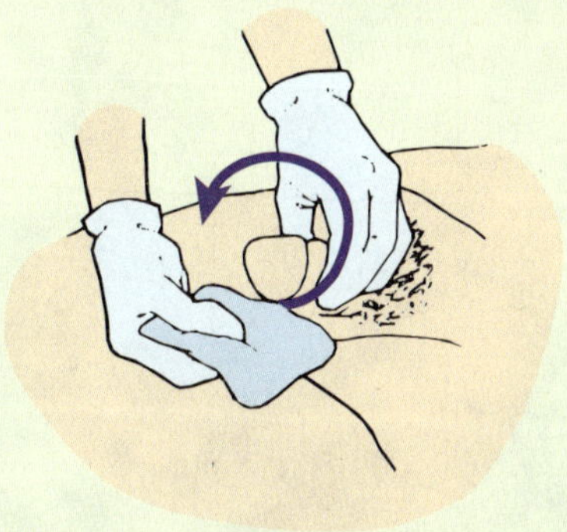

STEP1q(3)(d) Use circular motion to cleanse tip of penis.

SKILL 29-1 BATHING AND PERINEAL CARE—cont'd

STEP	RATIONALE
Clinical Decision Point: **Package directions for CHG products warn against use on mucous membranes. However, CHG solutions may be used to clean the external genitalia only.**	
(e) Return foreskin to its natural position. This is extremely important in patients with decreased sensation in their lower extremities.	Tightening of foreskin around shaft of penis causes local edema and discomfort; if foreskin is not returned to normal position, permanent urethral damage occurs. Patients with reduced sensation may not feel tightening of foreskin.
(f) Gently cleanse shaft of penis and scrotum by having patient abduct legs. Pay special attention to underlying surface of penis. Lift scrotum carefully and wash underlying skinfolds. Rinse and dry thoroughly.	Vigorous massage of penis may cause an erection. Underlying surface of penis is an area where secretions accumulate. Abduction of legs provides easier access to scrotal tissues. Secretions easily collect between skinfolds.
(g) Avoid placing tension on indwelling catheter if present and clean area around it thoroughly. Provide catheter care (see Chapter 34).	Cleansing along catheter from exit site reduces incidence of hospital-associated urinary tract infection.
(h) Ask patient to assume comfortable position; cover with bath blanket.	
r. Remove soiled gloves and dispose in trash. Perform hand hygiene before helping patient complete grooming (e.g., combing hair, applying makeup).	Prevents transmission of microorganisms.
s. Check function and position of external devices (e.g., indwelling urethral catheters, nasogastric tubes, IV lines).	Ensures that systems remain functional after bathing activities.
t. Raise side rail and lower bed, being sure that patient can reach call light.	Maintains patient's safety.
u. Replace top bed linen by pulling sheet and bedspread from foot of bed to cover patient before removing bath blanket. (You may change bed linens following bath, or you may defer to a later time; see Skill 29-2 or Box 29-16). Gather soiled linen and place in linen bag. Do not allow linen to contact uniform.	Maintains patient warmth and privacy. Reduces transmission of microorganisms.
v. Cleanse/disinfect basin, dry, and replace bathing equipment, including over-bed table (see agency policy). Turn bath basin upside down for storage. Do not use basin as storage bin for toiletries. Perform hand hygiene.	Limited research suggests that bath basins might be potential source of transmission of hospital-acquired infections (Johnson et al., 2009). However, using bath basin exclusively for bath water and being sure that basin is dried after use may help reduce reservoir capacity of basin. Use hospital-recommended disinfectant for cleansing bath basins.
w. Verify that patient can reach personal items and call light. Leave room as clean and comfortable as possible.	Clean environment promotes patient's comfort. Keeping call light and articles of care within reach promotes patient's safety.
2. Cleansing Cloths or Commercial Bag Bath/Cleansing Pack	
a. A cleansing pack contains 5 to 10 premoistened towels for cleansing (see illustrations).	Provides soothing heat.

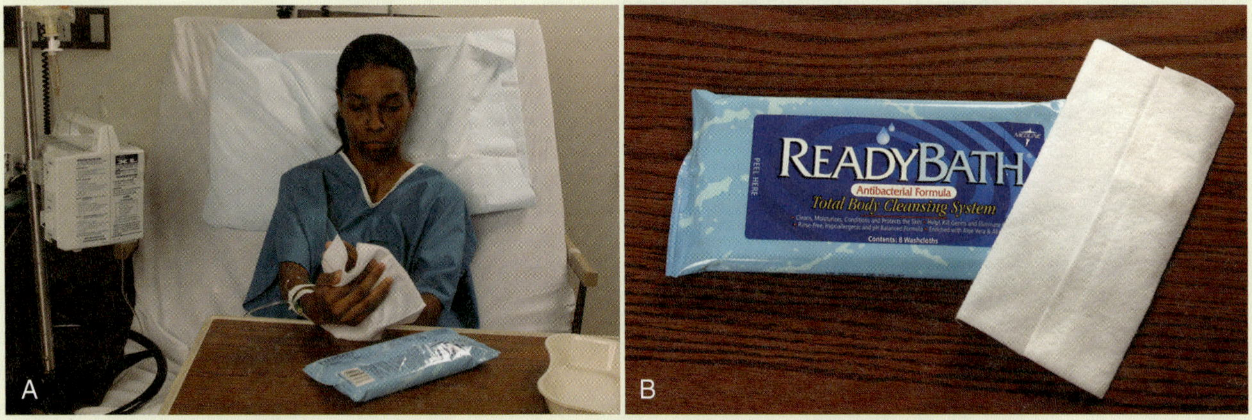

STEP 2a Bag bath. **A,** Patient uses individual wipes to bathe. **B,** Bag bath package.

STEP	RATIONALE
b. Use single towel for each general body part cleansed. Follow same order of cleansing as total or partial bed bath.	Reduces transmission of microorganisms.
c. Allow skin to air dry for 30 seconds. It is permissible to lightly cover patient with bath towel or blanket to prevent chilling.	Drying skin with towel removes emollient that is left behind after water/cleanser solution evaporates.
d. If there is excessive soiling (e.g., in perineal region), use an extra bag bath or conventional washcloths, soap, water, and towels.	To ensure removal of secretions.
3. Tub Bath or Shower	
a. Consider patient's condition and review orders for precautions concerning patient's movement or positioning.	Prevents accidental injury to patient during bathing.
b. Schedule use of shower or tub.	Prevents unnecessary waiting that causes fatigue.
c. Check tub or shower for cleanliness. Use cleaning techniques outlined in agency policy. Place rubber mat on tub or shower bottom. Place disposable bath mat or towel on floor in front of tub or shower.	Cleaning prevents transmission of microorganisms. Mats prevent slipping and falling.
d. Collect all hygienic aids, toiletry items, and linens requested by patient. Place within easy reach of tub or shower.	Placing items close at hand prevents possible falls when patient reaches for them.
e. Help patient to bathroom if necessary. Have patient wear robe and slippers to bathroom.	Assistance prevents accidental falls. Wearing robe and slippers prevents chilling.
f. Demonstrate how to use call signal for assistance.	Bathrooms are equipped with signaling devices in case patient feels faint or weak or needs immediate assistance. Patients prefer privacy during bath if safety is not jeopardized.
g. Place "occupied" sign on bathroom door.	Maintains patient's privacy.

Clinical Decision Point: **If patient is a fall risk, especially if victim of a previous fall, stay with him or her during the bath or stay just outside door or shower stall to prevent him or her from trying to get out of tub or shower alone.**

STEP	RATIONALE
h. Fill bath tub halfway with warm water. Check temperature of bath water, have patient test water, and adjust temperature if water is too warm. Explain which faucet controls hot water. If patient is taking shower, turn shower on and adjust water temperature before patient enters shower stall. Use shower seat or tub chair if needed (see illustration). Caution patient against use of bath oil in tub water.	Adjusting water temperature prevents accidental burns. Older adults and patients with neurological alterations (e.g., diabetes, spinal cord injury) are at high risk for burn as result of reduced sensation. Use of assistive devices facilitates bathing and minimizes physical exertion. Oil causes tub surfaces to become slippery.
i. Instruct patient not to remain in tub or shower longer than 10 to 15 minutes. Check on patient every 5 minutes or have NAP stay close by to check. Patients often try to get out of tubs without assistance, leading to falls.	Prolonged exposure to warm water causes vasodilation and pooling of blood in some patients, leading to light-headedness or dizziness.
j. Instruct patient to pull cord to summon assistance before trying to get out of tub or shower. Return to bathroom immediately when patient signals (knock before entering room). Have patient use safety bars when getting out of tub or shower.	Prevents slipping and falling.

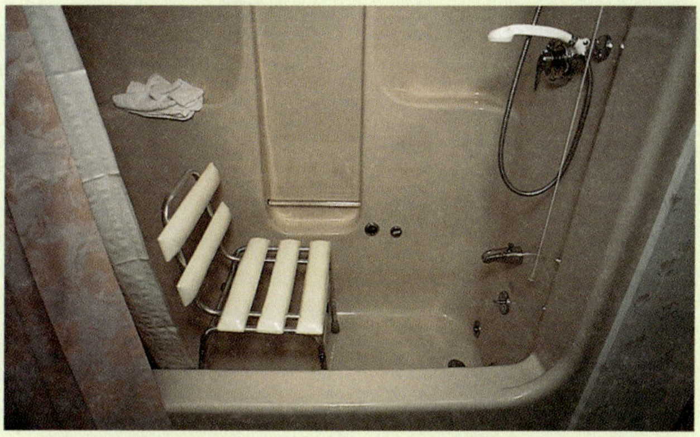

STEP 3h Shower seat for patient safety.

SKILL 29-1 BATHING AND PERINEAL CARE—cont'd

STEP	RATIONALE
k. For patient who is unsteady, drain tub of water before patient attempts to get out of it. Place bath towel over patient's shoulders. Help patient get out of tub as needed and help with drying.	Prevents accidental falls. Patient may become chilled as water drains.

Clinical Decision Point: **Weak or unstable patients need extra assistance getting out of a tub. Planning for additional personnel is essential before attempting to help patient from tub.**

STEP	RATIONALE
l. Help patient as needed to get dressed in a clean gown or pajamas, slippers, and robe. (In home setting patient may put on regular clothing.)	Maintains warmth to prevent chilling.
m. Help patient to room and comfortable position in bed or chair.	Maintains relaxation gained from bathing.
n. Clean tub or shower according to agency policy. Remove soiled linen and place in dirty-linen bag. Discard disposable equipment in proper receptacle. Place "unoccupied" sign on bathroom door. Return supplies to storage area.	Prevents transmission of infection through soiled linen and moisture.
o. Perform hand hygiene.	Reduces transfer of microorganisms.
EVALUATION	
1. Observe skin, paying particular attention to areas previously soiled, reddened, dry, or showing early signs of breakdown.	Techniques used during bathing leave skin clean and clear. Dry skin diminishes over time. If patient shows areas of redness, use Braden Scale to measure risk for pressure ulcers (see Chapter 37).
2. Observe or measure ROM during bath.	Measures joint mobility.
3. Ask patient to rate level of comfort.	Determines patient's tolerance of bathing activities.
4. Ask patient to rate level of fatigue.	Determines patient's tolerance of bathing activities.

RECORDING AND REPORTING

- Record procedure and observations (e.g., breaks in skin, inflammation, ulceration).
- Record type of bath, amount of assistance needed, and patient participation.
- Report any breaks in skin or ulcerations to nurse in charge or health care provider. These are serious in patients with altered circulation to lower extremities. Patient may need special foot-care treatments.

UNEXPECTED OUTCOMES AND RELATED INTERVENTIONS

- Areas of excessive dryness, itchiness, rashes, or pressure ulcers appear on skin.
  - Complete pressure ulcer assessment (see Chapter 37).
  - If using CHG soap it may be necessary to reduce frequency of bathing.
  - Apply moisturizing lotions or topical skin applications per agency policy.
  - Limit frequency of complete baths.
  - Obtain special bed surface if patient is at risk for skin breakdown.
- Joint ROM decreases.
  - Increase frequency of ROM exercises unless contraindicated.
  - Encourage more self-care by patient.
- Patient becomes excessively fatigued and unable to cooperate or participate in bathing.
  - Reschedule bathing to time when patient is more rested.
  - Leave pillow or elevate head of bed during bath for patient with breathing difficulties.
  - Notify health care provider if this is change in patient's fatigue level.
- Patient seems unusually restless or complains of discomfort.
  - Schedule patient rest periods.
  - Consider analgesia if patient complains of pain or discomfort before bath.
  - Consider use of patient-centered bathing techniques for patients with Alzheimer's or related dementia.
- Rectum, perineum, or genital area is inflamed or swollen or has foul-smelling odor.
  - Bathe perineal area frequently enough to keep clean and dry.
  - Obtain an order for sitz bath (see Chapter 37).
  - Apply protective barrier ointment or antiinflammatory cream.
  - Report findings to health care provider.

SKILL 29-2 MAKING AN OCCUPIED BED

DELEGATION CONSIDERATIONS

The skill of making an occupied bed can be delegated to nursing assistive personnel (NAP).The nurse directs the NAP about:

- Any positioning or activity restrictions for the patient.
- Looking for wound drainage, dressing material, drainage tubes, or intravenous (IV) tubing that becomes dislodged or is found in the linens.
- What to do if patient becomes fatigued.

EQUIPMENT (Figure 29-4)

- Linen bag
- Mattress pad (*optional* depending on facility practice; changed only when soiled)
- Bottom sheet (flat or fitted)
- Drawsheet *(optional)*
- Top sheet
- Blanket
- Bedspread
- Waterproof pads *(optional)*
- Pillowcases
- Bedside chair or table
- Clean gloves *(if linen soiled with drainage, excretions, secretions, or other body fluids)*
- Washcloth
- Antiseptic cleanser

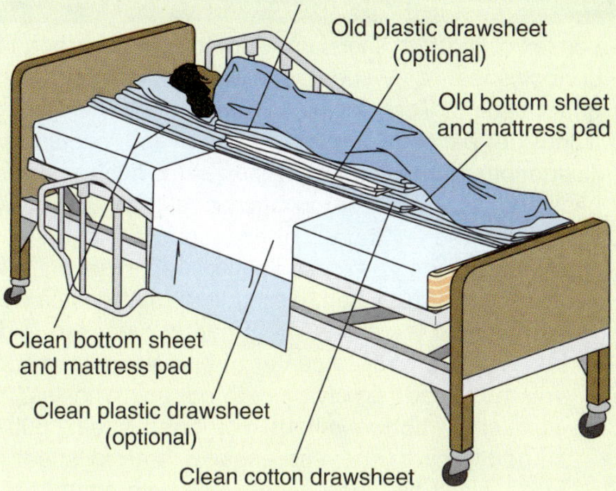

FIGURE 29-4 Equipment for making an occupied bed.

STEP	RATIONALE
ASSESSMENT	
1. Determine if patient has been incontinent or if excess drainage is present on linen.	Incontinence determines need for protective waterproof pads and use of gloves for changing linen.
2. Check chart for orders or specific precautions concerning movement and positioning.	Verifying ensures patient safety and use of proper body mechanics.
PLANNING	
1. Perform hand hygiene before obtaining and arranging needed linens and equipment on clean bedside table or cleared over-bed table. Arrange linen in order of use with items needed first on top. Do not let clean linen touch your uniform. Place linen bag within easy reach.	Assembling all equipment provides for smooth procedure and helps to increase patient's comfort. Placing linen on clean surface minimizes spread of infection. Uniform is less clean than clean linens.
2. Explain procedure to patient, noting that patient will be asked to turn on side and roll over layers of linen.	Explanation minimizes anxiety and promotes cooperation.
IMPLEMENTATION	
1. Pull room curtain around bed and close room door.	Maintains patient's privacy.
2. Raise bed to comfortable working level. Lower head of bed, keeping patient comfortable; lower side rail on side of bed where you are standing. Remove call light.	Proper positioning minimizes strain on back. It is easier to remove and apply linen evenly with bed in flat position. Provides easy access to bed and linen.
3. Loosen top linen at foot of bed.	Makes linen easier to remove.
4. Remove bedspread and blanket separately. If soiled, place in linen bag. If to be reused, fold into square and place over back of chair.	Reduces transmission of microorganisms.
5. Keep soiled lined away from uniform.	Reduces transmission of microorganisms.
6. Cover patient with bath blanket, placing It over top sheet. Have patient hold top edge of bath blanket or tuck it under patient's shoulders. Reach under blanket and remove top sheet. Place in linen bag.	Bath blanket provides warmth and keeps body parts covered during linen removal.
7. Help patient to side-lying position facing away from you. Encourage use of side rail to aid in turning. Adjust pillow under patient's head.	Provides space for removal and placement of clean linen. Side rail ensures patient safety.

Clinical Decision Point: **For patients with external medical devices check to make sure that repositioning does not place tension on the devices. If linen is grossly soiled with secretions, excretions, or waste or if linen is wet, apply gloves during linen change.**

SKILL 29-2 MAKING AN OCCUPIED BED—cont'd

STEP	RATIONALE
8. Loosen old bottom linens, moving from head to foot. Fanfold bottom sheet, drawsheet, and any cloth pads toward and under patient. Tuck edges of bottom linen being removed alongside patient's buttocks, back, and shoulders (see illustration). Remove any non-linen items such as disposable pads and discard in appropriate receptacle.	Prepares for removal of all bottom linen simultaneously. Provides maximum work space for placing clean linen. Later, when patient turns to other side, you can remove soiled linen easily.
9. Clean, disinfect, and dry mattress surface if needed.	Reduces transmission of microorganisms.
10. Apply clean linen to exposed half of bed in separate layers:	
a. If using mattress pad, place clean mattress pad on bed by folding it lengthwise with center crease in middle of bed. Fanfold layer to center of bed alongside patient. (If you reuse pad, simply smooth out any wrinkles.)	Applying linen over bed in successive layers minimizes energy and time used in bed making.
b. Next apply bottom sheet. For fitted sheet, pull sheet smoothly over mattress ends. If bottom sheet is not fitted, place flat sheet lengthwise with center crease in middle of bed and fanfold to center of bed alongside patient. Allow edge of flat sheet to hang about 25 cm (10 inches) over mattress edge. Be sure that lower hem of bottom sheet lies seam down and even with bottom edge of mattress (see illustration).	Proper positioning of linen on one side ensures that adequate linen is available to cover opposite side of bed. Keeping seam edges down eliminates irritation to patient's skin.
11. If flat sheet is used for bottom sheet, miter bottom flat sheet at head of bed:	Ensures that secure flat sheet will not loosen easily.
a. Face head of bed diagonally. Place hand away from head of bed under top corner of mattress, near mattress edge, and lift.	
b. With other hand tuck edge of bottom sheet smoothly under mattress so side edges of sheet above and below mattress meet when brought together.	
c. Face side of bed and pick up top edge of sheet at approximately 45 cm (18 inches) from top end of mattress (see illustration).	
d. Lift sheet and lay it on top of mattress to form neat triangular fold with lower base of triangle even with mattress side edge (see illustration).	
e. Tuck lower edge of sheet, which is hanging free, under mattress (see illustration).	
f. Hold portion of sheet covering side of mattress in place with one hand while with other hand picking up triangular linen fold and bringing it down over side of mattress. Tuck with palms down, without pulling triangular fold (see illustrations).	Mitered corners help sheet stay in place even if patient moves frequently in bed.

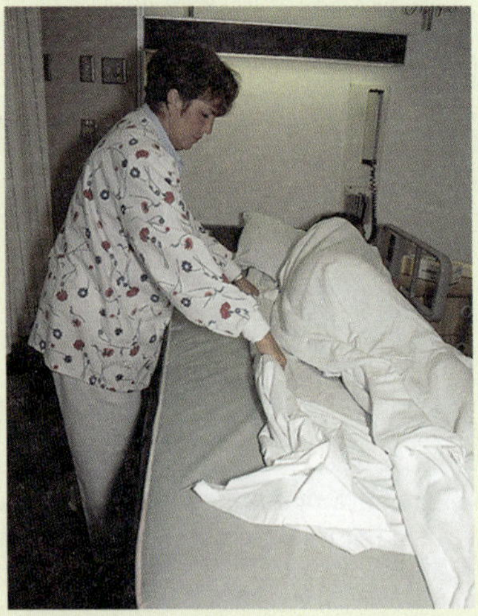

STEP 8 Old linen tucked under patient.

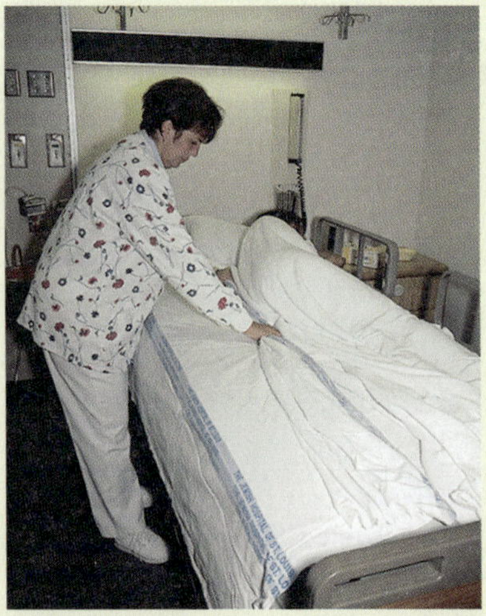

STEP 10b Clean linen applied to bed.

STEP	RATIONALE
12. Tuck remaining portion of sheet under mattress, moving toward foot of bed. Keep linen smooth.	Folds of linen are source of irritation.
13. If needed, open clean drawsheet so it unfolds in half. Lay centerfold along middle of bed lengthwise and position sheet so it will be under patient's buttocks and torso (see illustration). Fanfold top layer toward patient, with edge along patient's back. Smooth bottom layer out over mattress and tuck excess edge under mattress (keep palms down).	You use drawsheet to lift and reposition patient. Placement under patient's torso distributes most of patient's body weight over sheet.
14. If needed place waterproof pad over drawsheet with centerfold against patient's side. Fanfold top layer toward patient.	Protects bed linen from being soiled.
15. Advise patient that he or she will be rolling over a thick layer of linens. Ask patient to roll slowly toward you, over the layers of linen (see illustration). Help patient into comfortable position and raise side rail before moving to other side of bed.	Positions patient for removal of old linen and placement of new linens. Maintains patient's safety and body alignment during turning.
16. Move to opposite side of bed; lower side rail. Loosen edges of soiled linen from under mattress.	Exposes opposite side of bed for removal of soiled linen and placement of clean linen. Makes linen easier to remove.
17. Remove soiled linen by folding it into bundle or square with soiled side turned in. Hold linen away from your body and place in linen bag. Clean, disinfect, and dry mattress as needed.	Reduces transmission of microorganisms.
18. Pull clean, fan-folded linen smoothly over edge of mattress from head to foot of bed.	Smooth linen does not irritate patient's skin.
19. Help patient roll back into supine position. Reposition pillow.	Maintains patient's comfort.
20. Pull fitted sheet smoothly over mattress ends or miter top corner of bottom flat sheet if used (see Step 11). When tucking corner, be sure that sheet is smooth and free of wrinkles.	Wrinkles and folds cause irritation to skin.

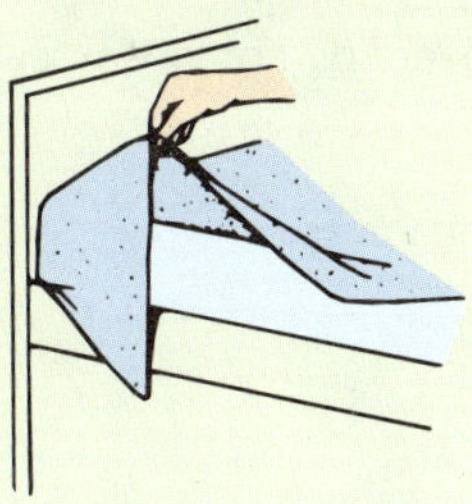

STEP 11c Top edge of sheet picked up.

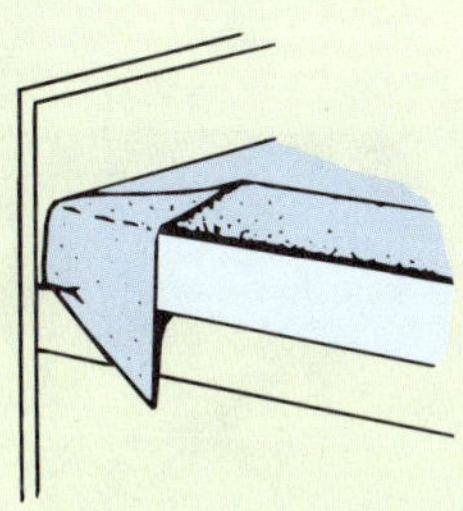

STEP 11d Sheet on top of mattress in triangular fold.

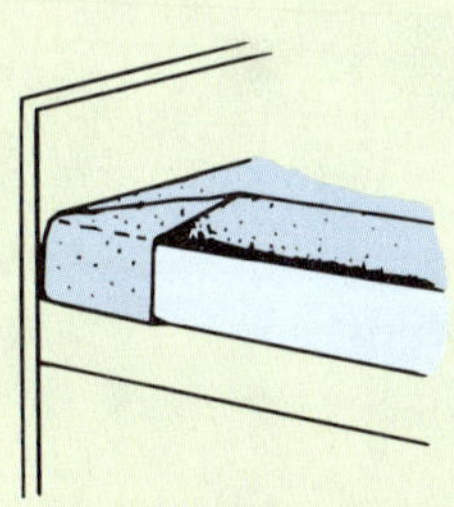

STEP 11e Lower edge of sheet tucked under mattress.

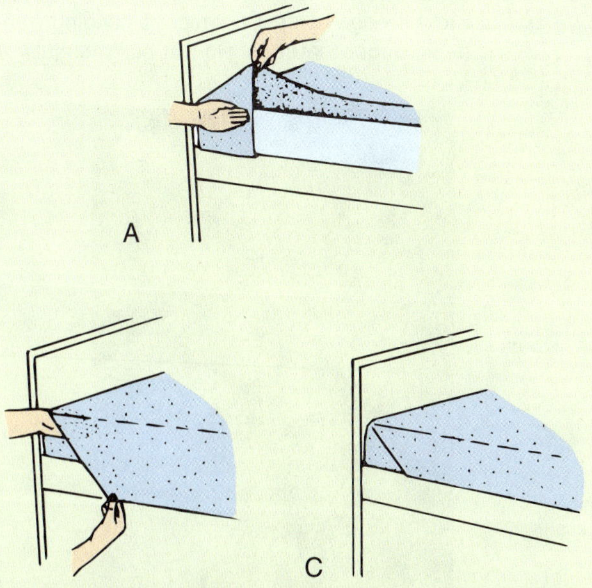

STEP 11f A and B, Triangular fold placed over side of mattress. **C,** Linen tucked under mattress.

SKILL 29-2 MAKING AN OCCUPIED BED—cont'd

STEP	RATIONALE
21. Facing side of bed, grasp remaining edge of bottom flat sheet. Lean back, keep back straight, and pull while tucking excess linen under mattress. Proceed from head to foot of bed. (Avoid lifting mattress during tucking to ensure fit.)	Proper use of body mechanics while tucking linen prevents injury.
22. Smooth fan-folded drawsheet out over bottom sheet. Tucking is optional; grasp edge of sheet with palms down, lean back, and tuck sheet under mattress. Tuck from middle to top and then to bottom. If used, also smooth out waterproof pad.	Tucking first at top or bottom pulls sheet sideways, causing poor fit.
23. Place top sheet over patient with centerfold lengthwise down middle of bed and seam side of hem facing up. Open sheet from head to foot and unfold over patient. Be sure that top edge of sheet is even with top edge of mattress.	Correctly positioning centerfold distributes sheet equally over bed. Sheet is folded over blanket or spread to form cuff; having seam up when placed results in seam side down when cuff formed.
24. Ask patient to hold clean top sheet or tuck sheet around patient's shoulders. Remove bath blanket and place in linen bag.	Sheet prevents exposure of body parts. Having patient hold sheet encourages his or her participation in care.
25. Place clean or reused bed blanket or bedspread on bed, placing it so crease runs lengthwise along middle of bed. Unfold it to cover patient. Make sure that top edge is parallel with edge of top sheet and 15 to 20 cm (6 to 8 inches) from edge of top sheet.	Place blanket to cover patient completely and provide adequate warmth.
26. Make cuff by turning edge of top sheet down over top edge of blanket or spread.	Protect patient's face from rubbing against blanket or spread.
27. Make horizontal toe pleat; stand at foot of bed and fanfold sheet and blanket 5 to 10 cm (2 to 4 inches) across bed. Pull sheet and blanket up from bottom to make fold approximately 15 cm (6 inches) from bottom edge of mattress.	Pressure ulcers develop on patient's toes and heels from feet rubbing against tight-fitting bed sheets.
28. Tuck in remaining portion of sheet and blanket or spread under foot of mattress. Tuck top sheet and blanket or spread together. Be sure that toe pleats are not pulled out.	Ensures that top covers do not loosen easily.
29. Make modified mitered corner with top sheet and blanket or spread (see illustration in Box 29-16). **a.** Pick up side edge of top sheet and blanket and spread approximately 45 cm (18 inches) from foot of mattress. Lift linen to form triangular fold and lay it on bed. **b.** Tuck lower edge of sheet, which is hanging free below mattress, under mattress. Do not pull triangular fold.	Provides a neat appearance.

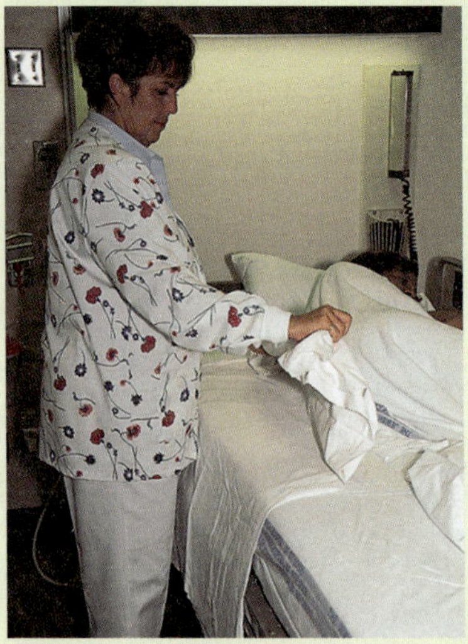

STEP 13 Optional drawsheet.

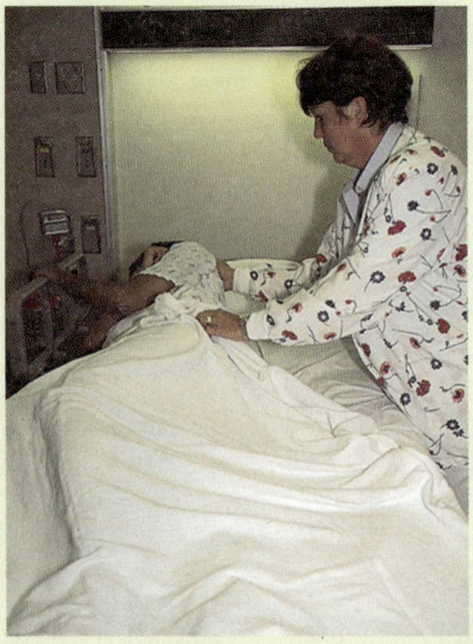

STEP 15 Helping patient roll over folds of linen.

STEP	RATIONALE
c. Pick up triangular fold and bring it down over mattress while holding linen in place alongside of mattress. Do not tuck tip of triangle.	Secures top linen but keeps even edge of blanket and top sheet draped over mattress.
30. Raise side rail. Make other side of bed; spread sheet, blanket, and bedspread out evenly. Fold top edge of spread over blanket and make cuff with top sheet (see Step 26); make modified mitered corner at foot of bed (see Step 29).	Side rail protects patient from accidental falls and aids patient's movement in bed.
31. Change pillowcase(s):	
a. Have patient raise head. While supporting neck with one hand, remove pillow. Allow patient to lower head.	Support of neck muscles prevents injury during flexion and extension of neck.
b. Remove soiled case by grasping pillow at open end with one hand and pulling case back over pillow with other hand. Place case in linen bag.	Pillows slide out easily, thus minimizing contact with soiled linen.
c. Grasp clean pillowcase at center of closed end. Gather case, turning it inside out over hand holding it. With same hand, pick up middle of one end of pillow. Pull pillowcase down over pillow with other hand. Do not hold pillow against your uniform while changing pillowcase.	Eases sliding of pillowcase over pillow. Prevents transfer of microorganisms from uniform to clean pillow case.
d. Be sure that pillow corners fit evenly into corners of pillowcase. Place pillow under patient's head.	Poorly fitting case constricts fluffing and expansion of pillow and interferes with patient comfort.
32. Place call light within patient's reach and return bed to comfortable position and in low horizontal position.	Ensures patient safety and comfort.
33. Open room curtains. Place personal items within easy reach on over-bed table or bedside stand. Ask patient if anything else is needed and if he or she is comfortable.	Promotes sense of well-being. Facilitates patient-centered care.
34. Place bag of soiled linen in appropriate location.	Prevents transmission of infection.
35. Remove and dispose of gloves if worn. Perform hand hygiene before leaving room.	Prevents transmission of microorganisms.
EVALUATION	
1. Inspect skin for areas of irritation.	Folds in linen cause pressure on skin.
2. Observe patient for signs of fatigue, dyspnea, pain, or discomfort.	Provides you with data about patient's level of activity tolerance and ability to participate in other procedures.

RECORDING AND REPORTING

- It is not necessary to record the making of an occupied bed.

UNEXPECTED OUTCOMES AND RELATED INTERVENTIONS

- Patient feels discomfort from linen fold.
  - Tighten sheets.
  - Change patient's position frequently.
- Patient's skin shows signs of breakdown.
  - Institute skin care measures to reduce risk for pressure ulcer (see Chapter 37).
  - Change patient's position more frequently.

KEY POINTS

- Various personal, social, cultural, and developmental factors influence patients' hygiene practices.
- Incorporate knowledge of the factors influencing an individual patient's hygiene practices into hygiene care.
- Assess a patient's physical and cognitive ability to perform hygiene self-care and provide care according to the patient's needs and preferences.
- Integrate other activities such as physical assessment, wound care, teaching, and ROM exercises while providing hygiene care.
- While providing daily hygiene needs, use communication skills and teaching to develop a caring relationship with the patient.
- Maintain privacy, comfort, and patient safety when providing hygiene care.
- Wear gloves during hygiene care when the risk for contacting body fluids or nonintact skin or mucosal surfaces is present; always wear gloves during perineal care and when performing oral care.
- When providing oral care for a debilitated or unconscious patient, take precautions to prevent aspiration.
- Providing oral care for at-risk patients such as those intubated can help decrease the incidence of pneumonia.

- Patients who are immobilized and poorly nourished and who have reduced sensation or peripheral circulation are at risk for altered skin integrity; these patients require special nail, foot, and skin care.
- Administer symptom-relief therapies for complaints such as pain or nausea before hygiene care to enable the patient to better tolerate and participate in care.
- Base evaluation of hygiene care on the patient's sense of comfort, relaxation, well-being, and understanding of hygiene techniques.

CLINICAL DECISION-MAKING EXERCISES

Mrs. Winkler's daughter is visiting her today at the extended care facility. Jamie, the nursing student, enters the room and finds Carol, Mrs. Winkler's daughter, preparing a basin of water for her mother to soak her feet. Jamie introduces herself to Carol. Carol states, "Mom needs a good pedicure, so I'm going to soak her feet in hot water before I clip her nails. She likes for me to polish her nails."

1. Which response or action by Jamie is the appropriate initial response to Carol's statement?
   a. Sitting down and help Mrs. Winkler and Carol pick out a nail polish color
   b. "Oh, no! You shouldn't soak her feet."
   c. Explaining why Mrs. Winkler's feet should not be soaked in hot water
   d. Explaining the proper technique to soak Mrs. Winkler's feet
2. Which assessment is most important for Jamie to perform before helping Mrs. Winkler and Carol continue with foot care?
   a. Measuring blood glucose level at the bedside
   b. Observing condition of feet and nails
   c. Asking Mrs. Winkler when she last had her toe nails cut
   d. Observing condition of skin in general

Jamie assesses Mrs. Winkler's feet and finds the following: dry skin, especially between toes and on heels; decreased touch and temperature sensation in both feet; long, curving nails; and a tender unbroken area on the left little toe.

3. Which of the following points does Jamie need to include when teaching Mrs. Winkler and her daughter Carol about foot care? (Select all that apply.)
   a. Use nail clippers to trim nails.
   b. File nail edges smooth.
   c. Dry feet carefully after washing, especially between toes.
   d. Never walk barefoot.
   e. Report minor foot injuries immediately for treatment.
   f. Use over-the-counter treatments for corn removal.
4. Jamie helps wash Mrs. Winkler's feet and applies a lanolin cream. What approach should Jamie take regarding trimming Mrs. Winkler's toenails?
   a. Collaborate with Mrs. Winkler's nurse to obtain a podiatrist consultation order
   b. Carefully cut the nails using nail scissors
   c. File the long, curving nails
   d. Ask Carol to trim the nails

evolve

Answers to Clinical Decision-Making Exercises can be found on the Evolve website.

QSEN ACTIVITY: EVIDENCE-BASED PRACTICE

Today the student nurse Jamie changes clinical rotations. She is orienting to the medical intensive care unit and shadowing one of the nurses there. Jamie observes that many of the patients in the unit are on ventilators. Throughout the morning she observes oral care being performed. She notices that different nurses perform the care in different ways. She recalls hearing previously in class about research regarding oral care, use of chlorhexidine, and ventilator-associated pneumonia. Jamie wants to be ready to provide evidence-based oral care for her next experience.

To clarify her search for evidence-based information, what would be Jamie's PICO question?

Where should Jamie look for the best evidence regarding her question?

evolve

Answers to QSEN Activities can be found on the Evolve website.

REVIEW QUESTIONS

1. You are helping a patient with heart failure bathe at the sink. During the bath the patient complains of being dizzy; you assess that the patient is breathing rapidly and the pulse is rapid. What is the most appropriate response?
   1. Ask the patient to hurry up and finish the bath quickly
   2. Call for help and help the patient return to bed
   3. Leave the patient alone to rest in the chair at the sink for a few minutes
   4. Instruct the patient to take deep breaths and try to relax
2. Which of the following actions would best help prevent skin breakdown in a patient who is incontinent of stool and very weak and drowsy?
   1. Check frequently for soiling.
   2. Wash the perineal area with strong soap and hot water.
   3. Place the call light within easy reach.
   4. Keep a pad under the patient.
3. A nurse is caring for a patient who has reduced sensation in both feet. Which of the following should the nurse do? (Select all that apply.)
   1. Avoid cleaning the feet until an order from the health care provider is received

2. Wash the feet with lukewarm water and then pat dry thoroughly
3. Apply moisturizing lotion to the feet, especially between the toes
4. File the toenails straight across

4. The nurse recognizes that her older-adult patient needs additional teaching about skin care when the patient says, "I should:
   1. Bathe no more than twice a week."
   2. Rinse well after using soap."
   3. Use warm (not hot) water for bathing."
   4. Drink plenty of fluids."
5. While planning morning care, which of the following patients would receive the highest priority to receive his or her bath first?
   1. A patient who just returned to the nursing unit from surgery and is resting comfortably
   2. A patient who prefers a bath in the evening when his wife visits and can help him
   3. A patient who is wet from perspiration because of a fever
   4. A patient who has just returned from diagnostic testing and complains of being very fatigued
6. The nurse caring for a male patient observes the nursing assistive personnel (NAP) performing perineal care for the patient. Which of the following observed actions indicates a need for further teaching for the NAP?
   1. The NAP did not wear gloves.
   2. The NAP retracted the foreskin before cleansing.
   3. The NAP used disposable cloths for each cleansing wipe.
   4. The NAP used a circular motion to cleanse from urinary meatus outward.
7. The nurse plans to talk with an African-American female patient about hair care to prevent traction alopecia. Which of the following does the nurse include in her teaching? (Select all that apply.)
   1. Hairstyles do not contribute to traction alopecia.
   2. Hair should be washed daily.
   3. Avoid using excessive amounts of heat for styling hair.
   4. Select shampoos that contain sulfates.
   5. Avoid using relaxer treatments too frequently.
8. Place in order the following steps when performing perineal care for a female patient.
   1. ____ Labia minora, urethral meatus, and vaginal orifice
   2. ____ Labia majora
   3. ____ Upper thighs
9. The nurse observes a patient with hearing aids trying to care for the aids. Which of the following statements or actions by the patient would indicate that the nurse needs to teach the patient proper care?
   1. "I leave my hearing aids in when I'm at the beauty shop under the hair dryer."
   2. She regularly uses a wax loop to remove cerumen from the hearing aids.
   3. "If I'm not wearing my hearing aid for a day or more, I remove the batteries."
   4. She performs hand hygiene before handling the hearing aids.
10. The nurse instructs a patient on how to correctly brush the teeth. Which of the following statements or actions by the patient would indicate that he or she has correctly learned proper technique?
   1. "I'll get a new toothbrush once a year."
   2. "I'll use a strong mouthwash with alcohol to help prevent infections."
   3. She was observed brushing inner and outer surfaces of teeth from gum to crown.
   4. She was observed holding the toothbrush with bristles at a 20-degree angle to the gum line.

evolve

Rationales for Review Questions can be found on the Evolve website.

1. 2; **2.** 1; **3.** 2, 4; **4.** 1; **5.** 3; **6.** 1; **7.** 3, 5; **8.** 3, 2, 1; **9.** 1; **10.** 3

REFERENCES

Alzheimer's Association: *Ten early signs and symptoms of Alzheimer's disease*, 2009, http://www.alz.org/alzheimers_disease_10_signs_of_alzheimers.asp#signs. Accessed March 24, 2013.

American Academy of Dermatology: *Changes in skin care soothe aging skin*, 2010, http://www.skincarephysicians.com/agingskinnet/winter_skin.html. Accessed August 7, 2012.

American Academy of Dermatology: *Dry skin: tips for relieving*, 2012a, http://www.aad.org/diseases-and-treatments/a---d/dry-skin/tips. Accessed January 19, 2014.

American Academy of Dermatology: *Handle with care: African-American hair needs special care to avoid damage*, 2012b, http://www.aad.org/stories-and-news/news-releases/handle-with-care-african-american-hair-needs-special-care-to-avoid-damage. Accessed August 14, 2012.

American Dental Association: *Mouth healthy: brushing your teeth*, 2012, http://www.mouthhealthy.org/en/az-topics/b/brushing-your-teeth.aspx. Accessed August 17, 2012.

American Diabetes Association: *Diabetes statistics*, 2012a, http://www.diabetes.org/diabetes-basics/diabetes-statistics/?loc=DropDownDB-stats. Accessed May 10, 2013.

American Diabetes Association: *Foot care*, 2012b, http://www.diabetes.org/living-with-diabetes/complications/foot-complications/foot-care.html. Accessed August 15, 2012.

American Podiatric Medical Association: *Foot health information*, 2012, http://www.apma.org/learn/FootHealth.cfm?ItemNumber=980. Accessed May 10, 2013.

Ayello EA, Fulmer T: Preventing pressure ulcers and skin tears. In Boltz M, et al, editors: *Evidence-based geriatric protocols for best practice*, ed 4, New York, 2012, Springer, p 298.

Centers for Disease Control and Prevention (CDC): *Head lice treatment*, 2010, http://www.cdc.gov/parasites/lice/head/treatment.html. Accessed September 2, 2012.

Centers for Disease Control and Prevention (CDC): *Tick removal*, 2011, http://www.cdc.gov/lyme/removal/index.html. Accessed September 2, 2012.

Chatham N, Caris C: *How to manage incontinence-associated dermatitis*, 2012, http://woundcareadvisor.com/how-to-manage-incontinence-associated-dermatitis/. Accessed May 10, 2013.

Climo MW, et al: The effect of daily bathing with chlorhexidine on the acquisition of methicillin-resistant *Staphylococcus aureus,* vancomycin-resistant *Enterococcus,* and health care–associated bloodstream infections: results of a quasi-experimental multicenter trial, *Crit Care Med* 37(6):1858, 2009.

Climo MW, et al: Effect of daily chlorhexidine bathing on hospital-acquired infection, *N Engl J Med* 368(6):533, 2013.

Cronenwett L, et al: Quality and safety education for nurses, *Nurs Outlook* 55(3):122, 2007.

Dixon JM, Carver RL: Daily chlorhexidine gluconate bathing with impregnated cloths results in statistically significant reduction in central line–associated bloodstream infections, *Am J Infect Control* 38(10):817, 2010.

Edelman CL, Mandle CL: *Health promotion throughout the lifespan*, ed 7, St Louis, 2010, Mosby.

Erikson E: *Childhood and society*, ed 2, New York, 1963, WW Norton.

Evans HL, et al: Effect of chlorhexidine whole-body bathing on hospital-acquired infections among trauma patients, *Arch Surg* 145(3):240, 2010.

Galanti GA: *Caring for patients from different cultures*, ed 4, Philadelphia, 2008, University of Pennsylvania Press.

Geraghty J: Introducing a new skin-care regimen for the incontinent patient, *Br J Nurs* 20(7):409, 2011.

Giger JN, editor: *Transcultural nursing: assessment and intervention*, ed 6, St Louis, 2013, Mosby.

Grap MJ, et al: Oral care interventions in critical care: frequency and documentation, *Am J Crit Care* 12(2):114, 2003.

Harris DJ, et al: Putting evidence into practice: evidence-based interventions for the management of oral mucositis, *Clin J Oncol Nurs* 12(1):141, 2008.

Harris M, Richards KC: The physiological and psychological effects of slow-stroke back massage and hand massage on relaxation in older people, *J Clin Nurs* 19(7):917, 2010.

Hockenberry MJ, Wilson D: *Wong's nursing care of infants and children*, ed 9, St Louis, 2011, Mosby.

Hoeffer B, et al: Assisting cognitively impaired nursing home residents with bathing: effects of two bathing interventions on caregiving, *Gerontologist* 46(4):524, 2006.

Johnson D, et al: Patients' bath basins as potential sources of infection: a multicenter sampling study, *Am J Crit Care* 18(1):31, 2009.

Jury LA, et al: Effectiveness of routine patient bathing to decrease the burden of spores on the skin of patients with *Clostridium difficile* infection, *Infect Control Hosp Epidemiol* 32(2):181, 2011.

Kassakian SZ, et al: Impact of chlorhexidine bathing on hospital-acquired infections among general medical patients, *Infect Control Hosp Epidemiol* 32(93):238, 2011.

Labeau SO, et al: Prevention of ventilator-associated pneumonia with oral antiseptics: a systematic review and meta-analysis, *Lancet Infect Dis* 11:845, 2011.

Meiner SE: *Gerontologic nursing*, ed 4, St Louis, 2011, Mosby.

Munro CL, et al: Chlorhexidine, toothbrushing, and preventing ventilator-associated pneumonia in critically ill adults, *Am J Crit Care* 18(4):428, 2009.

Munoz-Price LS, et al: Prevention of bloodstream infections by use of daily chlorhexidine baths for patients at a long-term acute care hospital, *Infect Control Hosp Epidemiol* 30(11):1031, 2009.

Munoz-Price LS, et al: Effectiveness of stepwise interventions targeted to decrease central catheter-associated bloodstream infections, *Crit Care Med* 40(5):1464, 2012.

National Cancer Institute (NCI): *Oral mucositis*, 2013, http://www.cancer.gov/cancertopics/pdq/supportivecare/oralcomplications/HealthProfessional/page5. Accessed March 24, 2013.

Oncology Nursing Society (ONS): *Putting evidence into practice: mucositis*, 2007, http://www.ons.org/outcomes/volume2/mucositis.shtml. Accessed August 8, 2012.

O'Horo JC, et al: The efficacy of daily bathing with chlorhexidine for reducing health care–associated bloodstream infections: a meta-analysis, *Infect Control Hosp Epidemiol* 33(3):257, 2012.

Padilha DMP, et al: Hand function and oral hygiene in older institutionalized Brazilians, *J Am Geriatr Soc* 55(9):1333, 2007.

Popovich KJ, et al: Effectiveness of routine patient cleansing with chlorhexidine gluconate for infection prevention in the medical intensive care unit, *Infect Control Hosp Epidemiol* 30(10):959, 2009.

Powers J, et al: Chlorhexidine bathing and microbial contamination in patients' bath 186 basins, *Am J Crit Care* 21(5):338, 2012.

Rader J, et al: The bathing of older adults with dementia, *Am J Nurs* 106(4):40, 2006.

Saxon SV, et al: *Physical change and aging: a guide for the helping professions*, ed 5, New York, 2010, Springer.

Sciubba JJ, Elston DM: *Denture stomatitis follow-up*, 2010, http://emedicine.medscape.com/article1075994-overview. Accessed August 24, 2012.

Snyders O, et al: Oral chlorhexidine in the prevention of ventilator-associated pneumonia in critically ill adults in the ICU: a systematic review, *S Afric J Crit Care* 27(2):48, 2011.

The Joint Commission (TJC): *National Patient Safety Goals*, Oakbrook Terrace, IL, 2014, The Commission. Available at http://www.jointcommission.org/standards_information/npsgs.aspx.

Touhy TA, Jett K: *Ebersole and Hess' gerontological nursing and healthy aging*, ed 3, St Louis, 2010, Mosby.

Touhy TA, Jett K: *Ebersole and Hess' toward healthy aging: human needs and nursing responses*, ed 8, St Louis, 2012, Mosby.

Wallace M, Shelkey M: Katz index of independence in activities of daily living (ADL), *Am J Nurs* 108(4):67, 2008.

Zullino DF, et al: Local back massage with an automated massage chair: several muscle and psychophysiologic relaxing properties, *J Altern Complement Med* 11(6):1103, 2005.

CHAPTER 30

Oxygenation

evolve WEBSITE

http://evolve.elsevier.com/Potter/essentials

- Video Clips
- Crossword Puzzle
- Audio Glossary

OBJECTIVES

- Describe the structure and function of the cardiopulmonary system.
- Identify the physiological processes of cardiac output, myocardial blood flow, coronary artery circulation, and respiratory gas exchange.
- Describe the relationship of cardiac output, preload, afterload, contractility, and heart rate.
- Diagram the electrical conduction system of the heart.
- Identify the physiological processes involved in ventilation, perfusion, and exchange of respiratory gases.
- Describe the effects of a patient's health status, age, lifestyle, and environment on tissue oxygenation.
- Identify and describe clinical outcomes as a result of disturbances in conduction, altered cardiac output, impaired valvular function, myocardial ischemia, and impaired tissue perfusion.
- Identify nursing interventions for promotion, maintenance, and restoration of cardiopulmonary function in the primary care, acute care, and restorative and continuing care settings.
- Identify and describe clinical outcomes for hyperventilation, hypoventilation, and hypoxemia.

KEY TERMS

afterload, p. 803
atelectasis, p. 807
atrioventricular (AV) node, p. 804
cardiac index, p. 803
cardiac output (CO), p. 803
cardiopulmonary rehabilitation, p. 830
cardiopulmonary resuscitation (CPR), p. 830
chest percussion, p. 827
chest physiotherapy (CPT), p. 827
chest tube, p. 828
depolarization, p. 804
diaphragmatic breathing, p. 831
diffusion, p. 800
dyspnea, p. 808
dysrhythmia, p. 805
hemoptysis, p. 812
hemothorax, p. 828
humidification, p. 823
hypercapnia, p. 807
hyperventilation, p. 802
hypoventilation, p. 802
hypoxemia, p. 802
hypoxia, p. 802
myocardial contractility, p. 803
myocardial infarction, p. 804
myocardial ischemia, p. 804
nebulization, p. 823
normal sinus rhythm (NSR), p. 804
orthopnea, p. 805
oxygen therapy, p. 819
perfusion, p. 800
pneumothorax, p. 828
postural drainage, p. 827
preload, p. 803
productive cough, p. 812
pursed-lip breathing, p. 831
repolarization, p. 804
respiration, p. 800
sinoatrial (SA) node, p. 803
stroke volume (SV), p. 803
surfactant, p. 808
ventilation, p. 800
vibration, p. 828
wheezing, p. 812

CASE STUDY *Mr. King*

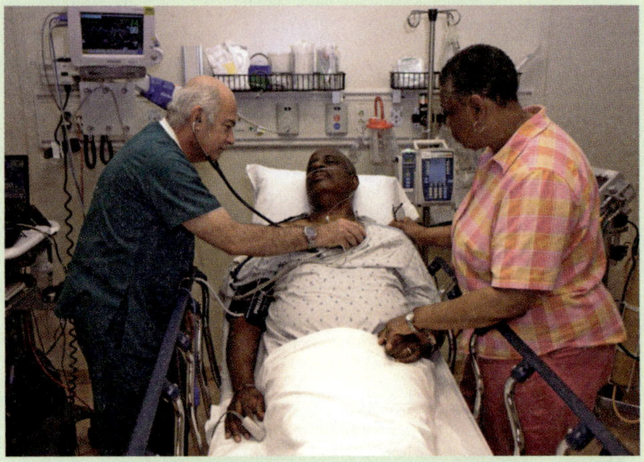

Mr. King, a 62-year-old man, entered the emergency department with a 6-day history of chest pain, shortness of breath, cough, and generalized malaise. His wife and son are with him. Mr. King works in sales and lives with his wife. He has a history of chronic obstructive pulmonary disease (COPD) and alcohol abuse but at present is not drinking. Mr. and Mrs. King have been heavy smokers for more than 40 years. Mr. King used to help out with the housework and loves to tinker in the garden; however, lately he has been unable to participate in any of the activities. His wife states, "All he seems to be able to do is sit in his chair and watch TV." Mr. King is admitted to the hospital for his breathlessness.

John Smith is the nurse assigned to Mr. King. He has experience in health assessment and patient teaching related to health promotion activities. After reviewing the medical record, John determines that Mr. King has health promotion needs such as smoking cessation and the need to add exercise to his daily routine. When John meets Mr. King and performs his morning assessment, he determines that Mr. King is in respiratory distress. It seems that every breath is a struggle for him and he is extremely anxious. Everything that John planned to do for Mr. King seems less important. Mrs. King is at his side, watching John's every move and demanding something to make her husband breathe easier.

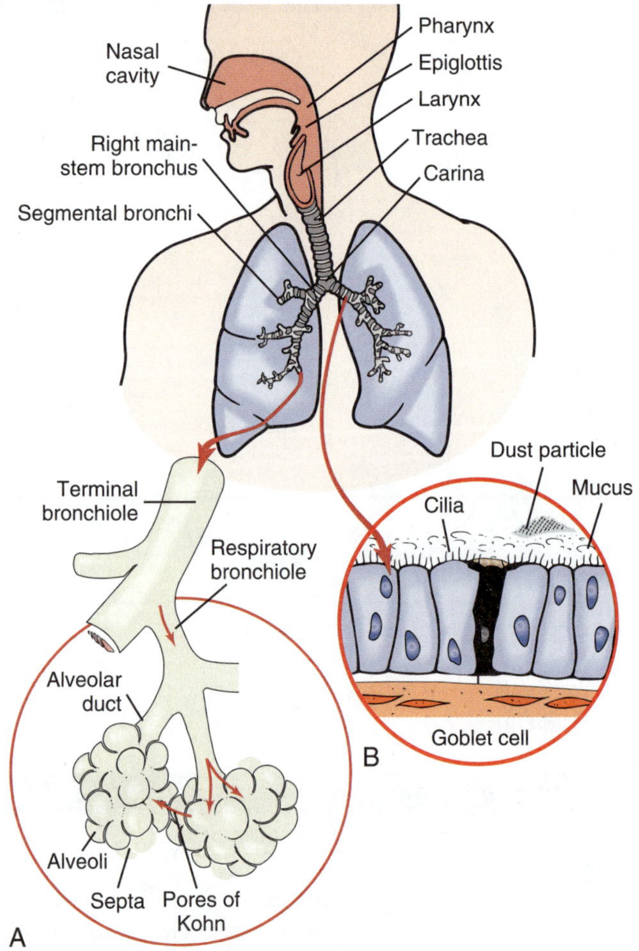

FIGURE 30-1 Structures of the respiratory tract. **A,** Pulmonary functional unit. **B,** Ciliated mucous membrane. (From Lewis SM, et al: *Medical surgical nursing: assessment and management of clinical problems,* ed 8, St Louis, 2011, Mosby.)

SCIENTIFIC KNOWLEDGE BASE

Oxygen is a basic human need. The heart and lungs supply the body with oxygen necessary for carrying out the respiratory and metabolic processes needed to sustain life. You frequently encounter patients who are unable to meet their oxygenation needs. This is often the result of ineffective gas exchange (lungs) or an ineffective pump (heart). Any condition that affects cardiopulmonary functioning directly affects the ability of the body to meet oxygen demands.

Cardiopulmonary Physiology

The function of the cardiopulmonary system is to provide oxygen to the tissues and remove carbon dioxide and waste products from the body. The primary functions of the lungs include **ventilation,** the movement of air in and out of the lungs, and **diffusion,** the movement of gases between air spaces and the bloodstream. **Respiration** is the exchange of oxygen and carbon dioxide during cellular metabolism. The heart supports **perfusion,** the movement of blood into and out of the lungs to the organs and tissues of the body.

Structure and Function of the Pulmonary System

The pulmonary system consists of two lungs, their airways, the chest walls, and the blood vessels that support them (Figure 30-1). The right lung is made up of three lobes: the upper, middle, and lower lobes. The left lung has two lobes: the upper and lower lobes. The trachea enters the thorax and bifurcates, or branches out, into the right and left mainstem bronchus. The bronchi branch into smaller and smaller bronchioles, similar to a tree. The last branch of the airways ends at the exchanging unit of the lung, the alveoli. The blood flows around the alveoli, allowing for diffusion of oxygen and carbon dioxide across the alveolar capillary membrane. The alveoli are lined with a phospholipid-rich substance,

BOX 30-1 NEURAL AND CHEMICAL REGULATION OF RESPIRATION

NEURAL REGULATION
Neural regulation maintains rhythm and depth of respiration and the balance between inspiration and expiration.

CEREBRAL CORTEX
Voluntary control of respiration delivers impulses to the respiratory motor neurons by way of the spinal cord. Voluntary control of respiration accommodates speaking, eating, and swimming.

MEDULLA OBLONGATA
Automatic control of respiration occurs continuously.

CHEMICAL REGULATION
Chemical regulation maintains appropriate rate and depth of respirations based on changes in the carbon dioxide (CO_2), oxygen (O_2), and hydrogen ion (H^+) concentration of the blood.

CHEMORECEPTORS
Chemoreceptors are located in the medulla, aortic body, and carotid body. Changes in chemical content of O_2, CO_2, and H^+ stimulate chemoreceptors, which in turn stimulate neural regulators to adjust the rate and depth of ventilation to maintain normal arterial blood gas levels. Chemical regulation occurs during physical exercise and in some illnesses. It is a short-term adaptive mechanism.

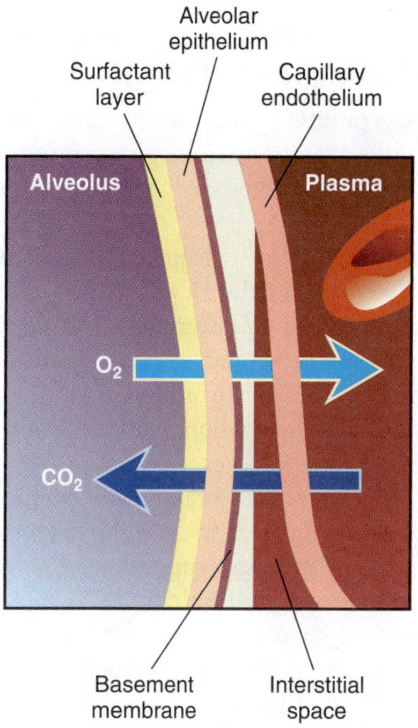

FIGURE 30-2 Diffusion: Gas-exchange membrane. (Modified from McCance K, Huether S: *Pathophysiology: the biologic basis for disease in adults and children,* ed 6, St Louis, 2010, Mosby.)

surfactant, which prevents the alveoli from collapsing on expiration. Surfactant is essential for normal lung function. Without adequate amounts of surfactant the alveoli would collapse on expiration, leading to impaired gas exchange.

Regulation of Ventilation. Successful ventilation depends on neuroreceptors and chemoreceptors in the lungs and central nervous system (CNS), muscles that support inspiration and exhalation, and lung elasticity. Control of ventilation provides for adequate oxygen to meet metabolic demands such as exercise, infection, or pregnancy. Ventilation promotes exhalation of metabolically produced carbon dioxide, which is a determinant of acid-base status (see Chapter 18).

Neural and chemical regulators control ventilation (Box 30-1). Neural regulation involves the CNS. The CNS sends signals to the chest wall musculature to control ventilation rate, depth, and rhythm. Chemical regulation involves the influence of chemicals such as carbon dioxide and hydrogen ions, which affect the rate and depth of ventilation.

Oxygen Transport. The delivery of oxygen depends on the amount of oxygen entering the lungs (oxygenation) from the atmosphere. Ventilation allows for movement of oxygen and carbon dioxide into and out of the lungs. Once oxygen has reached the alveoli, diffusion occurs. Oxygen crosses the alveolar-capillary membrane and is dissolved into the plasma (Figure 30-2). It then moves into the red blood cells (RBCs) and binds with hemoglobin molecules. Hemoglobin transports most oxygen and serves as a carrier for both oxygen and carbon dioxide. The hemoglobin molecule combines with oxygen to form oxyhemoglobin. The formation of oxyhemoglobin is easily reversible, allowing hemoglobin and oxygen to dissociate, which frees oxygen to enter tissues. The amount of dissolved oxygen in the plasma, the amount of hemoglobin, and the tendency of hemoglobin to bind with oxygen all influence the capacity of the blood to carry oxygen. Perfusion of oxygenated blood occurs in the capillary beds of the organs and tissues.

Carbon Dioxide Transport. The blood carries CO_2 in three ways: (1) dissolved in plasma, (2) as carbamino compounds, and (3) as bicarbonate. At the capillary level carbon dioxide diffuses from the cells into the plasma with 7% of CO_2 remaining dissolved in the plasma (PCO_2). The rest of the CO_2 rapidly moves into the RBCs and is hydrated into carbonic acid (H_2CO_3). The carbonic acid dissociates into hydrogen (H^+) and bicarbonate (HCO_3^-) ions. The H^+ ion binds to hemoglobin, which has released its oxygen, to form HHb and deoxyhemoglobin ($HbCO_2$). Twenty-three percent of CO_2 is transported as $HbCO_2$. The HCO_3^- ion moves out of the RBCs and back into the plasma (see Chapter 18). Seventy percent of CO_2 is carried as HCO_3^-, helping to maintain an electroneutral state. Once the CO_2 is transported by the venous blood to the lungs, diffusion occurs again. The CO_2 is highly soluble, and it quickly crosses the gas membrane into the alveoli. Through ventilation the CO_2 is expelled from the lungs into the atmosphere.

Alterations of the Pulmonary System: Factors Affecting Ventilation and Oxygen Transport

Illnesses and conditions that affect ventilation or oxygen transport cause alterations in respiratory functioning. The primary alterations are hypoxia, hypoxemia, hypoventilation, and hyperventilation.

Hypoxia. Hypoxia is inadequate tissue oxygenation with a deficiency in oxygen delivery or oxygen utilization at the cellular level. Mild hypoxia stimulates peripheral chemoreceptors to increase heart and respiration rates. The central mechanisms that regulate breathing fail in severe hypoxia, leading to irregular respiration, Cheyne-Stokes respiration, apnea, and respiratory and cardiac failure. The tissues most sensitive to hypoxia are the brain, heart, pulmonary vessels, and liver. Causes of hypoxia include the following:

- A lowered oxygen-carrying capacity, as in anemia or carbon monoxide poisoning
- Diminished concentrations of inspired oxygen, as in high altitudes and airway obstruction
- The inability of the tissues to extract oxygen from the blood, as in septic shock and cyanide poisoning
- Obstructive or restrictive diseases such as COPD, in which airways and alveoli lose elasticity and become inflamed
- Impaired ventilation from multiple rib fractures, chest trauma, spinal cord injury, neuromuscular disease, CNS depression
- Poor tissue perfusion with oxygenated blood, as in all types of shock
- Failure of the hemoglobin to release oxygen to the tissues, as with a left-shifted oxyhemoglobin dissociation curve

Signs and symptoms of hypoxia include tachycardia, peripheral vasoconstriction, dizziness, and mental confusion. Treatment may include cardiac and respiratory stimulant drugs, oxygen therapy, mechanical ventilation, and frequent analysis of blood gases.

Hypoxemia. Hypoxemia is an abnormal deficiency in the concentration of oxygen in arterial blood, a low partial pressure of oxygen (PaO_2). Chronic hypoxemia stimulates RBC production by the bone marrow, leading to secondary polycythemia.

Causes of hypoxemia include the following:

- Decreased diffusion of oxygen from the lung (alveoli) into the blood, as in pneumonia or atelectasis
- Decreased alveolar oxygen tension
- Shunting of blood from the right side of the heart to the left side without exchange of gases in the lungs, cardiac arrhythmias such as ventricular fibrillation, or asystole.

Symptoms of acute hypoxemia include changes in respiration (tachypnea, dyspnea); blood pressure (hypertension, hypotension); color (pallor, cyanosis); mental status (headache, anxiety, impaired judgment, confusion, euphoria, lethargy); motor function (loss of coordination, weakness, tremors, hyperactive reflexes, restlessness, stupor, coma [around 30 mm Hg], death); arrhythmias (tachycardia, bradycardia), diaphoresis, blurred or tunnel vision, and nausea/vomiting. Treatment for hypoxemia includes administration of oxygen and correction of the underlying cause.

Hypoventilation. Hypoventilation occurs when ventilation is inadequate to meet the oxygen demands of the body or to eliminate carbon dioxide. This results in hypoxia or hypercapnia, an arterial carbon dioxide ($PaCO_2$) level greater than 45 mm Hg, and respiratory acidosis. Causes of hypoventilation include:

- Impaired ventilation related to trauma, pain, infection, obstructive diseases, or fluid volume overload
- Alterations in neurological regulation of breathing
- Alterations in chemical regulation of breathing
- Collapse of alveoli related to severe atelectasis

As ventilation decreases, $PaCO_2$ is elevated. Clinical signs and symptoms of hypoventilation include dizziness, occipital headache on awakening, lethargy, disorientation, decreased ability to follow instructions, cardiac dysrhythmias, electrolyte imbalances, convulsions, and possible coma or cardiac arrest.

When caring for patients with COPD and chronically elevated $PaCO_2$ levels, remember that inappropriate administration of excessive oxygen may result in hypoventilation. Patients with COPD and hypercapnia (high carbon dioxide levels) adapt to the higher carbon dioxide level. The carbon dioxide–sensitive chemoreceptors are no longer sensitive to increased carbon dioxide as a stimulus to breathe. Their stimulus to breathe is a decreased PaO_2.

Administering excessive oxygen to patients with COPD satisfies the oxygen requirement of the body and negates the stimulus to breathe. High concentrations of oxygen (e.g., greater than 24% to 28% [1 to 3 L/min]) prevent the PaO_2 from falling. As a result, this suppresses the stimulus to breathe, resulting in hypoventilation. The excessive retention of carbon dioxide leads to respiratory acidosis and ultimately respiratory arrest. If untreated, a patient's status rapidly declines, and death is possible. Treatment for hypoventilation involves treating the underlying cause, improving tissue oxygenation, restoring ventilation, and achieving acid-base balance.

Hyperventilation. Hyperventilation is an increase in respiratory rate, resulting in excess amounts of carbon dioxide elimination. This results in a decrease in $PaCO_2$, or hypocapnia, and respiratory alkalosis. Causes of hyperventilation include severe anxiety, infection, head injury, medications, or acid-base imbalance. Acute anxiety and an increased respiratory rate may cause loss of consciousness from excess carbon dioxide exhalation. An increase of 1°F in body temperature causes a 7% increase in metabolic rate, thereby increasing carbon dioxide production. The clinical response is increased rate and depth of respiration. Hypoxia associated with pulmonary embolus or shock also results in hyperventilation.

Hyperventilation produces signs and symptoms, including tachycardia, shortness of breath, chest pain, dizziness, light-headedness, decreased concentration, paresthesia, circumoral and/or extremity numbness, tinnitus, blurred vision,

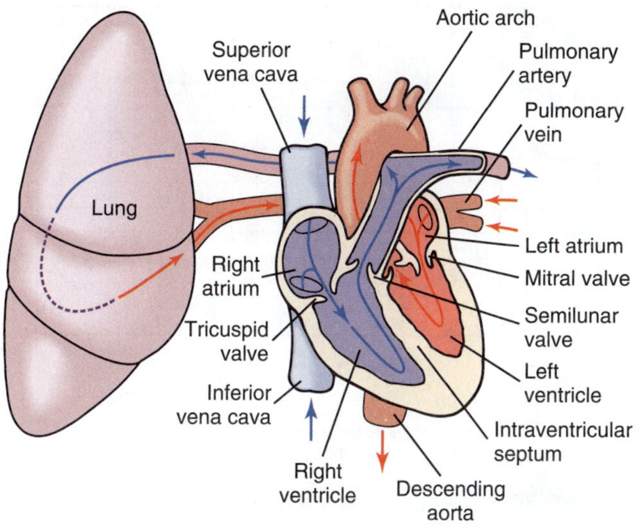

FIGURE 30-3 Schematic representation of blood flow through the heart. *Arrows* indicate direction of flow. (From Lewis SM, et al: *Medical surgical nursing: assessment and management of clinical problems,* ed 7, St Louis, 2007, Mosby.)

disorientation, and tetany (carpopedal spasm). Treatment for hyperventilation involves treating the underlying cause, improving tissue oxygenation, restoring ventilation, reducing respiratory rate, and achieving acid-base balance.

Structure and Function of the Circulatory System

The function of the circulatory system is to deliver oxygen, nutrients, and other substances to bodily tissues to support cellular life. Once cellular metabolism occurs, waste products accumulate. The system then removes waste products such as carbon dioxide and delivers them to the lungs and/or kidneys, where the wastes are eliminated. The pumping action of the heart is essential to support the circulatory system. The four heart valves (tricuspid, pulmonic, mitral, and aortic) ensure the one-way flow of blood through the heart (Figure 30-3).

Regulation of Blood Flow. There are multiple regulators of blood flow (Table 30-1). The heart muscle (myocardium) relaxes and contracts to support the regulation of blood flow. The contraction phase is called *systole,* in which blood is expelled from the ventricles into the systemic circulation. **Afterload** is the resistance to the ejection of blood from the left ventricle. The left ventricular pressure must be greater than the aortic pressure to eject blood from the heart. The relaxation phase is called *diastole,* in which blood fills the ventricles. **Preload** is the amount of blood at the end of ventricular diastole, or measured as end-diastolic pressure. Each contraction and relaxation consists of one cardiac cycle.

The amount of blood ejected from the left ventricle each minute is termed **cardiac output (CO).** A normal cardiac output for a healthy adult is 4 to 6 L/min. The cardiac output is calculated as follows:

$$\text{Cardiac output (CO)} = \text{Stroke volume (SV)} \times \text{Heart rate (HR)}$$

TABLE 30-1 REGULATION OF BLOOD FLOW

REGULATOR	DEFINITION
Cardiac output	Amount of blood ejected from the left ventricle per minute Normal range (adult): 4-6 L/min
Cardiac index	Measure of adequacy of the cardiac output: cardiac index equals cardiac output divided by patient's body surface area Normal range (adult): 2.5-4 L/min/m^3
Stroke volume	Amount of blood ejected from the ventricle with each contraction Normal range (adult): 50-75 mL per contraction
Preload	Amount of blood in the ventricles at end diastole
Afterload	Resistance of the ejection of blood from the left ventricle
Myocardial contractility	Ability of the heart to squeeze blood from the ventricles and prepare for the next contraction

Stroke volume (SV) is the amount of blood ejected from the ventricle with each contraction. The normal range for a healthy adult is 50 to 75 mL per contraction. The heart rate, or beats per minute, is regulated by the sympathetic and parasympathetic systems. Normal limits for heart rate are between 60 and 100 beats/min. **Myocardial contractility** is the ability of the heart to squeeze blood from the ventricles and prepare for the next contraction. This is difficult to measure because preload, afterload, and heart rate must remain constant. **Cardiac index** is a measure of adequacy of the cardiac output. It equals the cardiac output divided by the patient's body surface area. This calculation provides a caregiver with a more accurate calculation of blood flow by considering a patient's body surface area.

Conduction System. The conduction system generates impulses that initiate the electrical mechanical chain of events for a normal heartbeat. The rhythmic relaxation and contraction of the atria and ventricles depend on continuous, organized transmission of electrical impulses to the muscle. The conduction system generates, controls, and transmits these impulses (Figure 30-4). The autonomic nervous system influences the rate of impulse generation, the transmission speed through the conductive pathway, and the strength of contractions through sympathetic and parasympathetic (vagus nerve) nerve fibers in the atria and ventricles. The vagus nerve (parasympathetic) also innervates sinoatrial and atrioventricular nodes and is able to reduce the rate of impulse generation.

The conduction system originates with the **sinoatrial (SA) node,** the "pacemaker" of the heart. The SA node is in the

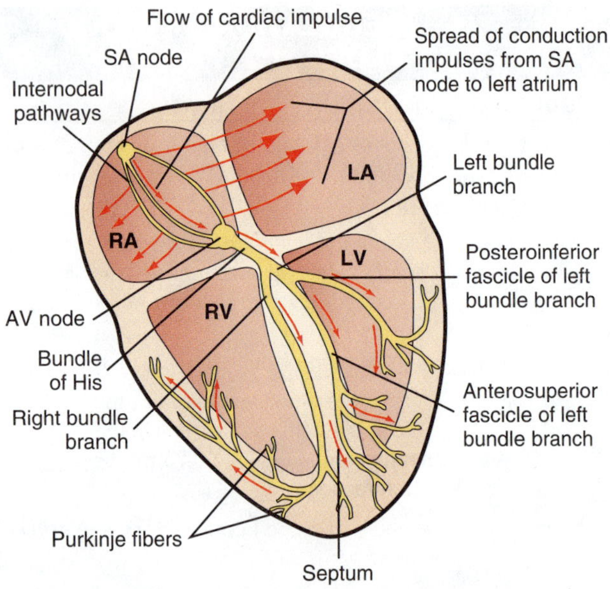

FIGURE 30-4 Conduction system of the heart. *AV,* Atrioventricular; *LA,* left atrium; *LV,* left ventricle; *RA,* right atrium; *RV,* right ventricle; *SA,* sinoatrial. (From Lewis SM, et al: *Medical surgical nursing: assessment and management of clinical problems,* ed 7, St Louis, 2007, Mosby.)

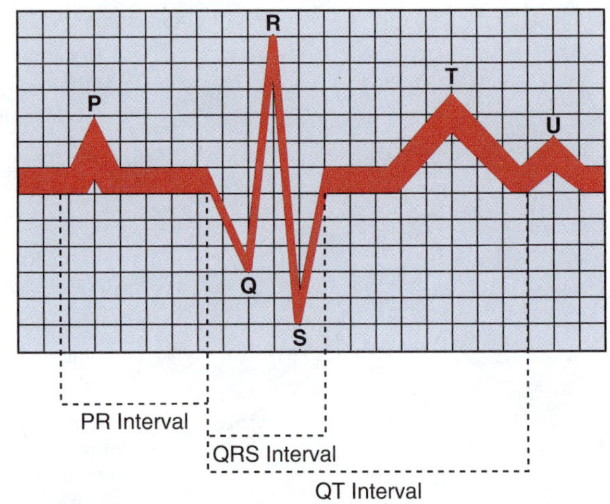

FIGURE 30-5 Normal electrocardiogram (ECG) pattern. The P wave represents depolarization of the atria. The QRS complex indicates depolarization of the ventricles. The T wave represents repolarization of the ventricles. The U wave, if present, may represent repolarization of the Purkinje fibers, or it may be associated with hypokalemia. The PR, QRS, and QT intervals reflect the length of the time it takes for the impulse to travel from one area of the heart to another. (From Lewis SM, et al: *Medical surgical nursing: assessment and management of clinical problems,* ed 7, St Louis, 2007, Mosby.)

right atrium next to the entrance of the superior vena cava. Impulses begin at the SA node at an intrinsic rate of 60 to 100 beats/min. The resting adult rate ranges from 60 to 80 beats/min. Electrical impulses are then transmitted along intraatrial pathways to the **atrioventricular (AV) node.** The AV node mediates impulse transmission between the atria and the ventricles. Delaying the impulse at the AV node before transmitting it through the bundle of His and ventricular Purkinje network assists atrial emptying.

An electrocardiogram (ECG) records the electrical activity of the conduction system as waves and complexes. An ECG monitors the regularity and path of the electrical impulse through the conduction system; however, it does not reflect the muscular work of the heart. The normal sequence of electrical impulses on the ECG is called **normal sinus rhythm (NSR)** (Figure 30-5). A normal ECG waveform consists of a P wave (atrial **depolarization**), QRS complex (ventricular depolarization), and T wave (ventricular **repolarization**). Health care providers interpret the size, appearance, and sequence of waves to identify dysrhythmias and recognize the area of the heart affected.

Alterations of the Circulatory System

Illnesses and conditions that affect cardiac rate, rhythm, strength of contraction, blood flow through the chambers, myocardial blood flow, and peripheral circulation alter cardiac functioning. Controllable risk factors for heart disease include smoking, uncontrolled hypertension, physical inactivity, obesity, uncontrolled diabetes, uncontrolled stress and anger, and high-density lipoprotein (HDL) and low-density lipoprotein (LDL) or bad cholesterol levels. Uncontrollable risk factors include the male gender, older age, a family history of heart disease, postmenopause, and a patient's ethnicity (CDC, 2012a). African-Americans, American Indians, and Mexican Americans are at greater risk than Caucasians for developing heart disease. Several genetic disorders lead to an increased risk of early heart attacks. Familial hypercholesterolemia is a genetic condition in which there are high levels of LDL from birth, occurring in about 1 in 500 people in the United States.

Decreased Cardiac Output. Failure of the myocardium to eject sufficient blood volume to the systemic and pulmonary circulations results in heart failure. Failure of the myocardial pump results from primary coronary artery disease (CAD), valvular disorders, cardiomyopathic conditions, conduction disorders and pulmonary disease.

Myocardial Ischemia. **Myocardial ischemia** happens when the coronary artery does not supply sufficient blood to the heart muscle (myocardium). Decreased perfusion to the myocardium results in chest pain, especially with activity. Angina or angina pectoris is the result of decreased blood flow to the myocardium as a result of coronary artery spasms or temporary constriction. When decreased myocardial blood perfusion is extensive or perfusion is completely blocked, the tissue becomes necrotic, and a **myocardial infarction** occurs. Myocardial infarction presents clinically as severe or crushing chest pain, jaw pain, left arm pain, breathlessness, diaphoresis, and hypotension (a fall in blood pressure).

Impaired Valvular Function. Valvular heart disease is an acquired or congenital disorder of a cardiac valve characterized by stenosis, which results in obstructed blood flow, or valvular degeneration and regurgitation, which results in backflow of blood. When stenosis occurs in the aortic and pulmonic valves, the adjacent ventricles work harder to move the ventricular volume beyond the stenotic valve. When regurgitation occurs, there is a backflow of blood into an adjacent chamber, which causes either pulmonary or systemic congestion.

Left-Sided Heart Failure. Left-sided heart failure is characterized by impaired functioning of the left ventricle. This is usually caused by increased preload (fluid volume overload) or afterload (increased systemic vascular resistance such as hypertension). If left ventricular failure is significant, the amount of blood ejected from the left ventricle drops greatly, resulting in decreased cardiac output. Patients may present with pulmonary congestion; as a result you will note crackles on auscultation and patient complaints of fatigue, dyspnea, and orthopnea (difficulty breathing while lying down).

Right-Sided Heart Failure. Right-sided heart failure results from impaired functioning of the right ventricle, which is typically caused by pulmonary disease or pulmonary hypertension. An increase in pressure in the pulmonary system causes increased resistance in the right ventricle. The right ventricle fails as a result of this pressure. The patient then develops venous congestion in the systemic circulation, and on assessment you often identify distended jugular veins and peripheral edema. Right-sided heart failure may also result from untreated or end-stage left-sided heart failure.

Hypovolemia. Hypovolemia is a reduced circulating blood volume resulting from extracellular fluid losses that occurs in conditions such as shock and severe dehydration. If the fluid loss is significant, the body tries to adapt by increasing the heart rate and constricting peripheral vessels to increase the volume of blood returned to the heart and the cardiac output.

Disturbances in Conduction. A dysrhythmia is a disturbance in the electrical impulse of the heart rhythm. Any rhythm not generated at the SA node is classified as such. Dysrhythmias are primary conduction disturbances that occur as a response to ischemia, valvular abnormalities, anxiety, and drug toxicity (e.g., digoxin toxicity). Dysrhythmias also occur as a result of excess caffeine, alcohol, or tobacco use; following cardiothoracic surgery; or as a complication of acid-base or electrolyte imbalance (see Chapter 18).

Dysrhythmias are classified by their site of origin and cardiac response (Table 30-2). The cardiac response can be an increase in heart rate such as tachycardia (greater than 100 beats/min), a decrease in heart rate such as bradycardia (less than 60 beats/min), premature (early beat) atrial or ventricular beats, or blocked (delayed or absent beat) atrial or ventricular beats. Dysrhythmias often affect the pumping mechanism of the heart.

TABLE 30-2 COMMON BASIC CARDIAC DYSRHYTHMIAS

RHYTHM CHARACTERISTICS	ETIOLOGY	CLINICAL SIGNIFICANCE	MANAGEMENT
Sinus Tachycardia			
Regular rhythm, rate 100-180 beats/min (higher in infants), normal P wave, normal QRS complex	Rate increase is a normal response to exercise, emotion, or stressors such as pain, fever, pump failure, hypovolemia, hyperthyroidism, and certain drugs (e.g., caffeine, nitrates, nicotine).	Patient with damaged heart may be unable to sustain increased workloads (increased myocardial oxygen consumption) brought on by persistent increases in heart rate; reduces myocardial perfusion.	Assess and support ABCs. Check vital signs. Consult expert clinician. Correct underlying factors; remove offending drugs.
Sinus Bradycardia			
Regular rhythm, rate <60 beats/min, normal P wave, normal PR interval, normal QRS complex	Rate decrease is a normal response to sleep or a well-conditioned athlete; abnormal drops in rate are caused by diminished blood flow to SA node, vagal stimulation, hypothyroidism, increased intracranial pressure, or certain drugs (e.g., digoxin, propranolol, procainamide).	Has clinical significance when associated with signs of impaired cardiac output and symptoms of dizziness, hypotension, syncope, chest pain.	Assess and support ABCs. Check vital signs. Consult expert clinician. Correct underlying causes; prepare for transcutaneous pacing; consider atropine; consider IV epinephrine or dopamine.

Continued

TABLE 30-2 COMMON BASIC CARDIAC DYSRHYTHMIAS—cont'd

RHYTHM CHARACTERISTICS	ETIOLOGY	CLINICAL SIGNIFICANCE	MANAGEMENT
Atrial Fibrillation (A-FIB)			
Irregular atrial activity resulting in an irregular ventricular response with resultant irregular cardiac rate and rhythm. No identifiable P wave. Rate determined by conduction of multiple atrial impulses across the AV node	Caused by aging, calcification of the SA node, electrolyte imbalances, valvular disturbances, or changes in myocardial blood supply	Loss of the atrial kick (portion of the cardiac output squeezed in the ventricles with a coordinated atrial contraction), pooling of blood in the atria, and development of microemboli. Patients complain of fatigue, a fluttering in the chest, and shortness of breath if ventricular response is rapid. Patients may have hypotension.	Assess and support ABCs. Check vital signs. Consult expert clinician. Prepare for synchronized cardioversion (shock delivered during the relative refractory period of the cardiac cycle). Prepare for rate control medication therapy such as diltiazem or beta-blockers. Treat underlying cause. Managed with blood thinners such as warfarin (Coumadin).
Ventricular Tachycardia			
Rhythm slightly irregular, rate 100-200 beats/min, P wave absent, QRS complex wide and bizarre, >0.12 sec	Caused by irritable ventricular foci firing repetitively, commonly caused by myocardial infarction	Often occurs before ventricular fibrillation; if condition persistent and rapid, causes decreased cardiac output because of decreased ventricular filling time. Patient may or may not have a pulse.	Assess and support ABCDs. Check vital signs. Consult expert clinician. Prepare for IV amiodarone over 10 min. Prepare for synchronized cardioversion (patient with a pulse). Prepare for CPR and unsynchronized cardioversion/defibrillation (patient without a pulse).
Ventricular Fibrillation			
Irregular and chaotic rhythm with no discernible waves or rate	Ventricles are quivering, not pumping	The patient is pulseless and apneic.	Immediate resuscitation is required. Begin ABCDs. In-hospital goals: Give rescue breaths and begin CPR within 1 min. Apply AED or defibrillator within 3 min and deliver unsynchronized shocks. Prepare to administer IV/IO epinephrine every 3-5 min (or vasopressin to replace the first or second epinephrine dose). Consider antiarrhythmics such as amiodarone or lidocaine.
Asystole			
Absence of electrical activity; no discernible rate or rhythm	Cardiac standstill	The patient is pulseless and apneic.	Immediate resuscitation is required. Begin ABCDs. Prepare to administer IV/IO epinephrine every 3-5 min (or vasopressin to replace the first or second epinephrine dose). Prepare to administer IV/IO atropine every 3-5 min (up to three doses).

Data from American Heart Association: *CPR*, 2010, http://www.Americanheart.org.
ABC, Airway, breathing, circulation; *ABCD*, airway, breathing, circulation, defibrillation; *AED*, automatic external defibrillator; *AV*, atrioventricular; *CPR*, cardiopulmonary resuscitation; *IO*, intraosseous; *IV*, intravenous.

Factors Affecting Oxygenation

Alterations in oxygenation result from a decrease in oxygen-carrying capacity of blood (e.g., anemia), an increase in the metabolic demands of the body (e.g., fever or infection), and any alteration that affects a patient's chest wall movement or the CNS.

Decreased Oxygen-Carrying Capacity. Ninety-seven percent of oxygen is carried on the hemoglobin molecule. Any process that decreases or alters hemoglobin such as anemia or inhalation of toxic substances decreases the oxygen-carrying capacity of blood. Anemia is the reduction in RBCs or decrease in hemoglobin, the oxygen-carrying protein of RBCs. Acute blood loss or chronic disease often results in anemia.

Carbon monoxide is the most common toxic inhalant decreasing the oxygen-carrying capacity of blood. Hemoglobin tends to bind with carbon monoxide 20 times more readily than with oxygen, creating a functional hypoxemia (Thibodeau and Patton, 2011). Because of the strength of the bond, it is not easy for carbon monoxide to dissociate (break away) from hemoglobin, making the hemoglobin unavailable for oxygen transport.

Decreased Inspired Oxygen Concentration. When the concentration of inspired oxygen declines, the oxygen-carrying capacity of the blood decreases. An upper or lower airway obstruction limiting delivery of inspired oxygen to alveoli causes a decrease in the fraction of inspired oxygen concentration (FiO_2). Decreased environmental oxygen (as occurs at high altitudes) or decreased delivery of inspired oxygen as the result of an incorrect oxygen concentration setting on respiratory therapy equipment also results in a decreased FiO_2.

Increased Metabolic Rate. Increases in metabolic activity of the body increase oxygen demand. Oxygen levels fall when the body is unable to meet an increased oxygen demand. An increased metabolic rate is a normal response of the body to pregnancy, wound healing, and exercise because the body is building tissue. Most people are able to meet increased oxygen demands and do not display signs of oxygen deprivation.

Fever increases the need of the tissues for oxygen. As a result, carbon dioxide production also increases. If a fever lasts for a period of time, the metabolic rate remains high, and the body begins to break down protein stores, resulting in muscle wasting and decreased muscle mass. Respiratory muscles such as the diaphragm and intercostals are also wasted. The body attempts to adapt to the increased carbon dioxide (hypercapnia) levels by increasing the rate and depth of respiration to eliminate the excess carbon dioxide. The patient's work of breathing increases, and the patient eventually displays signs and symptoms of hypoxemia, a decreased arterial oxygen level in the blood. Early clinical signs and symptoms of hypoxemia include:

- Anxiety
- Change in level of consciousness
- Restlessness
- Inability to concentrate
- Increased heart rate
- Increased respiratory rate and blood pressure
- Cardiac dysrhythmias such as premature ventricular contractions, premature atrial contractions, and sinus tachycardia

As the hypoxemia worsens some patients lose consciousness. Patients with pulmonary diseases are at greater risk for hypoxemia and hypercapnia, an elevated $PaCO_2$ level. Patient assessments often show an increased rate and depth of respiration and the use of pursed-lip breathing and accessory muscles of respiration.

Conditions Affecting Chest Wall Movement. Any condition that reduces chest wall movement decreases ventilation. If the diaphragm is unable to fully descend with breathing, the volume of inspired air decreases, delivering less oxygen to the alveoli and subsequently to tissues.

Musculoskeletal Abnormalities. Abnormalities in the thoracic region such as abnormal structural shapes and muscle disease contribute to decreased oxygenation and ventilation. Abnormal structural shapes impairing oxygenation include those that affect the rib cage such as pectus excavatum and those that affect the spinal column such as kyphosis. The angle of curvature in kyphosis can progress with time, resulting in severe hypoventilation and hypoxemia.

Muscle diseases such as muscular dystrophy affect oxygenation by decreasing diaphragmatic movement (i.e., the patient's ability to expand and contract the chest). This impairs ventilation and often causes atelectasis, hypercapnia, and hypoxemia.

Nervous System Diseases. Myasthenia gravis, Guillain-Barré syndrome, and poliomyelitis are examples of nervous system diseases that result in hypoventilation. These diseases impair nervous and muscular control, causing reduced ventilation (hypoventilation).

Disease or trauma involving the medulla oblongata and spinal cord of the CNS has the ability to impair respiration. When the medulla oblongata is affected, neural regulation of respiration is damaged, and abnormal breathing patterns develop. Damage to the spinal cord affects respiration in two ways. If the phrenic nerve is damaged, the diaphragm does not descend, thus reducing inspiratory lung volumes and causing hypoxemia. Cervical trauma at C3 to C5 level results in paralysis of the phrenic nerve. Spinal cord trauma below the fifth cervical vertebra usually leaves the phrenic nerve intact but damages nerves that innervate the intercostal muscles, preventing anteroposterior chest expansion.

Trauma. Trauma to the chest wall also impairs inspiration. The person with multiple rib fractures sometimes develops a flail chest, a life-threatening condition in which fractures cause instability in part of the chest wall. This causes paradoxical breathing in which the lung underlying the injured area contracts on inspiration and expands on expiration, making ventilation ineffective. Chest wall or upper abdominal incisions also decrease chest wall movement because incisional pain causes patients to inhale shallowly, which decreases chest wall movement.

NURSING KNOWLEDGE BASE

Your nursing knowledge prepares you to anticipate a patient's oxygenation needs. Knowledge of a patient's lifestyle patterns and developmental status allows you to anticipate cardiopulmonary problems.

Developmental Factors

The developmental stage of a patient and the normal aging process affect tissue oxygenation.

Premature Infants. Premature infants are at risk for hyaline membrane disease, which is caused by surfactant deficiency. **Surfactant** is a chemical in the lung that maintains the integrity of the alveoli, keeping the alveoli dry and preventing alveolar collapse. When surfactant is inadequate, the alveoli become stiff and fluid filled, which impedes the exchange of respiratory gases. The surfactant-synthesizing ability of the lung develops about the seventh month and is lacking in preterm infants born before or during the seventh month. Premature infants are at risk for development of respiratory illnesses such as respiratory syncytial virus (RSV) infection as a result of the underdevelopment of the lung.

Infants and Toddlers. Infants and toddlers are at risk for upper respiratory tract infections as a result of frequent exposure to other children and exposure to secondhand smoke. During the teething process some infants develop nasal congestion, which encourages bacterial growth and increases the risk for respiratory tract infection. Upper respiratory tract infections are usually not dangerous, and infants and toddlers recover with little difficulty. Infants and toddlers are also at risk for airway obstruction because of their tendency to place a foreign object in their mouth.

School-Age Children and Adolescents. School-age children and adolescents are exposed to respiratory infections and respiratory risk factors such as secondhand smoke and are at risk to experiment with cigarette smoking. A healthy child usually does not have adverse pulmonary effects from respiratory infections. However, a person who starts smoking in adolescence and continues to smoke into middle age has an increased risk for cardiopulmonary disease and lung cancer.

Young and Middle-Age Adults. Young and middle-age adults are exposed to many cardiopulmonary risk factors: an unhealthy diet, lack of exercise, stress, excessive use of highly caffeinated energy drinks, and cigarette smoking. Reducing these modifiable factors sometimes decreases a patient's risk for cardiac or pulmonary diseases.

Pregnancy causes changes in ventilation. As the fetus grows during pregnancy, the greater size of the uterus pushes abdominal contents up against the diaphragm. During the last trimester of pregnancy the inspiratory capacity declines, resulting in **dyspnea** on exertion and increased fatigue.

Older Adults. The cardiac and pulmonary systems change throughout the aging process (Table 30-3). Normal changes of aging place an older adult at risk for complications in oxygenation, particularly when hospitalized. Older adults are at increased risk for the development of influenza, community-acquired pneumonia, and RSV infection, which sometimes results in death (Centers for Disease Control and Prevention [CDC], 2012b).

Lifestyle Factors

Patients are exposed to numerous lifestyle factors that alone or combined affect cardiopulmonary function. Knowledge of these factors enables a nurse to consider the health promotion needs of patients.

Nutrition. Nutrition affects cardiopulmonary function in several ways. Good nutritional status supports the normal metabolic functions. A poor diet leads to risk factors affecting the heart and lungs such as obesity, hypertension, heart disease, and chronic lung disease.

Inadequate nutrition occurs when nutritional intake does not meet nutritional needs. Without essential nutrients, a patient may experience respiratory muscle wasting, resulting in decreased muscle strength and respiratory excursion. Cough efficiency is reduced secondary to respiratory muscle weakness, putting a patient at risk for retention of pulmonary secretions. A patient with chronic lung disease usually requires a diet higher in calories because of the increased work of breathing. A moderate-carbohydrate diet is recommended to prevent an increase in carbon dioxide production. Calories from carbohydrates should be no more than 50% of the daily allowance.

Overnutrition or the excess intake of nutrients most commonly leads to obesity. This leads to a decrease in lung expansion and an increase in oxygen demand to meet metabolic needs. Diets high in fat increase cholesterol and development of plaque in the coronary arteries, placing individuals at risk for CAD. Patients who have alterations in nutrition are also at risk for anemia. If the diet does not supply iron needed for hemoglobin synthesis, RBC synthesis is reduced, and oxygen-carrying capacity decreases.

Hydration. Fluid intake is essential for cellular health. Fluid intake depends on a patient's diet and disease processes that would require more or less water. Fluid volume overload or hypervolemia may lead to vascular congestion in patients with heart, kidney, or lung diseases. Dehydration or fluid volume deficit may result in dizziness; fainting, hypotension; a decrease in respiratory secretion production; or a thickening of respiratory secretions, making it difficult for a patient to expectorate secretions.

Exercise. Exercise increases the metabolic activity and oxygen demand of the body. The rate and depth of respiration increase, enabling a person to inhale more oxygen and exhale excess carbon dioxide. A physical exercise program has many benefits (see Chapter 27). People who exercise daily for 30 to 60 minutes have a lower heart rate, lower blood pressure, decreased cholesterol, increased blood flow, and greater oxygen extraction by working muscles. The addition of weight training has shown benefit in decreasing the work of the heart by increasing the efficiency of the other muscles of the body. Fully conditioned people are able to increase

TABLE 30-3 CHANGES IN THE AGING CARDIOPULMONARY SYSTEM

FUNCTION	PATHOPHYSIOLOGICAL CHANGE	KEY CLINICAL FINDINGS
Heart		
Muscle contraction	Ventricular wall thickened, collagen increased, and elastin decreased in the heart muscle	Decreased cardiac output
Blood flow	Heart valves, especially the mitral and aortic valves, become thicker and stiffen	Systolic ejection murmur
Conduction system	SA node becomes fibrotic from calcification; decrease in number of pacemaker cells in the SA node	Increased PR, QRS, and Q/T intervals; decreased amplitude of the QRS complex
Arterial vessel compliance	Vessels become calcified; loss of arterial distensibility, decreased elastin in the vessel walls, more tortuous vessels	Hypertension, with an increase in systolic blood pressure
Lungs		
Breathing mechanics	Decreased chest wall compliance and loss of elastic recoil Decreased respiratory muscle mass and strength	Prolonged exhalation phase Decreased vital capacity
Oxygenation	Increased ventilation-perfusion mismatch Decreased alveolar surface area and decreased carbon dioxide diffusion capacity	Decreased PaO_2 Decreased cardiac output Slightly increased PaO_2
Breathing control/breathing pattern	Decreased responsiveness of central and peripheral chemoreceptors to hypoxemia and hypercapnia	Decreased tidal volume Increased respiratory rate
Lung defense mechanisms	Decreased number of cilia Decreased immunoglobulin A (IgA) production and humoral and cellular immunity	Decreased airway clearance Increased risk for infection
Sleep and breathing	Decreased respiratory drive Decreased tone of upper airway muscles	Increased risk for arterial desaturation Increased risk for aspiration and infection Snoring/obstructive sleep apnea

PaO_2, Partial pressure of oxygen; *SA,* sinoatrial.

oxygen consumption by 10% to 20% because of increased cardiac output and efficiency of the myocardium.

Cigarette Smoking. Cigarette smoking is associated with a number of diseases, including heart disease, COPD, and lung cancer. Inhaled nicotine enables plaque to build up more quickly in the blood vessels, increases the risks for blood clots, and causes vasoconstriction in the coronary and peripheral vessels. The risk for lung cancer is 10 times greater for a person who smokes than for a nonsmoker. Exposure to secondhand smoke increases the risk for lung cancer in the nonsmoker and worsens other pulmonary problems such as asthma or COPD.

Substance Abuse. Excessive use of alcohol and other drugs impairs tissue oxygenation. A patient who has chronic substance abuse usually has a poor nutritional intake. This often causes a decreased intake from iron-rich foods, leading to a decrease in hemoglobin production. Excessive use of alcohol and certain other drugs depresses the respiratory center, reducing the rate and depth of respiration and the amount of inhaled oxygen. Substances that are inhaled or smoked cause direct injury to lung tissue, leading to permanent lung damage and impaired oxygenation. Intravenous drug use places a person at risk for infections of the heart (endocarditis or myocarditis), blood clots, and transmitted diseases such as human immunodeficiency virus (HIV).

Stress. Stress is a perceived threat that results in sympathetic stimulation (the fight-or-flight response). It often poses a demand that exceeds a patient's coping ability, both physically and emotionally. Continuous stress adversely affects a patient's health and well-being. A continuous state of stress increases the metabolic rate and oxygen demand of the body. The body responds to stress by an increased rate and depth of respiration and increased cardiac output. Stressors also alter the normal response to illness and pain. Stress causes an increased release of cortisol, which affects the metabolism of fat and creates a risk for CAD and hypertension. Stressors are also often triggers for asthma attacks. Most people are able to adapt to physical or emotional stressors. Some patients, particularly those with chronic illnesses or acute life-threatening illnesses, cannot tolerate the oxygen demands associated with stress.

Environmental Factors

The environment also influences oxygenation. The incidence of pulmonary disease is higher in smoggy, urban areas than in rural areas. In addition, a patient's workplace sometimes increases the risks for cardiopulmonary disease. Occupational pollutants include asbestos, talcum powder, dust, and airborne fibers. For example, tunnel workers exposed to dust from blasting, drilling, and rock transport have an increased risk for COPD. Construction workers may be at risk for asbestosis from asbestos exposure. This leads to pulmonary fibrosis, a restrictive lung disease, and may also lead to lung cancer.

CRITICAL THINKING

Synthesis

You will apply elements of critical thinking whenever you perform the nursing process with patients. Consider the scientific knowledge you have learned, your experience, critical thinking attitudes, and standards to ensure an individualized approach to patient care (Box 30-2).

Knowledge. When caring for patients with cardiopulmonary problems, you need to incorporate and apply knowledge from physiology and pathophysiology; pharmacology; nutrition; and fluid, electrolyte, and acid-base balance. Your knowledge of health promotion and disease prevention is essential. This prevents or helps to reduce at-risk behaviors and unhealthy lifestyles in your patients who are at risk for or have cardiopulmonary problems.

A patient can reduce his or her blood pressure by 25 points by changing his or her lifestyle. Instruct patients on lifestyle modifications such as weight reduction by following the low-sodium and low-fat DASH diet (U.S. Department of Health and Human Services, 2006). Also advise patients to increase their activity levels daily (minimum 30 minutes, 5 days/week) and to achieve a target blood pressure <135/85 mm Hg (NHLBI guidelines) or 140/90 mm Hg (JNC-8 Guidelines, Jones et al., 2014). The reduction of cardiovascular/renal morbidity and mortality and the reduction of LDL <100 mg/dL, total cholesterol (TC) <200 mg/dL, and HDL >60 mg/dL also lowers risk factors for cardiac disease. Your knowledge of risk factors for cardiopulmonary disease helps patients attain and maintain optimal cardiopulmonary function.

Experience. In the acute care setting you care for patients with acute aggravations of their disease. When your patients require nursing management in the community setting, they are usually stable, productive members of the community with little or no change in lifestyle. Use your experience in caring for patients with cardiopulmonary diseases to recognize clinical changes and select effective interventions. Most important, use the resources available in your work area to help you provide safe patient care.

Attitudes. You use critical thinking attitudes as you provide nursing care for patients with cardiopulmonary alterations. As a patient's advocate, determine if the patient is aware of his or her risk factors and then partner with him or her to find the best teaching approaches to reinforce learning or provide instruction. Do not be judgmental. Use discipline when providing health care information to your patients. For example, when deciding on the approach for a patient who has respiratory disease and still smokes, use the best-known teaching approaches. On the other hand, it is unlikely that an older adult with end-stage disease will be willing or able to stop smoking. In this case it is better to acknowledge that your patients already know the risks of smoking and why they should stop than to bombard them with teaching materials.

Perseverance is also important in finding effective patient-centered solutions. For example, when a patient has severe cardiac or pulmonary disease and limited income, your solutions for promoting health and maintaining patient independence are complex. Sometimes you need to continue to provide the same information at each visit. Often patients with chronic hypoxemia have a decreased short-term memory, and you need to reinforce information previously provided. Also consider involving family caregivers in any instructions you provide.

Standards. Nationally recognized organizations set forth best practices. The American Heart Association (AHA), American Lung Association (ALA), American Thoracic Society (ATS), American Cancer Society (ACS), and Agency

BOX 30-2 SYNTHESIS IN PRACTICE

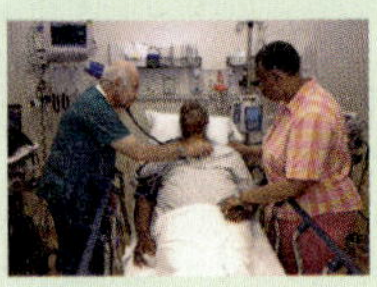

John's *knowledge* of the physiology of pulmonary conditions helps him care for Mr. King. Mr. King's history reveals risk factors in addition to a 40-year history of smoking 2 packs per day, and he still continues to smoke. John knows that the shortness of breath is because the infection is obstructing his alveolocapillary membrane, preventing oxygenation of blood in some parts of his lung. He also is aware of his preexisting COPD and the effects of his smoking. Because of John's *experience* working with patients who are addicted to inhaled nicotine, he recognizes the difficulty in quitting. He knows that the most effective time to encourage a patient to stop smoking is when he or she is in an acute care setting with an illness exacerbated by smoking.

John's *attitude* about his nursing care reflects his respect for the patient's autonomy and balances this with continually educating Mr. King about the risk factors of smoking. John knows the impact of support systems in helping patients cope with chronic illnesses. He uses creativity and independent thinking to incorporate community and family resources into the plan of care for Mr. King. John needs to inquire about his social supports and the availability in his community of programs to help him quit smoking. He reviews the *standards* set by the American Cancer Society to identify that tobacco use accounts for at least 30% of all cancer deaths and 87% of lung cancer deaths. He uses this and the resources at http://www.cancer.org to help educate Mr. King and his wife about cancer statistics and methods to quit smoking.

COPD, Chronic obstructive pulmonary disease.

for Healthcare Research and Quality (AHRQ) have specific guidelines for cardiopulmonary nursing care and disease management. The American Nurses Association (ANA) also has guidelines and standards for patient care. Each of these organizations reviews best practice standards and publishes its findings. Knowledge of the evidence that supports your practice enables you to provide safe and effective nursing care.

You use professional standards in the care of all patients. In the care of Mr. King, these standards help to determine the appropriate medical and nursing interventions for a patient with pneumonia.

NURSING PROCESS

ASSESSMENT

Make sure that nursing assessment of your patient's cardiopulmonary functioning includes data collected from the following areas:

- History of the patient's baseline and present cardiopulmonary function, past cardiopulmonary illnesses/surgeries, and measures the patient uses to improve breathing or heart function (e.g., medications, treatments, exercises)
- Physical examination of the patient's cardiopulmonary status (see Chapter 16)
- Review of laboratory and diagnostic test results

Nursing History. The nursing history focuses on your patient's ability to meet oxygen needs and control symptoms. Ask questions that help the patient describe symptoms. Box 30-3 gives examples of assessment questions for you to ask your patient with cardiopulmonary conditions.

Risk Factors. Investigate familial, occupational, and environmental risk factors. Review the patient's family history of cardiovascular or lung disease. Document which blood relatives have cardiopulmonary disease, the type of condition, and their present level of health or age at time of death. Other family risk factors to assess include the presence of infectious diseases, particularly tuberculosis (TB). Determine who in the patient's household has the disease and the status of the treatment.

Environmental exposure to many inhaled substances such as smog, cotton fibers, silicon, mold, cockroaches, secondhand smoke, and asbestos is closely linked to respiratory disease. Investigate exposures in the patient's home and workplace. Ask the following:

- Are there environmental conditions that affect your breathing where you work?
- Have you recently traveled to countries or areas of the United States where you have been exposed to uncommon respiratory diseases?
- What is/was your occupation? Were you exposed to chemicals or inhalants?

Assess the patient for other risk factors such as exercise habits, presence and frequency of stress, tobacco use, and diet. It helps to have patients record what they eat over a week's period of time to determine dietary habits and types of food eaten.

Fatigue. Fatigue is a subjective sensation reported as a loss of endurance. It is a common sign of prolonged exposure to stress and is often an early sign of worsening of an existing chronic cardiopulmonary disease. To provide a mechanism to objectively measure fatigue, use a visual analog scale (see Chapter 31) with a rating from 0 to 10, with 10 being the worst level of fatigue and 0 representing no fatigue. In addition, ask your patients questions about their perception of fatigue:

- When did you first notice the fatigue? What makes it get better or worse?

BOX 30-3 NURSING ASSESSMENT QUESTIONS

NATURE OF THE CARDIOPULMONARY PROBLEM

- Tell me the types of breathing problems you are having.
- Describe the problem you are having with your heart.
- Does it occur at a specific time of the day, during or after exercise, or all the time?

SIGNS AND SYMPTOMS

- How has your breathing pattern changed?
- Are you having sputum with coughing? Is this different?
- Tell me what the sputum looks like. Is it a different color from normal?
- Are you having any chest pain? Does the pain occur with breathing or activity?

ONSET AND DURATION

- If you are having chest pain, what causes the pain and how long does it last? Is this a different type of pain?
- When did you notice your sputum change in color and amount?
- When did your coughing increase? How does this differ from your usual pattern of coughing?

SEVERITY

- On a scale of 0 to 10, with 10 being the most severe, rate your shortness of breath.
- What helps your shortness of breath?
- On a scale of 0 to 10, with 0 being no pain and 10 the most severe pain, rate your chest pain. Is the severity of your pain different today?
- What do you do for this pain?

PREDISPOSING FACTORS

- Have you been exposed to another person who had a cold or the flu?
- Are you taking your prescribed medications?
- Do you smoke? Have you been exposed to secondhand smoke?
- Have you been doing any unusual exercises?

EFFECT OF SYMPTOMS ON PATIENT

- Do these symptoms affect your daily activities? If so, how?
- What impact do these symptoms have on your appetite, sleeping habits, activity status?

- Was the onset sudden or gradual? Is it related to any time of the day or constant throughout the day?
- Does it prevent you from doing what you want to do?

Pain. Cardiac pain does not occur with respiratory variations. It is most often substernal and typically radiates to the left arm and jaw in males. Some women have epigastric pain, complaints of indigestion, nausea or vomiting, or a choking feeling and dyspnea. Pericardial pain resulting from an inflammation of the pericardial sac is usually nonradiating and often occurs with inspiration or when leaning forward. Use a visual analog scale to help a patient describe the pain (see Chapter 32).

Pleuritic chest pain is peripheral and usually radiates to the scapular regions. Inspiratory maneuvers such as coughing, yawning, and sighing aggravate pleuritic chest pain. An inflammation or infection in the pleural space usually causes pleuritic chest pain. Patients often describe it as knifelike, lasting from 1 minute to hours and increasing with inspiration.

Musculoskeletal pain is often present following exercise, rib trauma, and prolonged coughing episodes. Inspiratory movements aggravate the pain and are easily confused with pleuritic chest pain.

When assessing pain in patients with cardiopulmonary disease, obtain information specific to cardiac or inspiratory pain. For example, ask your patient the following:

- Have you ever had pain in your chest? Explain.
- Where and when do you feel the pain? Does it radiate? Does it change with inspiration? Does this pain go away when you hold your breath?
- What does the pain feel like? Sharp, dull, stabbing? Does it change with inspiration or expiration?
- Does it occur at rest or with activity?
- How long does it last?
- What makes it better?

Breathing Patterns. Dyspnea is the subjective sensation of breathlessness as perceived by a patient. It is a clinical sign of hypoxia. Dyspnea is associated with symptoms such as exaggerated respiratory effort, use of the accessory muscles of respiration, nasal flaring, and marked increases in the rate and depth of respirations. Use a visual analog scale to help patients objectively assess their dyspnea, with 0 being no dyspnea and 10 being the worst dyspnea the patient has experienced. Measurement of dyspnea on the analog scale helps to show change in a patient's perception of breathlessness. Chronic dyspnea has long-term physical, psychological, and sociocultural consequences.

Dyspnea that occurs when a patient is sleeping is called paroxysmal nocturnal dyspnea (PND). The patient awakens in a panic, feels as if he or she is suffocating, and has a strong need to sit up to relieve the breathlessness. The cause of PND is probably resorption of fluid from dependent body areas when the patient is recumbent or reclining (Lewis et al., 2010).

Orthopnea is an abnormal condition in which a patient has difficulty breathing when lying down and has to use multiple pillows or sit to breathe. The number of pillows required for sleep (e.g., two or three) quantifies the presence and severity of orthopnea.

Wheezing is a high-pitched musical sound caused by high-velocity movement of air through a narrowed airway. It is present in asthma, acute bronchitis, or pneumonia. It occurs on inspiration, expiration, or both. Determine any precipitating factors such as respiratory infection, allergens, exercise, or stress.

Cough. Cough is a sudden, audible expulsion of air from the lungs. Coughing is a protective reflex to clear the trachea, bronchi, and lungs of irritants and secretions. Some patients with chronic sinusitis cough only in the early morning, while trying to sleep, or immediately after rising from sleep. This clears the airway of sputum resulting from sinus drainage. Patients with chronic bronchitis generally produce sputum all day, although the body produces greater amounts after rising from a semi-recumbent or flat position. A **productive cough** results in sputum production that is swallowed or expectorated. Carefully collect data about the type, amount, color, and quantity of sputum.

If a patient reports **hemoptysis** (bloody sputum), determine the source. Is it associated with coughing and bleeding from the upper respiratory tract, from sinus drainage, or from the gastrointestinal tract (hematemesis)? Describe the hemoptysis, including amount, color, duration of bleeding, and presence of sputum. When hemoptysis develops, note if the patient is on anticoagulants.

Respiratory Infections. Determine if your patient has had a Pneumovax or flu vaccine in the past (National Center for Immunization and Respiratory Diseases, 2011). Determine if the patient is on immunomodulators or immunosuppressant therapy or has asthma or COPD because these patients are at higher risk of developing respiratory infections. Ask about any known exposure to TB and the results of the tuberculin skin test, including type of test and date. Some patients with a history of intravenous drug use, blood transfusions, multiple unprotected sex partners, or a homosexual lifestyle are at a higher risk for developing HIV/acquired immunodeficiency syndrome (AIDS) infection. Patients may not display any symptoms of HIV/AIDS infection until they have an opportunistic infection or present with vague complaints of fatigue and malaise.

Medication Use. Assess your patient's knowledge and ability to correctly take medication (see Chapter 17). Include a family caregiver in your assessment if he or she assists with medication preparation or administration. Review what the patient understands about medication side effects and what or when to report to the health care provider. Common drugs monitored by measuring blood levels include theophylline and digitalis preparations.

Many herbals and over-the-counter (OTC) medications affect the heart rate and blood pressure and promote blood thinning. For example, the herb ma huang, a naturally occurring ephedrine, increases blood pressure and heart rate. Patients with cardiopulmonary disease should not use this herb. Patients with asthma should not use ephedrine-containing products such as bronchodilators because they cause increased bronchospasm and respiratory arrest. Ginseng, garlic capsules, and ginkgo biloba have properties similar to those of aspirin and decrease platelet aggregation.

Illicit drugs, particularly parenterally administered narcotics, often come diluted with talcum powder. This causes pulmonary disorders resulting from the irritant effect of talcum powder on lung tissues.

Older Adult Considerations. The older adult has a wide range of normal heart rate, from the 40s to more than 100 beats/min (Seidel et al., 2011). The older adult has a decreased cardiac output as a result of ventricular wall thickening and a decrease in elastin. Hypertension and a rise in systolic blood pressure are caused by calcified arterial vessels that have lost elastin. The older adult has a decline in oxygenation as a result of changes in the alveoli and a reduced surface area for gas exchange. Loss of functional cilia in the airway causes a decrease in the effectiveness of the cough, putting the older adult at increased risk for respiratory infections. Multiple questions may be tiring to older adults. Be aware of their breathing pattern and breathlessness.

Patient Expectations. Knowing what a patient expects regarding his or her health and its maintenance helps to determine goals of care, interventions, and use of patient education and home care resources.

You need to assess a patient's willingness to follow a treatment schedule. In addition, determine what your patient expects from caregivers. Does the patient expect health to improve, or does he or she expect supportive care? Does your patient want to be an active participant in care, or does he or she expect family caregivers to make decisions and provide care?

Physical Examination. The physical examination includes a detailed, organized, and systematic evaluation of the entire cardiopulmonary system (see Chapter 16) (Tables 30-4 to 30-6).

Be mindful of your patient's limitations such as breathlessness or fatigue. In some cases you have to complete your assessment in short sections to allow the patient to rest and recover. If your patient is breathless or fatigued, you may ask closed-ended questions with yes or no answers. Focus your initial assessment on your patient's immediate problems (Table 30-7).

Diagnostic Tests. Diagnostic tests determine adequacy of the cardiac conduction system, myocardial contraction, and blood flow. They also measure the adequacy of ventilation and oxygenation and visualize structures of the respiratory system. Some patients need an ECG, chest x-ray film examination, pulse oximetry, laboratory tests (e.g., arterial blood gas levels, complete blood count, sputum analysis, and cardiac enzyme levels), cardiac stress test, pulmonary function test, or cardiac catheterization.

TB skin testing is important to determine exposure to TB (Box 30-4). Patients from foreign countries often have received bacille Calmette-Guerin (BCG) vaccinations to prevent it and will have a positive TB skin test. Thus health care providers will often use the QuantiFERON-TB Gold test instead because it is more reliable in patients who have

TABLE 30-4 INSPECTION OF CARDIOPULMONARY STATUS

ABNORMALITY	CAUSE
Eyes	
Xanthelasma (yellow lipid lesions on eyelids)	Hyperlipidemia
Corneal arcus (whitish opaque ring around junction of cornea and sclera)	Abnormal finding in young to middle-age adults associated with hyperlipidemia (normal finding in older adults with arcus senilis)
Pale conjunctivae	Anemia
Cyanotic conjunctivae	Hypoxemia
Petechiae on conjunctivae	Fat embolus or bacterial endocarditis
Skin	
Peripheral cyanosis	Vasoconstriction and diminished blood flow
Central cyanosis	Hypoxemia (late sign)
Decreased skin turgor	Dehydration (normal finding in older adults as a result of decreased skin elasticity)
Dependent edema	Right- and left-sided heart failure
Periorbital edema	Kidney disease
Fingertips and Nail Beds	
Cyanosis	Decreased cardiac output or hypoxia; sometimes the result of decreased circulation to the affected limb or vasoconstriction secondary to cold
Splinter hemorrhages	Bacterial endocarditis
Clubbing	Chronic hypoxemia
Mouth and Lips	
Cyanotic mucous membranes	Decreased oxygenation (hypoxia)
Pursed-lip breathing	Chronic lung disease
Neck Veins	
Distention	Right-sided heart failure; fluid overload
Nose	
Flaring nares	Air hunger, dyspnea
Chest	
Retractions	Increased work of breathing, dyspnea
Asymmetry	Chest wall injury

TABLE 30-5 ASSESSMENT OF ABNORMAL CHEST WALL MOVEMENT

ABNORMALITY	CAUSE
Retraction: Visible sinking in soft tissues of chest that lie between and around firmer tissue (e.g., cartilaginous and bony ribs); retractions have specific beginning point and worsening, with need for increased inspiratory effort; possibly found at intercostal space, intraclavicular space, trachea, and substernally*	Any condition that causes increased inspiratory effort (e.g., airway obstruction, asthma, tracheobronchitis)
Paradoxical breathing: Asynchronous breathing; chest contraction during inspiration and expansion during expiration	Flail chest
Increased anteroposterior diameter	Senile emphysema or chronic obstructive pulmonary disease

*Infants can experience sternal and substernal retractions with only slight inspiratory effort because of chest pliability.

TABLE 30-6 RESPIRATORY PATTERNS

TYPE/PATTERN	RATE (BREATHS/MIN)	CLINICAL SIGNIFICANCE
Eupnea	12-20	Normal rate in the adult
Tachypnea	>20	Results from anxiety or response to pain or fever, respiratory failure, shortness of breath, or a respiratory infection; leads to respiratory alkalosis, paresthesia, tetany, and confusion
Bradypnea	<10	Results from sleep, respiratory depression, drug overdose, or central nervous system lesion
Apnea	Periods of no respiration lasting >15 seconds	Sometimes intermittent such as in sleep apnea or prolonged as in a respiratory arrest
Kussmaul's	Usually >35, may be slow or normal	Tachypnea pattern associated with metabolic imbalances such as diabetic slow or normal ketoacidosis, metabolic acidosis, or renal failure
Cheyne-Stokes	Abnormal pattern of breathing, varying between apnea and tachypnea	Caused by damage to respiratory system; lungs are compensating for changing serum partial pressures of oxygen and carbon dioxide

TABLE 30-7 FOCUSED PATIENT ASSESSMENT

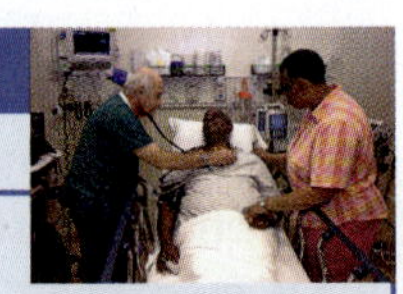

FACTORS TO ASSESS	QUESTIONS	PHYSICAL ASSESSMENT
Dependent edema	Do your legs swell every day? Are they swollen in the morning when you arise? Does the swelling get better if you put your feet up? Do you have trouble getting your socks and shoes on and off? Does your belt or waistband feel tighter?	Palpate amount of edema: trace to 4+. Observe for neck vein distention. Observe for breathlessness at rest and on exertion. Assess pedal and popliteal pulses. Observe for bilateral or unilateral edema.
Breathing pattern	When do you become short of breath? Are you able to do your own personal hygiene without getting tired? How far can you walk without getting short of breath? How many pillows do you use to sleep at night?	Observe breathing pattern. Observe patient perform activities of daily living. Observe patient ambulating. Determine distance walked without shortness of breath.
Airway patency	How often do you cough? Do you bring up any mucus when coughing? Is there anything that brings on your cough?	Observe for use of pursed-lip breathing. Observe patient in various positions. Monitor sputum for color, consistency, amount, and odor.

BOX 30-4 TUBERCULOSIS SKIN TESTING

- Skin testing determines the presence of *Mycobacterium tuberculosis.*
- The tuberculosis skin test (TST) requires an intradermal injection of 0.1 mL of tuberculin purified protein derivative (PPD) on the inner surface of the forearm (see Chapter 17). The injection produces a pale elevation of the skin (a wheal) 6 to 10 mm in diameter. Afterward the injection site is circled, and the patient is instructed not to wash off the circle.
- Tuberculin skin tests are read between 48 to 72 hours. If the site is not read within 72 hours, the patient must have another skin test.
- *Positive results:* A palpable, elevated, hardened area around the injection site, caused by edema and inflammation from the antigen-antibody reaction, measured in millimeters
- A reddened flat area is *not* a positive reaction, and you do not need to measure it.
- Tuberculosis testing in patients with altered immune function such as an older adult, an HIV-positive patient, or someone receiving chemotherapy is less reliable.

HIV, Human immunodeficiency virus.

received BCG vaccinations. Many patients usually will have an initial chest radiographic examination if their TB skin test is positive. Repeat chest radiographs are recommended only if a patient develops symptoms such as hemoptysis, weight loss, fatigue, or night sweats.

NURSING DIAGNOSIS

A patient with an altered level of oxygenation often has nursing diagnoses that are primarily of cardiovascular or pulmonary origin. You base each nursing diagnosis on specific defining characteristics and include the related etiology. The defining characteristics or signs and symptoms identified during your assessment validate the diagnostic label. Appropriate nursing diagnoses include but are not limited to the following:

- *Activity Intolerance*
- *Ineffective Airway Clearance*
- *Ineffective Breathing Pattern*
- *Decreased Cardiac Output*
- *Fatigue*
- *Impaired Gas Exchange*
- *Risk for Infection*
- *Acute Pain*

During the assessment process you collect data that accurately reflects a patient's needs. For example, your objective findings in a patient who comes to the clinic with a diagnosis of pneumonia include productive cough, breathlessness, crackles, tachypnea, changes in depth of respiration, and pleuritic pain. These findings support the diagnosis of *Ineffective Airway Clearance related to the presence of tracheobronchial secretions.* The ability of your patient to bring up sputum is a crucial part of treatment for pneumonia. Pleuritic pain interferes with a patient's ability to rest and impairs the ability to cough and clear the airway, resulting in worsening infection.

Another example of a related nursing diagnosis is *Activity Intolerance related to imbalance between oxygen supply and demand.* The objective findings include an inability to move secretions, restlessness, tachycardia, breathlessness, use of accessory muscles, and hypoxia (PaO_2 less than 60 mm Hg). Patients avoid physical effort because exercise often brings on more breathlessness. Consequently their level of fitness decreases, they become weak, and they have difficulty with normal activities of daily living. As a patient increases exercise tolerance, the degree of dyspnea and shortness of breath may diminish. Identifying the appropriate related factor enables you to design nursing interventions to maximize the balance between a patient's oxygen supply and demand.

PLANNING

Goals and Outcomes. Patients with impaired oxygenation require nursing care plans that are patient-centered, thus directed toward meeting their actual or potential oxygenation needs. Oxygenation goals for your patient often include providing a patent airway, improving oxygenation, and increasing the level of independence and tolerance for activity (see Care Plan).

All goals need to have measurable outcomes for you to be able to determine whether they have been met. These include objective data such as oxygen saturation levels, laboratory findings, chest radiographs, ECG patterns, blood pressure, and pulse. Quantify subjective findings such as the reported degree of breathlessness or pain on visual analog scales.

Patients have more than one nursing diagnosis, and often these diagnoses have an impact on one another (Figure 30-6). It is important to include any family caregiver and the patient in all care planning. Alterations in oxygenation are often chronic problems that affect the patient and family. The patient remains a member of the community despite the illness. Planning with the family and using community resources help patients adapt to activities of daily living.

Setting Priorities. Help the patient and family caregiver set priorities for care based on the patient's tolerance level. Ask the patient how he or she is feeling today and then determine which aspects of care are most important. If the patient is having pain, relief of pain is the priority over getting up in the chair or completing personal hygiene. Ask patients what they want to accomplish. If they are diaphoretic, they appreciate clean sheets and a bath after being medicated for pain.

Base your decision to delegate responsibility to nursing assistive personnel (NAP) on your assessment of the patient and the type of care the patient will receive. Consider which tasks are safe to delegate and within the skill set of the NAP and how the patient will feel about the care that you have delegated. The priority is to maintain or improve the patient's oxygenation and meet his or her needs. You are ultimately responsible for all total patient care.

CARE PLAN

Oxygenation

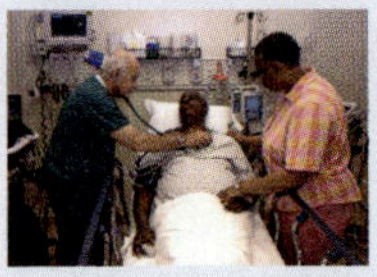

ASSESSMENT

John Smith begins his morning care for Mr. King, who is restless and anxious. As the day progresses, John notices that Mr. King's coughs are weaker, less sputum is produced, and Mr. King is becoming more fatigued.

ASSESSMENT ACTIVITIES	FINDINGS/DEFINING CHARACTERISTICS*
Ask Mr. King how long he has been short of breath.	He replies, "I have been **short of breath for 1 week,** and it has **gotten worse.**" His vital signs are pulse rate, 120 beats/min; temperature, 102°F; **increased respiratory rate, 36 breaths per minute;** blood pressure, 110/45 mm Hg, and **a SpO_2 of 82%.** Mr. King is short of breath as he answers questions.
Ask Mr. King how long he has had his cough and if it is a productive cough.	"I usually **cough** when I wake up in the morning. Three days ago I noticed that I **was coughing up thick mucus** that has not stopped."
Auscultate Mr. King's lung fields.	On auscultation there are **audible expiratory wheezes, crackles, and diminished breath sounds** over right lower lobe.
Ask Mr. King to produce a sputum sample.	**Sputum is thick and discolored (yellow-green).**

*__Defining characteristics__ are shown in **bold** type.

NURSING DIAGNOSIS: Ineffective Airway Clearance related to retained pulmonary secretions

PLANNING

GOAL

- Pulmonary secretions will return to baseline levels within 24 to 36 hours.
- Mr. King's oxygenation status will improve in 36 hours.

EXPECTED OUTCOMES (NOC)†

Respiratory Status: Gas Exchange

- Mr. King's sputum is clear, white, and thinner in consistency within 36 hours.
- Mr. King's lung sounds are at baseline within 36 hours.
- Mr. King's respiratory rate is between 16 and 24 breaths/min within 24 hours.
- Mr. King is able to clear airway secretions by coughing in 24 hours.
- Mr. King's SpO_2 is greater than 95% within 24 hours.
- Mr. King's perceptions of dyspnea improve.

†Outcomes classification label from Moorhead S, et al, editors: *Nursing outcomes classification (NOC),* ed 5, St Louis, 2013, Mosby.

INTERVENTIONS (NIC)‡	RATIONALE
Airway Management	
• Have Mr. King deep breathe and cough every 2 hours while awake.	A major complication of reduced mobility is retention of pulmonary secretions, which predisposes patient to atelectasis and pneumonia (Augustyn; 2007; Sedwick et al., 2012).
• Have Mr. King change position frequently if on bed rest. If able, have him ambulate 10 to 15 minutes every 4 hours (while awake) and encourage him to sit up in a chair as often as he is able to tolerate.	Body movement (e.g., ambulation, sitting upright, and frequent position changes) helps mobilize secretions and promote normal lung function (Staudinger et al., 2010).
• Encourage Mr. King to increase his fluid intake to 2800 mL/24 hours if his cardiac condition does not contraindicate it. Avoid caffeinated beverages and alcohol; recommend water.	Fluids help liquefy secretions for easier removal. Caffeinated and alcoholic beverages promote diuresis and dehydration. Water is an effective expectorant that is easily available and cost-effective.

‡Intervention classification labels from Bulechek GM, et al, editors: *Nursing interventions classification (NIC),* ed 6, St Louis, 2013, Mosby.

CARE PLAN—cont'd

Oxygenation

EVALUATION

NURSING ACTIONS	PATIENT RESPONSE/FINDING	ACHIEVEMENT OF OUTCOME
Ask Mr. King to keep track of his fluid intake. Assess respiratory secretions.	Mr. King has completed accurate intake list daily, averaging 2800 mL/hr. Coughing thin secretions.	Good daily fluid intake; secretions thin, white, and watery; outcome met.
Check flow sheet for number of times patient ambulated during the day.	Mr. King ambulated once every 8 hours.	Mr. King ambulates for about 5 minutes. Outcome not completely achieved.
Auscultate chest.	Lung sounds are clear.	Outcome met.
Ask Mr. King to keep track of deep breathing every 2 hours while awake.	Diary completed for each day. Mr. King has documented deep breathing every 2 hours while awake 85% of the time.	Secretions are thin, lung is clear, and there is no evidence of infection. Outcome met.

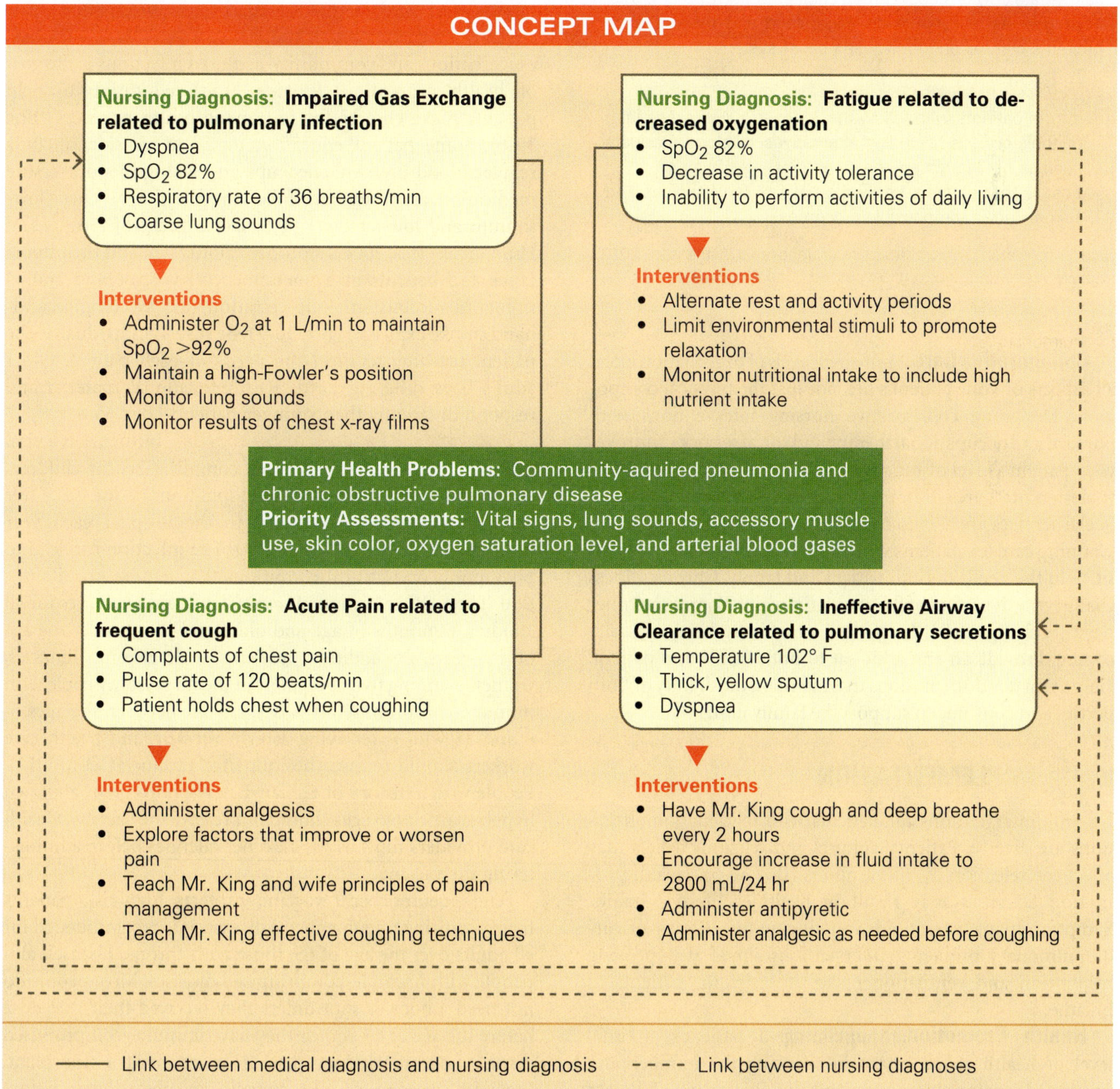

FIGURE 30-6 Concept map.

BOX 30-5 PATIENT-CENTERED CARE

As a nursing student you will encounter patients from different cultures, experiences, and religious faiths. A patient's beliefs affect how you care for your patient and his or her family. One example of a religious faith that affects direct care interventions is the Jehovah's Witnesses. It is a religion in which the individual believes in God and Jesus. Jehovah's Witnesses adhere to the *New World Translation of the Holy Scriptures,* and all of their beliefs are based on the Bible. Patients of the Jehovah's Witnesses faith accept many routine health care practices, such as exercise management and pain control therapies. They do not believe in faith healing, and seeking medical care is a personal choice. A common ethical dilemma is the Jehovah's Witnesses' avoidance of blood products, transfusions, and food that contains blood. Members quote, "It's blood—you must not eat," (Genesis 9:3-4) to support their choice not to receive blood. Your goal as a nurse is to understand and respect each patient's cultural and faith-based belief system.

IMPLICATIONS FOR PRACTICE

- Inform patients who follow the Jehovah's Witnesses faith of their options, including alternatives to blood products such as hetastarch and dextran.
- Ensure that patients know the risks of their choices and acknowledge the possible outcomes.

Data from Watchtower: official site of Jehovah's Witnesses, 2012, http://www.watchtower.org/. Accessed June 26, 2013.

BOX 30-6 PATIENT-CENTERED CARE

Patients with oxygenation problems often experience feelings of loss of control because they cannot control their breathing. Activities of daily living can become overwhelming for the patient because of his or her breathlessness. It is important to provide the patient the opportunity to participate in the care planning.

IMPLICATIONS FOR PRACTICE

- Include patient in care-planning activities.
- Ask patient how he or she would like the day to proceed.
- Allow time for patient to complete activities without feeling pressured.
- Encourage patient when he or she tries to complete activities and encounters problems.

Collaborative Care. Impaired levels of oxygenation affect all aspects of your patient's life, not just the physical component. Designing collaborative nursing interventions with physical and occupational therapy and social services improves your patient's level of functioning. Respiratory therapy helps to design measures to improve breathing and cough control. Social services are able to recommend support groups. When planning care for patients with impaired oxygenation, be sensitive to the needs of both patient and family. Chronic illness changes the dynamics of family relationships. Sometimes roles need to change, and the patient and family have difficulty coping. Provide an empathic ear to both family and patient. Help them develop solutions that maintain the dignity of both parties and continue to support the family unit.

IMPLEMENTATION

Nursing interventions for patients with oxygenation alterations are diverse. Patients' cultural and religious beliefs may affect the selection of interventions (Box 30-5). Health promotion activities may result in healthier lifestyle habits. Symptom management aids in reducing the severity of cardiopulmonary problems. Interventions aimed at improving respiration and ventilation makes it easier for patients to breathe.

Health Promotion. Maintaining a patient's optimal level of health is important in reducing the number and severity of cardiopulmonary symptoms. Prevention of disease exacerbations and community-acquired infections is the goal of health promotion. Provide health education to help patients make choices for improving health practices (Box 30-6). Some patient education topics to consider include regular blood pressure checkups and taking blood pressure medication as prescribed, following the DASH Diet (low-sodium and low-fat diet) (U.S. Department of Health and Human Services, 2006), a proper caloric diet, and the importance and benefits of a pneumococcal vaccine and annual influenza vaccine, smoking cessation, and avoiding second-hand smoke exposure (Box 30-7). Be sure to individualize the patient teaching to meet the needs of each patient. Older adults have differing needs with educational material and respond differently than younger patients (Box 30-8).

Influenza and Pneumococcal Vaccine. Influenza is a viral infection that can cause serious complications in children, older adults, and those with cardiopulmonary diseases. Over 226,000 patients are admitted to the hospital each year because of influenza (CDC, 2013). The infection can lead to pneumonia and critical conditions that require hospitalization. The CDC recommends annual influenza vaccines for all children 6 months of age and older and people over the age of 50 years. In addition, patients with chronic illnesses, women planning to be pregnant in the flu season, people with immune-compromised diseases, anyone between the ages of 6 and 18 who is receiving aspirin therapy, and health care workers should receive the influenza vaccine (CDC, 2013). People with a history of Gillian-Barré syndrome or a known hypersensitivity to eggs should not receive the vaccine. Health care providers must assess all other allergies before administering the vaccine.

The pneumococcal vaccine protects high-risk patients from acquiring pneumococcal disease. It is recommended for all adults over the age of 65, those with chronic diseases, and people with immune-compromised diseases. Most people do not need a booster shot unless they received their first dose before the age of 65 and/or they have immune-compromised diseases, chronic kidney disease, or received a transplant. Pregnant women should consult an obstetrician before

BOX 30-7 PATIENT TEACHING

Health Maintenance

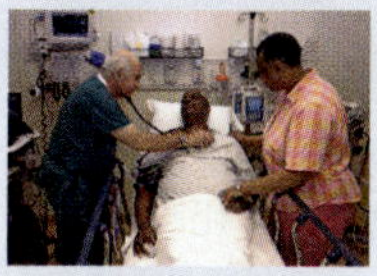

Mr. and Mrs. King are both interested in how to prevent hospitalizations in the future and what they can do to maintain their health. John Smith develops the following teaching plan to help the Kings meet their goals:

OUTCOME

On completion of the teaching session, Mr. and Mrs. King will verbalize the steps they need to take to improve their health maintenance and reduce the risk for future hospitalizations.

TEACHING STRATEGIES

- Establish rapport with the Kings and maintain eye contact during the teaching session.
- Use words that the Kings understand; avoid medical jargon when possible.
- Set goals in partnership with the Kings so they are realistic, meaningful, and achievable.
- With each significant point ask the Kings to repeat back the information you have given them.
- Provide an overview of chronic obstructive pulmonary disease and pneumonia, signs and symptoms of exacerbation, medications, and follow-up appointments.
- Encourage Mr. King to balance activity and rest. Report any changes in activity tolerance to his primary health care provider.
- Provide a written copy of the material taught for reinforcement and reference.
- Allow time for questions and answer honestly.
- Summarize the material.

EVALUATION STRATEGIES

- Ask Mr. and Mrs. King to verbalize what they learned.
- Ask Mr. King to describe in simple terms community-acquired pneumonia and chronic obstructive pulmonary disease and signs and symptoms of exacerbation.
- Ask the Kings to verbalize understanding of each medication that Mr. King will be taking.
- Ask Mr. and Mrs. King if they have any questions or need any additional information.

BOX 30-8 CARE OF THE OLDER ADULT

Oxygen Problem Manifestations

- Risk-factor modification is important, including smoking cessation, weight reduction, a low-cholesterol and low-salt diet, management of hypertension, and exercise.
- Coronary artery disease is the leading cause of death and disability in women older than 40 years of age.
- Older adults have more atypical signs and symptoms of coronary artery disease.
- The incidence of atrial fibrillation increases with age and is the leading contributing factor for stroke in the older adult.
- Healthy behavior changes sometimes slow or halt the progression of an older adult's disease. However, it is often more difficult to get older adults to change long-term unhealthy habits.
- Mental-status changes are often the first sign of respiratory problems in the older adult and include subtle increases in forgetfulness and irritability.
- An older adult often does not complain of dyspnea until it affects activities of daily living and then only if the activities are important to him or her.
- Use cough suppressants with caution because of changes in an older patient's cough mechanism. Cough suppression leads to retention of pulmonary secretions, plugged airways, and atelectasis.
- Chronic illness in an older adult sometimes results in unacceptable behavior patterns because of loss of control experienced with a chronic illness.

receiving either vaccine (National Center for Immunization and Respiratory Diseases, 2011).

Environmental Modifications. Avoiding exposure to secondhand smoke is important for patients with cardiopulmonary illnesses. Most public places and businesses have adopted a no-smoking policy or offer separate smoking areas. Provide counseling and support so that a patient who lives with secondhand smoke in the home understands its effects. Also assess environmental hazards in the workplace. Many health care institution dress codes prohibit the use of perfumes and colognes because they often affect patient breathing patterns and allergies. Discuss risk factors and ways to reduce exposure.

Acute Care. Patients with acute cardiopulmonary illnesses require nursing interventions directed toward halting the pathological process such as a respiratory tract infection. Nursing interventions also focus on shortening the duration and severity of the illness such as hospitalization with heart failure and preventing complications from illness or treatments such as hospital-acquired infection resulting from invasive procedures.

Dyspnea Management. Dyspnea is difficult to measure and treat, thus requiring individualized treatments for each patient. You usually need to implement more than one therapy. Initially you treat and stabilize the underlying processes that cause or worsen dyspnea and then you administer four additional therapies:

1. Medications (e.g., bronchodilators, steroids, mucolytics, antianxiety drugs)
2. Oxygen therapy as indicated
3. Physical techniques (e.g., cardiopulmonary reconditioning, breathing techniques, cough control)
4. Psychosocial techniques (e.g., relaxation techniques, biofeedback, meditation) to lessen the sensation of dyspnea

Oxygen Therapy. Some patients require oxygen therapy to keep a healthy level of tissue oxygenation. The goal of **oxygen therapy** is to prevent or relieve hypoxia. Any patient with impaired tissue oxygenation benefits from controlled oxygen administration. Oxygen is not a substitute for other treatments. Use it only when ordered and indicated. Oxygen is a drug. It is expensive and has dangerous side effects. As with any drug, continuously monitor the dosage or concentration. Routinely check the health care provider's orders to verify that the patient is receiving the prescribed oxygen concentration and flow rate. The six rights of medication administration also apply to oxygen administration (see Chapter 17).

Safety Precautions with Oxygen Therapy. Oxygen is a highly combustible gas and fuels fire readily. Although it does not spontaneously burn or cause an explosion, it can easily cause a fire to ignite if it contacts a spark from a cigarette or electrical equipment. Special procedures exist in health care settings for the safe handling and storage of oxygen equipment.

With increasing use of home oxygen therapy, patients and health care professionals need to be aware of these dangers of combustion. Promote safety by using the following measures (Medline Plus, 2012):

- Place "No smoking" signs on the patient's room door, over the bed, and in every room of the home where oxygen is used. Inform the patient, visitors, roommates, and all personnel that smoking is not permitted in areas where oxygen is in use.
- Determine that all electrical equipment in a health facility room or patient's home is functioning correctly and is properly grounded (see Chapter 28).
- Know the fire procedures and the location of the closest fire extinguisher.
- Check the oxygen level of portable tanks before transporting to ensure that there is enough oxygen in the tank.
- Store oxygen tanks in secure holders to prevent them from being knocked over.
- Store oxygen tanks 6 feet away from toys with electric motors, electric space heaters, fireplaces, electric blankets, hair dryers, or other appliances. Do not store in a trunk box or small closet.

Oxygen Supply. Within health care settings, oxygen tanks or a permanent wall-piped system supplies oxygen to a patient's bedside. Oxygen tanks are transported on wide-based carriers that allow the tank to be upright at the patient's bedside. Regulators control the amount of oxygen delivered. One common type of oxygen tank has an upright flowmeter with a flow-adjustment valve at the top. A second type is a cylinder indicator with a flow-adjustment handle.

Methods of Oxygen Delivery. Nasal cannula, nasal catheter, face mask, and the mechanical ventilator are all ways to deliver oxygen to a patient (Table 30-8; Box 30-9).

TABLE 30-8 OXYGEN DELIVERY SYSTEMS

DELIVERY SYSTEM	INDICATIONS	O_2 CONCENTRATION (FLOW RATE)	CONSIDERATIONS
Nasal cannula	Simple, comfortable device to deliver low-concentration O_2 (<6 L/min)	24% (1 L/min) 28% (2 L/min) 32% (3 L/min) 36% (4 L/min) 40% (5 L/min) 44% (6 L/min)	Flow rates more than 4 L/min often cause drying effect on mucosa; humidify oxygen; be alert for skin breakdown over ears and in nares; questionable efficiency in mouth breathers.
Transtracheal O_2 (TTO) cannula	For chronic lung diseases; small, intravenous-size catheter inserted directly into trachea	Flow rates range from ¼ to 1 L/min and range from 22%-45% (AARC, 2007); individualized to meet patient requirements	TTO requires greater patient supervision and has an increased risk for complications. There is no O_2 lost to atmosphere; patients achieve adequate oxygenation at lower rates (more efficient, less expensive, and produces fewer side effects); patients more likely to use O_2 because of mobility, comfort, and cosmetic improvement.
Oxygen masks	Administer O_2, humidity, or heated humidity		Be alert for skin breakdown around face and ears.
Simple face mask (Figure 30-7)	Short-term O_2 therapy	40%-60% (5-8 L/min)	Contraindicated for patients with carbon dioxide retention; effective for mouth breathers
Partial nonrebreather mask with reservoir bag	Delivers high concentrations of O_2	60%-95% (6-10 L/min)	Frequently inspect the bag to make sure that it is inflated.
Venturi mask	Can deliver precise, high-flow rates of O_2; adapters can be applied to increase humidification	24%-28% (4 L/min) 35%-40% (8 L/min) 50%-60% (12 L/min)	Mask must be removed when patient eats.

BOX 30-9 PROCEDURAL GUIDELINES

View Video!

Applying a Nasal Cannula or Oxygen Mask

DELEGATION CONSIDERATIONS

The skill of applying **(not setting or adjusting oxygen flow)** or adjusting a nasal cannula or oxygen mask can be delegated to nursing assistive personnel (NAP). However, the nurse is responsible for assessment of the patient's respiratory system and response to and setup of oxygen therapy, including adjustment of oxygen flow rate. The nurse directs the NAP by:

- Informing how to safely position and adjust the device (e.g., loosening the strap on oxygen mask) and clarifying its correct placement and positioning.
- Instructing to inform the nurse immediately about any vital-sign changes; about skin irritation from the cannula, mask, or straps; if patient reports pain or breathlessness; or if patient has decreased level of consciousness or increased confusion.
- Having personnel provide skin care around patient's ears and nose.

EQUIPMENT

Note: When device is used in the home, the home care equipment vendor provides the equipment. Oxygen-delivery device as ordered by patient's health care provider; oxygen tubing (consider extension tubing), humidifier if indicated, sterile water for humidifier, oxygen source, oxygen flowmeter, stethoscope, pulse oximeter, appropriate room signs

STEPS

1. Identify the patient using two identifiers (e.g., name and birthday or name and account number) according to agency policy. Compare identifiers with information on the patient's MAR or medical record.
2. Assess patient's respiratory status, including symmetry of chest wall expansion, chest wall abnormalities (e.g., kyphosis), temporary conditions (e.g., pregnancy, trauma) affecting ventilation, respiratory rate and depth, sputum production, and lung sounds.
3. Observe for patent airway and remove secretions by having patient cough and expectorate mucus or by suctioning.

***Clinical Decision Point:* Patients with sudden changes in their vital signs, level of consciousness, or behavior are often experiencing profound hypoxia. Patients who demonstrate subtle changes over time have worsening of a chronic or existing condition or a new medical condition.**

4. Obtain patient's most recent SpO_2 or arterial blood gas (ABG) values if available. Review patient's medical record for medical order for oxygen, noting delivery method, flow rate, and duration of oxygen therapy.
5. Explain to patient and family what happens during procedure and the purpose of oxygen therapy.
6. Perform hand hygiene.
7. Attach oxygen-delivery device (e.g., nasal cannula or mask) to oxygen tubing and attach to humidified oxygen source adjusted to prescribed flow rate (see illustration).
8. Apply oxygen delivery device.
   a. Position tips of nasal cannula, pointing in and down, into patient's nares and adjust elastic headband or plastic slide on cannula so it is snug and comfortable (see illustration).
   b. Apply an oxygen mask by placing over mouth and nose, and adjust elastic headband until mask fits snugly and comfortably over patient's face.
   c. Apply face tent loosely under patient's chin and over mouth and nose.
9. Maintain sufficient slack on oxygen tubing and secure to patient's clothes.
10. Observe for proper functioning of oxygen-delivery device.
    a. *Nasal cannula*: Cannula is positioned properly in nares with humidification functioning.
    b. *Reservoir nasal cannula/Oxymizer:* Fit as for nasal cannula. Position reservoir under patient's nose or have it worn as a pendant (see illustration).

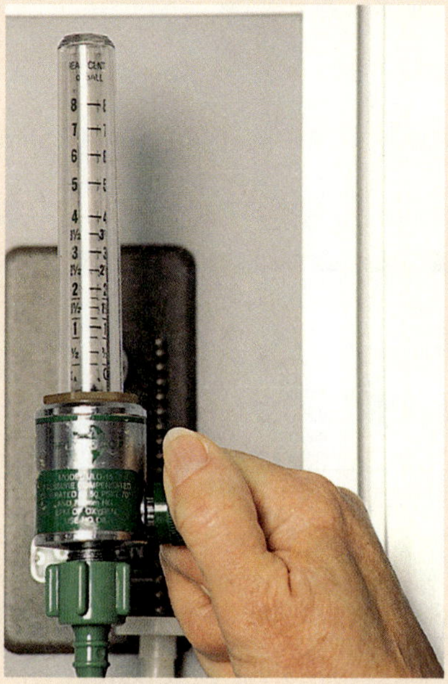

STEP 7 Adjusting flowmeter to prescribed oxygen flow rate.

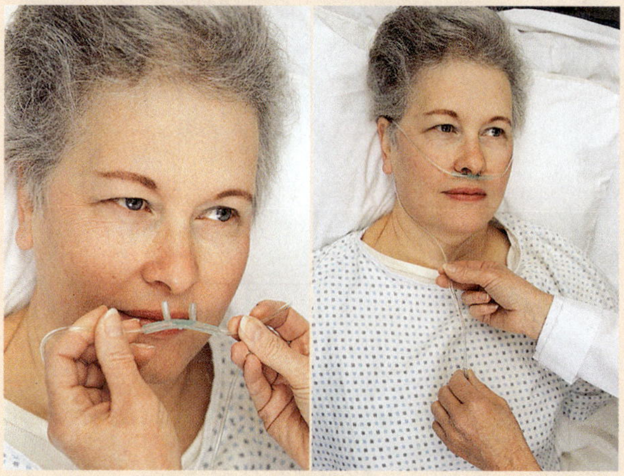

STEP 8a Applying nasal cannula and adjusting fit to patient comfort.

Continued

BOX 30-9 PROCEDURAL GUIDELINES—cont'd

View Video!

Applying a Nasal Cannula or Oxygen Mask

c. *Nonrebreathing mask:* Mask should create a tight seal over patient's mouth and nose. Valves on mask close so exhaled air does not enter reservoir bag (see illustration).

d. *Partial rebreathing mask:* Mask forms a tight seal over mouth and nose. Ensure that bag remains partially inflated.

e. *Venturi mask:* Mask forms tight seal over patient's mouth and nose (see illustration).

f. *Face tent:* Tent fits and a mist is always present (see illustration).

11. Verify setting on flowmeter and oxygen source for proper setup and prescribed flow rate.
12. Check cannula/mask every 8 hours. Keep humidification container filled at all times.
13. Monitor patient's response to changes in oxygen flow rate with pulse oximetry. **NOTE:** Monitor ABGs when ordered; however, obtaining ABG measurement is an invasive procedure, and ABGs are not measured frequently.
14. Observe for decreased anxiety, improved level of consciousness and cognitive abilities, decreased fatigue, absence of dizziness, decreased respiratory rate, improved color, improved oxygen saturation, and return to patient's baseline vital signs.
15. Check adequacy of oxygen flow each shift.
16. Observe patient's external ears, bridge of nose, nares, and nasal mucous membranes for evidence of skin breakdown.

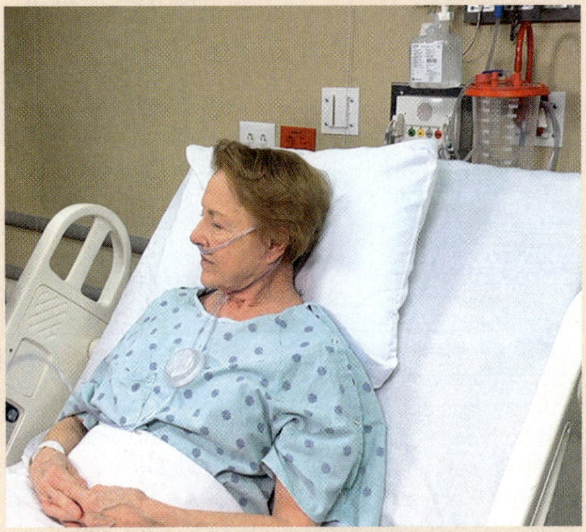

STEP 10b Reservoir nasal cannula/Oxymizer.

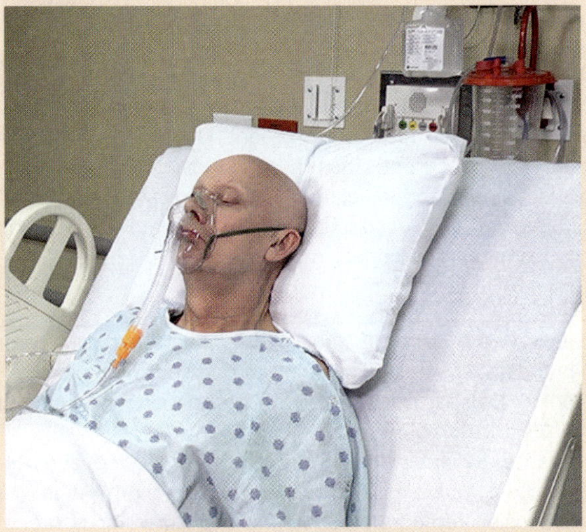

STEP 10e Venturi mask.

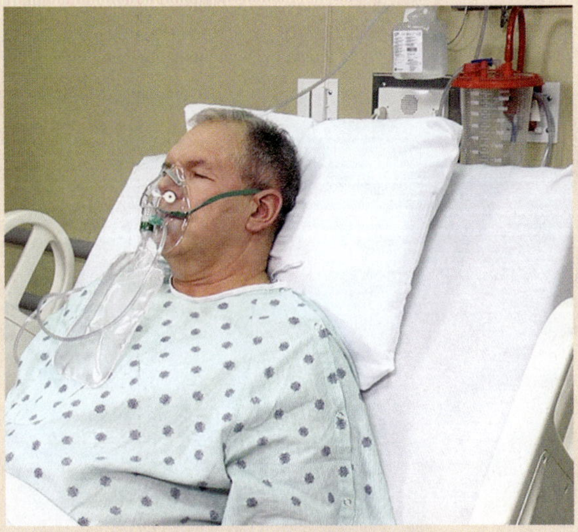

STEP 10c Nonrebreathing mask.

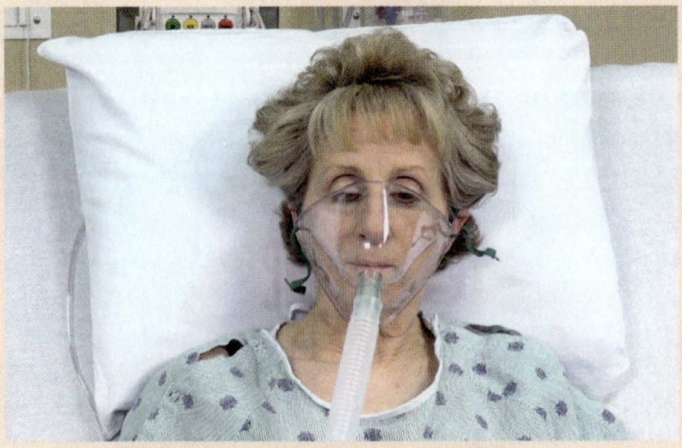

STEP 10f Face tent.

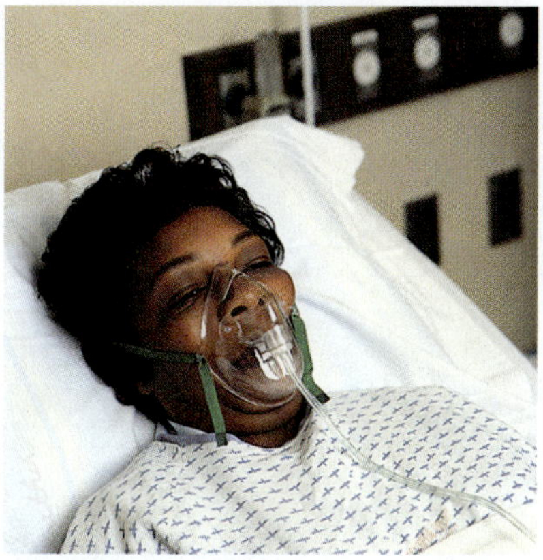

FIGURE 30-7 Simple face mask.

Home Oxygen. Indications for long-term home oxygen therapy include patients whose disease is stable with PaO_2 of 55 mm Hg or less (American Thoracic Society, 2013) or arterial oxygen saturation (SaO_2) of 88% or less on room air at rest, on exertion, or with exercise. When home oxygen is necessary, it is usually delivered by nasal cannula. If your patient has a permanent tracheostomy, a T tube or tracheostomy collar is necessary to provide humidification to the airway.

Three types of oxygen systems are used: compressed oxygen, liquid oxygen, and oxygen concentrators. In the home the major consideration is the oxygen-delivery source. Patients requiring home oxygen need extensive teaching to be able to continue oxygen therapy at home efficiently and safely. This includes oxygen safety, regulation of the amount of oxygen, and how to use the prescribed home oxygen-delivery system. The case coordinator or social worker usually assists with arranging for the home care nurse and oxygen vendor.

Mobilization of Pulmonary Secretions. The ability of a patient to mobilize pulmonary secretions is the difference between a short-term illness and a long recovery involving complications.

Hydration. Maintenance of adequate hydration promotes mucociliary clearance, the natural mechanism of the body for removing mucus and cellular debris from the respiratory tract. In patients with adequate hydration pulmonary secretions are thin, white, watery, and easily removable with minimal coughing. A fluid intake of 1500 to 2000 mL per day helps to keep pulmonary secretions thin and easy to expectorate unless contraindicated by cardiac condition.

Humidification. Humidification is necessary for patients receiving oxygen therapy at more than 4 L/min (AARC, 2007). Oxygen humidification via a nasal catheter, nasal cannula, or face mask is achieved by bubbling oxygen through water. When using humidity, make sure to use sterile saline for inhalation. In addition, make sure to change the solution according to agency procedures. Humidification is a source for hospital-acquired infections because the moist environment supports the growth of pathogens.

Nebulization. Nebulization uses the aerosol principle to suspend a maximum number of water drops or particles of the desired size in inspired air. This type of therapy is often used to deliver medications. The moisture added to the respiratory system through nebulization improves clearance and is used for administration of bronchodilators and mucolytic agents.

Maintenance of a Patent Airway. The airway is patent when the trachea, bronchi, and large airways are free from obstructions. You use three types of interventions to maintain a patent airway: coughing techniques, suctioning, and insertion of an artificial airway.

Coughing Techniques. Coughing maintains a patent airway by removing secretions from both the upper and lower airways. You evaluate cough effectiveness by sputum expectoration, a patient's report of swallowed sputum, or clearing of adventitious lung sounds. Encourage patients with chronic pulmonary diseases, upper respiratory tract infections, and lower respiratory tract infections to deep breathe and cough at least every 2 hours while awake. Encourage patients with a large amount of sputum to cough every hour while awake and awaken to cough every 2 to 3 hours while asleep until the acute phase of sputum production has ended.

Cascade Cough. With the cascade cough a patient takes a slow, deep breath and holds it for 2 seconds while contracting expiratory muscles. He or she then opens the mouth and performs a series of coughs throughout exhalation, thereby coughing at progressively lowered lung volumes. This technique promotes airway clearance and a patent airway in patients with large volumes of sputum.

Huff Cough. The huff cough stimulates a natural cough reflex and is generally effective only for clearing central airways. While exhaling, a patient opens the glottis by saying the word *huff.* With practice a patient inhales more air and is able to progress to the cascade cough.

Quad Cough. The quad cough technique is for patients without abdominal muscle control such as those with spinal cord injuries. While the patient breathes out with a maximal expiratory effort, the patient or you push inward and upward on the abdominal muscles toward the diaphragm, causing the cough.

Suctioning Techniques. When coughing does not effectively clear respiratory tract secretions, suctioning is indicated to clear the airways. The primary suctioning techniques are oropharyngeal, nasopharyngeal, orotracheal and nasotracheal, and tracheal suctioning through an artificial airway (see Skill 30-1).

Sterile technique is required for orotracheal and nasotracheal suctioning because the tip of the catheter enters the sterile tracheal airway. The mouth is considered clean; therefore the suctioning of oral and nasopharyngeal secretions requires only clean technique. When combining suction techniques, always suction oral secretions after suctioning the nasotrachea and trachea. Clinical assessment determines the frequency of suctioning. When you notice secretions by inspection or auscultation techniques, suctioning is required. A common practice in the past was to suction patients every

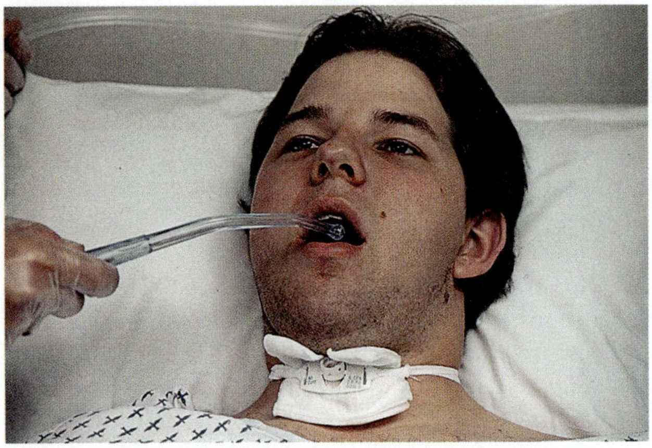

FIGURE 30-8 Oropharyngeal suctioning.

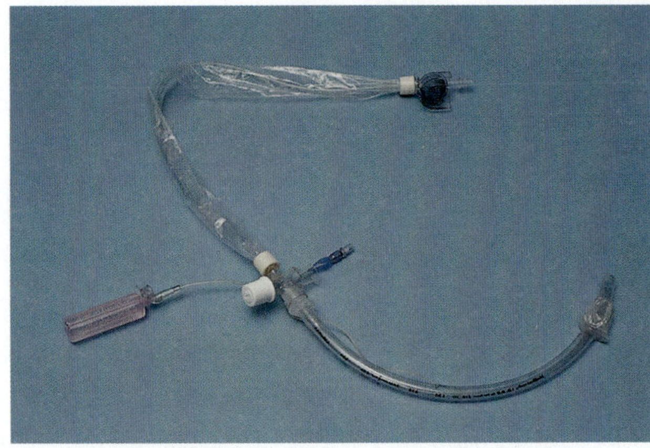

FIGURE 30-9 Ballard tracheal care closed suction.

1 to 2 hours; however, there is no evidence that this practice improves airway patency over suctioning on an as-needed basis.

Oropharyngeal and Nasopharyngeal Suctioning. Use oropharyngeal or nasopharyngeal suctioning to help a patient who is able to cough effectively but is unable to clear secretions by expectorating or swallowing. Use a Yankauer or tonsillar tip suction device for oropharyngeal suctioning (Figure 30-8). A Yankauer suction catheter is a rigid plastic catheter with one large and several small eyelets through which mucus is removed. The catheter is angled to facilitate removal of secretions from the mouth. Use the Yankauer suction catheter when oral secretions are thick and plentiful. Do not use it in the nares because of its size.

Orotracheal and Nasotracheal Suctioning. Orotracheal or nasotracheal suctioning is necessary when a patient is unable to cough and does not have an artificial airway (see Skill 30-1). You pass a catheter through the mouth or nose and then into the trachea. The nose is the preferred route because stimulation of the gag reflex is minimal. The procedure is similar to nasopharyngeal suctioning, but the catheter tip enters the trachea.

Tracheal Suctioning. Perform tracheal suctioning through an artificial airway such as a tracheostomy tube or endotracheal tube. Two tracheal suctioning methods include use of a single catheter for one-time use and closed suctioning, which includes a multiple-use catheter. The suction catheter in closed suctioning is encased in a plastic sheath and used for 24 to 48 hours (Figure 30-9). You use closed suctioning most often for patients who require mechanical ventilation because it continuously delivers oxygen during suctioning and keeps the delivery system sterile (Box 30-10).

Artificial Airways. An artificial airway is for a patient with decreased level of consciousness, airway obstruction, mechanical ventilation, or an inability to remove tracheobronchial secretions (see Skill 30-1). Patients with artificial airways who are also on mechanical ventilation need specific oral hygiene care (see Chapter 29). Routine oral hygiene with chlorhexidine reduces the patient's risk for ventilator-associated pneumonia (see Box 30-10).

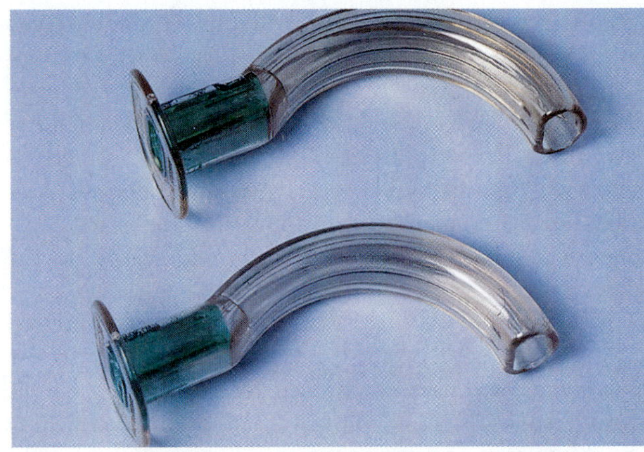

FIGURE 30-10 Artificial oral airways.

Oral Airway. The oral airway (Figure 30-10), the simplest type of artificial airway, prevents obstruction of the trachea by displacement of the tongue into the oropharynx. The oral airway extends from the teeth to the oropharynx, maintaining the tongue in the normal position. Determine proper oral airway size by measuring the distance from the corner of the mouth to the angle of the jaw just below the ear. The length is equal to the distance from the flange of the airway to the tip. You need to use the correct-size airway. If the airway is too small, the tongue will not stay in the anterior portion of the mouth; if too large, it will force the tongue toward the epiglottis and obstruct the airway.

Turn the curve of the airway toward the cheek and place it over the tongue while inserting the airway. When the airway is in the oropharynx, turn it so the opening points downward. Correctly placed, the airway moves the tongue forward, away from the oropharynx and the flange. The flat portion of the airway rests against the patient's teeth. Incorrect insertion merely forces the tongue back into the oropharynx.

Tracheal Airway. Tracheal airways include endotracheal, nasotracheal, and tracheal tubes (Box 30-11). These allow easy access to the trachea for deep tracheal suctioning.

BOX 30-10 EVIDENCE-BASED PRACTICE

PICO Question: In patients requiring mechanical ventilation, does the introduction of a ventilator care bundle compared with standard practices contribute to a reduction in ventilator-associated pneumonia (VAP)?

SUMMARY OF EVIDENCE

Ventilator-associated pneumonia (VAP) is pneumonia that develops 48 hours after mechanical ventilation via an endotracheal tube or respiratory tract and lung parenchyma. It is a complication in as many as 28% of patients who receive mechanical ventilation (Augustyn, 2007; Amanullah et al., 2013). Patients have increased fever, increased secretions, and pulmonary infiltrates (air spaces filled with fluid, exudate, or cells) seen on chest radiograph. Over time these infiltrates progressively increase, and the patient's lung functions decline.

The incidence of VAP increases with the duration of mechanical ventilation. The mortality rate for VAP is 27% to 76%. Higher mortality rates are seen with *Pseudomonas* or *Acinetobacter* than with other organisms.

Studies show that specific patient positioning techniques, oral care practices, and prompt extubation aid in reducing VAP incidence and mortality risk (Amanullah et al., 2013; Morrow, Kollef, and Casale, 2010; Siempos et al., 2010). Early-onset pneumonia occurs within the first 4 days of hospitalization, whereas late-onset VAP develops 5 or more days after admission and is usually associated with multidrug-resistant (MDR) organisms.

The Institute for Health Care Improvement Ventilator Bundle (IHCI, 2012) is a series of interventions related to ventilator care that, when implemented together, achieve significantly better outcomes than when implemented individually. The key components of the IHI Ventilator Bundle are:

- Elevation of the head of the bed (HOB)
- Daily "sedation vacations" and assessment of readiness to extubate
- Peptic ulcer disease prophylaxis
- Deep venous thrombosis prophylaxis
- Daily oral care with chlorhexidine

Studies on the frequency of ventilator circuit changes have found no increase in VAP with prolonged use.

APPLICATION TO NURSING PRACTICE

- Unless contraindicated, maintain HOB elevation between 30 and 45 degrees to reduce aspiration of oropharyngeal and/or gastric fluids, which reduces the risk for VAP.
- Avoid prolonged supine positioning. Pulmonary aspiration is increased by supine positioning and pooling of secretions above the ET tube cuff (Sedwick et al., 2012).
- Orotracheal and orogastric tubes are preferred over nasal devices to reduce the risk of VAP (Lacherade et al., 2010).
- Suction frequently to remove oropharyngeal and subglottic secretions to reduce the risk of early-onset VAP.
- Monitor cuff pressure frequently to ensure that there is an adequate seal to prevent aspiration of secretions (Lacherade et al., 2010).
- Provide daily oral care with chlorhexidine (IHCI, 2012).
- Always drain ventilator circuit condensation away from patient and into the appropriate receptacle (AARC, 2010). Drain the tubing hourly to prevent accumulation.
- Compared to supine positioning, studies have shown that simple positioning with HOB elevation to 30 degrees or higher significantly reduces gastric reflux and VAP.
- Keep patient's HOB bed raised between 30 and 45 degrees unless other medical conditions do not allow this to occur.

Because of the artificial airway, a patient no longer has normal humidification of the tracheal mucosa. Ensure that nebulization or an oxygen delivery system is supplying humidity to the airway. Humidification is protective and helps reduce the risk for airway plugging.

Maintenance or Promotion of Lung Expansion. Nursing interventions to maintain or promote lung expansion include positioning, incentive spirometry, chest physiotherapy, and chest tube management.

Positioning. Healthy people maintain adequate ventilation and oxygenation by frequent position changes. When a person has restricted mobility, it increases his or her risk for respiratory impairment. Frequent position changes are a simple and cost-effective method for reducing a patient's risk for pooled airway secretions and decreased chest wall expansion.

The most effective position for patients with cardiopulmonary diseases is the 45-degree semi-Fowler's position, using gravity to assist in lung expansion and reduce pressure from the abdomen on the diaphragm. Ensure that a patient does not slide down in bed, causing reduced lung expansion. When positioning a patient with unilateral lung disease such as a pneumothorax or atelectasis, position him or her with the healthy lung down. This promotes better perfusion of the healthy lung, improving oxygenation. In the presence of pulmonary abscess or hemorrhage, place the affected lung down to prevent drainage toward the healthy lung.

Incentive Spirometry. Incentive spirometry is a method of encouraging voluntary deep breathing by providing visual feedback to patients about inspiratory volume. It is an effective method for promoting deep breathing to prevent or treat atelectasis in the postoperative patient. Incentive spirometry encourages patients to breathe to their normal inspiratory capacities. A postoperative inspiratory capacity one half to three fourths of the preoperative volume is acceptable because of postoperative pain. Administration of pain medications before incentive spirometry helps a patient achieve deep breathing by reducing pain and splinting. There is no clinical benefit to using incentive spirometry in place of early ambulation. Encourage your postoperative patients to ambulate as soon as possible.

Flow-oriented incentive spirometers consist of one or more plastic chambers that contain freely moving colored balls. The patient inhales slowly with an even flow to elevate

BOX 30-11 PROCEDURAL GUIDELINES

View Video!

Closed (In-Line) Suctioning

DELEGATION CONSIDERATIONS

The skill of airway suctioning with a closed (in-line) suction catheter is not routinely delegated to nursing assistive personnel (NAP). In some situations such as suctioning a patient with a permanent tracheostomy tube, this procedure may be delegated. However, the nurse is responsible for assessing the patient's cardiopulmonary status. Before delegation the nurse informs NAP about:

- Any individualized aspect of care that pertains to suctioning such as position, duration of suction, and pressure settings.
- Expected quality, quantity, and color of secretions and to immediately report any changes to the nurse.
- A patient's anticipated response to suction and to immediately report to the nurse any changes in vital signs, complaints of pain, and changes in patient's respiratory status, mental status, or restlessness.

EQUIPMENT

Closed system or in-line suction catheter, suction machine; 6 feet of connecting tubing, clean gloves *(optional)*, mask *(optional)*, goggles *(optional)*, saline vial or syringe, face shield, clean towel, pulse oximeter, and stethoscope

STEPS

1. Perform assessment as in Skill 30-1.
2. Explain the procedure to patient and the importance of coughing during the suctioning procedure.
3. Help patient assume a position of comfort for both patient and nurse, usually semi-Fowler's or high-Fowler's position. Place towel across patient's chest.
4. Perform hand hygiene, apply clean gloves and face shield, and attach suction. **NOTE:** If risk for splash is present or patient is on respiratory precautions, mask and goggles might also be needed.
   a. In some settings the catheter is attached to the closed ventilator circuit by a respiratory therapist. If catheter is not already in place, open the closed-suction catheter package using aseptic technique, attach catheter to ventilator circuit by removing swivel adapter, and place catheter apparatus on endotracheal tube or tracheostomy tube. Connect Y on mechanical ventilator circuit to closed suction catheter with flex tubing (see illustration).
   b. Connect one end of connecting tubing to suction machine and other end to the end of a closed system or in-line suction catheter if not already done. Turn suction device on and set vacuum regulator to appropriate negative pressure (see manufacturer directions). Many closed-system suction catheters require slightly higher suction; consult manufacturer guidelines.
5. Hyperinflate and/or hyperoxygenate patient with bag-valve-mask or manual breathing mechanism on mechanical ventilator according to institution protocol/health care provider orders (usually 100% oxygen).
6. Unlock suction control mechanism if required by manufacturer. Open saline port and attach saline syringe or vial.
7. Pick up suction catheter enclosed in plastic sleeve with dominant hand.

Clinical Decision Point: The instillation of normal saline into the airway before closed in-line suctioning may not be appropriate for all patients and needs further investigation (see agency policy). Normal saline instillation in conjunction with artificial airway suctioning may lead to dispersion of microorganisms into the lower respiratory tract.

8. Insert catheter; use a repeating maneuver of pushing catheter and sliding (or pulling) plastic sleeve back between thumb and forefinger until you feel resistance or patient coughs.
9. Encourage patient to cough and apply suction by squeezing on suction control mechanism while withdrawing catheter. It is difficult to apply intermittent pulses of suction and nearly impossible to rotate the catheter compared with a standard catheter. Be sure to withdraw catheter completely into plastic sheath so it does not obstruct airflow.
10. Reassess cardiopulmonary status, including pulse oximetry, to determine need for subsequent suctioning or complications. Repeat Steps 5 through 9 one or two more times to clear secretions. Allow adequate time (at least 1 full minute) between suction passes for ventilation and reoxygenation.
11. When airway is clear, withdraw catheter completely into sheath. Be sure that colored indicator line on catheter is visible in the sheath. Squeeze vial or push saline syringe while applying suction to rinse inner lumen of catheter. Use at least 5 to 10 mL of saline to rinse the catheter until you clear it of retained secretions, which cause bacterial growth and increase the risk for infection. Lock suction mechanism, if applicable, and turn off suction.
12. If patient requires oral or nasal suctioning, perform Skill 30-1 with separate standard suction catheter.
13. Reposition patient.
14. Remove face shield and gloves and discard them and perform hand hygiene.
15. Compare patient's cardiopulmonary assessments before and after suctioning and observe airway secretions.

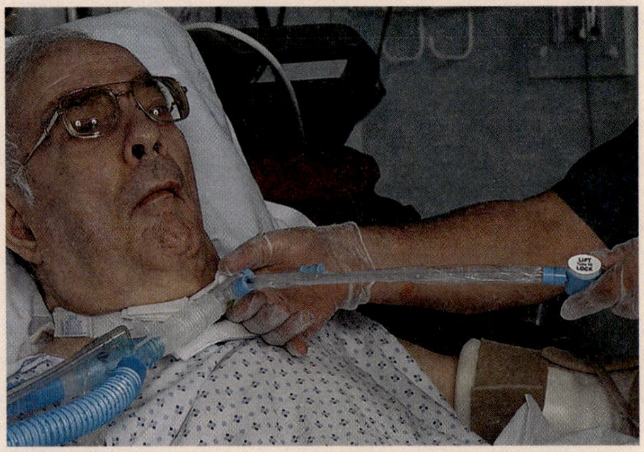

STEP 4a Suctioning tracheostomy with closed-system suction catheter.

ET, Endotracheal tube.

BOX 30-12 CHEST PHYSIOTHERAPY

Nursing and respiratory therapy collaborate with the health care provider to determine if chest physiotherapy (CPT) is best for a patient. Consultation also determines the position for the patient to assume during the procedure. Use the following guidelines to conduct physical assessment and subsequent decision making:

- Know patient's normal range of vital signs. Conditions requiring CPT such as atelectasis and pneumonia affect vital signs. The degree of change is related to the level of hypoxia, overall cardiopulmonary status, and tolerance for activity.
- Know the patient's medications. Certain medications, particularly diuretics and antihypertensives, cause fluid and hemodynamic changes. These decrease patient's tolerance for positional changes and postural drainage. Long-term steroid use increases patient's risk for pathological rib fractures and often contraindicates vibration.
- Know patient's medical history. Certain conditions such as increased intracranial pressure, spinal cord injuries, and abdominal aneurysm resection contraindicate the positional changes of postural drainage. Thoracic trauma or surgery also contraindicates percussion and vibration.
- Know patient's level of cognitive function. Participation in controlled cough techniques requires patient to follow instructions. Congenital or acquired cognitive limitations alter patient's ability to learn and participate in these techniques.
- Be aware of patient's exercise tolerance. CPT maneuvers are fatiguing. When patient is not used to physical activity, usually he or she has little tolerance for the maneuvers. However, with gradual increases in activity and planned CPT, patient tolerance for the procedure improves.

TABLE 30-9 POSITIONS FOR POSTURAL DRAINAGE

LUNG SEGMENT	POSITION OF PATIENT
Adult	
Left and right upper lobes	High-Fowler's
Apical Segments	
Right upper lobe—anterior segment	Supine with head elevated
Left upper lobe—anterior segment	Sitting on side of bed Supine with head elevated
Right upper lobe—posterior segment	Side-lying with right side of chest elevated on pillows
Left upper lobe—posterior segment	Side-lying with left side of chest elevated on pillows
Left and right middle lobes—anterior segment (right shown)	Three-fourths supine position with dependent lung in Trendelenburg's position
Right middle lobe—posterior segment	Prone with thorax and abdomen elevated
Both lower lobes—anterior segments	Supine in Trendelenburg's position
Left lower lobe—lateral segment	Right side-lying in Trendelenburg's position
Right lower lobe—lateral segment	Left side-lying in Trendelenburg's position
Right lower lobe—posterior segment	Prone with right side of chest elevated in Trendelenburg's position
Both lower lobes—posterior segment	Prone in Trendelenburg's position
Child	
Sitting on nurse's lap, leaning slightly forward flexed over pillow	
Bilateral—middle anterior segments	Sitting on nurse's lap, leaning against nurse
Bilateral lobes—anterior segments	Lying supine on nurse's lap, back supported with pillow

the balls and keep them floating as long as possible. This allows a maximally sustained inhalation.

Volume-oriented incentive spirometry devices have a bellows that rises to a predetermined volume by an inhaled breath. An achievement light or counter is used to provide feedback. Some devices do not turn the light on unless the bellows is at a minimum desired volume for a specified period of time.

Chest Physiotherapy. Chest physiotherapy (CPT) mobilizes pulmonary secretions (Box 30-12). CPT includes postural drainage, chest percussion, and vibration, followed by productive coughing or suctioning. CPT is for patients who produce more than 30 mL of sputum per day or have evidence of atelectasis by chest x-ray film.

Postural Drainage. Postural drainage is the use of positioning techniques to drain secretions from specific segments of the lungs and bronchi into the trachea. Table 30-9 includes some of the basic positions for postural drainage. Because some patients do not require postural drainage of all lung segments, adapt the procedure and position patients based on clinical assessment findings. For example, some patients with left lower lobe bronchiectasis or pneumonia require postural drainage of only the affected region, whereas a child with cystic fibrosis requires postural drainage of all segments.

Chest Percussion. Chest percussion involves striking the chest wall over the area of the lung being drained. You position each of your hands so that the fingers and thumb touch, cupping the hand (Figure 30-11). Percussion on the surface of the patient's chest wall sends waves of varying amplitude and frequency through the chest, changing the consistency and location of the sputum. You perform chest percussion by alternating hand motion against the chest wall (Figure 30-12). Perform percussion over a single layer of clothing, not over buttons, snaps, or zippers. The single layer of clothing prevents directly slapping the patient's skin. Thicker or multiple

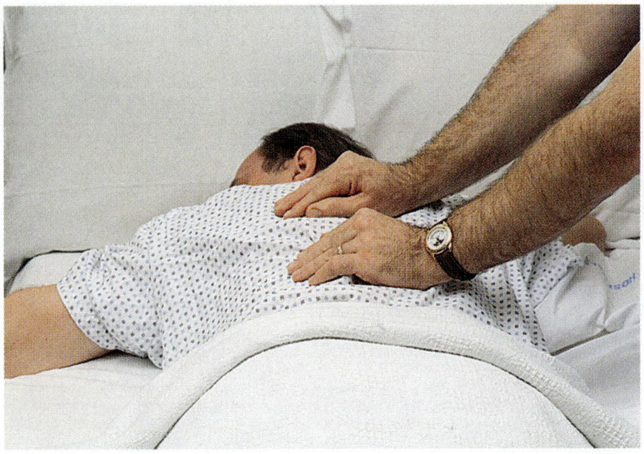

FIGURE 30-11 Hand position for chest wall percussion during physiotherapy.

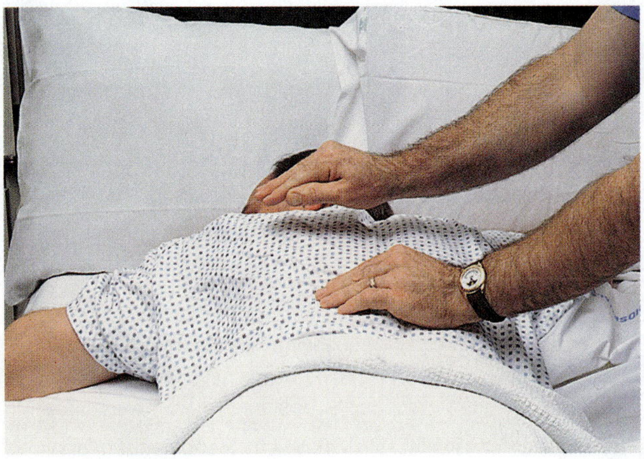

FIGURE 30-12 Chest wall percussion alternating hand motion against patient's chest wall.

layers of material dampen the vibrations. Be careful when percussing the lung fields not to percuss the scapular area, or trauma will occur to the skin and underlying musculoskeletal structures. Percussion is contraindicated in patients with bleeding disorders, osteoporosis, or fractured ribs. Percussion vests are now available in hospitals and the home setting to make chest percussion easier and more comfortable.

Vibration. Vibration is a fine, shaking pressure applied to the chest wall only during exhalation. This technique increases the velocity and turbulence of exhaled air, facilitating secretion removal. Vibration increases the exhalation of trapped air, shakes mucus loose, and induces a cough. You use vibration most often with patients with cystic fibrosis. It is not recommended for infants and young children.

Chest Tubes. A chest tube is a catheter inserted through the rib cage into the pleural space to remove air and/or fluids from the pleural space and reestablish normal intrapleural and intrapulmonic pressures. Chest tubes promote lung expansion and drain fluid or air from the pleural cavity after chest surgery or chest trauma and for pneumothorax, hemothorax, or an empyema (see Skill 30-2).

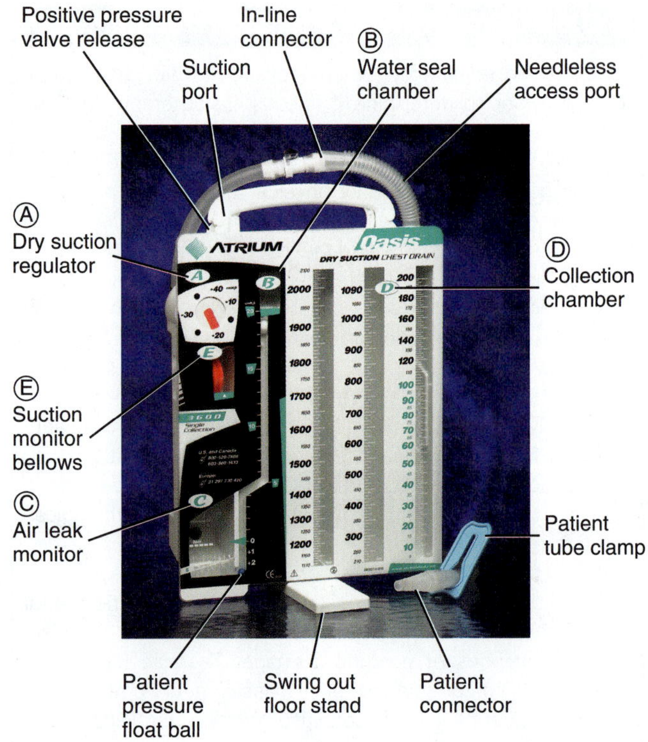

FIGURE 30-13 Dry Suction chest drainage system. (Courtesy Atrium Medical Corp.)

A pneumothorax is a collection of air or other gas in the pleural space. The gas causes the lung to collapse because it destroys the negative intrapleural pressure. This exerts a counter pressure against the lung, making it unable to expand. There are a variety of mechanisms for a pneumothorax. It occurs spontaneously, from chest trauma, or secondary to chronic lung disease. A patient with a pneumothorax feels sharp pain because atmospheric air irritates the parietal pleura. Dyspnea is common and worsens as the size of the pneumothorax increases.

A tension pneumothorax (i.e., a complete collapse of the lung) is a medical emergency resulting from a simple pneumothorax. Air is trapped in the pleural cavity between the chest wall and the lung. The volume of trapped air increases with each inspiration and is unable to escape with expiration, causing increased pressure on the lung, heart, and blood vessels of the thorax. A large-bore cannula or chest tube must be placed immediately to release the pressure.

Hemothorax is an accumulation of blood in the pleural cavity between the parietal and visceral pleurae, usually as the result of trauma. It produces a counter pressure and prevents the lung from full expansion. In addition to pain and dyspnea, signs and symptoms of shock develop if blood loss is severe.

Disposable chest drainage systems such as the Thora-Seal III or Pleur-Evac chest drainage system (DeKental) are one-piece molded plastic units that evacuate any volume of air or fluid with controlled suction (Figure 30-13). The first chamber in each system provides a water seal to prevent air from being drawn back into the pleural space. The second chamber collects fluid or blood. The third chamber is for suction, to facilitate removal of chest drainage and trapped air. The suction pressure causes gentle, continuous bubbling in the third chamber. Suction pressure is measured in centimeters of water. You usually set suction at −15 to −20 cm H_2O for adults. Children require lesser amounts of suction pressure.

The disposable units appear to be the system of choice because they are cost-effective and safe. Your knowledge of the basics of chest tube management and troubleshooting maneuvers reduces a patient's risk for complications.

Special Considerations. Clamping chest tubes is contraindicated when a patient is ambulating or being transported. Handle the chest drainage unit carefully and maintain the drainage device below the patient's chest. The health care provider may choose to clamp the tube temporarily to determine if the patient has fluid accumulation. This requires an order, and you must assess the patient frequently. If the tubing accidentally disconnects from the unit, instruct the patient to exhale as much as possible and cough. This maneuver rids the pleural space of as much air as possible. Quickly cleanse the tip of the tubing and reconnect the tubing to the unit. Clamping the chest tube is not recommended because it may result in a tension pneumothorax, a life-threatening event.

Chest Tube Removal. Removal of a chest tube requires patient preparation. An analgesic administered before removal helps to minimize discomfort and anxiety. Generally the health care provider removes the tube and places occlusive petrolatum gauze dressing over the wound. Monitor the patient's vital signs, lung sounds, and oxygen saturation (SpO_2). The most frequent sensations reported during removal of a chest tube include burning, pain, and a pulling sensation.

Noninvasive Ventilation. Noninvasive ventilation (NIV) maintains positive airway pressure and improves alveolar ventilation without the need for an artificial airway. In addition, this mechanical ventilator alternative reduces and reverses atelectasis, improves oxygenation, reduces pulmonary edema, and improves cardiac function. Positive airway pressure keeps the terminal airways (alveoli) partially inflated, reducing the risk for atelectasis. If atelectasis has occurred, positive pressure assists in reinflation. Because the alveoli remain partially inflated, there is a continuous exchange of respiratory gas; as a result the patient's oxygenation improves. In the cardiac patient NIV reduces pulmonary edema because the increased alveolar pressure forces interstitial fluid out of the lungs and back into the pulmonary circulation. In patients with altered cardiac function secondary to sleep apnea, NIV provides improved myocardial oxygenation and improved function. Substantial reductions in mortality and the need for subsequent ventilation support are associated with noninvasive ventilation in acute respiratory failure, especially in patients with COPD.

Continuous positive airway pressure (CPAP) maintains a steady stream of pressure throughout the patient's breathing cycle (Figure 30-14). It is very beneficial to a patient with sleep apnea. During sleep the upper airway collapses and prevents normal airflow. When the airflow is interrupted, there is a drop in the patient's oxygen saturation, and frequent awakenings occur. CPAP uses continuous positive pressure to keep the airway open and prevent upper airway collapse. As a result the patient breathes more normally, sleeps better, and has markedly reduced snoring. A CPAP setting of 5 cm H_2O provides 5 cm of pressure during inspiration and expiration. The usual CPAP setting is 5 to 20 cm of water. There are disadvantages to this device (Table 30-10).

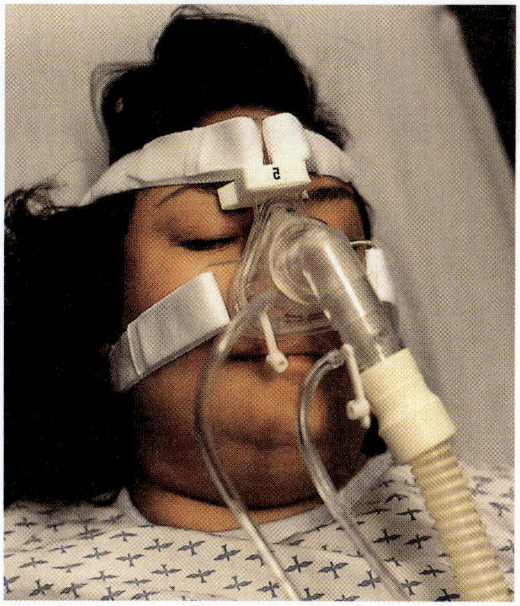

FIGURE 30-14 Mask suitable for either continuous positive airway pressure (CPAP) or bi-level positive airway pressure (BiPAP) device.

Bi-level positive airway pressure (BiPAP) works by providing assistance during inspiration and preventing airway closure during expiration. It provides two levels of pressure: inspiratory positive airway pressure (IPAP) and a lower expiratory positive airway pressure (EPAP). During inspiration BiPAP generates a preset positive-pressure support, which increases a patient's tidal volume and ultimately alveolar ventilation. This pressure support lowers when the patient begins exhaling, which allows for easier exhalation. As a result there is an increase in the functional residual capacity (the amount of air remaining in the lungs at the end of expiration), reduced airway closure, reexpansion of an atelectatic area, and improved oxygenation.

The goals of NIV include improved ventilation and sleep, enhanced quality of life, reduction of morbidity, improvement of physical and physiological function, and cost-effectiveness. You prepare family caregivers and patients who are candidates for noninvasive ventilation for discharge by using a multidisciplinary team.

Restoration of Cardiopulmonary Functioning. The American Heart Association publishes guidelines for cardiopulmonary care and resuscitation every 5 years. The organization outlines the standards for acute myocardial infarction

TABLE 30-10 PROBLEMS ASSOCIATED WITH CONTINUOUS POSITIVE AIRWAY PRESSURE

PROBLEM	CAUSE
Discomfort	Large tight-fitting mask fits over patient's nose. Oxygen flow rate causes dry mucous membranes.
Risks to skin integrity	Tight fit of the mask causes pressure and diaphoresis, which can cause a pressure ulcer. Patients need to remove the mask to relieve pressure.
Hypercapnia	Although CPAP improves alveolar function, which increases carbon dioxide clearance from the blood, it also causes air trapping. In some patients this causes a rise in carbon dioxide levels.
Gastric distention	CPAP forces more air into the stomach, which causes distention and discomfort in some patients. In addition, severe gastric distention impedes diaphragmatic motion and reduces lung volumes. It may be necessary to insert a nasogastric tube if this occurs.
Noise	Some patients find the machine very noisy. It interferes not only with sleep but also with leisure activities.

Data from Peter J, et al: Noninvasive ventilation in acute respiratory failure: a meta-analysis update, *Crit Care Med* 30(3):555, 2002; Woodrow P: Using non-invasive ventilation in acute wards, part I, *Nurs Stand* 18(1):39, 2003.
CPAP, Continuous positive airway pressure.

(AMI), acute stroke, near-fatal asthma, anaphylaxis, and cardiopulmonary arrest for children and adults (Peberdy et al., 2010).

Cardiac arrest is the result of severe and prolonged hypoxia. A cardiac arrest is a sudden cessation of cardiac output and circulation. When this occurs, the tissues do not receive oxygen, carbon dioxide is not transported from tissues, tissue metabolism becomes anaerobic, and metabolic and respiratory acidosis occurs. Permanent heart, brain, and other tissue damage occurs within 4 to 6 minutes.

Cardiopulmonary Resuscitation. A patient with an absent pulse and respiration is in cardiac arrest. If you determine that a patient has experienced cardiac arrest, begin **cardiopulmonary resuscitation (CPR).** CPR is a basic emergency procedure of artificial respiration and manual external cardiac massage. The sequence for CPR is C-A-B: chest compression, early defibrillation, establishing an airway and rescue breathing (Peberdy et al., 2010). Defibrillation is recommended within 5 minutes for an out-of-hospital sudden cardiac arrest and within 3 minutes for an in-hospital victim. The recommendation further states that, in addition to health care providers, specific lay individuals, police, firefighters, security personnel, ski patrol members, ferryboat crews, and airline flight attendants need training in CPR and the use of an automated external defibrillator (AED) (Peberdy et al., 2010) (Box 30-13).

BOX 30-13 AUTOMATED EXTERNAL DEFIBRILLATOR

- The automated external defibrillator (AED) is a device used to administer an electrical shock through the chest wall to the heart.
- The AED has a built-in computer that assesses the victim's heart rhythm and determines if defibrillation is needed.
- The rescuer delivers a shock to the victim after announcing, "Everyone stand back."
- The AED can be used by nonmedical personnel.
- Use of an AED strengthens the chain of survival. Every minute of a sudden cardiac death without defibrillation decreases the survival rate by 7% to 10% (American Heart Association, 2013).

The recommendation is to deliver chest compressions for 2 minutes in a child and then call 9-1-1. For adult victims the recommendation is to call 9-1-1 if you are alone, unless they have been involved in a drowning, drug overdose, or trauma; in these cases begin chest compressions immediately. The rate of compression for an adult, child, or infant is at least 100 compressions per minute. The ratio of compressions to breaths in one- and two-rescuer CPR for people 8 years or older and for one-rescuer child or infant is 30 compressions to 2 ventilations. You use a ratio of 15 compressions to 2 ventilations in infant and child two-rescuer CPR (Peberdy et al., 2010). When you cannot establish an airway, reassess proper head position and assess for airway obstruction. The 2010 guidelines for CPR *do not* recommend that lay rescuers perform blind sweeps of the mouth or abdominal thrusts (Peberdy et al., 2010).

Restorative and Continuing Care. Restorative and continuing care emphasize cardiopulmonary reconditioning as a structured rehabilitation program. **Cardiopulmonary rehabilitation** involves actively helping a patient achieve and maintain an optimal level of health through controlled physical exercise, nutrition counseling, relaxation and stress management techniques, prescribed medications, and oxygen administration. As physical reconditioning occurs, the patient's physical symptoms, anxiety, depression, or somatic concerns decrease. The patient and the rehabilitation team define the goals of rehabilitation.

Respiratory Muscle Training. Respiratory muscle training improves strength and endurance, resulting in improved activity tolerance. Respiratory muscle training can prevent respiratory failure in patients with COPD.

Breathing Exercises. Breathing exercises include techniques to improve ventilation and oxygenation. The three basic techniques are deep breathing and coughing exercises, pursed-lip breathing, and diaphragmatic breathing.

Pursed-lip breathing involves deep inspiration and prolonged expiration through pursed lips to prevent alveolar collapse. Instruct the patient to sit up and then take a deep breath and exhale slowly through pursed lips. Patients need to gain control of the exhalation phase so exhalation is longer than inhalation. The patient is usually able to perfect this technique by counting inhalation time and gradually increasing the count during exhalation.

Diaphragmatic breathing is more difficult and requires a patient to relax the intercostal and accessory respiratory muscles while taking deep inspirations. The patient concentrates on expanding the diaphragm during controlled inspiration. Teach the patient to place one hand flat below the breastbone above the waist and the other hand 2 to 3 cm below the first hand. Then ask him or her to inhale while the lower hand moves outward during inspiration. The patient observes for inward movement as the diaphragm ascends. Initially teach these exercises with the patient in the supine position and then practice while the patient sits and stands. The exercise is often used with the pursed-lip breathing technique.

EVALUATION

Patient Care. You evaluate nursing interventions and therapies by comparing a patient's progress to the goals and desired outcomes of the nursing care plan. When nursing measures directed to improve oxygenation are unsuccessful, modify the care plan by revising existing interventions or introducing new interventions. Do not hesitate to notify the health care provider about a patient's decline in oxygenation status. Prompt notification helps to avoid an emergency situation or even the need for CPR.

Management of Mr. King, a patient with COPD, depends on achieving three major goals: reduction of airflow obstruction, prevention or management of complications, and improvement in the patient's quality of life (Box 30-14).

Patients with chronic cardiopulmonary disease present a nursing challenge. They require frequent nursing interventions when they are acutely ill. With chronic diseases do not think in terms of recovery, but rather health maintenance. You are caring for patients with acute exacerbations of their chronic diseases. You will not see a dramatic cure, but your goal is to return the patient to his or her functional and cognitive status before this most recent exacerbation. You will be helping patients improve the quality of their lives in small but significant ways.

Patient Expectations. Individualize the goals that you set for a patient and make sure they are realistic. Some patients need to learn how to cope with chronic disease. Before any teaching program is effective, a patient must want to learn. Ask the patient if he or she would like to know more about respiratory illnesses, vaccinations, or smoking cessation. Inform the patient that it is possible to gain greater independence, improve mobility, decrease dyspnea, and decrease the frequency of acute respiratory infections. Presenting an individualized education program based on assessment data helps to ensure that the patient will comprehend, learn, use, and ultimately benefit from the education.

BOX 30-14 EVALUATION

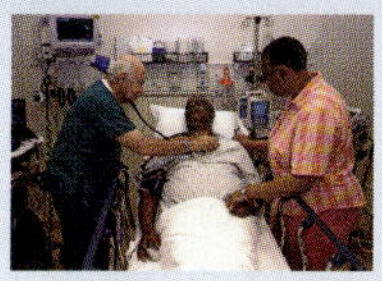

John cares for Mr. King throughout his hospital stay. Mr. King is afebrile, his white blood cells are within normal limits, and his sputum cultures are negative on day of discharge. He does not require supplemental oxygen use. He is able to describe ways to prevent respiratory infections because they aggravate airways and precipitate an episode of acute respiratory failure. Because he now practices pursed-lip breathing, his breathing is more controlled, relieving his subsequent anxiety.

While John is observing Mr. King preparing for discharge, it is quite evident that Mr. King is using the various breathing techniques that they have worked on together. The patient is able to go home with improved activities of daily living. His wife even appears less anxious and states that she feels as though for the first time they have taken a small step to improve the quality of their lives.

DOCUMENTATION NOTE

"Mr. King discharged to home. Able to state the purpose of breathing exercises and each medication, able to list causes and symptoms of respiratory tract infection. Has an appointment in 1 week with a community-based rehabilitation program. Scheduled to see his health care provider in 2 weeks. Prescriptions explained and given to patient. Accompanied to the exit. Left with wife and son."

SAFETY GUIDELINES FOR NURSING SKILLS

Ensuring patient safety is an essential role of the professional nurse. To ensure patient safety, communicate clearly with members of the health care team, assess and incorporate the patient's priorities of care and preferences, and use the best evidence when making decisions about your patient's care. When performing the skills in this chapter, remember the following points to ensure safe, individualized care.

- Patients with sudden changes in their vital signs, level of consciousness, or behavior are *possibly experiencing profound hypoxia.* Patients who demonstrate subtle changes over time have worsening of a chronic or existing condition or a new medical condition.

- *Perform tracheal suctioning before pharyngeal suctioning whenever possible.* The mouth and pharynx contain more bacteria than the trachea does. If there is an abundance of oral secretions present before beginning the procedure, suction mouth with oral suction device.
- *Use caution when suctioning patients with a head injury.* Suctioning elevates the intracranial pressure (ICP). Reduce this risk by hyperventilating prior to suctioning, which results in hypocarbia that in turn induces vasoconstriction. Vasoconstriction reduces the potential increase in ICP. It is recommended that you limit the introduction of a catheter to 2 times with each suctioning procedure.
- The routine use of normal saline instillation into the airway before endotracheal and tracheostomy suctioning is not recommended. Normal saline instillation in conjunction with endotracheal suction leads to the spread of microorganisms into the lower respiratory tract and decreases in oxygenation saturation (Pedersen et al., 2009). Current evidence shows normal saline is not effective in thinning secretions or improving removal of secretions. In certain circumstances, if it is necessary to stimulate a cough, normal saline may be indicated. This requires collaboration with the health care team.
- *Check your institutional policy before stripping or milking chest tubes.* Most institutions have stopped this practice because stripping the tube greatly increases intrapleural pressure, which can damage the pleural tissue and cause pneumothorax or worsen an existing pneumothorax. However, even though the literature is contradictory, you will perform stripping or milking in selected patients (e.g., fresh postoperative thoracic surgery or chest traumas). The rationale for selective use of stripping or milking is that the presence of clotted tube drainage decreases lung reexpansion and increases risk for tension pneumothorax. Thus the benefits of milking outweigh the risks in these special cases.

SKILL 30-1 SUCTIONING

View Video!

DELEGATION CONSIDERATIONS

The skills of nasotracheal and artificial airway suctioning are not routinely delegated to nursing assistive personnel (NAP). However, when a patient is assessed by the nurse to be stable, oral and permanent tracheostomy tube suctioning may be delegated. Before delegation the nurse instructs the NAP about:

- Any individualized aspects of care that pertain to suctioning such as position, duration of suction, and suction pressure settings.
- Signs and symptoms of hypoxemia or respiratory distress such as change in patient's respiratory status, confusion, and restlessness and to immediately report these signs to the nurse.
- Reporting changes in a patient's secretions such as quality, quantity, and color.

EQUIPMENT

- Appropriate-size suction catheter or closed-suction catheter (smallest diameter that will remove secretions effectively) or Yankauer catheter (oral suction)
- Nasal or oral airway (if indicated)
- Sterile gloves
- Clean gloves
- Pulse oximeter
- Stethoscope
- Clean towel or paper drape
- Portable or wall suction
- Mask, goggles, or face shield
- Connecting tube (6 feet)

If Not Using Closed-Suction Catheter

- Small Y-adapter (if catheter does not have a suction control port)
- Water-soluble lubricant
- Sterile basin
- Sterile normal saline solution or water (about 100 mL)

STEP	RATIONALE
ASSESSMENT	
1. Assess for risk factors for upper or lower airway obstruction, including obstructive lung disease; pulmonary infections; impaired mobility; sedation; decreased level of consciousness; seizures; presence of feeding tube; anatomy of nasopharynx and oral pharynx; decreased gag or cough reflex; decreased swallowing ability; allergies; sinus drainage; and head, neck, or chest trauma.	The presence of these risk factors impairs patient's ability to clear secretions from the airway and requires nasopharyngeal or nasotracheal suctioning. Physical signs and symptoms result from decreased oxygen to tissues and pooling of secretions in upper and lower airways.
2. Determine the presence of apprehension, anxiety, decreased ability to concentrate, lethargy, decreased level of consciousness (especially acute), increased fatigue, dizziness, behavioral changes (especially irritability), decreased oxygen saturation (from pulse oximetry), increased pulse rate, increased rate of breathing, decreased depth of breathing, elevated blood pressure, cardiac dysrhythmias, pallor, cyanosis, and dyspnea or use of accessory muscles.	Signs and symptoms are associated with hypoxia (low oxygen at the cellular or tissue level), hypoxemia (low oxygen tension in the blood), or hypercapnia (elevated carbon dioxide tension in the blood). Patients report sensations of pain and discomfort with the suctioning procedure; as a result, this increases their anxiety before suctioning. Anxiety and pain consume oxygen and in turn worsen the signs of hypoxia.

STEP	RATIONALE
3. Assess vital signs, including pulse oximetry (SpO_2) and, if on ventilator, peak inspiratory pressure and tidal volume.	Changes in vital signs can indicate respiratory distress.
4. Assess for signs and symptoms of upper and lower airway obstruction, including abnormal respiratory rate, wheezes, crackles, or gurgling on inspiration or expiration; restlessness; ineffective coughing; unilateral, segmental, or lobar absent or diminished breath sounds (in absence of pneumonectomy or lobectomy); tachycardia; hypertension or hypotension; cyanosis; decreased level of consciousness, especially acute; or excess nasal secretions, drooling, or gastric secretions or vomitus in the mouth (AARC, 2004).	Physical signs and symptoms result from decreased oxygen to tissues and pooling of secretions in upper and lower airways.
5. Determine additional factors that normally influence upper or lower airway function: recent surgery, ineffective or absent cough, chemical neuromuscular blockade, neuromuscular diseases, heart failure, pulmonary edema, adult respiratory distress syndrome, hyaline membrane disease, or diaphragmatic weakness or paralysis.	Allows nurse to identify patients at risk for airway obstruction needing endotracheal (ET) or tracheostomy tube suctioning.
6. Assess the following factors that influence character of secretions:	
a. Fluid status	Fluid overload increases amount of secretions. Dehydration promotes thicker secretions.
b. Lack of humidity	The environment influences secretion formation and gas exchange, necessitating airway suctioning when a patient cannot clear secretions effectively.
c. Infection (e.g., pneumonia)	Patients with respiratory infections are likely to have increased secretions that are thicker and sometimes more difficult to expectorate.
7. For endotracheal suctioning assess patient's peak inspiratory pressure when on volume-controlled ventilation or tidal volume during pressure-controlled ventilation.	Increased peak pressure or decreased tidal volume sometimes indicates airway obstruction (AARC, 2010).
8. Assess patient's need for suctioning and consider contraindications to nasotracheal suctioning (AARC, 2004): a. Facial traumas/surgery b. Acute head injury c. Bleeding disorders d. Nasal bleeding e. Epiglottitis or croup f. Laryngospasm g. Irritable airway h. Gastric surgery with high anastomosis	Consider these conditions only if suctioning appears to be hazardous. The passage of a catheter though the nasal route causes additional trauma, increased nasal bleeding, or severe bleeding in the presence of bleeding disorders. In the presence of epiglottitis, croup, laryngospasm, or irritable airway, the entrance of a suction catheter via the nasal route causes intractable coughing, hypoxemia, and severe bronchospasm, necessitating emergency intubation or tracheostomy.

Clinical Decision Point: **ET suctioning is necessary for patients with artificial airways. Most contraindications are relative to a patient's risk of developing adverse reactions or a worsening clinical condition as a result of the procedure. The decision to withhold suctioning to avoid possible adverse reaction may in fact be lethal (AARC, 2010).**

STEP	RATIONALE
9. Examine sputum microbiology data.	Certain bacteria are easy to transmit or require isolation because of virulence or antibiotic resistance.
10. Identify patient using two identifiers (e.g., name and birthday or name and account number) according to agency policy. Compare identifiers with information on patient's medication administration record (MAR) or medical record.	Ensures correct patient. Complies with The Joint Commission requirements for patient safety (TJC, 2014).
11. Assess patient's understanding of procedure.	Reveals need for patient instruction and encourages cooperation.
PLANNING	
1. Explain to patient how procedure will help clear airway and relieve breathing problems. Explain that temporary coughing, sneezing, gagging, or shortness of breath is normal during the procedure.	Encourages cooperation and minimizes risks, anxiety, and pain of procedure.

SKILL 30-1 SUCTIONING—cont'd

STEP	RATIONALE
2. Explain importance of coughing during procedure. Encourage patient to cough out secretions. Practice coughing if patient is able. Splint surgical incisions if necessary.	Facilitates secretion removal and reduces frequency and duration of future suctioning.
3. Help patient assume comfortable position (usually semi-Fowler's or sitting upright with head hyperextended unless contraindicated).	Reduces stimulation of gag reflex, promotes patient comfort and secretion drainage, and prevents aspiration.
4. Place towel or paper drape across patient's chest, if needed.	Reduces transmission of microorganisms by protecting gown from secretions.

IMPLEMENTATION

STEP	RATIONALE
1. Perform hand hygiene and apply mask, goggles, or face shield if splashing during suctioning is likely.	Reduces transmission of microorganisms.
2. Connect one end of connecting tubing to suction machine and place other end in convenient location near patient. Turn suction device on and set suction pressure to as low a level as possible to effectively clear secretions (AARC, 2010). Occlude end of suction tubing to check suction pressure.	Excessive negative pressure damages nasal, pharyngeal, and tracheal mucosa and induces greater hypoxia. Lowest possible suction pressure is recommended (less than 150 mm Hg in adults) (AARC, 2010; Pedersen et al., 2009).
3. If indicated, increase supplemental oxygen therapy to 100% or as ordered by health care provider. Encourage patient to breathe deeply.	Hyperoxygenation provides some protection from suction-induced decline in oxygenation. It is most effective in the presence of hyperinflation such as encouraging patient to deep breathe or increasing ventilator tidal volume (Pedersen et al., 2009).

Clinical Decision Point: **After suctioning is completed, readjust oxygen or ventilator settings to preprocedure level as ordered to avoid increased risk for oxygen toxicity and absorption, atelectasis from prolonged administration of high concentrations of oxygen, and increased carbon dioxide retention in patients with chronic obstructive lung diseases.**

STEP	RATIONALE
4. Prepare suction catheter.	
A. **One time–use catheter**	
(1) Open suction kit or catheter using aseptic technique. Keep kit or catheter on work surface. If sterile drape is available, place it across patient's chest or on over-bed table. Do not allow suction catheter to touch any nonsterile surfaces.	Maintains asepsis and reduces transmission of microorganisms.
(2) Stand on side of bed facing patient with your dominant hand next to the bed. Unwrap or open sterile basin and place on bedside table. Be careful not to touch inside of basin. Fill with about 100 mL sterile normal saline solution or water (see illustration).	Use saline or water to clean tubing after each suction pass.
(3) Open lubricant. Squeeze small amount onto the open sterile catheter package without touching package. **NOTE:** Lubricant is not necessary for artificial airway suctioning.	Prepares lubricant while maintaining sterility. Use water-soluble lubricant to avoid lipoid aspiration pneumonia. Excessive lubricant occludes catheter.

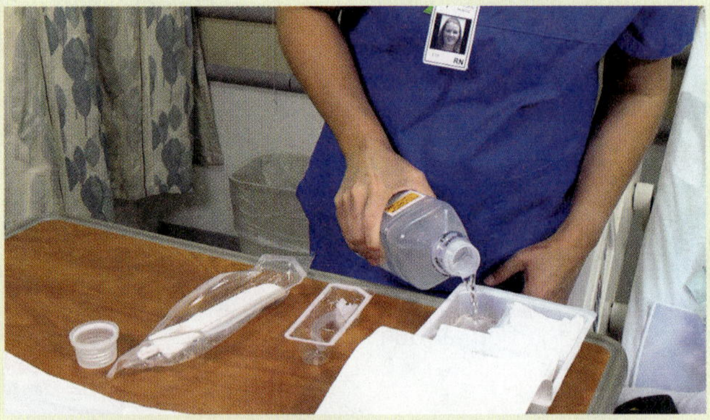

STEP 4A(2) Pouring sterile saline into tray.

STEP	RATIONALE
B. Closed (in-line) suction catheter Prepare catheter following steps in Box 30-11.	
5. Apply clean gloves for oropharyngeal suction. Apply sterile glove to each hand or a clean glove to nondominant hand and sterile glove to dominant hand for all other suction techniques.	Maintains appropriate aseptic technique.
6. Pick up suction catheter with dominant hand without touching nonsterile surfaces. Pick up connecting tubing with nondominant hand. Secure catheter to tubing (see illustration).	Maintains catheter sterility. Connects catheter to suction.
7. Suction a small amount of normal saline solution from basin.	Ensures equipment function. Lubricates internal catheter and tubing.
8. Suction airway.	
A. Oropharyngeal suctioning	
(1) Remove oxygen mask if present. Nasal cannula may remain in place. Keep oxygen mask near patient's face.	Allows access to patient's mouth while having access to oxygen delivery system.
(2) Insert Yankauer catheter along gum line to pharynx. With suction applied, move catheter around mouth until secretions are cleared. Encourage patient to cough. Replace oxygen mask as appropriate.	Intermittent suction prevents invagination of oral mucosa into suction catheter. Invagination of mucosa causes trauma to mucous membranes. Coughing moves secretions from lower to upper airways into mouth.
(3) Rinse catheter with water in basin until catheter and connecting tube are cleared of secretions.	Clearing secretions before they dry reduces probability of transmission of microorganisms and enhances delivery of preset suction pressures.
(4) Place catheter or Yankauer in clean, dry area for reuse with suction turned off. If patient is able to suction self, place within his or her reach with suction on.	Facilitates prompt removal of airway secretions for future suctioning.
B. Nasopharyngeal and nasotracheal suctioning	
(1) Increase oxygen flow rate for face masks as ordered. Have patient deep breathe slowly if possible.	Hyperoxygenation is recommended, especially in patients who are hypoxemic or at risk for hypoxemia (AARC, 2010).
(2) Lightly coat distal 6 to 8 cm (2 to 3 inches) of catheter tip with water-soluble lubricant.	Lubricates catheter for easier insertion.
(3) Remove oxygen delivery device (if applicable) with nondominant hand. Without applying suction and using dominant thumb and forefinger, gently but quickly insert catheter into naris as patient inhales. Following the natural course of the naris, slightly slant catheter downward or through mouth. Do not force through naris (see illustration).	Application of suction pressure while introducing catheter into trachea increases risk for damage to mucosa and risk for hypoxia because of removal of entrained oxygen present in airways.

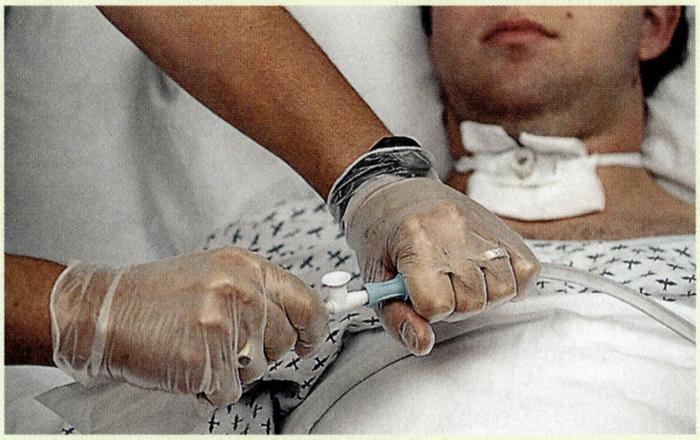

STEP 6 Attaching catheter to suction.

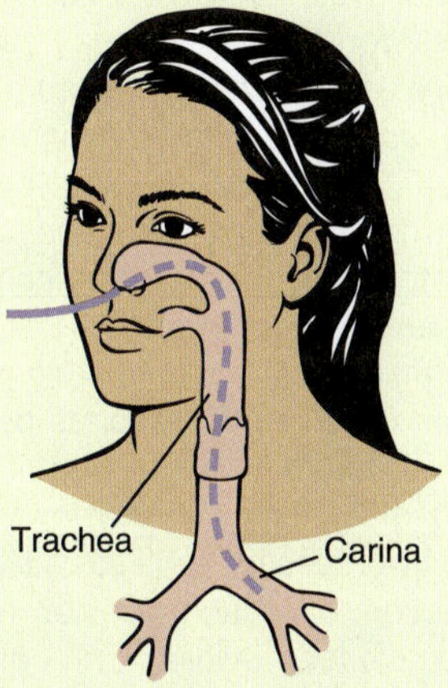

STEP 8B(3) Pathway for nasotracheal catheter progression.

SKILL 30-1 SUCTIONING—cont'd

STEP	RATIONALE
Clinical Decision Point: **Be sure to insert catheter as patient inhales, especially if inserting it into trachea, because epiglottis is open. Do not insert during swallowing or catheter will most likely enter esophagus. Never apply suction during insertion. Make sure that patient coughs. If patient gags or becomes nauseated, the catheter is most likely in the esophagus. Remove the catheter.**	
(a) *Nasopharyngeal suctioning:* In adults insert catheter about 16 cm (6 to 7 inches); in older children, 8 to 12 cm (3 to 5 inches); in infants and young children, 4 to 8 cm (2 to 3 inches). Rule of thumb is to insert catheter distance from tip of nose (or mouth) to angle of mandible.	Ensure that catheter tip reaches pharynx for suctioning.
(b) *Nasotracheal suctioning (without applying suction):* In adults insert catheter about 20 cm (8 inches); in older children, 16 to 20 cm (6 to 8 inches); and in young children and infants, 4 to 7.5 cm (1.6 to 3 inches) (see Step 8B(3)) (AARC, 2004).	Ensure that catheter tip reaches pharynx for suctioning.
Clinical Decision Point: **When there is difficulty passing the catheter, ask patient to cough or say "ash" or try to advance the catheter during inspiration. Both of these measures help to open the glottis to permit passage of the catheter into the trachea.**	
(c) If you have difficulty inserting catheter into trachea, have patient turn head to the right to help suction left mainstem bronchus; turn head to left to help suction right mainstem bronchus. If you feel resistance after insertion of catheter for maximum recommended distance, catheter has probably hit carina. Pull it back 1 to 2 cm (0.4 to 0.8 inches) before applying suction (AARC 2010).	Turning patient's head to side elevates bronchial passage on opposite side.
(4) With catheter tip in position (pharynx or trachea), apply intermittent suction for no longer than 10 seconds by placing and then releasing nondominant thumb over vent of catheter and slowly withdrawing catheter while rotating it back and forth between dominant thumb and forefinger. Encourage patient to cough. Replace oxygen device if applicable.	Intermittent suction and rotation of catheter when using a closed suctioning system reduce risk for injury to mucosa. If catheter "grabs" mucosa, remove thumb to release suction. Suctioning longer than 10 seconds causes cardiopulmonary compromise, usually from hypoxemia or vagal overload.
Clinical Decision Point: **Monitor vital signs and oxygen saturation throughout suction procedure. If the pulse drops more than 20 beats/min or increases more than 40 beats/min or if pulse oximetry falls below 90% or 5% from baseline, stop suctioning. Any deteriorating change in patient's physiological status during suctioning requires termination of the procedure, hyperoxygenation, and other appropriate interventions (e.g., position change).**	
(5) Rinse catheter and connecting tubing with normal saline or water until cleared.	Secretions that remain in suction catheter or connecting tubing decrease suctioning efficiency.
(6) Assess for need to repeat suctioning procedure. Observe for alterations in cardiopulmonary status. Allow adequate time (1 minute) between suction passes for ventilation and oxygenation. Do not perform more than two passes with catheter. Ask patient to deep breathe and cough.	Suctioning sometimes can induce hypoxemia, dysrhythmias, laryngospasm, and bronchospasm. Deep breathing ventilates and deoxygenates alveoli. Repeated passes clear airway of excessive secretions but also remove oxygen and induce laryngospasm.
C. Artificial airway suctioning	
(1) Hyperinflate and/or hyperoxygenate with 100% oxygen for 30 to 60 seconds by adjusting fractional inspired oxygen (FiO_2) setting on a mechanical ventilator or using an oxygen enrichment program on microprocessor ventilators (AARC, 2010). Manual ventilation of patient is not recommended; it is ineffective for providing 100% oxygen (AARC, 2010).	Preoxygenation converts a large proportion of resident lung gas to 100% oxygen to offset amount used in metabolic consumption while ventilation or oxygenation is interrupted and volume is lost during suctioning. Routine use of hyperinflation is not recommended because of possibility of trauma resulting from large volumes and high peak pressures (Pedersen et al., 2009).

STEP	RATIONALE
(2) If patient is receiving mechanical ventilation, open swivel adapter; or if necessary remove oxygen or humidity delivery device with nondominant hand.	Exposes artificial airway.
(3) Without applying suction, gently but quickly insert catheter using dominant thumb and forefinger into artificial airway (it is best to try to time catheter insertion into artificial airway with inspiration) until you meet resistance or until patient coughs; then pull back 1 cm (½ inch).	Application of suction pressure while introducing catheter into trachea increases risk for damage to tracheal mucosa and increased hypoxia related to removal of entrained oxygen present in airways. Pulling back stimulates cough and removes catheter from mucosal wall so catheter is not resting against tracheal mucosa during suctioning. Shallow suctioning is recommended to prevent tracheal mucosa trauma (AARC, 2010).

Clinical Decision Point: **If you are unable to insert catheter past the end of the ET tube, it is probably caught in the Murphy eye (i.e., side hole at the distal end of the ET tube that allows for collateral airflow in the event of tracheal mainstem intubation). If so, rotate the catheter to reposition it away from the Murphy eye or withdraw it slightly and reinsert with the next inhalation. Usually the catheter meets resistance at the carina. One indication that the catheter is at the carina is acute onset of coughing because the carina contains many cough receptors. Pull the catheter back 1 cm (½ inch) (AARC, 2010).**

STEP	RATIONALE
(4) Apply intermittent suction by placing and releasing nondominant thumb over vent of catheter; slowly withdraw catheter while rotating it back and forth between dominant thumb and forefinger (see illustration). Encourage patient to cough. Watch for respiratory distress.	Intermittent suction and rotation of catheter prevent injury to tracheal mucosal lining. If catheter "grabs" mucosa, remove thumb to release suction.

Clinical Decision Point: **If patient develops respiratory distress during the suction procedure, immediately withdraw catheter and supply additional oxygen and breaths as needed. In an emergency administer oxygen directly though the catheter. Disconnect suction and attach oxygen at prescribed flow rate through the catheter.**

STEP	RATIONALE
(5) If patient is receiving mechanical ventilation, close swivel adapter or replace oxygen delivery device.	Reestablishes artificial airway.
(6) Encourage patient to deep breathe if able. Some patients respond well to several manual breaths from the mechanical ventilator or bag-valve-mask.	Reoxygenates and reexpands alveoli. Suctioning sometimes causes hypoxemia and atelectasis.
(7) Rinse catheter and connecting tubing with normal saline until clear. Use continuous suction.	Removes catheter secretions, which can decrease suctioning efficiency and provide environment for microorganism growth.
(8) Assess patient's cardiopulmonary status for secretion clearance. Repeat Steps (1) through (7) to clear secretions. Allow adequate time (1 to 2 minutes) between suction passes for ventilation and oxygenation. Do not perform more than two passes with catheter.	Suctioning induces dysrhythmias, hypoxia, and bronchospasm and impairs cerebral circulation or adversely affects hemodynamic stability. A repeated pass with suction catheter clears airway of excessive secretions and promotes improved oxygenation.

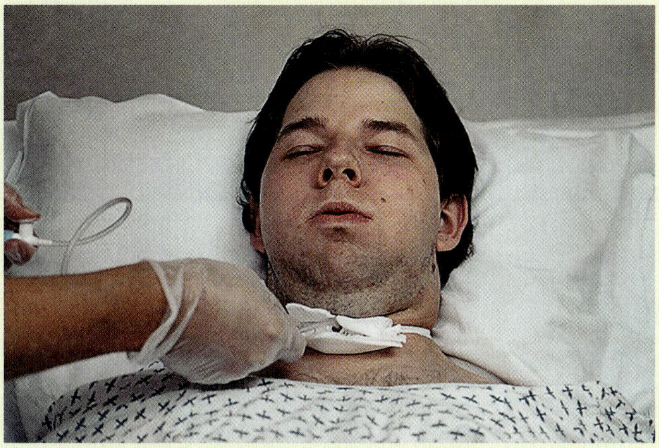

STEP 8C(4) Suctioning tracheostomy.

SKILL 30-1 SUCTIONING—cont'd

STEP	RATIONALE
9. When you have cleared pharynx and/or trachea sufficiently of secretions, perform oropharyngeal suctioning to clear mouth of secretions. Do not suction nose or artificial airway again after suctioning mouth.	Removes upper airway secretions. In general, more microorganisms are present in mouth. Upper airway is considered "clean," and lower airway is considered "sterile." Use same catheter to suction from sterile to clean areas but not from clean to sterile areas.
10. Remove towel, place in laundry or appropriate receptacle, and reposition patient. Wear clean gloves to provide oral hygiene or any other type of personal care.	Reduces transmission of microorganisms. Promotes comfort.
11. Discard catheter by enclosing it in glove and removing glove over catheter. Dispose of glove and perform hand hygiene.	Reduces transmission of microorganisms.
12. If indicated, readjust oxygen to original level because patient's blood oxygen level should return to baseline.	Prevents absorption atelectasis and oxygen toxicity while allowing patient time to reoxygenate blood.
13. Discard remainder of normal saline into appropriate receptacle. If basin is disposable, discard into appropriate receptacle. If basin is reusable, rinse it out and place it in storage area for soiled items in utility room.	Reduces transmission of microorganisms.
14. Remove face shield and discard into appropriate receptacle. Perform hand hygiene.	Reduces transmission of microorganisms.
15. Place unopened suction kit on suction machine table or at head of bed.	Provides immediate access to suction catheter for next procedure.
16. Help patient return to comfortable position.	
EVALUATION	
1. Measure patient's vital signs and perform cardiopulmonary assessment for hypoxia, and SpO_2 values. If patient is on a ventilator, compare FiO_2 and tidal volume.	Provides subjective confirmation that you relieved airway obstruction during suctioning procedure.
2. Observe airway secretions.	Provides data to document presence or absence of respiratory tract infection.
3. Observe patient's behaviors and ask patient if he or she is breathing easier and if there is less congestion.	Provides data to determine if you established patent airway.

RECORDING AND REPORTING

- Record the method of suctioning and the amount, consistency, color, and odor of secretions.
- Record patient's response to the suction procedure.
- Record and report the patient's presuctioning and postsuctioning cardiopulmonary status.

UNEXPECTED OUTCOMES AND RELATED INTERVENTIONS

- Worsening cardiopulmonary status
  - Limit length of time suctioning.
  - Determine need for presuctioning hyperoxygenation and hyperinflation.
  - Determine need for more frequent, shorter-duration suctioning.
  - Notify health care provider of changes.
- Return of bloody secretions
  - Determine amount of suction pressure used and adjust accordingly.
  - Evaluate frequency of suctioning and reduce if appropriate.
  - Determine other factors that lead to bloody secretions (e.g., prolonged bleeding time).
  - Provide more frequent oral hygiene.
- Unable to pass suction catheter through first naris attempted
  - Try other naris or oral route.
  - Insert nasal airway, especially if suctioning through patient's naris frequently.
  - Guide catheter along naris floor to avoid turbinates.
  - If obstruction is mucus, apply suction to relieve obstruction but do not apply it to mucosa. If you think obstruction is a blood clot, consult health care provider.
- Paroxysms of coughing (severe coughing attacks)
  - Administer supplemental oxygen.
  - Allow patient to rest between passes of suction catheter.
  - Consult health care provider regarding need for inhaled bronchodilators or topical anesthetics.
- Unable to obtain secretions
  - Determine adequacy of humidification of oxygen delivery device.
  - Evaluate patient's fluid status.
  - Determine need for chest physiotherapy.
  - Assess for signs of infection.

SKILL 30-2 CARE OF PATIENTS WITH CHEST TUBES

View Video!

DELEGATION CONSIDERATIONS

The skill of caring for a patient with chest tubes cannot be delegated to nursing assistive personnel (NAP). The nurse instructs NAP to:

- Properly position the patient with chest tubes to facilitate chest tube drainage and optimal functioning of the system.
- Safely ambulate and transfer the patient with chest drainage.
- Report any changes in vital signs, level of comfort, SpO_2, or excessive bubbling in water-seal chamber of drainage system.
- Immediately notify the nurse if there is a disconnection of the system, change in type and amount of drainage, bleeding, or sudden cessation of bubbling.

EQUIPMENT

- Disposable chest drainage system (see Figure 30-13)
- Suction source and setup (wall canister or portable)
  - Water-seal system: Add sterile water or normal saline solution to cover the lower 2.5 cm (1 inch) of water-seal U tube. Pour water or normal saline solution into the suction control chamber if suction is to be used (see manufacturer directions)
  - Waterless system: Add vial of 30- to 45-mL injectable sodium chloride or water (for diagnostic air-leak indicator), 20-mL syringe, 21-gauge needle, and antiseptic swab
- Clean gloves
- 2-inch tape
- Sterile gauze sponges
- Vital sign equipment and pulse oximeter

STEP	RATIONALE
ASSESSMENT	
1. Identify patient using two identifiers (e.g., name and birthday or name and account number) according to agency policy. Compare identifiers with information on patient's medication administration record (MAR) or medical record.	Ensures correct patient. Complies with The Joint Commission requirements for patient safety (TJC, 2014).
2. Perform hand hygiene and assess pulmonary status:	Signs and symptoms determine level of respiratory distress. Signs and symptoms of increased respiratory distress and/or chest pain are decreased breath sounds over the affected and nonaffected lungs, marked cyanosis, and asymmetrical chest movements.
a. Assess lung sounds over affected lung area and ask if patient feels chest pain or dyspnea (see Chapters 15 and 16). Observe chest movements and note if patient shows nonverbal signs of pain.	
b. Determine if patient has chest pain on inspiration.	
3. Obtain vital signs, SpO_2, and level of cognition.	Changes in pulse SpO_2 and blood pressure (hypotension) and tachycardia indicate infection, respiratory distress, or pain. Cognitive changes indicate hypoxia.
4. If possible, ask patient to rate level of comfort on a visual analog scale of 0 to 10.	Chest tubes are often painful and interfere with patient's mobility, coughing and deep breathing, and rehabilitation.
5. Observe:	
a. Chest tube dressing and site surrounding tube insertion.	Leakage of air into tissue presents as subcutaneous emphysema around tube insertion site or neck. Ensures that dressing is intact without air or fluid leaks and that area surrounding insertion site is free of drainage or skin irritation.
b. Tubing for kinks, dependent loops, or clots.	Maintains patent, freely draining system, preventing fluid accumulation in chest cavity. Presence of kinks, dependent loops, or clotted drainage increases patient's risk for infection, atelectasis, and tension pneumothorax.
c. Chest drainage system to ensure that it is upright and below level of tube insertion (see illustrations).	Facilitates drainage. Ensures that system is in position to function properly.
6. Assess patient's knowledge of chest tube care.	Encourages cooperation, minimizes risks and anxiety. Identifies teaching needs.
PLANNING	
1. Attach two hemostats for each chest tube to top of patient's bed with adhesive tape. Chest tubes are only clamped under specific circumstances per health care provider's order or nursing policy and procedure:	Hemostats have a covering to prevent hemostat from penetrating chest tube once changed. The use of these hemostats or other clamp prevents air from reentering pleural space.
a. To assess air leak (Table 30-11).	
b. To quickly empty or change disposable drainage system; performed by nurse who has received education in procedure.	

SKILL 30-2 CARE OF PATIENTS WITH CHEST TUBES—cont'd

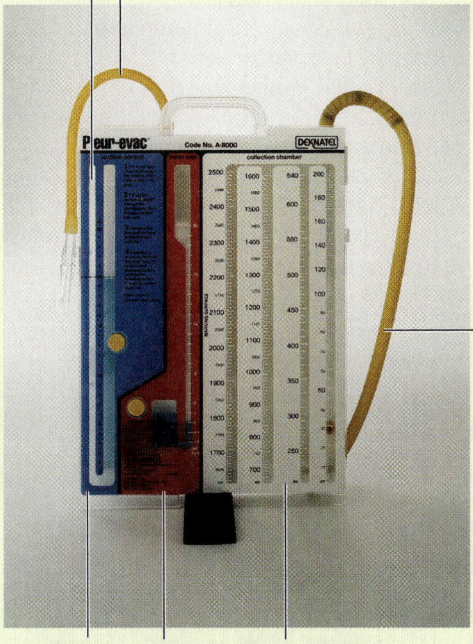

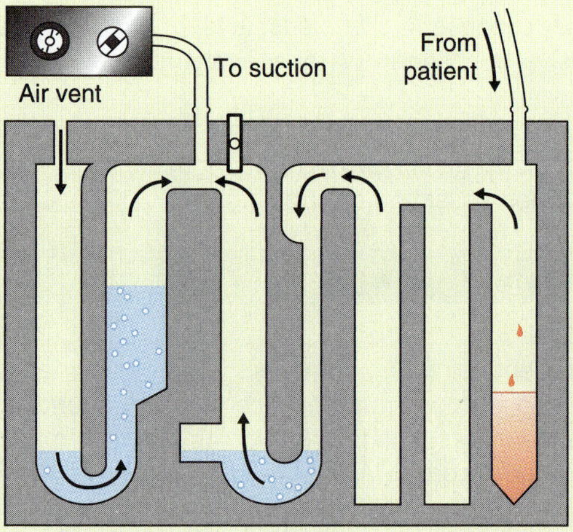

STEP 5c *Left,* Pleur-Evac drainage system, a commercial three-bottle chest drainage device. *Right,* Schematic of drainage device.

TABLE 30-11 EMERGENCY CARE WITH CHEST TUBES

ASSESSMENT	INTERVENTION
1. Air leak: can occur at insertion site, at connection between tube and drainage, or within drainage device itself. Continuous bubbling occurs in water-seal chamber and water seal.	Locate leak by clamping tube at different intervals along the tube. Leaks are corrected when constant bubbling stops. Unclamp tube, reinforce chest dressing, and notify health care provider immediately. Leaving chest tube clamped may cause collapse of lung, mediastinal shift, and eventual collapse of other lung from buildup of air pressure within the pleural cavity. If a leak is found in the drainage device, change it. Use adhesive tape at all connections.
2. Break in chest drainage device	Place the end of the chest tube in a bottle of sterile saline. Notify the health care provider immediately and change the drainage device according to manufacturer instructions.
3. Chest tube dislodgment	Apply pressure to chest tube site wound using petroleum gauze, a dry gauze dressing, and adhesive tape. Notify health care provider immediately and obtain a STAT order for a chest x-ray film examination. Prepare for health care provider to insert another chest tube.
4. Tension pneumothorax Signs and symptoms include: • Severe respiratory distress • Low oxygen saturation • Chest pain • Absence of breath sounds on affected side • Tracheal shift to unaffected side • Tachycardia	Assess chest tube for any clamping or kinking of the tubing. Notify the health care provider immediately and obtain a STAT order for a chest x-ray examination. Prepare for health care provider to insert another chest tube. Have emergency equipment in patient's room to prepare for resuscitation if needed.
5. Drainage suddenly stops	Assess chest tube for any clamping or kinking of the tubing. Notify health care provider immediately and obtain an order to gently milk the chest tube to reestablish chest drainage.

STEP	RATIONALE
c. To assess if patient is ready to have chest tube removed (which is done by health care provider's order); monitor patient for recurrent pneumothorax (see illustration).	
2. Position patient.	Permits optimal drainage of fluid and/or air.
a. Semi-Fowler's position to evacuate air (pneumothorax).	Air rises to highest point in chest. Pneumothorax tubes are usually placed on anterior aspect at midclavicular line, second or third intercostal space.
b. High-Fowler's position to drain fluid (hemothorax).	Permits optimal drainage of fluid. Posterior tubes are placed on midaxillary line, eighth or ninth intercostal space.
IMPLEMENTATION	
1. Perform hand hygiene and ensure that tube connection between chest and drainage tube is intact and taped.	Secures chest tube to drainage system and reduces risk for air leak causing breaks in airtight system.
a. Make sure that water-seal vent is not occluded.	Permits displaced air to pass into atmosphere.
b. Make sure that suction control chamber vent is not occluded when using suction. Waterless systems have relief valves without caps.	Provides safety factor of releasing excess negative pressure into atmosphere.
2. Coil excess tubing on mattress next to patient. Secure with rubber band, safety pin, or plastic clamp.	Prevents excess tubing from hanging over edge of mattress in dependent loop. It is possible for drainage to collect in loop and occlude drainage system (Centre for Reviews and Dissemination, 2008).
3. Adjust tubing to hang in straight line from top of mattress to drainage chamber.	Promotes drainage and prevents fluid or blood from accumulating in pleural cavity.
4. If chest tube is draining fluid, indicate time (e.g., 0900) that you began drainage on adhesive tape on drainage bottle or on write-on surface of disposable commercial system.	Provides baseline for continuous assessment of type and quality of drainage.
5. Perform hand hygiene.	Reduces transmission of microorganisms.
EVALUATION	
1. Monitor vital signs, breath sounds, and pulse oximetry as ordered. Inspect chest wall movement and note skin and mucous membrane color.	Provides ongoing data regarding change in respiratory status and level of oxygenation. Increase in respiratory distress, decrease in breath sounds, marked cyanosis, asymmetrical chest wall movements, presence of subcutaneous emphysema around insertion site or neck, hypotension, tachycardia, and/or mediastinal shift are critical and indicate a severe change in patient status such as excessive blood loss or tension pneumothorax. Notify health care provider immediately.
2. Observe:	
a. Chest tube dressing. Check dressing carefully; it can come loose from skin, although this is not always readily apparent.	Appearance of drainage is sometimes caused by an occluded tube, causing drainage to exit around tube.

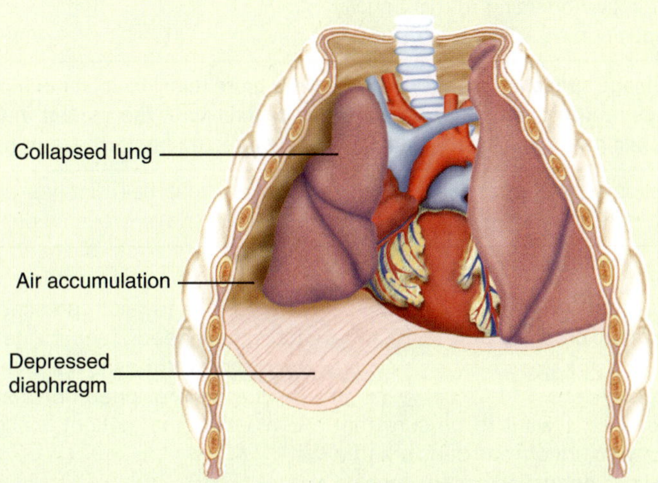

STEP 1c Pneumothorax. (From Seidel HM, et al: *Mosby's guide to physical examination*, ed 7, St Louis, 2011, Mosby.)

SKILL 30-2 CARE OF PATIENTS WITH CHEST TUBES—cont'd

STEP	RATIONALE
b. Tubing to be sure it is free of kinks and dependent loops.	Straight and coiled drainage tube positions are optimal for pleural drainage. However, when dependent loop is unavoidable, periodic lifting and draining of tube also promotes pleural drainage.
c. Chest drainage system to be sure it is upright and below level of tube insertion. Note presence of clots or debris in tubing. Monitor position of system relative to chest tube carefully, especially during patient transport.	Ensures that system is in position to function.
d. Water seal for fluctuations with patient's inspiration and expiration.	Water seal provides important diagnostic information about condition of patient's lung. If patient is breathing spontaneously, intrapleural pressure becomes more negative on inspiration and the water level will rise. During exhalation, the water level should return to baseline.
(1) Waterless system: Diagnostic indicator for fluctuations with patient's inspirations and expirations.	In the nonmechanically ventilated patient fluid rises in the water-seal chamber or diagnostic indicator with inspiration and falls with expiration. The opposite occurs in the patient who is mechanically ventilated. This indicates that system is functioning properly.
(2) Water-seal system: Bubbling in water-seal chamber.	When you initially connect system to patient, expect bubbles from chamber. These are from air that was present in system and in patient's intrapleural space. In many cases the bubbling stops after a short time. Fluid continues to fluctuate in water-seal chamber on inspiration and expiration until lung reexpands or system becomes occluded.
(3) Water-seal system: Bubbling is in suction control chamber (when suction is being used).	Suction control chamber has constant gentle bubbling. Tubing should be free of obstruction, and suction source should be turned to appropriate setting.
e. Type and amount of fluid drainage: Note color and amount of drainage. Be aware of what is normal amount of drainage for patient's condition:	Character of drainage reveals if condition is improving or if infection or hemorrhage is developing.
(1) In adult less than 100 mL/hr immediately after surgery in mediastinal chest tube; approximately 500 mL in the first 24 hours.	Dark-red drainage is normal only in postoperative period, turning serous with time.
(2) Between 100 and 300 mL of fluid drains in a pleural chest tube in an adult during the first 3 hours after insertion. This rate decreases after 2 hours; expect 500 to 1000 mL in first 24 hours. Drainage is grossly bloody during first several hours after surgery and then changes to serous. Sudden gush of drainage is often retained blood and not active bleeding and is usually the result of patient repositioning.	Reexpansion of lungs forces drainage into tube. Coughing also causes large gushes of drainage or air. Report excessive amounts and/or continued presence of frank bloody drainage the first several hours after surgery to health care provider, along with patient's vital signs and respiratory status.

Clinical Decision Point: **If drainage suddenly increases or if there is more than 100 mL/hr of bloody drainage (except for the first 3 hours after surgery), inform the health care provider and remain with the patient and assess vital signs, oxygen saturation by pulse oximetry, and cardiopulmonary status. This may indicate hemorrhage or perforation of the lung.**

STEP	RATIONALE
f. Waterless system: The suction control (float ball) indicates the amount of suction that patient's intrapleural space is receiving.	Suction float ball dictates amount of suction in system. It allows no more suction than dictated by its setting. If suction source is set too low, suction float ball cannot reach prescribed setting. In this case increase suction for float ball to reach prescribed setting.
3. Ask patient to rate level of comfort on scale of 0 to 10.	Indicates need for analgesia. Patient with chest tube discomfort hesitates to take deep breaths and as a result is at risk for pneumonia and atelectasis.
4. Use Teach Back—State to patient, "I want to be sure that you understand why I want you to sit upright and deep breathe and cough every hour." Revise your instruction now or develop plan for revised patient teaching to be implemented at an appropriate time if patient is not able to teach back correctly.	Evaluates what patient is able to explain or demonstrate.

RECORDING AND REPORTING

- Record and report patency of chest tubes; presence, type, and amount of drainage; presence of fluctuations; patient's vital signs; chest dressing status; amount of suction and/or water seal; patient's level of comfort.
- Record patients understanding of positioning and need to cough while the chest tube is in place.
- Document your evaluation of patient learning.

UNEXPECTED OUTCOMES AND RELATED INTERVENTIONS

- Air leak unrelated to patient respirations
  - Locate source (see Table 30-11).
  - Notify health care provider.
  - Drain tubing contents into drainage bottle. Coil excess tubing on mattress and secure in place or place in straight line down length of bed.
- Tension pneumothorax present
  - Determine that chest tubes are not clamped, kinked, or occluded. Obstructed chest tubes trap air in intrapleural space when air leak originates within patient.
  - Notify health care provider immediately.
  - Prepare immediately for another chest tube insertion. Obtain a flutter (Heimlich) valve or large-gauge needles for short-term emergency release of air in intrapleural space. Have emergency equipment (e.g., oxygen, code cart) near patient.
- Continuous bubbling in water-seal chamber, indicating that leak is between patient and water seal
  - Tighten loose connections between patient and water-seal system.
  - Cross-clamp chest tube closest to patient's chest. If bubbling stops, air leak is inside patient's thorax or at chest tube insertion site. Unclamp tube and notify health care provider immediately. Reinforce chest dressing. Leaving chest tube clamped causes tension pneumothorax and mediastinal shift.
  - Gradually move clamps down drainage tubing away from patient and toward drainage chamber, moving one clamp at a time. When bubbling stops, leak is in section of tubing or connection distal to clamp. Replace tubing or secure connections and release clamp.

KEY POINTS

- The primary functions of the heart are to deliver oxygenated blood and nutrients to the tissues in exchange for deoxygenated blood and to deliver deoxygenated blood to the lungs for oxygenation.
- Cardiac dysrhythmias are classified by cardiac activity and site of impulse origin.
- The primary functions of the lung are to transfer oxygen from the atmosphere into the alveoli and carbon dioxide out of the body as a waste product.
- Ventilation is the process of providing adequate oxygenation from the alveoli to the blood.
- The process of inspiration and expiration is achieved with changes in lung pressures and volumes.
- Respiration is controlled by the CNS and chemicals within the blood.
- Decreased hemoglobin levels alter a patient's ability to transport oxygen.
- Hypoventilation causes carbon dioxide retention.
- Hypoxia occurs if the amount of oxygen delivered to tissues is too low.
- The nursing assessment includes data about a patient's respiratory symptoms, environmental exposures, respiratory and cardiopulmonary risk factors, use of medications, and physical functioning.
- Breathing exercises improve ventilation, oxygenation, and sensations of dyspnea.
- Chest physiotherapy includes postural drainage, percussion, and vibration to mobilize pulmonary secretions.
- Coughing and suctioning techniques help to maintain a patent airway.
- Oxygen therapy improves levels of tissue oxygenation and is delivered by nasal cannula, nasal catheter, or oxygen mask.

CLINICAL DECISION-MAKING EXERCISES

Mr. King, a 62-year-old salesman with a history of COPD, is readmitted during the night shift. He was discharged 5 days ago. He has increased shortness of breath, fever, nonproductive cough, nausea, and malaise. You are assigned to care for Mr. King on the day shift. You receive report from the night registered nurse (RN) who provides the following information: vital signs include the following: blood pressure, 152/90 mm Hg; pulse, 102 beats/min; respiratory rate, 28 breaths/min; temperature, 102.8° F; SpO_2, 78%. During your rounds you assess Mr. King and observe that his breathing is labored and he is using the accessory muscles of respiration. His lungs have bibasilar *crackles and diminished breath sounds. He is complaining of increasing shortness of breath and right-sided chest pain and is diaphoretic.*

1. List two nursing assessments that you would perform immediately. Explain why.
2. What do the lungs sounds indicate?

The health care provider arrives at the patient's bedside. The patient's vital signs include the following: blood pressure, 152/90 mm Hg; pulse, 102 beats/min; respiratory rate, 28 breaths/min; temperature, 102.8° F; SpO_2, 78%. The health care provider orders a Venturi mask at 8 L/min to titrate to 92%, arterial blood gas determination, and a chest x-ray film examination.

3. What preparations do you make in anticipation of acute respiratory failure? List possible nursing interventions.

evolve

Answers to Clinical Decision-Making Exercises can be found on the Evolve website.

QSEN ACTIVITY: TEAMWORK AND COLLABORATION

You are collaborating with the admitting night nurse before taking over Mr. King's care.

What additional information do you need to receive from the night nurse when assuming his care? Explain why.

evolve

Answers to QSEN Activities can be found on the Evolve website.

REVIEW QUESTIONS

1. The difference between hypoxia and hypoxemia is:
   1. Hypoxemia is a low oxygen level at the cell.
   2. Hypoxia is a low oxygen level in the blood.
   3. Hypoxia is inadequate oxygen at the cellular level.
   4. Hypoxemia and hypoxia are the same concept.
2. A nurse is caring for a patient in respiratory distress. Which of the following is included in the assessment? (Select all that apply.)
   1. Use of accessory muscles of respiration
   2. Respiratory rate
   3. Alignment of clavicles
   4. Pulse oximetry
   5. Ability to converse
3. The normal electrical pathway of the heart is:
   1. AV node–SA node–ventricles.
   2. SA node–AV node–bundle of His–Purkinje fibers–ventricles.
   3. SA node–atria–AV node–bundle of His–Purkinje fibers–ventricles.
   4. SA node–AV node–Purkinje fibers–bundle of His–ventricles.
4. The most effective breathing techniques for a patient with COPD include:
   1. Orthopneic position.
   2. Pursed lip breathing.
   3. Diaphragmatic breathing.
   4. All of the above.
5. Afterload is defined as:
   1. The resistance of the ejection of blood from the left ventricle.
   2. The amount of blood ejected from the left ventricle each minute.
   3. Heart rate times stroke volume.
   4. The amount of blood at the end of ventricular diastole.
6. Which of the following characteristics are associated with ventilator-associated pneumonia (VAP)?
   1. Purulent secretions before intubation
   2. Fever and leukocytosis before intubation
   3. Clearing infiltrates on the chest radiograph 24 hours after initiation of mechanical ventilation
   4. Fever and progressive infiltrates on the chest radiograph 3 days after initiation of mechanical ventilation
7. Which of the following findings are consistent with an increased risk of developing ventilator-associated pneumonia (VAP)?
   1. An increased gag reflex
   2. Pooling of secretions in the oropharynx
   3. Increased force of cough
   4. Increased mucociliary clearance of secretions
8. Ventilator-associated pneumonia (VAP) is associated with colonization of the:
   1. Digestive system.
   2. Respiratory system.
   3. Respiratory and digestive systems.
   4. Upper airway and stomach.
9. The current compression rate for cardiopulmonary resuscitation (CPR) is at least:
   1. 100 beats/min.
   2. 75 beats/min.
   3. 80 to 100 beats/min.
   4. 60 beats/min.
10. Preload is:
    1. The same as the blood pressure.
    2. The amount of blood that is pumped from the right ventricle.
    3. The product of the heart rate and the stroke volume.
    4. The amount of blood at the end of ventricular diastole, or measured as end-diastolic pressure.

evolve

Rationales for Review Questions can be found on the Evolve website.

1. 3; 2. 1, 2, 4, 5; 3. 3; 4. 2; 5. 1; 6. 4; 7. 2; 8. 3; 9. 1; 10. 4

REFERENCES

Amanullah S, et al: *Ventilator-associated pneumonia overview of nosocomial pneumonias*, 2013, http://emedicine.medscape.com/article/304836-overview. Accessed February 15, 2014.

American Association of Respiratory Care (AARC): AARC clinical practice guideline: nasotracheal suction—2004 revision and update, *Respir Care* 49:1080, 2004.

American Association of Respiratory Care (AARC): AARC clinical practice guideline: oxygen therapy in the home or alternate site health care facility—2007 revision and update, *Respir Care* 52(1):1063, 2007.

American Association for Respiratory Care (AARC): AARC clinical practice guideline: endotracheal suctioning of mechanically ventilated patients with artificial airways, *Respir Care* 55(6):758, 2010.

American Heart Association: *Sudden cardiac arrest*, 2013, http://www.heart.org/idc/groups/heart-public/@wcm/@adv/documents/downloadable/ucm_301793.pdf. Accessed February 18, 2014.

American Thoracic Society: *Home oxygen therapy: appropriate candidates for long-term oxygen therapy*, 2013, available at http://www.thoracic.org/clinical/copd-guidelines../for-health-professionals/management-of-stable-copd/long-term-oxygen-therapy/home-oxygen-therapy.php. Accessed November 1, 2013.

Augustyn B: Ventilator-associated pneumonia: risk factors and prevention, *Crit Care Nurse* 27(4):32, 2007.

Centers for Disease Control and Prevention (CDC): *Heart disease risk factors*, 2012a, http://www.cdc.gov/HeartDisease/risk_factors.htm. Accessed June 26, 2013.

Centers for Disease Control and Prevention (CDC): *Respiratory syncytial virus*, 2012b, http://www.cdc.gov/rsv/. Accessed June 26, 2013.

Centers for Disease Control and Prevention (CDC): *2013-2014 Flu season*, 2013, http://www.cdc.gov/flu/about/season/upcoming.htm. Accessed February 15, 2014.

Centre for Reviews and Dissemination: The nursing management of chest drains: a systematic review, *Joanna Briggs Institute for Evidence-Based Nurs Midwifery* 3:5, 2008.

Institute for Health Care Improvement (IHCI): *Implement the IHI ventilator bundle*, 2012, http://www.ihi.org/knowledge/Pages/Changes/ImplementtheVentilatorBundle.aspx. Accessed June 26, 2013.

James PA, et al: 2014 evidence-based guideline for the management of high blood pressure in adults, report from the Panel members appointed to the eighth Joint National Committee (JNC8), *JAMA* 311(5):507, 2014.

Lacherade JC, et al: Intermittent subglottic secretion drainage and ventilator-associated pneumonia: a multicenter trial, *Am J Respir Crit Care Med* 182(7):910, 2010.

Lewis SM, et al: *Medical surgical nursing: assessment and management of clinical problems*, ed 8, St Louis, 2010, Mosby.

Medline Plus, US National Library of Medicine, National Institutes of Health: *Oxygen safety*, 2012, www.nlm.nih.gov/medlineplus/ency/patientinstructions/000049.htm. Accessed November 1, 2013.

Morrow LE, Kollef MH, Casale TB: Probiotic prophylaxis of ventilator-associated pneumonia: a blinded, randomized, controlled trial, *Am J Respir Crit Care Med* 182(8):1058, 2010.

National Center for Immunization and Respiratory Diseases: General recommendations on immunization: recommendations of the Advisory Committee on Immunization Practices (ACIP), *MMWR* 60(2):1, 2011.

Peberdy MA, et al: Part 9: post-cardiac arrest care: 2010 American Heart Association guidelines for cardiopulmonary resuscitation and emergency cardiovascular care, *Circulation* 122(18 Suppl 3):S768, 2010.

Pedersen CM, et al: Endotracheal suctioning of the adult intubated patient—what is the evidence? *Intensive Crit Care Nurs* 25(1):21–30, 2009.

Sedwick MB, et al: Using evidence-based practice to prevent ventilator-associated pneumonia, *Crit Care Nurse* 32(4):41, 2012.

Seidel HM, et al: *Mosby's guide to physical examination*, ed 7, St Louis, 2011, Mosby.

Siempos II, et al: Impact of the administration of probiotics on the incidence of ventilator-associated pneumonia: a meta-analysis of randomized controlled trials, *Crit Care Med* 38(3):954, 2010.

Staudinger T, et al: Continuous lateral rotation therapy to prevent ventilator-associated pneumonia, *Crit Care Med* 38(2):486, 2010.

The Joint Commission (TJC): *National Patient Safety Goals*, Oakbrook Terrace, IL, 2014, The Commission. Available at http://www.jointcommission.org/standards_information/npsgs.aspx.

Thibodeau GA, Patton KT: *Structure and function of the body*, ed 14, St Louis, 2011, Mosby.

US Department of Health and Human Services: *Your guide to lowering your blood pressure with DASH*, NIH publication No 06-4082, 2006, www.nhlbi.nih.gov/health/public/heart/hbp/dash/new_dash.pdf. Accessed November 1, 2013.

CHAPTER

31

Sleep

evolve WEBSITE

http://evolve.elsevier.com/Potter/essentials

- Crossword Puzzle
- Audio Glossary

OBJECTIVES

- Explain the effect the 24-hour sleep-wake cycle has on biological function.
- Discuss mechanisms that regulate sleep.
- Describe the normal stages of sleep.
- Explain the functions of sleep.
- Compare and contrast the characteristics of sleep for different age-groups.
- Identify factors that promote or disrupt sleep.
- Discuss characteristics of common sleep disorders.
- Conduct a sleep history.
- Describe interventions appropriate to promoting sleep for patients with various sleep disorders.
- Discuss differences in sleep interventions for patients of different age-groups.
- Describe ways to evaluate the effectiveness of sleep therapies.

KEY TERMS

biological clock, p. 847
cataplexy, p. 854
circadian rhythm, p. 847
excessive daytime sleepiness (EDS), p. 849
hypnotics, p. 863
insomnia, p. 852
melatonin, p. 863
narcolepsy, p. 854
nocturia, p. 851
nonrapid eye movement (NREM) sleep, p. 847
rapid eye movement (REM) sleep, p. 847
sedatives, p. 863
sleep, p. 849
sleep apnea, p. 852
sleep deprivation, p. 854

Physical and emotional health depend on adequate rest and sleep. Without proper amounts of rest and sleep, a person's ability to concentrate, make judgments, promote healing, and participate in daily activities decreases. To help a patient gain needed rest and sleep, you need to understand the nature of sleep, the factors influencing it, and the patient's sleep habits. Nurses care for patients who often have preexisting sleep disturbances and who develop sleep problems as a result of illness or being in the health care environment. You learn to use an individualized approach based on patients' personal sleep habits and patterns of sleep to provide effective sleep therapies.

SCIENTIFIC KNOWLEDGE BASE

Physiology of Sleep

Sleep is a cyclical physiological process that alternates with longer periods of wakefulness. The sleep-wake cycle influences and regulates body functions and behavioral responses.

CASE STUDY *Walter Murphy*

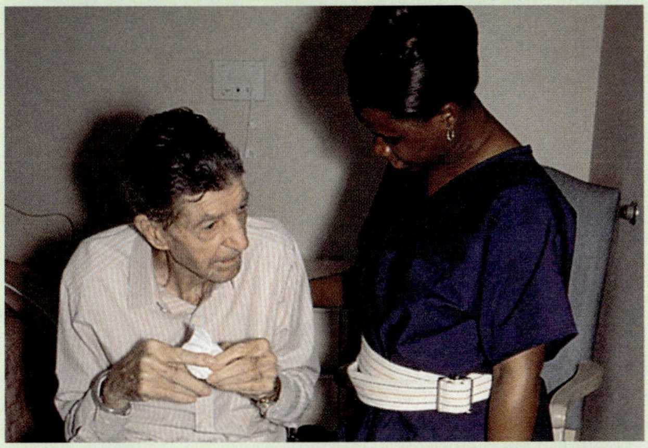

Walter Murphy is 82 years old and has resided in the local nursing home for the last 3 months. His wife, Mary, still lives at home but visits Mr. Murphy on a daily basis. Mr. Murphy is confined to a wheelchair as a result of osteoarthritis and a mild stroke he experienced 1 year ago. Even though he has physical limitations, he is alert and oriented. Over the last several weeks, Mary found her husband to be very sleepy when visiting him just before lunchtime. Mr. Murphy tells Mary that he has trouble falling asleep at night, and once he does fall asleep, he reawakens frequently during the night. Mary is concerned because her husband does not seem as alert or interested during her visit.

Anna is a 23-year-old nursing student assigned to the nursing home for her second semester in nursing school. She has had experience in nursing homes, having worked in one center as a nurse assistant during the last two summers. Anna's assignment is to care for Mr. Murphy over the next 4 weeks.

Circadian Rhythms. People experience cyclical rhythms as part of their everyday life. The most familiar rhythm is the 24-hour, day-night cycle known as the diurnal or **circadian rhythm.** The suprachiasmatic nucleus (SCN) nerve cells in the hypothalamus control the rhythm of the sleep-wake cycle and coordinate this cycle with other circadian rhythms (McCance et al., 2010). Circadian rhythms influence the 24-hour pattern of major biological and behavioral functions such as the predictable changing of body temperature, heart rate, blood pressure, hormone secretion, sensory acuity, and mood (Van der Zee et al., 2009).

Light and temperature affect all circadian rhythms, including the sleep-wake cycle. External factors such as social activities and environmental stressors also affect circadian rhythms. Every person has a **biological clock** that is normally synchronized by exposure to light and activity. This explains why some people fall asleep at 8 PM, whereas others go to bed at midnight or early in the morning. Different people also function best at different times of the day.

Hospitals or extended care facilities usually do not adapt care to an individual's sleep-wake cycle preferences. Typical hospital routines involve nurses needing to interrupt patients' sleep to assess their status or administer treatments. Poor quality of sleep results when a person's sleep-wake cycle changes. Reversals in the sleep-wake cycle such as when a person who is normally awake during the day falls asleep during the day often indicate a serious illness.

The normal sleep rhythm is synchronized with other body functions. For example, changes in temperature correlate with sleep patterns. When the sleep-wake cycle becomes disrupted (e.g., by working rotating shifts), other physiological functions change as well. For example, a new nurse who starts working the night shift experiences a decreased appetite and loses weight. Anxiety, restlessness, irritability, and impaired judgment are other common symptoms of sleep cycle disturbances. Failure to maintain an individual's usual sleep-wake cycle negatively influences his or her overall health.

Sleep Regulation. Sleep involves a series of physiological states maintained by highly integrated central nervous system (CNS) activity that is associated with changes in the peripheral nervous, endocrine, cardiovascular, respiratory, and muscular systems (McCance et al., 2010). Specific physiological responses and patterns of brain activity identify each sequence. Instruments such as the electroencephalogram (EEG), which measures electrical activity in the cerebral cortex; the electromyogram (EMG), which measures muscle tone; and the electrooculogram (EOG), which measures eye movements provide information about some structural physiological aspects of sleep.

The major sleep center in the body is the hypothalamus. Hypocretins (a form of peptide) secreted by the hypothalamus promote wakefulness and rapid eye movement (REM) sleep. Prostaglandin D_2, L-tryptophan, and growth factors control sleep (McCance et al., 2010).

Researchers believe that the ascending reticular activating system (RAS) located in the upper brainstem contains special cells that maintain alertness and wakefulness. The RAS receives visual, auditory, pain, and tactile sensory stimuli. Activity from the cerebral cortex (e.g., emotions or thought processes) also stimulates the RAS. Arousal, wakefulness, and maintenance of consciousness result from neurons in the RAS releasing catecholamines such as norepinephrine (Izac, 2006).

The homeostatic process (Process S), which primarily regulates the length and depth of sleep; and the circadian rhythms (Process C: "biological time clocks"), which influence the internal organization of sleep and timing and duration of sleep-wake cycles, operate simultaneously to regulate sleep and wakefulness (Daroff et al., 2012). Time of wake up is defined by the intersection of Process S and Process C (Figure 31-1).

Stages of Sleep. Normal sleep involves two phases: **nonrapid eye movement (NREM) sleep** and **rapid eye movement (REM) sleep** (Box 31-1). During NREM sleep an individual progresses through four stages during a typical 90-minute sleep cycle. The quality of sleep from stage 1 through stage 4 becomes increasingly deep. Lighter sleep is characteristic of stages 1 and 2, when a person is more easily arousable. Stages 3 and 4 involve a deeper sleep called

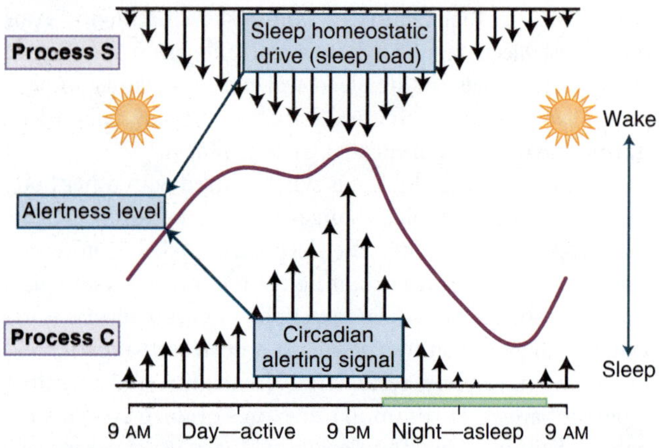

FIGURE 31-1 Two-process model of sleep regulation shows the time course of the homeostatic process *(Process S)* and the circadian process *(Process C)*. Process S rises during waking and declines during sleep. The intersection of Process S and Process C defines the time of wake-up. (From Daroff RB, et al: *Bradley's neurology in clinical practice,* ed 6, Philadelphia, 2012, Saunders.)

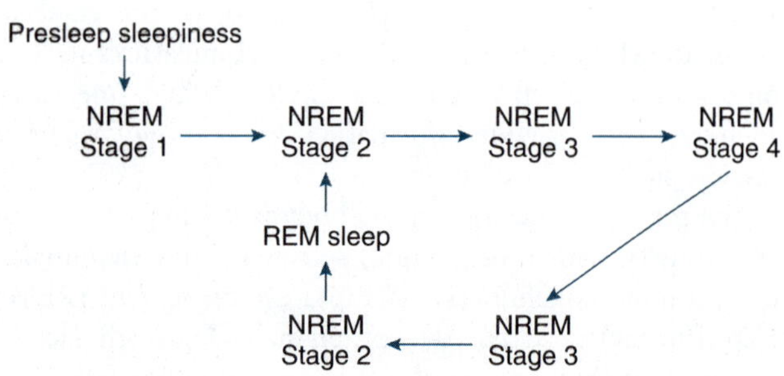

FIGURE 31-2 The stages of the adult sleep cycle.

BOX 31-1 STAGES OF THE SLEEP CYCLE

NREM STAGE 1

- Stage includes lightest level of sleep.
- Stage lasts a few minutes.
- Decreased physiological activity begins with gradual fall in vital signs and metabolism.
- Sensory stimuli such as noise easily arouse sleeper.
- If awakened, person feels as though daydreaming has occurred.

NREM STAGE 2

- Stage is period of sound sleep.
- Relaxation progresses.
- Arousal is still relatively easy.
- Stage lasts 10 to 20 minutes.
- Body functions continue to slow.

NREM STAGE 3

- It involves initial stages of deep sleep.
- Sleeper is difficult to arouse and rarely moves.
- Muscles are completely relaxed.
- Vital signs decline but remain regular.
- Stage lasts 15 to 30 minutes.

NREM STAGE 4

- It is deepest stage of sleep.
- It is very difficult to arouse sleeper.
- If sleep loss has occurred, sleeper spends considerable part of night in this stage.
- Vital signs are significantly lower than during waking hours.
- Stage lasts approximately 15 to 30 minutes.
- Sleepwalking and enuresis sometimes occur.

REM SLEEP

- Vivid, full-color dreaming occurs.
- Stage usually begins about 90 minutes after sleep has begun.
- Stage is typified by autonomic response of rapidly moving eyes, fluctuating heart and respiratory rates, and increased or fluctuating blood pressure.
- Loss of skeletal muscle tone occurs.
- Gastric secretions increase.
- It is very difficult to arouse sleeper.
- Duration of REM sleep increases with each cycle and averages 20 minutes.

NREM, Nonrapid eye movement; *REM,* rapid eye movement.

slow-wave sleep from which a person is more difficult to arouse. REM sleep is the phase at the end of each 90-minute sleep cycle. During REM sleep there is increased brain activity associated with rapid eye movements and muscle atonia. REM sleep is a phase at the end of each sleep cycle.

Sleep Cycle. Normally an adult's routine sleep pattern begins with a presleep period during which the person is aware only of a gradually developing sleepiness. This period normally lasts 10 to 30 minutes. Individuals experiencing difficulty falling asleep often remain in this stage for an hour or more.

Once asleep the person usually passes through four to six complete sleep cycles, each consisting of four stages of NREM sleep and a period of REM sleep. Each cycle lasts approximately 90 to 110 minutes (Chokroverty, 2010). The cyclical pattern usually progresses from stage 1 through stage 4 of NREM sleep, followed by a reversal from stage 4 to 3 to 2, ending with a period of REM sleep (Figure 31-2).

With each successive cycle, stages 3 and 4 of NREM sleep shorten, and the period of REM lengthens. REM sleep lasts up to 60 minutes during the last sleep cycle. Not all people progress consistently through the usual stages of sleep. For example, a sleeper fluctuates back and forth for short intervals between NREM stages 2, 3, and 4 before entering REM sleep. The amount of time spent in each stage varies. The number of sleep cycles depends on the total amount of time that the person spends sleeping.

Functions of Sleep

The primary function of sleep is unknown (Gilsenan, 2012). One theory suggests that it is a time of restoration and preparation for the next period of wakefulness (McCance et al., 2010). During NREM sleep biological functions slow. A healthy adult's normal heart rate throughout the day averages 70 to 80 beats/min. However, during sleep the heart rate normally falls to 60 beats/min or less, thus preserving cardiac function. Other biological functions that decrease during sleep are respirations, blood pressure, and muscle tone (McCance, et al., 2010).

Sleep allows the body to restore biological processes. During deep slow-wave (NREM stage 4) sleep, the body releases human growth hormone for the repair and renewal of epithelial and specialized cells such as brain cells (McCance et al., 2010). Protein synthesis and cell division for the renewal of tissues also occur during rest and sleep. The basal metabolic rate lowers during sleep, which conserves the energy supply of the body (Izac, 2006).

REM sleep appears to be important for early brain development, cognition, and memory (Hobson, 2009). Researchers associate REM sleep with changes in the brain, including cerebral blood flow and increased cortical activity. In addition, there is increased oxygen consumption and epinephrine release. These changes are associated with memory storage and learning (McCance et al., 2010).

The benefits of sleep often go unnoticed until a person develops a problem resulting from sleep deprivation. Sleep deprivation affects immune function, metabolism, nitrogen balance, protein catabolism, and quality of life. A loss of REM sleep often leads to confusion and suspicion. Prolonged sleep loss alters various body functions (e.g., mood, motor performance, memory, and equilibrium) (National Sleep Foundation, 2010). The annual direct cost of sleep-related problems in this country is 16 billion dollars. An additional 50 to 100 billion dollars are spent on indirect costs related to accidents, litigation, property damage, hospitalization, and death (University of Maryland Medical Center Sleep Disorders Center, 2013).

Dreams. The dreams of REM sleep are more vivid and elaborate than those of NREM sleep; and researchers believe them to be functionally important to learning, memory processing, and adaptation to stress (Kryger et al., 2011). REM dreams progress in content throughout the night from dreams about current events to emotional dreams of childhood or the past. Personality influences the quality of dreams (e.g., a creative person may have very vivid, unusual dreams; whereas a depressed person may have dreams of helplessness).

Dreams help people sort out immediate concerns or erase certain fantasies or nonsensical memories. Because most dreams are forgotten, many people have little dream recall and do not believe they dream at all. To remember a dream a person must consciously think about it on awakening. People who recall dreams vividly usually awaken just after a period of REM sleep.

NURSING KNOWLEDGE BASE

Sleep and Rest

When people are at rest, they usually feel mentally relaxed, free from anxiety, and physically calm. Rest does not imply inactivity, although everyone often thinks of it as settling down in a comfortable chair or taking a brief nap.

Sleep is a recurrent, altered state of consciousness that occurs for sustained periods. When people get proper sleep, they feel that their energy has been restored. Sleep provides time for the repair and recovery of body systems for the next period of wakefulness. Adequate quality and quantity of sleep contribute to optimum health.

Normal Sleep Requirements and Patterns

Neonates. Sleep duration and quality vary among people of all age-groups. The neonate and infant up to the age of 3 months average about 16 hours of sleep a day. Approximately 50% of this sleep is REM sleep, which stimulates the higher brain centers (Hockenberry and Wilson, 2011).

Infants. Infants usually develop a nighttime pattern of sleep by 3 months of age. They sometimes take several naps during the day but usually sleep an average of 9 to 11 hours during the night. Infants spend about 30% of sleep time in the REM cycle. Awakening commonly occurs early in the morning, although infants sometimes awaken during the night.

Toddlers and Preschoolers. By the age of 2 years children usually sleep through the night and take daily naps. Total sleep averages 12 hours a day. Some children stop taking naps altogether at age 3. It is common for toddlers to awaken during the night. The percentage of REM sleep continues to fall. Toddlers are often unwilling to go to bed at night. A preschooler sleeps an average of 12 hours a night (about 20% is REM). By the age of 5 the preschooler rarely takes daytime naps (Hockenberry and Wilson, 2011), except in cultures in which a siesta is the custom. The preschooler usually has difficulty relaxing or quieting down after long, active days and often has problems with bedtime fears, waking during the night, and nightmares.

School-Age Children. The school-age child usually does not require a nap. A 6-year-old averages 11 to 12 hours of sleep nightly, whereas an 11-year-old sleeps about 9 to 10 hours (Hockenberry and Wilson, 2011). Encouraging quiet activities usually persuades the 6- or 7-year-old to go to bed. The older child often resists sleeping because of an unawareness of fatigue or a need to be independent.

Adolescents. Adolescents need between 8½ and 9½ hours of sleep each night; however, the typical teenager gets about 7½ hours of sleep per night. At a time when sleep needs actually increase, the typical adolescent is subject to a number of changes that often reduce the time spent sleeping such as the time when school starts, after-school social events, part-time jobs, and extracurricular activities. The shortened sleep time in adolescents often results in excessive daytime sleepiness (EDS), which can reduce performance in school, increase risk of accidents, increase the use of alcohol, and lead to behavior and mood problems (Noland et al., 2009; Vallido et al., 2009). The prevalence rate of EDS (37.7%) is higher for adolescents who are addicted to using the internet compared with those who are not addicted (Choi et al., 2009).

Young Adults. Most young adults average 6 to 8½ hours of sleep a night, but this varies. Young adults rarely take regular naps. They spend approximately 20% of sleep time in REM sleep, which remains consistent throughout the remainder of life. Healthy young adults require adequate sleep to participate in daily busy activities. However, lifestyle demands and family relationships often lead to insomnia and the use of sleep medication. Pregnancy increases the need for rest and sleep. Common problems during the third trimester of pregnancy include restless legs syndrome (RLS), insomnia, periodic limb movements, and sleep-disordered breathing (Kryger et al., 2011).

Middle Adults. During middle adulthood the total time spent sleeping at night begins to decline. The amount of stage 4 sleep begins to fall, a decline that continues with advancing age. Health care workers often initially diagnose sleep disturbances among people in this age range even when the symptoms of a disorder have been present for several years. Because of stresses experienced in middle age, insomnia is a common occurrence. It is often experienced by menopausal women.

Older Adults. Complaints of sleeping difficulties increase with age. More than 50% of people age 65 and older report regular problems with sleep (Neikrug and Ancoli-Israel, 2010). Older adults spend more time in stage 1 and have less stages 3 and 4 NREM sleep; some older adults have almost no NREM stage 4 or deep sleep. Episodes of REM sleep tend to shorten, and there is less deep sleep and more lighter sleep. Older adults awaken more often during the night, and it takes more time for them to fall asleep. To compensate they increase the number of naps taken during the day.

An estimated 70% of older adults with insomnia have co-morbid psychiatric illness or medical conditions, take medications that disrupt sleep patterns, or use drugs or alcohol (Fiorentino and Martin, 2010). Cognitive therapy is a treatment option.

Factors Affecting Sleep

A number of factors (physical, psychological, and environmental) affect the quantity and quality of sleep. Often more than one factor combines to cause a sleep problem.

Physical Illness. Any illness or condition that causes pain, difficulty breathing, nausea, or mood problems such as anxiety or depression can result in sleep problems (Table 31-1). Individuals with such alterations have trouble falling or staying asleep. Illnesses also sometimes force patients to sleep in positions to which they are unaccustomed. For example, it is difficult for a patient with a leg in traction to rest comfortably.

Sleep-related breathing disorders are linked to increased incidence of nocturnal angina (chest pain), increased heart rate, electrocardiogram changes, high blood pressure, and risk of heart diseases and stroke (McCance et al., 2010). Hypertension often causes early-morning awakening and fatigue. Hypothyroidism decreases stage 4 sleep, whereas hyperthyroidism causes a person to take longer to fall asleep.

TABLE 31-1 ILLNESSES AND CONDITIONS THAT CAN ALTER SLEEP

ILLNESS/CONDITION	NATURE OF SLEEP ALTERATION
Respiratory disease (e.g., emphysema, asthma, bronchitis, allergic rhinitis, common cold)	Shortness of breath requires the use of two to three pillows to raise head and alters rhythm of breathing. Nasal congestion and sore throat impair breathing and ability to relax.
Coronary heart disease with episodes of chest pain and irregular heart rates	Heart disease causes frequent awakenings, sleep stage changes during sleep, and significant alterations in all stages of sleep.
Hypertension	Reduced length and depth of NREM sleep and a shortened REM latency period cause arousals and early morning awakening, resulting in fatigue.
Hypothyroidism	Decreases in slow-wave and REM sleep and increased movements during sleep contribute to daytime sleepiness.
Hyperthyroidism	Increase in metabolism causes insomnia resulting from increased time needed to fall asleep.
Nocturia (reduced bladder tone, diabetes, urethritis, prostate disease)	Waking at night to urinate results in difficulty returning to sleep.
Gastric reflux	Burning pain in lower esophagus or nocturnal coughing increases when lying flat in bed.
Depression	Early morning awakenings with inability to return to sleep are worsened by anxiety or agitation.
Perimenopause	Waking at night is caused by hot flashes and sweating.
Pain	Delay in sleep onset, increased waking from sleep, and decreased slow-wave activity during sleep result in poor sleep quality. Pain is worsened by increased sympathetic activity, resulting in high cardiac heart rate.

NREM, Nonrapid eye movement; *REM,* rapid eye movement.

Nighttime urination **(nocturia)** disrupts sleep and the sleep cycle. It is difficult to return to sleep after repeated awakenings that prevent a complete sleep cycle from occurring. Although this condition is most common in older people with reduced bladder tone or people with cardiac disease, diabetes, urethritis, or prostatic disease, it also affects a significant portion of younger people (Van Kerrebroeck, 2011).

RLS is a neurologic sensorimotor disorder that causes an irresistible urge to move the legs while they are at rest. Symptoms are most severe in the evening and night and can severely disrupt a patient's sleep (National Sleep Foundation, 2013b).

Drugs and Substances. A considerable number of drugs cause sleepiness, insomnia, or fatigue as a side effect (Box 31-2). Medications prescribed for sleep often cause more problems than benefits. L-tryptophan is a natural protein found in foods such as milk, cheese, and meats (e.g., turkey and chicken) and sometimes helps a person sleep. It is a precursor, or forerunner, to the neurotransmitter serotonin, which has a role in the sleep-wake cycle.

Lifestyle. A person's daily routine influences sleep patterns. For example, an individual who alternately works day and night shifts often has difficulty adjusting to the altered sleep schedule. Lifestyle changes that contribute to decreased quantity and quality of sleep include working an increased number of hours or at multiple jobs and spending more time watching television or being on the Internet. Other alterations in routine that disrupt sleep patterns include performing unaccustomed heavy work or exercise, engaging in late-night social activities, and changing evening mealtime. Travel across time zones is a common factor associated with insomnia.

Usual Sleep Patterns and Excessive Daytime Sleepiness. More than half (63%) of Americans need approximately 7½ hours of sleep a night but get only 6 hours and 55 minutes a weeknight (National Sleep Foundation, 2011a). This leads to EDS during the day that often results in impairment of waking function, poor work or school performance, accidents while driving or using equipment, and behavioral or emotional problems. A contributor to this is the use of technology close to bedtime such as watching television, talking or texting on a cell phone, playing video games, and surfing the Internet (National Sleep Foundation, 2011a).

Sleepiness becomes pathological when it occurs at times when people need or want to be awake. People who temporarily experience sleep deprivation as a result of an active social evening or lengthened work schedule usually feel sleepy the next day. However, they are sometimes able to overcome these feelings even though they have difficulty performing tasks and remaining attentive. Chronic lack of sleep is much more serious than temporary sleep deprivation and causes serious alterations in the ability to perform daily activities. EDS is most difficult to overcome during sedentary tasks (e.g., driving).

Emotional Stress. Worry over personal problems or situations interferes with sleep. Emotional stress causes tension and often leads to frustration when sleep does not come. Stress also causes a person to try too hard to fall asleep, to awaken frequently during the sleep cycle, or to

BOX 31-2 EFFECT OF MEDICATIONS AND OTHER SUBSTANCES ON SLEEP

HYPNOTICS
- Interfere with reaching deeper sleep stages
- Provide only temporary (1 week) increase in quantity of sleep
- Sometimes cause "hangover" feeling during day
- In some cases worsen sleep apnea in older adults

DIURETICS (ADMINISTERED LATE IN THE DAY)
- Cause nocturia, which leads to nighttime awakenings

ANTIDEPRESSANTS AND STIMULANTS
- Suppress REM sleep
- Decrease total sleep time

ALCOHOL
- Speeds onset of sleep and disrupts REM sleep
- Awakens person during night and causes difficulty returning to sleep

CAFFEINE
- Stimulant; prevents person from falling asleep
- Causes person to awaken during night

NICOTINE
- Causes decrease in sleep time
- Causes nighttime awakenings
- Causes difficulty staying asleep

BETA-ADRENERGIC BLOCKERS
- Cause nightmares and insomnia
- Cause awakening from sleep

BENZODIAZEPINES
- Increase sleep time
- Increase daytime sleepiness

OPIATES
- Suppress REM sleep
- Cause increased daytime drowsiness

ANTIHISTAMINES
- Cause drowsiness
- Cause insomnia when used in excess

ANTICONVULSANTS
- Decrease REM sleep
- Cause daytime drowsiness

REM, Rapid eye movement.

oversleep. Continued stress causes poor sleep habits in some cases.

Environment. The physical environment in which a person sleeps influences the ability to fall and remain asleep. Proper ventilation, a comfortable temperature, and a darkened or softly lit room are essential for restful sleep. The size, firmness, and position of a bed also affect sleep quality. Hospital beds are often harder than those at home. If a person usually sleeps with another individual, sleeping alone during times of illness causes wakefulness. However, sleeping with a restless or snoring bed partner also disrupts sleep. Noise easily disturbs older adults' sleep because most of their sleep is in lighter sleep stages. It is best for them to avoid using the bed for nonsleep activities such as snacking, watching television, or reading.

Hospitals across the country are evaluated for their quality of care using The Hospital Consumer Assessment of Healthcare Providers and Systems survey, called HCAHPS (Centers for Medicare and Medicaid Services, 2013). The survey measures patients' perspectives on hospital care following discharge. The survey encompasses nine key topics: communication with doctors, communication with nurses, responsiveness of hospital staff, pain management, communication about medicines, discharge information, cleanliness of the hospital environment, transition of care, and quietness of the hospital environment. Noise within hospitals can be a significant source of patient dissatisfaction.

In health care facilities the noise created by caregivers, equipment, and other patients is usually new or strange and causes a problem for them. This problem is greatest the first night a patient stays in a hospital or other facility, and often he or she experiences increased total wake time, increased awakening, and decreased REM sleep and total sleep time. Nursing activities are a source of increased sound levels. The intensive care setting is one of the loudest, where close proximity of patients, noise from confused and ill patients, and ringing of alarm systems and telephones make the environment very disruptive.

Exercise and Fatigue. A person who is moderately fatigued usually achieves restful sleep, especially if the fatigue results from enjoyable work or exercise. Exercise 2 or more hours before bedtime allows time for the body to cool and maintain a state of fatigue that promotes relaxation. On the other hand, excessive fatigue can make falling asleep difficult. It is common in adolescents who stay active with long hours involving school, extracurricular activities, and work.

Food and Caloric Intake. Following good eating habits is important for proper health, including sleep. Eating a large, heavy, and/or spicy meal within 3 to 4 hours of bedtime sometimes results in indigestion that interferes with sleep. Alcohol consumed in the evening has insomnia-producing and diuretic effects. Coffee, tea, cola, and chocolate contain caffeine and xanthines that cause sleeplessness as a result of CNS stimulation.

Weight loss or weight gain influences sleep patterns. Weight gain contributes to obstructive sleep apnea (OSA) because of the increased size of the soft tissue structures in the upper airway (Kryger et al., 2011). Weight loss causes insomnia and decreased amounts of sleep (Ross et al., 2011). Certain sleep disorders are the result of the semi-starvation diets popular in a weight-conscious society.

Sleep Disorders

Sleep disorders are conditions that, if untreated, cause disturbed nighttime sleep that results in the problems of insomnia; movement disorders; sleep-related breathing disorders; or EDS, also known as *hypersomnolence* (Kryger et al., 2011). Many adults in the United States have significant sleep problems from inadequacies in either the quantity or quality of their nighttime sleep and experience hypersomnolence on a daily basis (National Sleep Foundation, 2013c). The American Academy of Sleep Medicine has developed the International Classification of Sleep Disorders version 2 (ICSD-2), which classifies sleep disorders into eight major categories (Box 31-3).

In sleep-related movement disorders the person experiences simple stereotypical movements that disturb sleep. The Isolated Symptoms, Apparently Normal Variants, and Unresolved Issues category includes sleep-related symptoms that fall between normal and abnormal sleep. The Other Sleep Disorders category contains sleep problems that do not fit into other categories.

Insomnia. Insomnia is a symptom rather than the name of a disease and is common among patients suffering from depression (National Sleep Foundation, 2013c). It is experienced by patients who have chronic difficulty falling asleep, frequent awakenings from sleep, and/or a sleep or a nonrestorative sleep (Kryger et al., 2011). Insomnia leads to insufficient quantity and quality of sleep. However, a patient often gets more sleep than he or she realizes. Insomnia sometimes signals an underlying physical or psychological disorder. It is more common in older adults and females.

Often people experience transient or temporary insomnia as a result of situational stresses such as work or family problems. Insomnia sometimes recurs, but between episodes the patient is able to sleep well. However, a temporary case of insomnia caused by a stressful event has the ability to lead to chronic difficulty in getting enough sleep. Insomnia is often associated with poor sleep hygiene, which negates behaviors that promote sleep (Daroff et al., 2012). If the condition continues, the fear of not being able to sleep is enough to cause wakefulness. During the day a person with chronic insomnia feels sleepy, fatigued, depressed, and anxious. It is important to treat underlying emotional or medical problems that cause the insomnia.

Sleep Apnea. Sleep apnea is a disorder in which the individual is unable to breathe and sleep at the same time. There is a lack of airflow through the nose and mouth for periods from 10 seconds to 1 to 2 minutes in length. There are three types of sleep apnea: obstructive; central; and mixed apnea, which has both an obstructive and a central component.

The most common form is OSA, which is a cessation or stopping of airflow despite the effort to breathe. It occurs

BOX 31-3 CLASSIFICATION OF SELECT SLEEP DISORDERS

INSOMNIAS
- Adjustment sleep disorder (acute insomnia)
- Inadequate sleep hygiene
- Paradoxical insomnia
- Insomnia caused by mental disorder
- Behavioral insomnia of childhood
- Idiopathic insomnia
- Insomnia caused by medical condition

SLEEP-RELATED BREATHING DISORDERS

Central Sleep Apnea Syndromes
- Primary central sleep apnea
- Central sleep apnea caused by a drug or substance
- Central sleep apnea caused by a medical condition

Obstructive Sleep Apnea Syndromes
- Obstructive sleep apnea, adult
- Obstructive sleep apnea, pediatric

HYPERSOMNIAS OF CENTRAL ORIGIN
- Narcolepsy (four specified types)
- Menstrual-related hypersomnia
- Idiopathic hypersomnia with long sleep time
- Behaviorally induced insufficient sleep syndrome
- Hypersomnia caused by a medical condition

PARASOMNIAS

Disorders of Arousal
- Sleepwalking
- Sleep terrors

Parasomnias Usually Associated with REM Sleep
- Nightmare disorder
- REM sleep behavior disorder
- Sleep paralysis

Other Parasomnias
- Sleep-related groaning
- Sleep-related hallucinations
- Sleep-related eating disorder
- Sleep-related enuresis (bed-wetting)

CIRCADIAN RHYTHM SLEEP DISORDERS
- Delayed sleep phase type
- Advanced sleep phase type
- Jet lag type
- Shift work type
- Caused by a drug or substance

SLEEP-RELATED MOVEMENT DISORDERS
- Restless legs syndrome
- Periodic limb movements
- Sleep-related leg cramps
- Sleep-related bruxism (teeth grinding)

ISOLATED SYMPTOMS, APPARENTLY NORMAL VARIANTS, AND UNRESOLVED ISSUES
- Long sleeper
- Short sleeper
- Snoring
- Sleep talking
- Benign sleep myoclonus of infancy

OTHER SLEEP DISORDERS
- Physiological (organic) sleep disorders
- Environmental sleep disorder
- Sleep disorder not caused by a substance or physiological condition

Data from American Academy of Sleep Medicine: International classes of diseases and international classification of sleep disorders. In Kryger M, et al, editors: *Principles and practice of sleep medicine,* ed 5, St Louis, 2011, Saunders.

when muscles or soft structures of the oral cavity or throat relax during sleep. The upper airway becomes partially or completely blocked, and nasal airflow diminishes (hypopnea) or stops (apnea). The person tries to breathe because chest and abdominal movements continue, which often results in loud snoring sounds. When breathing is partially or completely diminished, the person becomes sufficiently hypoxic that he or she must awaken to breathe. Structural abnormalities such as a deviated septum, nasal polyps, narrow lower jaw, or enlarged tonsils sometimes predispose a patient to OSA. More than 18 million people in the United States are affected by OSA (National Sleep Foundation, 2013c). However, a large majority of people are undiagnosed and untreated because of lack of awareness by the public and health professionals (Ho and Brass, 2011).

Obesity is a major factor in OSA. Body weight, body mass index (BMI) in particular, has been shown to be the strongest risk factor for developing OSA. Large neck circumference and age are also increased risks. Individuals over 65 years of age are more frequently diagnosed with this sleep disorder. Research has shown an increased risk in African-American and Asians as compared with Caucasians (Ho and Brass, 2011).

Central sleep apnea (CSA) originates in the CNS. Pauses in breathing happen in the respiratory and pulmonary systems at the same time. The brain stops sending signals to muscles that control breathing. Conditions that are associated with CSA include stroke, degeneration of the cervical spine, obesity, and encephalitis. CSA is frequently seen in patients with congestive heart failure (A.D.A.M. Medical Encyclopedia, 2011).

EDS is a common complaint in people experiencing OSA. Untreated sleep apnea can lead to an increased risk of hypertension, diabetes, heart disease, and heart failure. Lifestyle changes, including a weight-reduction program in people who are obese, improved sleep hygiene, continuous positive airway pressure (CPAP), surgery, and dental appliances, are treatment options for OSA (Ho and Brass, 2011).

Narcolepsy. Narcolepsy is a rare CNS dysfunction of mechanisms that regulate sleep and wake states. EDS is the most common complaint associated with narcolepsy. During the day a person suddenly feels an overwhelming wave of sleepiness and falls asleep. It is possible for REM sleep to occur within 15 minutes of falling asleep. There are two narcolepsy states: with or without cataplexy. Cataplexy is a sudden muscle weakness during intense emotions such as anger or laughter that occurs at any time during the day. In a severe cataplectic attack, a patient loses voluntary muscle control and falls to the floor. It is not uncommon for narcolepsy to include frightening dreamlike experiences during transition from being awake to falling asleep.

A person with narcolepsy often falls asleep uncontrollably at inappropriate times. Unless you recognize this disorder, you mistake a person who suddenly and inappropriately falls asleep as someone who is lazy, disinterested, or possibly drunk. Typically symptoms first occur in adolescence and are sometimes confused with EDS. Narcolepsy is treated with stimulants that sometimes only partially increase wakefulness and reduce sleep attacks. Antidepressants are also prescribed to suppress cataplexy and other REM-related symptoms. Short daytime naps, no longer than 20 minutes, have been shown to reduce feelings of sleepiness. Regular exercise, eating light meals high in protein, deep breathing, chewing gum, and taking vitamins are other management methods (Kryger et al., 2011).

Sleep Deprivation. Many patients experience sleep deprivation as a result of a sleep disorder. It occurs from insufficient or disrupted sleep. Causes include illness (e.g., fever, difficulty breathing, or pain), emotional stress, medications, environmental disturbances (e.g., frequent interruptions in sleep during nursing care), and variability in the timing of sleep as a result of shift work.

With sleep deprivation, there is a decrease in the quantity and quality of sleep and an inconsistency in the timing of sleep. When sleep becomes interrupted or fragmented, changes in the normal sequencing of the sleep cycles occur. A cumulative sleep deprivation develops over time.

Individuals respond to sleep deprivation differently. Some patients experience a variety of physiological and psychological symptoms such as blurred vision, decreased reflexes, slow response time, confusion, and irritability. The severity of symptoms is often related to the duration of sleep deprivation. The most effective treatment for sleep deprivation is elimination or correction of environmental factors and patient care activities that disrupt the sleep pattern. Nurses play an important role in identifying treatable sleep-deprivation problems. Evidence suggests that sleep deprivation is associated with obesity, type II diabetes, poor memory, depression, digestive problems, and the development of cardiovascular disease (Ohlmann and O'Sullivan, 2009).

Parasomnias. The parasomnias are sleep disorders that can occur during arousal from REM or partial arousal from NREM sleep. They include sleep walking, night terrors, nightmares, teeth grinding, and bed-wetting. These are more common in children. An individual often experiences more than one parasomnia. Specific treatment for these disorders varies based on the underlying cause. However, in all cases it is important to support patients experiencing a disorder and maintain their safety.

CRITICAL THINKING

You will apply elements of critical thinking whenever you perform the nursing process with patients. Consider the scientific knowledge you have learned, your experience, critical thinking attitudes, and standards to ensure an individualized approach to patient care.

Synthesis

It is not uncommon for almost any patient to experience some type of sleep disorder, especially if sleeping in a new place. However, it is important not to overlook the problem or consider it as normal. Use of a critical thinking approach helps you to correctly identify the nature of a sleep problem and initiate appropriate nursing care. Apply your knowledge, experience, and appropriate critical thinking attitudes and standards to make the correct clinical judgments for patients (Box 31-4).

BOX 31-4 SYNTHESIS IN PRACTICE

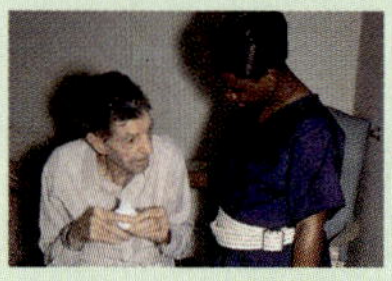

As Anna prepares to conduct an assessment of Mr. Murphy, she knows that it is important to consider sleep alterations in older adults. Because they typically have less deep sleep and more awakenings, it is important to consider which factors in the nursing home environment disrupt sleep. In addition, she has learned that the pain from Mr. Murphy's osteoarthritis is a contributing factor to his sleep disturbances. His immobility resulting from the stroke adds discomfort. Anna also plans to assess Mr. Murphy's medications carefully to determine if any drugs are adding to a sleep alteration.

From Anna's experience in a nursing home, she knows that a resident's sleep is often fragmented. Furthermore, she has read in a journal article that multiple factors affect sleep in the nursing home patient, including physical illness, dementia, depression, high prevalence of sleep-disordered breathing, chronic bed rest, circadian rhythm disturbances, and the noise and lighting of the nursing home environment. She wants to be sure that her assessment considers all potential factors influencing Mr. Murphy's sleep pattern. Because Mr. Murphy is in a nursing home, Anna determines whether environmental stimuli are disrupting his sleep. She evaluates whether he has a roommate who stays up late or has multiple visitors, the presence of electrical equipment at his bedside, and the likelihood of noise coming from an outside hallway.

Anna plans to include Mr. Murphy's wife in the assessment to learn more about her perceptions of changes in his behavior. A complete assessment needs to be clear and precise; thus Anna plans to talk with Mr. Murphy more than one time to gather the necessary information and keep her patient from becoming fatigued.

Knowledge. To make decisions about the nature and cause of a patient's sleep problems, it is important for you to synthesize knowledge regarding the physiology and functions of sleep and factors that affect it. Knowledge of the pathophysiology of select disease processes further helps in understanding the mechanisms for certain sleep problems. In addition, a thorough knowledge of pharmacological information is important because many medications that patients receive may contribute to sleeping difficulties.

Another important area of knowledge to synthesize is the patient's personal routine and cultural orientation. Infant care practices such as co-sleeping and the practice of regular siestas or naps are examples of cultural variations influencing sleep. Anticipate how such cultural factors ultimately influence an individual patient's ability to sleep.

Experience. You know of factors that have either disrupted or promoted your own ability to sleep. This personal experience is valuable when assessing patients' sleep problems or in selecting therapies for sleep promotion. Previous clinical experience with patients helps you to appreciate that environmental and lifestyle variations significantly affect the quality and quantity of sleep that a patient receives.

Attitudes. When dealing with sleep problems, it sometimes takes a long time to find effective therapies. For example, it is not easy to eliminate chronic insomnia in a short period. Perseverance and discipline are important critical thinking attitudes to use to help develop a plan of care with effective solutions to manage a patient's sleep problems. The problems that result from sleep disruption also often require creative approaches. Sometimes an original idea is necessary to minimize or control environmental stressors in a patient's sleep environment.

Standards. When learning about a patient's sleep problem, you use numerous intellectual standards in conducting the nursing assessment. Always conduct a detailed sleep assessment to understand the nature of the sleep problem and potential causes and solutions. A clear, precise, specific, and accurate assessment is very important so you establish an appropriate plan of care suited to the patient's specific sleep problem. Professional standards such as the Perianesthesia Nursing Standards, Practice Recommendations, and Interpretive Statements offer guidelines for care of patients with OSA (American Society of PeriAnesthesia Nurses, 2012). Because patient satisfaction based on HCAHPS scores has become a priority in hospitals, many nursing units are developing unit-based standards to promote sleep for patients.

NURSING PROCESS

ASSESSMENT

Assess a patient's sleep pattern to gather information about factors that usually influence sleep. Because sleep is a subjective experience, only the patient is able to report whether it is sufficient and restful. If a patient admits to or you suspect a sleep problem, gather a more detailed history. Aim your assessment at understanding the characteristics of any sleep problem and the patient's usual sleep habits so you incorporate ways for promoting sleep into nursing care.

Sources for Sleep Assessment. Patients are your best resource for describing a sleep problem and any change from their usual sleep and waking patterns. Parents or bed partners offer information on patients' sleep patterns that reveal the nature of certain disorders.

Obtain a child's sleep history from the parents. Older children often are able to relate the fears or worries that prevent them from falling asleep. If a child awakens frequently in the middle of bad dreams, parents are usually able to identify the problem without necessarily knowing the meaning of the dreams. Parents can describe typical behavior patterns that encourage or impair sleep. When children have chronic sleep problems, parents relate the duration of the problem, its progression, and the child's responses. It is a good idea for parents of an infant to keep a 24-hour log of their infant's waking and sleeping behavior over a period of several days.

Sleep History. Obtain a brief sleep history from patients on admission. Determine usual bedtime, normal bedtime rituals, preferred environment for sleeping, and what time the patient usually rises to plan care to support his or her positive sleep habits and patterns. Assess the quality and characteristics of sleep in greater depth when you suspect a sleep problem (Table 31-2).

Sleep Pattern and Quality. Begin the sleep history with the patient's self-reported sleep pattern. Most patients give a reasonably accurate estimate of their sleep patterns, particularly if any changes have occurred. An effective, subjective method for you to use for assessing sleep quality is the visual analogue scale (Lashley, 2004). Draw a straight horizontal line about 100 mm (4 inches) long. Opposing statements such as "best night's sleep" and "worst night's sleep" are at each end of the line. Ask the patient to place a mark along the horizontal line at the point that best matches their perception of the previous night's sleep. The distance of the mark along the line in millimeters offers a numerical value for satisfaction with sleep. Use the scale with the same patient repeatedly to show change in sleep over time. Do not use the scale to compare the quality of sleep for different patients.

A scale commonly used to assess the degree of daytime sleepiness or EDS is the Epworth Sleepiness Scale (National Sleep Foundation, 2011b). A patient completes 8 questions about the likeliness of being sleep during certain activities (e.g., watching television, sitting and talking with someone) on a scale of 0 (would never doze or sleep) to 3 (high chance of dozing or sleeping). A score of 10 or more is considered sleepy. A score of 18 or more is very sleepy. The scale is available at http://www.stanford.edu/~dement/epworth.html.

Always have patients describe their usual sleep pattern in case there are significant changes created by a sleep disorder. Ask the following questions:

- What time do you usually get in bed?
- What time do you usually fall asleep? Do you do anything special to help you fall asleep?

TABLE 31-2 FOCUSED PATIENT ASSESSMENT

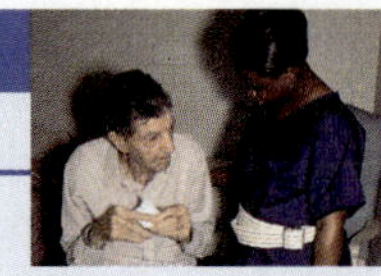

FACTORS TO ASSESS	QUESTIONS	PHYSICAL ASSESSMENT
Bedtime routines	How do you prepare for bed? Do you go to bed at the same time each night?	Observe for dark circles under patient's eyes. Observe the number of times the patient yawns.
Bedtime environment	How much light is in your bedroom at night? What is the temperature of your room during the night? Do you listen to music to go to sleep?	Ask patient or sleeping partner about multiple patient position changes during sleep or frequent reawakenings.
Current life events	What are your normal working hours? Have you experienced any recent changes in your job or home responsibilities? Which activities do you do to relax outside of work? What hobbies do you have?	Observe patient's ability to concentrate on the conversation.

- How many times do you wake up during sleep? Why do you think you awaken? What do you do about it?
- What time do you typically wake up?
- What time do you get out of bed, and how long do you stay up once you have awakened?
- What is the average number of hours you sleep?

Compare the assessment data with the pattern usually found for other patients of the same age and look for patterns that suggest problems. Sometimes patients with sleep problems show patterns very different from their usual one, and sometimes the change is relatively minor. Hospitalized patients usually need or want more sleep as a result of illness. However, some require less sleep because they are less active. Some patients who are ill think that it is important to try to sleep more than usual, eventually making sleeping difficult.

Description of Sleeping Problems. When a patient admits to or you suspect a sleep problem, ask open-ended questions to help the patient describe the problem more fully. A general description of the problem followed by more focused questions usually reveals specific sleep characteristics.

You need to understand the nature of the sleep problem, its signs and symptoms, its onset and duration, its severity, predisposing factors or causes, and the overall effect on the patient. Examples of assessment questions include the following:

1. *Nature of the problem:* Tell me what type of problem you have with your sleep. Tell me why you think you're not getting enough sleep. Describe for me a recent typical night's sleep. How is this sleep different from your usual sleep?
2. *Signs and symptoms:* Have you been told that you snore loudly? Do you have headaches when awakening? Does your child wake up from nightmares? Ask bed partner or parents whether patient has restful sleep or problems such as going to the bathroom frequently.
3. *Onset and duration:* When did you notice the problem? How long has this problem lasted?
4. *Severity:* How long does it take you to fall asleep? How often during the week do you have trouble falling asleep or staying asleep?
5. *Predisposing factors:* Tell me what you do just before going to bed. Have you recently had any changes at work, school, or home? How would you describe your current mood, and have you noticed any recent changes? Which medications or recreational drugs do you take regularly? Do you eat foods (e.g., spicy or greasy foods) or drink liquids (e.g., alcohol, caffeinated beverages) that disrupt your sleep? If so, how much do you eat or drink daily?
6. *Effect on patient:* How has the loss of sleep affected you? Do you feel well rested? Do you feel excessively sleepy or irritable or have trouble concentrating? Do you have trouble staying awake? Have you fallen asleep at inappropriate times? Ask a family member or friend: Have you noticed any changes in the patient's behavior since the sleep problem started?

Sleep Diary. Ask the patient and bed partner to keep a sleep-wake diary when it is obvious the patient is having serious sleep problems. Have them complete the diary daily until they are scheduled to be seen for their next health care visit; this will provide information on day-to-day variations in sleep-wake patterns over time. Entries in the diary often include 24-hour information on waking and sleeping activities such as exercise, work activities, mealtimes, and alcohol and caffeine intake. They should also include time and length of daytime naps, evening and bed routines, the time the patient tries to fall asleep, time and number of awakenings, and the time of morning awakening. If necessary, have the partner help to complete the sleep-wake diary. The diary is most helpful if the patient is motivated to complete it thoroughly. Using a tape recorder is a helpful option for patients with visual impairment or who have difficulty writing. Do not use the diary for hospital inpatients.

Physical Illness. Assess for any physical or psychological problems that affect a patient's sleep. A review of known medical conditions reveals symptoms (e.g., pain, nausea, shortness of breath, or fear) that interfere with the patient's normal sleep pattern. If a patient is scheduled for surgery, be sure to ask about a history of sleep apnea. Patients with sleep apnea who receive general anesthesia and pain medications after surgery have increased risk for developing airway obstruction during recovery. If the patient has recently undergone surgery, expect him or her to experience some disturbance in sleep.

Medications. Assess a patient's medication history, including over-the-counter and prescribed drugs. If he or she takes medications for sleep, gather information about the type and amount that he or she uses. Know the effects of medications on sleep (see Box 31-2).

Current Life Events. Changes in lifestyle disrupt a patient's sleep. A person's family situation or occupation offers clues to the nature of a sleep problem. Changes in job responsibilities, rotating shifts, and the recent birth of a child or loss of a family member sometimes contribute to a sleep disturbance. Questions about social activities, recent travel, or mealtime schedules also help clarify the sleep assessment.

Emotional and Mental Status. If a patient is anxious, fearful, or angry, mental preoccupations seriously disrupt sleep. In this situation a patient experiences emotional stress related to illness or situational crises. Ask patients to explore feelings about family relationships, job, or other meaningful situations.

Bedtime Routines. Ask how patients prepare for sleep. Assess habits that are beneficial compared with those that disturb sleep. You need to point out that a particular habit is interfering with sleep and help patients find ways to change or eliminate disruptive habits. For example, does the patient perform strenuous exercise within 2 hours of going to sleep? Does he or she usually spend 1 to 2 hours cooling down or relaxing before sleep?

Bedtime Environment. Ask patients to describe their preferred bedroom conditions. For example, ask if the patient keeps the bedroom dark or softly lit and closes the door. Some patients listen to a radio or watch television or prefer a quiet environment if noise prevents them from falling asleep. Also ask about room temperature and ventilation.

Assess the type of bed in which the person sleeps. Does he or she sleep in the same bed every night? Is the mattress comfortable? Does the patient need several pillows or cushions in bed to sit up during sleep? Does he or she use a lounge chair to sleep? Information about the sleeping environment helps you design better sleeping conditions.

Behaviors of Sleep Deprivation. Some patients are unaware of how their sleep problems are affecting their behavior. Observe for behaviors such as irritability, disorientation (similar to a drunken state), and slurred speech. If sleep deprivation has lasted a long time, psychotic behavior such as delusions and paranoia develop. For example, a patient reports seeing strange objects or colors in the room, or the patient acts afraid when you or other health personnel enter the room suddenly or without warning.

Older Adult Considerations. Older adults have a harder time falling asleep and more trouble staying asleep than do young adults. Sleep studies on older adults show a decline in REM sleep and an increase in nighttime awakenings. Research suggests that much of sleep disturbance in the elderly is attributed to physical and mental illnesses and medications used to treat them. Circadian rhythms that coordinate activities such as sleep change as the body ages. It is a common misconception that sleep needs decrease with aging. Older patients become sleepier in the early evening and wake earlier in the morning but still require the necessary 7 to 8 hours of sleep a day.

Older patients are more prone to RLS and should be assessed for the presence of this condition. Since increased age is associated with an increased incidence of chronic medical conditions, assessing for those associated with sleep disturbance is important. The elderly frequently experience losses such as retirement and death of a loved one, which may lead to emotional stress or depressive mood problems that effect sleep efficacy (National Sleep Foundation, 2009).

Patient Expectations. After assessing a patient's sleep history, determine his or her expectations regarding nursing care. Use a caring and skilled approach to assess the patient's sleep needs and preferences. For example, ask, "Now that I understand more about your sleep habits and the recent problems you've had, what do you expect from us regarding your care?" or "To improve your sleep, what do you think is most important that we do for you?" The patient sometimes has a different view about the relationship of sleep and health from your own. Examining patient expectations and preferences helps to clarify any misconceptions you have. Ask the patient which interventions he or she prefers and how to implement them. In the hospital setting some patients are more concerned about being sure that you are checking their condition routinely than about whether you wake them and disturb sleep.

NURSING DIAGNOSIS

Your assessment reveals clusters of data that include defining characteristics for a sleep problem or other nursing diagnoses that result from disturbed sleep. If you identify a sleep pattern disturbance, it is helpful for you to specify the exact condition. By determining the nature of a sleep disturbance, you can design more effective interventions. The following is a list of potential nursing diagnoses that you may identify for a patient with a sleep problem:

- *Anxiety*
- *Ineffective Breathing Pattern*
- *Acute Confusion*
- *Ineffective Coping*
- *Fatigue*
- *Insomnia*
- *Disturbed Sleep Problem*
- *Sleep Deprivation*
- *Ineffective Health Maintenance*
- *Readiness for Enhanced Sleep*

Your assessment also needs to identify the probable cause or related factor for the sleep disturbance such as a noisy environment, a high intake of caffeine, or stress involving work. The cause becomes the focus of interventions for minimizing or eliminating the problem. For example, a hospitalized patient who experiences insomnia as a result of a noisy sleeping environment benefits from a reduction in hospital equipment noise or minimizing interruptions. If the insomnia is related to worry over a threatened marital separation, your interventions involve introducing coping strategies. If you define the probable cause or related factors incorrectly, the patient will not benefit from your care.

PLANNING

Goals and Outcomes. After identifying all relevant nursing diagnoses for a patient (Figure 31-3), you develop a plan of care (see Care Plan). You develop an individualized care plan only after you understand how the nursing diagnosis relates to your patient's normal and current sleep pattern, his or her perception of the sleep problem, and the factors disrupting sleep. Together you and the patient develop realistic goals and outcomes. For example, the goal of "Patient will establish a healthy sleep pattern" includes outcomes such as "Patient falls asleep within a half hour of planned time" and "Patient has less than two awakenings during the night." This will be realistic if you know from your assessment that it now takes the patient an hour to fall asleep and that awakenings occur 3 or 4 times a night. The outcomes serve as measurable guidelines to determine goal achievement. An effective plan includes outcomes established over a realistic time frame that focus on the goal of improving the quality of sleep. This type of plan requires many weeks to accomplish.

Setting Priorities. Using the data you gathered about the nature of the patient's problem, you next identify priority strategies and interventions to promote sleep. Together you and the patient identify and select the strategies and interventions that are most likely to be beneficial in the home or health care setting. The plan of care includes priority strategies that support positive sleep habits and patterns that fit the patient's living environment, cultural orientation, and lifestyle. For example, the patient decides that purchasing a new mattress to increase comfort is the first step toward improving sleep. In a health care setting you plan treatments or routines together to give the patient more time to rest. For example, you turn and reposition a patient at the same time you give him or her medication or perform a treatment such as suctioning to limit the number of nurse-patient contacts. All staff caring for the patient need to know the plan so they

CARE PLAN

Insomnia

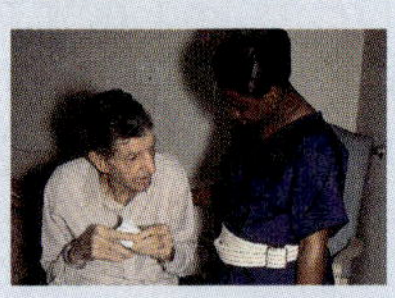

ASSESSMENT

Mr. Murphy is in a double room at the nursing home. Anna notices during the assessment that Mr. Murphy's roommate is frequently calling out to anyone who passes the room door. The roommate's television is also on. Mrs. Murphy comes to visit every day. She is concerned about how tired Mr. Murphy seems.

ASSESSMENT ACTIVITIES	FINDINGS/DEFINING CHARACTERISTICS*
Ask Mr. Murphy to describe the nature of his sleep problem. Ask Mr. Murphy to rate the quality of previous night's sleep.	Since being in the nursing home, he now reports, **"I have so much trouble falling asleep; it probably takes over an hour."** When asked if he awakens during the night, Mr. Murphy responds, "Are you kidding? No one can sleep here; something's always going on." Mr. Murphy admits to **waking up as many as 3 or 4 times during the night.** The patient estimates that he received maybe **4 hours of sleep the previous night. Mr. Murphy places a mark on the analog scale near "worst night's sleep."**
Ask Mr. Murphy to describe the usual bedtime routine that he practiced at home.	Anna learns that Mr. Murphy usually slept from 10:30 PM to 6:00 AM when he was at home, usually waking up once or twice during the night to urinate. He rarely had difficulty falling asleep; but, according to his wife, listening to music helped him relax.
Ask Mr. Murphy if he is having any other trouble that is contributing to his sleep problem.	He reports that he has some discomfort from the osteoarthritis and difficulty changing positions and getting comfortable. He rates pain at rest as a 4 on a scale of 0 to 10.
Assess Mr. Murphy for signs of sleep problems.	While Mr. Murphy describes his situation, he yawns frequently and states, "I really feel tired, **I have no energy**." He shifts his position in his wheelchair multiple times.

***Defining characteristics** are shown in **bold** type.

CARE PLAN—cont'd

Insomnia

NURSING DIAGNOSIS: Insomnia related to excessive environmental stimuli

PLANNING

GOAL	EXPECTED OUTCOMES (NOC)[†]
	Sleep
• Mr. Murphy will obtain a sense of restfulness following sleep within 1 month.	• Mr. Murphy has fewer than two self-reported awakenings during the night within 2 weeks. • Mr. Murphy reports being able to fall asleep within a half hour of going to bed within 2 weeks. • Mr. Murphy sleeps an average of 7 hours per night within 4 weeks.

[†]Outcomes classification labels from Moorhead S, et al, editors: *Nursing outcomes classification (NOC),* ed 5, St Louis, 2013, Mosby.

INTERVENTIONS (NIC)[‡]	RATIONALE
Sleep Enhancement	
• Have Mr. Murphy sit in the sunroom near the window for 30 to 60 minutes in the morning each day.	Bright light in the morning helps maintain the 24-hour circadian rhythm that regulates sleep-wake cycle (Chang et al., 2012).
• Discourage early morning and late afternoon napping or naps longer than 30 minutes.	Early morning and late afternoon napping interferes with sleeping (National Sleep Foundation, 2013a).
• Have an egg-crate–type mattress placed over bed mattress. Have staff position patient with extra pillows.	Increases comfort of sleeping position, enhancing relaxation, which promotes a sleep state.
• Encourage Mr. Murphy to decrease his fluids 2 to 4 hours before sleep.	Decreases number of times patient awakens to urinate (Touhy and Jett, 2011).
Relaxation Therapy	
• Arrange for Mr. Murphy to have a CD player with earphones to play music of his choice when first going to sleep.	Music therapy decreases situational anxiety and improves sleep efficiency (Bloch et al., 2010).
• Arrange for Mr. Murphy to have some of his favorite reading material at his bedside.	Reading before bedtime is a rest-promoting prebedtime activity.
Exercise Promotion	
• Have Mr. Murphy get regular exercise (e.g., have him propel down hallways in wheelchair for 5 minutes 4 times a day before dinner).	Regular exercise improves sleep quality.

[‡]Interventions classification label from Bulechek GM, et al, editors: *Nursing interventions classification (NIC),* ed 6, St Louis, 2013, Mosby.

EVALUATION

NURSING ACTIONS	PATIENT RESPONSE/FINDING	ACHIEVEMENT OF OUTCOME
Ask Mr. Murphy to use a visual analogue scale to rate the quality of his sleep at the end of each week.	At the end of the first week Mr. Murphy rates his quality of sleep as 6 out of 10. For the second week he rates his sleep at 8 out of 10.	Mr. Murphy is implementing sleep-hygiene measures. His sleep is improving because he rates his sleep as improving.
Ask Mrs. Murphy to evaluate her perceptions of Mr. Murphy's level of fatigue.	Mrs. Murphy states that her husband seems more awake, alert, and talkative when she visits. He does not nod off or nap in the early afternoon any more. She is also pleased that he enjoys doing the wheelchair exercises.	The sleep-hygiene measures along with the exercises have contributed to improved sleep for Mr. Murphy, resulting in decreased daytime fatigue.
Ask Mr. Murphy at the end of 4 weeks to keep a record for a week of the length of time he estimates sleeping.	Mr. Murphy reports that he falls asleep within 30 minutes and generally wakes up 2 to 3 times a night. He reports that he is sleeping 6 hours a night.	Mr. Murphy's use of relaxation therapy and music has improved his sleep.

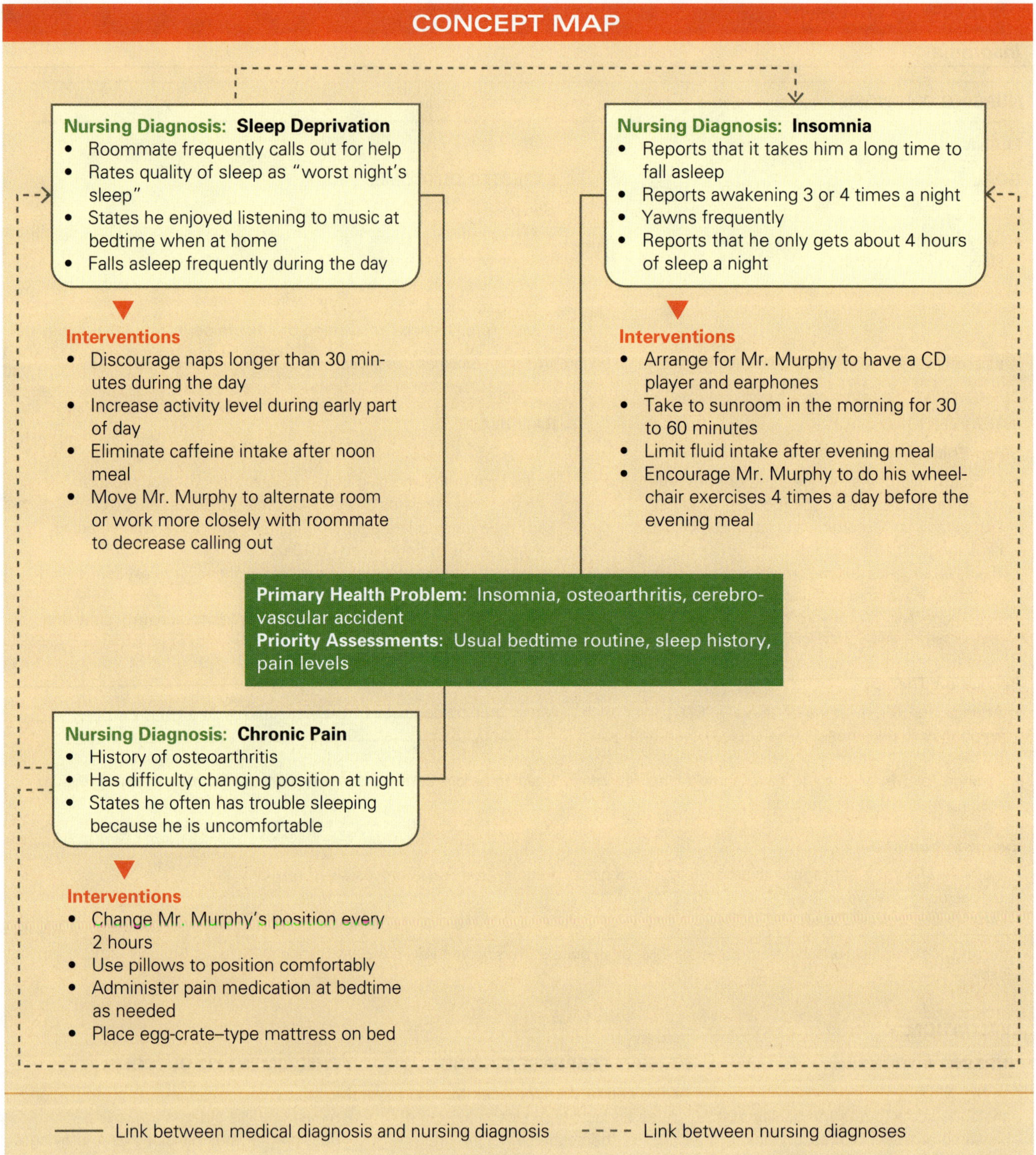

FIGURE 31-3 Concept map.

cluster activities at times to reduce awakenings. In a nursing home some plan rest periods around the activities of other residents.

Collaborative Care. The nature of a sleep disturbance determines whether referrals to additional health care providers are necessary. For example, if a sleep problem is related to a situational crisis or emotional problem, refer the patient to a psychiatric clinical nurse specialist, pastoral care professional, or clinical psychologist for counseling. This helps to ensure that you attend to the patient's problems not only in the health care setting but in the home as well. Sharing information with a home care nurse on patient discharge is useful in planning interventions to ensure that the patient gets adequate sleep when home. When chronic insomnia is the problem, a medical referral or referral to a sleep center is beneficial.

IMPLEMENTATION

Your nursing interventions for improving the quality of a person's sleep largely focus on health promotion. In an acute care setting your focus becomes managing the environment in a way that supports the patient's normal sleep habits and keeps the patient safe. When patients enter long-term care or nursing home environments, you need to make special considerations to promote adequate sleep and rest.

Health Promotion. Patients need adequate sleep and rest to maintain active and productive lifestyles. Your specific interventions promote a person's normal sleep and rest pattern.

Environmental Controls. All patients require a sleeping environment with a comfortable room temperature and proper ventilation, minimal noise, a comfortable bed, and proper lighting. Infants sleep best when the room temperature is 18° to 21° C (64° to 70° F) and they are covered with a light, warm blanket. Place healthy infants on their sides or backs when being put to sleep (American Academy of Pediatrics, 2012). The national "Back to Sleep" campaign has been very successful in teaching parents and infant caregivers to place infants on their backs for sleeping to reduce the incidence of sudden infant death syndrome (SIDS) (National Institute of Child Health and Human Development, 2013). Children and adults vary more in regard to comfortable room temperature but usually sleep best in cooler environments. Some prefer to sleep without covers. Older adults sometimes require extra blankets or covers or sleep wearing socks (Box 31-5).

Eliminate or reduce distracting noise so the bedroom is as quiet as possible. In the home the television or the ringing of the telephone disrupts a patient's sleep. The television is too stimulating to watch before sleep and should not be watched in bed or immediately before going to bed. Family members become important participants in care when each has a different schedule for going to sleep. It often requires the cooperation of several people living with the patient to reduce noise. Some patients sleep better with familiar inside noises such as the hum of a ceiling fan.

Make sure that the bed and mattress provide support and comfortable firmness. Place a bed board under the mattress to add support. Sometimes extra pillows help a person position more comfortably in bed. The position of the bed in the room also makes a difference for some patients.

For any patient prone to confusion or falls, safety is critical. In the home a small night-light helps the patient become oriented to the room environment before arising to go to the bathroom. Beds set lower to the floor reduce the risk for falls when a person stands. Remove clutter from the path a patient uses to walk from the bed to the bathroom. If a patient needs help in ambulating from the bed to the bathroom, have a small bell at the bedside to call family members.

BOX 31-5 CARE OF THE OLDER ADULT

Sleep Disturbances

SLEEP-WAKE PATTERN

- Maintain a regular rising time and bedtime.
- Eliminate early morning and late afternoon naps.
- If patient takes naps, limit to 20-30 minutes or less twice a day.
- Go to bed when sleepy.
- Use relaxation techniques and a regular bedtime routine to promote sleep.
- If unable to sleep in 15 to 30 minutes, get out of bed.

ENVIRONMENT

- Expose to natural light for 30 minutes to 2 hours daily, preferably soon after waking.
- Sleep where you sleep best.
- Keep noise to a minimum; use soft music to mask noise if necessary.
- Use night-light and keep path to bathroom free of obstacles.
- Set room temperature to preference; use blankets and socks to promote comfort.

MEDICATIONS

- Use sedatives and hypnotics as last resort and then use only short term if needed.
- Adjust medications being taken for other conditions and look for drug interactions that cause insomnia or EDS.

DIET

- Limit alcohol, caffeine, and nicotine in late afternoon and evening.
- Eat a light snack such as cereal and milk or cheese and crackers before bedtime.
- Decrease fluids 2 to 4 hours before sleep.

PHYSIOLOGICAL/ILLNESS FACTORS

- Elevate head of bed and provide extra pillows as preferred.
- Use analgesics 30 minutes before bed to ease aches and pains.
- Use prescribed medications to control symptoms of chronic conditions.

EDS, Excessive daytime sleepiness.

Patients vary in regard to the amount of light that they prefer at night. Infants and older adults sleep best in softly lit rooms. Do not have light shining directly on their eyes. Small table lamps or night-lights prevent total darkness. For older adults this reduces the chance of confusion when arising from bed. If streetlights shine through windows or when patients nap during the day, heavy shades, drapes, or slatted blinds are helpful.

Promoting Bedtime Routines. Bedtime routines and sleep-hygiene measures relax patients in preparation for sleep. It is important for people to go to sleep when they feel tired or sleepy. To develop good sleep hygiene at home, patients and their bed partners need to learn techniques that promote sleep and conditions that interfere with it (Box 31-6). Hospitalized patients should be encouraged to follow their at-home bedtime routine.

Newborns and infants benefit from quiet activities such as holding them snugly in blankets, talking or singing softly, and gently rocking. A bedtime routine (e.g., same hour for bedtime or quiet activity) used consistently helps toddlers and preschool children avoid delaying sleep. Parents need to reinforce patterns of preparing for bedtime. Reading stories, allowing children to sit in a parent's lap while listening to music or praying, and coloring are routines associated with preparing for bed.

BOX 31-6 PATIENT TEACHING

Improving Sleep

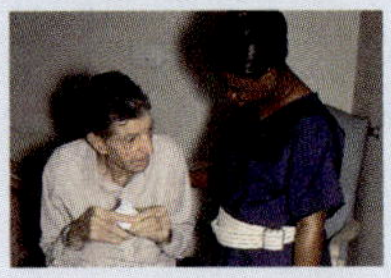

On one of her visits to the nursing home, Mary Murphy tells Anna, the nursing student, that she is having trouble sleeping and does not feel rested. Anna asks Mrs. Murphy to describe her current sleep habits. Using what she knows about sleep-hygiene measures, Anna then develops a teaching plan to help Mrs. Murphy improve her sleeping.

OUTCOME

At the end of the teaching session, Mrs. Murphy develops a plan that includes effective sleep-hygiene practices.

TEACHING STRATEGIES

- Discuss with Mrs. Murphy the need to practice sleep hygiene habits regularly.
- Caution Mrs. Murphy against delaying bedtime or sleeping long hours during weekends or holidays to maintain her normal sleep-wake cycle.
- Explain to her not to use the bedroom for watching television, snacking, or other nonsleep activity.
- Encourage Mrs. Murphy to take a warm bath before bedtime.
- Encourage Mrs. Murphy to walk for 30 minutes every morning.
- Instruct Mrs. Murphy to play soft relaxing music at bedtime to help her fall asleep.
- Demonstrate relaxation techniques to Mrs. Murphy.
- Advise Mrs. Murphy that, if she does not fall asleep within 20 minutes, she needs to get out of bed and do some quiet activity until feeling sleepy enough to go back to bed.
- Instruct Mrs. Murphy to avoid heavy meals for 3 hours before bedtime; a light snack, including protein and carbohydrates helps.
- Answer questions that Mrs. Murphy has about sleep problems.

EVALUATION STRATEGIES

- Ask Mrs. Murphy to describe three sleep hygiene habits.
- Have Mrs. Murphy demonstrate a relaxation technique to use to promote sleep.
- Ask Mrs. Murphy to identify an appropriate bedtime snack.
- Ask Mrs. Murphy to identify the benefits of listening to soothing music at bedtime .

Adults need to avoid excessive mental stimulation just before bedtime. Reading a light novel, watching a relaxing television program, or listening to music helps a person relax. Relaxation exercises and praying often induce calm in patients.

Promoting Comfort. People fall asleep only after feeling comfortable and relaxed. You recommend and use several measures to promote comfort such as encouraging the patient to wear loose-fitting nightwear and void before bedtime. Have family members give a relaxing back rub. Minor irritants keep people awake. Change diapers before placing infants in bed. An extra blanket prevents chilling when trying to fall asleep.

Have patients who suffer painful illnesses try a variety of measures at home to promote comfort. Application of dry or moist heat, use of supportive dressings or splints, and proper positioning with the use of extra pillows for support are very helpful. For patients with temporary acute pain (e.g., following surgery), it is sometimes advantageous to the patient and bed partner to let the patient sleep alone until the pain subsides. In addition, encourage the patient to take pain medications 30 to 60 minutes before going to bed.

You help patients with physical illness learn ways to control symptoms that disrupt sleep. For example, a patient with respiratory abnormalities needs to sleep with two pillows or in a semi-sitting position to ease the effort to breathe. The patient often benefits from taking prescribed bronchodilators before sleep to prevent airway obstruction.

Promoting Activity. In the home encourage patients to stay physically active during the day so they are more likely to sleep at night. Increasing daytime activity lessens problems with falling asleep. Always plan rigorous exercise at least 2 to 3 hours before bedtime.

Research indicates that exercise is beneficial, particularly for older adults, to improve nighttime sleep. General recommendations include increasing daytime activity or exercise (Reeve and Bailes, 2010). However, older adults with chronic diseases that influence their functional abilities are likely to have limited activity (Touhy and Jett, 2011). Recommend activities that are safe for older patients to perform. Walking, swimming, wheelchair propulsion, and cycling on a stationary bike are excellent for patients with limited physical impairment. Weight lifting using light weights (e.g., 2 to 5 lbs) is also excellent to build upper body strength and endurance. Activity and exercise often prove to be beneficial by improving activity endurance, mobility, and sense of well-being.

Stress Reduction. When patients feel emotionally upset, urge them to try not to force sleep. Otherwise insomnia often develops, and soon they will associate bedtime with the inability to relax. Encourage a patient who has difficulty falling asleep to get up and pursue a relaxing activity rather than staying in bed and thinking about sleep. When the emotional problem is ongoing and the patient finds little relief, encourage referral to an appropriate counselor.

Children often have problems going to bed and falling asleep. Have parents enter their children's rooms immediately after nightmares and talk to them briefly about their fears to provide a cooling-down period. Comforting children while they lie in their own bed is reassuring. Keeping a light on in the room also helps. Usually experts do not recommend that a child be allowed to sleep with parents; however, cultural traditions cause families to approach sleep practices differently (Box 31-7).

Bedtime Snacks. Some people enjoy bedtime snacks, whereas others cannot sleep after eating. A bedtime snack containing protein and carbohydrates such as cereal and milk or cheese and crackers, which contain L-tryptophan, may help to promote sleep. A full meal before bedtime often causes gastrointestinal upset and interferes with the ability to fall asleep.

Make sure that patients avoid drinking excess fluids or ingesting caffeine before bedtime. Coffee, tea, cola, and chocolate cause a person to stay awake or wake up throughout the night. Alcohol interrupts sleep cycles and reduces the amount of deep sleep. Coffee, tea, colas, and alcohol act as diuretics, which cause nocturia.

BOX 31-7 PATIENT-CENTERED CARE

Co-sleeping with children is a culturally preferred habit. It is more common in nonindustrialized countries. This practice is also common in the United States with Asian American and African-American families. Health care personnel in the United States discourage this practice because of safety issues. American culture promotes independence in childhood. Co-sleeping does not promote this independence; thus health care workers discourage it. As a nurse you need to be culturally sensitive when discussing co-sleeping practices with parents and developing sleeping plans for children.

IMPLICATIONS FOR PRACTICE

- Complete a thorough sleep assessment of the child and family.
- Discuss the risks of co-sleeping with parents. During the discussion remain culturally sensitive and respectful of the parents' views (Sobralske and Gruber, 2009).
- Co-sleeping affects the infant's normal sleep pattern by decreasing slow-wave sleep and increasing the number of nighttime arousals.
- Co-sleeping has been linked to increased risk for sudden infant death syndrome (SIDS) under certain conditions such as parental smoking or alcohol or drug use.
- Instruct parents to avoid using alcohol or drugs that impair arousal. Decreased arousal prevents the parents from waking up if the child is having problems.
- Co-sleeping should only occur with parents and child and not another adult or child.
- Avoid soft bedding surfaces. Infants and children become entangled or have their heads covered if the bed contains loose coverings, pillows, or stuffed toys.
- Encourage parents to use light sleeping clothes, keep the room temperature comfortable, and not bundle the child tightly or in too many clothes.

Pharmacological Approaches to Promoting Sleep. **Melatonin** is a neurohormone produced in the brain that helps control circadian rhythms. It is a popular nutritional supplement in the United States used to aid sleep. The recommended dose is 0.3 to 1 mg taken 2 hours before bedtime. Older adults with decreased levels of melatonin find it beneficial in aiding sleep (Kryger et al., 2011). Few studies have investigated whether melatonin supplements are safe and effective for long-term use (University of Maryland Medical Center, 2012), but the short-term use of melatonin is considered safe with infrequent mild side effects of nausea, headache, and dizziness (Larzelere et al., 2010). More research is needed. The drug is not FDA approved for sleep.

Sedatives and **hypnotics** are groups of drugs that induce and/or maintain sleep. However, long-term use of these drugs disrupts sleep and leads to more serious problems. Benzodiazepines are a common classification of drug used to treat sleep problems when a change in sleep hygiene is not effective. Examples of benzodiazepines include temazepam (Restoril), flurazepam (Dalmane), estazolam (ProSom), and triazolam (Halcion). Benzodiazepines may cause psychological and physical dependence, and physical withdrawal symptoms may occur if the drug is not carefully tapered following long-term use (University of Maryland Medical Center, 2012). The use of benzodiazepines in the older adult population is potentially dangerous. Long-term use and high doses in this population have been associated with suicidal ideation (Bosse et al., 2011).

The nonbenzodiazepine, benzodiazepine receptor agonists are newer medications that appear to have better safety profiles and fewer adverse effects than the benzodiazepines. They are also associated with a lower risk of abuse and dependence than the benzodiazepines, although abuse and dependence do occur. Examples of medications in this class include zolpidem (Ambien), zaleplon (Sonata), and eszopiclone (Lunesta) (University of Maryland Medical Center, 2012). A low dose of a short-acting medication such as zolpidem can be effective for short-term use (no longer than 2 to 3 weeks). Patients should avoid the use of alcohol while taking these drugs.

A new class of drugs called melatonin agonists promotes the onset of sleep by increasing levels of the natural hormone melatonin, which helps normalize circadian rhythm and sleep/wake cycles. Ramelteon (Rozerem) belongs to this drug class. Side effects may include daytime sleepiness, dizziness, and fatigue (University of Maryland Medical Center, 2012).

The use of nonprescription OTC sleeping medications is not advisable. Over the long term these drugs lead to further sleep disruption even when they initially seem effective. Help patients with interventions that do not require the use of drugs.

Regular use of any sleep medication leads to tolerance, and withdrawal causes rebound insomnia. Make sure that all patients understand the possible side effects of sleep medications. In 2007 the FDA released a warning related to complex sleep-related behaviors such as sleep driving or sleep eating that have occurred with prescription sleep medications

(U.S. FDA, 2007). Routine monitoring of patient response to sleeping medications is important.

Managing Specific Sleep Disturbances. Patients who suffer specific sleep disturbances likely benefit from the health promotion strategies discussed so far. Weight loss can be effective for the patient with OSA. It is important for the patient to follow an appropriate weight-reduction plan. In milder cases of OSA, body position during sleep is effective. One suggestion is to elevate the head of the bed (Touhy and Jett, 2011).

Acute Care. The nursing interventions described for health promotion are applicable to a patient requiring acute care. The nature of the acute care setting requires you to be creative in finding ways to maintain the patient's normal sleep pattern (Box 31-8).

Managing Environmental Stimuli. A challenge in the hospital is controlling noise. Because many patients spend only a short time in hospitals, it is easy to forget the importance of establishing good sleep conditions. In a hospital setting, plan nursing care activities to avoid waking patients. Try to schedule assessments, treatments, procedures, and routines for times when patients are awake. Perform nursing activities before the patient receives sleeping medication or begins to fall asleep. For example, you have a patient who has had surgery. Before the patient gets ready for bed, change the surgical dressing, reposition the patient, administer pain medication, and check vital signs. Give medications and draw blood during waking hours when possible. Plan with other departments and services to schedule therapies at intervals that give patients time to rest. Whenever it becomes necessary to wake a patient, do it as quickly as possible so the patient can fall back to sleep as soon as possible.

BOX 31-8 EVIDENCE-BASED PRACTICE

PICO Question: Does a sleep-hygiene protocol compared to standard unit routines create an environment conducive to sleep for older adult patients in a hospital setting?

SUMMARY OF EVIDENCE

Sleep is necessary for healing (Richardson et al., 2009). However, because of noise, lighting, and patient-care activities, hospital environments are not conducive to sleep (Gardner et al., 2009). Staff conversation and alarms are generally regarded as the most disturbing noises for patients' sleep in ICUs (Xie et al., 2009). Implementing a sleep-hygiene protocol is an effective strategy to improve sleep quality for hospitalized patients (LaReau, et al., 2008). A daily quiet time when patient-care activities are limited, pain medication is used, positioning is adjusted, noise is reduced, and light levels are decreased is helpful in promoting sleep.

APPLICATION TO NURSING PRACTICE

- Teach patients effective sleep hygiene measures (LaReau et al., 2008).
- Interventions shown to improve patients' sleep include earplugs, behavioral modification by nursing staff, and sound masking (use of ocean sounds or white noise) (Xie et al., 2009).
- Noise reduction strategies included cutting down the intensity of alarm sounds and talking, and switching off the phone, television and radio.
- Establish a "quiet time" (2 to 4 AM, 2 to 4 PM) protocol for a nursing unit (Xie et al., 2009).
- Keep patient doors closed at night to minimize noise (Gardner et al., 2009).
- Decrease light levels (Gardner et al., 2009).
- Cluster patient-care activities to provide uninterrupted periods of sleep (LaReau et al., 2008).
- Post a sign on the patient door informing caregivers of patient's uninterrupted sleep periods (LaReau et al., 2008).

Safety. Safety precautions are important for patients who wake up during the night to use the bathroom and for those with EDS. Set beds lower to the floor to lessen the chance of the patient falling when first standing. Remove clutter and move equipment from the path that a patient uses to walk from the bed to the bathroom. If a patient needs assistance in ambulating from the bed to the bathroom, make sure that the call light is within his or her reach. Be sure that the patient knows how to turn the light on correctly.

If patients normally use a continuous positive airway pressure (CPAP) machine at home because of sleep apnea, it is important that they bring their home equipment with them to the hospital and use it every night. This is even more important for patients with sleep apnea who have surgery and receive general anesthesia. In these patients the anesthesia in combination with pain medications used after surgery reduces the patient's defenses against airway obstruction. After surgery the patient achieves very deep levels of REM sleep that lead to muscle relaxation and airway obstruction (Hwang et al., 2008). These patients need ventilator support in the postoperative period because OSA is linked to increased postoperative respiratory complications. Make sure that the patients use their home CPAP equipment. Use pain medication carefully in these patients. Monitor the patient's breathing and oxygen saturation levels regularly (see Chapter 15). Notify the health care provider right away if the patient is difficult to arouse or is having trouble breathing.

Patients who experience EDS can fall asleep while sitting up in a chair or wheelchair. Position patients so they do not fall out of the chair when sleeping. Elevating their feet on an ottoman or small bench may help to position them safely. A pillow placed in the patient's lap offers some support. If a patient enjoys leaning over an over-bed table while sitting in a chair, be sure that the table is locked and secure. Avoid using safety belts because they are considered restraints (see Chapter 28).

Comfort Measures. You make the patient more comfortable in an acute care setting by providing personal hygiene before bedtime. A warm bath or shower is very relaxing. Offer patients restricted to bed the opportunity to wash their face and hands. Toothbrushing and care of dentures also help to prepare the patient for sleep. Have patients void before going to bed so they are not kept awake by a full bladder. While a patient prepares for bed, help to position him or her off any potential pressure sites. Offering a back rub or massage helps relax the patient.

Removal of irritating stimuli is another way to improve the patient's comfort for a restful sleep. Changing or removing moist dressings, repositioning drainage tubing, reapplying wrinkled thromboembolic hose, and changing tape on nasogastric tubes eliminate constant irritants to the patient's skin. When an intravenous (IV) site becomes irritated and painful, reinsertion of the IV line is usually recommended. Cleanse the perineal or anal area thoroughly for patients who are incontinent. Diaphoretic patients benefit from a cool bath and dry clothes or linens.

Restorative and Continuing Care. The quality of sleep in a long-term care or nursing home environment is often fragmented. Residents of a nursing home often suffer chronic disease, incontinence, and dementia and take multiple medications, all of which can disrupt sleep. Noise, light, and repositioning nursing home residents during linen changes are factors that cause patients to awaken. Besides care activities, nursing home residents themselves are very disruptive when they call out loudly to roommates or nursing staff.

In the long-term care environment many patients require rehabilitation or supportive care. The nature of their illnesses and treatment requirements disrupt sleep. For example, patients who are ventilator dependent likely get brief periods of sleep throughout the day rather than prolonged sleep because of disruptions from ventilator alarm sounds and the need for occasional suctioning.

Maintaining Activity. In the restorative care setting try to limit the time residents spend in bed. In the nursing home serve meals in the resident dining area. Otherwise residents should be up in a chair for meals and for personal hygiene activities. It is also important to keep the residents involved in social activities planned at the nursing home (e.g., card playing or arts and crafts). Regular exercise keeps people active and stimulated. It is also ideal to limit daytime napping to 30 minutes or less. Short naps taken in the midafternoon increase alertness and cognitive ability.

Residents with dementia often have disrupted sleep-wake cycles. They often become easily fatigued and experience periods of insomnia (Touhy and Jett, 2011). In this situation activities and visits need to be shortened to allow the patient to maintain an adequate energy level. If a patient wakes up during the night, keeping the lights at a low level and using soothing techniques such as quiet music or a back rub promote returning to sleep.

Reducing Sleep Disruption. Knowing the many factors that disrupt sleep in restorative care settings, you find ways to make the environment more favorable to sleep. Noise control is critical. Often staff within a nursing home speak louder because of residents' difficulties with hearing, even though raising one's voice does not improve hearing reception. Walking up close to a patient and talking in a normal but clear voice likely improves the patient's hearing and reduces the chance of waking a nearby roommate. Teach nursing assistive personnel to be more sensitive to the sources of noise that disrupt patients' sleep.

EVALUATION

Patient Care. Individualize your evaluation of therapies designed to promote sleep and rest (Box 31-9). Patients in relatively good health often do not need as much sleep as patients whose physical condition is poor.

If you have established realistic goals of care, the expected outcomes become guidelines for evaluating a patient's progress and response to interventions. Use evaluative measures shortly after trying a therapy. Use other evaluative measures after a patient awakens from sleep (e.g., asking a patient to describe the number of awakenings during the night). Together the patient and bed partner can usually provide accurate information. If the patient lives or sleeps alone, the evaluation may be unreliable.

BOX 31-9 EVALUATION

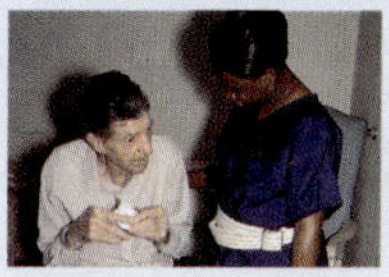

After 4 weeks at the nursing home, Anna has been able to have Mr. Murphy transferred to a new room and has been monitoring his progress. He has been in the new room for 2 weeks. Anna asks Mr. Murphy, "Tell me how our plan to improve your sleep has been working. Have the music and headphones been helpful?" Mr. Murphy replies, "Well, it has helped to be down here at the end of the hall. It still is a bit noisy, especially if the nurses are working with people across the way. I've used the headphones the last 2 weeks, and they've helped me relax and fall asleep in about 20 or 30 minutes." Anna questions Mr. Murphy further and learns that he is waking up 2 or 3 times during the night. However, during the last week he estimated getting about 6 hours of sleep, an improvement from a month ago. Mr. Murphy also reports that the staff has usually been good about reminding him to do his daily exercises with the wheelchair. He dislikes staying in his room and has tried to exercise as much as possible.

Anna wants to know Mr. Murphy's level of satisfaction with her care. She asks, "Have I met your expectations so far? If not, tell me how I can better help you." Mr. Murphy replies, "You've been great. I know you can't make this place like home. There's so much to think about when you're here. I think about my wife a lot." Anna responds, "Tell me more. What do you mean, 'There's so much to think about'?" Anna recognizes that psychological and physical stressors alter sleep. She decides to reassess Mr. Murphy to determine if additional nursing interventions are appropriate.

DOCUMENTATION NOTE

"Reports some improvement in overall sleep quality. Able to fall asleep within 20 to 30 minutes using headphones with music. Reports sleeping approximately 6 hours per night. Continues to experience awakenings, resulting from noise in outside hallway. Recommend closing room door at night to reduce noise further. Admits to thinking about his wife and other concerns. Will explore further with him."

When a patient does not meet expected outcomes, revise the nursing measures based on the patient's needs or preferences. Document his or her response to sleep therapies to maintain a continuum of care.

Patient Expectations. Review progress in the plan of care with your patient and determine if his or her expectations were met. Does the patient believe that your interventions were helpful and useful? Did you incorporate his or her typical sleep routine into the plan of care? For the hospitalized patient, did staff avoid unnecessary interruptions or excessive noise, giving the patient a chance to rest? The patient's perceptions are valuable sources of information regarding the overall success in improving the quality of the patient's sleep.

KEY POINTS

- Researchers think that sleep provides physiological and psychological restoration.
- The 24-hour sleep-wake cycle is a circadian rhythm that affects physiological function and behavior.
- The control and regulation of sleep depends on a balance between CNS regulators.
- During a typical night's sleep a person fluctuates between NREM stages 2, 3, and 4 before entering REM sleep. The amount of time in each stage varies.
- The number of hours of sleep needed by each person to feel rested varies.
- Long-term use of sleeping pills leads to difficulty in initiating and maintaining sleep.
- The hectic pace of a person's lifestyle, emotional and psychological stress, and drug and alcohol ingestion disrupt the sleep pattern.
- An environment with a darkened room, reduced noise, comfortable bed, appropriate temperature, and good ventilation promotes sleep.
- The most common type of sleep disorder is insomnia. Characteristics of insomnia include the inability to fall asleep, to remain asleep during the night, or to go back to sleep after waking up earlier than desired.
- Use your patient's self-report to determine if sleep is restful.
- When using environmental controls to promote sleep, consider the usual characteristics of the patient's home environment and normal lifestyle.
- Noise can disrupt sleep and enhance pain perception.
- The HCAHPS survey measures patients' perspectives on hospital care after discharge, including quietness of the hospital environment.
- A bedtime routine of relaxing activities prepares a person physically and mentally for sleep.
- Pain or other symptom control is essential to promoting the ability to sleep.
- One of the most important nursing interventions for promoting sleep is establishing periods for uninterrupted sleep.

CLINICAL DECISION-MAKING EXERCISES

During one of Mrs. Murphy's visits with Mr. Murphy, she tells Anna that her husband says that he cannot sleep in the nursing home despite the fact that he has been taking a hypnotic drug for 2 months to help him sleep. Mrs. Murphy believes that her husband is depressed, and she is very concerned that he has said he no longer desires to live.

1. How should Anna respond to Mrs. Murphy?
2. Anna is charged with developing a sleep-hygiene plan for Mr. Murphy. What should be included in the plan?

Anna has a class presentation to give as part of her clinical learning experience. She chooses the topic of sleep.

3. What content should she include in her presentation about sleep hygiene?

evolve

Answers to Clinical Decision-Making Questions can be found on the Evolve website.

QSEN ACTIVITY: QUALITY IMPROVEMENT

The nursing home decides to try to implement "quiet hours" or "quiet time" during the day to improve the residents' restfulness. Anna is involved in the project and decides to involve the nursing home residents in planning the implementation of the new policy.

Which critical attitudes is Anna demonstrating? What would be key steps to determining if the process for change is successful?

evolve

Answers to QSEN Activities can be found on the Evolve website.

REVIEW QUESTIONS

1. When developing a nursing care plan, which intervention would be most appropriate for a patient experiencing obstructive sleep apnea (OSA)?
   1. Develop a weight reduction plan
   2. Instruct patient to take an over-the -counter sleep aid
   3. Complete a health history
   4. Instruct patient to keep a sleep log
2. Which statement from a patient would indicate an understanding of behaviors that may disrupt sleep?
   1. "I will not watch television in bed."
   2. "Reading in bed will help me sleep."
   3. "A short nap late in the evening will lead to a more restful night of sleep."
   4. "A glass of wine before bed will help me relax and sleep through the night."

3. Which nursing intervention(s) best promote(s) effective sleep in an older adult? (Select all that apply.)
   1. Limit fluids 2 to 4 hours before sleep
   2. Ensure that room is completely dark
   3. Encourage walking an hour before going to bed
   4. Provide warm covers
4. A sleeping patient is very difficult to arouse. This indicates which stage in the sleep cycle?
   1. Stage 1 NREM
   2. Stage 2 NREM
   3. REM
   4. Transitioning from REM to NREM stage 2
5. Which patient statement would require the nurse to intervene?
   1. "I drink a cup of warm milk in the evening to help me sleep."
   2. "Long-term use of hypnotics will cure my insomnia."
   3. "I understand that the recommended dose of melatonin is 0.3 to 1 mg."
   4. "I plan to make 8 PM my regular bedtime."
6. When educating a new mother on normal infant sleep patterns, which statement would be accurate?
   1. Expect your infant to have developed a regular nighttime sleep pattern by the end of his first year.
   2. It will be unusual for your infant to wake in early morning hours.
   3. You can expect your infant to sleep an average of 16 hours a day.
   4. Infants usually sleep throughout the night.
7. The nurse is completing a sleep history for a patient being assessed for narcolepsy. Which symptom(s) does the patient most likely report? (Select all that apply.)
   1. Headache
   2. Nocturia
   3. Frightening dreamlike experiences
   4. Difficulty staying asleep
8. In providing education for a patient taking melatonin as a sleeping aid, which points should be included? (Select all that apply.)
   1. Should not be used indefinitely
   2. May cause nausea
   3. It is not regulated by the U.S. Food and Drug Administration (FDA)
   4. May cause night sweats
9. Which condition in the patient's history most likely contributes to the patient's diagnosis of obstructive sleep apnea (OSA)?
   1. Hyperthyroidism
   2. Gastric reflux
   3. Obesity
   4. Anorexia
10. Which priority nursing intervention would be appropriate to include in a plan of care to promote sleep for a hospitalized patient?
    1. Give patient a cup of coffee 1 hour before bedtime
    2. Assess vital signs every 4 hours
    3. Turn television on 15 minutes before bedtime
    4. Have patient follow at-home bedtime schedule

evolve

Rationales for Review Questions can be found on the Evolve website.

1. 1; 2. 1; 3. 1, 4; 4. 3; 5. 2; 6. 3; 7. 3; 8. 1, 2, 3; 9. 3; 10. 4

REFERENCES

A.D.A.M Medical Encyclopedia: *Central sleep apnea*, 2011, http://www.ncbi.nlm.nih.gov/pubmedhealth/PMH0004404/. Accessed December 23, 2013.

American Academy of Pediatrics (AAP): Changing concepts of sudden infant death syndrome: implications for infant sleeping environment and sleep position, *Pediatrics* 105:650, 2012.

American Society of PeriAnesthesia Nurses: *2012-2014 Perianesthesia Nursing Standards, Practice Recommendations and Interpretive Statements*, Cherry Hill, NJ, 2012, The Society.

Bosse C, et al: Suicidal ideation, death thoughts, and use of benzodiazepines in the elderly population, *Can J Commun Mental Health* 30(1):1, 2011.

Bloch B, et al: The effects of music relaxation on sleep quality and emotional measures in people living with schizophrenia, *J Music Ther* 41(1):27, 2010.

Centers for Medicare and Medicaid Services: *HCAHPS: patients' perspectives of care survey*, 2013, http://www.cms.gov/Medicare/Quality-Initiatives-Patient-Assessment-Instruments/HospitalQualityInits/HospitalHCAHPS.html. Accessed December 23, 2013.

Chang AM, et al: Human responses to bright light of different durations, *J Physiol* 590(Pt. 13):3103, 2012.

Choi K, et al: Internet overuse and excessive daytime sleepiness in adolescents, *Psychiatry Clin Neurosci* 63(4):455, 2009.

Chokroverty S: Overview of sleep and sleep disorders, *Indian J Med Res* 131:126–140, 2010.

Daroff RB, et al, editors: *Bradley's neurology in clinical practice*, ed 6, Philadelphia, 2012, Saunders.

Fiorentino L, Martin JL: Awake at 4 AM: treatment of insomnia with early morning awakenings among older adults, *Clin Psych J* 66(11):1161, 2010.

Gardner G, et al: Creating a therapeutic environment: a non-randomized controlled trial of a quiet time intervention for patients in acute care, *Int J Nurs Studies* 46:778, 2009.

Gilsenan I: Nursing interventions to alleviate insomnia, *Nurs Older People* 24(4):14, 2012.

Ho ML, Brass SD: Obstructive sleep apnea, *Neurol Int* 3(e15):60, 2011.

Hobson JA: REM sleep and dreaming: towards a theory of protoconsciousness, *Nature Rev/Neurosci* 10:803, 2009.

Hockenberry MJ, Wilson D: *Wong's nursing care of infants and children*, ed 9, St Louis, 2011, Mosby.

Hwang D, et al: Association of sleep-disordered breathing with postoperative complications, *Chest* 133(5):1128, 2008.

Izac SM: Basic anatomy and physiology of sleep, *Am J Electroneurodiagnostic Technol* 46:18, 2006.

Kryger MH, et al: *Principles and practice of sleep medicine*, ed 5, St Louis, 2011, Saunders.

LaReau R, et al: Examining the feasibility of implementing specific nursing interventions to promote sleep in hospitalized elderly patients, *Geriatr Nurs* 29(3):197, 2008.

Larzelere MM, et al: Complementary and alternative medicine usage for behavioral health indicators, *Prim Care Clin Office Pract* 37(2):213, 2010.

Lashley F: Measuring sleep. In Frank-Stromborg M, Olsen SJ, editors: *Instruments for clinical health-care research*, ed 3, Boston, 2004, Jones & Bartlett.

McCance KL, et al, editors: *Pathophysiology: the biologic basis for disease in adults and children*, ed 6, St Louis, 2010, Mosby.

National Institute of Child Health and Human Development: *Safe to sleep public education campaign*, 2013, http://www.nichd.nih.gov/sts/about/Pages/default.aspx. Accessed November 7, 2013.

National Sleep Foundation: *Aging and sleep*, Washington, DC, 2009, http://www.sleepfoundation.org/article/sleep-topics/aging-and-sleep. Accessed December 23, 2013.

National Sleep Foundation: *Depression and sleep*, 2010, http://sleepfoundation.org/article/sleep-topics/depression-and-sleep. Accessed July 11, 2013.

National Sleep Foundation: *Annual sleep in America poll exploring connections with communications technology use and sleep*, 2011a, http://www.sleepfoundation.org/article/press-release/annual-sleep-america-poll-exploring-connections-communications-technology-use-. Accessed July 24, 2012.

National Sleep Foundation: *Epworth sleepiness scale*, 2011b, http://www.sleepfoundation.org/sleep-scale. Accessed July 11, 2013.

National Sleep Foundation: *Napping*, 2013a, http://www.sleepfoundation.org/article/sleep-topics/napping. Accessed July 12, 2013.

National Sleep Foundation: *Restless legs syndrome (RLS) and sleep*, 2013b, http://www.sleepfoundation.org/article/sleep-related-problems/restless-legs-syndrome-rls-and-sleep. Accessed July 11, 2013.

National Sleep Foundation: *Sleep apnea and sleep*, Washington, DC, 2013c, The Foundation, available at http://www.sleepfoundation.org/article/sleep-topics/sleep-apnea-and-sleep. Accessed December 23, 2013.

Neikrug AB, Ancoli-Israel S: Sleep disorders in the older adult: a mini review, *Gerontology* 56:181, 2010.

Noland H, et al: Adolescents' sleep behaviors and perceptions of sleep, *J School Health* 79(5):224, 2009.

Ohlmann KK, O'Sullivan MI: The costs of short sleep, *AAOHN J* 57(9):381, 2009.

Reeve K, Bailes B: Insomnia in adults: etiology and management, *J Nurs Pract* 6(1):53, 2010.

Richardson A, et al: Development and implementation of a noise reduction intervention programme: pre- and post-audit of three hospital wards, *J Clin Nurs* 18:3316, 2009.

Ross C, et al: Association between insomnia symptoms and weight change in older women: caregiver osteoporotic fractures study, *J Am Geriatr Soc* 59(9):1697, 2011.

Sobralske MC, Gruber ME: Risks and benefits of parent/child bed sharing, *J Am Acad Nurse Pract* 21(9):474, 2009.

Touhy T, Jett K: *Ebersole & Hess' toward healthy aging: human needs and nursing response*, ed 8, St Louis, 2011, Mosby.

University of Maryland Medical Center: *Insomnia*, 2012, http://umm.edu/health/medical/altmed/condition/insomnia. Accessed December 26, 2013.

University of Maryland Medical Center Sleep Disorders Center: *Sleep disorders*, 2013, http://www.umm.edu/sleep/sleep_dis_main.htm. Accessed December 23, 2013.

US Food and Drug Administration: *FDA requests label change for all sleep disorder drug products*, 2007, http://www.fda.gov/newsevents/newsroom/press announcements/2007/ucm108868.htm. Accessed December 26, 2013.

Vallido T, et al: Sleep in adolescence: a review of issues for nursing practice, *J Clin Nurs* 18:1819, 2009.

Van der Zee EA, et al: The neurobiology of circadian rhythms, *Curr Opin Pulm Med* 14:534, 2009.

Van Kerrebroeck P: Nocturia: current status and future perspectives, *Curr Opin Obstet Gynecol* 23(5):376, 2011.

Xie H, Kang J, Mills GH: Clinical review: The impact of noise on patients' sleep and the effectiveness of noise reduction strategies in intensive care units, *Crit Care* 13(2):208, 2009.

CHAPTER

32

Pain Management

evolve WEBSITE

http://evolve.elsevier.com/Potter/essentials

- Video Clip
- Crossword Puzzle
- Audio Glossary

OBJECTIVES

- Discuss common misconceptions about pain.
- Describe the physiology of pain.
- Identify components of the pain experience.
- Assess a patient experiencing pain.
- Develop appropriate nursing diagnoses for a patient in pain.
- Describe guidelines for selecting and individualizing pain therapies.
- Describe applications for use of nonpharmacological pain therapies.
- Discuss nursing implications for administering analgesics.
- Describe interventions for the relief of acute pain following operative or medical procedures.
- Describe the sequence of treatments recommended in pain management for cancer patients.
- Evaluate a patient's response to pain therapies.

KEY TERMS

analgesics, p. 889
cutaneous stimulation, p. 887
endorphins, p. 871
epidural infusion, p. 892
guided imagery, p. 888
local anesthesia, p. 891
nociceptor, p. 870
opioid, p. 889
patient-controlled analgesia (PCA), p. 876
prostaglandins, p. 870
relaxation, p. 888
transcutaneous electrical nerve stimulation (TENS), p. 887

Providing comfort is central to the art of nursing. All patients bring physiological, sociocultural, spiritual, psychological, and environmental characteristics that influence how they interpret and experience comfort. An understanding of comfort gives you, as the nurse, a larger range of choices when selecting pain therapies. Pain management is more than administering analgesics. First you need to understand how the pain experience affects a patient's ability to function and then use therapies that meet the unique needs of patients (Pasero and McCaffery, 2011).

Congress declared 2000 to 2010 the Decade of Pain Control and Research, yet pain continues to be a leading public health problem in the United States. According to the American Bar Association (2009), pain management is a basic right of people who are seriously ill. The Joint Commission (TJC) (2005) amended the Patients' Bill of Rights, with

CASE STUDY *Mrs. Ellis*

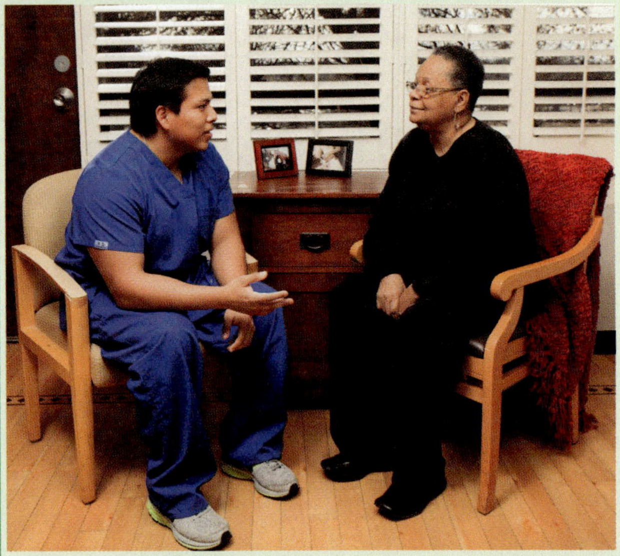

Mrs. Ellis is a 70-year-old African-American woman with hypertension, diabetes, and rheumatoid arthritis. She is receiving care following her recent hospitalization to control her diabetes. Her current health priority is the discomfort and disability associated with her rheumatoid arthritis. Arthritis has severely deformed her hands and feet. The pain in her feet is so severe that Mrs. Ellis often walks only short distances. The pain interferes with sleep and reduces her energy both physically and emotionally. As a result she does not leave her home often. She has lived alone since her husband's death 6 years ago.

Jim is a 26-year-old nursing student assigned to do home visits with the community health nurse. Jim conducts assessments, performs procedures, and teaches health promotion to a variety of patients with various illnesses. This is Jim's first experience caring for a patient with severe chronic pain.

a key component being the right to pain assessment and management. As a nurse you are legally and ethically responsible for managing patients' pain and suffering.

SCIENTIFIC KNOWLEDGE BASE

Nature of Pain

Pain is more than a single physiological sensation caused by a specific stimulus. It is subjective and highly individualized. The person having pain is the only authority on it. According to McCaffery's classic definition, "Pain is whatever the experiencing person says it is, existing whenever he says it does" (McCaffery, 1979). Acute pain is a physiological mechanism that protects an individual from a harmful stimulus. It warns of tissue damage and alerts the body to protect itself. Inability to express pain because of aphasia, airway intubation, or mental status changes does not mean that a patient is not having it. Careful pain assessment is critical. Some patients such as those with spinal cord injuries are

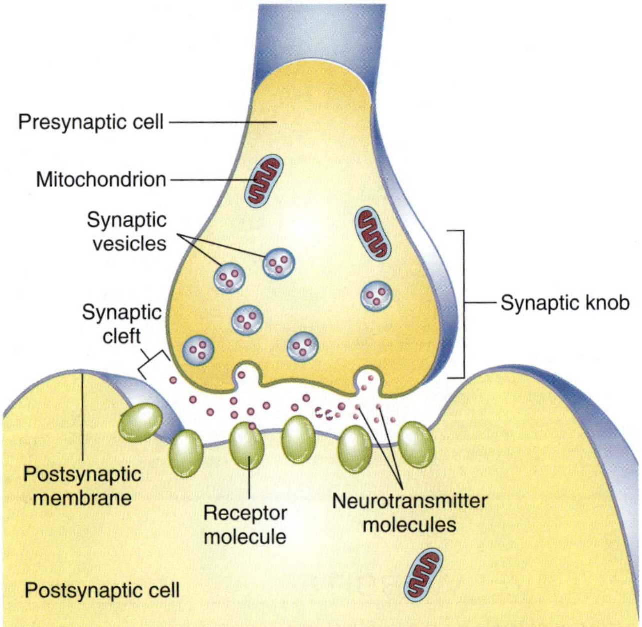

FIGURE 32-1 Chemical synapses involve transmitter chemicals (neurotransmitters) that signal postsynaptic cells. (From Patton KT, Thibodeau GA: *Anatomy & Physiology*, ed 7, St Louis, 2010, Mosby.)

unable to sense painful stimuli. You must take special precautions to protect them from additional injury (Pasero and McCaffery, 2011).

Physiology of Pain

There are four physiological processes of normal pain: transduction, transmission, perception, and modulation (Pasero and McCaffery, 2011). A patient in pain cannot discriminate among the processes. Understanding each process helps you recognize factors that cause pain and the rationale for therapies.

Transduction. Thermal (e.g., burn or frostbite), mechanical (e.g., surgical incision), or chemical (e.g., leakage of hydrochloric acid out of the stomach) injuries release stimuli that cause pain. Transduction converts energy produced by these stimuli into electrical energy. The process begins in the periphery when a pain-producing stimulus sends an impulse across a sensory peripheral pain nerve fiber (**nociceptor**), initiating an action potential. Once transduction is complete, transmission of a pain impulse begins.

Transmission. Cellular damage from thermal, mechanical, or chemical injury results in the release of excitatory neurotransmitters such as **prostaglandins**, histamine, bradykinin, and substance P (Figure 32-1). These pain-sensitizing substances surround the pain fibers in the extracellular fluid, spreading the pain message and causing an inflammatory response (Pasero and McCaffery, 2011). The pain stimulus enters the spinal cord via the dorsal horn and travels one of several routes until ending within the gray matter of the spinal cord. At the dorsal horn substance P is released, causing a synaptic transmission from the afferent (sensory) nerve to

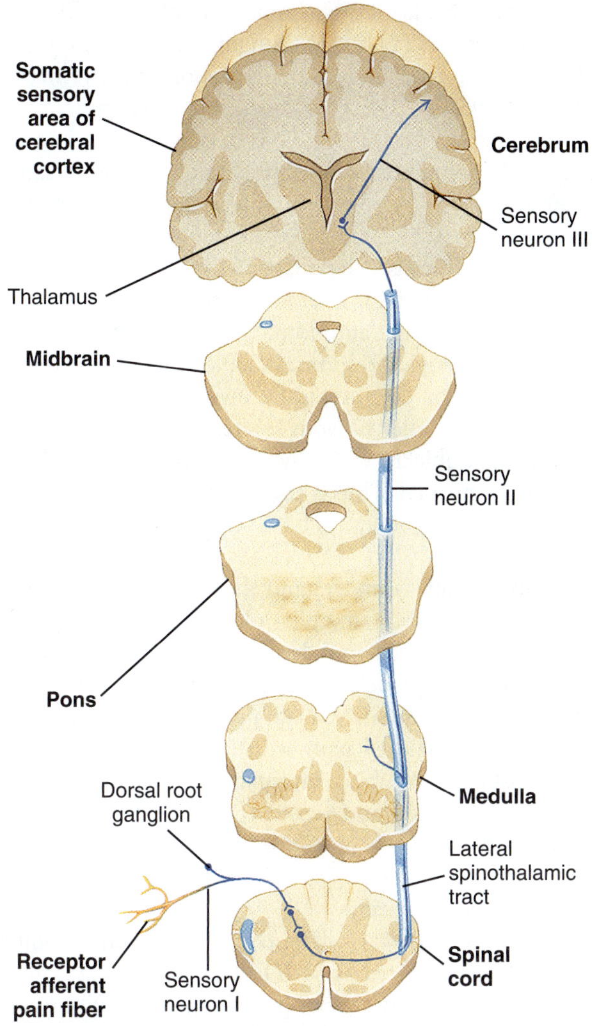

FIGURE 32-2 Spinothalamic pathway that conducts pain stimuli to the brain.

spinothalamic tract nerves, which cross to the opposite side (Pasero and McCaffery, 2011) (Figure 32-2).

Nerve impulses travel along afferent peripheral nerve fibers. Two types of peripheral nerve fibers conduct painful stimuli: the fast, myelinated A-delta fibers and the small, slow unmyelinated C fibers. The A fibers send sharp, localized, and distinct sensations that specify the source of the pain and detect its intensity. The small C fibers relay slower impulses that are poorly localized, visceral, and persistent. For example, after stepping on a nail, the person initially feels a sharp localized pain, which is the result of A-fiber transmission, or first pain. Within a few minutes the whole foot aches from C-fiber stimulation, or second pain.

Pain impulses travel up the spinal cord (see Figure 32-2). After the pain impulse ascends the spinal cord, the thalamus transmits information to higher centers in the brain, including the limbic, somatosensory cortex, and association cortex, where pain perception occurs.

Perception. As a pain impulse ascends to the brain, the central nervous system extracts information such as location, duration, and quality of the pain impulse. Psychological and cognitive factors interact with neurophysiological ones. The thalamus is the first structure in the brain to process the impulse. It sends the impulse to many areas in the brain, including the cerebral cortex, hypothalamus, and limbic system. Thus a person becomes aware of the experience of pain and attaches meaning to it. There is no one "pain center" in the brain that supports the complex nature of pain. Any factor that interrupts or influences normal pain perception such as normal fatigue, depression, or an analgesic affects a person's awareness and response to pain.

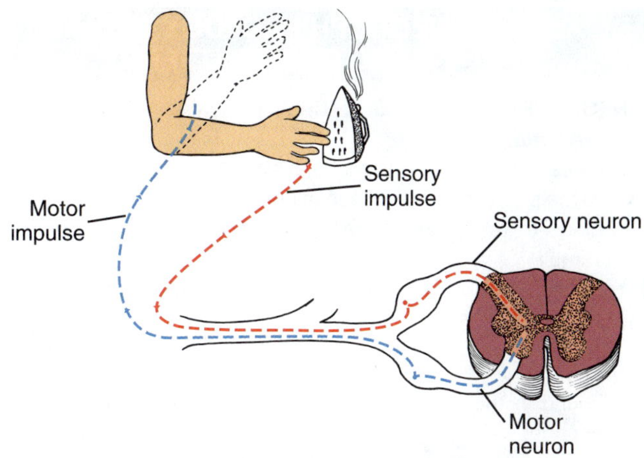

FIGURE 32-3 Protective pain reflex. Sensory impulse directly stimulates motor nerves, bypassing brain and causing withdrawal from pain stimulus.

Modulation. When a person perceives a harmful impulse, the brain releases inhibitory neurotransmitters such as endogenous opioids, serotonin, norepinephrine, and gamma-aminobutyric acid (GABA). The neurotransmitters hinder the transmission of pain to help produce an analgesic effect (Pasero and McCaffery, 2011).

A protective reflex response also occurs with pain (Figure 32-3). When a person is injured, a noxious stimulus from the skin travels along sensory neurons to the dorsal horn of the spinal cord where it synapses with spinal motor neurons. The impulse continues to travel along the spinal nerve to the skeletal muscle, causing the person to withdraw from the source of the pain.

Pain processes require an intact peripheral nervous system and spinal cord. Common factors that disrupt the pain experience include trauma, drugs, tumor growth, and metabolic disorders.

Neurotransmitters. Neurotransmitters are substances that affect the sending of nerve stimuli (Box 32-1). They either excite or inhibit nerve transmission. Excitatory neurotransmitters such as substance P send electrical impulses across the synaptic cleft between two nerve fibers, enhancing the transmission of the painful impulse. Inhibitory neurotransmitters such as **endorphins** decrease neuron activity without directly transferring a nerve signal through a synapse. Researchers believe that endorphins act indirectly by increasing or decreasing the effects of neurotransmitters. Pain perception is influenced by balancing neurotransmitters and by the

BOX 32-1 NEUROPHYSIOLOGY OF PAIN: NEUROTRANSMITTERS

NEUROTRANSMITTERS (EXCITATORY)

Bradykinin

- Released from plasma that leaks from surrounding blood vessels at the site of tissue injury
- Binds to receptors on peripheral nerves, increasing pain stimuli
- Binds to cells that cause the chain reaction producing prostaglandins

Substance P

- Found in the pain neurons of the dorsal horn (excitatory peptide)
- Needed to transmit pain impulses from the periphery to higher brain centers
- Causes vasodilation and edema

Serotonin

- Released from the brainstem and dorsal horn to inhibit pain transmission

Prostaglandins

- Generated through the breakdown of phospholipids in cell membranes
- Increase sensitivity to pain

NEUROTRANSMITTERS (INHIBITORY)

Endorphins, Enkephalins, and Dynorphins

- Natural supply of morphinelike substances in the body
- Activated by stress and pain
- Located within the brain, spinal cord, and gastrointestinal tract
- Cause analgesia when they attach to opiate receptors in the brain
- Present in high levels in people who have less pain than others with a similar injury

descending pain-control fibers originating from the cerebral cortex (Lehne, 2010).

Gate Control Theory of Pain. The gate control theory gives you a way to understand pain-relief measures. The gate control theory of Melzack and Wall (1996) suggests that gating mechanisms along the central nervous system can regulate and possibly block pain impulses. The gating mechanism occurs within the spinal cord, thalamus, reticular formation, and limbic system. The brain determines whether the gate will be open or closed, either increasing or decreasing the intensity of the ascending pain impulse. The theory suggests that pain impulses pass through when the gate is open and not while it is closed. Closing the gate is the basis for nonpharmacological pain-relief interventions. The gate control theory suggests the importance of psychological variables (thoughts and feelings) and physiological sensations in the perception of pain. Using psychological, physiological, and/or pharmacological interventions to close the gate lowers pain intensity. For example, therapies such as exercise, heat, cold, massage, and transcutaneous electrical nerve stimulation (TENS) are thought to release endorphins, which close the gate and reduce perception of pain (Melzack and Wall, 1996).

Physiological Responses. When acute pain impulses travel up the spinal cord toward the brainstem and thalamus, the autonomic nervous system is stimulated as part of the stress response. Acute pain of low-to-moderate intensity and superficial pain cause the fight-or-flight response of the general adaptation syndrome. Acute stimulation of the sympathetic branch of the autonomic nervous system results in transient physiological responses (Table 32-1). If pain is unrelenting, severe, or deep, typically involving visceral organs, the parasympathetic nervous system is activated. Most patients adapt quickly, with physical signs such as vital signs returning to normal. Thus a patient in pain, especially persistent pain, does not always have physical signs (Pasero and McCaffery, 2011).

It is important to understand that patients with chronic pain do not have the same physiological responses as those with acute pain. They do not demonstrate autonomic or sympathetic nervous system reactions. In addition, if you do not treat acute pain adequately, it can progress to chronic pain. It appears that unrelieved pain sensitizes and changes nerves (neuroplasticity), resulting in enhanced intensity, duration, and distribution of pain (Arnstein, 2007). These permanent neuroplastic changes contribute to the development of chronic pain syndromes. Chronic pain is not simply acute pain that lasts a long time.

Behavioral Responses. The response to pain is complex and variable, influenced by such factors as a person's culture, experiences with pain, meaning of pain, and ability to cope with stress. Be familiar with behavioral responses to pain. Clenching the teeth, facial grimacing, holding or guarding the painful part, and bent posture are common indications of acute pain. Chronic pain affects a patient's activity (eating, sleeping, hygiene, social interactions), thinking (confusion, forgetfulness, helplessness), or emotions (anger, depression, irritability, frustration) and quality of life and productivity (IOM, 2011). Recognizing a patient's unique response to pain is important in assessing the success of the pain-management plan. Some patients choose not to report pain if they believe that it inconveniences others or if it signals loss of self-control. Encourage your patients to accept pain-relieving measures so they remain active and involved in daily activities. In contrast, other patients seek relief before pain occurs, having learned that prevention is easier than treatment. Unless a patient openly reacts to pain, it is difficult to assess the nature and extent of the discomfort. Help patients communicate their pain response effectively and do not question their report of pain (Pasero and McCaffery, 2011).

Acute and Chronic Pain

Chronic pain is a common and expensive twenty-first century health care problem. Estimates are that over one million people in the United States suffer from chronic pain, at an annual cost of $560 to $630 billion (IOM, 2011). The two

TABLE 32-1 **PHYSIOLOGICAL REACTIONS TO ACUTE PAIN**

RESPONSE	CAUSE OR EFFECT
Sympathetic Stimulation*	
Dilation of bronchial tubes and increased respiratory rate	Provides increased oxygen intake
Increased heart rate	Provides increased oxygen transport
Peripheral vasoconstriction (pallor, elevation in blood pressure)	Elevates blood pressure with shift of blood supply from periphery and viscera to skeletal muscles and brain
Increased blood glucose level	Provides additional energy
Diaphoresis	Controls body temperature during stress
Increased muscle tension	Prepares muscles for action
Dilation of pupils	Affords better vision
Decreased gastrointestinal motility	Frees energy for more immediate activity
Parasympathetic Stimulation†	
Pallor	Causes blood supply to shift away from periphery
Muscle tension	Results from fatigue
Decreased heart rate and blood pressure	Results from vagal stimulation
Rapid, irregular breathing	Causes body defenses to fail under prolonged stress of pain
Nausea and vomiting	Causes return of gastrointestinal function
Weakness or exhaustion	Results from expenditure of physical energy

*Pain of low to moderate intensity and superficial pain.
†Severe or deep pain.

types of pain that you observe in patients are acute (transient) and chronic (persistent), which includes cancer and noncancer pain.

Acute/Transient Pain. Acute pain is protective, usually has an identifiable cause, is of short duration, and has limited tissue damage and emotional response. It is common after acute injury, disease, or surgery. Acute pain warns people of injury or disease; thus it is protective. It eventually resolves after the damaged tissue heals. Patients in acute pain are frightened, anxious, and expect relief quickly. Acute pain is self-limiting; therefore the patient knows that an end is in sight. Because it usually has an identifiable cause and is usually of short duration, health care providers are willing to treat it aggressively.

Acute pain seriously threatens a patient's recovery by hampering his or her ability to become active and involved in self-care. This results in prolonged hospitalization from complications such as physical and emotional exhaustion, immobility, sleep deprivation, delayed wound healing, and pulmonary complications. As long as acute pain persists, a patient focuses all of his or her energy on pain relief. Efforts aimed at teaching and motivating a patient toward self-care are often hampered until pain is managed successfully. If not adequately controlled, acute pain can progress to chronic pain (IOM, 2011). When you relieve acute pain, the patient is able to direct full attention toward recovery.

Chronic/Persistent Noncancer Pain. Unlike acute pain, chronic pain is not protective and thus serves no purpose. Chronic pain is prolonged, varies in intensity, and usually lasts longer (typically at least 6 months) than is typically expected or predicted (IOM, 2011). It does not always have an identifiable cause and leads to great personal suffering. Examples of chronic noncancer pain include arthritis, low back pain, myofascial pain, headache, and peripheral neuropathy. Chronic noncancer pain such as low back pain often results from nonprogressive or healed tissue injury. The pain is ongoing and often does not respond to treatment. Chronic pain is a major cause of psychological and physical disability, leading to problems such as job loss, sexual dysfunction, and social isolation. A person with chronic noncancer pain often does not show obvious symptoms and does not adapt to the pain. Associated symptoms include fatigue, insomnia, anorexia, weight loss, apathy, hopelessness, and anger. Health care providers are usually less willing to treat chronic pain with opioids, although a policy statement supports the use of opioids for it (Chou et al., 2009). In addition, the American Society of Anesthesiologists (2010) developed *Practice Guidelines for Chronic Pain Management*, which includes use of opioids. Often a person with chronic pain who consults with numerous health care providers is labeled a drug seeker, when he or she is actually seeking adequate pain relief. Nurses need to discourage patients from having multiple health care providers for treating pain and refer them to specialists. Pain centers use nonpharmacological and pharmacological strategies for a holistic approach to pain management (Pasero and McCaffery, 2011).

Chronic Episodic Pain. Pain that occurs sporadically over an extended period of time is episodic pain. Pain episodes last for hours, days, or weeks. Examples are migraine headaches and pain related to sickle cell crisis.

Cancer Pain. Not all patients with cancer have pain. For those who do, as many as 90% are able to have their pain managed with simple measures (Lehne, 2010). Some patients with cancer have acute and/or chronic pain. The pain is nociceptive and/or neuropathic. Cancer pain is usually caused by tumor progression and related pathological processes, invasive procedures, treatment toxicities, infection, and physical limitations. A patient senses pain at the actual tumor site or distant to the site, called *referred pain*. Always completely assess reports of new pain by a patient with existing pain. Although the treatment of cancer pain has improved, undertreatment continues. One study has shown that women over 65 years of age representative of a cultural minority, with earlier-stage disease, cared for at home, and with high-school education or less are at highest risk of having uncontrolled cancer pain (Fairchild, 2010).

Idiopathic Pain. Idiopathic pain is chronic pain in the absence of an identifiable physical or psychological cause or pain perceived as excessive for the extent of an organic pathological condition. An example of idiopathic pain is complex regional pain syndrome (CRPS). Research is needed to better identify the cause of idiopathic pain, thus leading to more effective treatment (Pasero and McCaffery, 2011).

NURSING KNOWLEDGE BASE

Knowledge, Attitudes, and Beliefs

Knowledge of nurses and other health care providers affects pain management. Often they have preconceptions about patients in pain. Some do not believe that their patients are experiencing pain unless a patient shows objective signs of pain. These assumptions about patients in pain influence your nursing assessment and seriously limit your ability to offer pain relief. Too often nurses allow misconceptions about pain (Box 32-2) to affect their willingness to provide pain relief. Many nurses avoid acknowledging patients' pain because of fear of contributing to medication addiction. These fears and beliefs lead to mistrust, increased patient recovery time, complications and mortality, psychological problems, and cost (Pasero and McCaffery, 2011). Nurses with more than 6 years of experience, higher job motivation, and perceived higher levels of pain-care skills have been shown to be better patient advocates in providing pain management (Vaartio et al., 2009).

The failure of health care providers to assess pain accurately and consistently results in poor pain management and increased patient suffering. National and international organizations have made efforts to correct this problem (AHCPR, 1992; APS, 2012). TJC (2013) has a pain standard that requires health care workers to assess all patients for pain on a regular basis. Many health care institutions have adopted this standard by recommending that pain be assessed as the "fifth vital sign" (APS, 2012). It is important that you develop an awareness of pain when you care for patients. Assess for pain in every patient, select proper therapies, and evaluate the effects of your actions in relieving patients' pain.

BOX 32-2 COMMON BIASES AND MISCONCEPTIONS ABOUT PAIN

- Patients who are knowledgeable about opioids and make regular efforts to obtain them are drug seeking (addicted).
- There is no reason for patients to hurt when you cannot find a physical cause for pain.
- Administering analgesics regularly leads to patients' tolerance and physical drug dependence.
- The amount of tissue damage in an injury accurately indicates pain intensity.
- Health care workers are the best judge of the existence and severity of pain.
- Pain threshold and tolerance are the same for everyone.
- Pain is a natural outcome of growing old.
- Pain perception, or sensitivity, decreases with age.
- You use physical or behavioral signs of pain to verify the existence and severity of pain.
- Patients who fall asleep really do not have pain.

Factors Influencing Pain

To accurately assess and then treat a patient's pain, you need to understand the various factors that influence the pain experience.

Physiological Factors

Age. Developmental differences influence how patients of all ages react to pain. Infants demonstrate pain through crying, changes in vital signs, facial expression, and extremity movement (Herr et al., 2011). Children have trouble understanding pain and any treatments or procedures that cause pain. Children without full vocabularies have difficulty verbally describing and expressing pain to parents or caregivers. Toddlers and preschoolers are unable to recall explanations about pain, or they associate it with experiences that occur in various situations. A child's temperament affects coping with pain.

Typically children are grossly undermedicated for pain. They often describe treatments and procedures as the most difficult part of being sick or in a hospital. Analgesic doses are often too small or given too infrequently to be effective. It is necessary for you to understand a child's response to pain. If a child is too young to speak, observe behavioral changes such as irritability, loss of appetite, unusual quietness, disturbed sleep patterns, restlessness, and rigid posturing as signs of pain (IOM, 2011). If a behavior such as crying changes after a child receives an analgesic, pain was probably the cause of the behavior (Herr et al., 2011).

Pain in adolescents is usually related to an acute condition, considering the high rate of motor vehicle accidents and injuries resulting from violence in this age-group. Pain assessment and any patient education regarding treatments with adolescents must consider the cognitive development and language skills and growth and development needs.

Adults suffer from pain from acute and chronic conditions. Health care providers may be less accepting of reports of severe pain from younger adults than older adults. There may be an expectation of higher tolerance of pain in adults. Concern about drug-seeking behaviors and prescription drug abuse is also common among health care providers (Pasero and McCaffery, 2011).

Pain is not a natural part of aging. Likewise pain perception does not decrease with age. However, older adults have a greater likelihood of developing pathological conditions, which are accompanied by pain. The person in pain, his or her family, and health care providers frequently take these conditions for granted or underestimate the pain. Serious impairment in functional status often accompanies pain in older adults. It potentially reduces mobility, activities of daily living (ADLs), social activities, and activity tolerance (Pasero and McCaffery, 2011).

The ability of older patients to interpret pain is complicated. They use words such as *hurting* or *aching* instead of the word *pain* to describe their pain. Older adults sometimes also have more than one painful site. They often hesitate to discuss their pain because of concerns about bothering their health care providers. Frequently older adults adopt a fatalistic attitude toward pain and think that they simply must endure it. These barriers contribute to their inadequate pain management. A patient with cognitive impairment or who is nonverbal (aphasic or mental status changes) has trouble communicating pain and providing a detailed description. You must attempt to assess pain by observing physical and behavioral cues (Herr et al., 2011).

Multiple diseases and vague symptoms affecting similar parts of the body further complicate the ability of older adults to interpret pain. When older patients have more than one source of pain, be sure to gather detailed assessments. Different diseases cause similar symptoms. For example, the patient who has had a below-knee amputation continues to perceive pain from the foot that has been amputated (phantom pain) and has suture-line pain from the surgery. The patient who has had a stroke sometimes has pain in the paralyzed arm and in areas of the body unaffected by the stroke (IOM, 2011).

Fatigue. Fatigue heightens pain perception. If it occurs along with sleeplessness, the perception of pain is even greater. Patients describe fatigue as feeling tired, weak, worn-out, heavy, slow, or having no energy or get-up-and-go. When a healthy person is tired because of day-to-day activities, the fatigue can be relieved by sleep and rest. Cancer-related fatigue is different. Cancer patients become more tired after less activity (e.g., even something as simple as unloading a bag of groceries or cooking a simple meal) than people who do not have cancer (National Cancer Institute [NCI], 2013).

Neurological Function. A patient's neurological function influences his or her pain experience. Any factor that interrupts or influences normal pain reception or perception (e.g., spinal cord injury, peripheral neuropathy) affects a patient's awareness of and response to pain.

Gender. Research on pain in men and women demonstrates differences in occurrence and response to pain related to gender. Chronic pain conditions occur more in women than men. This is related to the fact that some chronic pain conditions such as endometriosis occur only in women and some such as chronic fatigue syndrome and fibromyalgia occur predominately in women. Complaints of headache and joint pain are more common in women than men. This may be related to hormonal effects and inadequate coping strategies. Women also report adverse drug reactions to pain medications more frequently than men (IOM, 2011).

Social Factors

Attention. The degree to which a patient focuses attention on pain influences pain perception. Increased attention has been associated with increased pain, whereas distraction has been associated with decreased pain. You apply this concept when you use nonpharmacological pain-relief therapies such as listening to music and rhythmical breathing. By focusing a patient's attention and concentration on other stimuli, you help turn his or her focus away from the pain. Usually increased tolerance for pain lasts only during the time of distraction.

Previous Experience. All people learn from painful experiences. Previous experience includes pain that a patient has experienced personally and pain that a patient has heard about from someone else. Prior experience does not mean that a person accepts pain more easily in the future. Frequent episodes of pain without relief or bouts of severe pain produce anxiety or fear. In contrast, if a person repeatedly experiences the same type of pain that was successfully relieved in the past, it is easier for him or her to interpret the sensation. As a result the person is better prepared to take steps to relieve the pain. A patient who has had no experience with a particular type of pain sometimes has an impaired ability to cope with it. You prepare patients with a clear explanation of the type of pain that he or she will experience and the methods to reduce it (Vallerand et al., 2007).

Family and Social Support. Patients depend on the support and assistance of family members or friends when coping with pain. Family members sometimes have misconceptions about pain and pain management. Some think patients should wait as long as possible before receiving pain medication and fear the possibility of addiction. It is your responsibility to educate the patient, family, and public about the importance of early assessment and treatment of pain (Pasero and McCaffery, 2011). The presence of a loved one usually minimizes loneliness and fear when a patient is experiencing pain. Absence of social support often makes the pain experience more stressful. The presence of parents is especially important for children in pain. Patients of different sociocultural groups have different expectations of people to whom they report their pain.

Spiritual Factors. Spirituality is an active searching for meaning to situations in which one finds oneself. Spiritual questions include, "Why has this happened to me?" "Why am I suffering?" Often spiritual concerns include the loss of

BOX 32-3 PATIENT-CENTERED CARE

Pain has both personal and cultural meanings. This influences the verbal expression of pain, individual reaction to pain, and pain treatment preferences. Disparities in pain perception, assessment, and treatment occur in all settings.

IMPLICATIONS FOR PRACTICE

- Undertreatment of pain is a risk often related to cultural differences.
- Ask a patient which word she or he prefers to use to describe pain. Many patients use *hurt* or *ache* to describe mild or moderate pain, reserving the word *pain* for severe discomfort.
- Use language-specific pain-intensity tools; these tools are available in many languages.
- Cultural responses to pain are often divided into two categories: stoic and emotive. One is not better than the other. Health care providers need to appreciate cultural variations of verbal and nonverbal responses to pain to accurately assess it.
- Health care providers are more likely to respond to communication about pain by an individual of the same cultural background and have less understanding of pain in patients from a different culture.
- Recognize that communicating pain is not always acceptable within a culture.
- The meaning of pain differs among people of different cultures. Some people view pain as a punishment for the past, a part of life, or something to endure to enter heaven or progress to the next life.
- Biological variations of drug metabolism, dosing requirements, therapeutic response, and adverse effects are a function of race and ethnicity. It is important to assess the response to analgesics and not assume that an inadequate response is a nonadherence issue.
- Health care providers' beliefs about cultural groups and attitude toward pain influence pain management. Self-awareness of potential cultural bias is essential to provide adequate pain management.

Data from Pasero C, McCaffery M: *Pain assessment and pharmacologic management,* St Louis, 2011, Mosby; Narayan MC: Culture's effects on pain assessment and management, *Am J Nurs* 110(4):38, 2010.

independence and becoming a burden to one's family. Be sensitive to a patient's spiritual needs and consider referral to a pastoral care professional (see Chapter 21).

Cultural Factors. Culture influences how people perceive the causes and meaning of pain. Their cultural background influences their reaction to and expression of pain. Understanding cultural background and personal characteristics helps you more accurately assess pain and its meaning for patients (Box 32-3). People from some cultures appear to have a higher pain tolerance and avoid vocalizing to express their pain, whereas other cultures are more expressive with moaning and crying. The words used to describe pain may vary in other cultures. When the patient does not speak the same language as you, you may find that their language does not have a word equivalent to "pain." Understanding your own values, personal biases, and assumptions about pain helps you become culturally sensitive to others (Narayan, 2010). Many references are available from reputable sources to identify cultural-specific responses to pain.

Psychological Factors

Meaning of Pain. The meaning that a patient attributes to pain affects the pain experience. Patients perceive pain differently if it suggests a threat, loss, punishment, or challenge. The degree and quality of pain perceived by a patient are related to its meaning (Narayan, 2010).

Anxiety. High anxiety levels increase pain perception, and pain causes anxiety. Autonomic arousal patterns are similar in pain and anxiety. Patients who worry about symptoms that are minor or do not exist have health anxiety. The presence of health anxiety in patients who have chronic pain negatively influences their response to pain and its associated treatments (Bruckenthal, 2008). Nurses act to reduce health anxiety levels to lower pain perception.

Depression. The incidence of depression is very high in patients with chronic pain. They experience many losses such as their ability to enjoy life, be in control, work, socialize, and be independent (Jann and Slade, 2007). Suicidal thoughts are relatively common; therefore you need to routinely assess for suicidal tendencies (Menefee-Pujol, Katz, and Zacharoff, 2007). As a nurse be aware of the possibility of depression in patients with persistent pain and suggest a referral if symptoms of major depression emerge.

Coping Style. Pain can be lonely for some. Frequently patients feel a loss of control over their environment or the outcome of events. Coping style influences the ability to cope with pain. Patients with internal loci of control perceive themselves as having personal control over their environments and the outcome of events. They ask questions, desire information, and like choices of treatment. In contrast, patients with external loci of control perceive other factors in their environments such as nurses as being responsible for the outcome of events. These patients tend to be less demanding, follow directions, and are more passive in managing their pain. They want specific instructions but become anxious if you give them too much information (Vallerand et al., 2007). Frequently those with internal loci of control report less severe pain than those with external loci. This concept is applied in the use of **patient-controlled analgesia (PCA).**

CRITICAL THINKING

Synthesis

You will apply elements of critical thinking whenever you perform the nursing process with patients. Consider the scientific knowledge you have learned, your experience, critical thinking attitudes, and standards to ensure an individualized approach to patient care (Box 32-4).

Knowledge. It is important that you apply knowledge about the physiology of pain, along with the physiology of any underlying disease processes, to understand a patient's

BOX 32-4 SYNTHESIS IN PRACTICE

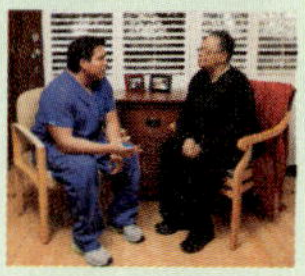

Jim is preparing for tomorrow's home care visit with Mrs. Ellis. He reviews what he has learned about pain physiology and the pathophysiology of rheumatoid arthritis. This allows him to anticipate the need to carefully assess to what extent pain limits Mrs. Ellis's ability to walk and perform activities of daily living.

Jim plans to assess the location, duration, and aggravating and relieving factors influencing Mrs. Ellis's pain and any behavioral symptoms he observes. He plans to determine the pain scale that Mrs. Ellis prefers to assess the baseline for the severity of her pain. Because Mrs. Ellis is 70, Jim reviews gerontological principles and knows that he needs to take time to establish a trusting relationship to encourage the complete description of the pain experience. Jim recalls previous experiences with patients in chronic pain and interventions used to relieve pain. He remembers his own experiences with pain after suffering a broken arm during a soccer game. These experiences make him sensitive to the personal and dynamic nature of each individual's pain experience.

Jim considers the AHRQ and APS guidelines for the management of chronic pain. He wants to carefully clarify with Mrs. Ellis the extent to which the chronic arthritic pain and the acute exacerbations have affected her life. If Jim is to help her with pain relief and health promotion activities, he needs to learn as much as he can about Mrs. Ellis's lifestyle and the support systems that are available for her. Because Mrs. Ellis lives alone, Jim wants to assess if family or friends who can offer assistance live nearby.

pain response, type of pain, and interventions needed for pain management. Knowledge and application of communication skills enhance the thoroughness of a pain assessment. Once you have a clear picture of the physiological nature of a patient's condition, synthesis of knowledge regarding his or her psychological and sociocultural perspective becomes critical for an individualized approach to care. In addition, an understanding of pharmacological and nonpharmacological therapies helps you to work with a patient and health care provider in selecting pain therapies (Pasero and McCaffery, 2011).

Experience. Caring for patients who have pain is an important part of a nurse's clinical experience. Because pain is so common, you soon learn that patients vary widely in their expressions of pain. The degree of pain affects their behaviors and the actions they take to find relief. Such experience either positively or negatively affects your willingness to begin pain interventions. Furthermore, your own experience with pain emphasizes the importance of having someone who is supportive and understanding. Reflecting on the experiences of caring for those in pain helps you search for better approaches for each new patient you meet.

Attitudes. Critical thinking attitudes ensure that you make decisions that are fair and responsible. When a patient is in pain, you need perseverance to find an approach that offers him or her some degree of relief. Quick solutions without follow-up aggravate a patient's discomfort. Learn as much as possible about a patient's pain, try various interventions, and continue different creative approaches until you discover an effective one. Accept a patient's report of pain (Pasero and McCaffery, 2011), even if you question the severity of the pain reported. At times you are concerned about patients trying to fool you. By acting according to your professional standards and guidelines and accepting each patient's self-report of pain, you are demonstrating the attitude of integrity. You are also taking responsibility for providing optimal pain management to your patients by using these standards and guidelines.

Standards. The application of intellectual standards is particularly important when completing an accurate pain assessment. A clear, precise, and accurate description of a patient's pain is essential. Ensure that information related to factors influencing a patient's pain is relevant and complete. In addition, have an open mind and listen to all sources affected by his or her experience (patient, family, and friends) to gain a clear picture of what pain means for the patient. This ensures inclusion of all criteria needed for accurate evaluation of the patient's pain experience.

Professional standards, guidelines, and position statements such as those developed by the AHRQ through the National Guidelines Clearinghouse, the American Pain Society (APS), the World Health Organization (WHO), and the American Society of Pain Management Nurses (ASPMN) guide health care professionals in pain management. Originally developed in 2001 and recently released as a fact sheet, TJC (2012) offers three standards for health care organizations to follow in pain management:

- Recognize the right of patients to appropriate assessment and management of pain.
- Screen patients for pain during their initial assessment and, when clinically required, during ongoing, periodic reassessments.
- Educate patients suffering from pain and their families about pain management.

Apply these guidelines when making decisions about pain therapies.

NURSING PROCESS

ASSESSMENT

The comprehensive assessment of pain aims to gather information about the cause of a person's pain and determine its effect on his or her ability to function. Accurate and factual pain assessment is necessary for determining a patient's responses, arriving at proper nursing diagnoses, and selecting appropriate therapies (Table 32-2). Pain assessment is one of the most frequent and difficult activities you perform. It is important to carefully interpret pain cues and remember that psychological and physical components of pain influence a patient's reaction to it.

When assessing pain, be sensitive to a patient's level of discomfort and determine which level will allow your patient to function. For example, ask a patient in pain, "Which level

TABLE 32-2 FOCUSED PATIENT ASSESSMENT

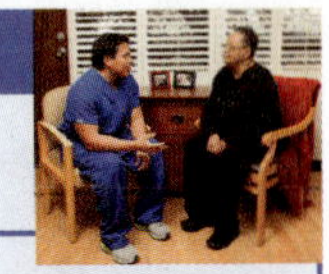

FACTORS TO ASSESS	QUESTIONS	PHYSICAL ASSESSMENT
Location of pain	Where is the pain located? Can you point to where the pain is?	Depending on area of pain, use inspection to determine if body part is swollen, discolored, or warm to touch. Have patient use hand to locate area where pain originates and then spreads. Use light palpation over area identified by patient.
Aggravating factors	Does your pain get worse when you move? Do you do other things that make your pain worse? Does anything make the pain better?	When positioning body part aggravates pain, determine if range of motion is altered. Observe patient's facial expression and movement when patient attempts activity that typically aggravates pain.

TABLE 32-3 IMPLICATIONS OF PAIN ASSESSMENT FOR NURSING INTERVENTIONS

ASSESSMENT CRITERIA (PQRSTU)	NURSING INTERVENTIONS
Palliative or Provocative factors—What makes your pain worse or better?	Avoid activities that cause or aggravate pain. Teach patient or family to avoid these activities.
Quality—How do you describe your pain?	Suggest changing pharmacological interventions if the quality of pain (neuropathic vs. nociceptive) changes.
Relief measures—What do you take at home to gain pain relief?	Use measures that patient uses to relieve pain as long as they are safe and appropriate.
Region (location)—Show me where you hurt.	Position patient off affected area. Apply local treatments (e.g., elastic bandage, cold, heat, splinting) directly over painful site.
Severity—On a scale of 0 to 10, with 10 being worst, how bad is your pain now?	Change or revise interventions, depending on success of one intervention in reducing severity.
Timing (onset, duration, and pattern)—Is your pain constant, intermittent, or both?	Administer analgesics so peak action occurs when pain is most acute (e.g., during dressing change or exercise therapy).
U (effect of pain on patient)—What are you not able to do because of your pain?	Schedule activities that are important to patient during time of day when he or she feels pain least.

of pain on a scale of 0 to 10 (with 10 being worst pain ever) allows you to walk down the hall?" If the patient answers that walking is possible when it is at a level of 2, you then focus efforts on decreasing pain to that level. If pain is acutely severe, it is unlikely that the patient will provide detailed information. During an episode of acute pain you primarily assess its location, severity (what the pain feels like now), and quality. Collect a more detailed assessment when the patient is more comfortable, using the PQRSTU characteristics of pain (Table 32-3). A more comprehensive pain assessment takes time; you do this when the patient becomes more alert and attentive.

Pain is not static but always changing. Monitor it on a regular basis along with other vital signs. Many institutions now treat pain as the fifth vital sign. Pain assessment is *not* simply a number. Relying solely on a number is unsafe (APS, 2012). Although pain assessment is a nursing function, nursing assistive personnel (NAP) also screen for pain and are responsible for informing registered nurses immediately when a patient is having pain. This allows a nurse to confirm the assessment and provide appropriate therapy.

For patients with chronic pain focus assessment on the emotional impact and meaning of the experience and on its history and context. In addition, assessment includes level of function because it is sometimes impossible to achieve complete pain relief. The AHCPR has recommended that families of patients with cancer learn how to assess pain so they promote continuity of effective pain management (Box 32-5) (Jacox et al., 1994). In the home setting family members' involvement in pain assessment offers patients and families control over their experience. Be aware of possible errors in pain assessment. Bias (overestimating or underestimating level of pain), vague or unclear assessment questions, and use of unreliable or invalid pain assessment tools do not provide accurate data. Family estimates of the patient's pain are not always accurate. Use them only when the patient is unable to verbalize pain intensity.

Patient's Expression of Pain. A patient's self-report of pain is the single most reliable indicator of its existence and intensity (Pasero and McCaffery, 2011). However, patients often fail to report or discuss pain. To complicate assessment, nurses frequently believe that patients will report pain if they

BOX 32-5 ROUTINE CLINICAL APPROACH TO PAIN ASSESSMENT AND MANAGEMENT (ABCDE)

A ***Ask*** about pain regularly.
Assess pain systematically.
B ***Believe*** patient and family in their report of pain and what relieves it.
C ***Choose*** pain control options appropriate for patient, family, and setting.
D ***Deliver*** interventions in timely, logical, and coordinated fashion.
E ***Empower*** patients and their families.
Enable them to control their course to the greatest extent possible.

From Jacox A, et al: *Management of cancer pain,* Clinical Practice Guideline No. 9, AHCPR Pub No. 94-0592, Rockville, MD, March 1994, Agency for Health Care Policy and Research, US Department of Health and Human Services, Public Health Service.

have it, but patients often think that the health care providers know about their pain because that is their job. Do not assume that patients are pain free if they do not volunteer their pain intensity. It is important to regularly *ask* patients about pain. In addition, pay attention to the nonverbal ways that patients communicate discomfort (Pasero and McCaffery, 2011). Pain is individualistic. If patients sense that you doubt their pain exists, they share little information with you. Establish a caring relationship that allows for open communication. Refrain from using the phrase *complaining of pain* when discussing a patient's pain. It is better to use words such as *stating, telling,* or *reporting,* which is what the patient is doing.

Patients Unable to Self-Report Pain. Patients unable to communicate effectively often require special attention during assessment. Some examples are the following:

- Infants and children
- Patients who are critically ill and/or unconscious
- Patients with dementia
- Patients who are mute or aphasic
- Patients with an intellectual disability
- Patients at the end of life

These patients all require different assessment approaches. However, be alert for subtle behaviors that indicate pain (Box 32-6). Note a patient's vocal response (e.g., moaning, crying, or gasping), facial movements (e.g., grimacing, clenched teeth, or tightly closed eyes), and body movements (e.g., restlessness, increased hand and finger movements, or pacing), or inactivity. Also assess social interaction. Does the patient avoid conversation or social contacts? Does he or she have a short attention span? Infants, children, and patients with cognitive impairments require simple assessment approaches involving close observation for changes in behavior. Monitor critically ill patients receiving medications that paralyze their muscles because these medications prevent them from being able to communicate their pain verbally or behaviorally. Often proxy pain ratings (i.e., the rating of pain by family members, friends, or those who care for patients or observe their behavior), are useful (Herr et al., 2011). Do not assume that a patient is pain free if he or she is unable to report pain to you.

Characteristics of Pain. Only a patient can describe pain characteristics. Each characteristic presents implications for how you help to manage a patients' pain. The PQRSTU model is an effective tool for assessing pain in adults and determining interventions to relieve the pain (see Table 32-3).

Timing (Onset, Duration, and Pattern). Ask questions to determine the start, duration, and time sequence of pain. When did it begin? How long has it lasted? Does it occur at the same time each day? How often does it recur? It is sometimes easier to diagnose the nature of pain by identifying time factors. The onset of sudden and severe pain is easier to assess than gradual, mild discomfort. Knowing the time cycle of a patient's pain helps you intervene before the pain occurs or worsens.

Precipitating Factors. Determine the specific events or conditions that precipitate or aggravate pain. Ask the patient to describe activities that cause pain such as sitting, bending over, drinking coffee or alcohol, urination, swallowing, or emotional stress. Ask the patient to demonstrate actions that cause painful responses such as coughing or turning in a certain manner. After identifying specific factors, it is easier to plan interventions to avoid worsening the pain.

Quality. There is no common pain vocabulary in general use. Patients describe pain in their own way. Patients of American descent often use *hurt* and *ache* to describe their pain, reserving the word *pain* for severe discomfort. Knowing the quality of pain helps to select appropriate therapies to treat it. When assessing the quality of pain, do not provide descriptive words for a patient. Assessment is more accurate if a patient describes the sensation in his or her own words after open-ended questions. For example, say, "Tell me what your pain feels like." The only time you offer to list descriptive terms is when the patient is unable to describe pain.

There is some consistency in the way patients describe certain types of pain. People often describe the pain of a myocardial infarction (heart attack) as crushing or viselike. Some people describe the pain of a surgical incision as sharp and stabbing. Neuropathic pain is burning or electric-like. When a patient's descriptions fit the pattern forming in your assessment, you are able to make a clearer analysis of the nature and type of pain. This leads to more appropriate pain management (e.g., you treat nociceptive and neuropathic pain differently).

Relief Measures. Make sure that you know if a patient has an effective way of relieving pain such as changing position, using ritualistic behavior (pacing, rocking, or rubbing), eating, praying, or applying heat or cold to a painful site. A patient's methods are often ones that you can use for treatment. Determine if patients use relief measures safely in their home. Patients gain trust when they know you are willing to try their relief measures. They also gain a sense of control over the pain instead of the pain controlling them.

BOX 32-6 EVIDENCE-BASED PRACTICE

PICO Question: Which best practices in pain management for adults with substance use disorders are effective in pain relief compared with traditional pharmacological therapies?

SUMMARY OF EVIDENCE

In 2012 the American Society for Pain Management Nursing (ASPMN) updated its position statement and clinical practice recommendations on managing pain in patients with substance use disorders. In collaboration with the International Nurses Society on Addictions, they state that all patients experiencing pain deserve the right to respect, dignity, and high-quality pain management. Stigmatization, misconceptions, and access to skilled providers are barriers that these patients encounter (Oliver et al., 2012).

APPLICATION TO NURSING PRACTICE

Summary of Recommendations

For all patients with low, moderate, or high risk for addiction:

- Use 10-step Universal Precautions plan for pain.
  1. Pain diagnosis
  2. Psychological assessment
  3. Informed consent
  4. Treatment agreement
  5. Assessment of pain and function before and after interventions
  6. Trial of opioid medications with or without adjunctive medications
  7. Evaluation of pain and function
  8. Consistent assessment of the five "As" of pain medications: analgesia, activity, adverse effects, aberrant behavior, and affect
  9. Regular review of the treatment plan
  10. Documentation of response to plan
- Consider multimodal and integrative therapy options.
- Limit legal liability by using standardized assessment tools and procedures.

For patients at moderate risk (in addition to previous recommendations):

- Use appropriate nonopioid medication and nonpharmacological pain-management interventions as much as possible.
- Do not substitute sedatives for analgesics.
- Do not treat opioid dependence with opioid agonists since this could lead to acute withdrawal.
- Taper medications no longer needed to minimize symptoms of withdrawal.
- Develop a plan for treatment and potential relapse.
- Involve pain and addiction specialists for inpatient management.

For patients at high risk (in addition to previous recommendations):

- Assess patient for drug and alcohol withdrawal and treat as appropriate.
- Provide therapy for patients with whom inappropriate use of prescribed or illicit drugs is suspected or verified.
- Consider termination of treatment for patients who refuse to cooperate with treatment for their substance use disorder.

For nurses, prescribers, and institutions:

- Stay current on new evidence in the areas of pain-management and substance-use disorders.
- Advocate for your patients and provide evidence-based care without bias.
- Use safe prescribing policies with individualization as necessary.
- Monitor processes for quality and efficacy (Oliver et al., 2012).

Assessment also includes identification of all health care providers (e.g., physician, acupuncturist). Patients with chronic pain are more likely to try alternative health care methods.

Region/Location. To assess pain location, ask a patient to point to all areas of discomfort. To localize the pain more specifically, have the patient trace the area from the most severe point outward. This is difficult to do if pain is diffuse, involves several sites, or involves large parts of the body. Use a drawing showing the location of pain as the baseline if the pain changes. Use anatomical landmarks and descriptive terminology to record the pain location (e.g., "Pain is in the right upper abdominal quadrant"). Pain classified by location is superficial or cutaneous, deep or visceral, localized or diffuse, or referred or radiating.

Severity. One of the most subjective and therefore most useful characteristics for reporting pain is its severity or intensity. Nurses use a variety of pain scales to help patients communicate pain intensity. Many are available in foreign languages. Examples of pain intensity scales include the verbal descriptor scale (VDS), the numerical rating scale (NRS), and the visual analog scale (VAS) (Figure 32-4). Use

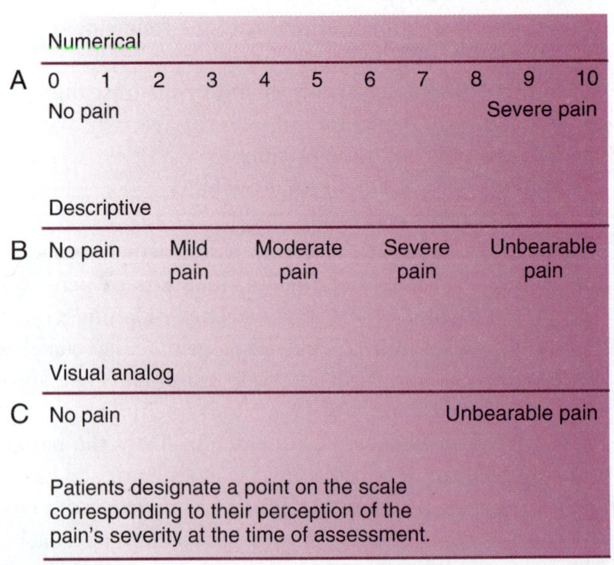

FIGURE 32-4 Sample pain scales. **A,** Numerical. **B,** Descriptive. **C,** Visual analog.

a scale to measure the current severity of a patient's pain. In addition, ask patients to rate their average pain and the worst pain they have had over the past 24 hours. This helps to determine an average pain intensity that allows you to see trends.

An NRS requires patients to rate pain on a line scale of 0 to 10, with 0 representing no pain and 10 representing the worst pain the patient can imagine. These scales work best when assessing pain intensity before and after a therapy (e.g., ambulation or an analgesic). A VDS consists of a line with three to six word descriptors equally spaced along the line. Show the patient the scale and ask him or her to choose the descriptor that best represents the severity of pain. A VAS consists of a straight line without labeled subdivisions. The straight line shows a continuum of intensity and has labeled end points (no pain to pain as bad as it could possibly be). The patient indicates pain by marking the appropriate point on the line (Pasero and McCaffery, 2011).

A good pain scale is easy to use, understandable, and not time consuming. If a patient is able to read and understand a scale easily, the description of pain is more accurate. If patients use a hearing aid or glasses, be sure that they are using them when answering pain-assessment questions or marking the pain scale. Descriptive scales are useful in assessing pain severity and evaluating changes in a patient's condition. Once you select a scale that works for a patient, be sure to use it consistently. Do not use pain-scale ratings to compare one patient to another but only to compare one patient's current pain level to what it was previously.

Several pain scales are available to assess pain in children. Wong and Baker (1988) developed the FACES Pain Rating Scale to assess pain in children (Figure 32-5). The scale shows six cartoon faces ranging from the very happy, smiling face for "no pain" to increasingly less happy faces to the final sad, tearful face for "worst pain." Children as young as 3 years of age can use the scale. The advantage is that patients do not have to interpret the meaning of numbers or adjectives. The faces clearly and quickly depict the concept of pain or discomfort (Pasero and McCaffery, 2011). Another tool designed to measure pain intensity in children is the Oucher pain scale (Beyer et al., 1992). The Oucher consists of two separate scales: the 0 to 100 scale on the left for older children and the six-picture photographic scale on the right for younger children (Figure 32-6). There are Oucher scales for several common ethnic populations. Photographs of the face of a child (in increasing levels of discomfort) are designed to cue children into understanding what pain is and its severity. The child merely points to the selection, simplifying the task of describing the pain. There are additional pain rating tools for older children with verbal skills, neonates, and infants.

Effect of Pain on Patient. Pain alters a person's lifestyle and psychological well-being. For example, chronic/persistent pain causes suffering, loss of control, loneliness, and an impaired quality of life. To understand a patient's pain experience, ask the patient what the pain prevents him or her from doing. Patients who live with daily pain or who have prolonged pain during a hospitalized illness are less able to participate in routine activities, which often leads to physical deconditioning. This deconditioning can slow recovery of the hospitalized patient. Assessment reveals the extent of the disability and the adjustments that will be necessary for participation in self-care (Box 32-7). Establish goals to provide sufficient pain relief to restore the ability to do those activities. Successful pain management results in improved function.

Concomitant Symptoms. Concomitant symptoms occur with pain and usually increase pain intensity. These include nausea, headache, dizziness, urge to urinate, constipation, depression, and restlessness. Certain types of pain have predictable symptoms. For example, severe rectal pain often causes constipation. These symptoms are as much a problem to a patient as the pain itself.

Patient Expectations. Patients rely on their caregivers to recognize and alleviate their physical discomfort. This may involve using a skilled and caring approach, trying a variety of comfort measures, and serving as an advocate for patients. You demonstrate caring when you tailor care to an individual's needs. Always ask patients what they expect regarding their comfort needs. This includes asking not only which interventions they prefer but also how they think you should administer them and how often. It is important to understand if patients expect full pain relief or if they simply hope to have their discomfort reduced. Full pain relief is often not possible. You must explain this to patients and clarify the level of comfort you can provide so their expectations are realistic.

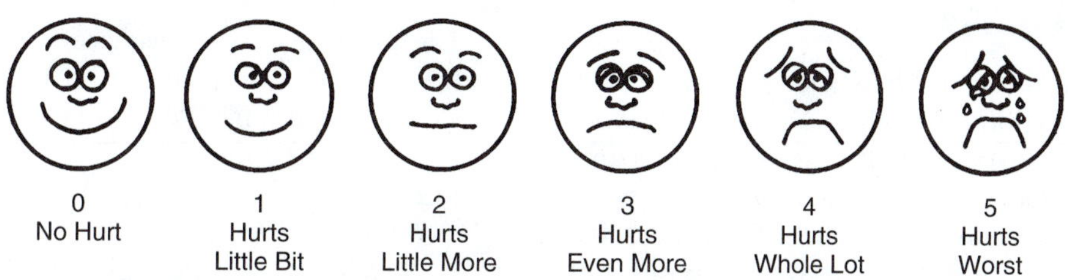

FIGURE 32-5 Wong-Baker FACES Pain Rating Scale. (From Hockenberry MJ, Wilson, D: *Wong's nursing of infants and children,* ed 9, St Louis, 2011, Mosby.)

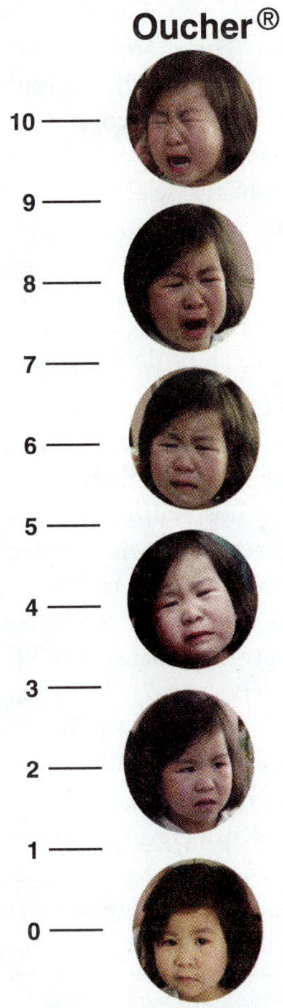

FIGURE 32-6 Asian girl version of Oucher pain scale. (The Asian versions of the Oucher scale [male and female] were developed and copyrighted in 2003 by CH Yeh [University of Pittsburgh] and CH Wang, Taiwan.)

BOX 32-7 ASSESSING THE INFLUENCE OF PAIN ON ACTIVITIES OF DAILY LIVING

SLEEP
- Does the patient have difficulty falling asleep?
- Does pain awaken the patient at night?
- Are sleeping pills or other aids needed?

HYGIENE
- Does pain hinder the patient's ability to bathe, dress, or perform other hygiene measures independently?
- Are family members or friends available or needed to help?

EATING
- Is the patient able to manipulate eating utensils?
- Can the patient chew and swallow without discomfort?

SEXUAL FUNCTIONING
- Do physical conditions such as arthritis or back pain prevent the patient from assuming usual positions during intercourse?
- Does pain or fatigue reduce the patient's desire for sex?
- Is the patient fearful that pain will increase as the result of intercourse?

HOME MANAGEMENT AND WORK ACTIVITIES
- Is the patient able to perform usual housework chores?
- Does the patient's job require physical activity, and does pain limit activity now?
- If pain is related to emotional stress, does the job involve tension-filled decision making?
- Does the patient need to stop activities momentarily to relieve pain?

SOCIAL ACTIVITIES
- Does the patient regularly socialize?
- To what extent has pain disrupted activities?

When your patients ask for assistance because of pain, they expect you to respond promptly.

Documentation. Carefully assess and routinely document your patient's report of pain and the effectiveness of interventions. Use the assessment tool that is appropriate for your patient and always use the same tool to reassess the patient's pain.

NURSING DIAGNOSIS

You identify accurate nursing diagnoses for patients in pain by thorough data collection and analysis. You make an accurate diagnosis after reviewing all of the assessment data and identifying patterns of the defining characteristics. For the diagnosis of *Acute Pain*, you might assess the patient for withdrawal from interacting with others, rigid posturing, moaning, and verbalization of discomfort. In contrast, you make the diagnosis of *Anxiety* by observing the patient's facial tension and appearance, poor eye contact, restlessness, and verbalization of feeling scared. The two diagnoses have similar defining characteristics, but you sort out other defining characteristics (e.g., coded report on a pain scale) to identify patterns to distinguish *Acute Pain* from *Anxiety.*

The related factor for the diagnostic statement focuses on the specific nature of a patient's problem. *Acute Pain related to physical trauma* and *Acute Pain related to natural childbirth processes* require very different nursing interventions. Successful identification of related factors ensures that you direct nursing therapies toward relieving the patient's discomfort.

The following nursing diagnoses are applicable for patients with acute or chronic pain:
- *Risk for Caregiver Role Strain*
- *Ineffective Coping*
- *Fatigue*
- *Impaired Physical Mobility*
- *Acute Pain*
- *Chronic Pain*
- *Bathing Self-Care Deficit*
- *Dressing Self-Care Deficit*
- *Risk For Situational Low Self-Esteem*
- *Social Isolation*

PLANNING

Goals and Outcomes. Develop an individualized plan of care for each nursing diagnosis identified (see Care Plan). Work with a patient and family to set realistic expectations for pain relief. Make sure that the patient understands that complete pain relief is not guaranteed but it will be attempted. Individualize realistic goals for pain relief and levels of function with measurable outcomes (Pasero and McCaffery, 2011). For example, if a patient's baseline assessment reveals a pain severity consistently between 7 and 8 on the VAS, a realistic goal is for the patient to achieve the level of comfort that permits the patient to function. A pain severity outcome of 2 or 3 out of 10 usually allows for improved function or even full pain relief. No pain-rating number offers an absolute guideline for a patient's perceived level of comfort. However, pain ratings of 7 or higher on a 0 to 10 pain scale require urgent action by members of the health care team. In the example for the goal, "The patient will achieve a satisfactory level of pain relief within 24 hours," the following are possible outcomes:

- Reports pain at 3 or less
- Uses relaxation techniques before dressing change
- Able to dress self without a self-report of increased discomfort

CARE PLAN

Chronic Pain

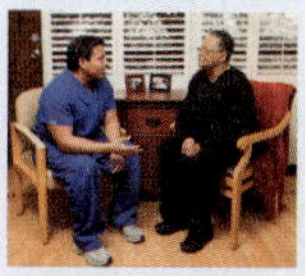

ASSESSMENT

When Jim enters Mrs. Ellis's four-room apartment, he finds the home to be in some disarray. Mrs. Ellis is sitting in the recliner in her living room, with clothing on the floor and soiled dishes on the nearby table. She reports that the pain she has been experiencing has made it very difficult to use her hands and walk between rooms. She is able to get to the bathroom, but it causes her to become fatigued. Her pain is constant and localized in the joints of her hands and knees.

ASSESSMENT ACTIVITIES	FINDINGS/DEFINING CHARACTERISTICS*
Ask Mrs. Ellis to select the pain scale that she prefers and rate her current pain intensity.	She rates the pain at the level of **3 on the FACES Pain Scale of 0 to 10.**
Ask Mrs. Ellis to rate her pain intensity when it is most severe.	She rates the pain at 6 on the FACES Pain Scale of 0 to 10.
Ask Mrs. Ellis what she does to control her pain.	She currently takes aspirin for the pain; but the pain **prevents her from being able to fall asleep;** and, when she does fall asleep, she **often reawakens at night.**
Ask Mrs. Ellis if she has noticed any problems or side effects taking the aspirin.	She reports "burning in the stomach" when she takes the aspirin.
Observe Mrs. Ellis standing and walking to the kitchen. Measure the pain severity.	She has **difficulty standing and an unsteady gait, with pain** at a level of 4.
Ask Mrs. Ellis if she has friends or neighbors available to help her.	She states, "I hate to be a bother, although my next-door neighbor has offered to help in the past."

*__Defining characteristics__ are shown in **bold** type.

NURSING DIAGNOSIS: Chronic Pain related to joint inflammation

PLANNING

GOAL	EXPECTED OUTCOMES (NOC)[†]
	Pain Level
• Mrs. Ellis will report a sense of pain relief within 1 week.	• Mrs. Ellis reports pain at 2 on the FACES Pain Scale of 0 to 10 following relaxation therapy and heat application.
	Pain: Disruptive Effects
• Mrs. Ellis will ambulate with less discomfort on self-report within 14 days.	• Mrs. Ellis demonstrates ability to rise to standing position without help within 1 week. • Mrs. Ellis demonstrates ability to walk from room to room with a walker with steady gait and at a pain severity of 3 or less in 2 weeks.
• Mrs. Ellis will be able to perform activities of daily living with less discomfort within 14 days.	• Mrs. Ellis is able to wash dishes and clean house at a pain severity of 3 or less in 2 weeks.

[†]Outcomes classification label from Moorhead S et al, editors: *Nursing outcomes classification (NOC)*, ed 5, St Louis, 2013, Mosby.

Continued

CARE PLAN—cont'd

Chronic Pain

INTERVENTIONS (NIC)‡	RATIONALE
Analgesic Administration	
• Discuss the possibility of starting a disease-modifying antirheumatic drug (DMRAD) (e.g., methotrexate), a biological response modifier (BRM) (e.g., infliximab [Remicade]), a nonsteroidal antiinflammatory drug (NSAID) (e.g., ibuprofen), or an analgesic (e.g., acetaminophen) with Mrs. Ellis's primary health care provider.	Different medications are used to control the pain and symptoms of rheumatoid arthritis. DMRADs cause immunosuppression; DMRADs, NSAIDs, and BRMs decrease inflammation; and DMRADs, NSAIDs, and analgesics relieve pain (Arthritis Foundation, 2012).
• Consult with health care provider to allow Mrs. Ellis to take analgesics around the clock (e.g., every 4 hours) and plan activities such as ambulating, performing self-care activities, or going to sleep 30 minutes after a dose. Instruct her to take medication with a light snack or meal and a full glass of water. During instruction tell her that the drug relieves pain.	Opioids should be administered on a fixed schedule, with each dose given before pain returns (Lehne, 2010). Medication exerts peak effect when patient begins activities. Administration with meals and water reduces chance of gastrointestinal upset. An added positive effect occurs when the patient understands the action and purpose of the analgesic and believes that the medication will relieve pain.
Cutaneous Stimulation	
• Have Mrs. Ellis place a sturdy stool in shower stall and run warm water continuously over joints of hands and feet.	Heat reduces pain by improving blood flow and reducing stiffness of inflamed tissues (Barclay, 2007).
• Have Mrs. Ellis apply moist, warm compresses to joints of hands 3 times a day before dressing or other self-care activities.	Cutaneous stimulation activates mechanoreceptor A-beta fibers, thus inhibiting transmission of pain by releasing inhibitory neurotransmitters (Barclay, 2007).
Referral	
• Refer Mrs. Ellis to a physical therapist to determine possible use of the walker or other assistive devices.	Physical therapists teach effective exercise and ambulation techniques to reduce pain and conserve energy.

‡Intervention classification labels from Bulechek GM et al, editors: *Nursing interventions classification (NIC)*, ed 6, St Louis, 2013, Mosby.

EVALUATION

NURSING ACTIONS	PATIENT RESPONSE/FINDING	ACHIEVEMENT OF OUTCOME
Observe Mrs. Ellis's ability to stand and walk from living room to kitchen.	Mrs. Ellis is able to ambulate with walker from living room to kitchen; gait is slow but steady.	Mrs. Ellis is successfully ambulating with steady gait.
Ask Mrs. Ellis if she experiences discomfort during dressing and bathing.	Mrs. Ellis has less discomfort from bathing after using warm water over joints. Dressing is still causing some discomfort when manipulating buttons on clothing.	Cutaneous stimulation is providing some pain relief. Consider referring to occupational therapy to adapt clothes fasteners requiring less hand mobility.
Ask Mrs. Ellis to rate pain on FACES Pain Scale 30 minutes after analgesic is administered.	Mrs. Ellis rates pain at a level of 2 after receiving analgesic.	Mrs. Ellis continues to have discomfort but less severe than preintervention level.

An effective method for planning care is a concept map (Figure 32-7). Patients who are in pain frequently have interrelated problems. As one problem worsens, other aspects of a patient's level of health also change. A concept map shows links or relationships among multiple nursing diagnoses, a patient's medical diagnosis, and associated interventions. This helps you learn how assessment findings and interventions can apply to more than one diagnosis so you can form a holistic plan of care.

It is always important to remember that a successful plan of care requires development of a therapeutic relationship with a patient/family and a focus on education regarding pain. Helping patients learn how to manage their pain is an important goal of care. You help best by seeing each patient as a total person, listening carefully to concerns, attending promptly to his or her needs, and respecting any response to pain. In the successful nurse-patient relationship, you recognize that a patient knows more about his or her own pain and is an important partner in identifying successful pain-relieving strategies.

Setting Priorities. When setting priorities in pain management, consider the type of pain that a patient is having and how it affects various body functions. Work with a patient to select interventions that are most appropriate for priority

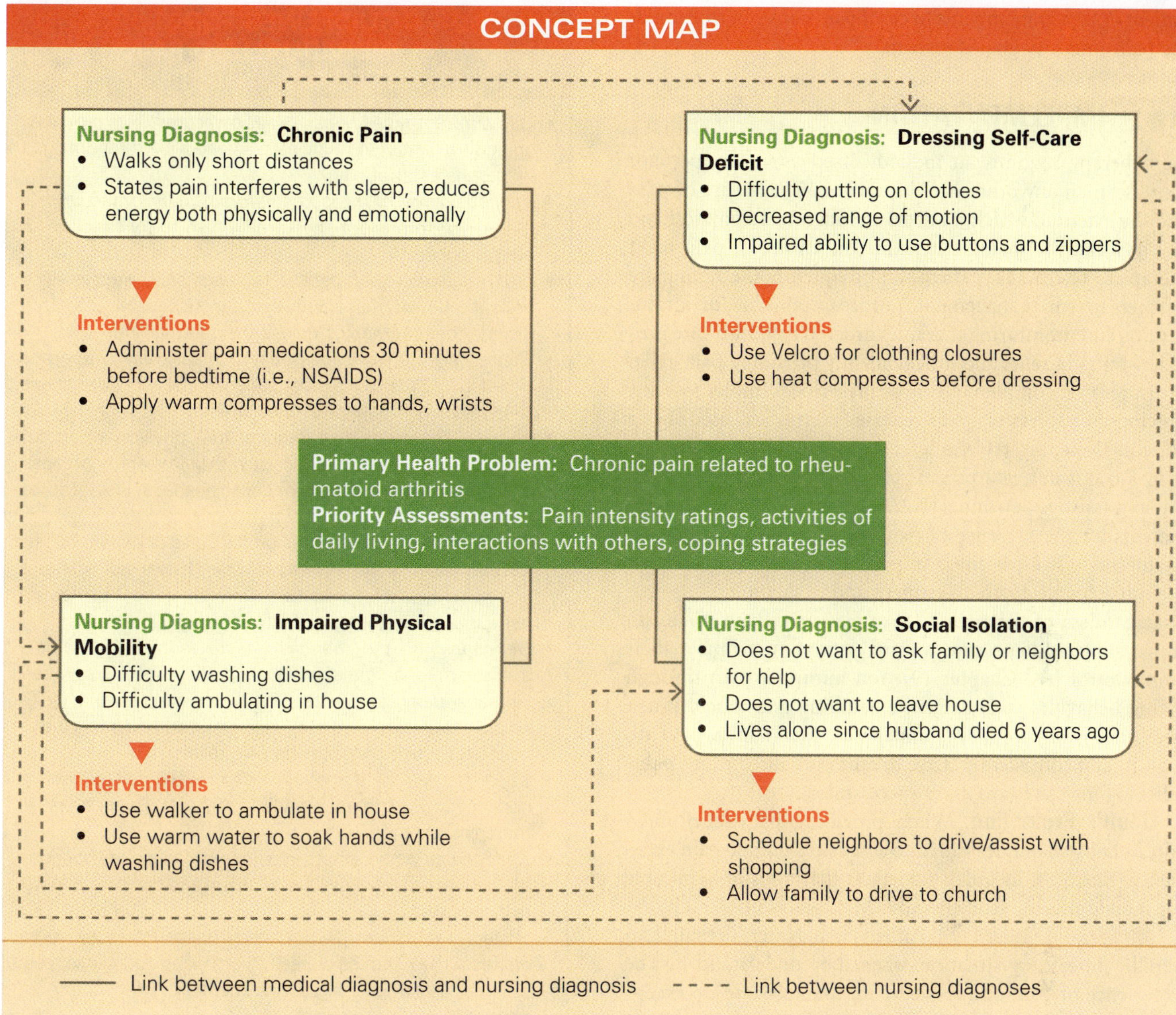

FIGURE 32-7 Concept map. *NSAIDs,* Nonsteroidal antiinflammatory drugs.

needs. For example, if a patient's acute pain is under control, focus attention on improving his or her appetite or ability to sleep. However, if the pain continues to be severe, preventing you from implementing other interventions, immediate pain relief becomes your priority. Priorities change as a patient's pain experience changes.

Collaborative Care. A comprehensive plan of care involves using the resources of a patient's family and friends. The family often gives care in the home and thus needs to be prepared to assess a patient's pain and administer therapies safely. Discharge teaching in an acute care setting prepares a patient and family to understand the nature and extent of the patient's pain, the choice of therapies, and how to safely administer therapies. Family members or friends who show a disinterest or prejudice toward pain slow a patient's recovery. Additional resources in planning care include nurse and physician specialists, Doctors of Pharmacology (PharmDs), physical therapists, occupational therapists, licensed massage therapists, medical social workers, and clergy. An oncology nurse specialist understands therapies for chronic cancer pain. Physician pain specialists are experts on invasive therapies. PharmDs are knowledgeable about pharmacological treatments for pain. Physical therapists plan exercises that strengthen or relax muscle groups and lessen pain. Occupational therapists devise splints to support painful body parts. Licensed massage therapists offer massage that may relax muscles and block perceptions of pain. Clergy offer strategies to relieve spiritual pain. If an agency does not have the resources to manage a patient's pain, refer the patient to the health care provider or agency that can provide the care needed.

Because patients are often transferred between departments of the same institution and sometimes between different institutions, documentation of the pain-management plan is important for continuity of care. Record all discharge teaching and referrals implemented. A notation of whom the patient or family member is to call if pain consistently exceeds the pain-intensity goal is essential.

IMPLEMENTATION

Pain therapy requires an individualized approach, perhaps more so than any other health problem. The nature of pain and the extent to which it affects an individual's physical and psychosocial well-being determine the choice of pain-relief therapies. The nurse, patient, and frequently the family are partners in pain management. You are responsible for administering and monitoring therapies ordered by health care providers for pain relief and independently providing pain-relief measures that complement those prescribed. Implement any previously successful pain-relieving remedies used by a patient. Generally try the least invasive and safest therapy first. Do not delegate pain assessment and management to nursing assistive personnel (NAP). However, NAP may screen patients for the presence of pain by asking them if they are having pain. If a patient is in pain, the NAP reports this to the nurse for in-depth assessment and evaluation.

Regardless of the type of therapies used, your ability to show compassionate care toward patients maximizes their pain control (see Chapter 19). You minimize pain through caring behaviors such as gentle handling and touch. When you successfully convey compassion, maintain a patient's dignity, and consistently strive to minimize discomfort, pain-relieving measures are more successful.

Health Promotion. When providing pain-relief measures, choose therapies suited to a patient's unique pain experience. Box 32-8 includes guidelines that are still applicable for individualizing pain therapy (McCaffery, 1979).

Maintaining Wellness. Patients are better prepared to handle almost any situation when they understand it. The experience of pain and related pain therapies are no exception. However, patients with moderate-to-severe pain are not always able to participate in the decision-making process until their pain is controlled at an acceptable level. Once you achieve pain relief, you are able to begin patient teaching.

Patients actively participate in their own well-being whenever possible. Common holistic health approaches include wellness education, regular exercise, rest, attention to good hygiene practices and nutrition, and management of interpersonal relationships. Offer nonpharmacological and pharmacological therapies when a person develops pain. Several nonpharmacological interventions are available and can be initiated independently by nurses.

Measures that promote a sense of well-being by minimizing or avoiding discomfort include warm baths, massage, and a schedule of adequate rest. Chapter 31 discusses the effect that pain has on a patient's sleep pattern and ways to promote better sleep habits. Help patients find ways to plan rest periods before participating in exhausting activities. Patients with chronic pain need to rest before any social activities in the home.

Some pain disables and immobilizes a person enough to impair the ability to perform self-care activities. As a result, a patient also experiences social isolation, depression, and changes in self-concept. Change in function means a significant loss to a patient. Help patients and families learn to discuss their feelings about the loss so they can find ways to cope with pain and the lifestyle it imposes (see Chapter 23).

Pain from an injury or disabling illness often limits a patient's mobility. In this case you target health promotion at retaining function. Instruct patients and families in the safe and proper use of elastic bandages, braces, and splints that protect body parts. When a patient has chronic, disabling pain, instruct family members in proper positioning techniques and ways to assist the patient with ambulation.

Refer patients who have difficulty eating, bathing, grooming, and dressing to an occupational therapist. Some agencies

BOX 32-8 GUIDELINES FOR INDIVIDUALIZED PAIN THERAPY

- *Use different types of pain-relief measures.* This produces an additive effect in reducing pain and allows for changes in the character of pain.
- *Provide pain-relief measures before pain becomes severe.* It is easier to prevent severe pain than to try to relieve it after it occurs.
- *Use measures that patient believes are effective.* The patient's beliefs make pain therapy successful; therefore include these remedies unless they are harmful.
- *Some patients have ideas about measures to use and times to use them.* Consider patient's ability or willingness to participate in pain-relief measures.
- Suggest measures that require little physical effort for patients unable to actively assist with pain therapy because of fatigue or altered levels of consciousness. Do not force participation.
- *Choose pain-relief measures on the basis of patient behavior that reflects the severity of pain.* Never administer a potent analgesic for mild pain. Only the patient can determine the potency of an effective therapy.
- *Depending on the therapy, ensure that you attempt a sufficient trial before abandoning it.* Pharmacological interventions particularly often need around-the-clock (ATC) administration for several days to attain and maintain therapeutic level and thus provide pain relief.
- *Keep an open mind about ways to relieve pain.* Rejecting nonconventional therapy leads to mistrust. Be sure that all therapies are safe.
- *Keep trying.* When efforts at pain relief fail, do not abandon the patient but reassess the situation and consider alternative therapies.
- *Protect the patient.* Pain therapy does not cause more distress than the pain itself; you want to relieve pain without disabling the patient mentally, emotionally, or physically.
- *Educate the patient about pain.* Explain the cause of pain, times when you will give analgesics, and alternative therapies.

Data from McCaffery M: *Nursing management of the patient with pain,* ed 2, Philadelphia, 1979, Lippincott.

require a health care provider's order to begin occupational therapy. Devices designed to maintain function, even when finger movement or grasp is impaired, help. The therapist attaches eating utensils, a comb, or a toothbrush to extension devices that have enlarged handles or splints for easy use. Velcro fasteners on clothing allow patients to remove or apply clothing without assistance.

Some patients with pain avoid sexual activity. However, pain does not negate the need for sexual warmth. Patients learn to express themselves sexually by assuming alternative positions during intercourse and learning more about ways to make their partner feel sexually stimulated. Caution patients that some pain medications decrease libido and may cause impotency.

Nonpharmacological Pain-Relief Measures. There are a number of nonpharmacological or complementary therapies for pain relief, including massage, guided imagery, music, biofeedback, meditation, hypnosis, prayer, journaling, exercise, therapeutic touch, acupuncture, and relaxation techniques. Several of these therapies require special training to perform, including biofeedback and acupuncture. You use other therapies such as massage and relaxation techniques that lessen the reception and perception of pain. Use these therapies in combination with pharmacological measures. The AHCPR guidelines for acute pain management (1992) cite nonpharmacological interventions appropriate for patients who:

- Find such interventions appealing.
- Express anxiety or fear.
- Benefit from avoiding or reducing drug therapy.
- Are likely to experience and need to cope with a prolonged interval of postoperative pain.
- Have incomplete pain relief with use of pharmacological therapies.

Do not exclude patients using pharmacological measures from use of nonpharmacological therapies.

Reducing Pain Reception and Perception. One simple way to promote comfort is to remove or prevent painful stimuli. This is especially important for patients who are immobilized or have difficulty expressing themselves. For example, tighten and smooth wrinkled bed linen and be sure to position patients off tubing and other equipment. Change wet dressings or bed linen immediately. Do not allow tubing from a Foley catheter to become kinked because bladder distention is uncomfortable. When repositioning patients, lift them in bed with safe patient-handling techniques. Do not pull when positioning them in correct anatomical alignment. Avoid exposing the skin to irritants such as diarrheal stool or wound drainage. Many of these measures are easy for family members to learn. Removing noxious stimuli is especially important for patients who are immobile. You can prevent pain by anticipating painful activities (e.g., ambulation or turning). Before performing a procedure, consider the patient's condition, aspects of the procedure that are painful, and ways to avoid causing pain. It takes simple consideration of the patient's comfort and a little extra time to avoid pain-producing situations.

Anticipatory Guidance. Modifying anxiety directly associated with pain relieves pain and adds to the effects of other pain-relief measures. Giving patients detailed descriptions of all medical procedures and expected postprocedural discomfort and giving instruction for decreasing treatment- and mobility-related pain decrease self-reported pain, analgesic use, and postoperative length of stay. Provide patients sufficient procedural and sensory information (e.g., prick of the needle during blood draw or burning during urinary catheter insertion) to satisfy their interests and enable them to assess, evaluate, and communicate pain.

Distraction. The reticular activating system inhibits painful stimuli if a person receives sufficient or excessive sensory input. With meaningful sensory stimuli a patient is able to ignore or become unaware of pain. Pleasurable sensory stimuli reduce pain perception by the release of endorphins. Distraction directs a patient's attention to something else, thus reducing the awareness of pain. Distraction works best for short, intense pain lasting a few minutes such as during an invasive procedure or while waiting for an analgesic to work. Useful forms of distraction include singing, praying, describing photos out loud, telling jokes, and playing games. Music is helpful for treating acute or chronic pain, stress, anxiety, and depression (Allred et al., 2010). It diverts a person's attention and creates a relaxation response. Music therapy uses all forms of music but always let patients select the type of music they prefer. Therapeutic sessions offer sound, silence, space, and time and are best when lasting 20 to 30 minutes (Hughes, 2008). Patients use earphones to enhance their concentration on the music. Evidence shows that music decreases the use of analgesics in some postoperative patients (Engwall and Duppils, 2009).

Cutaneous Stimulation. Stimulation of the skin helps to relieve pain. A massage, warm bath, ice bag, and **transcutaneous electrical nerve stimulation (TENS)** are simple ways to reduce pain perception (Wright, 2012). How **cutaneous stimulation** works is unclear, but it may cause release of endorphins, thus blocking transmission of painful stimuli. The gate control theory suggests that cutaneous stimulation activates larger, faster A-beta sensory nerve fibers that are sensitive to touch, pressure, and warmth. This decreases pain transmission through small diameter A-delta and C fibers. Synaptic gates thus close to pain transmission (Menefee-Pujol, et al., 2007).

Cutaneous stimulation gives patients and families some control over pain symptoms and treatment in the home. Using it properly helps to reduce muscle tension, resulting in less pain. When using cutaneous stimulation methods, eliminate environmental noise, help a patient to assume a comfortable position, and explain the purpose of the therapy. Do not use cutaneous stimulation directly on sensitive skin areas (e.g., burns, bruises, skin rashes, inflammation, or underlying bone fractures).

Massage is effective for producing physical and mental relaxation, reducing pain, and enhancing the effectiveness of pain medication. Massaging the back, shoulders, hands, and/or feet for 3 to 5 minutes relaxes muscles and promotes sleep.

Cutshall et al. (2010) reported a significant decrease in pain, anxiety, and tension in patients with cardiac problems who received a 20-minute massage. In older adults slow back massage and a 20-minute hand massage relieved pain, anxiety, tension, and insomnia (Harris and Richards, 2010). Massage conveys caring, and family members are able to learn how to do this easily.

Cold and heat applications relieve pain and promote healing (see Chapter 37) (Box 32-9). The choice to use heat or cold is based on the origin of the pain and the patient's past preferences and experiences with pain relief using these methods. For example, moist heat relieves the pain from a tension headache, and a cold pack reduces acute pain from inflamed joints. The use of heat or cold applications in the acute care setting requires a health care provider's order. When using any form of heat or cold application, instruct a patient to avoid injury to the skin by checking the temperature and not applying it directly to the skin. Older adults, confused patients, and patients with spinal cord or other neurological injuries and decreased sensation are at risk for burns from heating pads and similar devices.

TENS is a form of stimulation of the skin with a mild electrical current passed through external electrodes. The electrodes are placed directly over or near the site of pain. A patient turns on a battery-powered transmitter to create a tingling electrical current when feeling pain. TENS is useful in managing postoperative pain and reducing pain caused by postoperative procedures (e.g., removing drains) (Barclay, 2007). High-stimulation intensity has been shown to have better effects than low-stimulation intensity in patients with knee osteoarthritis. The research evidence on the use of TENS for pain relief is often conflicting, partly because of problems with the way research studies have been designed (Wright, 2012). However, TENS is safe, noninvasive, nonaddictive, inexpensive, and easy to use. It requires a health care provider's order.

Relaxation and Guided Imagery. Relaxation and **guided imagery** allow patients to alter affective-motivational and cognitive pain perception. **Relaxation** is mental and physical freedom from tension or stress that provides individuals a sense of self-control. Potential physiological and behavioral changes associated with relaxation include decreased pulse, blood pressure, and respirations; heightened awareness; decreased oxygen consumption; a sense of peace; and decreased muscle tension and metabolic rate. However, research is unclear about the benefits because there is great variation in the dose-response relationship (change in an individual resulting from different levels of the therapy) and the individual differences that might influence response to relaxation interventions (Kwekkeboom and Gretarsdottir, 2006). Relaxation strategies include meditation, yoga, Zen, guided imagery, and progressive relaxation. Sometimes a combination is needed to achieve pain relief. The techniques require periodic reinforcement through encouragement and coaching.

For effective relaxation a patient needs to participate and cooperate. Teach relaxation techniques only when a patient is not anxious or in acute discomfort or severe pain and thus is able to concentrate. Explain the technique in detail. It sometimes takes several teaching sessions before patients effectively minimize pain. They can practice relaxation training indefinitely and usually with no side effects. Remove any noises or other irritating stimuli such as bright lights from the environment. Have a patient sit in a comfortable chair in proper alignment or lie in bed. A light sheet or blanket keeps the patient warm and comfortable. Describe common sensations that he or she will experience (e.g., a decrease in temperature, a feeling of heaviness, or numbness of a body part). The patient uses these sensations as feedback. Acting as the coach, guide the patient slowly through the steps of the exercise.

In guided imagery a patient creates an image in the mind, concentrates on that image, and gradually becomes less aware of pain. Initially ask the patient to think of a pleasant scene or experience that promotes using all senses. The patient describes the image, and you record it for later use. Use only specific information given by the patient and make no changes in the image. The following is an example of a portion of a guided imagery exercise:

> Imagine yourself lying on a cool bed of grass with the sounds of water trickling over stones in a nearby stream. It's a warm

BOX 32-9 PATIENT TEACHING

Application of Moist Heat

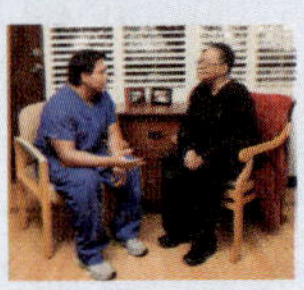

If your patient would benefit from the application of moist heat for pain relief, as was recommended for Mrs. Ellis, develop a teaching plan that ensures pain relief with no adverse effects.

OUTCOME

At the end of the teaching session patient demonstrates proper application of moist heat for pain relief to affected areas.

TEACHING STRATEGIES

- Plan teaching session in quiet environment at time that is convenient for patient.
- Avoid teaching during times of moderate-to-severe pain.
- Teach patient about expected outcomes of use of moist heat to relieve chronic pain related to rheumatoid arthritis.
- Ask patient to demonstrate how to apply moist heat to painful areas.
- To avoid burns, warn patient against using water that is too hot or making the compress too hot.
- Summarize what you taught and clarify questions or concerns.

EVALUATION STRATEGIES

- Use Teach Back techniques such as asking open-ended questions to have patient restate what has been taught.
- Have patient demonstrate how to apply moist heat to painful areas.
- Have patient verbalize why it is necessary to avoid using water or a compress that is too hot.

day. You turn to see a patch of blue wildflowers in bloom, and you smell their fragrance.

Sit close enough so the patient can hear you but not so close that you are intrusive. A calm, soft voice helps the patient focus more completely on the suggested image. While relaxing the patient focuses on the image, and you speak continuously. If the patient shows signs of agitation, restlessness, or discomfort, stop the exercise and begin later when he or she is more at ease.

Progressive relaxation exercises involve the combination of controlled breathing exercises and a series of contractions and relaxation of muscle groups. A patient begins by breathing slowly and diaphragmatically, allowing the abdomen to rise slowly; the chest remains still while fully expanding. Often a patient closes the eyes to focus on the exercise. When the patient establishes a regular breathing pattern, coach him or her to locate any area of muscular tension, think about how it feels, gently tense the muscles, and then completely relax them. This creates the sensation of removing all discomfort and stress. Gradually the patient relaxes the muscles without first tensing them. After he or she achieves full relaxation, pain perception is lowered, and anxiety toward the pain experience becomes minimal. If the patient becomes agitated or uncomfortable, stop the exercise. If the patient reports difficulty relaxing part of the body, slow the progression of the exercise and concentrate on the tensed body part. If the patient reports increased pain, focus on relaxing areas of muscle tension instead of consciously tensing the muscle. The patient may stop the exercise at any time. With practice the patient learns to perform relaxation exercises independently. Relaxation techniques are particularly effective for chronic pain, labor pains, and relief of procedure-related pain. The techniques are less effective for episodes of acute or severe pain.

Acute Care

Pharmacological Pain Therapy. All pharmacological agents require a health care provider's order. Your judgment in the use and management of analgesics with or without other pain therapies ensures the best pain relief possible. A systematic approach to pain assessment and appropriate treatment choices ensures a quick response for managing patient discomfort.

Analgesics. The most common treatment for pain relief is **analgesics.** However, health care providers still tend to undertreat patients because of incorrect drug information, concerns about addiction, anxiety over errors in using opioid analgesics, and administration of less medication than was ordered (D'Arcy, 2008). Make sure that you understand the drugs available for pain relief and their pharmacological effects. Reassure patients that treatment of pain is necessary to aid recovery and that addiction is highly unlikely when analgesics are taken correctly.

There are three types of analgesics: (1) nonopioids, including acetaminophen and nonsteroidal antiinflammatory drugs (NSAIDS); (2) **opioids** (traditionally called *narcotics*); and (3) adjuvant or coanalgesics, a variety of medications that enhance analgesics or analgesic properties that were originally unknown (Pasero and McCaffery, 2011).

Acetaminophen (Tylenol) is considered one of the most tolerated and safest analgesics available. It has no antiinflammatory effects, and its action is unknown. Its major adverse effect is toxicity to the liver. It is in a variety of over-the-counter (OTC) cold, flu, and allergy remedies. The maximum 24-hour dose is 4 g (the same limitation as aspirin). It is often combined with opioids (e.g., oxycodone [Percocet], hydrocodone [Vicodin], and tramadol [Ultracet] because it reduces the dose of opioid needed).

Nonselective NSAIDs such as aspirin and ibuprofen provide relief for mild-to-moderate acute intermittent pain such as that from headache or muscle strain. Treatment for mild-to-moderate postoperative pain begins with an NSAID unless contraindicated (Pasero and McCaffery, 2011). NSAIDs most likely inhibit synthesis of prostaglandins (Lehne, 2010) and thus cellular response to inflammation. Most NSAIDs act on peripheral nerve receptors to reduce transmission of pain stimuli. Unlike opioids, NSAIDs do not depress the central nervous system, nor do they interfere with bowel and bladder function (Pasero and McCaffery, 2011). However, chronic NSAID use in older adults is not recommended because it is associated with gastrointestinal bleeding and renal insufficiency. Some patients with asthma or an allergy to aspirin are also allergic (cross-sensitivity) to other NSAIDs (Kaufman, 2010).

Opioid or opioid-like analgesics are prescribed for moderate-to-severe pain. Examples include codeine, morphine, hydromorphone (Dilaudid), and fentanyl. These analgesics act on higher centers of the brain and spinal cord by binding with opiate receptors to modify pain perception. A rare adverse effect of opioids in opioid-naïve patients (patients who have used opioids around the clock *less* than approximately 1 week) is respiratory depression. Respiratory depression is only clinically significant if there is a decrease in the rate *and* depth of respirations from a patient's baseline assessment (Pasero and McCaffery, 2011). Patients who breathe deeply rarely have clinical respiratory depression. Sedation always occurs before respiratory depression. Closely monitor for sedation in opioid-naïve patients. If a patient develops respiratory depression, administer naloxone (Narcan) (0.4 mg diluted with 9 mL saline) intravenous (IV) push at a rate of 0.5 mL every 2 minutes until the respiratory rate is greater than 8 breaths/min with good depth. Evaluate patients who receive naloxone every 15 minutes for 2 hours because its duration is less than that of the opioid and respiratory depression can return. Additional adverse effects of opioids include nausea, vomiting, constipation, itching, urinary retention, and altered mental processes.

One way to maximize pain relief while potentially decreasing drug use is to administer analgesics on an around-the-clock (ATC) rather than a prn basis. The American Pain Society (2003) supports ATC administration if pain is anticipated for the majority of the day. There are also a variety of extended- or controlled-release oral opioid formulations (dosing intervals of 8, 10, 12, or 24 hours) and transdermal patches (dosing interval of 72 hours). These formulations

BOX 32-10 NURSING PRINCIPLES FOR ADMINISTERING ANALGESICS

KNOW PATIENT'S PREVIOUS RESPONSE TO ANALGESICS

- Determine whether patient obtained relief.
- Ask whether a nonopioid was as effective as an opioid.
- Identify previous doses and routes of administration to avoid under treatment.
- Determine whether patient has allergies.
- Know if patient is at risk for using NSAIDs (e.g., history of gastrointestinal [GI] bleed or renal insufficiency) or opioids (e.g., history of obstructive sleep apnea).

SELECT PROPER MEDICATIONS WHEN MORE THAN ONE IS ORDERED

- Use nonopioid analgesics or opioid combination drugs (e.g., oxycodone with acetaminophen) for mild-to-moderate pain.
- You can give opioids with nonopioids.
- In older adults avoid combinations of opioids.
- Fentanyl patches, morphine, or hydromorphone are opioids of choice for long-term severe pain.
- Intravenous medications act more quickly and usually relieve severe, acute pain within 1 hour, whereas oral medications take as long as 2 hours to relieve pain.
- Avoid intramuscular analgesics, especially in older adults.
- For chronic pain give oral extended-release formulations for longer, more sustained relief.

KNOW ACCURATE DOSAGE

- Remember that patients with severe pain generally need higher doses of analgesics.
- Adjust doses as appropriate for children and older patients.
- Large doses of opioids are acceptable in opioid-tolerant patients but not opioid-naïve patients.
- When titrating opioids it is important to titrate to effect or to uncontrollable side effects.
- Dosage typically requires adjustment over time.

ASSESS RIGHT TIME AND INTERVAL FOR ADMINISTRATION

- Administer analgesics as soon as pain occurs and before it increases in severity.
- An around-the-clock (ATC) administration schedule is best.
- Give analgesics *before* pain-producing procedures or activities.
- Know average peak and duration of action for drug so you time drug administration to peak when pain is most intense.
- Give extended-release opioid formulations on an ATC basis and not prn.
- Avoid abruptly stopping opioids in patients who are opioid tolerant.

CHOOSE RIGHT ROUTE

- Oral route is preferred; intravenous route is preferred if patient is unable to swallow or has GI problems.
- Avoid intramuscular and subcutaneous administration because these routes are painful and absorption is not reliable.

Modified from Pasero, C, McCaffery M: *Pain assessment and pharmacological management,* St Louis, 2011, Mosby.
NSAIDs, Nonsteroidal antiinflammatory drugs.

maintain constant serum opioid concentration, minimizing toxic and subtherapeutic concentrations (Lehne, 2010). They also lessen the severity of end-of-dose pain, allowing a patient to sleep through the night and reduce "clock watching" by patients.

When you convert a patient from an IV to an oral form of the same opioid, understand that the dose of the oral opioid is usually much higher than the IV dose because of the first-pass effect (Pasero and McCaffery, 2011). When a patient takes oral opioids, the opioids first go to the liver, where most (but not all) of the medication is inactivated. Thus the body needs larger doses of oral opioids to achieve the same level of pain relief as the same opioid given intravenously. Know the comparative potencies of analgesics in oral and injectable form. Also know the route of administration that is most effective for a patient to achieve controlled, sustained pain relief. Equianalgesic charts (i.e., charts converting one opioid to another or parenteral forms of opioids to oral forms) are available on nursing units or in the pharmacy. Nurses on succeeding shifts need to know the route of administration most effective for a patient so the patient achieves controlled, sustained pain relief.

Adjuvants or coanalgesics are drugs (e.g. steroids, anticonvulsants, antidepressants, and muscle relaxants) originally developed to treat conditions other than pain, but the drugs have analgesic properties. For example, tricyclic antidepressants (e.g., nortriptyline), anticonvulsants (e.g., gabapentin), and infusional lidocaine successfully treat neuropathic pain. Corticosteroids relieve pain associated with inflammation and bone metastasis. Adjuvants have analgesic properties, enhance pain control, or relieve other symptoms associated with neuropathic pain such as anxiety, depression, and nausea. You give these alone or with analgesics (Pasero and McCaffery, 2011). Sedatives, antianxiety agents, and muscle relaxants have no analgesic effect; however, they often cause drowsiness and impaired coordination, judgment, and mental alertness.

The proper use of analgesics requires careful assessment, application of pharmacological principles, and common sense (Box 32-10). Not all patients react the same way to analgesics. For example, an NSAID is as effective as an opioid for some patients but not others. An orally administered analgesic usually brings the same relief as an injectable form.

Children require careful calculation of drug doses (see Chapter 17). Equianalgesia charts that convert recommended adult doses to children's doses are available. These charts consider age and body size. Older adults also require special considerations (Box 32-11).

Patient-Controlled Analgesia. Patients benefit from having control over their pain therapy. Patient-controlled

BOX 32-11 **CARE OF THE OLDER ADULT**

Principles of Pain Management in the Older Adult

- Pain is *not* a normal part of aging. Presence of pain requires aggressive assessment and management.
- Older adults are at high risk for pain-inducing situations.
- Several pain-producing conditions sometimes coexist.
- Older adults are often fearful that pain will result in loss of independence, making them a burden to their family.
- Age-related changes in pain perception are most likely not clinically significant (American Geriatrics Society, 2009).
- Older patients experience faster onset, longer duration of action and adverse effects from analgesics because of lower serum protein levels and reduced liver, renal, and cardiac function.
- Older adults may be more sensitive to the analgesic and adverse effects of opioids. Thus start with low doses of opioids and increase the dose slowly as needed (Pasero and McCaffery, 2011).
- When choosing an opioid, avoid propoxyphene (Darvon, Darvocet) in older patients because of possible cardiovascular and neurological adverse effects (AGS, 2009).
- There is an increased risk for gastric and renal toxicity from NSAIDs among older adults.

NSAIDs, Nonsteroidal antiinflammatory drugs.

analgesia (PCA) is a safe method for a variety of painful conditions, including but not limited to postoperative, traumatic, sickle cell crisis, cancer, and burns (Pasero and McCaffery, 2011). It is a drug-delivery system that allows patients to self-administer opioids such as morphine, hydromorphone, and fentanyl with minimal risk of overdose, when they want them, and without repeated parenteral injections (see Skill 32-1). The goal is to maintain a constant plasma level of analgesic to avoid the problems of prn dosing. Systemic PCA traditionally involves IV or subcutaneous administration; however, a controlled analgesia device for oral medications, medication on demand (MOD), is now available. The MOD device allows patients to access single doses of their own oral prn medications, including opioids and other analgesics at the bedside (Rosati et al., 2007).

PCA infusion pumps are portable and computerized and contain a cassette or chamber for a syringe. It delivers a small preset dose of opioid. To receive a demand dose, a patient pushes a button attached to the PCA device. Systems are designed to deliver a specified number of doses every 1 to 4 hours (depending on the pump settings) given every 5 to 15 minutes (programmable) to avoid overdoses. On-demand doses typically add 1 mg of morphine every 10 minutes, with a limit set for every hour or every 4 hours (Lehne, 2010). Most pumps have locked safety systems that prevent tampering by patients or family members and are generally safe to be managed in the home. The typical PCA prescription relies on a series of "loading" doses (e.g., 3 to 5 mg of morphine repeated every 5 to 10 minutes until initial pain diminishes). A low-dose basal infusion (0.5 to 1 mg/hr) at night allows uninterrupted sleep; this option is commonly used throughout the day for cancer pain. Use continuous basal infusions with caution in opioid-naïve patients during the first 24 to 48 hours after surgery because of the possibility of respiratory depression from the combination of anesthetics with opioids (Pasero and McCaffery, 2011).

Benefits of PCA include the following:

- Patients have control over pain.
- Pain relief does not depend on nurses' availability.
- Patients tend to take less medication.
- Small doses of opioids delivered at short intervals stabilize serum drug concentrations for sustained pain relief.

Patient preparation and teaching are critical to the safe and effective use of PCA. Patients having surgery receive teaching and demonstration of the PCA pump before surgery if the health care provider orders PCA use. They need to understand PCA and be able to physically locate and press the button to deliver the dose (Pasero and McCaffery, 2011). Therefore PCA therapy is not appropriate for patients who are confused, have altered levels of consciousness, or are unable to understand how to use the equipment. Be sure to instruct family members not to "push the button" for patients. Use Authorized Agent Controlled Analgesia (AACA) guidelines to authorize a family member or nurse to administer the analgesic when appropriate (Wuhrman et al., 2006). In these cases you select one family member or significant other to be the patient's primary pain manager (Pasero and McCaffery, 2011). The ASPMN developed the position statement on unauthorized proxy dosing by PCA in 2006.

Check the patient's IV line or subcutaneous needle placement and PCA device regularly to ensure proper functioning. Certain pumps track cumulative dosages and print out the information when needed. Document drug doses carefully and record any wasted or unused opioid. Monitor the patient for adverse drug effects and pain-management effectiveness. Use of PCA gives you and the patient more flexibility in pain management.

Perineural Local Anesthetic Infusion. Perineural infusion pumps are an option for managing pain for a variety of inpatient and outpatient adult and pediatric surgical procedures. An unsutured catheter from a surgical wound placed near a nerve or groups of nerves connects to a pump containing a local anesthetic (bupivacaine or ropivacaine). You set the pump on demand or continuous mode, and it is usually left in place for 48 hours. Patients learn how to discontinue the pump at home by pulling out the catheter and bringing it to their next health care provider visit.

Local Anesthetics. The loss of sensation to a localized body part is termed **local anesthesia.** Health care providers use local anesthetic (e.g., lidocaine, bupivacaine, or ropivacaine) during brief surgical procedures such as removing a skin lesion or suturing a wound. Local anesthetics are applied topically on skin and mucous membranes or are injected subcutaneously or intradermally to anesthetize a body part. The drugs produce temporary loss of sensation by inhibiting nerve conduction. Local anesthetics also block motor and autonomic functions, depending on the amount used and the location and depth of an injection. Smaller sensory nerve fibers are more sensitive to local anesthetics than large motor fibers. Thus a patient loses sensation before losing motor function; conversely motor function returns before sensation.

Local anesthetics cause side effects, depending on their absorption into the circulation. Itching or burning of the skin or a localized rash is common after topical applications. Application to vascular membranes increases the chance of systemic effects such as a change in heart rate. Protect patients from injury until full sensory and motor function return. They can easily injure themselves without knowing it. You need to educate patients receiving local anesthesia by explaining insertion sites and warning them that they will temporarily lose sensory function. Further reassure patients by explaining the application of the anesthetic and the sensations that they will experience. Injection is painful unless the health care provider first numbs the injection site. Prepare patients for such discomfort. Before a patient receives an anesthetic, assess for any medication allergies. To monitor systemic effects, assess vital signs.

Epidural Analgesia. Epidural analgesia is a form of regional anesthesia and an effective therapy for the treatment of postoperative, labor and delivery, and chronic cancer pain (Chumbley and Thomas, 2010). It permits control or reduction of severe pain without the sedative effects of opioids, and it reduces a patient's overall opioid requirement. Epidural analgesia is short or long term, depending on a patient's condition and life expectancy. Short-term epidural analgesia is especially effective for pain after intrathoracic, abdominal, and orthopedic surgery. Long-term epidural therapy is effective for pain unresponsive to oral or parenteral medications. The advantages of epidural analgesia include the following:

- Production of excellent analgesia
- Occurrence of minimal sedation
- Long-lasting pain relief with fewer opioid doses
- Facilitation of early ambulation
- Avoidance of repeated injections
- No significant effect on sensation
- Little effect on blood pressure or heart rate
- Fewer pulmonary complications or improved pulmonary function

Epidural analgesia is administered into the epidural space to block a group of sensory nerve fibers. It is administered through a catheter, which is usually placed in the operating room, postanesthesia care unit, or intensive care unit. The patient lies in the fetal position (lateral decubitus) to open the space between the vertebrae. The health care provider administers a local anesthetic into the skin at the needle insertion site and then inserts a blunt-tip needle into the level of the vertebral interspace nearest to the area requiring analgesia (usually L4-L5). The health care provider advances a plastic catheter into the epidural space and then removes the needle (Figure 32-8). The remainder of the catheter is secured with an occlusive dressing and taped up the back of the patient. A temporary catheter is sometimes connected to tubing positioned along the spine and over the patient's shoulder. You can place the end of the catheter on the patient's chest for easier access. Permanent catheters are tunneled through the skin and exit at the patient's side. Assessment of the insertion site and patency of the tubing are important nursing responsibilities (Pasero and McCaffery, 2011).

The epidural catheter is connected to a continuous **epidural infusion** pump, a port, or a reservoir; or it is capped off for bolus injections. In many hospitals only anesthesiologists or nurse anesthetists administer epidural anesthesia. However, registered nurses certified in this procedure also administer it in some settings. In addition, some institutions allow patients to deliver epidural analgesic doses (patient-controlled epidural analgesia) via a pump. To reduce the risk for accidental epidural injection of drugs intended for IV use, always place a brightly colored intermittent injection cap on the catheter tubing. TJC (2006) recommends labeling a catheter "epidural catheter" or using color-coded catheters to prevent accidental connections of IV tubing to the epidural catheter. Hospitals use tubing that has no access ports to minimize accidental introduction of IV medications. Administer continuous infusions through electronic infusion devices for

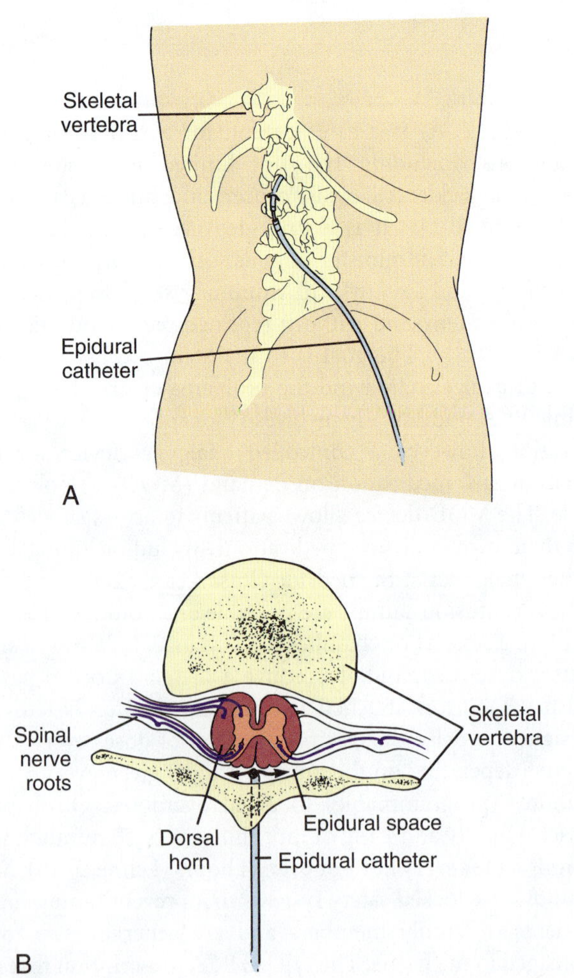

FIGURE 32-8 A, Epidural catheter inserted into L4-L5 space. **B,** Anatomical drawing of epidural space.

proper control. Because of the catheter location, follow strict surgical aseptic technique when handling tubing to prevent a potentially fatal infection. Notify a health care provider immediately if any signs or symptoms of infection or pain at the insertion site develop (Pasero and McCaffery, 2011).

Medications used commonly for epidural analgesia include preservative-free solutions of morphine sulfate, hydromorphone, fentanyl, sufentanil citrate, bupivacaine, and clonidine. Sometimes your patient receives the combination of two of these solutions. Do not administer supplemental doses of opioids or sedative/hypnotics because of possible additive central nervous system effects. Epidural medications block transmission of pain stimuli in the spinal cord (Pasero and McCaffery, 2011).

Nursing implications for managing epidural analgesia are numerous (Table 32-4). Monitoring for drug effects differs, depending on whether infusions are intermittent or continuous. Some complications of epidural opioid use are respiratory depression (rare), nausea and vomiting, urinary retention, constipation, orthostatic hypotension, and pruritus (Lehne, 2010). When you start patients on epidural analgesia, monitoring occurs as often as every 15 minutes, including assessment of respiratory rate, respiratory effort, and skin color. Often pulse oximetry is a standard measurement as well. If a patient remains stable, monitoring takes place every hour (see agency policy). Inform patients about the potential for respiratory depression and instruct them to notify you if breathing difficulty develops. If respiratory depression develops, turn off the infusion immediately.

Patients with Cancer Pain. Some cancer pain is stubborn and difficult to treat. It becomes so debilitating that patients will try anything to gain relief. The AHCPR developed clinical practice guidelines for the management of cancer pain that have been updated and continue to be a reference today (AHRQ, 2010; Jacox et al., 1994). The guidelines treat cancer pain in a more comprehensive and aggressive manner, thus providing patients and families more options for pain relief. Figure 32-9 is a flowchart depicting cancer pain management from assessment to various treatment measures. The best choice of treatment often changes when a patient's condition and the characteristics of pain change. Both nonpharmacological and pharmacological therapies are beneficial.

Various medications and routes of administration provide relief for patients with cancer pain. Long-acting or controlled-release medications are very successful. These controlled-released medications (e.g., morphine [MS Contin, RoxanolSR] and oxycodone [OxyContin] relieve pain for 8 to 12 hours). A 72-hour fentanyl patch is also available. You can manage most cancer pain with oral or patch medications.

Administering analgesics to treat cancer-related pain requires applying principles different from those used to treat acute pain. WHO (1990) has recommended a three-step approach to managing cancer pain (Figure 32-10). Therapy begins with NSAIDs and/or adjuvants and progresses to strong opioids if pain persists. Side effects of opioids such as nausea and constipation are treated aggressively so patients are able to continue using them. Patients usually become tolerant to their side effects, with the exception of constipation. Health care providers should routinely order stimulant laxatives, not simple stool softeners, to prevent and treat constipation.

When a patient with cancer first has pain, it is best to begin with a higher dosage than what will be routinely needed. This provides a patient with immediate pain relief. The health care provider then slowly decreases the dosage to the amount that successfully controls pain. Patients receiving long-term opioids often develop a drug tolerance. Therefore they require higher dosages to attain pain relief. Higher dosages are not

TABLE 32-4 NURSING CARE OF PATIENTS WITH EPIDURAL INFUSIONS

GOAL	ACTIONS
Prevent catheter displacement	Secure catheter (if not connected to implanted reservoir) carefully to skin.
Maintain catheter function	Check external dressing around catheter site for dampness or discharge. (Leak of cerebrospinal fluid may develop.) Use transparent, adhesive dressing to aid inspection. Inspect catheter for breaks.
Prevent infection	Use aseptic technique when caring for catheter. Do *not* routinely change dressing over site. Change tubing every 24 hours or per agency policy.
Monitor for respiratory depression	Monitor vital signs, especially respirations, per policy. Use pulse oximetry and apnea monitoring when necessary. Maintain head of bed at 30 to 45 degrees.
Prevent undesirable complications	Assess for pruritus (itching) and nausea and vomiting. Administer antihistamines and antiemetics as ordered. Verify that tubing is connected to epidural catheter; label appropriately.
Maintain urinary and bowel function	Monitor intake and output. Assess bladder and bowel for distention. Assess for discomfort, frequency, and urgency.

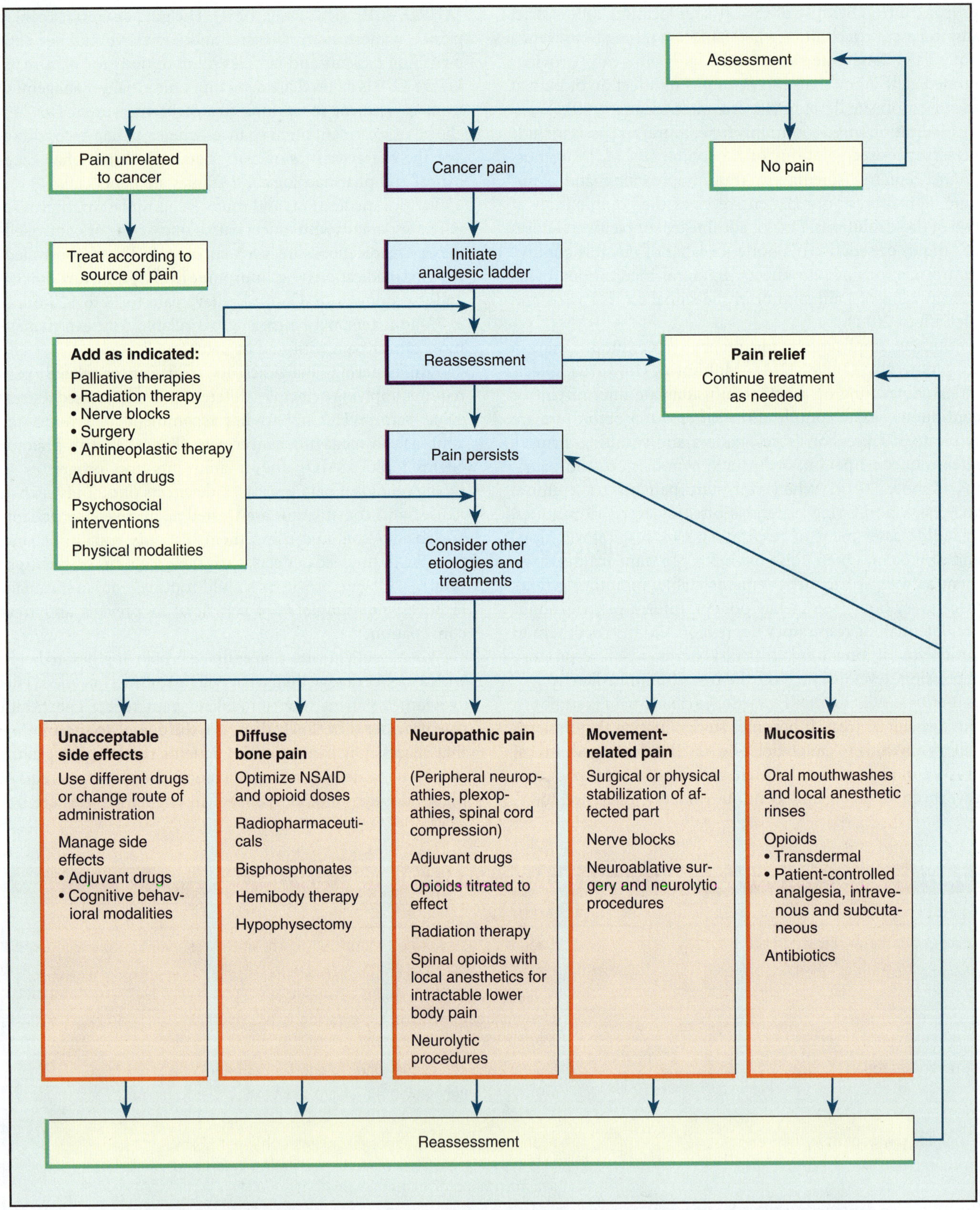

FIGURE 32-9 Flowchart: continuing pain management in patients with cancer. *NSAID*, Nonsteroidal antiinflammatory drug. (From Jacox A, et al: *Management of cancer pain,* Clinical Practice Guideline No. 9, AHCPR Pub No. 94-0592, Rockville MD, March 1994, Agency for Health Care Policy and Research, Public Health Service, US Department of Health and Human Services.)

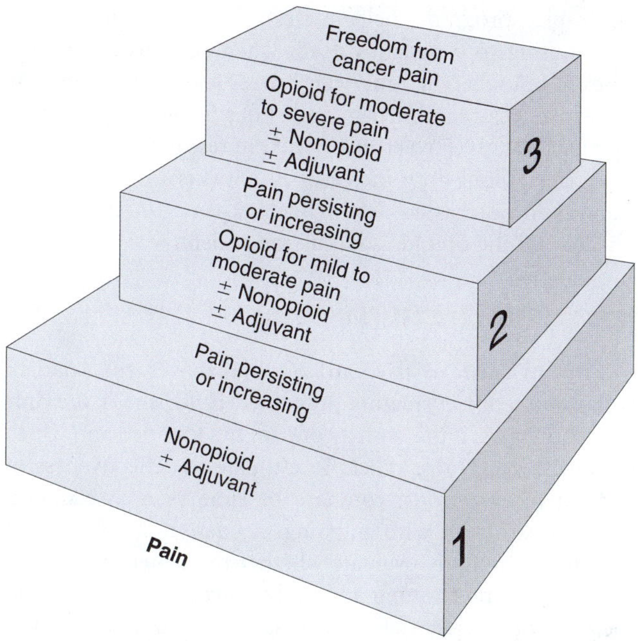

FIGURE 32-10 World Health Organization analgesic ladder is three-step approach to treating cancer pain: ± adjuvant, with or without adjuvant medications. (From http://www.who.int/cancer/palliative/painladder/en/. Accessed September 18, 2013.)

lethal because most patients also develop tolerance to life-threatening side effects (McCaffery and Pasero, 1999).

For patients with cancer the aim of drug therapy is to anticipate and prevent or minimize pain. Therefore it is necessary to give required analgesic dosages regularly, even when pain subsides. Regular administration maintains blood levels for ongoing pain control. However, patients still have flares of pain or "breakthrough pain" that requires additional bolus doses of medication (rescue doses). Breakthrough pain is a transient flare of moderate-to-severe pain superimposed on continuous or persistent pain. A decrease in the duration of pain relief or an increase in the intensity of pain relief provided by the regular analgesia therapy and the need for an increased number of rescue doses are indications that a patient needs a higher opioid dose (McCaffery and Pasero, 1999). A transmucosal fentanyl "unit" now exists to treat breakthrough pain in opioid-tolerant patients. Swab the fentanyl unit in the mouth over the buccal mucosa and gums. The unit stays intact to dissolve in the mouth, not to be chewed. Allow to absorb over a 15-minute period. Use no more than two units per breakthrough pain episode (Pasero and McCaffery, 2011); thereafter notify the health care provider.

Transdermal drug systems administer drugs (e.g., fentanyl) via a patch placed on the skin. Patches are useful when patients are unable to take drugs orally. Self-adhesive patches deposit the opioid into the subcutaneous tissue. The subcutaneous tissue releases the drug slowly over time at predetermined rates for 48 to 72 hours. This results in effective analgesia throughout the day and night. Inform patients that it sometimes takes 12 to 16 hours for analgesia to take effect when they first begin to use an analgesic patch (Pasero and McCaffery, 2011). Therefore it is important for you to obtain an order for an immediate-release opioid for any breakthrough pain. Heat causes more rapid drug absorption. For this reason warn patients to avoid external heat such as heating pads, hot showers, and prolonged exposure to the sun while using patches. Only patients who have chronic stable pain and who have routinely received 40 mg or more of morphine (or its equivalent) daily on an ATC basis for a week or more are candidates for the fentanyl patch.

Another measure for treating severe persistent cancer pain is morphine given by continuous IV drip or intermittently by a PCA pump. Continuous infusions provide uniform pain control at lower dosages. Thus there are fewer side effects. Continuous-drip morphine is given in acute care settings and the home. An infusion control pump delivers morphine intravenously to ensure safe and accurate administration. Each agency has guidelines for morphine dose and infusion rates.

When a patient receives continuous-drip morphine, assess the IV site to ensure that it is patent and without complications (e.g., no redness, swelling, or drainage). A central line catheter such as a Groshong or Hickman catheter, an implanted venous access port, or a peripherally inserted central catheter (PICC) is usually best for long-term IV infusion. When a patient starts on continuous IV morphine, you need to prevent overdose and central nervous system depression. Record baseline blood pressure and respiratory rates before the infusion begins. Monitor the patient closely for the first hour of the infusion and then according to agency policy. If the patient's blood pressure or respirations decrease, reduce the infusion rate according to the health care provider's order or agency policy. Small IV doses of naloxone can be ordered for severe respiratory depression and to increase respiratory rate and depth but not to reverse the pain relief (refer to agency policy). Patients who are placed on continuous analgesic infusions are opioid tolerant; thus respiratory depression is rare.

Restorative and Continuing Care. Patients in need of restorative care for pain usually have chronic persistent pain that is unrelenting. You continue to use nonpharmacological measures that are effective for individual patients. However, additional pharmacological measures designed to give patients better long-term pain control are required. The goal is to use a comprehensive approach in supporting the patient and family.

Opioid Infusions. In the home or extended care settings, patients use ambulatory infusion pumps for opioid infusions. The pumps are lightweight and compact and allow free movement. A pump is battery powered and worn in a pouch attached to a belt or harness. The bag of medication and parenteral fluid fits inside the pump. A dose of opioid, delivered continuously over 24 hours, is usually slowly infused intravenously through a PICC or a subclavian placed catheter (see Chapter 18). Both catheters are left in place for an extended period of time. Sometimes pain medication is infused subcutaneously with a small catheter that the patient inserts into subcutaneous tissue and replaces every 72 hours. The ambulatory pumps differ from PCA devices, which deliver only small, preset doses of medication. The patient and family learn to manage the pump, observe for drug side effects, and maintain function of the catheter that delivers the medication. Because the patient is managed initially on the opioid in the hospital before going home, the risk for side effects is not as great. The home care nurse routinely visits to be sure that patients or family members manage the pump correctly.

Failure of Pain Control Medications with Chronic Pain. The use of opioid therapy for chronic noncancer pain has increased dramatically. The concept of breakthrough pain in patients with this pain is poorly understood (Manchikanti et al., 2011). The issues related to failure of pain-control medications in managing chronic noncancer pain include high doses of long-acting opioids, high usage rates, overuse, misuse and abuse of prescription opioids, adverse drug events, and rising treatment costs. The impact of breakthrough pain in patients with chronic noncancer pain may include decreased quality of life, physical deconditioning, loss of productivity and work, and withdrawal from activities and social situations. Although treatment of breakthrough pain in cancer patients has been well supported in the literature, additional investigation is necessary in the area of chronic noncancer pain (Manchikanti et al., 2011).

Palliative Care. Palliative care offers treatments to help patients live, perhaps years, with a variety of incurable conditions, including persistent pain. The goals of palliative care are to relieve suffering and support the best possible quality of life for patients with chronic and life-threatening conditions and their family members (National Consensus Project, 2013). Palliative care is not the same as end-of-life or hospice pain management.

Patients with chronic pain require a different approach to pain management than patients with acute pain. Unfortunately health care providers cannot eliminate all pain, and learning to live with daily pain is not easy. It is important for patients with chronic pain to gain control of their pain versus allowing the pain to control them. Consider making a referral to the palliative care team when you care for patients diagnosed with incurable conditions that have persistent pain. These teams are composed of a variety of health care professionals who help patients achieve the level of pain control that allows them to function and enjoy life (National Consensus Project, 2013). The patient is an active participant in pain management. Without patient involvement, adequate pain control is not possible.

Hospice. Hospice programs care for the terminally ill by helping patients continue to live at home in comfort and privacy with the help of a health care team. The emphasis is on quality of life over quantity, and pain control is a priority. Under the guidance of hospice nurses, families learn to monitor patients' symptoms and become the primary caregivers. Some hospice patients become hospitalized such as in the event of a brief acute care crisis or family problem. Chapter 26 discusses hospice in detail.

Hospice programs help nurses overcome their fears of contributing to a patient's death when administering large doses of opioids. The American Nurses Association supports aggressive treatment of pain and suffering even if it hastens a patient's death (Fowler, 2010). Recent research suggests that moderate opioid dose increases in patients who are terminally ill do not hasten death (Bengoechea et al., 2010). The disease, not the opioid, is killing the patient.

EVALUATION

Patient Care. With regard to pain management, a patient is the source for evaluating outcomes. He or she is the only one who knows if the severity of pain has lessened and which therapies bring most relief. To evaluate the effectiveness of nursing interventions, compare baseline pain assessments before treatments with ongoing evaluation findings after treatment. Similarly evaluate whether the patient's response to pain (e.g., positioning and body movements or ability to socialize or perform self-care) has changed (Box 32-12). Compare actual outcomes with expected outcomes (see Care Plan) to determine if your patient met his or her goal. Is the

BOX 32-12 EVALUATION

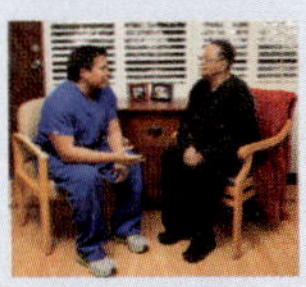

Two weeks after his last visit Jim returns to evaluate Mrs. Ellis's progress. Her niece is present, visiting. Mrs. Ellis reports that she has gone to see the nurse practitioner, who prescribed an NSAID for her arthritic pain. She has not filled the prescription yet and is still taking her aspirin. She continues to have some gastrointestinal irritation after taking the aspirin. Jim has the chance to observe Mrs. Ellis use a warm compress on her hands and wrists. She applies the heat correctly, and the niece helps correctly. After 15 minutes Mrs. Ellis rates her pain on the FACES Pain Scale as 3. She states that the heat is soothing. During the visit Mrs. Ellis gets up to go to the kitchen using her walker, which she obtained from the physical therapist. Jim notes that, although it takes her time to stand, her gait is steadier. He confirms that the niece can be called when Mrs. Ellis needs help at home. Mrs. Ellis shows Jim that she has her niece's phone number posted in the kitchen next to the phone. She also notes that her neighbor has offered help with shopping.

DOCUMENTATION NOTE

"Reports receiving some pain relief from using heat on hands. Rates pain at level 3 on the FACES Pain Scale after applying warm compresses. Niece is able to help correctly with procedure. Appears less fatigued and is ambulating with steadier gait, using walker. Continues to have gastric irritation following use of aspirin. Identified her niece as one whom she can call when she needs assistance, and her neighbor will help with shopping. Recommended that she have niece pick up NSAID prescription at pharmacy as soon as possible. Explained need to replace aspirin with NSAID. Will evaluate effectiveness of NSAID at next visit in 2 weeks."

NSAID, Nonsteroidal antiinflammatory drug.

patient able to perform the activities that pain had prevented? Continuous evaluation allows you to determine whether the patient needs new or revised therapies and if new nursing problems have developed. It is important to discuss the patient's ongoing pain-management needs with family members and health care providers who will be involved in the patient's care on discharge or transfer.

Patient Expectations. Subtle behaviors such as a gentle smile or a sigh of relief indicate the level of a patient's satisfaction with pain relief. However, it is important for you to *ask* patients if you have met their expectations. Do not ask them if they are satisfied with their pain management because patients often answer "yes" even when their pain is severe. Instead say to a patient, "Tell me how well you think your pain medicine is helping you" or "You agreed to try relaxation to lessen your abdominal pain. Tell me, how has this worked for you?" If a patient's expectations have not been met, you need to spend more time understanding his or her desires. Working closely with the patient enables you to help the patient set realistic expectations that will be met within the limits of his or her condition and treatment. It is also important to review the current pain-management plan and suggest changes as appropriate.

The HCAHPS (Hospital Consumer Assessment of Healthcare Providers and Services) survey is a national, standardized, publicly reported survey of patients' perspectives of hospital care. Data from HCAHPS provide a standard for comparing hospitals. HCAHPS scores influence how hospitals are reimbursed by the Centers for Medicare & Medicaid Services. Two of the 18 HCAHPS survey items focus on patients' perceptions of how well hospital staff manage their pain (HCAHPS, 2012).

SAFETY GUIDELINES FOR NURSING SKILLS

To ensure patient safety communicate clearly with members of the health care team, assess and incorporate a patient's priorities of care and preferences, and use the best evidence when making decisions about your patient's care. When performing the skills in this chapter, remember the following points to ensure safe, individualized patient care:

- Be vigilant during the entire process of medication administration. Ensure that your patients receive the appropriate medications by following the six rights (see Chapter 17). Know why each medication is ordered for your patient. Understand what you need to do before, during, and after medication administration. Evaluate the effectiveness and assess for adverse effects after your patients take their medications.
- Take care of yourself. You think as clearly and critically as possible if you are healthy. Healthy behaviors such as getting adequate sleep, making healthy food choices, and coping with stress in positive ways help you better process information and make safe decisions during medication administration.
- Set up and prepare medications in distraction-free areas.

SKILL 32-1 PATIENT-CONTROLLED ANALGESIA

View Video!

DELEGATION CONSIDERATIONS

The skill of patient-controlled analgesia cannot be delegated to nursing assistive personnel (NAP). The nurse directs the NAP to:

- Notify the nurse if the patient complains of pain or has signs of becoming oversedated.
- Notify the nurse if the patient has questions about the patient-controlled analgesia (PCA) process or equipment.
- Never administer a PCA dose for the patient.

EQUIPMENT

- PCA system
- Identification label and time tape (may already be attached and completed by pharmacy)
- Alcohol swab
- Adhesive tape
- Clean gloves when applicable
- Equipment for vital signs and pulse oximeter

STEP	RATIONALE
ASSESSMENT	
1. Assess patient's cognitive ability, including level of consciousness, memory, and ability to answer questions (see Chapter 16).	Determines if patient is able to use PCA for pain management.
2. Assess character of patient's pain, including location, duration, severity, quality, and predisposing and relieving factors.	Reveals source and nature of pain and factors that may increase it.
3. Assess for physical, behavioral, and emotional signs and symptoms of pain or discomfort.	Combination of signs and symptoms reveals source and nature of pain.

SKILL 32-1 PATIENT-CONTROLLED ANALGESIA—cont'd

STEP	RATIONALE
4. Assess patency of intravenous (IV) access and surrounding tissue for inflammation or swelling.	A patent IV line is necessary for safe administration of pain medication. Confirmation of placement of IV catheter and integrity of surrounding issues ensures that medication is administered safely.
5. Check accuracy and completeness of medication administration record (MAR) or computer printout with health care provider's order for patient's name, name of medication, dose, frequency of medication (continuous or demand or both), and lockout period.	Health care provider order required for administration of opioid mediation. Ensures that patient receives right medications.
6. Have a second registered nurse (RN) confirm health care provider's order and correct setup of PCA (see agency policy). The second RN independently checks health care provider's order and the machine and does not simply look at the first RN's setup.	Prevents medication errors.
7. Check patient's history for drug allergies. Be aware that nausea is not an allergic reaction and it can be treated; itching alone is not an allergic reaction and is common to opioid use. Itching is also treatable and does not rule out the use of PCA.	Avoids placing patient at risk for allergic reaction.
PLANNING	
1. Collect appropriate equipment.	Ensures an organized procedure.
2. Review medication information in drug reference manual or consult with pharmacist if uncertain about any medications to be administered.	Understanding medications before administering them prevents medication errors.
3. Explain purpose and demonstrate function of PCA to patient and family (see illustration).	Allows patient participation in care and independence in pain control. Preoperative education about PCA therapy improves postoperative pain relief (ASPMN, 2006).
4. Check infuser and patient-controlled module for accurate labeling or evidence of leaking.	Avoids medication error. Damage to system can occur; inspect to avoid injury or harm to patient, self, or others.
5. Program computerized PCA pump to deliver prescribed medication dose and lockout interval (see illustration).	Ensures safe, therapeutic drug administration.
6. Draw curtains around patient's bed or close door to room.	Maintains patient privacy.
7. Position patient comfortably for procedure. Maintain any position restrictions. Venipuncture or central line site needs to be accessible.	Comfortable position enhances effectiveness of analgesia.

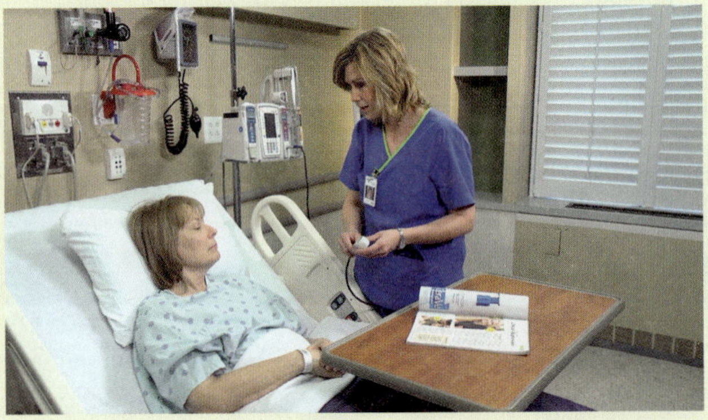

STEP 3 Explain purpose and demonstrate function of PCA.

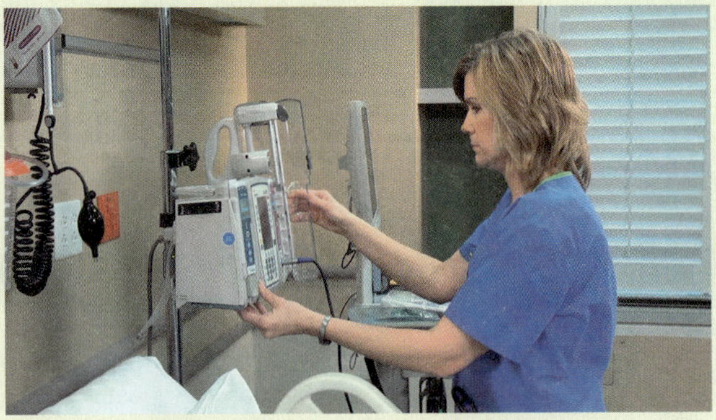

STEP 5 Programming PCA pump.

STEP	RATIONALE
IMPLEMENTATION	
1. Perform hand hygiene. Apply clean gloves.	Reduces transmission of microorganisms.
2. Follow the six rights of medication administration to be sure of correct medication. Identify patient using two identifiers (e.g., name and birthday or name and account number) according to agency policy. Compare identifiers with information on patient's MAR or medical record.	Ensures correct patient. Complies with The Joint Commission requirements for patient safety (TJC, 2014).
3. Attach drug reservoir to infusion device and prime tubing.	Locks system and prevents air from infusing into IV tubing.
4. Attach needleless adapter to tubing adapter of patient-controlled module.	Needed to connect with IV line.
5. Wipe injection port of maintenance IV line with alcohol if using a closed port.	Topical antiseptic minimizes entry of surface microorganisms during needle insertion.
6. Insert and secure needleless adapter into injection port nearest patient.	Establishes route for medication to enter main IV line. Prevents delay of medication delivery to patient. Needleless systems prevent needlestick injuries.
7. Administer loading dose of analgesia as prescribed; administer manually or program into PCA pump.	Establishes initial dose of analgesic to achieve pain control.
8. Discard gloves and supplies in appropriate containers. Dispose of empty cassette or syringe in compliance with institutional policy. Perform hand hygiene.	Reduces transmission of microorganisms. The Federal Controlled Substances Act regulates the control and dispensation of opioids for all institutions.
9. If PCA is discontinued before device is completely empty, record drug wastage on PCA MAR as another RN observes (see agency policy). Note date, time, amount of drug wasted, and reason for wastage.	Two RNs must witness wastage of opioids (narcotics) and sign the record to meet requirements of the Controlled Substances Act for scheduled drugs.
10. Most PCA systems need a secondary IV infusion running at TKO (to keep open) rate. Be sure that infusion is running properly before leaving room.	To maintain patency of vein between PCA intermittent (bolus) doses.
EVALUATION	
1. Use pain-rating scale to evaluate patient's pain intensity according to agency policy.	Determines response to PCA dosing.

Clinical Decision Point: **Documenting "PCA in use" or" PCA effective" is not an adequate record of the patient's pain level.**

STEP	RATIONALE
2. Observe patient for nausea or itching.	Common side effects of opiates.
3. Observe for signs of adverse reactions, especially excessive sedation. Monitor level of sedation (ability to arouse), respirations (rate and depth), pulse and blood pressure, and pulse oximetry every 2 hours for the first 12 hours.	Patient is at highest risk the first 12 hours of use. Excess sedation precedes respiratory depression.
4. According to agency policy, evaluate number of attempts (number of times patient pushed the button), delivery of demand doses (number of times drug actually given), and basal dose if ordered.	Helps to evaluate effectiveness of PCA dose and frequency in relieving pain. Maintains compliance with Controlled Substances Act.
5. Use Teach Back— State to the patient, "I want to be sure I explained to you how to use the PCA system when you experience pain. Can you show me how to use this device?" Revise your instruction now or develop plan for revised patient teaching to be implemented at an appropriate time if patient is not able to teach back correctly.	Evaluates what the patient is able to explain or demonstrate.

RECORDING AND REPORTING

- Record drug, dose, and time that PCA is initiated on MAR. Note lockout time, demand, and basal dose.
- Record regular assessments of patient pain, vital signs, and oxygen saturation.
- Record amount of drug delivered and amount wasted.
- Document your evaluation of patient learning.

SKILL 32-1 PATIENT-CONTROLLED ANALGESIA—cont'd

UNEXPECTED OUTCOMES AND RELATED INTERVENTIONS

- Patient verbalizes continued or worsening discomfort or displays nonverbal behaviors indicative of pain, suggesting that underlying condition has changed or patient is undermedicated.
  - Perform complete pain reassessment.
  - Inspect IV site for possible catheter occlusion or infiltration.
  - Consult with health care provider.
- Patient is not readily arousable.
  - Stop PCA, elevate head of bed unless contraindicated, and assess vital signs. Do not leave patient's bedside.
  - Notify health care provider and/or call for help.
  - Prepare to administer an opioid-reversing agent (naloxone [Narcan]).
- Patient unable to manipulate PCA device to maintain pain control.
  - Consult with health care provider regarding alternative medication route.
  - Discuss with health care provider possible basal (continuous) dose.
  - Assess patient support system for significant other who can responsibly manipulate PCA device as an authorized PCA agent.

KEY POINTS

- Acute pain, a protective mechanism that warns a person of tissue injury, is completely subjective.
- Misconceptions about pain lead to undertreatment of the patient's pain.
- A patient's age, gender, anxiety level, culture, previous experience, and meaning of pain influence the pain experience.
- The difference between acute and chronic pain involves the duration of discomfort, physical signs and symptoms, and the patient's perceptions regarding relief.
- Assessment of a patient's pain must be comprehensive and performed to understand the extent to which pain affects the person's ability to function.
- A patient's family and friends are a key resource in pain assessment.
- You individualize pain therapy by collaborating closely with a patient and often the family, using assessment findings, trying a variety of therapies, and maintaining the patient's well-being.
- Eliminating sources of painful stimuli is a basic nursing measure for promoting comfort.
- Nonpharmacological therapies are effective in altering patient perception of pain, promoting muscle relaxation, and giving a patient control over pain.
- When administering opioids know that respiratory depression is only clinically significant if there is a decrease in the rate *and* depth of respirations from a patient's baseline assessment.
- For patients unable to self-report pain be alert for subtle behaviors that indicate it.
- Using a regular ATC schedule for analgesic administration is more effective than an as-needed schedule.
- A PCA device gives patients pain control with a low risk for overdose.
- Your primary role in caring for a patient who receives local anesthesia is protecting the patient from injury.
- The goal of therapy for patients with chronic pain is to anticipate and prevent pain.
- When a patient is receiving epidural analgesia, do not administer supplemental doses of opioids or sedative/hypnotics because of possible additive central nervous system effects.

CLINICAL DECISION-MAKING EXERCISES

Jim returns to evaluate Mrs. Ellis's progress over the past month. He asks her to rate her arthritic pain on the FACES Pain Scale of 0 to 10. Mrs. Ellis rates it as 2. She states that, although her joints are still stiff and tender when she awakens in the morning and after she sits for long periods, the pain is not as sharp in her hands and knees. Mrs. Ellis reports that she saw her nurse practitioner 2 weeks ago and has been referred to physical therapy for supportive hand splints. She is continuing to use the warm compresses 3 times a day. Mrs. Ellis reports that she has been having "stomach pains." Jim asks her to rate her stomach pain on the scale of 0 to 10. Mrs. Ellis rates them as 3. She further states that she cannot point to the exact location of the stomach pain. Mrs. Ellis states that the nurse practitioner has prescribed an NSAID for pain control and ordered it around the clock, but she has not been to the pharmacy to pick up her prescription yet. So she continues taking her aspirin. When questioned about why she has not picked up the NSAID prescription, Mrs. Ellis states that she did not want to bother her neighbor again since he already takes her to the grocery store every 2 weeks. She further states that she plans to pick up the prescription when she goes to the grocery store the next time. Jim asks her if any family members are able to help her at home or with errands. Mrs. Ellis reports that her niece calls her several times a week and her cousin takes her to church once a week. During the visit Jim gets the chance to observe Mrs. Ellis walk to the kitchen. He notes that, although it takes her time to stand, her gait is steadier. She is ambulating with the walker that the physical therapist recommended. When asked, Mrs. Ellis also states the she falls asleep more easily if she takes her medication 30 minutes before going to bed.

1. Based on the assessment findings, describe Mrs. Ellis's pain status using the PQRSTU model of pain assessment.
2. Which kind of pain is Mrs. Ellis describing in reference to her "stomach pains"? Why would this concern you?
3. What is the priority nursing diagnosis for Mrs. Ellis?
4. Which plan would you recommend related to her aspirin and the new NSAID prescription?
5. Given Mrs. Ellis's history and age, which nonpharmacological nursing intervention could Jim recommend that she use to help alleviate the pain?

evolve

Answers to Clinical Decision-Making Exercises can be found on the Evolve website.

QSEN ACTIVITY: PATIENT-CENTERED CARE

As Jim continues to work with Mrs. Ellis, he becomes concerned about her safety related to living alone and having significant physical limitations. He suggests that she ask her niece or cousin to help her by coming to visit her in her home routinely. Mrs. Ellis responds immediately that she does not want to be a burden to her family. However, she does agree that her niece seems willing to help her.

How can Jim include the niece in a patient-centered approach to Mrs. Ellis's pain management?

evolve

Answers to QSEN Activities can be found on the Evolve website.

REVIEW QUESTIONS

1. A 24-year-old patient is admitted to the trauma unit with a diagnosis of a fractured femur after a motor vehicle accident. He states that he has pain in the injured leg. What should be the first action taken by the nurse?
   1. Administer the lowest dose of pain medication
   2. Assess the characteristics of the pain
   3. Call the orthopedic surgeon
   4. Complete the admission assessment
2. A 7-year-old pediatric patient tells you that he is in pain. The patient rates the pain as 4 on the Faces Pain Scale of 0 to 10. His mother, who is in the room, states that her son is having pain at a level of 8 on the 0 to 10 scale. Which is the most accurate assessment of the pain?
   1. The patient is the best resource for assessing the pain and should receive the appropriate pain medication.
   2. The patient is the best resource for assessing the pain but should not receive the pain medication because his pain level is only 4 out of 10.
   3. The primary health care provider is the best resource for assessing the pain and should be called to determine if the pain medication should be administered.
   4. The family member is the best resource for assessing the pain, and the patient should receive the maximum dose of pain medication ordered.
3. Your patient developed respiratory depression after her first dose of intravenous (IV) morphine. After giving 0.2 mg of naloxone (Narcan) IV push, the patient's respiratory rate and depth are within normal limits. Which action do you take now?
   1. Leave the patient alone to sleep
   2. Discontinue all pain medications ordered
   3. Administer another dose of naloxone in 1 hour
   4. Assess the patient's vital signs every 15 minutes for 2 hours
4. A patient with a history of stroke 4 years ago resulting in aphasia (inability to verbally express thoughts) returns to the surgical unit after a cholecystectomy. The surgeon ordered an intravenous pain medication every 4 hours as needed (prn) for postoperative pain. The best nursing intervention related to pain control after surgery would be to:
   1. Administer the pain medication when the patient becomes restless.
   2. Wait until the patient verbalizes that he is experiencing pain to administer the pain medication.
   3. Assess the patient's level of pain with a Faces Pain Scale.
   4. Administer the pain medication every 4 hours.
5. One hour after administering the first dose of an intravenous opioid to your postoperative patient, about which of the following assessments should you be most concerned?
   1. Respiratory rate of 6 breaths/min
   2. Oxygen saturation of 95%
   3. Heart rate of 70
   4. Blood pressure of 140/72
6. Your patient is being discharged home on an around-the-clock opioid for chronic rheumatoid arthritis pain. You would expect an order for which of the following classes of medications to accompany this order?
   1. Laxative
   2. Antibiotic
   3. Stool softener
   4. Proton pump inhibitor
7. Which of the following instructions for use of a patient-controlled analgesia (PCA) pump is most important when educating the patient and family before implementation?
   1. Notify the nurse when you need to push the button.
   2. Only the patient should push the button.
   3. A spouse can push the button when the patient is asleep.
   4. Wait for the pain to become severe before pushing the button.
8. Your patient is recovering from knee surgery and states that her pain level is 5 on a 0- to-10 pain scale. She

received a dose of medication 15 minutes ago. Which interventions may be beneficial for this patient at this time? (Select all that apply.)
1. Massage her back.
2. Help her be repositioned on her side.
3. Tell her that she cannot have any more pain medication at this time because she may become addicted to it.
4. Take a few minutes and talk to her about the pictures of her family that she brought with her.

9. You are caring for a patient who receives an opioid analgesic and a corticosteroid for breast cancer that has spread to the bones. The patient's husband inquires about the purpose of the corticosteroid. What is your best answer?
1. The steroid prevents further spread of the cancer.
2. The steroid is an adjuvant to reduce inflammation.
3. The steroid is an NSAID for enhancing pain control.
4. The steroid is a nonopioid analgesic.

10. Which of the following nursing interventions can improve the effectiveness of relaxation? (Select all that apply.)
1. When using guided imagery, explain the technique in detail.
2. Make the environment stimulating by being sure that lights are turned on.
3. Describe any sensations that patients will experience as they begin to relax.
4. Explain the relaxation technique when the patient's pain is most severe.

evolve

Rationales for Review Questions can be found on the Evolve website.

1. 2; **2.** 1; **3.** 4; **4.** 3; **5.** 1; **6.** 1; **7.** 2; **8.** 1, 2, 4; **9.** 2; **10.** 1, 3

REFERENCES

Agency for Health Care Policy and Research (AHCPR), Acute Pain Management Guideline Panel: *Acute pain management in infants, children and adolescents: operative or medical procedures and trauma*, Clinical Practice Guideline, AHCPR Pub No. 92-0032, Rockville, MD, 1992, Agency for Health Care Policy and Research, Public Health Service, US Department of Health and Human Services.

Agency for Healthcare Research and Quality (AHRQ): *Cancer pain management (general)*, updated 2010, http://guideline.gov/content.aspx?id=23895. Accessed October 15, 2013.

Allred K, et al: The effect of music on postoperative pain and anxiety, *Pain Manage Nurs* 11(1):15, 2010.

American Bar Association: *Legal guide for the seriously ill*, 2009, http://apps.americanbar.org/abanet/media/release/news_release.cfm?releaseid=849. Accessed October 15, 2013.

American Geriatrics Society (AGS): Pharmacological management of persistent pain in older persons, *J Am Geriatr Soc* 57:1331, 2009.

American Pain Society (APS): *Principles of analgesic use in the treatment of acute and cancer pain*, ed 5, Glenview, IL, 2003, The Society.

American Pain Society (APS): *APS Press Room, Media Backgrounder*, July 2012, http://www.americanpainsociety.org/about-aps/Press-Room/about-aps-press-room.html. Accessed October 15, 2013.

American Society of Anesthesiologists (ASA): Practice guidelines for chronic pain management, *Anesthesiology* 112:1, 2010.

American Society for Pain Management Nursing (ASPMN): Patient-controlled analgesia: authorized agent controlled analgesia, a position statement, *Pain Manag Nurs* 7(4):134, 2006.

Arnstein P: Learning to "live with" chronic pain: lessons from Mrs. Tandy, *Adv Pract Nurs eJ* 7(1), 2007, http://www.medscape.com/viewarticle/557719. Accessed December 9, 2013.

Arthritis Foundation: *Medications for rheumatoid arthritis*, 2012, http://www.arthritistoday.org/about-arthritis/types-of-arthritis/rheumatoid-arthritis/treatment-plan/medication-overview/ra-medications.php. Accessed October 15, 2013.

Barclay L: Physical therapy modalities helpful for the family clinician to know, *Medscape Medical News*, 2007, http://www.medscape.org/viewarticle/567325. Accessed December 9, 2013.

Bengoechea I, et al: Opioid use at the end of life and survival in a hospital at home unit, *J Palliat Med* 13(9):10799, 2010.

Beyer J, et al: The creation, validation, and continuing development of the Oucher: a measure of pain intensity in children, *J Pediatr Nurs* 7(5):335, 1992.

Bruckenthal P: *Risk factors associated with the onset of persistent pain*, 2008, http://www.medscape.org/viewarticle/576473. Accessed September 3, 2012.

Chou R, et al: Clinical guidelines for the use of chronic opioid therapy in chronic noncancer pain, *J Pain* 10(2):113, 2009.

Chumbley G, Thomas S: Care of the patient receiving epidural analgesia, *Nurs Stand* 25(9):35, 2010.

Cutshall SM, et al: Effect of massage therapy on pain, anxiety, and tension in cardiac surgical patients: a pilot study, *Complement Ther Clin Pract* 16(2):92, 2010.

D'Arcy Y: Meeting the challenges of acute pain management, *Neurol Neurosurg* 2008, http://www.medscape.org/viewarticle/574105. Accessed December 9, 2013.

Engwall M, Duppils GS: Music as a nursing intervention for postoperative pain: a systematic review, *J PeriAnesth Nurs* 24(6):370, 2009.

Fairchild A: Under-treatment of cancer pain, *Curr Opin Support Palliat Care* 4(1):11, 2010.

Fowler MDM: *Guide to the code of ethics for nurses*, Silver Spring, MD, 2010, American Nurses Association.

Harris M, Richards KC: The physiological and psychological effects of slow-stroke back massage and hand massage on relaxation in older people, *J Clin Nurs* 19(7-8):917, 2010.

Herr K, et al: Pain assessment in the patient unable to self-report: position statement with clinical practice recommendations, *Pain Manag Nurs* 12(4):230, 2011.

Hospital Consumer Assessment of Healthcare Providers and Services (HCAHPS): *HCAHPS fact sheet*, 2012, hcahpsonline.org/files/HCAHPS%20 Fact%20sheet%20May%202012.pdf.

Hughes RG, editor: *Patient safety and quality: an evidence-based handbook for nurses*, prepared with support from the Robert Wood Johnson Foundation, AHRQ Publication No. 08-0043, Rockville, MD, 2008, Agency for Healthcare Research and Quality.

Institute of Medicine (IOM): *Relieving pain in America: a blueprint for transforming prevention, care, education, and research*, Washington, DC, 2011, National Academies Press.

Jacox A, et al: *Management of cancer pain*, Clinical Practice Guideline No. 9, AHCPR Pub No. 94-0592, Rockville, MD, 1994, Agency for Health Care Policy and Research, US Department of Health and Human Services, Public Health Service.

Jann M, Slade J: Antidepressant agents for the treatment of chronic pain and depression, *Pharmacotherapy* 27(11):1571, 2007.

Kaufman G: Basic pharmacology of nonopioid analgesics, *Nurs Stand* 24(30):55, 2010.

Kwekkeboom KL, Gretarsdottir E: Systematic review of relaxation interventions for pain, *J Nurs Scholarship* 38(3):269, 2006.

Lehne R: *Pharmacology for nursing care*, ed 7, Philadelphia, 2010, Saunders.

Manchikanti L, et al: Breakthrough pain in chronic noncancer pain: fact, fiction, or abuse, *Pain Physician* 14: E103, 2011.

McCaffery M: *Nursing management of the patient with pain*, ed 2, Philadelphia, 1979, Lippincott.

McCaffery M, Pasero C: *Pain: clinical manual*, ed 2, St Louis, 1999, Mosby.

Melzack R, Wall P: *The challenge of pain*, ed 2, London, 1996, Penguin.

Menefee-Pujol LA, Katz NP, Zacharoff KL: *PainEDU.org manual: a pocket guide to pain management*, ed 3, Newton, MA, 2007, Inflexxion.

Narayan MC: Culture's effects on pain assessment and management, *AJN* 110(4):38, 2010.

National Cancer Institute (NCI): *Fatigue (PDQ)*, 2013, http://www.cancer.gov/cancertopics/pdq/supportivecare/fatigue/Patient. Accessed October 15, 2013.

National Consensus Project: *Clinical practice guidelines for quality palliative care*, ed 3, 2013, http://www.nationalconsensusproject.org/NCP_Clinical_Practice_Guidelines_3rd_Edition.pdf. Accessed October 15, 2013.

Oliver J, et al: American Society for Pain Management Nursing Position Statement: pain management in patients with substance use disorders, *Pain Manage Nurs* 13(3):169, 2012.

Pasero C, McCaffery M: *Pain assessment and pharmacologic management*, St Louis, 2011, Mosby.

Rosati J, et al: Evaluation of an oral patient-controlled analgesia device for pain management in oncology inpatients, *J Supportive Oncol* 5(9):448, 2007.

The Joint Commission (TJC): *Patients' bill of rights and responsibilities*, amended 2005, http://www.usafa.edu/10abw/10mdg/cc/support/patient_BillofRights.pdf. Accessed February 4, 2013.

The Joint Commission (TJC): *Tubing misconnection: a persistent and potentially deadly occurrence*, Sentinel Event Alert, 36, 2006, http://www.jointcommission.org/sentinel_event_alert_issue_36_tubing_misconnections%E2%80%94a_persistent_and_potentially_deadly_occurrence/. Accessed October 15, 2013.

The Joint Commission (TJC): *Facts about pain management*, 2012, http://www.jointcommission.org/assets/1/18/Pain_Management.pdf. Accessed October 15, 2013.

The Joint Commission (TJC): *Comprehensive accreditation manual for hospital standards: the official handbook*, Oak Brook, IL, 2013, The Commission.

The Joint Commission (TJC): *National Patient Safety Goals*, Oakbrook Terrace, IL, 2014, The Commission. Available at http://www.jointcommission.org/standards_information/npsgs.aspx.

Vaartio H, et al: Nursing advocacy in procedural pain care, *Nurs Ethics* 16(3):340, 2009.

Vallerand A, et al: Knowledge of and barriers to pain management in caregivers of cancer patients receiving homecare, *Cancer Nurs* 30(1):31, 2007.

Wong DL, Baker CM: Pain in children: comparison of assessment scales, *Pediatr Nurs* 14(1):9, 1988.

World Health Organization (WHO): *Cancer pain relief and palliative care*, Report of a WHO expert committee, WHO Technical Report Series No. 804, Geneva, Switzerland, 1990, WHO.

Wright A: *Exploring the evidence for using TENS to relieve pain*, Nursing Times.Net, March 9, 2012, http://www.nursingtimes.net/exploring-the-evidence-for-using-tens-to-relieve-pain/5042395.article. Accessed October 15, 2013.

Wuhrman E, et al: *Authorized and unauthorized ("PCA by PROXY") dosing of analgesic infusion pumps*, 2006, http://www.aspmn.org/organization/documents/PCAbyProxy-final-ew_004.pdf. Accessed October 15, 2013.

CHAPTER 33

Nutrition

evolve WEBSITE

http://evolve.elsevier.com/Potter/essentials

- Video Clip
- Crossword Puzzle
- Audio Glossary

OBJECTIVES

- Explain the importance of a balance between energy intake and output.
- List the end products of carbohydrate, protein, and lipid metabolism.
- Explain the significance of saturated, unsaturated, and polyunsaturated lipids in nutrition.
- Describe the basic food groups and their value in planning meals for good nutrition.
- Explain dietary guidelines.
- Discuss the major areas of nutritional assessment.
- Identify nutritional problems and describe a patient at risk for these problems.
- Establish a plan of care to meet the nutritional needs of a patient.
- Discuss methods for feeding patients who require assistance with oral intake.
- Describe the procedure for initiating and maintaining enteral tube feedings.
- Describe the procedure for initiating and maintaining parenteral nutrition.

KEY TERMS

amino acids, p. 905
anabolism, p. 907
anthropometry, p. 915
basal metabolic rate (BMR), p. 907
body mass index (BMI), p. 911
carbohydrates, p. 905
catabolism, p. 907
dietary reference intakes (DRIs), p. 908
dysphagia, p. 915
enteral nutrition (EN), p. 924
gluconeogenesis, p. 907
glycogenesis, p. 907
ideal body weight (IBW), p. 915
jejunostomy tube, p. 928
lipid, p. 906
medical nutrition therapy (MNT), p. 930
metabolism, p. 907
minerals, p. 906
monounsaturated fatty acid, p. 906
nitrogen balance, p. 905
nutrient, p. 905
parenteral nutrition (PN), p. 928
polyunsaturated fatty acid, p. 906
saturated fatty acid, p. 906
unsaturated fatty acid, p. 906
vitamins, p. 906

Nutrition is a basic component of health and is essential for normal growth and development, tissue maintenance and repair, cellular metabolism, and organ function. The human body needs an adequate supply of nutrients for essential functions of cells.

Scientific principles regarding nutrition and the role of various nutrients in metabolism and health form a basis for the nutritional plan of care that you develop with your patients. Disease processes, age, gender, and activity all affect use of nutrients and nutritional requirements.

CASE STUDY *Mrs. Gonzalez*

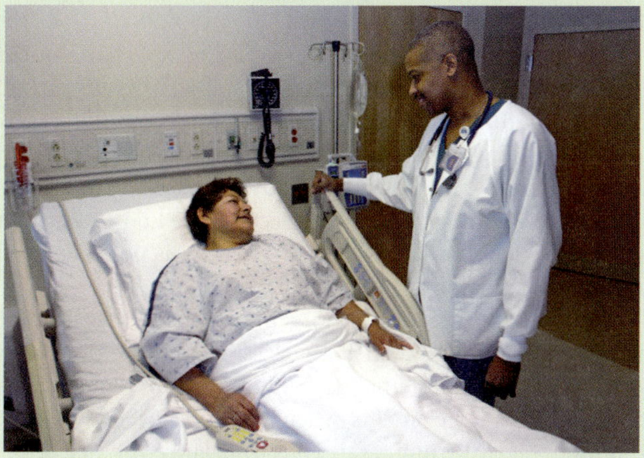

Mrs. Gonzalez is a 65-year-old Hispanic woman who comes to the emergency department with slurred speech, right facial droop, and weakness in her upper and lower right-side extremities. She is admitted to the hospital with a diagnosis of acute stroke. Mrs. Gonzalez lives alone in a senior apartment complex. She has a daughter and two teenage grandchildren who live in another town nearby.

Mrs. Gonzalez is awake and alert in her hospital room but is drooling from the right side of her mouth. When she tries to drink water, she starts to cough. The physician ordered nothing by mouth (NPO). The evaluation by the speech-language pathologist (SLP) indicates inadequate clearance of food and liquid from the vocal folds and aspiration of thickened liquids. Mrs. Gonzalez has trouble swallowing with oropharyngeal dysphagia. The SLP recommends enteral (EN) feedings and speech and swallowing therapy to help her return to oral feedings.

Matt is a nursing student assigned to Mrs. Gonzalez. As he prepares to assess her, he recalls information about the effect of dysphagia on nutrition and rehabilitation. He will assess Mrs. Gonzalez's weight and weight history, diet history, and cultural customs. Matt knows to consult with a registered dietitian (RD) to assess Mrs. Gonzalez's nutritional status and help with nutritional interventions. Matt and the RD will work as team members along with the SLP and physician to help Mrs. Gonzalez in her speech and swallowing rehabilitation.

Matt is responsible for initiating the tube feedings after Mrs. Gonzalez's small-bore nasogastric (NG) feeding tube is inserted. The RD recommends a feeding plan that will meet her nutritional needs. Matt will continue to work with the RD in preventing problems and monitoring for safe and effective delivery of her EN feeding.

Pharmaceutical agents prescribed to treat disease also interact with nutrients and foods.

SCIENTIFIC KNOWLEDGE BASE

Principles of Nutrition

The body requires food to provide energy for movement, maintenance of body temperature, growth and development, cellular metabolism, synthesis and repair of tissues, and organ function. The gastrointestinal (GI) system contains a number of organs and structures that nourish the body through the ingestion of food. Each organ or structure in the GI tract has a specific function aimed toward preparing food for the digestion and absorption of its nutrients.

Nutrients. A **nutrient** is a chemical substance that provides nourishment and affects metabolic and nutritive processes. The essential nutrients include carbohydrates, proteins, lipids, vitamins, minerals, and water. Only carbohydrates, proteins, and lipids provide energy. Vitamins and minerals are catalysts for the use of nutrients for energy. Minerals and water regulate body processes.

Carbohydrates. **Carbohydrates** are composed of carbon, hydrogen, and oxygen. They are starches and sugars obtained mainly from plant foods, with the exception of lactose, which is found in milk (milk sugar). Carbohydrates contribute as much as 90% of the total caloric intake in parts of the world where grains are a major food source. Carbohydrates are a source of energy, providing 4 kilocalories per gram (kcal/g).

Another type of carbohydrate is fiber. Fiber is the structural part of plants and is sometimes called *nonstarch polysaccharides*. It also includes some nonpolysaccharides such as lignins and tannins. Human digestive enzymes cannot break down fiber. Therefore it does not contribute calorically to the diet. Each fiber has a different structure. Most fibers contain monosaccharides, which differ in regards to types and bonds. Fiber is either soluble or insoluble. Soluble fiber becomes a gel in water and delays GI transit time; because of this, soluble fiber helps prevent diarrhea in patients receiving tube feedings. Insoluble fiber does not change in water and accelerates intestinal transit; this is helpful in preventing constipation in patients taking pain medication.

Proteins. **Amino acids** are the building blocks of proteins and are made of hydrogen, oxygen, carbon, and nitrogen. They are the most important components of proteins in the human body and are essential for synthesis of body tissue in growth, maintenance, and repair. The body is unable to synthesize some amino acids such as essential amino acids. It can only obtain these from daily food sources. Proteins are a source of energy, providing 4 kcal/g.

The required daily intake of protein varies according to age. For example, infants under 6 months of age require 2.2 g/kg daily. Adolescents require 1 g/kg daily. Most healthy adults require only about 0.8 g/kg of body weight per day. In disease such as in patients with major burns, protein requirements double or triple. Pregnant women require an additional 30 g, and lactating women an additional 20 g above the usual daily need.

Protein is composed of 16% nitrogen. The body uses nitrogen for building, repair, and replacement of body tissues. The achievement of equal nitrogen input and output is called **nitrogen balance.** When intake of nitrogen is greater than output, the patient is in positive nitrogen balance. The body needs a positive nitrogen balance for growth, maintenance of lean muscle mass and vital organs, and wound healing. When output of nitrogen is greater than intake, negative nitrogen balance occurs. Negative nitrogen balance occurs in infection, sepsis, fever, burns, starvation, and trauma. Protein provides energy; however, because of the essential role of protein in growth, maintenance, and repair, a diet needs to provide adequate kilocalories from nonprotein sources. When there is insufficient carbohydrate in the diet to meet the energy needs of the body, protein stores are used as an energy source.

Fats. Fats **(lipids)** are compounds that are insoluble in water but soluble in organic solvents such as ethanol and acetone. Fats are made up of triglycerides and fatty acids. Lipids are a source of energy, providing 9 kcal/g.

Triglycerides are made up of three fatty acids attached to a glycerol. Approximately 98% of the lipids in foods and 90% of the lipids in the human body are in the form of triglycerides. Triglycerides contribute to high blood levels of certain lipoproteins linked to cardiovascular diseases.

A **saturated fatty acid** contains as much hydrogen as it is able to hold. A **monounsaturated fatty acid** is able to take up another hydrogen atom, and a **polyunsaturated fatty acid** is able to take up many more hydrogen atoms and become hydrogenated or saturated fat. Ingestion of saturated fatty acids appears to increase blood cholesterol levels. Ingestion of **unsaturated fatty acids** has a minimal effect on blood cholesterol. Monounsaturated fatty acids appear to lower blood cholesterol levels. Fatty acids are usually not purely saturated, unsaturated, or polyunsaturated. Most animal fats have high proportions of saturated fatty acids; most vegetable fats have higher amounts of unsaturated and polyunsaturated fatty acids (e.g., safflower oil is about 75% polyunsaturated, olive oil about 25%). Trans fatty acids are created when vegetable oils are hydrogenated in food processing; they raise "bad" cholesterol while lowering "good" cholesterol.

There are also essential fatty acids (EFAs). The two primary EFAs are linoleic acid (an omega-6 fatty acid) and linolenic acid (an omega-3 fatty acid). EFAs have many roles in the body, including the production of cell membranes and hormones. The metabolism of EFAs has effects on the regulation of blood pressure, blood clot formation, and immune response.

Vitamins. **Vitamins** are organic substances present in small amounts in foods and are essential for normal metabolism. They serve as coenzymes or catalysts in cellular enzyme reactions. The body is unable to synthesize vitamins in the required amounts and depends on dietary intake. The exception to this is vitamin K, which the body synthesizes by bacteria in the intestine. Although vitamins are contained in many foods, processing, storage, and preparation all affect them. Vitamin content is usually highest in foods that are fresh and used quickly after minimal exposure to heat, air, or water. Certain vitamins, including beta-carotene and vitamins A, C, and E (Nix, 2013), are being studied in their role as antioxidants. They neutralize substances called *free radicals,* which produce oxidative damage to body cells and tissues. Vitamins are water soluble and fat soluble.

Water-soluble vitamins (C and B complex) are stored in limited amounts for short periods of time, requiring daily consumption. Although they are not stored, toxicity can still occur from excessive intake. Water-soluble vitamins are absorbed easily from the GI tract.

Fat-soluble vitamins (A, D, E, and K) are able to be stored in the body for longer periods; however, dietary intake is still necessary, with some exceptions. Vitamin K is in dark, leafy green vegetables; but the body also produces it within the large intestine. In addition, the body produces vitamin D as a response to sunlight exposure. Because the body has a high storage capacity for these vitamins, toxicity is possible when a person takes large doses of them.

Minerals. **Minerals** are inorganic elements that catalyze biochemical reactions. They are classified as macrominerals when the daily requirement is 100 mg or more and microminerals or trace elements when the body needs less than 100 mg daily. Macrominerals help to balance the pH of the body, and specific amounts are necessary in the blood and cells to promote acid-base balance. Interactions occur among trace minerals. For example, excess of one trace mineral sometimes causes deficiency of another. This deficiency then allows for or worsens the deficiency of another.

Vitamins and minerals are best obtained from a healthy diet. When deficiencies or potential deficiencies exist, they can also be provided through supplementation. However, vitamin and mineral supplements may not always be beneficial, especially when taken in excess amounts that may be toxic.

Water. Normal cell function depends on an aqueous environment, so water is an important nutrient. Water has the following functions in the body: transporting nutrients and waste products; providing a structure to large molecules (protein, glycogen); promoting metabolic reactions; serving as solvent, lubricant, and cushion; regulating body temperature; and maintaining blood volume.

Water makes up 60% to 70% of the total body weight. A lean person's body contains a higher percentage of water than an obese person's body. Infants have the greatest percentage of total body weight as water; older adults have the least. Infants and older adults are most vulnerable to water deprivation or water loss.

The human body requires 1.5 mL of water for every kilocalorie of energy used. The ingestion of liquids and solid foods such as fresh fruits and vegetables aids the body in meeting fluid needs. The body also produces water when food is oxidized during digestion.

Thirst is a protective mechanism that alerts an oriented person to the need for fluids. It is a less reliable guide for infants and patients who are confused because they are unable to communicate that they are thirsty.

Digestion. The process of digestion begins in the mouth, where mastication, or chewing, breaks down food into smaller particles, and amylase in saliva begins to break down starches. Mucus lubricates food particles for their passage through the esophagus into the stomach. Churning movements of the stomach mix food particles with hydrochloric acid in the stomach. The body produces gastric lipase and amylase to begin fat and starch digestion. Digestive proteins, or enzymes, in the GI system break food particles into a simpler form. The small intestine digests and absorbs most nutrients, whereas the large intestine absorbs electrolytes and water, thus helping to maintain the electrolyte balance of the body (see Chapter 18).

Absorption. The small intestine is the primary site of absorption of simple nutrients. It is lined with villi, which project into the lumen and greatly increase the surface area available for absorption. The upper duodenum absorbs cholesterol, vitamins E and K, folic acid, riboflavin, and thiamin. The lower duodenum and upper jejunum absorb glucose, amino acids, minerals, and fats; and the lower jejunum and ileum absorb sucrose, lactose, and maltose. Understanding sites of absorption explains the nature of diseases that affect intestinal function.

Intestinal contents move by peristaltic action into the large intestine. The large intestine absorbs water and electrolytes. The body excretes other nutrients remaining in the intestinal contents when they reach the large intestine as waste products. The body loses nutrients when intestinal motility is increased (i.e., diarrhea). This occurs because diarrhea causes the nutrients to move through the small intestine too quickly for complete absorption.

Metabolism. Metabolism refers to all of the bodily biochemical and physiological processes. Through metabolism nutrients are converted into necessary substances for cell function. The two basic types of metabolism are anabolism and catabolism. Anabolism is the production of more-complex chemical substances by synthesis of nutrients needed to build or repair body tissue. Catabolism is the breakdown of body tissues into simpler substances. Although catabolism produces some energy, both processes require energy, which comes from food or stored sources.

Carbohydrate, protein, and fat produce chemical energy and maintain a dynamic balance of tissue buildup and breakdown. The chemical energy produced by metabolism is converted to other types of energy by different tissues. Muscle contraction involves mechanical energy, the nervous system involves electrical energy, and the mechanisms of heat production involve thermal energy. These forms of energy all begin in metabolism.

Absorbed nutrients travel to the liver, where major metabolic processes occur. The liver also regulates energy through its control of glucose metabolism. Glucose is the primary fuel for the body. The liver and muscles store glucose in the form of glycogen via a process called glycogenesis. Lipogenesis converts glucose to fat for storage. Insulin and glucagon act as regulatory hormones to promote glucose storage or use. Insulin promotes glucose use, and glucagon promotes glucose storage. During states in which energy needs exceed glycogen storage, the body breaks down fat and amino acids for conversion to glucose via a process called gluconeogenesis.

The basal metabolic rate (BMR) represents the energy needs of a person at rest after awakening. Energy needs are based on BMR along with activity level, energy required to break down food, and energy required for healing during illness. Energy balance occurs when energy requirements equal energy intake. In general, when energy needs exceed intake, a person loses weight. If intake exceeds energy needs, a person gains weight.

Storage. The body stores energy as adipose tissue. Glycogen is stored in small reserves in liver and muscle tissue, and protein is stored in muscle mass. When body energy demands exceed dietary sources, the body uses stored (fat) energy. When the body has unused energy, it is stored principally in fat. Fat-soluble vitamins are also stored in limited reserves (6 to 8 months), and the body releases them to meet the needs when dietary intake is insufficient. Most water-soluble vitamins are stored for only 3 to 5 days.

Elimination. The intestinal contents move through the large intestine by peristalsis (see Chapter 35). As the contents move toward the rectum, water is resorbed through the mucosa. The end products of digestion include cellulose and similar fibrous substances that the body is unable to digest. The body also eliminates sloughed cells from the intestinal walls, mucus, digestive secretions, water, and microorganisms.

Dietary Guidelines

A number of agencies and organizations in the United States regularly publish and update dietary guidelines. The guidelines change as nutritional researchers discover new knowledge.

Food Guidelines. The ChooseMyPlate program was developed by the U.S. Department of Agriculture (USDA) (Figure 33-1) to replace the food pyramid (USDA, 2013). ChooseMyPlate aims to help the American population choose healthier foods and confront the obesity epidemic by providing a basic, visual guide for making food choices for a healthy lifestyle. The USDA also developed a number of educational tools that are accessible through their website: http://www.choosemyplate.gov/print-materials-ordering.html. Choose my Plate, along with the U.S. Department of

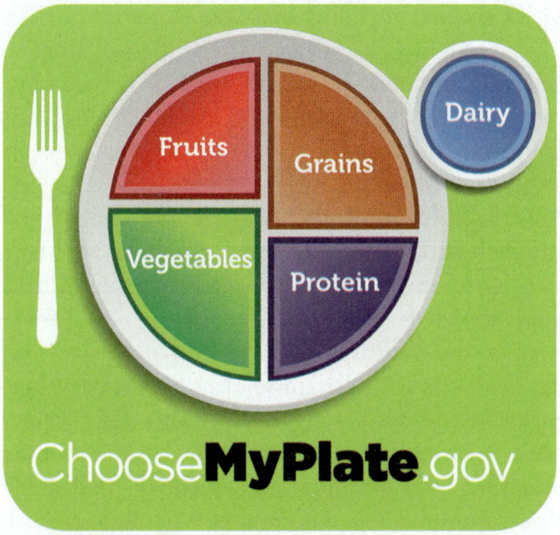

FIGURE 33-1 ChooseMyPlate. (From US Department of Agriculture: ChooseMyPlate, 2011.)

BOX 33-1 2010 DIETARY GUIDELINES FOR AMERICANS: KEY RECOMMENDATIONS FOR THE GENERAL POPULATION

- Adopt a balanced eating pattern with a variety of nutrient-dense food and beverages among the basic food groups.
- Maintain body weight in a healthy range.
- Encourage physical activity and decrease sedentary activities.
- Encourage fruits, vegetables, whole-grain products, and fat-free or low-fat milk.
- Reduce amount of foods containing sugars.
- Eat moderate amount of lean meats, poultry, and eggs.
- Keep total fat intake between 20% and 35% of total calories, with most fats coming from polyunsaturated or monounsaturated fatty acids.
- Choose and prepare foods and beverages with little added sugars or sweeteners.
- Choose and prepare foods with little salt while at the same time eating potassium-rich foods.
- Limit intake of alcohol to moderate use (i.e., one drink daily for women and two drinks daily for men).
- Use food-safety principles of clean, separate, cook, and chill to prevent microbial foodborne illness.

Data from USDA and USDHHS: *Dietary guidelines for Americans, 2010.* Report of Dietary Guidelines Advisory Committee on dietary guidelines for Americans 2010, http://www.cnpp.usda.gov/dietaryguidelines.htm. Accessed August 17, 2012.

Health and Human Services 2010 Dietary Guidelines for Americans (USDA and USDHHS, 2010) place a stronger emphasis on reducing calorie consumption and increasing physical activity for the more than one third of children and more than two thirds of adults in the United States who are overweight or obese (Box 33-1). Previous dietary guidelines focused on the healthy general population; however, the 2010 Dietary Guidelines are for Americans over the age of 2 years, including those at risk for chronic disease. The Dietary Guidelines offer an excellent set of standards in the selection of food. To plan healthy diets, however, it is important to match the Dietary Guidelines with the food preferences of different racial and ethnic groups, vegetarians, and others.

Dietary Reference Intakes. In 1997 the Food and Nutrition Board of the National Institute of Medicine/National Academy of Sciences, in partnership with Health Canada, initiated **dietary reference intakes (DRIs)** in response to the increased public use of nutritional supplements. The DRIs are nutrient reference values developed by the Institute of Medicine (IOM, 2009). The values are intended to serve as a guide for good nutrition and provide the scientific basis for the development of food guidelines such as recommended amounts of vitamins in both the United States and Canada. There are four components to the DRIs: estimated average requirement (EAR), recommended dietary allowances (RDAs), adequate intakes (AIs), and tolerable upper intake levels (ULs). The EAR is the recommended amount of a nutrient that appears sufficient to maintain a specific body function for 50% of the population based on age and gender. The RDA is the average needs of 98% of the population, not the exact needs of an individual. The AI is the suggested intake for individuals based on observed or experimentally determined estimates of nutrient intakes by groups and is provided when there is insufficient evidence to set RDAs. The tolerable UL is the highest level that likely poses no risk for adverse health events. It is not a recommended level of intake (IOM, 2009).

Other Dietary Guidelines. Other professional organizations have published dietary guidelines. Examples are the American Cancer Society Guidelines on Nutrition and Physical Activity for Cancer Prevention, the American Diabetes Association (ADA, 2008), and the American Heart Association Guidelines for Heart-Healthy Eating (AHA, 2010). These guidelines are similar to the Dietary Guidelines for Americans. Medical nutrition therapy (MNT) uses nutritional therapy and counseling to manage diseases (American Dietetic Association, 2010). Standards now exist that clearly designate the standard of care for promotion of optimal nutrition in all health care patients (Kushi et al., 2012).

In 1997 the USDHHS and the Public Health Service (PHS) began a consensus process that resulted in establishing nutritional goals and objectives for *Healthy People 2020* (USDHHS, 2010). *Healthy People 2020* continues the overall goal to promote health and reduce chronic disease related to diet and weight. The initiative is the United States' contribution to the "Health for All" strategy of the World Health Organization (WHO, 2010) (Box 33-2). The challenge is to motivate consumers to put these objectives into practice. Health professionals play a key role in promoting healthy dietary practices.

NURSING KNOWLEDGE BASE

There are sociological, cultural, psychological, and emotional aspects to eating and drinking in all societies. Holidays and events are celebrated with food, food is brought to those who are grieving, and food is used for medicinal purposes. We also recognize cultural and religious food differences (Box 33-3). Food is incorporated into family traditions and rituals, and appearance is often associated with eating behaviors. An understanding of your patients' values, beliefs, and attitudes about food and how those values affect food purchase, preparation, and intake will allow you to help your patients make healthy food choices.

Nutritional requirements depend on many factors. Individual caloric and nutrient requirements vary by stage of development, body composition, activity levels, conditions such as pregnancy and lactation, and the presence of disease. RDs use predictive equations that take into account some of these factors to estimate patient's nutritional requirements.

BOX 33-2 EXAMPLES OF NUTRITION OBJECTIVES FOR *HEALTHY PEOPLE 2020*

WEIGHT AND GROWTH

- Increase proportion of adults who are at a healthy weight (BMI 18.5 to 24.9).
- Reduce proportion of adults who are obese.
- Reduce proportion of children (2-11 years) who are overweight or obese.

FOOD AND NUTRIENT CONSUMPTION

- Decrease saturated fat intake in population 2 years and older.
- Increase the variety of vegetable and fruit intake in the population 2 years and older.
- Increase intake of grain products and consumption of calcium in the population 2 years and older.
- Reduce daily intake of sodium in the population 2 years and older.

IRON DEFICIENCY AND ANEMIA

- Reduce prevalence of iron deficiency in children and childbearing women.
- Reduce prevalence of anemia in pregnant women in third trimester to 20%.

SCHOOLS, WORK SITES, AND NUTRITION COUNSELING

- Increase work-site nutrition education and weight-management program offerings.
- Offer nutritional assessment and individualized planning at primary care sites.
- Increase percentage of schools that offer nutritious foods and beverages outside of school meals.
- Increase the number of states with nutrition standards for food and beverages provided to preschool-age children in child care.

FOOD SECURITY

- Increase food security to 94% of households.

Data from U.S. Department of Health and Human Services: *Healthy People 2020,* 2010, http://www.healthypeople.gov/hp2020/objectives. Accessed September 29, 2013.

BOX 33-3 PATIENT-CENTERED CARE

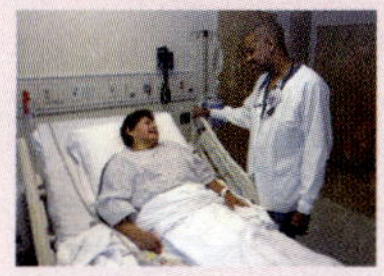

Matt reads about the influence of an individual's culture on nutrition. This includes ethnic food preferences, the personal meaning of certain foods, availability of food by geographic area, economic resources for food preferences, and social norms that influence when and what a person eats. Matt learns that all of these factors influence food habits and eating patterns. Foods often have symbolic meanings and are associated with births, deaths, religion, and social occasions. Special ethnic dishes or foods are served at ceremonies, holidays, and family celebrations. Recipes for these special dishes or foods are passed from generation to generation. There has been an "Americanization" of some of the special dishes and eating patterns. Regular use of traditional foods is seen more frequently in older members of a family than in younger members. The younger family members generally use these foods more on holidays or for special events.

Matt wants to know more about Mrs. Gonzalez's food preferences and eating patterns. Eventually she will return to oral feeding as her swallowing becomes safer. He learns from her family that they typically get their protein from dry beans, cheeses, meats, fish, and eggs. Their grain intake is generally corn made into tamales and tortillas, although many families still make these with flour. Rice and wheat products are other sources of fiber. They frequently eat chili peppers and deep-green and yellow vegetables, along with a variety of fruits such as guava, papaya, mango, and other citrus fruits. Matt and the dietitian identify foods that Mrs. Gonzalez enjoys that will help provide a balanced diet as her ability to swallow improves.

IMPLICATIONS FOR PRACTICE

- Matt asks Mrs. Gonzalez about food she likes to prepare and serve at home and gathers input from her daughter as well.
- Matt identifies fluids that Mrs. Gonzalez enjoys despite the current need to thicken them.
- Matt works with the dietitian to incorporate some of Mrs. Gonzalez's favorite foods into her diet within the guidelines of her restrictions.
- Matt helps Mrs. Gonzalez identify ways to decrease fat intake and increase vegetables and fruit in her daily meals to ensure that she receives a well-balanced diet.

Data from Nix S: *Williams' basic nutrition and diet therapy*, ed 14, St Louis, 2013, Mosby; and Touhy and Jett: *Ebersole and Hess' toward healthy aging: human needs and nursing response*, ed 8, St Louis, 2012, Mosby.

Alternative Food Patterns

Individuals follow special patterns of food intake based on religion, cultural background, ethics, health beliefs, or concern about the environment. Such special diets do not necessarily provide more or less nutritional benefit than diets based on ChooseMyPlate or other nutritional guidelines. Adequate nutritional intake depends on balanced consumption of all required nutrients. The vegetarian diet is an example of a dietary pattern that is commonly consumed because of religious or personal beliefs. It is primarily plant based and includes the elimination of many animal-based foods. Vegetarians are grouped into several categories. Ovolactovegetarians avoid meat, fish, and poultry but eat eggs and milk. Lactovegetarians drink milk but avoid eggs and other animal-based foods. Vegans eat only foods of plant origin. Individuals consuming the vegan diet are susceptible to vitamin B_{12} and protein deficiency. Vegans supplement their diets with vitamin B_{12} and carefully choose foods to ensure ingestion of essential amino acids. Knowledge of high–biological value protein versus low–biological value protein sources ensures intake of all of the essential amino acids.

Developmental Needs

Infants Through School-Age. Infancy is marked by rapid growth and high protein, vitamin, mineral, and energy requirements. Infants need an energy intake of approximately 108 kcal/kg of body weight in the first half of infancy and 98 kcal/kg in the second half (Nix, 2013). Infants need approximately 100 to 120 mL/kg/day of fluid because a large portion of total body weight is water.

Breastfeeding. The American Academy of Pediatrics (AAP) (2012) strongly supports breastfeeding. The benefits include reduced food allergies and intolerances, fewer infant infections, and easier digestion. In addition, breast milk is convenient, fresh, always the correct temperature, and economical because it is less expensive than formula. It also provides increased time for mother and infant interaction.

Formula. Infant formulas contain the approximate nutrient composition of human milk. Infants should not have regular cow's milk during the first year of life. Evidence shows infants receiving cow's milk have lower intake of iron, linoleic acid, and vitamin E and excessive amounts of sodium, potassium, and protein. It may also cause a small amount of GI bleeding and increase risk for milk-product allergies (Mahan, Escott-Stump, and Raymond, 2012). The AAP recommends breast milk or formula as the major source of food for up to 1 year in age. Honey and corn syrup are potential sources of botulism toxin and should not be used in an infant's diet. The toxin is potentially fatal in children under 1 year of age (Mahan, Escott-Stump, and Raymond, 2012).

Introduction to Solid Food. Although breast milk remains the major source of nutrition, parents usually begin to introduce solid foods to their infants at 4 to 6 months of age. Iron-fortified cereals are typically the first semisolid food to be introduced and are an important nonmilk source of protein. Health care providers recommend that parents introduce new foods one at a time, approximately 4 to 7 days apart, to identify any allergies. Teach parents to introduce new foods before giving milk or other foods to avoid satiety (Hockenberry and Wilson, 2011).

The growth rate slows during toddler years, requiring fewer kilocalories but an increased amount of protein in relation to body weight. As a result appetite often decreases at 18 months of age. Toddlers exhibit strong food preferences and become picky eaters. Small, frequent meals consisting of breakfast, lunch, and dinner with three interspersed high–nutrient density snacks help improve nutritional intake (Hockenberry and Wilson, 2011). Calcium and phosphorus are important for healthy bone growth.

Toddlers need to drink whole milk until the age of 2 years to make sure that there is adequate intake of fatty acids necessary for brain and neurological development. Certain foods such as hot dogs, candy, nuts, grapes, raw vegetables, and popcorn often cause choking deaths and need to be avoided. Preschoolers' (3 to 5 years) dietary requirements are similar to those of toddlers. They consume slightly more than toddlers, and nutrient density is more important than quantity.

School-age children, 6 to 12 years old, grow at a slower and steadier rate, with a gradual decline in energy requirements per unit of body weight. Despite the better appetites and more varied food intake of school-age children, you need to assess their diets carefully for adequate protein and vitamins A and C. There has been a consistent decrease in physical activity level and increase in consumption of high-calorie readily available food, leading to an increase in childhood obesity (Han et al., 2010)

Adolescents. During adolescence energy needs increase to meet greater metabolic demands of growth. Daily requirement of protein also increases. Calcium is essential for the rapid bone growth of adolescence, and girls need a continuous source of iron to replace menstrual losses. Boys also need adequate iron for muscle development. Iodine supports increased thyroid activity, and use of iodized table salt ensures availability. B-complex vitamins are necessary to support heightened metabolic activity. Nutritional deficiencies often occur in adolescent girls as a result of dieting and use of oral contraceptives. Snacks provide approximately 25% of a teenager's total dietary intake. Fast food is common and adds extra salt, fat, and kilocalories. Skipping meals or eating meals with wrong choices of snacks contributes to nutrient deficiency and obesity (Hockenberry and Wilson, 2011).

Young and Middle-Age Adults. The demands for most nutrients are reduced as the growth period ends. Mature adults need nutrients for energy, maintenance, and repair. Energy needs usually decline over the years. Obesity becomes a problem as a result of decreased physical exercise, dining out more often, and increased ability to afford more luxury foods. Adult women who use oral contraceptives often need extra vitamins. Iron and calcium intake continues to be important.

Pregnancy. Poor nutrition during pregnancy causes low birth weight in infants and decreases chances of survival. The nutritional status of a mother at the time of conception is important. The energy requirements of pregnancy are related to a mother's body weight and activity. Protein intake throughout pregnancy needs to increase to 60 g daily. Calcium intake is especially critical in the third trimester, when fetal bones are mineralized. Supplemental iron provides for increased maternal blood volume, fetal blood storage, and blood loss during delivery.

Folic acid intake is particularly important for deoxyribonucleic acid (DNA) synthesis and the growth of red blood cells. Inadequate intake is associated with increased risk of fetal abnormalities (Schlenker and Roth, 2011). It is now recommended that women of child-bearing age consume 400 mcg of folic acid daily, increasing to 600 mcg daily during pregnancy.

Lactation. A woman who is lactating needs 500 kcal/day above the usual kcal allowance because the production of milk increases energy requirements. Protein requirements during lactation are also greater than the protein requirement during pregnancy. There is an increased need for vitamins A and C. Daily intake of water-soluble vitamins (B and C) is necessary to ensure adequate levels in breast milk. Fluid intake needs to be adequate but not excessive. Women who are lactating also need to avoid caffeine, alcohol, and drugs because they are excreted in breast milk.

BOX 33-4 CARE OF THE OLDER ADULT

Dietary Teaching

- Eat a balanced diet that contains a variety of foods. Avoid too much fat, cholesterol, sugar, and sodium or salt.
- Eat foods that have adequate amounts of starch and fiber such as fruits and vegetables and whole-grain cereals and breads.
- Consult with pharmacist about potential for medication and food interactions (e.g., be aware that grapefruit and grapefruit juice may decrease the absorption of specific medications).
- Drink adequate fluids because thirst sensation diminishes, often leading to inadequate fluid intake or dehydration. Water requirements do not decrease with age.
- If unable to eat meat because of cost or difficulty chewing, find alternate sources of protein.
- Cream soups and meat-based vegetable soups are nutrient-dense sources of protein.
- Cheese, eggs, and peanut butter are also useful high-protein alternatives.
- Drink milk for calcium and vitamin D to protect against osteoporosis (a decrease of bone mass density). Provide calcium supplements if lactose intolerance is present.
- Take vitamin and nutrient supplements as recommended.

Older Adults. Adults 65 years and older have a decreased need for calories because metabolic rate slows with age, although they continue to have similar needs for vitamins and minerals. This makes it even more important that older adults have well-balanced diets and ingest foods with high nutritional value. Numerous factors influence the nutritional status of older adults. Living on a fixed income often reduces the amount of money available to buy food. The older adult is often on a therapeutic diet or has difficulty eating because of physical symptoms, lack of teeth, or dentures or is at risk for drug-nutrient interactions. The diet of older adults needs to contain choices from all food groups and often requires a vitamin and mineral supplement (Box 33-4).

The USDHHS's Administration on Aging (AOA) requires states to provide nutritional screening services for older-adult patients who benefit from home-delivered or congregate meal services. Older adults who are homebound and have chronic illness have additional nutritional risks. Frequently they live alone with few or no social or financial resources to help them obtain or prepare nutritionally sound meals. Increased nutritional screening by the nurse results in early recognition of potential nutritional deficiencies and needed treatment of these deficiencies. Undernourishment of older adults often results in health problems that lead to admission to acute care hospitals or long-term care facilities.

Overweight and Obesity

The problems of individuals who are overweight and obese are at epidemic levels in the United States. From 2009 to 2010 35.7% of U.S. adults were obese, and those ages 60 and over were more likely to be obese than younger adults (Ogden et al., 2012). A combination of factors contribute to the problem, including energy imbalance between calories consumed and calories expended, genetics, and metabolic and lifestyle factors. **Body mass index (BMI)** which is calculated from height and weight in children and adults is a reliable indicator of body fat. BMI is calculated by dividing weight in kilograms (kg) by height in meters squared (m^2). A BMI range of 18.5 to 24.9 is recommended for optimal health. A BMI greater than 24.9 is considered overweight, and a BMI greater than 29.9 is considered obese. Obesity places individuals at higher risk for coronary artery disease, some cancers, diabetes mellitus, degenerative joint disease, and hypertension. Other factors such as lack of access to healthy food and inadequate health care also contribute to the development of obesity (Schlenker and Roth, 2011).

The proportion of children 5 through 17 years of age who are obese is 5 times higher in 2008 and 2009 than in 1973 and 1974 (Roger et al., 2012). Childhood obesity contributes to medical problems related to the cardiovascular system, endocrine system, and mental health. Prevention of childhood obesity is considered the best approach to reverse this trend. Family education is an important component of decreasing the prevalence of this problem. Promote healthy food choices and eating in moderation along with increased physical activity (Han et al., 2010).

CRITICAL THINKING

Synthesis

You will apply elements of critical thinking whenever you perform the nursing process with patients. Consider the scientific knowledge you have learned, your experience, critical thinking attitudes, and standards to ensure an individualized approach to patient care (Box 33-5).

Knowledge. Application of knowledge from nutritional principles and the basic and social sciences form your knowledge base related to nutritional care. Information that comes from interviewing and observing a patient and the responses you obtain during nursing interventions guide you toward application of knowledge. For example, your patient reports a dietary pattern of avoiding cabbage. This pattern could arise from physiological discomfort (gas-forming food), psychological issues (forced to eat cabbage as a child), sociological reasons (associated with lower socioeconomic class), ethnicity (not readily available in the country of origin), teaching- or learning-related reasons (never taught how to prepare cabbage), or mythology (a food that contains harmful chemicals). Consider these factors when planning a nutritious diet.

Experience. Just as multiple factors influence your patients' choices of dietary practices, multiple factors also influence your dietary patterns. Individuals who have nutritional or health problems change their long-standing dietary practices to enhance health. In helping a patient change dietary patterns, draw on examples from your own experience. Perhaps you attempted to change a dietary practice or

BOX 33-5 SYNTHESIS IN PRACTICE

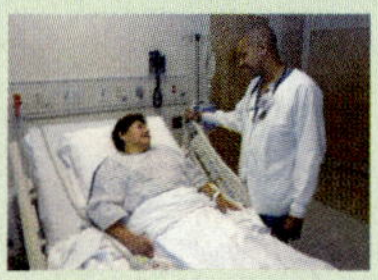

As Matt prepares to assess Mrs. Gonzalez, he recalls information about nutrition and its effect on rehabilitation, especially the importance of adequate calorie, protein, and fluid intake in patients who have had a stroke. He focuses on Mrs. Gonzalez's need for adequate nutrition, which for now is safely delivered via enteral feeding tube, and he monitors her tolerance of the therapy. He wants to ensure that it is providing the energy that she needs to heal and adequately rehabilitate to come as close to her norm as possible. He consults with a registered dietitian to make sure that the regimen is meeting her needs for macronutrients, micronutrients, and fluid.

Matt visits with the speech pathologist to assess the progress she is making in terms of swallowing safely. He explores whether it is expected that she will be able to resume oral intake soon or whether longer-term enteral feeding through a gastrostomy tube will be needed. A video swallow study demonstrates safe swallowing of a dysphagia diet with nectar-thick liquids. Matt acknowledges that Mrs. Gonzales has little interest in oral intake at this time; therefore he explores with her foods that she finds appealing and is interested in trying. Experience has taught Matt that economic and cultural preferences influence her food choices. He is aware that she may not receive the fluid she needs since her fluids must be thickened for her safety in swallowing. Matt also knows that, as the tube feeding is decreased and oral intake improves, she may still need to have fluid delivered via her feeding tube to make sure that she receives adequate fluid until her dietary restrictions are lifted.

have a family member who requires a special diet. Previous experiences with therapeutic diets or behavioral changes help you identify nursing interventions that will be successful for the patient.

Attitudes. Integrity and discipline are critical thinking skills that are beneficial during nutritional assessment and counseling. Although you encounter patients whose dietary practices are dramatically different from yours, you help all patients attain a nutritionally balanced diet. In addition, you care for patients whose dietary patterns are not healthful. Changes in dietary practices often occur over time. Perseverance is necessary in educating patients to understand the impact of unhealthy food choices.

Standards. The use of professional standards such as the DRIs, the USDA's MyPlate, dietary guidelines, and *Healthy People 2020* objectives provide guidelines for assessing and maintaining patients' nutritional status. Other professional standards by the AHA (2010; Roger et al., 2012), the American Diabetes Association (ADA, 2008), the American Cancer Society (Kushi et al., 2012), and the American Society for Parenteral and Enteral Nutrition (ASPEN, 2009; Choban et al., 2013; Mueller et al., 2011) are available. These standards are evidence based and are updated as needed based on new research findings.

NURSING PROCESS

ASSESSMENT

Screening. Nutritional screening is part of your initial assessment of a patient. Screening is a quick method of identifying malnutrition or risk for malnutrition (Ukleja et al., 2010). Nutritional screening tools commonly include objective measures such as height, weight, weight change, primary diagnosis, and the presence of comorbidities (Ukleja et al., 2010). A single objective measure alone does not predict a person's nutritional risk. Combine multiple objective measures with subjective measures related to nutrition to screen for nutritional risk. Health care institutions commonly use the initial nursing assessment as a nutritional screening. Certain nutritional risk factors such as unintentional weight loss, the presence of a modified diet, or the presence of nutritional impact symptoms (i.e., nausea, vomiting, diarrhea, constipation) are triggers for a nutritional consultation.

There are several standardized nutritional screening tools for you to use in the outpatient setting. One example is the Subjective Global Assessment (SGA), which is a validated clinical method that uses patient history, weight, and physical assessment data to evaluate nutritional status (Charney, 2008). The SGA is a simple, inexpensive technique that predicts nutrition-related complications.

Nutritional Assessment. If a patient is at risk for nutritional problems, refer him or her to an RD for a more in-depth nutritional assessment. Nutritional assessment is different from nutritional screening. The RD completes a nutritional assessment, which includes an in-depth exploration of medical history, dietary history, physical examination, anthropometric measurements, and laboratory data (Table 33-1). This process often leads to the identification and diagnosis of nutritional issues. Nutritional assessment includes the determination of nutrient and protein needs. In an acute care setting the RD is available to make these calculations. In an outpatient setting an RD is not always available to complete a nutritional assessment.

Diet History. The diet history focuses on habitual intake of food and liquids and information about preferences, allergies, and digestive problems (Box 33-6). Open-ended questions encourage a patient to provide more information on food intake during the interview. For example, ask a patient who reports that she avoids dairy products, "Tell me what led you to avoid dairy products?" The patient's answer to this question leads to physiological, psychological, sociological, religious, cultural, or food preference factors that you further explore.

Ask the patient to keep a detailed record of food intake over 3 days, including one weekend day, to determine a typical eating pattern and whether routine intake is meeting DRIs. Three-day food records require the use of measuring cups

TABLE 33-1 FOCUSED PATIENT ASSESSMENT

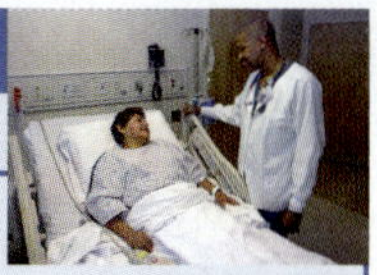

FACTORS TO ASSESS	QUESTIONS	PHYSICAL ASSESSMENT
Food and nutrient intake	How many meals a day do you eat? What times do you normally eat meals and snacks? What portion sizes do you eat at each meal? Are you on a special diet because of a health problem? Who purchases and prepares the food?	Inspect oral cavity for physical barriers to eating (e.g., tooth decay, poor-fitting dentures). Inspect condition of skin, hair, and nails. Assess skin turgor.
Patterns and dietary history	Which types of food do you like? Are you allergic to any foods? What type of problems do you have with these foods? Have you noticed any changes in taste? Do you have any problems with chewing or swallowing?	Observe patient swallowing. Observe percentage of food consumed from meal tray.
Changes in weight	Has your appetite changed? Have you noticed a change in your weight? Was this change anticipated (e.g., were you on a weight-reduction diet)?	Weigh patient and analyze for changes. Observe patient's muscle tone. Inspect oral cavity for signs of malnutrition such as cheilosis, stomatitis, and dry lesions at corners of mouth (see Table 33-2).
Skin	Have you noticed any changes in your skin such as scaliness, dryness, or bruising? Do you use skin moisturizers regularly?	Observe skin for color, moisture, changes in pigment, or bruising (see Table 33-2).

BOX 33-6 INFORMATION CONTAINED IN A DIET HISTORY

- Twenty-four-hour diet recall of the day
  - Use of enteral or parenteral nutrition
  - Food consumed for breakfast, lunch, dinner, and snacks
  - Number of meals and snacks a day
  - Timing of meals and snacks
  - Use of nutritional supplements, vitamins, minerals, and herbal products
- Dietary restrictions
  - Medically prescribed diets
  - Modified-consistency diets
  - Weight reduction, vegetarian, macrobiotic, vegan, or fad diets
- Food preferences, allergies, and aversions
  - Foods that cause indigestion, diarrhea, or gas
- Chewing or swallowing difficulties (examine the mouth)
  - Use of dentures (have patient remove dentures to examine the mouth)
  - Presence of tooth decay
  - Presence of xerostomia, mucositis, or mouth sores
- Usual bowel movements
  - Presence of constipation or diarrhea
  - Duration of constipation or diarrhea
  - Symptoms of malabsorption such as clay-colored or frequent fatty stools
- Meal procurement and preparation responsibility
  - Appetite changes
  - Weight history, including percentage of weight lost over period of time lost

Modified from Nix S: *Williams' basic nutrition and diet therapy,* ed 14, St Louis, 2013, Mosby.

and scales. Instruct your patients to record the specific type of foods and the exact amounts ingested. Information on a patient's activity level and presence of disease is necessary to estimate energy needs. For example, a patient who has a fever or has experienced severe trauma has high caloric demands, even though the activity level is limited. Estimated energy need, as calculated through prediction equations, is compared to actual caloric intake, obtained through calorie counts. A calorie count uses records of observed amounts of food consumed from a patient's meal trays as documented by the nursing or nutrition staff to estimate total calories and protein consumed daily. Consult with an RD to determine a calorie count or energy requirements.

Medication History. Prescribed and over-the-counter medications have the potential for drug-nutrient interactions. Knowing which medications your patients take is important when meeting their nutritional needs. Consultation with a pharmacist determines the specific risks for nutrient-drug interactions for your patients.

Older Adult Considerations. Multiple age-related factors often affect nutritional status in older adults. The presence of chronic illness, anorexia, slowed digestion and peristalsis, decreased physical and cognitive function, ability to feed self, medication side effects, loss of dentition, and reduced saliva production may all contribute to development of malnutrition.

The Mini Nutritional Assessment (MNA) (Figure 33-2) was developed as a nutritional screening tool for the older-adult population. This 18-item tool has two sections: screening and assessment. The screening section contains six questions related to decline in food intake, weight

Nestlē Nutrition Institute

Mini Nutritional Assessment MNA®

Last name: First name:

Sex: Age: Weight, kg: Height, cm: Date:

Complete the screen by filling in the boxes with the appropriate numbers. Total the numbers for the final screening score.

Screening

A Has food intake declined over the past 3 months due to loss of appetite, digestive problems, chewing or swallowing difficulties?
0 = severe decrease in food intake
1 = moderate decrease in food intake
2 = no decrease in food intake ☐

B Weight loss during the last 3 months
0 = weight loss greater than 3 kg (6.6 lbs)
1 = does not know
2 = weight loss between 1 and 3 kg (2.2 and 6.6 lbs)
3 = no weight loss ☐

C Mobility
0 = bed or chair bound
1 = able to get out of bed / chair but does not go out
2 = goes out ☐

D Has suffered psychological stress or acute disease in the past 3 months?
0 = yes 2 = no ☐

E Neuropsychological problems
0 = severe dementia or depression
1 = mild dementia
2 = no psychological problems ☐

F1 Body Mass Index (BMI) (weight in kg) / (height in m^2)
0 = BMI less than 19
1 = BMI 19 to less than 21
2 = BMI 21 to less than 23
3 = BMI 23 or greater ☐

IF BMI IS NOT AVAILABLE, REPLACE QUESTION F1 WITH QUESTION F2.
DO NOT ANSWER QUESTION F2 IF QUESTION F1 IS ALREADY COMPLETED.

F2 Calf circumference (CC) in cm
0 = CC less than 31
3 = CC 31 or greater ☐

Screening score
(max. 14 points) ☐☐

12-14 points:	Normal nutritional status
8-11 points:	At risk of malnutrition
0-7 points:	Malnourished

Ref. Vellas B, Villars H, Abellan G, et al. *Overview of the MNA® - Its History and Challenges.* J Nutr Health Aging 2006;10:456-465.
Rubenstein LZ, Harker JO, Salva A, Guigoz Y, Vellas B. *Screening for Undernutrition in Geriatric Practice: Developing the Short-Form Mini Nutritional Assessment (MNA-SF).* J. Geront 2001;56A: M366-377.
Guigoz Y. *The Mini-Nutritional Assessment (MNA®) Review of the Literature - What does it tell us?* J Nutr Health Aging 2006; 10:466-487.
Kaiser MJ, Bauer JM, Ramsch C, et al. *Validation of the Mini Nutritional Assessment Short-Form (MNA®-SF): A practical tool for identification of nutritional status.* J Nutr Health Aging 2009; 13:782-788.

For more information: www.mna-elderly.com

FIGURE 33-2 Mini Nutritional Assessment (MNA). (Copyright© Nestle, 1994, Revision 2009. N67200 12/99 10M.)

loss, mobility, stress, and BMI. The health care practitioner completes the assessment portion if the patient scores 11 or less (Guigoz et al., 1996). The 12-item assessment includes specific medical history and eating habits and some anthropometric measurements. A score of less than 17 points indicates protein-energy malnutrition (PEM) (Guigoz and Vellas, 1999; Guigoz et al., 1996). Research found that the MNA is a useful tool to predict pressure ulcer development in older adults. Early identification of risk for pressure ulcers in older adults allows you to plan interventions to improve nutritional status (Yatabe et al., 2013).

Patients at Risk for Nutritional Problems. Assess any patient with a condition that interferes with the ability to ingest, digest, or absorb adequate nutrients. Use a standardized tool to assess nutritional risks when possible. Congenital anomalies and surgical revisions of the GI tract interfere with normal function. Patients receiving only intravenous infusion of 5% to 10% dextrose are at risk for nutritional deficiencies. Older adults, infants, or people who are malnourished are at greatest risk.

Physical Examination. Examine the patient for signs of actual or potential nutritional alterations (Table 33-2). You can conduct a portion of the exam while performing or assisting the patient with hygiene. The skin and hair are primary areas that reflect nutrient and hydration deficiencies. Be alert for rashes; dry, scaly skin; poor skin turgor; skin lesions; hair loss; easily pluckable hair; hair without luster; and an unhealthy scalp.

Anthropometry. Anthropometry is a systematic measurement of the size and makeup of the body using height and weight as the principal measures. Height and weight measurements typically are obtained during a patient's admission to any health care setting. If a patient is unable to stand, estimate height by measuring the patient's length with a tape measure while the patient lies supine. Assess weight with bed scales and then compare height and weight with usual measurements, called *usual body weight (UBW)*, and standard norms for normal height-weight relationships, called ideal body weight (IBW). Serial measures of weight over time provide more useful information than one measurement. When collecting serial measurements of weight, weigh the patient about the same time each day, on the same scale, and with the same amount of clothing. In some patients a weight change of 2 lbs in 24 hours is significant because 1 lb is roughly equivalent to 500 mL of fluid. BMI, which is the height-to-weight index, is discussed in the section on Overweight and Obesity.

Laboratory Values. No single laboratory or biochemical test is diagnostic for malnutrition. Factors that frequently alter test results include fluid balance, liver function, kidney function, and the presence of disease. Laboratory values useful in nutritional assessment include complete blood count (CBC), albumin, prealbumin (transferrin), electrolytes, blood urea nitrogen, 24-hour urine urea nitrogen (UUN), creatinine, glucose, cholesterol, and triglycerides. Individual laboratory measures alone are not specific enough to indicate nutritional risk; therefore they are combined with multiple objective measures to determine malnutrition. A low red blood cell count and depressed hemoglobin value indicate anemia. The hemoglobin, hematocrit, electrolyte, and blood urea nitrogen values also help to reflect the state of hydration. Serum proteins such as prealbumin and albumin levels are affected by inflammatory states and reflect the severity of disease rather than nutritional status (Davis et al., 2012). Nitrogen balance, which is measured through laboratory analysis of a 24-hour UUN, is important to establish adequacy of protein and calorie intake (see the discussion of protein in this chapter).

Dysphagia. Dysphagia refers to difficulty with swallowing. It occurs as a result of damage to muscles and nerves and obstructive causes (Box 33-7). The complications of dysphagia vary, including aspiration pneumonia, dehydration, decreased nutritional status, and weight loss. Dysphagia leads to disability or decreased functional status, increased length of stay and cost of care, increased likelihood of discharge to institutionalized care, and increased mortality (Tanner, 2010).

Several indicators warn you that your patient has dysphagia. Signs of dysphagia include cough; change in voice tone or quality after swallowing; abnormal movements of the mouth, tongue, or lips; and slow, weak, imprecise, or uncoordinated speech. Abnormal gag, delayed swallowing, incomplete oral clearance or pocketing, regurgitation, pharyngeal

BOX 33-7 CAUSES OF DYSPHAGIA

MYOGENIC (MUSCLE)
- Myasthenia gravis
- Aging
- Muscular dystrophy
- Polymyositis

NEUROGENIC (NERVE)
- Stroke
- Cerebral palsy
- Guillain-Barré syndrome
- Multiple sclerosis
- Amyotrophic lateral sclerosis (Lou Gehrig disease)
- Diabetic neuropathy
- Parkinson's disease

OBSTRUCTIVE
- Benign peptic stricture
- Lower esophageal ring
- Candidiasis
- Head and neck cancer
- Inflammatory masses
- Trauma/surgical resection
- Anterior mediastinal masses
- Cervical spondylosis

OTHER
- Gastrointestinal or esophageal resection
- Rheumatological disorders
- Connective tissue disorders
- Vagotomy

TABLE 33-2 PHYSICAL SIGNS OF NUTRITIONAL STATUS

BODY AREA	NORMAL APPEARANCE	INDICATORS OF MALNUTRITION
General appearance	Alert, responsive	Listless, apathetic, cachectic
Weight	Normal for height, age, body build	Overweight, obese, or underweight (special concern for underweight); weight trend, including weight loss over period of time
Posture	Erect; arms and legs straight	Sagging shoulders, sunken chest, humped back
Muscles	Well-developed, firm, good tone; some fat under skin	Flaccid, poor tone, undeveloped, tender; "wasted" appearance; impaired ability to walk
Nerve conduction and mental status	Good attention span, not irritable or restless, normal reflexes, psychological stability	Inattentive, irritable, confused, burning and tingling of hands and feet (paresthesia), loss of position and vibratory sense, weakness and tenderness of muscles (may result in inability to walk), decrease or loss of ankle and knee reflexes
Gastrointestinal function	Good appetite and digestion, normal regular elimination, no palpable (perceptible to touch) organs or masses	Anorexia, indigestion, constipation or diarrhea, symptoms of malabsorption, liver or spleen enlargement; distention, firmness, audible air with percussion
Cardiovascular function	Normal heart rate and rhythm, no murmurs, normal blood pressure for age	Rapid heart rate (above 100 beats/min, tachycardia), enlarged heart, abnormal rhythm, elevated blood pressure
General vitality	Endurance, energetic, sleeps well, vigorous	Easily fatigued, no energy, falls asleep easily, looks tired, apathetic
Hair	Shiny, lustrous, firm, not easily plucked; healthy scalp	Stringy, dull, brittle, dry, thin and sparse, depigmented, easily plucked
Skin (general)	Smooth, slightly moist, good color	Rough, dry, scaly, pale, pigmented, irritated, bruises, petechiae
Face and neck	Skin color uniform; smooth, healthy appearance; not swollen	Greasy, discolored, scaly, swollen, skin dark over cheeks and under eyes, lumpiness or flakiness of skin around nose and mouth
Lips	Smooth, good color, moist, not chapped or swollen	Dry, scaly, swollen, redness and swelling (cheilosis); angular lesions at corners of mouth, fissures, or scars (stomatitis)
Mouth, oral mucous membranes	Reddish-pink mucous membranes in oral cavity	Swollen, deep red or magenta oral mucous membranes; oral lesions
Gums	Good pink color, healthy, red, no swelling or bleeding	Spongy, bleed easily, marginal redness, inflamed, receding
Tongue	Good pink color or deep reddish in appearance, not swollen or smooth, surface papillae present, no lesions	Swelling, scarlet and raw, magenta color, beefy (glossitis), hyperemic and hypertrophic papillae, atrophic papillae
Teeth	No pain, no sensitivity	Missing teeth, broken teeth
Eyes	Bright, clear, shiny; no sores at corner of eyelids, membranes moist and healthy pink color, no prominent blood vessels or mound of tissue or sclera, no fatigue circles beneath	Eye membranes pale (pale conjunctivae), redness of membrane (conjunctival injection), dryness or infection, Bitot's spots, redness and fissuring of eyelid corners (angular palpebritis), dryness of eye membrane (conjunctival xerosis), dull appearance of cornea (corneal xerosis), soft cornea (keratomalacia)
Neck (glands)	No enlargement	Thyroid or lymph nodes enlarged
Nails	Firm, pink	Spoon-shaped (koilonychia), brittle, ridged
Legs and feet	No tenderness, weakness, or swelling; good color	Edema, tender calf, tingling, weakness, lesions
Skeleton	No malformations	Bowlegs, knock-knees, chest deformity at diaphragm, beaded ribs, prominent scapulas

Data from Nix S: *Williams' basic nutrition and diet therapy,* ed 14, St Louis, 2013, Mosby.

pooling, drooling, delayed or absent trigger of swallow, and inability to speak consistently are other signs of dysphagia. Patients with dysphagia do not usually exhibit overt signs such as coughing when food enters the airway. *Silent aspiration,* or aspiration that occurs without a cough, is a common cause of complications.

Dysphagia causes decreases in food intake, which often leads to malnutrition caused by inability to consume an adequate volume of food. The period of adjustment to new dietary restrictions and the rehabilitation period affect intake for long periods of time. Malnutrition resulting from inadequate protein, calorie, and micronutrient intake significantly slows down recovery. Early nursing screening with a dysphagia screening protocol significantly decreases the risk for aspiration pneumonia in patients (Garon et al., 2009).

Dysphagia Screening. Dysphagia screening quickly identifies problems with swallowing so you can refer at-risk patients for a more in-depth assessment (see Skill 33-1). Dysphagia screening includes medical record review and observation of a patient at a meal for change in voice quality, posture and head control, percentage of meal consumed, eating time, drooling of liquids and solids, cough during/after a swallow, facial or tongue weakness, difficulty with secretions, pocketing, and presence of voluntary and dry cough. Screening tools such as the Bedside Swallowing Assessment, Burke Dysphagia Screening Test, Acute Stroke Dysphagia Screen, and the Standardized Swallowing Assessment have been validated in patients with dysphagia. These tools evaluate holding, leakage, coughing, choking, breathlessness, and quality of voice. They are designed for multidisciplinary use by registered nurses (RNs), RDs, physicians, or SLPs (Edmiaston et al., 2010).

Patient Expectations. Patients who require assistance with nutritional problems have a variety of expectations. It is important for you to learn what a patient expects in terms of resuming a normal diet or learning to adjust to a therapeutic diet. Patients with impairments in upper-arm mobility often require assistance with activities such as preparing meals, setting up the meal tray or plate, or being fed. Other patients expect information on the availability and use of assistive devices to increase independence with meals. A consultation with occupational therapy helps patients obtain assistive devices and provides education on their proper use. You will often need to teach patients who have impaired vision how to feed themselves.

NURSING DIAGNOSIS

Following nursing assessment, cluster relevant defining characteristics to determine whether actual or potential nutritional problems exist. An alteration occurs when the body does not ingest a nutrient in sufficient quantity, when it poorly digests or does not completely absorb nutrients, or when total daily caloric needs are deficient or excessive. The following are examples of nursing diagnoses appropriate for patients with nutritional alterations:

- *Risk for Aspiration*
- *Diarrhea*
- *Adult Failure to Thrive*
- *Deficient Knowledge (Nutrition)*
- *Imbalanced Nutrition: Less Than Body Requirements*
- *Imbalanced Nutrition: More Than Body Requirements*
- *Readiness for Enhanced Nutrition*
- *Risk for Imbalanced Nutrition: More Than Body Requirements*
- *Impaired Swallowing*
- *Feeding Self-Care Deficit*

During your assessment, identify the probable cause or related factor for the nutritional problem. Make sure that the nursing diagnosis is as precise as possible. Related factors need to be accurate so you will select the appropriate interventions. For example, you suspect an overweight patient has nutrient deficiencies. The nursing assessment identifies dietary patterns that have contributed to obesity. A more focused assessment examines the adequacy of all food groups and finds that the patient often consumes high-fat foods and an inadequate amount of fruits and vegetables. In this situation you use the nursing diagnosis *Imbalanced Nutrition: Less Than Body Requirements related to excess intake from poor eating habits.* Interventions include providing appropriate balanced diets and supplements or specialized nutritional support during episodes of acute illness. In contrast, if the assessment revealed the related factor to be more associated with inadequate physical activity, the diagnosis is *Imbalanced Nutrition: Less Than Body Requirements related to excess intake in relation to physical activity.* Your interventions then focus on proper diet as well as an exercise program.

PLANNING

During planning you select nursing interventions intended to improve a patient's nutritional status and the monitoring and evaluation to determine the effectiveness of those interventions. The input of all disciplines involved in patient care is necessary for planning nutritional interventions. Reflect on the causes of the patient's malnutrition or risk for malnutrition. Individualize all intervention to the patient's needs and take into consideration his or her comfort and preferences. Although variables exist between and among patients, common nutritional goals include symptom management, weight maintenance, and preservation of functional status. The use of modified diets, the addition of oral nutritional supplements, or the initiation of more complex and costly enteral nutrition (EN) or parenteral nutrition (PN) is sometimes required to improve nutritional status. Consider the cost of these modifications and patient and family caregiver burden before beginning an intervention. The services of social workers are very beneficial in situations in which patients are not able to afford an intervention.

Goals and Outcomes. The goal in caring for patients with nutritional alterations is to improve their nutritional

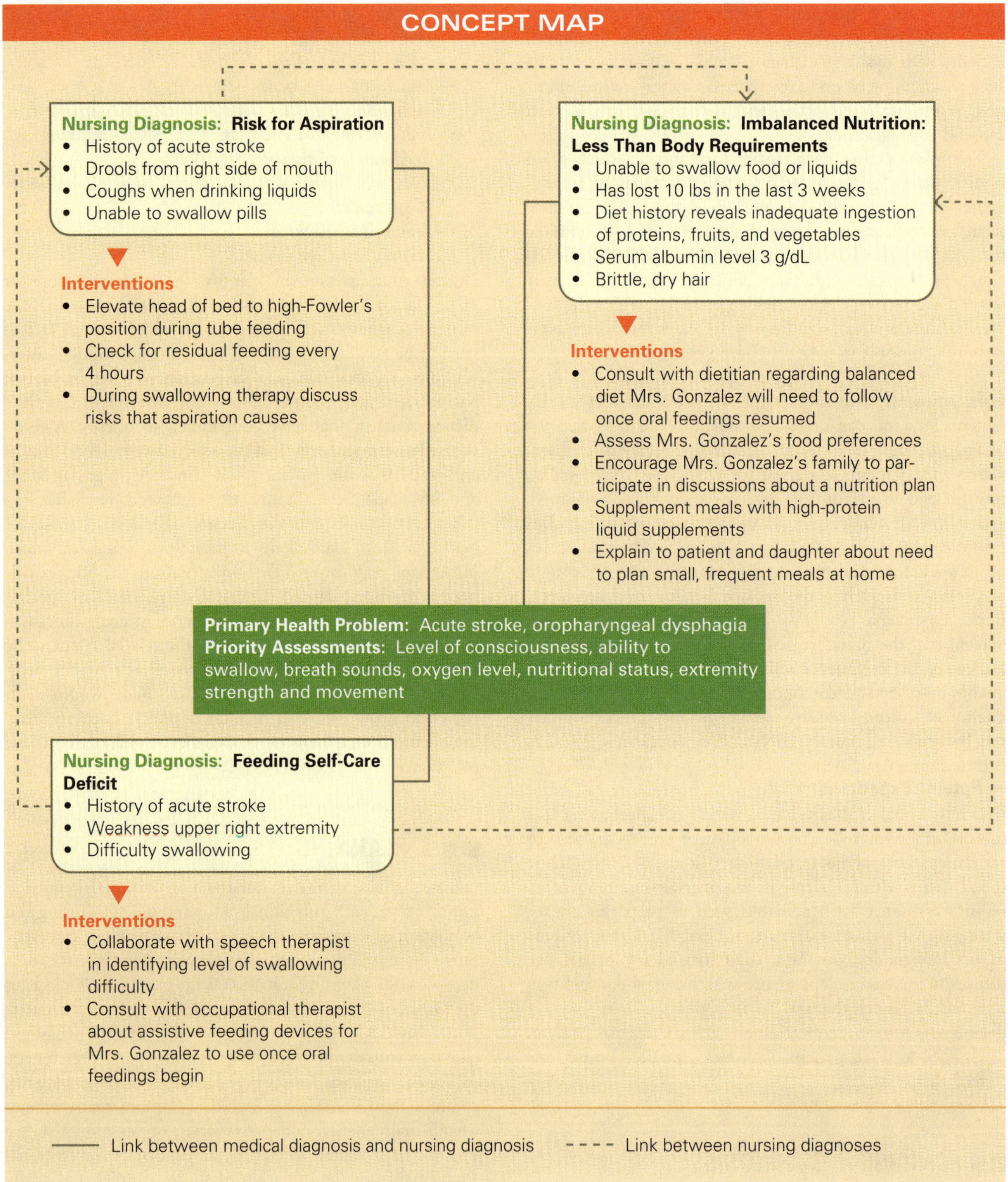

FIGURE 33-3 Concept map.

status. Consider the relationship between your patient's nursing diagnoses when determining appropriate goals and outcomes for your patient (Figure 33-3). If the nutritional diagnosis is *Imbalanced Nutrition: Less Than Body Requirements,* a goal will be for the patient to gain weight or to ingest adequate nutrients. If a patient is obese, a goal of care is to safely achieve weight reduction. Determine specific, individualized goals by identifying patient behaviors that have led to the nutritional alteration (see Care Plan). Correction of poor dietary patterns is a long-term rather than a short-term goal.

CARE PLAN

Nutrition

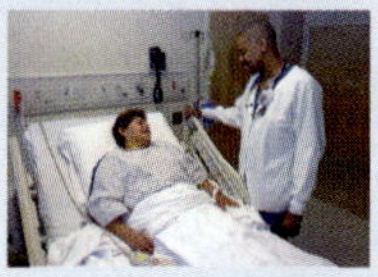

ASSESSMENT

Mrs. Gonzalez has had a stroke. Matt knows that strokes often cause dysphagia, which increases the risk for aspiration. Mrs. Gonzalez's diet history reveals that she ate balanced meals 3 times daily, including at least three servings of fruits and vegetables, and that she was eating adequately and had not lost weight before her stroke. Her health care provider orders tube feedings through a nasally inserted feeding tube. Mrs. Gonzalez states, "I just don't know about a tube. I wish my doctor would just let me eat."

ASSESSMENT ACTIVITIES	FINDINGS/DEFINING CHARACTERISTICS*
Assess Mrs. Gonzalez's ability to swallow safely and the risk for aspiration.	Mrs. Gonzalez was diagnosed with **acute stroke.** She starts to **cough when she tries to drink water.** The speech-language pathologist's (SLP)'s evaluation shows that Mrs. Gonzalez is **unable to swallow safely and is likely to aspirate oral intake.** The SLP has diagnosed her with **oropharyngeal dysphagia.**
Evaluate Mrs. Gonzalez's physical status, emphasizing her gastrointestinal status.	Her abdomen is soft and nondistended. She is not prone to diarrhea or constipation. Her bowel sounds are active.
Monitor Mrs. Gonzalez's respiratory status.	Lung sounds are clear. Respirations are regular at a rate of 12 breaths/min. She has no shortness of breath. Oxygen saturation is 96% on room air.
Assess Mrs. Gonzalez's nutritional status and needs.	Baseline albumin, blood glucose, renal function, and electrolyte levels are within normal limits.

***Defining characteristics** are shown in **bold** type.

NURSING DIAGNOSIS: Risk for Aspiration

PLANNING

GOAL

- Mrs. Gonzalez will receive adequate nutrition without aspiration by discharge.
- Mrs. Gonzalez will regain swallowing ability assisted by speech therapy training as soon as possible by discharge.

EXPECTED OUTCOMES (NOC)[†]

Nutritional Status: Nutrient Intake

- Mrs. Gonzalez's weight at discharge is within 2 lbs of admission weight.
- Mrs. Gonzalez does not exhibit signs of aspiration before discharge.
- Mrs. Gonzalez's albumin and prealbumin levels remain normal before discharge.
- Mrs. Gonzalez progresses to an oral diet before discharge to the restorative care facility.

[†]Outcomes classification label from Moorhead S et al, editors: *Nursing outcomes classification (NOC)*, ed 5, St Louis, 2013, Mosby.

INTERVENTIONS (NIC)[‡]	RATIONALE
Aspiration Precautions	
• Position Mrs. Gonzalez with head of bed elevated a minimum of 30 degrees.	Head of the bed elevated a minimum of 30 to 45 degrees decreases the risk for aspiration (AACN, 2012; Metheny and Frantz, 2013).
• Check tube placement before each use and at least every 4 to 6 hours.	Feeding tube misplacement increases the risk for aspiration (Bourgault and Halm, 2009; Metheny, Davis-Jackson, and Stewart, 2010).
• Check gastric residual volume and monitor abdominal status (e.g., for gastric distention or firmness) every 4 to 6 hours and prn for signs of discomfort.	Gastric residual volume indicates if gastric emptying is delayed. Delayed gastric emptying increases the risk for aspiration (AACN, 2012; Bankhead et al., 2009).
• Continue with speech therapy and follow recommendations per provider order. Make sure that patient is properly positioned and supervised during oral intake trials.	Regularly provided speech therapy helps patient regain the ability to swallow foods and liquids. Speech therapy includes trials of various consistencies of foods and liquids. Aspiration of food and liquids can lead to pneumonia.

Continued

CARE PLAN—cont'd

Nutrition

INTERVENTIONS (NIC)[‡]	RATIONALE
Nutrition Therapy	
• Insert feeding tube as ordered.	Enteral tube feeding allows for safe provision of nutrients while swallowing is rehabilitated with the assistance of the SLP.
• Initiate enteral tube feeding per health care provider orders.	The tube feeding is initiated at a low rate of infusion and increased slowly to allow for maximum tolerance.
• Advance tube feeding to goal rate, monitoring for tolerance.	Abdominal discomfort, large gastric residual volume, and diarrhea may be signs of feeding intolerance and need to be evaluated (Bankhead et al., 2009; McClave et al., 2009).

[‡]Intervention classifications labels from Bulechek, Butcher, and Dochterman, editors: *Nursing interventions classification (NIC)*, ed 6, St Louis, 2013, Mosby.

EVALUATION

NURSING ACTIONS	PATIENT RESPONSE/FINDING	ACHIEVEMENT OF OUTCOME
Monitor Mrs. Gonzalez's respiratory status.	Mrs. Gonzalez's lung sounds are clear, and she has no symptoms of aspiration.	Mrs. Gonzalez's lungs remain free of signs of aspiration.
Assess Mrs. Gonzalez for abdominal distention and bowel sounds.	Mrs. Gonzalez admits that she has occasional constipation, and her abdomen is slightly distended. She has bowel movements after fiber is added and fluid is increased.	Bowel movements are regular, and abdomen is soft and nondistended.
Weigh Mrs. Gonzalez weekly.	Mrs. Gonzalez's weight is ½ lb less than her admission weight.	Mrs. Gonzalez's weight is maintained.
Monitor laboratory values.	Prealbumin remains 20 mg/dL, and albumin is 4 g/dL.	Prealbumin and albumin values are maintained within normal limits.

Short-term goals usually involve achieving calorie or nutrient targets on a daily or weekly basis. It is important to explore patients' feelings about their weight and food and to help them set realistic and achievable goals. Goals are achieved through a prescribed diet, patient education, and helping a patient develop new behaviors that will enable him or her to achieve an adequate nutritional status.

Individualized planning for nutrition is critical. Mutually planned goals among the patient, RD, and nurse ensure success. Patients often have unrealistic expectations about nutritional needs or dieting in reference to weight gain or loss. Help them understand this concept by asking them to reflect on their rate of weight gain or loss. Changes in weight usually occur over months or years unless an acute illness has occurred. Patients become discouraged when they do not see rapid achievement of weight goals. Help a patient set realistic outcomes. For example, the following outcomes focus on achieving a weight-loss goal:

- Patient loses ½ to 1 lb per week.
- Patient's daily fat intake is less than 30% of total calories.
- Patient eliminates sugared beverages from diet.
- Patient increases fruit and vegetable servings in diet to five servings per day.

Setting Priorities. Patients at risk for nutritional problems have a plan of care aimed at improving nutritional status. However, many factors influence setting priorities so a patient receives proper nourishment. For example, if a patient is on oral intake, symptom control may be a priority (e.g., nausea or pain) before he or she feels comfortable to eat. Physiological factors such as fear or depression often influence a person's willingness to eat. If this is the situation, discussing a patient's concerns takes precedence over starting mealtime. Food is important for all people; but, when illness disrupts appetite or the ability to eat, anticipate what is most important to help your patient achieve good nutrition.

The development of the care plan requires collaboration of the health care team, the patient, and the family caregivers. Family and caregivers are often involved in food purchase and preparation. The nutritional plan of care will not succeed without their commitment to, involvement in, and understanding of nutritional goals.

Collaborative Care. Patients' nutritional needs extend beyond the acute hospital setting and into the home or rehabilitation care setting, requiring collaboration of health care professionals. Professionals who help provide care include the RD, nutritional support clinical nurse specialist, pharmacists, and medical health care providers. Consult with an SLP, RD, pharmacist, social worker, and/or occupational therapist when doing discharge planning that includes ongoing nutritional assessment and interventions to meet nutritional needs. Some patients with physiological conditions causing more severe cases of malnutrition require EN or PN to meet fluid, electrolyte, and nutritional needs.

Patients and family members need to learn the skills to administer nutritional therapies safely and effectively. Home care nurses play an important role in helping patients and families with the need for dietary changes and administration concerns, monitoring and problem prevention related to EN and PN feeding, and related lifestyle changes. Long-term nutritional management is a challenge that requires collaboration among the patient, family, and health care team.

IMPLEMENTATION

Health Promotion. You play a major role in promoting healthy dietary practices. Using tools such as the ChooseMyPlate program helps patients with food choices, menu planning, and dietary patterns. You also educate patients about food labels and their meanings. An area of particular importance is education about product claims that are misleading: some "reduced-fat" foods still have significant amounts of fat, some "lite" foods still contain considerable calories, and "low cholesterol" does not always mean low fat.

Increasing numbers of patients are acknowledging their weight and seeking weight-loss strategies. A high percentage of those who attempt to lose weight are unsuccessful, regaining lost weight over time. Diet and exercise compliance affects success with weight loss. Many individuals are willing to pay for weight-loss programs if the program meets individual needs. Information on weight-loss diets is available everywhere, from the bookstore to the Internet. However, there is a lack of good evidence evaluating the effectiveness of commercial weight-loss programs. A successful weight-loss plan involves sustainable lifestyle modifications that include physical activity, self-monitoring, portion control, and knowledge of energy content of food.

One diet that is highly effective in promoting health is The Dietary Approaches to Stop Hypertension (DASH) eating plan, which is based on research by the National Heart, Lung and Blood Institute (NHLBI) (USDHHS, 2006). This diet has been shown to effectively reduce blood pressure with foods low in saturated fat, cholesterol, and total fat. The DASH diet includes fruits, vegetables, fat-free or low-fat milk and milk products, whole grain products, fish, poultry, and nuts. It is also rich in protein and fiber. The DASH diet offers menus and recipes for two levels of daily sodium intake—2300 and 1500 milligrams per day. The lower 1500-mg sodium diet lowers blood pressure more quickly and is recommended by the Institute of Medicine (USDHHS, 2006). The DASH diet helps to reduce a person's risk for getting heart disease by helping to reduce blood pressure and lower LDL ("bad") cholesterol. Go to the following link for additional information: http://www.nhlbi.nih.gov/health/public/heart/hbp/dash/new_dash.pdf.

Food safety is a commonly overlooked aspect of health promotion. Contaminated and undercooked food products, especially eggs and meats, often result in severe debilitating and even fatal illnesses (Table 33-3). Patient education is one method of improving safe food practices for patients and their families (Box 33-8). Food safety is also an important nursing consideration if EN tube feeding is used to provide nutrition for the patient in the home setting.

Acute Care. It is common for oral intake to decrease during periods of stress. This occurs as a result of the anorexic effects of stress-induced hormones. It is important to monitor a patient's nutrient intake, identify influences that reduce appetite, and plan interventions to increase intake.

One disruptive influence on intake in acute care is diagnostic testing. Some blood and radiographic studies require a patient to receive nothing by mouth (NPO). Therefore the patient's food and liquids are withheld until testing is completed. This disrupts mealtimes, and sometimes patients are too fatigued to eat, become dehydrated, or experience discomfort related to the test. Continue to assess the patient's nutritional status. Patients who continue to be NPO and receive only standard intravenous fluids for more than 4 to 7 days are at nutritional risk, especially if they had reduced intake before admission.

Emotional stress also influences food intake. Patients who are worried about their families, finances, employment, or illness are not always able to eat or eat enough to compensate for the effect of stress on metabolism.

Medications may also affect intake and in some cases the use of nutrients. Some medications cause reduced appetite, slowed motility and constipation, anorexia, or malabsorption. For example, opioids (e.g., morphine sulfate, Codeine) used for pain relief can be very constipating. Medication-induced and condition-related nausea, vomiting, and diarrhea also greatly affect intake. This is common with chemotherapy for cancer treatment. Taste changes often occur with chemotherapy, diuretics, and mineral preparations such as zinc. Work with an RD to help a patient select foods that are tolerated and do not worsen the nausea or other symptoms. Sometimes medications need to be provided to decrease nausea or pain, and other medications can be changed or their administration altered.

Symptoms associated with illness often have a major effect on appetite. Pain, nausea, and shortness of breath make it difficult for patients to chew, swallow, and tolerate stomach filling. Often patients refuse to eat to avoid the associated discomfort. Patients who are ill, have had surgery, or have been NPO for a long period of time often have specialized dietary needs. The lack of taste of diets that are low in sodium or fat may lead to reduced dietary intake. In this situation you need to weigh the benefits associated with the therapeutic diet

TABLE 33-3 **FOOD SAFETY**

FOODBORNE DISEASE	ORGANISM	FOOD SOURCE	SYMPTOMS*
Botulism	*Clostridium botulinum*	Improperly home-canned foods, smoked and salted fish, ham, sausage, shellfish	Symptoms vary from mild discomfort to death in 24 hours, initially nausea and dizziness, progressing to motor (respiratory) paralysis
Escherichia coli	*Escherichia E. coli* O157:H7	Undercooked meat (ground beef)	Severe cramps, nausea, vomiting, diarrhea (may be bloody), renal failure; appear 1-8 days after eating, last 1-7 days
Listeriosis	*Listeria L. monocytogenes*	Soft cheese, meat (hot dogs, pate, lunch meats), unpasteurized milk, poultry, seafood	Severe diarrhea, fever, headache, pneumonia, meningitis, endocarditis; appear 3-21 days after infection
Perfringens enteritis	*Clostridium C. perfringens*	Cooked meats, meat dishes held at room or warm temperature	Mild diarrhea, vomiting; appear 8-24 hours after eating, last 1-2 days
Salmonellosis	*Salmonella S. typhi S. paratyphi*	Milk, custards, egg dishes, salad dressings, sandwich fillings, polluted shellfish	Mild-to-severe diarrhea, cramps, vomiting; appear 12-24 hours after ingestion, last 1-7 days
Shigellosis	*Shigella S. dysenteriae*	Milk, milk products, seafood, salads	Mild diarrhea to fatal dysentery; appear 7-36 hours after ingestion; last 3-14 days
Staphylococcus	*Staphylococcus S. aureus*	Custards, cream fillings, processed meats, ham, cheese, ice cream, potato salad, sauces, casseroles	Severe abdominal cramps, pain, vomiting, diarrhea, perspiration, headache, fever, prostration; appear 1-6 hours after ingestion, last 1-2 days

From Nix S: *Williams' basic nutrition and diet therapy*, ed 14, St Louis, 2013, Mosby.
*Symptoms are generally most severe for youngest and oldest age-groups.

BOX 33-8 **PATIENT TEACHING**

Food Safety

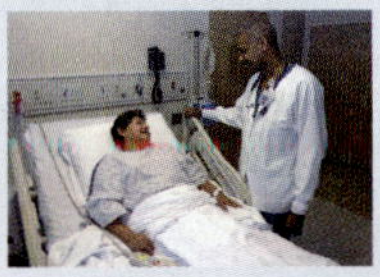

As Matt discusses measures he is taking to maintain the safety of Mrs. Gonzalez's feeding, her daughter Maria asks Matt questions about food safety in general. Matt recognizes that as a nurse he has opportunities to provide education in many different formats. He relates that the very young, older adults, patients with chronic illness, and patients who are immunosuppressed are at increased risk for foodborne illnesses (see Table 33-3). As Mrs. Gonzalez improves and begins to tolerate oral feeding, Matt consults with the registered dietitian, and together they develop a teaching plan regarding food safety for the foods that his patient's family will be preparing at home.

OUTCOME

At the end of the teaching session Mrs. Gonzalez's family is able to state measures to reduce foodborne illnesses.

TEACHING STRATEGIES

- Instruct Mrs. Gonzalez's family on ways to avoid foodborne illnesses:
  - Wash hands, food-preparation surfaces, and utensils with hot, soapy water.
  - Cook meat, poultry, fish, and eggs until well done (180° F).
  - Wash fresh fruits and vegetables thoroughly.
  - Do not eat raw meat or unpasteurized milk or juices.
  - Do not use food past expiration date.
  - Refrigerate foods at 40° F within 2 hours of cooking.
  - Keep foods properly refrigerated.
  - Thaw frozen foods in the refrigerator.
  - Discard food that you suspect is spoiled.
  - Do not use wooden cutting boards. Instead use plastic laminate or solid surface cutting boards that can be disinfected.
  - Wash dishcloths, dishtowels, and sponges regularly with bleach or use paper towels.
  - Clean inside of refrigerator and microwave regularly with bleach or soap.

EVALUATION STRATEGIES

- Ask Mrs. Gonzalez's family to state six measures to prevent foodborne illnesses.
- Observe Mrs. Gonzalez's daughter Maria at home for safe practices if making a home visit.

Modified from Nix S: *Williams' basic nutrition and diet therapy*, ed 14, St Louis, 2013, Mosby.

against the detrimental effects of weight loss and malnutrition. Table 33-4 describes commonly prescribed diets for patients in health care settings.

Food presentation also affects appetite. Hot foods that are cold or cold foods that are warm are not appetizing. Overcooked or undercooked foods are unappealing. A meal tray precariously balanced on a crowded, soiled over-bed table does not enhance a meal. Removing the tray lid outside of a patient's room helps to decrease distress in patients sensitive to odors (e.g., patients with nausea). Pay attention to details in food presentation, meal scheduling, and a patient's symptoms to enhance food intake. You help stimulate a patient's appetite through environmental adaptations, consultation with an RD, attention to food preferences, and patient and family counseling.

Providing a Comfortable Environment. Provide an environment conducive to eating. Offer a means for hand hygiene, such as a warm washcloth, before a meal. Make sure that the patient's room is free of reminders of treatments and odors. Provide mouth care when necessary to remove unpleasant tastes. Plan to administer analgesics or antiemetics early enough so patients are more comfortable to eat at mealtime. Position the patient comfortably so the meal is more enjoyable. If a patient refuses a portion of the meal, make every effort to replace it with a suitable alternative.

Assisting Patients with Feeding. Some patients are unable to feed themselves adequately because of the severity of their illness, fatigue, or debilitation of their condition. Improve patient feeding by carefully protecting their dignity and actively involving them. Encourage the patient to eat a small amount of food at a comfortable pace when helping with feeding. Provide independence through the use of adaptive devices (Figure 33-4) or finger foods. Position the patient in a chair or high-Fowler's position to improve swallowing and digestion. Allow him or her time to empty the mouth after every spoonful, attempting to match the speed of feeding to the patient's readiness. Encourage patients to direct the order in which they wish to eat food items. Mealtime is a good time to instruct patients and their families about the selection of appropriate foods and the importance of a balanced diet.

Patients with visual deficits also need special assistance. Patients with decreased vision are able to feed themselves independently when they are given adequate information. Identify the food location on the plate as if it were a clock (e.g., meat at 9 o'clock and vegetable at 3 o'clock). Tell the patient where the beverages are located in relation to the plate. Be sure that other care providers set the meal tray and plate in the same manner. Patients with impaired vision are more independent during mealtimes with the use of large-handled adaptive utensils, which are easier to grip and manipulate.

Dysphagia. A certified SLP identifies patients at risk for dysphagia and makes recommendations for dysphagia therapy. The SLP administers trials of several consistencies of foods and fluids to obtain a comprehensive assessment of a patient's phases of swallowing. Fluoroscopy aids in this assessment. The SLP determines the degree of dysfunction

TABLE 33-4 THERAPEUTIC DIETS

DIET	DESCRIPTION
Clear liquid	Broth, bouillon, coffee, tea, carbonated beverages, clear fruit juices, gelatin, popsicles
Full liquid	As for clear liquid with addition of smooth-textured dairy products (e.g., ice cream, yogurt drinks, milk), custards, refined cooked cereals, vegetable juice, pureed vegetables, all fruit juices
Dysphagia-stages, thickened liquids; pureed	As for liquids with addition of scrambled eggs; pureed meats, vegetables, and fruits; mashed potatoes and gravy
Mechanical soft	As for all liquids with addition of ground or finely diced meats, flaked fish, cottage cheese, cheese, rice, potatoes, pancakes, light breads, cooked vegetables, cooked or canned fruits, bananas, soups, peanut butter
Soft/low residue	Addition of low-fiber, easily digested foods such as pastas, casseroles, moist tender meats, and canned cooked fruits and vegetables; desserts, cakes, and cookies without nuts or coconut
High fiber	Addition of fresh uncooked fruits, steamed vegetables, bran, oatmeal, and dried fruits
Low sodium	4-g (no added salt), 2-g, 1-g, or 500-mg sodium diets; vary from no added salt to severe sodium restriction (500-mg sodium diet) that requires selective food purchases
Low cholesterol	300 mg/day cholesterol, in keeping with American Heart Association guidelines for serum lipid reduction
Diabetic	Nutrition recommendations by the American Diabetes Association: focus on total energy and a balanced intake of carbohydrates from fruits, vegetables, whole grains, legumes and low-fat milk; fats, and proteins; caloric recommendations vary to accommodate patients' metabolic demands
Gluten Free	Eliminates wheat, oats, rye, barley, and their derivatives
Regular	No restrictions unless specified

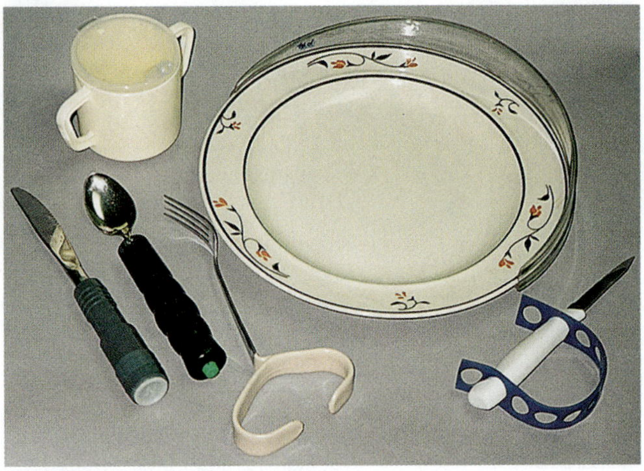

FIGURE 33-4 Assist devices for self-feeding.

and aspiration risk. Treatment recommendations focus on consistencies of foods and fluids and the use of swallowing therapies.

Dysphagia Diet Management. Patients with dysphagia are at risk for aspiration and need more help with feeding and swallowing. Provide a rest period before eating. Position the patient in an upright, seated position in a chair or raise the head of the bed to 90 degrees (Hughes, 2011). Have the patient slightly flex the head to a chin-down position to help prevent aspiration. If the patient has unilateral weakness, teach the patient and caregiver to place food in the stronger side of the mouth. Determine the viscosity of foods that the patient tolerates best through the use of trials of different consistencies of foods and fluids. Thicker fluids are generally easier to swallow. The American Dietetic Association published the National Dysphagia Diet Task Force's (NDDTF's) National Dysphagia Diet to provide uniformity of diets provided to patients with dysphagia (NDDTF, 2002). There are four levels of diet: dysphagia pureed, dysphagia mechanically altered, dysphagia advanced, and regular. The four levels of liquid are thin liquids (low viscosity), nectar-like liquids (medium viscosity), honey-like liquids (viscosity of honey), and spoon-thick liquids (viscosity of pudding) (Academy of Nutrition and Dietetics, 2012; NDDTF, 2002).

Feed the patient with dysphagia slowly, providing smaller-size bites, and allow the patient to chew thoroughly and swallow the bite before taking another. Frequently assess the patient's chewing and swallowing throughout the meal. Allow the patient time to empty the mouth after each spoonful, matching the speed of feeding to the patient's readiness. If the patient begins to cough or choke, remove the food immediately.

Patients with Disabilities. Allow patients with disabilities that interfere with independent food intake to do as much as possible for themselves. When necessary, prepare the meal tray, cutting food into bite-size pieces, buttering bread, and pouring liquids. Use special eating utensils if necessary or as recommended by occupational therapy. Patients with decreased motor skills may be more independent during mealtimes with the use of large-handled adaptive utensils. Some patients become fatigued during the course of the meal, leading to suboptimal intake. Provide assistance at the end of meals as needed. Evaluate the results of self-feeding on the basis of food intake. Recognize and commend patient success.

Interventions for Those Unable to Meet Nutritional Needs Orally. Guidelines help the health care professional set goals and plan care for the patient who is unable to maintain adequate nutrition by the oral route (Bankhead et al., 2009). These guidelines focus on enhancing oral nutrition by mouth as a first priority. This involves modifying food choices to increase the nutritional value of food ingested, administering medication to relieve nausea or pain if it interferes with oral intake, adjusting mealtimes or helping with the process of eating as indicated. When these interventions are insufficient to improve oral intake or when oral intake is not deemed safe, enteral nutrition (EN) should be considered to maintain adequate nutrition. PN should be considered only when nutritional support via the GI tract is not safe, when the bowel must be rested, or when nutritional needs cannot be met. Research has demonstrated that EN is preferred over PN because it improves use of nutrients, is generally safer for patients, maintains gut structure and function, decreases the risk for infection and sepsis, and is less expensive (Bankhead et al., 2009; McClave et al., 2009). Work with the patient, family, and other health care team members to maintain adequate nutrition in the safest, most physiological and cost-effective manner possible.

Enteral Tube Feedings. **Enteral nutrition (EN)** refers to administration of nutrients and fluid into the stomach or intestinal tract via a feeding tube. NG feedings are delivered through a feeding tube introduced through the nose and into the stomach. Nasointestinal feedings are delivered through a feeding tube inserted through the nose and into the small intestine (duodenum or jejunum). When patients have nasopharyngeal obstructions or are not candidates for nasally placed tubes or when the need for EN is anticipated to be longer than several weeks, feeding tubes may be inserted directly into the stomach (gastrostomy) or jejunum (jejunostomy) (Table 33-5). A variety of enteral feeding formulas are available, including products either with or without fiber. Special enteral formulas are available, including products such as for those with renal or hepatic disease, those who have had trauma or recent GI surgery, and those who need adequate protein but reduced calories. Specific additives such as protein or fiber products are sometimes included in the nutritional regimen. When provided in amounts to meet a patient's protein and calorie needs, many products also meet the patient's RDIs. As a rule enteral formulas do not meet most patients' needs for fluid, and additional water must be provided. Consult with an RD to ensure a patient's nutritional and fluid needs are met. The skills presented in this chapter focus on the administration of nutritional feedings directly into the GI tract with the goal of restoring and maintaining the patient's nutritional status.

Skill 33-2 describes insertion of a small-bore feeding tube. Feeding tubes are referred to as being nasally placed because

TABLE 33-5 COMPARISON OF ENTERAL FEEDING TUBES

TUBE	FEATURES	NURSING CONSIDERATIONS
Gastrostomy	Placed surgically (laparoscopic or open) with an endoscope or fluoroscopy Held in place internally with a balloon or a semisolid "bolster" or "bumper"-type end Uses external disc to prevent tube from migrating internally Uses low-profile tubes for patients who are conscientious of their body image or may be prone to pull at tube	Monitor external tube length as guide for placement. Internal migration can block the pylorus, leading to gastric retention, patient discomfort, and emesis or large residual volumes. Check for tube tightness if person gains weight or is bloated or distended. If external disc is too tight, circulation is restricted, and skin breakdown often occurs. Use small gauze dressing under external disc. It may be used for stomach decompression. Usual gastric returns are expected. If tube is placed high in stomach, repositioning patient may help obtain returns. Use adaptor for administration through low-profile tubes.
Jejunostomy	Placed surgically with an endoscope or fluoroscopy Held in place by sutures, Dacron cuff or small-volume balloon	Ability to use for gravity bolus feeding (meal-like feedings) is limited because jejunum lacks storage capacity of stomach. Monitor external tube length to watch for internal or external migration. High gastric-like residual volumes are not expected.
Gastrojejunostomy	Has gastric and small-bowel ports Low-profile gastrojejunostomy tubes that have small-bowel access may be used	Label port to be used for feeding and medications. Gastric port typically is used for decompression. Jejunal port is used for feeding. Monitor gastric returns. Gastric returns may indicate that jejunal port has flipped into stomach and is no longer appropriate for jejunal feeding.

that is the route most frequently used, primarily because the nose provides a natural stability for tubes. However, feeding tubes are sometimes placed orally if there has been trauma to the nose or if a patient already has an endotracheal tube placed in the mouth. Avoid large-bore NG tubes for primary use as a feeding tube because they carry an increased risk for aspiration and are more irritating to the nasopharyngeal and esophageal mucosa (McGinnis, Worthington, and Lord, 2010). Occasionally the large-bore tube, initially inserted for gastric decompression, is used to initiate enteral feeding because it is already in place. If the feeding continues for more than a few days, consult with the health care provider about placement of a small-bore feeding tube. Small-bore feeding tubes create less discomfort for a patient. For an adult most of these tubes are 8 to 12 Fr and 43 to 55 inches long. A stylet is often used during insertion of a small-bore tube to stiffen it and removed when the correct position of the tube is confirmed.

Feeding Tube Insertion. When a patient cannot safely swallow food or take adequate amounts of food orally but can digest and absorb nutrients, a small-bore feeding tube is placed nasally into the stomach or small intestine (see Skill 33-2). When making the decision regarding enteral access, the health care provider considers the patient's rate of gastric emptying, GI anatomy, risk for gastric reflux and aspiration, anticipated duration of requirement for enteral access, and disease state. Nasal tubes are associated with sinusitis, otitis, vocal cord paralysis, pressure ulcers of the nose and sinuses, and the potential for displacement. Thus you do not use them for long-term enteral access. Feeding tubes that end in the stomach are used for gravity bolus or continuous infusion feedings. The small intestine does not have the storage capability of the stomach, and therefore a tube feeding administered into the small intestine is delivered more slowly and continuously with an infusion pump.

Aspiration into the lung can occur from secretions or other material in the oral pharyngeal area, or it may occur as a result of reflux of gastric content, including tube feeding formula. Aspiration of material foreign to the lung irritates the bronchial mucosa and provides growth material for pneumonia or other infections. Some of the common conditions that increase the risk for aspiration include severity of illness and interventions that compromise the gag reflex. Specific factors that increase a patient's risk for aspiration include sedation, mechanical ventilation, nasotracheal suctioning, neurologic compromise, an altered level of consciousness, lying flat, hemodynamic instability, and sepsis (Makic et al., 2011). To reduce the risk of aspiration, keep the head of the bed elevated at least 30 or preferably 45 degrees unless medically contraindicated (Bankhead et al., 2009; Metheny and Frantz, 2013). Most health care providers order measurement of gastric residual volume (GRV) every 4 to 6 hours in patients receiving continuous feedings and immediately before a feeding in patients receiving intermittent feedings (Bankhead et al., 2009). However, the amount of GRV in a patient's stomach is not predictive of aspiration. Aspiration has been shown to occur with 5 to 500 mL of GRV (McClave et al., 2005).

BOX 33-9 EVIDENCE-BASED PRACTICE

PICO Question: In hospitalized patients receiving enteral tube feeding, does the use of evidence-based strategies prevent inadvertent tubing misconnections?

SUMMARY OF EVIDENCE

Enteral feeding tube misconnections can result in solutions being delivered through inappropriate delivery systems, causing serious and even fatal consequences for patients. The enteral feeding system can inadvertently be connected to equipment such as intravascular lines, peritoneal dialysis catheters, tracheostomy tube cuffs, or medical gas tubing (Guenter, Hicks, and Simmons, 2009). For example, the delivery of enteral tube feeding formula into an intravascular catheter can have immediate fatal consequences. The Joint Commission issued a sentinel event alert to address this serious issue, citing over 300 reported cases involving a variety of misconnection errors (TJC, 2006). Millin and Brooks (2010) suggest that misconnection likely occurs more often than that which is reported because the misconnection is blamed on human error instead of on device failure. One factor that can help reduce the potential for these errors includes product redesign such as tubing connection redesign, including standardizing connector size, bright-colored solid or striped tubing, and "enteral feeding only" stickers (Guenter, Hicks, and Simmons, 2009). Nurses must be vigilant to ensure that solutions are connected to the appropriate delivery devices and follow agency guidelines and procedures to prevent any adverse events that could lead to patient harm.

APPLICATION TO NURSING PRACTICE

- Ensure that all connections are appropriate; never force connections (Millin and Brooks, 2010).
- Ensure that each device is clearly labeled.
- Don't rely on color coding to identify connections because color coding is not universal (Millin and Brooks, 2010).
- Don't modify or adapt intravenous or feeding devices (Millin and Brooks, 2010).
- Ensure good communication during patient transfer and handoffs, including tracing all connections (Millin and Brooks, 2010).
- Make sure that staff (and patients as indicated) are properly educated about new devices (Guenter, Hicks, and Simmons, 2009).
- Educate visitors and nonclinical staff not to reconnect disconnected lines but to seek clinical assistance instead.
- Follow agency policy and procedure for reporting any near misses or adverse events (Millin and Brooks, 2010).

The North American Summit on Aspiration in the Critically Ill Patient made the following recommendations regarding GRV: (1) stop feedings immediately if aspiration occurs; (2) withhold feedings and reassess patient tolerance to feedings if GRV is over 500 mL; and (3) evaluate the patient for aspiration and use nursing measures to reduce the risk for aspiration if GRV is between 200 and 500 mL (Bankhead et al., 2009; McClave et al., 2009). When GRVs are high, evaluate the patient's abdominal status for distention, firmness, tympany, and discomfort. Also assess bowel status for constipation or diarrhea. One of the most important steps is to evaluate a patient's tolerance of tube feeding, because an increased acceptance of a higher GRV often maximizes delivery of adequate nutrition (Makic et al., 2011).

Ensure that enteral feedings are correctly connected to an enteral feeding tube (Box 33-9). The outdated bedside method of testing placement of a feeding tube by injecting air into the tube while listening over the stomach with a stethoscope is ineffective. The gold standard for determining tube location is radiographic confirmation. Assessing the color and pH of gastric aspirate for ongoing monitoring of tube location has been shown to be effective and less costly (Box 33-10) (AACN, 2012; Proehl et al., 2011). Monitoring the length of a tube that is external from the nose or abdomen is very helpful in detecting tube displacement.

Gastrostomy/Jejunostomy Tubes and Tube Feedings. When patients cannot tolerate nasally or orally placed tubes or when EN is anticipated to be needed for more than several weeks, tubes may be placed percutaneously into the GI tract through the abdomen. A surgeon inserts a G-tube through a small incision in the left upper quadrant of the stomach either laparoscopically or with an open surgical technique. This type of feeding tube is held in place internally by a balloon, pigtail design, or other design. A G-tube may also be placed with an endoscope and is also called a *percutaneous endoscopic gastrostomy (PEG) tube.* A PEG tube is held in place because of its design (Figure 33-5). You administer feedings into the stomach via a G-tube using gravity bolus in small volumes or continuously by a slow infusion. Because gastrostomy tubes (G-tubes) permit more options for feeding delivery and thus more freedom and flexibility

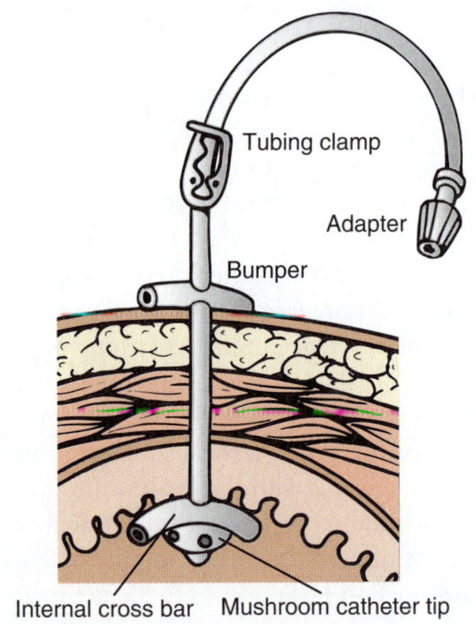

FIGURE 33-5 Percutaneous endoscopic gastrostomy tube.

BOX 33-10 PROCEDURAL GUIDELINES

Verifying Enteral Tube Placement by Obtaining Gastrointestinal Aspirate for pH Measurement via Large-Bore and Small-Bore Feeding Tubes: Intermittent and Continuous Feeding

DELEGATION CONSIDERATIONS

The skill of measuring pH in gastrointestinal (GI) aspirate cannot be delegated to nursing assistive personnel (NAP). The nurse directs the NAP to:

- Immediately inform the nurse if patient's respirations change or patient complains of shortness of breath, coughing or choking.
- Immediately inform the nurse if the patient vomits.

EQUIPMENT

60 mL catheter-tipped syringe, pH test paper (scale of 1.0 to 11.0 or greater), tap or sterile water (see agency policy), paper towel, small medication cup, clean gloves

STEPS

1. Identify conditions that increase risk for spontaneous tube migration or dislocation: altered level of consciousness; retching, vomiting, or coughing; nasotracheal suction.
2. Observe for change in length of the external portion of tube (as determined by movement of the marked portion of the tube) (AACN, 2009).
3. Review routine chest and abdominal x-ray reports to determine if the radiologist has assessed feeding tube location (AACN, 2009).
4. Review patient's medication record for orders for continuous feeding or a gastric acid inhibitor or proton pump inhibitor.
5. Review patient's record for history of prior tube displacement.
6. Identify patient using two identifiers (e.g., name and birthday or name and account number) according to agency policy.
7. Verify tube placement at the following times:
    a. For intermittently fed patients, test placement immediately before feeding (usually a period of at least 4 hours will have elapsed since previous feeding). More frequent checking has been associated with increased clogging of small-bore tubes.
    b. For continuously tube-fed patients, test placement following agency policy. AACN (2009) recommends that continuous feedings be stopped for several hours to obtain reliable pH readings because enteral formula buffers the pH of gastric secretions. It may be helpful to measure when feedings are interrupted for procedures or diagnostic studies.
    c. Wait at least 1 hour after medication administration by tube or mouth. Premature aspiration of contents removes unabsorbed medication, reducing dose delivered to patient. Medication also interferes with pH testing and appearance of aspirate (Gilbertson, Rogers and Ukoumunne, 2011; Simmons and Abdallah, 2012).
8. Perform hand hygiene and apply clean gloves.
9. Draw up 30 mL of air into syringe. Disconnect or unplug feeding tube and attach syringe tip to end of feeding tube. Flush tube with 30 mL of air before attempting to aspirate fluid. It is likely more difficult to aspirate fluid from the small intestine than from the stomach. Repositioning patient from side to side is helpful. More than one bolus of air through the tube is necessary in some cases. Burst of air aids in aspirating fluid more easily.
10. Draw back on syringe slowly and obtain 5 to 10 mL of gastric aspirate. Observe appearance of aspirate (see illustration).
11. Gently mix aspirate in syringe. Expel a few drops into a clean medicine cup. Dip the pH strip into the fluid or apply a few drops of the fluid to the strip (see illustration). Compare the color of the strip with the color on the chart provided by the manufacturer.

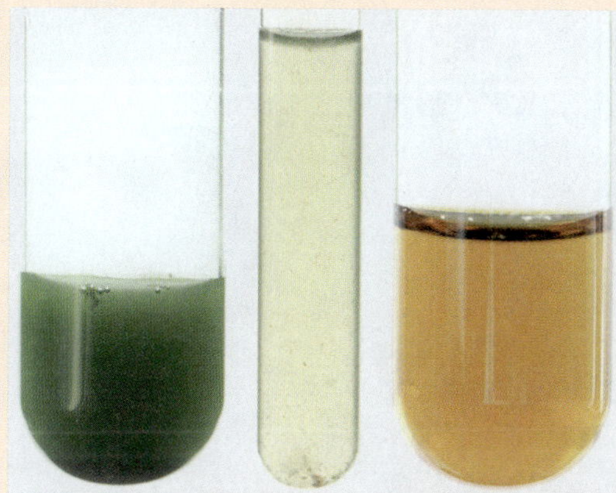

STEP 10 Gastrointestinal contents. *From left to right,* Stomach, Intestine, Airway. (Courtesy Dr. Norma Metheny, Professor, St. Louis University School of Nursing.)

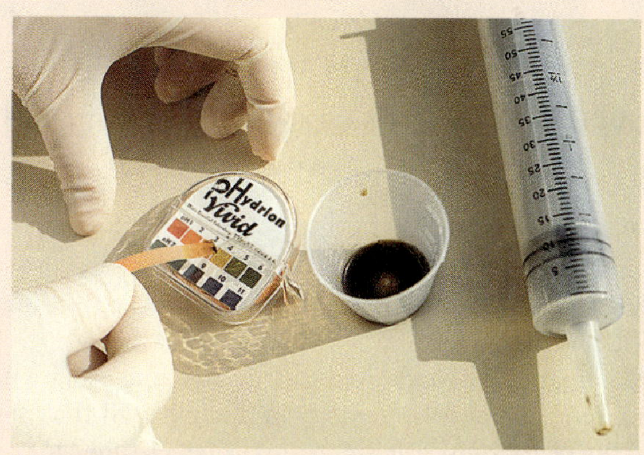

STEP 11 Comparing pH strip with color chart.

    a. Fasting (at least 4 hours) gastric fluid pH is usually 5 or less, even in patients receiving gastric acid inhibitors (Bankhead et al., 2009; AACN, 2009).
    b. Fluid from nasointestinal tube of fasting patient usually has pH greater than or equal to 6.0 (Bankhead et al., 2009; AACN, 2009).
    c. Patient with continuous tube feeding often has pH of 5.0 or higher (AACN, 2009).
    d. pH of pleural fluid from tracheobronchial tree is generally greater than 6.0.

Continued

BOX 33-10 PROCEDURAL GUIDELINES—cont'd

Verifying Enteral Tube Placement by Obtaining Gastrointestinal Aspirate for pH Measurement via Large-Bore and Small-Bore Feeding Tubes: Intermittent and Continuous Feeding

Clinical Decision Point: **If, after repeated attempts, it is not possible to aspirate fluid from a tube that was originally established by x-ray film examination to be in desired position and (a) there are no risk factors for tube dislocation, (b) there is no change in external marked tube length, and (c) patient is not experiencing difficulty, assume that tube is placed correctly (Bankhead et al., 2009; Stepter, 2012).**

12. After testing for pH and after checking for gastric residual (see Skill 33-3) flush feeding tube. Draw up 30 mL of water into syringe. Insert tip of syringe into end of feeding tube. Slowly instill irrigating solution. Irrigation prevents clogging of tube (Bankhead et al., 2009).
13. Remove syringe and reinstitute tube feeding or administer medication as ordered.
14. Remove gloves and discard supplies. Perform hand hygiene.

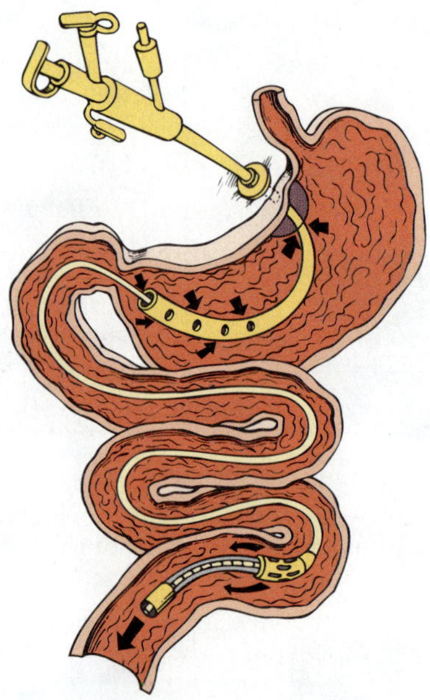

FIGURE 33-6 Endoscopic insertion of jejunostomy tube.

for patients, they should be considered for longer-term feeding instead of jejunal tubes whenever possible (Bankhead et al., 2009).

When patients have delayed gastric emptying or have had gastric resection or other surgery in the upper GI tract such as a pancreatectomy, a **jejunostomy tube** (J-tube) may be inserted to deliver nutrition (see Skill 33-3). Feedings delivered via J-tube are usually delivered even more slowly (e.g., over a period of hours overnight) because the jejunum lacks the storage and regulated emptying capacity of the stomach. J-tubes are inserted directly into the small intestine through a percutaneous incision, or they may be inserted through a gastrostomy opening into the small intestine. Gastrojejunostomy tubes are tubes that have access to both the stomach and the small intestine. The gastric port may be used for decompression of accumulated stomach content while feeding is delivered into the jejunal port (Figure 33-6). You need to know which port is gastric and which port is jejunal.

It is important to take measures to prevent and monitor for feeding tube displacement. G-tubes that migrate internally sometimes block the pylorus or exit from the stomach to the small intestine. This results in increased GRV, discomfort, emesis, and/or leaking around the tube. Application of an external disk helps to prevent migration of a G-tube. Tubes that are too tight impair circulation between the external disc and the insertion site and can quickly lead to breakdown of the site. Daily cleaning and evaluation of the site helps detect problems. Take measures to prevent displacement of a feeding tube, including taping it to the abdomen or tucking it into clothing for security as indicated or even applying an abdominal binder if necessary. Displacement of a tube can lead to infusion of fluid into the peritoneal space, which leads to serious complications Check your agency policy regarding tube displacement. Perform site care and assessment of the insertion site daily for abdominally placed tubes.

Providing Parenteral Nutrition. **Parenteral nutrition (PN)** is the administration of a solution consisting of glucose, amino acids, minerals, electrolytes, trace elements, and vitamins through a peripheral or central venous catheter (CVC). Administration of PN is used when the GI tract cannot be used or cannot absorb nutrients in sufficient amounts to provide adequate nutrition. There is an increased risk for infection when administering PN because it requires intravascular access and because of the high concentration of glucose in PN solutions. Using the GI tract for nutrition provides many physiological benefits that are not realized when the GI tract is not used. PN is also significantly more costly than EN. The health care team evaluates the need for PN on a daily basis. The goal is to move toward the use of the GI tract for oral intake or EN as soon as possible (Bankhead et al., 2009; McClave et al., 2009).

PN solutions that contain 10% dextrose or greater are hyperosmolar (i.e., highly concentrated) and irritate small peripheral veins. As a result, PN at this concentration must be administered through CVCs where the blood flow is very rapid. This is called *central PN*. PN solutions with osmolality less than 900 mOsm may be administered through peripheral veins. Peripheral PN is usually used only for a short period because it is still irritating to the blood vessels. In addition, it is challenging to meet a patient's nutritional needs with these less concentrated solutions. A PN solution is formulated to meet a patient's specific nutritional needs and is adjusted as needed based on a patient's laboratory values and metabolic and nutritional status. A PN solution may or may not contain fat emulsion (lipid). Some patients receive no fat emulsion or receive fat emulsion only 2 or 3 times per week, depending on their specific needs.

If a PN prescription includes fat emulsion, it is sometimes combined with the other nutrients to make a total nutrient admixture (TNA), or the fat can be provided in a separate bag. Do not administer TNA if you observe oil droplets or an oily or creamy layer on the surface of the solution. The lipid emulsion may be administered peripherally or via a larger blood vessel (centrally) below an in-line filter, bypassing the filter, unless the filter is of an appropriate size to accommodate the size of the fat molecule. The infusion rate is 0.5 to 1 mL/min for the first 30 minutes the first time it is administered. Reactions to lipid infusion include dyspnea, cyanosis, vomiting, headache, and/or chest pain. If a reaction occurs, stop the infusion and notify the health care provider immediately. If the patient tolerates the slow lipid infusion, advance the rate as ordered by the health care provider.

Initiating Parenteral Nutrition. PN therapy requires a CVC inserted into the superior vena cava via the subclavian vein or, less ideally, the jugular vein. The administration of PN can also be given via a peripherally inserted central catheter (PICC) (ASPEN, 2009; INS, 2011). Nurses assist physicians who place CVCs. Specially trained nurses insert PICCs (see agency policy) (see Chapter 18). A chest x-ray film confirms the location of the CVC when it is initially placed and when misplacement is suspected. Instead of a catheter, patients have a long-term central venous access device (CVAD) such as a tunneled catheter or an implanted port. When administering PN, be sure the formula ordered is being delivered into a catheter or CVAD that terminates in the appropriate position. This requires you to assess and detect a catheter that may have become displaced.

Before beginning an infusion, inspect the solution and check the contents carefully to make sure that it is formulated according to the health care provider order. The solution is provided at a specified rate using an infusion pump over the course of the day to meet the patient's nutritional needs. PN is usually started at a lower rate (e.g., 40 to 60 mL/hr) and advanced to meet the patient's goal rate as tolerance is demonstrated. Patients receiving PN at home frequently administer the entire daily solution over 10 or 12 hours at night. This allows the patient to disconnect from the infusion each morning, flush the central line, and have independent mobility during the day.

Caring for the Patient Receiving Parenteral Nutrition. Nursing care for the patient receiving PN focuses on seven major nursing goals: (1) preventing infection; (2) maintaining the PN system; (3) preventing metabolic, electrolyte, or fluid balance complications; (4) ensuring that the patient's nutritional and fluid needs are being met; (5) evaluating the continued need for PN or if oral intake or EN may be initiated and, if not; (6) planning for home PN if this is indicated; and (7) supporting the patient and family during major lifestyle changes.

Primary methods to prevent infection include meticulous aseptic technique during insertion; use and care of the CVC and dressing; use of an in-line intravenous filter; and maintaining secure, uncontaminated tubing connections (ASPEN, 2009; INS, 2011). Make sure PN solutions do not exceed their 24-hour infusion limit. If you are using a CVC that has multiple lumens, use a port that is exclusively dedicated for the PN. Label the port for PN, and do not infuse other solutions or medications through the port (INS, 2011). During CVC dressing changes, always wear a mask to reduce the risk of introducing airborne contaminants. Assess the insertion site for signs of infection. If the site itself must be touched, wear a sterile glove. Change the CVC dressing per institution policy and anytime it becomes wet, loose, or contaminated. Chlorhexidine gluconate (CHG) solution is the preferred solution for skin antisepsis as part of CVC site care (INS, 2011). However, 1% to 2% tincture of iodine, iodophor, and 70% alcohol may also be used. Scrub the catheter hub or port with alcohol or CHG using friction before each use or entrance into the system (CDC, 2011; INS, 2011). An in-line 0.22-μm filter is typically used to remove air and particulate matter such as bacteria with fat emulsion (lipid) administered closer to the patient so it will not go through the filter. If fat emulsion is included in the solution, a larger filter (0.5 μm) is used as the molecule is larger in size.

Monitor patients receiving PN closely to assess for tolerance, the need for adjustments to the solution, and efficacy of the nutrition provided. Analyze frequent laboratory measurements for metabolic or electrolyte abnormalities and assess fluid balance, weight trend, and the ability to heal during administration. Laboratory monitoring includes frequent blood glucose testing because the high dextrose (glucose) content of the solution easily leads to hyperglycemia and requires supplemental insulin as needed (Phillips, 2010) (Figure 33-7 and Box 33-11). A sudden cessation of the high-dextrose solution often leads to a low blood sugar or hypoglycemia. To reduce the risk of hypoglycemia, taper the solution before it is discontinued, especially if the patient is not currently receiving another incoming source of carbohydrate. Be alert for changes in vital signs or fluid balance and abnormal laboratory results that indicate osmotic diuresis and dehydration, infection (e.g., an increased temperature or white blood cell count), electrolyte imbalance or hyperglycemia, and clinical symptoms of high or low blood glucose. Report any unusual symptoms to the health care provider.

Restorative and Continuing Care

Diet Therapy in Disease Management. Patients discharged from a hospital with diet prescriptions often need dietary education to plan meals that meet specific therapeutic requirements. Restorative care includes immediate postsurgical, posthospitalization, and routine medical care. Therefore

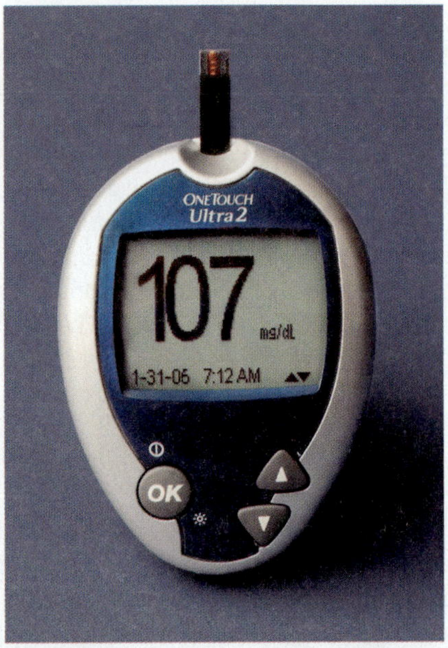

FIGURE 33-7 Blood glucose monitor. (Courtesy LifeScan, Inc., Milpitas, CA.)

integrate preparation for the restorative aspect of patient care within the acute care setting.

Medical Nutrition Therapy. Optimal nutrition is important in health and illness, but the specific dietary intake pattern that results in optimal nutrition is modified for patients with particular diseases. **Medical nutrition therapy (MNT)** is the use of specific nutritional therapies to treat an illness, injury, or condition. MNT is necessary to assist the ability of the body to metabolize certain nutrients, correct nutritional deficiencies related to a disease, and eliminate foods that exacerbate disease symptoms. Patients with specific diseases often need modified dietary intake patterns to achieve good nutrition. These include GI diseases such as irritable bowel syndrome and malabsorption syndromes, metabolic disorders such as diabetes mellitus and hypoglycemia, cardiovascular diseases, renal diseases, and cancers. Diet modifications need to correspond with the ability of the body to metabolize certain nutrients, correct nutritional deficiencies, and eliminate harmful foods from the diet. In all cases work with the physician or health care provider and RD when planning and implementing modified diets.

Home Care. Sometimes specialized nutritional therapies such as EN and PN continue beyond the hospital setting to the home setting. In these cases it is important to determine a feeding regimen that best meets a patient's lifestyle. In addition, the regimen must meet the patient's nutritional and fluid needs based on the clinical condition and be compatible with the type of feeding tube. For example, meal-like or bolus feedings administered over the length of time of a comfortable meal (e.g., 20 to 30 minutes if the tube terminates in the stomach or delivered over 10 to 12 hours at night for jejunal feedings) frees a patient of a pump during the day. As a home care nurse you are often the only care provider who sees the patient on a regular basis. You provide education for patients or family caregivers so they can administer PN or EN; assess the catheter or feeding tube; assess tolerance and adequacy of the nutritional and fluid regimen by monitoring weight, hydration status, or glucose level; watch for signs of infection; and help with troubleshooting and problem prevention. GRVs are typically not measured in adult patients receiving EN at home. You can withdraw gastric contents if the patient is very uncomfortable to avoid emesis and if indicated by the health care provider. If you do this, assess the patient's bowel status.

You help a patient transition to oral intake when indicated by making suggestions for adjusting the nutritional regimen according to the health care provider order. Support the patient receiving EN or PN in being as independent and maintaining control of his or her own life as much as possible while maintaining safety and a therapeutic regimen. The need for nutritional support is accompanied by major lifestyle changes for both the patient and the family. You serve as an advocate for your patient by investigating best options for his or her lifestyle and whether the nutrition and fluid provided adequately meets your patient's needs.

EVALUATION

Patient Care. Ongoing evaluation measures the effectiveness of your plan of care in meeting a patient's nutritional needs. Allow enough time to evaluate your patient's progress because nutritional improvement takes time.

Evaluation of clinical progress includes objective data such as weight gain or improved laboratory parameters and subjective data such as a patient reporting improvement in food choices or self-reporting improved intake (Box 33-12). When clinical progress does not occur, determine whether the interventions were not effective, not done or accepted by the patient, not realistic or appropriate, or affected by unanticipated or unidentified factors (see Care Plan).

If outcomes are not met, reassess the patient to determine if you missed any important data. Some patients need reeducation if they have forgotten or misunderstood essential skills or knowledge. In addition, attempt to validate that the patient is in agreement with the goals and is willing and able to follow the nutritional plan of care.

Patient Expectations. Nutritional interventions often depend on a patient's willingness and ability to change behavior patterns and learn new patterns. If a patient is not fully committed to the expected changes, the interventions will not always be successful. Some patients also find it difficult to change behavior and are less motivated with the passage of time. It is important to remember to individualize the nutrition care plan and focus on the patient.

Most patients respond well to the opportunity to make informed choices. Explaining the reasons for the behavioral change and providing a patient options for how to achieve the change help him or her make the change. If necessary provide education in several brief sessions to maximize the retention of information.

BOX 33-11 PROCEDURAL GUIDELINES

Blood Glucose Monitoring

DELEGATION CONSIDERATIONS

The skill of blood glucose monitoring can be delegated to nursing assistive personnel (NAP) if the patient's condition is stable. However, the nurse is responsible for the assessment of the patient and analysis of the results of testing. The nurse directs the NAP by:

- Explaining appropriate sites to use for puncture and when to obtain glucose levels.
- Reviewing expected levels and when to report to the nurse unexpected glucose levels.

EQUIPMENT

Antiseptic swab, cotton ball, sterile lancet or blood-letting device, blood glucose meter (e.g., Accucheck III, OneTouch), blood glucose reagent strips (brand determined by meter used), clean gloves, paper towel

STEPS

1. Assess patient's understanding of procedure and purpose of blood glucose monitoring. Determine if patient understands how to perform test and the importance of glucose monitoring.
2. Determine if specific conditions need to be met before or after sample collection (e.g., with fasting, after meals, after certain medications, before insulin doses). In addition, determine if risks exist for performing skin puncture (e.g., low platelet count, anticoagulant therapy, bleeding disorders).
3. Assess area of skin to be used as puncture site. Inspect fingers or forearm for edema, inflammation, cuts, or sores. Alternative site for children is the heel. Avoid areas of bruising and open lesions, as well as the hand on the side of a mastectomy.
4. Review health care provider's order for time or frequency of measurement.
5. For patient with diabetes who performs test at home, assess ability to handle skin-puncturing device. If a family caregiver measures in the home, test his or her competency. If patient chooses, he or she may wish to continue self-testing while in hospital.
6. Explain procedure and purpose to patient and/or family. Offer patient and family opportunity to practice testing procedures. Provide resources/teaching aids for patient and family caregiver.
7. Identify patient using two identifiers (e.g., name and birthday or name and account number) according to agency policy) (TJC, 2014). Compare identifiers with information on patient's MAR or medical record.
8. Perform hand hygiene before procedure. Instruct adult to perform hand hygiene with soap and warm water, rinsing thoroughly if able. Food residue on skin can alter blood glucose results.
9. Position patient comfortably in chair or in semi-Fowler's position in bed.
10. Remove reagent strip from container; tightly seal cap. Check code on test strip vial. Use only test strips recommended for glucose meter. Some newer meters do not require code and/or have disk or drum with 10 or more test strips.
11. Insert strip into glucose meter (refer to manufacturer directions) and make necessary adjustments (see illustration). Do not bend strip. Meter turns on automatically. If monitor is not activated when reagent strip is inserted, turn on glucose monitor.

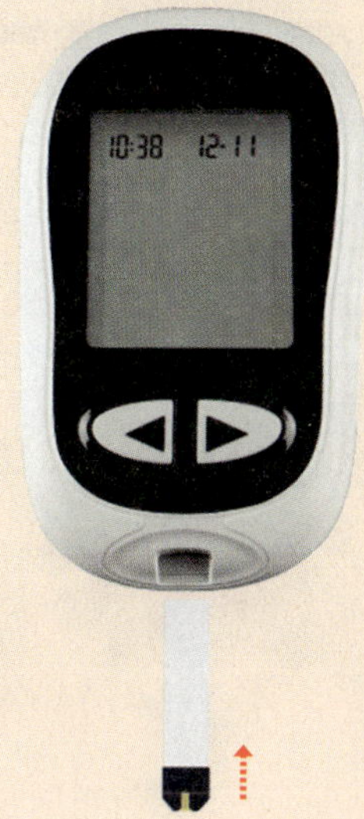

STEP 11 Load test strip into meter. (Courtesy of the manufacturer.)

12. Remove unused reagent strip from meter and place on paper towel or clean, dry surface with test pad facing up (see manufacturer directions).
13. Meter displays code on screen that must match code from test strip vial. Press proper button on meter to confirm matching codes. Meter is ready for use.
14. Perform hand hygiene and apply clean gloves.
15. Prepare single- or multiple-use lancet device. **NOTE:** Some meters recommend that this step be completed before preparing test strip. Remove cap from lancet device; insert new lancet. Some lancet devices have disk or cylinder that rotates to new lancet.
    a. Twist off protective cover on tip of lancet. Replace cap of lancet device.
    b. Cock lancet device, adjusting for proper puncture depth.
16. Choose puncture site. Puncture site should be vascular. In adult select lateral side of finger; be sure to avoid central tip of finger, which has more dense nerve supply (Pagana and Pagana, 2013). Hold finger that you will puncture in dependent position. Do not milk or massage finger site because this may hemolyze specimen and introduce excess tissue fluid (Pagana and Pagana, 2013).
17. Clean site with antiseptic swab, and *allow it to dry completely*.
18. Hold area to be punctured in a dependent position, and hold tip of lancet perpendicular to puncture site. Press release button on device (see illustration). Some devices allow you to see blood sample forming. Remove device.

Continued

BOX 33-11 PROCEDURAL GUIDELINES—cont'd

Blood Glucose Monitoring

19. Wipe away first droplet of blood with cotton ball. (See manufacturer directions for meter used.)
20. Lightly squeeze puncture site (without touching) until large droplet of blood has formed (see illustration). Repuncturing is necessary if large enough drop does not form to ensure accurate test results. (See manufacturer directions regarding how blood is applied.)
21. Be sure that meter is still on. Bring test strip in meter to drop of blood. The blood wicks onto test strip (see manufacturer instructions). Some meters (such as OneTouch [LifeScan]) require blood sample to be applied to test strip already in meter.
22. Once the drop of blood is applied, meter automatically calculates reading. The blood glucose test result appears on screen (see illustration). Some devices "beep" when completed. Do not scrape blood onto test strips or apply blood to wrong side of test strip. This prevents accurate glucose measurement.
23. Turn meter off. Some meters turn off automatically.
24. Dispose of test strip, lancet, and gloves in proper receptacle.
25. Perform hand hygiene.
26. Discuss test results with patient and encourage questions and participation in care.
27. Document glucose results and describe response, including presence or absence of pain or excessive oozing of blood at puncture site.
28. Report blood glucose levels out of target range and take appropriate action for hypoglycemia or hyperglycemia.
29. Evaluate puncture site for bleeding or tissue injury. Compare glucose meter reading with normal blood glucose levels and previous test results.

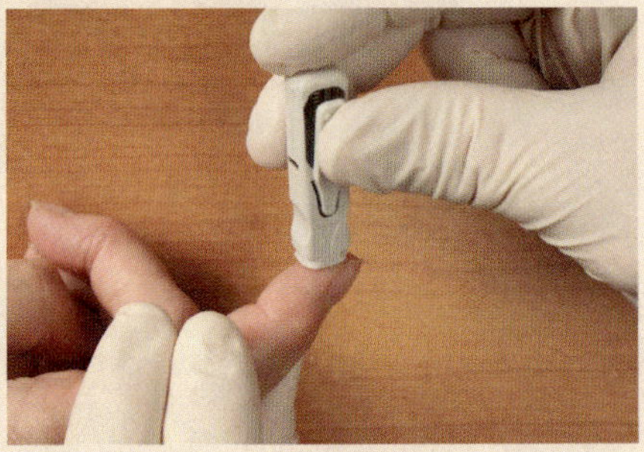

STEP 18 Prick side of finger with lancet.

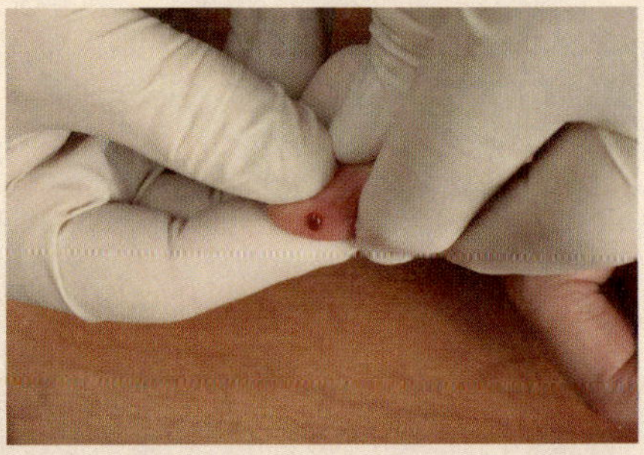

STEP 20 Squeeze puncture site until large droplet of blood is formed.

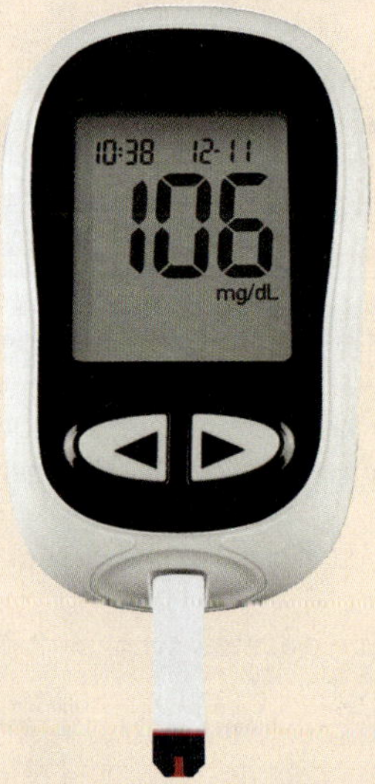

STEP 22 Results appear on meter screen. (Courtesy of the manufacturer.)

BOX 33-12 EVALUATION

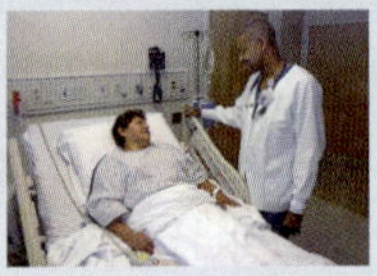

Matt sees Mrs. Gonzalez before discharge to a restorative care facility for rehabilitation before returning home. As Mrs. Gonzalez begins to eat again, Matt encourages her to eat first and then infuses her feeding right after meals as she increases the amounts that she can eat. Her feeding volumes decrease as her oral intake increases. He also encourages her to ingest adequate volumes of fluid so her feeding tube is no longer needed. Mrs. Gonzalez is now able to consume all of her required fluid and nutrients with a ground diet and nectar-thickened liquids. Matt removes the feeding tube in preparation for her transport to the new facility.

Matt advises Mrs. Gonzalez to continue the current plan of care and emphasizes that it is important to continue speech therapy. He discusses the importance of compliance with diet modifications until swallowing function returns completely.

DOCUMENTATION NOTE

"Swallows without signs of aspirating. Oral intake of mechanically altered diet and fluid meets 100% of estimated needs according to dietitian. To be followed by restorative care facility."

SAFETY GUIDELINES FOR NURSING SKILLS

Ensuring patient safety is an essential role of the professional nurse. To ensure patient safety, communicate clearly with members of the health care team, assess and incorporate the patient's priorities of care and preferences, and use the best evidence when making decisions about your patient's care. When performing the skills in this chapter, remember the following points to ensure safe, individualized care:

- Label enteral equipment with patient name, room number, formula name, rate, date and time of initiation, and nurse initials (Bankhead et al., 2009).
- Ensure "right patient, right formula, right tube" by matching formula and rate to feeding order and verifying that enteral tubing set connects formula to feeding tube (Bankhead et al., 2009).
- Elevate the head of the bed a minimum of 30 to 45 degrees unless medically contraindicated for patients receiving enteral feedings (Metheny and Frantz, 2013).
- Trace all lines and tubing back to patient to ensure that you have only enteral-to-enteral connections (Bankhead et al., 2009; Guenter et al., 2008).
- Monitoring tube placement is essential in early detection of tube misplacement. Auscultation is not a reliable method for verification of NG or nasointestinal tube placement because a tube inadvertently placed in the lungs, pharynx, or esophagus also transmits a sound similar to that of air entering the stomach (Proehl et al., 2011; Simmons and Abdallah, 2012).
- Food safety is especially important in providing EN. Feeding products and equipment used to deliver them are good growth media for bacteria. Clean, dry, and store syringes as two pieces to prevent moisture accumulation. Keep other equipment clean and dry and change according to agency protocol. Use freshly obtained tap water as the flush and fluid administration solution unless normal saline is ordered or agency protocol is to use sterile water for immunocompromised patients (ASPEN, 2009).
- Refer to manufacturer guidelines to determine hang time for enteral feedings. Maximum hang time for formula is 8 hours in an open system; 24 to 48 hours in a closed, ready-to-hang system (if it remains closed). There is increased risk for bacterial growth in feedings that exceed the recommended hang time.
- Follow enteral feedings with fluid administration or flushes to prevent tube clogging and ensure that the patient is receiving adequate fluid intake. Use freshly obtained tap water as the flush and fluid administration solution unless normal saline is ordered or agency protocol is to use sterile water for immunocompromised patients (ASPEN, 2009).
- Medications administered via the feeding tube should be in liquid form whenever possible or well crushed and adequately diluted. Do not mix medications. Administer water before and after administering each medication. If a tube does clog, warm water is more effective in unclogging tubes than other agents such as cola or cranberry juice (Bankhead et al., 2009).
- Administer continuous EN and PN with an infusion pump.

SKILL 33-1 ASPIRATION PRECAUTIONS

View Video!

DELEGATION CONSIDERATIONS

The skill of following aspiration precautions while feeding a patient can be delegated to nursing assistive personnel (NAP). However, the nurse is responsible for the assessment of a patient's risk for aspiration and determination of positioning. However, NAP may feed patients after receiving instruction in aspiration precautions. The nurse instructs NAP to:

- Position patient with head elevated a minimum of 30 degrees (45 to 90 degrees preferred) to decrease aspiration risk.
- Use aspiration precautions while feeding patients who need assistance.
- Report to the nurse in charge any onset of coughing, gagging, a wet voice, or oral pocketing of food.

EQUIPMENT

- Chair or electric bed (to allow patient to sit upright)
- Thickening agents as designated by SLP (rice, cereal, yogurt, gelatin, commercial thickening agent)
- Tongue blade
- Medication cup and 50 mL of water
- Penlight
- Equipment for oral hygiene (see Chapter 29)
- Pulse oximeter
- Oral suction equipment (see Chapter 30)
- Clean gloves

STEP	RATIONALE
ASSESSMENT	
1. Perform nutritional assessment.	Patients at risk for aspiration from dysphagia often alter their eating patterns and select foods with less nutritional value because they are easier to eat, or they sometimes ingest less in general because of difficulty eating and/or drinking.
2. Assess patients for aspiration risk factors (see Box 33-7) and for signs and symptoms of dysphagia (e.g., cough, pharyngeal pooling, change in voice after swallowing). Use dysphagia screening tool if available.	Patients at risk include those who have neurological or neuromuscular diseases and those who have had trauma to or surgical procedures of the oral cavity or throat.

SKILL 33-1 ASPIRATION PRECAUTIONS—cont'd

STEP	RATIONALE
3. Observe patient during previous mealtimes for signs of dysphagia and allow him or her to attempt to feed self. Observe patient consume various consistencies of foods and liquids. Note at end of meal if patient fatigues.	Helps detect abnormal eating patterns such as frequent clearing of throat or prolonged eating time. Chewing and sitting up for feeding bring on onset of fatigue (Meiner, 2011). Fatigue increases risk for aspiration.
4. Ask patient about any difficulties with chewing or swallowing various textures of food.	Patients are likely to aspirate certain foods more than others.
5. Assess mental status: alertness, orientation, and ability to follow simple commands (e.g., open your mouth)	If orientation and command following are impaired, there is a higher risk of aspiration (Leder et al., 2009).
6. If patient is alert, have him or her attempt to swallow 50 mL of water in 5-mL allotments. Stop if patient begins to choke.	The Kidd water test is an accurate predictor of dysphagia (Kidd et al., 1993).
7. Assess patient's oral health, level of dental hygiene, missing teeth or poorly fitting dentures (apply clean gloves if needed).	Poor oral hygiene can result in decayed teeth, plaque, and periodontal disease and cause growth of bacteria in the mouth that can be aspirated (Eisenstadt, 2010).
PLANNING	
1. Instruct patient and/or family caregiver about what you are going to do and why.	Increases patient cooperation and prepares family caregiver for being able to assist.
2. Explain to patient why you are observing him or her while he or she eats.	Signs or symptoms associated with aspiration indicate the need for further evaluation of swallowing such as a fluoroscopic swallow study (White et al., 2008).
3. Provide a 30-minute rest period before feeding time.	Swallowing difficulty is less likely in a well-rested patient (Metheny, 2011).
IMPLEMENTATION	
1. Perform hand hygiene.	Reduces transmission of microorganisms.
2. Provide thorough oral hygiene, including brushing of tongue, before meal.	Risk for aspiration pneumonia has been associated with poor oral hygiene (Eisenstadt, 2010).
3. Position patient upright (90 degrees) in bed or in highest position allowed by medical condition during meals, or position in chair. Have patient assume chin-tuck position.	Chin-tuck or chin-down position helps reduce aspiration. Supine position increases probability of aspiration (Eisenstadt, 2010).
4. Apply pulse oximeter to patient's finger; monitor during feeding.	A decrease in oxygen saturation sometimes indicates aspiration (Weinhardt, 2008).
5. Using penlight and tongue blade, gently inspect mouth for pockets of food (apply gloves as needed).	Pockets of food in mouth indicate difficulty swallowing (Remig and Weeden, 2012). Patient is usually unaware of pocketing (Chang and Roberts, 2011).
6. Add thickener to thin liquids to create desired consistency per SLP assessment. Encourage patient to feed self.	Thin liquids such as water and fruit juice are difficult to control in the mouth and pharynx and are more easily aspirated (Garcia et al., 2010). Promotes independence and may help patient initiate a more natural swallow.
7. Remind patient to not tilt head backward when eating or while drinking.	Extension of neck may cause food and liquid to be misdirected into airway (Ney et al., 2009).
8. If patient unable to feed self, place ½ to 1 teaspoon of food on unaffected side of mouth, allowing utensil to touch mouth or tongue.	Small bites help patient's ability to swallow (Grodner et al., 2012). Provides tactile cue to food being eaten; avoids pocketing of food on weaker side, which may increase risk of aspiration (Brady, 2008).
9. Provide verbal coaching; remind patient to chew and think about swallowing. a. Open your mouth. b. Feel the food in your mouth. c. Chew and taste the food. d. Raise your tongue to the roof of your mouth. e. Think about swallowing. f. Close your mouth and swallow. g. Swallow again. h. Cough to clear airway.	Verbal cueing keeps patient focused on normal swallowing. Positive reinforcement enhances patient's confidence in ability to swallow.

STEP	RATIONALE
10. Avoid mixing food of different textures in same mouthful. Alternate liquids and bites of food. Refer to RD if patient has difficulty with a particular consistency.	Gradual increase in types and textures combined with constant monitoring ensures that patient is able to eat safely. Single textures are easier to swallow than multiple textures. Alternating solids with liquids removes food residue in mouth (Ney et al., 2009).
11. Observe for throat clearing, coughing, choking, gagging, and drooling of food; suction airway as necessary.	These are indications that suggest dysphagia and risk for aspiration (DeFabrizio and Rajappa, 2010).
12. Minimize distractions and do not rush patient. Allow time for adequate chewing and swallowing. Provide rest periods as necessary during meal.	Environmental distractions and conversations during mealtime increase risk for aspiration (Chang and Roberts, 2011). Avoiding fatigue decreases risk for aspiration.
13. Ask patient to remain sitting upright for at least 30 to 60 minutes after meal.	Remaining upright after meals or snack reduces chance of aspiration by allowing food particles remaining in pharynx to clear (Frey and Ramsberger, 2011).
14. Provide oral hygiene after meals.	Oral hygiene reduces plaque and secretions containing bacteria that can cause pneumonia (Eisenstadt, 2010; Frey and Ramsberger, 2011).
15. Remove gloves if worn. Return patient's tray to appropriate place and perform hand hygiene.	Reduces spread of microorganisms.
EVALUATION	
1. Observe patient's ability to swallow food and fluids of various textures and thickness without choking.	Indicates whether aspiration risk is increased with thin liquids or foods.
2. Monitor pulse oximetry readings for high-risk patients during eating.	Deteriorating oxygen saturation levels may indicate aspiration.
3. Monitor patient's intake and output, calorie count, and food intake.	Aids in detection of malnutrition and dehydration.
4. Weigh patient daily or weekly per order.	Determines if weight is stable and reflects adequate caloric level.
5. Observe patient's oral cavity after meal to detect pockets of food.	Determines presence of pockets of food when meal has included foods of various textures.

RECORDING AND REPORTING

- Document the following in patient's medical record: patient's tolerance of liquids and various food textures, amount of assistance required, position during meal, absence or presence of any symptoms of dysphagia during eating, and amount eaten.
- Report any coughing, gagging, choking, or swallowing difficulties to nurse in charge or health care provider.
- Communicate with other staff that patient has dysphagia such as in patient's medical record, on Kardex or plan of care, and during hand-off communication.

UNEXPECTED OUTCOMES AND RELATED INTERVENTIONS

- Patient coughs, gags, complains of food "stuck in throat," or has wet quality to voice when eating.
  - Stop feeding immediately and place patient on NPO. Notify health care provider and suction as needed.
- Patient avoids certain textures of food.
  - Change consistency and texture of food.
- Patient experiences weight loss.
  - Discuss findings with health care provider and/or RD about increasing frequency of meals or providing oral nutritional supplements.

SKILL 33-2 INSERTING A NASOGASTRIC OR NASOINTESTINAL FEEDING TUBE

DELEGATION CONSIDERATIONS

The skill of inserting a nasogastric (NG) or nasointestinal (NI) feeding tube cannot be delegated to nursing assistive personnel (NAP). The nurse guides the NAP to:

- Assist patient with positioning during tube insertion.
- Perform oral hygiene before the procedure for patient comfort and to cleanse the oral cavity.

EQUIPMENT

Tube Insertion

- Small bore NG tube or NI feeding tube with or without stylet (select smallest diameter possible: 8 to 10 Fr)
- 60-mL or larger slip tip, Luer-Lok, or catheter-tip syringe
- Stethoscope and pulse oximeter
- Tube fixation device or hypoallergenic tape
- Transparent dressing
- *Option:* When using tape to secure NG tube or transparent membrane, have skin barrier protectant and tincture of benzoin available
- pH indicator strip (scale 1.0 to 11.0)
- Glass of water and straw if patient able to swallow safely and focus on swallowing during tube insertion
- Towel (hand towel may be adequate)
- Emesis bag or basin
- Facial tissues
- Clean gloves
- Suction equipment in case of aspiration
- Penlight to check placement in nasopharynx
- Tongue blade

Tube Removal

- Disposable pad, facial tissues, clean gloves, disposable plastic bag or receptacle

STEP	RATIONALE
ASSESSMENT	
1. Verify health care provider's order for type of tube and enteric feeding schedule.	Health care provider's order is needed to place feeding tube.
2. Assess patient's knowledge of procedure.	Encourages cooperation, reduces anxiety, and minimizes risks. Identifies teaching needs.
3. Review patient's medical history for contraindications such as basilar skull fracture, nasal problems, nosebleeds, facial trauma, nasal surgery, deviated septum, anticoagulant therapy, coagulopathy, or recent upper GI surgery.	Nasoenteric tubes may be contraindicated in patients with recent nasal surgery, basilar skull fractures, facial traumas, and nosebleeds and those receiving anticoagulation.

Clinical Decision Point: **If a patient is at risk for intracranial passage of a tube, avoid the nasal route. Insertion of a gastrostomy or jejunostomy tube is an alternative.**

STEP	RATIONALE
4. Have patient close each nostril alternately and breathe. Examine each naris for patency and skin breakdown. Also ask for patient preference for tube placement.	Identifies most appropriate naris to use for success in the tube insertion. Some patients have a preference for naris used, and participation enhances success of the therapeutic relationship.
5. Assess for bowel sounds, abdominal pain or tenderness, and abdominal distention.	Signs may indicate medical problems that contraindicate feedings. Absence of bowel sounds indicates decreased or absent peristalsis and increased risk for aspiration.
6. Assess patient's mental status (ability to cooperate with procedure), presence of cough and gag reflex, ability to swallow, and presence of an artificial airway.	These are risk factors for inadvertent tube placement into tracheobronchial tree (Krenitsky, 2011).
PLANNING	
1. Identify patient using two identifiers (e.g., name and birthday or name and account number) according to agency policy.	Ensures correct patient. Complies with The Joint Commission requirements for patient safety (TJC, 2014).
2. Consider measures to ease patient discomfort for the procedure such as something to grasp for distraction. If numbing agent (e.g., lidocaine gel) is ordered, administer it per naris per institutional protocol.	Nasal tube insertion can be uncomfortable; distraction can help ease this discomfort (Shaw and Lamdin, 2011; Uri et al., 2011). The naris is typically the most uncomfortable portion of the tube insertion. Lidocaine gel may provide some relief of this discomfort (Ducharme and Matheson, 2003; Uri et al., 2011).
3. Explain procedure to patient as well as how to communicate during intubation by raising index finger to indicate discomfort.	Reduces anxiety to promote cooperation. Provides a way of communicating during insertion. Observations of nonverbal cues of patient comfort level are important.

STEP	RATIONALE
IMPLEMENTATION	
1. Perform hand hygiene. Position patient in sitting or high-Fowler's position unless contraindicated. If patient is comatose, raise head of bed as tolerated at least 45 degrees. If necessary, have an assistant help with positioning a confused or comatose patient. If patient needs to remain supine, place in reverse Trendelenburg's position.	Reduces transmission of microorganisms. Positioning reduces risk for pulmonary aspiration in event patient should vomit. Forward head position assists with closure of airway and passage of tube into esophagus.
2. Apply pulse oximeter and measure vital signs.	Permits objective assessment of respiratory status during tube insertion.
3. Position yourself so you can comfortably advance the feeding tube with your dominant hand without straining to reach across or cause discomfort to patient. This may involve lowering a side rail so you are nearer to patient.	Helps to effectively and safely insert the tube without causing strain to patient or yourself.
4. Place towel over patient's chest. Keep facial tissues in reach.	Provides clean work area on chest and is more esthetic. Prevents soiling of gown. Insertion of tube often causes tearing.
5. Determine length of tube to be inserted and mark location with tape or indelible ink: **a.** Measure distance from tip of nose to earlobe to xyphoid process of sternum (see illustration). **b.** Add additional 20 to 30 cm (8 to 12 inches) for NI tube.	Using appropriate measurement technique estimates depth of insertion of tube for proper placement. Since internal structures may vary, further verification of placement is necessary after the tube is placed. Occasionally further insertion or slight withdrawal of the tube may be indicated based on findings of tube verification.
6. Prepare NG or NI tube for intubation:	
a. If tube has a guidewire or stylet, inject 10 mL of water from the catheter tip or Luer-Lok syringe into it.	Ensures that tube is patent. Aids in guidewire or stylet removal. Activates lubricant coating of tube if present.
b. Position guidewire securely against weighted tip and ensure that connections are snugly fitted together.	Promotes smooth passage of tube into GI tract. Improperly positioned stylet could induce trauma.
7. Prepare tube fixation device or membrane dressing or cut hypoallergenic tape 10 cm (4 inches) long.	Anchors tube following insertion.
8. Apply clean gloves.	Reduces transmission of microorganisms.
9. Apply water-soluble lubricant to end of tube. If tube is coated with water-activated lubricant, dip tip into glass of room temperature water, keeping it very clean.	Water activates lubricant on coated tube. Lubricant facilitates passage of tube and helps protect against damage to dry nasal tissues.
10. Hand alert patient a glass of water with straw or piece of crushed ice (if able to swallow).	Asking patient to swallow water facilitates tube passage.

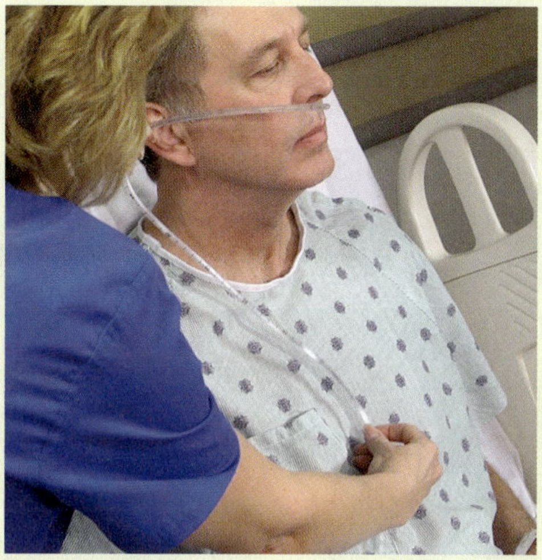

STEP 5A Determine length of tube that you will insert.

SKILL 33-2 INSERTING A NASOGASTRIC OR NASOINTESTINAL FEEDING TUBE—cont'd

STEP	RATIONALE
11. Explain the step and gently insert tube through nostril to back of throat (posterior nasopharynx). May cause patient to gag. Aim back and down toward ear (see illustration).	Natural contours ease passage of tube into GI tract.
12. Have patient flex head toward chest after tube has passed through nasopharynx.	Closes off glottis and reduces risk for tube entering trachea.
13. Encourage patient to swallow small sips of water or ice chips. Advance tube as patient swallows. Rotate tube 180 degrees while inserting.	Swallowing facilitates passage of tube past oropharynx. Rotating may decrease friction.
14. If patient is unable to swallow safely or follow directions, watch his or her breathing pattern as you insert tube. You do not want to advance the tube during inspiration or during a cough since it is more likely to enter the respiratory tract. Monitor pulse oximetry readings.	Many times a nasally placed feeding tube is ordered for patients because they cannot swallow safely. Asking them to swallow may actually increase the risk of entering the respiratory tract. Watch for cues of distress to help detect and prevent inadvertent respiratory placement. Sometimes patients do not cough or exhibit distress even if the tube enters the lung. Therefore accurate verification of placement is essential before any use.
15. Advance tube as patient swallows until it has passed the desired length as long as it advances without resistance.	Resistance may indicate kinking of the tube or anatomic irregularity. Advancing despite resistance could cause injury to patient.

Clinical Decision Point: **Do not force the tube. If you meet resistance or if patient starts to cough, choke, or oxygen saturation drops, stop advancing the tube and pull it back approximately to the naris and start over.**

STEP	RATIONALE
16. Check position of tube in back of throat with penlight and tongue blade.	Tube may be coiled, kinked, or entering trachea.
17. Temporarily anchor tube to nose with small piece of tape.	Movement of tube stimulates gagging. Allows you to assess general position of tube before permanent anchoring.
18. Attach syringe to end of feeding tube and obtain gastric aspirate: assess amount, color, and quality of returns. Measure pH of returns (see Box 33-10, Steps 9 to 11).	Properly obtained pH of 1.0 to 4.0 is a good indication of gastric placement (Bourgault and Halm, 2009; Proehl et al., 2011).
19. After you obtain gastric aspirates, secure the tube, avoiding pressure on nares. Use one of following options to secure the tube:	A properly secured tube allows patient more mobility, reduces potential for displacement, and prevents trauma to nasal mucosa.
a. Apply tube fixation device with shaped adhesive patch:	Secures tube and reduces friction on naris.
(1) Apply wide end of patch to bridge of nose (see illustration).	
(2) Slip connector around feeding tube as it exits nose (see illustration).	

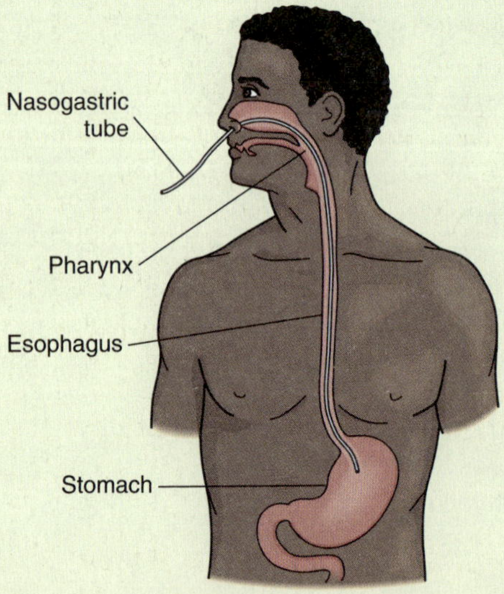

STEP 11 NG tube inserted through nose and esophagus into stomach.

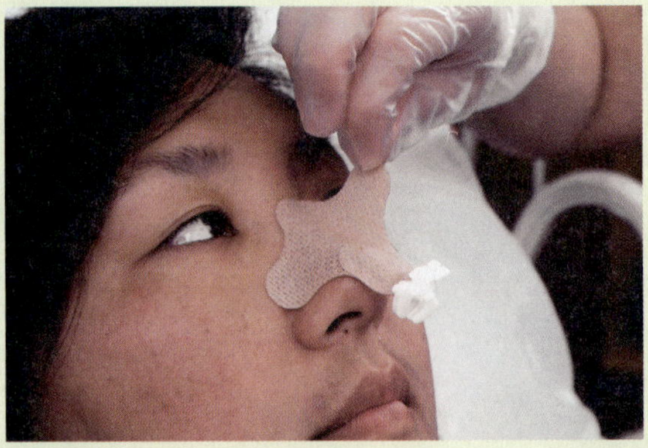

STEP 19a(1) Applying tube fixation device to bridge of nose.

STEP	RATIONALE
b. Apply hypoallergenic tape to nose:	
(1) Optional: Apply tincture of benzoin or other skin adhesive on tip of patient's nose and allow it to become "tacky."	Helps tape adhere better. Protects skin.
(2) Split one end of the prepared tape strip lengthwise 5 cm (2 inches).	
(3) Wrap each of the 5-cm strips in opposite directions around tube as it exits nose (see illustration), taking care that it is not secured against side of naris naris too tightly.	Securing tape to naris can cause tissue damage if taped too tightly.
(4) Optional: Use transparent dressing to secure tube to cheek (see illustration). Be sure skin is clean and non-oily. Apply dressing to cheek, then apply second dressing, overlapping the first to make sure tube is secure.	Securing tube on cheek relieves downward pulling of tube against naris, which increases chance of pressure ulcer.
20. Fasten tube to patient gown (see illustration) using clip or piece of tape. Allow for adequate head movement. Do not use safety pin.	Reduces traction on tube and its securement (McGinnis, 2011). Safety pin can unfasten and injure patient.
21. Keep the head of the bed elevated at least 30 degrees unless contraindicated. For intestinal tube placement, position patient on right side when possible until radiological confirmation of correct placement. Remove gloves and perform hand hygiene.	Promotes patient comfort. Placing patient on the right side promotes passage of tube into the small intestine.

Clinical Decision Point: **Leave guidewire or stylet in place until x-ray verifies tube position. Never try to reinsert a partially or fully removed stylet or guidewire; this could perforate the tube and injure the patient.**

STEP	RATIONALE
22. Obtain x-ray film of abdomen.	X-ray film examination is currently the most accurate method to determine feeding tube placement (Tho et al., 2011).

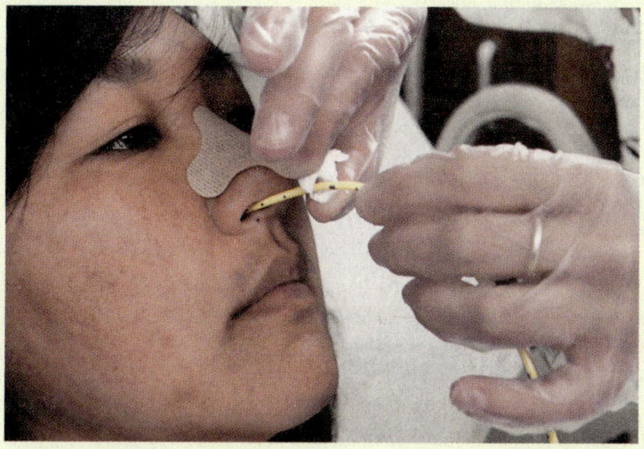

STEP 19a(2) Slip connector around feeding tube.

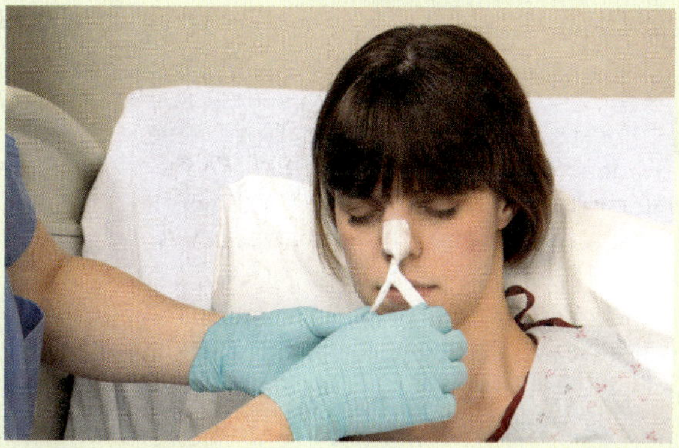

STEP 19b(3) Wrapping tape to anchor nasoenteral tube.

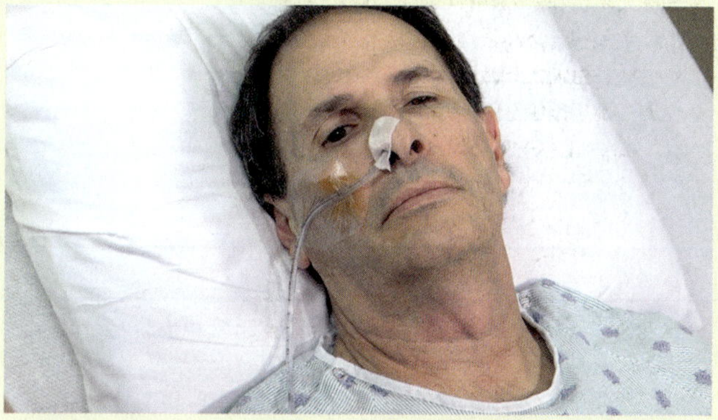

STEP 19b(4) Tube attached with transparent dressing.

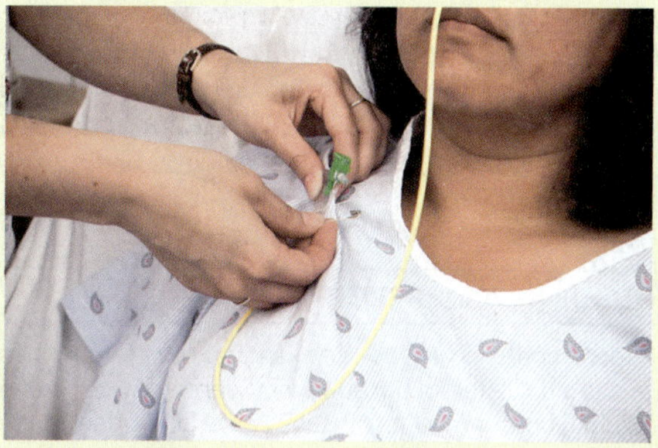

STEP 20 Fastening feeding tube to patient's gown.

SKILL 33-2 INSERTING A NASOGASTRIC OR NASOINTESTINAL FEEDING TUBE—cont'd

STEP	RATIONALE
23. After proper tube position is verified, measure the amount of tube that is external and mark the exit of the tube at the naris with indelible marker as a guide for displacement.	Although the maintenance of the mark at the same location is not absolute confirmation that the tube has not become displaced, it can alert the nurse of displacement when the mark is further out than the area of the naris. Any time the mark is observed to be further external, the placement of the tube must be verified so it is still safe for the prescribed infusion.
24. Apply clean gloves and administer oral hygiene (see Chapter 29). Clean tubing at nostril with washcloth dampened in mild soap and water.	Promotes patient comfort and integrity of oral mucous membranes.
25. Remove gloves, dispose of equipment, and perform hand hygiene.	Reduces transmission of microorganisms.
TUBE REMOVAL	
1. Verify health care provider's order for tube removal.	
2. Identify patient using two identifiers (e.g., name and birthday or name and account number) according to agency policy.	Ensures correct patient. Complies with The Joint Commission requirements for patient safety (TJC, 2014).
3. Gather equipment and explain procedure to patient.	
4. Perform hand hygiene. Apply clean gloves.	Reduces transmission of microorganisms.
5. Position patient in high Fowler's position unless contraindicated.	Reduces risk of pulmonary aspiration in the event patient vomits.
6. Place disposable pad or towel over patient's chest. Disconnect tube from feeding administration set (if present).	Prevents mucus and gastric secretions from soiling patient's clothing. Prevents formula from spilling from tube as it is removed.
7. Remove tape or tube fixation device from patient's nose. Unclip tube from patient's gown.	Allows tube to be removed easily.
8. Instruct patient to take deep breath and hold it.	Prevents inadvertent aspiration of gastric contents while tube is removed.
9. Kink end of tube securely by folding it over on itself. Then completely withdraw tube by pulling it out steadily and smoothly. Dispose in proper receptacle.	Prevents residual leaking of fluid in tube. Minimizes patient discomfort. Prevents transmission of microorganisms.
10. Offer tissues to patient to blow nose. Provide oral hygiene.	Cleans nasal passages of remaining secretions. Promotes patient comfort.
11. Remove gloves and perform hand hygiene.	Reduces transmission of microorganisms.
EVALUATION	
1. Observe patient's response to NG or NI tube intubation. Have patient speak. Monitor vital signs, pulse oximetry, and abdominal status. *Option:* You may use capnography in critical care settings to determine if tip of tube is in trachea or lung.	A patient who is comfortable, is able to speak, and does not exhibit signs of distress is more likely to have a correctly placed tube.
2. Confirm x-ray film results with health care provider.	Verifying proper tube position is essential before instilling anything into the tube such as fluid or enteral feedings.
3. Remove the guidewire or stylet after x-ray film verification of correct placement.	Verifies tube position.
4. Routinely evaluate location of exit site marking on tube and amount of tube external. Monitor color and pH of fluid withdrawn from the NG or NI tube when checking gastric residual volume.	Helps to reveal if end of tube has changed position. However, it is possible that tube changed position inside the GI tract with no external evidence of the change.
5. After tube removal, assess patient's level of comfort.	Ensures continued patient comfort.

RECORDING AND REPORTING

- Record and report type, size, and length of tube placed; location of distal tip of tube when confirmed by x-ray film examination; amount of tube external when properly placed; and patient's tolerance of procedure.
- Record and report any type of unexpected outcome and interventions performed.
- Record removal of tube and patient's tolerance.

UNEXPECTED OUTCOMES AND RELATED INTERVENTIONS

- Tube becomes displaced.
  - Stop any feeding infusion.
  - Aspirate GI contents and measure pH.
  - Remove displaced tube and insert and verify placement of new tube.
  - Assess reason for tube displacement and take appropriate measures to reduce potential displacement when tube is repositioned or reinserted.
  - If there is a question of aspiration, obtain chest x-ray film.
- Patient has aspirated stomach contents into respiratory tract as evidenced by coughing, dyspnea, decrease in oxygen saturation.
  - Position patient on side to facilitate drainage of oral secretions. Encourage patient to cough and expel secretions.
  - Suction patient nasotracheally or orotracheally if patient is unable to cough to try to remove aspirated substance.
  - Auscultate lung status and monitor vital signs to identify changes and serve as guide for further changes.
  - Immediately report change in patient condition to the health care provider; prepare for repeat chest x-ray.
- Patient complains of sore throat from dry, irritated mucous membranes.
  - Perform oral hygiene more frequently.
  - Ask health care provider whether patient can suck on ice chips, throat lozenges, or local anesthetic medication.

SKILL 33-3 ADMINISTERING ENTERAL NUTRITION VIA NASOENTERIC, GASTROSTOMY, OR JEJUNOSTOMY TUBES

DELEGATION CONSIDERATIONS:

The skill of administering enteral nutrition may be delegated to trained nursing assistive personnel (NAP) (check agency policy). However, the nurse must verify tube placement and patency and that the feeding product and fluid (water) to be administered are correct. The nurse must monitor the patient for effectiveness and tolerance of the feeding being delivered. The nurse instructs NAP to:

- Elevate the head of the bed to a minimum of 30 degrees (preferably 45 degrees) or sit patient up in bed or a chair.
- Report any difficulty infusing the feeding or discomfort voiced by patient.
- Report any coughing, choking, discomfort, or vomiting.
- Maintain ordered feeding rate; infuse the feeding as ordered.
- Provide frequent oral hygiene.

EQUIPMENT

- Disposable feeding bag and tubing or ready-to-hang system
- 60-mL Luer-Lok or catheter-tip syringe
- Stethoscope
- pH indicator strip (scale of 1.0 to 11.0)
- Enteral infusion pump (required for continuous or intestinal feedings)
- Prescribed enteral feeding
- Normal saline or tap water
- Clean gloves
- Equipment to obtain blood glucose by fingerstick

STEP	RATIONALE
ASSESSMENT	
1. Assess patient's clinical status to determine need for enteral tube feedings (see Skill 33-2).	Identifies patients who need tube feedings before they become nutritionally depleted.
2. Assess patient for food allergies or intolerances.	Prevents patient from developing localized or systemic allergic responses.
3. Perform physical assessment of abdomen, including auscultation of bowel sounds.	Absent bowel sounds are not a contraindication to feeding, but you need to report a change from baseline in abdominal examination, particularly if tenderness or distention is present, to ordering health care provider to determine if tube feeding can proceed safely (Bankhead et al., 2009; McClave et al., 2009).
4. Obtain baseline weight and review serum electrolytes and blood glucose measurements. Assess patient for fluid volume excess or deficit, electrolyte abnormalities, and metabolic abnormalities such as hyperglycemia.	Provides objective data to measure responses to and effectiveness of feedings.
5. Verify health care provider's order for type of formula, rate, route, and frequency.	Ensures that you administer correct formula in appropriate volume.
6. For feeding tubes placed through the abdominal wall, assess the insertion site for breakdown, irritation, drainage discomfort, or presence of an external disc that it is not excessively snug. Monitor that the amount external remains the same as when it was originally placed.	Infection, pressure from gastrostomy tube, or drainage of gastric secretions cause skin breakdown. A disc that is too snug does not allow adequate circulation and may lead to breakdown at the site. Internal tube migration may block the pylorus and cause patient distress.

SKILL 33-3 ADMINISTERING ENTERAL NUTRITION VIA NASOENTERIC, GASTROSTOMY, OR JEJUNOSTOMY TUBES—cont'd

STEP	RATIONALE
PLANNING	
1. Identify patient using two identifiers (e.g., name and birthday or name and account number) according to agency policy.	Ensures correct patient. Complies with The Joint Commission requirements for patient safety (TJC, 2014).
2. Explain procedure to patient.	Decreases patient anxiety.
IMPLEMENTATION	
1. Perform hand hygiene and apply clean gloves.	Reduces transmission of microorganisms and potential contamination of enteral formula.
2. Obtain formula to administer:	
a. Verify correct formula and check expiration date; note condition of container.	Ensures that you administer correct feeding and checks integrity of formula. Tube feedings administered within the designated shelf life from a container without cracks or breaks reduces patient's risk for obtaining tube feeding–borne GI infections. Prevents leakage of tube feeding.
b. Have tube feeding at room temperature.	Cold formula causes gastric cramping and discomfort because the mouth and esophagus did not warm the liquid.
3. Prepare formula for administration.	
a. Use aseptic technique when handling the feeding system or touching the can tops, container openings, spike, and spike port.	Ensures that feeding system, including the bag, connections, and tubing, is free of contamination to prevent bacterial growth (Bankhead et al., 2009; Lau and Girard, 2011).
b. Shake formula container well (prepackaged or can). Clean top of canned formula with alcohol swab before opening it (Bankhead et al., 2009). For a closed system, connect administration tubing to prepared feeding container. If using an open system, connect administration tubing to feeding container and then pour formula from brick pack or can into administration bag using clean technique (see illustration).	Ensures integrity of formula; prevents transmission of microorganisms.
c. Label bag with feeding formula, patient name, date, time, and initials. Open clamp on tubing and fill tubing with formula to remove air (prime tubing). Clamp off tubing with roller clamp. Hang bag or container on feeding pump pole.	Filling the tubing with formula prevents excess air from entering GI tract once infusion begins.
4. Place patient in high-Fowler's position or elevate head of bed at least 30 degrees (preferably 45 degrees).	Elevated head helps prevent aspiration (AACN, 2012; Metheny and Frantz, 2013).

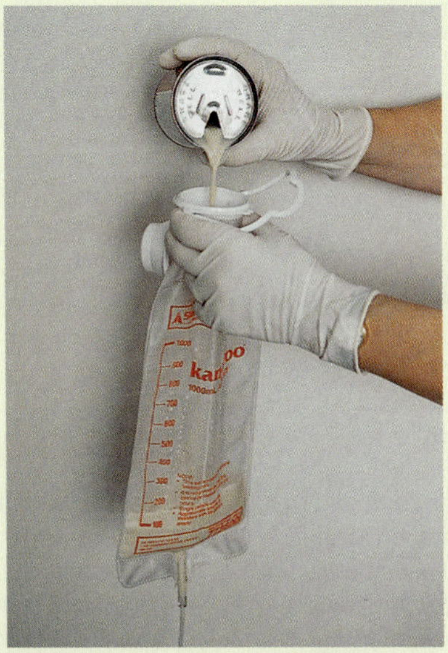

STEP 3b Pour formula into feeding container.

STEP	RATIONALE
5. Verify tube placement.	
a. Nasoenteric tube: See Box 33-10. Attach syringe and aspirate 5 mL of gastric contents. Observe appearance of aspirate and note pH.	Verifies if tip of tube is in stomach or intestine. Feedings instilled into a misplaced tube can cause serious injury or death. Return of fluids prevents fluid and electrolyte imbalance.
b. Gastrostomy tube: Attach syringe and aspirate 5 mL of gastric returns (see Box 33-10); observe appearance and check pH as indicated.	Fluid from gastric tube of patient who has fasted for at least 4 hours usually has a pH of 1.0 to 4.0, especially when patient is not receiving a gastric acid inhibitor. Continuous administration of tube feedings elevates pH (Simmons and Abdallah, 2012).
c. Jejunostomy tube: Aspirate 5 mL of intestinal secretions (see Box 33-10); observe appearance. If significant amounts are returned or resemble gastric returns, check pH.	Presence of intestinal fluid indicates that the end of the tube is in the small intestine (i.e., duodenum or jejunum). If fluid tests acidic on pH test or looks like gastric fluid, displacement of the tube into the stomach may have occurred.
6. Check gastric residual volume (GRV) (see illustration).	
a. Draw up 10 to 30 mL of air into syringe and connect syringe to end of feeding tube. Inject air slowly. Pull back slowly and aspirate the total amount of gastric contents that you can aspirate.	GRV may not be easy to obtain through a small-bore feeing tube. The 60 mL syringe prevents gastric tube collapse (Makic et al., 2011).

Clinical Decision Point: **A number of factors affect measurement accuracy of GRV, including size of gastric tube, position of the tube port in the gastric antrum, patient's position, and whether tube location is near the gastroesophageal junction. Best evidence suggests that a single high GRV should be monitored for the following hour, but enteral feeding should not be stopped or withheld for an isolated GRV (see agency policy) (Makic et al., 2011).**

STEP	RATIONALE
b. Return aspirated contents to stomach unless volume is greater than 250 mL (check agency policy) (Metheny, 2010).	Prevents loss of nutrients and electrolytes in discarded fluid. Some questions exist regarding safety of returning high volumes of fluid into stomach (Metheny, 2010).
c. Do not administer feeding when a single GRV measurement exceeds 500 mL or when two measurements taken 1 hour apart each exceed 250 mL (Bankhead et al., 2009) (check agency policy).	Some controversy exists regarding ability of elevated GRVs to identify risk for pulmonary aspiration. However, frequent interruptions of feeding based on GRV levels is a recognized reason for failure to meet nutritional goals (Bankhead et al., 2009; DeLegge, 2011).

Clinical Decision Point: **Intestinal residual is usually very small, so if residual volume is greater than 10 mL, displacement of tube into stomach may have occurred. Notify health care provider.**

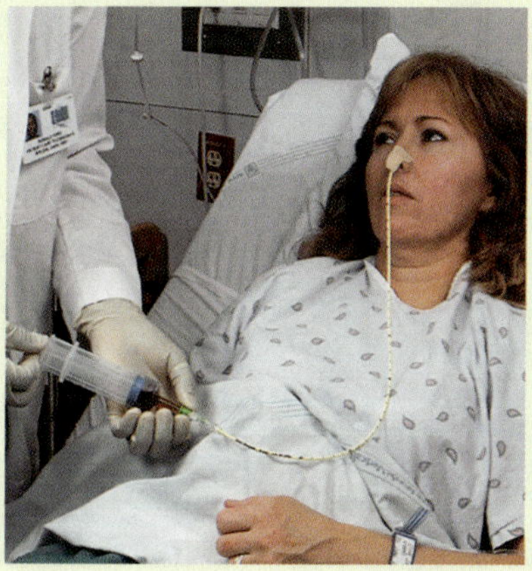

STEP 6 Check for gastric residual (small-bore tube).

SKILL 33-3 ADMINISTERING ENTERAL NUTRITION VIA NASOENTERIC, GASTROSTOMY, OR JEJUNOSTOMY TUBES—cont'd

STEP	RATIONALE
7. Flush feeding tube.	Ensures that tube is clear and decreases risk for occlusion (Bankhead et al., 2009). Irrigation is routinely performed before, between, and after final medication; before each intermittent feeding; and before initial continuous feeding.
a. After measuring GRV, kink feeding tube to prevent leakage of fluid. Draw up 30 mL of water into syringe. Do not use irrigation fluids from bottles that are used on other patients.	Amount of water will flush length of tube. Water is most effective for preventing tube clogging (Bankhead et al., 2009; Dandeles and Lodolce, 2011).
b. Insert tip of syringe into end of feeding tube. Release kink and slowly instill irrigation solution (see illustration).	Irrigation fluid clears tubing.
c. If unable to instill water, reposition patient on left side and try again.	Tip of tube may be against stomach wall.
d. When water has been instilled, remove syringe. Cap tube.	Tubing is clear.
8. Before attaching feeding administration set to feeding tube, trace tube to its point of origin. Label administration set, "Tube Feeding Only."	Avoids misconnections between feeding set and intravenous systems or other medical tubing or devices (Bankhead et al., 2009; Simmons et al., 2011).
9. Initiate an intermittent gravity feeding.	
a. Pinch proximal end of feeding tube and remove cap. Connect distal end of administration set tubing to end of feeding tube. Set rate by adjusting roller clamp on tubing or by placing on a feeding pump.	Reduces air introduced to stomach. Helps ensure food safety.
b. Allow bag to empty gradually over 30 to 45 minutes (see illustration) (the length of time of a comfortable meal). Immediately follow feeding with water (e.g., 1 cup, per orders) to clean bag and feeding tube, prevent feeding tube from clogging, and provide patient with adequate fluid. Cover end of bag with cap. Keep bag as clean as possible. Change bag every 24 hours.	Gradual emptying of tube feeding by gravity reduces risk for abdominal discomfort, vomiting, or diarrhea induced by bolus or too-rapid infusion of tube feedings. It is the patient's meal and should be delivered in the amount of time that a well-tolerated meal is eaten. Helps decrease bacterial growth.
10. Continuous-infusion feeding	
a. Remove cap and connect feeding tube to distal end of administration set tubing.	Reduces air introduced into stomach.

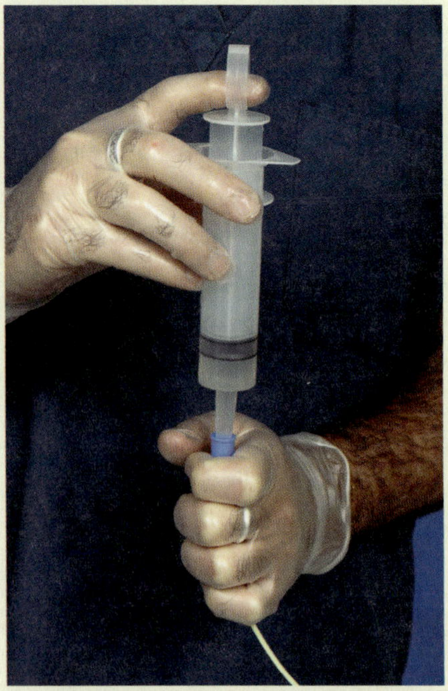

STEP 7b Irrigate feeding tube.

STEP	RATIONALE
b. Thread tubing through infusion pump for enteral feedings, set rate on pump and turn on (see illustration).	Delivers continuous feeding at steady rate and pressure. Alarms sound for increased resistance.

***Clinical Decision Point:* Maximum hang time for formula is 12 hours in an open system and 24 to 48 hours in a closed, ready-to-hang system (if it remains closed). Refer to manufacturer guidelines.**

STEP	RATIONALE
11. Advance rate of tube feeding and concentration of feeding gradually per health care provider orders.	Feedings may be advanced slowly for patients who have not had good nutrition for a period of time or who are at risk for refeeding syndrome or intolerance. Feeding rate advancement should be individualized, based on patient clinical conditions (McClave et al., 2009). Gradual advancement to goal rates also helps to prevent diarrhea intolerance (Bankhead et al, 2009).
12. Flush feeding tube with 30 mL of water every 4 hours during continuous feeding and after an intermittent feeding. Collaborate with registered dietitian and provider regarding recommended total free water requirement per day and obtain health care provider order.	Clears tubing of formula and prevents clogging of tube (Bankhead et al., 2009). Provides patient with source of water to help maintain fluid and electrolyte balance.
13. When patient is receiving intermittent tube feedings, cap or clamp end of feeding tube when not being used.	Prevents air from entering stomach between feedings and limits microbial contamination of system.
14. Rinse bag and tubing with warm water whenever feedings are interrupted. Use a new administration set every 24 hours.	Rinsing bag and tubing with warm water clears old tube feedings and reduces bacterial growth.
15. For abdominally placed tubes, clean the insertion site daily and as needed. A small breathable dressing may be used as a dressing. The site is usually left open to air. It may be helpful to secure the tubing to the patient's abdomen per patient preference.	Decreases risk for infection. Breathable dressing promotes air exchange and reduces moisture at the site. Secures tube and may reduce trauma or potential for tube misplacement.
16. Dispose of supplies and perform hand hygiene.	Reduces transmission of organisms.

EVALUATION

STEP	RATIONALE
1. Measure and assess GRV per agency policy, usually every 4 to 6 hours, and ask if nausea or abdominal cramping is present.	Provides input regarding GI tolerance of tube feeding.
2. Monitor fingerstick blood glucose if indicated (usually at least every 6 hours until maximum administration rate is reached and maintained for 24 hours) per health care provider order.	Like oral intake, may impact glucose level of those who are prone to high blood glucose levels, especially patients with diabetes mellitus.

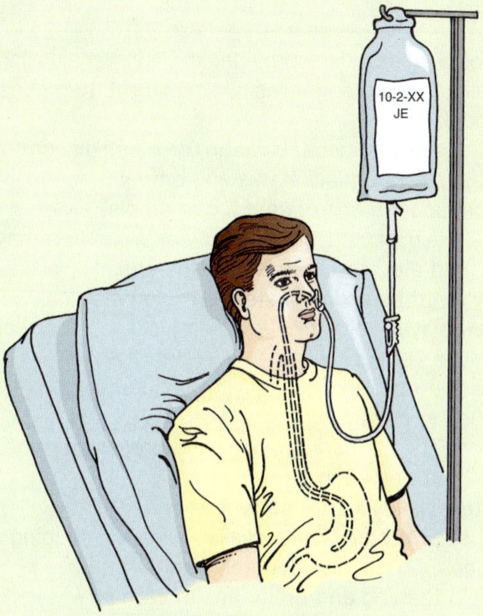

STEP 9b Administer feeding.

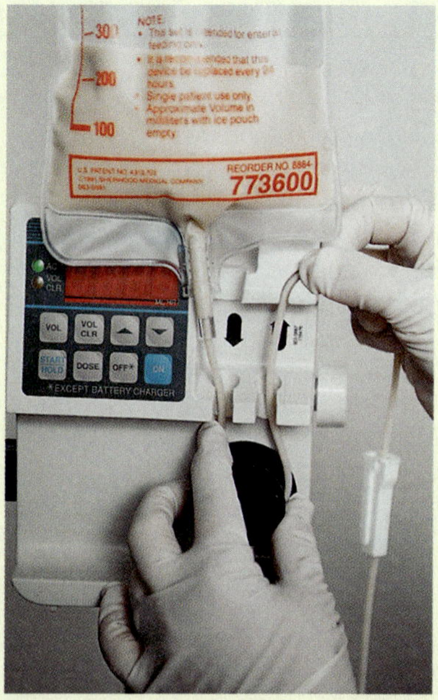

STEP 10b Connect tubing through infusion pump.

SKILL 33-3 ADMINISTERING ENTERAL NUTRITION VIA NASOENTERIC, GASTROSTOMY, OR JEJUNOSTOMY TUBES—cont'd

STEP	RATIONALE
3. Monitor intake and output at least every 8 hours and calculate daily totals.	Intake and output are indications of fluid balance or fluid volume excess or deficit. Excessive stool output may indicate poor nutritional absorption. If there is more output than intake, share with provider because more fluid intake may be needed to prevent dehydration.
4. Weigh patient daily until he or she reaches and maintains maximum administration rate for 24 hours; then weigh patient 3 times per week.	Weight gain is indicator of improved nutritional status; however, sudden gain or loss of more than 2 lbs in 24 hours usually indicates fluid variation.
5. Monitor laboratory values.	Determines correct administration of formula rate and strength and indicates patient's nutritional and hydration status. Imbalances may occur when feeding someone who has had poor nutrition (e.g., refeeding syndrome) (Bankhead et al., 2009).
6. Observe patient's respiratory status.	Change in respiratory status may indicate aspiration of oral secretions or tube feeding.
7. Observe patient's level of comfort.	Reduced gastric emptying leads to abdominal discomfort.
8. Auscultate bowel sounds and monitor abdominal status for distention, firmness, tympany, or general discomfort. Monitor bowel status daily.	Distention, firmness, and tympanic sounds with auscultation may indicate impaired peristalsis (e.g., constipation).
9. Observe nasoenteral tube insertion site for skin integrity. For tubes placed through the abdominal wall, observe insertion site for skin integrity and symptoms of infection, injury, or tightness of the tube, which may lead to tissue damage.	Irritation of tube and presence of gastric or intestinal secretions can lead to skin breakdown. Tightness of the external skin disc can lead to tissue damage and skin injury at the insertion site. Keep site clean and dry.

RECORDING AND REPORTING

- Record amount and type of feeding, method of infusion, patient's response to tube feeding, patency of tube, and condition of skin at tube insertion site.
- Record volume of formula and any additional water in intake and output area of patient's medical record.
- Report to health care provider excess GRV or patient symptoms of GI or respiratory distress.

UNEXPECTED OUTCOMES AND RELATED INTERVENTIONS

- The patient experiences frequent diarrhea (more than three loose stools in 24 hours) after feeding is initiated.
  - Assess consistency and frequency of stool. Initial loose stools may not be unexpected, but ongoing loose stool must be investigated.
  - Notify health care provider because stool cultures for infections such as *Clostridium difficile* or bacterial contamination of feeding might be indicated (McClave et al., 2009).
  - Monitor fluid and electrolyte status.
  - Ensure that administration technique is not contributing to food safety issues.
  - Discuss medications with pharmacist for potential causes of loose stools.
  - Provide perianal skin care.
- Gastric residual exceeds 250 mL or cutoff per agency policy.
  - Reassess residual volume 1 hour after you stop the feeding (check agency policy) to determine if volume has lessened or increased.
  - Notify health care provider if GRV remains high (typically hold feeding if residual >250 mL two consecutive checks).
  - Assess for nausea, bloating, or other discomfort.
  - Assess abdominal status and bowel function, including constipation or frequent loose stools.
  - Maintain patient in semi-Fowler's position; have head of bed elevated at least 30 degrees.
- Patient vomits and aspirates formula when gastric emptying is delayed, or formula is administered too rapidly and produces vomiting.
  - Position patient in side-lying position.
  - Suction airway.
  - Notify health care provider and prepare for chest x-ray.
- Feeding tube becomes clogged.
  - Attempt to flush tube with water.
  - Special products are available for unclogging feeding tubes; do not use soda or cranberry juice.
  - Hold feeding and notify health care provider.
  - Maintain patient in semi-Fowler's or Fowler's position.

KEY POINTS

- Eating a balanced diet of carbohydrates, protein, lipids, vitamins, microminerals, and macrominerals provides the essential nutrients to carry out the normal physiological functioning of the body.
- Ideal body weight is maintained when energy intake as food or fluids equals energy requirements.
- Digestion is the mechanical and chemical process by which food is broken down into its simplest form for absorption. Digestion and absorption occur mainly in the small intestine.
- DRIs, the basis for diet selection, were formulated for population groups, not individuals.
- Guidelines for dietary change advocate reduced intake of fat, saturated fat, salt, refined sugar, and cholesterol and increased intake of complex carbohydrates and fiber.
- Age, developmental stages, and clinical conditions affect the requirements for essential nutrients. Periods of rapid growth increase the need for protein, vitamins, and minerals.
- Because improper nutrition affects all body systems, nutritional assessment includes a review of total physical assessment findings.
- Special hospital diets alter the composition, texture, digestibility, and residue of foods to suit a patient's particular needs.
- EN is for patients who are unable to ingest food safely or adequately but are able to digest and absorb nutrition via the GI tract.
- EN preserves intestinal structure and function and enhances immunity.
- PN supplies essential nutrients in appropriate amounts through a concentrated nutrient solution administered into the superior vena cava and is used when nutrition via the GI tract is not possible or cannot effectively meet patient needs.
- Medical nutrition therapy is a recognized treatment modality for both acute and chronic disease states.

CLINICAL DECISION-MAKING EXERCISES

As Matt initially works with Mrs. Gonzalez, the patient has difficulty asking questions and expressing her concerns. Matt visits with her and her family to help learn what her concerns may be. As a result of his investigation, he recognizes that eating and food preparation have been very important in her life and in her role as mother for her family.

1. What information might Matt provide to help Mrs. Gonzalez know why she is not allowed to eat by mouth at present, why she has a feeding tube, and what she might expect?
2. How can Matt best monitor the adequacy of her feeding and tolerance to her enteral feeding regimen?
3. As Mrs. Gonzalez' ability to swallow improves and she begins to take nutrition by mouth, how can Matt help her improve her oral intake while ensuring the safety and effectiveness of what she is able and willing to eat?

evolve

Answers to Clinical Decision-Making Exercises can be found on the Evolve website.

QSEN ACTIVITY: SAFETY

Matt is currently doing his clinical rotation on a medical nursing unit that cares for many patients with feeding tubes. He observes a nurse on the unit who is not following the agency protocol for checking feeding tube placement.

What should Matt do in this situation?

evolve

Answers to QSEN Activities can be found on the Evolve website.

REVIEW QUESTIONS

1. The nurse is teaching a patient about a healthy diet. Which nutrients would the nurse teach the patient to include?
   1. Protein, carbohydrate, fat, vitamins, and minerals
   2. Protein, carbohydrate, little or no fat, a water-soluble vitamin, and mineral supplements
   3. Protein, carbohydrate, trans fats, vitamins, and minerals
   4. Protein, carbohydrate, saturated fats, a fat-soluble vitamin, and mineral supplements
2. In reviewing a patient's chart, the nurse notes that the patient's serum albumin level is 2.5 g/dL and the BMI is 35. In analyzing the laboratory values, the nurse identifies which problem for the patient?
   1. This patient is underweight.
   2. This patient is malnourished.
   3. This patient needs a nitrogen balance study.
   4. This patient is obese.
3. Which factor related to nutrition does the nurse need to consider when planning care of patients in different age-groups and stages of life?
   1. Pregnant patients have the same nutritional requirements as nonpregnant patients.
   2. Adolescents no longer need calcium for bone growth.
   3. Elderly patients may not need as many calories as younger patients.
   4. Infants should remain on breast milk or formula only for the first year of life.
4. Which information should the nurse teach a patient to prevent foodborne illness? (Select all that apply.)
   1. Refrigerate foods at 40° F within 2 hours of cooking.
   2. Cook meat, poultry, fish, and eggs until well done (180° F).

3. Do not use food past expiration date.
4. Foods may be safely thawed on the kitchen counter overnight.
5. Oak cutting boards provide a solid surface for chopping foods.
6. Wash fresh fruits and vegetables thoroughly.

5. An older-adult patient is admitted with a history of recent weight loss of 20 lbs over the last 6 months. The patient wears dentures, has lactose intolerance, and is allergic to shellfish. Which finding in the medical history indicates the patient is at high risk for poor nutrition?
   1. Shellfish allergy
   2. Lactose intolerance
   3. 20-lb weight loss
   4. Dentures
6. Which interventions by the nurse promote nutrition for a patient whose oral intake is less than required? (Select all that apply.)
   1. Offering antinausea medication after meals
   2. Suggesting substitutions, such as nutritious snacks, to enhance nutritional value
   3. Encouraging frequent small meals
   4. Telling the patient he will need for parenteral nutrition if he doesn't eat better
7. When nutrition support is indicated for your patient, which of the following would be an appropriate factor for the use of parenteral nutrition (PN) instead of enteral tube feeding?
   1. It has less serious complications.
   2. It can be started immediately in an existing intravenous line.
   3. It can be used when the gastrointestinal tract does not function adequately to absorb nutrients.
   4. It should be used when the patient's advanced directive indicates that no aggressive measures such as a feeding tube are to be used.
8. Which measure should the nurse take to ensure safety while the patient is receiving feeding via a nasally placed gastric feeding tube?
   1. Administer medications together to reduce the amount of fluid you need to flush the tube
   2. Ensure that the tube is well secured and that no more tube is external than when the tube was originally placed and determined to be in good position whenever you are with the patient and at least every 4 hours
   3. Listen while a bolus of air is injected to ascertain placement before you administer medication into the tube
   4. Consider that the amount of feeding and fluid that are administered for this patient must be adequate to meet his or her needs because they are the same amounts that you have been using for other patients
9. Which point is important for the nurse to include in the plan of care to monitor the patient's tolerance to enteral tube feeding?
   1. Strict guidelines for residual volumes
   2. Serum albumin level
   3. Lack of feeding tube misplacement
   4. Abdominal assessment and monitoring of bowel status
10. What are the major concerns for the nurse caring for a patient receiving parenteral nutrition (PN)?
   1. Infection and hyperglycemia
   2. Hyponatremia and hypoglycemia
   3. Diarrhea or constipation
   4. Hypoxia and dehydration

evolve

Rationales for Review Questions can be found on the Evolve website.

1. 1; 2. 4; 3. 3; 4. 1, 2, 3, 6; 5. 3; 6. 2, 3; 7. 3; 8. 2; 9. 4; 10. 1

REFERENCES

Academy of Nutrition and Dietetics: *Nutrition care manual*, 2012, http://www.nutritioncaremanual.org. Accessed August 24, 2012.

American Academy of Pediatrics (AAP): Policy statement: breastfeeding and the use of human milk, *Pediatrics* 129(3):496, 2012.

American Association of Critical Care Nurses (AACN): AACN Practice Alerts: Prevention of aspiration, *Crit Care Nurse* 32(3):71, 2012.

American Association of Critical Care Nurses (AACN): *Verification of feeding tube placement (blindly inserted)*, 2009, AACN, http://www.aacn.org/WD/Practice/Docs/PracticeAlerts/Verification_of_Feeding_Tube_Placement_05-2005.pdf. Accessed November 30, 2013.

American Diabetes Association (ADA): Position statement: nutrition recommendations and interventions for diabetes—2008, *Diabetes Care* 31(Suppl 1):2140, 2008.

American Dietetic Association: Position of the American Dietetic Association: integration of medical nutrition therapy and pharmacotherapy, *J Am Diet Assoc* 110(6):950, 2010.

American Heart Association (AHA): *Diet and lifestyle recommendations revision*, 2010, http://www.heart.org/HEARTORG/GettingHealthy/Diet-and-Lifestyle-Recommendations_UCM_305855_Article.jsp. Accessed October 3, 2013.

American Society for Parenteral and Enteral Nutrition (ASPEN) Board of Directors: Guidelines for the use of parenteral and enteral nutrition in adult and pediatric patients, *JPEN J Parenter Enteral Nutr* 33:255, 2009.

Bankhead R, et al: ASPEN Enteral nutrition practice recommendations, *J Parenter Enteral Nutr* 33(2):122, 2009. DOI: 10.1177/0148607108330314.

Bourgault AM, Halm MA: Feeding tube placement in adults: safe verification method for blindly inserted tubes, *Am J Crit Care* 18(1):73, 2009.

Brady A: Managing the patient with dysphagia, *Home Health Nurse* 26(1):41, 2008.

Centers for Disease Control and Prevention (CDC): *Guidelines for the prevention of intravascular catheter-related infections*, 2011, http://www.cdc.gov/hicpac/pdf/guidelines/bsi-guidelines-2011.pdf. Accessed November 12, 2013.

Chang C, Roberts B: Strategies for feeding patients with dementia, *Am J Nurs* 111(4):36, 2011.

Charney P: Nutrition screening vs nutrition assessment: how do they differ? *Nutr Clin Pract* 23(4):366, 2008.

Choban P, et al: ASPEN clinical guidelines: nutrition support of hospitalized adult patients with obesity, *J Parenter Enteral Nutr* published online August 23, 2013. DOI: 10.1177/0148607113499374. Accessed October 11, 2013.

Dandeles LM, Lodolce AE: Efficacy of agents to prevent and treat enteral feeding tube clogs, *Ann Pharmacother* 45:676, 2011.

Davis CJ, et al: The use of prealbumin and C-reactive protein for monitoring nutrition support in adult patients receiving enteral nutrition in an urban medical center, *J Parenter Enteral Nutr* 36:197, 2012.

DeFabrizio M, Rajappa A: Contemporary approach to dysphagia management, *J Nurse Pract* 6(9):625, 2010.

DeLegge DH: Managing gastric residual volumes in the critically ill patient: an update, *Curr Opin Nutr Metab Care* 14:193, 2011.

Ducharme J, Matheson K: What is the best topical anesthetic for nasogastric insertion? A comparison of lidocaine gel, lidocaine spray, and atomized cocaine, *J Emerg Nurs* 29(5):421, 2003.

Edmiaston J, et al: Validation of a dysphagia screening tool in acute stroke patients, *Am J Crit Care* 19(4):357, 2010.

Eisenstadt ES: Dysphagia and aspiration pneumonia in older adults, *J Am Acad Nurse Pract* 22:17, 2010.

Frey K, Ramsberger G: Comparison of outcomes before and after implementation of a water protocol for patients with cerebral vascular accident and dysphagia, *J Neurosci Nurs* 43(3):165, 2011.

Garcia JM, et al: Quality of care issues for dysphagia: modification involving oral fluids, *J Clin Nurs* 19:1618, 2010.

Garon BR, et al: Silent Aspiration: Results of 2000 video fluoroscopic evaluations, *J Neurosci Nurs* 41(4):178, 2009.

Gilbertson HR, Rogers EJ, Ukoumunne OC: Determination of a practical pH cutoff level for reliable confirmation of nasogastric tube placement, *J Parenter Enteral Nutr* 35(4):540, 2011. DOI: 10.1177/0148607110383285.

Grodner M, et al: *Foundations and clinical application of nutrition: a nursing approach*, ed 4, St Louis, 2012, Mosby.

Guenter P, et al: Enteral feeding misconnections: a consortium position statement, *The Joint Commission J Qual Patient Safety* 34(5):285, 2008.

Guenter P, Hicks R, Simmons D: Enteral feeding misconnections: an update, *Nutr Clin Pract* 24(3):325, 2009. DOI: 10.1177/0884533609335174.

Guigoz YB, et al: Assessing the nutritional status of the elderly: the Mini Nutritional Assessment as part of the geriatric evaluation, *Nutr Rev* 54(1 Pt 2):S59, 1996.

Guigoz Y, Vellas B: The Mini Nutritional Assessment (MNA) for grading the nutritional state of elderly patients: presentation of the MNA, history and validation, *Nestle Nutr Workshop Ser Clin Perform Programme* 1:3, 1999.

Han JC, et al: Childhood obesity, *Lancet* 375:1737, 2010.

Hockenberry MJ, Wilson D: *Wong's nursing care of infants and children*, ed 9, St Louis, 2011, Mosby.

Hughes S: Management of dysphagia in stroke patients, *Nurs Older People* 23:3, 2011.

Infusion Nurses Society (INS): Infusion Nursing Standards of Practice, revised 2011, *J Infusion Nurs* 34(1S):S1, 2011.

Institute of Medicine (IOM): *Dietary reference intakes*, 2009, http://fnic.nal.usda.gov/dietary-guidance/dietary-reference-intakes/dri-tables. Accessed August 21, 2012.

Kidd D, et al: Aspiration in acute stroke: a clinical study with videofluoroscopy, *Q J Med* 86:825, 1993.

Kushi LH, et al: American Cancer Society guidelines on nutrition and physical activity for cancer prevention: reducing the risk for cancer with health food choices and physical activity, *CA Cancer J Clin* 67:30, 2012.

Krenitsky J: Blind bedside placement of feeding tubes: treatment or threat? *Pract Gastroenterol* XXXV:32, 2011.

Lau MT, Girard J: Ensuring safer enteral feeding, *Nurs Manage* 42(12):39, 2011.

Leder S, et al: Answering orientation questions and following single-step verbal commands: effect on aspiration status, *Dysphagia* 24:290, 2009.

Makic MBF, et al: Evidence-based practice habits: putting more sacred cows out to pasture, *Crit Care Nurse* 31:38, 2011.

Martino R, et al: The Toronto Bedside Swallowing Screening Test (TOR-BSST): development and validation of a dysphagia screening tool for patients with stroke, *Stroke* 40:555, 2009.

Mahan L, Escott-Stump S, Raymond J: *Krause's Food and nutrition care process*, ed 13, St Louis, 2012, Saunders.

McClave SA, et al: Guidelines for the provision and assessment of nutritional support therapy in the adult critically ill patient: Society of Critical Care Medicine (SCCM) and American Society for Parenteral and Enteral Nutrition (ASPEN), *J Parenter Enteral Nutr* 33(3):277, 2009.

McGinnis C: The feeding tube bridle: one inexpensive, safe, and effective method to prevent inadvertent feeding tube dislodgement, *Nutr Clin Pract* 26(1):70, 2011.

McGinnis CM, Worthington P, Lord LM: Nasogastric versus feeding tubes in critically ill patients, *Crit Care Nurse* 30(6):80, 2010.

Meiner S: *Gerontologic Nursing*, ed 4, St Louis, 2011, Mosby.

Metheny NA: Inconclusive evidence regarding the volume of gastric aspirate that can be safely reintroduced following residual volume measurements, *Evidence-based Nurs* 13:71, 2010.

Metheny NA: Preventing aspiration in older adults with dysphagia, *Med-Surg Matters* 20(5):6, 2011.

Metheny NA, Frantz RA: Head-of-bed elevation in critically ill patients: a review, *Crit Care Nurse* 33(3):53, 2013.

Metheny NA, Davis-Jackson J, Stewart BJ: Effectiveness of an aspiration risk-reduction protocol, *Nurs Res* 59(1):17, 2010. DOI: 1097/NNR.obo13e3181c3ba05.

Millin CJ, Brooks M: Reduce—and report—enteral feeding tube misconnections, *Nursing* 40(11):59, 2010.

Mueller C, et al: ASPEN Clinical Guidelines: Nutrition screening, assessment and intervention in adults, *JPEN J Parenter Enteral Nutr* 35(1):16, 2011.

National Dysphagia Diet Task Force (NDDTF): *National dysphagia diet: standardization for optimal care*, Chicago, 2002, American Dietetic Association.

Ney D, et al: Senescent swallowing: impact, strategies and interventions, *Nutr Clin Pract* 24:395, 2009.

Nix S: *Williams' basic nutrition and diet therapy*, ed 14, St Louis, 2013, Mosby.

Ogden CL, et al: *Prevalence of obesity in the United States, 2009-2010*, NCHS data brief, no 82, Hyattsville, MD, 2012, National Center for Health Statistics.

Pagana KD, Pagana TJ: *Mosby's diagnostic and laboratory test reference*, ed 11, St Louis, 2013, Mosby.

Phillips LD: *Manual of IV therapeutics: evidence-based practice for infusion therapy*, ed 5, Philadelphia, 2010, FA Davis.

Proehl JA, et al: Emergency nursing resource: gastric tube placement verification, *J Emerg Nurs* 37(4):357, 2011.

Remig V, Weeden A: Medical nutrition therapy for neurologic disorders. In Mahan LK, Escott-Stump S, Raymond JL, editors: *Krause's food nutrition and the nutrition care process*, ed 13, Philadelphia, 2012, Saunders.

Roger VL, et al: On behalf of the American Heart Association Statistics Committee and Stroke Statistics Subcommittee. Heart disease and stroke statistics—2012 update: a report from the American Heart Association, *Circulation* 125(1):e2, 2012.

Schlenker ED, Roth SL: *Williams' Essentials of nutrition and diet therapy*, ed 10, St Louis, 2011, Mosby.

Shaw S, Lamdin R: Nurses have an ethical imperative to minimize procedural pain, *Kai Tiaki Nurs N Zealand* 17(7):12, 2011.

Simmons D, et al: Tubing misconnections: normalization of deviance, *Nutr Clin Pract* 26:28, 2011.

Simmons SR, Abdallah LM: 2012 Bedside assessment of enteral tube placement: aligning practice with evidence, *Am J Nurs* 112(2):40, 2012.

Stepter CR: Maintaining placement of temporary enteral feeding tubes in adults: a critical appraisal of the evidence, *MedSurg Nurs* 21(2):61, 2012.

Tanner DC: Lessons from nursing home dysphagia malpractice litigation, *J Gerontol Nurs* 36(3):41, 2010.

The Joint Commission (TJC): *Sentinel practice alert*, Issue 36, April 3, 2006, https://www.premierinc.com/quality-safety/tools-services/safety/topics/tubing-misconnections/downloads/jcaho-sentinel-event-issue-36.pdf. Accessed November 12, 2013.

The Joint Commission (TJC): *National Patient Safety Goals*, Oakbrook Terrace, IL, 2014, The Commission. Available at http://www.jointcommission.org/standards_information/npsgs.aspx.

Tho PC, et al: Implementation of the evidence review on best practice for confirming the correct placement of nasogastric tube in patients in an acute care hospital, *Int J Evid Based Healthc*, 9(1):51-60, 2011.

Ukleja A, et al: Standards for nutrition support: adult hospitalized patients, *Nutr Clin Pract* 25(4):403, 2010.

Uri O, et al: Lidocaine gel as an anesthetic protocol for nasogastric tube insertion in the ED, *Am J Emerg Med* 29:386, 2011.

US Department of Agriculture (USDA): *ChooseMyPlate*, 2013, available at http://www.choosemyplate.gov/ Accessed November 27, 2013.

US Department of Agriculture (USDA) and US Department of Health and Human Services (USDHHS): *Dietary guidelines for Americans*, 2010, Report of Dietary Guidelines Advisory Committee on dietary guidelines for Americans 2010, http://www.cnpp.usda.gov/dietaryguidelines.htm. Accessed August 17, 2012.

US Department of Health and Human Services (USDHHS): *National Institutes of Health National Heart, Lung, and Blood Institute: Your guide to lowering blood pressure with the DASH eating plan*, NIH Publication No. 06-4082, Revised April 2006, http://www.nhlbi.nih.gov/health/public/heart/hbp/dash/new_dash.pdf. Accessed November 30, 2013.

US Department of Health and Human Services (USDHHS): *Healthy people 2020*, 2010, http://www.healthypeople.gov. Accessed September 29, 2013.

Weinhardt J: Accuracy of a bedside dysphagia screening: a comparison of registered nurses and speech therapists, *Rehabil Nurs* 33(6):247, 2008.

White G, et al: Dysphagia: cause, assessment, and management, *Geriatrics* 63(5):15, 2008.

World Health Organization (WHO): *Food security*, 2010. http://www.who.int/trade/glossary/story028/en/. Accessed October 3, 2013.

Yatabe MS, et al: Mini nutritional assessment as a useful method of predicting the development of pressure ulcers in elderly inpatients, *J Am Geriatric Soc* 61:1698, 2013.

CHAPTER

34

Urinary Elimination

evolve WEBSITE

http://evolve.elsevier.com/Potter/essentials

- Crossword Puzzle
- Audio Glossary

OBJECTIVES

- Explain the structures of the urinary system, including function and role in urine formation and elimination.
- Identify factors that commonly influence urinary elimination.
- Discuss common alterations associated with urinary elimination.
- Obtain a nursing history from a patient with an alteration in urination.
- Perform a physical assessment related to urinary elimination.
- Describe characteristics of normal and abnormal urine.
- Describe nursing implications of common diagnostic tests of the urinary system.
- Identify nursing diagnoses associated with alterations in urinary elimination.
- Discuss nursing measures to promote normal urination and control incontinence.
- Discuss nursing measures to reduce urinary tract infections.
- Apply an external catheter and insert a urinary catheter.
- Measure postvoid residual using a bladder scan.

KEY TERMS

bacteremia, p. 953
bacteriuria, p. 953
catheterization, p. 972
cystitis, p. 953
dysuria, p. 953
graduated measuring container, p. 963
hematuria, p. 952
micturition, p. 953
postvoid residual, p. 971
proteinuria, p. 952
pyelonephritis, p. 953
residual urine, p. 971
stoma, p. 954
suprapubic catheter, p. 974
ureterostomy, p. 957
urinal, p. 971
urinary diversion, p. 954
urinary incontinence (UI), p. 953
urinary reflux, p. 952
urinary retention, p. 953
urine hat, p. 963
urometer, p. 963
urosepsis, p. 953
voiding, p. 953

Providing effective nursing care requires you to support patients as they respond to threats to their physical, psychological, spiritual, and emotional health. A basic human function is urinary elimination, a function that can be compromised by a wide variety of illnesses and conditions. It is your role to assess urinary tract function and support bladder emptying. During acute illnesses patients sometimes require urinary catheterization for close monitoring of urine output or to facilitate bladder emptying when bladder function is compromised. Some patients require long-term urethral or suprapubic indwelling catheters when the bladder fails to empty effectively. You also implement measures to minimize risk for infection when bladder function is impaired or urinary drainage tubes are required. Nurses in all health care settings play a key role in teaching patients about bladder health and supporting them to improve or become continent.

CASE STUDY ***Mrs. Vallero***

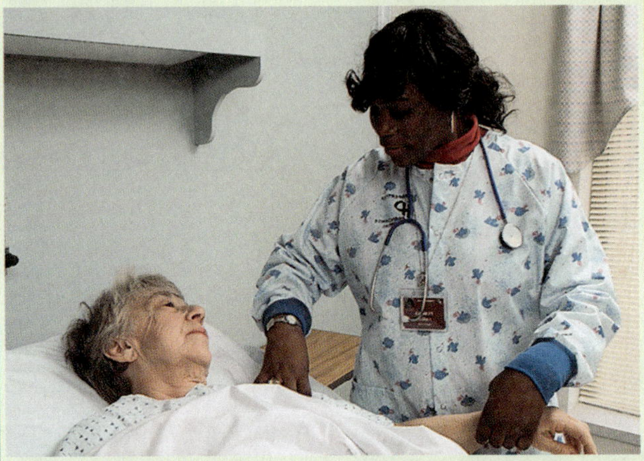

Mrs. Vallero is a 75-year-old woman. She has been hospitalized for 4 days because of heart failure, fluid retention, and poorly controlled diabetes. She has a history of urinary incontinence and repeated episodes of urinary retention related to diabetes neuropathy. At the 3 PM shift report, Sandy, the nursing student, learns that the Mrs. Vallero's indwelling urinary catheter was removed 2 days ago and replaced within 12 hours because of frequent small-volume voiding of less than 100 mL, frequent episodes of small-volume incontinence, lower abdominal pain, and a postvoid residual of 600 mL. A second voiding trial was started this morning, and the patient has had no recorded urine output since 7 AM when the catheter was removed. While making rounds, Sandy talks with Mrs. Vallero, who states that she has only "dribbled" urine and is worried because "I thought this was all under control." Mrs. Vallero's nurse notified the health care provider of current assessment findings. A bladder scan revealed 400 mL of retained urine, and an order was obtained for intermittent catheterization. The registered nurse on the day shift catheterized Mrs. Vallero at 3 PM for 400 mL of pale, clear yellow urine.

SCIENTIFIC KNOWLEDGE BASE

Urinary elimination is the last step in the removal and elimination of excess water and the by-products of body metabolism. Adequate elimination depends on the coordinated function of the ureters, bladder, and urethra (Figure 34-1). The kidneys filter waste products of metabolism from the blood. The ureters transport urine from the kidneys to the bladder. The bladder holds urine until the volume in the bladder triggers a sensation of urge, indicating the need to pass urine. When the brain gives the bladder permission to empty, the bladder contracts, the urinary sphincter relaxes, and urine leaves the body through the urethra.

Anatomy and Physiology of the Urinary Tract

Kidneys. The kidneys lie on either side of the vertebral column behind the abdominal peritoneum and against the deep muscles of the back level with the twelfth thoracic and third lumbar vertebrae. Normally the left kidney is higher than the right because of the anatomical position of the liver.

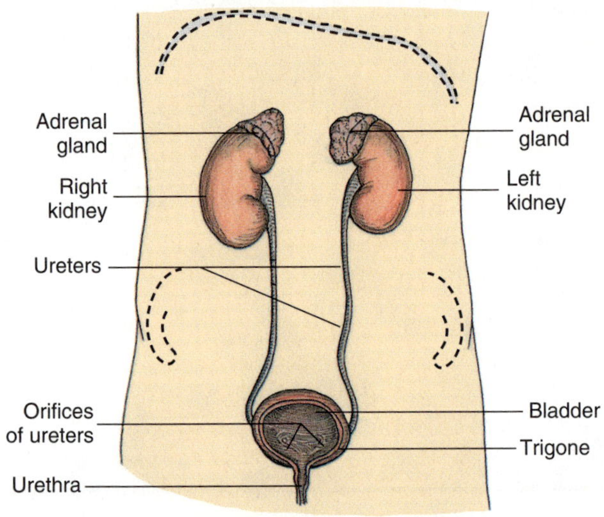

FIGURE 34-1 Organs of the urinary system.

Nephrons, the functional unit of the kidneys, remove waste products from the blood and play a major role in the regulation of fluid and electrolyte balance. Each nephron contains a cluster of capillaries called the *glomerulus*. The glomerulus filters water, glucose, amino acids, urea, uric acid, creatinine, and major electrolytes. Large proteins and blood cells do not normally filter through the glomerulus. Suspect glomerular injury when protein **(proteinuria)** or blood **(hematuria)** is found in the urine.

Not all glomerular filtrate is excreted as urine. Approximate 99% is resorbed into the plasma by the proximal convoluted tubule of the nephron, the loop of Henle, and the distal tubule. The remaining 1% is excreted as urine. The delicate balance of fluid and electrolytes is maintained during the resorption process (Huether and McCance, 2012). The kidneys normally produce 1 to 2 L of urine daily (Huether and McCance, 2012). Many factors influence the production of urine such as fluid intake, physical activity, and body temperature.

Ureters. A ureter is attached to each kidney pelvis and carries urinary wastes to the bladder. Urine draining from the ureters to the bladder is sterile. Peristaltic waves cause the urine to enter the bladder in spurts rather than steadily. Contractions of the bladder during micturition compress the lower portion of the ureters to prevent urine from back flowing into them (Huether and McCance, 2012). Obstruction of urine flow through the ureters such as by a kidney stone can cause a back flow of urine **(urinary reflux)** into the ureters and pelvis of the kidney, causing distention (hydroureter/hydronephrosis), infection from stasis, and in some cases permanent damage to sensitive kidney structures and function.

Bladder. The urinary bladder is a hollow, distensible, muscular organ that holds urine. When empty, the bladder lies in the pelvic cavity behind the symphysis pubis. In the male the bladder rests against the rectum, and in the female it rests against the anterior wall of the uterus and vagina. The bladder expands as it fills with urine. Normally the pressure in the bladder during filling remains low; this prevents the dangerous backward flow of urine into the ureters and kidneys. In a pregnant woman the developing fetus pushes against the bladder, reducing capacity and causing a feeling of fullness.

Urethra. Urine travels from the bladder through the urethra and passes to the outside of the body through the urethral meatus. The urethra passes through a thick layer of skeletal muscles called the *pelvic floor muscles.* These muscles stabilize the urethra and contribute to urinary continence. The external urethral sphincter, composed of striated muscles, contributes to voluntary control over the flow of urine (Huether and McCance, 2012). The female urethra is approximately 3 to 4 cm (1.18 to 1.5 inches) long, and the male urethra is about 18 to 20 cm (7 To 7.8 inches) long (Huether and McCance, 2012). The shorter length of the female urethra increases risk for urinary tract infection (UTI) because of close access to the bacteria-contaminated perineal area.

Act of Urination

Urination, **micturition,** and **voiding** are all terms that describe the process of bladder emptying. Micturition is a complex interaction between the bladder, urinary sphincter, and central nervous system. Several areas in the brain are involved in bladder control: the cerebral cortex, thalamus, hypothalamus, and brainstem. There are two micturition centers in the spinal cord; one coordinates inhibition of bladder contraction, and the other coordinates bladder contractility. As the bladder fills and stretches, bladder contractions are inhibited by sympathetic stimulation from the thoracic micturition center. Normal bladder capacity in adults is approximately 300 to 600 mL. With a strong sensation of urge and when in the appropriate place to void, the central nervous system sends a message to the micturition centers stopping sympathetic stimulation and starting parasympathetic stimulation from the sacral micturition center. The urinary sphincter relaxes, and the bladder contracts. When the time and place are inappropriate, the brain sends messages to the micturition centers to contract the urinary sphincter and relax the bladder muscle.

Factors Influencing Urination

Physiological factors, psychosocial conditions, and diagnostic or treatment-induced factors can all affect normal urinary elimination (Box 34-1). Knowledge of these factors enables you to anticipate possible elimination problems and intervene when they develop.

Common Urinary Elimination Problems

The most common urinary elimination problems involve the inability to store urine or to fully empty urine from the bladder. Problems can result from infection; irritable or overactive bladder; obstruction of urine flow; impaired bladder contractility; or issues that impair innervation to the bladder, resulting in sensory or motor dysfunction.

Urinary Retention. **Urinary retention** is the inability to partially or completely empty the bladder. Acute or rapid-onset urinary retention stretches the bladder, causing feelings of pressure, discomfort/pain, and tenderness over the symphysis pubis; restlessness; and sometimes diaphoresis. Patients often have no urine output over several hours and in some cases experience frequency, urgency, small-volume voiding, or incontinence of small volumes of urine. Chronic urinary retention has a slow, gradual onset during which patients may report decreased voiding volumes, straining to void, frequency, urgency, incontinence, and sensations of incomplete emptying. Complete urinary retention occurs when there is no voiding; during partial retention, the bladder never empties completely. Incontinence caused by urinary retention is called *overflow incontinence.* The pressure in the bladder exceeds the ability of the sphincter to prevent the passage of urine, and the patient dribbles urine (Table 34-1). *In the case study Mrs. Vallero has signs of urinary retention. She has had diabetes mellitus for over 35 years, and it is likely that neuropathy has contributed to the inability of her bladder to empty completely.*

Urinary Tract Infections. UTIs are the most common health care–acquired infections; 80% of these infections result from the use of an indwelling urinary catheter (Lo et al., 2009). *Escherichia coli,* a bacterium commonly found in the colon, is the most common causative pathogen (Gupta et al., 2011). Risk for a UTI increases in the presence of an indwelling catheter, any instrumentation of the urinary tract, urinary retention, urinary and fecal incontinence, and poor perineal hygiene practices.

Bacteriuria (bacteria in the urine) can lead to serious upper UTI (pyelonephritis) and life-threatening bloodstream infection **(bacteremia** or **urosepsis).** Symptoms of a lower UTI (bladder) include burning or pain with urination **(dysuria)** or irritation of the bladder **(cystitis)** characterized by urgency, frequency, incontinence, suprapubic tenderness, and foul-smelling, cloudy urine. Older adults often experience *delirium,* a change in mental status. In some cases there is obvious blood in the urine (hematuria). If infection spreads to the upper urinary tract **(pyelonephritis),** patients frequently experience fever (39°C [102.2°F]), chills, diaphoresis, flank pain, and lower back pain (Gray and Moore, 2009).

Urinary Incontinence. **Urinary incontinence (UI)** is defined by the International Continence Society as the "involuntary loss of urine" (Haylen et al., 2009). The most common forms of UI are urge or urgency UI (strong desire to void associated with involuntary loss of urine) and stress UI (involuntary loss of urine associated with an increase in intraabdominal pressure such as with coughing or exercise). Mixed UI occurs when stress and urgency symptoms are both present. Stress UI results from weakness or injury to the urinary sphincter or pelvic floor muscles. The urethra cannot stay closed because pressure increases in the bladder as a

BOX 34-1 FACTORS INFLUENCING URINARY ELIMINATION

GROWTH AND DEVELOPMENT

- Children cannot voluntarily control voiding until 18 to 24 months of age when myelination is complete.
- Readiness for toilet training includes the ability to recognize the feeling of bladder fullness, hold urine for 1 to 2 hours, and communicate the sense of urgency.
- Older adults may experience a decrease in bladder capacity, increased bladder irritability, and an increased frequency of bladder contractions during bladder filling.
- In older adults the ability to hold urine between the initial desire to void and an urgent need to void decreases.
- Older adults are at increased risk for urinary incontinence as a result of chronic illnesses and factors that interfere with mobility, cognition, and manual dexterity.

SOCIOCULTURAL FACTORS

- Cultural and gender norms vary. North Americans expect toilet facilities to be private, whereas some cultures accept communal toilet facilities.
- Religious or cultural norms may dictate who is acceptable to assist in elimination practices.
- Social expectations (e.g., school recesses, work breaks) can interfere with timely voiding.

PSYCHOLOGICAL FACTORS

- Anxiety and stress sometimes affect a sense of urgency and increase frequency of voiding.
- Anxiety can impact bladder emptying because of inadequate relaxation of the pelvic floor muscles and urinary sphincter.
- Depression can decrease the desire for urinary continence.

PERSONAL HABITS

- The need for privacy and adequate time to void can influence the ability to adequately empty the bladder.

FLUID INTAKE

- If fluids, electrolytes, and solutes are balanced, increased fluid intake increases urine production.
- Alcohol decreases the release of antidiuretic hormones, thus increasing urine production.
- Fluids containing caffeine and other bladder irritants can prompt unsolicited bladder contractions, resulting in frequency, urgency, and incontinence.

PATHOLOGICAL CONDITIONS

- Diabetes mellitus, multiple sclerosis, and stroke can alter bladder contractility and the ability to sense bladder filling. Patients experience either bladder overactivity or deficient bladder emptying.
- Arthritis, Parkinson's disease, dementia, and chronic pain syndromes can interfere with timely access to a toilet.
- Spinal cord injury or intervertebral disk disease (above S-1) can cause the loss of urine control because of bladder overactivity and impaired coordination between the contracting bladder and urinary sphincter.
- Prostatic enlargement (e.g., benign prostatic hyperplasia [BPH]) can cause obstruction of the bladder outlet, which results in urinary retention.

SURGICAL PROCEDURES

- Local trauma during lower abdominal and pelvic surgery sometimes obstructs urine flow, requiring temporary use of an indwelling urinary catheter.
- Anesthetic agents and other agents given during surgery can decrease bladder contractility and/or sensation of bladder fullness, causing urinary retention (Elsamara and Ellsworth, 2012).

MEDICATIONS

- Diuretics increase urinary output by preventing resorption of water and certain electrolytes.
- Some drugs change the color of urine (e.g., phenazopyridine—orange, riboflavin—intense yellow).
- Aniticholinergics (e.g., atropine, overactive bladder [OAB] agents) may increase the risk for urinary retention by inhibiting bladder contractility (Lehne, 2010).
- Hypnotics and sedatives (e.g., analgesics, antianxiety agents) may reduce the ability to recognize and act on the urge to void.

DIAGNOSTIC EXAMINATIONS

- Cystoscopy may cause localized trauma of the urethra, resulting in transient (1-2 days) dysuria and hematuria.
- Whenever the sterile urinary tract is catheterized, there is a risk for infection.

result of increased abdominal pressure. Urgency UI is caused by involuntary contractions of the bladder that cause leakage of urine. Overflow UI is associated with acute or chronic urinary retention. Functional UI is caused by factors that prohibit or interfere with a patient's access to the toilet or other acceptable receptacle for urine. It is a significant problem for older adults who experience problems with mobility or the dexterity to manage their clothing and toileting behaviors. Functional UI may also be caused by poor motivation for continence as seen in severe depression or by cognitive decline that has impaired the ability to sense and act on the urge to void in an appropriate manner. Functional UI can be associated with underlying stress, urge, or mixed UI. In many cases functional incontinence is the direct result of caregivers not responding in a timely manner to requests for help with toileting. See Table 34-1 for a summary of the types, characteristics, and selected nursing interventions for UI.

Urinary Diversions. Patients who have their bladder removed (cystectomy) because of cancer or significant bladder dysfunction (e.g., related to radiation injury or neurogenic dysfunction with frequent UTI) require surgical procedures that divert urine to the outside of the body through an opening in the abdominal wall called a **stoma. Urinary**

TABLE 34-1 TYPES OF URINARY INCONTINENCE

DEFINITION	CHARACTERISTICS	SELECTED NURSING INTERVENTIONS
Transient Incontinence		
Incontinence caused by medical conditions that in many cases are treatable and reversible	Common reversible causes include: • Delirium and/or acute confusion • Inflammation (e.g., urinary tract infection [UTI], urethritis) • Medications (diuretics) (Hall et al., 2012) • Excessive urine output (e.g., hyperglycemia, congestive heart failure) • Mobility impairment from any cause • Fecal impaction • Depression • Acute urinary retention	With new-onset or increased incontinence look for reversible causes. Notify health care provider of any suspected reversible causes.
Functional Incontinence		
Loss of continence from causes outside the urinary tract; usually related to functional deficits such as altered mobility and manual dexterity, cognitive impairment, or environmental barriers	Toilet access restricted by: • Sensory impairments (e.g., vision) • Cognitive impairments (e.g., delirium, dementia, severe retardation) • Altered mobility (e.g., hip fracture, arthritis, chronic pain, spastic paralysis associated with multiple sclerosis; slow movements associated with Parkinson's disease, hemiparesis) • Altered manual dexterity (e.g., arthritis, upper-extremity fracture) • Environmental barriers (e.g., caregiver not available to help with transfers, pathway to bathroom not maneuverable with walker, tight clothing that is difficult to remove, incontinence briefs)	Ensure adequate lighting in bathroom. Provide individualized toileting program designed for degree of cognitive impairment: habit training program, scheduled toileting program, prompted voiding program. Provide mobility aids (e.g., raised toilet seats, toilet grab bars). Clear toilet area to allow access for a walker or wheelchair. Suggest use of elastic waist pants without buttons or zippers. Stress that call bell always be within reach. Use incontinence containment product that patient can easily remove such as a pull-up type pant or a pad that can be moved aside easily for voiding.
Overflow Urinary Incontinence		
Involuntary loss of urine caused by an overdistended bladder; often related to bladder outlet obstruction or poor bladder emptying caused by weak or absent bladder contractions	• Distended bladder on palpation • High postvoid residual • Frequency • involuntary leakage of small volumes of urine • Nocturia	Interventions are individualized related to the severity of the urinary retention, ability of bladder to contract, and kidney damage. **Mild retention with some bladder function** • Timed voiding • Double voiding • Monitor postvoid residual per health care provider's direction • Intermittent catheterization **Severe retention, no bladder function** • Intermittent catheterization • Indwelling catheterization
Stress Urinary Incontinence		
Involuntary leakage of small volumes of urine associated with increased intraabdominal pressure related to either urethral hypermobility or an incompetent urinary sphincter (e.g., weak pelvic floor muscles, trauma after childbirth, radical prostatectomy)	• Small volume loss of urine with coughing, laughing, exercise, walking, getting up from a chair • Usually does not leak urine at night when sleeping	As directed by health care provider, instruct patient in pelvic muscle exercises (Kegel).

Continued

TABLE 34-1 TYPES OF URINARY INCONTINENCE—cont'd

DEFINITION	CHARACTERISTICS	SELECTED NURSING INTERVENTIONS
Urge Urinary Incontinence		
Involuntary passage of urine often associated with strong sense of urgency related to overactive bladder (involuntary bladder contractions) caused by neurological problems, bladder inflammation, or bladder outlet obstruction	May experience one or all of the following symptoms: • Urgency • Frequency • Nocturia • Difficulty or unable to hold urine once urge to void occurs • Leaks on way to bathroom • Leaks larger volumes of urine, sometimes enough to wet outer clothing • Dribbling small amounts on way to bathroom • Strong urge/leaks when hears water running, washes hands, drinks fluids	Ask patient about symptoms of a UTI. Avoid bladder irritants (e.g., caffeine, artificial sweeteners, alcohol). As directed by health care provider, instruct patient in pelvic muscle exercises. As directed by health care provider, instruct patient in urge inhibition exercises. As directed by health care provider, instruct patient in bladder training. If ordered by health care provider, monitor patient symptoms and for presence of side effects of antimuscarinic medications.
Reflex Urinary Incontinence		
Involuntary loss of urine occurring at somewhat predictable intervals when patient reaches specific bladder volume related to spinal cord damage between C1 to S2.	• Diminished or absent awareness of bladder filling and urge to void • Leakage of urine without awareness • May not completely empty bladder because of dyssynergia of the urinary sphincter (i.e., inappropriate contraction of the sphincter when the bladder contracts, causing obstruction to urine flow) • **CAUTION:** Patients with reflex incontinence are at risk for developing autonomic dysreflexia, a life-threatening condition that causes severe elevation of blood pressure and pulse rate and diaphoresis.	Follow prescribed schedule for emptying the bladder either through voiding or by intermittent catheterization. Use urine containment products: condom catheter, undergarments, pads, briefs. Monitor for signs and symptoms of urinary retention and UTI. Monitor for autonomic dysreflexia; this is a medical emergency requiring immediate intervention. Notify health care provider immediately.

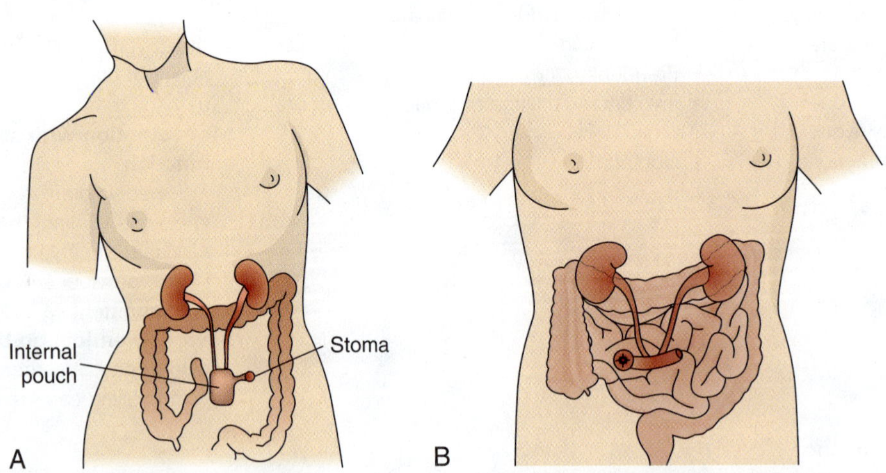

FIGURE 34-2 Types of incontinent and continent urinary diversions. **A,** Continent urinary reservoir. **B,** Urostomy (ileal conduit).

diversions are constructed from a section of intestine to create a storage reservoir or conduit for urine. Diversions are temporary or permanent, continent or incontinent.

There are two types of continent urinary diversions. The continent urinary reservoir (Figure 34-2, *A*) is created from a distal portion of the ileum and proximal portion of the colon. The ureters are embedded in the reservoir, which is placed under the abdominal wall. A narrow ileal segment is brought out through the abdominal wall to form a small stoma. The ileocecal valve creates a one-way valve in the pouch. A catheter is inserted through the stoma to empty urine from the pouch. Patients need to catheterize the pouch 4 to 6 times a day for the rest of their lives.

The other type of continent urinary diversion, an orthotopic neobladder, uses an ileal pouch to replace the bladder. Anatomically the pouch is in the same position as the bladder was before removal, allowing a patient to void through the urethra using the Valsalva technique.

An ileal conduit or ureterostomy is a permanent incontinent urinary diversion created by transplanting the ureters into a closed-off portion of the intestinal ileum. The other end of the ureters come out onto the abdominal wall, forming a stoma (Figure 34-2, *B*). Patients have no sensation or control over the continuous flow of urine through the ileal conduit, requiring the effluent (drainage) to be collected in a pouch.

Nephrostomy tubes are small tubes tunneled through the skin into the renal pelvis. These tubes are placed to drain the renal pelvis when the ureter is obstructed. Patients go home with these tubes and need careful teaching about site care and signs of infection.

NURSING KNOWLEDGE BASE

Urinary elimination is a basic body function that includes a variety of psychological and physiological needs. Physiological and psychosocial nursing care is essential when illness or disability interferes with meeting these needs. Patient-centered care requires an understanding beyond anatomy and physiology of the urinary system.

Infection Control and Hygiene

The urinary tract is sterile. Use infection control principles to help prevent the development and spread of UTIs. You need to follow the principles of asepsis when carrying out procedures involving the urinary tract or external genitalia. Perineal hygiene is an essential component of care (see Chapter 29) when there is an alteration in the usual pattern of urinary elimination.

Developmental Considerations

A patient's ability to control micturition changes during the life span. The neurological system is not well developed until 2 or 3 years of age. Until this time the small child is not able to associate sensation of filling and urge with urination. When the child recognizes feelings of urge, can hold urine for 1 or 2 hours, and is able to communicate a need to eliminate, toilet training becomes successful. Continence starts during daytime hours. Children who wet the bed at night without awakening from sleep have what is called *nocturnal enuresis.* In some cases they experience this nighttime incontinence until late in childhood.

Pregnancy causes many changes in the body, including the urinary tract. In early and late pregnancy urinary frequency is common. Hormonal changes and the pressure of the growing fetus on the bladder cause increased urine production and shrinking bladder capacity.

BOX 34-2 PATIENT-CENTERED CARE

Urinary elimination is a private human activity. You need to incorporate sensitivity and awareness of factors that affect care when caring for patients from divergent cultures and religions who have urinary elimination problems. Variations within a cultural group are common; thus you assess and care for each patient individually. Many cultures have specific beliefs and practices related to elimination, privacy, and gender-specific care.

IMPLICATIONS FOR NURSING PRACTICE

- Whenever possible, provide for a same-gender caregiver for cultures that emphasize female modesty and ban nonrelated males and females from touching such as Iranian, Jewish Orthodox, Korean, Hindu, and Vietnamese (Beji et al., 2010; Purnell, 2009).
- Privacy is important in many cultures; thus pay careful attention to closing doors, bedside curtains, and draping.
- Be certain that patients understand instructions and patient education when English is not their primary language (see Chapter 11). Provide a professional interpreter as needed.
- Certain cultures such as Hindus and Muslims observe meticulous hygiene practices that designate the left hand to perform unclean procedures such as genitourinary hygiene. Perform hand hygiene before touching the patient and use your right hand when possible. Use the left hand to handle the urinal and/or secretions.
- Some cultures continue to practice female genital circumcision, which often includes removal of all or part of the clitoris, partial or complete removal of the labia minora, or total removal of the clitoris and labia minora and sewing together the labia majora, leaving only a small opening for urine and menses (AAP, 2010).

Psychosocial Implications

Self-concept, culture, and sexuality are all closely related concepts that are affected when a patient has elimination problems. Self-concept changes over one's life span and includes body image, self-esteem, roles, and identity (see Chapter 23). Sometimes children resist urinating on the toilet and associate their urine and feces as extensions of self, thus not wanting to flush them away. The process of micturition is often a private event and requires you to be sensitive to a need for privacy. Incontinence is frequently devastating to self-image and self-esteem. When your patient asks for help for such a private and personal activity, it can be perceived as embarrassing or being treated like a child, or it may threaten the patient's sense of self-determination. Culture often dictates gender-specific roles when it comes to care of elimination issues. It may be inappropriate for a male to touch or even talk about elimination matters with a woman (Box 34-2).

CRITICAL THINKING

Synthesis

You will apply elements of critical thinking whenever you perform the nursing process with patients. Consider

BOX 34-3 SYNTHESIS IN PRACTICE

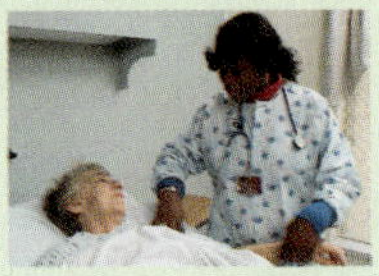

As Sandy prepares to assess Mrs. Vallero, she remembers that urinary problems are common in older adults who have diabetes. Advanced age does not cause incontinence. She recalls that patients with urinary retention sometimes leak or "dribble" urine and are inaccurately diagnosed as incontinent. She knows that patients generally void at least every 6 hours and that Mrs. Vallero's recent catheterization, her decreased mobility, and history of diabetes increase her risk for urinary retention, incontinence of small amounts of urine, and urinary tract infection. In addition, she knows that she needs to assess if Mrs. Vallero feels the urge to urinate. She determines that no one has taken Mrs. Vallero to the bathroom recently. Sandy also needs to find out more about her patient's urination patterns at home because Mrs. Vallero has verbalized anxiety about her present voiding patterns.

Through previous clinical experiences, Sandy learned that palpation of the abdomen over a distended bladder causes some discomfort, often creating an urge to urinate. Mrs. Vallero says she has a little *dolor* (pain) and grimaces slightly when Sandy palpates her abdomen.

the scientific knowledge you have learned, your experience, critical thinking attitudes, and standards to ensure an individualized approach to patient care. Successful critical thinking requires synthesis of knowledge, experience, attitudes, and professional standards. To make an appropriate nursing diagnosis and develop an individualized plan of care, all elements need to be integrated (Box 34-3).

Knowledge. During your patient's assessment, take into consideration your knowledge about the urinary system. Integrate knowledge from nursing and other disciplines. Many factors affect the urinary tract. For example, older adults often experience a change in mental status in response to UTIs; men experience stress UI caused by damage to the urinary sphincter after surgery for prostate cancer; and caffeine intake and the use of a diuretic frequently increases urinary urgency and frequency. Patients who are normally continent sometimes become incontinent after developing impaired mobility.

Experience. Urinary elimination problems are common in all health care settings. Reflect on previous and personal experiences to help you determine a patient's elimination needs. Perhaps you cared for an incontinent patient who develops a skin rash secondary to incontinence. Reflection on past experiences prompts you to start using a moisture barrier ointment as a preventive and protective skin care measure. Your experience with a UTI helps you understand a patient's frustration and embarrassment caused by frequency, urgency, and dysuria. Caring for other older adults with a functional disability helps you anticipate patient needs related to toileting.

Attitudes. Application of critical thinking attitudes is an important component of caring for a patient with urinary elimination problems. Approach patients with a confident attitude but at the same time remain open to the opinions of other clinicians. A disciplined approach to infection control principles when performing urinary catheterization decreases a patient's risk for catheter-associated UTI (CAUTI). When assessing the needs of older adults with incontinence, persevere in getting the whole story, especially their continence status before acute care admission. It makes a significant difference when designing an appropriate plan of care.

Standards. When you care for a patient with an alteration in urinary elimination, it is important to apply standards of critical thinking. When assessing and planning care for a patient with incontinence, it is important to identify patient needs accurately, determine that the interventions are relevant to identified needs, and ensure that the plan of care is broad enough to capture the whole problem. It is appropriate to administer an antibiotic for a UTI, knowing that the UTI has aggravated the incontinence; but the plan would not be complete without addressing problems with toilet access and patient teaching about UTI prevention. Use standards of care such as the *HICPAC Guideline for the Prevention of Catheter-Associated Urinary Tract Infections* (http://www.cdc.gov/hicpac/pdf/cauti/cautiguideline2009final.pdf) or those developed by the Wound, Ostomy, Continence Nurses Society (www.wocn.org) related to the care of incontinence-related skin problems, ostomies, and incontinence.

NURSING PROCESS

ASSESSMENT

When completing a patient assessment, thoroughly assess all aspects of the patient and critically analyze findings to ensure patient-centered diagnosis and care. To identify urinary elimination problems, use your scientific and nursing knowledge, conduct a nursing history of the patient's problem, perform a physical examination, assess the patient's urine, and review information from diagnostic tests and examinations.

Nursing History. The nursing history includes a review of the patient's elimination patterns, symptoms of urinary alterations, and assessment of factors affecting normal urination.

Pattern of Urination. Ask a patient about daily voiding patterns, including frequency and times of day, normal volume at each voiding, and history of recent changes. Frequency of voiding varies among individuals, depending on fluid intake, medications such as diuretics, and the use of bladder irritants such as caffeine. Be sure to ask if the patient is awakened from sleep with an urge to void and how many times this occurs. It is normal for patients who awaken at night because of noise, pain, or nighttime treatments to experience an urge to void. Information about the pattern of urination is necessary to establish a baseline for comparison.

Symptoms of Urinary Alterations. Assessment of symptoms specific to urinary alterations is an essential part of the nursing history. During assessment ask the patient about the presence of symptoms listed in Table 34-2. Also determine whether the patient is aware of conditions or factors that precipitate or aggravate the symptoms.

Factors Affecting Voiding. Focused assessment enables you to gather data relevant to your patient's elimination pattern and identify factors that impact the ability to void normally (Table 34-3). Throughout your nursing assessment it is important to consider a patient's frame of reference related to any illness or urinary problem. Assess the patient's understanding of urinary problems, expectations of what you will do, and what the patient can do independently. Do not assume that, because a patient has a diagnosis of cognitive impairment, the individual cannot understand or participate in care. Be aware of cultural differences related to the very private act of urination and how it affects nursing assessment and care.

Because urination is often considered a private matter, some patients find it difficult to talk about their voiding habits. Approach patients in a professional manner and assure them that you will maintain their confidentiality. Some postoperative patients or patients receiving medications that affect bladder function become concerned that something is wrong when you assess voiding amount and frequency every 2 hours. Patients receiving intravenous (IV) fluids do not always realize that they have an increased need for urination. Sensitivity to patient misconceptions quickly identifies areas for patient education.

Older Adult Considerations. Normal aging causes changes in the urinary tract and the rest of the body that increase the risk for bladder dysfunction (see Box 34-1; Box 34-4). Prostatic enlargement in older men causes obstruction of urine flow from the bladder, resulting in incomplete bladder emptying, urgency, frequency, UTIs, and damage to the upper urinary tract from urinary retention. Patterns of urine production often change as a result of a shift in circadian rhythm of water secretion. Some older adults produce more than 50% of their urine at night, causing nocturia (Newman and Wein, 2009). Other changes in the urinary tract that have the potential to cause problems with elimination include a decreased ability to delay voiding, increased incidence of overactive bladder, a loss of bladder contractility increasing the risk for urinary retention, and a decrease in estrogenization of perineal tissue in women that increases the risk of UTI (Newman and Wein, 2009).

Physical Assessment. A physical assessment provides you with data to best determine patient needs. Assessment of the urinary system helps you identify signs and severity of urinary problems and monitor responses to medical and nursing interventions. The primary areas to assess include the kidneys, bladder, external genitalia, urethral meatus, and perineal skin (see Chapter 16).

BOX 34-4 CARE OF THE OLDER ADULT

Bladder Dysfunction

- The prevalence of overactive bladder (OAB) (urgency, urge incontinence, frequency, and nocturia) increases with age (Harris and Smith, 2010).
- The risk for urinary incontinence increases in patients with cognitive impairment, mobility limitations, and chronic illnesses (stroke, diabetes, degenerative joint, Parkinson's disease, heart failure, dementia) (Gomelsky and Dmochowski, 2011; Lee et al., 2009).
- Nocturia increases with aging, increasing the risk for disturbed sleep patterns and falls (Gomelsky and Dmochowski, 2011).
- Evaluate all possible causes of new-onset incontinence, which includes taking medications that affect cognition, alertness, mobility, or voiding. Older adults tend to take more medications; some (e.g., antihypertensives, cholinesterase inhibitors, antidepressants, sedatives) limit the bladder's ability to hold urine or empty adequately (Hagglund, 2009; Lee et al., 2009).
- Carefully assess older adults taking an antimuscarinic medication to treat urgency, urge incontinence, and OAB for mental status changes. Side effects of these medications include cognitive impairment in older adults (Wagg et al., 2010).
- Implement plans to maximize self-care and continence (e.g., toileting program, mobility aides, assistance with hygiene) when caring for older adults with impaired mobility and incontinence.
- Teach older women with stress incontinence about pelvic muscle exercises. There is no age limit on their effectiveness.
- The sensation of thirst decreases with aging. Remind older adults to drink adequate amounts of water (Touhy and Jett, 2010).

Kidneys. When the kidneys become infected or inflamed, they become tender, and flank pain usually develops. You assess for tenderness by gently percussing the costovertebral angle (the angle formed by the spine and twelfth rib).

Bladder. In adults the bladder rests below the symphysis pubis. When distended with urine, it rises above the symphysis pubis along the midline of the abdomen. A very full bladder extends to the umbilicus. On inspection you may observe a swelling or convex curvature of the lower abdomen. On gentle palpation of the lower abdomen, a full bladder is palpated as smooth and rounded. When a full bladder is palpated, patients report a sensation of urinary urge tenderness or even pain. Use percussion to identify a full bladder. Gently tap the abdomen along the midline starting just above the umbilicus. You identify the edge of the bladder by percussion sounds that change to a dull note. If you suspect an overfull bladder, further assess the patient with a bladder scanner, a portable ultrasound that measures the volume of urine in the bladder. Using a bladder scanner minimizes

TABLE 34-2 COMMON SYMPTOMS OF URINARY ALTERATIONS

DESCRIPTION	COMMON CAUSES
Urgency	
An immediate and strong desire to void that is not easily deferred	Full bladder Urinary tract infection Inflammation or irritation of the bladder Overactive bladder
Dysuria	
Pain or discomfort associated with voiding	Urinary tract infection Inflammation of the prostate Urethritis Trauma to the lower urinary tract Urinary tract tumors
Frequency	
Voiding more than 8 times during waking hours and/or at decreased intervals such as less than every 2 hours	High volumes of fluid intake Bladder irritants (e.g., caffeine) Urinary tract infection Increased pressure on bladder (e.g., pregnancy) Bladder outlet obstruction (e.g., prostate enlargement, pelvic organ prolapse) Overactive bladder Uncontrolled diabetes mellitus or diabetes insipidus
Hesitancy	
Delay in the start of the urinary stream when voiding	Anxiety (e.g., voiding in public restroom) Bladder outlet obstruction (e.g., prostate enlargement, urethral stricture)
Polyuria	
Voiding excessive amounts of urine	High volumes of fluid intake Uncontrolled diabetes mellitus Diabetes insipidus Diuretic therapy
Oliguria	
Diminished urinary output in relation to fluid intake	Fluid and electrolyte imbalance (e.g., dehydration) Kidney dysfunction or failure Increased secretion of antidiuretic hormone (ADH) Urinary tract obstruction
Nocturia	
Awakened from sleep by the urge to void	Excessive intake of fluids (especially coffee or alcohol before bedtime) Bladder outlet obstruction (e.g., prostate enlargement) Overactive bladder Medications (e.g., diuretic taken in the evening) Cardiovascular disease (e.g., hypertension) Urinary tract infection
Dribbling	
Leakage of small amounts of urine despite voluntary control of micturition	Bladder outlet obstruction (e.g., prostatic enlargement) Incomplete bladder emptying Stress incontinence
Hematuria	
Presence of blood in urine Gross hematuria—blood easily seen in the urine Microscopic hematuria—blood not visualized but measured on urinalysis	Tumors (e.g., kidney, bladder) Infection (e.g., glomerular nephritis, cystitis) Urinary tract calculi Trauma to urinary tract
Retention	
Acute retention: Suddenly unable to void when bladder is adequately full or overfull Chronic retention: Bladder does not empty completely during voiding, and urine retained in bladder	Bladder outlet obstruction (e.g., prostatic enlargement, urethral obstruction) Absent or weak bladder contractility (e.g., neurological dysfunction such as caused by diabetes, multiple sclerosis, lower spinal cord injury) Side effects of certain medications (e.g., anesthesia, anticholinergics, antispasmodics, antidepressants)

TABLE 34-3 FOCUSED PATIENT ASSESSMENT

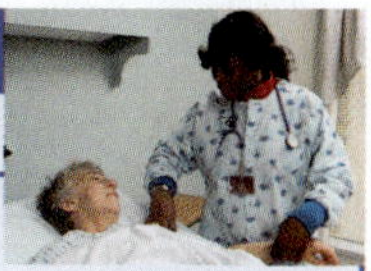

FACTORS TO ASSESS	QUESTIONS	PHYSICAL ASSESSMENT
Fluid intake	Do you have any fluid restrictions? How much do your normally drink in 24 hours? Are you decreasing your fluid intake because you need to use the toilet too often? How often do you drink beverages that contain caffeine? (e.g., coffee, tea, alcohol, soft drinks)	Observe skin and mucous membranes for adequate hydration. Obtain intake and output over 24 hours.
Urinary symptoms	Are you experiencing a sudden urge to urinate, burning or painful urination, frequent urination, difficulty urinating, excessive urination, the need to urinate at night, dribbling or blood in the urine, straining when you urinate, leaking urine on the way to the bathroom, or leaking urine when you cough or sneeze (see Table 34-2)? Do you feel like you have completely emptied your bladder after you have urinated? When did you last urinate? Do you use a product to contain urine leakage? (adult brief, undergarment, pad)	Observe urine for: • Red color • Cloudiness • Foul odor • Amount with each voiding Assess vital signs for fever and tachycardia. Assess 24-hour intake and output. Start a bladder diary to record frequency and episodes of incontinence. Inspect the abdomen for distention. Inspect the perineal skin for evidence of incontinence-associated dermatitis. Palpate the bladder for tenderness or distention. Determine postvoid residual by bladder scan if available.
Medication usage	Which medications do you take? Include prescription, over-the-counter, and herbal supplements.	Assess for signs of fluid and electrolyte disturbances (see Chapter 18).
	Have you recently been treated with a blood pressure medicine or diuretic?	Inspect urine for pale color and dilute concentration. Start a bladder diary to record frequency and episodes of incontinence.
	Are you taking pain medicine?	Assess output for decreased frequency and amount. Palpate the bladder for distention. Assess bowel pattern for constipation.
Functional ability	Do you have trouble getting to the bathroom or toilet on time? What type of help do you need at home when using the bathroom? Do you have trouble removing your clothing to use the toilet? Do you have difficulty cleaning yourself after urinating?	Observe patient's ability to get up or out of bed and walk safely to the bathroom. Observe patient's ability to safely get on and off the toilet. Observe patient's ability to remove clothing for toileting and perform hygiene. Assess patient's ability to understand instructions related to toileting (cognition, language, culture).
Environment	Does anything prevent you from getting to the bathroom on time?	Assess for adequate lighting in the bathroom; easy access to a nurse call light; clear path to the bathroom, especially if a walker is used; and prompt response of nursing assistive personnel to patient requests for toileting.
Medical history that possibly affects the urinary system	Do you have a history of a urinary tract infection, urinary incontinence, urinary retention, prostate disease, neurological disease (multiple sclerosis, Parkinson's disease, spinal cord injury, stroke, dementia, pelvic organ prolapse), diabetes mellitus? Do you have any difficulty feeling the need to urinate?	Start a bladder diary to record frequency, amount, and episodes of incontinence.
Recent surgery and critical illness (Some anesthesia affects sensory and motor function of the bladder.)	Do you feel the urge to urinate? Have you urinated since your surgery? Did you have a catheter before or after surgery?	Assess intake and output record for adequate frequency and amounts of voiding. Using a bladder scan, assess for urinary retention (see Box 34-5).

BOX 34-5 PROCEDURAL GUIDELINE

Using a Bladder Scanner to Measure Postvoid Residual

DELEGATION CONSIDERATIONS

The skill of measuring bladder volume by bladder scan can be delegated to nursing assistive personnel (NAP). The nurse determines the timing and frequency of the bladder scan measurement and interprets the measurements obtained. The nurse also assesses a patient's ability to use the toilet before measurement of postvoid residual (PVR) and assesses the abdomen for distention if urinary retention is suspected. The nurse directs NAP to:

- Follow manufacturer recommendations for the use of the device.
- Measure PVR volumes 10 minutes after helping patient void.
- Report and record bladder scan volumes.

EQUIPMENT

Bladder scanner, ultrasound gel, cleaning agent for scanner head such as an alcohol pad

STEPS

1. Discuss procedure with patient. If the measurement is for PVR, ask patient to void and measure and record voided urine volume. Complete scanning within 10 minutes after a patient voids.
2. Raise bed to appropriate working height. Help patient to supine position with head slightly elevated. If side rails are raised, lower side rail on working side.
3. Expose patient's lower abdomen.
4. Turn on the scanner per manufacturer guidelines.
5. Set the gender designation per manufacturer guidelines. Designate women with a history of a hysterectomy as male.
6. Wipe the scanner head with an alcohol pad or other cleanser and allow to air dry.
7. Palpate patient's symphysis pubis (pubic bone). Apply a generous amount of ultrasound gel (or if available a bladder scan gel pad) to the midline abdomen 2.5 to 4 cm (1 to 1.5 inches) above the symphysis pubis. The ultrasound gel ensures adequate transmission and thus accurate measurement.
8. Place the scanner head on the gel, making sure that the scanner head is oriented per manufacturer guidelines.
9. Apply light pressure, keep the scanner head steady, and point it slightly downward toward the bladder. Press and release the scan button (see illustration).
10. Verify accurate aim (refer to manufacturer guidelines). Complete the scan and print the image (if needed) (see illustration).
11. Remove ultrasound gel from patient's abdomen with a paper towel.
12. Remove ultrasound gel from scanner head and wipe with alcohol pad or other cleanser; let air dry.
13. Help patient to a comfortable position. Lower bed and place side rails accordingly.

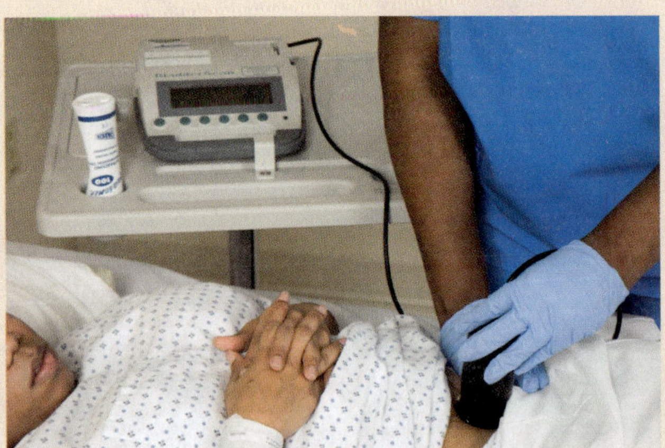

STEP 9 Point scanner head slightly downward toward bladder.

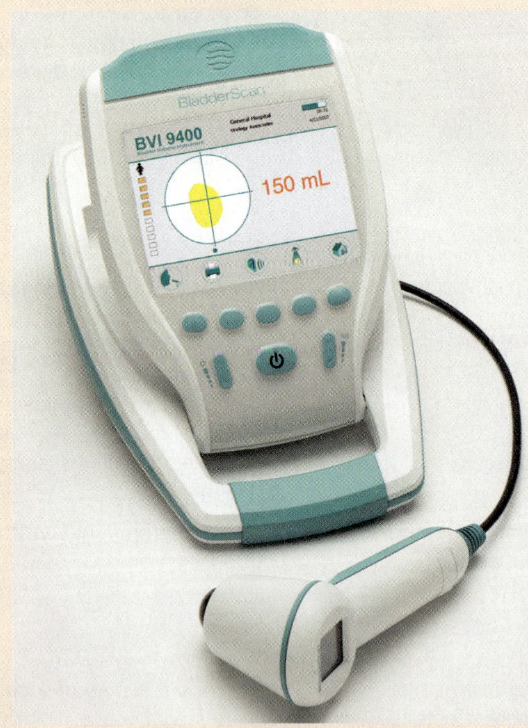

STEP 10 Bladder scan image. (Courtesy Verathon Inc.)

unnecessary catheterization and associated risk for UTI (Box 34-5).

External Genitalia and Urethral Meatus. Careful and sensitive inspection of the external genitalia and urethral meatus yield important data. Normally there should be no drainage or inflammation. To best examine the female patient, position her in the dorsal recumbent position to provide full exposure of the genitalia. Observe the labia majora for swelling, redness, tenderness, rashes, lesions, or evidence of scratching. Using a gloved hand retract the labial folds. The labia minora is normally pink and moist. The urethral meatus appears as an irregular opening or slit close to the vaginal opening. Look for drainage and lesions and ask the patient if there is discomfort. If there is drainage, note the color and consistency. The vaginal tissue of postmenopausal woman may be dryer and less pink than in younger women.

Examine the penis. Look for any redness or irritation. If the man is uncircumcised, retract the foreskin or ask the patient to do so. The foreskin normally moves easily back to expose the glans penis. In some cases the foreskin becomes tight and cannot be retracted (phimosis), increasing risk for inflammation and infection. The urethral meatus is a slitlike opening just below the tip of the penis. Inspect the glans penis and meatus for discharge, lesions, and inflammation. Following inspection, return the foreskin to the unretracted position. Retracted foreskins cause dangerous swelling (paraphimosis) of the penis (Seidel et al., 2011).

Assess the urinary meatus of patients with an indwelling catheter for infection, such as catheter-related damage and presence of inflammation and discharge. Pulling and traction on catheters damages the urinary meatus by creating pressure on the urethra and meatus. In some severe cases the catheter erodes through the meatus to the vagina or through the glans and shaft of the penis. Early detection of trauma results in prompt intervention and prevention of further injury.

Perineal Skin. Regularly assess skin exposed to moisture, especially urine, for signs of moisture-associated damage. Observe for erythema in areas exposed to moisture and skin erosion. Also assess patients when they tell you they are experiencing burning, itching pain (Gray et al., 2012).

Assessment of Urine. To assess a patient's urine, measure the patient's fluid intake and urinary output (I&O) and observe the characteristics of the urine.

Intake and Output. You assess I&O to evaluate bladder emptying, renal function, and fluid and electrolyte balance. Although often written as part of a health care provider's order, placing a patient on I&O is also nursing judgment. Obtaining accurate I&O measurement often requires cooperation and assistance from a patient and family. Intake measurements need to include all oral liquids and semiliquids, enteral feedings, and any parenteral fluids (see Chapter 18). Output measurement includes urine and any other fluid that leaves the body that can be measured such as vomitus, gastric drainage tubes, and wound drains.

Urinary output is a key indicator of kidney and bladder function. A change in urine volume is significant, often indicating fluid imbalance, kidney dysfunction, or decreased blood volume. If a patient has an indwelling catheter after surgery, you assess the patient's hourly urinary output to indirectly measure circulating blood volume. Immediately assess your patient for signs of blood loss and notify the health care provider if the urinary output falls below 30 mL/hr. Urinary output indicates bladder function. Evaluate patients who have not voided for longer than 3 to 6 hours and have had fluid intake recorded for urinary retention. In some patients just helping them to a normal position to void prompts voiding. Assess for any extreme increase or decrease in urine volume. You need to further assess your patient and notify the health care provider if a patient's urine output is less than 30 mL/hr for more than 2 consecutive hours or if your patient has excessive urine output (polyuria).

You measure urine volume with containers that have volume measurement markings. Use a **graduated measuring container** after a patient voids in a bedside commode, bedpan, or urinal or after emptying urine from a catheter drainage bag. **Urine hats** (Figure 34-3) collect urine in a toilet, allowing for patient privacy in the bathroom. Some patients with catheters have a specialized drainage bag with a **urometer** attached between the drainage tubing and drainage bag that allows for accurate hourly urine measurement (Figure 34-4).

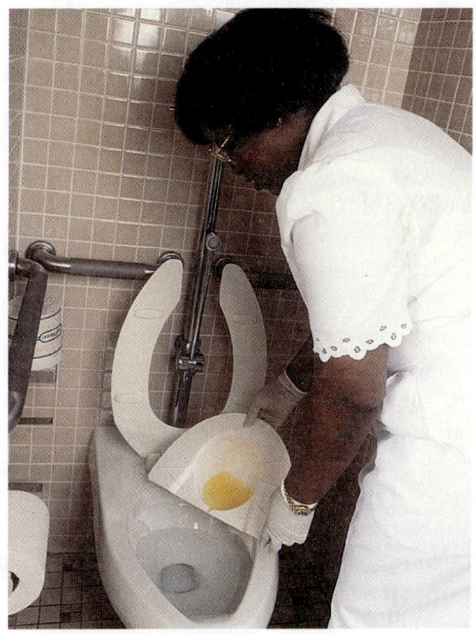

FIGURE 34-3 Urine hat.

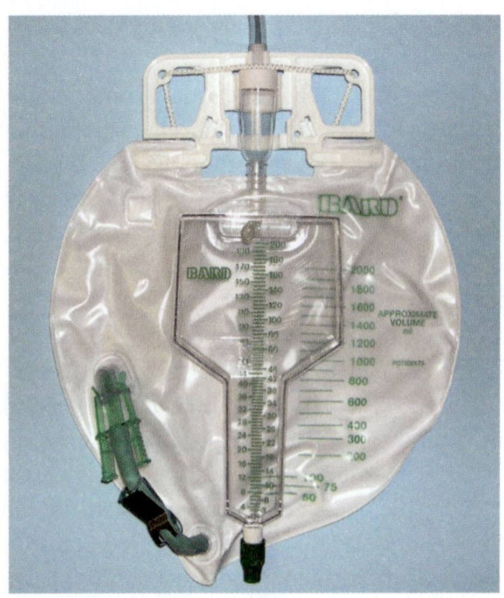

FIGURE 34-4 Urometer. (Courtesy Michael Gallager, RN, BSN, MSN, OSF, Saint Francis Medical Center, Peoria, IL.)

Empty drainage bags every 8 hours or as needed and record the amount on a patient's I&O record. When emptying catheter drainage bags, make sure that the drainage tube is reclamped and secured. Each patient needs to have a graduated receptacle for individual use to prevent potential cross-contamination. Label each container with the patient's name. Rinse the container after each use to minimize odor and bacterial growth.

Characteristics of Urine. Inspect a patient's urine for color, clarity, and odor. Monitor and document any changes.

Color. Normal urine ranges in color from pale yellow (like straw) to amber depending on its concentration. Urine is usually more concentrated in the morning or with fluid volume deficits. As a patient drinks more fluids, urine becomes less concentrated, and the color lightens. Patients taking diuretics commonly void dilute urine while the medication is active.

Hematuria is never a normal finding. Bleeding from the kidneys or ureters usually causes urine to become dark red; bleeding from the bladder or urethra usually causes bright red urine. Hematuria and blood clots commonly cause urinary catheter blockage.

Various medications and foods change the color of urine. For example, patients taking phenazopyridine, a urinary analgesic, void urine that is bright orange. Eating beets, rhubarb, and blackberries causes red urine. The kidneys excrete special dyes used in IV diagnostic studies, which discolor the urine. Patients with liver disease who have high concentrations of bilirubin (urobilinogen) often have dark amber urine. Report unexpected color changes to the health care provider.

Clarity. Normal urine appears transparent at the time of voiding. Urine that stands several minutes in a container becomes cloudy. Sometimes a patient's first voided urine of the day is cloudy because the urine is stored in the bladder overnight; urine normally clears on the next voiding. Patients with bacteria and white blood cells in their urine usually have thick and cloudy urine. In patients with renal disease, freshly voided urine often appears cloudy because of protein concentration.

Odor. Urine has a characteristic ammonia odor. The more concentrated the urine, the stronger the odor. As urine remains standing (e.g., in a collection device), more ammonia breakdown occurs, and the odor becomes stronger. A foul odor often indicates a UTI. Some foods such as asparagus and garlic can change the odor of urine.

Laboratory and Diagnostic Testing. You are responsible for collecting urine specimens for laboratory testing. The type of test determines the method of collection. Label all specimens with the patient's name, date, time, and type of collection. You also need to complete laboratory requisition forms with specific information required by the testing laboratory. Most urine specimens need to reach the laboratory within 2 hours of collection or be preserved according to the laboratory protocol (Pagana and Pagana, 2011). Urine that stands in a container at room temperature without the required preservative grows bacteria and experiences changes that affect the accuracy of the test. You need to follow agency infection control policies and Standard Precautions when handling urine specimens (see Chapter 14). Urine specimens commonly collected include first morning specimen, random urine specimen, timed urine specimen, double voided specimen, and urine for culture and sensitivity. To obtain urine that is freshly voided, you need to ask the patient to double void. Ask the patient to empty the bladder, then send the second voided specimen to the laboratory. To obtain urine as free of bacterial contamination as possible, a midstream, clean-catch urine specimen is sometimes required.

Urinalysis. When a routine urinalysis is ordered, you usually collect a random or first morning specimen. A routine urinalysis requires no special preparation and is collected either by the patient voiding into an appropriate clean container or by urethral catheterization. Specimens can be obtained from an indwelling catheter as long as the specimen port, not the drainage bag, is used. The urinalysis includes a number of tests that are used for screening and are diagnostic for such things as fluid and electrolyte disturbances, UTI, presence of blood, and other metabolic problems (Table 34-4). In some health care settings you test urine using reagent strips. You need to follow manufacturer instructions when performing the test and reading the strips. Dip the reagent strip into fresh urine, and observe for color changes on the strip. You compare the colors on the strip with a color chart on the reagent strip container. Be sure to examine each color at the exact time indicated on the container.

Timed Urine Tests. Timed testing requires urine collection and testing either at a specific time of day or urine collected over a specific time period. These tests measure bodily substances that may be excreted at higher levels at specific times of the day such as glucose 2 hours after a meal or substances that are to be measured over a specific time period such as sodium, potassium, and chloride as indicators of fluid and electrolyte disturbance (Pagana and Pagana, 2011). In most 24-hour specimen collections you discard the first voided specimen and start collecting urine in a special container that already has a preservative added. Depending on the test, you need to keep the urine container cool by placing it in a container of ice. You provide patient education, including an explanation of the test, an emphasis on the need to collect all urine voided during the prescribed time period, and how to avoid contaminating the specimen with stool or toilet paper. Carefully document the start and stop time of the test, as requested by the laboratory, to improve testing accuracy.

Clean-Catch Midstream Specimen. You need to collect a clean-catch midstream specimen when you want to obtain a specimen relatively free of contaminating microorganisms. Instruct your patient how to cleanse the urinary meatus effectively. A clean-catch urine specimen kit includes a sterile cup and disinfectant wipes. Illustrated instructions are often included. Review with female patients how to clean the meatus by wiping front to back. They need to cleanse the meatus 2 to 3 times and use a separate clean wipe or clean section of a wipe each time. Instruct male patients to retract

TABLE 34-4 **ROUTINE URINALYSIS VALUES**

MEASUREMENT (NORMAL VALUE)	INTERPRETATION
pH (4.6 to 8.0)	pH level indicates acid-base balance. Acid pH helps protect against bacterial growth. Urine that stands for several hours becomes alkaline from bacterial growth.
Protein (up to 8 mg/100 mL)	Protein is normally not present in urine. The presence of protein is a very sensitive indicator of kidney function. Damage to the glomerular membrane (such as in glomerulonephritis) allows for the filtration of larger molecules such as protein to seep through.
Glucose (not normally present)	Patients with poorly controlled diabetes have glucose in the urine because of inability of tubules to resorb high serum glucose concentrations (>180 mg/100 mL). Ingestion of high concentrations of glucose causes some glucose to appear in urine of healthy persons.
Ketones (not normally present)	With poor control of type 1 diabetes, patients experience breakdown of fatty acids. End products of fatty acid metabolism are ketones. Patients with dehydration, starvation, or excessive aspirin ingestion also have ketonuria.
Blood	A positive test for occult blood occurs when intact erythrocytes, hemoglobin, or myoglobin is present. Damage to the glomerulus or tubules causes blood cells to enter urine. Trauma or disease of lower urinary tract also causes hematuria.
Specific gravity (1.0053 to 1.030)	Specific gravity tests measure concentration of particles in urine. High specific gravity reflects concentrated urine, and low specific gravity reflects diluted urine. Dehydration, reduced renal blood flow, and increase in ADH secretion elevate specific gravity. Overhydration, early renal disease, and inadequate ADH secretion reduce specific gravity.
Microscopic examination RBCs (up to 2)	Damage to glomeruli or tubules allows RBCs to enter the urine. Trauma, disease, presence of urethral catheters, or surgery of the lower urinary tract also causes RBCs to be present.
WBCs (0-4 per low-power field)	Elevated numbers indicate inflammation or infection.
Bacteria (not normally present)	Bacteria in the urine usually indicates infection or colonization (presence of bacteria and the patient shows no symptoms of infection).
Casts (not normally present)	Casts are microscopic cylindrical bodies that look like objects within the renal tubule. Types include hyaline, WBCs, RBCs, granular cells, and epithelial cells. Their presence indicates renal disease.
Crystals (not normally present)	Crystals indicate increased risk for the development of renal calculi (stone). Some patients with high uric acid levels (gout) develop uric acid crystals.

Data from Pagana KD, Pagana TJ: *Mosby's diagnostic and laboratory test reference*, ed 10, St Louis, 2011, Mosby.
ADH, Antidiuretic hormone; *RBCs*, red blood cells; *WBCs*, white blood cells.

their foreskin if not circumcised and cleanse the meatus in a circular motion, moving from the center of the meatus to the outside. After cleansing, the patient opens the sterile urine cup. Caution your patient not to touch the inside of the cup. To collect the specimen, instruct your patient to start voiding in the toilet or other receptacle, stop the stream, position the sterile cup to collect urine, and then continue voiding into the cup. When finished, you or your patient puts the lid on the cup, and you send the specimen to the laboratory for testing.

Urine for Culture and Sensitivity. Urine specimens collected for culture and sensitivity determine the presence of bacteria and identify the appropriate antibiotic needed to treat a specific bacteria. You collect the specimen using clean-catheter midstream urine or by sterile catheterization (see Skill 34-1). Collect the specimen in patients with indwelling urinary catheters using the specimen port, not the drainage bag. You catheterize the stoma of a patient with a urinary diversion to obtain an accurate specimen. In some cases a preliminary report is available in 24 hours, but usually 48 to 72 hours are need for bacterial growth and sensitivity testing (Pagana and Pagana, 2011).

Diagnostic Examinations. The urinary system is one of the few organ systems accessible to accurate diagnostic study by radiographic techniques. Studies are either simple and noninvasive or complex and invasive (Table 34-5).

Many of the nursing responsibilities related to diagnostic testing of the urinary tract are common to most studies. The responsibilities before testing include:

- Ensure that a signed consent is completed (check agency policy).
- Assess if a patient has allergies or has experienced a previous reaction to a contrast agent (Schabelman and Witting, 2010).

TABLE 34-5 **COMMON DIAGNOSTIC TESTING**

PROCEDURE	DESCRIPTION	SPECIAL NURSING CONSIDERATIONS
Noninvasive Procedures		
Abdominal roentgenogram (plain film; kidney, ureter, bladder (KUB) or flat plate)	X-ray film of the abdomen to determine the size, shape, symmetry, and location of the structures of the lower urinary tract Common uses: Detect and measure the size of urinary calculi	No special preparation
Computerized axial tomography (CT) scan	Detailed imagery of the abdominal structures provided by computerized reconstruction of cross-sectional images Common uses: Identify anatomical abnormalities, renal tumors, cysts, calculi, and obstruction of the ureters	**Preparation:** • Cleansing bowel (see agency or health care provider protocol). • Assess for allergy to shellfish (iodine) or previous reaction to contrast media (if contrast is ordered). • Restrict food and fluid up to 4 hours before test (see agency or health care provider protocol). **After procedure:** • Encourage fluids to promote excretion of dye. • Assess for delayed hypersensitivity reaction to the contrast media. **Patient teaching:** • Explain that patient will be placed on a special bed that will move through a tunnel-like imaging chamber. He or she needs to lie still when instructed by the technician. Some patients feel claustrophobic.
Intravenous pyelogram (IVP)	Imaging of the urinary tract that views the collecting ducts and renal pelvis and outlines the ureters, bladder, and urethra (After intravenous injection of contrast media [iodine-based that converts to a dye], a series of x-ray films are taken to observe the passage of urine from the renal pelvis to the bladder.) Common uses: Detect and measure urinary calculi, tumors, hematuria, obstruction of the urinary tract	**Preparation:** • Assess for allergies. • Assess for dehydration. • Cleanse bowel (see agency or health care provider protocol). • Restrict food and fluid up to 4 hours before test (see agency or health care provider protocol). **After procedure:** • Assess for delayed hypersensitivity to the contrast media. • Encourage fluids after the test to dilute and flush dye from the patient. • Assess urine output. Less than 30 mL/hr increases risk for contrast-induced nephropathy. **Patient teaching:** • Facial flushing is a normal response during dye injection. Patients often feel dizzy, warm, or nauseated.
Ultrasound renal bladder	Imaging of the kidneys, ureters, and bladder using sound waves Identifies gross structural abnormalities and estimates the volume of urine in the bladder Common uses: Detect masses, obstruction, presence of hydronephrosis or hydroureter, abnormalities of bladder wall, and calculi; measuring postvoid residual	Patients need to come to the study with a full bladder.

TABLE 34-5 COMMON DIAGNOSTIC TESTING—cont'd

PROCEDURE	DESCRIPTION	SPECIAL NURSING CONSIDERATIONS
Invasive Procedures		
Endoscopy-cystoscopy	Introduction of a cystoscope through the urethra into the bladder to provide direct visualization, specimen collection, and/or treatment of the bladder and urethra (In most cases the procedure is performed using local anesthesia, but under certain circumstances general anesthesia or conscious sedation may be used.) Common uses: Microscopic hematuria; detect bladder tumors and obstruction of the bladder outlet and urethra	When applicable, follow agency protocol for preoperative preparation (see Chapter 39). Patient teaching: Urine is sometimes pink tinged after the test. Assess for signs and symptoms of urinary tract infection.

Data from Gray M, Moore, KN: *Urologic disorders*, St Louis, 2009, Mosby; Pagana, KD, Pagana, TJ: *Mosby's diagnostic and laboratory test reference*, ed 10, St Louis, 2011, Mosby.

- Administer bowel-cleansing agents as ordered; check agency policy.
- Ensure a patient adheres to the appropriate pretest diet (clear liquids) or nothing by mouth (NPO).

Responsibilities after testing include:

- Assess I&O.
- Assess voiding and urine (color, clarity, presence of blood, dysuria, problems emptying).
- Encourage fluid intake, especially if using radiopaque dye.

NURSING DIAGNOSIS

A thorough assessment of a patient's urinary elimination function reveals patterns of data that allow you to make relevant and accurate nursing diagnoses. Use critical thinking to reflect on knowledge of previous patients and the application of knowledge of urinary function. Identification of the defining characteristics leads you to select appropriate nursing diagnoses (see Chapter 9). An important part of formulating nursing diagnoses is identifying the relevant causative or related factor. Specifying related factors for each diagnosis allows selection of individualized nursing interventions (Ackley and Ladwig, 2011). For example, *Toileting Self-Care Deficit* related to impaired transfer ability or impaired mobility guides the selection of nursing interventions that remove barriers to toilet access. *Toileting Self-Care Deficit* related to cognitive impairment guides the selection of nursing interventions such as a prompted-voiding program or habit-training program. Some nursing diagnoses common to patients with urinary elimination problems include the following:

- *Functional Urinary Incontinence*
- *Reflex Urinary Incontinence*
- *Stress Urinary Incontinence*
- *Urge Urinary Incontinence*
- *Risk for Urge Urinary Incontinence*
- *Risk for Infection*
- *Toileting Self-Care Deficit*
- *Impaired Urinary Elimination*
- *Readiness for Enhanced Urinary Elimination*
- *Urinary Retention*

PLANNING

You plan nursing care using a process that integrates what you have assessed to be the patient's problem, your nursing knowledge related to the problem, and evidenced-based standards of nursing care (see Care Plan).

Goals and Outcomes. Goals and outcomes for urinary elimination problems need to be realistic and individualized. Patients often have more than one nursing diagnosis, and these diagnoses often affect one another (Figure 34-5). Evaluate the relationships among these diagnoses and establish patient-centered goals and outcomes in collaboration with the patient and family. For example, a realistic patient goal for a patient with *Toileting Self-Care Deficit* related to impaired mobility status is: Patient will be able to independently use the toilet. An appropriate outcome is: Patient safely transfers to the toilet. To achieve this outcome you identify a number of interventions such as ensuring that the patient's call bell is within reach and providing assistive devices such as a raised toilet seat, support rails next to the toilet, and easy access to the urinal when in bed.

Setting Priorities. Establish priorities of care based on a patient's immediate physical and safety needs, patient expectations, and readiness to perform some self-care activities. For example, a patient with a long-term indwelling catheter is admitted to acute care with a severe UTI. The patient expects to resume self-care of the catheter. However, because of the severity of the infection and the patient's condition, you perform all catheter care at this time. The priorities are

CARE PLAN

Urinary Retention

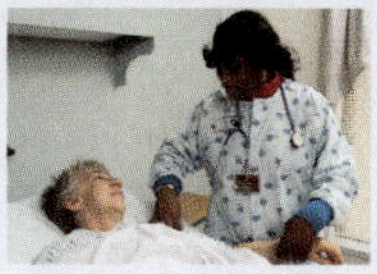

ASSESSMENT

Mrs. Vallero was unable to void 8 hours after catheter removal, and a bladder scan showed retained urine. She was straight catheterized, and 500 mL of urine was obtained. It is now 4 hours since the catheterization. She has been drinking fluids, including hot tea and water, to increase her chances of urinating on her own. She complains of a feeling of pressure over her lower abdomen and has been dribbling small amounts of urine.

ASSESSMENT ACTIVITIES	FINDINGS/DEFINING CHARACTERISTICS*
Inspect the abdomen for distention and gently palpate for bladder distention every 2 hours on the even hours.	Able to palpate bladder, indicating **bladder distention.** During palpation patient states she has **sensation of bladder fullness.**
Assess patient's voiding pattern, including volume at each voiding, frequency, times of day, and history of any changes.	She complains of **dribbling frequently** and being **unable to urinate.**

*__Defining characteristics__ are shown in **bold** type.

NURSING DIAGNOSIS: Urinary Retention related to deficient detrusor (bladder muscle) contraction strength and recent removal of indwelling urinary catheter

PLANNING

GOAL	EXPECTED OUTCOMES (NOC)[†]
	Urinary Elimination
• Mrs. Vallero will be able to void every 2-3 hours within 1 week.	• Mrs. Vallero will void greater than 150 mL each time.
	Urinary Continence
	• Mrs. Vallero will verbalize no episodes of dribbling or incontinence.
	Symptom Severity
	• Mrs. Vallero will verbalize relief of lower abdominal discomfort.

[†]Outcomes classification label from Moorhead S et al, editors: *Nursing outcomes classification (NOC)*, ed 5, St Louis, 2013, Mosby.

INTERVENTIONS (NIC)[‡]	RATIONALE
Urinary Retention Care	
• Remind Mrs. Vallero to use the toilet every 2 to 3 hours while awake (timed voiding).	Timed voiding is a primary treatment for elevated bladder volumes when there is diminished or loss sensation of bladder filling (Gray and Moore, 2009; Wyndaele et al., 2009).
• Instruct Mrs. Vallero to keep a diary of her voiding time and amount and when she experiences urine leakage.	Keeping a record of urinary output is important to confirm voiding in small amounts and the degree of incontinence (Newman and Wein, 2009).
• Encourage Mrs. Vallero to use strategies that stimulate voiding such as drinking a warm beverage before voiding, taking a warm shower or bath, listening to running water when attempting to void, or pouring warm water over the perineal area when on the toilet.	These strategies help in relaxation of the pelvic floor muscles and to stimulate bladder contractions (Gray and Moore, 2009).
• Instruct Mrs. Vallero to double void.	Instructing patients to void and then void again in 3 to 5 minutes allows the bladder to rest in between bladder contractions (Gray and Moore, 2009).
• Measure postvoid residual (PVR) by bladder scan at ordered intervals.	Monitoring PVR after catheter removal can prevent dangerous and painful urinary retention (Newman and Wein, 2009).

[‡]Intervention classification labels from Bulechek GM et al, editors: *Nursing interventions classifications (NIC)*, ed 6, St Louis, 2013, Mosby.

CARE PLAN—cont'd

Urinary Retention

EVALUATION

NURSING ACTIONS	PATIENT RESPONSE/FINDING	ACHIEVEMENT OF OUTCOME
Ask Mrs. Vallero about her urge to void, sensation of bladder fullness, and dribbling episodes.	Mrs. Vallero denies dribbling episodes, and she has a decreased urgency to urinate.	Dribbling episodes and sense of urgency relieved.
Have Mrs. Vallero keep a log of her pattern of elimination, including urine output volumes with each voiding, during the 1-week period.	Mrs. Vallero states that she and her family have measured her urine and most output is greater than 150 mL.	Urinary output is greater than 150 mL with each void.
Ask Mrs. Vallero if she continues to have lower abdominal pain.	Mrs. Vallero denies lower abdominal pain at this time. States that since she has urinated more at a time she no longer has discomfort.	Lower abdominal discomfort is absent.

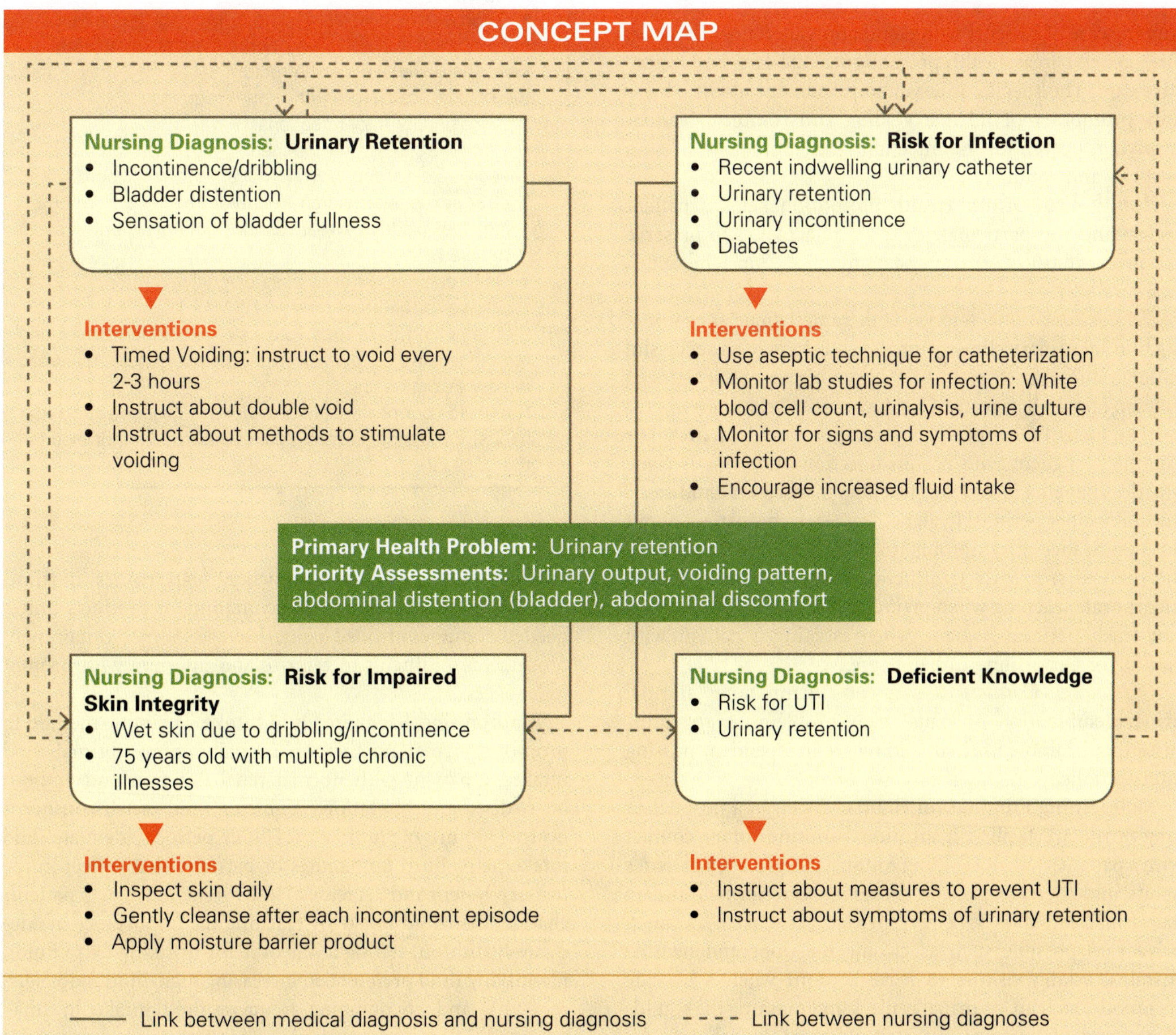

FIGURE 34-5 Concept map.

to treat the infection, prevent reinfection, and teach the patient how to resume care of the catheter to prevent future infections.

Collaborative Care. You use the expertise of the health care team and incorporate the team into the plan when planning individualized care. For example, when planning care for a patient with urge UI, you incorporate the expertise of a continence nurse specialist to help the patient learn techniques to inhibit the urinary urge and strengthen pelvic floor muscles; an occupational therapist to help the patient learn efficient and safe toilet transfers; a physical therapist to help with strengthening exercises of the lower extremities; and a social worker to obtain assistive devices in the home. Include the family in planning when applicable, especially when a primary caregiver is identified. Your active and thoughtful role in planning these interventions results in a patient's progress toward improved urinary elimination.

IMPLEMENTATION

Nursing care of patients with elimination alterations focus on three general areas: health promotion, acute care, and restorative care. The specific interventions include patient education, promotion of normal voiding and complete bladder emptying, prevention of infection, and promotion of skin integrity and comfort.

Health Promotion. Health promotion helps a patient understand and participate in self-care activities to preserve and protect healthy urinary system function. You achieve this in several ways.

Patient Education. Success of therapies aimed at optimizing normal urinary elimination depends in part on successful patient education (Box 34-6). Although many patients need to learn about all aspects of healthy urinary elimination, it is best to focus on a specific elimination problem first. For example, a patient who has an infection and poor hygiene practices benefits most from teaching focused on handwashing and proper perineal hygiene. You teach this patient about the significance of symptoms that indicate another UTI and the need to seek early treatment to prevent serious illness. Incorporate teaching when giving nursing care. For example, you teach perineal hygiene when assisting a patient with bathing or performing catheter care.

Promoting Normal Micturition. Maintaining normal urinary elimination prevents many problems. Many measures that promote normal voiding are independent nursing interventions.

Maintaining Elimination Habits. When in a hospital or long-term care facility, institutional routines often conflict with a patient's normal voiding routine. Integrating a patient's habits into the care plan promotes a more normal voiding pattern. Elimination is a very private act. Create as much privacy as possible such as closing the door and bedside curtains; asking visitors to leave a room when a bedside commode, bedpan, or urinal is used; and masking the sounds of voiding with running water. Respond to requests for assistance with toileting as quickly as possible. Embarrassing accidents are easily avoided when help comes in time. Avoid the use of incontinence containment products unless needed for uncontrolled urine leakage. Some containment products are difficult to remove and interfere with prompt toilet access.

Maintaining Adequate Fluid Intake. A simple method to promote normal micturition is maintaining optimal fluid intake. A patient with normal renal function and without heart disease or alterations requiring fluid restriction needs up to 2300 mL of fluid in a 24-hour period. Adequate fluid intake helps flush out solutes or particles that collect in the urinary system and decrease bladder irritability. Help patients change their fluid intake by teaching the importance of adequate hydration, setting a schedule for drinking extra fluids, identifying fluid preferences, increasing high-fluid foods such as fruits, and encouraging frequent fluid intake in small volumes. To prevent nocturia suggest that a patient avoid drinking fluids 2 hours before bedtime.

BOX 34-6 HEALTH PROMOTION/RESTORATION: PATIENT EDUCATION FOR A HEALTHY BLADDER

1. Maintain adequate hydration.
   - Drink 6-8 glasses of water a day. Spread it out evenly throughout the day.
   - Avoid or limit drinking beverages that contain caffeine (coffee, tea, chocolate drinks, soft drinks).
   - To decrease nocturia, avoid drinking fluids 2 hours before bedtime.
   - Do not limit fluids if you experience incontinence. Concentrated urine may irritate the bladder and increase bladder symptoms.
2. Keep good voiding habits.
   - Women: Sit well back on the toilet seat, avoid "hovering over the toilet," and make sure that the feet are flat on the floor.
   - Void at regular intervals, usually every 3-4 hours, depending on fluid intake.
   - Avoid straining when voiding or moving the bowels.
   - Take enough time to empty the bladder completely.
3. Keep the bowels regular. A rectum full of stool may irritate the bladder, causing urgency and frequency.
4. Prevent urinary tract infections.
   - Women: Cleanse the perineum from front to back after each voiding and bowel movement; void before and after sexual intercourse to prevent bacteria from entering the bladder; wear cotton undergarments; avoid bubble baths.
   - Drink enough water to pass pale yellow urine.
   - Shower or bathe regularly.
5. Stop smoking to reduce your risk for bladder cancer and for developing a cough, which can contribute to stress urinary incontinence.
6. Report to your health care provider any changes in bladder habits, frequency, urgency, pain when voiding, or blood in the urine.

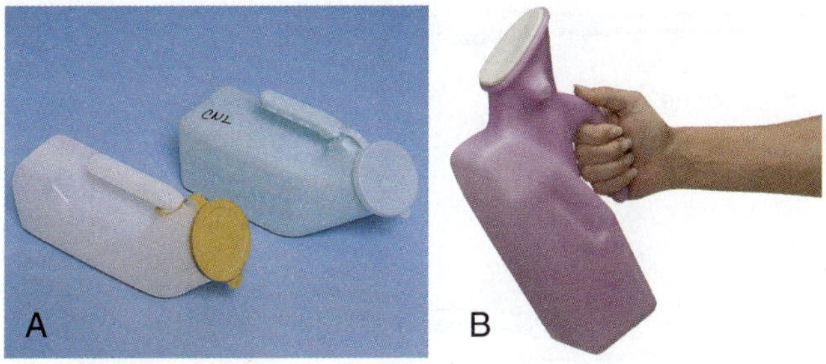

FIGURE 34-6 Types of male (**A**) and female (**B**) urinals. (**B** Courtesy Briggs Medical Service Co.)

Promoting Complete Bladder Emptying. It is normal for a small volume of urine to remain in the bladder after micturition. When the bladder does not empty completely, and **residual urine** volumes are high, there is risk for incontinence and dangerous urinary retention. Urinary retention increases the risk for UTI and damage to the kidneys. Adequate bladder emptying depends on feeling an urge to urinate, contracting the bladder, and the ability to relax the urethral sphincter. Help patients assume the normal position for voiding to promote relaxation and stimulate bladder contractions. Squatting is the normal anatomical position for female voiding. Women empty the bladder better when sitting on the toilet or bedside commode with the feet on the floor. If a patient cannot use a toilet, position her on a bedpan (see Chapter 35). After bedpan use, help the patient perform perineal hygiene (see Chapter 29). A man voids more easily while standing. If the patient is unable to reach a toilet, have him stand at the bedside and void into a **urinal** (a plastic or metal receptacle for urine) (Figure 34-6, *A*). Always assess mobility status and determine if he can stand safely. At times one or more nurses need to help a male patient stand. If the patient is unable to stand at the bedside, you need to help him use the urinal in bed. Some patients need the nurse to position the penis completely within the urinal and hold the urinal in place or help the patient hold the urinal. Once the patient finishes voiding, carefully remove the urinal and perform perineal hygiene (see Chapter 29). Most urinals are used by men, but some are specially designed for women (Figure 34-6, *B*). The female urinal has a larger opening at the top with a defined rim that helps position the urinal closely against the genitalia.

Other measures improve bladder emptying (Box 34-7). To promote relaxation and stimulate bladder contractions, use sensory stimuli (e.g., turning on running water, putting a patient's hand in a pan of warm water, or stroking the female patient's inner thigh) and provide privacy. To improve bladder emptying, encourage patients to wait until the urine flow completely stops when voiding, encourage them to attempt a second void (double voiding), and encourage them to attempt voiding according to the clock, not urge. This is called *timed voiding*. Do not implement the Credé method or manual compression of the bladder (i.e., placing the hands over the bladder and compressing it to assist in emptying) until consulting with the health care provider. In the presence of high

BOX 34-7 PATIENT TEACHING

Urinary Retention Care

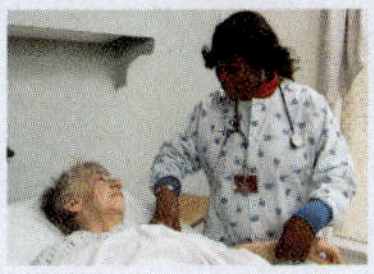

Mrs. Vallero is concerned about regaining her urinary function. Sandy develops the following teaching plan for her regarding her urinary retention.

OUTCOME

At the end of the teaching session Mrs. Vallero will describe approaches to promote normal urinary elimination habits.

TEACHING STRATEGIES

- Establish rapport with Mrs. Vallero.
- Find out what Mrs. Vallero already knows about good practices for urinary health.
- Use the correct terms for the anatomy that you discuss but explain them so Mrs. Vallero knows what they are.
- Provide appropriate visual diagrams and written materials for Mrs. Vallero.
- Instruct her how to monitor her own urinary output.
- Instruct Mrs. Vallero about adequate fluid intake, incorporating her fluid preferences.
- Describe the importance and technique of timed and double voiding.
- Reinforce correct perineal hygiene measures to reduce the risk for urinary tract infection.
- Provide Mrs. Vallero with pertinent signs and symptoms of infection to report to her health care provider.

EVALUATION STRATEGIES

- Ask Mrs. Vallero to verbalize her understanding of normal urinary function.
- Ask Mrs. Vallero to describe her normal voiding routine; evaluate if her stated routine supports healthy urination habits.

postvoid residuals or a complete inability of the bladder to empty, either intermittent or indwelling urinary catheterization is often required.

Preventing Infection. UTIs are one of the most common infections encountered in a primary care practice (Gupta et al., 2011). As a nurse, you play a key role in implementing evidenced-based practices to avoid this common and potentially dangerous infection. Some key interventions include promoting adequate fluid intake, perineal hygiene, and voiding at regular intervals. In women you encourage wiping front to back after voiding and defecation, avoiding perfumed perineal washes and spays, avoiding bubble baths and tight clothing, voiding before and after sexual intercourse, and wearing cotton underwear. If a patient has a problem with urine leakage, you need to stress the importance of hygiene. Patients who use containment products need to use products that are designed for urine and wick wetness away from the body. They also need to avoid prolonged periods of urine wetness.

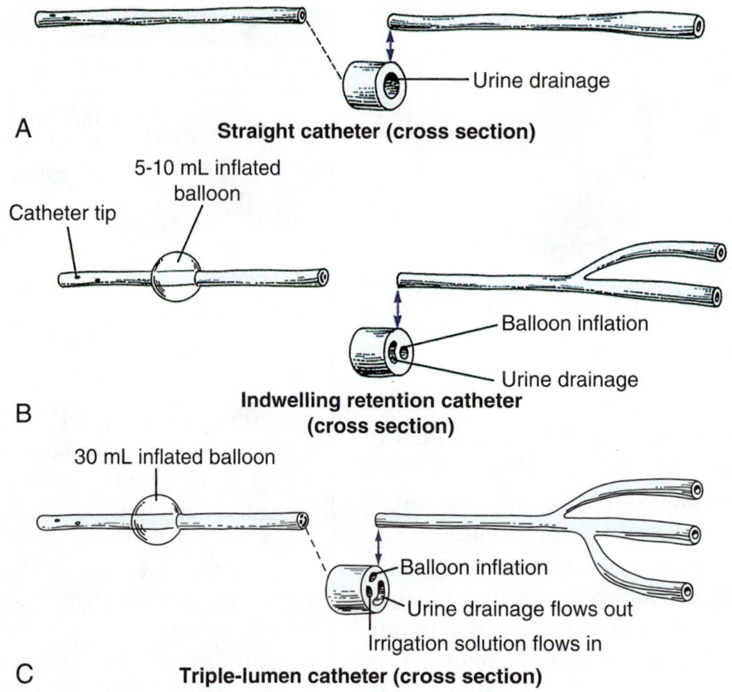

FIGURE 34-7 **A,** Straight catheter (cross section). **B,** Indwelling retention catheter (cross section). **C,** Triple-lumen catheter (cross section).

Acute Care. Patients with acute illness, surgery, or impaired urinary tract function usually require interventions that support urinary elimination.

Catheterization. Urinary catheterization is the placement of a tube through the urethra into the bladder to drain urine. This is an invasive procedure that requires a medical order and in institutional settings aseptic technique (Gould et al., 2009; Lo et al., 2009). Skill 34-1 lists steps for performing female and male urethral catheterization.

Urinary catheterization is either short term (2 weeks or less) or long term (more than 1 month) (Parker et al., 2009). Conditions that require the use of a short- or long-term urinary catheter include the need for accurate monitoring of urine output, perioperative or postoperative care after urologic or gynecological procedures, and inadequate emptying of the bladder because of an obstruction or neurological condition. Excessive accumulation of urine in the bladder is painful for the patient; increases the risk for UTI; and can cause backward flow of urine up the ureters to the kidneys, causing kidney damage. UI often requires indwelling catheterization if the leaking urine interferes with wound healing (Cottenden et al., 2009). Intermittent catheterization is used to measure postvoid residual when a bladder scanner is not available or as a way to manage chronic urinary retention.

Types of Catheters. Urinary catheters differ based on the number of catheter lumens. Some have balloons to keep the indwelling catheter in place and some have a closed drainage system. Urinary catheters are made with one to three lumens (Figure 34-7). You use single-lumen catheters (see Figure 34-7, *A*) for intermittent/straight catheterization (i.e., the insertion of a catheter for one-time bladder emptying). Double-lumen catheters, designed for indwelling catheters, provide one lumen for urinary drainage and a second lumen that is used to inflate a balloon that keeps the catheter in place (see Figure 34-7, *B*). Use triple-lumen catheters (see Figure 34-7, *C*) for continuous bladder irrigation or when it is necessary to instill medications into a patient's bladder. One lumen drains the bladder, a second lumen inflates the balloon, and a third lumen delivers irrigation fluid into the bladder.

A health care provider chooses a catheter on the basis of factors such as latex allergy, history of catheter encrustation, and susceptibility to infection. Indwelling catheters are made of latex or silicone. Latex catheters with special coatings reduce urethral irritation (Cottenden et al., 2009). All silicone catheters have a larger internal diameter and are often helpful in patients who require frequent catheter changes because of encrustation (Newman and Wein, 2009). Antimicrobial catheters are coated with silver or an antibiotic. Current evidence shows they reduce the incidence of CAUTI for short-term use, but to date there are insufficient data to support their use in long-term catheter users (Parker et al., 2009). Intermittent/straight catheters are made of rubber (softer and more flexible) or polyvinyl chloride (PVC). Patients who self-catheterize have a large selection of catheters, some with special coatings that do not require lubrication and others that are self-contained systems consisting of a prelubricated catheter and packaged with a preconnected drainage bag.

Catheter Sizes. The size of a urinary catheter is based on the French (FR) scale, which reflects the internal diameter of the catheter. Most adults with an indwelling catheter use a size 14-16 Fr to minimize trauma and risk for infection. Larger catheter diameters increase the risk for urethral trauma (Parker et al., 2009). Patients use larger sizes in special

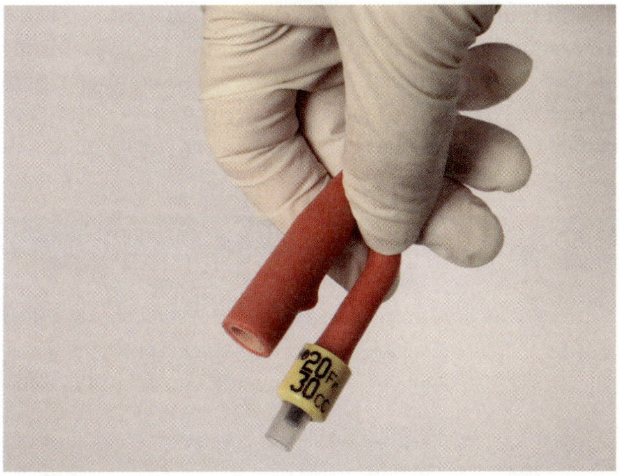

FIGURE 34-8 Size of catheter and balloon printed on catheter.

circumstances such as after urological surgery or in the presence of gross hematuria. Use smaller sizes for children such as a 5-6 Fr for infants, 8-10 Fr for children, and 12 Fr for young girls.

Indwelling catheters come in a variety of balloon sizes from 3 mL (for a child) to 30 mL for continuous bladder irrigation (CBI). The size of the balloon is usually printed on the catheter port (Figure 34-8). The recommended balloon size for an adult is a 10-mL balloon (the balloon is 5 mL and requires 10 mL to fill completely). Current evidence shows long-term use of larger balloons (30 mL) is associated with increased patient discomfort, irritation and trauma, increased risk of catheter expulsion, and incomplete emptying of the bladder because of urine that pools below the level of the catheter drainage eyes (Cottenden et al., 2009; Newman and Wein, 2009).

Catheter Changes. You individualize catheter changes for patients requiring long-term catheterization (i.e., urinary retention or critical illness) (Gould et al., 2009; Willson et al., 2009). In many cases you need to change catheters every 4 to 6 weeks. Change long-term catheters if they leak or become blocked and before obtaining a sterile specimen for urine culture. Avoid use of long-term catheterization because of its association with the increased risk of UTI. Make every attempt to remove catheters as soon as a patient can void.

Closed Drainage Systems. An indwelling catheter is attached to a closed-system drainage bag to collect the continuous flow of urine. Do not separate the drainage system unless absolutely necessary to avoid introducing pathogens (Figure 34-9). Always hang the bag below the level of the bladder on the bed frame or a chair so urine drains down, out of the bladder. Do **not** let the bag touch the floor or secure it on a side rail. When a patient ambulates, carry the bag below the level of the patient's bladder. The only exception to this rule is when a catheter is attached to a specially designed drainage bag (belly bag) that a patient wears across the abdomen. A one-way valve prevents the back flow of urine into the bladder. To keep the drainage system patent, check for kinks or bends in the tubing, avoid positioning a patient

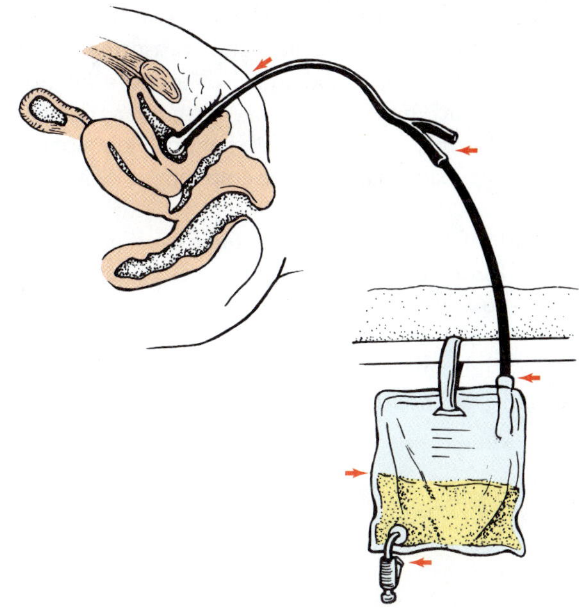

FIGURE 34-9 Potential sites *(arrows)* for introduction of infection.

on drainage tubing, prevent tubing from becoming dependent, and observe for clots or sediment that block the catheter or tubing.

Routine Catheter Care. Patients with indwelling catheters require regular perineal hygiene, especially after bowel movements, to reduce the risk for CAUTI (Gould et al., 2009). In many institutions patients receive catheter care every 8 hours as the minimal standard of care (see Chapter 29). You gently separate the labia of a female or retract the foreskin (if uncircumcised) of a male to clearly visualize the urethral meatus when cleansing a patient with an indwelling catheter. Note any discharge, odor, or inflammation. Grasp the catheter with two fingers to prevent unnecessary traction on the catheter. Using a washcloth, soap, and water, start cleansing close to the urinary meatus and move outward for about 10 cm (4 inches) in a circular motion to remove any secretions that adhere to the catheter (Figure 34-10). Be sure to remove all traces of soap and replace the foreskin if pulled back. Replace the catheter securement device as necessary (see Skill 34-1). Empty the drainage bag when it is half full and record output. An overfull drainage bag creates tension and pulls on the catheter, resulting in trauma to the urethra and/or urinary meatus (Cipa-Tatum et al., 2011). See Boxes 34-8 and 34-9 for evidence-based nursing interventions to prevent CAUTI.

Catheter Removal. A hospital-acquired UTI (HAUTI) is one of the never events identified by the Centers for Medicare and Medicaid Services (CMS) (Saint et al., 2009). Removing an indwelling catheter promptly, after it is no longer needed is a key intervention that decreases the incidence and prevalence of HAUTI. See Skill 34-1 for the steps to remove a catheter. Monitor patients' voiding and urine output after catheter removal by using a voiding record or bladder diary. A bladder diary records the time and amount of each voiding, including any incontinence. Use a bladder scan when needed to monitor bladder functioning and measuring postvoid residual (see Box 34-5). Abdominal pain and distention, a sensation of incomplete emptying, incontinence, constant dribbling of urine, and voiding in very small amounts indicates possible inadequate bladder emptying, which requires intervention.

The risk of UTI increases with the use of an indwelling catheter (Parker et al., 2009). Symptoms of infection can develop 2 to 3 or more days after catheter removal. Patients need to be informed of the risk for infection, prevention measures, and signs and symptoms that need to be reported to the nurse and health care provider.

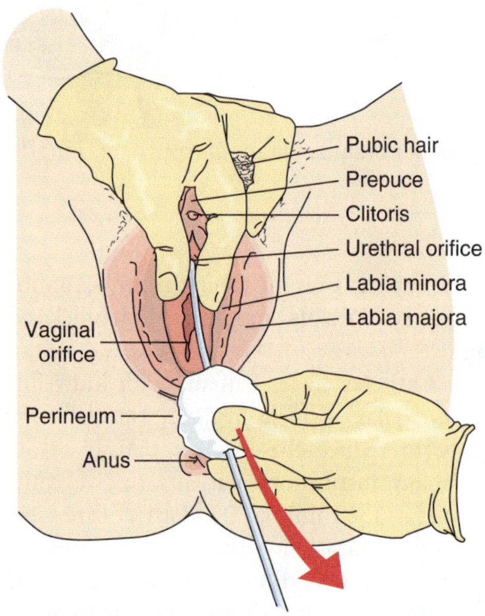

FIGURE 34-10 Cleansing the catheter during catheter care. (From Sorrentino SA, Remmert LA: *Mosby's textbook for nursing assistants*, ed 8, St Louis, 2012, Mosby.)

Suprapubic Catheters. A **suprapubic catheter** is a urinary drainage tube inserted surgically into the bladder through the abdominal wall above the symphysis pubis (Figure 34-11). The catheter is sutured to the skin, secured with an adhesive material, or retained in the

BOX 34-8 PREVENTING CATHETER-ASSOCIATED URINARY TRACT INFECTIONS

- Use aseptic technique with sterile equipment when inserting urinary catheters into patients in an acute care hospital.
- Secure indwelling catheters to prevent movement and pulling on the catheter.
- Maintain a closed urinary drainage system.
- Maintain an unobstructed flow of urine through the catheter, drainage tubing, and drainage bag.
- Keep the urinary drainage bag below the level of the bladder at all times.
- Avoid dependent loops in urinary drainage tubing.
- Prevent the urinary drainage bag from touching or dragging on the floor.
- When emptying the urinary drainage bag, use a separate measuring receptacle for each patient. Do not let the drainage spigot touch the receptacle.
- Before transfers or activity, drain all urine from tubing into bag and empty drainage bag.
- Empty the drainage bag when half full.
- Perform routine perineal hygiene daily and after soiling.
- Obtain urine samples using the sampling port. Cleanse the port with disinfectant. Use a sterile syringe/cannula.
- Ensure quality improvement programs alert providers when a patient has a catheter and include regular educational programming about catheter care.

Data from Gould CV et al: *Guideline for prevention of catheter-associated urinary tract infections,* 2009, http://www.cdc.gov/hicpac/cauti/001_cauti.html. Accessed February 9, 2014.

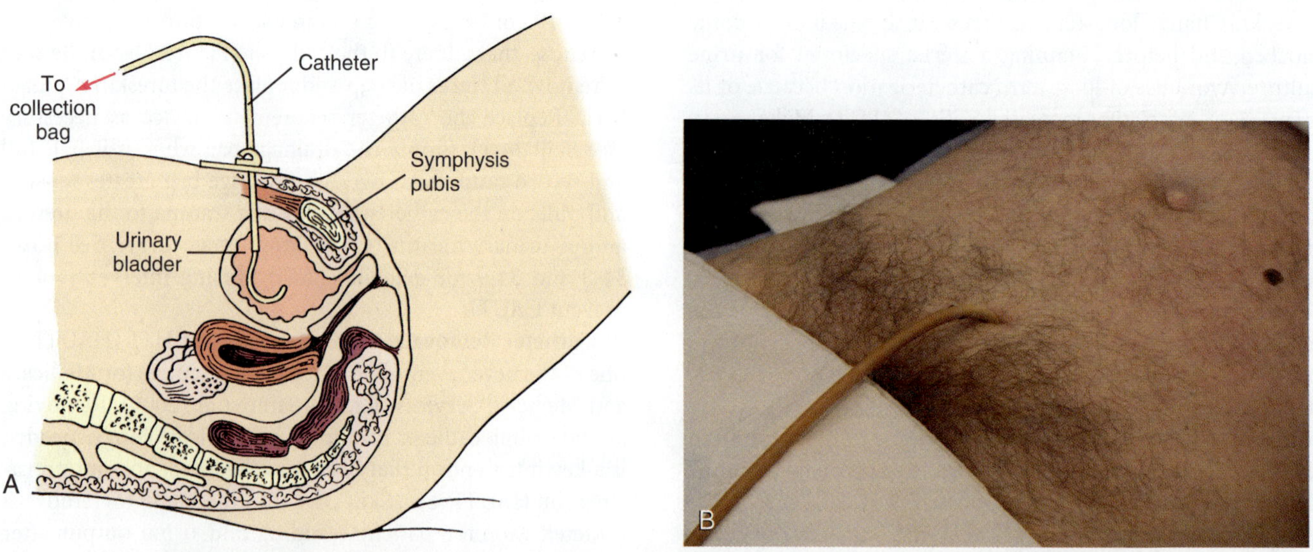

FIGURE 34-11 A, Placement of suprapubic catheter above the symphysis pubis. **B,** Suprapubic catheter without a dressing.

bladder with a fluid-filled balloon similar to an indwelling catheter.

Suprapubic catheters are placed when there is blockage of the urethra (e.g., enlarged prostate, urethral stricture, after urological surgery) and in situations when a long-term urethral catheter causes irritation or discomfort or interferes with sexual functioning.

Care of a suprapubic catheter involves daily cleansing of the insertion site and catheter. The same care for the tubing and drainage bag of a urethral catheter applies for a suprapubic catheter. Assess the insertion site for signs of inflammation and growth of over-granulation tissue. If insertion is new, expect slight inflammation as part of normal wound healing; however, monitor the site carefully because inflammation also indicates infection. Over-granulation tissue can develop at the insertion site as a reaction to the catheter. In some instances intervention is needed. Site care follows principles of applying a dry dressing, and institutional policy indicates if aseptic or sterile technique is required (see Chapter 37).

Condom Catheters. The external catheter, also called a *condom catheter* or *penile sheath,* is a soft, pliable condomlike sheath that fits over the penis, providing a safe and noninvasive way to contain urine. Most external catheters are made of soft silicone that aids in reducing friction and are clear to allow for easy visualization of skin under the catheter. Latex catheters are used by some patients. Verify that a patient does not have a latex allergy before applying this type of catheter. Condom-type external catheters are held in place by either an adhesive coating of the internal lining of the sheath, a double-sided self-adhesive strip, brush-on adhesive applied to the penile shaft, or in rare cases an external strap or tape. They may be attached to a small-volume (leg) drainage bag or a large-volume (bedside) urinary drainage bag, both of which need to be kept lower than the level of the bladder. The condom-type external catheter is suitable for patients who are incontinent and have complete and spontaneous bladder emptying. Condom catheters come in a variety of styles and sizes. Refer to manufacturer guidelines to ensure the best fit and correct application. See Box 34-10 for the steps in applying a condom catheter. Condom catheters are associated with less risk for UTI than indwelling catheters; thus they are an excellent option for a male with UI (Newman and Wein, 2009). For men who cannot be fitted for a condom catheter, there are other externally applied catheters. One type attaches to the glans penis using hydrocolloid strips that stay in place for multiple days and allows intermittent/straight catheterization (Kyle, 2011). Another option available is a reusable condomlike device that is held in place by specially designed underwear.

Urinary Diversions. Immediately after surgery a patient with an incontinent urinary diversion wears a pouch to collect the effluent (drainage). The pouch keeps the patient clean and dry, protects the skin from damage, and provides a barrier against odor. Urinary pouches with an antireflux flap are opaque or clear, drainable one-piece or two-piece pouches, with cut-to-fit or precut wafers. You need to change the pouch every 4 to 6 days (Richbourg et al., 2008). Each pouch may be connected to a bedside drainage bag for use at night.

When changing a pouch, gently cleanse the skin surrounding the stoma with warm tap water using a washcloth and pat dry (Geng et al., 2009). Measure the stoma and cut the opening in the pouch. Apply the pouch after removing the protective backing from the adhesive surface. Press firmly into place over the stoma. Observe the appearance of the stoma and surrounding skin. The stoma is normally red and moist and is located in the right lower quadrant of the abdomen. It is important for the patient to have the correct type and fit of an ostomy pouch. A specialty ostomy nurse is an essential resource when selecting the right appliance so the pouch fits snugly against the surface of the skin

BOX 34-9 EVIDENCE-BASED PRACTICE

PICO Question: Does the implementation of evidence-based nursing protocols decrease the occurrence of urinary tract infections (UTIs) in hospitalized patients with indwelling urinary catheters?

SUMMARY OF EVIDENCE

Catheter-associated UTI (CAUTI) is responsible for 30% or more of infections in the acute care setting and increases length of hospital stay, morbidity, mortality, and cost (Bernard, Hunter, and Moore, 2012). In 2009 the Centers for Disease Control and Prevention (CDC) updated their *Guideline for Prevention of Catheter-Associated Urinary Tract Infections* (Gould et al., 2009). The CDC organized measures to reduce CAUTI into major areas that include appropriate use, proper insertion and maintenance techniques, quality improvement programs and ongoing surveillance for CAUTI, and related causative factors. Current research supports these guidelines. Of particular concern is continued inappropriate catheter practices in high-risk hospitalized older adults. Fakih et al. (2010) showed that elderly patients admitted through the emergency department were more likely than younger patients to have a urinary catheter inserted that did not meet institutional guidelines and disproportionately increased their risk for UTI. Current evidence supports the effectiveness of nurse-driven protocols in reducing unnecessary catheter insertion, the duration of catheter use, and the incidence of CAUTI (Bernard, Hunter, and Moore, 2012; Voss, 2009). However, Fink et al. (2012) found varied implementation of CAUTI prevention measures in acute care hospitals.

APPLICATION TO NURSING PRACTICE

- Become familiar with guidelines related to CAUTI prevention and care.
- Be aware of indications for catheter insertion and advocate for a patient if the indications do not meet accepted guidelines.
- Collaborate with health care providers to remove catheters when medical indications no longer exist.
- Become a patient advocate in your institution through careful adherence to CAUTI preventive practices.

BOX 34-10 PROCEDURAL GUIDELINES

Applying a Condom Catheter

DELEGATION CONSIDERATIONS

The skill of application of a condom catheter can be delegated to nursing assistive personnel (NAP). The nurse instructs NAP to:

- Be sensitive to privacy needs of patients.
- Immediately report any redness, swelling, or skin irritations or breakdown of glans penis or penile shaft.
- Follow manufacturer directions for applying the condom catheter and securing the device.

EQUIPMENT

Condom catheter (includes securing device such as internal adhesive, strap, or tape), collection bag, basin with warm water, towel and washcloth, clean gloves, scissors, hair guard or paper towel, bath blanket, and sheet

STEPS

1. Identify patient using two identifiers (e.g., name and birthday or name and account number) according to agency policy.
2. Perform hand hygiene.
3. Assess urinary elimination patterns, patient's ability to empty bladder effectively, and degree of continence.
4. Assess patient's mental status, knowledge about the procedure, and ability to self-apply device. Explain procedure.
5. Provide for privacy by closing room door or bedside curtain. Raise bed to working height and lower side rail on working side.
6. Prepare condom catheter (prescribed size and type) and drainage bag and tubing (see manufacturer directions). Most manufacturers provide a measuring guide and instructions.
7. Help patient to a supine or sitting position. Place bath blanket over upper torso; fold a sheet over lower torso so only penis is exposed.
8. Apply clean gloves; provide perineal care (see Chapter 29) and dry thoroughly. If patient is uncircumcised, ensure that foreskin is in the normal nonretracted position. Do not apply barrier cream.
9. Assess penis for erythema, rashes, and/or open areas. Apply condom catheters only to intact skin (Newman and Wein, 2009).
10. Clip hair at base of penile shaft as necessary. Do not shave the pubic area. Some manufacturers provide a hair guard, which you place over the penis before applying the device. An alternative to a hair guard is to tear a hole in a paper towel, place it over the penis, and remove after application of the device (Kyle, 2011).
11. Apply condom catheter. With nondominant hand grasp penis along shaft. With dominant hand hold condom sheath at tip of penis and smoothly roll sheath onto penis. Allow 2.5 to 5 cm (1 to 2 inches) of space between tip of penis and end of catheter (see illustration).
12. Secure condom catheter according to manufacturer directions:
    a. Outer securing strip-type catheter: Spiral wrap penile shaft with supplied elastic adhesive. Do not overlap strip, and ensure elastic strip is be snug but not tight (see illustration). **NOTE: Never use adhesive tape.**
    b. Self-adhesive catheter: Apply gentle pressure on penile shaft for 10 to 15 seconds to secure.
13. Connect drainage tubing to end of condom catheter. Be sure that condom is not twisted. Connect catheter to large-volume drainage bag or leg bag.
14. Help patient to a safe, comfortable position. Lower bed and place side rails accordingly.
15. Dispose of contaminated supplies, remove gloves, and perform hand hygiene.
16. Inspect penis with condom catheter in place within 15-30 minutes after application for any swelling, discoloration, or discomfort. Observe for patency of urinary drainage system, characteristics of urine, condition of penis, and proper placement of condom catheter.
17. Remove and reapply daily following the previous steps unless an extended-wear device is used. For removal, wash the penis with warm, soapy water and gently roll the sheath and adhesive off the penile shaft (Kyle, 2011).

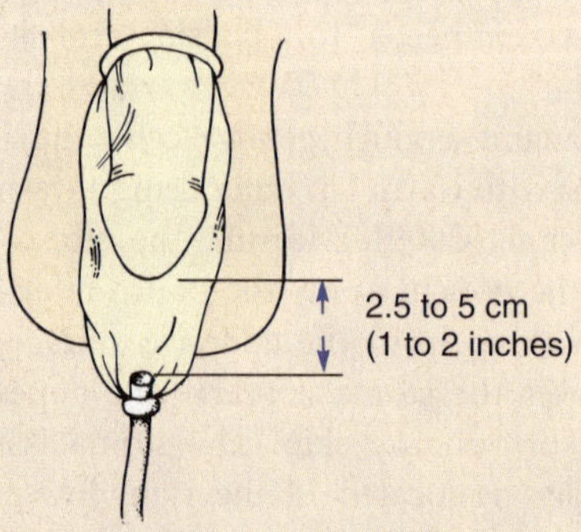

STEP 11 Distance between end of penis and tip of condom.

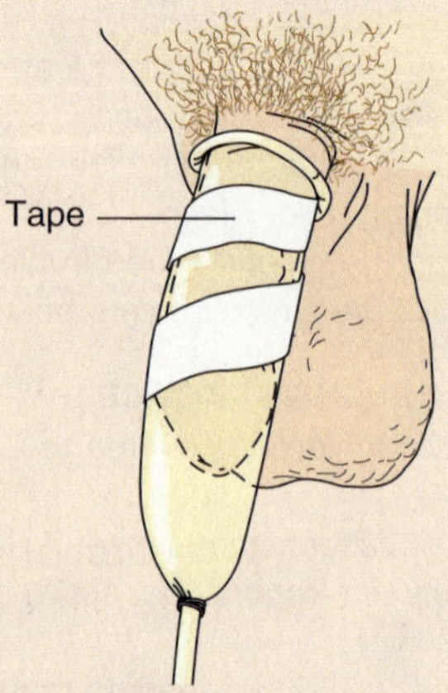

STEP 12a Apply elastic tape in spiral fashion to secure condom catheter to penis.

around the stoma, preventing damaging leakage of urine (see Chapter 35).

Patients with continent urinary diversions do not have to wear an external pouch. However, you need to teach a patient that has a continent urinary reservoir how to intermittently catheterize the pouch. Patients need to be able and willing to do this 4 to 6 times a day for the rest of their lives. After creation of an orthopic neobladder, patients have frequent episodes of incontinence until the neobladder slowly stretches and the urinary sphincter is strong enough to contain the urine. To achieve continence, a patient needs to follow a bladder-training schedule and perform pelvic muscle exercises (Geng et al., 2010). The postoperative care of patients having continent urinary diversions varies widely with the surgical techniques used, and it is important to learn the surgeon's preferred routine or health care facility procedures before caring for these patients.

Medications. Some medications effectively treat urgency UI. The most commonly used are called *antimuscarinics* and include darifenacin, oxybutynin, solifenacin, fesoterodine, tolterodine, and tropsium (Lehne, 2010). The most common adverse effects of the antimuscarinics are dry mouth, constipation, and blurred vision. In some cases these medications cause a change in mental status in older adults (Andersson et al., 2009). Mirabegron, a beta 3-adrenoceptor agonist, is a newer agent that does not have the same adverse effects as the antimuscarinics but causes problems with blood pressure in some patients (Andersson, 2013). Currently there are no medications other than off-label vaginal estrogen to treat stress UI in postmenopausal women (Shamliyan et al., 2012). Be familiar with all the medications your patients take. Be sure you understand why your patient is taking the medications and the potential side effects of each medication.

When caring for a patient newly starting an antimuscarinic, monitor the patient for medication effectiveness, watching for a decrease in UI symptoms such as urgency, frequency, and urgency. A bladder diary that records the time of voiding and any incontinent episodes is one of the best ways to do this. In addition, you need to regularly assess the patient for side effects, including monitoring for constipation, straining during bowel movements, and changes in stool consistency.

Restorative Care. Some techniques improve a patient's control over bladder emptying and restore some degree of urinary continence. These techniques are commonly referred to as *behavioral therapy* and include lifestyle changes, pelvic floor muscle training (PFMT), bladder retraining, and a variety of toileting schedules. In some cases, when the bladder does not empty, patients or caregivers learn to catheterize intermittently. Whenever there is a risk for urine leakage, skin care is an essential component of the plan of care. Adequate urine containment and skin protection promote patient comfort and dignity.

Lifestyle Changes. Teach patients a number of lifestyle modifications to improve bladder function and decrease incontinence. In addition to interventions listed earlier in this chapter under health promotion, teach patients about foods and fluids that cause bladder irritation and increase symptoms of frequency, urgency, and incontinence. Teach patients to avoid common irritants such as artificial sweeteners, spicy foods, citrus products, and caffeine (Jura et al., 2011; Lohsiriwat et al., 2011). Discourage intake of large volumes of fluid in one sitting. Constipation also frequently affects bladder symptoms; implement measures to promote bowel regularity (see Chapter 35). Encourage patients with edema to elevate their feet for a few hours in the afternoon to help reduce nighttime voiding frequency.

Pelvic Floor Muscle Training. Evidence supports that patients with urgency, stress, and mixed UI experience improvement and can eventually achieve continence when treated with PFMT (Shamliyan et al., 2012). PFMT involves teaching patients how to identify and contract the pelvic floor muscles in a structured exercise program (Newman and Wein, 2009). This exercise program is commonly called *Kegel exercises* and is based on therapy first developed by obstetrician gynecologist Dr. Arnold Kegel in the 1940s. The exercises are considered as first-line treatment for women with stress UI, urge UI, and mixed UI (Dumoulin and Hay-Smith, 2010). The exercises work by increasing the pressure in the urethra, strengthening the pelvic floor muscles, and inhibiting unwanted bladder contractions. Many patients benefit from verbal instructions on how to do the exercises (Box 34-11). Consult with a specialist who uses computerized equipment and provides a visual display of muscle activity *(biofeedback)* for patients who are unable to correctly contract the appropriate muscles.

Bladder Retraining. Bladder retraining is a behavioral therapy designed to help patients control bothersome urinary urgency and frequency. Patients learn about their bladder and techniques to suppress urgency. They collaborate with their health care providers to develop a toileting schedule based on their bladder diary. The toileting schedule slowly increases the interval between voiding. Patients need regular support and positive reinforcement during the retraining period. They learn to inhibit the urge to void by taking slow and deep breaths to relax and then performing 5 to 6 quick strong pelvic muscle exercises (flicks) in quick succession (Newman and Wein, 2009). Only highly motivated and cognitively intact patients are candidates for this therapy. You support patients by reinforcing their schedule and providing emotional encouragement.

Toileting Schedules. A key component of any treatment plan for UI is regular toilet access. Toileting schedules need to be individualized based on a patient's type of incontinence and functional disability (e.g., cognitive impairment). Toileting schedules can be implemented in any care setting and are your first plan of action when you determine a patient is incontinent. Timed voiding or scheduled toileting is toileting based on a fixed schedule; it is not based on a patient's urge to void. You set the schedule based on a time interval (i.e., every 2 to 3 hours) or times of day such as before and after meals. It is very successful in adults with moderate-to-severe cognition and mobility impairments. Habit training is a toileting schedule based on a patient's usual voiding pattern. The

BOX 34-11 PATIENT TEACHING

Teaching Pelvic Muscle Exercises (Kegel Exercises)

OUTCOME

At the end of the teaching session the patient is able to demonstrate how to perform pelvic muscle exercises.

TEACHING STRATEGIES

1. Use pictures to teach the patient pelvic anatomy and the location of the pelvic muscles.
2. Teach patient to identify and contract the correct muscle.
   - Women: Instruct the patient to squeeze the anus as if to hold in gas or to insert a finger into the vagina and feel the muscle squeeze around her finger.
   - Men: Instruct the patient to stand in front of a mirror, squeeze the anus as if to hold in gas, and watch to see if the penis moves up and down as he contracts the pelvic floor muscles.
   - Tell the patient to avoid contracting the abdomen, buttocks, or thighs when contracting the pelvic muscles.
3. Teach pelvic muscle contraction exercises.
   - Quick flicks: Squeeze the muscle for 2-3 seconds and relax.
   - Sustained contractions: Squeeze the muscle for 5-10 seconds and relax after each contraction for 10 seconds.
4. Teach patient to maintain a daily exercise schedule.
   - Perform three to five quick flicks followed by five to ten sustained contractions.
   - Repeat these exercises 3-4 times a day.

EVALUATION STRATEGIES

- Ask patient to describe how to do pelvic muscle exercises.
- Observe while patient performs pelvic muscle exercises.
- Assess for symptoms of UI and determine if they are improving.

usual times that a patient voids are identified from a bladder diary. The patient is toileted at these times. Prompted voiding is a program of toileting designed for patients with mild or moderate cognitive impairment. Caregivers ask the patient if he or she is wet or dry, give positive feedback for dryness, prompt the patient to toilet, and reward the patient for desired behavior. Although very successful, this toileting program requires a consistent motivated caregiver, a cooperative patient, and evidence that the patient will void when toileted at least 50% of the time or more (Newman and Wein, 2009).

Intermittent Catheterization. Some patients experience chronic inability to completely empty the bladder because of neuromuscular damage related to multiple sclerosis, diabetes, spinal cord injury, and urinary retention caused by outlet obstruction. To minimize the risk of UTI, patients or caregivers are taught to catheterize the bladder using clean technique. In institutions where there is increased risk for exposure to multiple pathogens, intermittent catheterization follows the principles of asepsis as discussed earlier in the chapter.

BOX 34-12 EVALUATION

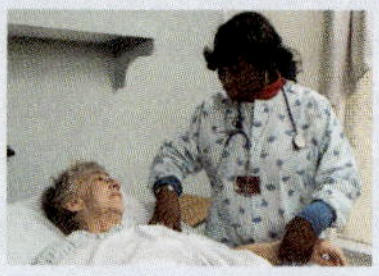

Sandy talks with Mrs. Vallero the next evening. The patient's care plan incorporates timed voiding, oral fluids, and use of double voiding. She palpates Mrs. Vallero's bladder and then assists her to the toilet. After being sure that she is comfortable and leaving the call light in place, Sandy instructs her to double void. She returns to measure Mrs. Vallero's urinary output and evaluates for bladder residual using ultrasound bladder scan.

DOCUMENTATION NOTE

"Patient reports sensation of bladder fullness. Abdomen soft, sensation of bladder fullness over suprapubic area on light palpation. Assisted to bathroom. Gait was slightly unsteady and slow. Breathing was easy and regular. Double voiding technique reinforced. Patient voided 400 mL of clear, pale yellow urine. Stated, 'I don't feel so full now.' Returned to bed. Postvoid residual volume 10 mL using portable ultrasound."

Teach patients and caregivers the importance of adequate fluid intake, signs of infection, and about their individualized catheterization schedule. The goal for intermittent catheterization is drainage of 400 mL of urine, and you individualize the schedule to meet this goal.

Skin Care. Incontinence-associated dermatitis (IAD) is defined as "erythema and edema of the surface of the skin, sometimes accompanied by bullae with serous exudates, erosion, or secondary cutaneous infection" (Gray et al., 2012). It is caused when urine irritates the skin as a result of skin overhydration, increased pH, and friction injury during movement (Gray et al., 2012). Exposure to stool and urine increases the risk for skin injury. Key components for IAD prevention and treatment include gentle skin cleansing with a no-rinse pH balanced cleanser, skin moisturization, and application of a moisture barrier product (Doughty et al., 2012). In some cases patients develop a topical fungal infection that requires treatment with a steroid/antifungal cream or ointment. Typically these patients present with erythema with raised red spots or satellite lesions located near the edge. Patients often state they have intense itchiness. The problem is intensified in patients such as infants or adults who wear absorbent products to absorb urine.

EVALUATION

Patient Care. To evaluate your patient's care plan, use the expected outcomes developed during planning to determine whether interventions were effective (Box 34-12). This evaluation process is dynamic. Use information gathered to modify the plan of care to meet expected outcomes. Evaluate for changes in a patient's voiding pattern and/or presence of symptoms such as dysuria, urinary retention, and UI. If a behavioral plan is in effect, evaluate patient/caregiver compliance with the plan such as toileting according to the schedule or the number of incontinent episodes. Reinforce patient education and explore potential barriers when your patient has difficulty following a behavioral plan.

Patient Expectations. Your patient is the best source of evaluation of outcomes and responses to nursing care. Include patients during evaluation. Encourage patients to express in their own words if their preferences and needs were met. Make revisions based on their feedback. Remember that urinary problems affect a patient physically, emotionally, psychologically, spiritually, and socially. You need to carefully evaluate a patient's self-image, social interactions, sexuality, and emotional status.

SAFETY GUIDELINES FOR NURSING SKILLS

SAFETY CONSIDERATIONS

Ensuring patient safety is an essential role of the professional nurse. To ensure patient safety, communicate clearly with members of the health care team, assess and incorporate the patient's priorities of care and preferences, and use the best evidence when making decisions about your patient's care. When performing the skills in this chapter, remember the following points to ensure safe, individualized care:

- Follow principles of medical and surgical asepsis when performing catheterizations, helping patient with toileting needs, and handling urine specimens.
- Identify patients at risk for latex allergies.
- Identify patients with allergies to povidone-iodine (Betadine). Provide alternatives such as chlorhexidine.

SKILL 34-1 INSERTING AND REMOVING STRAIGHT/INTERMITTENT OR INDWELLING CATHETERS

DELEGATION CONSIDERATIONS

The skill of inserting a straight/intermittent or indwelling catheter cannot be delegated to nursing assistive personnel (NAP). The nurse directs NAP to:

- Assist with patient positioning, focus lighting for the procedure, empty urine from collection bag, and assist with perineal care.
- Report postprocedure patient discomfort, fever, or catheter leakage.
- Report abnormal color, odor, or urine amount.

EQUIPMENT

Catheter Insertion

- Catheter kit containing the following sterile items: (Catheter kits vary; thus it is important to check the list of contents on the package.)

  Straight/Intermittent Catheterization Kit
  - Single-lumen catheter (commonly 12-14 Fr)
  - Drapes (one fenestrated—has an opening in the center, one with no opening)
  - Sterile gloves
  - Lubricant
  - Cleansing solution incorporated in an applicator or to be added to cotton balls (forceps to pick up cotton balls)
  - Specimen container and label

  Indwelling Catheterization Kit
  - Double-lumen catheter (Some kits contain a catheter with attached drainage bag; others contain only a catheter; others have no catheter.)
  - Drapes (one fenestrated—has an opening in the center, one with no opening)
  - Lubricant
  - Cleansing solution incorporated in an applicator or to be added to cotton balls (forceps to pick up cotton balls)
  - Prefilled syringe with sterile water for balloon inflation
  - Sterile drainage tubing and bag (Some kits come preconnected; others do not, and a separate package is required.)
  - Sterile gloves
  - Specimen container and label
- Sterile drainage tubing and bag (if not included in kit)
- Device to secure catheter (catheter strap or other device)
- Extra sterile gloves and catheter (optional)
- Bath blanket
- Waterproof absorbent pad
- Clean gloves, basin with warm water, soap or perineal cleanser, washcloth, and towel for perineal care
- Additional lighting as needed (such as a flashlight or procedure light)
- Measuring container for urine
- Bladder scanner (if available)

Catheter Removal

- Clean gloves
- Waterproof pad
- Bath blanket
- Soap, washcloth, towel, and basin filled with warm water
- 10-mL or larger syringe without needle (Information on balloon size [mL] is printed directly on balloon inflation valve [see Figure 34-9].)
- Graduated cylinder to measure urine
- Toilet, bedside commode, urine "hat," urinal, or bedpan
- Bladder scanner (if available and indicated)

SKILL 34-1 INSERTING AND REMOVING STRAIGHT/INTERMITTENT OR INDWELLING CATHETERS—cont'd

STEP	RATIONALE
ASSESSMENT	
1. Review patient's medical record, including health care provider's order and nurses' notes. Note previous catheterizations, including catheter size, response of patient, and time of catheterization.	Identifies purpose of inserting catheter such as for measurement of residual urine or specimen collection, previous catheter size, and potential difficulty with catheter insertion.
2. Identify patient using two identifiers (e.g., name and birthday or name and account number) according to agency policy. Compare identifiers with information on patient's MAR or medical record.	Ensures correct patient. Complies with The Joint Commission requirements for patient safety (TJC, 2014).
3. Review the medical record for any pathological conditions that will possibly impair passage of the catheter (e.g., enlarged prostate gland in men, urethral strictures).	Obstruction of urethra often prevents passage of catheter into the bladder.
4. Ask patient and check medical record for allergies.	Identifies allergy to components of catheterization kit and/or catheter (e.g., antiseptic, tape, latex).
5. Assess patient's weight, level of consciousness, developmental level, ability to cooperate, and mobility.	Determines positioning for catheterization and indicates how much assistance is needed to properly position patient, ability of patient to cooperate during procedure, and level of explanation needed.
6. Patient's gender and age.	Determines catheter size.

Clinical Decision Point: **Large catheters often damage the urethra and urinary meatus, increase bladder irritability, and cause urine to leak around the catheter because of spasm (Cottenden et al., 2009). Use the smallest size catheter possible to minimize trauma and patient discomfort (Gould et al., 2009).**

STEP	RATIONALE
7. Assess patient's knowledge and prior experience with catheterization and feelings about procedure.	Reveals need for patient instruction and/or support.
8. Assess bladder for fullness by palpating it over symphysis pubis or use bladder scanner if available (see Box 34-5).	Determines if bladder is full or overfull.
9. Perform hand hygiene, apply clean gloves. Inspect perineal area for anatomical landmarks, erythema, drainage or discharge, and odor. Remove gloves and perform hand hygiene.	Assessment of female perineal landmarks improves accuracy and speed of catheter insertion.
PLANNING	
1. Collect appropriate equipment.	
2. Explain procedure to patient.	Promotes cooperation and decreases anxiety.
3. Arrange for extra nursing personnel to assist as necessary.	More than one person is needed to help position patients who are weak, frail, obese, or confused.
IMPLEMENTATION	
1. Perform hand hygiene.	Reduces transmission of microorganisms.
2. Provide privacy by closing room door and bedside curtain.	Protects patient confidentiality.
3. Raise bed to appropriate working height. If side rails in use, raise side rail on opposite side of bed and lower side rail on working side.	Promotes good body mechanics. Use of side rails promotes patient safety.
4. Place waterproof pad under patient.	Prevents soiling bed linen.

Clinical Decision Point: **Obtain assistance to position and support weak, frail, or confused patients.**

STEP	RATIONALE
5. Position and drape patient:	
A. **Female Patient**	
(1) Assist to dorsal recumbent position (supine with knees flexed). Ask patient to relax thighs to externally rotate hip joints.	Provides good visualization of perineal structures and decreases risk for fecal contamination.
(2) Alternate female position: Position side-lying (Sims') position with upper leg flexed at knee and hip. Ensure that rectal area is covered with drape to reduce risk of contamination. Support patient with pillows if necessary to maintain position.	Alternate position is more comfortable if patient cannot abduct leg at hip joint (e.g., patient has arthritic joints or contractures).

STEP	RATIONALE
(3) It is helpful to place blanket diamond fashion over patient, with one corner at patient's neck, side corners over each arm and side, and last corner over perineum (see illustration).	Protects patient dignity by avoiding unnecessary exposure of body parts.
B. **Male Patient**	
(1) Position supine with legs extended and thighs slightly abducted.	Comfortable position for patient that aids in visualization of penis.
(2) Cover upper part of body with small sheet or bath blanket. Cover lower extremities with sheet or blanket, exposing only genitalia (see illustration).	Protects patient dignity by avoiding unnecessary exposure of body parts.
6 Apply clean gloves. Wash perineal area with soap and water and dry (see Chapter 29). Identify urinary meatus. Remove and discard gloves; perform hand hygiene.	Hygiene before catheter insertion removes secretions, urine, and feces that could contaminate the sterile field and increase risk for catheter-associated urinary tract infection (CAUTI).
7. Position light to illuminate genitals or have assistant available to hold light source to visualize urinary meatus.	Adequate visualization of urinary meatus helps with speed and accuracy of catheter insertion.
8. *Perform hand hygiene.*	
9. Open catheterization kit (some products have double wrapping requiring removal of outer wrapper or plastic covering; others require pealing back a paper top). Place opened kit on clean bedside table or, if possible, between patient's open legs. Patient size and positioning dictate exact placement.	Provides easy access to supplies during catheter insertion.
10. If present, open inner sterile wrap covering box using sterile technique (see Chapter 14).	Inner sterile wrap serves as a sterile field. Straight catheterization trays do not routinely come with double wrapping.
A. **Straight/Intermittent Catheterization:** All needed supplies are in sterile tray. You can use the tray that contains supplies for urine collection.	
B. **Indwelling Catheterization Open System:** Open the separate package containing the drainage bag, check to make sure that clamp on drainage port is closed, and place drainage bag and tubing so they are easily accessible. Open outer package of sterile catheter, maintaining sterility of inner wrapper.	An open drainage bag system requires separate sterile packaging for sterile catheter, drainage bag and tubing, and insertion kit.

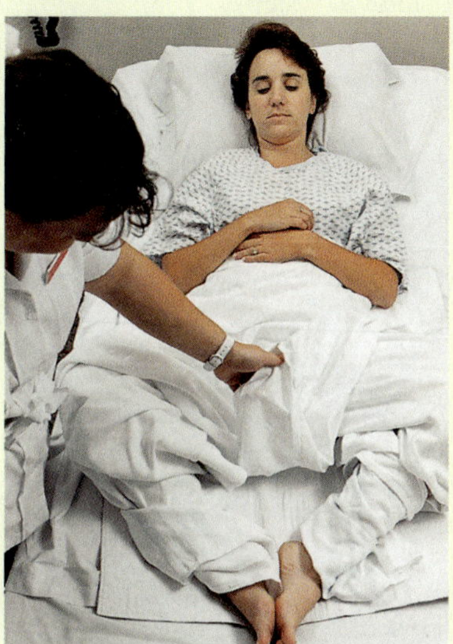

STEP 5A(3) Draping female for catheterization.

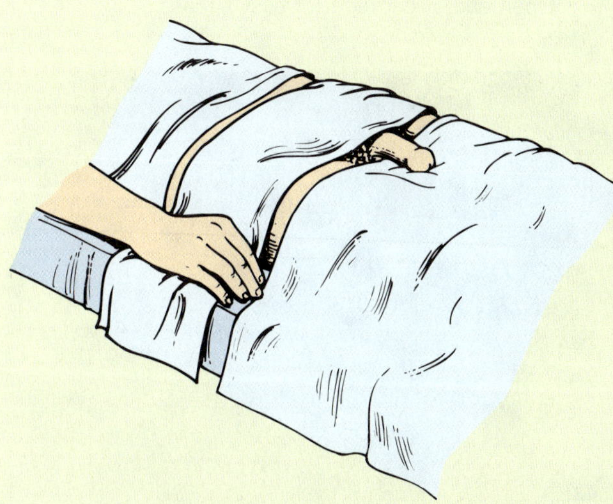

STEP 5B(2) Draping male for catheterization.

SKILL 34-1 INSERTING AND REMOVING STRAIGHT/INTERMITTENT OR INDWELLING CATHETERS—cont'd

STEP	RATIONALE
C. **Indwelling Catheterization Closed System:** All supplies are in sterile tray. Once you put on sterile gloves, check to make sure that clamp on drainage bag is closed.	Closed drainage bag systems have catheter preattached to drainage tubing and bag.

Clinical Decision Point: **The sequence of supplies in a kit varies. In some kits the sterile gloves are below the square sterile drape. In this case you pick up the square drape from the tray by the edges and allow it to unfold without touching unsterile surfaces. Fold away the top edge (sterile side up, hands on the shiny underside) to form a cuff over both hands and carefully place the drape. Then put on your sterile gloves and place the fenestrated drape. Use supplies in order to prevent contamination of underlying supplies.**

STEP	RATIONALE
11. Apply sterile gloves. Drape perineum, keeping gloves sterile.	Sterile drapes provide sterile field over which nurse work during catheterization.
A. **Drape Female**	
(1) Pick up square drape and allow it to unfold without touching unsterile surfaces. Allow top edge of drape to form cuff over both hands. Place drape with shiny side down on bed between patient's thighs. Slip cuffed edge just under buttocks as you ask patient to lift hips. Take care not to touch contaminated surfaces with sterile gloves.	You maintain sterility of gloves and workspace when creating cuff over sterile gloved hands.
(2) Pick up fenestrated sterile drape. Allow drape to unfold without touching unsterile surfaces. Allow top edge of drape to form cuff over both hands. Drape over perineum, exposing labia (see illustration).	Opening in drape creates sterile field around labia.
B. **Drape Male:** Pick up square drape and allow it to unfold without touching unsterile surfaces. Place over thighs with shiny side down, just below penis. Place fenestrated drape with opening centered over penis (see illustration).	
12. Arrange supplies on sterile field, maintaining sterility of gloves. Place sterile tray with cleaning medium (premoistened swab sticks or cotton balls, forceps, and solution) lubricant, catheter, and prefilled balloon inflation syringe (indwelling catheterization only) on sterile drape.	Provides easy access to supplies during catheter insertion and helps to maintain aseptic technique. Appropriate placement is determined by size of patient and position during catheterization.
a. Open package of sterile antiseptic solution; pour cleansing solution over sterile cotton balls. Some kits contain package of premoistened swab sticks instead. Open end of package for easy access.	Use of sterile supplies and antiseptic solution reduces risk of CAUTI (Gould et al., 2009).

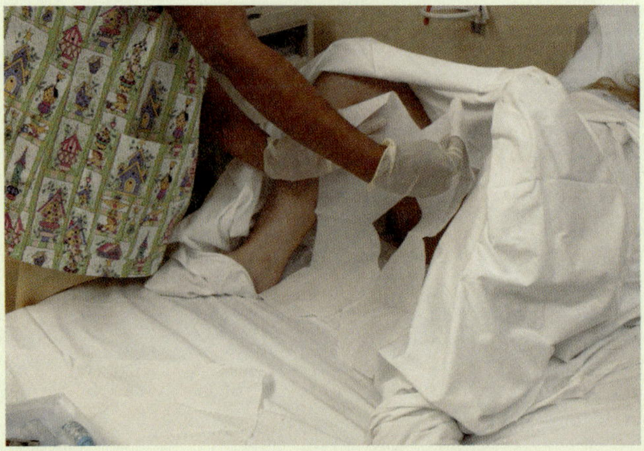

STEP 11A(2) Place sterile fenestrated drape (with opening in center) over perineum with labia exposed.

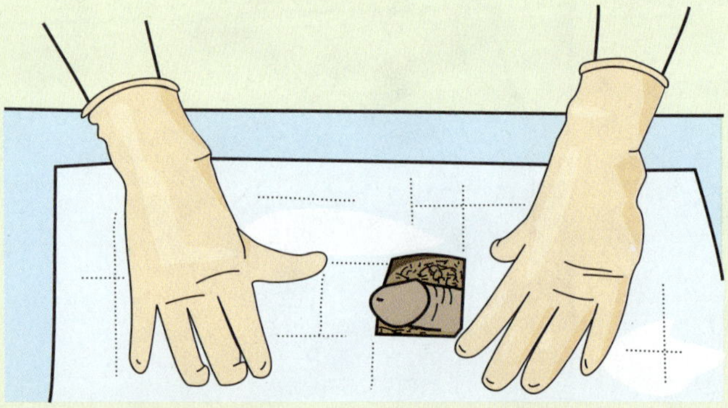

STEP 11B Draping male with fenestrated drape.

STEP	RATIONALE
b. Open sterile specimen container if urine specimen required.	Makes container accessible to receive urine from catheter if specimen is needed.
c. Indwelling catheterization: Open inner sterile wrapper of catheter. If part of kit, remove tray with catheter and attached drainage bag and place on sterile drape. Many kits are a closed system, and catheter is already preattached. Make sure that clamp on drainage port of bag is closed.	

Clinical Decision Point: **Observe contents of catheter trays. Indwelling catheter trays vary. Some have preattached catheters; others need to be attached but are part of the sterile tray; others do not have catheter of drainage system as part of the tray.**

STEP	RATIONALE
d. Open packet of lubricant (lubricant in some kits comes in a syringe) and squeeze out on sterile field. Lubricate catheter by dipping it into water-soluble gel 2.5 cm to 5 cm (1 to 2 inches) for women and 12.5 to 17.5 cm (5 to 7 inches) for men (see illustration).	Lubrication minimizes trauma to urethra and discomfort during catheter insertion. Male catheter needs enough lubricant to cover length of catheter inserted.

Clinical Decision Point: **It is essential to check manufacturer instructions before inserting an indwelling catheter. Some manufacturers do not recommend pretesting the inflation balloon. Pretesting by inflation/deflation of balloon may lead to formation of ridges in balloon, potentially causing trauma on insertion.**

STEP	RATIONALE
13. Cleanse urethral meatus:	
A. Female Patient	
(1) Gently separate labia with fingers of nondominant hand (now contaminated) to fully expose urinary meatus.	Optimal visualization of urethral meatus is possible.
(2) Maintain position of nondominant hand and keep labia spread throughout procedure.	Allows for better visualization of urinary meatus. If the labia closes, the area becomes contaminated and you need to repeat the cleansing procedure.
(3) Holding forceps in dominant hand, pick up one cotton ball or one swab stick at a time. Clean labia and urinary meatus from clitoris toward anus. Use new cotton ball or swab for each area that you cleanse. Cleanse by wiping far labial fold, near labial fold, and directly over center of urethral meatus (see illustration).	Front to back cleansing is cleaning from area of least contamination toward highly contaminated area (see Chapter 37). Dominant gloved hand remains sterile.
B. Male Patient	
(1) With nondominant hand (now contaminated), retract foreskin (if uncircumcised) and gently grasp penis at shaft just below glans. Hold shaft of penis at right angle to body. This hand remains in this position for remainder of procedure.	When grasping shaft of penis, avoid pressure on dorsal surface to prevent compression of urethra. Positioning penis at this 90-degree angle to the patient straightens out curvature of male urethra and eases insertion (Mendez-Probst, 2012).

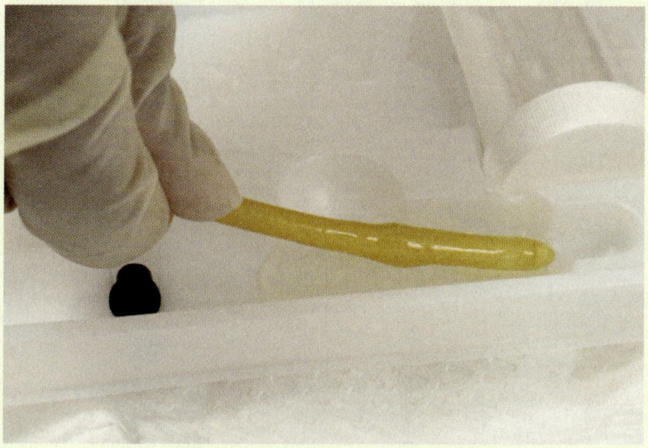

STEP 12d Lubricating catheter.

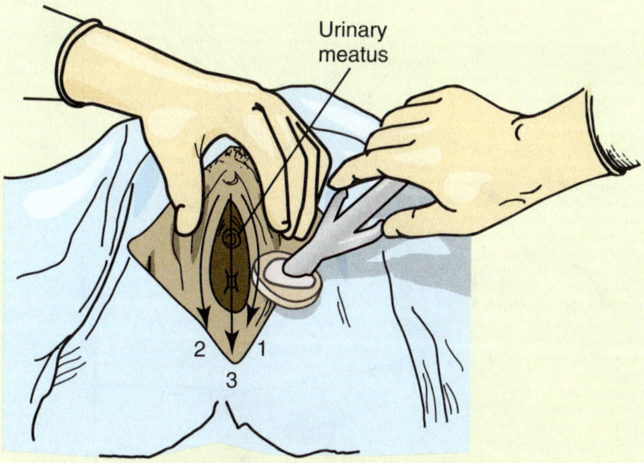

STEP 13A(3) Cleansing female perineum.

SKILL 34-1 INSERTING AND REMOVING STRAIGHT/INTERMITTENT OR INDWELLING CATHETERS—cont'd

STEP	RATIONALE
(2) With uncontaminated dominant hand, cleanse meatus with cotton balls/swab sticks using circular strokes, beginning at meatus and working outward in spiral motion. Repeat 3 times using clean cotton ball/stick each time (see illustration).	Circular cleansing pattern follows principles of medical asepsis (see Chapter 37).
14. Pick up and hold catheter 7.5 to 10 cm (3 to 4 inches) inches from catheter tip with catheter loosely coiled in palm of hand. If catheter is not attached to drainage bag, make sure to position urine tray so end of catheter can be placed there once insertion begins.	Holding catheter near tip allows for easier manipulation and better control of catheter during insertion. Coiling catheter in palm prevents distal end from striking a nonsterile surface.
15. Insert catheter:	
A. **Female Patient**	
(1) Ask patient to bear down gently and slowly insert catheter through urethral meatus (see illustration).	Bearing down helps visualize urinary meatus and promotes relaxation of external urinary sphincter, aiding in catheter insertion.
(2) Advance catheter a total of 5 to 7.5 cm (2 to 3 inches) in adult **or until urine flows out of catheter.** When urine appears, advance catheter another 2.5 to 3 cm (1 to 2 inches). Do not use force to insert catheter.	Urine flow indicates that catheter tip is in bladder.
(3) Release labia but maintain secure hold on catheter.	Prevents accidental dislodgement of catheter.

Clinical Decision Point: **If no urine appears, catheter may be in vagina. If misplaced, leave catheter in vagina as landmark indicating where not to insert and insert another sterile catheter. Never attempt to reinsert the used catheter.**

STEP	RATIONALE
B. **Male Patient**	
(1) Lift penis to position perpendicular (90 degrees) to patient's body and gently apply upward traction to penis (see illustration).	Straightens urethra to ease catheter insertion.
(2) Ask patient to bear down as if to void and slowly insert catheter through urethral meatus.	Relaxation of external sphincter aids in insertion of catheter.
(3) Advance catheter 17 to 22.5 cm (7 to 9 inches) or until urine flows out end of catheter.	Length of the male urethra varies. Flow of urine indicates that tip of catheter, but not necessarily balloon portion of indwelling catheter, is in bladder.

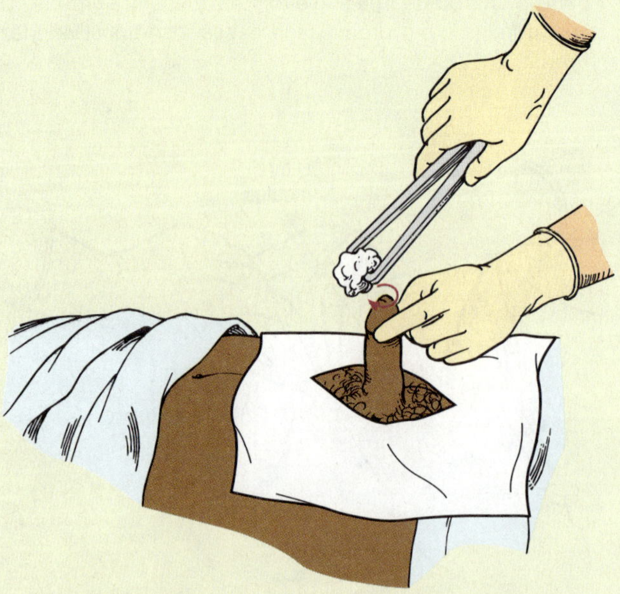

STEP 13B(2) Cleansing male urinary meatus.

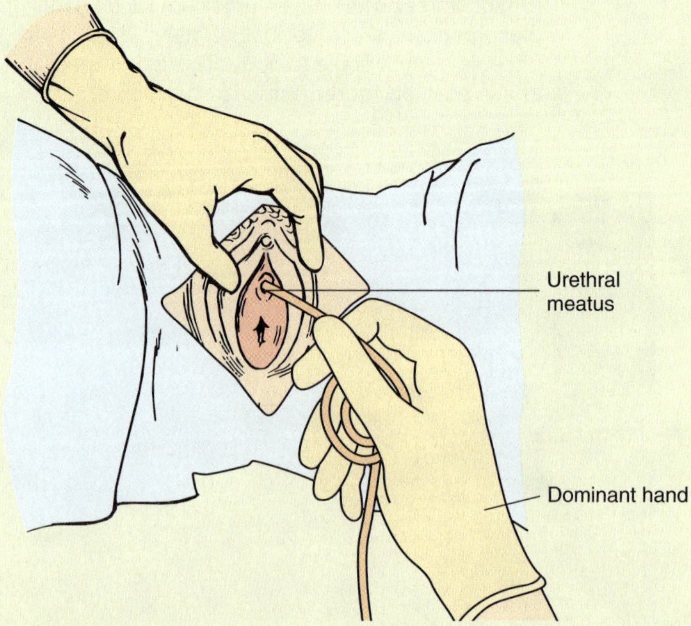

STEP 15A(1) Inserting catheter into female urinary meatus.

STEP	RATIONALE
(4) Stop advancing with a straight catheter. When urine appears in an indwelling catheter, advance it to bifurcation (inflation and deflation port exposed) (see illustration).	There is natural resistance as the catheter passes through the U-shaped bulbar urethra. Further advancement of catheter to bifurcation of drainage and balloon inflation port ensures that balloon portion of catheter is not in prostatic urethra (D'Cruz et al., 2009; Geng et al., 2012; Mendez-Probst et al., 2012; Newman and Wein, 2009).

Clinical Decision Point: **If there is resistance or pain when advancing the catheter, DO NOT USE FORCE and stop catheter advancement. Ask patient to take slow, deep breaths to promote relaxation. Hold catheter gently in place without forcing. After a few seconds the sphincter often relaxes, allowing you to advance the catheter. An inability to advance a catheter may mean an enlarged prostate or some other obstruction of the urethra.**

STEP	RATIONALE
(5) Lower penis and hold catheter securely in nondominant hand.	Prevents accidental dislodgement of catheter.
16. Allow bladder to empty fully unless institution policy restricts maximum volume of urine drained (see agency policy).	No definitive evidence exists regarding whether there is benefit in limiting maximal volume drained.

Clinical Decision Point: **In the case of acute urinary retention (rapid onset) when the volume of urine is known to be excessive (greater than 1 L), notify the health care provider for guidance related to gradual bladder decompression to avoid possible decompression-induced hematuria (Mendez-Probst, 2012).**

STEP	RATIONALE
17. Collect urine specimen as needed by holding end of catheter over cup. Fill to desired level. Label and bag specimen according to agency policy. Send specimen to laboratory as soon as possible.	Obtains sterile specimen for culture analysis. Fresh urine specimen ensures more accurate findings (Pagana and Pagana, 2011).
18. Straight/Intermittent Catheterization: When urine flow stops, withdraw catheter slowly and smoothly until removed.	
19. Indwelling Catheterization: Inflate catheter balloon **with fluid amount designated by manufacturer.**	Do not overinflate or underinflate indwelling catheter balloons to prevent occlusion of catheter drainage holes, balloon distortion, and bladder irritation (Geng et al., 2012, Newman and Wein, 2009). Catheter balloons are only filled with sterile water. Other solutions might precipitate and occlude the fill tubing and catheter balloon fill valve (Mendez-Probst et al., 2012).

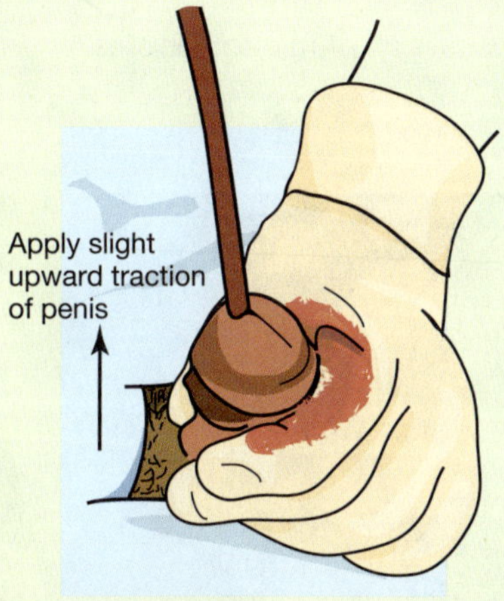

STEP 15B(1) Position of penis perpendicular to body for catheter insertion.

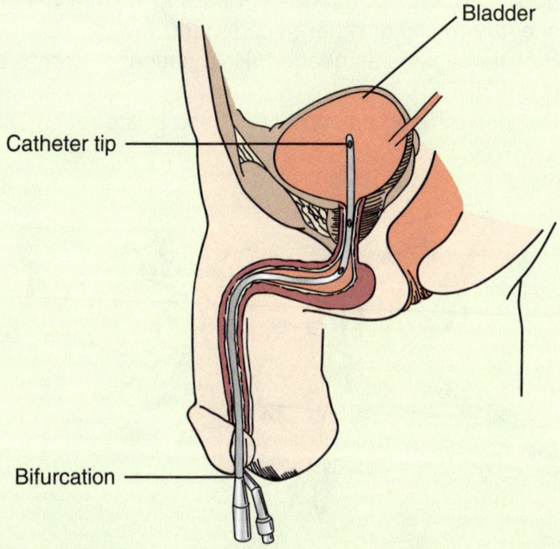

STEP 15B(4) Male anatomy with correct catheter insertion to bifurcation of drainage and balloon inflation port.

SKILL 34-1 INSERTING AND REMOVING STRAIGHT/INTERMITTENT OR INDWELLING CATHETERS—cont'd

STEP	RATIONALE
a. Continue to hold catheter with nondominant hand.	Holding on to catheter before inflating balloon prevents expulsion of catheter from urethra.
b. With free dominant hand connect prefilled syringe to injection port at end of catheter.	
c. Slowly inject total amount of solution (see illustration).	
d. After inflating catheter balloon, release catheter from nondominant hand. *Gently* pull catheter until resistance is felt. Then advance catheter slightly.	Withdrawing catheter places catheter balloon at base of bladder; slight advancement reduces risk of excessive pressure (Geng et al., 2012).
e. Connect drainage tubing to catheter if it is not already preconnected.	

***Clinical Decision Point:* If patient complains of sudden pain during inflation of a catheter balloon or you feel resistance when inflating the balloon, stop inflation, allow the fluid from the balloon to flow back into the syringe, advance catheter further, and reinflate balloon. The balloon may have been inflating in the urethra.**

STEP	RATIONALE
20. Secure catheter with catheter strap or other securement device. Allow enough slack to allow leg movement and avoid any traction on catheter (see illustration). Attach securement device at tubing just above catheter bifurcation.	Securing indwelling catheter reduces risk of urethral trauma, urethral erosion, CAUTI, or accidental removal (Cipa-Tatum et al., 2011; Gould et al., 2009).
A. **Female Patient:** Secure catheter tubing to inner thigh, allowing enough slack to prevent tension.	
B. **Male Patient:**	
(1) Secure catheter tubing to top of thigh or lower abdomen (with penis directed toward chest). Allow slack in catheter so movement does not create tension on catheter.	
(2) If retracted, replace foreskin over glans penis.	Leaving foreskin retracted can cause discomfort and dangerous edema.
21. Clip drainage tubing to edge of mattress. Position drainage bag lower than bladder by attaching to bed frame. Do not attach to side rails of bed or place on floor (see illustration).	Drainage bags that are below the level of the bladder ensure free flow of urine, thus decreasing risk for CAUTI (Gould et al., 2009). Bags attached to movable objects such as a side rail increase risk for urethral trauma caused by pulling or accidental dislodgement (Gould et al., 2009).
22. Check to make sure that there is no obstruction to urine flow. Coil excess tubing on bed and fasten to bottom sheet with clip or other securement device.	Obstruction prevents free flow of urine and decreases risk for CAUTI (Gould et al., 2009).
23. Provide hygiene as needed. Help patient to comfortable position.	
24. Dispose of used equipment in appropriate receptacles.	Reduces transmission of microorganisms.

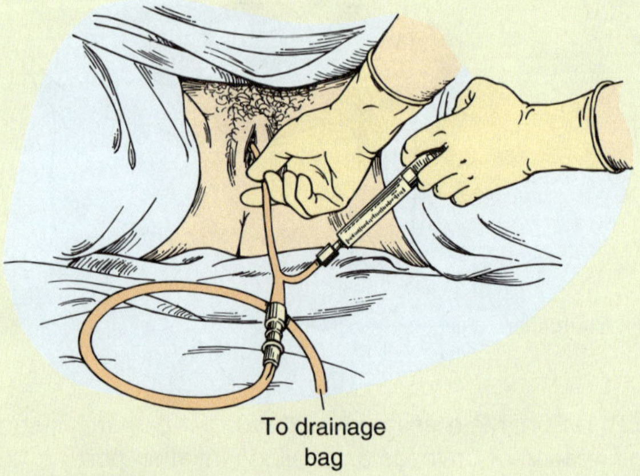

STEP 19c Inflating balloon (indwelling catheter).

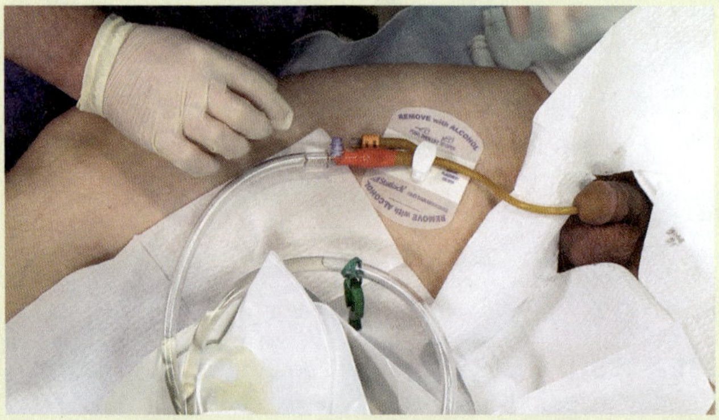

STEP 20 Catheter securement device.

STEP	RATIONALE
25. Label specimen container for culture, place in biohazard container, and send to laboratory.	Ensures prompt diagnostic analysis.
26. Measure urine and record.	
27. Remove gloves and perform hand hygiene.	
28. Removal of indwelling Foley catheter:	
a. Perform hand hygiene, put on clean gloves, and provide privacy.	Procedure requires use of medical asepsis.
b. Prepare patient:	
(1) Provide explanation of procedure.	
(2) Position patient with waterproof pad under buttocks and cover with bath blanket, exposing only genital area and catheter. Position females in dorsal recumbent position and male patients in supine position.	Shows respect for patient dignity by only exposing genital area and catheter.
(3) Remove catheter securement device and free drainage tubing.	
c. If needed, provide hygiene of genital area with soap and water (see Chapter 29).	Current evidence does not consistently show antiseptic cleaners decrease risk for CAUTI (Gould et al., 2009).
d. Move syringe plunger up and down to loosen and withdraw plunger to 0.5 mL. Insert hub of syringe into inflation valve (balloon port). Allow balloon fluid to drain into syringe by gravity. Make sure that entire amount of fluid is removed by comparing removed amount to volume needed for inflation. The amount of fluid in the balloon may be printed on catheter.	Partially inflated balloon traumatizes the urethral wall during removal. Passive drainage of catheter balloon prevents formation of ridges in balloon. These ridges can cause discomfort or trauma during removal.
e. Pull catheter out smoothly and slowly. Encourage patient to use controlled breathing to relax. Examine catheter to ensure that it is whole. Catheter should slide out easily. Do not use force. If you note any resistance, repeat Step 28d to remove remaining water. Notify health care provider if balloon does not deflate completely.	Promotes patient comfort and safety. Controlled breathing distracts patient and relaxes muscles.
f. Wrap contaminated catheter in waterproof pad. Unhook collection bag and drainage tubing from bed.	Prevents transmission of microorganisms.
g. Reposition patient as necessary. Provide hygiene as needed. Lower level of bed and position side rails accordingly.	Promotes patient safety and comfort.
h. Empty, measure, and record urine present in drainage bag. Discard in appropriate receptacle. Perform hand hygiene.	Records urinary output.
i. Encourage patient to maintain or increase fluid intake (unless contraindicated).	Maintains normal urine output.

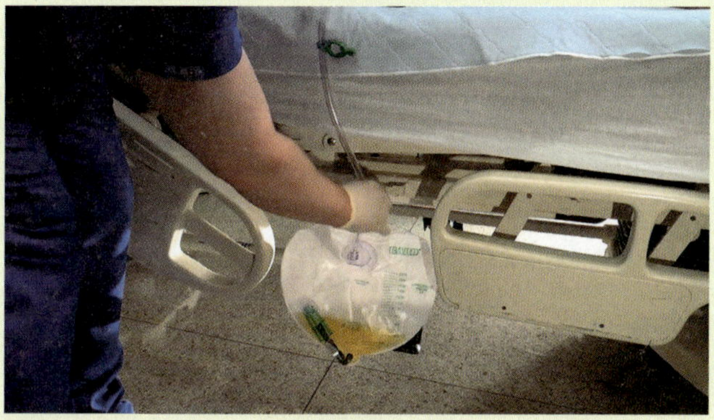

STEP 21 Drainage bag below level of bladder, connected to bed frame.

SKILL 34-1 INSERTING AND REMOVING STRAIGHT/INTERMITTENT OR INDWELLING CATHETERS—cont'd

STEP	RATIONALE
j. Initiate voiding record or bladder diary. Instruct patient to report when urge to void occurs and that all urine needs to be measured. Make sure that patient understands how to use collection container.	Evaluates bladder function.
k. Ensure easy access to toilet, commode, bedpan, or urinal. Place urine "hat" on toilet seat if patient is using toilet. Place call bell within easy reach.	
EVALUATION	
1. Palpate bladder for distention.	Determines if distention is relieved.
2. Ask patient to describe level of comfort.	Determines if patient's sensation of discomfort or bladder fullness has been relieved.
3. Indwelling Catheter: Observe character and amount of urine in drainage system.	Determines if urine is flowing adequately.
4. Indwelling Catheter: Determine that there is no urine leaking from catheter or tubing connections.	Prevents injury to patient's skin and ensures closed sterile system.
5. Observe time and measure amount of first voiding after catheter removal.	Indicates return of bladder function after catheter removal.
6. Evaluate patient for signs and symptoms of urinary tract infection.	Any patient with an indwelling catheter, who has recently had a catheter removed, or who has been recently catheterized is at risk for infection.
7. Use teach back. State to patient, "I want to be sure that I explained why the catheter is in place and why you should not pull on the catheter or drainage tube. Can you tell me why the catheter is in place and why you should not pull on the catheter or tubing?" Revise your instruction now or develop plan for revised patient teaching to be implemented at an appropriate time if patient is not able to teach back correctly.	Evaluates what patient is able to explain or demonstrate.

RECORDING AND REPORTING

- Report and record type and size of catheter inserted, amount of fluid used to inflate balloon, characteristics of urine, amount of urine, reasons for catheterization, specimen or residual collection, patient's response to procedure, and teaching topics.
- Document your evaluation of patient learning.
- Report and record time of catheter removal and time, amount, and characteristics of first voiding.
- Report hematuria, dysuria, inability or difficulty voiding, or incontinence after catheter removal.
- Record intake and output.

UNEXPECTED OUTCOMES AND RELATED INTERVENTIONS

- Patient states has bladder discomfort and/or notices catheter leaking.
  - Check catheter for occlusion of flow. Make sure that there is no traction or pulling and there are no kinks in catheter tubing.
  - Assess for signs of infection.
  - Notify health care provider. Patient may be experiencing bladder spasms or symptoms of a urinary tract infection.
- Patient exhibits one or more of the following: fever, chills, burning sensation, flank pain, back pain, hematuria, painful urination, urgency, frequency, lower abdominal pain, change in mental status, lethargy (Hooton et al., 2010).
  - Monitor vital signs and urine output.
  - Document characteristics of the urine (i.e., color, odor, clarity).
  - Report findings to health care provider; signs and symptoms may indicate a urinary tract infection.
- Patient is unable to void after catheter removal, has a sensation of not emptying, strains to void, or experiences small voiding amounts with increasing frequency.
  - Assess for bladder distention and perform bladder ultrasound (if available) to assess for excessive urine volume in bladder.
  - Assist to a normal position for voiding.
  - If patient is unable to void within 6 to 8 hours of catheter removal and/or experiences abdominal pain, notify health care provider.

KEY POINTS

- Voiding is a complex interaction among the bladder, urinary sphincter, and central nervous system.
- Symptoms common to urinary disturbances include urgency, dysuria, frequency, hesitancy, polyuria, oliguria, nocturia, dribbling, hematuria, and urinary retention.
- Many factors affect voiding such as fluid intake, medications, functional ability, environment, medical problems outside the urinary tract, and dysfunction within the urinary tract.
- UTIs are very common infections. Teach patients healthy bladder habits such as maintaining a healthy fluid intake, good perineal hygiene, and voiding at regular intervals.
- You will usually use a 14 to 16 Fr catheter with a 10-mL balloon when inserting an indwelling catheter in adults to minimize trauma and risk for infection.
- Any patient with an indwelling catheter or who has recently had a catheter is at risk for a UTI.
- Use strict asepsis when caring for a patient with a closed bladder drainage system.
- Incontinence is classified as functional, urge, stress, reflex, and overflow. Each type of incontinence has specific nursing interventions.
- A key component to any treatment plan for UI is regular toilet access.

CRITICAL DECISION-MAKING EXERCISES

Mrs. Vallero is now voiding and her postvoid residual urine measurements are less than 20 mL. Her latest urine testing showed that she did not have a urinary tract infection (UTI). She has an overactive bladder and neurogenic bladder (because of her diabetes). She tells you that that she is afraid of voiding in bed during the night and gets up numerous times "just in case." Mrs. Vallero tells Sandy that she has limited her outside activities because of being afraid of "having an accident and wetting myself." She says that nothing can be done for her because "incontinence is a normal part of getting old."

1. Formulate a priority nursing diagnosis for the patient.
2. Develop a corresponding goal and plan of care for question 1.
3. How would you respond to Mrs. Vallero's statement that urinary incontinence is a normal part of aging?
4. Keeping in mind that Mrs. Vallero has a history of urinary retention and diabetes, what is the most important health information you need to provide at this time?

evolve

Answers to Clinical Decision-Making Exercises can be found on the Evolve website.

QSEN ACTIVITY: QUALITY IMPROVEMENT

The patient care unit is evaluating a quality improvement (QI) project focused on reducing catheter-associated urinary tract infections (CAUTIs) (a never event). Urinary tract infections (UTIs) are common health care–associated infections. A high percentage of hospital-acquired UTIs are caused by urinary catheterization, resulting in longer hospital stays, increased costs, and increased mortality.

Which nursing care activities would Sandy, the nursing student, expect to find on the QI tool, and which data would indicate that the QI project was successful?

evolve

Answers to QSEN Activities can be found on the Evolve website.

REVIEW QUESTIONS

1. Place the following steps for insertion of an indwelling catheter in a female patient in appropriate order.
   1. Insert and advance catheter.
   2. Lubricate catheter.
   3. Inflate catheter balloon.
   4. Cleanse urethral meatus.
   5. Drape patient with the sterile square and fenestrated drapes.
   6. When urine appears advance another 2.5 to 5 cm.
   7. Prepare sterile field and supplies.
   8. Gently pull catheter until resistance is felt.
   9. Attach drainage tubing.
2. A patient's health care provider orders a postvoid residual urine volume by either bladder scan or straight catheterization. The patient states an inability to void. What is your *initial* nursing intervention?
   1. Implement measures to stimulate voiding.
   2. Catheterize the patient and record the amount of urine obtained.
   3. Measure bladder volume with the bladder scan and record the volume.
   4. Notify the health care provider that the patient cannot void.
3. Which nursing intervention decreases the risk for catheter-associated urinary tract infection (CAUTI)?
   1. Daily cleansing the urinary meatus with antiseptic solution
   2. Hanging the urinary drainage bag below the level with the bladder
   3. Changing the urinary drainage bag daily
   4. Irrigating the urinary catheter with sterile water
4. Which nursing action helps prevent trauma in a male patient with an indwelling urinary catheter?
   1. Applying a catheter securement device
   2. Washing the catheter with soap and water

3. Keeping the foreskin retracted while the catheter is in
4. Securing the drainage bag to patient's walker

5. What is the recommended catheter and balloon size for an indwelling catheter for an adult patient with urinary retention?
   1. 10 Fr, 3 mL
   2. 14 Fr, 30 mL
   3. 16 Fr, 10 mL
   4. 20 Fr, 10 mL
6. An elderly woman with dementia is incontinent of urine. She ambulates with a cane, has poor short-term memory, and never alerts staff that she has an urge to void. The staff do not usually see her using the toilet. What is the best nursing intervention for this patient?
   1. Offer her a bedpan every 2 hours.
   2. Start a scheduled toileting program.
   3. Recommend an indwelling catheter.
   4. Start a bladder-retraining program.
7. Describe normal findings on a nursing assessment of voided urine.
8. The urine flow has stopped in a patient's indwelling urinary catheter, and the nurse assesses tenderness and distention over the lower abdomen. What is your initial nursing action?
   1. Check the drainage tubing for kinks.
   2. Encourage patient to drink fluids.
   3. Remove the catheter.
   4. Notify the health care provider.
9. What does a nurse teach a female patient recovering from a urinary tract infection about prevention? (Select all that apply.)
   1. Keep the bowels regular.
   2. Limit water intake to 1 to 2 glasses a day.
   3. Wear cotton underwear.
   4. Cleanse the perineum from front to back.
10. A healthy 50-year-old male has a history of prostate disease. Which nursing assessment question *best* indicates that he is not emptying his bladder completely and has overflow incontinence?
    1. Do you leak urine when you cough or sneeze?
    2. Do you need help getting to the toilet?
    3. Do you dribble urine constantly?
    4. Does it burn when you pass your urine?

evolve

Rationales for Review Questions can be found on the Evolve website.

1. 5, 7, 2, 4, 1, 6, 3, 8, 9; **2.** 1; **3.** 2; **4.** 1; **5.** 3; **6.** 2; **7.** See Evolve; **8.** 1; **9.** 1, 3, 4; **10.** 3

REFERENCES

Ackley BJ, Ladwig GB: *Nursing diagnosis handbook: a guide for planning care*, ed 7, St Louis, 2011, Mosby.

American Academy of Pediatrics (AAP): Ritual genital cutting of female minors, *Pediatrics* 125(5):1088, 2010.

Andersson K: New developments in the management of overactive bladder: focus on mirabegron and onabutulinumtoxin A, *Ther Clin Risk Manag* 9:161, 2013.

Andersson K, et al: Pharmacological treatment of urinary incontinence. In Abrams P, et al, editors: *Incontinence*, ed 4, Paris, France, 2009, Health Publications.

Beji NK, et al: Overview of the social impact of urinary incontinence with a focus on Turkish women, *Urol Nurs* 30(6):327, 2010.

Bernard MS, Hunter KF, Moore KN: A review of strategies to decrease the duration of indwelling urethral catheters and potentially reduce the incidence of catheter-associated urinary tract infections, *Urol Nurs* 32(1):29, 2012.

Cipa-Tatum J, et al: Urethral erosion: a case for prevention, *J Wound Ostomy Continence Nurs* 38(5):581, 2011.

Cottenden A, et al: Management using continence products. In Abrams P, et al, editors: *Incontinence*, ed 4, Paris, France, 2009, Health Publications.

D'Cruz R, et al: Catheter balloon-related urethral trauma in children, *J Paediatr Child Health* 45:564, 2009.

Dumoulin C, Hay-Smith J: Pelvic floor muscle training versus no treatment, or inactive control treatments, for urinary incontinence in women, *Cochrane Database Syst Rev* 20(1):CD005654, 2010.

Doughty D, et al: Incontinence-associated dermatitis consensus statements, evidence-based guidelines for preventions and treatment, and current challenges, *J Wound Ostomy Continence Nurs* 39(3):303, 2012.

Elsamara SE, Ellsworth P: Effects of analgesic and anesthetic medications on lower urinary tract function, *Urol Nurs* 32(2):60, 2012.

Fakih MG, et al: Urinary catheters in the emergency department: very elderly women are at high risk for unnecessary utilization, *Am J Infect Control* 38(9):683, 2010.

Fink R, et al: Indwelling urinary catheter management and catheter-associated urinary tract infection prevention practices in Nurses Improving Care for Healthsystem Elders hospitals, *Am J Infect Control* 10:1, 2012.

Geng V, et al: Good practice in health care incontinent urostomy, *Eur Assoc Urol Nurses* 2009, http://files.sld.cu/urologia-enfermeria/files/2012/06/eaun_iu_guidelines_en_2009_lr.pdf. Accessed February 9, 2014.

Geng V, et al: Good practice in health care continent urinary diversion, *Eur Assoc Urol Nurses* 2010, http://www.uroweb.org/fileadmin/user_upload/EAUN/EAUN_Guidelines/0628EAUN_Guideline_2010_HR.PDF. Accessed February 9, 2014.

Geng V, et al: Evidence-based guidelines for best practice in urological health care: catheterisation indwelling catheters in adults urethral and suprapubic, *Eur Assoc Urol Nurses* 2012, http://www.uroweb.org/fileadmin/EAUN/guidelines/EAUN_Paris_Guideline_2012_LR_online_file.pdf. Accessed February 9, 2014.

Gomelsky A, Dmochowski RR: Urinary incontinence in the aging female, *Aging Health* 7(1):79, 2011.

Gould CV, et al: *Guideline for prevention of catheter-associated urinary tract infections*, 2009, http://www.cdc.gov/hicpac/cauti/001_cauti.html. Accessed February 9, 2014.

Gray M, Moore KN: *Urologic disorders: adult and pediatric care*, St Louis, 2009, Mosby.

Gray M, et al: Incontinence-associated dermatitis: a comprehensive review and update, *J Wound Ostomy Continence Nurs* 39(1):61, 2012.

Gupta K, et al: International clinical practice guidelines for the treatment of acute uncomplicated cystitis and pyelonephritis in women: a 2010 update by the Infectious Disease Society of America and the European Society for Microbiology and Infectious Diseases, *Clin Infect Dis* 52(5):e103, 2011, http://cid.oxfordjournals.org/content/52/5/561.full. Accessed February 9, 2014.

Hagglund D: A systematic literature review of incontinence care for persons with dementia: the research evidence, *J Clin Nurs* 19:303, 2009.

Hall SA, et al: Associations of commonly used medications with urinary incontinence in a community-based sample, *J Urol* 188(1):183, 2012.

Harris C, Smith PP: Overactive bladder in the older woman, *Clin Geriatr* 18(9):41, 2010.

Haylen BT, et al: An International Urogynecological Association (IUGA)/International Continence Society (ICS) joint report on the terminology for female pelvic floor dysfunction, *Neurourol Urodyn* 29(1):4, 2009.

Hooton TM, et al: Diagnosis, prevention, and treatment of catheter-associated urinary tract infection in adults: 2009 international clinical practice guidelines from the Infectious Diseases Society of America, *Clin Infect Dis* 50:625, 2010.

Huether SE, McCance KL: *Understanding pathophysiology*, ed 5, St Louis, 2012, Mosby.

Jura YH, et al: Caffeine intake, and the risk of stress, urgency and mixed urinary incontinence, *J Urol* 185(5):1775, 2011.

Kyle G: The use of urinary sheaths in male incontinence, *Br J Nurs* 20(6):338, 2011.

Lee PG, et al: The co-occurrence of chronic diseases and geriatric syndromes: the health and retirement study, *J Am Geriatr Soc* 57:511, 2009.

Lehne RA: *Pharmacology for nursing care*, ed 7, St Louis, 2010, Saunders.

Lo E, et al: Strategies to prevent catheter-associated urinary tract infections in acute care hospitals, *Infect Control Hosp Epidemiol* 30(4):404, 2009.

Lohsiriwat S, et al: Effect of caffeine on bladder function in patients with overactive bladder symptoms, *Urol Ann* 3(1):14, 2011.

Mendez-Probst CE, et al: Fundamentals of instrumentation and urinary tract drainage, In Wein A, et al, editors: *Campbell-Walsh urology*, ed 10, Philadelphia, 2012, Saunders.

Newman DK, Wein AJ: *Managing and treating urinary incontinence*, ed 2, Baltimore, 2009, Health Professions Press.

Pagana KD, Pagana TJ: *Mosby's diagnostic and laboratory test reference*, ed 10, St Louis, 2011, Mosby.

Parker D, et al: Nursing interventions to reduce the risk of catheter-associated urinary tract infection, *J Wound Ostomy Continence Nurs* 36(1):23, 2009.

Purnell LD: *Guide to culturally competent heath care*, ed 2, Philadelphia, 2009, FA Davis.

Richbourg L, et al: Ostomy wear time in the United States, *J Wound Ostomy Continence Nurs* 35(5):504, 2008.

Saint S, et al: Catheter-associated urinary tract infection and the Medicare rule changes, *Ann Intern Med* 150(12):877, 2009.

Schabelman E, Witting M: The relationship of radiocontrast, iodine, and seafood allergies: a medical myth exposed, *J Emerg Med* 39(5):701, 2010.

Seidel HM, et al: *Mosby's guide to physical examination*, ed 7, St Louis, 2011, Mosby.

Shamliyan T, et al: *Nonsurgical treatments for urinary incontinence in adult women: diagnosis and comparative effectiveness*, Comparative Effectiveness Review No. 36 (Prepared by the University of Minnesota Evidence-based Practice Center under Contract No. HHSA 290-2007-10064-I.) AHRQ Publication No. 11(12)-EHC074- EF. Rockville, MD, 2012, Agency for Healthcare Research and Quality, http://www.effectivehealthcare.ahrq.gov/ehc/products/169/1021/CER36_Urinary-Incontinence_execsumm.pdf. Accessed February 9, 2014.

The Joint Commission (TJC): *National Patient Safety Goals*, Oakbrook Terrace, IL, 2014, The Commission. Available at http://jointcommission.org/standards_information/npsgs.aspx.

Touhy TA, Jett KF: *Ebersole and Hess' gerontological nursing & healthy aging*, St Louis, 2010, Mosby.

Voss AMB: Incidence and duration of urinary catheters in hospitalized older adults before and after implementing a geriatric protocol, *J Gerontol Nurs* 35(6):35, 2009.

Wagg A, et al: Review of cognitive impairment with antimuscarinic agents in elderly patients with overactive bladder, *Int J Clin Pract* 64(9):1279, 2010.

Willson M, et al: Evidence-based report card: nursing interventions to reduce the risk of catheter-associated urinary tract infection. Part 2: Staff education, monitoring, and care techniques, *J Wound Ostomy Continence Nurs* 36(2):137, 2009.

Wyndaele JJ, et al: Neurologic urinary and faecal incontinence. In Abrams P, et al, editors: *Incontinence*, ed 4, Paris, France, 2009, Health Publications.

CHAPTER 35

Bowel Elimination

evolve WEBSITE

http://evolve.elsevier.com/Potter/essentials

- Video Clips
- Crossword Puzzle
- Audio Glossary

OBJECTIVES

- Explain the physiology of digestion, absorption, and bowel elimination.
- Discuss physiological and psychological factors that influence bowel elimination.
- Describe common physiological alterations in bowel elimination.
- Assess a patient's bowel elimination pattern.
- Perform a fecal occult blood test.
- List nursing diagnoses related to alterations in bowel elimination.
- Administer an enema.
- Remove a fecal impaction.
- List nursing measures aimed at promoting normal elimination and defecation.
- Describe nursing care required to manage a fecal diversion.

KEY TERMS

cathartics, p. 1010
colon, p. 994
colonoscopy, p. 1002
constipation, p. 994
defecation, p. 994
diarrhea, p. 996
enema, p. 1011
fecal impaction, p. 996
fecal incontinence, p. 997
fecal occult blood test (FOBT), p. 1002
feces, p. 994
flatus, p. 994
hemorrhoids, p. 997
ileus, p. 1011
laxatives, p. 1010
melena, p. 1001
ostomy, p. 997
peristalsis, p. 993
stoma, p. 997

Regular bowel elimination is essential to maintain a healthy body. Alterations in bowel elimination are often early signs or symptoms of problems either within the gastrointestinal (GI) or other body systems. Because bowel function depends on the balance of several factors, elimination patterns and habits vary among individuals.

Individuals of any age sometimes experience changes in intestinal elimination. These changes are often the result of illness, medications, diagnostic testing, or surgical intervention. Aging when accompanied by chronic illness, cognitive decline, decreased mobility, and a decrease in food and fluid intake changes digestive system function; but aging alone does not necessarily alter the digestive process. Alterations in intestinal elimination respond to both preventive and supportive nursing care.

SCIENTIFIC KNOWLEDGE BASE

Anatomy and Physiology of the Gastrointestinal Tract

The GI tract is a series of hollow mucous membrane–lined muscular organs that begin at the mouth and end at the

CASE STUDY *Mr. Gutierrez*

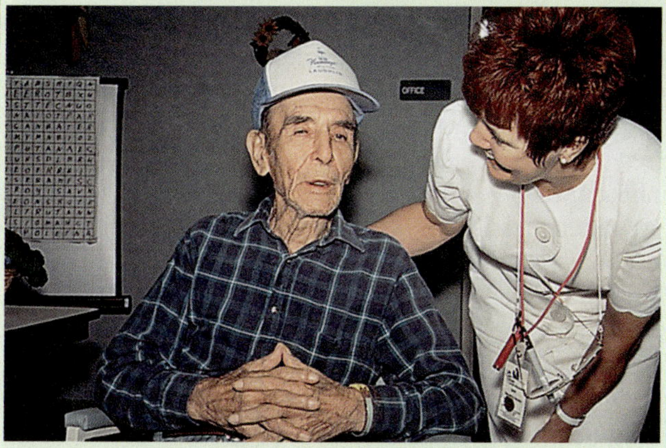

Mr. Gutierrez resides in an assisted-living apartment of a long-term care center. He keeps busy in his small garden plot and enjoys other activities of the center such as nightly card/bingo games and outings to major league baseball games and local museums. He is 82 years old and widowed and has lived in this area of the care center for over 3 years. His family, with whom he is quite close, is scattered across the country. He has one niece who lives in the same town. Mr. Gutierrez believes that he is in good health. As long as he eats green chili peppers every day, he believes that he will remain healthy. Because he has a small kitchen in his apartment, he is able to make some of his favorite foods. His diet consists of flour and corn tortillas, beans, and rice. He likes most meats, but he prefers chicken and *asado* (made with pork). For breakfast he usually has huevos rancheros. He has been hospitalized only twice, once for the flu and once for placement of a pacemaker. He presently takes three medications: digoxin, Zestril, and Metamucil.

This afternoon Mr. Gutierrez has telephoned his niece for the fourth time. He reports, "My bowels are locked up and haven't moved in the last 2 days." He ate a big meal the previous evening and now reports feeling "all gassed up." His niece tried to explain about eating foods containing fiber and more vegetables. She reminded Mr. Gutierrez that the nursing student was coming later this afternoon and he could talk to the student about his problem.

Vickie is the nursing student assigned to Mr. Gutierrez. She has been seeing him once a week for 5 weeks as a part of a home health care clinical experience. They have developed a good rapport. Mr. Gutierrez's self-identified problems with his bowels are a frequent topic of conversation.

anal orifice. The functions of the GI tract are to break down ingested food for use by body cells and promote the absorption of fluid and nutrients. It is a complex system, and changes in any one part alter the function of other parts (Figure 35-1).

Mouth. The mouth mechanically and chemically breaks down nutrients into usable size and form. The teeth chew food, breaking it down into a size suitable for swallowing. Saliva, produced by the salivary glands in the mouth, dilutes and softens the food in the mouth for easier swallowing. Enzymes in saliva begin the breakdown of food.

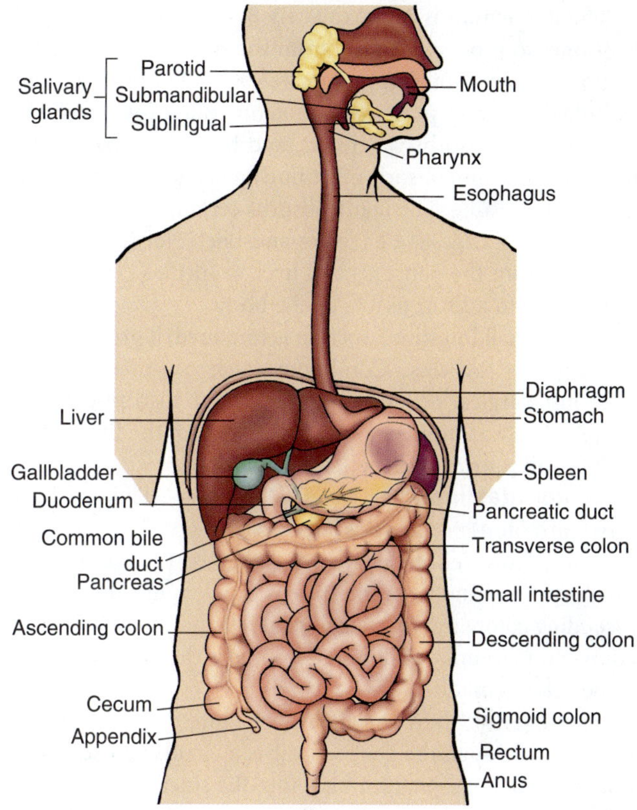

FIGURE 35-1 Gastrointestinal system. (From Monahan FD, Neighbors M: *Medical-surgical nursing,* ed 2, Philadelphia, 1998, Saunders.)

Esophagus. As food enters the upper esophagus, it passes through the upper esophageal sphincter, a circular muscle that prevents air from entering the esophagus and food from refluxing into the throat. The bolus of food travels down the esophagus with the aid of **peristalsis,** which is a contraction that propels food through the length of the GI tract. The food moves down the esophagus and reaches the cardiac sphincter, which lies between the esophagus and the upper end of the stomach. The sphincter prevents reflux of stomach contents back into the esophagus.

Stomach. The stomach performs three tasks: storing the swallowed food and liquid, mixing food with digestive juices, and regulating the emptying of its contents into the small intestine. The stomach produces and secretes hydrochloric acid (HCl), mucus, the enzyme pepsin, and intrinsic factor. Pepsin and HCl facilitate the digestion of protein. Mucus protects the stomach mucosa from acidity and enzyme activity. Intrinsic factor is essential in preparing vitamin B_{12} for absorption in the ileum.

Small Intestine. Movement within the small intestine, occurring by peristalsis, facilitates both digestion and absorption. Food comes into the small intestine as a semifluid material and mixes with digestive juices. Resorption in the small intestine is so efficient that, by the time the fluid reaches the end of the small intestine, it is semisolid in consistency. The small intestine is divided into three sections: the duodenum, the jejunum, and the ileum.

The duodenum is approximately 8 to 11 inches long and continues to process the fluid from the stomach. The second section, the jejunum, is approximately 8 feet long and absorbs carbohydrates and proteins. The ileum is approximately 12 feet long and absorbs water, fats, and bile salts. The duodenum and jejunum absorb most nutrients and electrolytes in the small intestine. The ileum absorbs certain vitamins, iron, and bile salts. Digestive enzymes and bile enter in the small intestine from the pancreas and liver to further break down nutrients into a form usable by the body.

When small intestine function is impaired, it greatly alters the digestive process. Conditions such as inflammation, infection, surgical resection, or obstruction disrupt peristalsis, reduce absorption, or block the passage of the fluid. Electrolyte and nutrient deficiencies then develop.

Large Intestine. The lower GI tract is called the *large intestine* (colon) because it is larger in diameter than the small intestine. However, its length (1.5 to 1.8 m [5 to 6 feet]) is much shorter. The large intestine is divided into the cecum, ascending colon, transverse colon, descending colon, sigmoid colon, and rectum (see Figure 35-1). It is the primary organ of bowel elimination.

The digestive fluid enters the large intestine by waves of peristalsis through the ileocecal valve, a circular muscle layer that prevents regurgitation back into the small intestine. The muscular tissue of the colon allows it to accommodate and eliminate large quantities of waste and gas (flatus). The colon has three functions: absorption, secretion, and elimination. It resorbs a large volume of water (up to 1.5 L) and significant amounts of sodium and chloride daily. The amount of water absorbed depends on the speed at which colonic contents move. Normally the fecal matter becomes a soft, formed solid or semisolid mass. If peristalsis is abnormally fast, there is less time for water to be absorbed, and the stool is watery. If peristaltic contractions slow, water continues to be absorbed, and a hard mass of stool forms, resulting in constipation.

Peristaltic contractions move contents through the colon. Intestinal content is the main stimulus for contraction. Mass peristalsis pushes undigested food toward the rectum. These mass movements occur only 3 or 4 times daily, with the strongest during the hour after mealtime.

The rectum is the final portion of the large intestine. Normally it is empty of waste products (feces) until just before defecation. The rectum contains vertical and transverse folds of tissue that help to control expulsion of fecal contents during defecation. Each fold contains veins that can become distended from pressure during straining. This distention results in hemorrhoid formation.

Anus. The body expels feces and flatus from the rectum through the anus. Contraction and relaxation of the internal and external sphincters, which are innervated by sympathetic and parasympathetic nerves, aid in the control of defecation. The anal canal contains a rich supply of sensory nerves that allow people to tell when there is solid, liquid, or gas that needs to be expelled and aids in maintaining continence.

Defecation. The physiological factors essential to bowel function and defecation include normal GI tract function, sensory awareness of rectal distention and rectal contents, voluntary sphincter control, and adequate rectal capacity and compliance (Huether et al, 2012). Normal defecation begins with movement in the left colon, moving stool toward the anus. When stool reaches the rectum, the distention causes relaxation of the internal sphincter and an awareness of the need to defecate. At the time of defecation the external sphincter relaxes, and abdominal muscles contract, increasing intrarectal pressure and forcing the stool out. Normally defecation is painless, resulting in passage of soft, formed stool. Straining while having a bowel movement indicates that the patient may need changes in diet or fluid intake or that there is an underlying disorder in GI function.

NURSING KNOWLEDGE BASE

To manage your patient's elimination problems, you need to understand normal elimination and factors that promote, impede, or cause alterations in elimination such as constipation, diarrhea, and fecal incontinence (Box 35-1). Supportive nursing care respects each patient's privacy and emotional needs, and interventions designed to promote normal bowel elimination minimize discomfort.

Any alteration in bowel elimination is embarrassing for a patient. Because of the sensitivity that many patients experience with bowel elimination and its associated sounds and odors, be very sensitive about how you communicate, especially nonverbally. A patient may perceive changes in facial expression as disgust. In addition, be aware of a patient's need for privacy during elimination.

Patients with chronic diseases of the GI system often have numerous hospitalizations, perhaps multiple surgeries, and significant changes in eating habits and lifestyles. They are often on complicated medication schedules that are taxing both physically and financially. Their desire for wellness sometimes leads them to consider alternative forms of medical treatment such as vitamin or herbal supplements. Always remain accepting of a patient's health care choices.

Some patients with chronic GI diseases require an ostomy, which involves the surgical creation of a stoma on the abdomen for the passage of stool. An ostomy results in body image changes and loss of control over a very basic body function. It takes time to adjust to an ostomy; but learning how to care for the ostomy and having a reliable pouching system that prevents leakage of the fecal output and odor help the patient to make this adjustment. A trained ostomy nurse should be asked to see the patient with a new ostomy if one is available.

Bowel Elimination Problems

Alterations in bowel elimination are caused by a variety of factors. Some of the more common ones are described in the following paragraphs.

Constipation. Constipation is defined as having fewer than three bowel movements per week, >25% of which are hard and require straining to evacuate the fecal matter (Spinzi, 2009). Constipation is most often caused by changes in diet, medications, mobility, inflammation, environmental factors

BOX 35-1 FACTORS INFLUENCING BOWEL ELIMINATION

AGE

- Infants have a smaller stomach capacity, less secretion of digestive enzymes, and more rapid intestinal peristalsis. The ability to control defecation does not occur until 2 to 3 years of age.
- Adolescents experience rapid growth and increased metabolic rate. There is also rapid growth of the large intestine and increased secretion of gastric acids to dissolve food fibers and act as a bactericide against swallowed organisms.
- Older adults may have decreased chewing ability. Partially chewed food is not digested as easily. Peristalsis declines, and esophageal emptying slows. This impairs absorption by the intestinal mucosa. Muscle tone in the perineal floor and anal sphincter weakens, causing difficulty in controlling defecation (NIDDK, 2012).

DIET

- Regular daily food intake promotes peristalsis.
- High-fiber foods (e.g., fruits, greens, and other vegetables) and whole grains (cereals and breads) promote peristalsis and defecation by creating bulk.
- Low-fiber foods (e.g., pasta, white rice, white bread, cheese) slow peristalsis.
- Gas-producing foods (e.g., broccoli, cauliflower, onions, dried beans) stimulate peristalsis.
- People with lactose intolerance lack the enzyme lactase, which is needed to digest the simple sugars in milk. Such intolerance leads to diarrhea and cramping.
- People with gluten intolerance experience pain, bloating, diarrhea, or constipation.

POSITION DURING DEFECATION

- A sitting position allows a person to lean forward, exert intraabdominal pressure, and contract thigh muscles for normal defecation.
- Older adults or those with chronic pain or immobility may have difficulty sitting down on or rising from a toilet seat. Modifications such as an elevated toilet seat and chair arms on the sides of the toilet may help to promote regular bowel elimination.
- Immobilized patients required to use a bedpan while lying down cannot contract muscles to defecate.

PREGNANCY

- As pregnancy advances and the fetus enlarges, this exerts pressure on the rectum. Constipation commonly occurs.

DIAGNOSTIC TESTS

- Certain examinations involving visualization of gastrointestinal (GI) structures require the emptying of bowel contents. Patients receive nothing by mouth (NPO) or only clear liquids, bowel evacuants, and enema administration to cleanse the bowel before the test. This is called *bowel prep* and temporarily interferes with normal elimination.
- Barium examinations require ingestion of barium, a mixture that can cause constipation unless the barium is eliminated soon after a test.

FLUID INTAKE

- When there is adequate fluid intake (1.5-2 L/day), the body absorbs fluid into the fecal mass and increases bulk for easier passage.
- Warm beverages and fruit juices soften stool and increase peristalsis.
- Caffeinated drinks in moderation may stimulate peristalsis.

ACTIVITY

- Immobilization depresses colon motility.
- Regular physical exercise promotes peristalsis.

PSYCHOLOGICAL FACTORS

- Stress, anxiety, or fear initiates parasympathetic impulses, causing the acceleration of digestion and peristalsis. Diarrhea and gaseous distention result.
- Emotional depression decreases peristalsis and leads to constipation.

PERSONAL HABITS

- Personal habits such as failing to respond to the need to defecate and lack of privacy interfere with normal elimination patterns and lead to constipation.
- Hospitalized patients often share toilet facilities or use bedpans or bedside commodes. The resulting embarrassment causes them to ignore the urge to defecate.

PAIN

- Hemorrhoids, rectal surgery, and abdominal surgery cause a patient to suppress defecation because of pain; constipation develops.

MEDICATIONS

- Laxatives and cathartics soften stool and promote peristalsis.
- Antidiarrheal agents inhibit peristalsis.
- Opiates and anticholinergic drugs depress peristalsis and cause constipation.
- Antibiotics alter normal bowel flora and often produce diarrhea.
- Drugs that contain iron sometimes turn the stool black. Antacids cause a white discoloration. Anticoagulants can cause frank or occult blood in the stool.

SURGERY AND ANESTHESIA

- General anesthetics cause slowing or halting of peristalsis.
- Surgery involving bowel manipulation may temporarily stop peristalsis, creating a condition called *paralytic ileus,* which lasts for hours or days and resolves spontaneously.

(e.g., unavailability of toilet facilities or lack of privacy), and lack of knowledge about regular bowel habits. It is not a physiological response to aging, but changes in mobility and co-morbidities that occur with aging make this condition more prevalent in the elderly (Spinzi, 2009). Regardless of etiology, intestinal motility slows, causing prolonged exposure of the fecal mass to the intestinal wall. Liquid from the feces continues to be absorbed, leaving the stool hard and dry (Box 35-2).

Constipation has significant health implications. Straining during defecation causes problems for patients with recent abdominal, gynecological, or rectal surgery. An effort to pass a stool can cause stress and pain in the surgical site. In addition, patients with cardiovascular disease, diseases causing elevated intraocular pressure (glaucoma), and increased intracranial pressure need to prevent constipation and avoid straining to have a bowel movement.

BOX 35-2 COMMON CAUSES OF CONSTIPATION

- Irregular bowel habits and ignoring the urge to defecate
- Chronic illnesses (e.g., Parkinson's disease, multiple sclerosis, rheumatoid arthritis, chronic bowel diseases, depression, eating disorders)
- Low-fiber diet high in animal fats (e.g., meats and carbohydrates); low fluid intake
- Stress (e.g., illness of a family member, death of a loved one, divorce)
- Physical inactivity
- Medications, overuse of laxatives
- Changes in life or routine such as pregnancy, aging, and travel
- Neurological conditions that block nerve impulses to the colon (e.g., stroke, spinal cord injury, tumor)
- Chronic bowel dysfunction (e.g., colonic inertia, irritable bowel)

Data from National Institute of Diabetes, Digestive and Kidney Diseases (NIDDK): *Health information for the public,* 2012, http://www.niddk.nih.gov. Accessed October 23, 2013.

Impaction. Fecal impaction results from unrelieved constipation. The patient is unable to expel the hardened feces retained in the rectum. In severe impaction the hardened fecal mass extends up into the sigmoid colon. Patients at greatest risk for impaction include those who are confused or unconscious, weak, or unaware of the need to defecate or those who have experienced an interruption in nerve supply to the bowel. An obvious sign of impaction is the inability to pass a stool for several days, despite a repeated urge to defecate. Continuous oozing of liquid stool after several days with no fecal output may indicate an impaction. Loss of appetite, abdominal distention and cramping, nausea and/or vomiting, and rectal pain also occur.

Diarrhea. Diarrhea is an increase in the number of stools and the passage of liquid, unformed stools (Table 35-1). It is associated with disorders affecting digestion, absorption, and secretion in the GI tract. Some of the most common causes are infection, inflammation, and food intolerance (Huether et al., 2012). Intestinal contents pass too quickly through the small intestine and colon to allow for the usual absorption of fluid and nutrients. Dehydration leading to fluid and electrolyte and acid-base imbalances can result from diarrhea. Older adults and the very young are at the greatest risk for dehydration (Box 35-3). Persistent diarrhea may cause skin breakdown in the perianal region.

A common cause of diarrhea in health care facilities is *Clostridium difficile,* in which symptoms range from mild to severe diarrhea. This infection is acquired by use of

TABLE 35-1 CONDITIONS THAT CAUSE DIARRHEA

CONDITION	PHYSIOLOGICAL EFFECTS
Intestinal infection (streptococcal or staphylococcal enteritis)	Inflammation of intestinal mucosa, increased mucus secretion
Food allergies	Abnormal digestion of food elements, increased mucus secretion
Food intolerance (lactose, gluten, high fat, coffee, alcohol, spicy foods)	Abnormal digestion of food elements, increased mucus secretion
Tube feedings	Hyperosmolarity of some enteral solutions results in diarrhea because hyperosmolar fluids draw fluids into the gastrointestinal tract
Medications	
Iron supplements	Irritation of intestinal mucosa
Antibiotics	Loss of normal flora, susceptibility to opportunistic infection
Laxatives (short term)	Increased intestinal motility and irritability
Inflammatory bowel disease (colitis, Crohn's disease)	Inflammation and ulceration of intestinal walls, reduced absorption of fluids, increased intestinal motility
Surgical alterations	
Gastrectomy	Loss of reservoir function of stomach, improper absorption because food moves into duodenum too quickly
Intestinal resection	Reduced length of intestine, reduced amount of absorptive surface
Emotional stress (anxiety)	Increased intestinal motility

antibiotics that depress natural intestinal flora, allowing an overgrowth of *C. difficile,* and by contact with the *C. difficile* organism. The best ways to prevent the occurrence and spread of *C. difficile* is cautious use of antibiotics and rigorous hand hygiene with soap and water (Cohen et al., 2010). Communicable foodborne pathogens also cause diarrhea. Simple handwashing after using the bathroom and before and after meal preparation and careful cleansing and storing of fresh produce and meats help to reduce foodborne illnesses.

Fecal Incontinence. Fecal incontinence is the inability to control the passage of feces and gas from the anus. It may be a temporary or permanent condition. Fecal incontinence is underreported because of shame or a sense that nothing can be done about it, but it affects up to 20% of community-living adults and nearly 50% of nursing home residents (Leung and Rao, 2009). It is embarrassing and may cause social isolation and loss of intimacy. A person may be mentally alert but physically unable to avoid uncontrolled defecation. Impairment of anal sphincter function or control may cause incontinence. Conditions that create frequent, large-volume, watery stools predispose to fecal urgency and incontinence. Like diarrhea, incontinence predisposes a patient to skin breakdown. Management of fecal incontinence requires a complete understanding of the causes.

Flatulence. Flatulence (having accumulated gas) is one of the most common GI disorders. It refers to a sensation of bloating and abdominal distention accompanied by excess gas. As gas accumulates in the lumen of the intestines, the bowel wall stretches and distends. Normally intestinal gas escapes through the mouth (belching) or the anus. However, when intestinal motility is reduced as a result of such things as medications, general anesthetics, abdominal surgery, or immobilization, flatulence may become severe, causing abdominal distention and sharp pain.

Hemorrhoids. Hemorrhoids are dilated, engorged veins in the lining of the rectum. Increased venous pressure resulting from straining at defecation, pregnancy, and chronic illnesses such as congestive heart failure and chronic liver disease are causative factors. A hemorrhoid forms either within the anal canal (internal) or through the opening of the anus (external). Passage of hard stool causes hemorrhoid tissue to stretch and bleed. Hemorrhoid tissue becomes inflamed and tender, and patients complain of itching and burning. Because pain worsens during defecation, the patient sometimes ignores the urge to defecate, resulting in constipation.

Intestinal Diversions. Certain diseases or surgical alterations make the normal passage of intestinal contents throughout the small and large intestine difficult or inadvisable. When these conditions are present, a temporary or permanent opening (stoma) is surgically created by bringing a portion of the intestine out through the abdominal wall. These surgical openings are called an *ileostomy* or *colostomy*, depending on which part of the intestinal tract is used to create the stoma (Figures 35-2 and 35-3). Newer surgical techniques allow more patients to have portions of their small and large intestine removed and the remaining portions to be reconnected so they can continue to defecate through the anal canal.

Ostomies. The location of an ostomy determines stool consistency. The more intestine remaining, the more formed and normal the stool. For example, an ileostomy bypasses the entire large intestine, creating frequent, liquid stools. A person with a sigmoid colostomy has a more formed stool.

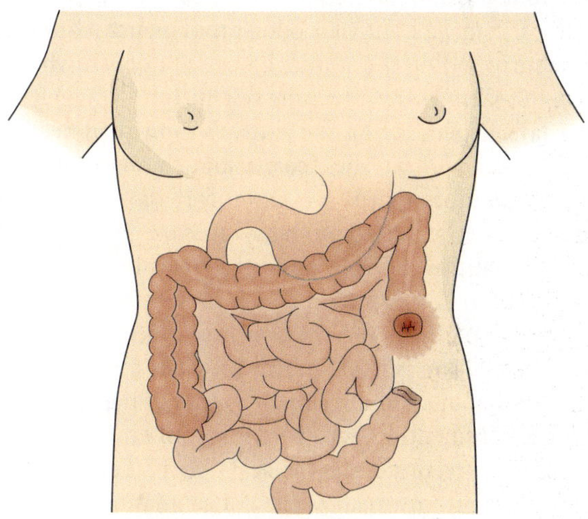

FIGURE 35-2 Sigmoid colostomy.

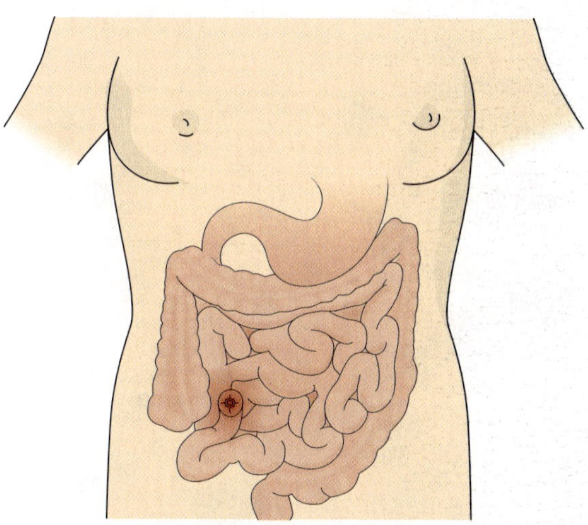

FIGURE 35-3 Ileostomy.

BOX 35-3 SIGNS OF DEHYDRATION

Signs of dehydration in adults include the following:
- Thirst
- Less frequent urination than usual
- Dark-colored urine
- Dry skin
- Fatigue
- Dizziness
- Light-headedness

Signs of dehydration in infants and young children include the following:
- Dry mouth and tongue
- No tears when crying
- No wet diapers for 3 hours or more
- Sunken eyes, cheeks, or soft spot in the skull
- High fever
- Listlessness or irritability

Loop ostomies are frequently performed on an emergency basis and are reversible stomas that may be constructed in the ileum or the colon. The surgeon pulls a loop of intestine onto the abdomen and places a plastic rod, bridge, or rubber catheter temporarily under the bowel loop to keep it from slipping back. He or she then opens the bowel and sutures it to the skin of the abdomen. The loop ostomy has two openings through the stoma. The proximal end drains fecal effluent, and the distal portion drains mucus.

An end colostomy consists of a stoma formed by bringing a piece of intestine out through a surgically created opening in the abdominal wall, turning it down like a turtleneck and suturing it to the abdominal wall (Figure 35-2). The intestine distal to the stoma is either removed or sewn closed (called *Hartmann's pouch*) and left in the abdominal cavity. End ostomies may be permanent or reversible. The rectum may be left intact or removed.

Managing a stoma that produces frequent passage of liquid stool (e.g., an ileostomy) can be challenging. Skin protection is important because of the liquid and caustic nature of the output, which may cause irritant dermatitis. The more common peristomal skin problems are contact dermatitis, fungal infections, or folliculitis (Goldberg et al., 2010). An ostomy is managed with an odor-proof pouch with a skin barrier surrounding the stoma. Empty the pouch when it is ⅓ to ½ full. Change the pouching system approximately every 3 to 7 days, depending on the patient's individual needs.

Other Procedures. The ileoanal pouch anastomosis is a surgical procedure that is an option for some patients who need to undergo a colectomy (removal of the colon) for treatment of ulcerative colitis or familial polyposis. In this procedure the colon is removed, a pouch is created from the end of the small intestine, and the pouch is attached to the anus (Figure 35-4). The ileoanal pouch provides for collection of waste material in a fashion similar to that of the rectum. The patient is continent of stool because stool evacuates via the anus. When surgeons create the ileal pouch, they also make a temporary ileostomy to allow the pouch anastomosis to heal.

A continent ileostomy involves creating a pouch from the small intestine. This procedure is rarely done now; however, there are still patients who had this procedure in the past. The pouch has a continent stoma on the abdomen created with a valve that can be drained only when the patient places a large catheter into the stoma. The patient empties the pouch several times a day.

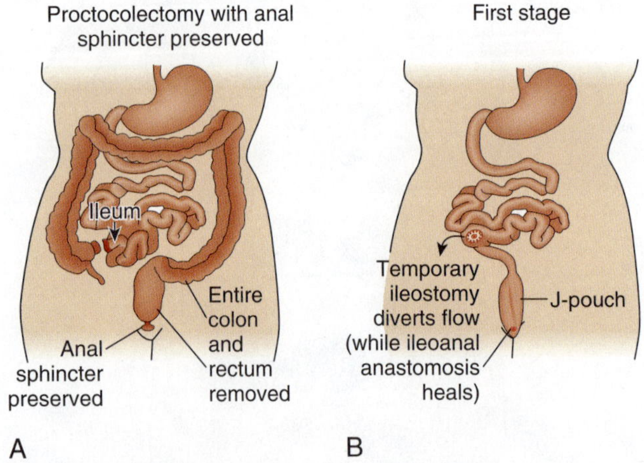

FIGURE 35-4 Ileal pouch anal anastomosis.

The antegrade continence enema (ACE) procedure is usually done in children with fecal soiling associated with neuropathic or structural abnormalities of the anal sphincter. A continence valve with an opening on to the abdomen is surgically created in the intestine so the patient or caregiver can insert a tube and give himself or herself an enema that comes out through the anus. Colonic evacuation begins about 10 to 20 minutes after the patient receives the enema fluid.

CRITICAL THINKING

Synthesis

You apply elements of critical thinking whenever you perform the nursing process with a patient. Consider the scientific knowledge you have learned, your experience, critical thinking attitudes, and standards to ensure an individualized approach to patient care (Box 35-4).

BOX 35-4 SYNTHESIS IN PRACTICE

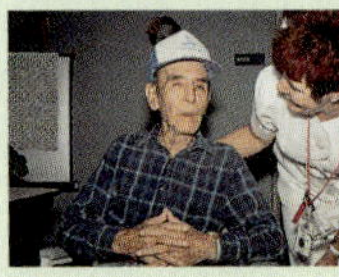

As Vickie prepares to assess Mr. Gutierrez, she reflects back on experiences with other patients in the home setting. She recalled one patient in particular who had elimination problems resulting from a diet consisting mainly of high-fat and high-carbohydrate foods. She believes that her involvement with that patient is likely to help in the care of Mr. Gutierrez.

Vickie also reviews her class notes on the anatomy and physiology of the gastrointestinal (GI) system. Given Mr. Gutierrez's age, Vickie reviews the physiological changes that aging produces within the digestive system. These changes include loss of teeth, taste bud atrophy, decreased secretion of gastric acid, and a slight decrease in small intestine motility.

Vickie thoroughly assesses Mr. Gutierrez's dietary intake by using a 24-hour diet recall. Being familiar with Mr. Gutierrez's Hispanic heritage, Vickie anticipates certain food preferences and needs to assess these. She knows that Mr. Gutierrez does not like the food served at the long-term care center and frequently requests "home-cooked" tortillas and green chili peppers from his niece.

The symptoms that Mr. Gutierrez exhibits (i.e., no bowel movement in 2 days and a feeling of bloating) are associated with several different problems. Vickie plans a thorough and precise assessment, being sure to rule out any abdominal discomfort or other symptoms expected from elimination problems. Because problems with bowel elimination have been an ongoing concern for Mr. Gutierrez, Vickie uses her assessment to identify nursing diagnoses and outline goals of care. She needs to avoid preconceived ideas regarding constipation in older adults. She must remain open to all of the possibilities concerning changes in GI functioning.

Knowledge. Reflect on knowledge regarding normal anatomy and physiology of the GI tract and specific GI alterations. This information helps you more accurately focus your nursing assessment and identify alterations when they exist. Even insignificant alterations in bowel elimination produce significant health problems for patients. For example, diarrhea leads to electrolyte imbalances, dehydration, and rectal soreness.

Abdominal pain is one of the most common complaints of patients who seek health care. Apply knowledge of the nature of pain (see Chapter 32) and pain assessment to analyze elimination problems. This helps to determine if the pain causes the symptoms associated with altered bowel elimination or if the bowel elimination problem results in pain or discomfort.

Functional bowel disorders make up the most frequently reported GI complaints. It is important that you have the knowledge from anatomy and physiology and information from the psychosocial sciences to understand and consider the psychological aspects associated with these diseases to provide appropriate care.

The intake of certain foods also reflects a patient's culture or beliefs. Foods in various cultures have different status relating to religion, availability, cost, and tradition. Understand the patient's cultural heritage and the role diet plays in health promotion and maintenance (see Chapter 20). When caring for patients from other cultures and ethnic groups, modifications of care are frequent. This is particularly important when you care for patients' elimination needs (Box 35-5).

Experience. Elimination alterations are common for many patients who seek health care. In the acute care environment numerous variables, including diet changes, medications, fluid restrictions, decreased activity, and diagnostic tests and surgery, cause major alterations to bowel function. You provide better care to patients by reflecting on your previous experiences involving patients with similar alterations and lifestyle habits affecting elimination.

Attitudes. Apply all of the attitudes of critical thinking when caring for patients with elimination problems (see Chapter 8). Creativity comes into play, especially when patients need adjustments in their diet and exercise planning or when caring for patients with an intestinal diversion. Similarly perseverance is important in selecting effective diet therapies or finding the right medication regimen for patients with constipation or diarrhea. Confidence is an important factor in providing care to patients with bowel diversions or resections. Often these patients are very ill and in significant pain. Your confidence with moving and positioning a patient, managing ostomy care, and managing pain places the patient at ease and facilitates the recovery process.

Standards. To establish regular bowel habits, patients require consistency in bowel care and training. It is possible to establish regular bowel habits by setting standards for appropriate nutritional and elimination support. For example, the Association for Parenteral and Enteral Nutrition (ASPEN) has specific guidelines for nutritional support (see Chapter 33). The Wound, Ostomy and Continence Nurses Society (Goldberg et al., 2010) has specific standards for ostomy care. Regardless of age or disease state, maintenance of bowel function and integrity is essential to well-being.

When assessing a patient's abdominal pain, make sure that your findings are reported and documented clearly, accurately, and in a timely manner. Although the intellectual standards for critical thinking apply to all symptoms, thorough pain assessment is difficult because it is subjective in nature but essential. Numerous problems are detectable based on the nature of abdominal pain. Collaborate with health care providers as you assess your patients and identify appropriate plans of care.

Patients with alterations in bowel elimination, especially incontinence, are frequently embarrassed and need to be treated with respect by all health care providers. It is your responsibility to ensure that each patient's privacy is carefully protected and their physical care is provided in a respectful, competent, and timely manner.

BOX 35-5 PATIENT-CENTERED CARE

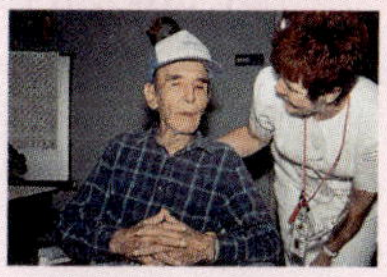

As Vickie prepares to care for Mr. Gutierrez, she learns that people from different cultures have different beliefs and practices. She knows that Mr. Gutierrez keeps many of his cultural practices, and it is important that she understand early in his care how his culture and customs may impact her care plan. Elimination needs are very personal, and Vickie knows that she needs to respect and be sensitive to her patient's elimination practices.

IMPLICATIONS FOR PRACTICE

- When assisting patient with bowel elimination needs or if the patient has an ostomy, accommodate the need for gender-congruent care if a patient expresses modesty and a need for privacy. Learn each patient's expectations.
- In any culture the presence and care of an ostomy presents unique challenges. New ostomies require monitoring and observation. A patient's cultural orientation may find the procedure more invasive and embarrassing.
- Most cultures consider bowel and urinary secretions as not fit for public display. However, exposure of the lower torso, which is needed for ostomy care, is generally avoided among Africans, Hispanics, Asians, Arabic, Hindus, Muslims, Orthodox Jewish, and Amish groups.
- Provide for distinct hygienic practices observed by certain cultures such as Hindus and Muslims that designate the left hand to perform unclean procedures such as bowel elimination. Wash your hands thoroughly before touching the patient.
- Promote patients' understanding of the procedure to be done. Apply health literacy principles.
- Use an interpreter if needed.
- Repeat explanations because patient's anxiety about the loss of privacy can pose a distraction.

NURSING PROCESS

The needs and problems of patients experiencing alterations in bowel elimination are distinct and numerous. Incorporate a caring approach and use appropriate communication techniques throughout the nursing process.

ASSESSMENT

Assessment of bowel elimination requires you to focus on any problems a patient has affecting the GI system. A patient's ability to chew food, recent intake of both solids and liquids, personal eating habits, and level of stress all influence bowel function. Include this information in your assessment.

Health History. In determining a patient's bowel habits, remember that "normal" is unique to each individual. Apply this knowledge in preparing questions for the patient interview to determine the presence and extent of GI alterations. Family members are usually helpful if the patient is unable to provide necessary information. Organize much of the nursing history around factors that affect bowel elimination (Seidel et al., 2011):

1. Determine your patient's usual pattern of bowel elimination. Usual frequency and time of day are important, but also determine if any changes in elimination patterns have occurred. Ask the patient to make suggestions about why this change occurred.
2. Get the patient's description of usual characteristics of stool. Determine if the stool is normally watery or formed and soft or hard and the typical color. Ask the patient to describe the shape of a normal stool and the number of stools per day. Use a scale such as the Bristol Stool Form Scale to obtain an objective measure of stool characteristics (Figure 35-5).
3. Identify specific routines followed to promote normal elimination. Examples are drinking warm liquids, laxatives, eating specific foods, or making the effort to defecate at the same time each day. If your patient uses a specific routine that is appropriate, consider incorporating the routine in your plan of care.
4. Assess how the patient manages constipation at home (e.g., the use of enemas, laxatives, herbal preparations, or special foods before having a bowel movement). Ask how often he or she uses any of these interventions for constipation.
5. Determine the presence of a bowel diversion. If the patient has an ostomy, assess the frequency of fecal drainage, character of feces, type of pouching system used, and which routine of care works well for the patient.
6. Identify changes in appetite. Include changes in your patient's eating patterns and a change in weight, either loss or gain. If a change in weight is reported, inquire if the patient planned the weight change such as weight loss with a diet.
7. Ask about diet history, including the patient's dietary preferences. Is mealtime regular or irregular, and does the patient eat certain foods infrequently? This enables you to determine the intake of grains, fruits, meats, and vegetables.

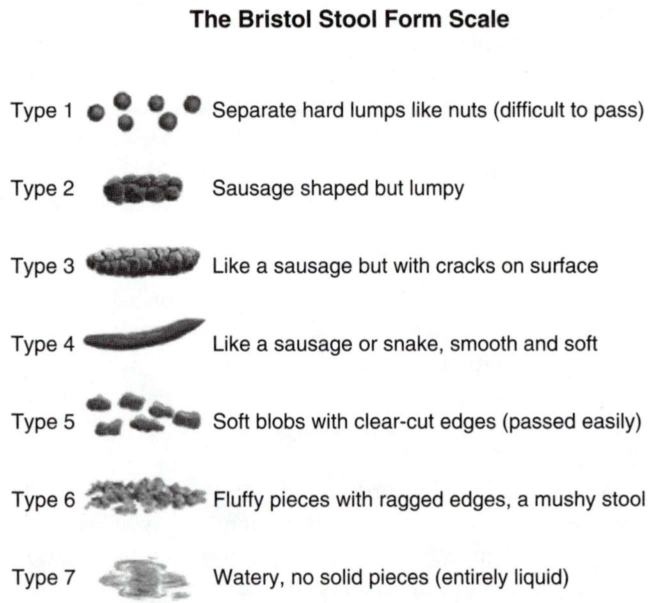

FIGURE 35-5 Bristol Stool Form Scale. (Used with permission. *Bristol Stool Form Scale guideline,* 2013, http://aboutconstipation.org/site/about-constipation/treatment/stool-form-guide. Accessed September 20, 2013.)

8. Obtain a daily fluid intake, including the type and amount of fluid. Have the patient estimate the amount using common household measurements. Ask him or her to give you a 24-hour diet recall during your assessment. You may also want to ask the patient to complete a 72-hour food intake diary for the next visit.
9. Obtain a history of surgery or illnesses affecting the GI tract. This information often helps to explain if a patient has the ability to maintain or restore normal elimination patterns and if there is a family history of cancer involving the GI tract (Box 35-6).
10. Ask about medication history, including over-the-counter and herbal medications. Determine whether the patient takes medications that alter defecation or fecal characteristics.
11. Assess the patient's emotional state, including tone of voice and mannerisms, which reveal significant behaviors indicating stress.
12. Assess the patient's exercise history. Obtain a description of the type, frequency, and amount of daily exercise.
13. Gather a history of pain or discomfort. Ask the patient whether there is a history of abdominal or anal pain. The location and nature of pain help to locate the source of a problem (see Chapter 32).
14. If the patient complains of diarrhea, determine the number of stools per day, the consistency, and how

BOX 35-6 SCREENING FOR COLORECTAL CANCER

RISK FACTORS

- Age: Over 50
- Family history: Colorectal cancer, familial adenomatous polyposis, hereditary nonpolyposis colon cancer (Lynch syndrome)
- Personal history: Colorectal cancer or colorectal polyps, inflammatory bowel disease (IBD)
- Race: African-Americans have highest colon cancer rates
- Diet: High intake of animal fats or red meat and low intake of fruits and vegetables
- Obesity and physical inactivity
- Smoking and heavy alcohol consumption
- Type 2 diabetes

WARNING SIGNS

- Change in bowel habits (e.g., diarrhea, constipation, narrowing of stool lasting more than few days)
- Rectal bleeding or blood in stool
- Sensation of incomplete evacuation
- Unexplained abdominal or back pain

AMERICAN CANCER SOCIETY SCREENING GUIDELINES FOR THE EARLY DETECTION OF COLORECTAL CANCER IN AVERAGE-RISK ASYMPTOMATIC PEOPLE*

Men and women Age 50+	Fecal occult blood test (FOBT) done on multiple samples at home	Annual, starting at age 50
	Fecal immunochemical test (FIT) done on multiple samples at home	Annual, starting at age 50
	Flexible sigmoidoscopy	Every 5 years, starting at age 50
	Double-contrast barium enema	Every 5 years starting at age 50
	Computed tomography, colonography	Every 5 years, starting at age 50
	Colonoscopy	Every 10 years, starting at age 50

*These procedures are ordered by a health care provider, depending on availability of resources and patient needs. If positive findings result from the flexible sigmoidoscopy, barium enema, or colonography, follow-up with a colonoscopy should be done.

Data from: American Cancer Society (ACS): *Cancer facts and figures 2012,* http://www.cancer.org/acs/groups/content/@epidemiologysurveilance/documents/document/acspc-031941.pdf. Accessed October 4, 2013.

long the problem has been present. Ask about causative factors such as recent illness, new medications, and dietary changes or travel outside the country in the past month. Assess for signs and symptoms of dehydration.

15. Assess the patient's mobility and dexterity. Determine your patient's ability to toilet independently or whether he or she needs assistive devices. Does the patient rely on a family caregiver in the home?

Older Adult Considerations. When assessing an elderly patient it is important to know and understand the changes that occur because of the aging process. Far too often nurses do not acknowledge an older adult's problems with intestinal elimination as an important consideration in their care. Remember that what appears at the outset to be a trivial complaint may be a significant problem physically and/or psychologically.

Physical Assessment. Assess the status of GI function to detect factors that affect elimination. Focus your patient assessment to identify problems associated with bowel elimination (Table 35-2). You need to conduct an examination of the oral cavity, abdomen, and external anal opening. If fecal impaction is suspected, a rectal examination may be done (see Chapter 16). When a digital examination is necessary, inspect the fecal material on the glove for several characteristics (Table 35-3). If there are no feces on the glove, ask the patient to describe a typical stool, noting recent changes. The patient or family caregiver is the most knowledgeable about changes. You also determine whether the patient passes a large amount of gas or little gas.

Laboratory and Diagnostic Examinations

Laboratory Tests. There are no blood tests to specifically diagnose most GI disorders, but hemoglobin and hematocrit may be done to determine if anemia from GI bleeding is present. Liver function tests and serum amylase to assess for hepatobiliary diseases and pancreatitis are possible tests that may be ordered by the health care provider.

Fecal Specimens. Analysis of fecal contents also detects alterations in GI functioning. Careful handling of a specimen is important to prevent exposure to infectious microorganisms. Follow Standard Precautions (see Chapter 14) when collecting and sending specimens to the laboratory. A patient is often capable of obtaining the specimen without assistance if properly instructed. Make sure that the patient understands not to mix feces with urine or water. He or she defecates into a clean, dry bedpan or special container placed under the toilet seat.

Laboratory tests for blood in the stool, ova and parasites, and stool cultures require only a small sample. Blood in the stool or melena causes stool to turn black and sticky; thus the term *tarry stools.* Collect approximately 1 inch of formed stool or 15 to 30 mL of liquid diarrhea stool. Tests for measuring the output of fecal fat require a patient to collect stools for 3 to 5 days. You need to save all fecal material throughout the test period. Stool specimen tests for ova and parasites may require a chemical fixative. Fresh specimens are best for revealing parasites or larvae; therefore collected specimens should be taken directly to the laboratory for immediate examination. A stool culture to test for bacteria in the feces should also go the laboratory quickly for the most accurate result.

After obtaining a specimen, tightly seal the container, place in the proper biohazard bag, complete laboratory requisition forms, and record all specimen collections in the patient's medical record. Avoid delays in sending specimens to the

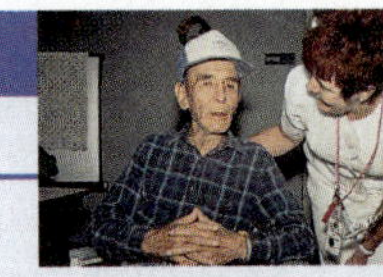

TABLE 35-2 **FOCUSED PATIENT ASSESSMENT**

FACTORS TO ASSESS	QUESTIONS	PHYSICAL ASSESSMENT
Chewing	Do you have difficulty chewing? Do you have any mouth pain? Do you wear any dental devices such as dentures or partial replacement of teeth?	Inspect condition of teeth, tongue, gums, and mouth. Observe for fit of dentures or other dental devices, observing for sores or pressure areas from these devices. Observe patient eating meal; determine patient's ability to eat all types of foods.
Mobility	**In Ambulatory Patients** Do you exercise regularly? How often do you exercise? What type of exercise do you do? How active are you? **For Patients With Restricted Mobility** Are you able to use the toilet independently? How much help do you need for toileting?	Observe patient's gait. Observe patient's ability to help with transfer, sit down on and get up from toilet, and activity.
Abdomen	Do you have gas, feel bloated, or have any pain or discomfort? Can you point to the area of pain or discomfort on your abdomen? Is the pain or discomfort always in the same place?	Observe all four abdominal quadrants, noting the presence of scars, masses, venous patterns, stomas, lesions, and peristaltic waves. Auscultate all four quadrants for the presence of bowel sounds; note if sounds are normal (gurgling), absent, or abnormal (high-pitched, or tinkling). Gently palpate all four quadrants, noting areas of distention, masses, or pain. When pain is present, note the location.
Anal sphincter function	Can you feel if you are distended?	Inspect anal sphincter at rest and perform digital examination while asking patient to contract and relax sphincter. **NOTE:** A small amount of stool is normal; large amount of stool or hard stool indicates impaired emptying of bowel.

laboratory. Some tests require the stool to be warm. When stool specimens stand at room temperature, bacteriological changes occur that alter test results.

A common test is the **fecal occult blood test (FOBT),** or guaiac test, which measures microscopic amounts of blood in the feces (Box 35-7). It is a useful screening test for colon cancer as recommended by the American Cancer Society (ACS) but is not conclusive since other GI disorders can also cause bleeding (see Box 35-6). Two types of FOBT are currently used: the most commonly used guaiac FOBT and the fecal immunochemical test (FIT). The FIT test requires no preparation or dietary restrictions, but it is more expensive; thus the FOBT is more commonly used. You or the patient need to repeat the test at least 3 times on three separate bowel movements while the patient refrains from ingesting foods and medications that cause a false-positive or false negative result. The FOBT is done in the patient's home or health care provider's office. All positive tests should be followed up with flexible sigmoidoscopy or colonoscopy (ACS, 2012).

When your patients are going to have an FBOT, it is important to instruct them to avoid eating red meat for 3 days before testing. Although the health care provider should be consulted before asking a patient to stop any medication, if there are no contraindications the patient should be instructed to stop taking aspirin, ibuprofen, naproxen, or other nonsteroidal antiinflammatory drugs for 7 days because these could cause a false-positive test result. Vitamin C supplements and citrus fruits and juices should be stopped 3 days before the test because they can cause a false-negative result (ACS, 2012).

Diagnostic Examinations. For patients experiencing alterations in the GI system, there are various radiological and diagnostic tests (Box 35-8). Some of these examinations such as a **colonoscopy** require bowel preparation (bowel prep) for the test to be completed successfully. A bowel-cleansing program may be difficult or unpleasant for a patient, and the nurse needs to provide education and support to ensure an optimal test result.

Patient Expectations. When you assess a patient's expectations of care, it is helpful to anticipate his or her need for privacy and respect it. Bowel elimination problems are embarrassing for some. Ask the patient what is important to ensure that you give care in a personal and professional way.

When determining the patient's expectations, consider his or her normal bowel pattern. Some patients wish to have activities planned to maintain their normal routines. If what

TABLE 35-3 FECAL CHARACTERISTICS

CHARACTERISTIC	NORMAL	ABNORMAL	ABNORMAL CAUSE
Color	Infant: Yellow Adult: Brown	White or clay Black or tarry (melena) Red Pale and oily	Absence of bile Iron ingestion or GI bleeding GI bleeding, hemorrhoids, ingestion of beets Malabsorption of fat
Odor	Malodorous; may be affected by certain foods	Noxious change	Blood in feces or infection
Consistency	Soft, formed	Liquid Hard	Diarrhea, reduced absorption Constipation
Frequency	Varies: Infant 4 to 6 times daily (breastfed) or 1 to 3 times daily (bottle-fed) Adult twice daily to 3 times a week	Infant more than 6 times daily or less than once every 1 to 2 days Adult more than 3 times a day or less than once a week	Hypermotility or hypomotility
Shape	Resembles diameter of rectum	Narrow, pencil shaped	Obstruction, increased peristalsis
Constituents	Undigested food, dead bacteria, fat, bile pigment, cells lining intestinal mucosa, water	Blood, pus, foreign bodies, mucus, worms	Internal bleeding, infection, swallowed objects, irritation, inflammation, infestation of parasites
		Oily stool	Malabsorption syndrome, enteritis, pancreatic disease, surgical resection of intestine
		Mucus	Intestinal irritation, inflammation, infection, or injury

GI, Gastrointestinal.

BOX 35-7 PROCEDURAL GUIDELINES

Measuring Fecal Occult Blood

DELEGATION CONSIDERATIONS

The skill of performing a guaiac fecal occult blood test (FOBT) can be delegated to nursing assistive personnel (NAP). The nurse is responsible for assessing the significance of the findings. You may need to send the specimen to the laboratory (see agency policies). The nurse instructs the NAP to:

- Notify the nurse if frank bleeding occurs after obtaining the sample.

EQUIPMENT

Hemoccult test paper, Hemoccult developer, wooden applicator, and clean gloves. (Check expiration dates on developer and test paper before using.)

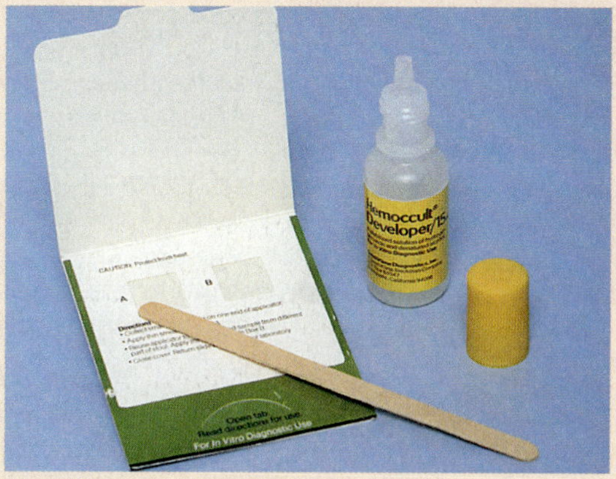

STEP 4 Equipment needed for fecal occult blood testing.

STEPS

1. Identify patient using two identifiers (e.g., name and birthday or name and account number) according to agency policy. Compare identifiers with information on patient's MAR or medical record.
2. Explain purpose of test and ways patient can help. Patient can collect own specimen if possible.
3. Perform hand hygiene and apply clean gloves.
4. Use tip of wooden applicator (see illustration) to obtain small portion of stool specimen. Be sure that specimen is free of toilet paper and not contaminated with urine.
5. Perform Hemoccult slide test:
   a. Open flap of slide and, using wooden applicator, thinly smear stool in first box of guaiac paper. Apply second fecal specimen from different portion of stool to second box of slide (see illustration).

Continued

BOX 35-7 PROCEDURAL GUIDELINES—cont'd

Measuring Fecal Occult Blood

b. Close slide cover and turn packet over to reverse side (see illustration). After waiting 3 to 5 minutes, open cardboard flap and apply 2 drops of developing solution on each box of guaiac paper. A blue color indicates positive guaiac, or presence of fecal occult blood.
c. Interpret color of the guaiac paper after 30 to 60 seconds.
d. After determining if patient's specimen is positive or negative, apply 1 drop of developer to quality control section and interpret within 10 seconds.
e. Dispose of test slide in proper receptacle.

6. Wrap wooden applicator in paper towel, remove gloves, and discard in proper receptacle.
7. Perform hand hygiene.
8. Record results of test; note any unusual fecal characteristics. (Submit only one sample per day.)

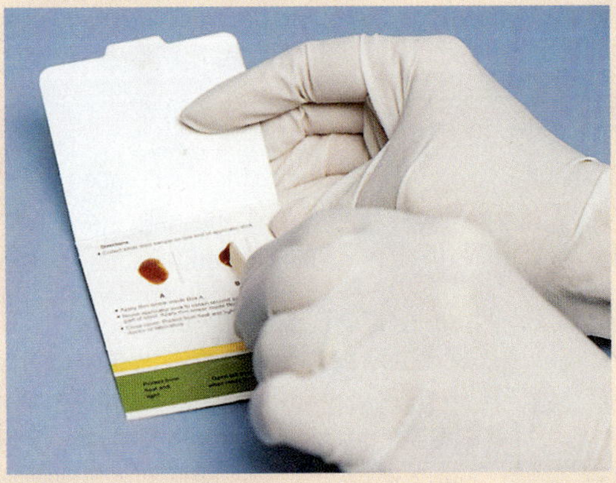

STEP 5a Application of fecal specimen on guaiac paper.

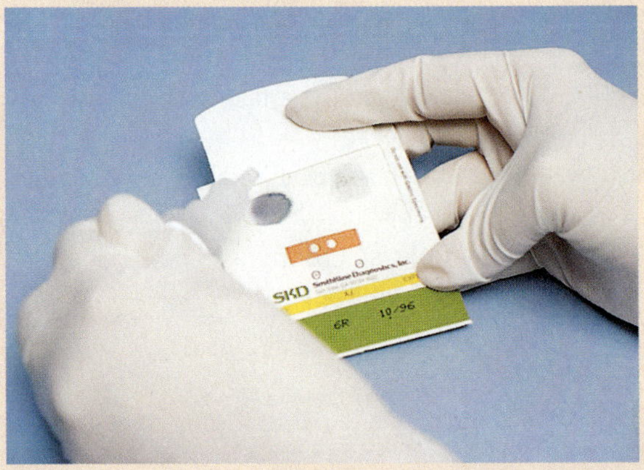

STEP 5b Application of Hemoccult developing solution on guaiac paper on reverse side of test kit.

BOX 35-8 RADIOLOGICAL AND DIAGNOSTIC TESTS

DIRECT VISUALIZATION

Endoscopy

Examinations such as a gastroscopy or colonoscopy use a lighted fiberoptic tube to directly visualize the upper gastrointestinal (GI) tract (upper endoscopy) or large intestine (colonoscopy). The fiberoptic tube contains a lens, forceps, and brushes for biopsy. If an endoscopy identifies a lesion such as a polyp, the polyp can be removed, and a biopsy will be done. These tests are done under sedation, usually in outpatient centers. Patients receive instructions about the preparation needed for the tests at the time they are scheduled for the procedure. Bowel preparation is necessary before a colonoscopy can be performed successfully.

INDIRECT VISUALIZATION

Anorectal Manometry

Measures the pressure activity of internal and external anal sphincters and reflexes during rectal distention, relaxation during straining, and rectal sensation.

Plain Film of Abdomen/Kidneys, Ureter, Bladder (KUB)

Simple x-ray film of the abdomen requiring no preparation.

Barium Swallow/Enema

X-ray film examination using an opaque contrast medium (barium, which is swallowed) to examine the structure and motility of the upper GI tract, including pharynx, esophagus, and stomach.

Barium instilled through the anal opening via an enema provides visualization of the structures of the lower GI tract. Usually a bowel preparation with laxatives is ordered before the procedure.

Ultrasound Imaging

Technique that uses high-frequency sound waves to echo off body organs, creating a picture of the GI tract.

Computed Tomography (CT) Scan or CT (Virtual Colonoscopy)

X-ray film examination of the body from many angles using a scanner analyzed by a computer. An oral contrast solution for the patient to drink may be ordered before the test. Intravenous contrast solution may be injected during the test to improve visualization. This does not replace the colonoscopy because it does not allow for removal of polyps and biopsies.

Colonic Transit Study

A patient swallows a capsule containing radiopaque markers. He or she maintains a high-fiber diet for 5 days and refrains from medications that affect bowel function. On the fifth day x-ray film examination is performed.

Magnetic Resonance Imaging

A noninvasive examination that uses magnet and radio waves to produce a picture of the inside of the body.

is "normal" to a patient is unhealthy or promotes negative health practices, you must educate the patient and work with him or her to adopt healthier routines.

Because there is a direct link between nutrition and bowel elimination, consider the patient's cultural choices of foods and fluids. Sometimes the patient has to make concessions about certain food selections. Methods of preparation are also a concern, especially if tradition, access, and cost are deciding factors.

NURSING DIAGNOSIS

Gather data from the nursing assessment, validate the data, and analyze clusters of defining characteristics to identify relevant nursing diagnoses. Reflecting on each of your data sources is necessary to determine the correct diagnosis. Defining characteristics identified during your assessment sometimes apply to more than one diagnosis; therefore be clinically skillful in determining patterns that reveal the diagnosis that best fits the patient's situation.

For example, a patient reports not having a bowel movement for several days. This defining characteristic applies to the diagnosis of *Constipation* and *Perceived Constipation*. The difference is that on examination the patient with *Constipation* has a dry, hard stool with abdominal or rectal fullness. In contrast, the patient with *Perceived Constipation* has an expectation of having a stool daily, when in fact the stools are quite normal. A variety of nursing diagnoses are relevant for patients with altered bowel elimination. Some examples follow (NANDA International, 2012):

- *Disturbed Body Image*
- *Bowel Incontinence*
- *Constipation*
- *Perceived Constipation*
- *Risk for Constipation*
- *Diarrhea*
- *Nausea*
- *Dysfunctional Gastrointestinal Motility*
- *Deficient Knowledge (Nutrition)*
- *Acute Pain*
- *Toileting Self-Care Deficit*

It is important to establish the correct "related to" factor for a diagnosis. For example, with the diagnosis of *Constipation* you distinguish between related factors of nutritional imbalance, exercise, medications, and emotional problems. Selection of the correct related factors for each diagnosis ensures that you implement the appropriate nursing interventions.

PLANNING

Goals and Outcomes. After you identify nursing diagnoses, determine how they are related to the patient's current status (Figure 35-6). Then you and the patient set goals and expected outcomes to direct interventions. When possible these goals and outcomes incorporate the patient's elimination routines or habits as much as possible and reinforce those that promote health. In addition, consider the patient's preexisting health concerns. For example, one method of reducing the risk for constipation is to achieve the goal of "establishing a normal defecation pattern" by increasing fluids and bulk to the patient's diet. An outcome would be that the patient "passes a soft, formed stool within 48 hours." However, if your patient is at risk for developing congestive heart failure, you need to tailor the intervention of increasing fluid intake to the patient's cardiac function. For this reason it might take longer to achieve the outcome.

The goals and expected outcomes that you establish need to be realistic. The outcomes provide measurable behaviors or physiological responses that indicate progress toward the goal of a normal bowel elimination pattern. Design nursing interventions to achieve the outcomes of care.

Setting Priorities. Defecation patterns vary among individuals. For this reason you and the patient work together to plan effective interventions to meet elimination needs and priorities (see Care Plan). A realistic time frame to establish a normal defecation pattern for one patient is sometimes very different for another. In addition, if the patient has a new ostomy resulting from cancer, the priority of coping with cancer and its treatment precedes the patient's need to become independent in managing the care of the bowel diversion. In addition, when a bowel diversion is necessary, coping with changes in body image is a high priority for both the patient and family.

Collaborative Care. Other health care team members are important resources for the patient and family. You sometimes refer a patient with chronic constipation to a dietitian to plan a nutritionally balanced diet that incorporates the patient's food preferences and lifestyle.

Involving the family in the plan of care is important. When patients are disabled or debilitated, family members often become the primary caregivers. Patient and family education is important to promote understanding of ways to establish normal bowel function. If access to proper nutrition is a concern, referrals to community organizations that deliver meals to the home (e.g., Meals on Wheels and church groups) or provide transportation for patients are beneficial.

A clinical nurse specialist or wound, ostomy, and continence nurse specialist provides guidance in the care and management of ostomies and problems involving incontinence or skin breakdown. Use professionals from a variety of health care disciplines to provide safe, effective care.

IMPLEMENTATION

Health Promotion. Factors that normally promote bowel elimination are appropriate interventions for helping patients develop normal bowel habits. It is important to teach your patient about the benefits and effects of a balanced diet, regular exercise, and stress management and how to integrate each into a bowel routine. Teach your patients to try to develop a routine time for bowel evacuation. A good time is after a morning or evening meal when your patient does not feel rushed. Establishing a consistent time for bowel hygiene is just one practice to avoid constipation (Box 35-9).

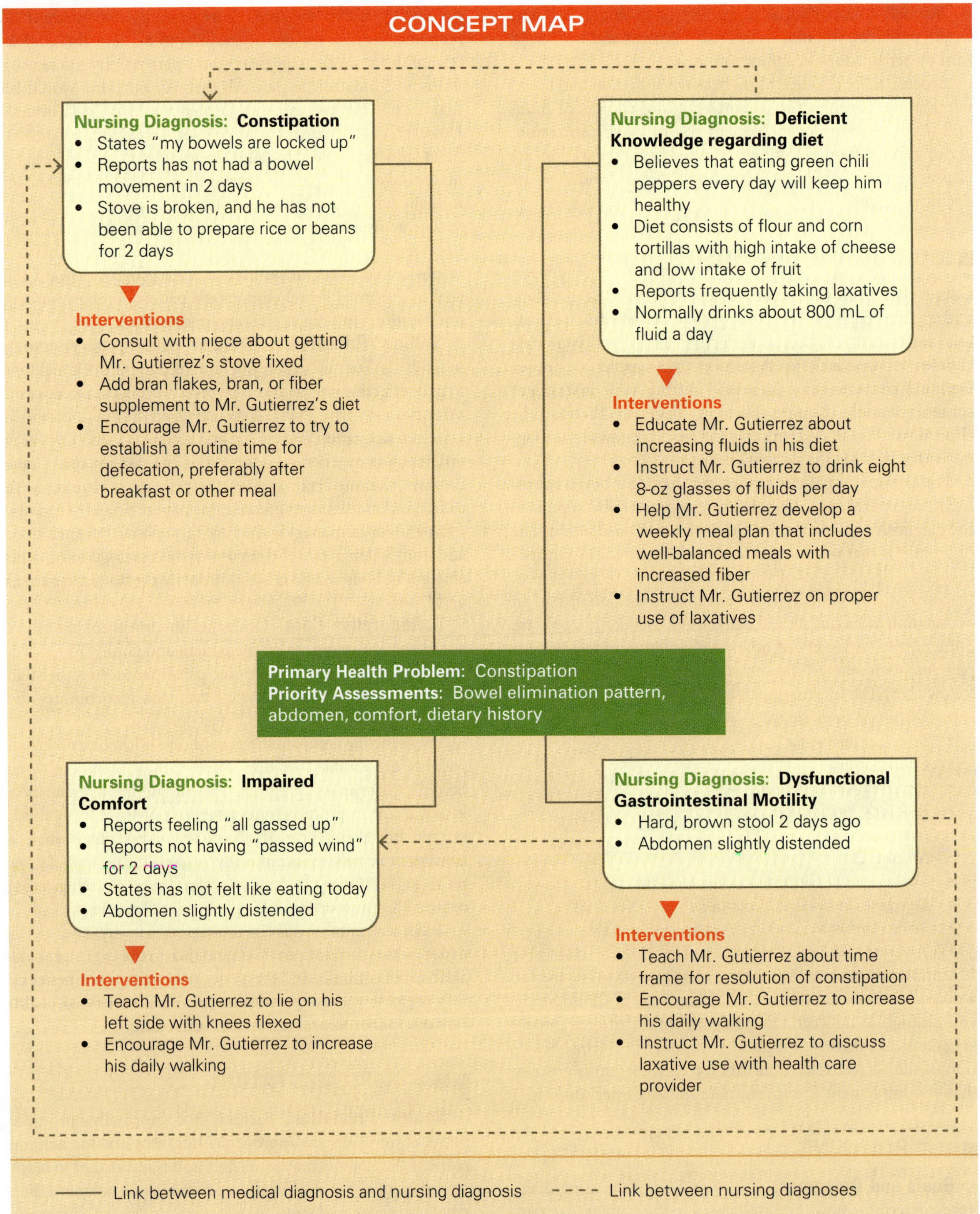

FIGURE 35-6 Concept map.

CARE PLAN

Constipation

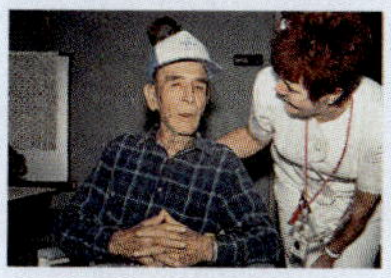

ASSESSMENT

Vickie and Mr. Gutierrez have been able to communicate without difficulty. Mr. Gutierrez complains of feeling "full of gas" but has not "passed any wind" in the last 2 days. His stove has not been working well, and he has been unable to prepare rice and beans. Based on the nursing history, Vickie estimates that Mr. Gutierrez normally drinks about 800 mL of fluid daily.

ASSESSMENT ACTIVITIES	FINDINGS/DEFINING CHARACTERISTICS*
Determine when Mr. Gutierrez had his last bowel movement.	Mr. Gutierrez had his **last bowel movement 2 days ago. The stool was brown in color and hard.** "I took a laxative last night, and I think I need an enema."
Determine Mr. Gutierrez's medication history.	A medication history shows that Mr. Gutierrez **frequently resorts to taking laxatives.**
Establish Mr. Gutierrez's dietary habits.	Mr. Gutierrez eats a **high intake of corn tortillas and cheese and a low intake of fruits.** Mr. Gutierrez also states, "I really **haven't felt like eating today and have not eaten much for the last 4 days,** and I need to move my bowels."

*__Defining characteristics__ are shown in **bold** type.

NURSING DIAGNOSIS: Constipation related to less than adequate fluid and dietary intake and chronic laxative use

PLANNING

GOAL	EXPECTED OUTCOMES (NOC)†
	Bowel Elimination
• Mr. Gutierrez will establish and maintain a normal defecation pattern within 1 month.	• Mr. Gutierrez has a bowel movement within 48 hours. • Mr. Gutierrez's abdomen is soft, nondistended, and nontender within 24 hours. • Mr. Gutierrez passes soft, formed stools at least every 3 days.
	Nutritional Status: Food and Fluid Intake
• Mr. Gutierrez will identify practices that reduce risk for or prevent constipation within 2 weeks.	• Mr. Gutierrez identifies need to increase the fiber content of his diet within 1 week. • Mr. Gutierrez discontinues laxative use and uses fiber supplements when needed. • Mr. Gutierrez identifies need to drink eight 8-ounce glasses of fluids a day within 3 days.

†Outcomes classification labels from Moorhead S et al, editors: *Nursing outcomes classification (NOC)*, ed 5, St Louis, 2013, Mosby.

INTERVENTIONS (NIC)‡	RATIONALE
Constipation/Impaction Management	
• Instruct Mr. Gutierrez in a weekly menu plan, including foods high in fiber: brown rice, beans and rice, tomatoes, and wheat tortillas.	High-fiber foods increase the bulk of the fecal contents, which in turn increases peristalsis and improves the movement of intestinal contents through the gastrointestinal (GI) tract (Spinzi, 2009).
• Add bran flakes, bran, or fiber supplement to Mr. Gutierrez's diet.	Bran as flakes or fiber supplements adds bulk to the feces and increases the number of soft-formed stools. Dietary fiber, either through diet or supplement, reduces the need for laxatives (Lewis et al., 2011).
• Consult with Mr. Gutierrez's niece and long-term care center to have patient's stove repaired.	Cooking facilities are necessary for preparation of selected food preferences.
• Educate Mr. Gutierrez about use of liquids to promote softening of stool and defecation.	Fluids help to keep fecal mass soft and increase stool bulk, causing increase in colon peristalsis (www.niddk.nih.gov).

Continued

CARE PLAN—cont'd

Constipation

• Encourage Mr. Gutierrez to try to establish a routine time for defecation (e.g., after breakfast or other meal).	With aging there may be some normal changes in rectal sensation, and the body needs larger volumes to elicit the sensation to defecate. The normal mass-movement response to eating, which results in movement of colon contents approximately 1 hour after a meal, helps to establish routine bowel habits (Lewis et al., 2011).

‡Intervention classification labels from Bulechek GM, et al, editors: *Nursing interventions classification (NIC),* ed 6, St Louis, 2013, Mosby.

EVALUATION

NURSING ACTIONS	PATIENT RESPONSE/FINDING	ACHIEVEMENT OF OUTCOME
Review Mr. Gutierrez's diary of foods and ask him about his intake as well.	Mr. Gutierrez described likes and dislikes but admits to eating high-fat foods and few fruits and vegetables. Fluid intake averaged 1400 mL daily for a week.	Mr. Gutierrez's intake of high-fiber foods is still limited. Fluid intake is improving.
Ask Mr. Gutierrez about his pattern of elimination over the last 2 weeks and laxative use.	Mr. Gutierrez says, "I'm not having so much trouble going." He states that he thinks he now goes about every 2 days. Mr. Gutierrez has not used any laxatives for a week.	He has bowel movements approximately every 2 days. He is successfully avoiding use of laxatives.
During follow-up visit examine patient's abdomen and observe stool (if possible).	Patient reports that stool is formed but is "not hard like before." Abdomen is soft and nontender with no distention.	Stool is softer. His abdomen is less distended.

BOX 35-9 HEALTH PROMOTION

Bowel Hygiene

Helping patients and their families in healthy food selection and preparation practices helps to reduce the risks of gastrointestinal (GI) disorders. There is increasing evidence that weight control with a body mass index of 25 or below; a diet rich in fruits, vegetables, and whole grains and low in fat and red meat; and daily exercise reduce risk for colorectal cancers, digestive diseases, and other cancers (ACS, 2012). Give consideration to whether a patient is able to afford the foods recommended. In addition to solid foods, the patient with elimination problems needs to drink 1.5-2 L of fluids daily if not contraindicated by other medical conditions.

APPLICATION TO NURSING PRACTICE

- Recommend fluid intake of at least 1.5 L per day.
- Teach patients to limit alcohol because of its diuretic properties and not to count any alcoholic beverage as part of their daily intake of fluids.
- Suggest a high-fiber diet (25 to 30 g per day) to reduce constipation; as fiber passes through the colon, it retains fluid. As a result, bulkier and softer stools develop. In addition, the waste moves through the colon more easily and results in more regular bowel movements.
- Teach patients to use a combination of insoluble and soluble fiber (e.g., bran, fruits, and vegetables) to prevent constipation.
- Assess patient's ability to afford foods.
- Encourage physical activity in combination with adequate fluid intake and high-fiber diet to manage constipation. Walking once or twice a day for 30 minutes is sufficient.
- Explain need to use laxatives with caution. A stepwise progression of laxatives is recommended: first bulk-forming laxatives, followed by stool softeners and osmotic stimulants. Use suppositories and/or enemas if the diet, fluid, and laxative regimen is not successful.

Diet. A well-balanced diet that includes several servings of fruits and vegetables and whole grain foods daily and an adequate fluid intake promotes normal bowel function. A patient with an ileostomy may need a lower-residue diet if he or she has a high output of fecal effluent. Patients with GI disorders or food intolerances need the help of a nutritionist to devise a diet that meets their specific needs and promotes normal bowel function.

Exercise. An age-specific exercise program also helps patients maintain a healthy bowel pattern. Regular exercise such as walking, biking, or swimming 30 minutes daily promotes normal GI motility. Have a patient who experiences a period of immobilization from illness ambulate as soon as possible within the activity restrictions set by the health care provider.

Timing and Privacy. One of the most important habits you teach your patients regarding bowel habits is to take time for defecation. Ignoring the urge to defecate and not taking time to defecate completely are common causes of constipation. To establish regular bowel habits, a patient needs to respond to the urge to defecate. Prompt response helps the patient reduce episodes of constipation.

Defecation is most likely to occur after meals. If a patient attempts to defecate during the time when mass colonic peristalsis occurs, the chances of successfully evacuating the rectum are greater. If a patient is restricted to bed or requires assistance in ambulating, recommend use of a bedside commode or a bedpan or have a caregiver help the patient reach the bathroom. Patients need prompt assistance before the urge disappears.

Some patients have previously established routines to help them with defecation. When patients are hospitalized, health promotion habits become disrupted. Encourage patients to maintain as many of these regular practices as possible. Privacy is often a concern for patients. Health care providers should knock before entering a patient's room. Privacy curtains should be used, especially for patients who reside in semiprivate rooms or shared living areas. Remain acutely aware of the patient's need for modesty and privacy.

Promotion of Normal Defecation. To help patients evacuate contents normally and without discomfort, recommend interventions that stimulate the defecation reflex or increase peristalsis. Helping the patient into an upright sitting position increases pressure on the rectum and facilitates use of intraabdominal muscles. Patients who have had surgery or have muscular weakness or mobility limitations benefit from the use of elevated toilet seats. Regular toilets may be too low for patients to lower themselves to a sitting position because of pain or altered mobility. With an elevated seat the patient exerts less effort to sit and stand.

Acute Care. When patients become acutely ill the GI system is often affected. Simple changes in activity levels, sleeping patterns, diet, and medications directly affect regular bowel habits. Surgical intervention creates additional elimination problems for the patient in acute care (e.g., discomfort from an abdominal incision, absent or decreased GI peristalsis, or increased accumulation of intestinal gas following surgery). Whenever possible help the patient to the toilet or bedside commode and allow for privacy for a bowel movement. This facilitates the return of normal bowel habits.

Positioning on Bedpan. A patient restricted to use of a bedpan for defecation usually needs help. Sitting on a bedpan is uncomfortable and awkward. Help position the patient comfortably. Two types of bedpans are available (Figure 35-7). The regular bedpan, made of hard plastic, has a curved smooth upper end and a sharper-edged lower end and is about 5 cm (2 inches) deep. A fracture pan is used for patients with low-extremity fractures or any patient for whom raising hips to get on a bedpan is too painful. It has a shallow upper

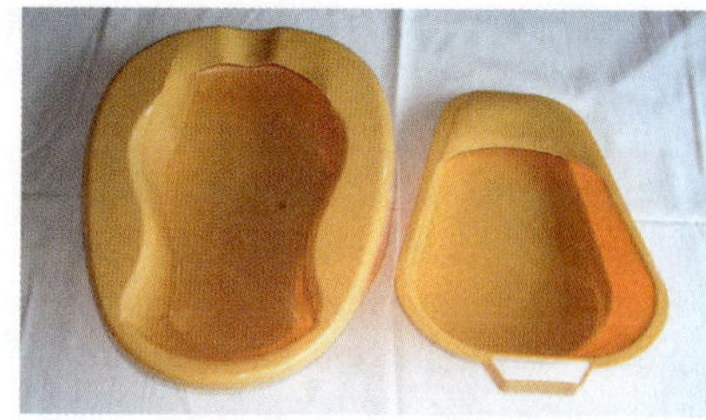

FIGURE 35-7 Types of bedpans. *From left:* Regular bedpan and fracture pan.

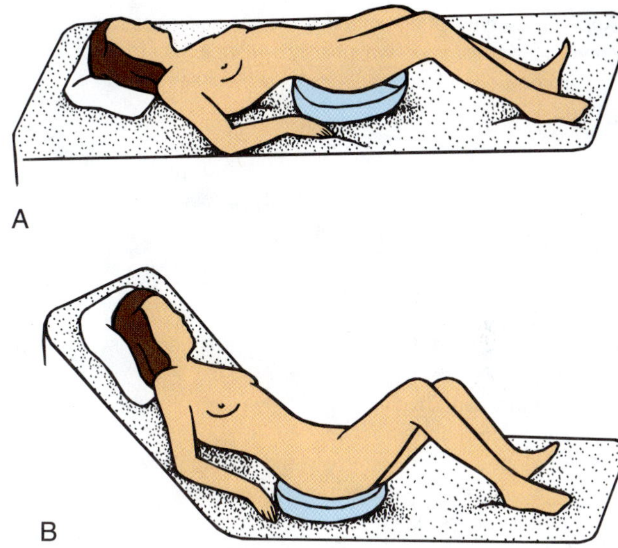

FIGURE 35-8 Positions on bedpan. **A,** Improper positioning of patient. **B,** Proper position reduces patient's back strain.

end about 2.5 cm (1 inch) deep. The shallow end of the pan fits under the buttocks toward the sacrum, and the deeper end goes just under the upper thighs. The pan needs to be high enough so the stool can enter the pan.

The most important element for you to consider in positioning or assisting a patient to use a bedpan is prevention of muscle strain and discomfort (Box 35-10). Never place a patient on a bedpan and then leave the bed flat unless activity restrictions demand it. This forces the patient to hyperextend the back to lift the hips onto the pan (Figure 35-8, *A*). It is often necessary to have the bed flat when placing a patient on a bedpan. Rolling the patient on to the bedpan is the most comfortable way to position a patient with impaired mobility. After it is positioned under the patient, raise the head of the bed 30 to 45 degrees (Figure 35-8, *B*). Patients who have overhead trapeze frames are able to lift themselves by grasping the trapeze bar. Always be sure to come back to the patient frequently to see if he or she is ready to get off. The patient who is sedated or cognitively impaired could fall asleep on the bedpan and develop serious pressure damage to the buttocks if left on it for a prolonged period of time.

For the more mobile patient a bedside commode is a safe, effective alternative to a bedpan. Its use is less exhausting and allows the patient to assume a more normal or familiar position for defecation.

BOX 35-10 PROCEDURAL GUIDELINES

Assisting Patient On and Off a Bedpan

DELEGATION CONSIDERATIONS

The skill of assisting a patient onto a bedpan can be delegated to nursing assistive personnel (NAP). The nurse assists the NAP in the proper way to position patients who have mobility restrictions. The nurse also instructs the NAP in how to position patients who have therapeutic equipment present such as drains, intravenous catheters, or traction.

EQUIPMENT

Appropriate type of clean bedpan; toilet tissue; specimen container (if necessary); washbasin; washcloths; towels; soap; waterproof, absorbent pads; clean drawsheet *(optional)*; clean gloves

STEPS

1. Assess patient's level of mobility, strength, ability to help, and presence of any condition (e.g., orthopedic) that interferes with use of bedpan.
2. Explain technique that you will use in turning and positioning to the patient.
3. Offer bedpan after meals because patient may have an urge to defecate at that time.
4. Perform hand hygiene and apply clean gloves.
5. Close room curtain for privacy.
6. Raise bed to comfortable working height. Position patient high in bed with head elevated 30 degrees (unless contraindicated).
7. Fold back top linen to patient's knees.
8. Help with positioning an independent patient: Raise side rails. Instruct patient to bend knees, place weight on feet, grasp side rails, and lift hips while you slip bedpan into place.
9. Dependent patient: Raise side rail on side of bed opposite from nurse. Lower head of bed flat and roll patient onto side facing away from nurse. Apply powder lightly to lower back and buttocks *(optional)*. Place bedpan firmly against buttocks (see illustration *A*). Push bedpan down into mattress with open rim toward patient's feet (see illustration *B*). Keeping one hand against bedpan, place other hand on patient's hip (see illustration *C*). Ask patient to roll onto pan, flat on bed. With patient positioned comfortably, raise head of bed 30 degrees.
10. Place rolled towel under lumbar curve of patient's back if needed for support.
11. Place call light and toilet tissue within patient's reach and keep side rails up as needed. Give patient time to defecate.
12. Remove bedpan as patient lifts hips up or carefully rolls off pan and to side. Hold pan firmly as patient moves.
13. Help to cleanse anal area. Wipe from pubic area toward anus. Replace top covers.
14. If you are collecting a specimen or recording urine output, do not dispose of tissue in bedpan. Dispose of in proper recepticle.
15. Have patient wash and dry hands.
16. Empty contents of pan, rinse, and store. Dispose of gloves and perform hand hygiene.
17. Inspect stool for color, amount, consistency, odor, or presence of abnormal substances. Document findings.

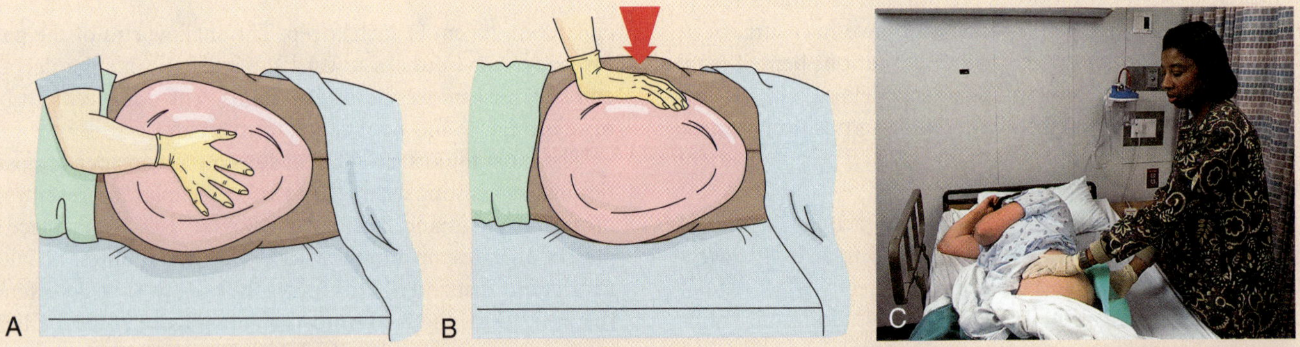

STEP 9 Place one hand against bedpan; place other hand around patient's hip.

Medications. Some medications initiate and facilitate stool passage. Laxatives and cathartics have the short-term action of emptying the bowel. These agents are also used to cleanse the bowel for patients undergoing GI tests and abdominal surgery. Although the terms *laxative* and *cathartic* are often used interchangeably, cathartics generally have a stronger and more rapid effect on the intestines.

Although patients usually take medications orally, laxatives prepared as suppositories may act more quickly because of their stimulant effect on the rectal mucosa. Suppositories such as bisacodyl act within 30 minutes. Give the suppository shortly before the patient's usual time to defecate or immediately after a meal. Teach patients about the potential harmful effects of overuse of laxatives such as impaired bowel motility and decreased response to sensory stimulus. Make sure that the patient understands that laxatives are not to be used long term for maintenance of bowel function.

Before recommending a laxative, it is important to assess for signs of a fecal impaction. The impaction must be removed before laxative therapy is initiated.

Laxatives and cathartics are classified by the method by which the agent promotes defecation. They are listed here in the order in which they should be used with the patient.

- Bulk-forming agents, also known as *fiber supplements,* generally are considered the safest and least irritating to the intestine. They absorb water in the intestine and make the stool softer and bulkier. The fecal bulk stretches the intestinal walls, stimulating peristalsis. Passage of stool occurs in 12 to 24 hours. These agents must be taken with water and should be used with patients who have an adequate food and fluid intake. Patients may note increased gas formation and flatus when they first start taking these laxatives, but this will abate after 4 to 5 days.
- Emollient laxatives soften the fecal mass and make it easier to evacuate. These agents are also called *stool softeners.*
- Osmotic laxatives pull fluid into the bowel to soften the stool and distend the bowel to stimulate peristalsis. Some are saline based; and others contain lactulose, sorbitol, and polyethylene glycol.
- Stimulant laxatives cause local irritation to the intestinal mucosa, increase intestinal motility, and inhibit resorption of water in the large intestine. The rapid movement of feces causes retention of water in the stool. The drugs cause formation of a soft-to-fluid stool in 6 to 8 hours and usually contain bisacodyl or senna.

Some newer drugs are being used currently for chronic constipation or motility disorders. It is too soon to tell if these medications will be effective and safe for long-term treatment, but they are not used for the relief of occasional constipation.

The most commonly used antidiarrheal agents are loperamide or diphenoxylate with atropine. Antidiarrheal agents decrease intestinal muscle tone to slow the passage of feces. As a result the body absorbs more water through the intestinal walls. However, the cause of diarrhea must be determined before effective treatment can be ordered by the health care provider. For example, if an infection is the causative factor, an antibiotic may be used for treatment; or, if inflammation is the cause, steroids may be given.

Nasogastric Tube for Gastric Decompression. At times following abdominal or pelvic surgery an ileus or temporary cessation of peristalsis occurs. A patient cannot eat or drink fluids without causing abdominal distention, nausea, and vomiting. The insertion of a nasogastric (NG) tube into the stomach serves to decompress the stomach, keeping it empty until normal peristalsis returns (see Skill 35-1). An NG tube is a pliable tube that is inserted through the patient's nose, through the nasopharynx, and into the stomach. The tube has a hollow lumen that allows the removal of gastric secretions and the introduction of solutions into the stomach. The Levin and Salem sump tubes are most commonly used for stomach decompression. The Levin tube is a single-lumen tube with holes near the tip. You connect the tube to a drainage bag or an intermittent suction device to drain stomach secretions. The Salem sump tube is preferable for stomach decompression. The tube has two lumina: one for removal of gastric contents and one to provide an air vent. A blue "pigtail" is the air vent that connects with the second lumen. When you connect the main lumen of the sump tube to suction, the air vent permits free, continuous drainage of secretions. *Never clamp the air vent if tube is connected to suction, and never use for irrigation.*

NG tube insertion does not require sterile technique. Clean technique is adequate. The procedure is uncomfortable; patients experience a burning sensation as the tube passes through the sensitive nasal mucosa. One of the greatest nursing care challenges is keeping the patient comfortable because the tube is a constant irritation to mucosa. Routinely assess the condition of the nares and mucosa for inflammation and excoriation. Supportive care includes changing soiled tape or fixation devices daily when they become soiled, keeping the nares lubricated and clean, and providing frequent mouth care to minimize dehydration from mouth breathing.

Enemas. An enema is an instillation of a solution into the rectum and sigmoid colon. It is given primarily to promote defecation by stimulating peristalsis. The volume of fluid instilled breaks up the fecal mass, stretches the rectal wall, and begins the defecation reflex. Enemas are also a vehicle for drugs that exert a local effect on rectal mucosa.

The most common use for an enema is temporary relief of constipation. Other indications include removing impacted feces, emptying the bowel before diagnostic tests, some surgical procedures, and beginning a program of bowel training. Discourage patients from relying on enemas to maintain bowel regularity. Enemas do not treat the cause of constipation. As with overuse of laxatives, frequent use may affect normal defecation reflexes.

Cleansing enemas promote complete evacuation of feces from the colon. They act by stimulating peristalsis through the infusion of a large volume of solution or through local irritation of the mucosa of the colon. Cleansing enemas include tap water, normal saline, low-volume hypertonic saline, and soapsuds solution. Each solution exerts a different osmotic effect, causing the movement of fluids between the colon and interstitial spaces beyond the intestinal wall. Infants and children should only be given normal saline enemas because they are at greater risk for fluid imbalance (see Chapter 18).

Tap water is hypotonic and exerts a lower osmotic pressure than fluid in interstitial spaces. After infusion into the colon, tap water escapes from the bowel lumen into interstitial spaces. The net movement of water is low; the infused volume stimulates defecation before large amounts of water leave the bowel. Do not repeat tap-water enemas because water toxicity or circulatory overload develops if the body absorbs large amounts of water.

Physiologically normal saline is the safest solution to use because it exerts the same osmotic pressure as fluids in interstitial spaces around the bowel. The volume of infused saline stimulates peristalsis. Giving normal saline enemas does not create the danger of excess fluid absorption. Add ordered soap solution to tap water or saline to create the additional

BOX 35-11 PROCEDURAL GUIDELINES

Digital Removal of Stool

DELEGATION CONSIDERATIONS

The skill of digitally removing stool cannot be delegated to nursing assistive personnel (NAP). In some institutions only physicians and APNs perform this procedure. The nurse instructs the NAP:

- To provide perineal care and other necessary hygiene following each bowel movement.
- To observe any evacuated stool for color and consistency.

EQUIPMENT

Bedpan, waterproof pad, water-soluble lubricant, washcloths, towels, soap, and clean gloves

STEPS

1. Identify patient using two identifiers (e.g., name and birthday or name and account number) according to agency policy. Compare identifiers with information on patient's MAR or medical record.
2. Perform hand hygiene. Pull curtains around bed, obtain patient's baseline vital signs, assess level of comfort, and palpate for abdominal distention before procedure.
3. Explain procedure and help patient lie on the left side in Sims' position with knees flexed and back toward you.
4. Drape trunk and lower extremities with bath blanket and place waterproof pad under buttocks. Keep bedpan next to patient.
5. Apply clean gloves; lubricate index finger of dominant hand with water-soluble lubricant.
6. Instruct patient to take slow, deep breaths. Gradually and gently insert index finger into rectum and advance finger slowly along rectal wall.
7. Gently loosen fecal mass by massaging around it. Work finger into hardened mass.
8. Work feces downward toward end of rectum. Remove small pieces one at a time and discard into bedpan.
9. Periodically reassess patient's pulse and look for signs of fatigue. Stop procedure if pulse rate drops significantly (check agency policy) or rhythm changes.
10. Continue to clear rectum of feces and allow patient to rest at intervals.
11. After completion wash and dry buttocks and anal area.
12. Remove bedpan; inspect feces for color and consistency. Dispose of feces. Remove gloves by turning them inside out and discard.
13. Help patient to toilet or on bedpan if urge to defecate develops.
14. Perform hand hygiene.
15. Record results of procedure by describing fecal characteristics and amount.
16. Follow procedure with enemas or cathartics as ordered by health care provider.
17. Reassess patient's vital signs and level of comfort and observe status of abdominal distention.

effect of intestinal irritation. Only pure castile soap is safe. Harsh soaps or detergents cause bowel inflammation.

Hypertonic solutions infused into the bowel exert osmotic pressure that pulls fluids into the colon. The colon fills with fluid, and the resultant distention promotes defecation. Patients unable to tolerate large volumes of fluid benefit most from this type of enema. A hypertonic solution of 120 to 180 mL (4 to 6 oz) is usually effective. The Fleet enema is the most common.

A health care provider sometimes orders a high or low cleansing enema. The terms *high* and *low* refer to the height and pressure with which you deliver the fluid. You give high enemas to clean the entire colon. A low enema cleans only the rectum and sigmoid colon. After you infuse the enema, ask the patient to turn from the left lateral to the dorsal recumbent and over to the right lateral position. The position changes help fluid reach the large intestine.

Oil-retention enemas lubricate the rectum and colon. The feces absorb the oil and become softer and easier to pass. To enhance action of the oil, the patient retains the enema for several hours if possible.

Certain enemas contain medications. An example is sodium polystyrene sulfonate (Kayexalate), used to treat patients with dangerously high serum potassium levels. Skill 35-2 outlines the steps for enema administration.

Digital Removal of Stool. For patients with an impaction, the fecal mass is sometimes too large to pass voluntarily. If enemas fail, the mass needs to be broken up digitally. Patients with an impaction frequently have a continuous oozing of liquid stool because liquid passes around the impacted feces. This procedure is done only when all other measures have failed (Box 35-11).

The procedure is uncomfortable for the patient. Excess rectal manipulation irritates the mucosa and can cause bleeding. There is also risk of stimulation of the vagus nerve, which can result in a reflex slowing of the heart rate. Because of the potential complications of the procedure, some institutions restrict nurses from removing impactions digitally. Before you perform the procedure, check your agency policy regarding a health care provider's order.

Continuing and Restorative Care. Before a patient is able to return home or is transferred to an extended care facility, you need to help establish regular elimination patterns. Bowel retraining is one essential step in regaining independence.

Bowel Training. A bowel-training program helps patients who still have some neuromuscular control to achieve normal defecation. The training program involves setting up a daily routine. By attempting to defecate at the same time each day and using measures that promote defecation, the patient gains control of bowel reflexes. The program requires time, patience, and consistency. The health care provider determines the patient's physical readiness and ability to benefit from bowel training.

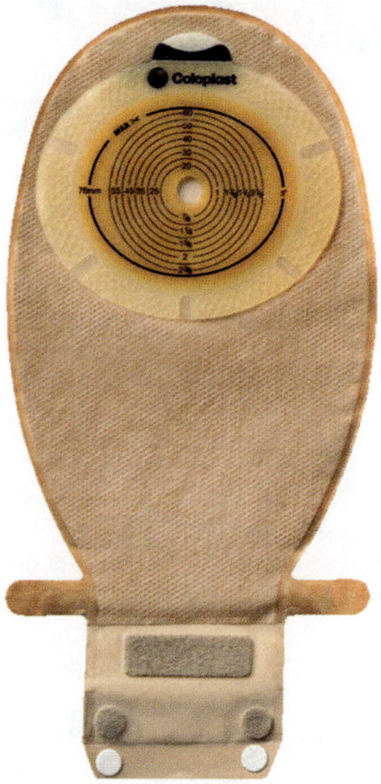

FIGURE 35-9 One-piece pouch with Velcro closure. (Courtesy Coloplast, Minneapolis, MN)

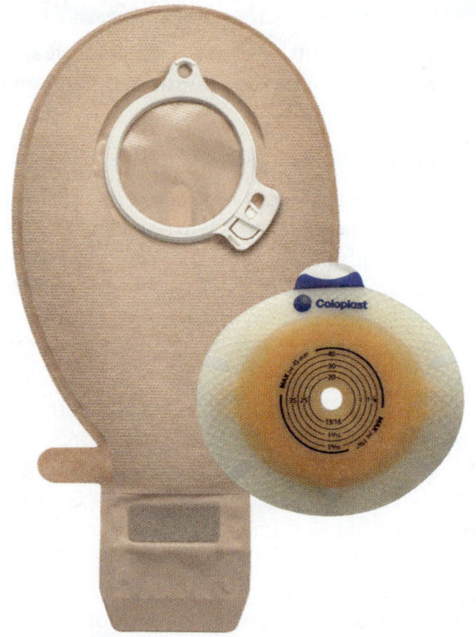

FIGURE 35-10 Two-piece pouching system with separate skin barrier and attachable pouch. (Courtesy Coloplast, Minneapolis, MN)

Ostomy Care. Immediately after a surgical diversion it is necessary to place a pouch over the newly created stoma because in some ostomies output of effluent begins soon after surgery. The pouch collects all effluent and protects the skin from irritating dermatitis. A proper pouch fits comfortably, with its skin barrier covering the skin surface around the stoma and creating a good seal. The postoperative pouch is transparent to allow visibility of the stoma.

For up to 6 weeks the new stoma may be edematous. The stoma itself often has a series of small stitches around its perimeter. Apply a pouch and skin barrier that fits right around the stoma and protects the surrounding skin. Take care to avoid disrupting the suture line. It may be several days after surgery before bowel function returns. In the case of an ileostomy, the patient has frequent liquid stools when peristalsis returns. With a colostomy the fecal output may be loose in the first few days after surgery, but a more formed stool would be expected after the patient is eating again.

Many types of pouches and skin barriers are available (Goldberg et al., 2010). Some pouches have skin barriers attached and are one-piece pouching systems (Figure 35-9). Some of these one-piece pouches already are precut to size by the manufacturer, whereas others you custom cut to size for the patient's stoma measurement. Other systems have two separate pieces (Figure 35-10). Attach the pouch to the skin barrier by attaching it to the flange (a plastic ring) on the barrier. Often you have to custom cut the skin barrier to the patient's specific stoma size. For two-piece systems use the skin barrier with flange corresponding to the size of the ring on the pouch, making sure that both pieces are from the same manufacturer. Understand how to use each of these different pouching systems before attempting to teach ostomy care to the patient. If possible, change the pouch when the stoma is less active, usually before meals. Have the patient participate in the procedure as much as possible. The patient needs to learn to recognize the normal appearance of a stoma. Skill 35-3 describes the steps for pouching an ostomy.

A patient with an ostomy suffers a change in body image. The appearance of the stoma and accompanying effluent and odor can cause psychological stress. For the patient with a new ostomy, it is important for you to encourage self-care and acceptance of the ostomy (Box 35-12). Early involvement in self-care promotes confidence. Even simple tasks such as holding pieces of equipment during stoma pouching and learning to open and close the pouch help the patient begin to adjust to bodily changes. Whenever possible, have an ostomy nurse provide care and teaching for the patient with a new stoma (Box 35-13). In addition, patients may benefit from information and encouragement from an ostomy support group.

Care of Hemorrhoids. Many patients experience discomfort from alterations in elimination. The patient with hemorrhoids has pain when hemorrhoidal tissue is directly irritated from passage of hard stool. The primary goal for the patient with hemorrhoids is soft-formed stools. Treatment includes proper diet, fluids, and regular exercise. Application of heat provides temporary relief to swollen hemorrhoids. A sitz bath is an effective means of heat application (see Chapter 37).

When hemorrhoids are present, it is important to prevent trauma to tissues. Use caution when inserting rectal thermometers, suppositories, or rectal tubes. Make sure that you can see the anal opening and never use force with insertion. A generous amount of lubricating jelly reduces friction. The

BOX 35-12 EVIDENCE-BASED PRACTICE

PICO Question: In adult patients with ostomies, what is the effect of patient education about ostomy care on the patient's quality of life?

SUMMARY OF EVIDENCE

Placement of an ostomy following colorectal cancer causes individuals to experience a change in body image. Individuals must adjust both physically and psychologically following the ostomy. Research found that quality of life was lowest 2 months after surgery but improved to almost preoperative levels at 12 months (Ito et al., 2012). Ito et al. (2012) also found that physical and social functioning was lower in individuals as they tried to incorporate ostomy care tasks into their daily life. Individuals continue to have long-term concerns 5 or more years after an ostomy that impacts their adjustment and quality of life (Sun et al., 2013). These concerns included clothing adaptations, dietary concerns, activity limitations and adaptations, leakage, seal and adhesive issues, and skin and odor issues. Individuals with ostomies who received ostomy care education look for ways to adjust their lives. Family caregivers also benefit from ostomy care education because they provide assistance to their loved ones (Palma, et al., 2012).

APPLICATION TO NURSING PRACTICE

- Nurses with specialized knowledge and training can provide education to individuals before surgery that can help with postoperative adjustment (Ito et al., 2012).
- Home health services during the first few months following ostomy placement improve individuals' adjustment.
- Help patients develop long-term support systems to cope with their ostomies (Sun et al., 2013).
- Provide support for family caregivers of individuals with ostomies on an ongoing basis (Palma et al., 2012).
- Provide long-term education and support for individuals with ostomies (Sun et al., 2013).

BOX 35-13 PATIENT TEACHING

The Patient with an Ostomy

OUTCOME

Patient/caregiver can demonstrate changing an ostomy pouch.

TEACHING STRATEGIES

- Provide a comprehensive list of the products needed to care for the ostomy.
- Provide patient/caregiver with supplies to last 1 to 2 weeks and the contact number of the closest medical supply store.
- Demonstrate how to empty the pouch and have patient begin emptying it while still in the hospital.
- Show patient/caregiver the step-by-step approach for changing an ostomy pouch.
- Provide at least one opportunity for patient/caregiver to change the ostomy pouch while patient is in hospital.
- Set up visits with an ostomy nurse or home care nurse and provide contact numbers.
- Provide detailed discharge instructions for skin care, driving, lifting, resuming exercise, and when to contact the health care provider.

EVALUATION STRATEGIES

- Observe patient/caregiver empty and change the ostomy pouch.
- Ask patient/caregiver to state signs of peristomal skin irritation and how to relieve it.
- Ask patient/caregiver about expected output from stoma and when to call health care provider.

patient may be able to insert a suppository without causing pain if he or she has done this before as part of his or her routine of care.

Maintenance of Skin Integrity. The patient with diarrhea or fecal incontinence is at risk for skin breakdown when fecal contents remain on the skin (see Chapter 37). The same problem exists for the patient with an ostomy that drains liquid stool. Liquid stool is usually acidic and contains digestive enzymes. Irritation from repeated wiping with toilet tissue causes skin breakdown. To prevent skin irritation, cleanse and dry the skin immediately after soiling occurs.

Instruct the patient or caregiver about cleansing the perineal area with a no-rinse perineal cleanser and warm water or a prepackaged perineal wipe after each passage of stool. When caring for a patient who is debilitated, incontinent, and unable to ask for assistance, check frequently for defecation. Cleanse the skin. Protect the skin around the anal area with barrier ointments. Baby powder or cornstarch is contraindicated because it does not provide a barrier to protect the skin. Check the skin for rashes that could indicate a yeast infection. Patients with incontinence who are taking antibiotics are particularly susceptible to these infections. The rash is raised and deep red with satellite lesions. The patient may complain of itching. This rash should be reported promptly so topical treatment can be started.

EVALUATION

Patient Care. Evaluate the effectiveness of nursing interventions for the patient with alterations in bowel elimination by determining success in meeting his or her expected outcomes and goals of care. Optimally the patient is to eliminate soft-formed stools regularly. In addition, he or she gains the information necessary to establish a normal elimination pattern (Box 35-14).

Evaluate success of the plan by having the patient describe his or her elimination pattern following therapy. Also make it a point to evaluate the character of the patient's stool. A return to a more normal, regular elimination pattern can take time. Periodically reevaluate the patient. Patients who defecate every 1 to 2 days and have a soft, nondistended abdomen with soft formed stool are desirable findings.

BOX 35-14 EVALUATION

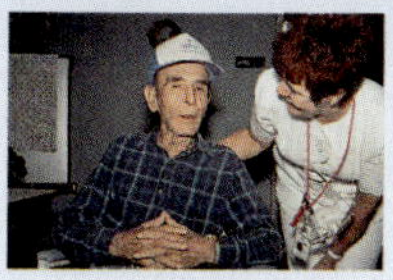

Vickie returns to see Mr. Gutierrez 2 weeks later. She is eager to determine if Mr. Gutierrez has made changes in his diet and if his problems with bowel elimination have been progressing. She is also eager to learn if the niece has helped to have Mr. Gutierrez's stove repaired.

Mr. Gutierrez tells Vickie that he has been eating bran cereal in the morning, has been eating rice and/or beans for dinner, and has added one fruit each day to his diet. He has been walking twice a day through the long-term care center. Although he does not have a bowel movement each day, his stools are much softer and easier to pass, and he says that he is less concerned. He has not taken a laxative since last talking with Vickie.

DOCUMENTATION NOTE

"Bowel elimination is improving. Abdomen is soft and nondistended. After discussing the teaching plan, has agreed to alter his eating habits to include more fiber, fruit, and fluids. Although concern over bowel habits has not ceased, does state he feels 'in better control' and has decreased laxative use. Niece assisted in having stove repaired."

Evaluate the adjustment of a patient to an ostomy during self-care. Inspect the patient's peristomal skin, looking for impairment in skin integrity. Your evaluation also includes observing the patient change and empty an ostomy pouch. Evaluate the stool formation in the patient with a colostomy because he or she may become constipated and should not have hard stools. A liquid-to-semiformed stool with an ileostomy is considered normal. Assess the patient's emotional state with regard to the ostomy and provide support as needed.

Patient Expectations. Using patient expectations identified during assessment, determine the patient's level of satisfaction with nursing care. Does the patient believe that you provided care respectfully, offering privacy and support when necessary? Is he or she satisfied with the elimination pattern established? Are stools easier to manage?

Your goal for the patient with an ostomy is to achieve a realistic level of self-care and maintain or reinforce a healthy body image. When discussing these issues with the patient, determine if the patient's participation in care helped him or her accept the ostomy. Were expectations of the patient unrealistic? Did the patient feel like a partner in care? Learning about the patient's level of satisfaction with care goes a long way toward helping future patients.

SAFETY GUIDELINES FOR NURSING SKILLS

Ensuring patient safety is an essential role of the professional nurse. To ensure patient safety, communicate clearly with the members of the health care team, assess and incorporate the patient's priorities of care and preferences, and use the best evidence when making decisions about your patient's care. When performing the skills in this chapter, remember the following points to ensure safe, individualized patient care:

- If a patient has cardiac disease or is on cardiac or hypertensive medication, obtain pulse rate before an enema because manipulation of rectal tissue stimulates the vagus nerve and can cause a sudden decline in pulse rate, which can increase patient's risk for fainting while on the bedpan, commode, or toilet.
- Instruct patients who self-administer enemas to use the side-lying position. Administering an enema with the patient sitting on the toilet is unsafe because it is impossible to safely guide the tubing into the rectum.
- Keep patient in sitting high-Fowler's position during nasogastric intubation to prevent aspiration.

SKILL 35-1 INSERTING AND MAINTAINING A NASOGASTRIC TUBE FOR GASTRIC DECOMPRESSION

DELEGATION CONSIDERATIONS

The skill of inserting and maintaining a nasogastric (NG) tube cannot be delegated to nursing assistive personnel (NAP). The nurse directs the NAP to:

- Measure and record the drainage from an NG tube.
- Provide oral and nasal hygiene measure.
- Perform selected comfort measures such as positioning or offering ice chips if allowed.
- Use the correct technique to anchor the tube to the patient's gown during routine care to prevent accidental displacement.

EQUIPMENT

- 14- or 16-Fr NG tube (smaller-lumen catheters are not used for decompression in adults because they must be able to remove thick secretions)
- Water-soluble lubricant
- Clean gloves
- pH test strips (measure gastric aspirate acidity); use paper with a range of 1.0 to 11.0 or higher
- Tongue blade
- Flashlight
- Emesis basin

SKILL 35-1 INSERTING AND MAINTAINING A NASOGASTRIC TUBE FOR GASTRIC DECOMPRESSION—cont'd

- Asepto bulb or catheter-tipped syringe
- Commercial fixation device
- Clip or safety pin and rubber band
- Marking pen
- Clamp, drainage bag, or suction machine with pressure gauge if wall suction is to be used
- Towel
- Glass of water with straw
- Normal saline
- Facial tissues
- Tincture of benzoin *(optional)*
- Stethoscope
- Suction equipment

STEP	RATIONALE
ASSESSMENT	
1. Perform hand hygiene and apply clean gloves.	Reduces transmission of microorganisms.
2. Inspect condition of patient's nasal and oral cavity. Dispose of gloves.	Baseline condition of nasal and oral cavity determines need for special nursing hygiene measures after tube placement.
3. Ask if patient has had history of nasal surgery and note if deviated nasal septum is present.	Alerts nurse to possible obstruction. Insert tube into ***uninvolved*** nasal passage. Procedure may be contraindicated if surgery is recent.
4. Auscultate for bowel sounds. Palpate patient's abdomen for distention, pain, and rigidity.	In presence of diminished or absent bowel sounds, auscultate abdomen at least 1 minute in each quadrant (Seidel et al., 2011). Documents baseline for any abdominal distention, gastrointestinal (GI) ileus, and general GI function, which later serves as comparison once tube is inserted.
5. Assess patient's level of consciousness and ability to follow instructions.	Determines patient's ability to assist in procedure.
6. Determine if patient has had an NG tube insertion in the past and which naris was used.	Patient's previous experience complements any explanations.
7. Verify health care provider's order for type of NG tube to be placed and whether tube is to be attached to suction.	Procedure requires health care provider's order. Adequate decompression depends on NG suction.
PLANNING	
1. Prepare equipment at the bedside. Have available an NG tube fixation device or a 10-cm (4-inch) piece of tape with one end split in half to form a V.	Ensures well-organized procedure. Tape is used to initially hold tube in place after insertion.
2. Identify patient using two identifiers (e.g., name and birthday or name and account number) according to agency policy. Compare identifiers with information on patient's MAR or medical record.	Ensures correct patient. Complies with The Joint Commission requirements for patient safety (TJC, 2014).
3. Position patient in high-Fowler's position with pillows behind head and shoulders. Raise bed to a horizontal level comfortable for the nurse.	Promotes patient's ability to swallow during procedure. Good body mechanics prevent injury to nurse.
IMPLEMENTATION	
1. Perform hand hygiene. Apply clean gloves.	Reduces transmission of microorganisms.
2. Place bath towel over patient's chest; give facial tissues to patient. If necessary, allow patient to blow nose. Place emesis basin within reach.	Prevents soiling of patient's gown. Tube insertion through nasal passages may cause tearing and coughing with increased salivation.
3. Pull curtain around bed or close room door. Wash bridge of nose with soap and water or alcohol swab.	Provides privacy. Removes oils from nose to allow fixation device or tape to adhere.
4. Stand on patient's right side if right-handed, left side if left-handed.	Allows easiest manipulation of tubing.
5. Instruct patient to relax and breathe normally while occluding one naris. Repeat this action for other naris. Select nostril with greater airflow.	Tube passes more easily through naris that has more airflow.

STEP	RATIONALE
6. Measure distance to insert tube:	
a. *Traditional method:* Measure distance from tip of nose to earlobe to xiphoid process (see illustration).	Approximates distance from naris to stomach; distance varies with each patient. Tube tip should enter stomach.
b. *Hanson method:* First mark 50-cm (20 inches) point on tube; then do traditional measurement. Tube insertion should be to midway point between 50 cm (20 inches) and traditional mark.	
7. Mark end point designating length of tube to be inserted with marking pen.	Marks amount of tube to be inserted from naris to stomach.
8. Curve 10 to 15 cm (4 to 6 inches) of end of tube tightly around index finger and release.	Curving tube tip aids insertion and decreases stiffness of tube.
9. Lubricate 7.5 to 10 cm (3 to 4 inches) of end of tube with water-soluble lubricating gel.	Minimizes friction against nasal mucosa and aids insertion of tube. Water-soluble lubricant is less toxic if aspirated.
10. Alert patient that procedure is to begin.	Decreases patient anxiety and increases patient cooperation.
11. Initially instruct patient to extend neck back against pillow; insert tube slowly through naris with curved end pointing downward (see illustration).	Facilitates initial passage of tube through naris and maintains clear airway for open naris.
12. Continue to pass tube along floor of nasal passage, aiming down toward ear. When you feel resistance, apply gentle downward pressure to advance tube (do not force past resistance).	Minimizes discomfort of tube rubbing against upper nasal turbinates. Resistance is caused by posterior nasopharynx. Downward pressure helps tube curl around corner of nasopharynx.
13. If resistance is met, try to rotate tube and see if it advances. If still resistant, withdraw tube, allow patient to rest, relubricate tube, and insert into other naris.	Forcing against resistance can cause trauma to mucosa. Helps relieve patient's anxiety.

Clinical Decision Point: **If unable to insert tube in either naris, stop procedure and notify health care provider.**

STEP	RATIONALE
14. Continue insertion of tube until just past nasopharynx by gently rotating tube toward opposite naris.	
a. Once past nasopharynx, stop tube advancement, allow patient to relax, and provide tissues.	Relieves patient's anxiety; tearing is natural response to mucosal irritation, and excessive salivation may occur because of oral stimulation.
b. Explain to patient that next step requires that patient swallow. Give patient glass of water unless contraindicated.	Sipping water aids passage of NG tube into esophagus.
15. With tube just above oropharynx, instruct patient to flex head forward, take a small sip of water, and swallow. Advance tube 2.5 to 5 cm (1 to 2 inches) with each swallow of water. If patient is not allowed fluids, instruct to dry swallow or suck air through straw. Advance tube with each swallow.	Flexed position closes off upper airway to trachea and opens esophagus. Swallowing closes epiglottis over trachea and helps move tube into esophagus. Swallowing water reduces gagging or choking. Water can be removed later from stomach by suction.

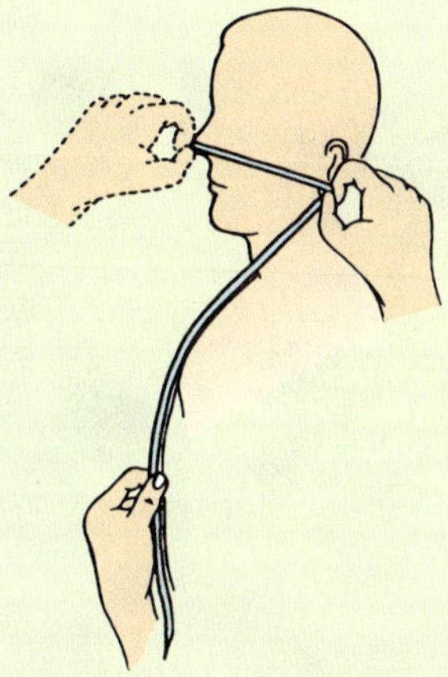

STEP 6a Technique for measuring distance to insert NG tube.

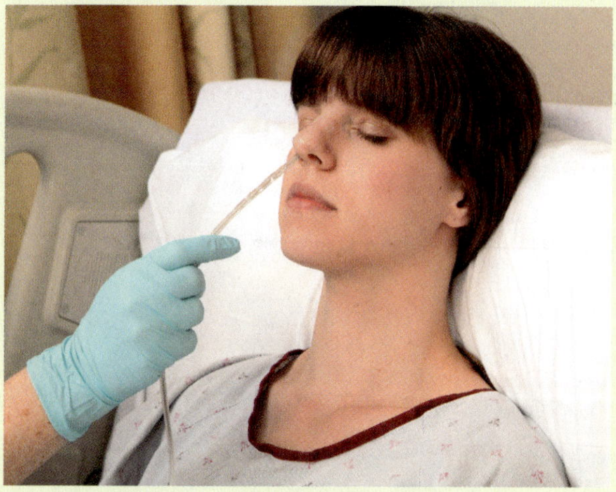

STEP 11 Insert NG tube with curved end pointing downward.

SKILL 35-1 INSERTING AND MAINTAINING A NASOGASTRIC TUBE FOR GASTRIC DECOMPRESSION—cont'd

STEP	RATIONALE
16. If patient begins to cough, gag, or choke, withdraw slightly and stop tube advancement. Instruct patient to breathe easily and take sips of water.	Tubing may accidentally enter larynx and initiate cough reflex, and withdrawal of tube reduces risk for laryngeal entry. Swallowing water eases gagging, which you must give cautiously to reduce risk for aspiration.

***Clinical Decision Point:* If vomiting occurs, help patient clear airway; oral suctioning may be needed. Stop procedure.**

STEP	RATIONALE
17. Retry insertion. If patient continues to cough, pull tube back slightly.	Tube may enter larynx and obstruct airway.
18. If patient continues to gag or complains that tube feels as though it is coiling in back of throat, check back of oropharynx with flashlight and tongue blade. If tube is coiled, withdraw it until tip is back in oropharynx. Reinsert with patient swallowing.	Tube may coil around itself in back of throat and stimulate gag reflex.
19. After patient relaxes, continue to advance tube with swallowing until you reach mark on tube, which signifies that tube is at desired distance. Temporarily anchor tube to patient's cheek with piece of tape until tube placement is verified.	Tip of tube should be within stomach to decompress properly. Anchoring tube prevents accidental displacement while tube placement is verified.
20. Verify tube placement: Check agency policy for preferred methods of checking tube placement.	
a. Ask patient to talk.	Patient is unable to talk if NG tube has passed through vocal cords.
b. Inspect posterior pharynx for presence of coiled tube.	Tube is pliable and can coil up in back of pharynx instead of advancing into esophagus.
c. Place towel under end of NG tube and attach Asepto or catheter-tipped syringe to end of tube and aspirate by gently pulling back on syringe to obtain gastric contents. Observe color (see illustration).	Gastric contents are usually cloudy and green but may be off-white, tan, bloody, or brown in color. Aspiration of contents provides means to measure fluid pH and thus determine tube tip placement in GI tract. Other common aspirate colors include yellow or bile-stained aspirate (duodenal placement) and saliva-appearing aspirate (may or may not occur from esophagus) (Hockenberry and Wilson, 2011; Lewis et al., 2011).
d. Use gastric (Gastroccult) pH paper and measure pH of aspirate with color-coded pH paper with range of whole numbers from 1.0 to 11.0 or greater (see illustration).	A properly obtained pH of 1.0 to 4.0 is a good indication of gastric placement (Bourgault and Halm, 2009; Proehl et al., 2011). Intestinal aspirates usually have a pH greater than 4.0, whereas respiratory secretions usually have a pH greater than 6.0 (Durai, Venkatraman, and Ng, 2009).

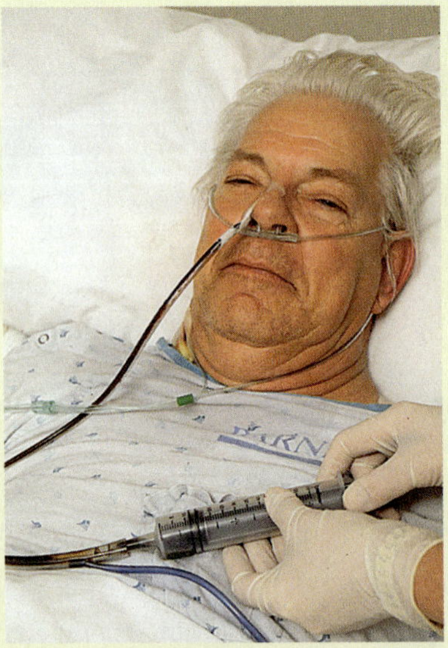

STEP 20c Aspiration of gastric contents.

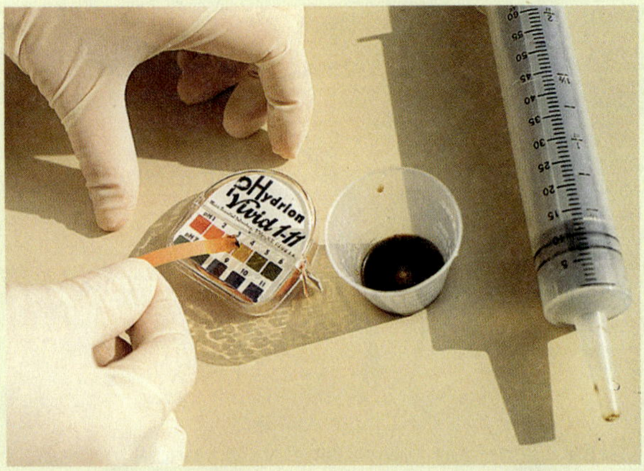

STEP 20d Checking pH of gastric aspirate.

STEP	RATIONALE
e. Have ordered x-ray film examination of chest/abdomen performed.	X-ray examination is best method to verify initial placement of tube.
f. If tube is not in stomach, advance another 2.5 to 5 cm (1 to 2 inches) and repeat Steps 20a to d to check tube position.	Tube must be in stomach to provide decompression.
21. Anchor tube, avoiding pressure on nares.	
a. Clamp end of tube or connect it to suction machine after tube is properly inserted and positioned.	Drainage bag is used for gravity drainage. Intermittent suction is most effective for decompression. Patient going to operating room or for diagnostic tests often has tube clamped.
b. Apply tube fixation device with shaped adhesive patch (see illustration).	
(1) Apply wide end of patch to bridge of nose.	
(2) Slip connector around NG tube as it exits nose.	
c. Tape tube to nose; avoid putting pressure on naris.	Prevents tissue necrosis. Tape anchors tube securely.
(1) Apply small amount of tincture of benzoin to tip of nose and allow to become "tacky" *(optional).*	Benzoin prevents loosening of tape if patient perspires.
(2) Split one end of the prepared 10-cm (5-inch) strip of tape 5 cm (2 inches).	
(3) Carefully wrap each of the 5-cm strips in opposite directions around tube as it exits nose (see illustration).	
d. Fasten end of NG tube to patient's gown by using clip or by looping rubber band around tube in slipknot and pinning rubber band to gown. Provide slack for head movement. Do not attach pin to NG tube itself.	Reduces pressure on naris if tube moves.
e. When using Salem sump tube, keep pigtail above level of stomach.	Prevents siphoning action that clogs tube.
f. Unless health care provider orders otherwise, head of bed should be elevated 30 to 45 degrees.	Helps prevent esophageal reflux and resultant aspiration. Minimizes irritation of tube against posterior pharynx.
g. Explain to patient that sensation of tube should decrease somewhat with time.	Adaptation to continued sensory stimulus occurs.
h. Remove gloves, discard, and perform hand hygiene.	Reduces transmission of microorganisms.
22. Once placement is confirmed by x-ray:	
a. Place a mark, either a red mark or piece of tape, on tube to indicate where tube exits nose.	Mark or tube length is to be used as guide to indicate whether displacement may have occurred.
b. *Option:* Measure tube length from naris to connector as alternative method.	
c. Document tube length in patient record.	

***Clinical Decision Point:* Never reposition the NG tube of a gastric surgery patient, because repositioning could rupture the suture line.**

23. Attach NG tube to suction as ordered. Usual setting is low intermittent.	Suction creates gastric decompression.

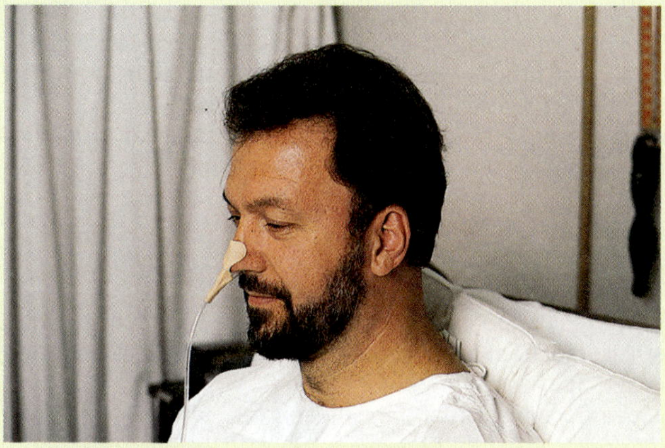

STEP 21b Patient with tube fixation device.

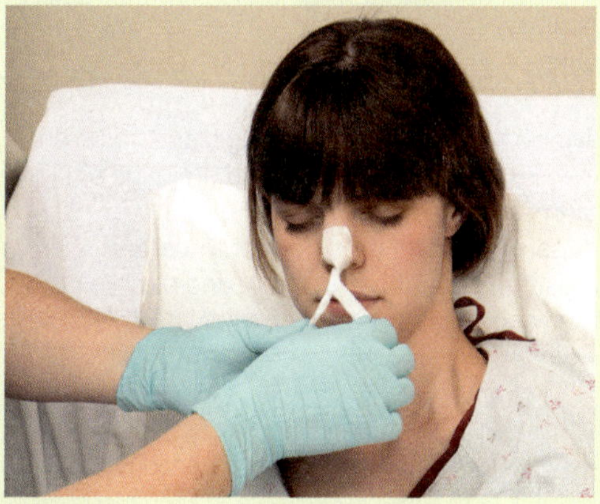

STEP 21c(3) Tape is crossed over and around NG tube.

SKILL 35-1 INSERTING AND MAINTAINING A NASOGASTRIC TUBE FOR GASTRIC DECOMPRESSION—cont'd

STEP	RATIONALE
24. Tube irrigation:	
a. Perform hand hygiene and apply clean gloves.	Reduces transmission of microorganisms.
b. Check for tube placement in stomach (see Step 20d). Temporarily clamp tube or reconnect to connecting tube and remove syringe.	Prevents accidental entrance of irrigating solution into lungs.
c. Draw up 30 mL of normal saline into Asepto or catheter-tip syringe.	Use of saline minimizes loss of electrolytes from stomach fluids.
d. Kink end of NG tube. Disconnect clamp or remove connecting tubing. Lay end of connection tubing on towel.	Reduces soiling of patient's gown and bed linen.
e. Insert tip of irrigating syringe into end of NG tube. Release tube. Hold syringe with tip pointed at floor and inject saline slowly and evenly. Do not force solution.	Position of syringe prevents introduction of air into vent tubing, which could cause gastric distention. Solution introduced under pressure can cause gastric trauma.

Clinical Decision Point: **Do not introduce saline through blue "pigtail" air vent of Salem sump tube.**

STEP	RATIONALE
f. If resistance occurs, check for kinks in tubing. Turn patient onto left side. Report repeated resistance to health care provider.	Tip of tube may lie against stomach lining. Repositioning on left side may dislodge tube away from stomach lining. Buildup of secretions causes distention.
g. After instilling saline, immediately aspirate by pulling back slowly on syringe to withdraw fluid. If amount aspirated is greater than amount instilled, record difference as output. If amount aspirated is less than amount instilled, record difference as intake.	Irrigation clears tubing; thus stomach should remain empty. Fluid remaining in stomach is measured as intake.
h. Reconnect NG tube to drainage or suction. (If solution does not return, repeat irrigation.)	Reestablishes drainage collection; may repeat irrigation or repositioning of tube until NG tube drains properly.
i. Remove gloves and perform hand hygiene.	Reduces transmission of microorganisms.
25. Removal of NG tube:	
a. Verify order to remove NG tube.	Health care provider's order required for procedure.
b. Auscultate abdomen for presence of bowel sounds.	Verifies the return of peristalsis.
c. Explain procedure to patient and reassure that removal is less distressing than insertion.	Minimizes anxiety and increases cooperation. Tube passes out smoothly.
d. Perform hand hygiene and apply clean gloves.	Reduces transmission of microorganisms.
e. Turn off suction and disconnect NG tube from drainage bag or suction. Remove tape or fixation device from bridge of nose and unpin tube from gown.	Have tube free of connections before removal.
f. Stand on patient's right side if right-handed, left side if left-handed.	Allows easiest manipulation of tube.
g. Hand patient facial tissue; place clean towel across chest. Instruct patient to take and hold a deep breath.	Patient may wish to blow nose after tube is removed. Towel may keep gown from getting soiled. Airway is temporarily obstructed during tube removal.
h. Clamp or kink tubing securely and pull tube out steadily and smoothly into towel held in other hand while patient holds breath.	Clamping prevents tube contents from draining into oropharynx. Reduces trauma to mucosa and minimizes patient's discomfort. Towel covers tube, which is an unpleasant sight. Holding breath helps to prevent aspiration.
i. Measure amount of drainage and note character of content. Dispose of tube and drainage equipment into proper container.	Provides accurate measure of fluid output. Reduces transfer of microorganisms.
j. Clean naris and provide mouth care.	Promotes comfort.
k. Position patient comfortably and explain procedure for drinking fluids if not contraindicated.	Depends on health care provider's order. Sometimes patients are allowed nothing by mouth (NPO) for up to 24 hours. When fluids are allowed, oral intake usually begins with a small amount of ice chips each hour and increases as patient is able to tolerate more.
l. Remove gloves and perform hand hygiene.	Reduces transmission of microorganisms.

STEP	RATIONALE
26. Clean equipment and return to proper place. Place soiled linen in utility room or proper receptacle.	Proper disposal of equipment prevents spread of microorganisms and ensures proper exchange procedures.
EVALUATION	
1. Observe amount and character of contents draining from NG tube. Ask if patient feels nauseated.	Determines if tube is decompressing stomach of contents.
2. Inspect condition of naris and nose.	Evaluates onset of skin and tissue irritation.
3. Observe position of tubing.	Determines if tension is being applied to nasal structures.
4. Ask if patient feels sore throat or irritation in pharynx.	Evaluates level of patient's discomfort.
5. Use Teach Back—State to the patient, "I want to be sure I explained why you need the NG tube and the importance of letting me know if you are nauseated." Revise your instruction now or develop plan for revised patient teaching to be implemented at an appropriate time if patient is not able to teach back correctly.	Evaluates what the patient is able to explain or demonstrate.

RECORDING AND REPORTING

- Record length, size, and type of gastric tube inserted; time of insertion; and through which nostril it was inserted. Also record patient's tolerance to procedure, confirmation of tube placement, character of gastric contents, pH value, whether tube is clamped or connected to suction, and amount of suction supplied.
- Record amount of normal saline instilled and amount of gastric aspirate removed. Record amount and character of contents draining from NG tube every shift.
- Record removal of tube as "intact," patient's tolerance of procedure, and final amount and character of NG drainage.
- Document your evaluation of patient learning.

UNEXPECTED OUTCOMES AND RELATED INTERVENTIONS

- Patient's abdomen is distended or painful.
  - Assess patency of tube.
  - Irrigate tube.
  - Verify that suction is on as ordered.
- Patient complains of sore throat from dry, irritated mucous membranes.
  - Perform oral hygiene more frequently.
  - Ask health care provider whether patient can suck on ice chips or throat lozenges.
- Patient develops irritation or erosion of skin around nares.
  - Provide frequent skin care to area.
  - Retape tube to avoid pressure on naris.
  - Consider reinsertion and switching tube to other naris. Consult with health care provider.
- Patient develops signs and symptoms of pulmonary aspiration: fever, shortness of breath, or pulmonary congestion.
  - Perform complete respiratory assessment.
  - Notify health care provider.
  - Obtain chest x-ray film examination as ordered.
  - Clamp tubing and do not flush it or put any medications through it until tube placement is verified.

SKILL 35-2 ADMINISTERING A CLEANSING ENEMA

View Video!

DELEGATION CONSIDERATIONS

The skill of administering an enema can be delegated to nursing assistive personnel (NAP); check agency policy. It is the nurse's responsibility to assess the patient for specific considerations such as need for alternative positioning, comfort, and stable vital signs before the procedure. Instruct NAP about:

- Proper ways to position patients who have mobility restrictions.
- Positioning of patients with therapeutic equipment such as drains, intravenous (IV) catheters, or traction present.
- Reporting signs and symptoms of patient not tolerating the procedure and when to stop it, including abdominal pain (more than a pressure sensation), abdominal cramping, abdominal distention, or rectal bleeding.
- The expected outcome of the enema and to immediately inform the nurse if blood is present in the stool or around the rectal area, any change in patient vital signs, or new symptoms so the nurse is able to further assess the patient.

EQUIPMENT

- Clean gloves
- Water-soluble lubricant
- Waterproof, absorbent pads
- Bath blanket
- Toilet tissue
- Bedpan, bedside commode, or access to toilet
- Basin, washcloths, towel, and soap
- IV pole

SKILL 35-2 ADMINISTERING A CLEANSING ENEMA—cont'd

Enema Bag Administration

- Enema container with tubing and clamp attachment
- Appropriate-size rectal tube:
  - Adult: 22 to 30 Fr
  - Child: 12 to 18 Fr
- Correct volume of warmed solution:
  - Adult: 750 to 1000 mL
  - Child:
    - 150 to 250 mL, infant
    - 250 to 350 mL, toddler
    - 300 to 500 mL, school-age child
    - 500 to 700 mL, adolescent

Prepackaged Enema

- Prepackaged enema container with rectal tip (Figure 35-11).

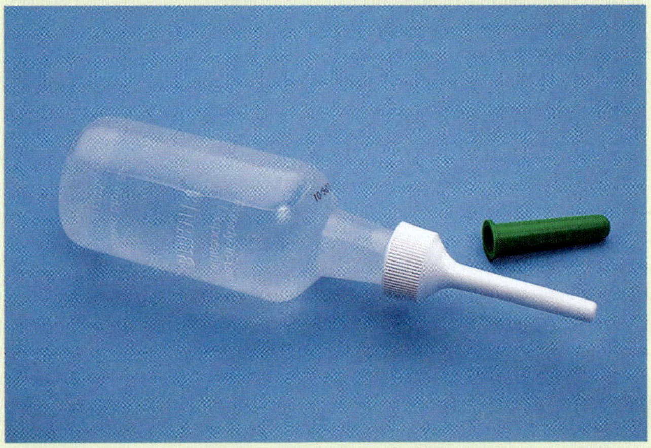

FIGURE 35-11 Prepackaged enema container with rectal tip.

STEP	RATIONALE
ASSESSMENT	
1. Review health care provider's order for type of enema and number to administer.	Enemas require health care provider's order. Determines number and type of enema that you give.
2. Assess status of patient: last bowel movement, normal versus most recent bowel pattern, presence of hemorrhoids, mobility, presence of abdominal pain.	Determines factors indicating need for enema and influencing type of enema used. Also establishes baseline for bowel function.
3. Review medical record for presence of increased intracranial pressure; glaucoma; or recent abdominal, rectal, or prostate surgery.	These conditions contraindicate use of enemas.
4. Inspect abdomen for presence of distention.	Provides baseline for determining effectiveness of enema.
5. Determine patient's level of understanding of purpose of enema.	Allows you to plan for appropriate teaching measures.

Clinical Decision Point: **"Enemas until clear" order means that you repeat enemas until patient passes fluid that is clear of fecal matter. Check agency policy, but usually patients receive no more than three consecutive enemas to avoid disruption of fluid and electrolyte balance. It is essential to observe contents of solution passed. Consider results "clear" when no solid fecal material exists but the solution is sometimes colored.**

STEP	RATIONALE
PLANNING	
1. Collect appropriate equipment.	
2. If enema is medicated, check accuracy and completeness of each medication administration record (MAR) with the health care provider's written order. Check patient's name, type of enema, and time for administration. Compare MAR with label of enema solution.	The order is the most reliable source and only legal record of drugs or procedure that the patient is to receive. Ensures that patient receives the correct enema solution.
3. Identify patient using two identifiers (e.g., name and birthday or name and account number) according to agency policy. Compare identifiers with information on patient's MAR or medical record.	Ensures correct patient. Complies with The Joint Commission requirements for patient safety (TJC, 2014).
4. Assemble enema bag with appropriate solution and ordered medication and rectal tube if enema administration set does not have tube integrated into kit.	Proper equipment promotes best outcome from procedure.

STEP	RATIONALE
IMPLEMENTATION	
1. Provide privacy by closing curtains around bed or closing door.	Reduces embarrassment for patient.
2. Place bedpan or commode in easily accessible position. If patient will be expelling contents in toilet, ensure that toilet is free. (If patient will be getting up to bathroom to expel enema, place patient's slippers and bathrobe in easily accessible position.)	Try to avoid incontinence of stool and enema fluid to avoid discomfort and psychological stress.
3. Raise bed to appropriate working height. Raise side rail on opposite side of bed from where you plan to stand.	Promotes good body mechanics and patient safety.
4. Perform hand hygiene and apply clean gloves.	Reduces transmission of microorganisms.
5. Help patient into left side-lying (Sims') position with right knee flexed. Children may also be placed in dorsal recumbent position.	Positioning allows enema solution to flow downward by gravity along natural curve of sigmoid colon and rectum, thus improving retention of solution.

Clinical Decision Point: **Patients with poor sphincter control are unable to retain all of the enema solution and require placement of a bedpan under the buttocks. Administering an enema with patient sitting on the toilet is unsafe because the curved rectal tubing can abrade the rectal wall.**

STEP	RATIONALE
6. Place waterproof pad under hips and buttocks.	Prevents soiling of linen.
7. Cover patient with bath blanket, exposing only rectal area, clearly visualizing anus. Separate buttocks and examine perianal region for abnormalities, including hemorrhoids, anal fissure, and rectal prolapse (protrusion of colon through the anal opening).	Provides warmth, reduces exposure of body parts, and allows patient to feel more relaxed and comfortable. Findings influence approach to insert enema tip. Prolapse contraindicates an enema.
8. Administer enema:	
A. **Enema bag**	
(1) Add warmed solution to enema bag: warm tap water as it flows from faucet, place saline container in basin of hot water before adding saline to enema bag. Check temperature of solution by pouring small amount of solution over inner wrist.	Hot water burns intestinal mucosa. Cold water causes abdominal cramping and is difficult to retain.
(2) If soapsuds enema is ordered, add castile soap.	
(3) Raise container, release clamp, and allow solution to flow long enough to fill tubing.	Removes air from tubing.
(4) Reclamp tubing.	Prevents further loss of solution.
(5) Lubricate 6 to 8 cm (2½ to 3 inches) of tip of rectal tube with lubricating jelly.	Allows smooth insertion of rectal tube without risk for irritation or trauma to mucosa.
(6) Gently separate buttocks and locate anus. Instruct patient to relax by breathing out slowly through mouth.	Breathing out promotes relaxation of external anal sphincter.
(7) Insert tip of enema tube slowly by pointing tip in direction of patient's umbilicus. Length of insertion varies: Adult and adolescent: 7.5 to 10 cm (3 to 4 inches); child: 5 to 7.5 cm (2 to 3 inches); infant: 2.5 to 3.75 cm (1 to 1½ inches).	Careful insertion prevents trauma to rectal mucosa from accidental lodging of tube against rectal wall. Insertion beyond proper limit causes bowel damage.

Clinical Decision Point: **If pain occurs or resistance is felt during the procedure, stop and discuss with health care provider. Do not force tube into rectum.**

STEP	RATIONALE
(8) Hold tubing in rectum constantly until end of fluid instillation.	Prevents expulsion of rectal tube during bowel contractions.
(9) Open regulating clamp and allow solution to enter slowly while holding container at patient's hip level.	Rapid instillation stimulates evacuation of rectal tube and can cause cramping.

SKILL 35-2 ADMINISTERING A CLEANSING ENEMA—cont'd

STEP	RATIONALE
(10) Raise height of enema container slowly to appropriate level above anus: 30 to 45 cm (12 to 18 inches) for high enema, 30 cm (12 inches) for regular enema, 7.5 cm (3 inches) for low enema. Instillation time varies, depending on volume of solution you administer (e.g., 1 L may take 10 min) (see illustration). You may use an IV pole to hold an enema bag once you get a slow flow of fluid established.	Allows for continuous, slow instillation of solution; raising container too high causes rapid instillation and possible painful distention of colon. High pressure causes rupture of bowel in infant.
(11) Lower container or clamp tubing if patient complains of cramping or if fluid escapes around rectal tube.	Temporarily stopping instillation prevents cramping, which prevents patient from retaining all fluid, altering effectiveness of enema.
(12) Clamp tubing after you instill all solution.	Prevents air from entering rectum.
B. Prepackaged disposable container	
(1) Remove plastic cap from rectal tip. Apply more jelly as needed to prelubricated tip.	Lubrication provides for smooth insertion of rectal tube without causing rectal irritation or trauma.
(2) Gently separate buttocks and locate rectum. Instruct patient to relax by breathing out slowly through mouth.	Breathing out promotes relaxation of external rectal sphincter.
(3) Expel any air from enema container.	Introducing air into colon causes further distention and discomfort.
(4) Insert tip of bottle gently into rectum toward umbilicus (see illustration). • *Adult/adolescent:* 7.5 to 10 cm (3 to 4 inches) • *Child:* 5 to 7.5 cm (2 to 3 inches) • *Infant:* 2.5 to 3.75 cm (1 to 1½ inches)	Gentle insertion prevents trauma to rectal mucosa.
(5) Squeeze bottle until all solution has entered rectum and colon. Instruct patient to retain solution until urge to defecate occurs, usually 2 to 5 minutes.	Hypertonic solutions require only small volumes to stimulate defecation.

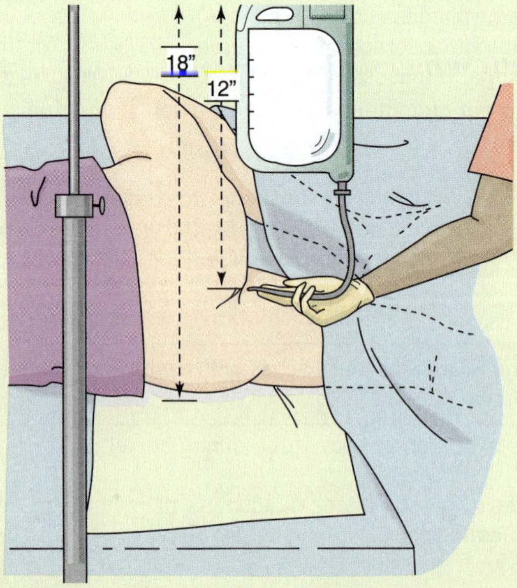

STEP 8A(10) An enema is given in Sims' position. The intravenous (IV) pole is positioned so enema bag is 12 inches above anus and approximately 18 inches above mattress (depending on patient's size). (From Sorrentino SA: *Mosby's textbook for nursing assistants*, ed 8, St Louis, 2012, Mosby.)

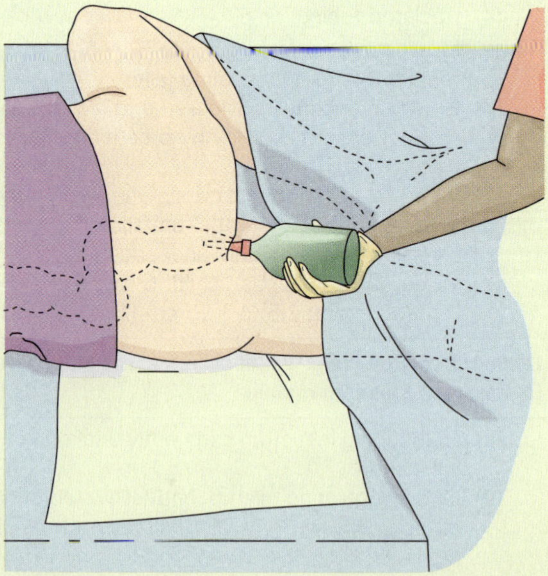

STEP 8B(4) With patient in left lateral Sims' position, insert tip of commercial enema into rectum. (From Sorrentino SA: *Mosby's textbook for nursing assistants*, ed 8, St Louis, 2012, Mosby.)

STEP	RATIONALE
9. Place layers of toilet tissue around tube at anus and gently withdraw rectal tube.	Provides for patient's comfort and cleanliness.
10. Explain to patient that feeling of distention and some abdominal cramping are normal. Ask patient to retain solution as long as possible while lying quietly in bed. (For infant or young child, gently hold buttocks together for few minutes.)	Solution distends bowel. Length of retention varies with type of enema and patient's ability to contract rectal sphincter. Longer retention promotes more effective stimulation of peristalsis and defecation.
11. Discard enema container and tubing in proper receptacle or rinse bag out thoroughly with warm soap and water if container is reusable.	Reduces transmission and growth of microorganisms.
12. Help patient to bathroom or help to position patient on bedpan.	Normal sitting position promotes defecation.
13. Help patient as needed in washing anal area with warm water, premoistened perineal wipe, or no-rinse perineal cleanser (if you administer perineal care, use clean gloves).	Fecal contents irritate skin. Hygiene promotes patient's comfort.
14. Remove and discard gloves and perform hand hygiene.	Reduces transmission of microorganisms.
EVALUATION	
1. Observe character of feces and solution evacuated (caution patient against flushing toilet before inspection). Inspect color, consistency, amount of stool, odor, and fluid passed.	Determines if stool is evacuated or fluid is retained. Note abnormalities such as presence of blood or mucus.
2. Assess condition of abdomen; cramping, rigidity, or distention indicates a serious problem.	Determines if distention is relieved. Excess volume distends or damages bowel.
3. Use Teach Back—State to the patient, "I want to be sure I explained the correct position for an enema. Can you show me how you would lie down?" Revise your instruction now or develop plan for revised patient teaching to be implemented at an appropriate time if patient is not able to teach back correctly.	Evaluates what the patient is able to demonstrate.

RECORDING AND REPORTING

- Record type and volume of enema given, time administered, characteristics of results, and patient's tolerance to procedure in nurses' notes.
- Report failure of patient to defecate and any adverse effects to health care provider.
- Document your evaluation of patient learning.

UNEXPECTED OUTCOMES AND RELATED INTERVENTIONS

- Abdomen becomes rigid and distended, and patient complains of severe pain.
  - Stop enema.
  - Notify health care provider.
  - Obtain vital signs.
- Abdominal pain or cramping develops.
  - Slow rate of instillation; have patient take slow, deep breaths.
- Bleeding develops.
  - Stop enema.
  - Notify health care provider.
  - Remain with patient and obtain vital signs.

SKILL 35-3 POUCHING AN OSTOMY

View Video!

DELEGATION CONSIDERATIONS

The skill of pouching a new ostomy cannot be delegated to nursing assistive personnel (NAP). In some agencies care of an established ostomy (4 to 6 weeks or more after surgery) can be delegated to NAP (see agency policy). The nurse informs the NAP about:

- The expected amount, color, and consistency of drainage from the ostomy.
- The expected appearance of the stoma.
- Special equipment needed to complete procedure.
- When to report changes in the patient's stoma and surrounding skin integrity.

SKILL 35-3 POUCHING AN OSTOMY—cont'd

EQUIPMENT

- Skin barrier/pouch—clear, drainable one-piece or two-piece, cut to fit or precut size
- Pouch closure device such as a clip if needed
- Ostomy measuring guide
- Adhesive remover *(optional)*
- Clean gloves
- Washcloth
- Towel or disposable waterproof barrier
- Basin with warm tap water
- Scissors
- Waterproof bag for disposal of pouch
- Stethoscope
- Tape or ostomy belt *(optional)*
- Gown and goggles if there is a risk of splash when emptying the pouch *(optional)*

STEP	RATIONALE
ASSESSMENT	
1. Perform hand hygiene and apply gloves. Auscultate for bowel sounds.	Reduces transmission of microorganisms. Documents presence of peristalsis. Absence of sounds may be a warning sign of problems.
2. Observe existing skin barrier and pouch for leakage and length of time in place. Pouch should be changed every 3 to 7 days, not daily (Goldberg et al., 2010). Depending on type of pouching system used (such as opaque pouch), you may have to remove pouch to fully observe stoma. Clear pouches permit viewing of stoma without their removal.	Assesses effectiveness of pouching system and allows for early detection of potential problems. To minimize skin irritation, avoid unnecessary changing of entire pouching system; but, if the effluent is leaking under the wafer, change it because skin damage from effluent causes more skin trauma than early removal of wafer. Repeated leaking may indicate need for different type of pouch.

***Clinical Decision Point:* Repeated leaking may indicate need for different type of pouch. If ostomy pouch is leaking, change it. Taping or patching it to contain effluent leaves the skin exposed to chemical or enzymatic irritation.**

STEP	RATIONALE
3. Observe amount of effluent in pouch and empty pouch if it is more than one-third to one-half full. Open clip and drain contents of pouch into container for measurement of output. Note consistency of effluent and record intake and output.	Pouches must be emptied when they are one-third to one-half full because weight of pouch may disrupt seal of adhesive on skin. Monitors fluid balance and return of bowel function after surgery.
4. Observe stoma for location, color, swelling, trauma, and healing or irritation of peristomal skin. Assess type of stoma. Determine if it is budded, flush with skin level, or retracted below skin level (see illustrations). Remove and dispose of gloves.	Stoma characteristics are one of the factors to consider in selecting appropriate pouching system. Convexity in skin barrier is often necessary with flush or retracted stoma.
5. Observe abdomen for best type of pouching system. Consider: **a.** Abdominal contour **b.** Presence of scars or incisions **c.** Location and type of stoma	Determines pouching system selection. Abdominal contours, scars, or incisions affect type of system and adhesion to skin surface.

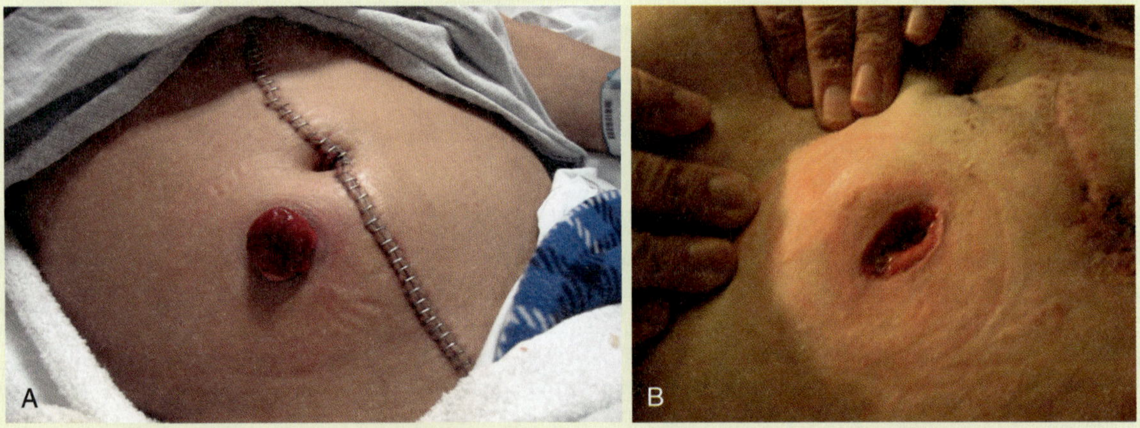

STEP 4 A, Budded stoma. **B,** Retracted stoma. (Courtesy Jane Fellows.)

STEP	RATIONALE
6. Explore patient's attitude toward learning self-care and identify others who will be helping patient after leaving hospital.	Facilitates teaching plan and timing of care to coincide with availability of caregivers.
PLANNING	
1. Identify patient using two identifiers (e.g., name and birthday or name and account number) according to agency policy.	Ensures correct patient. Complies with The Joint Commission requirements for patient safety (TJC, 2014).
2. Explain procedure to patient; encourage patient's interaction and questions.	Lessens patient's anxiety and promotes patient's participation.
3. Assemble equipment and close room curtains or door.	Optimizes use of time; provides privacy.
IMPLEMENTATION	
1. Position patient in semireclining position. (**Note:** Some patients with established ostomies prefer to stand.) If possible provide patient a mirror for observation.	When patient is semireclining, there are fewer skin wrinkles, which allows for ease of application of pouching system.
2. Perform hand hygiene and apply clean gloves.	Reduces transmission of microorganisms.
3. Place towel or disposable waterproof barrier across patient's lower abdomen.	Protects bed linen; maintains patient's dignity.
4. If not done during assessment, remove used pouch and skin barrier gently by pushing skin away from barrier. An adhesive remover may be used to facilitate removal of skin barrier. Dispose in waterproof bag.	Reduces skin trauma. Improper removal of pouch and barrier can cause peristomal skin irritation or breakdown.
5. Cleanse peristomal skin gently with warm tap water with a washcloth; do not scrub skin. If you touch stoma, minor bleeding is normal. Pat skin dry. When pouching an ileostomy, place disposable washcloth over stoma.	Avoid soap. It leaves residue on skin, which may irritate skin; and pouch does not adhere to wet skin. Ileostomies leak continuously in some patients.
6. Measure stoma (see illustration). Expect size of stoma to change for first 4 to 6 weeks after surgery.	Allows for proper fit of pouch that protects peristomal skin.
7. Trace pattern on pouch/skin barrier (see illustration).	Prepares for cutting opening in pouch.
8. Cut opening on skin barrier wafer (see illustration).	Customizes pouch to provide appropriate fit over stoma.
9. Remove protective backing from adhesive (see illustration).	Prepares skin barrier for placement.
10. Apply pouch over stoma (see illustration). Press firmly into place around stoma and outside edges. Have patient hold hand over pouch to apply heat to secure seal.	Pouch adhesives are heat and pressure sensitive and hold more securely at body temperature.
11. Close end of pouch with clip or integrated closure. Remove drape from patient.	Ensures pouch is secure. Contains effluent.
12. Properly dispose of used pouch and remove drape from patient.	Avoids odor in room.
13. Remove gloves. Perform hand hygiene.	Reduces transmission of microorganisms.

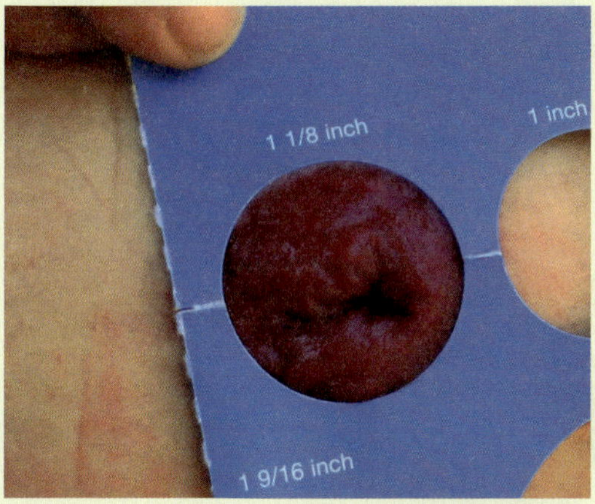

STEP 6 Measure stoma. (Courtesy Coloplast, Minneapolis, MN.)

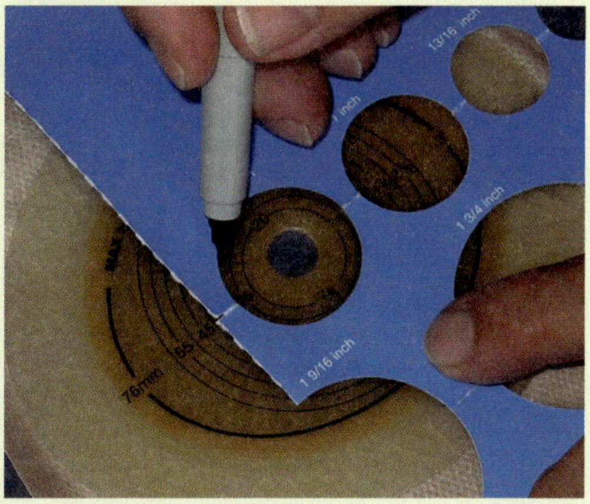

STEP 7 Trace measurement on skin barrier. (Courtesy Coloplast, Minneapolis, MN.)

SKILL 35-3 POUCHING AN OSTOMY—cont'd

STEP	RATIONALE
EVALUATION	
1. Observe condition of skin barrier and adherence to abdominal surface.	Determines presence of leaks.
2. Observe appearance of stoma, peristomal skin, abdominal contours, and suture line during pouch change.	Provides information if another type of pouching system or additional skin care products are needed.

Clinical Decision Point: **If peristomal skin is raw, blistered, or weeping, the skin surface is moist, and the pouch does not adhere, making the patient vulnerable to more severe skin breakdown. Consult the ostomy care nurse before proceeding with placing a pouch over moist, damaged skin.**

STEP	RATIONALE
3. Observe characteristics of stool.	Determines status of peristalsis and bowel elimination.
4. Observe patient's, family caregiver's, or significant other's willingness to view stoma and ask questions about procedure.	Determines level of adjustment and understanding of stoma care and pouch application. Allows planning for future education needs and progress toward acceptance of altered body image.
5. Use Teach Back—State to the patient, "I want to be sure I explained how to apply your pouch over your stoma. Can you show me how you will do this at home?" Revise your instruction now or develop plan for revised patient teaching to be implemented at an appropriate time if patient is not able to teach back correctly.	Evaluates what the patient is able to demonstrate.

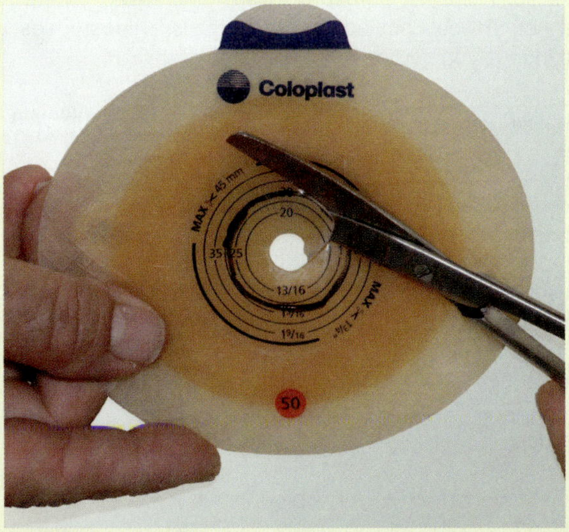

STEP 8 Cut opening in wafer. (Courtesy Coloplast, Minneapolis, MN.)

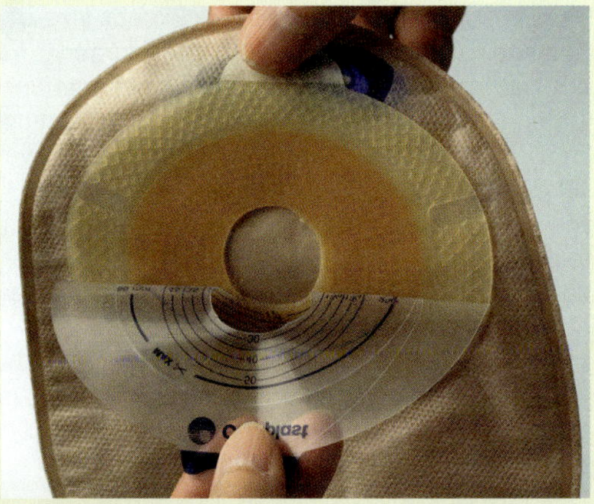

STEP 9 Remove protective backing. (Courtesy Coloplast, Minneapolis, MN.)

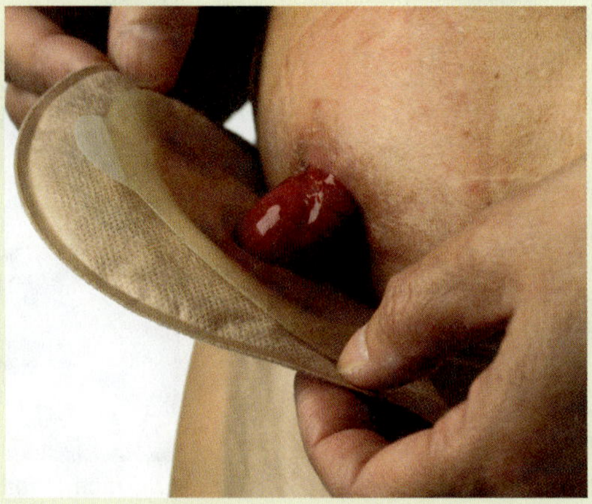

STEP 10 Apply pouch over stoma. (Courtesy Coloplast, Minneapolis, MN.)

RECORDING AND REPORTING

- Document type of pouch and skin barrier applied.
- Record amount and appearance of stool or drainage in pouch, size of stoma, color of stool, texture, condition of peristomal skin, and sutures.
- Document abdominal distention and excessive tenderness.
- Record patient's level of participation and need for teaching.
- Report any of the following to nurse in charge and/or health care provider:
  - Abnormal appearance of stoma, suture line, peristomal skin, character of output,
  - No flatus in 24 to 36 hours and no stool by third day
- Document your evaluation of patient learning.

UNEXPECTED OUTCOMES AND RELATED INTERVENTIONS

- Skin around stoma is irritated, blistered, or bleeding or a rash is noted. May be caused by undermining of pouch seal by fecal contents, allergic reaction, or fungal skin eruption.
  - Remove pouch more carefully.
  - Change pouch more frequently or use different type of pouching system.
  - Consult ostomy care nurse.
- Necrotic stoma is manifested by purple or black color, dry instead of moist texture, failure to bleed when washed gently, or tissue sloughing.
  - Report to nurse/health care provider.
  - Document appearance.
- Patient refuses to view stoma or participate in care.
  - Obtain referral for ostomy care nurse.
  - Allow patient to express feelings.
  - Encourage family support.

KEY POINTS

- Mechanical breakdown of food elements, GI motility, and selective absorption and secretion of substances by the large intestine influence the character of feces.
- Food high in fiber content and an increased fluid intake keep feces soft.
- Daily exercise is important to maintenance of normal bowel function.
- The greatest dangers from diarrhea are dehydration and fluid and electrolyte imbalance.
- A patient with a fecal diversion (colostomy or ileostomy) requires teaching in the care of the stoma and support in adjusting to the change in body image and function.
- The location of an ostomy influences the consistency of stool.
- Assessment of an elimination pattern focuses on bowel habits, an analysis of factors that normally influence defecation, a review of recent changes in elimination, and a physical examination.
- An FOBT or a FIT is a test to determine if blood is present in a stool sample. It is a screening tool for colon cancer and is frequently done annually as a part of a routine physical on those who are over 50 years of age.
- Consider frequency of defecation, fecal characteristics, effect of foods on GI function, and patient's food preferences when selecting a diet promoting normal elimination.
- Proper administration of an enema requires the slow instillation of the correct volume of a solution.
- Dangers during digital removal of stool include traumatizing the rectal mucosa and promoting vagal stimulation.
- Skin breakdown occurs after repeated exposure to liquid stool; prevention of this is an important nursing responsibility.

CLINICAL DECISION-MAKING EXERCISES

Mr. Gutierrez has had surgery for rectal cancer and has a colostomy. He is going to be discharged from the hospital soon. He is adamant that he wishes to go back to his assisted-living facility. However, he walks with a walker and the assistance of one person and has attempted to empty his ostomy pouch but has difficulty opening and closing it because of weakness in his hands. He has not participated in changing his pouch. He is eating small meals but not taking fluids by mouth because he reports getting full if he drinks too much.

1. Who should be involved in planning for Mr. Gutierrez's discharge?
2. Which services need to be coordinated to ensure the patient's safe discharge from the hospital?

3. Which patient education goals must be met before discharge?

evolve
Answers to Clinical Decision-Making Exercises can be found on the Evolve website.

QSEN ACTIVITY: TEAMWORK AND COLLABORATION

Vickie continued to keep in touch with Mr. Gutierrez's niece while he was in the hospital and visited him several times. He reluctantly agreed to go to a skilled nursing facility for a couple of weeks for continued ostomy care, teaching, and physical therapy. She learns that he is able to open and close his ostomy pouch and can empty the pouch with minimal assistance. Mr. Gutierrez and his niece have had several visits from the ostomy nurse at the hospital, and she gave them written instructions for his care. The family requests that Vickie continue with her visits since she has a good relationship with the patient and he responds well to her.

How can Vickie best prepare to continue caring for her patient although she has little experience in ostomy care other than what she has received in her classroom learning?

evolve
Answers to QSEN Activities can be found on the Evolve website.

REVIEW QUESTIONS

1. The nurse should do which of the following when placing a bedpan under an immobilized patient?
   1. Have another caregiver lift the patient's hips off the bed and slide the bedpan under the patient
   2. Roll the patient on his or her side, place the bedpan against the buttocks, and roll the patient on his or her back while holding the bedpan in place under the buttocks
   3. Adjust the head of the bed so it is lower than the feet and use gentle but firm pressure to push the bedpan under the patient
   4. Raise the patient's bed to a sitting position and have two caregivers lift the patient while the nurse slides the bedpan under him or her
2. A patient has not had a bowel movement for 5 days. Now the patient has small amounts of liquid stool seepage and complains of "rectal pressure." Based on this scenario, which problem should the nurse suspect?
   1. An intestinal obstruction
   2. Irritation of the intestinal mucosa
   3. Gastroenteritis
   4. A fecal impaction
3. During an enema the patient complains of cramping abdominal pain that he or she rates as a 6 out of 10. Which action should the nurse take first?
   1. Stop the instillation
   2. Slow down the rate of instillation
   3. Obtain vital signs
   4. Tell the patient to bear down as he or she would when having a bowel movement
4. Which points would the nurse include when doing patient teaching for a patient with chronic complaints of constipation? (Select all that apply.)
   1. Increase fiber and fluids in the diet.
   2. Use a low-volume enema daily.
   3. Take laxatives twice a day.
   4. Exercise for 30 minutes every day.
   5. Schedule time to use the toilet at the same time every day.
   6. Eat a high-carbohydrate, low-fat diet.
5. When caring for a patient with a new colostomy on the first postoperative day, which of the following tasks would be appropriate to teach the patient?
   1. How to change the pouch
   2. How to empty the pouch
   3. How to open and close the pouch
   4. What kind of diet he or she should be eating in the hospital
6. Diarrhea may be a result of which of the following conditions in the intestinal tract?
   1. Infection, inflammation, food intolerance
   2. Loss of sphincter control, infection, decreased peristalsis
   3. Inflammation, decreased peristalsis, fecal impaction
   4. Food intolerance, fecal impaction, loss of sphincter control
7. Place the steps for changing an ostomy pouch in the correct order.
   1. Close the end of the pouch.
   2. Measure the stoma.
   3. Cut the hole in the wafer.
   4. Press the pouch into place over the stoma.
   5. Remove the old pouch.
   6. Trace the correct measurement onto the back of the wafer.
   7. Assess the stoma and the skin around it.
   8. Cleanse and dry the peristomal skin.
8. Which of the following symptoms are warning signs of possible colorectal cancer according to American Cancer Society guidelines? (Select all that apply.)
   1. Change in bowel habits
   2. Blood in the stool
   3. A larger-than-normal bowel movement
   4. Unexplained abdominal or back pain
   5. Muscle cramps
   6. Incomplete emptying of the colon
   7. Mucus in the stool

9. The nurse is teaching the patient to obtain a specimen for fecal occult blood testing (FOBT) at home. Which is the correct way for the patient to collect the specimen?
   1. Three fecal smears from one bowel movement
   2. One fecal smear from an early-morning bowel movement
   3. One fecal smear from three separate bowel movements
   4. Three fecal smears when blood can be seen in the bowel movement
10. When a patient has fecal incontinence, which point is important for the nurse to instruct to all caregivers?
   1. Cleanse the skin with antibacterial soap and apply baby powder.
   2. Use diapers and heavy padding on the bed.
   3. Cleanse the skin with a no-rinse cleanser and apply a barrier ointment.
   4. Help the patient to toilet once every hour.

evolve

Rationales for Review Questions can be found on the Evolve website.

1. 2; **2.** 4; **3.** 1; **4.** 1, 4, 5; **5.** 3; **6.** 1; **7.** 5, 8, 7, 2, 6, 3, 4, 1; **8.** 1, 2, 4; **9.** 3; **10.** 3

REFERENCES

American Cancer Society (ACS): *Cancer facts and figures 2012*, 2012, http://www.cancer.org/acs/groups/content/@epidemiologysurveilance/documents/document/acspc-031941.pdf. Accessed October 4, 2013.

Bourgault AM, Halm MA: Feeding tube placement in adults: safe verification method for blindly inserted tubes, *Am J Crit Care* 18(1):73, 2009.

Cohen SH, et al: Clinical practice guidelines for *Clostridium difficile* infection in adults: 2010 update by the Society for Healthcare Epidemiology of America (SHEA) and the Infectious Diseases Society of America (IDSA), *Infect Control Hosp Epidemiol* 31(5):431, 2010.

Durai M, Venkatraman R, Ng P: Nasogastric tubes 1: insertion technique and confirming the correct position, *Nurs Times* 105(16):12, 2009.

Goldberg M, et al: *Management of the patient with a fecal ostomy: best practice guidelines for clinicians*, Mt Laurel, NJ, 2010, Wound, Ostomy, Continence Nurses Society.

Hockenberry MJ, Wilson D: *Wong's nursing care of infants and children*, ed 9, St Louis, 2011, Mosby.

Huether SE, et al: *Understanding pathophysiology*, ed 5, St Louis, 2012, Mosby.

Ito N, et al: Prospective longitudinal evaluation of quality of life in patients with permanent colostomy after curative resection for rectal cancer, *J Wound Ostomy Continence Nurs* 39(2):172, 2012.

Leung F, Rao S: Fecal incontinence in the elderly, *Gastroenterol Clin North Am* 38(3):503, 2009.

Lewis S, et al: *Medical-surgical nursing: assessment and management of clinical problems*, ed 8, St Louis, 2011, Mosby.

NANDA International: *NANDA International nursing diagnoses: definitions and classifications, 2012-2014*, Oxford, UK, 2012, Wiley-Blackwell.

National Institute of Diabetes, Digestive and Kidney Diseases (NIDDK): *Health information for the public*, 2012, http://www.niddk.nih.gov. Accessed October 2012.

Palma E, et al: An observational study of family caregivers' quality of life caring for patients with a stoma, *Gastroenterol Nurs* 35(2):99, 2012.

Proehl JA, et al: Emergency nursing resource: gastric tube placement verification, *J Emerg Nurs* 37(4):357, 2011.

Seidel HM, et al: *Mosby's guide to physical examination*, ed 7, St Louis, 2011, Mosby.

Spinzi G: Constipation in the elderly, *Drugs Aging* 26(6):469, 2009.

Sun V, et al: Surviving colorectal cancer: long-term, persistent ostomy-specific concerns and adaptations, *J Wound Ostomy Continence Nurs* 40(1):67, 2013.

The Joint Commission (TJC): *National Patient Safety Goals*, Oakbrook Terrace, IL, 2014, The Commission. Available at http://www.jointcommission.org/standards_information/npsgs.aspx.

CHAPTER

36

Immobility

evolve WEBSITE

http://evolve.elsevier.com/Potter/essentials

- Video Clip
- Crossword Puzzle
- Audio Glossary

OBJECTIVES

- Describe mobility and immobility.
- Discuss the importance of no-lift policies for patients and health care providers.
- Discuss the appropriate decision-making process when choosing equipment needed for safe patient handling and movement.
- Identify changes in metabolic rate associated with immobility.
- Describe common physical and physiological changes associated with immobility.
- Discuss factors that contribute to pressure ulcer formation.
- Describe psychosocial and developmental effects of immobilization.
- Complete a nursing assessment of an immobilized patient.
- Develop a nursing care plan for an immobilized patient.
- List appropriate nursing interventions for an immobilized patient.
- Evaluate nursing care for an immobilized patient.

KEY TERMS

activities of daily living (ADLs), p. 1036
activity tolerance, p. 1038
anthropometric measurements, p. 1039
bed rest, p. 1035
body alignment, p. 1033
bone resorption, p. 1036
disuse osteoporosis, p. 1036
diuresis, p. 1035
footdrop, p. 1036
hypostatic pneumonia, p. 1035
immobility, p. 1035
instrumental activities of daily living (IADLs), p. 1056
ischemia, p. 1036
joint contracture, p. 1036
mobility, p. 1038
negative nitrogen balance, p. 1035
orthostatic hypotension, p. 1035
osteoporosis, p. 1036
pathological fractures, p. 1036
thrombus, p. 1036

SCIENTIFIC KNOWLEDGE BASE

The capacity to move around freely in the environment is a critical element for health as previously discussed in Chapter 27. It serves many purposes and requires the functioning of the nervous and musculoskeletal systems. Understanding the movements and functions of muscles in maintaining posture and movement and implementing evidence-based knowledge and safe patient handling are essential to protecting the safety of both patients and nurses.

Movement

When the musculoskeletal and nervous systems work in concert, the result is movement or coordinated body mechanics. Before evidence-based research, principles that nurses learned from physics regarding the lifting or moving of inanimate objects were applied to moving or lifting patients. This frequently resulted in injuries to patients, nurses, or other health care workers. Today nurses use information about body alignment, balance, gravity, and risk assessments when

CASE STUDY *Mr. Paul Rogers*

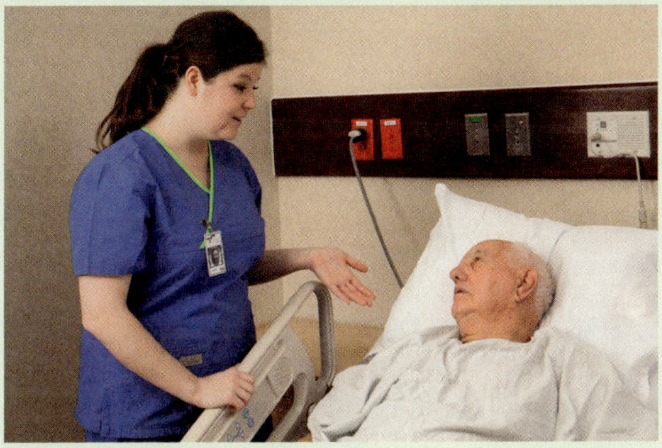

Mr. Paul Rogers, a 91-year-old widower, was admitted to the orthopedic unit for a right total knee replacement after experiencing several years of severe pain and limited mobility because of osteoarthritis of that knee. He is to be out of bed using a walker as tolerated but is still receiving an opioid for postoperative pain. He is 2 days postsurgery. He has had type 2 diabetes mellitus for the past 15 years and is on anticoagulant therapy because of his joint replacement. There is no history of smoking or use of alcohol. He lives by himself since the death of his wife 4 years ago but has a son and daughter who live within a 25-minute drive. Both are married and visit him several times during the week. His weight is 185 lbs, and he is 6 feet 1 inch tall. He cooks for himself following the prescribed diet "OK," but did admit that he likes his cake, ice cream, and sweets. His daughter tries to monitor his blood sugar and brings meals on the weekends that follow the diabetic diet guidelines.

Abby Goodman, a 20-year-old nursing student, is assigned to Mr. Rogers for the week. Abby has reviewed the care for a patient who has received a joint replacement, including mobility restrictions. She has also reviewed possible nursing diagnoses for patients undergoing the surgery that are appropriate for Mr. Rogers because of his age, impaired mobility, and medications.

providing care and moving patients. In some facilities nurses use algorithms derived from evidence-based research to determine the safest method to transfer a patient from one location to another or to reposition their patients safely.

Body Alignment and Balance

The terms *body alignment* and *posture* are similar and refer to the positioning of the joints, tendons, ligaments, and muscles while standing, sitting, and lying. **Body alignment** means that the individual's center of gravity is stable. Correct body alignment reduces strain on musculoskeletal structures, aids in maintaining adequate muscle tone, promotes comfort, and contributes to balance and conservation of energy. Without balance control, the center of gravity is displaced, thus creating a risk for falls. Individuals require balance for maintaining a static position (e.g., sitting) and moving (e.g., walking). The concepts related to the physiology and regulation of movement and to body mechanics are presented in Chapter 27.

Pathological Influences on Mobility

The following is a brief presentation of four pathological influences that can affect a patient's mobility.

Postural Abnormalities. These can be acquired or congenital and interfere with the functioning of the musculoskeletal system. This altered functioning may result in pain, impaired alignment or mobility, or both. Knowledge about the characteristics, causes, and treatment of common postural abnormalities is necessary for lifting, transfer, and positioning (Table 36-1). The plan of care may also require participation of other health care team members such as physical therapists for optimal patient outcomes.

Muscle Abnormalities. Injuries and disease can lead to numerous alterations in musculoskeletal function. For example, patients with muscular dystrophy experience progressive, symmetrical weakness and wasting of skeletal muscle groups, with increasing disability and deformity (McCance and Huether, 2010).

Damage to the Central Nervous System. Damage to any component of the central nervous system that regulates voluntary movement results in impaired body alignment, balance, and mobility. Trauma from a head injury, ischemia from a stroke or brain attack (cerebrovascular accident [CVA]), or bacterial infection such as meningitis can damage the cerebellum or the motor strip in the cerebral cortex. Damage to the cerebellum causes problems with balance, and motor impairment is directly related to the amount of destruction of the motor strip.

Direct Trauma to the Musculoskeletal System. Direct trauma to the musculoskeletal system results in bruises, contusions, sprains, and fractures. A fracture is a disruption of bone tissue continuity. Fractures most commonly result from direct external trauma, but they also occur as a consequence of some deformity of the bone (e.g., pathological fractures of osteoporosis or osteogenesis imperfecta). Young children are usually able to form new bone more easily than adults and, as a result, have fewer complications after a fracture. Treatment often includes positioning the fractured bone in proper alignment and immobilizing it to promote healing and restore function. Even this temporary immobilization results in some muscle atrophy, loss of muscle tone, and joint stiffness.

NURSING KNOWLEDGE BASE

Nurses need to know (1) how to apply their understanding of movement and immobility in the clinical setting so they can determine the safest way to move patients, and (2) the effect of immobility on the physiological and psychosocial aspects of patient care.

Safe Patient Handling

Nurses are exposed to the hazards related to lifting and transferring patients in many settings such as hospitals and

TABLE 36-1 POSTURAL ABNORMALITIES

ABNORMALITY	DESCRIPTION	CAUSE	POSSIBLE TREATMENTS*
Torticollis	Inclining of head to affected side, in which sternocleidomastoid muscle is contracted	Congenital or acquired condition	Surgery, heat, support, or immobilization, depending on cause and severity; gentle ROM
Lordosis	Exaggeration of anterior convex curve of lumbar spine	Congenital condition Temporary condition (e.g., pregnancy)	Spine-stretching exercises (based on cause)
Kyphosis	Increased convexity in curvature of thoracic spine	Congenital condition Rickets, osteoporosis Tuberculosis of spine	Spine-stretching exercises, sleeping without pillows, using bed board, bracing, spinal fusion (based on cause and severity)
Scoliosis	Lateral S- or C-shaped spinal column with vertebral rotation; unequal heights of hips and shoulders	Sometimes a consequence of numerous congenital, connective tissue, and neuromuscular disorders	Approximately half of children with scoliosis require surgery Nonsurgical treatment with braces and exercises
Congenital hip dysplasia	Hip instability with limited abduction of hips and occasionally adduction contractures (head of femur does not articulate with acetabulum because of abnormal shallowness of acetabulum)	Congenital condition (more common with breech deliveries)	Maintenance of continuous abduction of thigh so head of femur presses into center of acetabulum Abduction splints, casting, surgery
Knock-knee (genu valgum)	Legs curved inward so knees come together as person walks	Congenital condition Rickets	Knee brace; surgery if not corrected by growth
Bowlegs (genu varum)	One or both legs bent outward at knee, which is normal until 2-to-3 years of age	Congenital condition Rickets	Slowing rate of curving if not corrected by growth With rickets, increase of vitamin D, calcium, and phosphorus intake to normal ranges
Clubfoot	*95%:* Medial deviation and plantar flexion of foot (equinovarus) *5%:* Lateral deviation and dorsiflexion (calcaneovalgus)	Congenital condition	Casts, splints such as Denis Browne splint, and surgery (based on degree and rigidity of deformity)
Footdrop	Inability to dorsiflex and invert foot because of peroneal nerve damage	Congenital condition Trauma Improper position of immobilized patient	None (cannot be corrected) Prevention through physical therapy Bracing with ankle-foot orthotic (AFO)
Pigeon toes	Internal rotation of forefoot or entire foot; common in infants	Congenital condition Habit	Growth; wearing reversed shoes

Data from McCance K, Huether SE: *Pathophysiology,* ed 6, St Louis, 2010, Mosby.
ROM, Range of motion.
*Severity of condition and cause dictate treatment, which is individualized to patient's needs.

long-term care facilities. Manually lifting and transferring patients contributes to the high incidence of work-related musculoskeletal problems and back injuries in nurses and other health care staff (Nelson, Motacki, and Menzel, 2009). Current evidence shows that many nurses frequently transfer to different positions and leave the profession because of work-related injuries (ANA, 2012). Implementing evidence-based interventions and programs (e.g., lift teams) reduces the number of work-related injuries, which improves the health of the nurse and reduces indirect costs to the health care agency (e.g., workers' compensation and replacing injured workers). The American Nurses Association (ANA) has been advocating for safe patient handling since initiating the policy in 1992 and establishing standards in 2012 (ANA, 2012). The Association of Safe Patient Handling Professionals (ASPHP, www.asphp.org/certification/) is offering certifications for health care professionals and hospitals. The focus here should be on safe handling and transfer to avoid injury to patients and nurses (see also Chapter 27).

Today several states have laws that mandate safe patient handling in health care agencies or are in the process of passing legislation. Health care agencies are implementing comprehensive safe patient-handling programs in all parts of the country. They include the following elements: an ergonomics assessment protocol for health care environments, patient assessment criteria, algorithms for patient handling and movement, special equipment kept in convenient locations to help transfer patients, back-injury resource nurses, an "after-action review" or Safety Huddles that allows the health care team to apply knowledge about safe patient moving in different settings, and a no-lift policy (Nelson et al., 2009).

Immobility

A patient's mobility can be restricted for therapeutic reasons such as when bed rest is ordered. Therapeutic reasons for **bed rest** include decreasing the oxygen needs of the body, reducing cardiac workload, reducing pain, and allowing the debilitated or ill patient to rest. The duration of bed rest depends on the type and nature of the illness or injury and the patient's prior state of health. Factors that further contribute to the extent of a patient's **immobility** include length and severity of illness, presence of pain, cognitive and emotional status such as depression, and physical condition. It is essential to remember that the hazardous effects of immobility are imposed on each of the systems of a patient's body (Box 36-1) (McCance and Huether, 2010). The greater the extent and longer the duration of immobility, the more pronounced the effects.

Respiratory Changes. Decreased lung expansion, generalized respiratory muscle weakness, and dependent stasis of secretions occur with immobility. These conditions often contribute to the development of atelectasis (collapse of alveoli) and **hypostatic pneumonia** (inflammation of the lung from stasis or pooling of secretions). General muscle weakness reduces a patient's ability to cough. Mucus accumulates, particularly when the patient lies supine, providing an excellent medium for bacterial growth. The result may be hypostatic pneumonia.

Metabolic Changes. Immobility disrupts normal metabolic functioning, decreasing the metabolic rate and altering the metabolism of carbohydrates, proteins, and fats. A patient's basal metabolic rate (BMR) decreases in response to reduced cellular energy because of the decreased ability of the body to produce insulin and metabolize glucose. The body then begins to break down its protein stores for energy, resulting in a **negative nitrogen balance** and increased oxygen demands. However, in the presence of an infection, immobilized patients have an increased BMR. Fever and wound repair add to cellular oxygen requirements; this is discussed further in Chapter 37.

Fluid and Electrolyte Balances. Major shifts in blood volume occur in immobile patients. **Diuresis** (increased urine excretion) occurs as a result of increased blood flow to the kidneys and expanded circulating blood volume. Diuresis causes the body to lose electrolytes such as potassium and sodium and reduces serum calcium levels. Immobility increases calcium resorption (loss) from bones, causing a release of excess calcium into circulation or hypercalcemia, which may result in pathological fractures if the patient's kidneys cannot respond appropriately.

BOX 36-1 PATHOPHYSIOLOGY OF IMMOBILITY

PHYSIOLOGICAL OUTCOMES

- ↓ Basal metabolic rate
- ↓ Gastrointestinal motility
  - ↓ Nutrients/fluids
  - ↓ Appetite
- Shift in electrolyte balance
- ↓ O_2 availability/ischemia
  - ↓ O_2/CO_2 exchange
  - ↑ Respiratory muscle weakness
  - ↓ Lung expansion
  - ↑ Atelectasis/hypostatic pneumonia
- ↓ Cardiac output
  - ↑ Cardiac workload
  - ↑ Oxygen demand
  - ↑ Dependent edema
  - ↑ Clot formation (deep vein thrombosis)
- ↑ Muscle atrophy
  - ↓ Strength/flexibility/endurance
  - ↑ Joint contractures
- ↑ Disuse osteoporosis
- ↑ Bone resorption

PSYCHOLOGICAL OUTCOMES

- ↑ Stressors
- ↑ Depression
  - ↓ Self-identity
  - ↓ Self-esteem
- ↑ Behavioral changes
- ↑ Changes in sleep-wake cycles
- ↓ Coping successes
- ↑ Isolation
- ↑ Passive behaviors
- ↑ Sensory deprivation/overload

DEVELOPMENTAL OUTCOMES

- ↑ Dependence
- ↑ Regression in development

Gastrointestinal Changes. An immobile patient is at risk for constipation from lack of activity and hypercalcemia, which depresses peristalsis. Constipation is sometimes so severe that fecal impaction occurs (see Chapter 35). Left untreated, a partial or complete bowel obstruction occurs.

Cardiovascular Changes. Orthostatic hypotension occurs in patients on bed rest and after prolonged sitting. **Orthostatic hypotension** is an increase in heart rate of more than 15% and a drop of 15 mm Hg or more in systolic blood pressure or a decrease of 10 mm Hg in diastolic blood pressure when the patient rises from a lying or sitting position to a standing position (McCance and Huether, 2010). A decreased circulating fluid volume, pooling of blood in the lower extremities, and a decreased autonomic response occur, resulting in decreased venous return, decreased central venous pressure and stroke volume, and a drop in systolic blood pressure when the immobilized patient first stands (McCance and Huether, 2010). Prolonged bed rest increases the workload of the heart, producing a need for more oxygen.

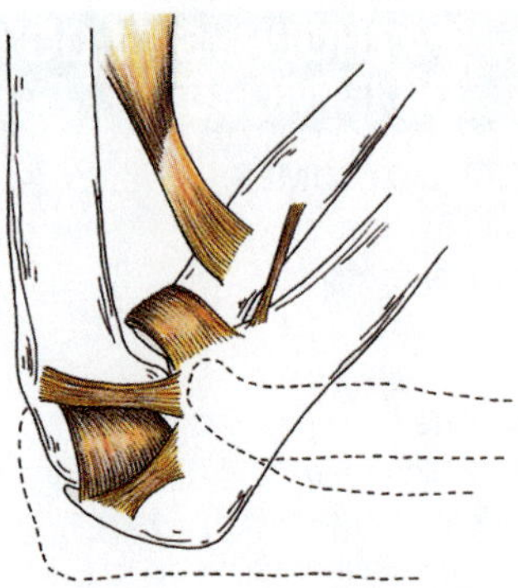

FIGURE 36-1 Flexion contracture of elbow resulting in permanent flexion of joint. Normally the elbow is able to extend to a 90-degree angle *(dotted line)* and a 180-degree angle *(not shown).*

Immobilized patients are at risk for deep vein thrombosis (DVT). A **thrombus** is an accumulation of platelets, fibrin, clotting factors, and cellular elements of the blood attached to the interior wall of a vein or artery, sometimes occluding the lumen of the vessel. Three factors contribute to venous thrombus formation: (1) loss of integrity of the vessel wall (e.g., injury), (2) abnormalities of blood flow (e.g., slow blood flow in calf veins associated with bed rest because of pressure from the mattress and/or decreased pumping action of the skeletal muscles of the legs from not walking), and (3) alterations in blood constituents (e.g., a change in clotting factors or increased platelet activity). These three factors are referred to as Virchow's triad (McCance and Huether, 2010). A DVT places a patient at risk for pulmonary emboli, a life-threatening complication.

Musculoskeletal Changes. The body loses muscle strength when muscles are inactive. The rate of muscle decline varies with the degree of immobility, but it is rapid while mobility and weight bearing are restricted. These effects are devastating to patients who are marginally functional with their **activities of daily living (ADLs).**

As immobility progresses and muscles are not exercised, muscle mass continues to decrease. The muscle atrophies, and the size of the muscle decreases. Immobility affects the leg muscles the most, which explains the difficulty that older patients have in getting up from a chair after periods of bed rest.

Immobility causes two skeletal changes: a joint contracture and disuse osteoporosis. A **joint contracture** is a preventable, abnormal, and possibly permanent condition characterized by fixation of the joint. Disuse, atrophy, and shortening of muscle fibers and surrounding joint tissues cause joint contracture. When a contracture occurs, the joint cannot maintain full range of motion (ROM) (Figure 36-1). Contractures leave joints in nonfunctional positions, as seen in patients who are permanently curled in a fetal position.

One common and debilitating contracture is **footdrop** (Figure 36-2). When footdrop occurs, the foot is permanently in plantar flexion. Patients are no longer able to walk when this occurs.

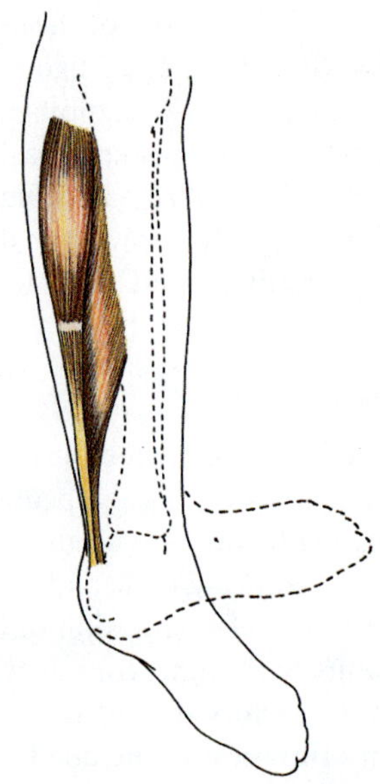

FIGURE 36-2 Footdrop. Ankle is fixed in plantar flexion.

Disuse osteoporosis is a disorder characterized by **bone resorption.** Immobilization increases the rate of bone resorption, which results in reduced bone tissue density. This increases a patient's risk for **pathological fractures.** If patients have **osteoporosis** at the time of admission, nurses must recognize that they are at high risk for accelerated bone loss if immobilized.

Integument Changes. The direct effect of pressure on the skin by immobility is compounded by metabolic changes. Older adult patients and patients with paralysis have a greater risk for developing pressure ulcers (see Chapter 37). When a patient lies in bed or sits in a chair, the weight of the body is on bony prominences. The longer the pressure is applied, the longer the period of **ischemia** (i.e., temporary decrease of blood flow to tissue), and therefore the greater the risk for skin breakdown. Because of the change of circulation, any break in the integrity of the skin is difficult to heal in the immobilized patient.

Urinary Elimination Changes. In the upright position urine flows from the renal pelvis into the ureter to the bladder because of gravity. When a patient is in bed, the kidneys and ureters move toward a more level plane, and urine tries to move from the kidney to the bladder against gravity. Because the peristaltic contractions of the ureters are not strong enough to overcome gravity, the renal pelvis fills before urine enters the ureters. This condition, called *urinary stasis,* increases the patient's risk for urinary tract infection (UTI) and renal calculi or calcium stones. These stones lodge in the renal pelvis and pass through the ureters. Immobilized patients are at risk for calculi because of altered calcium metabolism and the resulting hypercalcemia (see Chapter 34).

Psychosocial Effects

Immobilization reduces a patient's independence and creates a sense of loss. As a result, emotional, intellectual, sensory, and sociocultural responses occur. The most common emotional changes are depression, social isolation, sleep-wake disturbances, and impaired coping.

Some immobilized patients become depressed because of changes in self-concept (see Chapter 23). Depression is an affective disorder characterized by exaggerated feelings of sadness, melancholy, dejection, worthlessness, emptiness, helplessness, and hopelessness. It results from worrying about present and future levels of health, finances, and family needs. Because immobilization removes patients from their daily routines, they have more time to worry about disability. Worrying quickly increases patients' depression, causing withdrawal. Withdrawn patients often do not want to participate in their own care and are unwilling to take part in other activities, thereby aggravating any immobile condition.

Immobilized patients require vigilant nursing care such as repositioning at least every 2 hours or more often to avoid physical complications. Because of the need for frequent repositioning, it is important to organize care activities together, including nursing and medical interventions, to ensure that the patient gets sufficient sleep (see Chapter 31). Disruption of normal sleeping patterns causes further behavioral changes and affects coping patterns.

Long-term immobility or bed rest affects usual coping patterns. Some immobilized patients withdraw and become passive. The passive patient demonstrates little interest in achieving independence or participating in care. Assess the patient's normal coping mechanisms and develop a nursing care plan that is based on patient strengths and encourages patient input as much as possible.

Developmental Effects

Developmental effects of immobility more commonly affect the very young and the older adult. The immobilized young or middle-age adult experiences few, if any, developmental changes.

When an infant, toddler, or preschooler is immobilized, it is usually because of trauma or the need to correct a congenital skeletal abnormality. Prolonged immobilization delays the child's motor skill and intellectual development (Hockenberry and Wilson, 2010). Growth is frequently uneven.

Prolonged immobilization alters adolescent growth patterns as well. In addition, adolescents who experience immobility often are behind peers in gaining independence and accomplishing certain skills such as obtaining a driver's license, a major milestone for many teenagers. Social isolation is another concern for this age-group when immobilization occurs, although computers and smartphones reduce this concern considerably.

A healthy adult patient who is briefly immobile may not experience the hazards of immobility; but, if the immobilization is prolonged or the patient has one or more chronic conditions, all physiological systems are at risk. In addition, the role of the adult often changes with regard to the family or social structure. Some adults lose their jobs, which affects their self-concept.

Immobilization in older adult patients increases their physical dependence on others and accelerates functional losses in physiological systems (Touhy and Jett, 2010). Immobilization in this patient group usually results from a degenerative disease, neurological trauma, or chronic illness. For some patients immobilization occurs gradually and progressively; whereas for others, especially those who have had a CVA, loss of mobility is sudden. Develop nursing care plans that encourage patient independence in as many self-care activities as possible.

CRITICAL THINKING

Critical thinking is a synthesis of many elements to which you have been exposed thus far (i.e., knowledge, experience, attitudes, and standards). All of these are also infused with data from patients.

Synthesis

You apply elements of critical thinking whenever you perform the nursing process with a patient. Consider the scientific knowledge you have learned, your experience, critical thinking attitudes, and standards to ensure an individualized approach to patient care. Gather information from a variety of sources when caring for patients. Integrating knowledge and experience makes it possible to determine physical, psychosocial, and developmental needs of immobilized patients. The needs of the immobile patient are multiple and indeed complex.

Knowledge. Knowledge of pathophysiology helps you anticipate how patients are affected by limitations in mobility. These limitations are sometimes the direct result of musculoskeletal alteration such as a broken ankle or deconditioning from a chronic health problem such as heart failure. Your assessment of any limitation should focus on the pathophysiological changes that you expect so the plan of care will be comprehensive and help prevent complications.

Understand the importance of a patient's culture and traditions regarding activity (e.g., does the person's culture require that he or she exercise with another person, or are there certain times of day that are reserved for prayer and activities such as exercise are not permitted?) (Box 36-2). Also apply knowledge of patients' developmental stages to determine their current functional and mobility status and health care needs. Application of knowledge gained from the study of human growth and development is essential for accurately assessing patient needs and selecting appropriate interventions for mobility alterations.

Information of the physiological changes associated with immobility enables you to identify complications and intervene appropriately. Concepts for patient teaching are based on developmental stages and are vital in preparing patients for rehabilitation following immobilization.

Experience. Taking care of patients who had mobility restrictions in the past allows you to anticipate patients' needs for comfort, pain control, positioning, and support of ADLs. Experiential learning also occurs during visits to a physical

BOX 36-2 PATIENT-CENTERED CARE

Cultural factors influence many aspects of patients' lives, including time orientation, health care practices, and nutrition. Not as much attention has been given to the impact of cultural factors on mobility and exercise. You know that being immobile, even for a short period of time, can result in a number of hazards for the patient. Therefore knowing the patient's cultural practices helps you plan care.

Unhealthy lifestyles are associated with socioeconomic factors such as social class, education, geographic location, and income. This is the case with physical activity and obesity. In addition, not having social support and certain ethnic customs may cause people to be inactive.

IMPLICATIONS FOR PRACTICE

- Help patients plan physical activities that are culturally appropriate (Purnell, 2009).
- Make exercise programs that are flexible, affordable, and accommodate family and community culture yet keep patients safe from negative patient outcomes (Purnell, 2009).
- Incorporate cultural beliefs and desired patient outcomes when designing the plan of care (Lim et al., 2009).

therapy unit in the hospital or in the community. Your experience with a variety of exercise strategies helps develop health promotion activities or rehabilitation plans for assigned patients.

Attitudes. Design creative solutions to improve a patient's mobility status. Speak with other health care providers to determine the best setting to provide care. Collaboration and creativity help to establish an individualized rehabilitation program. The attitude of perseverance is essential for coordinating patient care and working with patients experiencing psychological and developmental changes resulting from immobilization. Use discipline and be thorough in your approach, considering patients' needs once they return home and how family caregivers can become involved.

Standards. Promote a patient's independence while adhering to the prescribed rehabilitation plan and maintaining safety. Since 2003 in the *Position Statement on Elimination of Manual Patient Handling to Prevent Work-Related Musculoskeletal Disorders,* the ANA has prompted the use of evidence-based research on which to develop policies for safe patient handling (ANA, 2012). The leadership of the ANA (2012) set standards for safe patient handling and continues to review and revise these policies to help nurses develop policies and procedures for the safe use of transfer and positioning equipment within their facilities. Such policies result in decreased injuries to nurses and patients (ANA, 2012).

Discharge instructions must be clear and explicit. Always use the ethical standard of autonomy in supporting patients in making decisions about their discharge needs. To evaluate discharge teachings, have patients demonstrate required actions to ensure that they understand them completely and can perform them correctly, therefore validating the quality of the teaching sessions.

Synthesis of knowledge, experience, attitudes, and standards is important in developing an individualized care plan with the immobilized patient. This plan of care helps to prevent complications, promote rehabilitation, and expedite discharge.

NURSING PROCESS

ASSESSMENT

Mobility assessment focuses on patients' past and present mobility and its potential effects. Table 36-2 presents a focused patient assessment of immobility, pain associated with movement, and activity tolerance.

Mobility. Assessment of a patient's **mobility** focuses on the musculoskeletal system and includes range of motion, muscle strength, activity tolerance, gait, and posture. Observing the patient's posture while sitting and standing and assessing gait helps to determine the type of assistance the patient requires for ambulation or transfer (i.e., notice which method the patient uses to push up from a chair or if the patient grabs onto objects to steady himself or herself) (see Chapter 27).

Assessment of ROM is important as a baseline measurement to compare and evaluate whether loss in joint mobility has occurred. Refer to Table 36-3 when assessing a patient's ROM. Be sure to assess all joints in the body. Ask questions about and physically examine the patient for stiffness, swelling, pain, limited movement, and unequal movement. Patients whose mobility is restricted require ROM to reduce the hazards of immobility. Therefore determine the type of ROM exercise a patient is able to perform. ROM exercises are active (the patient moves all joints through their ROM unassisted), passive (the patient is unable to move independently, and the nurse moves each joint through its ROM), or somewhere in between. For example, provide support for a weak patient while the patient performs most of the movement. Some patients are able to move some joints actively, whereas the nurse passively moves others.

The major musculoskeletal changes expected during assessment of an immobilized patient include decreased muscle strength, loss of muscle tone and mass, and contractures. Patients with musculoskeletal injuries or chronic conditions require careful palpation of joints and extremities to minimize discomfort. Because immobilized patients are weakened, determine if difficulty in moving joints is the result of fatigue or decreased ROM. Remember that the patient's total musculoskeletal system must be evaluated, from the head and neck down to the toes. Any limitation not identified early can result in the patient developing a permanent complication that will impact mobility in the future.

Activity tolerance is the type and amount of exercise or work that a person is able to perform. Assessment of activity tolerance is necessary when planning activity such as walking, ROM exercises, or ADLs. Activity tolerance assessment includes data from physiological, emotional, and

TABLE 36-2 **FOCUSED PATIENT ASSESSMENT**

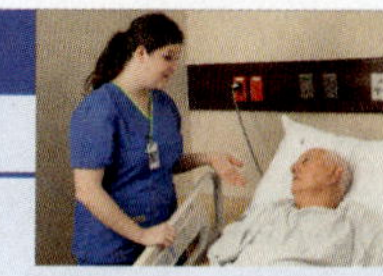

FACTORS TO ASSESS	QUESTIONS	PHYSICAL ASSESSMENT
Mobility	Do you have any difficulty walking or getting around? Do you have problems with steps? Do you have a history of connective tissue disorders or fractures, or have you had damage to your ligaments or tendons?	Observe patient's gait as he or she walks. Observe patient sit and rise from chair. Observe patient while performing self-care activities.
Pain	Do you have any pain or discomfort on movement? Ask patient to rate pain on a 0-10 pain scale. Please tell me about your pain. When did it start? How long does it last? Can you get relief? Would you like your pain medication before I help you walk?	Observe for objective signs of pain such as grimacing; moaning; increasing respiratory rate, pulse, and blood pressure. Inspect joints for redness or swelling, indicating potential inflammatory process. Watch if patient favors one leg or knee when walking, sitting, or changing position. Use appropriate pain scale for patients who cannot verbalize their pain.
Endurance and activity	Are you feeling tired now? Are you having difficulty with bathing or washing yourself, getting to the bathroom, or dressing yourself because you feel weak? Are you having shortness of breath, either when resting or moving; palpitations; light-headedness or dizziness?	Observe for signs of fatigue. Observe patient's performance of ADLs. Observe patient for pallor; obtain baseline vital signs. Monitor oxygen saturation before and after activity.

ADLs, Activities of daily living.

developmental domains (see Chapter 27). This assessment is applicable in all clinical settings.

As activity is incorporated into the plan of care, monitor patients' tolerance and assess for dyspnea, fatigue, chest pain, and/or a change in heart rate or blood pressure. The weak or debilitated patient is unable to sustain even slight changes in activity because of the increased demand for energy. Seemingly simple tasks such as eating and moving in bed often result in extreme fatigue. When the patient experiences decreased activity tolerance, carefully assess how much time he or she needs to recover. Decreasing recovery time indicates improving activity tolerance.

People who are depressed, worried, or anxious are frequently unable to tolerate exercise. Depressed patients tend to withdraw rather than participate. Patients who worry or are frequently anxious expend a tremendous amount of mental energy and often report feeling fatigued. Because of this they also experience physical and emotional exhaustion.

Periods of prolonged immobility or bed rest cause major physiological, psychological, and social effects. These effects are gradual or immediate and vary from patient to patient. The greater the extent and the longer the duration of immobility, the more pronounced the consequences. The patient with complete mobility restrictions is continually at risk for the hazards of immobility. Therefore you must assess each body system for these risks related to the hazards of immobility, regardless of age.

Respiratory System. Perform a respiratory assessment at least every 2 hours for acutely ill patients with restricted activity. Monitor the patient's respiratory rate and oxygen saturation. Inspect chest wall movements for symmetry and auscultate the lungs to identify regions of diminished breath sounds. Focus auscultation for adventitious lung sounds on the dependent lung field because pulmonary secretions tend to accumulate in the lower lobes. If a patient has an atelectatic area (an area of collapsed alveoli), breath sounds are asymmetrical. A complete respiratory assessment identifies the presence of secretions and is used to determine nursing interventions necessary to maintain optimal respiratory function.

Metabolic System. When assessing a patient's metabolic functioning, measure intake and output and review laboratory data to evaluate fluid and electrolyte status. Assess the patient's nutritional status to determine the risk for nitrogen imbalance. A patient whose mobility is restricted often has a reduced appetite, altered gastrointestinal function, and a reduced capacity to self-feed.

Anorexia commonly occurs in immobilized patients. Assess food intake and the environment for unpleasant odors or noises that interfere with appetite. You can avoid nutritional imbalances if you learn the patient's previous dietary patterns and food preferences early in the immobilization (see Chapter 33).

Anthropometric measurements include height, weight, mid upper-arm circumference, and triceps skinfold measurements. Mid upper-arm circumference and triceps skinfold measurements can also be taken at regular intervals to determine loss of muscle mass. A decrease in mid upper-arm circumference measured in centimeters or triceps skinfold measured in millimeters indicates a decline in muscle mass. After the initial assessment take this measurement every 2 to 4 weeks, depending on the patient's age, previous physical condition, and the amount of immobility.

TABLE 36-3 RANGE-OF-MOTION EXERCISES

BODY PART	TYPE OF JOINT	TYPE OF MOVEMENT	RANGE (DEGREES)	PRIMARY MUSCLES
Neck, cervical spine	Pivotal	*Flexion:* Bring chin to rest on chest.	45	Sternocleidomastoid
		Extension: Return head to erect position.	45	Trapezius
		Hyperextension: Bend head back as far as possible.	10	Trapezius
		Lateral flexion: Tilt head as far as possible toward each shoulder.	40-45	Sternocleidomastoid
		Rotation: Turn head as far as possible in circular movement.	180	Sternocleidomastoid, trapezius
Shoulder	Ball and socket	*Flexion:* Raise arm from side position forward to position above head.	45-60	Coracobrachialis, deltoid
		Extension: Return arm to position at side of body.	180	Latissimus dorsi, teres major, triceps brachii
		Hyperextension: Move arm behind body, keeping elbow straight.	45-60	Latissimus dorsi, teres major, deltoid
		Abduction: Raise arm to side to position above head with palm away from head.	180	Deltoid, supraspinatus
		Adduction: Lower arm sideways and across body as far as possible.	320	Pectoralis major
		Internal rotation: With elbow flexed, rotate shoulder by moving arm until thumb is turned inward and toward back.	90	Pectoralis major, latissimus dorsi, teres major, subscapularis
		External rotation: With elbow in full circle, move arm until thumb is upward and lateral to head.	90	Infraspinatus, teres major
		Circumduction: Move arm in full circle. (Circumduction is combination of all movements of ball-and-socket joint.)	360	Deltoid, coracobrachialis, latissimus dorsi, teres major
Elbow	Hinge	*Flexion:* Bend elbow so lower arm moves toward its shoulder joint and hand is level with shoulder	150	Biceps brachii, brachialis, brachioradialis
		Extension: Straighten elbow by lowering hand.	150	Triceps brachii
Forearm	Pivotal	*Supination:* Turn lower arm and hand so palm is up.	70-90	Supinator, biceps brachii
		Pronation: Turn lower arm so palm is down.	70-90	Pronator teres, pronator quadratus
Wrist	Condyloid	*Flexion:* Move palm toward inner aspect of forearm.	80-90	Flexor carpi ulnaris, flexor carpi radialis
		Extension: Move fingers and hand posterior to midline.	80-90	Extensor carpi radialis brevis, extensor carpi radialis longus, extensor carpi ulnaris
		Hyperextension: Bring dorsal surface of hand back as far as possible.	80-90	Extensor carpi radialis brevis, extensor carpi radialis longus, extensor carpi ulnaris
		Abduction (radial deviation): Bend wrist laterally toward fifth finger.	Up to 30	Flexor carpi radialis, extensor carpi radialis brevis, extensor carpi radialis longus
		Adduction (ulnar deviation): Bend wrist medially toward thumb.	30-50	Flexor carpi ulnaris, extensor carpi ulnaris

TABLE 36-3 **RANGE-OF-MOTION EXERCISES—cont'd**

BODY PART	TYPE OF JOINT	TYPE OF MOVEMENT	RANGE (DEGREES)	PRIMARY MUSCLES
Fingers	Condyloid hinge	*Flexion:* Make fist.	90	Lumbricales, interosseus volaris, interosseus dorsalis
		Extension: Straighten fingers.	90	Extensor digiti quinti proprius, extensor digitorum communis, extensor indicis proprius
		Hyperextension: Bend fingers back as far as possible.	30-60	Extensor digitorum
		Abduction: Spread fingers apart laterally.	30	Interosseus dorsalis
		Adduction: Bring fingers together laterally.	30	Interosseus volaris
Thumb	Saddle	*Flexion:* Move thumb across palmar surface of hand.	90	Flexor pollicis brevis
		Extension: Move thumb straight away from hand.	90	Extensor pollicis longus, extensor pollicis brevis
		Abduction: Extend thumb laterally (usually done when placing fingers in abduction and adduction).	30	Abductor pollicis brevis and longus
		Adduction: Move thumb back toward hand.	30	Adductor pollicis obliquus, adductor pollicis transversus
		Opposition: Touch thumb to each finger of same hand.		Opponens pollicis, opponens digiti minimi
Hip	Ball and socket	*Flexion:* Move leg forward and up.	90-120	Psoas major, iliacus, sartorius
		Extension: Move leg behind body.	90-120	Gluteus maximus, semitendinosus, semimembranosus
		Hyperextension: Move leg behind body.	30-50	Gluteus maximus, semitendinosus, semimembranosus
Knee	Hinge	*Abduction:* Move leg laterally away from body.	30-50	Gluteus medius, gluteus minimus
		Adduction: Move leg back toward medial position and beyond if possible.	30-50	Adductor longus, adductor brevis, adductor magnus
		Internal rotation: Turn foot and leg toward other leg.	90	Gluteus medius, gluteus minimus, tensor fasciae latae
		External rotation: Turn foot and leg away from other leg.	90	Obturatorius internus, obturatorius externus, quadratus femoris, piriformis, gemellus superior and inferior, gluteus maximus
		Circumduction: Move leg in circle.	120-130	Psoas major, gluteus maximus, gluteus medius, adductor magnus
		Flexion: Bring heel back toward back of thigh.	120-130	Biceps femoris, semitendinosus, semimembranosus, sartorius
		Extension: Return leg to floor.	120-130	Rectus femoris, vastus lateralis, vastus medialis, vastus intermedius
Ankle	Hinge	*Dorsal flexion:* Move foot so toes are pointed upward.	20-30	Tibialis anterior
		Plantar flexion: Move foot so toes are pointed downward.	45-50	Gastrocnemius, soleus
Foot	Gliding	*Inversion:* Turn sole of foot medially.	10 or less	Tibialis anterior, tibialis posterior
		Eversion: Turn sole of foot laterally.	10 or less	Peroneus longus, peroneus brevis
Toes	Condyloid	*Flexion:* Curl toes downward.	30-60	Flexor digitorum, lumbricalis pedis, flexor hallucis brevis
		Extension: Straighten toes.	30-60	Extensor digitorum longus, extensor digitorum brevis, extensor hallucis longus
		Abduction: Spread toes apart.	15 or less	Abductor hallucis, interosseus dorsalis
		Adduction: Bring toes together.	15 or less	Adductor hallucis, interosseus plantaris

If an immobilized patient has a wound, the speed of healing indicates how well the body delivers nutrients to the tissues for use (see Chapter 37). The normal progression of wound healing indicates that the metabolic needs of the injured tissues are met.

Cardiovascular System. Cardiovascular assessment of the immobilized patient includes monitoring blood pressure, apical and peripheral pulses, and observing the venous system by checking capillary refill and noting skin color. Because of the risk for orthostatic hypotension, measure blood pressure when a patient moves from lying to a sitting or standing position. These measurements document the patient's tolerance to postural changes and are vital to know during transferring the patient from one position or location to another.

Also assess apical and peripheral pulses. Lying down increases cardiac workload and results in an increased pulse rate. In some patients, particularly older adults, the heart does not tolerate the added workload, and a form of cardiac failure develops. A third heart sound, heard at the apex, is an early indication of congestive heart failure. Monitoring peripheral pulses allows you to evaluate the ability of the heart to pump blood. Immediately document and report the absence of a peripheral pulse in the lower extremities to the patient's health care provider, especially if the pulse was present previously.

Edema sometimes develops in patients who have had a tissue injury or whose heart is unable to handle the increased workload of bed rest. Because edema moves to dependent body regions as a result of gravity, assessment of the immobilized patient includes the sacrum, legs, and feet. If the heart is unable to tolerate the increased workload, peripheral body regions such as the hands, feet, nose, and earlobes are colder than central body regions.

Because DVT is a hazard of immobility, assess the venous system. A dislodged venous thrombus, called an embolus, can travel through the circulatory system to the lungs and impair circulation and oxygenation. Venous emboli that travel to the lungs are sometimes life threatening. More than 90% of all pulmonary emboli begin in the deep veins of the lower extremities (Copstead-Kirkhorn and Banasik, 2010).

Assess the venous system for DVT. To assess for DVT, remove the patient's antiembolic stockings or sequential compression device (SCD) once every 8 hours or according to agency policy and observe the calves and thighs for unilateral leg swelling, redness, warmth, and tenderness. Ask the patient about calf pain. Assessing for Homans' sign (i.e., discomfort in the upper calf during forced dorsiflexion of the foot) is not considered an accurate predictor of DVT. Some believe that forceful dorsiflexion may dislodge a clot if one is present, and some facilities prohibit this assessment. Measure bilateral calf circumference and record it daily as an alternative assessment for DVT. To do this, mark a point on each calf 10 cm down from the midpatella. Measure the circumference each day using this mark for placement of the tape measure. Unilateral increases in calf circumference are an early indication of thrombosis (Black and Hawks, 2009). If the patient has a history of DVT, measurement of the thighs should also be conducted daily since the upper thigh is a common site for clot formation. It should be noted that approximately half of all patients with DVTs are asymptomatic.

Skin Integrity. Continually assess the skin for signs of pressure ulcer formation, especially over bony prominences. *All* immobilized patients are at high risk for developing pressure ulcers, regardless of age. Use of valid, objective scales such as the Braden Scale or the Gosnell Scale provides a patient's risk for pressure ulcer formation. The type of risks then directs the interventions most appropriate to prevent or treat ulcers and an objective measure for increasing risk (Chapter 37).

Elimination System. Assess a patient's elimination status during each shift and the total intake and output every 24 hours (see Chapter 34). Inadequate intake and output or fluid and electrolyte imbalances increase the risk for renal system impairment, ranging from recurrent infections to kidney failure. Dehydration also increases the risk for skin breakdown, thrombus formation, respiratory infections, and constipation.

Assessment of elimination also includes auscultation for bowel sounds, the frequency and consistency of bowel movements, and the patient's typical urine and bowel elimination patterns (see Chapter 35). Accurate assessment and identification of patient problems enable you to intervene before constipation leads to fecal impaction and urinary incontinence occur.

Psychosocial Condition. Changes in psychosocial status usually occur slowly. Observe for changes in emotional status (e.g., depression) and behavioral changes. Common reactions to immobilization include boredom and feelings of isolation, depression, and anger. Observe for changes in a patient's emotional status and listen carefully to family if they report emotional changes. Examples of change that indicate psychosocial concerns are a cooperative patient who becomes less cooperative or an independent patient who asks for more help than is necessary. Continual communication with family members is vital because they can identify and report changes in a patient's personality that you or other caregiving team members may not recognize.

Assess patients' readiness to improve their level of independence. Be prepared to adapt teaching and motivational strategies to meet their expectations and needs.

Identify and correct any changes in a patient's sleep-wake cycle such as difficulty falling asleep or frequent awakenings (see Chapter 31). Many sleep disruptions are preventable with an assessment of prior sleep habits and early intervention when you suspect problems. Consider instituting a "quiet-time" rule to promote rest. Nurses can prevent or minimize most stimuli that interrupt the sleep-wake cycle (e.g., nursing activities, a noisy environment, or discomfort). Some medications such as analgesics, sleeping pills, or cardiovascular drugs also cause sleep disturbances.

Observe for changes in the use of normal coping mechanisms to adapt to immobilization. Decreasing coping ability causes patients to become disoriented, confused, or depressed. Identifying how the patient usually copes with loss is vital (see Chapters 25 and 26). Change in a person's mobility status, whether permanent or not, produces a grief reaction.

Development. Assessment of the immobilized patient must include developmental considerations. Assess a young child's developmental stage before immobilization and determine whether the child is able to meet developmental tasks and is progressing normally. Developmental delays or regression occur with prolonged bed rest. Reassure parents that these developmental changes are usually temporary.

Immobilization of a family member changes the family's functioning. The family's response to this change often leads to problems, stress, and anxieties. Children seeing parents who are immobile sometimes have difficulty understanding what is happening and have difficulty coping. A decline in developmental functioning of a patient of any age needs prompt investigation to determine why the change occurred and interventions that can return the patient to an optimal level of functioning as soon as possible (see Chapter 22).

Older Adult Considerations. Immobility has a significant effect on the older adult's level of health, independence, and functional status. Your assessment enables you to determine his or her ability to meet needs independently and adapt to developmental changes such as declining physical functioning and altered family and peer relationships (Box 36-3). As the person grows older, activity tolerance changes. Muscle mass is reduced, and posture and the composition of bones change. There are often changes in the cardiorespiratory system such as decreased maximum heart rate and decreased lung compliance that affect the intensity of exercise. As age progresses some older individuals still exercise but do so at a reduced intensity. The more inactive a patient is, the more pronounced are these activity changes.

BOX 36-3 CARE OF THE OLDER ADULT

Improving Overall Well-being for Older Adults via Exercise and Physical Activity

Research has indicated that physical activity and exercise have many benefits when started early in life. But it has been shown that when older adults, even those with chronic conditions, participate in aerobic and resistance exercise training, they benefit as well. Therefore include such activities in your plan of care and encourage the older adult to continue them after discharge (ACSM, 2009).

- Older adults, even those with chronic health conditions and sedentary lifestyles, can benefit from aerobic and resistance exercise training (ACSM, 2009).
- Guidelines for exercises that can be continued after discharge are available to share with older adults so they can begin an exercise program, regardless of their physical limitations.
- Including aerobic and resistance exercise training in the older adult's daily routine helps to reduce the occurrence of depression and improve/maintain cognitive functioning.

Chapter 27 provides some general guidelines.

Pain also affects a person's mobility. Pain is subjective, and its severity is frequently based on self-reported assessments. In the older adult frequent assessment for pain is essential, and it is important not to rely solely on self-reported measures. Include physiological and behavioral assessments for pain (Chapter 32). When you notice a change in your older adult patient's activity level, a more extensive pain assessment and readjustment of pain medication may be necessary (Box 36-4).

Abrupt changes in personality often have a physiological cause such as surgery, a medication reaction, a pulmonary embolus, or an acute infection. For example, compromised older patients have confusion as their primary symptom with

BOX 36-4 EVIDENCE-BASED PRACTICE

PICO Question: Does the reliability of assessment of older adults' pain improve with use of pain scales compared to relying solely on self-reported pain for hospitalized older patients?

SUMMARY OF EVIDENCE

Studies have shown that pain is a common occurrence with older adults and that unfortunately it is commonly undertreated. The reasons for this include the belief that pain is just a normal part of aging, misconceptions about addiction to pain medications, and a lack of routine pain assessment of the elderly (Flaherty, 2012). Persistent pain has been associated with functional impairments, falls, slow rehabilitation, depression, anxiety, decreased socialization, and increased health cost. Thus management of the geriatric patients' pain must be achieved (AGS, 2009). Three tools have been found to be highly effective when used to assess pain with older adult patients: the Numeric Rating Scale, the Verbal Descriptor Scale, and the Faces Pain Scale–Revised. All three were used in community and acute and long-term care settings and could be used with cognitively impaired older adults (Pasero and McCaffery, 2011). By using these scales consistently, the pain in hospitalized older adults can be assessed properly and managed effectively (Herr, 2010). Once pain is effectively managed, a patient's ability and willingness to become mobile and active often increases, and the risk for falling is reduced.

APPLICATION TO NURSING PRACTICE

- Assess for pain as frequently as you do the other vital signs (Flaherty, 2012).
- Evaluate the management of the pain control; if inadequate, advocate for another intervention (e.g., another medication or dose) (AGS, 2009).
- Evaluate the pain management regimen in relation to patient activities such as PT and ambulation, and modify pain interventions to increase patient comfort during activity.
- Use one of the three pain scales to assess your patient's level of pain, even if he or she also has cognitive impairments (Pasero and McCaffery, 2011).
- Use the same scale consistently for the most effective management of the patient's pain (Herr, 2010).

an acute UTI or fever. Identifying confusion is an important component of your assessment. Acute confusion in older adults is not normal, and a thorough nursing assessment is the priority. Impaired mobility in the older adult also increases the risk for falls; therefore you must also assess for your older patient's risk for falls by using a valid instrument such as the Hendrich II Fall Risk Model (Touhy and Jett, 2010).

Assessment also includes the patient's home and community to identify factors that are risks to the patient's mobility and safety, regardless of the individual's age (see Chapter 28).

NURSING DIAGNOSIS

Assessment reveals clusters of data that indicate if a patient is at risk or if a mobility problem exists. The clusters of data include pertinent defining characteristics that support the nursing diagnoses.

A patient who is experiencing an alteration in mobility often has one or more nursing diagnoses. The two diagnoses most directly related to mobility problems are *Impaired Physical Mobility* and *Risk for Disuse Syndrome.* The diagnosis of *Impaired Physical Mobility* applies to the patient who has some limitation but is not completely immobile. The diagnosis of *Risk for Disuse Syndrome* applies to the patient who is immobile and at risk for multisystem problems because of inactivity. Beyond these diagnoses, the list of potential diagnoses is extensive because immobility affects multiple body systems. An immobilized or partially immobilized patient can have one or more of the following nursing diagnoses:

- *Ineffective Airway Clearance*
- *Risk for Constipation*
- *Risk for Disuse Syndrome*
- *Risk for Falls*
- *Impaired Physical Mobility*
- *Risk for Impaired Skin Integrity*
- *Risk for Deficient Fluid Volume*
- *Impaired Urinary Elimination*

The list of potential nursing diagnoses related to immobility is more extensive when alterations in physical, psychosocial, or developmental functioning occur. Often these problems are interrelated, and it is imperative that nursing care focus on all dimensions.

Unfortunately most often the physiological dimension is the major focus of nursing care for patients with impaired mobility, and the psychosocial and developmental dimensions are neglected. Yet all dimensions are important to health. During immobilization some patients experience decreased social interaction and stimuli. These patients frequently use the call bell to request minor physical attention when their real need is greater socialization. Nursing diagnoses for health needs in developmental areas reflect changes from the patient's normal activities. Immobility may lead to a developmental crisis if the patient is unable to resolve problems and continue to mature.

BOX 36-5 SYNTHESIS IN PRACTICE

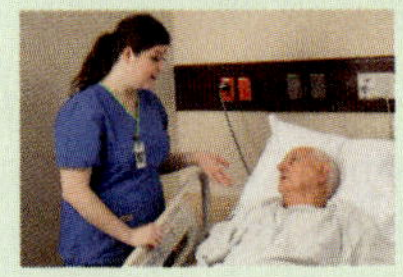

As Abby prepares for Mr. Rogers' assessment, she reviews the pathophysiology regarding the hazards of immobility. She gathers knowledge about total knee-replacement surgery and the expected postoperative physical therapy and rehabilitative measures. During a previous clinical experience Abby cared for a patient who received a cardiac valve and was given anticoagulant therapy. She knows that the postoperative medication that Mr. Rogers is receiving is also an anticoagulant and that, after surgery, Mr. Rogers' bleeding times must be monitored very closely. The therapeutic range must be maintained to prevent clots in the deep veins, but he must also be monitored for any overt or covert episodes of bleeding. Abby learned the importance of pain relief and the challenge this may present with an older patient.

Movement is important for both the operative knee and his general well-being. She reviews the information about the passive continuous motion (PCM) machine that Mr. Rogers will have on while in bed to help bend and straighten his operative leg. He will also wear antiembolic stockings to prevent venous stasis.

Abby knows that she needs to respect Mr. Rogers' need to be independent and desire to participate in his care as much as possible. She realizes their difference in age and understands that Mr. Rogers probably has his "own way of doing things." She approaches this clinical experience with patience and creativity and plans to implement individualized care to increase Mr. Rogers' activity level, keep him as independent as possible, prevent hazards of immobility, and help him progress through the acute phase of his care by addressing his need for acute pain relief.

Selecting appropriate related factors for each diagnosis allows you to intervene appropriately. For example, *Impaired Physical Mobility* related to lower extremity weakness versus general fatigue requires different nursing approaches. Individualize nursing diagnoses for selecting patient-centered goals and interventions (Box 36-5).

PLANNING

Plan for therapeutic interventions and recognize how the patient's multiple nursing diagnoses interact with and impact on one another (Figure 36-3). As you plan care synthesize information from resources such as knowledge of the role of respiratory and physical therapy, standards such as skin-care guidelines from the Agency for Healthcare Research and Quality (AHRQ) and the Wound, Ostomy and Continence Nurses Society (WOCN), protocols for patients at risk for falls, attitudes such as creativity and perseverance, and past experiences with immobilized patients. Critical thinking ensures that the patient's plan of care integrates all that you know about the individual and key critical thinking elements. Professional standards are especially important to consider

CONCEPT MAP

Nursing Diagnosis: Acute Pain
- States pain is 9 when first asked
- Facial expressions indicate experience of pain
- Elevated heart rate when lying on the right side

Interventions
- Explain to Mr. Rogers he has medication ordered before going to physical therapy
- Discuss acceptable level of comfort (4 or less) and explain importance of reducing pain on healing

Nursing Diagnosis: Impaired Physical Mobility
- Change in walking
- Use of walker postoperatively
- Reduced range of motion in right knee

Interventions
- Collaborate with physical therapist to reinforce exercises when Mr. Rogers is back on unit
- Monitor Mr. Rogers' use of walker to ensure he is using it properly
- Make sure Mr. Rogers is ready for his physical therapy sessions
- Monitor Mr. Rogers' skin for any signs of pressure or impaired circulation
- Have Mr. Rogers deep breathe and cough every 2 hours while awake

Primary Health Problem: Total right knee replacement
Priority Assessments: Pain level related to surgery and activity, level of consciousness related to pain medications, change in mobility related to surgery on knee, safety needs related to medications and use of assistive devices for ambulation

Nursing Diagnosis: Risk for Falls
- Orthostatic hypotension
- Weakness of right leg
- Dizziness as side effect of pain medication
- Fatigue from physical therapy
- New environment

Interventions
- Teach Mr. Rogers to move positions slowly
- Place cell bell within reach
- Monitor vital signs before assisting Mr. Rogers out of bed
- Alert staff of Mr. Rogers' potential for falls
- Work with Mr. Rogers to increase strength of muscles
- Keep room clear of any clutter; use night light

Nursing Diagnosis: Deficient Knowledge—medication risks
- Increased chance of bleeding
- Reports not knowing foods with increased vitamin K
- Concerned about recovery period

Interventions
- Teach Mr. Rogers about signs and symptoms of bleeding internally and not to use sharps
- Teach Mr. Rogers diet restrictions to reduce bleeding risk
- Explain risk of injury when taking anticoagulants

—— Link between medical diagnosis and nursing diagnosis   - - - - Link between nursing diagnoses

FIGURE 36-3 Concept map.

when you develop a plan of care since they often establish scientifically proven guidelines for selecting effective nursing interventions.

Active care planning focused on prevention of physical, psychosocial, and developmental complications is essential. For example, providing for ROM and patient repositioning is a first step in preventing serious complications such as pneumonia or contractures. In addition, routine monitoring of patients' skin condition using an objective measurement such as the Braden Scale helps avoid deterioration leading to infection or sepsis. Attention to detail in care planning is critical.

Goals and Outcomes. Patients at risk for hazards of immobility require nursing care plans directed at meeting their actual and potential needs (see Care Plan). It is important to develop patient-centered goals aimed at preventing or reducing the hazards of immobility. Set realistic expectations for care and include the patient and family when possible. Set goals that are individualized, realistic, and measurable. The goals focus on preventing mobility problems or risks for falls.

A family who does too much or too little in an attempt to help the patient seriously impedes the patient's progress. Watching a family member walk slowly and with effort seems

CARE PLAN

Impaired Physical Mobility

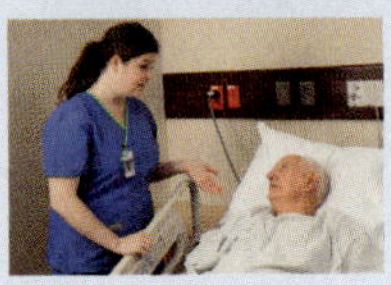

ASSESSMENT

Mr. Rogers is 2 days' postsurgery, and Abby knows that her patient has type 2 diabetes mellitus, is on anticoagulants because of the joint-replacement surgery, and has limited mobility. She believes that he is at risk for complications related to the hazards of immobility and for falls. His pain affects his ability to participate in physical therapy.

ASSESSMENT ACTIVITIES	FINDINGS/DEFINING CHARACTERISTICS*
Review demographics of Mr. Rogers.	Mr. Rogers is **91 years of age.**
Assess Mr. Roger's level of pain on a scale of 0 to 10, with 0 being no pain and 10 being the worst.	Mr. Roger's states, "**My right knee hurts an 8** when I come from physical therapy or when I walk with the walker too much after lunch or dinner."
Ask Mr. Rogers if he is light-headed when moving from a lying to a sitting position and when moving from the bed to standing with walker.	Mr. Rogers said, "**I get dizzy when I move around,** but then I'm OK." "**I have to hold on to the walker** because my **right knee still hurts and is weak** and I **feel like I need the support.**"
Ask Mr. Rogers to stand at bedside.	Mr. Rogers is able to stand but **requires a walker.**

*__Risk factors__ are shown in **bold** type.

NURSING DIAGNOSIS: Risk for Falls

PLANNING

GOAL	EXPECTED OUTCOMES (NOC)[†]
	Fall Prevention Behavior
• Mr. Rogers will remain free from falls while recuperating from knee-replacement surgery.	• Mr. Rogers consistently uses safe transfer procedures.
• Mr. Rogers consistently uses assistive device correctly.	• Mr. Rogers can demonstrate the proper use of his walker for mobility and equipment for safe transfer procedures by the time of his discharge to a rehabilitation facility.
	Pain Level
• Mr. Rogers achieves pain control.	• Mr. Rogers consistently reports his level of pain at 4 (mild) or below following pain medication. • Mr. Rogers communicates if the plan is not successful in relieving his pain.
• Mr. Rogers uses nonpharmacologic methods to help him reach a level of comfort.	• Mr. Rogers will be able to demonstrate two nonpharmacological methods to help reduce his level of pain.

[†]Outcomes classification labels from Moorhead S et al., editors: *Nursing outcomes classification (NOC),* ed 5, St Louis, 2013, Elsevier.

CARE PLAN—cont'd

Impaired Physical Mobility

INTERVENTIONS (NIC)[‡]	RATIONALES
Pain Management	
• Administer and monitor local infiltration analgesia as ordered.	Shown to enhance recovery when used in pain management for knee replacement (Ibrahim et al., 2013).
• Explain to Mr. Rogers the importance of achieving an acceptable level of comfort or relief for his pain.	Unrelieved acute pain can have physiological and psychological consequences that facilitate negative patient outcomes (Evans et al., 2009).
• Once Mr. Rogers's level of comfort has been established with infusion pump and ordered medications, teach him relaxation and distraction to help reduce his pain.	Nonpharmacological interventions should be used to supplement, not replace, pharmacological interventions (APS, 2009).
Fall Prevention	
• Collaborate with physical therapy in instructing on proper use of walker during ambulation.	Assistive device can increase risk for falls unless used correctly.
• Use safe patient handling during transfer from bed to chair.	Prevents injury to nurse and patient.

[‡]Interventions classification label from Bulechek GM et al., editors: *Nursing interventions classification (NIC),* ed 6, St Louis, 2013, Elsevier.

EVALUATION

NURSING ACTIONS	PATIENT RESPONSE/FINDING	ACHIEVEMENT OF OUTCOME
Ask Mr. Rogers to rate his pain on a scale of 0 ("no pain") to 10 ("worse pain ever") when he speaks to nurses about his pain level.	Mr. Rogers rated his pain as a 3 to 4 with analgesic pump infusing and listening to classical music on his headphones.	Pain control is satisfactory with use of analgesia and distraction.
Continue to observe Mr. Rogers for nonverbal signs of pain.	Mr. Rogers displayed no nonverbal signs of pain.	Pain control is satisfactory and will also help to reduce risk of falls.
Observe Mr. Rogers transfer from sitting on the bed to a standing position, then ambulate with the walker and sit in a stationary chair in his room using proper technique.	Mr. Rogers was able to stand up from the bed with the assistance of the walker and ambulate to the chair in the corner of the room without reporting weakness or feeling dizzy.	Mr. Rogers was able to change positions, transfer, and ambulate without reporting feelings of loss of balance or actually losing his balance, thereby reducing his risk of falling.
Observe Mr. Rogers for signs of loss of balance while moving from bed/chair to ambulating with a walker in the hall,	Mr. Rogers was able to ambulate with walker without any episode of falling or loss of balance.	Mr. Rogers was able to complete physical therapy sessions and ambulate in hallway with walker without any incident of falling while in agency.
	Mr. Roger's increased his mobility after surgery.	The increased mobility after surgery helped to decrease complications associated with immobility.

cruel, and some families excessively perform tasks that patients need to learn to do for themselves. Patients often suffer immobility for a long time. Develop goals and expected outcomes to help the patient achieve his or her highest level of mobility and ensure progressive improvement over time.

Setting Priorities. The effect that problems have on the patient's mental and physical health determines the urgency of any problem. Set priorities when planning care to ensure that immediate needs are met first. This is particularly important when patients have multiple diagnoses. For example, relieve the patient's pain first before implementing aggressive mobility activities. Because you can delegate many of the skills associated with care of the immobile patient such as turning and applying antiembolic stockings, it is easy to overlook *potential* complications until they occur. It is especially important in priority setting that you do not overlook potential complications such as pressure ulcers or disuse syndrome and that you address these complications as part of the care plan. Therefore be vigilant in assessing and monitoring patients, reinforcing prevention techniques, and supervising nursing assistive personnel in carrying out activities aimed at preventing complications of immobility.

Collaborative Care. It is wise to use a collaborative approach when providing care with and for a patient with impaired mobility. For example, physical therapists are a resource for planning ROM or strengthening exercises, and occupational therapists are a means for planning ADLs. Wound care specialists and respiratory therapists are experts at preventing pressure ulcers and respiratory complications, respectively, as they relate to immobility. Proper nutrition is essential for wound healing and prevention of skin breakdown; therefore a registered dietitian contributes significantly to the plan of care, especially if the patient is older or experiencing nutritional difficulties. You may also need to refer the patient to a mental health advanced practice nurse, licensed social worker, or psychologist to assist with coping or psychosocial issues.

Discharge planning begins when a patient first enters the health care system. In anticipation of the patient's discharge from an agency, make appropriate referrals to a case manager or a discharge planner to ensure the patient's needs are met at home. Consider the patient's home environment when planning therapies to maintain or improve mobility and reduce the risk of falls. Referrals to home care or outpatient therapy are often needed. This should include assessing the patient's mobility within the community (e.g., how the patient with limited mobility will get to and return from the required health care appointments).

IMPLEMENTATION

Nursing interventions for the completely or partially immobilized patient focus on health promotion and prevention of complications. Many patients with limited mobility function in the home or assisted-living settings; thus they require active intervention to prevent complications that might necessitate hospitalization. Specific interventions in the acute care setting focus on reducing severity of complications that have developed (e.g., by positioning and transferring patients correctly). In restorative and continuing care direct your interventions at regaining and maximizing functional mobility and independence.

Health Promotion. Health promotion activities aim to keep individuals mobile and include prevention of work-related injuries, fall prevention measures, and exercise. The work by Nelson et al. (2009) has helped to significantly reduce nurses' work-related injuries associated with lifting or moving patients. The researchers have established a series of algorithms to be used to lift and transfer patients safely and without injury to the health care provider or the patient.

Fall prevention measures are implemented when a patient is identified as at risk for falls. The Morse Fall Scale provides a valid and reliable tool available from the Veteran Administration Fall Prevention Program (Morse, 2009). It can be used in acute and long-term patient care facilities and addresses risk factors such as the patient's history of falling, secondary diagnosis, ambulatory aid, intravenous/heparin lock, gait/transferring, and mental status. When a fall is prevented, the mobility of the patient is not compromised.

Structured exercise programs for immobile patients improve their endurance, strength, overall health, and feelings of well-being. Chapter 27 presented in greater detail the importance of exercise and activity for general well-being. Exercise is recommended before surgery for patients expected to have mobility restrictions after surgery. Putting exercise into the care plan for patients on bed rest or who have had surgery helps to reduce risks of immobility. Start by having patients stretch; perform ROM; and, when allowed, set specific goals such as "walk 20 feet 3 times a day." When the actual distance is stated, patients can keep track of their progress.

Older patients need special consideration. Disuse and disease account for much of the functional decline in the older adult population. However, this is not a developmental norm of aging. By incorporating exercise into the older patient's care plan and collaborating with the physical therapist, it is possible to prevent disuse syndrome for these patients.

Respiratory System. Aim interventions for the respiratory system at promoting expansion of the chest and lungs, preventing stasis of pulmonary secretions, and maintaining a patent airway.

Promoting Expansion of the Chest and Lungs. Regular exercise and activities such as changing the position of patients at least every 2 hours allows the dependent lung regions to reexpand, maintains the elastic recoil property of the lungs, and clears the dependent lung regions of pulmonary secretions (see Chapter 30). Your assessment determines if patients need more-frequent exercising and position changes.

Preventing Stasis of Pulmonary Secretions. Stagnant secretions accumulating in the bronchi and lungs of the immobilized patient lead to the growth of bacteria and the subsequent development of pneumonia. Changing the patient's position reduces stagnation of secretions, rotates the dependent lung, and mobilizes secretions.

Make sure that the immobile patient has a fluid intake of at least 2000 mL per day, if not contraindicated, to help keep mucociliary clearance intact. In patients free from infection and with adequate hydration, pulmonary secretions appear thin, watery, and clear. It is easy for the patient to remove these secretions with coughing. Without adequate hydration secretions become thick, tenacious, and difficult to remove. One method for removing pulmonary secretions is chest physiotherapy (CPT). The use of this technique drains secretions from specific segments of the bronchi and lungs into the trachea and helps the patient expel the secretions by coughing (see Chapter 30). Combine coughing with the deep-breathing exercises and have the patient do these on a regular schedule.

Metabolic System. Adequate nutrition is essential to prevent tissue breakdown for a patient of any age who is immobile. Therefore the plan of care must be designed to incorporate enough carbohydrates, proteins, and fats to combat the effects of immobility. Carbohydrates meet energy requirements; proteins are necessary for tissue repair and to counter negative nitrogen balance. Fats prevent further breakdown of nutritional stores. Determine the patient's specific caloric and diet prescription from the nutritional assessment. Collaborate with the registered dietitian for any dietary restrictions related to other medical conditions or for patients not consuming the necessary nutrients. The nutritional deficit results in complications such as pressure ulcers, which could be fatal for the older patient (see Chapter 33).

Cardiovascular System. Design health promotion nursing therapies to minimize or prevent thrombus formation.

Preventing Thrombus Formation. Proper positioning used with other therapies (e.g., anticoagulants and antiembolic stockings) helps reduce thrombus formation. Provide appropriate patient education to patients who are on anticoagulation therapy (Box 36-6). When positioning patients, use caution to prevent pressure on the posterior knee and deep veins in the lower extremities. Teach patients to avoid crossing the legs, sitting for prolonged periods of time, wearing tight clothing that constricts the legs or waist, putting pillows under the knees, and massaging the legs.

ROM exercises reduce the risk for contractures and also help to prevent thrombi (see Table 36-3). Activity causes contraction of the skeletal muscles, which exerts pressure on the veins to promote venous return. This reduces venous stasis. Specific exercises that help prevent thrombophlebitis are ankle pumps, foot circles, hip rotation, and knee flexion. Ankle pumps, sometimes called *calf pumps*, include alternating plantar flexion and dorsiflexion. Foot circles require the patient to rotate the ankle. While the patient is supine (lying on back) or sitting, he or she rotates the hip joint by rotating the entire leg and pointing the toes inward and outward. Knee flexion involves alternately extending and flexing the knee. These exercises are usually done each hour while awake and are aimed at preventing thrombi; they are sometimes called *antiembolic exercises*.

Musculoskeletal System. The immobilized or partially immobilized patient needs to exercise to prevent excessive muscle atrophy, decreased endurance, and joint contractures. The amount of activity required to prevent physical disuse syndromes is only about 2 hours in a 24-hour period; therefore schedule exercise regularly throughout the day based on individual patient needs and tolerance.

If the patient is unable to move any part or all of the body, perform passive ROM exercises for all immobilized joints at least 3 or 4 times a day unless contraindicated. Teach family caregivers how to provide these exercises in the home. If one extremity is paralyzed, teach the patient to perform passive ROM on the paralyzed limb and encourage him or her to engage in active ROM with all other extremities (see Table 36-3). Encourage patients to use mobile extremities during ADLs (e.g., dressing) as much as possible. The bath is an excellent time to perform ROM.

The best nursing intervention is establishing an individualized progressive exercise program. A progressive exercise program gradually increases the patient's physical activity to reverse the deconditioning associated with immobility. Teaching is an important aspect for patients with limited mobility (see Box 36-6). Depending on the setting and resources available, collaborate with physical therapy to help set up the exercise program.

Skin Integrity. The major risk to the skin from restricted mobility is the formation of pressure ulcers. Early identification of high-risk patients (e.g., wheelchair-bound patients, stroke patients) helps to prevent them. Interventions aimed at prevention are positioning, skin care, and the use of pressure-relief devices. Change the immobilized patient's position according to his or her activity level, perceptual ability, status of peripheral circulation, treatment protocols, and daily routines (see Chapter 37). For example, a person in a wheelchair learns to move the buttocks and hips up and off of the wheelchair seat every 15 to 20 minutes. Although turning is essential, it is sometimes necessary to use devices

BOX 36-6 PATIENT TEACHING

Decreasing Risk of Bleeding

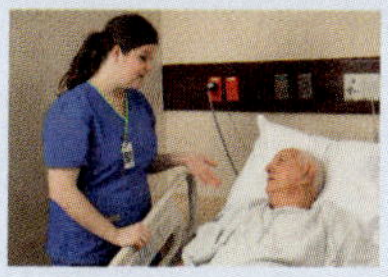

Mr. Rogers is taking an oral anticoagulant medication. Abby examined the evidence-based research on bleeding related to oral anticoagulant medications and realized that her patient could be at risk for this serious complication (Cunningham et al., 2011). Therefore she decided to teach him how to recognize the signs of this complication if it should occur after he is discharged from the hospital.

OUTCOME

At the end of the teaching session Mr. Rogers lists three signs of internal bleeding for which he should call his health care provider immediately. He also lists five activities to avoid while taking the oral anticoagulant (e.g., taking aspirin or other over-the-counter medications, using a regular razor to shave, or operating an electric saw).

TEACHING STRATEGIES

- Plan his teaching session at a time when he is rested, his pain is controlled, and there is reduced noise in the environment.
- Speak clearly and slowly, making sure that she is facing Mr. Rogers.
- Keep the teaching session short and reinforce the important points several times during the session.
- Use letters in plain script large enough for Mr. Rogers to read easily, and list the main points.

EVALUATION STRATEGIES

- Use focused questions to evaluate Mr. Rogers' understanding of what he should and should not eat or which medications he must not take while taking the oral anticoagulant.
- Ask Mr. Rogers to list three signs that may indicate that he is bleeding internally.
- Ask Mr. Rogers what he would do if he noticed any of the signs of bleeding.

for relieving pressure. Normally the time that a mobile patient sits uninterrupted in a chair is 1 hour or less, but this time interval must be individualized. Uninterrupted pressure causes skin breakdown. Teach patients who are able to move to shift their weight every 15 to 20 minutes. Make sure that chair-bound patients have a pressure-reducing device for the chair (AHRQ, 2011).

Elimination System. Health promotion interventions for maintaining optimal urinary functioning are to keep the patient well hydrated without causing bladder distention and the reflux of urine into the ureters and renal pelvis. This helps to prevent renal calculi and UTIs. Timely toileting prevents bladder distention. Make sure that the patient's urine is light yellow and comparable in amount to the fluid intake by monitoring total fluid intake and output each shift or each day when in the home.

A patient who continually dribbles urine and whose bladder is distended likely has reflex incontinence. If the immobilized patient does not have voluntary control of bladder elimination, bladder retraining is necessary. Teaching patients how to perform Kegel exercises is effective (see Chapter 34). It may become necessary to insert a straight or indwelling Foley catheter (see Chapter 34) if the patient experiences ongoing bladder distention.

Record the frequency and consistency of bowel movements. A diet rich in fruits and vegetables helps to facilitate normal peristalsis. Insoluble fiber is necessary to facilitate both the passage of stool and adequate water intake. Make sure that the patient has at least 6 to 8 glasses of water daily, unless contraindicated, to help promote bowel elimination. If a patient is unable to maintain normal bowel patterns, initiate a bowel-training program; and the health care provider may order stool softeners, cathartics, or enemas (see Chapter 35).

Psychosocial Problems. Health promotion for the immobilized patient requires anticipation of changes in psychosocial status and intervention with preventive measures. Provide routine and informal socialization for the patient. Help family caregivers learn the importance of keeping patients involved in decisions about their care and engaging them in conversation and self-help activities. Plan activities to give patients in health care settings the opportunity to interact with the staff. If possible, place these patients in a room with other mobile patients. If the patient remains in a private room, ask staff members to visit periodically throughout waking hours. Provide stimuli to maintain orientation and entertain the patient.

Encourage patients to wear their glasses or dentures and to shave or apply makeup. These are normal activities to enhance body image. Encourage him or her to perform as much self-care as possible. Make sure that hygiene and grooming articles are within easy reach so the patient can attend to personal needs.

Developmental Changes. Plan care to stimulate the patient, especially a young child, mentally and physically. Incorporate play activities into the nursing care plan. For example, puzzles help patients develop fine-motor skills. Place an immobilized child in a room with children of the same age who are mobile unless a contagious disease is present (Hockenberry and Wilson, 2010). Health promotion for older adults requires matching mobility needs with the patient's developmental limitations. Older adults benefit when exercise routines are mildly progressive. Walking, aquatic exercise, swimming, and gardening are good ways to promote ROM and endurance.

Acute Care. Patients in acute care settings demonstrate more rapid and pronounced complications of immobility because of the presence of multisystem involvement. In these patients design nursing interventions to reduce the impact of immobility on body systems and prepare the patient for restorative and continuing care. Use interventions combined with those outlined in the health promotion section to return the patient to an optimal level of function.

Respiratory System. Encourage patients to cough and deep breathe every 1 to 2 hours while awake. This action expands all lobes of the lungs and prevents atelectasis. Coughing reduces the stasis of pulmonary secretions. Some immobile patients, particularly after surgery, need to use an incentive spirometer to aid in deep breathing (see Chapter 30).

Postoperative patients who have undergone general anesthesia especially need to cough and deep breathe to prevent atelectasis and stasis of secretions. Timely pain management for incision discomfort is essential. Patients cough more effectively when their pain is under control. If a patient becomes drowsy from medication, actively reinforce coughing and deep breathing. Encouraging early ambulation helps prevent multiple pulmonary complications.

Maintaining a Patent Airway. Immobilized patients and those on bed rest are generally weakened. The cough reflex gradually becomes inefficient as the weakness progresses. If the patient is too weak or unable to cough up secretions, maintain the patient's airway by using suctioning techniques (see Chapter 30). This usually involves oral or nasotracheal suctioning and suctioning of artificial airways. Suspect hypostatic bronchopneumonia if the patient develops a productive cough with greenish-yellow sputum, fever, and pain on breathing.

Cardiovascular System. After prolonged bed rest patients usually have an increased heart rate, a decrease in pulse pressure, and a drop in blood pressure with an increase in fainting when rising to a sitting or standing position (Black and Hawks, 2009). Attempt to have the patient move as soon as the physical condition allows, even if this only involves dangling at the bedside or moving to a chair. This activity maintains muscle tone and increases venous return. Isometric exercises (i.e., activities that involve muscle tension without muscle shortening) do not have any beneficial effect on preventing orthostatic hypotension, but they improve activity tolerance (see Chapter 27).

When transferring from a supine position into a chair, move the patient gradually. First obtain a baseline blood pressure and pulse with the patient in the supine position. Then raise the patient to a high-Fowler's position and measure blood pressure and pulse again to detect decreases in blood pressure or elevations in pulse. Leave the patient in this position for 2 minutes to allow the body to adapt. Monitor him or her for dizziness or light-headedness. The patient is now ready to sit at the side of the bed with the feet on the floor. If there is no dizziness, help the patient to a chair. When transferring an immobile patient for the first time, make sure to use the appropriate safe patient handling and movement algorithm (Figure 36-4) (Nelson, 2013).

It is also important to direct nursing interventions at reducing cardiac workload. When a patient moves up in bed or strains on defecation, a Valsalva maneuver occurs. During a Valsalva maneuver the patient holds his or her breath and strains, increasing intrathoracic pressure, which decreases venous return and cardiac output. When the strain is released,

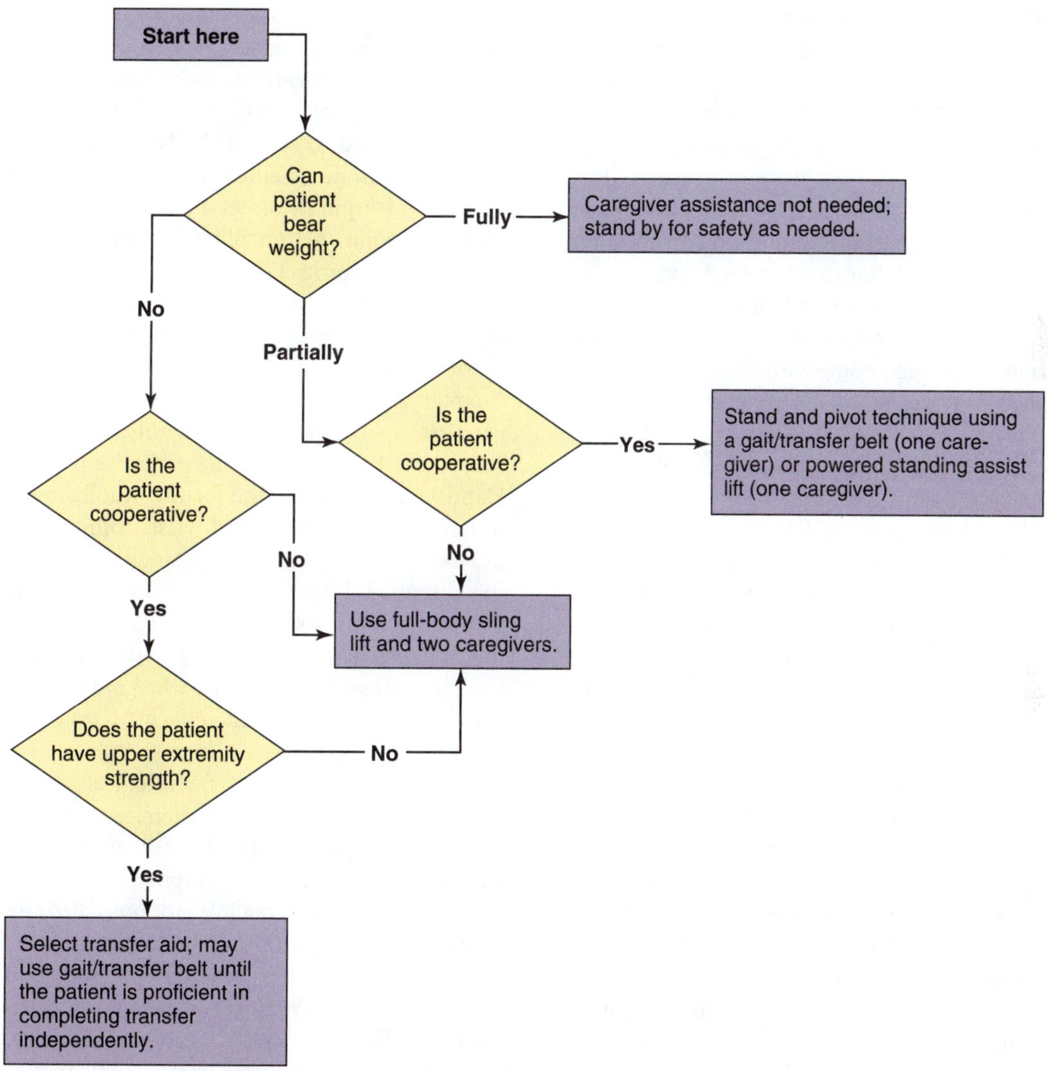

- For seated transfer aid, must have chair with arms that recess or are removable.
- For full-body sling lift, select a lift that was specifically designed to access a patient from the car (if the car is the starting or ending destination).
- If patient has partial weight-bearing capacity, transfer toward stronger side.
- Toileting slings are available for toileting.
- Mesh slings are available for bathing.
- During any patient transferring task, if any caregiver is required to lift more than 35 lbs of a patient's weight, the patient should be considered to be fully dependent, and assistive devices should be used for the transfer.

FIGURE 36-4 Algorithm used to transfer patient to and from bed to chair, chair to toilet, chair to chair, or car to chair. (From Nelson A: *Safe patient handling and movement algorithms,* 2006, VISN8 Patient Safety Center, http://www.visn8.va.gov/patientsafetycenter/safepthandling/safepatienthandlingassessment_algorithms_121112.doc. Accessed November 19, 2013.)

venous return and cardiac output immediately increase, and systolic blood pressure and pulse pressure rise. These pressure changes produce a reflex bradycardia that can be associated with sudden cardiac death, particularly in patients with heart disease. Teach the patient to breathe out while moving or being lifted up in bed to avoid straining.

Because DVT is a hazard of immobility, interventions that reduce the risk for thrombus formation in the immobilized patient such as leg exercises, encouraging fluids, and position changes must be incorporated into the plan of care. Instruct preoperative patients in leg exercises before their surgery (see Chapter 39). Other interventions such as antiembolic elastic stockings and SCD require a health care provider's order.

Elastic stockings help to maintain pressure on the muscles of the lower extremities and therefore promote venous return. Make sure to measure the patient's lower extremities correctly to ensure proper fit and apply the stockings properly (Box 36-7). Remove and reapply them at least every 8 hours or according to agency policy. Improper application of stockings can lead to decreased circulation in the lower extremities. Always observe the status of circulation to the extremities (see Chapter 16) and be sure stockings do not roll down leg. Patients are usually discharged home with these stockings. Be sure that they learn how to apply them correctly and how to observe the status of circulation to the extremities. Instruct patients on the signs of allergic reactions, thrombophlebitis, or skin irritation so they can report changes to their health care provider.

SCDs consist of inflatable plastic sleeves wrapped around the legs and secured with Velcro. The sleeves are connected to an air pump that alternately inflates and deflates, providing rhythmic, external extremity compression (Box 36-8). Use of SCDs on the legs decreases venous stasis by increasing venous return. Postoperative patients are encouraged to ambulate even when SCD therapy is in use. Remove SCDs for ambulation.

Immobilized patients are frequently on prophylactic (preventive) low-dose heparin therapy to minimize the risk for venous thromboembolism. Heparin is an anticoagulant that suppresses clot formation. This therapy requires a health care provider's order. Newer low-molecular-weight (LMW) heparins such as ardeparin and enoxaparin are being prescribed in place of older forms of unfractionated heparin. The LMW heparins have a more predictable anticoagulant effect. The drugs are given subcutaneously, usually every 12 hours until the risk for DVT declines. LMW heparin compared with unfractionated heparin reduces the occurrence of major hemorrhage as a side effect (Lewis et al., 2011). Local irritation such as erythema, hematoma, and urticaria at injection sites is common. However, it is still wise to monitor the patient for signs of bleeding (e.g., increased bruising, guaiac-positive stools, and bleeding gums). Report any occurrence of hemorrhage immediately.

When you suspect DVT, do not massage the area; report assessment findings to the health care provider immediately; and elevate the leg, with no pressure on the area of the leg with the suspected thrombus. If the patient complains of shortness of breath or severe chest pain, suspect a pulmonary embolus. Immediately place the patient in high-Fowler's position and check his or her oxygen saturation. This complication is life threatening and requires prompt medical attention and activation of the Rapid Response Team if required by agency policy.

Musculoskeletal System. The immobilized patient needs to get some exercise to prevent excessive muscle atrophy and joint contractures. For patients on bed rest, incorporate active ROM exercises into their daily schedules. Patients with impaired nervous, skeletal, or muscular system functioning and significant weakness often require help to attain and maintain body alignment.

Several devices are available for maintaining proper patient positioning (see Chapter 27, Table 27-3). Pillows are commonly used to support body alignment. Before using a pillow, determine whether it is the proper size and consistency. A thick pillow under a patient's head causes excessive cervical flexion. A thin pillow under bony prominences is inadequate to protect skin and tissue from damage. When additional pillows are unavailable, use folded sheets, blankets, or towels as positioning aids. The 30-degree lateral position is for patients at risk for pressure ulcer development (see Chapter 37). Elevate the patient's calves on pillows to avoid pressure on the heels. A trochanter roll prevents external rotation of the hips when the patient is in a supine position. Hand rolls maintain the hand, thumb, and fingers in a functional position. Hand-wrist splints are individually molded for the patient to maintain proper alignment of the thumb. A trapeze bar is a triangular device that hangs from a securely fastened overhead bar that is attached to the patient's bed frame. It is a useful device for helping to increase patient independence when moving in bed, maintain upper body strength, and reduce friction from movement in bed.

Some orthopedic and neurological conditions require more frequent passive ROM exercises to restore the injured joint or extremity to maximal function. Patients with such conditions use automatic equipment for passive ROM exercises. The continuous passive motion (CPM) machine moves an extremity within a prescribed range for a specific period. This method is beneficial when the patient gradually increases ROM of a particular joint. For example, it is used for patients who have had total knee–replacement surgery. It is applied immediately after surgery and is only removed when the patient is receiving physical therapy. Over time the patient progresses from its use to flexion and extension of the joint without the aid of the CPM (Figure 36-5).

Active ROM exercises also maintain function of the musculoskeletal system. Have patients participate in active ROM and collaborate with physical therapy if needed to establish an individualized progressive exercise program when possible. A progressive exercise program gradually increases the patient's physical activity to reverse the deconditioning associated with immobility. Progressive exercise programs are successful in patients with musculoskeletal, neurological, cardiopulmonary, renal, and other chronic diseases.

BOX 36-7 PROCEDURAL GUIDELINES

View Video!

Applying Antiembolic Elastic Stockings

DELEGATION CONSIDERATIONS

You can delegate the skill of applying antiembolic elastic stockings to nursing assistive personnel (NAP). The nurse instructs the NAP to inform the nurse:

- If patient complains of leg pain or leg swelling.
- If patient has any skin irritation.

Also instruct the NAP to inform the patient:

- To avoid activities that promote venous stasis (e.g., crossing legs, wearing garters).
- To elevate legs while sitting and before applying stockings to improve venous return.
- Not to massage legs.
- To avoid wrinkles in the stockings.

EQUIPMENT

Tape measure, elastic support stockings

STEPS

1. Identify patient using two identifiers (e.g., name and birthday or name and account number) according to agency policy.
2. Assess patient for risk factors in Virchow's triad:
   a. *Hypercoagulability:* All patients with clotting disorders, fever, dehydration, pregnancy and first 6 weeks' postpartum if the woman was confined to bed, and oral contraceptive use (especially if patient smokes)
   b. *Venous wall abnormalities:* Local trauma, orthopedic surgeries, major abdominal surgery, varicose veins, atherosclerosis
   c. *Blood stasis:* Immobility, obesity, pregnancy
3. Observe for signs, symptoms, and conditions that contraindicate use of antiembolic elastic stockings. Signs and symptoms include:
   a. Dermatitis or open skin lesion.
   b. Recent skin graft.
   c. Decreased circulation in lower extremities as evidenced by cyanotic, cool extremities and gangrenous conditions affecting the lower limb(s).
4. Assess and document condition of patient's skin and circulation to legs (i.e., presence of pedal pulses; edema, temperature, and discoloration of skin; lesions or abrasions).
5. Obtain physician's or health care provider's order.
6. Assess patient's or family caregiver's understanding of application of antiembolic elastic stockings.

***Clinical Decision Point:* Clinical signs of thrombophlebitis vary according to the size and location of the thrombus. Signs and symptoms of superficial thrombosis include palpable veins and surrounding area that is tender to the touch, reddened, and warm. Temperature elevation and edema may or may not be present. Signs and symptoms of deep vein thrombosis (DVT) include swollen extremity; pain; warm, cyanotic skin; and temperature elevation. However, up to 80% of patients are asymptomatic. Homans' sign (pain in the calf on dorsiflexion of the foot) is no longer considered a reliable assessment. Fewer than 20% of patients have a positive Homans' sign (Black and Hawks, 2009).**

7. Use tape measure to measure patient's legs to determine proper stocking size (follow package directions).
8. Explain procedure and reasons for applying stockings.
9. Perform hand hygiene. Provide hygiene to patient's lower extremities as needed.
10. Position patient in supine position.
11. Apply elastic stockings:
    a. Turn elastic stocking inside out up to heel by placing one hand into stocking, holding heel. Pull top of stocking with the other hand inside out over foot of stocking to heel.
    b. Place patient's toes into the foot of elastic stocking, making sure that stocking is smooth (see illustration).

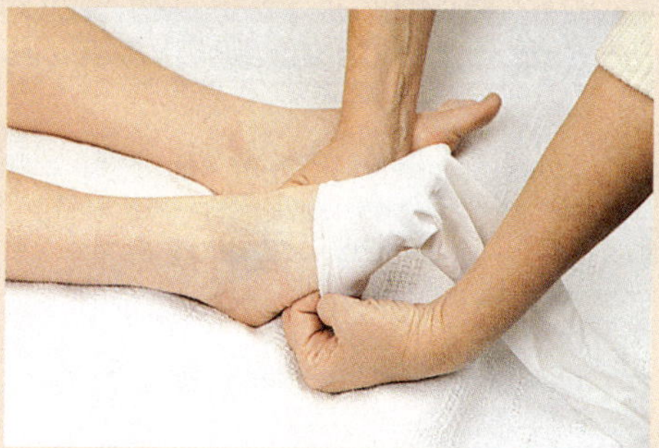

STEP 11b Place toes into foot of stocking.

    c. Slide remaining part of stocking over patient's foot, being sure that toes are covered. Make sure that foot fits into toe and heel position of stocking (see illustration).

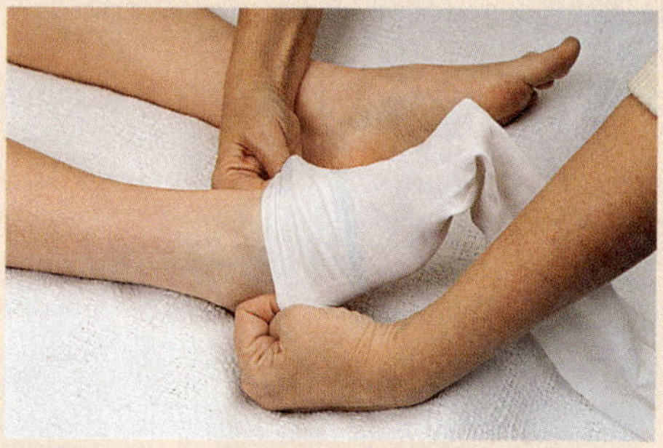

STEP 11c Slide heel of stocking over foot.

    d. Slide top of stocking up over patient's calf until it is completely extended. Be sure that stocking is smooth and that no ridges or wrinkles are present, particularly behind knee (see illustration).

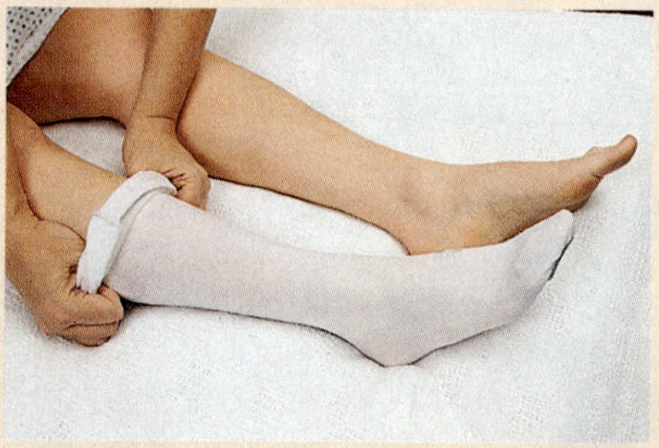

STEP 11d Slide stocking up leg until completely extended.

    e. Instruct patient not to roll stockings partially down.

Continued

BOX 36-7 PROCEDURAL GUIDELINES—cont'd

View Video!

Applying Antiembolic Elastic Stockings

12. Reposition patient for comfort and perform hand hygiene.
13. Remove stockings at least once every 8 hours.
14. Inspect stockings for wrinkles or constriction.
15. Inspect elastic stockings to determine that there are no wrinkles, rolls, or binding.
16. Observe circulatory status of lower extremities. Observe color, temperature, and condition of skin. Palpate pedal pulses.
17. Observe patient's response to wearing antiembolic elastic stockings.
18. Observe patient or caregiver applying stockings.

BOX 36-8 PROCEDURAL GUIDELINES

Applying Sequential Compression Devices

DELEGATION CONSIDERATIONS

You can delegate the skill of applying sequential compression devices (SCDs) to nursing assistive personnel (NAP). The nurse is responsible for assessing circulation in the extremities. Instruct the NAP to notify nurse:

- If patient complains of leg pain.
- If discoloration develops in extremities.

EQUIPMENT

SCD insufflator with air hoses attached, adjustable Velcro compression stockings/SCD sleeve, hygiene supplies

STEPS

1. Assess patient for need for sequential compression stockings (see Box 36-7).
2. Obtain baseline assessment data about the status of circulation, pulse, and skin integrity on patient's lower extremities before initiating sequential compression stockings.
3. Identify patient using two identifiers (e.g., name and birthday or name and account number), according to agency policy.
4. Perform hand hygiene. Provide hygiene to patient's lower extremities as needed.
5. Assemble and prepare equipment.
6. Arrange SCD sleeve under patient's leg according to leg position indicated on inner lining of the sleeve (see illustration).

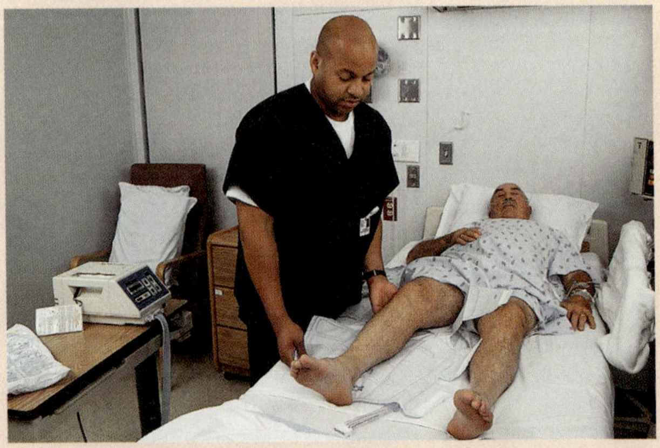

STEP 6 Correct leg position on inner lining.

   a. Back of patient's ankle should line up with ankle on inner lining of the sleeve.
   b. Position back of knee with popliteal opening (see illustration).

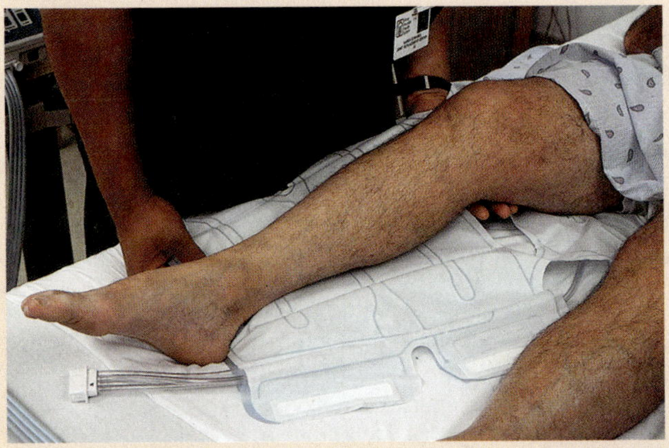

STEP 6b Position back of patient's knee with popliteal opening.

7. Wrap SCD sleeve securely around patient's leg.
8. Verify fit of SCD sleeves by placing two fingers between patient's leg and sleeve (see illustration).

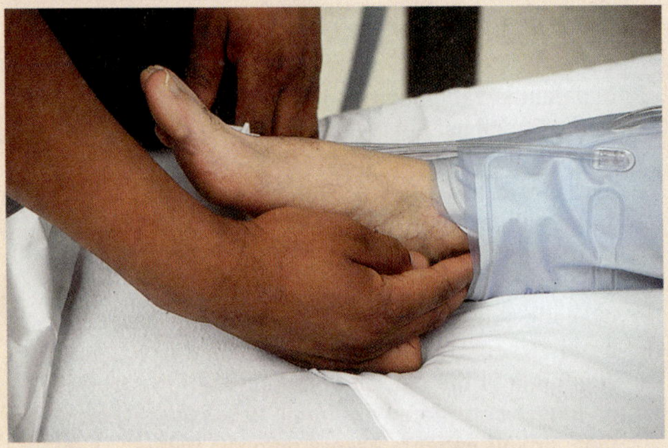

STEP 8 Check fit of SCD sleeve.

BOX 36-8 **PROCEDURAL GUIDELINES—cont'd**

Applying Sequential Compression Devices

9. Attach sleeve of SCD connector to plug on mechanical unit. Arrows on compressor line up with arrows on plug from mechanical unit (see illustration).
10. Turn mechanical unit on. Green light indicates that unit is functioning.
11. Observe functioning of unit for one complete cycle.
12. Reposition patient for comfort and perform hand hygiene.
13. Remove compression stockings at least once every 8 hours.
14. Monitor skin integrity and circulation to patient's lower extremities as ordered or as recommended by SCD manufacturer.

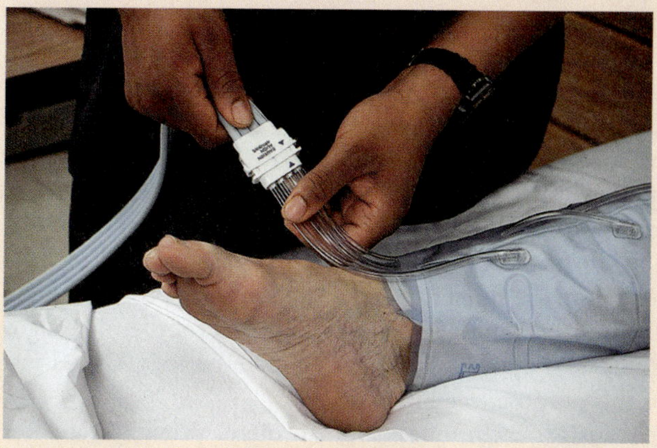

STEP 9 Align arrows when connecting to mechanical unit.

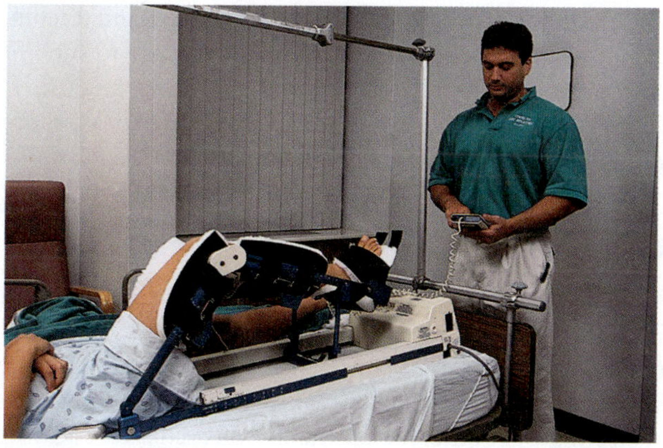

FIGURE 36-5 Continuous passive range-of-motion machine.

Integumentary System. The major risk to skin integrity from restricted mobility is the formation of pressure ulcers. Continuous use of tools such as the Braden Scale to monitor high-risk patients helps prevent pressure ulcers (see Chapter 37). Interventions aimed at preventing prolonged pressure should prevent or delay the development of the ulcers until the patient is able to move more freely or be out of bed. Change the immobilized patient's position according to the patient's activity level, perceptual ability, treatment protocols, and daily routines. Although turning every 1 to 2 hours is recommended for preventing ulcers, it is sometimes necessary to use support surfaces (e.g., mattresses) for relieving pressure. Usually the time that a patient sits uninterrupted in a chair is limited to 1 hour. This interval is shortened in patients who are at very high risk for skin breakdown. Teach patients to shift their weight every 15 to 20 minutes. Chair-bound patients use pressure-relief cushions (AHRQ, 2011).

Psychosocial Problems. Establish a balance among rest, the physiological effects of bed rest, and the patient's psychosocial needs. Keep assessments to a minimum in a stable patient who is able to turn in bed unassisted. More seriously ill patients need medications, assessments, and skin care during the night. Coordinate nursing care to prevent as many interruptions as possible between 10 PM and 7 AM. For example, administer medications and assess vital signs as the patient is turned or receives special skin care. If the plan of care is not improving coping patterns, collaborate with a mental health and advanced practice nurse, counselor, social worker, spiritual adviser, or other health care professional and incorporate their recommendations into the plan of care.

Nurses provide stimuli to maintain a patient's orientation. If possible place the patient in a room with others who are mobile and interactive. If a private room is required, ask staff members to visit throughout the shift to provide meaningful interaction. Access to daily news helps patients keep track of events and time. Bedside conversations at appropriate moments familiarize the patient with nursing activities, meals, and visiting hours. Books help occupy the patient when he or she is alone. The patient can participate in craft activities; and radio, television, or computers provide stimulation and help pass the time.

Involve patients in their care whenever possible. For example, have the patient determine when the bed should be made. Some patients rest better during the night when fresh sheets are put on in the evening rather than in the morning. Keep hygiene and grooming articles within easy reach. Encourage patients to wear their glasses or artificial teeth and to shave or apply makeup. These activities help maintain body image, thus improving the patient's outlook.

Developmental Changes. Immobilization or restricted mobility of an older adult requires complex care and innovative approaches because older adults are at risk for cognitive changes and depression as a result of immobilization, chronic illnesses, and medications. It is important to focus on activities to promote cognitive awareness of the patient's surroundings (see Chapter 22). Give explanations before starting care and have the patient make decisions about care. Plan nursing care to allow the older adult patient to perform as many ADLs as possible by allowing extra time for routine activities. Not only are older adults more susceptible to the hazards of immobility, but the consequences of immobility appear more quickly and become severe more rapidly.

Safe Patient Handling and Movement. Before attempting any movement or transfer always explain the process and equipment being used to the patient in terms that is appropriate for his or her developmental stage. Patients unable to move themselves safely from one location to another must depend on the nursing staff to choose the appropriate piece of equipment with which to facilitate that transfer. The algorithms developed by Nelson et al. (2009) were designed just for this purpose (see Figure 36-4).

Transfer Techniques. Nurses often provide care for immobilized patients whose position must be changed, who must be moved up in bed, or who must be transferred from a bed to a chair or from a bed to a stretcher. As noted earlier, body mechanics alone do not protect the nurse from injury to the musculoskeletal system when moving, lifting, or transferring patients. Although nurses use many transfer techniques, knowledge of ergonomics and safe patient handling is crucial in maintaining caregiver and patient safety (see Chapter 27).

Assess every situation that involves patient handling and movement to minimize risk of injury. After completing the assessment, use an algorithm to guide decisions about safe patient handling. Use the patient's strength when lifting, transferring, or moving when possible. Involving the patient has the added bonus of increasing participation in self-care, thus promoting a sense of accomplishment. In addition to handling patients safely, nurses need to assume an active role in their workplaces to ensure that a culture of safety exists and that appropriate patient-handling equipment is readily available (ANA, 2012).

Moving and Transferring Patients. A safe transfer is the first priority. Patients require various levels of assistance to move up in bed, move to the side-lying position, or sit up at the side of the bed. For example, a young, healthy woman needs only a little support as she sits at the side of the bed for the first time after childbirth, whereas an older man needs help from two or more nurses to do the same task 1 day after abdominal surgery.

Always ask the patient to help to the fullest extent possible. To determine what he or she is able to do alone and how many people are needed to help move the patient in bed, assess the patient to determine whether the illness contradicts exertion (e.g., cardiovascular disease). Next determine whether he or she comprehends what is expected. For example, a patient recently medicated for postoperative pain is too lethargic to understand instruction; thus to ensure safety two nurses are necessary to move him or her. Then determine the comfort level of the patient. It is important to evaluate your personal strength and knowledge of the procedure. Finally determine whether the patient is too heavy or immobile for you to move alone (Nelson et al., 2009). Through the use of assessment tools and patient movement algorithms, you determine the safest method by which to move the patient. Chapter 27 and Skills 27-1 and 27-2 describe the steps commonly used in moving patients in bed and transferring them to a sitting position at the side of the bed.

Restorative and Continuing Care. The goal of restorative and continuing care for the immobilized patient is to maximize independence, increase endurance, and prevent injury. Restorative interventions focus on instrumental activities of daily living (IADLs) such as shopping, preparing meals, banking, taking medications, and ADLs. Often patients with mobility issues are transferred to rehabilitation centers to work on improving IADLs. Make sure to provide the rehabilitation center with a complete report to ensure patient safety and continuity of care (The Joint Commission, 2014).

Use many of the same interventions as described in the health promotion and acute care sections, but the emphasis now is on working collaboratively to help patients adjust in the home or in an extended-care facility. Sometimes occupational or physical therapy is ordered. Work collaboratively with these professionals and reinforce exercises and teaching. Common items used to help the patient adapt to mobility limitations include walkers; canes; wheelchairs; and assistive devices such as toilet seat extenders, reaching sticks, special eating utensils, and clothing with Velcro closures.

EVALUATION

Patient Care. Evaluate interventions for reducing the risks of immobility by comparing the patient's actual response to the expected outcomes for each goal. If expected outcomes are not achieved, revise the plan of care. Base the success in meeting each outcome on the use of evaluative measures such as ROM status, exercise tolerance, skin integrity, and fluid intake.

Evaluate outcomes designed to demonstrate normal function of specific systems and prevent complications (Box 36-9). For example, are the lungs clear; are any areas of skin showing signs of skin breakdown; is the patient regularly performing leg exercises? Evaluation provides evidence of whether you are meeting the outcomes set with the patient during the planning phase of care. If the answers to the questions indicate that outcomes are being met, the plan is working; if not, you need to reassess and revise the plan with input from the patient.

Patient Expectations. People often take movement for granted. Patients who are immobile and dependent on others for some or all of their needs sometimes become overly dependent or try to do too much themselves too early. Finding the balance between independence and dependence is a difficult task. Patients want control over their mobility that is personally satisfactory. For patients who are completely dependent on others for care, control over how and when things are done is very important. Do they believe that they are treated with dignity? Do caregivers treat them as adults? Patients who are dependent on others for care

BOX 36-9 EVALUATION

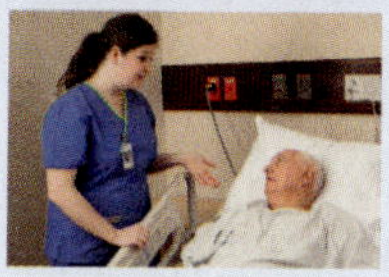

It has been 5 days since Mr. Rogers' knee-replacement surgery. He is becoming more independent. He is reporting his pain at a level of 4 on the pain scale while on the local anesthesia infusion pump. He will be discharged to his home and will continue outpatient physical therapy 3 times a week.

During his stay in the hospital Abby taught Mr. Rogers the importance of following the American Diabetes Association (ADA) diet. In addition, she worked with the patient and his physical therapist in deciding which exercises he will perform at home. Abby also made sure that Mr. Rogers' children understood his medications and exercises so they could work with him as well. Mr. Rogers must concentrate on increasing the strength of his upper extremities, reducing his weight by following an ADA diet as prescribed by his primary health care provider, and keeping up with his physical activities and exercises.

DOCUMENTATION NOTE

"Mr. Rogers discharged via car to home accompanied by son. Surgical incision dry, and staples intact. Patient presently reports pain at a level of 4 on a scale of 0 to 10. Has been able to demonstrate exercises as taught, is able to use a walker, and verbalized that he will be going to PT three times a week as an outpatient. He will be transported to PT sessions by Medivan each way. Mr. Rogers was also given instructions about his anticoagulant, pain medications, and diabetic diet. He is to call the orthopedic surgeon for a follow-up appointment in 2 weeks."

sometimes see their demands as the only control they have over their lives.

For most patients with mobility problems, lack of control is often a major issue. Do they think that staff are considerate, and do staff protect their privacy? Are patients' preferences taken into consideration when planning care? Do caregivers talk to them or ignore them? It is helpful to remember that lack of movement is often associated with punishment in our society. We give children "time-outs," teens are "grounded," and people who do not receive promotions are seen as failures because they have not advanced to another position. Therefore it is important to recognize that immobility possibly leads to fear, anger, grief, withdrawal, or hostility. If you are sensitive to these reactions and help the patient work through them instead of responding negatively, you can make a big difference in the patient's outcomes.

KEY POINTS

- Normal physical mobility depends on intact and functioning nervous and musculoskeletal systems.
- Findings from evidence-based nursing research indicate that safe patient handling prevents injuries to nurses and patients when moving and transferring patients.
- The risk for disabilities related to immobilization depends on the extent and duration of the immobilization and the patient's overall level of health.
- Immobility results from illness or trauma or is prescribed for therapeutic reasons; it presents hazards in the physical, psychological, and developmental dimensions.
- Pressure ulcers, although often preventable, are one of the most common physical hazards of immobility.
- Effects of immobility include depression, behavioral changes, changes in the sleep-wake cycle, decreased coping abilities, and developmental delays.
- Assessment focuses on range of joint motion, musculoskeletal status, complete physical examination for potential adverse effects in all body systems, and psychosocial and developmental effects.
- Patient movement algorithms serve as assessment tools and guide safe patient handling and movement.
- Appropriate friction-reducing assistive devices and mechanical lifts need to be used for patient transfers when applicable.
- No-lift policies benefit all members of the health care system: patients, nurses, and administration.
- Adequate hydration measures reduce immobility-related complications in the respiratory and elimination systems.
- Elastic antiembolic stockings and SCDs improve venous return and help prevent the potentially life-threatening complication of DVT.
- The primary evaluation criterion for nursing care in the developmental dimension for immobilized patients is the prevention of any measurable decline in functioning or delay in development.
- Early mobilization helps to decrease the effects of bed rest.

CLINICAL DECISION-MAKING EXERCISES

Abby, the nursing student, continues to provide care for Mr. Rogers and his family. They have many questions about Mr. Rogers' care and recovery. She talks with Mr. Rogers and his family to decrease their anxiety and improve their understanding of Mr. Rogers' care.

1. Mr. Rogers stated that his wife had a heart valve problem and was on a blood thinner. He asks you, "Why am I getting one?" How would you answer his question?
2. Identify four additional actions that will reduce the risk for clot formation in Mr. Rogers' condition.
3. His son says, "My dad is so frail. Why can't he just rest in bed instead of going to physical therapy?" How would you answer Mr. Rogers's son?

evolve

Answers to Clinical Decision-Making Questions can be found on the Evolve website.

QSEN ACTIVITY: QUALITY IMPROVEMENT

Abby had Mr. Rogers as her patient in the acute postoperative period.

If Mr. Rogers was unable to place any weight on his leg with the knee replacement and she had to transfer him out of bed to the bedside chair, which process should she implement that validates her QSEN safety competency?

evolve

Answers to QSEN Activities can be found on the Evolve website.

REVIEW QUESTIONS

1. When planning care for the older patient on complete bed rest, it is important to:
   1. Provide the patient's care in the following sequence: psychosocial, psychological, and physiological.
   2. Allow the patient to participate within the limits of his or her physical condition and tolerance.
   3. Assign a staff member to provide all of the patient's physical care and needs while on bed rest.
   4. Complete the patient's treatments and morning care as quickly as possible and all at one time.
2. Which patient is at greatest risk for developing the adverse effects of immobility?
   1. A 15-year-old immobilized in traction and in isolation because of burns from a car accident
   2. A 31-year-old with a walking cast on her left leg learning to use crutches with partial weight bearing
   3. A 55-year-old 3 days after surgery for a right hip replacement receiving physical therapy twice daily
   4. A 69-year-old admitted for elective surgery with a Braden Scale score of 21
3. A 74-year-old patient is restricted to bed following a motor vehicle accident. He has a fractured pelvis. The doctor has ordered sequential compression hose. Which factors should you assess before application? (Select all that apply.)
   1. Lower extremity strength
   2. Pedal pulses
   3. Condition of skin over calves and thighs
   4. Temperature of skin
4. Which of the following nursing interventions takes priority if the nurse suspects that the patient has a pulmonary embolus?
   1. Notifying the health care provider, checking the patient's vital signs, assessing for signs of deep vein thrombosis (DVT)
   2. Checking the patient's oxygen saturation and vital signs, raising the head of the bed to high Fowler's unless contraindicated, having someone call the health care provider
   3. Giving prescribed pain medication, monitoring vital signs, reassessing pain in 30 minutes to see if relieved
   4. Assessing for evidence of DVT, documenting presence of any signs, notifying health care provider
5. The family of the patient asks the nurse, "Do you think our father should walk so much on his new hip? He is 79 years old, and he just had surgery the day before yesterday." What is the nurse's best response?
   1. "He's better walking around than just staying in bed and maybe getting a blood clot."
   2. "You should ask his surgeon. He's the one who wrote the activity orders."
   3. "He looks good to me. I wouldn't worry if I were you."
   4. "You seem concerned. Is there something specific that you have questions about?"
6. The nurse is supervising nursing assistive personnel (NAP) on the unit. To make sure that the NAP understand the importance of using the appropriate assistive device when moving patients, the nurse emphasizes that:
   1. When the assistive device is not available, patient care must still be given but use care when lifting.
   2. The NAP must follow the policy manual or noncompliance will result in a reprimand.
   3. The best outcome when moving a patient is that neither the patient nor the staff member is injured.
   4. NAP can use their own judgment whether or not to use the assistive devices on their shift.
7. A newly licensed registered nurse is unsure as to which assistive device to use to transfer a patient with left-side paralysis from his bed into the bedside chair. Which of the following actions would be most appropriate for the nurse to take?
   1. Do not use any device at this time but use the principles of body mechanics learned in school to make the transfer safely by herself.
   2. Seek the assistance of a nursing assistive personnel (NAP) to lift-turn–and sit the patient in the chair while the nurse supervises the transfer.
   3. Check the algorithm for bed-to-chair-transfer in the unit procedure manual and choose the device based on the decision tree.
   4. Since the nurse is unsure, do not make the transfer and document in the patient's chart that the transfer could not be made safely because of the lack of inservice.
8. Immobility can affect the patient in many ways. Which of the following patient behaviors may indicate that being immobile is impacting the patient's stage of development?
   1. The toddler in traction who cries when the parent leaves the room but stops crying in a few minutes and plays with a toy
   2. The teenager in a body cast who is constantly on his smart phone texting his classmates or working on his laptop computer
   3. The graduate college student who is on complete bed rest and constantly complaining about the "dog food"

that was served for lunch or the "rock-hard pillow" on his bed

4. The older adult who had bilateral knee replacements and makes jokes about "setting off the alarms" the next time she goes through the airport metal detectors

9. Which of the following interventions is most appropriate to reduce the formation of pressure ulcers?
   1. Have the patient sitting in a chair shift his weight every 15 to 20 minutes
   2. Reposition every immobile patient in bed every 2 hours
   3. Make sure that immobile patients have high-carbohydrate, low-protein, low-fat diets
   4. Perform active and passive range-of-motion exercise every shift to promote circulation

10. Which of the following are physiological outcomes of immobility?
    1. Increased metabolism
    2. Reduced cardiac workload
    3. Decreased lung expansion
    4. Decreased oxygen demand

evolve

Rationales for Review Questions can be found on the Evolve website.

1. 2; 2. 1; 3. 2, 3, 4; 4. 2; 5. 4; 6. 3; 7. 3; 8. 3; 9. 1; 10. 3

REFERENCES

Agency for Healthcare Research and Quality (AHRQ): *Pressure ulcer prevention and treatment*, 2011, http://hstat.nlm.nih.gov/hq/Hquest/screen/TestBrowse/t/1049658066834/s/40521. Accessed August 8, 2012.

American College of Sports Medicine (ACSM): Position stand: exercise and physical activity for older adults, *Med Sci Sports Exerc* 41(7):1510, 2009.

American Geriatrics Society (AGS) Panel on the Pharmacological Management of Persistent Pain in Older Persons: Pharmacological management of persistent pain in older adults, *J Am Geriatr Soc* 58(8):1331, 2009.

American Nurses Association (ANA): *ANA leads initiative to develop national safe patient handling standards*, 2012, http://wwwnursingworld.org/HomepageCategory/NursingInsider/Initiative-to-Develop-National-Safe-Patient-Handling-Standards.html. Accessed August 27, 2012.

American Pain Society (APS): *Pain: current understanding of assessment, management and treatments*, 2009, http://www.americanpainsociety.org/uploads/pdfs/npc/npc.pdf. Accessed July 2013.

Bhavani-Shankar K, Oberol JS: Management of postoperative pain, *UpToDate*, 2013, http://www.uptodate.com/contents/management-of-postoperative-pain#H2. Accessed October 30, 2013.

Black J, Hawks J: *Medical-surgical nursing: clinical management for positive outcomes*, ed 8, Philadelphia, 2009, Elsevier.

Copstead-Kirkhorn LEC, Banasik JL: *Pathophysiology*, ed 4, Philadelphia, 2010, Saunders.

Cunningham A, et al: An automated database case definition for serious bleeding related to oral coagulant use, *Pharamcoepidemiol Drug Safety* 20:560, 2011, wileyonlinelibrary.com. Accessed August 23, 2012.

Evans C, et al: Impact of surgery on immunologic function: comparison between minimally invasive techniques and conventional laparotomy for surgical resection of colorectal tumors, *Am J Surg* 197:238, 2009.

Flaherty E: Pain assessment for older adults, try this. In *Best Practices in Nursing Care to Older Adults*, issue 7, New York, revised 2012, New York University College of Nursing, The Hartford Institute for Geriatric Nursing, http://consultgerirn.org/uploads/File/trythis/try_this_7.pdf. Accessed November 7, 2013.

Herr K: Pain in the older adult: an imperative across all health care settings, *Pain Manage Nurs* 11(suppl 2):S1, 2010.

Hockenberry M, Wilson D: *Wong's nursing care of infants and children*, ed 9, St Louis, 2010, Mosby.

Ibrahim MS, et al: An evidence-based review of enhanced recovery interventions in knee replacement surgery, *Ann R Coll Surg Engl* 95(6):386, 2013.

Lewis L, et al: *Medical-surgical nursing: assessment and management of clinical problems*, ed 8, St Louis, 2011, Elsevier.

Lim J, et al: *A cultural health belief model to understand health behaviors and health-related quality of life between Latina and Asian-American breast cancer survivors*, Paper presented at the 13th annual conference for the Society for Social Work and Research, January 16-18, 2009, Washington, DC, http://sswr.confex.com/sswr/2009/webprogram/Paper10556.html. Abstract accessed February 1, 2009.

McCance K, Huether S: *Pathophysiology: the biologic basis for disease in adults and children*, ed 6, St Louis, 2010, Mosby.

Morse JM: *Preventing patient falls*, ed 2, New York, 2009, Springer.

Nelson A: *Safe patient handling and movement algorithms*, 2006, VISN8 Patient Safety Center, http://www.visn8.va.gov/patientsafetycenter/safePtHandling. Accessed July 2013.

Nelson A, Motacki K, Menzel N: *The illustrated guide to safe patient handling and movement*, New York, 2009, Springer.

Pasero C, McCaffery M: *Pain assessment and pharmacologic management*, St Louis, 2011, Elsevier.

Purnell L: *Guide to culturally competent health care*, ed 2, Philadelphia, 2009, FA Davis.

The Joint Commission (TJC): *National Patient Safety Goals*, Oakbrook Terrace, IL, 2014, The Commission. Available at http://www.jointcommission.org/standards_information/npsgs.aspx.

Touhy T, Jett K: *Ebersole and Hess'* gerontological nursing and healthy aging, ed 3, St Louis, 2010, Mosby.

CHAPTER 37

Skin Integrity and Wound Care

evolve WEBSITE

http://evolve.elsevier.com/Potter/essentials

- Video Clips
- Crossword Puzzle
- Audio Glossary

OBJECTIVES

- Describe risk factors for pressure ulcer development.
- List the National Pressure Ulcer Advisory Panel (NPUAP) pressure ulcer stages.
- Discuss the response of the body during each phase of the wound healing process.
- Describe wound assessment criteria: anatomical location, size, type and percentage of wound tissue, volume and color of wound drainage, and condition of surrounding skin.
- Differentiate healing by primary and secondary intention.
- Discuss common complications of wound healing.
- Explain factors that impair or promote wound healing.
- Describe the purposes of and precautions taken with applying dressings and binders.
- Describe the mechanism of action of wound care dressings.
- Describe the differences in therapeutic effects of heat and cold.
- Complete an assessment for a patient with impaired skin integrity.
- List nursing diagnoses associated with impaired skin integrity.
- Develop a nursing care plan for a patient with impaired skin integrity.
- Evaluate outcomes of nursing care using appropriate criteria for a patient with impaired skin integrity.

KEY TERMS

abrasion, p. 1072
binders, p. 1084
blanchable hyperemia, p. 1062
compress, p. 1090
debride, p. 1080
dehiscence, p. 1066
ecchymosis, p. 1073
eschar, p. 1063
evisceration, p. 1066
friction, p. 1062
granulation tissue, p. 1064
hematoma, p. 1066
hemostasis, p. 1066
induration, p. 1070
laceration, p. 1064
maceration, p. 1077
nonblanchable hyperemia, p. 1062
pressure ulcer, p. 1061
primary intention, p. 1064
reactive hyperemia, p. 1062
secondary intention, p. 1064
shear, p. 1062
sitz bath, p. 1090
tissue ischemia, p. 1062

CASE STUDY ***Mr. Ahmed***

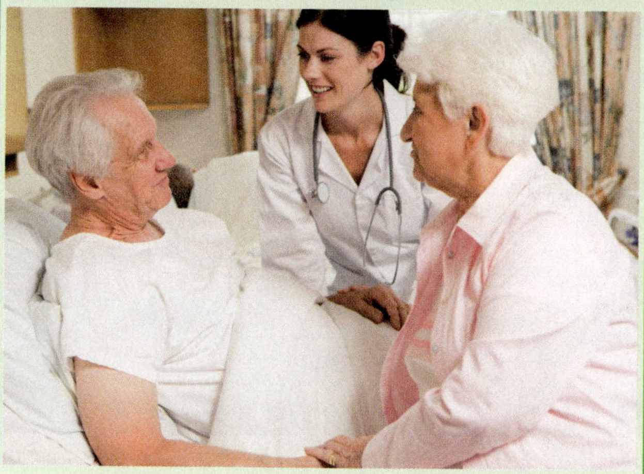

(Monkey Business Images/Thinkstock.)

Mr. Omar Ahmed, a 76-year-old accountant with a medical history of type 2 diabetes mellitus and hypertension, had coronary artery bypass surgery 6 months ago. While at home he became weak and rarely got out of his bed; he was unable to eat and has lost more than 20 lbs over the last 2 months. Mr. Ahmed was admitted to the hospital because of the change in his health status. While hospitalized he is diagnosed with pneumonia. As a precaution he is placed on telemetry monitoring. His mobility is limited because of his weakness, difficulty breathing, and acutely ill state. Mr. Ahmed is retired. He lives in a one-family home with his wife. Their children and grandchildren live nearby and visit often. He complains that his "bottom hurts" from lying in bed. Lynda is in her final year of nursing school and is assigned to care for Mr. Ahmed the week before his discharge.

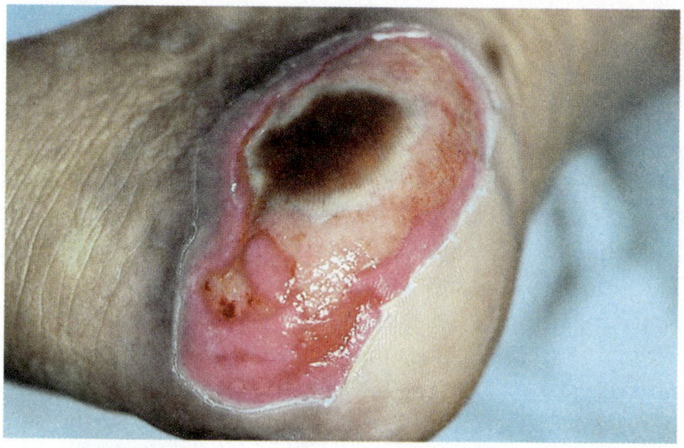

FIGURE 37-1 Pressure ulcer with tissue necrosis.

SCIENTIFIC KNOWLEDGE BASE

Pressure Ulcers

Pressure ulcer (formerly called *pressure sore, decubitus ulcer,* or *bedsore*) is the term that describes impaired skin integrity resulting from pressure (WOCN, 2010) (Figure 37-1). The European Pressure Ulcer Advisory Panel (EPUAP) and National Pressure Ulcer Advisory Panel (NPUAP) (2009) define a pressure ulcer as a localized injury to the skin and/or underlying tissue, usually over a bony prominence, as a result of pressure or pressure in combination with shear. Although a number of contributing or confounding factors are associated with pressure ulcers, the significance of these factors is currently not fully understood. A patient with decreased mobility, inadequate nutrition, excessive skin moisture, decreased sensory perception, or decreased activity is at risk for pressure ulcer development. Statistics vary, but in the United States pressure ulcer prevalence ranges from 14% to 17% (Pieper, 2012). Because pressure ulcers often develop quickly when a patient becomes ill, it is important to identify high-risk patients to target appropriate prevention interventions (Box 37-1).

BOX 37-1 EVIDENCE-BASED PRACTICE

PICO Question: Which interventions are most effective to reduce pressure ulcer development in patients who are hospitalized?

SUMMARY OF EVIDENCE

The development of pressure ulcers is a serious quality-of-care issue in all health care settings. A patient with a pressure ulcer has an increased mortality risk when compared with a patient with intact skin. The development of a pressure ulcer interferes with recovery, causes pain and infection, and often prolongs a patient's hospital stay. The Centers for Medicare and Medicaid Services (CMS) will no longer reimburse an acute care facility if a patient with intact skin develops a stage III or IV pressure ulcer while hospitalized. Thus it is essential for hospitals to implement skin-care protocols from a quality and fiscal standpoint. Pressure ulcers are preventable in many cases when hospitals develop and implement a comprehensive skin-care program (McInerney, 2008). A comprehensive program includes skin and risk assessment on admission to the health care facility and on an ongoing basis, quarterly collection of prevalence and incidence data, prevention and intervention protocols based on evidence-based guidelines, and a multidisciplinary team focused on prevention and early intervention. Current evidence also supports the use of organized skin-care rounds, decision algorithms (e.g., skin-care protocols), product bundles, and ongoing education for the nursing staff (Barker et al., 2013; Kelleher, Moorer, and Makic, 2012; McInerney, 2008).

APPLICATION TO NURSING PRACTICE

- Complete a thorough skin and risk assessment on all patients on admission to the health care setting and continue assessments regularly throughout the hospital stay.
- Use the results of the skin and risk assessment to plan topical therapy based on evidence-based guidelines (Barker et al., 2013).
- Develop algorithms or protocols that help nurses use assessment information to develop the appropriate prevention care plan.
- Collect prevalence and incidence data about pressure ulcers on nursing units to identify areas of practice that require attention.
- Consult with an interdisciplinary team to prevent pressure ulcers and promote their early treatment.

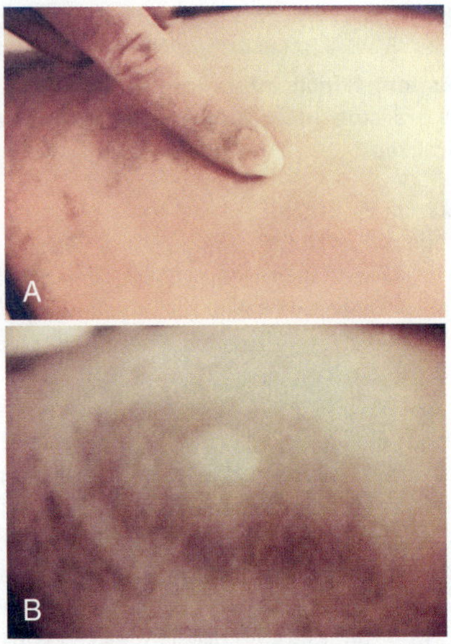

FIGURE 37-2 **A,** Check for blanching by applying fingertip pressure. **B,** Area of blanchable hyperemia.

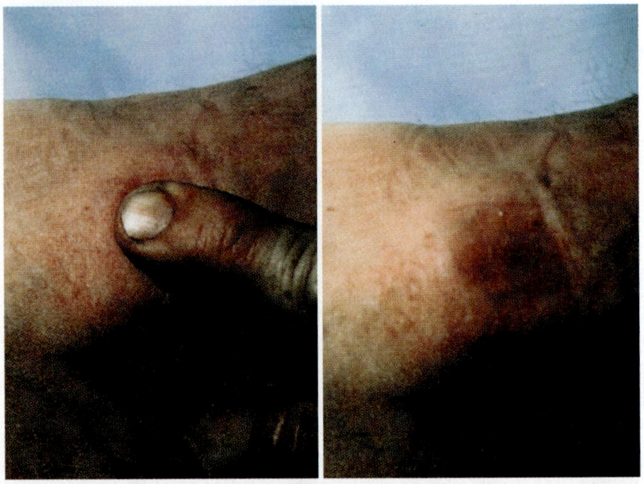

FIGURE 37-3 Nonblanchable hyperemia: area is darker than surrounding skin and does not blanch with fingertip pressure.

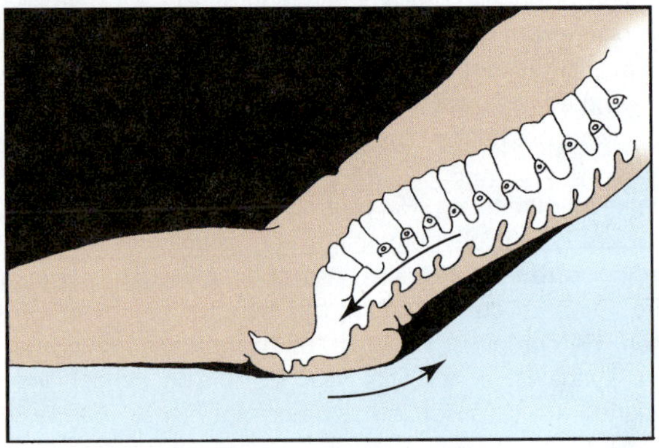

FIGURE 37-4 Shearing force.

Tissue ischemia (i.e., decreased blood flow to tissue) usually results in tissue death and occurs when capillary blood flow is obstructed, as in the case of pressure. When pressure is relieved in a relatively short time, reactive hyperemia occurs. **Reactive hyperemia** is a redness of the skin resulting from dilation of the superficial capillaries (WOCN, 2010). Reactive hyperemia blanches. In **blanchable hyperemia** the area that appears red and warm blanches (turns lighter in color) following fingertip palpation (Figure 37-2). This hyperemia usually resolves without tissue loss if pressure is reduced or eliminated. Blanchable hyperemia is harder to assess in patients with dark skin. The discoloration or redness is warm to touch and is often purple/blue or violet instead of red in darkly pigmented skin (Nix, 2012).

Nonblanchable hyperemia is redness that persists after palpation and indicates tissue damage (Figure 37-3). When you press a finger against the red or purple area, it does not turn lighter in color. This indicates deep tissue damage and is commonly the first stage of pressure ulcer development. This stage of skin injury is sometimes reversible if the pressure is relieved and the tissue protected.

Deeper tissue destruction occurs in some ulcers. The skin separates from the underlying granulation tissue at the wound margins. This is known as *undermining*. Undermining creates large areas of tissue damage below the surface of the skin and less damage at the surface. With continuous pressure over the area, deep-tissue destruction continues, which often results in larger pockets of necrotic tissue beneath the opening of the main wound that resemble a tunnel; this is referred to as *tunneling*. Some wounds have more than one tunnel.

Factors Contributing to Pressure Ulcer Formation. In addition to pressure, other factors increase a patient's risk for developing pressure ulcers. External factors include shear, friction, and moisture; internal factors include nutrition, infection, and age.

Shear. The force exerted against the skin while the skin remains stationary and the bony structures move is called **shear.** For example, when the head of the bed is elevated, gravity causes the bony skeleton to pull toward the foot of the bed while the skin remains against the sheets (Figure 37-4). The underlying tissue blood vessels become stretched and bent, impairing blood flow to the deep tissue. Ulcers occur with large areas of undermining and less damage at the skin surface.

Friction. **Friction** is surface damage caused by the skin rubbing against another surface that often results in an abrasion. An abrasion is the loss of the epidermis, the top layer of the skin. The body surfaces most at risk for friction are the elbows and heels because abrasion of these surfaces occurs when they are rubbed against the sheets during repositioning. Friction abrades or rubs the skin similar to a mild burn and is sometimes referred to as a *sheet burn* (Pieper, 2012).

Moisture. Skin moisture increases the risk for ulcer formation. Moisture softens the skin and reduces its resistance to other physical factors such as pressure or shear. Moisture comes from many sources such as wound drainage, perspiration, and/or fecal and urinary incontinence. Skin moisture and wetness from incontinence frequently cause skin breakdown (Gray et al., 2011).

Nutrition. Poor nutrition, specifically severe protein deficiency, increases the risk of the breakdown of soft tissue and alters fluid and electrolyte balance. Patients with protein loss have hypoalbuminemia. Low protein levels cause edema or swelling, which contributes to problems with the transportation of oxygen and nutrients (Pieper, 2012). When serum albumin levels fall drastically (e.g., below 3 g/100 mL), patients experience a shift of fluid from the extracellular fluid volume to the tissues, resulting in edema (Pieper, 2012). Edema increases the risk for pressure ulcer formation because of the changing pressures in the capillary circulation and capillary bed, resulting in decreased blood supply and retention of waste products in the edematous tissue.

Infection. Infection results from the presence of pathogens in the body. A patient with an infection usually has a fever. Infection and fever increase the metabolic needs of the body, making already hypoxic tissue more susceptible to ischemic injury. In addition, fever results in diaphoresis and increased skin moisture, which further predispose the patient to skin breakdown.

Age. The dermis becomes thinner in older adults. This makes the skin appear paper thin and nearly transparent and increases the risk for skin tears. Thus the older patient's skin is more vulnerable to pressure, shear, and friction (Pieper, 2012). Neonates and young children (i.e., younger than 5 years old) are also at higher risk for pressure ulcer occurrence (Coha et al., 2012).

Origins of Pressure Ulcers. Pressure exerted against the skin surface causes pressure ulcers; usually a bone and the surface of the bed compress the skin. However, pressure ulcers also occur on any skin surface where pressure applied against the skin exceeds capillary closure pressure. Classic research identified that normal capillary pressure (i.e., the amount of pressure needed to keep the capillary open) ranges from 12 to 32 mm Hg, depending on the location in the capillary (Landis, 1930). When the intensity of the pressure exerted on the capillary exceeds 12 to 32 mm Hg, the vessel occludes, causing ischemic injury to the tissues it normally feeds. However, pressure to the tissue does not routinely result in pressure ulceration. Two other concepts, duration of the pressure and tissue tolerance, play a role.

High pressure over a short time and low pressure over a long time cause skin breakdown. Thus duration influences the effects of pressure; the longer pressure is applied, the more likely it is that tissue loss will occur. Tissue tolerance also plays an important role in pressure ulcer development. The integrity of the skin and the supporting structures influence the ability of the skin to redistribute the pressure. The factors mentioned previously (i.e., shear, friction, moisture, and the internal factors such as nutrition, infection, and age) alter the ability of the skin and supporting tissue to respond to the pressure (Pieper, 2012).

Pressure Ulcer Classification. One method to classify pressure ulcers is to stage them according to tissue layer involvement. EPUAP and NPUAP (2009) support the following staging system:

- **Stage/Category I:** Intact skin with nonblanchable redness of a localized area, usually over a bony prominence. Darkly pigmented skin may not have visible blanching; its color may differ from that of the surrounding area. The area may be painful, firm, soft, warmer, or cooler compared to adjacent tissue. Category I may be difficult to detect in individuals with dark skin tones. May indicate "at risk" persons. (Figure 37-5, *A*).
- **Stage/Category II:** Partial-thickness loss of dermis presenting as a shallow open ulcer with a red-pink wound bed without slough. May also present as an intact or open/ruptured serum-filled blister (Figure 37-5, *B*). Presents as a shiny or dry shallow ulcer without slough or bruising. This category should not be used to describe skin tears, tape burns, incontinence-associated dermatitis, maceration, or excoriation. Bruising indicates deep-tissue injury.
- **Stage/Category III:** Full-thickness tissue loss. Subcutaneous fat may be visible; but bone, tendon, or muscle is not exposed. Slough may be present but does not obscure the depth of tissue loss. May include undermining and tunneling (Figure 37-5, *C*). The depth of a stage/category III pressure ulcer varies by anatomical location. The bridge of the nose, ear, occiput, and malleolus do not have (adipose) subcutaneous tissue; and stage/category III ulcers can be shallow. In contrast, areas of significant adiposity can develop extremely deep stage/category III pressure ulcers. Bone/tendon is not visible or directly palpable.
- **Stage/Category IV:** Full-thickness tissue loss with exposed bone, tendon, or muscle. Slough or eschar may be present. Often includes undermining and tunneling (Figure 37-5, *D*). The depth of a stage IV pressure ulcer varies by anatomical location. The bridge of the nose, ear, occiput, and malleolus do not have (adipose) subcutaneous tissue; and these ulcers can be shallow. Stage/category IV ulcers can extend into muscle and/or supporting structures (e.g., fascia, tendon, or joint capsule), making osteomyelitis or osteitis likely to occur. Exposed bone/tendon is visible or directly palpable.
- **Unstageable:** Full-thickness tissue loss—depth unknown. Full-thickness tissue loss in which the actual depth of the ulcer is completely obscured by slough (yellow, tan, gray, green, or brown) and/or eschar (tan, brown, or black) in the wound bed (Figure 37-5, *E*). Until enough slough and/or eschar are removed to expose the base of the wound, the true depth cannot be determined; but it is either stage/category III or IV. Stable (dry, adherent, intact without erythema or fluctuance) eschar on the heels serves as "the natural (biological) cover of the body" and should not be removed.
- **Suspected Deep-Tissue Injury—Depth Unknown:** Purple or maroon localized area of discolored intact skin or blood-filled blister caused by damage of underlying soft tissue from pressure and/or shear (Figure 37-5, *F*). The area may be preceded by tissue that is painful, firm, mushy,

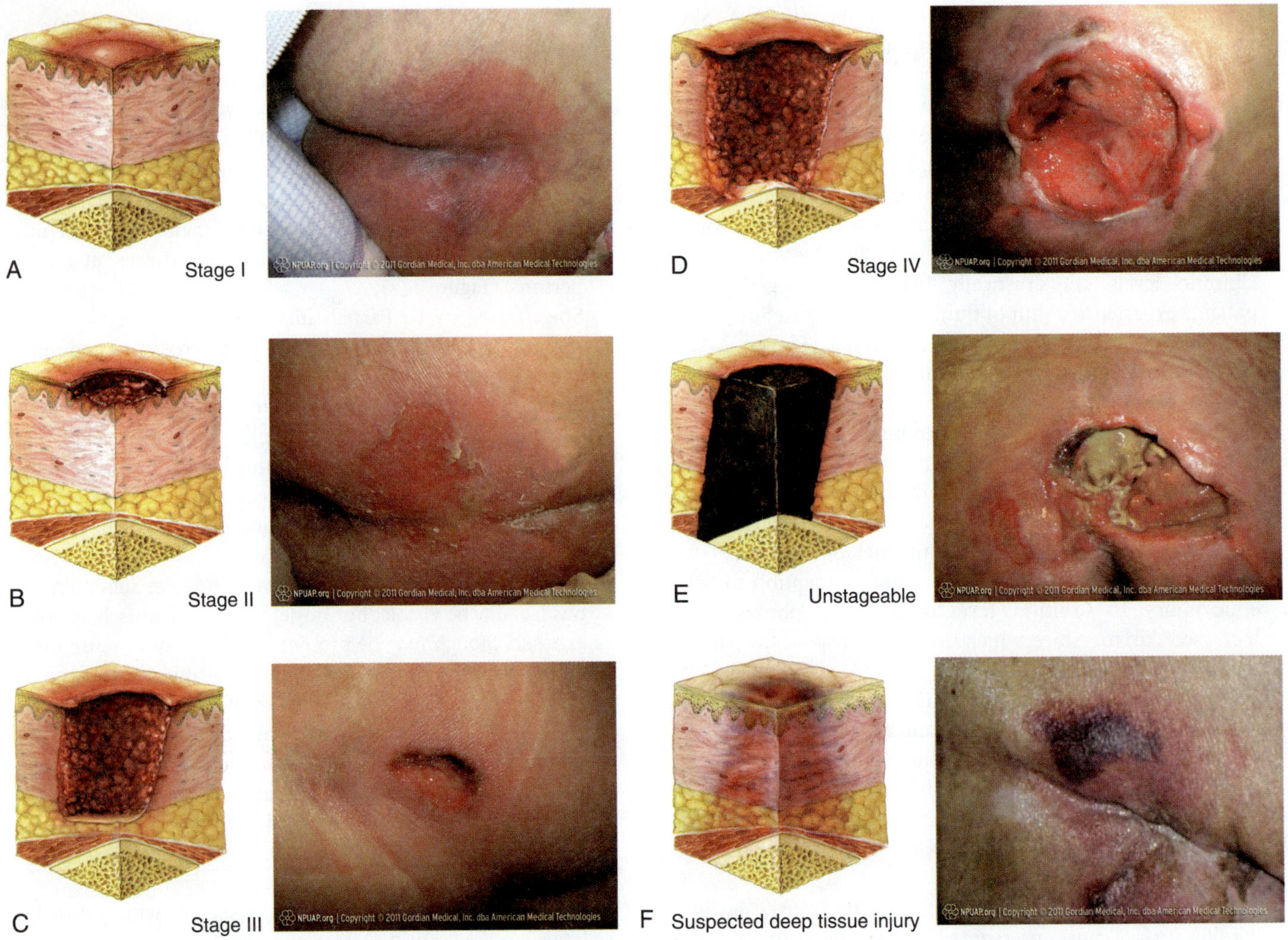

FIGURE 37-5 Diagram of stages. **A,** Stage I pressure ulcer. **B,** Stage II pressure ulcer. **C,** Stage III pressure ulcer. **D,** Stage IV pressure ulcer. **E,** Unstageable wound. **F,** Suspected deep-tissue injury. (Used with permission of the National Pressure Ulcer Advisory Panel. Copyright ©NPUAP.)

boggy, warmer, or cooler compared to adjacent tissue. Deep-tissue injury may be difficult to detect in individuals with dark skin tones. Evolution may include a thin blister over a dark wound bed. The wound may further evolve and become covered by thin eschar. Evolution may be rapid, exposing additional layers of tissue even with optimal treatment.

Wound assessment (regardless of cause) includes the following parameters: anatomical location, extent of tissue involvement (full or partial thickness loss), size (dimensions and depth of wound), tissue type (viable or nonviable) and percentage of wound tissue (e.g., viable versus nonviable), volume and color of wound exudate, and condition of surrounding skin (Nix, 2012). These measures help evaluate the progress of the wound, drive decision making, and evaluate wound healing.

Wound Healing Process

All wounds heal through an orderly series of integrated physiological responses. Multiple factors promote or impede wound healing (Box 37-2). A wound with little or no tissue loss such as a clean surgical incision heals by **primary intention.** The skin edges approximate, or close together, and the risk for infection is minimal. In contrast, a wound involving loss of tissue such as a severe **laceration** or a chronic wound such as a pressure ulcer heals by **secondary intention.** The skin edges cannot come together because of the extensive tissue loss, and healing occurs gradually. A layer of **granulation tissue,** which is red, moist tissue consisting of blood vessels and connective tissue, covers the wound base; wound contraction brings the wound edges together; and the wound closes with scar formation. There are also instances in which a surgical wound is initially closed in the deep-tissue layers; however, the subcutaneous fat and skin layers are left open. This method of wound closure is called *tertiary intention* or *delayed primary closure.* The wound heals with a layer of granulation tissue at the edges and base, and several days after the initial wounding the health care provider brings the wound edges together with sutures or adhesive closures. An example of a wound closure by delayed primary closure

BOX 37-2 FACTORS INFLUENCING WOUND HEALING

AGE

- Blood circulation and oxygen delivery to the wound, clotting, and the inflammatory response are sometimes impaired in the very young and older adults. Risk for infection is greater in these populations.
- Cell growth and differentiation in reconstruction are slower with advancing age.
- Scar tissue never regains the tensile strength of noninjured skin, increasing the risk for altered body part function in older adults.
- Age affects all phases of wound healing. A decline in the number of white blood cells places older adults at greater risk for a wound infection. A slowdown is common in the deposition of collagen in reepithelialization.

NUTRITION

- Tissue repair and infection resistance depend on a balanced diet. Surgery, severe wounds, serious infections, and preoperative nutritional deficits increase nutritional requirements.
- Nutrients provide raw materials needed for cellular activities that contribute to wound healing.

IMMUMOSUPPRESSION

- In the presence of immunosuppression, the repair process is more susceptible to infection.

OBESITY

- The less abundant supply of blood vessels in adipose tissue impairs delivery of nutrients and cellular elements needed for healing. Obesity increases the risk for dehiscence.

EXTENT OF WOUND

- Wounds with extensive tissue loss heal by secondary intention and remain open for a prolonged period of time.

TISSUE PERFUSION

- Oxygen fuels the cellular function needed for tissue repair. Chronic tissue hypoxia impairs collagen synthesis and reduces tissue resistance to infection.

SMOKING

- By-products of smoking reduce oxygenation and thus reduce fibroblast activity.

DIABETES MELLITUS

- The patient with diabetes has small-vessel disease that impairs tissue perfusion; thus oxygen delivery is poor.
- An elevated blood glucose level (hyperglycemia) impairs macrophage function. Risk for infection is increased because of hyperglycemia and poor wound healing.
- Patients with diabetes demonstrate the following problems with wound healing: reduced collagen synthesis, decreased wound strength, and impaired white blood cell functioning. These adverse effects are at least in part caused by poor glycemic control.

RADIATION

- Radiation therapy, which eventually results in fibrosis and vascular scarring, interferes with postoperative wound healing when surgery is delayed more than 4 to 6 weeks and irradiated tissues become fragile and poorly perfused.

WOUND STRESS

- Sustained stress (e.g., vomiting, abdominal distention, coughing) disrupts wound layers and tissue repair.

Modified from Doughty DL, DeFriese Sparkes B: Wound healing physiology in acute and chronic wounds. In Bryant RA, Nix DP, editors: *Acute and chronic wounds: current management concepts,* ed 4, St Louis, 2012, Mosby.

occurs when a patient has a ruptured appendix. In some cases the surgeon is unsure if the appendix had microperforations that caused subsequent spilling of the intestinal contents into the abdomen and wound. Thus the surgeon leaves the incision open for up to 4 to 5 days following surgery. He or she then evaluates the wound; and, if after 4 to 5 days there are no clinical signs of infection, he or she closes the wound with either adhesive strips or sutures.

Wounds heal by one of two mechanisms: partial-thickness wound repair or full-thickness wound repair. Partial-thickness wound repair is necessary when there is loss of only the epidermis and/or part of the dermis such as wound healing by primary intention. Full-thickness wound repair is necessary when there is loss of the epidermis, dermis, and possible extension into subcutaneous layers, bone, and/or muscle.

Partial-Thickness Wound Repair. The body repairs wounds that heal by primary intention and shallow wounds that involve loss of only the epidermis and perhaps some of the dermis by resurfacing the wound with new epidermal cells. The wounds go through several phases of wound healing.

Inflammatory Response. Erythema and edema are the first response, bringing white blood cells to the site. The wounded area appears red and swollen. If the exudate, or discharge, that brings the white blood cells to the area is allowed to dry, a scab forms. This response is limited and usually subsides in less than 24 hours (Doughty and Sparks-DeFriese, 2012).

Epidermal Repair. Epidermal cells begin migration across the wound, originating from the epidermal cells at the wound edges or the epidermal appendages. Peak epithelial proliferation occurs between 24 and 72 hours after injury. Wounds kept in a moist environment heal in approximately 4 days as opposed to 7 days when kept dry because new epithelial cells migrate across a moist surface. If a wound is dry, the cells need to find moisture below the skin surface (Doughty and Sparks-DeFriese, 2012).

Dermal Repair. The epidermis thickens, anchors to adjacent cells, and resumes normal function. The new epidermis is pink, dry, and fragile. If dermal repair is necessary, it occurs concurrently with epidermal repair.

Full-Thickness Wound Repair. Full-thickness wounds involve tissue loss and extend to at least the subcutaneous layer. A full-thickness wound is either acute (a surgical wound) or chronic (a pressure ulcer). Healing of a full-thickness acute wound such as a surgical incision proceeds by primary intention; healing of a full-thickness chronic wound such as a pressure ulcer proceeds by secondary intention. The key events differ between a chronic wound healing by secondary intention and an acute wound healing by primary intention.

Hemostasis Phase. A full-thickness wound healing by primary intention first goes through the hemostasis phase, which controls bleeding. Platelets cause coagulation and vasoconstriction. The platelets break down and release growth factors, which appear to initiate the entire wound-healing process (Holloway et al., 2011). Bleeding and hemostasis do not occur in wounds healing by secondary intention, thus compromising the repair process (Doughty and Sparks-DeFriese, 2012).

Inflammation Phase. The goal of this phase is to establish a clean wound bed and obtain bacterial balance. The inflammatory response brings white blood cells to the area, cleaning up the site and releasing additional growth factors. This phase lasts approximately 3 days in an acute clean wound such as a surgical incision. However, in a chronic wound healing by secondary intention this phase is prolonged and often lasts longer than 3 days.

Proliferative Phase. The key events in the proliferative phase are production of new tissue, epithelialization, and contraction. In wound healing by primary intention, new capillary networks form to provide oxygen and nutrients for new tissue and contribute to the synthesis of collagen. As collagen fibers and capillary networks continue to synthesize and increase in size, the wound begins to contract. The last component of this phase is epithelialization, in which the epithelial cells migrate and cover the defect. It is important to note that epithelialization occurs faster in a moist environment, supporting the role of moist wound dressings in wound care. In healing by secondary intention in a chronic wound such as a pressure ulcer, the proliferative phase is prolonged. As granulation tissue forms to fill in the defect, it is followed by contraction and epithelialization, the final phase. Contraction is much more important in secondary intention wounds because it reduces the amount of granulation tissue needed to fill the defect (Doughty and Sparks-DeFriese, 2012).

Remodeling Phase. The remodeling phase, which lasts up to 1 year, reorganizes the collagen to produce a more elastic, stronger collagen for the scar tissue. The tensile strength of the scar tissue is never more than 80% of the tensile strength in nonwounded tissue (Doughty and Sparks-DeFriese, 2012). The remodeling process is the same for wounds healing by primary and secondary intention.

Complications of Wound Healing

Wound healing frequently has complications. When caring for patients with wounds, you need to assess a patient's wound-healing process while observing for complications.

Hemorrhage. Bleeding from an acute wound is normal during and immediately after initial trauma, but **hemostasis,** which is cessation of bleeding by vasoconstriction and coagulation, usually occurs within several minutes. Hemorrhage occurring later possibly indicates a slipped surgical suture, a dislodged clot, infection, or the erosion of a blood vessel by a foreign object (e.g., a drain). Hemorrhage is external or internal. Symptoms of internal bleeding are hypovolemic shock and swelling of the affected body part. A **hematoma** is a localized collection of blood under the tissue, often appearing as a bluish swelling or mass. External hemorrhaging is obvious because dressings covering the wound quickly become saturated with blood. Surgical drains are sometimes used to drain blood.

Infection. Bacterial wound infection prevents healing by increasing tissue damage and altering the healing process. The chances of wound infection are greater when the wound contains dead or necrotic tissue, when foreign bodies are in or near the wound, and when the blood supply and local tissue defenses are lower than normal.

A contaminated or traumatic wound infection develops within 2 to 3 days; a surgical wound infection develops within 4 to 5 days. Locally drainage is often yellow, green, or brown and odorous, depending on the causative organism. The wound edges appear tense, swollen, and painful, with redness extending beyond the immediate wound edge. Systemic signs include fever, general malaise, and an elevated white blood cell count.

Dehiscence. When an acute wound fails to heal properly, the layers of skin and tissue separate. This most commonly occurs before collagen formation (3 to 11 days after injury). **Dehiscence** is the partial or total separation of layers of skin and tissue above the fascia in a wound that is not healing properly. Obese patients have a high risk for dehiscence because of constant strain on their wounds and the poor vascularity of fatty tissue. It occurs most often in abdominal surgical wounds after a sudden strain such as coughing, vomiting, or sitting up in bed. Patients often report feeling as though something has given way. When serosanguineous drainage increases from a wound, be alert for dehiscence.

Evisceration. **Evisceration** occurs when wound layers separate below the fascial layer and visceral organs protrude through the wound opening. It is a medical emergency requiring placement of sterile towels soaked in sterile saline over the extruding tissues to reduce chances of bacterial invasion and drying before surgical repair occurs.

NURSING KNOWLEDGE BASE

A major aspect of nursing care is the maintenance of skin integrity and wound care. Nursing research has an important role in developing guidelines for pressure ulcer care and prevention.

Prediction and Prevention

In 2003 the Wound, Ostomy and Continence Nurses Society (WOCN) developed the *Guidelines for Prevention and Management of Pressure Ulcers;* these guidelines were reviewed and updated in 2010. A panel of nurse experts performed extensive searches on the most up-to-date literature on pressure ulcers and established a level of evidence rating that provides the best available evidence in the prevention and management of pressure ulcers. This guideline was accepted by the guideline resource component of the Agency for Healthcare Research and Quality (AHRQ). Included in these guidelines are predictive tools for pressure ulcer development that identify patients at highest risk for their development. Patients identified to be at risk need a care plan that addresses and reduces identified risk factors. Patients with little risk for pressure ulcer development do not require a care plan that addresses skin breakdown and thus do not have the unnecessary expense of preventive treatments.

One reliable and predictive tool is the Braden Scale. The Braden Scale is made of six subscales: sensory perception, moisture, activity, mobility, nutrition, and friction and shear (Table 37-1). A hospitalized adult with a score of 16 or below and an older adult at 18 or below are at risk for pressure ulcer development (Ayello and Braden, 2002; Bergstrom et al., 1998). This instrument is highly reliable in identifying patients at greatest risk for pressure ulcers (Bergstrom et al., 1987a, 1987b, 1998).

CRITICAL THINKING

Synthesis

You apply elements of critical thinking whenever you perform the nursing process with patients. Consider the scientific knowledge you have learned, your experience, critical thinking attitudes, and standards to ensure an individualized

TABLE 37-1 BRADEN SCALE FOR PREDICTING PRESSURE SORE RISK

	1	2	3	4
SENSORY PERCEPTION				
Ability to respond appropriately to pressure-related discomfort	1. **Completely limited:** Unresponsive (does not moan, flinch, or grasp) to painful stimuli as a result of diminished level of consciousness or sedation *or* Limited ability to feel pain over most of body	2. **Very limited:** Responds only to painful stimuli Cannot communicate discomfort except by moaning or restlessness *or* Has sensory impairment that limits ability to feel pain or discomfort over half of body	3. **Slightly limited:** Responds to verbal commands but cannot always communicate discomfort or need to be turned *or* Has some sensory impairment, which limits ability to feel pain or discomfort in one or two extremities	4. **No impairment:** Responds to verbal commands Has no sensory deficit that limits ability to feel or voice pain or discomfort
MOISTURE				
Degree to which skin is exposed to moisture	1. **Constantly moist:** Skin kept moist almost constantly (e.g., by perspiration, urine) Dampness detected every time patient is moved or turned	2. **Very moist:** Skin often but not always moist Linen must be changed at least once a shift	3. **Occasionally moist:** Skin occasionally moist, requiring an extra linen change approximately once per day	4. **Rarely moist:** Skin usually dry; linen change only required at routine intervals
ACTIVITY				
Degree of physical activity	1. **Bedfast:** Confined to bed	2. **Chairfast:** Ability to walk severely limited or nonexistent Cannot bear own weight and/or must be assisted into chair or wheelchair	3. **Walks occasionally:** Walks occasionally during day, but for very short distances, with or without assistance Spends majority of each shift in bed or chair	4. **Walks frequently:** Walks outside room at least twice a day and inside room at least once every 2 hours during waking hours

Continued

TABLE 37-1 BRADEN SCALE FOR PREDICTING PRESSURE SORE RISK—cont'd

MOBILITY				
Ability to change and control body position	1. **Completely immobile:** Does not make even slight changes in body or extremity position without assistance	2. **Very limited:** Makes occasional slight changes in body or extremity position but unable to make frequent or significant changes independently	3. **Slightly limited:** Makes frequent though slight changes in body or extremity position independently	4. **No limitations:** Makes major and frequent changes in position without assistance
NUTRITION				
Usual food intake pattern	1. **Very poor:** Never eats a complete meal Rarely eats more than one third of any food offered Eats two servings or less of protein (meat or dairy products) per day Takes fluids poorly Does not take a liquid dietary supplement *or* Is NPO and/or maintained on clear liquids or IV feeding for more than 5 days	2. **Probably inadequate:** Rarely eats a complete meal and generally eats only about half of any food offered Protein intake includes only three servings of meat or dairy products per day Occasionally takes a dietary supplement *or* Receives less than optimal amount of liquid diet or tube feeding	3. **Adequate:** Eats over half of most meals Eats a total of four servings of protein (meat, dairy products) each day Occasionally refuses a meal but usually takes a supplement if offered *or* Is on a tube-feeding or TPN regimen that probably meets most nutritional needs	4. **Excellent:** Eats most of every meal Never refuses a meal Usually eats a total of four or more servings of meat and dairy products Occasionally eats between meals Does not require supplementation
FRICTION AND SHEAR				
	1. **Problem:** Requires moderate to maximal assistance in moving Complete lifting without sliding against sheets impossible Frequently slides down in bed or chair, requiring frequent repositioning with maximal assistance Spasticity, contractions, or agitation leads to almost constant friction	2. **Potential problem:** Moves feebly or requires minimal assistance During a move skin probably slides to some extent against sheets, chair, restraints, or other devices Maintains relatively good position in chair or bed most of the time but occasionally slides down	3. **No apparent problem:** Moves in bed and chair independently and has sufficient muscle strength to sit up completely during move Maintains good position in bed or chair at all times	

IV, Intravenous; *NPO,* nothing by mouth; *TPN,* total parenteral nutrition.

Instructions: Score patient in each of the six subscales; add all subscales for overall score. Level of risk: Not at risk >18, mild risk 15-18, moderate risk 13-14, high risk 10-12, and very high risk < 9.

approach to patient care. When you care for patients who have pressure ulcers, integrate information from all health-related sciences and knowledge from courses, experiences, and appropriate standards of practice into the management of your patient's wounds (Box 37-3).

Knowledge. Performing a pressure ulcer risk assessment requires you to use a validated risk assessment tool. Understanding the importance of risk factors that lead to pressure ulcer development allows you to plan appropriate interventions to reduce or eliminate risk factors to pressure ulcer development.

Knowing normal physiology of wound healing lets you implement the appropriate nursing measures to facilitate healing. In addition, knowledge of the normal healing process

BOX 37-3 SYNTHESIS IN PRACTICE

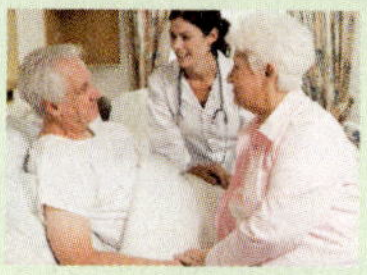

Lynda reviews the nursing admission assessment and she finds that Mr. Ahmed was admitted with a pressure ulcer. The ulcer is a stage II, 1- × 2-inch (2.5- × 3.5-cm) × ⅛-inch-deep partial-thickness wound over his sacral area. There is no necrotic tissue; and the wound bed has red, moist tissue. When Lynda prepares to conduct a skin assessment on Mr. Ahmed, she recalls information about how pressure ulcers develop and guidelines for skin assessment for patients with darkly pigmented skin. She focuses on determining changes in Mr. Ahmed's skin integrity.

Lynda observed care of a patient with a stage IV pressure ulcer during an experience in an extended care facility. From that experience she increased her knowledge about the debilitating effects of pressure ulcers. In addition, she was able to practice skin assessment techniques during her previous clinical experience.

helps you recognize complications requiring intervention. In choosing interventions consider the type of wound, the pain associated with it, conditions that affect healing, and a patient's psychological well-being.

Experience. You are better able to assess a patient's wound when you are able to draw from your experiences and recognize normal characteristics of wound healing. This is especially important when a patient has factors that impede wound healing such as peripheral vascular disease, poor nutrition, or reduced mobility. When caring for a patient who develops problems with wound healing, learn the clinical signs of complications. This is especially important when caring for a patient with darkly pigmented skin (Box 37-4).

Attitudes. Be observant when caring for a patient who is acutely ill. At times nurses overlook assessment of skin, wound integrity, or skin breakdown because of other perceived priorities such as respiratory or cardiac status. Assume responsibility and ensure that you include meticulous skin assessment and pressure ulcer prevention measures in a patient's plan of care. Skin assessment is important whenever a patient's health status changes (WOCN, 2010). Be aware that skin breakdown is sometimes unavoidable. However, the sooner you assess for and identify the risk factors for skin breakdown and plan interventions, the less severe the impaired skin integrity should be.

In the immediate postoperative period, some patients require well–thought out modifications of wound-care techniques. You usually do not change the initial dressing, but you are responsible for ensuring that the dressing remains dry and intact. With knowledge about pressure ulcers, wounds, and normal wound healing, use creative measures to reduce the risks of impaired skin integrity and promote wound healing.

Standards. The WOCN wrote the 2003 pressure ulcer guidelines and updated them in 2010 to support clinical practice by providing consistent research-based clinical decisions

BOX 37-4 PATIENT-CENTERED CARE

Skin assessment is an important element in early detection of the development of pressure ulcers. Changes in skin color that can be easily identified in light-colored skin may not be easily observed in skin with skin with darker pigmentation. Erythema also may be hard to detect in dark-skinned patients. In a light-skinned patient irritation may cause redness. But in a dark-skinned person it may cause an increase or decrease in pigmentation with no redness visible. Include a thorough assessment, looking for changes in skin texture, temperature, and warmth when assessing a patient with dark skin.

IMPLICATIONS FOR PRACTICE IN ASSESSING THE PERSON WITH DARK SKIN PIGMENTATION

- Examine skin when pressure is both applied and removed because the color can remain unchanged when pressure is applied. When pressure is applied to light-colored skin, blanching can occur that may demonstrate potential skin destruction.
- Assess for color changes at the site of pressure, which differ from those in patients with light skin color.
- With a gloved finger feel the area of potential skin damage because the skin in the injured area may feel cool to touch, indicating potential skin damage. Circumscribed area of intact skin is often warm to touch. As tissue changes color, intact skin feels cool to the touch.
- If a patient previously had a pressure ulcer, that location may be lighter in skin color.
- Localized area of involved skin may be purple/blue or violet (eggplant) instead of red.
- Edema may occur with induration and may appear shiny and taunt.
- Patient may complain of discomfort at a site that is predisposed to pressure ulcer development.

Data from Bennett MA: Report of the task force on the implications for darkly pigmented intact skin in the prediction and prevention of pressure ulcers, *Adv Wound Care* 8(6):34, 1995; Nix D: Skin and wound inspection and assessment. In Bryant RA, Nix DP, editors: *Acute and chronic wounds: current management concepts*, ed 4, St Louis, 2012, Mosby.

(Box 37-5). In addition, wound care protocols such as surgical wound management vary by agency policy. Know your agency policy and practices regarding the use of skin care products, dressing materials, and frequency of dressing change.

NURSING PROCESS

ASSESSMENT

Baseline and continual focused assessment data provide critical information about the patient's skin integrity and the increased risk for pressure ulcer development or impaired wound healing (Table 37-2). Although multiple factors affect skin integrity, it is important that you identify and assess the factors relevant for your patients.

Pressure Ulcers. Perform assessment of a patient for risk of development of pressure ulcers using one of the

BOX 37-5 PRESSURE ULCER PREVENTION POINTS

ASSESSMENT

1. Assess individual risk for developing pressure ulcers.
2. Perform a risk assessment (using a tool such as the Braden Scale) on entry to a health care setting and repeat on a regularly scheduled basis or when there is a significant change in a patient's condition.
3. Assess for intrinsic/extrinsic risk factors such as general medical conditions (e.g., diabetes, stroke, cardiopulmonary disease), significant weight loss, increased length of stay in a facility, and critically ill patients in the intensive care unit.
4. Inspect skin and bony prominences at least daily.
5. Assess for history of prior ulcer and/or pressure of current ulcer since this places patient at increased risk for additional pressure ulcers.

SKIN CARE AND EARLY TREATMENT

1. Continue preventive measures even when a patient has a pressure ulcer to prevent additional pressure areas from developing.
2. Clean and dry skin after each incontinent episode.
3. Use incontinence skin barriers such as creams, ointments, pastes, and film-forming skin protectants as needed to protect and maintain intact skin.
4. Use turning or lift sheets or devices to turn or transfer patients.
5. Maintain head of bed at or below 30 degrees or at the lowest level of elevation consistent with patient's medical condition.
6. Avoid vigorous massage over bony prominences.

SUPPORT SURFACES/PRESSURE REDUCTION

1. Place at-risk individuals on a pressure-reduction surface and not on an ordinary hospital mattress.
2. Schedule regular and frequent turning and repositioning for bed- and chair-bound individuals. Turn at least every 2 to 4 hours on a pressure-reducing mattress or at least every 2 hours on a non-pressure–reducing mattress.
3. Reposition individuals who are chair bound every hour if they are unable to perform pressure-relief exercises every 15 minutes.

NUTRITION

1. Offer individuals with nutritional and pressure ulcer risks a minimum of 30-35 kcal/kg of body weight per day with 1.25-1.5 g/kg/day protein and 1 mL of fluid intake per kcal per day.
2. Refer individuals with nutritional and pressure ulcer risks to a registered dietitian.

PATIENT/CAREGIVER EDUCATION

1. Educate patient/caregiver about the causes and risk factors for pressure ulcer development and ways to minimize risk.
2. Include information on the following:
   a. Etiology of and risk factors for pressure ulcers
   b. Importance of performing regular inspection of the skin especially over bony prominences
   c. Keeping the skin clean and dry
   d. Selection/use of support surfaces
   e. Measures to reduce friction from the sheet such as lifting rather than dragging across the bed
   f. Demonstration of positioning to decrease risk for tissue breakdown
   g. Promptly reporting health care changes and nutritional problems to health care providers

Data from Wound, Ostomy and Continence Nurses Society: *Guideline for prevention and management of pressure ulcers,* WOCN Clinical Practice Guidelines Series, Mount Laurel, NJ, 2010, The Society.

established predictive tools such as the Braden Scale. Do this on admission to the agency, 24 to 48 hours after admission, at regular intervals, and when there is a significant change in a patient's condition. Ongoing assessment is important because a patient's condition may change quickly. Subsequent assessments identify changes that increase a patient's risk for pressure ulcer development. In addition to assessing for potential risk factors, perform a thorough skin assessment on a daily basis to identify problems early and develop patient-centered interventions (see Skill 37-1). Prompt identification of patients at risk for or with skin integrity problems helps nurses use resources appropriately and reduce patients' risks. When patients are identified as being at risk for pressure ulcers, specific prevention and ulcer treatment strategies are included in the plan of care.

Skin. Assessment for tissue pressure damage includes visual and tactile inspection of the skin. Baseline assessment determines a patient's normal skin characteristics and any actual or potential areas of breakdown. This is especially important with high-risk patients such as those with diabetes, stroke, or serious malnutrition. The skin of an older-adult patient is more fragile and has an increased risk for skin breakdown (Box 37-6). Pay particular attention to areas exposed to casts, traction, or splints.

Assess all areas of the skin from head to toe, paying attention to any reddened areas or breaks in skin integrity. Document the assessment. When you notice hyperemia, document location, size, and color and reassess the area after 1 hour. If you suspect nonblanchable hyperemia, outline the affected area with a marker to make reassessment easier. Nonblanchable hyperemia is an early indicator of impaired skin integrity, but damage to the underlying tissue is sometimes more progressive. Palpate the tissues next to the observed area to gather further data about **induration** (hardening of tissue caused by edema or inflammation) and damage to the skin and underlying tissues.

Assess patients with lightly pigmented skin for blanching with return to normal skin tones. Also note changes in color, temperature, and hardness of the surrounding skin and tissues. Use visual and tactile inspection over the body areas

TABLE 37-2 **FOCUSED PATIENT ASSESSMENT**

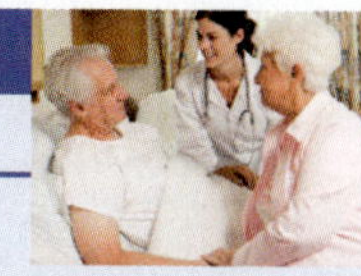

FACTORS TO ASSESS	QUESTIONS	PHYSICAL ASSESSMENT
Adequacy of patient's sensory perception	Do you feel me pinching the skin on your left hip? Can you feel me rubbing your left lower leg?	Apply painful stimuli to various body locations. If patient is unable to respond by affirming that he or she feels the stimuli, the patient has limited sensory perception.
Moisture	Does the bed sheet under your buttocks feel moist?	Routinely observe patient's bed linens for moisture. Observe patient's skin, noting if it is dry (rarely moist) or seldom damp (occasionally moist) or if skin is often but not always wet (moist). Observe for wound drainage.
Activity	Can you get out of bed by yourself to use the toilet? Are you able to get out of the bed or chair by yourself? Are you able to change your position in bed by yourself?	Check whether patient is incontinent of urine and stool. Assess patient's ability to walk at least once every 2 hours while awake (walks frequently) or whether patient is only able to ambulate short distances. Observe if patient is able to independently change positions in bed.
Nutrition	Were you able to eat the entire tray of food at breakfast? Are you hungry at mealtime? How much of your tray of food were you able to eat at the last meal?	Observe patient eating: Does patient need assistance? Determine if patient takes most of the meal and if intake is balanced (excellent nutrition). Assess the amount of food the patient eats at meals for adequate nutrition such as whether patient finishes over half of meals or is on tube feedings or TPN.
Friction and shear	When you are sitting up in the bed, do you find that you slide down toward the foot of the bed? Do you need assistance in moving up in bed or chair?	Assess if patient moves in bed and chair independently and maintains a good position at all times (no apparent problem). Determine if patient requires moderate-to-maximum assistance in moving and if the patient slides down in the bed and/or chair, which indicates a problem.

TPN, Total parenteral nutrition.

BOX 37-6 **CARE OF THE OLDER ADULT**

Issues Related to Skin Integrity

- There is decreased barrier function, thus less protection from excessive moisture, shear, friction and pressure.
- Aging skin experiences decreased epidermal turnover; thus healing requires more time.
- The thinning of the dermis and flattening of the dermal-epidermal junction that occur in aging predispose the older adult's skin to tearing.
- There is decreased inflammatory reaction, thus more susceptibility to infection.
- Sensory perception is reduced; thus ability to detect pain on initial injury is lessened.

Data from Wysocki A: Anatomy and physiology of skin and soft tissue. In Bryant RA, Nix DP, editors: *Acute and chronic wounds: current management concepts,* ed 4, St Louis, 2012, Mosby.

most frequently at risk for pressure ulcer development (Figure 37-6). When a patient lies in bed or sits in a chair, pressure occurs over bony prominences. Body surfaces subjected to the greatest weight or pressure such as the sacrum or ischium are at increased risk for pressure ulcer formation.

Mobility. Assessment includes documenting level of mobility, the potential effects of impaired mobility on skin integrity, and data regarding the quality of muscle tone and strength. For example, determine if a patient is able to lift the weight off the ischial tuberosities and roll to a side-lying position. Some patients have adequate range of motion (ROM) to independently move into a more protective position, but others do not. Finally assess the patient's activity tolerance (see Chapter 27).

Nutritional Status. Malnutrition is associated with overall morbidity and mortality. Best practice involves monitoring nutritional status as part of the total assessment (WOCN,

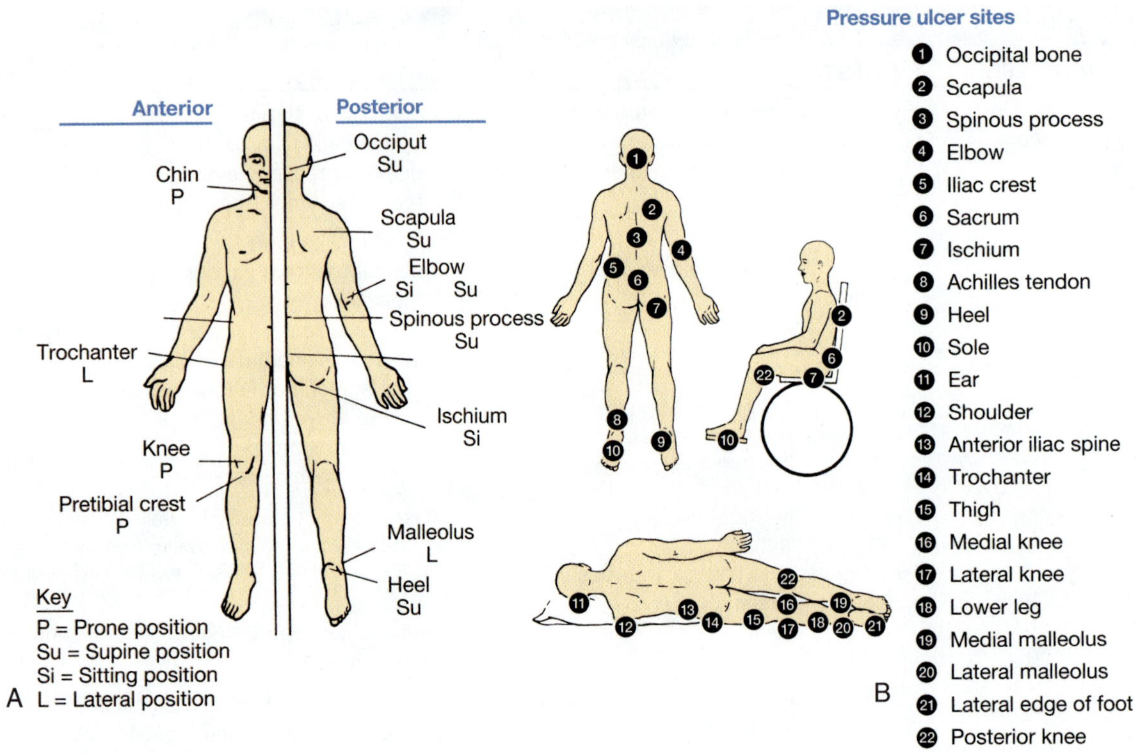

FIGURE 37-6 **A,** Bony prominences most frequently underlying pressure ulcers. **B,** Pressure ulcer sites. (From Trelease CC: Developing standards for wound care, *Ostomy Wound Manage* 20:46, 1988.)

BOX 37-7 NUTRITIONAL ASSESSMENT AND MANAGEMENT OF PRESSURE ULCERS: WOCN 2010 GUIDELINE RECOMMENDATIONS

Screen for nutritional deficiencies at admission to care setting and if patient's condition changes (see Chapter 33).

Include the following parameters in the assessment:

- Current and usual weight
- History of significant weight loss
- Nutritional intake versus needs, incorporating protein, calorie, and fluid needs
- Adequacy of nutritional intake (i.e., calories, protein, and fluid)
- Signs of dehydration (i.e., skin turgor, urine output, elevated sodium)
- Medical/surgical history or interventions that influence nutritional intake or absorption of nutrients

Data from Wound, Ostomy and Continence Nurses Society: *Guideline for prevention and management of pressure ulcers,* WOCN Clinical Practice Guidelines Series, Mount Laurel, NJ, 2010, The Society.

2010) (Box 37-7) (see Chapter 33). Inadequate caloric intake causes weight loss and a decrease in subcutaneous tissue, allowing bony prominences to compress and restrict circulation. Assess patients' nutritional status using a variety of approaches (e.g., monitoring intake and output, completing a 3-day calorie count, assessing serum albumin) to identify those who need nutritional support.

Wounds. Assessment of a patient's wound varies from one health care setting to another. Accurate and regular assessments of a patient's wounds drive treatment decisions and provide a baseline to evaluate the status of the wounds (WOCN, 2010).

Emergency Setting. In an emergency the type of wound determines the criteria for inspection. After you stabilize a patient's cardiopulmonary status (see Chapter 30), inspect the wound for bleeding. An abrasion, or loss of the dermis, is usually superficial with little bleeding but some weeping (plasma leakage from damaged capillaries). A laceration is damage to the dermis and epidermis and is a torn, jagged wound. The depth and location of the laceration affect the extent of bleeding, with serious bleeding possible in lacerations greater than 5 cm (2 inches) long or 2.5 cm (1 inch) deep.

Puncture wounds bleed in relation to the depth and size of the wound; internal bleeding and infection are the primary dangers. Inspect the wound for contaminant material such as soil, broken glass, shreds of cloth, and foreign substances clinging to penetrating objects. Next assess the size of the wound and the need for suturing or surface protection. When an injury results from trauma from a dirty penetrating object, determine if the patient has received a tetanus toxoid injection within the last 10 years.

Stable Setting. Once an acute wound is stable after surgery or treatment, assess progress toward healing. If a dressing covers the wound and there are orders not to change it, inspect the dressing and any external drains. If a dressing appears saturated with drainage, reinforce the secondary dressing and notify the patient's primary nurse and health care provider immediately. Saturated dressings provide an excellent environment for bacterial growth; and you need to inform the health care provider of the color, odor, and estimate of drainage amount.

When you plan a dressing change, consider giving the patient an analgesic at least 30 minutes before exposing a wound. Refer to notes documenting pain levels during previous dressing changes. Discuss pain levels at previous dressing changes with your patient to determine the appropriate pain-management interventions. Avoid accidentally removing or displacing underlying drains.

First inspect the appearance of the wound, noting the anatomical location; size; approximation of wound edges; presence and quality of exudate; type of the tissue in an open wound; skin integrity around the wound; and signs of dehiscence, evisceration, or infection. Measure the length, diameter, and depth of every wound with a centimeter measuring guide. Note any **ecchymosis,** skin discoloration, or bruising caused by blood leakage into subcutaneous tissues after trauma to underlying vessels. The outer edges of a wound normally appear inflamed for the first 2 to 3 days, but this slowly disappears. When an infection develops, the wound edges are usually brightly inflamed, warm, tender, and swollen.

Next assess the character of wound drainage by noting the amount, color, odor, and consistency. The amount of drainage depends on the location and extent of the wound. A simple method for estimating the volume of wound drainage is to report the number and type of dressings used and saturated over an interval of time. The color and consistency of drainage vary, depending on its components. Types of drainage include the following:

1. *Serous:* Clear, watery plasma
2. *Sanguineous:* Fresh bleeding
3. *Serosanguineous:* Pale, more watery, a combination of plasma and red cells; may be blood streaked
4. *Purulent:* Thick, yellow, green, or brown, indicating the presence of dead or living organisms and white blood cells

If drainage has a pungent or strong odor, an infection is likely. Document the integrity of the wound and the character of the drainage, describing the appearance by observable characteristics.

The presence of drains is another important assessment. A drain is used in a surgical wound if a health care provider expects a large amount of drainage. Drains lie within tissue, extend from the skin, and are connected to a drainage bag or suction apparatus or allowed to drain into a dressing. Most drains attach to a collection device. First observe the security of the drain and its location with respect to the wound. Next note the character and amount of drainage if there is a collecting device. Pay particular attention to the flow of drainage through the tubing and notify the health care provider of any sudden decrease that indicates a blocked drain or an increase indicating bleeding or infection.

In the case of a surgical wound, inspect the staples, sutures, or wound closures for irritation and note whether the wound edges are intact. After the first few days when normal swelling around closures usually has subsided, continued swelling sometimes indicates overly tight closures, which increases the risk for wound separation or dehiscence.

When a wound exhibits swelling, separation of its edges, or redness in the periwound area, it is important to evaluate for the presence of cellulitis. Use light palpation to detect localized areas of tenderness or collection of drainage. Wearing gloves, gently place your fingertips along the wound edges. If pressure causes fluid to be expressed from the wound, note the character of the drainage and collect a wound culture if needed. Sensitivity to such palpation is normal, but extreme tenderness indicates infection.

Pain assessment is an important component of wound assessment for detecting complications and planning for future wound care (see Chapter 32). Serious discomfort during inspection or palpation of the wound suggests underlying problems, whereas discomfort related to dressing removal or application calls for administration of analgesics before future dressing changes.

Wound Cultures. If you detect clinical symptoms that suggest a wound infection such as increased erythema; increase in the amount and/or change in character of exudate; odor; increased local warmth or systemic signs of infection such as fever, chills, or an increased white cell count, the collection of a wound culture is indicated. The swab technique is most commonly used. Cultures are obtained to direct antibiotic selection (Stotts, 2012). Never collect a wound culture sample from old drainage because resident colonies of bacteria grow in the exudate. Thus clean the wound to remove skin flora first. Aerobic organisms grow in superficial wounds exposed to the air, whereas anaerobic organisms tend to live in body cavities. Box 37-8 describes the procedure you use to collect an aerobic specimen. To collect an anaerobic specimen deep in a body cavity, use a sterile 10-mL syringe with a 22-gauge needle. Aspirate 5 mL of air into the syringe. After cleaning the skin with a disinfectant and allowing it to dry, insert a needle into the wound and aspirate wound drainage while moving the needle back and forth in two-to-four areas of the wound. Withdraw the needle from the wound and expel any air from the syringe. Inject contents from the syringe into a special vacuum container with culture medium. In some institutions you place a cork over the needle to prevent entrance of air and send the syringe to the laboratory.

Patient Expectations. When your patient has a pressure ulcer or a chronic wound, the course of treatment is often costly and lengthy. Because your patient needs to be involved with wound-care management, it is important to know his or her expectations. A patient who unrealistically expects rapid wound healing is easily discouraged and may not follow the treatment plan. Likewise a patient who knows that the process is lengthy may unrealistically expect the area to heal without scarring. Knowing these expectations helps you provide individualized care and helps a patient modify expectations when needed.

NURSING DIAGNOSIS

A patient with actual or risk for *Impaired Skin Integrity* usually has one or more nursing diagnoses related to the condition. Assessment reveals clusters of data that indicate whether actual or a risk for *Impaired Skin Integrity* exists. After gathering appropriate assessment data, cluster defining characteristics to establish nursing diagnoses. For example, the destruction of the surface of the skin clearly allows you to diagnose *Impaired Skin Integrity.* The identification of nursing diagnoses related to wound healing helps you anticipate the need for supportive or preventive care. Many nursing diagnoses are potentially relevant to your patient who requires wound care:

- *Risk for Infection*
- *Impaired Bed Mobility*
- *Impaired Physical Mobility*
- *Imbalanced Nutrition: Less Than Body Requirements*
- *Acute Pain*
- *Chronic Pain*
- *Impaired Skin Integrity*
- *Risk for Impaired Skin Integrity*
- *Ineffective Peripheral Tissue Perfusion*

Assess for related factors that contribute to each diagnostic statement. These related factors become the focus of your interventions. For example, the patient with *Impaired Skin Integrity related to a surgical incision* requires a different set of interventions than the patient with *Impaired Skin Integrity related to pressure and nutritional deficiency.* A patient whose surgical incision has increased drainage requires different and perhaps more frequent skin cleansing and dressings to manage additional drainage.

BOX 37-8 RECOMMENDATION PROCEDURE FOR SWAB WOUND-CULTURE TECHNIQUE

1. Prepare to collect specimen using sterile technique (before administering antibiotics).
2. Clean wound surface 1 cm^2 with an antiseptic solution.
3. Moisten swab with normal saline.
4. While applying pressure, rotate applicator within 1-2 cm^2 of clean wound tissue (try to draw out tissue fluid).
5. When tip is saturated, insert into appropriate sterile container.
6. Complete laboratory slip providing clinical data, which includes wound site, time collected, and prior antibiotics.
7. Transport specimen quickly, within 1 hour, to laboratory to keep the specimen stable.

Modified from European Pressure Ulcer Advisory Panel and National Pressure Ulcer Advisory Panel: *Treatment of pressure ulcers: quick reference guide,* Washington DC, 2009, National Ulcer Advisory Panel, http://www.npuap.org/wp-content/uploads/2012/03/Final_Quick_Treatment_for_web_2010.pdf. Accessed December 7, 2013; and Stotts NS: Wound infection: diagnosis and management. In Bryant RA, Nix DP, editors: *Acute and chronic wounds: current management concepts,* ed 4, St Louis, 2012, Mosby.

PLANNING

Plan therapeutic interventions for your patients with actual or potential risks to skin integrity (Care Plan and Figure 37-7). Design your therapies according to severity of risks to the patient. Individualize the plan according to the patient's developmental stage and level of health.

Goals and Outcomes. You need to develop patient-centered goals aimed at preventing or reducing impaired skin

CARE PLAN

Impaired Skin Integrity

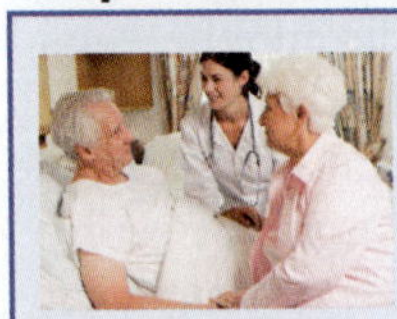

ASSESSMENT

Mr. Ahmed has limited activity tolerance. He does not tolerate position changes and wants to stay in a semi-Fowler's position at all times. He complains of a painful, burning sensation in his sacral region. An ulcer is present that measures 1 × 2 inches with a depth of ⅛ inch.

ASSESSMENT ACTIVITIES	FINDINGS/DEFINING CHARACTERISTICS*
Identify the support surface that appropriately decreases pressure on Mr. Ahmed's skin.	Mr. Ahmed **thinks that he cannot tolerate positions that relieve or reduce pressure to his skin.** Mr. Ahmed says, "I'm uncomfortable in any position except when I'm sitting up in bed."
Determine if Mr. Ahmed can tolerate small shifts of his body weight while in bed.	Mr. Ahmed can redistribute his body weight away from the pressure ulcer **with slight shifts of his weight, allowing adequate blood flow to the pressure ulcer.**

CARE PLAN—cont'd

Impaired Skin Integrity

ASSESSMENT ACTIVITIES	FINDINGS/DEFINING CHARACTERISTICS*
Inspect and palpate wound.	**Wound assessment: 1- × 2-inch partial-thickness ulcer over sacral area with a red, moist base. Reddened skin around the wound.** On palpation underlying skin is soft and indurated.
Conduct a calorie count.	Mr. Ahmed is eating fewer than 1600 calories daily.

*__Defining characteristics__ are shown in **bold** type.

NURSING DIAGNOSIS: Impaired Skin Integrity related to pressure over bony prominence in sacral region

PLANNING

GOAL	EXPECTED OUTCOMES (NOC)†
	Tissue Integrity: Skin & Mucous Membranes
• Mr. Ahmed's wound will show movement toward healing in 2 weeks.	• Wound decreases in diameter in 7 days. • There is no evidence of further wound formation in 3 days.

†Outcomes classification label from Moorhead S, et al, editors: *Nursing outcomes classification (NOC),* ed 5, St Louis, 2013, Mosby.

INTERVENTIONS (NIC)‡	RATIONALE
Pressure Management	
• Post and implement a turning schedule.	Repositioning redistributes pressure (Bryant and Nix, 2012; WOCN, 2010).
• Obtain and place a low-air-loss overlay over patient's mattress.	Redistributes amount of pressure on bony prominences (Nix and Mackey, 2012).
Wound Care	
• Cleanse wound and skin around wound; dry skin.	Removes debris from the wound bed without damaging healthy tissue (Rolstad, Bryant, and Nix, 2012).
• Apply hydrocolloid dressing to wound per order; extend dressing 1½ inches beyond wound edges.	Hydrocolloid dressings support moist wound healing and protect the wound (Rolstad, Bryant, and Nix, 2012).
Nutrition Management	
• Collaborate with dietitian to determine appropriate number of calories and types of nutrients needed to promote wound healing.	Adequate nutrition such as increased calorie count, protein intake, and vitamins aids in wound healing (WOCN, 2010).

‡Intervention classification labels from Bulechek GM, et al, editors: *Nursing interventions classification (NIC),* ed 6, St Louis, 2013, Mosby.

EVALUATION

NURSING ACTIONS	PATIENT RESPONSE/FINDING	ACHIEVEMENT OF OUTCOME
Observe wound to determine healing progress: measure wound diameter and depth; note condition of skin around wound; observe appearance of wound drainage and tissue at each dressing change.	Ulcer is 1 × 1 inch. Serous drainage is present. Wound tissue remains red and moist.	Improved tissue type. Reduction in wound size.
Palpate underlying skin around wound.	Underlying skin around wound remains intact with no palpable tissue change.	No evidence of advancing pressure ulcer or tissue damage.
Ask Mr. Ahmed if he has discomfort or sensations of tingling or burning at wound site.	Mr. Ahmed denies any new sensations at wound site.	No evidence of new tissue damage.
Ask Mr. Ahmed about his food intake.	Mr. Ahmed reports that his appetite is increasing and he is eating most of his meals.	Nutritional intake is improved.
Review calorie count over last week.	Calorie count denotes steady increase in daily calorie consumption.	

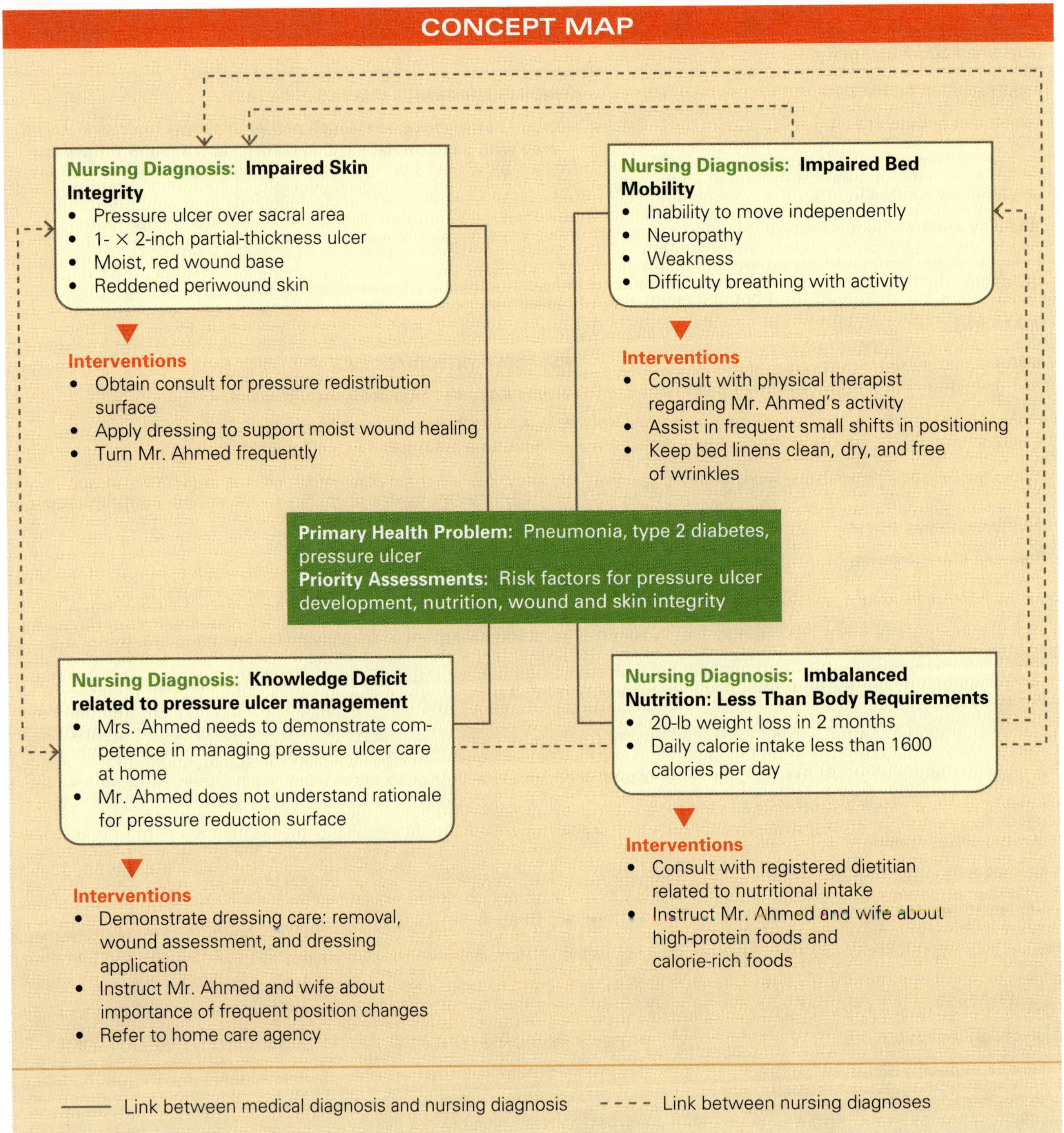

FIGURE 37-7 Concept map.

integrity or promoting wound healing. Individualize care planning for the patient, taking into consideration his or her most immediate needs. Assess all patients for the risk for skin breakdown and perform skin and wound assessments daily. Integrate information from the pressure ulcer risk and skin assessments into the plan of care and write attainable goals such as "Patient will not develop further skin breakdown" and "Patient's wounds will demonstrate healing." Include the patient and family in the assessment process so they begin to see their contribution to reducing risk factors.

Setting Priorities. When planning care, establish priorities based on comprehensive assessment data, goals, and expected outcomes. Acute needs are immediate. However, you also need to prioritize preventive interventions and implement them in a timely manner. Maintenance of skin integrity and promotion of wound healing prevent additional health care issues. Skin and wound priorities include ongoing assessment of pressure ulcer risk and wound status and providing interventions to control or eliminate contributing factors of pressure, shear, friction, moisture, and infection.

Consider other patient factors when setting priorities, including everyday activities and family factors. These factors are important for patients in institutional and home settings. Sometimes you need the help of another health care team member such as a physical or occupational therapist when considering mobility needs.

Collaborative Care. With the trend toward earlier discharge from health care settings, it is important to consider a patient's plan for discharge. Discharge planning begins when a patient enters the health care system. Anticipating a patient's discharge from an acute care institution and referral to a skilled nursing care facility or home care agency is necessary to help a patient remain mobile or regain mobility at home.

Patients and their families often need to continue wound management after discharge. Thus they need to discuss the likelihood that the patient will return home needing the assistance of home health nurses or transfer to a skilled nursing facility for more care and observation.

Consult with a case manager to plan for the necessary resources for support once a patient is discharged. Include a physical therapist for evaluation of a patients' ability to transfer and walk up stairs (if there are stairs in the home). Consult with a registered dietitian to assess a patient's nutritional status and help with nutrition interventions.

IMPLEMENTATION

Health Promotion. Health promotion for a surgical patient involves instruction about increasing protein intake before surgery and learning ways to reduce strain on surgical incision after surgery (see Chapter 39). Early identification of high-risk patients helps prevent pressure ulcers. Prevention minimizes the effect of risk factors and contributing factors on pressure ulcer development (see Box 37-5). Nursing interventions for prevention of pressure ulcers include topical skin care, positioning, and the use of support surfaces.

Topical Skin Care. Perform skin assessment daily, paying special attention to bony prominences. Do not massage reddened areas because reddened areas indicate tissue injury. Massage to these areas further injures the tissue by causing damage to the tissue capillaries. Examine your patient's skin for signs of dryness, cracking, edema, or excessive moisture. When cleansing the skin, use a mild cleansing agent. Soap causes dryness, which increases the risk for skin infection. Skin lubrication helps keep the skin intact; consider using a moisturizer on a routine basis (WOCN, 2010). Because intact skin is the initial defense for preventing skin breakdown, keep your patient's skin clean and dry. Many types of products are available for skin care; match their uses to the specific needs of your patient.

Use an incontinence cleanser for a patient who is incontinent of stool or urine. To protect the skin apply a moisture-barrier product (generally petrolatum or dimethicone based) liberally to the exposed area. The moisture barrier provides skin protection from the irritating effects of stool or urine and allows you to clean the next incontinent episode easily.

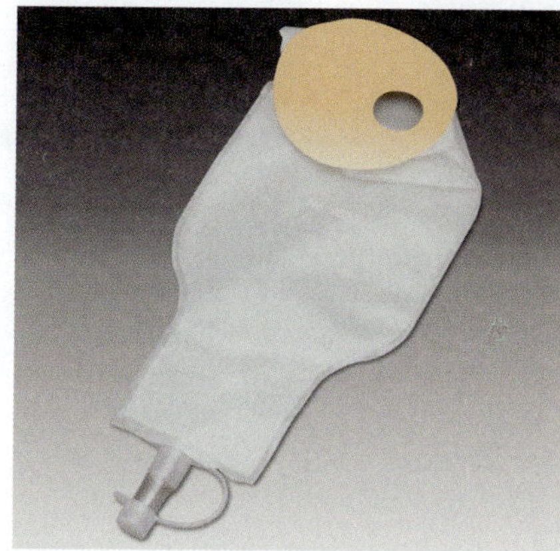

FIGURE 37-8 Hollister® Fecal Incontinence Collector. (Permission to use this copyrighted material has been granted by the owner, Hollister Inc.)

Apply the moisture-barrier ointment after each cleansing. For skin that has become exposed or stripped from incontinence, use a barrier paste that adheres to the irritated area and will not be removed with each cleansing. Offer a patient frequent access to the toilet to prevent fecal and urinary incontinence. You can contain fecal incontinence with a fecal incontinence collector (Figure 37-8), in which an adhesive skin barrier is attached to a drainable pouch applied around the anus to collect liquid stool. Use a fecal incontinence collector when a patient is experiencing frequent liquid bowel movements and has intact perianal skin. Other external collection devices include male external catheters applied to the shaft of the penis to collect urine. You can use underpads and diapers to protect skin in patients incontinent of stool and urine. Most underpads and diapers have a plastic outer lining that holds moisture against the skin. They irritate the skin if left under patients for prolonged periods of time. Select underpads or diapers that are absorbent to wick incontinence moisture away from the skin rather than trap it against the skin, which causes **maceration** (softening of the skin caused by moisture) (WOCN, 2010). When providing skin care to a patient who is incontinent, the health care team first assesses and treats the cause of the incontinence and then decides on protection and/or collection interventions.

Positioning. Positioning interventions reduce pressure and shear (Box 37-9). Repositioning frequency is determined by tissue tolerance, level of activity and mobility, general medical condition, overall treatment objectives, and support surface (EPUAP and NPUAP, 2009). Therefore a standard turning interval of 1 to 2 hours does not prevent pressure sore development in some patients. The WOCN (2010) recommends reducing shear by keeping a patient's head of bed below the 30-degree angle, using assistive devices when turning or transferring patients, using the bed gatch or footboard, and using the 30-degree lateral position (Figure 37-9).

When a patient is able to sit in a chair, reposition him or her every hour (EPUAP and NPUAP, 2009). In the sitting position the pressure on the ischial tuberosities is greater than

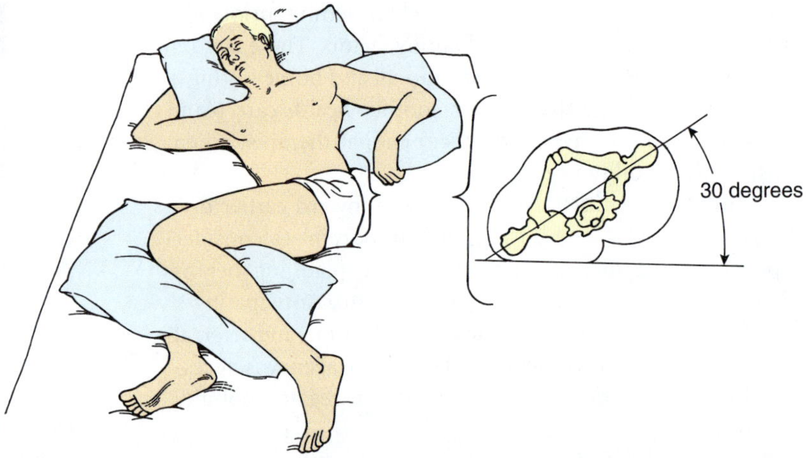

FIGURE 37-9 Thirty-degree lateral position. (Adapted from Bryant RA, Nix DP, editors: *Acute and chronic wounds: current management concepts,* ed 4, St Louis, 2012, Mosby.)

BOX 37-9 WOCN 2010 PRESSURE–REDUCTION/RELIEF RECOMMENDATIONS

- Use turn sheets, trapeze bars, and lift equipment to help with mobility.
- Maintain the elevation of the head of the bed to 30 degrees or less for the supine position to prevent shear.
- Reposition and turn regularly and frequently.
- Use positioning devices to avoid placing the patient on the pressure ulcer or other areas at risk for pressure ulceration.
- When side lying, use a 30-degree laterally inclined position to relieve pressure over the trochanter.

Data from Wound, Ostomy and Continence Nurses Society: *Guideline for prevention and management of pressure ulcers,* WOCN Clinical Practice Guidelines Series, Mount Laurel, NJ, 2010, The Society.

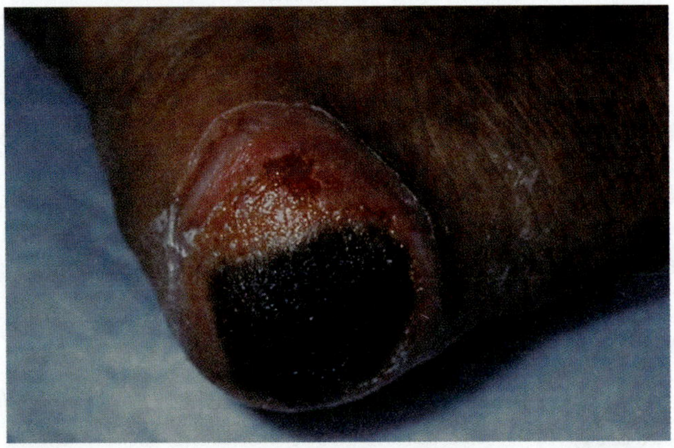

FIGURE 37-10 Formation of pressure ulcer on heel resulting from external pressure from mattress of bed. (Courtesy Janice Colwell, RN, MS, CWOCN, FAAN, Clinical Nurse Specialist, University of Chicago Medicine.)

when in the supine position. In addition, assist or teach patients with the ability to shift weight to reposition every 15 minutes. In addition, have the patient sit on gel or an air cushion to redistribute weight, decreasing the amount of weight on the ischial tuberosities.

A patient's heels are an area of concern because of the small surface area (Figure 37-10). Keep heels off the bed with a pillow under the lower leg or by the use of a heel protector (Bryant and Nix, 2012).

Support Surfaces. Support surfaces decrease the amount of pressure exerted over bony prominences by maximizing contact (allowing the body to touch the entire surface) and thereby redistributing weight over a large area. Support surfaces include mattresses, overlays, framed specialty beds, chair pads, table pads, and crib mattresses or pads (Table 37-3). In addition to redistributing pressure, many of the support surfaces reduce shear and friction and decrease moisture.

Select an appropriate support surface based on your assessment findings. A flow diagram (Figure 37-11) helps you in clinical decision making. When using a support surface, make sure that there are minimal layers of bed linens between a patient and the surface. Position a patient as close as possible to the surface for it to be effective. Remember, even when using a support surface, you still need to reposition a patient. Once a support surface is in use, reevaluate a patient on a frequent basis to determine the continued need and the effectiveness of the product. Patient and caregiver education on the importance and use of the support product is essential (Box 37-10).

Nutrition. Nutrition is fundamental to normal cell activity and tissue repair and regeneration. Although it is important for all patients, it is of particular importance for a patient with a wound to prevent severe or prolonged depletion of nutrients that can impact healing (Stotts, 2012). Complete a nutritional assessment on a patient who has a wound, collecting important data such as relevant patient history and laboratory data. Normal wound healing requires adequate intake of protein, fat, and carbohydrates. Consider consulting with a registered dietitian to obtain a thorough evaluation of a patient's nutritional status and identify related interventions to improve nutritional intake.

TABLE 37-3 SUPPORT SURFACES

CATEGORIES	MECHANISM OF ACTION	INDICATIONS
Low-Air-Loss System Available in a full bed or as an overlay	Pressure-redistribution device: A pump provides slow, continuous air flow, allowing for even distribution in the porous mattress and continuous air flow across the skin. The patient's weight is distributed more evenly for pressure redistribution.	Prevention of skin breakdown in patients who cannot be turned or have existing skin breakdown
Foam Available as an overlay or in a full mattress	Pressure redistribution Available in elastic or memory foam	High-risk patients
Static Air-Filled Overlay Available as overlay	Interconnected air-filled cells inflated to appropriate level: Pressure redistribution	High-risk patients
Air-Fluidized Bed Available as bed	Bed frame with silicone-coated beads that become fluidized when air is pumped through the beads: Pressure redistribution, antishear, antifriction surface	Patients with burns or multiple stage III or IV pressure ulcers; protection of new grafts and flaps
Kinetic Therapy Bed	Rotates in a regular pattern to facilitate pulmonary hygiene; some beds also provide low-air-loss therapy	Patients who are at risk for or have developed atelectasis and/or pneumonia

BOX 37-10 GUIDELINES FOR PATIENT EDUCATION REGARDING THERAPEUTIC SURFACES

- Explain the rationale for use of support surfaces. Be sure that patient and family know that this reduces pressure on the bony prominences by redistributing the pressure between the surface and patient's skin.
- Teach patient and family the importance of minimal layers of linen or absorbent pads between patient and surface.
- Instruct in the importance of frequent position changes, demonstrating small shifts of weight.
- Demonstrate to patient and caregiver the procedure for lateral positioning at a 30-degree angle and the use of pillows to support various positions.

BOX 37-11 WOUND-HEALING PRINCIPLES

1. Control or eliminate causative factors.
   a. Offload pressure.
   b. Reduce friction and shear.
   c. Protect from moisture.
2. Provide systemic support to reduce existing and potential cofactors.
   a. Optimize nutrition.
   b. Provide adequate hydration.
   c. Reduce edema.
   d. Control blood glucose levels.
3. Maintain physiological wound environment.
   a. Prevent and manage infection.
   b. Cleanse wound.
   c. Remove nonviable tissue (debridement).
   d. Maintain appropriate level of moisture.
   e. Eliminate dead space.
   f. Control odor.
   g. Eliminate or minimize pain.
   h. Protect periwound skin

From Rolstad BS, Bryant RA, Nix DP: Topical management. In Bryant RA, Nix, DP, editors: *Acute and chronic wounds: current management concepts,* ed 4, St Louis, 2012, Mosby.

Acute Care

Pressure Ulcers. Address wound-management principles in an orderly fashion (Box 37-11). Provide appropriate wound management, including managing pressure, shear, friction, and moisture (see Skill 37-2). Provide systemic support to enhance your patient's wound healing. Co-morbidities such as cardiovascular or pulmonary disease decrease the amount of oxygen-rich hemoglobin available for delivery to injured tissue. Oxygen is necessary for wound healing and resistance to infection. Interventions that maximize oxygen levels include pulmonary hygiene interventions and administering low-flow supplemental oxygen (see Chapter 30).

Wound healing also depends on adequate nutrition. Protein intake is necessary to support the development of new blood vessels and collagen synthesis. Carbohydrates, fats, and vitamins provide energy for cellular function. Interventions to support adequate nutritional intake include a nutritional referral and appropriate dietary supplements.

Certain medications (e.g., steroids) and medical conditions (e.g., diabetes) negatively influence wound healing. Because hyperglycemia impairs wound healing, blood glucose control is essential.

A stable wound environment and appropriate treatment are necessary to promote healing (Table 37-4). To maintain a

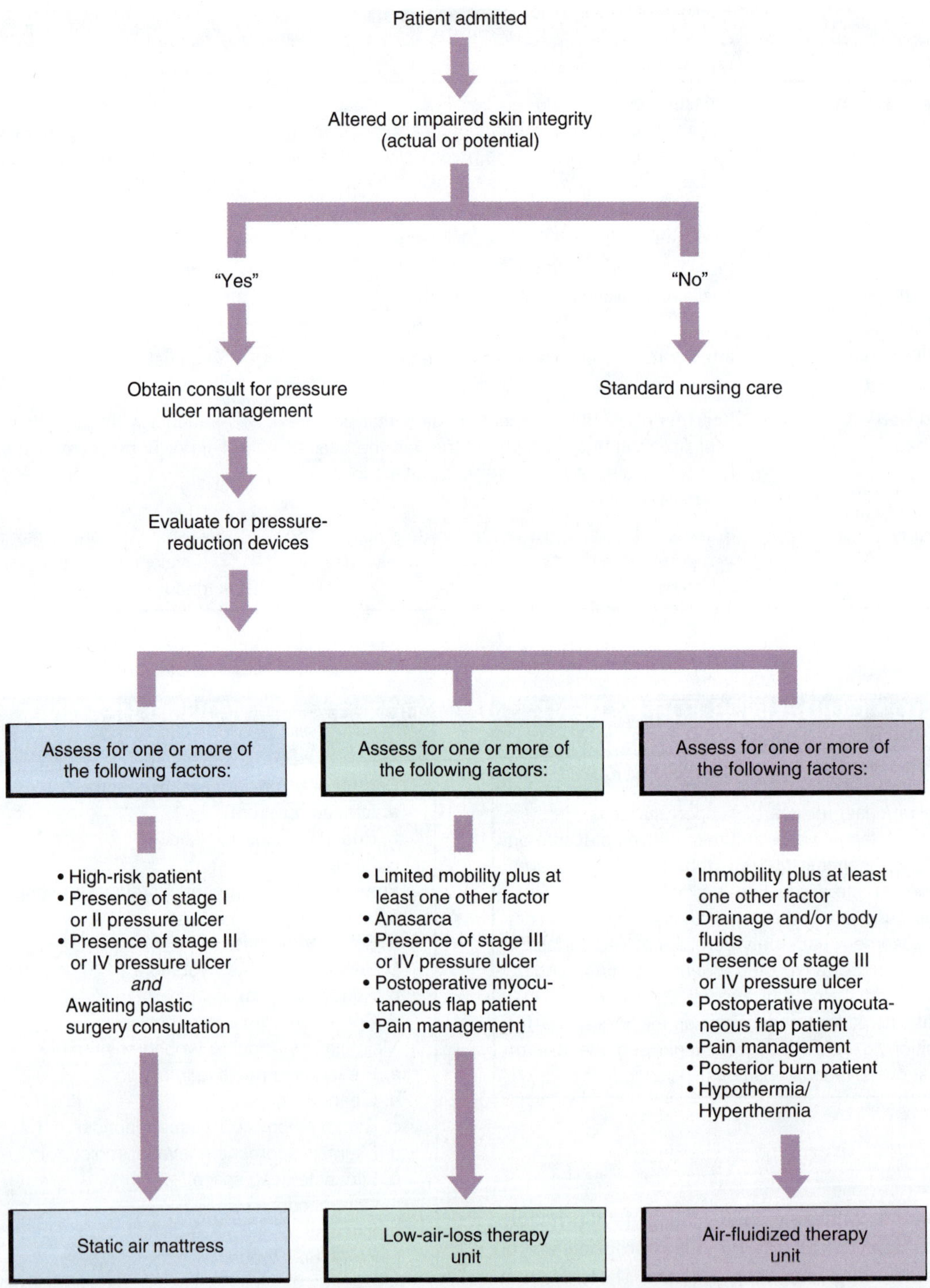

FIGURE 37-11 Flow diagram for ordering specialty surfaces. (Modified from Thomas C: Specialty beds: decision making made easy, *Ostomy Wound Manage* 23:51, 1989.)

stable environment it is important to control infection and promote cleansing, **debride** (remove) necrotic tissue, provide exudate management, control dead space, and provide wound protection. Assess a patient with a pressure ulcer for signs and symptoms of a wound infection: redness, warmth of surrounding tissue, odor, and the presence of exudate. If any of these signs is present, consult with the health care team to determine if you need to culture the wound and if systemic or topical antibiotics are indicated.

Cleanse pressure ulcers at each dressing change to promote removal of wound debris and bacteria from the wound surface (WOCN, 2010). Cleanse dirty wounds by irrigation. Clean wounds require only gentle flushing with normal saline solution.

TABLE 37-4 TREATMENT OPTIONS BY ULCER STAGE

ULCER STAGE	ULCER STATUS	DRESSING	COMMENTS*	EXPECTED CHANGE	TREATMENTS
I	Intact	None	Allows visual assessment.	Resolves slowly without epidermal loss over 7-14 days.	Turning schedule. Support hydration. Nutritional support. Pressure redistribution mattress or chair cushion.
		Transparent dressing	Protects from shear. Do not use in the presence of excessive moisture.		
		Hydrocolloid	May not allow visual assessment.		
II	Clean, granular base	Composite film	Limits shear.	Heals through reepithelialization.	See previous stage. Manage incontinence.
		Hydrocolloid	Change when seal of dressing breaks, maximal wear time 7 days.		
		Hydrogel	Provides moist environment.		
III	Clean, granular base	Hydrocolloid	See stage II.	Heals through granulation and reepithelialization.	See previous stages. Evaluate pressure redistribution needs.
		Foam	Apply over wound to protect and absorb moisture.		
		Calcium alginate	Use when there is significant exudate. Cover with secondary dressing.		
		Gauze	Use with normal saline or other prescribed solution. Wring out excess solution; unfold to make contact with wound.		
		Growth factors	Used with gauze per manufacturer instructions		
IV	Clean	Hydrogel	See stage II, clean.	Heals through granulation and reepithelialization.	Surgical consultation often necessary for closure. See stages I, II, and III.
		Calcium alginate	See stage III, clean.		
		Gauze plus ordered solution	Used with ordered solution; must unfold to make contact with wound; fill all dead space with gauze		
		Growth factors	Used with gauze		
Unstageable	Wound covered with eschar	Adherent film	Facilitates debridement.	Eschar lifts at edges as debridement progresses.	See previous stages. Surgical consultation may be considered for debridement.
		Gauze plus ordered solution	Delivers solution and wicks wound drainage and softens eschar	Eschar softens.	
		Enzymes	Facilitates debridement	Eschar softens.	
		None	If eschar is dry and intact, no dressing is used, allowing eschar to act as physiological cover; may be indicated for treatment of heel eschar.		

*As with *all* occlusive dressings, wounds should *not* be clinically infected.

Necrotic tissue slows wound healing because it is a source for infection and a barrier for epithelialization. After consulting with a health care provider or wound care specialist, plan a method of debridement. Types of debridement include mechanical, chemical, sharp, and autolytic (Ramundo, 2012).

A moist wound environment supports wound healing; however, excessive wound moisture macerates the wound edges and interferes with wound healing. Select a dressing that absorbs excessive moisture while providing the wound with necessary hydration. Eliminate dead space by loosely filling all cavities with dressings. You need to fill wound cavities to support the growth of granulation tissue and discourage infection.

It is important to involve a patient's family or caregiver in management of pressure ulcers and their treatment. Frequently patients require dressing changes after discharge. The patient's family or caregiver is an excellent source for dressing support and identification of possible wound-healing complications (Box 37-12).

BOX 37-12 PATIENT TEACHING

Pressure Ulcer Dressing Change

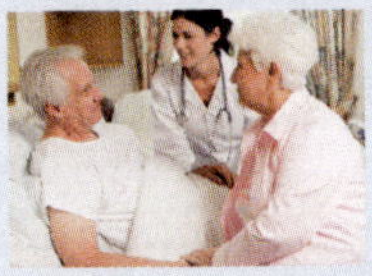

In preparation for Mr. Ahmed's discharge, Lynda develops a teaching plan for Mrs. Ahmed to teach her how to change Mr. Ahmed's pressure ulcer dressing.

OUTCOME

At the end of the teaching session Mrs. Ahmed changes Mr. Ahmed's dressing correctly.

TEACHING STRATEGIES

- Avoid using words that Mrs. Ahmed will not understand.
- Provide a brief description of what will be taught to both Mr. and Mrs. Ahmed. Include Mr. Ahmed in all of the teaching, even though he is unable to see the wound.
- Bring an extra dressing to the bedside to show Mr. and Mrs. Ahmed what the dressing looks like; explain how it works and how to apply it.
- Use a pictorial guide of a pressure ulcer to help Mrs. Ahmed understand what the wound looks like and how it will change in appearance as it heals.
- Plan one session in which Mrs. Ahmed will watch a demonstration of the wound being cleansed and the dressing applied. Plan a second session during which she will do a return demonstration.

EVALUATION STRATEGIES

- Ask Mrs. Ahmed questions as she does the procedure to evaluate her understanding of each step.
- Ask Mrs. Ahmed what she will evaluate at each dressing change.
- Observe Mrs. Ahmed changing the dressing and cleansing the wound. Observe any body language that indicates how she is feeling while doing the procedure. Provide reinforcement as needed.

Wounds

First Aid for Wounds. Use first-aid measures for wound care in emergency settings. Under more stable conditions you use a variety of interventions for wound healing. However, when a patient suffers a traumatic wound, first-aid interventions include promoting hemostasis, cleansing the wound, and protecting the wound from further injury.

Hemostasis. After assessing the type and extent of the wound, control bleeding from a laceration by applying direct pressure to the wound with a sterile or clean dressing. After bleeding subsides, an adhesive dressing strip or gauze dressing taped over the laceration allows skin edges to close and a blood clot to form. If a dressing becomes saturated with blood, add another layer of dressing, continue to apply pressure, and elevate the affected part. A health care provider sutures serious lacerations in an emergency clinic or hospital.

If a penetrating object such as a knife blade is in a patient's body, do not remove the object. Removal causes massive, uncontrolled bleeding. Apply pressure around the object but not on it or on surrounding tissues.

Cleansing. Gentle cleansing of a wound removes contaminants that serve as sources of infection. However, vigorous cleaning causes bleeding or further injury. For abrasions, minor lacerations, and small puncture wounds, rinse the wound in running water, gently cleanse with mild soap and water, rinse, and apply an over-the-counter antiseptic. When a laceration is bleeding profusely, only brush away surface contaminants and concentrate on hemostasis until the patient reaches a clinic or hospital.

Protection. Protect the wound by applying a sterile or clean dressing and immobilize the body part. A light dressing applied over minor wounds prevents entrance of microorganisms. In the case of small abrasions, it is acceptable to leave the wound open to air so a scab forms.

The more extensive the wound, the larger the dressing required. In a home emergency a clean towel or diaper is often the best dressing. A bulky dressing applied with pressure minimizes movement of underlying tissues and helps to immobilize the entire body part. A dressing or cloth wrapped around a penetrating object immobilizes it adequately.

Dressings. The use of dressings requires an understanding of wound healing and factors influencing healing. A variety of dressing materials are available commercially. The choice of dressing and how it is applied influence wound healing. The proper dressing does not allow a full-thickness wound to become dry with scab formation. When this occurs, the dermis dehydrates and crusts. As a result a barrier forms against normal epidermal cell growth, slowing wound healing. Furthermore, dryness increases discomfort. Ideally a dressing provides a moist environment to promote normal epidermal cell migration. The proper dressing also absorbs drainage to prevent bacterial growth and wound drainage from coming in contact with intact skin.

For surgical wounds that heal by primary intention, dressings are commonly removed as soon as drainage stops.

Frequently the health care provider removes the dressing 24 to 48 hours after surgery, which coincides with initial epithelialization.

Purpose. A dressing serves several purposes. It discourages the exposure of a wound to microorganisms. However, if a wound has minimal drainage, the natural formation of a fibrin seal eliminates the need for a dressing. A pressure dressing promotes hemostasis by exerting localized, downward pressure over an actual or potential bleeding site. A moist dressing lightly packed into the wound fosters normal healing by eliminating dead space in underlying tissues. Assess skin color, pulses in distal extremities, patient comfort, and any changes in sensation to ensure that pressure dressings do not interfere with circulation.

A dry dressing promotes healing by allowing the wound to heal by primary intention and absorbing minimal oozing of wound drainage. When a wound is healing by secondary intention, use a dressing to provide a moist environment. Moisten the gauze with a solution, usually normal saline, wring it out, and unfold and lightly pack it into the wound. The purpose of a moist gauze dressing is to act as a sponge, absorbing excessive wound drainage while providing a moist environment. Change the dressing when it is saturated or if it begins to dry out. Always cover a moist dressing with a dry, secondary dressing.

A firmly taped or wrapped dressing supports or immobilizes a body part, minimizing movement of the underlying incision and traumatized tissues. Finally a dressing promotes thermal insulation to the wound surface and protects it from the dehydrating effects of air.

Type. Dressings vary by type of material and mode of application (dry or moist). They are easy to apply, comfortable, and made of materials that promote wound healing.

Gauze is the most common dressing type. It does not interact with wound tissue and thus causes little wound irritation. It is available in different textures and shapes such as square, rectangle, and rolls of various lengths and widths. Gauze dressings are best for wounds with moderate drainage, deep wounds, undermining, and tunnels. Apply gauze either moist or dry. A moist gauze dressing is saturated with the prescribed solution, wrung out, opened, and placed onto the wound tissue. The moistened gauze increases the absorptive ability of the dressing to collect exudate. Cover the moist gauze with a secondary layer of dry gauze. Be sure that the moist gauze does not cover normal skin to prevent maceration. The moist dressing is changed on a scheduled basis to prevent drying of the gauze.

Transparent film dressings are clear sheets coated on one side with an adhesive. The adhesive side does not stick to the wound because of the moisture and traps moisture over the wound bed, providing a moist environment. The film is impermeable to fluid but semipermeable to oxygen. This type of dressing is used as a primary dressing in wounds with minimal tissue loss that have very little wound drainage. The dressing is applied to extend approximately 1½ inches beyond the wound to allow for adherence. Change the dressing when the seal is broken.

Hydrocolloid dressings are made of gelling agents and have an adhesive wound surface. They come in a variety of sizes and shapes and are used to cover wounds, extending the hydrocolloid dressing at least 1½ inches beyond the wound margin. Hydrocolloids form a gel as they interact with the wound surface. Because they are occlusive, they protect the wound from surface contaminants, and you can leave them over a wound for several days. When removed, you will note a gel over the wound base; the gel maintains a moist environment to support healing and washes away during wound cleansing.

Hydrogel dressings are available in sheets or in a gel in a tube (amorphous). They contain a high percentage of water and are indicated for wounds that require moisture, either a wound with granulation (maintaining the moist wound environment needed for healing) or a wound that has a high percentage of necrotic tissue (the hydrogel facilitates debridement by softening the dead tissue). Hydrogels maintain moisture in some wounds for 1 to 3 days.

Negative-pressure wound therapy (NPWT) uses negative pressure to help wound healing (Figure 37-12). NPWT supports wound healing by evacuating wound fluids, stimulating granulation tissue formation, reducing the bacterial burden of a wound, and maintaining a moist wound environment (Netsch, 2012). Apply NPWT by fitting the foam or dressing to the shape of the wound and placing a drainage/suction tube in the interior or on top of the dressing. Seal the dressing and the tube with a transparent dressing and connect the tube to a prescribed amount of negative pressure, which creates suction. The suction pulls all air out of the wound and creates an airtight seal. This therapy provides removal of excess wound fluid to stimulate granulation tissue and decrease wound bacteria (see Skill 37-3). Connect the suction tubing to a container that collects the wound fluid. NPWT is changed on a scheduled basis, usually every 48 hours. Current

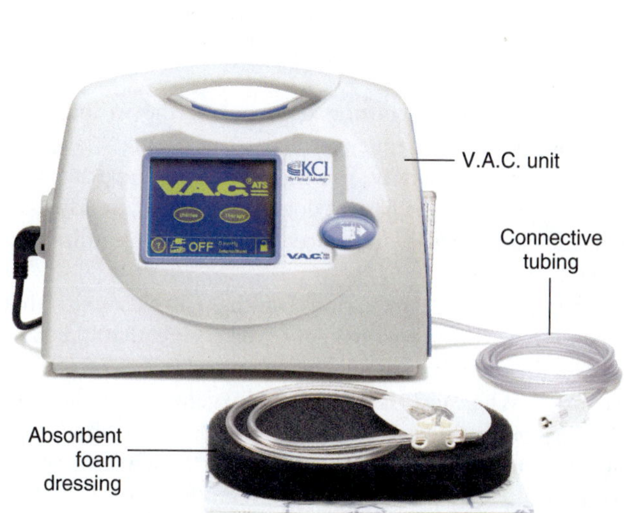

FIGURE 37-12 The V.A.C. ATS® NPWT system. *Top to bottom:* V.A.C. system itself, connective tubing to go between V.A.C. system and dressing, absorbent foam dressing. *NPWT,* Negative-pressure wound therapy. (Courtesy KCI Licensing, San Antonio, TX.)

evidence shows that this therapy often reduces healing time in chronic wounds and results in early grafting of wounds (Netsch, 2012).

Changing Dressings. To prepare to change a dressing, you need to know the type of dressing, any underlying drains used, and the type of supplies needed for wound care. You can adjust the type and amount of dressings if the amount of drainage changes or a wound becomes deeper. Notifying the health care provider of any change is essential.

The order for changing a dressing usually indicates the dressing type, frequency of changing, and solution or ointment you will apply. An order to "reinforce dressing prn" (add dressings without removing existing ones as needed) is common immediately after surgery when a health care provider does not want accidental disruption of the suture line or loss of hemostasis. A patient's medical or operating room record usually reveals whether drains are present. After the initial dressing change, communicate on the care plan the type of dressing materials and solutions to use and the type and location of drains.

Use aseptic technique during dressing change procedures (see Chapter 14). It is also essential for a patient to understand the steps of the procedure beforehand to reduce anxiety. Describe normal signs of the healing process and offer to answer questions about the procedure or wound.

If a patient needs to care for a wound at home, demonstrate dressing changes and provide an opportunity for the patient and family to practice. In the home wound healing stabilizes so sterile technique is usually unnecessary. However, patients need to learn clean technique. Make sure that the patient is able to change a dressing independently or with assistance from a family member before discharge unless home care will be provided. Skill 37-4 outlines the steps for applying moist saline dressings.

Securing Dressings. Use tape, ties, or dressings and cloth binders to secure a dressing over a wound site. **Binders** are dressings made of large pieces of material to fit a specific body part. An arm sling is an example of a binder. A binder reduces stress on a wound.

The choice of anchoring depends on the wound size, location, drainage, frequency of dressing changes, and the patient's level of activity. You most often use tape strips to secure dressings if the patient does not react to tape. Hypoallergenic paper, plastic, and woven fabric tapes minimize skin reactions.

Tape is available in various widths. Choose a size that secures the dressing sufficiently. Make sure that the tape crosses the dressing and adheres to several inches of skin on each side. When securing the dressing, gently press the tape, exerting pressure away from the wound. Never apply tape over irritated skin. Apply a skin barrier to the skin around the wound so the tape is secured to the skin barrier rather than to sensitive skin. To remove tape safely, loosen the end and gently release the tape from the patient's skin by pressing the skin away from the tape.

To avoid repeated removal of tape from sensitive skin, secure dressings with reusable Montgomery ties (see Skill 37-4, Step 16). Each tie consists of a long strip; half contains an adhesive backing to apply to the skin, and the other half folds back and contains a cloth tie that you tie across a dressing and untie at dressing changes. A long dressing may require two or more sets of Montgomery ties. To provide even support to a wound and immobilize a body part, apply elastic gauze or cloth dressings and binders over a dressing.

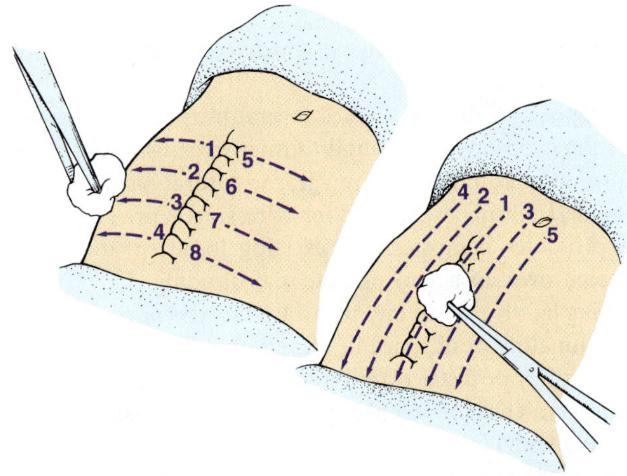

FIGURE 37-13 Methods for cleansing wound site.

Comfort Measures. Any wound can be painful, depending on the extent of tissue injury. You use several techniques to minimize discomfort. Interventions for pain reduction during dressing changes include allowing "time-outs" during painful procedures, scheduling dressing changes when a patient is feeling best, soaking dried dressings before removal, avoiding aggressive packing, positioning and supporting the wound area for comfort, and considering using low adhesive or nonadhesive dressings (Hopf, Sapshak, and Junkin, 2012).

Wound Cleansing. Wound cleansing removes surface bacteria, preventing the invasion of healthy tissue. Normal saline effectively cleans when delivered to the wound site with adequate force to agitate and wash away bacteria (Rolstad, Bryant, and Nix, 2012). Do not use povidone-iodine (e.g., Betadine), hydrogen peroxide, and acetic acid to irrigate a clean, granular wound. These solutions are toxic to fibroblasts, a key cellular component in wound healing. Apply the following concepts when cleaning wounds:

1. Cleanse in a direction from the least contaminated area to the most contaminated such as from the wound or incision to the surrounding skin (Figure 37-13) or from an isolated drain site to the surrounding skin (Figure 37-14).
2. Use light friction when applying antiseptics locally to the skin.
3. When irrigating, allow the solution to flow from the least contaminated to the most contaminated area.

Wound Irrigation. Irrigation is a way of cleansing wounds of exudate and debris. You use an irrigating syringe to flush the area with a constant flow of solution. Irrigations are useful for cleaning open, deep wounds or sensitive or inaccessible body parts. Administer the prescribed solution

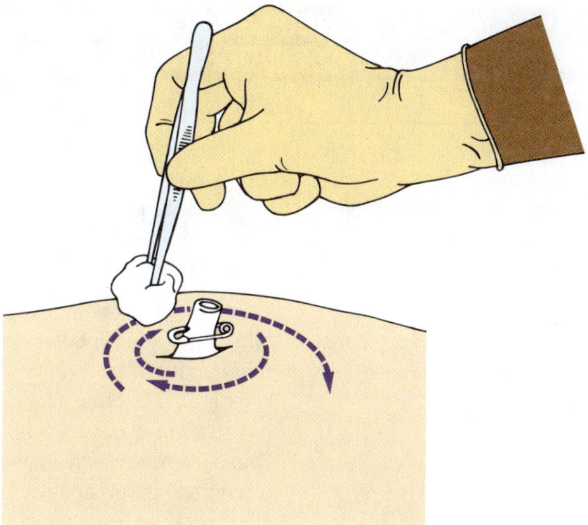

FIGURE 37-14 Cleansing drain site.

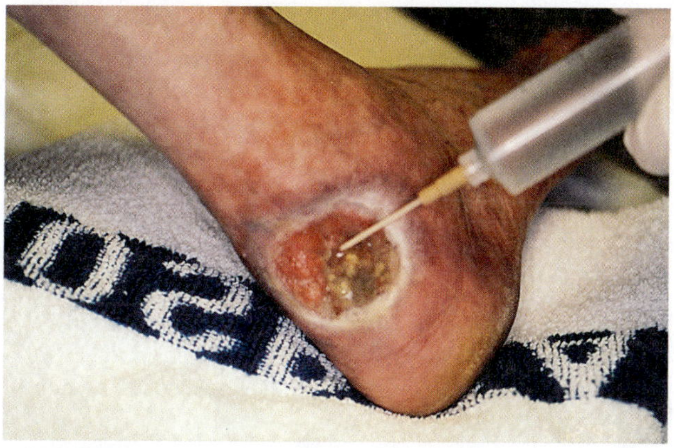

FIGURE 37-15 Wound irrigation using 35-mL syringe to facilitate removal of necrotic tissue.

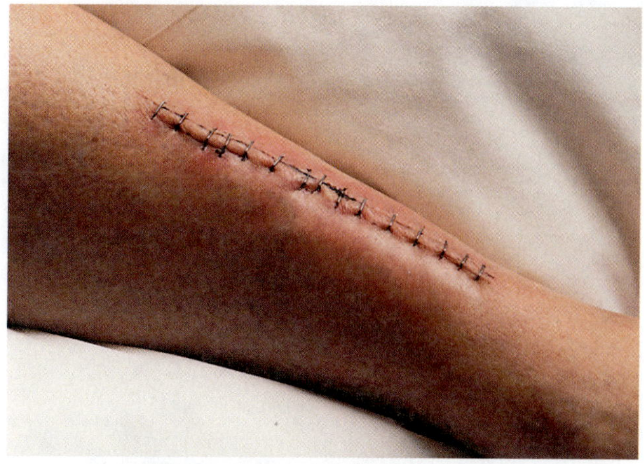

FIGURE 37-16 Wound closed with staples.

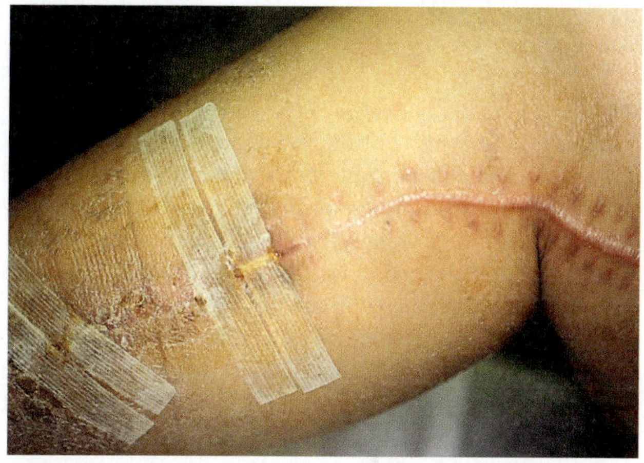

FIGURE 37-17 Steri-Strips placed over incision for closure.

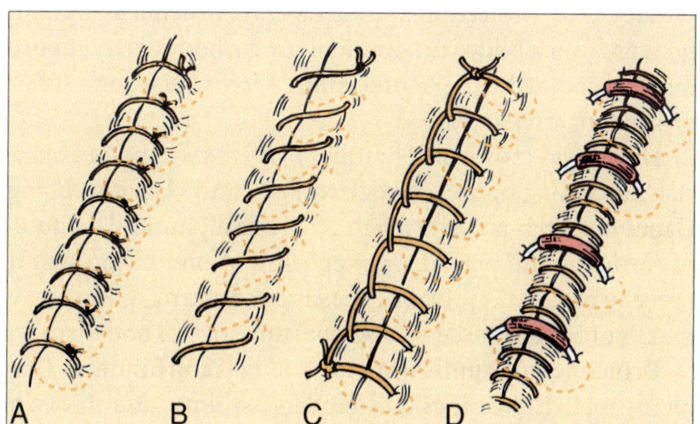

FIGURE 37-18 Examples of suturing methods. **A,** Intermittent. **B,** Continuous. **C,** Blanket continuous. **D,** Retention.

(usually normal saline) at body temperature to enhance comfort and provide local cleansing application.

When irrigating a clean wound, use sterile technique and an irrigation system with a safe level of pressure (4 to 15 psi) to prevent trauma to the newly formed granulation tissue (WOCN, 2010). This method provides an ideal solution pressure for cleansing wounds while minimizing tissue trauma (Figure 37-15). Make sure that the syringe tip is over but not sticking into the wound. Skill 37-5 lists steps for wound irrigation.

Suture Care. A surgeon closes a wound by bringing the edges as close together as possible to reduce the formation of scar tissue while minimizing trauma and tension and controlling bleeding. Sutures are threads or wires made of silk, steel, cotton, nylon, and polyester (Dacron) and are used to sew body tissues together. Dacron sutures minimize scar formation. Surgeons frequently use steel staples, a type of outer skin closure, because they result in less tissue trauma while providing extra strength (Figure 37-16). Wounds can also be closed with Steri-Strips, a sterile tape applied along both sides of a wound to keep the edges closed (Figure 37-17).

Be familiar with the types of suture methods (Figure 37-18). Policies vary among institutions as to who removes sutures. If you remove sutures, a health care provider's order is necessary.

Drainage Evacuation. When drainage interferes with healing, drainage evacuation is achieved by using a drain or

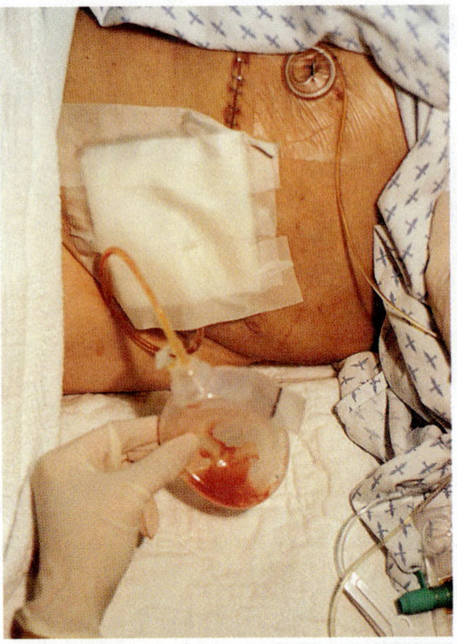

FIGURE 37-19 Jackson-Pratt drain and reservoir.

a drainage tube with continuous suction. Drainage evacuators are convenient, portable units that connect to tubular drains within a wound bed and exert a safe, constant, low-pressure vacuum to remove and collect drainage (Figure 37-19). Ensure that suction is exerted and that all connection points between the evacuator and tubing are intact. The evacuator collects drainage that is assessed for volume and character. When the evacuator fills, measure output by emptying the contents into a graduated cylinder and immediately reset the evacuator to apply suction.

Bandages and Binders. A simple gauze dressing is often not enough to immobilize or provide support to a wound. Bandages and binders applied over or around dressings provide extra protection and therapeutic benefits by creating pressure over a body part, immobilizing a body part, supporting a wound, reducing or preventing edema, securing a splint, or securing dressings.

Dressings are available in rolls of various widths and materials, including gauze, elasticized knit, and elastic webbing. Gauze dressings are lightweight, mold easily around contours of the body, and permit air circulation to underlying skin to prevent maceration. Elastic dressings conform well to body parts but are also used to exert pressure over a body part.

Principles for Application of Bandages and Binders. Correctly applied dressings and binders do not cause injury to underlying or nearby body parts or create discomfort for the patient. Before applying a dressing or binder, perform the following steps:

1. Inspect the skin for abrasions, edema, discoloration, or exposed wound edges.
2. Cover exposed wounds or open abrasions with a sterile dressing.
3. Assess the condition of underlying dressings and change if soiled.
4. Assess the skin of underlying body parts that are distal to the dressing for signs of circulatory impairment (coolness, pallor or cyanosis, diminished or absent pulses, swelling, numbness, and tingling) to provide a means for comparing changes in circulation after dressing application.

Table 37-5 outlines the principles of dressing and binder application. After you apply a dressing, assess, document, and immediately report any changes in circulation, comfort level, body function such as ventilation, and skin integrity. After you apply a dressing, loosen or readjust it as necessary, but seek an order before loosening or removing a dressing applied by a health care provider. Explain to the patient that any dressing or binder will feel relatively firm or tight; assess the dressing carefully to be sure that it is applied properly and is providing therapeutic benefit and replace dressings when they become soiled.

Binder Application. Binders are especially designed for the body part to be supported. The most common types of binders are an abdominal binder and sling (Box 37-13).

TABLE 37-5 PRINCIPLES FOR BANDAGE AND BINDER APPLICATION

PRINCIPLE	RATIONALE
Position body part you will be dressing in comfortable position of normal anatomical alignment.	Dressings cause restriction in movement. Immobilization in normal functioning position reduces risks of deformity or injury.
Prevent friction between and against skin surfaces by applying gauze or cotton padding.	Skin surfaces in contact with one another (e.g., between toes, under breasts) rub against one another to cause abrasion or chafing. Dressings over bony prominences rub against skin to cause breakdown.
Apply dressings securely to prevent slippage during movement.	Friction between dressing and skin causes skin breakdown.
When bandaging extremities, apply dressing first at distal end and progress toward trunk.	Gradual application of pressure from distal toward proximal portion of extremity promotes venous return and minimizes risk for edema or circulatory impairment.
Apply dressings firmly, with equal tension exerted over each turn or layer. Avoid excessive overlapping of dressing layers.	Equal tension prevents unequal pressure distribution over dressing body part. Localized pressure causes circulatory impairment.
Position pins, knots, or ties away from wound or sensitive skin areas.	Pins and ties used to secure dressings and binders exert localized pressure and irritation.

BOX 37-13 PROCEDURAL GUIDELINES

Applying Abdominal Binder

DELEGATION CONSIDERATIONS

The skill of applying an abdominal binder can be delegated to nursing assistive personnel (NAP). However, the nurse is responsible for the assessment of the area where the binder will be applied and the patient's comfort level after application.

EQUIPMENT

Abdominal binder, clean gloves, pins or metal fasteners as indicated by type of binder used

STEPS

1. Observe patient with need for support of thorax or abdomen. Observe ability to breathe deeply and cough effectively.
2. Identify patient using two identifiers (e.g., name and birthday or name and account number) according to agency policy. Review medical record if medical prescription for particular binder is necessary and reasons for application.
3. Inspect skin for actual or potential alterations in integrity. Observe for irritation, abrasion, skin surfaces that rub against one another or allergic response to adhesive tape used to secure binder.
4. Inspect any surgical dressing for drainage.
5. Assess patient's comfort level, using analog scale of 0 to 10 (see Chapter 32), and note any objective signs and symptoms of pain.
6. Gather necessary data regarding size of patient and appropriate binder.
7. Explain procedure to patient.
8. Perform hand hygiene and apply gloves (if likely to contact wound drainage).
9. Close curtains or room door.
10. Apply binder.
    a. Position patient in supine position with head slightly elevated and knees slightly flexed.
    b. Fanfold far side of binder toward midline of binder.
    c. Instruct and help patient roll away from you toward raised side rail while firmly supporting abdominal incision and dressing with hands.
    d. Place fanfolded ends of binder under patient.
    e. Instruct or help patient roll over folded ends toward you.
    f. Unfold and stretch ends out smoothly on far side of bed.
    g. Instruct patient to roll back into supine position.
    h. Adjust binder so supine patient is centered over binder using symphysis pubis and costal margins as lower and upper landmarks.
    i. Close binder. Pull one end of binder over center of patient's abdomen. While maintaining tension on that end of binder, pull opposite end over center and secure with Velcro closure tabs, metal fasteners, or horizontally placed safety pins (see Figure 37-20).
    j. Assess patient's comfort level.
    k. Adjust binder as necessary.
11. Remove gloves and perform hand hygiene.
12. Observe site for skin integrity, circulation, and characteristics of the wound. (Periodically remove binder and surgical dressing to assess wound characteristics.)
13. Evaluate comfort level of patient, using analog scale of 0 to 10 and noting any objective signs and symptoms of pain.
14. Evaluate patient's ability to ventilate properly, including deep breathing and coughing.

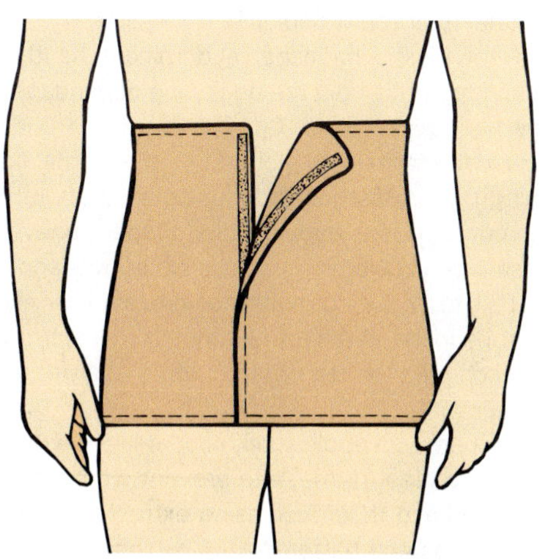

FIGURE 37-20 Abdominal binder secured with Velcro.

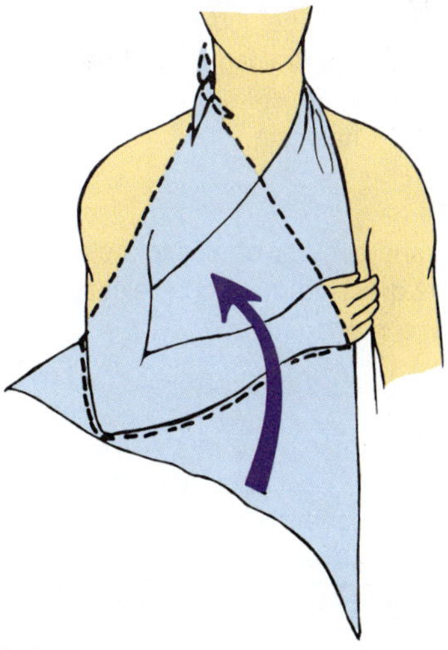

FIGURE 37-21 Application of a sling.

Abdominal Binder. An abdominal binder supports large incisions that are vulnerable to stress when the patient moves or coughs. It is a rectangular piece of cotton or elasticized material with many tails attached to the two longer sides or long extensions on each side to surround the abdomen (Figure 37-20).

Slings. Slings support arms with muscular sprains or fractures. A commercially made sling consists of a long sleeve that extends to the elbow and a strap that fits around the neck. In the home patients can use a large triangular piece of cloth as a sling. The patient sits or lies supine for a sling application (Figure 37-21). Instruct him or her to bend the affected arm, bringing the forearm straight across the chest. The open sling fits under the patient's arm and over the chest, with the base of the triangle under the wrist and the point of the triangle at the elbow. One end of the sling fits around the back of the neck. Bring the other end up over the affected arm while supporting the extremity. Tie the two ends at the side of the neck so the knot does not press against the cervical spine. You can fold the loose fold at the elbow evenly around the elbow and pin it. To prevent the formation of dependent edema, make sure that the lower arm is always supported at a level above the elbow.

Bandage Application. Rolls of dressing secure or support dressings over irregularly shaped body parts. Each roll has a free outer end and a terminal end at the center. The rolled portion of the dressing is its body, and you place its outer surface against the patient's skin or dressing. Box 37-14 describes essential points when applying an elastic bandage.

Heat and Cold Therapy. The local application of heat and cold to an injured body part provides therapeutic benefits. However, before using these therapies, understand normal body responses to local temperature variations, assess the integrity of the body part, determine the patient's ability to sense temperature variations, and ensure proper operation of equipment. You are legally responsible for the safe administration of all heat and cold applications.

Body Responses to Heat and Cold. Exposure to heat and cold causes systemic and local responses. Systemic responses occur through heat-loss mechanisms (sweating or vasodilation) or mechanisms promoting heat conservation (vasoconstriction or piloerection) and heat production (shivering) (see Chapter 15). Local responses to heat and cold occur through stimulation of temperature-sensitive nerve endings within the skin.

The adaptive ability of the body creates the major problem in protecting patients from injury resulting from temperature extremes. A person initially feels an extreme change in temperature but within a short time hardly notices the temperature variation. This phenomenon is dangerous because a person insensitive to heat and cold extremes is at risk for serious tissue injury. Recognize patients most at risk for injuries from heat and cold applications (Table 37-6).

Local Effects of Heat and Cold. Heat and cold stimuli create different physiological responses. The choice of heat or cold therapy depends on the local responses desired for wound healing (Table 37-7).

Heat generally is therapeutic. However, if it is applied for 1 hour or more, a reflex vasoconstriction reduces blood flow as the body attempts to control heat loss from the area. The periodic removal and reapplication of local heat restores vasodilation. Continuous exposure to heat damages epithelial

BOX 37-14 PROCEDURAL GUIDELINES

Applying Elastic Bandages

DELEGATION CONSIDERATIONS

The application of elastic bandages cannot be delegated to nursing assistive personnel (NAP). The nurse directs NAP to:

- Report if patient has drainage, numbness, or tingling around the dressing area.
- Report if patient has pain.

EQUIPMENT

Correct width and number of elastic dressings; clips, adhesive tape, or mesh dressing to secure elastic dressing; gloves if wound drainage is present

STEPS

1. Identify patient using two identifiers (e.g., name and birthday or name and account number) according to agency policy. Review patient's medical record and order for application of elastic dressing.
2. Inspect areas to be dressed for the following:
   a. Intact skin
   b. Abrasions
   c. Draining wounds
   d. Skin discoloration
3. Note circulation to the area requiring an elastic bandage.
   a. Palpate skin, noting temperature, color.
   b. Palpate pulse, noting pulse quality.
   c. Observe extremity for edema or dehydration.
4. Determine level of function of affected extremity.
5. Assess level of pain severity to area (scale of 0 to 10).
6. Explain procedure to patient.
7. Perform hand hygiene and apply gloves if indicated.
8. Close curtains or room door.
9. Hold roll of elastic bandage in dominant hand and use other hand to tightly hold the beginning of bandage at distal body part.
10. Apply bandage from distal point toward proximal boundary, stretching the dressing slightly, using a variety of bandage turns to cover various body shapes. Prevent uneven dressing tension or circulatory impairment by overlapping turns by one-half to two-thirds width of dressing roll. **NOTE:** Be sure that bandage is smooth (without creases).
11. Secure each roll with clip or tape before applying additional roll(s).
12. When finished with application, secure last elastic roll with clip, adhesive tape, or mesh to prevent wrap from becoming dislodged and thus decreasing extremity support.
13. Remove gloves and perform hand hygiene.
14. Evaluate circulation to dressing area every 4 hours.
    a. Palpate distal pulse.
    b. Palpate skin, noting temperature every 4 hours.
    c. Observe skin color.
15. Determine patient's level of comfort using analog scale of 0 to 10 and noting any objective signs and symptoms.
16. Observe for changes from baseline assessment in level of extremity function.

TABLE 37-6 CONDITIONS THAT INCREASE RISK FOR INJURY FROM HEAT AND COLD APPLICATION

CONDITION	RISK FACTORS
Very young; older adults	Thinner skin layers in children and older adults increase risk for burns; older adults have reduced sensitivity to pain.
Open wounds, broken skin	Subcutaneous tissue is more sensitive to temperature variations.
Areas of edema or scar formation	There is reduced sensation to temperature stimuli because of scar formation.
Peripheral vascular disease (e.g., diabetes, arteriosclerosis)	Body extremities are less sensitive to temperature and pain stimuli because of circulatory impairment and local tissue injury; cold application further compromises blood flow.
Confusion or unconsciousness	There is reduced perception of sensory or painful stimuli.
Spinal cord injury	Alterations in nerve pathways prevent reception of sensory or painful stimuli.

cells, causing redness, localized tenderness, and even blistering of the skin.

Prolonged exposure of the skin to cold results in a reflex vasodilation. The inability of the cell to receive adequate blood flow and nutrients results in tissue ischemia. The skin initially takes on a reddened appearance, followed by a bluish-purple mottling with numbness and a burning type of pain. Tissues actually freeze from exposure to extreme cold.

Factors Influencing Heat and Cold Tolerance. The response of the body to heat and cold therapies depends on the following factors:

1. *Duration of application:* A person is better able to tolerate short exposures to any temperature extremes.
2. *Body part:* The neck, inner aspect of the wrist and forearm, and perineal regions are more sensitive to temperature variations. The foot and the palm of the hand are less sensitive.
3. *Damage to body surface:* Exposed skin layers are more sensitive to temperature variations.
4. *Prior skin temperature:* The body responds best to minor temperature adjustments.
5. *Body surface area:* A person is less tolerant of temperature changes over a large area of the body.
6. *Age and physical condition:* The very young and old are most sensitive to heat and cold. If a patient's physical condition reduces the reception or perception of sensory stimuli, the tolerance to temperature extremes is high, but the risk for injury is also high.

Assessment for Temperature Tolerance. Before applying heat or cold therapies, first observe the area that you will treat

TABLE 37-7 THERAPEUTIC EFFECTS OF HEAT AND COLD APPLICATIONS

PHYSIOLOGICAL RESPONSE	THERAPEUTIC BENEFIT	EXAMPLES OF CONDITIONS TREATED
Heat Therapy		
Vasodilation Reduced blood viscosity Reduced muscle tension Increased tissue metabolism Increased capillary permeability	Improve blood flow to injured body part Promote delivery of nutrients and removal of wastes Improve delivery of leukocytes and antibiotics to wound site Promote muscle relaxation Reduce pain from spasm or stiffness Increase blood flow Provide local warmth Promote movement of waste products and nutrients	Arthritis or degenerative joint disease Localized joint pain or muscle strains Low back pain Menstrual cramping Hemorrhoidal, perianal, and vaginal inflammation Local abscesses
Cold Therapy		
Vasoconstriction Local anesthesia Reduced cell metabolism Increased blood viscosity Decreased muscle tension	Reduce blood flow to injured site, preventing edema formation Reduce inflammation Reduce localized pain Reduce oxygen needs of tissues Promote blood coagulation at injury site Relieve pain	Immediately after direct trauma (e.g., sprains, strains, fractures, muscle spasms) Superficial laceration or puncture wound Minor burn After injections Arthritis or joint trauma

so you are able to evaluate therapy-related skin changes. Alterations in skin integrity such as abrasions, open wounds, edema, bruising, bleeding, or localized areas of inflammation increase the risk for thermal injury. Identify conditions that contraindicate heat or cold therapy. *Do not* apply heat over an active area of bleeding (risk for continued bleeding) or an acute localized inflammation such as appendicitis (risk for rupture). If the patient has cardiovascular problems, do not apply heat to large portions of the body because massive vasodilation disrupts blood supply to vital organs. Cold is contraindicated if the site of injury is edematous or the patient has impaired circulation or is shivering (may intensify shivering and reduce blood flow).

Also assess the patient's sensory function and ability to recognize when heat or cold becomes excessive. If a patient has peripheral vascular disease, observe circulation to the extremities. If a patient is confused or unresponsive, observe skin temperature, circulation, and integrity frequently after therapy begins. Finally assess the condition of all equipment used, checking for cracked cords, frayed wires, damaged insulation, exposed heating components, leaks, and evenness of temperature distribution.

Patient Education and Safety. Before application of heat or cold therapy, make sure that the patient understands its purpose, the symptoms of temperature exposure, and the precautions taken to prevent injury. Box 37-15 provides safety guidelines for applying heat and cold therapy.

Applying Heat and Cold. A prerequisite to using heat or cold application is a health care provider's order, which includes the body site to be treated and the type, frequency, and duration of application. The correct temperature to use for heat and cold applications varies according to agency policy.

Choice of Moist or Dry. You administer heat and cold applications in dry or moist forms. Consider the type of wound or injury, location of the body part, and presence of drainage or inflammation when selecting dry or moist applications.

Warm Moist Compresses. A warm, moist compress improves circulation, relieves edema, and promotes concentration of pus and drainage. A **compress** is a piece of gauze dressing moistened in a prescribed warmed solution. A pack is a larger cloth or dressing applied to a larger body area.

Heat from warm compresses evaporates quickly. To maintain a constant temperature, change the compress frequently or apply a waterproof heating pad over the compress. Because moisture conducts heat, make sure that the temperature setting of the device is lower for a moist compress than for a dry application. A layer of plastic wrap or a dry towel insulates the compress and retains heat. Moist heat promotes vasodilation and evaporation of heat from the surface of the skin. For this reason a patient feels chilly. Control drafts and keep the patient covered with a blanket or robe.

Warm Soaks. Immersion of a body part in a warmed solution promotes circulation, lessens edema, increases muscle relaxation, and allows application of medicated solution. You also administer a soak by wrapping the body part in dressings and saturating them with the warmed solution.

Position the patient comfortably, place waterproof pads under the area you plan to treat, and heat the solution to the patient's tolerance. Check the temperature by placing a small amount of solution on the inside of your forearm. Adjust the temperature if the solution is too warm or not warm enough before applying it to a patient. After immersing the body part, cover the container and extremity with a towel to reduce heat loss. It is usually necessary to remove the cooled solution and the body part and add heated solution after about 10 minutes. The challenge is to keep the solution at a constant temperature. Never add a hotter solution while the body part remains immersed. After any soak, dry the body part thoroughly to prevent maceration.

Sitz Bath. The patient who has had rectal surgery or an episiotomy during childbirth or who has painful hemorrhoids or vaginal inflammation benefits from a **sitz bath,** a bath in which only the pelvic area is immersed in warm fluid. The patient sits in a special tub or chair or in a basin that fits on the toilet so the legs and feet remain out of the water. Immersing the entire body causes widespread vasodilation and negates the effect of local heat to the pelvic area.

The desired temperature for a sitz bath depends on whether the purpose is to promote relaxation or clean a wound. It is often necessary to carefully add warm water during the procedure, which usually lasts 20 minutes. A disposable basin contains an attachment that resembles an enema bag and allows the gradual introduction of warmer water.

Prevent overexposure by draping bath blankets around the patient's shoulders and thighs and controlling drafts. Make sure that the patient is able to sit in the basin or tub with feet flat on the floor and without pressure on the sacrum or thighs. Because exposure of a large portion of the body to

BOX 37-15 SAFETY GUIDELINES FOR APPLYING HEAT OR COLD THERAPY

- Explain the sensations that patient will feel during the procedure.
- Instruct patient to report changes in sensation or discomfort immediately.
- Provide a timer, clock, or watch so patient is able to help you time the application.
- Keep the call light within patient's reach.
- Refer to institution policy and procedure manual for safe temperatures.
- Do not allow patient to adjust temperature settings.
- Do not allow patient to move an application or place his or her hands on the wound site.
- Do not place patient in a position that prevents movement away from the temperature source.
- Do not leave patient who is unable to sense temperature changes or move from the temperature source unattended.

heat causes extensive vasodilation, assess the patient's pulse and facial color and ask whether he or she feels light-headed or nauseated.

Commercial Hot Packs. Commercially prepared, disposable hot packs apply warm, dry heat to an injured area. Striking, kneading, or squeezing the pack mixes chemicals that release heat. Package directions recommend the time for heat application.

Hot-Water Bottles. The hot-water bottle is an economical means of applying heat to an injured body part. Many patients use them in the home. Give patients and family members the following instructions about the safe use of water bottles:

1. Ensure that there are no leaks. Fill the bottle with warm tap water, secure the cap, and turn the bottle upside down.
2. Fill the bag only two-thirds full, expel air at the top, and secure the cap. The bag is then easier to mold over a body part.
3. Wipe off moisture on the outside of the bag.
4. Never apply a water bottle directly to the skin surface. Cover it with a towel or pillowcase.
5. Keep the bottle in place for 20 to 30 minutes.

Electric Heating Pads. Another conventional form of heat therapy is the heating pad, an electric coil enclosed within a waterproof pad covered with cotton or flannel cloth. The pad is connected to an electric cord that has a temperature-regulating unit for a high, medium, or low setting. Advise patients to avoid using the high setting and to never lie on the pad. Also advise them not to insert a safety pin through a heating pad to avoid electrical shock.

Cold Moist Compresses. The procedure for applying cold moist compresses is the same as that for warm compresses. Apply cold compresses for 20 minutes at a temperature of 15° C (59° F) to relieve inflammation and swelling. Compresses are clean or sterile. Observe for adverse reactions such as burning or numbness, mottling of the skin, redness, extreme paleness, or a bluish skin discoloration.

Cold Soaks. The procedure for preparing cold soaks and immersing a body part is the same as for warm soaks. The desired temperature for a 20-minute soak is 15° C (59° F). Take precautions to protect the patient from chilling.

Ice Bag or Collar. For a patient who has a muscle sprain, localized hemorrhage, or hematoma or has undergone dental surgery, an ice bag is ideal to prevent edema formation, control bleeding, and anesthetize the body part. Use the bag correctly:

1. Fill the bag with water, secure the cap, invert to check for leaks, and pour out the water.
2. Fill the bag two-thirds full with crushed ice so it molds easily over a body part.
3. Release air from the bag by squeezing its sides before securing the cap (because excess air interferes with conduction of cold).
4. Wipe off excess moisture.
5. Cover the bag with a flannel cover, towel, or pillowcase.
6. Apply the bag to the injury site for 20 to 30 minutes; you may reapply it in an hour.

Commercial Cold Packs. Commercially prepared, single-use ice packs come in various sizes and shapes. When you squeeze or knead the pack, an alcohol-based solution is released inside to create the cold temperature. The soft outer coverings are usually safe to apply directly to the skin surface.

Restorative and Continuing Care. Some chronic wounds are the result of underlying pathological conditions that continue long after wound healing occurs. Healing for a pressure ulcer or a chronic wound is lengthy and requires continuity of care from the acute care setting to the restorative care setting. In this setting you use many of the principles and interventions detailed in the acute care section. Continue diligent assessment to identify patients at risk for impaired skin integrity and institute preventive measures as needed.

Despite efforts with wound care, wound healing will not occur if the patient is malnourished. Tissue repair requires more protein, carbohydrates, fats, vitamins, minerals, water, and oxygen than normal tissue metabolism (see Chapter 33). In addition, the delivery of nutritional substances to tissues depends on a healthy circulatory system. Malnutrition causes an insufficient supply of the necessary nutritional elements and alterations in blood vessel integrity. Work closely with registered dietitians to provide a well-balanced diet and educate patients about the importance of good dietary habits. The surgical patient who is well nourished and has no complications requires at least 0.8 g of protein per kilogram daily for nutritional maintenance. For patients weakened or debilitated by illness, supportive nutritional therapies are necessary. Supplemental tube feedings (enteral feedings) introduce nutrients directly into the gastrointestinal tract. If a patient is unable to tolerate enteral feedings, a health care provider often orders parenteral (intravenously administered) nutrition.

The patient with a wound that restricts mobility or has the potential to compromise the function of a joint sometimes requires additional physical and/or occupational therapy. Work closely with a physical therapist to monitor a patient's activity and tolerance for exercise. It is important to optimize activity within a patient's physical limitations and return function as rapidly as possible.

EVALUATION

Patient Care. You evaluate nursing interventions for reducing and treating pressure ulcers by determining a patient's response to nursing therapies and determining whether you achieved each goal (Box 37-16). The primary goals are to prevent injury to the skin and tissues, reduce further injury to the skin and underlying tissues, and restore skin integrity. Also evaluate specific interventions designed to promote skin integrity and teach the patient and family how to reduce future threats to skin integrity. In addition, evaluate a patient's and family's need for additional support services and initiate the referral process when needed.

BOX 37-16 EVALUATION

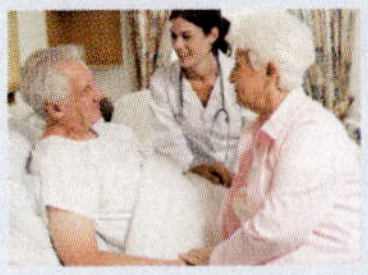

Lynda has completed her clinical experience with Mr. Ahmed. His pressure ulcer is still present, but it is reduced in size and demonstrates progress toward healing. No other sites of nonblanchable erythema are noted, and the rest of his skin remains intact. He is going to be discharged to his home in 2 days. Lynda taught Mrs. Ahmed how to do the dressing changes and how to assess her husband's skin for signs of increased risk for or actual further skin breakdown. On her last day of this clinical experience, Lynda referred her patient to a home care agency. Lynda, with the help of her instructor, devised a plan of care for the home; Lynda and her instructor are meeting with the home care nurse today when she visits Mr. and Mrs. Ahmed in the hospital.

DOCUMENTATION NOTE

"Small amount of serous drainage from stage II pressure ulcer on sacrum. Wound is 1 × 1 inch × ½ inch deep, with red tissue. Mrs. Ahmed cleansed the wound with normal saline and applied a hydrocolloid dressing. Maintained aseptic technique and correctly assessed skin. Mrs. Ahmed reminds her husband to change his position every 1½ to 2 hours. Awaiting visit from home care nurse."

Patient Expectations. A patient and caregiver need to understand how to prevent or treat pressure ulcers. Some patients enter into the wound-healing phase with unrealistic expectations regarding duration of care. Collect evaluation data about a patient's perception of wound-care management. Patients with chronic wounds receive care in their home settings and have certain expectations about their level of comfort, lifestyle, independence, and privacy. Therefore determine from the patient whether you respected and met his or her expectations.

SAFETY GUIDELINES FOR NURSING SKILLS

Ensuring patient safety is an essential role of the professional nurse. To ensure patient safety, communicate clearly with members of the health care team, assess and incorporate the patient's priorities of care and preferences, and use the best evidence when making decisions about your patient's care. When performing the skills in this chapter, remember the following points to ensure safe, individualized patient care.

- When assessing skin, reposition a patient to view all areas of the skin. Depending on a patient's mobility, condition, and size, consider asking a member of the health care team to help reposition the patient to avoid trauma or harm to the patient or caregiver.
- Skin that has not been wounded is always stronger than healed skin. When a patient has a previous history of pressure ulcer or skin damage, the healed area presents a greater risk for skin breakdown than healthy, unwounded skin.
- Modify the frequency of skin assessment to match a patient's risk.
- Modify the frequency of wound assessment based on wound condition.
- Modify skin care and pressure ulcer prevention interventions to match a patient's risk.
- Chronic diseases, especially vascular disease and diabetes, increase a patient's risk for pressure ulcer development and impede healing of wounds.
- If the potential for contamination from spray exists when cleaning a wound, use goggles and moisture-proof gowns.

SKILL 37-1 ASSESSMENT OF PATIENT FOR PRESSURE ULCER: RISK AND SKIN ASSESSMENT

View Video!

DELEGATION CONSIDERATIONS

The skill of assessment of adults for risk for pressure ulcers and skin assessment cannot be delegated to nursing assistive personnel (NAP). The nurse informs NAP to report:

- Any redness or break in the patient's skin.
- Any abrasion from assistive devices.
- Changes in patient's frequency of incontinence.

EQUIPMENT

- Risk assessment tool (e.g., Braden Scale)
- Skin assessment tool
- Documentation record
- Clean gloves

STEP	RATIONALE
ASSESSMENT	
1. Explain procedure.	Information promotes patient cooperation and reduces anxiety.
2. Perform hand hygiene. Close door or bedside curtains.	Reduces transmission of microorganisms. Maintains patient privacy.
3. Identify patient's risk for pressure ulcer formation using Braden Scale; assign a score for each of the six subscales (see Table 37-1).	Identifies patients at risk for developing pressure ulcers, allowing you to initiate individualized preventive interventions (Ayello and Braden, 2002).
4. Obtain risk score and evaluate based on patient's overall condition.	Score predicts need for interventions to prevent skin breakdown (see Table 37-1).
5. Conduct systematic skin assessment of all areas from head to toes. Apply clean gloves. Assess patient's entire body, especially at-risk areas of skin breakdown, including back of head, shoulders, ribs, hips, sacral region, ischia, inner and outer knees, inner and outer ankles, heels, and feet (see Figure 37-6)	Bony prominences are at high risk for skin breakdown because of high pressures exerted on these areas when patient is immobile. A finding of redness or impairment in skin integrity necessitates planning appropriate interventions.
6. Assess the following potential sites for skin breakdown:	
a. Ears and nares	Cartilage that nasal cannulas or tubing compresses develops pressure necrosis.
b. Lips	Oral airway and endotracheal tubes exert pressure if left in place for prolonged time periods.
c. Tube sites (e.g., gastrostomy or nasogastric tubes, Foley catheters, Jackson-Pratt drains)	Tubes exert pressure if taped snugly against skin or if there is stress at insertion site. If moisture is present around tube insertion sites, leakage of bodily fluids compromises skin integrity.
d. Orthopedic and positioning devices (e.g., casts, braces, cervical collar)	Improperly fitted or applied devices have potential to cause pressure on adjacent skin and underlying tissue.
7. Assess all skin surfaces for the following:	
a. Absence of superficial skin layers	Damage of superficial skin layers indicates injury from friction or moisture. The area is moist and sore to the touch.
b. Blisters	Suggest skin damage from friction and/or inappropriate tape removal. Blisters occur when top layer of skin is pulled or rubbed, separating epidermis from dermis.
c. Any loss of epidermis and dermis	Indicates damage to skin. Determine cause of this damage and begin interventions to prevent further damage.
IMPLEMENTATION	
1. If any risk factors receive low scores on the risk assessment tool, consider one or more of the interventions listed in Box 37-5.	Identified risk factors can be eliminated or reduced by instituting appropriate interventions.
2. Help patient change positions during assessment.	Different positions (e.g., prone, supine, side-lying) are used when completing skin assessment.
3. When you note a reddened area, check for the following:	
a. Skin discoloration (e.g., redness in light-tone skin; purplish or bluish in darkly pigmented skin) (see Box 37-4)	May indicate that tissue was under pressure.
b. Blanchable erythema	Indicates potential pressure damage that will resolve.
c. Nonblanchable erythema	Indicates potential damage to blood vessels and tissue damage. Once blood vessels are damaged, the red area does not lighten in color because tissue and blood vessels are inflamed.
d. Pallor or mottling	Persistent hypoxia in tissues alters circulation, and pallor or mottling may occur.
4. Remove gloves, perform hand hygiene, and reposition patient.	Reduces transmission of microorganisms.
EVALUATION	
1. Evaluate patient's skin daily, especially areas at high risk for breakdown (check agency policy).	Helps you determine success of prevention measures.
2. Compare current risk score with previous scores.	Allows you to determine patient progress and evaluate effectiveness of individualized plan of care.

SKILL 37-1 ASSESSMENT OF PATIENT FOR PRESSURE ULCER: RISK AND SKIN ASSESSMENT—cont'd

RECORDING AND REPORTING

- Record risk score, frequency of risk assessment, and appearance of skin, especially pressure points; describe positioning and turning schedule; describe preventive skin interventions; report changes in skin-care protocol; document consultation from skin/wound care specialists.

UNEXPECTED OUTCOMES AND RELATED INTERVENTIONS

- Skin becomes mottled, reddened, or blistered.
  - Position patient off affected area, keeping head of bed below 30-degree angle.
  - Obtain health care provider's order for skin care or pressure-reduction or pressure-relieving mattresses.
- Pressure areas become discolored or indurated or exhibit temperature changes.
  - Consult nurse specialist to revise skin care regimen for patient.
  - Consider pressure-relieving or reduction mattress.

SKILL 37-2 TREATING PRESSURE ULCERS

DELEGATION CONSIDERATIONS

The skill of pressure ulcer treatment cannot be delegated to nursing assistive personnel (NAP). The nurse instructs the NAP to:

- Position patient off affected area, keeping head of bed below 30-degree angle.

EQUIPMENT

- Clean gloves (check agency policy regarding use of sterile gloves)
- Goggles and cover gown *(optional)*
- Plastic bag for dressing disposal
- Measuring device
- Sterile cotton-tipped applicators
- Topical agent (as ordered)
- Cleansing agent (as ordered)
- Sterile solution container
- Washbasin, washcloths, towels
- Dressing of choice
- Hypoallergenic tape (if needed)
- Documentation records

STEP	RATIONALE
ASSESSMENT	
1. Identify patient using two identifiers (e.g., name and birthday or name and account number) according to agency policy.	Ensures correct patient. Complies with The Joint Commission requirements for patient safety (TJC, 2014).
2. Assess patient's level of comfort and need for pain medication. Administer analgesic as needed.	Although not all wounds are painful, in general most acute and chronic wounds cause moderate-to-severe pain (Hopf et al., 2012).
3. Determine if patient has allergies to latex or topical agents.	Latex gloves and topical agents contain elements that cause localized skin reactions if patient has allergies.
4. Review order for topical agent or dressing.	Ensures that proper medication and treatment are administered to right patient.
5. Close room door, perform hand hygiene, and apply clean gloves.	Provides privacy and prevents accidental exposure to body fluids.
6. Position patient to remove dressings if present before assessing skin. Assess each of patient's pressure ulcer(s) and surrounding skin to determine ulcer characteristics and continue ongoing wound assessment per agency policy. This is often done during dressing change.	Provides patient comfort and allows you to visualize wounds entirely.
a. *Wound location:* Describe body site where wound is located.	
b. *Stage of wound:* Describe extent of tissue destruction (see Figure 37-5).	Staging is a way of assessing a pressure ulcer, based on the depth of tissue destruction.

Clinical Decision Point: **To correctly stage a pressure ulcer, you need to be able to see the base of the wound. Therefore pressure ulcers that are covered with necrotic tissue cannot be staged until the eschar is debrided (EPUAP and NPUAP, 2009; WOCN, 2010). Document that the ulcer is unstageable if eschar is present.**

STEP	RATIONALE
c. Wound size: Measure length, width, and depth of wound per agency protocol. Measure depth of pressure ulcer using sterile cotton-tipped applicator or other device that allows measurement of wound depth. Place applicator gently into deepest portion of pressure ulcer until it touches bottom. Using a marker, mark place on applicator where it reaches top of the wound and remove applicator from ulcer. Measure distance from tip of applicator to mark with measuring tape or ruler to determine depth of pressure ulcer (see illustration).	Consistency in how wound is measured is important for determining wound progress (Nix, 2012).
d. *Presence of undermining:* Measure depth of undermining tissue. Use sterile cotton-tipped applicator to measure depth; if needed, gently probe under skin edges with gloved finger.	Wound depth determines amount of tissue loss.
e. *Condition of wound bed:* Describe type and percentage of tissue in wound bed.	Approximate percentage of each type of tissue in wound provides critical information on progress of wound healing and choice of dressing. A wound with high percentage of black tissue requires debridement, yellow tissue or slough tissue indicates presence of an infection, and granulation tissue indicates that wound is beginning to heal.
f. *Volume of exudate:* Describe amount, characteristics, odor, and color.	Amount and type of exudate often indicate type and frequency of dressing changes.
g. *Condition of skin around wound:* Note color, temperature, edema, moisture, and condition of skin around ulcer. Modify assessment technique based on patient's individual skin color (see Box 37-4).	Skin condition at ulcer edge may indicate progressive tissue damage. Maceration on skin around wound often shows need to alter choice of wound dressing.
h. *Wound edges:* Assess status of edges of wound.	Provides information about epithelialization, chronicity, and etiology.
7. Assess need for revisions to therapy during each dressing change (WOCN, 2010).	Changes in appearance of wound can indicate that topical therapy or type of dressing should be adjusted to continue to promote wound healing.
8. Remove gloves, discard appropriately, and perform hand hygiene.	Reduces transmission of microorganisms. Different wounds may be contaminated by different organisms. Failure to repeatedly perform hand hygiene can cause cross-wound contamination.
9. Assess for factors affecting wound healing such as nutrition, poor perfusion, immunosuppression, or infection.	Identified factors affect treatment decisions.
10. Assess patient's and caregiver's understanding of prevention, treatment, and factors contributing to recurrence of pressure ulcers (WOCN, 2010).	Involves patient and family to ensure patient-centered care, enhance wound healing, and prevent further skin breakdown.

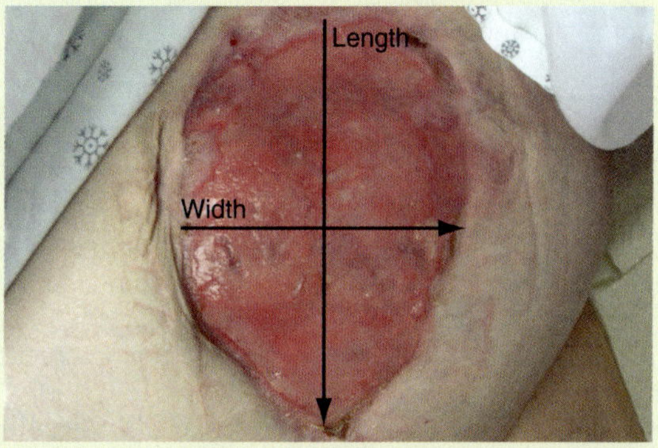

STEP 6c Measuring wound length and width. (From Bryant RA, Dix NP, editors: *Acute and chronic wounds: current management concepts,* ed 4, St Louis, 2012, Mosby.)

SKILL 37-2 TREATING PRESSURE ULCERS—cont'd

STEP	RATIONALE
PLANNING	
1. Explain procedure to patient and family. Individualize teaching plan for older-adult patients, taking into account normal aging changes that affect learning.	Preparatory explanations relieve anxiety, correct misconceptions about the ulcer and its treatment, and offer an opportunity for patient and family education.
2. Prepare the following necessary equipment and supplies:	
a. Washbasin, warm water, washcloth, and bath towel.	Used to bathe surrounding skin.
b. Normal saline or other wound-cleansing agent in sterile solution container.	Ulcer surface must be cleansed before application of topical agents and a new dressing.
Clinical Decision Point: **Use only noncytotoxic agents to clean ulcers.**	
c. Prescribed topical agent (e.g., enzymatic agents, topical antibiotic). Follow manufacturer instructions on package insert carefully.	Enzymes debride dead tissue to clean ulcer surface and are not applied to healthy tissue. Topical antibiotics are used to decrease the bioburden of the wound and should be considered for use if no healing is noted after 2 to 4 weeks of optimal care (WOCN, 2010).
Clinical Decision Point: **If using an enzymatic debriding agent, do not use wound-cleansing agents with metals.**	
d. Select an appropriate dressing and tape based on pressure ulcer characteristics, purpose for which dressing is intended, and patient care setting (see Table 37-4).	Dressing needs to maintain a moist environment for the wound while keeping surrounding skin dry (Rolstad et al., 2012).
3. Position patient to allow dressing removal and position plastic bag for dressing disposal.	Area needs to be accessible for dressing change. Proper disposal of old dressing promotes proper handling of contaminated waste.
IMPLEMENTATION	
1. Close room door or bedside curtains. Perform hand hygiene and apply clean gloves. Explain to patient what you will be doing. Bring supplies to bedside and open sterile packages and topical solution containers.	Maintains patient privacy. Provides patient with explanation of what will occur. Have supplies for easy application so you can use them without contaminating them; reduces transmission of microorganisms.
2. Remove bed linen and patient's gown to expose ulcer and surrounding skin. Keep remaining body parts draped.	Prevents unnecessary exposure of body parts.
3. Perform hand hygiene and apply clean gloves. Wear goggles, mask, and moisture-proof gown if potential for contamination from spray exists when cleaning wound.	Reduces transmission of microorganisms.
4. Remove old dressings and discard. Cleanse ulcer thoroughly with normal saline or prescribed wound-cleansing agent. Gently wash and dry periwound skin.	Cleaning skin surface reduces bacteria.
5. Remove gloves, perform hand hygiene, and apply new pair of gloves.	Maintains aseptic technique during cleaning, measuring, and applying dressings. Refer to institutional policy regarding use of clean or sterile gloves.
6. Clean wound thoroughly with normal saline or prescribed wound-cleaning agent from least contaminated to most contaminated areas.	Cleansing wound removes exudate and reduces surface bacteria.
7. Apply topical agents if prescribed, using sterile cotton-tipped applicators or gauze.	
a. Enzymes:	Follow manufacturer directions for frequency of application. Be aware of which solutions inactivate the enzymes and avoid their use in wound cleaning.
(1) Using a wooden tongue blade, apply small amount of enzyme debridement ointment directly to necrotic areas on base of pressure ulcer. Do not apply enzyme to surrounding skin.	Proper distribution of ointment ensures effective action. Some enzymes can cause transient erythema and irritation when in contact with intact skin (Ramundo, 2012).
(2) Place moist gauze dressing directly over ulcer and tape in place. Follow specific manufacturer recommendation for type of dressing material to use to cover a pressure ulcer when using enzymatic agent.	Protects wound and prevents removal of ointment during turning or repositioning.

STEP	RATIONALE
b. Antibacterials: If using an antibiotic preparation, apply per order and cover with gauze pad. Generally preparation is applied every 12 hours.	Reduces bacterial growth.
8. Apply prescribed wound dressing:	
a. Hydrogel agents:	
(1) Cover surface of ulcer with thick layer of amorphous hydrogel using applicator or gloved hand or cut a sheet to fit wound base.	Provides moist environment, facilitating wound healing.
(2) Apply secondary dressing such as dry gauze, hydrocolloid, or transparent dressing over gel to completely cover ulcer.	Holds hydrogel against wound surface because hydrogel amorphous form (in tube) or sheet form does not adhere to wound and requires secondary dressing to hold it in place.
(3) If using impregnated gauze, pack loosely into wound; cover with secondary gauze dressing and tape.	Loosely packed dressing delivers gel to wound base and allows wound debris to be trapped in gauze.
c. Calcium alginates:	Use in heavily draining wounds.
(1) Pack wound lightly with alginate using sterile cotton-tipped applicator or gloved finger.	Dressing swells and increases in size; tight packing can compromise blood flow to the tissues.
(2) Apply secondary dressing such as dry gauze, foam, or hydrocolloid over alginate and tape in place.	Holds alginate against wound surface.
9. Reposition patient comfortably off pressure ulcer.	Avoids accidental removal of dressings.
10. Remove gloves and dispose of soiled supplies. Perform hand hygiene.	Reduces transmission of microorganisms.
EVALUATION	
1. Observe skin surrounding ulcer for inflammation, edema, and tenderness.	Determines progress of wound healing. Expect clean pressure ulcer to show evidence of movement toward healing within 2 to 4 weeks.
2. Inspect dressings and exposed ulcers, observing for drainage, foul odor, and tissue necrosis. Monitor patient for signs and symptoms of infection, including fever and elevated white blood cell (WBC) count.	Ulcers can become infected.
3. Compare subsequent ulcer measurements.	Allows standardized objective comparison of serial measurements to assess wound healing.
4. Use one of the scales designed to measure wound healing such as PUSH Scale (Nix, 2012) or Bates-Jensen Wound Assessment Tool (Harris et al., 2010).	Provides standard method of data collection that demonstrates wound progress or lack thereof.

RECORDING AND REPORTING

- Record appearance of ulcer in patient's record; describe type of topical agent used, dressing applied, and patient's response; report any deterioration in ulcer appearance to nurse in charge or health care provider.

UNEXPECTED OUTCOMES AND RELATED INTERVENTIONS

- Skin surrounding ulcer becomes macerated.
  - Reduce exposure of surrounding skin to topical agents and moisture.
  - Select a dressing that has increased moisture-absorbing capacity.
- Ulcer becomes deeper with increased drainage and/or development of necrotic tissue.
  - Review current wound care management.
  - Consult with multidisciplinary team regarding changes in wound care regimen.
  - Obtain wound cultures.
- Pressure ulcer extends beyond original margins.
  - Monitor for systemic signs and symptoms of poor wound healing such as abnormal laboratory results (WBC, hemoglobin/hematocrit, serum albumin, serum prealbumin, total proteins), weight loss, and fluid imbalance).
  - Assess and revise current turning schedule.
  - Consider different pressure-relieving devices (see Table 37-3).

SKILL 37-3 NEGATIVE-PRESSURE WOUND THERAPY

DELEGATION CONSIDERATIONS

The skill of negative pressure wound therapy (NPWT) cannot be delegated to nursing assistive personnel (NAP). The nurse instructs NAP to:

- Use caution when repositioning or turning a patient to avoid displacement of tubing.
- Report changes in the patient's temperature or level of comfort.
- Report changes in the integrity of the NPWT unit or dressing.

EQUIPMENT

- NPWT system (requires health care provider's order) (see Figure 37-12)
- NPWT dressing (gauze or foam, see manufacturer recommendations; transparent dressing; adhesive drape)
- NPWT suction device
- NPWT tubing for connection between unit and dressing
- Three pairs of gloves, clean and sterile
- Scissors, sterile
- Waterproof bag for disposal
- Skin protectant/stomahesive/hydrocolloid dressings/skin barrier
- Protective gown, mask, goggles (used when spray from wound is a risk)

STEP	RATIONALE
ASSESSMENT	
1. Identify patient using two identifiers (i.e., name and birthday or name and account number) according to agency policy. Compare identifiers with information on MAR or medical record.	Complies with The Joint Commission requirements for patient safety (TJC, 2014).
2. Assess location, appearance, and size of wound to be dressed.	Allows you to gather information regarding status of wound healing, presence of complications, and type of supplies and assistance needed to apply NPWT dressing.
3. Review health care provider's orders for frequency of dressing change, type of foam to use, and amount of negative pressure to be used.	Health care provider orders frequency of dressing changes and special instructions.
4. Assess patient's level of comfort using scale of 0 to 10.	Patient who is comfortable during procedure is less likely to move suddenly, causing wound or supply contamination.
5. Assess patient's and family member's knowledge of purpose of dressing.	Identifies patient's learning needs. Prepares patient and family if dressing needs to be changed at home.
PLANNING	
1. Collect equipment and arrange at bedside.	Organizes procedure.
2. Explain procedure to patient.	Relieves anxiety and promotes understanding of healing process.
3. Position patient to allow access to wound site.	Facilitates application of dressing.
4. Plan dressing change to occur 30 minutes after analgesic is administered.	Provides time for pain medication to reduce or relieve patient's pain at wound site.
IMPLEMENTATION	
1. Close room door or cubicle curtains.	Provides for patient privacy and reduces transmission of organisms.
2. Position patient, expose wound site, and cover patient.	Draping provides access to wound while minimizing exposure. Positioning ensures patient comfort during procedure.
3. Cuff top of disposable waterproof bag and place within reach of work area.	Cuff prevents accidental contamination of top of outer bag.
4. Perform hand hygiene and put on clean gloves. If risk for spray exists, apply protective gown, goggles, and mask.	Reduces transmission of infectious organisms from soiled dressings to nurse's hands.
5. Follow manufacturer directions for removal and replacement; each NPWT unit varies slightly. Push off button on NPWT system.	Deactivates therapy.
6. Raise tubing connectors above level of NPWT unit. Engage clamp on dressing tubing.	Allows for proper drainage of fluid in drainage tubing.
7. Separate canister and dressing tubing at connection junctions.	
8. Allow therapy unit to pull any drainage in canister tubing into canister; engage clamp on canister tubing.	

STEP	RATIONALE
9. Gently stretch transparent film horizontally and slowly pull up from skin.	Reduces stress on suture line or wound edges and reduces irritation and discomfort.
10. Remove dressing. Observe appearance of drainage on dressing. Dispose of soiled dressings in waterproof bag. Keep soiled dressings away from patient's sight. Remove gloves by pulling them inside out and dispose of them in waterproof bag. Perform hand hygiene.	Determines dressings needed for replacement. Avoids accidental removal of drains. Reduces transmission of microorganisms.
11. Apply sterile or clean gloves. Irrigate wound with normal saline or other solution ordered by health care provider. Gently blot to dry (see Skill 37-5).	Irrigation removes wound debris and cleanses wound bed.
12. Measure and assess wound as ordered: at baseline, first dressing change, weekly, and discharge from therapy. Remove and discard gloves. Perform hand hygiene.	Provides objective measure of wound healing progress.

Clinical Decision Point: **Obtain cultures during the dressing change if there are local signs of infection: pus, change in odor or character of exudate, redness, induration, or change in wound odor (Stotts, 2012).**

STEP	RATIONALE
13. Depending on type of wound, apply new sterile or clean gloves.	Fresh sterile wounds require sterile gloves. Chronic wounds may require clean technique. Do not use the same gloves worn to remove old dressing because cross-contamination may occur.
14. Prepare wound edges with skin preparation product to enhance dressing seal and protect periwound skin.	
15. Select appropriate dressing, depending on wound type and stage of healing. Use sterile scissors to cut dressing to wound size, making sure to fit size and shape of wound. Fill wound with wound dressing.	Several wound dressings are used for NPWT, including open cell foam, silicone tubing wrapped with gauze, honeycomb-configured nonadherent matrix, and non-woven superabsorbent polymer (Netsch, 2012).
16. Place wound dressing gently all the way into undermined, tunneled, or sinus area. A 1- to 2-cm amount of wound dressing should be withdrawn from opening of undermined, tunneled, or sinus area (Netsch, 2012) (see illustration).	Fills entire wound, preventing dead space. Achieves even distribution of negative pressure (Netsch, 2012).
17. Cover with adherent transparent dressing (see illustration). Mark on adherent dressing the number of wound filler pieces used (Netsch, 2012).	Provides airtight seal. Ensures that all wound filler pieces are removed at next dressing change.
18. Trim transparent dressing to cover wound and overlap onto intact healthy surrounding skin (see illustration).	Ensures that wound is properly covered and negative-pressure seal can be achieved.
19. Open all clamps and place suction device per manufacturer directions. Connect to suction device.	Each company's devices have different types of suction and connections.
20. Adjust suction settings according to order. Check seal to be sure that there are no air leaks.	Air leaks indicate that suction is not achieved, and all air leaks needs to be addressed.
21. Change canister as needed; check manufacturer information.	
22. Discard soiled dressing-change materials properly. Remove gloves. Perform hand hygiene.	Reduces transmission of microorganisms.

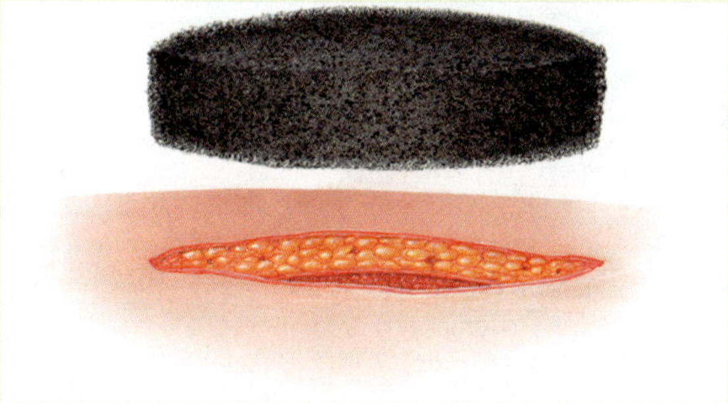

STEP 16 Dressing application. Properly sized foam dressing to cover wound.

A

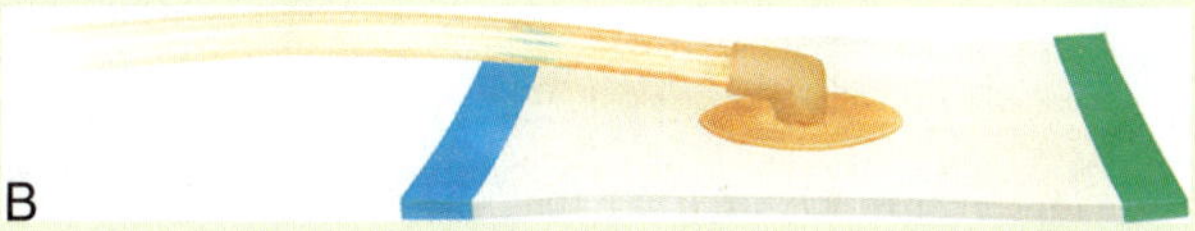

B

STEP 17 A, Transparent dressing. **B,** Secure tubing to foam and transparent dressing unit. (Courtesy KCI Licensing, San Antonio, TX.)

SKILL 37-3 NEGATIVE-PRESSURE WOUND THERAPY—cont'd

STEP	RATIONALE
23. Inspect NPWT unit to verify that negative pressure is achieved. **a.** Verify that display screen reads THERAPY ON. **b.** Be sure that clamps are open and tubing is patent. **c.** If leak is present, use strips of transparent film to patch areas around edges of wound.	Negative pressure is reached when airtight seal is achieved.
24. Help patient to comfortable position.	Enhances patient comfort and relaxation.
EVALUATION	
1. Inspect condition of wound on ongoing basis; note drainage and odor.	Determines status of wound healing.
2. Ask patient to rate pain on scale of 0 to 10.	Determines patient's level of comfort following procedure.
3. Verify airtight dressing seal and correct negative pressure setting.	Determines patient's level of comfort following procedure.
4. Measure wound drainage output in canister on regular basis.	Monitors fluid balance and wound drainage.
5. Observe patient's or family member's ability to perform dressing change.	Indicates that patient and family learning has occurred.

RECORDING AND REPORTING

- Record wound appearance, color and characteristics of any drainage, presence of wound healing, and patient tolerance to procedure. Record date and time of new dressing on the dressing as per agency policy.
- Report any brisk, bright red bleeding; evidence of poor wound healing; evisceration or dehiscence; and possible wound infection.

UNEXPECTED OUTCOMES AND RELATED INTERVENTIONS

- Wound appears inflamed and tender, drainage has increased, and odor is present.
  - Notify health care provider.
  - Obtain wound culture.
- Patient reports increase in pain.
  - If using black foam, switch to white foam.
- Patient needs more analgesic support when NPWT unit is initiated.
  - Reduce negative pressure.
- Negative pressure seal has broken.
  - Take preventive measures; before applying transparent dressing, clip hair around wound; avoid wrinkles in transparent dressing; and avoid use of adhesive remover because it leaves a residue that interferes with adherence.
  - Reinforce with transparent dressing strips.

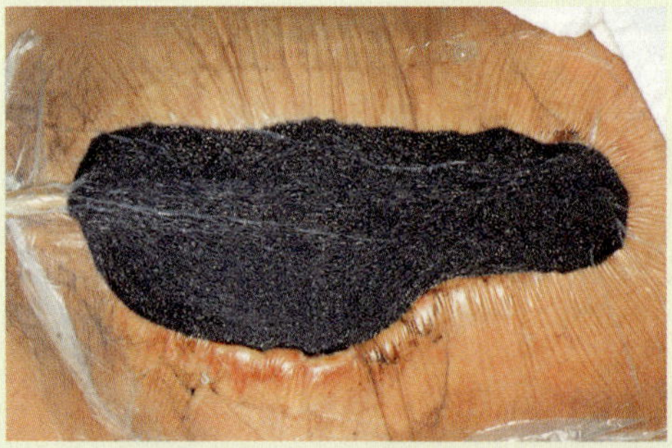

STEP 18 Foam dressing covered by transparent dressing with suction in place. (Courtesy KCI Licensing, San Antonio, TX.)

SKILL 37-4 APPLYING DRESSINGS: DRY, MOIST, AND TRANSPARENT

View Video!

DELEGATION CONSIDERATIONS

The skill of applying dressings to acute new wounds and those that require sterile technique or a moist dressing cannot be delegated to nursing assistive personnel (NAP). In some states you can delegate certain aspects of wound care. This sometimes includes the changing a dry dressing or changing the top dressing. The nurse always completes the *assessment* of the wound. The nurse instructs the NAP about:

- Any unique modifications of the skill such as the need for special tape or methods to secure the dressing.
- The need to immediately report increased erythema, drainage, redness in the skin around the wound, or increased pain in the area, which may indicate signs of infection or poor wound healing.

EQUIPMENT

- Clean and sterile gloves (check agency policy regarding use of sterile gloves)
- Sterile dressing set (scissors, forceps) (may be *optional;* check agency policy)
- Sterile drape *(optional)*
- Dressings: Sterile fine mesh 4 × 4 gauze flats, abdominal (ABD) pads, roll gauze, and transparent dressing
- Sterile basin *(optional)*
- Antiseptic ointment (as prescribed)
- Cleansing solution (as prescribed)
- Sterile normal saline or prescribed solution
- Tape, ties, or dressing as needed (include nonallergenic tape if necessary)
- Protective waterproof underpad
- Waterproof bag
- Adhesive remover *(optional)*
- Measurement device (optional): Tape measure, camera *(optional)*
- Protective gown, mask, goggles (used when spray from wound is a risk)
- Additional lighting if needed (e.g., flashlight, treatment light)

STEP	RATIONALE
ASSESSMENT	
1. Identify patient using two identifiers (e.g., name and birthday or name and account number) according to agency policy. Explain procedure.	Ensures correct patient. Complies with The Joint Commission requirements for patient safety (TJC, 2014).
2. Assess size of wound to be dressed (see Skill 37-2).	Helps in planning for proper type and amount of supplies needed.
3. Assess location of wound.	Determines dressing type needed and if assistance is needed to hold dressings in place.
4. Ask patient to rate pain using scale of 0 to 10.	Removal of dressing can be painful; patient may require pain medication before dressing change to allow peak effect of drug during procedure.
5. Assess patient's knowledge of purpose of dressing change.	Determines level of support and explanation that patient requires.
6. Assess need and readiness for patient or family member to participate in dressing wound.	Prepares patient or family member if dressing must be changed at home.
7. Review medical orders for dressing change procedure.	Indicates type of dressing or applications to use.
8. Identify patients with risk factors for wound-healing problems (e.g., aging, prematurity, obesity, diabetes, compromised circulation, poor nutritional status, immunosuppressive drugs, irradiation in area of wound, steroids).	Risk factors have potential to affect wound healing and resistance to pathogens (Doughty and Sparks-DeFriese, 2012).
PLANNING	
1. Explain procedure to patient.	Decreases patient's anxiety.
2. Position patient to allow access to area to be dressed.	Facilitates application of dressing.
3. Plan dressing change to occur 30 to 60 minutes following administration of analgesic if analgesic is needed.	Dressing change is better tolerated by patient if pain medication has been administered at least 30 minutes before dressing change.
4. Gather all necessary supplies and bring to bedside.	
IMPLEMENTATION	
1. Close room or cubicle curtains. Perform hand hygiene. Apply gown, goggles, and mask if risk for spray exists.	Provides for privacy and reduces transmission of microorganisms.
2. Position patient comfortably and drape to expose only wound site. Instruct patient not to touch wound or sterile supplies.	Draping provides access to wound yet minimizes unnecessary exposure.

SKILL 37-4 APPLYING DRESSINGS: DRY, MOIST, AND TRANSPARENT—cont'd

STEP	RATIONALE
3. Place disposable bag within reach of work area. Fold top of bag to make cuff. Put on clean gloves. Put on gown, goggles, and mask if risk for splashing exists.	Ensures easy disposal of soiled dressings. Prevents contamination of outer surface of bag. Prevents transmission of microorganisms.
4. Remove tape: Gently pull parallel to skin, toward dressing, and hold down skin. If over hairy areas, remove in direction of hair growth. Remove remaining adhesive from skin.	Pulling tape toward dressing reduces stress on suture line or wound edges, irritation, and discomfort.
5. With clean-gloved hand or forceps remove dressings. Carefully remove outer secondary dressing first and then remove inner primary dressing that is in contact with the wound bed. If drains are present, slowly and carefully remove dressings one layer at a time. Keep soiled undersurface from patient's sight.	Purpose of primary dressing is to remove necrotic tissue and exudate. Avoids accidental removal of drain. Appearance of drainage may be upsetting to patient.
6. Inspect wound for color, edema, drains, exudate, and integrity (see illustration). Observe appearance of drainage on dressing. Assess for odor. Gently palpate wound edges for drainage, bogginess, or patient report of increased pain. Measure wound size (length, width, and depth [if indicated]) (see Skill 37-2).	Provides assessment of drainage and condition of wound. Indicates movement toward healing (Nix, 2012).

Clinical Decision Point: **Dressings that are heavily saturated with exudate indicate a need to add more absorbent dressings to the wound. Assess the wound for any changes in color, drainage, odor, or edema.**

STEP	RATIONALE
7. Describe appearance of wound and any indicators of wound healing to the patient.	Wounds may appear unsettling and frightening to patients; it is helpful for patient to know that wound appearance is as expected and that healing is taking place.
8. Dispose of soiled dressings in disposable bag. Remove gloves by pulling them inside out. Dispose of gloves in bag. Perform hand hygiene.	Reduces transmission of microorganisms.
9. Open sterile dressing tray or individually wrapped sterile supplies. Place on bedside table.	Sterile dressings remain sterile while on or within sterile surface. Preparation of all supplies prevents break in technique during dressing change.
10. Open prescribed cleansing solution and pour over sterile gauze.	Keeps supplies sterile. Solution may be packaged to spray or pour directly on wound. Microorganisms move from nonsterile environment through dressing package to dressing itself by capillary action.

Clinical Decision Point: **If sterile drape or gauze packages become wet from solution, repeat preparation of supplies.**

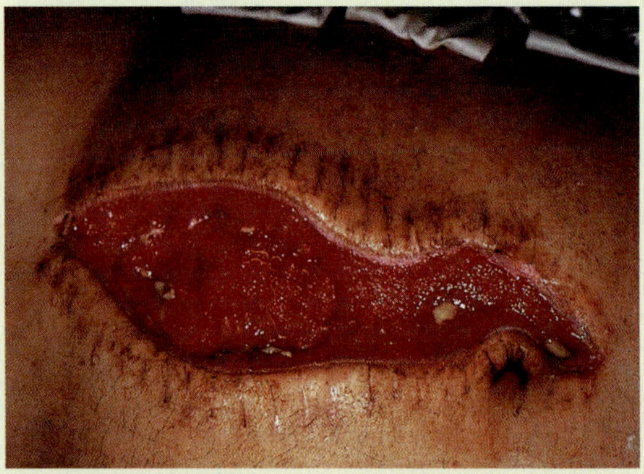

STEP 6 Abdominal wound with beefy red granulation tissue present and attached wound edges. (From Bryant RA, Dix NP, editors: *Acute and chronic wounds: current management concepts,* ed 4, St Louis, 2012, Mosby.)

STEP	RATIONALE
11. Put on gloves, clean or sterile, depending on institution policy.	Sterile gloves allow handling of sterile supplies without contamination. Follow guidelines of health care institution related to clean versus sterile gloves. There is insufficient research to support either sterile or clean gloves as being more effective in decreasing infection and improving wound healing (WOCN, 2011).
12. Cleanse wound:	
a. Use separate swab for each cleansing stroke or spray wound surface.	Prevents contaminating previously cleaned area.
b. Clean from least contaminated to most contaminated area, with center of wound least contaminated.	Cleaning in this direction prevents introduction of organisms into wound.
c. Clean around drain (if present), using circular stroke starting near drain and moving outward and away from insertion site.	Correct aseptic technique in cleaning prevents contamination of wound.
13. Use dry gauze to blot in same manner as in Step 12 to dry wound.	Drying reduces excess moisture, which could eventually harbor microorganisms. Transparent dressings do not adhere to damp surfaces.
14. Apply antiseptic ointment if ordered.	Helps reduce growth of microorganisms.
15. Apply dressings to incision or wound site:	Dressing protects wound, prevents infection, and provides comfort.
a. Dry Dressing	
(1) Apply loose woven gauze as contact layer.	Promotes proper absorption of drainage.
(2) Cut 4 × 4 gauze to fit around drain if present or use precut split drain.	Secures drain and promotes drainage absorption at site.
(3) Apply additional layers of gauze as needed.	Layering ensures proper coverage and optimal absorption.
(4) Apply thicker woven pad (e.g., Surgipad, ABD dressing).	This type of dressing is often used for postoperative wounds.
b. Moist Dressing	
(1) Moisten gauze dressing with prescribed solution.	

Clinical Decision Point: **Open or unfold the gauze that will be placed directly against the wound bed. Sometimes "packing strip" may be used to pack the wound (see illustration *A* for Step 15b[2]). When using packing strip, with sterile scissors cut the amount of dressing that you anticipate to be used to pack the wound. Do not let the packing strip touch the side of the bottle. Pour prescribed solution over the gauze or strip to moisten it; wring out excess fluid. Contact layer must be moist to increase absorptive abilities of dressing.**

STEP	RATIONALE
(2) Wring out excess fluid and apply moist fluffed gauze or packing strip directly onto wound surface; do not let gauze touch surrounding skin (see illustration *A*).	Moist gauze absorbs drainage and wicks wound debris (Rolstad, Bryant, and Nix, 2012).

Clinical Decision Point: **If wound is deep, gently lay moistened gauze over wound surface with forceps until all surfaces are in contact with moist gauze and the wound is loosely filled. Fill the wound but avoid packing the wound too tightly or having the gauze extend beyond the top of the wound (see illustration *B,* Step 15b[2]).**

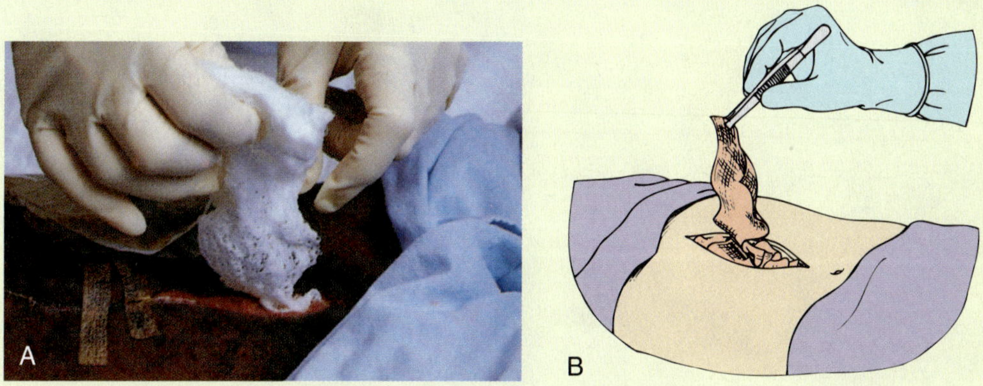

STEP 15b(2) A, Packing wound. **B,** Wound packed loosely until wound is filled.

SKILL 37-4 APPLYING DRESSINGS: DRY, MOIST, AND TRANSPARENT—cont'd

STEP	RATIONALE
(3) Make sure that any dead space from sinus tracts, undermining, or tunneling is loosely packed with gauze.	Do not overpack wound too tightly; it can cause wound trauma (Rolstad et al., 2012).
(4) Apply dry, sterile gauze over moistened gauze.	Dry layer absorbs excessive moisture from wound.
(5) Cover packed wound with secondary dressing such as an ABD pad, Surgipad, or gauze. Tape in place.	Protects wound from entrance of microorganisms.
c. **Transparent Dressing**	
(1) Apply dressing according to manufacturer directions. Do not stretch film during application. Avoid wrinkles in film.	Wrinkles provide tunnel for exudate to accumulate.
16. Secure dressing with roll gauze (for circumferential dressings) (see illustration *A*), tape, or Montgomery ties or straps (see illustration *B*), or binder.	Supports wound and ensures placement and stability of dressing.

Clinical Decision Point: **If areas of redness appear from tape, paper tape or alternatives such as elastic dressing, Kerlix, or a binder may be used to secure dressing. Sometimes strips of a hydrocolloid dressing are placed on the skin under the Montgomery ties to protect the skin from the adhesive.**

STEP	RATIONALE
17. Remove gloves and gown (if worn) and dispose of in bag. Dispose of all supplies. Remove goggles if worn.	Reduces transmission of microorganisms. Clean environment enhances patient comfort.
18. Help patient to comfortable position.	Promotes patient's sense of well-being.
19. Perform hand hygiene.	Reduces transmission of microorganisms.
EVALUATION	
1. Inspect condition of wound and presence of any drainage.	Determines rate of healing.
2. Have patient rate level of pain during procedure.	Pain is often an early indication of wound complication or result of dressing pulling tissue.
3. Inspect condition of dressing at least every shift.	Determines status of wound drainage.
4. Ask patient to describe steps and techniques of dressing change.	Evaluates patient's learning.

RECORDING AND REPORTING

- Record appearance of wound; color; presence and characteristics of exudate; change in wound characteristics, especially drainage amount; type and amount of dressings applied; and tolerance of patient to dressing change.
- Report unexpected appearance of wound drainage or accidental removal of drain, bright red bleeding, or evidence of wound dehiscence or evisceration.
- Write your initials, date, and time of dressing change on a piece of tape in ink (not marker) and place on dressing.

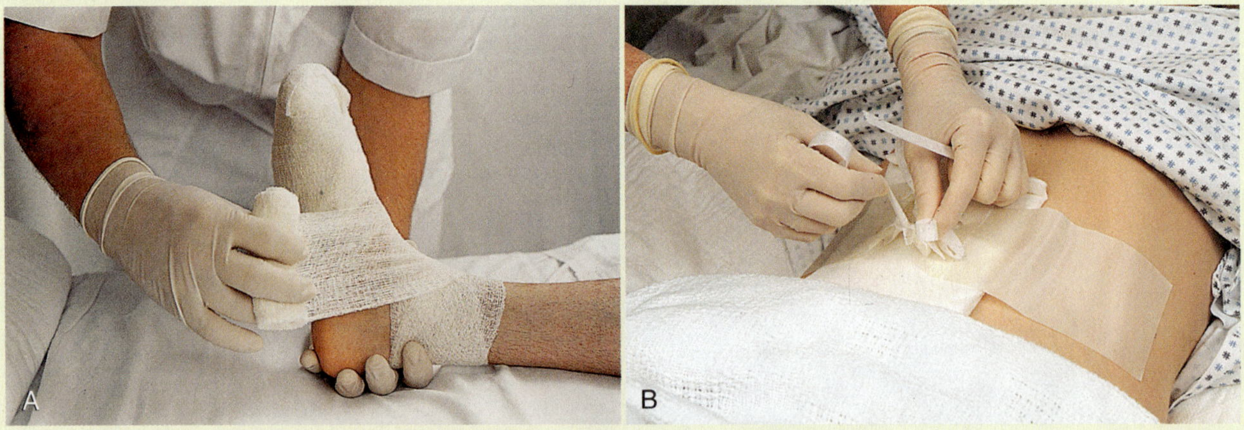

STEP 16 **A,** Application of roll gauze. **B,** Securing Montgomery ties.

UNEXPECTED OUTCOMES AND RELATED INTERVENTIONS

- Wound drainage increases.
  - Increase frequency of dressing changes.
  - Notify health care provider, who may consider alternative dressing method.
- Wound bleeds during dressing change.
  - Assess patient medication history and history of bleeding disorder.
  - If excessive, may need to apply pressure.
  - Observe color and amount of drainage.
  - Notify health care provider.
- Patient reports sensation that "something has given way under the dressing."
  - Remove dressing and inspect wound for dehiscence or evisceration.
  - Protect wound. Cover with sterile moist dressing.
  - Instruct patient to lie still.
  - Remain with patient to monitor vital signs.
  - Notify health care provider.
- Skin around wound margins becomes red, macerated, or excoriated.
  - Avoid allowing outer layer of wet-to-dry dressing to become too moist.
  - Notify health care provider.
  - Consult with wound care specialist on the appropriate dressing to use.
  - Securing method for dressing is causing irritation.
  - Change to paper tape.

SKILL 37-5 PERFORMING WOUND IRRIGATION

View Video!

DELEGATION CONSIDERATIONS

The skill of wound irrigation cannot be delegated to nursing assistive personnel (NAP). In some settings you can delegate the cleansing of chronic wounds using clean technique to NAP. It is the responsibility of the nurse to assess the wound and evaluate wound care interventions before any delegation. The nurse instructs the NAP to:

- Report any changes in patient's comfort level, wound drainage, increase in temperature, or any bright red drainage.
- Report the wound color, presence of bleeding, or drainage when a wound is cleansed.

EQUIPMENT

- Irrigant/cleansing solution (volume 1 to 2 times the estimated wound volume)
- Irrigation delivery system, depending on amount of pressure desired
- Sterile 35-mL irrigation syringe with sterile soft angiocatheter or 19-gauge needle (WOCN, 2010)
- Clean and sterile gloves
- Waterproof underpad if needed
- Dressing supplies
- Disposable waterproof bag
- Gown, goggles, mask for risk for spray
- Wound assessment supplies

STEP	RATIONALE
ASSESSMENT	
1. Identify patient using two identifiers (e.g., name and birthday or name and account number) according to agency policy. Explain procedure.	Ensures correct patient. Complies with The Joint Commission requirements for patient safety (TJC, 2014).
2. Review health care provider's order for irrigation of open wound and type of solution to be used.	Open-wound irrigation requires medical order, including type of solution(s) to use.
3. Assess recent documentation of signs and symptoms related to patient's open wound:	
a. Extent of impairment of skin integrity, including size of wound (measure length, width, and depth). Wounds are measured in centimeters and in the following order: length, width, and depth.	Determines volume of irrigation solution needed. Data also used as baseline to indicate change in condition of wound.
b. Drainage from wound (amount and color). Amount can be measured by part of dressing saturated or in terms of quantity (e.g., scant, moderate, copious).	Expect amount to decrease as healing takes place. Serous drainage is clear like plasma; sanguineous or bright red drainage indicates fresh bleeding; serosanguineous drainage is pink; purulent drainage is thick and yellow, pale green, or white.
c. Odor. Must state whether or not there is odor.	Strong odor indicates infectious process.
d. Wound color.	Color represents balance between necrotic tissue and new scar tissue. Proper selection of wound products based on color of wound facilitates removal of necrotic tissue and promotes new tissue growth (Rolstad et al., 2012).
e. Consistency of drainage.	Type and color of drainage depends on wound moisture and type of organisms present.

SKILL 37-5 PERFORMING WOUND IRRIGATION—cont'd

STEP	RATIONALE
f. Culture reports.	Chronic wounds heal by secondary intention, and they are often colonized with bacteria.
g. Dressing: Dry and clean; evidence of bleeding, profuse drainage.	Provides an initial assessment of present wound drainage.
4. Assess comfort level or pain on scale of 0 to 10 and identify symptoms of anxiety.	Discomfort may be related directly to wound or indirectly to muscle tension or immobility. Anxiety results from multiple factors (e.g., surgery, diagnosis, awaiting pathology reports) and anticipation of unknown nursing interventions (e.g., first wound irrigation).
5. Assess patient for history of allergies to antiseptics, tapes, or dressing material.	Known allergies suggest application of a sample of prescribed antiseptic as skin test before flushing wound with large volume of solution or selection of different tape or dressing material.
PLANNING	
1. Explain procedure of wound irrigation and cleansing and bring all supplies to bedside.	Providing information and being prepared reduces patient's anxiety.
2. Administer prescribed analgesic 30 to 60 minutes before starting wound irrigation procedure if necessary.	Promotes pain control and permits patient to move more easily and be positioned to facilitate wound irrigation.
3. Position patient.	
a. Position comfortably to permit gravitational flow of irrigating solution through wound and into collection receptacle (see illustration).	Directing solution from top to bottom of wound and from clean to contaminated area prevents further infection. Position patient during planning stage, keeping in mind bed surfaces needed for later preparation of equipment.
b. Position patient so wound is vertical to collection basin. Place container of irrigant/cleaning solution in basin of hot water to warm solution to body temperature.	Warmed solution increases comfort and reduces vascular constriction response in tissues.
c. Place padding or extra towel in the bed.	Protects bedding.
d. Expose only wound.	Prevents chilling of patient.
IMPLEMENTATION	
1. Perform hand hygiene.	Reduces transmission of microorganisms.
2. Form cuff on waterproof biohazard bag and place it near bed.	Cuffing helps to maintain large opening, thereby permitting placement of contaminated dressing without touching refuse bag itself.
3. Close room door or bed curtains.	Maintains privacy.
4. Apply gown, goggles, and mask.	Protects nurse from splashes or sprays of blood and body fluids.
5. Apply clean gloves and remove soiled dressing and discard in waterproof bag. Discard gloves. Perform hand hygiene.	Reduces transmission of microorganisms.
6. Prepare equipment; open sterile supplies.	
7. Apply sterile gloves.	Prevents transfer of microorganisms to wound surface.

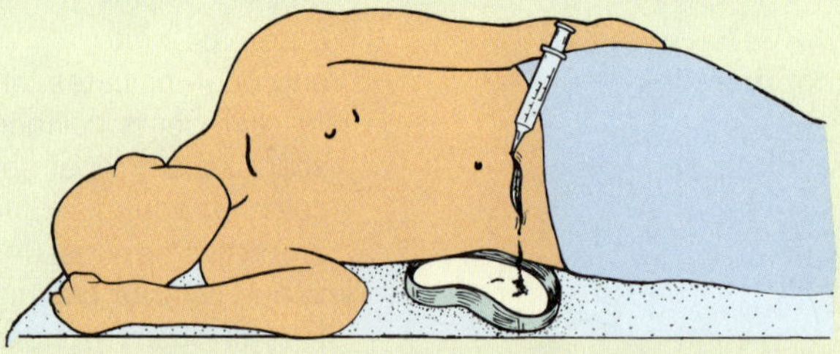

STEP 3a Position of patient for abdominal wound irrigation.

STEP	RATIONALE
8. To irrigate wound with wide opening:	
a. Fill 35-mL syringe with irrigation solution.	Flushing wound helps remove debris and facilitates healing by secondary intention.
b. Attach 19-gauge angiocatheter.	Provides ideal pressure for cleaning and removal of debris (Rolstad et al., 2012).
c. Hold syringe tip 2.5 cm (1 inch) above upper end of wound and over area being cleaned.	Prevents syringe contamination. Careful placement of syringe prevents unsafe pressure of flowing solution.
d. Using continuous pressure, flush wound; repeat Steps 8a, b, and c until solution draining into basin is clear.	Clear solution indicates that all debris has been removed.
9. To irrigate deep wound with very small opening:	
a. Attach angiocatheter to filled irrigating syringe.	Catheter permits direct flow of irrigant into wound. Expect wound to take longer to empty when opening is small.
b. Gently insert tip of catheter and pull out about 1 cm (½ inch).	Removes tip from fragile inner wall of wound.

***Clinical Decision Point:* Do not force catheter into the wound because this could cause tissue damage.**

STEP	RATIONALE
c. Using slow, continuous pressure, flush wound.	Provides adequate force to remove debris without damaging healthy tissue (Ramundo, 2012).

***Clinical Decision Point:* CAUTION: Splashing may occur during this step.**

STEP	RATIONALE
d. Remove and refill syringe. Reconnect to catheter and repeat until solution draining into basin is clear.	

***Clinical Decision Point:* Pulsatile high-pressure lavage may be the irrigation of choice for necrotic wounds. The amount of irrigant depends on the size of the wound. Keep pressure settings on the device between 8 and 15 psi. Do not use pulsatile high-pressure lavage on exposed blood vessels, muscle, tendon, and bone. Do not use this type of irrigation with graft sites and use it with caution in patients receiving anticoagulant therapy (Ramundo, 2012).**

STEP	RATIONALE
10. When indicated, obtain cultures after cleaning with nonbacteriostatic saline.	

***Clinical Decision Point:* Consider culturing a wound if it has a foul, purulent odor; inflammation surrounds the wound; a nondraining wound begins to drain; or patient is febrile.**

STEP	RATIONALE
11. Dry wound edges with gauze; dry patient if shower or whirlpool is used.	Prevents maceration of surrounding tissue from excess moisture.
12. Apply appropriate dressing (see Skill 37-4).	Maintains protective barrier and healing environment for wound.
13. Remove gloves, mask, goggles, and gown.	Prevents transfer of microorganisms.
14. Help patient to comfortable position.	
15. Dispose of equipment and soiled supplies and perform hand hygiene.	Reduces transmission of microorganisms.

EVALUATION

STEP	RATIONALE
1. Observe type of tissue in wound bed.	Identifies wound healing progress and determines type of wound cleaning and dressing needed.
2. Inspect dressing periodically.	Determines patient's response to wound irrigation and need to modify plan of care.
3. Evaluate skin integrity.	Determines if extension of wound has occurred.
4. Observe patient for signs of discomfort.	Patient's pain should not increase as a result of wound irrigation.
5. Observe for presence of retained irrigant.	Retained irrigant is medium for bacterial growth and subsequent infection.

RECORDING AND REPORTING

- Record wound irrigation and patient response in progress notes.
- Immediately report any evidence of fresh bleeding, sharp increase in pain, retention of irrigant, or signs of shock to attending health care provider.

SKILL 37-5 PERFORMING WOUND IRRIGATION—cont'd

UNEXPECTED OUTCOMES AND RELATED INTERVENTIONS

- Bleeding or serosanguineous drainage appears.
  - Flush wound during next irrigation using less pressure.
  - Notify health care provider of bleeding.
- Opening in suture line extends.
  - Notify health care provider.
  - Reevaluate amount of pressure to use for next wound irrigation.
- Retained fluid and debris appear.
  - Increase amount of fluid used during irrigation.
  - Increase amount of pressure when flushing wound.
  - Make sure that wound is clear of retained fluid and debris before applying dressing.

KEY POINTS

- Wounds with partial-thickness tissue loss heal by epidermal repair, and full-thickness wounds heal by forming scar tissue.
- A clean surgical incision with little tissue loss heals by primary intention.
- When there is extensive tissue loss, a wound heals by secondary intention.
- Healing of full-thickness wounds proceeds through four overlapping phases: hemostasis, inflammation, proliferation, and remodeling.
- The chances of wound infection are greater when the wound contains dead or necrotic tissue, when foreign bodies lie on or near the wound, and when blood supply and tissue defenses are reduced.
- Physical stress from vomiting, coughing, or sudden muscular contraction causes separation of wound edges, dehiscence.
- Wound assessment includes anatomical location, size (dimensions and depth of wound), type and percentage of wound tissue, volume and color of wound drainage, and condition of surrounding skin.
- Wound drains remove secretions within tissue layers to promote wound closure.
- Never collect a wound culture from old drainage.
- Principles of wound management include controlling or eliminating the cause, providing systemic support to reduce existing and potential cofactors, and maintaining a physiological wound environment.
- A moist environment supports wound healing.
- When cleaning wounds or drain sites, clean from the least to the most contaminated area.
- Apply a dressing or binder in a manner that does not impair circulation or irritate the skin.
- The safe use of heat or cold therapy requires an assessment of the patient's sensory function, identification of risk factors, and understanding of the physiological effects of heat and cold.
- An acute sprain, fracture, or bruise responds best to cold applications.
- Warm applications are effective for improving circulation to wound sites and promoting muscle relaxation.

CLINICAL DECISION-MAKING EXERCISES

1. Mr. Ahmed has a pressure ulcer over his sacral area. After reviewing his case study, what is the major contributing factor to the development of this pressure ulcer? Name two interventions that would be appropriate for reducing or eliminating the contributing factor. Explain the rationale for your answer.
2. Mr. Ahmed has a stage II pressure ulcer. What information does the assessment of a stage II pressure ulcer provide, which other assessments are important when assessing the pressure ulcer, and why are these assessments important?
3. On assessing the patient for risk of development of a pressure ulcer using the Braden Scale, you note that Mr. Ahmed scores very low on the moisture subscale. You determine that the patient has had frequent bowel movements and is incontinent of liquid stool at least 2 times in 24 hours. What are some possible interventions that you plan for Mr. Ahmed to protect his skin from fecal incontinence?

evolve

Answers to Clinical Decision-Making Exercises can be found on the Evolve website.

QSEN ACTIVITY: EVIDENCE-BASED PRACTICE

Lynda finished her clinical rotation on the medical surgical unit and is now on a pediatric intensive care unit. She is assigned to work with Claudia, an experienced nurse. Lynda and Claudia are caring for a 4-year-old child who has leukemia and is hospitalized with neutropenia (dangerously low white blood cell count) resulting from chemotherapy. The child has developed a small pressure ulcer on her right heel since being hospitalized. As Lynda and Claudia discuss different pressure ulcer prevention and treatment options for critically ill children, they develop the following PICO question: In acutely ill hospitalized children, which interventions are most effective in preventing and treating pressure ulcers? Lynda and Claudia need to complete a literature review to answer their question.

Which possible key terms could they use while searching an online database to find research studies and professional guidelines that will help them answer their question?

evolve

Answers to QSEN Activities can be found on the Evolve website.

REVIEW QUESTIONS

1. When repositioning a patient with several risk factors for developing a pressure ulcer, the nurse notices redness over the sacral area. After helping the patient to a side-lying position, the nurse presses a finger over the red area, and the area blanches. What is the significance of this finding?
   1. The patient has sensitive skin and requires the use of a special bed linen.
   2. The redness indicates cellulitis, and antibiotics need to be ordered.
   3. The reddened area may be from unrelieved pressure and could resolve with repositioning.
   4. This is a stage II pressure ulcer requiring a wound-care dressing for healing.
2. A nurse is planning care for a patient who has a red area that blanches when assessed. Which of the following interventions are appropriate? (Select all that apply.)
   1. Massage the area to improve the local circulation.
   2. Reposition the patient off the area.
   3. Reassess the area after the patient is off the area for 1 hour.
   4. Request nonbleached sheets for this patient's bed.
   5. Place a cold pack under the area and reassess in 1 hour.
   6. Inform the health care team of impending pressure ulcer development.
3. What is the mechanism of injury of a pressure sore?
   1. Blood vessel damage from repeated injections causing tissue loss
   2. Continual exposure of the skin to fecal or urinary incontinence
   3. Compression of the skin by two hard surfaces for a prolonged period of time
   4. Excessive dryness of the epidermis, stripping the skin and causing damage to the dermis
4. What is the most appropriate topical management of a wound filled with red granulation tissue and intact periwound skin healing by secondary intention?
   1. A moist wound dressing
   2. An antibiotic cream applied twice a day
   3. Whirlpool treatments to debride the granulation tissue
   4. A treatment plan that allows the wound to be exposed to air for 15 minutes twice a day
5. When obtaining a wound culture specimen to determine the presence of a wound infection, the nurse correctly collects the specimen from:
   1. The necrotic tissue.
   2. The wound drainage.
   3. The drainage on the dressing.
   4. Clean, healthy-looking tissue.
6. Two days after undergoing abdominal surgery, the patient with a closed abdominal wound reports a sudden "pop" after coughing. When the nurse examines the surgical wound site, the sutures are no longer holding the incisional edges together, there is a gap in the incision, and pieces of small bowel are noted at the bottom of the now opened wound. Which is the correct intervention?
   1. Allowing the area to be exposed to air until all drainage has stopped
   2. Placing several cold packs over the area, protecting the skin around the wound
   3. Covering the area with sterile saline-soaked towels and immediately notifying the surgical team
   4. Covering the area with sterile gauze, placing a tight binder over the area, and asking the patient to remain in bed for 30 minutes
7. Nursing interventions to manage a patient who is experiencing fecal and urinary incontinence include which of the following? (Select all that apply.)
   1. Using a large absorbent diaper, changing when saturated
   2. Keeping the buttocks exposed to air at all times
   3. Using an incontinence cleanser, followed by application of a moisture-barrier ointment
   4. Offering frequent ambulation and help to the toilet
8. The patient asks the nurse what a hydrocolloid dressing is and why and how it is used. How should the nurse best describe a hydrocolloid dressing?
   1. A seaweed derivative that is highly absorptive; can control wound moisture; and will be changed as needed, depending on the amount of wound drainage
   2. Premoistened gauze, containing an antibiotic solution that can be wrung out and placed into a wound, changed every 12 hours
   3. A debriding enzyme that is used to remove necrotic tissue, is used on the surface of the wound, extends about 1 inch onto intact skin, and is changed every 12 hours
   4. A bandage that forms a gel that interacts with the wound surface, providing moisture and protection, and is changed approximately every 3 days
9. A patient recently underwent a small bowel resection and developed a cough after surgery. The patient's abdominal girth is large, and coughing puts stress on the abdominal incision. Which device could be placed around this patient's abdomen to reduce the stress on the incision?
10. A patient undergoes emergency surgery for a ruptured diverticulum. At the time of surgery it is determined to

allow the wound to heal by secondary intention because there was fecal spillage into the abdominal cavity. Once the wound base shows no evidence of infection and the entire wound is filled with granulation tissue, it is determined that negative-pressure wound therapy would be the appropriate wound intervention because:

1. It provides wound protection from bacteria or other contaminants, preventing overgrowth of bacteria in the wound base.
2. It is a system that provides continuous irrigation under negative pressure in the wound bed, stimulating granulation tissue.
3. It is a wound-management system that uses negative pressure to the wound to promote and accelerate healing.
4. It is a method to clean the wound bed of necrotic tissue without the use of toxic solutions.

evolve

Rationales for Review Questions can be found on the Evolve website.

1. 3; **2.** 2, 3; **3.** 3; **4.** 1; **5.** 4; **6.** 3; **7.** 3, 4; **8.** 4; **9.** Abdominal binder; **10.** 3

REFERENCES

Ayello EA, Braden B: How and why do pressure ulcer risk assessment, *Adv Skin Wound Care* 15(3):125, 2002.

Barker AL, et al: Implementation of pressure ulcer prevention best practice recommendations in acute care: an observational study, *Int Wound J* 10(3):313, 2013.

Bergstrom N, et al: A clinical trial of the Braden Scale for predicting pressure sore risk, *Nurs Clin North Am* 22(2):417, 1987a.

Bergstrom N, et al: The Braden Scale for predicting pressure sore risk, *Nurs Res* 36:205, 1987b.

Bergstrom NL, et al: Predicting pressure ulcer risk: a multisite study of the predictive validity of the Braden Scale, *Nurs Res* 47(5):261, 1998.

Bryant RA, Nix DP: Developing and maintaining a pressure ulcer prevention program. In Bryant RA, Nix DP, editors: *Acute and chronic wounds: current management concepts*, ed 4, St Louis, 2012, Mosby.

Coha T, et al: Skin care needs of the pediatric and neonatal patient. In Bryant RA, Nix DP, editors: *Acute and chronic wounds: current management concepts*, ed 4, St Louis, 2012, Mosby.

Doughty DB, Sparks-Defriese B: Wound healing physiology. In Bryant RA, Nix DP, editors: *Acute and chronic wounds: current management concepts*, ed 4, St Louis, 2012, Mosby.

European Pressure Ulcer Advisory Panel (EPUAP) and National Pressure Ulcer Advisory Panel (NPUAP): *Prevention of pressure ulcers: quick reference guide*, Washington DC, 2009, National Ulcer Advisory Panel, http://www.epuap.org/guidelines/Final_Quick_Prevention.pdf. Accessed December 7, 2013.

Gray M, et al: Moisture associated skin damage: overview and pathophysiology, *J Wound Ostomy Continence Nurs* 38(3):233, 2011.

Harris C, et al: Bates-Jensen wound assessment tool: pictorial guide validation project, *J Wound Ostomy Continence Nurs* 37(3):253, 2010.

Holloway S, et al: Acute and chronic wound healing. In Baranoski S, Ayello EA, editors: *Wound care essentials: practice principles*, ed 3, Philadelphia, 2011, Lippincott Williams & Wilkins.

Hopf HW, Sapshak D, Junkin S: Managing wound pain. In Bryant RA, Nix DP, editors: *Acute and chronic wounds: current management concepts*, ed 4, St Louis, 2012, Mosby.

Kelleher AD, Moorer A, Makic MF: Peer-to-peer nursing rounds and hospital acquired pressure prevalence in a surgical intensive care unit: a quality improvement project, *J Wound Ostomy Continence Nurs* 39(2):152, 2012.

Landis EM: Micro-injection studies of capillary blood pressure in human skin, *Heart* 15:209, 1930.

McInerney JA: Reducing hospital-acquired pressure ulcer prevalence through a focused prevention program, *Adv Skin Wound Care* 21(2):75, 2008.

Netsch DS: Negative pressure wound therapy. In Bryant RA, Nix DP, editors: *Acute and chronic wounds: current management concepts*, ed 4, St Louis, 2012, Mosby.

Nix DP: Skin and wound inspection and assessment. In Bryant RA, Nix DP, editors: *Acute and chronic wounds: current management concepts*, ed 4, St Louis, 2012, Mosby.

Nix DP, Mackey DM: Support surfaces. In Bryant RA, Nix DP, editors: *Acute and chronic wounds: current management concepts*, ed 4, St Louis, 2012, Mosby.

Pieper B: Pressure ulcers: impact, etiology, and classification. In Bryant RA, Nix DP, editors: *Acute and chronic wounds: current management concepts*, ed 4, St Louis, 2012, Mosby.

Ramundo JM: Wound debridement. In Bryant RA, Nix DP, editors: *Acute and chronic wounds: current management concepts*, ed 4, St Louis, 2012, Mosby.

Rolstad BS, Bryant RA, Nix DP: Topical management. In Bryant RA, Nix DP, editors: *Acute and chronic wounds: current management concepts*, ed 4, St Louis, 2012, Mosby.

Stotts NA: Wound infection: diagnosis and management. In Bryant RA, Nix DP, editors: *Acute and chronic wounds: current management concepts*, ed 4, St Louis, 2012, Mosby.

The Joint Commission (TJC): *National Patient Safety Goals*, Oakbrook Terrace, IL, 2014, The Commission. Available at http://www.jointcommission.org/standards_information/npsgs.aspx.

Wound, Ostomy and Continence Nurses Society (WOCN): *Guideline for prevention and management of pressure ulcers*, WOCN Clinical Practice Guidelines Series, Mount Laurel, NJ, 2010, The Society.

Wound, Ostomy and Continence Nurses Society (WOCN): *Clean vs. sterile dressing techniques for management of chronic wounds: a fact sheet*, Mount Laurel, NJ, 2011, WOCN.

CHAPTER

38

Sensory Alterations

evolve WEBSITE

http://evolve.elsevier.com/Potter/essentials

- Crossword Puzzle
- Audio Glossary

OBJECTIVES

- Differentiate the processes of reception, perception, and reaction to sensory stimuli.
- Compare the relationship of sensory function with an individual's level of wellness.
- Discuss common causes and effects of sensory alterations.
- Discuss common sensory changes that occur with aging.
- Identify factors to assess in determining a patient's sensory status.
- Describe behaviors indicating sensory alterations.
- Develop a plan of care for patients with sensory deficits.
- Describe nursing interventions with rationales that promote effective communication with patients who have sensory alterations.
- Describe conditions in the health care agency or patient's home that you adjust to promote meaningful sensory stimulation.
- Discuss ways to maintain a safe environment for patients with sensory alterations.

KEY TERMS

accommodation, p. 1113
age-related macular degeneration, p. 1112
auditory, p. 1111
cataracts, p. 1112
diabetic retinopathy, p. 1112
glaucoma, p. 1112
gustatory, p. 1111
Meniere's disease, p. 1114
olfactory, p. 1111
ototoxic, p. 1113
presbycusis, p. 1113
presbyopia, p. 1114
proprioception, p. 1111
refractive errors, p. 1122
sensory deficits, p. 1112
sensory deprivation, p. 1112
sensory overload, p. 1112
tactile, p. 1111
tinnitus, p. 1113

People are unique because they are able to sense a variety of stimuli in their environment. Stimulation comes from many sources in and outside of the body, particularly through the senses of sight (visual), hearing **(auditory)**, touch **(tactile)**, smell **(olfactory)**, and taste **(gustatory)**. Additional senses include pressure, pain, temperature, vibration, and position **(proprioception)** (Meiner, 2011). People learn about the environment from healthy sensory organs. Patients need to adapt to their environment when their sensory function is altered. As a nurse you need to recognize when patients are at risk for developing sensory problems and help meet their needs when they have sensory alterations. Your nursing care helps patients learn to alter their environment for improved safety.

SCIENTIFIC KNOWLEDGE BASE

Normal Sensation

People feel and react to sensations when their nervous systems are intact. Perception or awareness depends on a region of

CASE STUDY ***Mrs. Alicea***

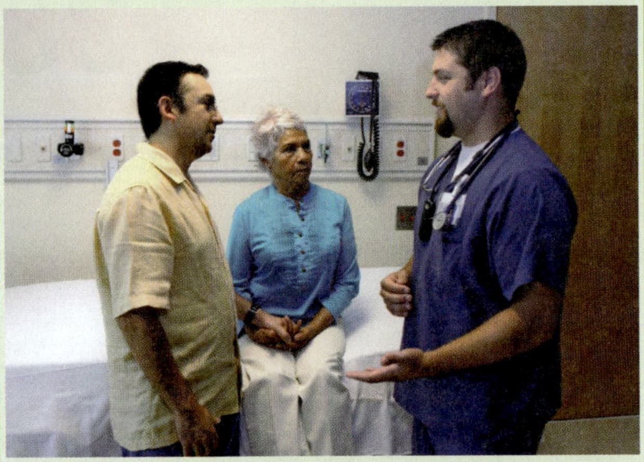

Mrs. Alicea is a 73-year-old woman who is at the senior health center for her routine 6-month checkup. She has been visiting the senior center on a regular basis for the past 8 years. She has lived alone since her husband died 1 year ago. She lives in a single-story, four-room home a few miles away from the health center. Her son, Rico, lives 5 minutes away. Rico drives Mrs. Alicea to her health care visits. Six months ago Mrs. Alicea reported progressive hearing loss. Today when she enters the clinic she reports "having trouble seeing."

Peter Morris, a nursing student assigned to the senior health center, is learning to conduct assessments and develop health promotion plans for patients at the senior center. For the past month Peter has been attending his clinical rotation at the center and participating in teaching health promotion activities. He is enjoying this rotation because he is learning more about geriatric patients and finding that they are very independent and have productive lifestyles.

the cerebral cortex where specialized brain cells interpret the quality and nature of each sensory stimulus. Sensory experiences include reception, perception, and reaction. People react to stimuli that are most meaningful to them. Sensory alterations occur when people attempt to react to every stimulus within their environment or when stimuli are lacking.

Types of Sensory Alterations

Many factors influence the capacity to receive or perceive sensations (Box 38-1). In your nursing experience you care for patients with a variety of sensory problems such as **sensory deficits, sensory deprivation,** and **sensory overload.** When patients have more than one sensory alteration, their ability to function and relate within the environment becomes impaired.

Sensory Deficits. Sensory deficits such as low vision and blindness are very common forms of disability. Four major diseases frequently cause impaired vision in Americans age 40 and over. They are **age-related macular degeneration, glaucoma, cataracts,** and **diabetic retinopathy** (Touhy and Jett, 2012). A sensory deficit occurs when problems with sensory reception or perception exist (Box 38-2). Patients are not able to receive certain stimuli (e.g., light and sound), or stimuli are distorted (e.g., blurred vision from cataracts and abnormal taste sensation from xerostomia). A sudden sensory loss caused by injury or as a side effect to medications (Box 38-3) causes fear, anger, and feelings of helplessness. Some patients withdraw socially to cope with the loss (Touhy and Jett, 2014). In addition, a patient's safety is threatened because of the inability to respond normally to stimuli. When a deficit is chronic or develops gradually, a patient learns to rely on unaffected senses. Some senses even become more acute to compensate for an alteration. Sensory deficits frequently cause patients to change their behaviors in adaptive or maladaptive ways. For example, a patient who is blind develops an acute sense of hearing and learns to use a cane to adapt to visual challenges, whereas a patient who cannot hear "bluffs" his way through a conversation instead of admitting that he did not hear what was said.

Sensory Deprivation. Sensory deprivation occurs when inadequate quality or quantity of stimuli impairs perception. It has different causes such as reduced sensory input (hearing loss), confusion, and a restricted environment (bed rest). Sensory deprivation sometimes produces cognitive changes such as the inability to solve problems, poor task performance, and disorientation. It also can cause affective changes (e.g., boredom, restlessness, increased anxiety, emotional lability) and/or perceptual changes (e.g., reduced attention span, disorganized visual and motor coordination, confusion of sleeping and waking states).

Children often become more anxious, displaying restlessness, difficulty with problem solving, and depression when they experience sensory deprivation (Hockenberry and Wilson, 2011). In adults the symptoms of sensory deprivation are similar to those of psychological illness, confusion, severe electrolyte imbalance, or the influence of psychotropic drugs. Thus accurate diagnosis of sensory deprivation is crucial.

Sensory Overload. When a person receives multiple sensory stimuli, the brain has difficulty distinguishing the stimuli, leading to sensory overload. A person with sensory overload no longer perceives the environment in a way that makes sense. Overload prevents a meaningful response to stimuli. As a result, thoughts race, attention moves in many directions, and restlessness occurs. The patient demonstrates panic, confusion, and aggressiveness. Sleep loss is common. Sensory overload causes a state similar to that of sensory deprivation.

Patients of all ages who are acutely ill easily develop sensory overload in the health care environment. Constant pain; noise from equipment; and the nursing activities of turning, repositioning, and administering treatments bombard patients with stimuli. Some patients are more sensitive to sensory overload than others. Behavioral changes are easily confused with mood swings or disorientation. Constant reorientation and control of excessive stimuli become an important part of a patient's care.

BOX 38-1 FACTORS THAT INFLUENCE SENSORY FUNCTION

AGE

Infants

- Binocular vision begins at 6 weeks and is well established by 4 months. During the second year of life infants discriminate shapes, objects, and colors.
- Neonates respond to loud noises. Within a year infants visually locate the source of noises.
- Newborns react to strong odors such as alcohol and vinegar by turning their heads. They can identify their own mother's milk.

Children

Refractive errors are the most common types of visual disorders in children and are treated with corrective lenses. Serious visual impairment affects a child's ability to play and socialize. Children are usually frightened and confused by a sudden or progressive loss of sight. Parents and children need support to help them adjust to the disability (Hockenberry and Wilson, 2011).

Adults

Visual changes include presbyopia and the need for glasses for reading (ages 40 to 50). In addition, the cornea, which helps with light refraction to the retina, becomes flatter and thicker. These aging changes lead to astigmatism. Pigment is lost from the iris; and collagen fibers build up in the anterior chamber, which increases the risk for glaucoma by decreasing the resorption of intraocular fluid.

Older Adults

Atrophy of the cerumen glands causes thicker and dryer wax, which is more difficult to remove and may completely obstruct the auditory canal (Touhy and Jett, 2014). Obstructive causes are reversible, but changes in the structure and function of the inner ear that occur as older adults grow older are not. Age-related hearing changes include **presbycusis,** characterized by decreased hearing acuity, speech intelligibility, and pitch discrimination. Low-pitched sounds are easiest to hear, but it is difficult to hear conversation over background noise. It is also difficult to discriminate consonants (*f, s, th, ch, sh, b, p, k,* and *t*). Speech sounds are distorted, and there is a delayed reception and reaction to speech.

Visual changes often include reduced visual fields, increased glare sensitivity, impaired night vision, reduced **accommodation,** reduced depth perception, and reduced color discrimination. Many of these symptoms occur because the pupils in the older adult take longer to dilate and constrict secondary to weaker iris muscles. Color vision decreases because the retina is duller and the lens yellows. Eventually older adults may require 3 times as much light to see things as they did when they were in young adulthood (Touhy and Jett, 2014).

Olfactory changes begin around age 50 and include a loss of cells in the olfactory bulb of the brain and a decrease in the number of sensory cells in the nasal lining. Reduced sensitivity to odors is common. A small decrease in the number of taste cells occurs with aging, beginning around age 60. Reduced sour, salty, and bitter taste discrimination is common. The ability to detect sweet tastes seems to remain intact (Touhy and Jett, 2014).

Proprioceptive changes in some older adults include an increased difficulty with balance, spatial orientation, and coordination. These changes make it difficult to avoid obstacles and prevent an accident from happening when fast action is necessary. The automatic response to protect and brace oneself when falling is slower.

Older adults sometimes experience tactile changes, including declining sensitivity to pain, pressure, and temperature secondary to peripheral vascular disease and neuropathies.

MEDICATIONS

Ototoxic medications (see Box 38-3) such as analgesics, antibiotics, or diuretics affect hearing acuity, balance, or both, with the most common symptom being **tinnitus** (ringing in the ears). Ototoxicity causes a progressive or continuing hearing loss that in many patients goes unnoticed until the ability to understand speech is affected (American Speech-Language-Hearing Association, 2014a). Hearing loss is not always permanent, depending on the extent of damage and the length of time that the drug is given. Patients with renal failure have an increased sensitivity to ototoxic drugs.

ENVIRONMENT

Excessive environmental stimuli result in sensory overload marked by confusion, disorientation, and inability to make decisions. Restricted environmental stimulation leads to sensory deprivation. Poor quality of environment worsens sensory impairment.

PREEXISTING ILLNESSES

Disorders such as peripheral vascular disease and stroke alter peripheral tissue perfusion and affect tactile information. Diabetic neuropathy is one of the most common complications of diabetes and can result in retinal edema, detachment, and blindness (Meiner, 2011).

SMOKING

Chronic tobacco use atrophies the taste buds and affects olfactory function.

NOISE LEVELS

Constant exposure to high noise levels causes hearing loss.

NURSING KNOWLEDGE BASE

In the United States between 25% and 40% of people over age 65 have a hearing impairment; the incidence increases with age (Touhy and Jett, 2014). Approximately 90% of adults older than 80 years have hearing loss (Touhy and Jett, 2012), 285 million people are visually impaired worldwide, and 39 million are blind (WHO, 2013). Older people are at increased risk of several eyes diseases, including age-related macular degeneration, cataracts, and glaucoma. It is estimated that

BOX 38-2 COMMON SENSORY DEFICITS

VISUAL
- **Presbyopia:** Gradual decline in ability of the lens to accommodate or to focus on close objects. Reduces ability to see near objects clearly.
- *Cataract:* Clouding of the lens in the eye that affects vision. Interferes with passage of light through the lens and reduces the light that reaches the retina. Cataracts usually develop gradually and often result in cloudy or blurry vision, glare, double vision, and poor night vision (National Eye Institute, 2009).
- *Dry eyes:* Result when tear glands produce too few tears, resulting in itching, burning, or even reduced vision.
- *Glaucoma:* A slowly progressive increase in intraocular pressure that causes progressive pressure against the optic nerve. At first vision stays normal, and there is no pain. If left untreated there may be a loss of peripheral (side) vision (Touhy and Jett, 2014).
- *Diabetic retinopathy:* Pathological changes of the blood vessels of the retina secondary to increased pressure, resulting in hemorrhage, macular edema, and reduced vision or vision loss.
- *Age-related macular degeneration:* Occurs when the macula (specialized portion of the retina responsible for central vision) degenerates as a result of aging and loses its ability to function efficiently. An early sign includes distortion that causes edges or lines to appear wavy. The disease causes the progressive loss of central vision. Peripheral vision remains intact (Touhy and Jett, 2014).

HEARING
- *Presbycusis:* A common progressive hearing disorder in older adults.
- *Cerumen accumulation:* Buildup and hardening of earwax in the external auditory canal causes conduction deafness.

BALANCE
- *Dizziness and disequilibrium:* Common condition in older adulthood, usually resulting from vestibular dysfunction and precipitated by change in position of the head to the rest of the body.
- **Meniere's disease:** Cause is unknown, but diagnosis is based on medical history interview; physical examination; and clinical symptoms of progressive low-frequency hearing loss, vertigo, tinnitus, and a full feeling or pressure in the affected ear (Meiner, 2011).

TASTE
- *Xerostomia:* Decrease in salivary production that leads to thicker mucus and a dry mouth. Interferes with the ability to eat and leads to appetite and nutritional problems.

NEUROLOGICAL
- *Peripheral neuropathy:* Most commonly associated with diabetes. Other causes include alcoholism, peripheral vascular disease, traumatic injury, medication effects, infections, and immune system diseases. Characterized by symptoms that include numbness and tingling of the affected area and stumbling gait.
- *Hemiplegia:* Caused by a thrombus, hemorrhage, or embolus affecting a blood vessel leading to or within the brain. Creates altered proprioception with marked incoordination and imbalance. Loss of sensation and motor function in extremities controlled by the affected area of the brain also occurs.

BOX 38-3 EXAMPLES OF MEDICATIONS REPORTED TO CAUSE OTOTOXICITY

ANTIBIOTICS
- Aminoglycosides
- Macrolides
- Vancomycin

SALICYLATES
- Aspirin

NSAIDS
- Ibuprofen

DIURETICS
- Ethacrynic acid
- Furosemide
- Bumetanide

ANTINEOPLASTIC AGENTS
- Cisplatin
- Carboplatin

From Mudd PA, Meyers AD: Ototoxicity, 2012, http://emedicine.medscape.com/article/857679-overview#a1. Accessed February 10, 2014.
NSAID, Nonsteroidal antiinflammatory drug.

one in five Americans will be over the age of 65 by 2050 (Touhy and Jett, 2012). Therefore the incidence of age-related decline in sensory function will continue to increase. The loss of major sensory input usually has profound consequences on patients' independence. As a nurse, stay informed of new health care and nursing knowledge as it pertains to the older-adult population and the effects of diverse sensory changes.

Vision and hearing alterations often have profound consequences for function and quality of life of older adults. A loss of sensory input often creates feelings of grief, anger, depression, and loss of self-esteem (Touhy and Jett, 2014). Self-esteem disturbances frequently lead to social isolation and withdrawal from social activities (Meiner, 2011). Your knowledge about the effects of sensory loss on your patients allows you to promote their healthy aging. Assess how a sensory impairment influences a patient's self-concept, mood, and ability to communicate and function in the everyday world. Patient education about prevention and treatment of diseases affecting vision and hearing, available social services, assistive devices, and the need for annual physical examinations helps provide the older patient with better coping abilities and health maintenance.

Managing patients with sensory alterations challenges you to apply nursing research and information from your practice to help patients participate in their environment, remain socially interactive, and continue to be productive. In addition, your application of critical thinking principles helps you promote patients' sensory function and protect them from possible injury (Box 38-4).

BOX 38-4 EVIDENCE-BASED PRACTICE

PICO Question: Do patients who are critically ill sleep better when a "quiet-time" protocol is implemented in an intensive care unit?

SUMMARY OF EVIDENCE

Excessive sensory stimulation in health care facilities often has negative psychological and physical effects on patients during hospitalization. For example, excess noise stimulates the cardiovascular system, decreases oxygen saturation, disrupts sleep, and impairs the ability to fight infections (Dennis et al., 2010). The number of patient rooms and the design of a unit, patient acuity, and health care professionals' conversations influence noise levels in health care facilities (Li et al., 2011). The continuous monitoring of patient's vital signs and the noise that monitoring devices produce can also be disturbing and create sensory overload. Current evidence supports that implementing protocols that require periods of time during which nurses reduce light and other environmental stimuli decreases peak sound and average noise levels (Dennis et al., 2010; Li et al., 2011). Quiet-time protocols also tend to enhance the amount of time and frequency that patients sleep, reduce interruptions in sleep, and improve the quality of sleep (Dennis et al., 2010; Li et al., 2011). Although it is challenging to create times without distractions in a busy intensive care unit, implementation of a quiet-time protocol can benefit patients.

APPLICATION TO NURSING PRACTICE

- Assess all patients for signs of sensory overload such as anxiety and restlessness.
- Identify sources of noise on the unit such as equipment and machines.
- Develop strategies to reduce noise to an acceptable level.
- Modify your work flow to establish a restful environment for patients to sleep.
- Establish a routine for patient care.
- Collaborate with hospital staff to provide patients with quiet time.
- Educate patients and families about the goal of quiet time to create a peaceful and healing environment.

BOX 38-5 SYNTHESIS IN PRACTICE

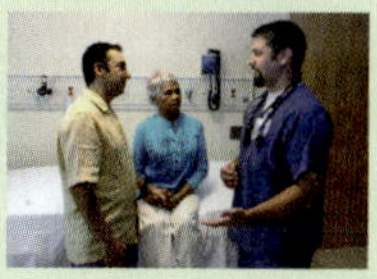

While Peter prepares to assess Mrs. Alicea, he recalls what he has learned about the pathophysiology of eye disorders. He focuses on the "warning signs" of eye problems, determining which, if any, of the signs Mrs. Alicea has experienced. Because Mrs. Alicea reports hearing and visual losses, Peter considers the communication approaches best suited for conducting a successful assessment. He plans to position himself so Mrs. Alicea is able to see his face clearly. Peter also will speak slowly and enunciate words clearly, giving time for Mrs. Alicea to respond to questions. Avoiding questions answered by "yes" or "no" will require Mrs. Alicea to provide more detailed answers, ensuring that she heard Peter's questions correctly.

Peter respects Mrs. Alicea's cultural background and explores implications for the delivery of culturally sensitive care. When beginning the interview, some Mexican-Americans engage in "small talk" before discussing the serious aspects of the interview, because being direct is considered rude and self-disclosure is for those whom the individual knows well (Owen et al., 2013). It will thus be important for Peter to express caring and respect for Mrs. Alicea and provide time for small talk to be successful in gathering a complete assessment. Family is highly valued and is the main focus of social identification within the Mexican culture (Owen et al., 2013). Rico will play a key role in Mrs. Alicea's ability to maintain self-care. Peter plans to determine if Rico is the primary individual who helps Mrs. Alicea complete instrumental activities of daily living (IADLs) and other activities.

Peter's own grandmother has bilateral cataracts. He reflects on how she adjusted to her visual loss to continue activities she enjoys. He learned in class that you can make a variety of adaptations to maximize the sensory functions that a patient still has. Peter plans to discover if Mrs. Alicea has made any adaptations in her home environment. Creativity is an important attitude to exercise.

CRITICAL THINKING

Synthesis

You will apply elements of critical thinking whenever you perform the nursing process with patients. Consider the scientific knowledge you have learned, your experience, critical thinking attitudes, and standards to ensure an individualized approach to patient care (Box 38-5). As you apply the nursing process for patients with sensory alterations, anticipate the kind of information necessary to form good clinical judgments. A combination of past patient care experiences and the application of scientific and nursing knowledge helps you develop an individualized plan of care for a patient.

Knowledge. A number of factors cause sensory alterations. Knowledge of these factors and of anatomy and physiology and the normal components of a sensory experience helps you understand how a particular alteration affects a patient's function. Knowing the pathophysiological changes of sensory organ disorders also helps you anticipate how sensory changes affect a patient. When you identify characteristics of sensory alterations and the interventions to minimize them, you are able to implement a comprehensive and individualized plan of care.

Depending on a patient's problem, use your knowledge of communication principles (see Chapter 11) to select the best communication method. Patients with hearing impairments require different communication approaches to obtain a complete and accurate nursing assessment and deliver interventions effectively. You also need to have a working knowledge of pharmacology because a variety of medications affect sensory function. Being able to anticipate the side effects of medications allows you to prepare patients for possible sensory changes.

Experience. Many of us have experienced altered sensory function personally or while interacting with family, friends, or patients. Previous personal or clinical experiences with sensory changes help you anticipate a patient's care needs. How do individuals adapt to hearing aids and glasses? What adjustments do they make to function safely in their homes? Which communication techniques are necessary when speaking to individuals with hearing impairment? Such experiences help you choose successful nursing interventions when caring for patients in a variety of health care settings.

Attitudes. Critical thinking attitudes lead you to become a more disciplined thinker. Creativity is often necessary to find the right solutions for your patient's problems. For example, living in a nonstimulating home environment can cause sensory deprivation. Work with your patient to develop changes in the environment to improve the quality of stimulation and reduce the patient's risk for injury. Curiosity applies when a patient shows unexplained behavioral changes. Asking why and being curious help you assess a less obvious sensory problem.

Standards. An important ethical standard to follow when assisting patients with sensory alterations is preservation of autonomy (see Chapter 6). For a patient to regain independence, do not override autonomy with the principle of beneficence. Although professionals believe they know what is best, remember patients have to live with the sensory alteration and adapt to the consequences of their own choices. The Joint Commission (TJC), along with the Americans with Disabilities Act (ADA), requires health care institutions to address the needs of patients with sensory alterations and provide interpretation services as necessary to establish understanding and maintain confidentiality (TJC, 2014). Evidence-based standards of care and practice such as those from the American Academy of Ophthalmology (2011) and the American Speech-Language-Hearing Association (2014b) provide criteria for screening sensory problems and establishing standards for competent, safe, effective care and practice.

NURSING PROCESS

ASSESSMENT

When assessing your patients, consider age and other factors that influence sensory function. Collect a complete nursing history by examining how a sensory deficit affects your patient's lifestyle, self-care ability, psychosocial adjustment, health promotion habits, and safety. In addition, focus the assessment on the quality and quantity of stimuli within a patient's environment.

Patients at Risk. Conduct a sensory assessment for any patient at risk for sensory alterations. These patients include those living in a confined environment such as a nursing home. Although most nursing homes or centers offer meaningful stimulation through group activities, environmental design, and mealtime gatherings, there are exceptions. Patients isolated in a health care setting or at home because of conditions such as active tuberculosis or severe immune system depression are often isolated in a private room and frequently experience sensory deprivation. Other patients who are immobilized by bed rest, physical impediments (e.g., casts or traction), or chronic disability are unable to experience all the normal sensations of free movement and are at risk for sensory deprivation. Always remain alert for any behavioral changes common to sensory deprivation.

Hospital environments are full of sensory stimuli. This does not mean that all hospitalized patients experience sensory overload. Carefully assess patients subjected to high stress levels (e.g., intensive care unit [ICU] environment, long-term hospitalization, and multiple therapies). Be aware that patients can have a combination of a sensory deficit and overload simultaneously. For example, a child in a pediatric intensive care unit experiences sensory deficit because the room has no windows but also experiences sensory overload from noise that occurs around the clock at the nurse's station.

Older Adult Considerations. Older adults are a high-risk group because of normal physiological changes associated with aging. However, be careful not to automatically assume that a patient's sensory problem is related to advancing age. For example, adult sensorineural hearing loss is often caused by exposure to excess and prolonged noise or metabolic, vascular, and other systemic alterations. Some older patients are unaware of sensory changes or are reluctant to share information for fear of the consequences (Touhy and Jett, 2012).

Sensory Status. Include an assessment of the nature and characteristics of sensory alterations in the nursing history. Assessment categories include the type and extent of sensory impairment, the onset and duration of symptoms, and whether there are factors that aggravate or relieve symptoms. Often you observe such characteristics by watching a patient perform routine activities of daily living (ADLs) in the home or health care setting. Table 38-1 provides examples of factors to assess, relevant questions to address with your patient, and appropriate physical assessment strategies.

Patient's Lifestyle. Learn about a patient's perception of a sensory loss to find out how his or her quality of life has been influenced. Ask patients to describe any problems that the sensory alteration creates for their normal daily routines and lifestyle. Does a sensory alteration change your patient's ability to retain social relationships, continue performing at work or school, or function within the home?

Socialization. The amount and quality of contact with family members or friends determines whether a patient with sensory alterations becomes isolated. Assess if a patient lives alone and whether family, friends, or neighbors frequently visit. The absence of visitors to the home or a health care setting creates a sense of monotony that contributes to social isolation. Also assess a patient's social skills and level of satisfaction in the support given by family and friends.

Self-Care Management. A patient's functional ability incorporates ADLs (e.g., grooming, bathing, dressing, and toileting) and instrumental activities of daily living (IADLs)

TABLE 38-1 FOCUSED PATIENT ASSESSMENT

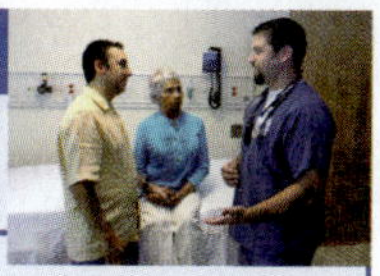

FACTORS TO ASSESS	QUESTIONS	PHYSICAL ASSESSMENT
Sensory status	Do you have problems with your ears, hearing, balance, vision, or sensing touch? If so, when did the difficulty begin? Did it begin gradually or suddenly? Is it constant, or does it come and go? How would you describe it? What are your preferences for treatment? If appropriate, would you wear glasses to improve your vision or hearing aids to improve communication?	Assess patient's hearing, balance, vision, and sense of touch (see Chapter 16). Observe patient behaviors during conversation and while watching patient perform IADLs and ADLs.
Self-care management in home and community care settings	Are you able to prepare a meal or write a check (for patients with visual alterations)? Is there a certain pitch that you have trouble hearing such as conversation on the telephone or the telephone ringing (for patients with hearing impairments)? Are you able to dress or bathe safely using warm water (for patients with decreased tactile sensation)?	Observe patient in the home, in the kitchen while preparing a meal. Observe patient's ability to communicate effectively. Observe patient during dressing and bathing.
Health promotion practices	How do you clean your ears? Do you have difficulty caring for your glasses, hearing aids, or contact lenses? Do you wear safety glasses, eye shields, or ear noise protective gear when appropriate?	Find out when patient last had an eye or ear screening. Observe ear/eye routine care. Check for appropriate eye protection with eye shields and safety glasses or face shields.

ADLs, Activities of daily living; *IADLs,* instrumental activities of daily living.

(e.g., grocery shopping, writing a check, and using a phone). If a sensory alteration impairs your patient's functional ability, planning for discharge from a health care setting and providing resources within the home become necessary. You need to consider the activities that patients normally do for themselves and how the sensory alteration impairs their functioning.

Psychosocial Adjustment. Because some patients are unaware of or unwilling to discuss behavioral changes, family and friends are often the best resources when determining if sensory changes have altered a patient's behavior. Assess if the patient has shown any recent mood swings such as outbursts of anger, depression, or fear. Does the patient avoid interactions with others? Sensory alterations also often cause changes in orientation and ability to concentrate.

Health Promotion Practices. Assess the daily routines that patients follow in maintaining sensory function. The information determines a patient's need for education or referral to appropriate resources.

Hazards. Make sure that the home environment is healthy, comfortable, and safe. A thorough home assessment helps you provide options for ways to make the home safe. First assess the home setting, including the outdoors and all rooms in the home, for any hazards that increase the risk for injury (e.g., poorly lit stairs, obstacles in walking paths, uneven sidewalks). A home safety checklist is usually available in most home care agencies. The type of sensory alteration makes some home features more hazardous than others. Patients with impaired vision require more light. Patients who are blind often need information written in braille. Patients with hearing deficits sometimes require safety alarms with visual signals. Those with severe hearing impairments need to have a telecommunication device for the deaf (TDD). The TDD has a keyboard and displays numbers and letters that provide messages to the hearing impaired from another TDD. The ADA requires any health care facility that receives Medicare funding to have TDDs for the hearing impaired (Touhy and Jett, 2014).

Assess for any factors in a health care setting that will be dangerous to the patient. Assess a patient's hospital room for clutter, unnecessary equipment, and obstacles in the path leading to the bathroom. Also ask the patient about barriers or obstacles that the patient perceives as potentially dangerous.

Meaningful Stimuli. Meaningful stimuli reduce the incidence of sensory deprivation. In the home check for the use of bright colors, comfortable furnishings, adequate lighting, good ventilation, and clean surroundings. Also observe for presence of pets, family pictures, television, a clock, or a calendar. Note if patients have roommates, visitors, or any personal items such as pictures. A patient becomes disoriented in a barren environment that gives few signals for normal sensory perception. Meaningful stimuli influence the patient's alertness and the ability to participate in self-care.

Environment. Excessive environmental stimuli causes sensory overload. In an acute care setting the frequency of observations, tests, and procedures is often stressful to the patient. Assess the location of a patient's room. If it is near repetitive or loud noises (e.g., nurses' station or supply room), the patient is at risk for sensory overload. In addition, explore a loud television, a roommate, or a bright room light as possible contributing factors. Patients who are in pain, traction, or restricted by a cast are also at risk for excessive stimulation. Your responsibility as a nurse is to identify and reduce or eliminate excessive stimuli.

Communication Methods. Assess if patients have trouble speaking, understanding, reading, or writing to understand the quality of their communication. Next, ask patients which communication method they prefer. Patients with existing sensory deficits often develop alternative ways of communicating. Some patients with hearing impairments read lips, use sign language, wear a hearing aid, or read and write notes. Patients with visual impairments learn to detect voice tones and inflections to identify the emotional tone of a conversation. To assess communication methods, sit facing the patient, speaking in a normal tone. Disorganized speech, a long period of silence, or a patient who continually asks you to repeat your sentences indicates a sensory deficit in the patient. Some patients also show signs and symptoms of confusion or respond in an inappropriate manner because of their hearing impairment.

Physical Examination. Patients with known or suspected sensory deficits resulting from visual and hearing losses, spinal cord injury, or peripheral neuropathies require complete and detailed sensory examinations (see Chapter 16). Assessing the extent of sensory loss allows you to focus your review on behaviors of sensory deficits (Table 38-2). If your examination suggests a sensory deprivation, observation during history taking, physical examination, or care provides additional information about a person's condition. Observe a patient's physical appearance, measure cognitive ability, and assess emotional stability. At this time also remember that factors other than sensory deprivation or overload cause impaired perception (e.g., medications, pain, or electrolyte imbalances).

Patient Expectations. When conducting an assessment, review a patient's expressed needs. Many patients have a definite plan as to how they want their care delivered. Some expect you to provide equipment for them so they can properly care for their sensory aids (eyeglasses or hearing aids). Asking patients what they expect helps you to initiate effective strategies and provide access to resources. Eliciting patient values and preferences is also an essential skill of patient-centered care (Box 38-6). Some patients request that family members or friends help with their care. Begin by asking, "What do you expect from the nursing staff to feel that you are receiving good care?" and "Now that I better understand what affects your ability to see/hear, what do you expect in the care that we will be providing for you?"

TABLE 38-2 BEHAVIORS INDICATING SENSORY DEFICITS

BEHAVIOR INDICATING DEFICIT (CHILDREN)	BEHAVIOR INDICATING DEFICIT (ADULTS)
Vision	
Self-stimulation, including eye rubbing, body rocking, sniffing, arm twirling; hitching (using legs to propel while in sitting position) instead of crawling	Poor coordination, squinting, underreaching or overreaching for objects, persistent repositioning of objects, impaired night vision, accidental falls
Hearing	
Frightened when unfamiliar people approach, no reflex or purposeful response to sounds, failure to be awakened by loud noise, slow or absent development of speech, greater response to movement than to sound, avoidance of social interaction with others	Blank looks, decreased attention span, lack of reaction to loud noises, increased volume of speech, positioning head toward sound, smiling and nodding head in approval when someone speaks, using other means of communication such as lip reading or writing, complaints of ringing in ears
Touch	
Inability to perform developmental tasks related to grasping objects or drawing, repeated injury from handling harmful objects (e.g., hot stove, sharp knife)	Clumsiness, overreaction or underreaction to painful stimulus, failure to respond when touched, avoidance of touch, sensation of pins and needles, numbness
Smell	
Difficult to assess until child is 6 or 7 years old; difficulty discriminating unpleasant odors	Failure to react to noxious or strong odors, increased body odor, decreased sensitivity to odors
Taste	
Inability to tell whether food is salty or sweet, possible ingestion of strange-tasting things	Change in appetite, excessive use of seasoning and sugar, complaints about taste of food, weight change
Position Sense	
Clumsiness, extraneous movement, excessive arm swinging in those with hyperactivity or learning difficulty	Poor balance and spatial orientation, shuffling gait, reduced response to bracing self when falling, more precise and deliberate movements

NURSING DIAGNOSIS

After assessment, review all available data and look critically for patterns and defining characteristics that suggest a health problem relating to sensory alterations. For example, seeking to be alone; being uncommunicative; verbalization or observation of discomfort in social situations; and a sad, dull affect are defining characteristics of *Social Isolation*. Validate your findings to ensure accuracy of the diagnosis. Examples of nursing diagnoses that apply to patients with sensory alterations include the following:

- *Anxiety*
- *Fear*
- *Impaired Physical Mobility*
- *Hopelessness*
- *Risk for Injury*
- *Deficient Knowledge*
- *Impaired Social Interaction*
- *Bathing Self-Care Deficit*
- *Risk for Falls*

Next determine the factor that likely causes the patient's health problem. The etiology or "related to" factor of a nursing diagnosis needs to be accurate to ensure that you select appropriate interventions. For example, if impacted cerumen is the cause of a patient's hearing alteration, following a protocol for cerumen removal improves auditory perception (Touhy and Jett, 2014). If a patient's auditory alteration is related to altered sensory reception from nerve deafness, nursing interventions of alternative communication methods are more successful in minimizing the patient's hearing impairment.

BOX 38-6 PATIENT-CENTERED CARE

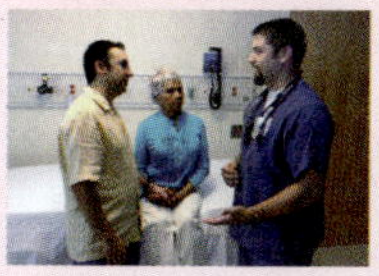

Peter is aware that people who are Hispanic/Latino are the largest minority group in the United States. However, he is uncertain if disparities in sensory alteration exist across ethnicities. Therefore, before he meets with Mrs. Alicea on his next clinical day, he takes some time to read about sensory alterations in the Latino population.

Peter learns that Hispanic/Latino individuals in the United States have higher rates of visual impairment and blindness than members of other ethnic groups. Visual field loss has a negative impact on health-related quality of life (Li et al., 2010). Peter uses this information to develop a patient-centered plan of care that focuses on Mrs. Alicea's visual impairment.

IMPLICATIONS FOR PRACTICE

- Assess what Mrs. Alicea already knows about her condition (Sudore and Schillinger, 2009).
- Ask Mrs. Alicea, "What questions do you have about your condition?"
- Encourage Mrs. Alicea to discuss the effect of her visual impairment on her health-related quality of life.
- Ask Mrs. Alicea how she is coping with visual alterations.
- Ask Mrs. Alicea about her social networks and supportive relationships.
- Elicit and respect Mrs. Alicea's preferences in her plan of care.
- Ask Mrs. Alicea to teach back or demonstrate what was taught (Sudore and Schillinger, 2009).

PLANNING

Patients with sensory alterations have many needs (Figure 38-1). The plan of care you develop depends on your assessment of the patient's sensory perception and acceptance of the sensory alteration and how well he or she has adjusted to the loss (see Care Plan).

Goals and Outcomes. During planning develop an individualized plan of care for each nursing diagnosis. Partner with your patient to develop a realistic plan that

CARE PLAN

Risk for Injury

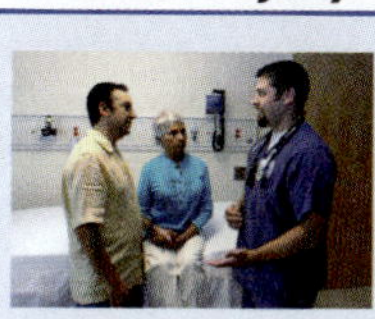

ASSESSMENT

Mrs. Alicea comes to the clinic reporting "having trouble seeing." Peter notes that Mrs. Alicea appears unsteady when standing. He knows that people with vision impairments are at risk for impaired balance and slow reaction time, contributing to a greater fall risk. Peter plans to assess Mrs. Alicea's changes in vision more closely to identify interventions to decrease her risk for injury related to visual alterations.

ASSESSMENT ACTIVITIES	FINDINGS/DEFINING CHARACTERISTICS*
Ask Mrs. Alicea to describe her vision changes.	Mrs. Alicea states, "When I try to read or sew, my **vision is blurred,** even with my glasses. I have **difficulty judging distance between objects, which is worse at night.**"
Ask Mrs. Alicea to describe any life changes that have occurred since the changes in vision.	Mrs. Alicea states, "I'm having **difficulty reading** and moving around the house. **I can't judge the steps clearly,** and my son has been helping me more with household chores."

Continued

CARE PLAN—cont'd

Risk for Injury

ASSESSMENT ACTIVITIES	FINDINGS/DEFINING CHARACTERISTICS*
Assess Mrs. Alicea's visual acuity.	Mrs. Alicea's corneas appear opaque, and there is a reduction in accommodation.
Ask Mrs. Alicea the results of her last visit with the ophthalmologist.	Mrs. Alicea reports that it has been about 2 years since she has been to an eye doctor. Mrs. Alicea states, "At my last visit, I was told that I had a cataract."
Conduct a home hazard assessment.	The home has **dim lighting, stairs without handrails,** and **numerous throw rugs on floors.**

*__Defining characteristics__ are shown in **bold** type.

NURSING DIAGNOSIS: Risk for Injury

PLANNING

GOAL	EXPECTED OUTCOMES (NOC)†
	Risk Control: Visual Impairment
• Mrs. Alicea's home environment will be safe and free of hazards within 4 weeks.	• Mrs. Alicea reports an increased sense of home safety and independence within 2 weeks. • Mrs. Alicea and her son make recommended changes to home environment within 4 weeks.

†Outcomes classification labels from Moorhead S, et al, editors: *Nursing outcomes classification (NOC)*, ed 5, St Louis, 2013, Mosby.

INTERVENTIONS (NIC)‡	RATIONALE
Environmental Management: Safety	
• Recommend that Mrs. Alicea's son Rico install a nonglare work surface in the kitchen area.	Sensitivity to glare increases because of clouding of the lens and vitreous, which results in scattering of light that passes through the lens.
• Recommend that Rico install incandescent lights in the home.	The intensity of lighting needs to be three times as powerful for older adults to produce the same visual acuity as for younger people (Touhy and Jett, 2014).
• Help Rico identify potential trip hazards such as throw rugs and suggest that they either be modified or removed.	Removal of trip hazards prevents falls and promotes a safe environment.
Fall Prevention	
• Teach Rico methods to improve environmental safety such as installing handrails along stairs, securing carpeting, removing throw rugs, and painting stairs.	A decrease in visual acuity and depth perception places a patient at risk for falls in the presence of environmental hazards (Touhy and Jett, 2012).
• Suggest that Rico place a nonslip surface such as a nonskid mat in the bathtub and shower.	Mrs. Alicea is at a higher risk for falling in the shower and bathtub because of visual impairments and difficulties with depth perception. Nonskid surfaces prevent falling in bathtubs and showers.

EVALUATION

NURSING ACTIONS	PATIENT RESPONSE/FINDING	ACHIEVEMENT OF OUTCOME
During her next visit to the health center, ask Mrs. Alicea if she has experienced any trips or falls since modifications to her home were made. Ask Rico if his mother is having any difficulties moving through her home.	Mrs. Alicea states that she has not fallen or tripped since Rico made the suggested modifications to her home. Rico states his mother is able to walk through her home with a steady, purposeful gait.	Outcome met.
Conduct a home visit and reassess the home environment.	Rico has changed all light bulbs in the halls and stairways. He removed all throw rugs and painted edges of stairs bright white. Kitchen work surface has not changed yet.	Home environment has improved. Rico needs help identifying contractors to help him change the work surface in the kitchen to decrease glare.

‡Interventions classification label from Bulechek GM, et al, editors: *Nursing interventions classification (NIC)*, ed 6, St Louis, 2013, Mosby.

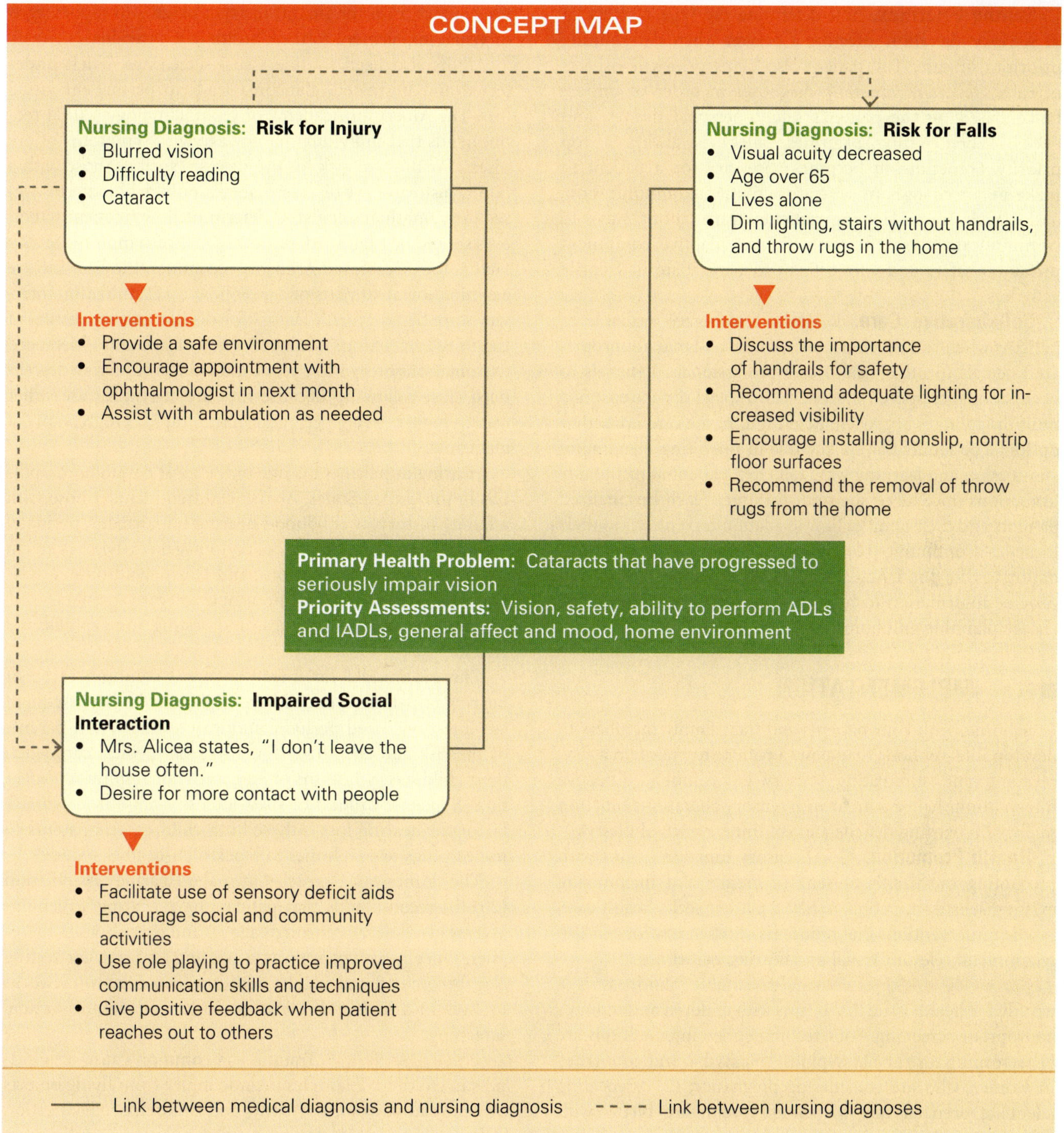

FIGURE 38-1 Concept map. *ADLs,* Activities of daily living; *IADLs,* instrumental activities of daily living.

incorporates what you know about the patient's sensory problems and the extent to which he or she can maintain or improve sensory function. Make sure that goals not only meet a patient's immediate needs but also strive toward rehabilitation. Goals and outcomes need to be realistic and measurable. Some sensory alterations are short term, requiring only temporary interventions. Permanent sensory alterations require long-term goals, with a series of outcomes that the patient reaches over time. For example, if a patient suffers an injury causing blindness, the long-term goal of "managing self-care within the home" requires numerous short-term outcomes and outcomes that show progressive advancement. Examples of outcomes include "Patient ambulates safely within the home in 2 weeks" and "Patient performs ADLs with minimal assistance within 4 weeks."

Setting Priorities. You determine the type and extent of sensory alteration affecting a patient when determining priorities of care. The patient also helps prioritize aspects of care. Generally you rank diagnoses in order of importance based on the patient's safety, personal desires, and needs. When setting priorities, safety is always a top priority. Sometimes it becomes necessary for a patient to make major changes in self-care activities, communication, and socialization. Helping patients learn about ways to communicate more effectively or use adaptive equipment promotes safety and allows them to participate in favorite activities.

Collaborative Care. Review all resources available to patients when you develop a plan of care and make appropriate referrals to other health care professionals. Referrals to occupational or speech therapists and social service ensure a multidisciplinary approach. Referral to home care is another option. The family plays a key role in providing meaningful stimulation and learning ways to help a patient adjust to any limitations once he or she returns home. Teach hospitalized patients and their families how to adapt interventions to their lifestyles. Community resources such as the American Foundation for the Blind, American Red Cross, and the Lions Club provide information to help patients and families with discharge planning and home needs.

IMPLEMENTATION

Collaborate with your patients and their family members to develop interventions that allow a patient to maintain a safe, pleasant, and stimulating sensory environment. Effective interventions help a patient with sensory alterations function safely with existing deficits and continue a normal lifestyle.

Health Promotion. Good sensory function begins with promoting the health of sensory organs and maximizing existing sensory function. When a patient seeks health care, provide interventions that reduce risk for sensory losses. Also recommend relevant visual and hearing guidelines.

Screening and Prevention. Preventable blindness is a worldwide health issue that begins with children and requires appropriate screening. Four recommended interventions are (1) screening for rubella, syphilis, chlamydia, and gonorrhea in women who are considering pregnancy; (2) advocating adequate prenatal care to prevent premature birth (with the danger of exposure of the infant to excessive oxygen); (3) administering eye prophylaxis in the form of erythromycin ointment approximately 1 hour after an infant's birth; and (4) periodic screening of all children, especially newborns through preschoolers, for congenital blindness and visual impairment caused by **refractive errors** and strabismus (Hockenberry and Wilson, 2011).

The most common visual problem during childhood is a refractive error such as nearsightedness. The school nurse is usually responsible for vision testing of school-age and adolescent children. Your role as a nurse is one of detection, education, and referral. Parents need to know the signs of visual impairment such as failure to react to light and reduced eye contact from the infant. Instruct parents to report signs of visual impairment to their health care provider.

Adults also need routine visual screenings. If left undetected and untreated, glaucoma leads to permanent visual loss. The American Academy of Ophthalmology (2011) recommends that individuals at any age with symptoms of eye disease or those at risk for eye disease (such as those with a family history of eye disease, diabetes, or high blood pressure) see their ophthalmologist to determine how frequently their eyes should be examined. In the absence of symptoms or risk factors for disease, the Academy recommends a baseline eye examination at 40 years of age. Follow-up examination interviews are based on risk factors for disease and the results of the initial screening. Adults 65 years of age and older need examinations every 1 to 2 years. Individuals of African descent need close follow-up because they are at risk for an earlier onset, higher incidence, and more rapid progression of glaucoma.

Hearing impairment is one of the most common disabilities in the United States. At-risk children include those with a family history of childhood hearing impairment, perinatal infection (rubella, herpes, or cytomegalovirus), low birth weight, chronic ear infections, and Down syndrome. Advise pregnant women of the importance of early prenatal care, avoidance of ototoxic drugs, and testing for syphilis and rubella.

Chronic middle ear infections are a common cause of hearing impairment in children. Children who have frequent ear infections need periodic auditory testing. Warn parents of the risk and encourage them to seek medical care when their child has symptoms of an earache or respiratory infection. Exposure to loud or high-intensity noise is also a risk factor for hearing loss. Advise both children and parents to use earplugs or earphones to block high-decibel sounds.

The American Speech-Language-Hearing Association (2014b) recommends that patients have hearing screenings at least every decade through age 50 and every 3 years thereafter. Once a patient reports a hearing loss, regular testing also becomes necessary. In addition, a patient who works or lives in a high-noise level environment requires annual screening.

Preventive Safety. Trauma is a common cause of blindness in children. Examples include injury from flying objects or penetrating wounds. Parents and children need education about ways to avoid eye trauma such as avoiding use of toys with long, pointed projections and instructing children not to run while carrying pointed objects. Instruct patients that they can find safety equipment in sports and department stores.

Adults are at risk for eye injury while playing sports and working in jobs involving exposure to chemicals or flying objects. The Occupational Safety and Health Administration (OSHA) (n.d.) has guidelines for workplace safety. Employers must have employees wear eye goggles and/or use equipment that reduces risk for injury. Occupational health nurses reinforce the use of protective devices. In addition, nurses need to routinely assess patients for noise exposure and participate

BOX 38-7 CARE OF HEARING AIDS

- Make sure that fingers are dry and clean before handling hearing aids.
- Insert and remove hearing aid over a soft surface.
- Place battery in hearing aid before you turn it on.
- Remove hearing aid battery when not in use and store in a marked container in a safe place.
- Protect hearing aids from water and excessive heat or cold.
- Use a soft, dry cloth to wipe hearing aids and a soft brush to clean difficult to reach areas.

Modified from Touhy TA, Jett A: *Ebersole and Hess' Gerontological nursing & healthy aging,* ed 3, St Louis, 2014, Mosby.

in providing hearing conservation classes for teachers, students, and patients.

Use of Assistive Aids. Patients with sensory deficits often require use of assistive aids. Patients who wear corrective lenses, eyeglasses, or hearing aids need to keep them accessible, functional, and clean (Box 38-7) (see Chapter 29). Sometimes a family member or friend also needs to know how to clean and care for the aids. Those who wear contact lenses who do not clean their lenses appropriately, use contaminated lens storage cases or contact lens solutions, or use homemade saline are at risk for serious eye infections. Reinforce proper lens care in any health maintenance discussions.

A wide variety of cosmetically acceptable hearing aids that enhance a person's hearing ability are currently available. Patients often need encouragement and support to explore assistive devices. Because hearing aids are expensive, explore potential financial resources with your patients. Offer them printed information on hearing loss, the benefits of hearing aid use, and how to use the hearing aid (Meiner, 2011). Family members or friends who support the use of the aid often influence the patient to use the aid as instructed. However, some patients are reluctant to wear hearing aids for a variety of reasons. When patients report that they have hearing aids but do not wear them, investigate potential reasons such as the appearance of the hearing aid, poor fit, difficulty in seeing or working with a small object, and lack of patient education about the hearing aid. When a patient has a new hearing aid, provide adequate education. Patients usually begin wearing the hearing aid for 15 to 20 minutes and gradually increase the time until they can wear it for 10 to 12 hours. If your patient is having problems tolerating a hearing aid, refer him or her to an audiologist and suggest that he or she explore other types of hearing aids.

Promoting Meaningful Stimulation. You help patients make their environments more stimulating by making adaptations that incorporate the normal physiological changes that accompany sensory deficits (Box 38-8). For example, as patients age, their pupils lose the ability to adjust, creating a sensitivity to glare. You reduce this sensitivity by having family members install nonglare surfaces in the home.

BOX 38-8 PROMOTING SENSORY STIMULATION

- Reduce glare by eliminating waxed floors and shiny surfaces exposed to bright sunlight, installing tinted glass or sheer curtains over large windows, and using soft and diffused lighting.
- Teach use of assistive devices to improve visual acuity (e.g., pocket magnifiers, telescopic-lens eyeglasses, large-print books, clocks, watches).
- Recommend introducing brighter colors (e.g., red, orange, yellow) into the home environment so patients are able to differentiate between surfaces and room objects.
- Explain how to maximize hearing reception or minimize effects of hearing loss by increasing amplification on televisions or radios and using recorded music in low-frequency sound.
- Promote sense of taste through good oral hygiene, serving well-seasoned and differently textured foods, chewing food thoroughly, and avoiding blending or mixing foods.
- Enhance the sense of smell by removing unpleasant odors from the environment and introducing pleasant smells such as mild room deodorizers or fragrant flowers.

Some patients experience reduced tactile sensations in a limited portion of their body. Touch therapy helps to stimulate existing function. If the patient is willing to be touched, hair brushing and combing, a backrub, and touching the arms or shoulders increase tactile contact. Turning and positioning also improve the quality of tactile sensation.

Establishing Safe Environments. Patients become less secure within their home and workplace when they have a sensory alteration. Make recommendations for improving safety within a patient's living environment without restricting independence. The nature of an actual or potential sensory loss determines the safety precautions necessary. Security is necessary for a person to feel independent. Inform patients that organizing informal network agreements with neighbors often have a positive effect on home safety and security concerns (Touhy and Jett, 2012).

Visual Adaptations. Safety is a concern when patients experience decreases in visual acuity, peripheral vision, adaptation to the dark, or depth perception. With reduced peripheral vision a patient cannot see panoramically because the outer visual field is less discrete. With reduced depth perception, a person is unable to judge how far away objects are located. This is a special danger when he or she walks down stairs or over uneven surfaces. A home safety assessment helps you identify hazards in the patient's living environment. Remove clutter such as footstools or electrical cords. Install thresholds over uneven floor surfaces between rooms. Arrange furniture so a patient is able to move about easily without fear of tripping or running into objects. Make sure that all flooring is in good repair and remove all throw rugs. Stairwells need to be well lighted, and securely fastened handrails extending the full length of both sides of the stairs are preferable.

Front and back entrances to the home and work areas need good lighting. Light fixtures need high-wattage bulbs with wider illumination. A light switch located at the top and bottom of stairwells is an additional safety element. Replace fluorescent lighting with incandescent lights.

Driving is a particular safety hazard for older adults with visual alterations. A sensitivity to glare creates a problem for driving at night with headlights. Reduced peripheral vision prevents a driver from seeing cars in the next lane. Reduced vision complicated by a decrease in reaction time, reduced hearing, and decreased strength in the legs and arms frequently limit the older adult's driving skills. To minimize risk, encourage older patients to drive only in familiar areas and not during rush hour. Urge them to drive defensively and avoid driving at night or at dusk. Older adults need to drive slowly but not so slowly that they create a safety hazard for other drivers.

Some patients have problems seeing dials or controls on electrical appliances and equipment. Use color contrasts such as tape, paint, or fingernail enamel to highlight dials. Have patients describe their usual daily activities to find opportunities for color coding to prevent accidents related to visual impairments.

Hearing Adaptations. Individuals need to hear environmental sounds such as fire alarms, alarm clocks, phones, or doorbells. Change or amplify the sound of these devices to a more low-pitched, buzzer-like quality. Signaling devices such as a flashing light on a phone allow patients with hearing impairments greater independence. Lamps designed to turn on in response to sounds such as doorbells, burglar alarms, smoke detectors, and babies crying are also available. Advise family and friends who call the patient regularly to let the phone ring for a longer period.

Smell and Tactile Adaptations. The patient with a reduced sensitivity to odors is often unable to smell leaking gas, a smoldering cigarette, fire, or tainted food. Make sure that a patient uses smoke detectors and takes precautions such as checking ashtrays or placing cigarette butts in water. Also advise the patient to check food package dates and inspect the appearance of food. Patients with reduced tactile sensation need to use hot and cold water bottles or heating pads cautiously and *never* use the high setting. Make sure that the temperature on the home water heater is no higher than 120° F.

Communication. It is important for individuals to be able to interact with people around them. The type of sensory loss influences the methods and styles of communication you use during interactions with patients. Some patients with hearing impairments are able to speak normally. To communicate clearly with patients who have hearing impairments, family and friends need to learn to move away from background noise, rephrase rather than repeat sentences, be positive, and have patience. On the other hand, some deaf patients have serious speech alterations. Patients who are deaf use sign language, read lips, write with pad and pencil, or learn to use a computer for communication (Box 38-9).

Acute Care. Some hospitalized patients are treated for sensory deficits (e.g., acute eye infection), and some have preexisting sensory problems. You need to know a patient's health history to appropriately support self-care activities while promoting a safe environment.

BOX 38-9 PATIENT TEACHING

Communication Strategies for Interacting with Patients Who Have Hearing Impairments

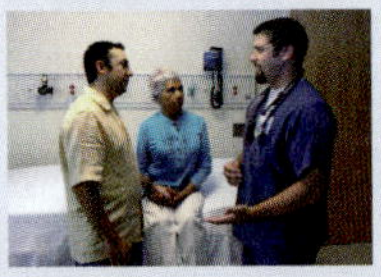

Rico tells Peter that he is concerned about communicating well with his mother now that she has both hearing and vision deficits. Peter understands that hearing impairment is a debilitating problem for many older adults; but interventions by health care providers, family, and friends help patients maintain communication. Peter investigates strategies for interacting with patients who have dual impairments. Using this information, he develops the following teaching plan for Rico:

OUTCOME

At the end of the teaching session, Rico verbalizes four strategies that he can use to improve communication with his mother.

TEACHING STRATEGIES

- Explain to Rico that he needs to face his mother directly and maintain good eye contact throughout the interaction (National Institute on Aging, 2013).
- Explain to Rico that communication is improved when there is good lighting and there is no glare in his mother's visual field (National Institute on Aging, 2013).
- Inform Rico to speak at a reasonable speed and not to shout (National Institute on Aging, 2013).
- Teach Rico to talk clearly toward his mother's best or normal ear and to use facial expressions or gestures to give conversational clues (National Institute on Aging, 2013).
- Explain to Rico that, when he is not understood, he should repeat himself using different words (National Institute on Aging, 2013).
- Teach Rico to make sure that his mother's hearing aids are in place and she is wearing her glasses when needed (Touhy and Jett, 2014).
- Tell Rico to pause between sentences or phrases to confirm understanding (Touhy and Jett, 2014).
- Tell Rico that he should be patient and stay positive and relaxed (National Institutes on Aging, 2013).
- Explain to Rico that comprehension is enhanced when background noise is minimized or eliminated (National Institute on Aging, 2013).
- Tell Rico to ask his mother how he can help (National Institute on Aging, 2013).

EVALUATION STRATEGIES

- Ask Rico to verbalize at least four communication approaches to use with his mother.
- Have Rico role play and use some of the communication strategies that you discussed.

Orientation to the Environment. Completely orient patients with sensory impairments to the immediate health care environment. Always keep your name tag visible, address the patient by name, explain the patient's location, and frequently include the time and date in conversations. Reduce the tendency for patients to become confused by offering short and simple, repeated explanations and reassurance. Encourage family and friends not to argue with or contradict a confused patient but to explain calmly their location, identity, and time of day.

Patients with serious visual impairments need to feel comfortable knowing the boundaries of their environment. The patient needs to walk through a room and feel the walls to establish a sense of direction. Remember to approach a patient who is blind from the front. Explain the location of objects within the room such as chairs or equipment. It is important to keep all objects in the same place and position. Moving an object even a short distance creates a safety hazard. You need to reorient the patient frequently by describing the location of key items. Place necessary objects such as the call light, patient-controlled analgesia (PCA) button, glasses, water, or facial tissue in front of patients to prevent falls caused by reaching. Ask the patient how to arrange objects so ambulation is easier. Remove clutter and unnecessary equipment. Always keep the path to the bathroom clear.

Safety Measures. Help patients with acute visual impairments walk (Figure 38-2). Stand on the patient's dominant, stronger, or uninjured side. The patient grasps your elbow or upper arm. You then walk one-half step ahead and slightly to the patient's side. His or her shoulder is directly behind your shoulder. Relax and walk at a comfortable pace. Warn the patient when approaching doorways and tell him or her whether the door opens in or out. Do not leave a patient with visual impairment alone in an unfamiliar area. If the patient has unstable mobility, use a gait belt during walking (see Chapter 27).

Communication. Strategies to enhance communication include providing adequate lighting and rearranging furniture so you can face a patient while talking. When communicating with patients, always actively listen and provide adequate time for patients with sensory deficits to respond (Touhy and Jett, 2014). Alert the entire multidisciplinary team when a patient has a sensory alteration. Note the most effective way to communicate with the patient in the patient's medical record.

Controlling Sensory Stimuli. Patients need time for rest and freedom from stress caused by frequent monitoring and repeated tests. Reduce sensory overload by organizing the plan of care to control for excessive stimuli. Combining activities such as dressing changes, bathing, and vital sign assessment in one visit prevents a patient from becoming overly fatigued. Coordination with other departments reduces the time needed for tests and examinations. The patient needs time for rest and quiet. Perform routine nursing procedures as quietly as possible. Encourage a family member to sit quietly with a patient or involve him or her in an undemanding repetitive activity such as combing hair.

Try to control extraneous noise in and around a patient's room such as television volume and visitors. Turn off bedside equipment not in use. Close a patient's room door if necessary. Hospital staff need to control loud laughter or conversation at the nurses' station. In addition to controlling excess stimuli, try to introduce meaningful stimulation that makes the environment pleasing and comfortable (Box 38-10).

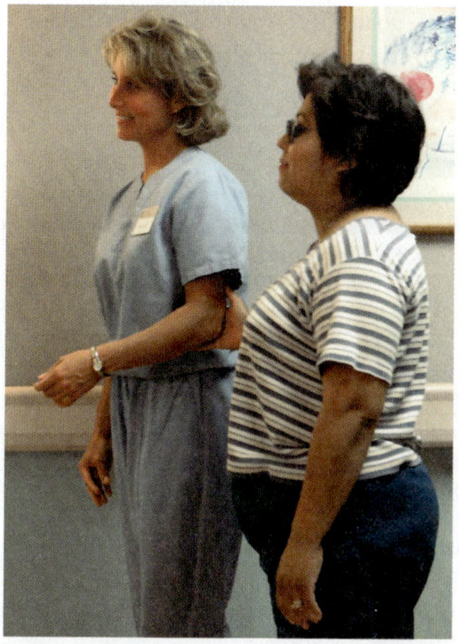

FIGURE 38-2 Nurse assists visually impaired patient with ambulation. (From Sorrentino SA, Remmert LN: *Mosby's textbook for nursing assistants*, ed 8, St Louis, 2012, Mosby.)

BOX 38-10 INTRODUCING STIMULI INTO THE CARE SETTING

VISUAL

- Open the drapes to the patient's room.
- Raise the head of the bed and draw back dividing curtains or partitions.
- Provide attractive decorations on tables or cabinets such as fresh flowers, plants, a picture, or greeting cards.
- Provide talking books and large-print reading material.

AUDITORY

- Sit down and speak with the patient. Make the conversation meaningful.
- Turn on a radio with the type of music the patient enjoys. A favorite radio or television program is stimulating.

TASTE AND SMELL

- Provide attractive, taste-appealing meals. Be sure that tableware and glasses are clean. Make sure that warm foods are served warm and cold foods are served cold.
- Provide a variety of textures, aromas, and flavors to enhance the patient's appetite.

Restorative and Continuing Care. After patients have experienced a sensory loss, they need to adjust to continue a normal lifestyle. Many of the interventions previously discussed under health promotion are adaptable for the home setting. The home environment needs to be healthy, comfortable, and safe. Suggest changes in a person's home environment after you assess the home setting for any hazards that increase the risk for injury.

Promoting Self-Care. Patients who have had surgery related to a sensory deficit need a plan of care that allows them to return safely to their home environment. Most patients have same-day surgical procedures (see Chapter 39). Family members or friends need to understand how the patient's sensory impairment affects the ability to perform ADLs and IADLs and the factors that lessen or worsen sensory problems. IADLs require a higher level of cognitive and physical functioning than ADLs and include such tasks as cleaning, yard maintenance, shopping, and money management (Touhy and Jett, 2012). Community resources discussed in the planning section are useful.

Patients with sensory impairments are often able to continue independent self-care activities. For meals you arrange food on the plate and condiments, salad, or drinks around the plate according to numbers on the face of a clock (Figure 38-3). The patient becomes oriented to the items after the family member explains the location of each. Patients need help to arrange self-care items such as clothing, hygiene, food supplies, and utensils in a consistent location to continue managing daily care activities.

A patient with visual impairments also needs help to reach the bathroom safely. Safety bars need to be installed near the toilet. A bar that is a different color from the wall is easier to see. Never place towels on safety bars because this interferes with a person's grasp.

If tactile sense is decreased, zippers or Velcro strips, pullover sweaters or blouses, and elasticized waists are easier for the patient to use. If the patient has a partial paralysis, you dress the affected side first. Some patients also need assistance with basic grooming such as brushing, combing, shaving, and shampooing hair. Make referrals to and collaborate with physical and/or occupational therapy to ensure that patients are able to function at an optimal level.

Socialization. Interacting with others becomes a burden for many patients with vision and hearing impairments. A patient with a hearing loss sometimes becomes embarrassed and exhausted after asking people to continuously repeat what they say. Patients often lose the motivation to engage in social activities, resulting in a deep sense of loneliness. Introduce therapies to reduce loneliness, particularly in older adults (Box 38-11). Family members need to learn to focus on a person's ability rather than his or her disability. Never assume that a person with a hearing or visual impairment does not wish to speak.

EVALUATION

Patient Care. It is important to evaluate whether care measures maintain or improve a patient's ability to interact and function within the environment (see Care Plan; Box 38-12). The patient is the source for evaluating outcomes. The nature of a patient's sensory alterations influences how you evaluate the outcome of care. When caring for a patient with a hearing deficit, use proper communication techniques and then evaluate whether he or she has gained the ability to hear or interact more effectively. When a patient does not achieve expected outcomes, you need to change interventions or alter the patient's environment.

For all patients it is important to evaluate the integrity of the sensory organs and the ability to perceive stimuli. This often involves a simple vision or hearing evaluation by asking a patient to perform a self-care skill. Be sure to determine if patients are following recommended therapies and meeting mutually set goals. If nursing care has been directed at improving or maintaining sensory acuity, asking a patient to

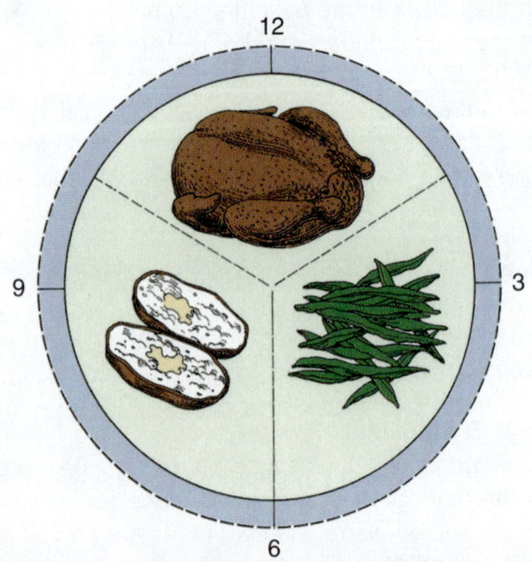

FIGURE 38-3 Arrange food on a plate and orient patient to placement based on numbers on a clock face.

BOX 38-11 CARE OF THE OLDER ADULT

Therapies to Reduce Loneliness

- Spend time with a person in silence or conversation.
- When it is culturally appropriate, use physical contact such as holding a hand or embracing a shoulder to convey caring.
- Help older adults keep contact with people important to them.
- Recommend alterations in living arrangements if physical isolation is a factor.
- Provide information about support groups or groups that provide assistive services.
- Link a person with organizations attuned to the social needs of older adults.
- Introduce the idea of bringing a companion such as a pet into the home when appropriate.

BOX 38-12 EVALUATION

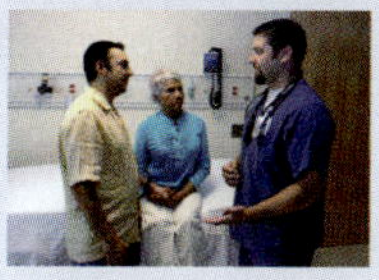

One month has passed since Mrs. Alicea's last visit to the senior health care center. Today Peter sits down and talks with both Mrs. Alicea and Rico. He learns that Mrs. Alicea is no longer having problems with glare because Rico changed the lights in the house to incandescent bulbs. Rico also reports that he plans to install sheer curtains that Mrs. Alicea chose last week in the living room. Mrs. Alicea also tells Peter that Rico has made a "few changes around the house," including rearranging furniture, securing some throw rugs while removing others, and removing the extension cords. After purchasing a magnifier at a local drug store, Mrs. Alicea is able to read the newspaper and medication labels more easily.

On examination Mrs. Alicea's visual acuity continues to reveal blurring when she tries to read an informational pamphlet. Her pupils continue to respond slowly to accommodation. Peter asks if she has made an appointment with her ophthalmologist. She confirms that the appointment is within the next 2 weeks.

Mrs. Alicea confides, "Overall I think the ideas we talked about last time helped me. I feel a little better about getting around the house and doing the things I like to do." When asked if he has noticed any changes in his mother's actions, Rico states, "She seems less fearful of falling."

DOCUMENTATION NOTE

"Visited clinic this morning as scheduled. Implemented measures at home to improve visual acuity and sensitivity to glare. Son supportive in making necessary home environment changes. Plans to make additional ones. Appointment with ophthalmologist in 2 weeks."

explain or demonstrate a newly learned self-care skill is an effective evaluative measure.

Patient Expectations. It is important to learn if patients think they are receiving appropriate care. A sensory deficit is potentially embarrassing and threatens a person's self-image. Does the patient feel comfortable relating to you? Was he or she able to maintain the plan of care for assistive devices? Did the patient think you were exhibiting a caring, professional approach? Asking patients if nursing care successfully met their expectations provides valuable knowledge when you care for other patients with similar sensory problems.

KEY POINTS

- Sensory perception depends on a region in the cerebral cortex where specialized brain cells interpret the quality and nature of sensory stimuli.
- Because a patient learns to rely on unaffected senses after a sensory loss, you design interventions to preserve function of these senses.
- Aging results in a gradual decline of acuity in all senses.
- Environmental stimuli in a hospital such as in an intensive care unit place a patient at risk for sensory overload.
- The extent of support from family members and significant others influences the quality of sensory experiences.
- Assessment of sensory function includes a physical examination and measurement of functional abilities.
- The presence of cerumen in the external auditory canal is a common cause of hearing loss in older adults.
- Sensory losses create loneliness and impair the ability to socialize.
- An assessment of environment includes identifying hazards, sources of meaningful stimulation, and the amount of stimuli.
- Prenatal screening and childhood immunizations prevent sensory alterations in the newborn and child.
- The care plan for patients with sensory alterations includes participation by family members.
- Patients with visual impairments need to learn boundaries within the environment to ambulate safely.
- Patients with existing hearing deficits are able to learn alternative ways to communicate.
- Nursing care for patients with sensory alterations includes using stronger sensory stimuli, compensating with other senses, and modifying the environment to maximize remaining sensory function.
- To prevent sensory overload, control stimuli, orient the patient to the environment, and promote rest by minimizing interruptions.
- Safety is a top concern when setting priorities for patients who experience sensory deprivation.

CLINICAL DECISION-MAKING EXERCISES

At Mrs. Alicea's last visit to the senior center, she reported that she feels more comfortable moving around the house, but Peter also learns that she does not leave the house often. She reports feeling alone much of the time. She tells Peter that she is having more problems hearing. Peter knows that Mrs. Alicea has hearing aids. He also knows that hearing aids are essential for communication and safety, so Peter decides to ask Mrs. Alicea if she wears hers. She reports that she doesn't wear them every day.

1. Discuss possible reasons that explain why Mrs. Alicea is reluctant to wear her hearing aids.
2. Identify some suggestions that Peter could share with Mrs. Alicea to influence her adaption to hearing aid use.
3. Based on these data, Peter develops a nursing diagnosis of *Impaired Social Interaction related to hearing deficits.* Identify one goal, two expected outcomes, and three related

nursing interventions that will help the patient meet the identified goals and outcome.

evolve

Answers to Clinical Decision-Making Exercises can be found on the Evolve website.

QSEN ACTIVITY: SAFETY

At the end of his clinical day, Peter is leaving the senior health center when he observes a loose throw rug at the top of the stairway at the entrance. Peter discussed home safety interventions with Mrs. Alicea; however, he is concerned about environmental modifications needed to make the health center safer for patients with sensory deficits. Peter considers to whom he should talk and whether his actions will make a difference. He decides to communicate his observations and concerns to his nursing instructor. Together they complete an environmental risk assessment, outline a plan to create an elder-friendly community health center, and communicate their observations and strategies to the health care team.

Did Peter display the knowledge, skills, and attitudes of what it means to be a competent nurse? Explain your answer. How did Peter's critical thinking attitude affect patient safety?

evolve

Answers to QSEN Activities can be found on the Evolve website.

REVIEW QUESTIONS

1. Which of the following guidelines do you need to follow when caring for patients with hearing impairments? (Select all that apply.)
   1. Position your patient so a light is on the person's face.
   2. Restate with the same words when you are not understood.
   3. When changing topics, preface the change by stating the topic.
   4. Verify that the information being given has been clearly understood.
   5. Use nonverbal approaches: gestures, visual aids, and written materials.
2. A nurse completes an assessment on an older adult with sensory alterations. During the examination the patient reports that he lives alone. Which of the following is a priority follow-up question?
   1. Do you have access to public transportation?
   2. How often do your friends and family visit?
   3. What time do you go to bed in the evening?
   4. What are your preferences for treatment?
3. A nurse is helping a visually impaired patient walk. Which of the following statements correctly describes how to guide a person with visual impairments? (Select all that apply.)
   1. Ask the patient to grasp your elbow or upper arm.
   2. Walk one step ahead and in front of the patient.
   3. Stand on the patient's dominant, stronger, or uninjured side.
   4. Use a gait belt if the patient has unstable mobility.
   5. Ask the patient to lead you in walking at a comfortable pace.
4. A school nurse is conducting a hearing screening program to identify children with possible hearing deficits. Which behavioral assessment finding is commonly found in children with hearing impairments?
   1. Slow or absent development of speech
   2. Clumsiness and failure to respond when touched
   3. Self-stimulation, including eye rubbing, body rocking, and arm twirling
   4. Inability to perform developmental tasks related to grasping objects or drawing
5. Which patient is most likely to experience sensory deprivation?
   1. A 62-year-old woman with a hearing impairment who lives in an assisted-living facility
   2. A 22-year-old isolated in the hospital because of immune system suppression related to chemotherapy
   3. A 76-year-old woman with visual impairments who attends recreational activities at the senior health care center
   4. An 11-year-old boy who is deaf and uses sign language to communicate with his friends, family, and teachers
6. A nurse is performing a home care assessment on a patient suspected of having a hearing impairment. The highest priority for the nurse at the onset of the interview is:
   1. To perform a physical examination.
   2. To understand that the patient will be uncooperative.
   3. To ask the patient or family what helps the person hear best.
   4. To share resources for the hearing impaired and refer as appropriate.
7. A nurse completes an assessment of a 72-year-old patient who comes to the clinic for the first time. During the examination the patient reaches for a glass of water and knocks it off the table. The patient is also observed squinting and reports a history of accidental falls. The nurse's assessment best indicates:
   1. A visual deficit.
   2. A hearing deficit.
   3. Sensory overload.
   4. Sensory deprivation.
8. A 76-year-old acutely ill woman who is in constant pain has been in the intensive care unit for 1 week. She is on a cardiac monitor and undergoes repeated tests daily. She has been restless and disoriented and is constantly touching her tubes and dressings. Considering the type of sensory alterations the patient most likely is experiencing, which nursing measures will help her function and

relate effectively within the environment? (Select all that apply.)

1. Ask the patient's family and friends to visit more frequently.
2. Constantly reorient the patient to the environment and reality.
3. Explain unusual sounds and prepare the patient for procedures in advance.
4. Reestablish normal sleep-wake cycle and encourage frequent rest periods.
5. Arrange for the patient to have a roommate and a room closer to the nurse's station.

9. A 75-year-old woman has macular degeneration. The home care nurse is conducting a home environment screening. Which of the following interventions will help the patient function safely with existing deficits and maintain a normal lifestyle? (Select all that apply.)
   1. Recommend that the patient move to a long-term care facility.
   2. Ask the patient to demonstrate or explain newly learned self-care skills.
   3. Encourage the use of brightly colored throw rugs throughout the home.
   4. Recommend that the patient organize informal network agreements with neighbors.
   5. Offer suggestions of ways to decorate a room and paint hallways so the patient is able to differentiate surfaces and objects in a room.

10. Which of the following interview questions best helps to ensure that the nurse is making patient-centered clinical decisions required for safe nursing care when completing a patient assessment?
    1. Do you use any devices to improve your hearing/vision?
    2. Which type of sounds or tones do you have difficulty hearing?
    3. Do you work or participate in any activities that have the potential for vision/hearing injury?
    4. What are your values, preferences, and expectations with regard to your sensory impairment?

evolve

Rationales for Review Questions can be found on the Evolve website.

1. 3, 4, 5; 2. 2; 3. 1, 3, 4; 4. 1; 5. 2; 6. 3; 7. 1; 8. 2, 3, 4; 9. 2, 4, 5; 10. 4

REFERENCES

American Academy of Ophthalmology: *Don't lose sight of your eye health*, 2011, http://www.geteyesmart.org/eyesmart/eye-health-news/press-releases/20110128.cfm. Accessed February 10, 2014.

American Speech-Language-Hearing Association: *Ototoxic medications (medication effects)*, 2014a, http://www.asha.org/public/hearing/Ototoxic-Medications/. Accessed February 10, 2014.

American Speech-Language-Hearing Association: *Who should be screened for hearing loss?* 2014b, http://www.asha.org/public/hearing/Who-Should-be-Screened/. Accessed February 10, 2014.

Dennis CM, et al: Benefits of quiet time for neuro-intensive care patients, *J Neurosci Nurs* 42(4):217, 2010.

Hockenberry MJ, Wilson D: *Wong's nursing care of infants and children*, ed 9, St Louis, 2011, Mosby.

Li Y, et al: Visual impairment and health-related quality of life among elderly adults with age-related eye diseases, *Qual Life Res* 20(6):845, 2010.

Li SY, et al: Efficacy of controlling night-time noise and activities to improve patients' sleep quality in a surgical intensive care unit, *J Clin Nurs* 20(3/4):396, 2011.

Meiner SE: *Gerontologic nursing*, ed 4, St Louis, 2011, Mosby.

National Eye Institute: *Facts about cataracts*, 2009, http://www.nei.nih.gov/health/cataract/cataract_facts.asp. Accessed February 10, 2014.

National Institute on Aging: *Age page: hearing loss*, 2013, US Department of Health and Human Services, http://www.nia.nih.gov/health/publication/hearing-loss. Accessed February 10, 2014.

Occupational Safety and Health Administration (OSHA): *Eye and face protection*, n.d., US Department of Labor, http://www.osha.gov/SLTC/eyefaceprotection/index.html. Accessed February 10, 2014.

Owen DC, et al: Mexican Americans. In Giger JN, editor: *Transcultural nursing: assessment & intervention*, ed 6, St Louis, 2013, Mosby.

Sudore RL, Schillinger D: Interventions to improve care for patients with limited health literacy, *J Clin Outcomes Manage* 16(1):20, 2009.

The Joint Commission (TJC): *2014 Hospital accreditation standards*, Oakbrook, IL, 2014, The Commission.

Touhy TA, Jett A: *Ebersole & Hess' Toward health aging: human needs and nursing response*, ed 8, St Louis, 2012, Mosby.

Touhy TA, Jett A: *Ebersole & Hess' Gerontological nursing and healthy aging*, ed 3, St Louis, 2014, Mosby.

World Health Organization (WHO): *Visual impairment and blindness*, 2013, http://www.who.int/mediacentre/factsheets/fs282/en/index.html. Accessed February 10, 2014.

CHAPTER 39

Surgical Patient

evolve WEBSITE

http://evolve.elsevier.com/Potter/essentials

- Video Clip
- Crossword Puzzle
- Audio Glossary

OBJECTIVES

- Explain the concept of perioperative nursing care.
- Differentiate among classifications of surgery and types of anesthesia.
- List factors to include in the preoperative assessment of a surgical patient.
- Design a patient-centered preoperative teaching plan.
- Prepare a patient for surgery.
- Explain the differences in caring for a patient undergoing outpatient surgery versus a patient undergoing inpatient surgery.
- Discuss safety initiatives applied throughout the perioperative patient experience.
- Describe intraoperative factors that affect a patient's postoperative course.
- Identify factors to assess in a patient in postoperative recovery.
- Describe the rationale for nursing interventions designed to prevent postoperative complications.

KEY TERMS

antiembolic stockings, p. 1148
atelectasis, p. 1131
bronchospasm, p. 1136
circulating nurse, p. 1150
conscious sedation, p. 1152
embolism, p. 1131
general anesthesia, p. 1152
laryngospasm, p. 1136
malignant hyperthermia, p. 1135
moderate sedation/analgesia, p. 1152
nasogastric (NG) tube, p. 1148
operating room, p. 1149
outpatient, p. 1130
paralytic ileus, p. 1156
perioperative nursing, p. 1130
postanesthesia care unit (PACU), p. 1153
preanesthesia care unit, p. 1149
preoperative teaching, p. 1144
presurgical care unit (PSCU), p. 1149
pulmonary hygiene, p. 1136
regional anesthesia, p. 1152
scrub nurse, p. 1150
sequential compression stockings, p. 1148

Perioperative nursing includes care given before (preoperative), during (intraoperative), and after (postoperative) surgery. Surgery takes place in a variety of settings, including hospitals, ambulatory surgery centers, clinics, health care providers' offices, and even mobile units. Minor surgeries are performed on an **outpatient** basis, with patients entering a health care setting, undergoing surgery, and being discharged the same day. Many surgical patients enter a health care setting as outpatients for preoperative screening and testing and are admitted to a hospital after surgery. Patients requiring extensive preoperative care are admitted to a hospital before surgery. The principles of caring for perioperative patients are the same, regardless of the setting.

CASE STUDY *Mr. Korloff*

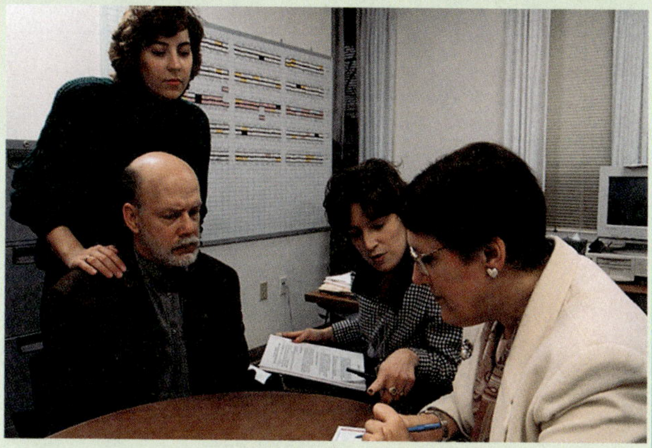

Mr. Korloff is a 53-year-old man who has had abdominal pain for 2 months. Following a series of diagnostic tests, he is now scheduled for elective laparoscopic gallbladder surgery. Mr. Korloff is originally from Russia and has lived in the United States for 10 years. He speaks English relatively well but still speaks in Russian when family is present. He is a vice president for an international business firm. He is widowed and has two adult daughters, both born in Russia before coming to the United States. The daughters are married and live in the same neighborhood as Mr. Korloff. However, both have full-time jobs.

Sue Collins is a nursing student assigned to the preadmission center at the local hospital where she has been working for 2 weeks. She is completing her last clinical rotation and will graduate in 1 month. Sue is 30 years old, is married, and has no children. She plans to seek employment in a hospital on a general surgery floor after graduation. Sue's father recently had surgery for prostate cancer.

This chapter synthesizes many concepts and skills previously presented in this text. You will recognize these previously learned areas such as patient education, oxygenation, and elimination and apply this information when caring for surgical patients in the preoperative and postoperative phases.

SCIENTIFIC KNOWLEDGE BASE

Classification of Surgery

Surgical procedures are classified according to the seriousness, urgency, and purpose of surgery (Table 39-1). For example, a breast biopsy, done for diagnostic purposes, is classified as urgent and done on an outpatient basis. Knowing the classification helps you to plan appropriate preoperative and postoperative care for each patient.

Surgical Risk Factors

Numerous factors create risks for a person undergoing surgery. Knowledge regarding the physiology of the stress response (see Chapter 25) and factors that affect a patient's response to the stress of surgery is necessary to anticipate patient needs for preoperative preparation, teaching, and postoperative care.

Smoking. There is a significant association between smoking and postoperative pulmonary complications, specifically pneumonia and **atelectasis.** Chronic smoking increases the amount and thickness of mucus secretions in the lungs. After surgery a patient who smokes has greater difficulty clearing the airways of mucus and needs to practice deep breathing and coughing exercises (see Chapter 30). Smoking also increases the risk for circulatory and infectious complications (Kiernan, 2012).

Age. Very young and older patients are at greater surgical risk as a result of an immature or a declining physiological status. Maintaining a patient's normal body temperature is a concern during surgery. When compared with adults, infants have a proportionately greater surface area and less subcutaneous fat, placing them at risk for wide temperature variations. In addition, general anesthetics inhibit shivering, a protective reflex to maintain body temperature; and anesthetics cause vasodilation, which results in heat loss. During surgery an infant also has difficulty maintaining a normal circulatory blood volume. The total blood volume of infants is considerably less than that of older children and adults, creating a risk for both dehydration and overhydration.

Nutrition. Normal tissue repair and resistance to infection depend on adequate nutrition. Surgery increases the need for nutrients. After surgery a patient requires at least 1500 kcal/day to maintain energy reserves. Additional protein; carbohydrates; zinc; and vitamins A, B, C, and K are necessary for proper wound healing (see Chapters 33 and 37). Patients who are malnourished are more likely to have poor tolerance of anesthesia, negative nitrogen balance, delayed postoperative recovery, infection, and delayed wound healing (Black and Hawks, 2009).

Obesity. A patient who is obese usually has reduced ventilatory capacity because of the upward pressure against the diaphragm caused by an enlarged abdomen. There is also an increased risk for aspiration during the administration of anesthesia (Kiernan, 2012). The recumbent and supine positions required on the operating bed (table) for surgery further limit a patient's ventilation. The increased workload of the heart and atherosclerotic blood vessels often results in compromised cardiovascular function. Because of these physiological changes, patients who are obese often have difficulty resuming normal physical activity after surgery. Hypertension, coronary artery disease, type 2 diabetes mellitus, and heart failure are common in this population. They are also more susceptible to developing **embolism,** atelectasis, and pneumonia after surgery than patients who are not obese (Black and Hawks, 2009).

In addition, excess weight placed on skin over bony prominences restricts blood flow and poses risk for impaired skin integrity. Obesity increases the risk of poor wound healing and wound infection because fatty tissue contains a poor blood supply, which slows the delivery of essential nutrients and antibodies needed for healing. It is often difficult to close a surgical wound when a patient is obese because of the thick adipose layer. The risk for wound dehiscence and evisceration is increased because of these factors (see Chapter 37).

TABLE 39-1 CLASSIFICATION FOR SURGICAL PROCEDURES

TYPE	DESCRIPTION	EXAMPLE
Seriousness		
Major	Involves extensive reconstruction or alteration in body parts; poses great risks to well-being	Coronary artery bypass, colon resection, removal of larynx, resection of lung lobe
Minor	Involves minimal alteration in body parts; often designed to correct deformities; involves minimal risks compared with major procedures	Cataract extraction, facial plastic surgery, tooth extraction
Urgency		
Elective	Performed on basis of patient's choice; not essential and is not always necessary for health	Bunionectomy, facial plastic surgery, breast reconstruction
Urgent	Necessary for patient's health, can prevent additional problems from developing (e.g., tissue destruction, impaired organ function); not necessarily an emergency	Excision of cancerous tumor, removal of gallbladder for stones, vascular repair for obstructed artery (e.g., coronary artery bypass)
Emergency	Must be done immediately to save life or preserve function of body part	Repair of perforated appendix, repair of traumatic amputation, control of internal hemorrhaging
Purpose		
Diagnostic	Surgical exploration that allows health care provider to confirm diagnosis; sometimes involves removal of tissue for further diagnostic testing	Exploratory laparotomy (incision into peritoneal cavity to inspect abdominal organs), breast mass biopsy
Ablative	Amputation or removal of diseased body part	Amputation, removal of appendix, cholecystectomy
Palliative	Relieves or reduces intensity of disease symptoms; does not produce cure	Colostomy, removal of necrotic tissue, resection of nerve roots
Reconstructive/restorative	Restores function or appearance to traumatized or malfunctioning tissues	Internal fixation of fractures, scar revision
Procurement for transplant	Removal of organs and/or tissues from a person pronounced brain dead for transplantation into another person	Kidney, cornea, or liver transplant
Constructive	Restores function lost or reduced as result of congenital anomalies	Repair of cleft palate, closure of atrial septal defect in heart
Cosmetic	Performed to improve personal appearance	Blepharoplasty to correct eyelid deformities; rhinoplasty to reshape nose

Obstructive Sleep Apnea. Obstructive sleep apnea (OSA) increases the risk for perioperative respiratory complications such as oxygen desaturation and apnea. OSA is a syndrome of periodic complete or partial obstruction of the upper airway during sleep (see Chapter 31). Always instruct patients diagnosed with OSA to bring their continuous positive airway pressure machine for use after surgery. Many patients have undiagnosed OSA and can be screened before surgery with simple questions regarding snoring, apnea during sleep, frequent arousals during sleep, morning headaches, daytime somnolence, and chronic fatigue (Phillips, 2012; Nugent, Phy, and Raj, 2012).

Immunocompetence. Radiation and chemotherapeutic drugs used to treat cancer, immunosuppressive agents used to prevent rejection after organ transplantation, and steroids used to treat inflammatory conditions make the body vulnerable to infection. All of these therapies, in addition to disorders affecting the immune system such as acquired immunodeficiency syndrome (AIDS), suppress the immune system of the body. Immunosuppression increases the risk for infection following surgery. For example, a patient with cancer has radiation therapy to reduce the size of a cancerous tumor before surgery to remove the tumor. Radiation causes fibrosis and vascular scarring in the radiated area. The tissues become fragile and poorly oxygenated, increasing the risk for wound infection. Ideally surgery takes place 4 to 6 weeks after the completion of radiation treatments to avoid wound-healing problems.

Fluid and Electrolyte Balance. The body responds to surgery as a form of trauma. As a result of the adrenocortical stress response, hormonal reactions cause sodium and water retention and potassium loss within the first 2 to 5 days after surgery (see Chapter 18). Severe protein breakdown creates a negative nitrogen balance. The severity of the stress response influences the degree of fluid and electrolyte imbalance. More extensive surgery is associated with more severe physiological stress. Patients with preexisting renal, fluid and electrolyte, gastrointestinal, respiratory, or cardiovascular problems are at greatest risk for operative complications. For example, a patient who is dehydrated from vomiting before surgery is at greater risk for hypovolemic shock.

Pregnancy. When caring for a pregnant patient, consider the needs of both the pregnant woman and her unborn fetus. Surgery is only for urgent or emergent reasons such as appendicitis or trauma. The enlarged uterus displaces abdominal organs and distorts landmarks, making surgery more complex. Anesthetics and medications cause fetal abnormalities during the first trimester. During pregnancy the following maternal physiological changes occur that increase the complexity of patient care (Rothrock, 2011):

1. Cardiac output and respiratory tidal volume increase to keep up with the increase in metabolism and blood pressure decreases, making interpretation of vital signs and recognition of hypovolemic shock more difficult.
2. The high level of progesterone relaxes the lower esophageal sphincter (LES) and decreases gastrointestinal motility, which slows gastric emptying, resulting in an increased risk for aspiration of stomach contents.
3. Near term there is an increase in white blood cells beyond the normal range for that of nonpregnant women who have no infection.
4. There is an increased risk for deep vein thrombosis as a result of increased fibrinogen levels and decreased clotting time.

In addition, a pregnant patient and her family experience increased psychological stress because of fear of fetal loss or deformity. The perioperative team addresses these concerns.

NURSING KNOWLEDGE BASE

Perioperative Communication

Perioperative nurses recognize the importance of providing continuity of care for the surgical patient using the nursing process. In some settings perioperative nurses assess a patient's health status before surgery, identify specific patient needs, teach and counsel, attend to a patient's needs in the operating room (OR), and follow a patient's recovery. In other words, one nurse follows a patient throughout the operative experience. However, most commonly different nurses care for a patient during each phase of the surgical experience. The process of communicating patient information between perioperative nurses during the transfer of care is essential to ensure continuity of care. Transitions from one care provider to another place patients at risk for injuries and errors. A standardized approach to hand-off communication between perioperative nurses minimizes these risks. The components of a safe and effective sign-out often uses the acronym *ANTICipate* (Box 39-1). In addition to a standardized process, mistakes can be reduced through the use of effective communication skills such as awareness of nonverbal behaviors, active listening, and understanding the effects and emotions of others in the OR setting (Cvetic, 2011) (see Chapter 11).

BOX 39-1 HAND-OFF COMMUNICATION IN THE OPERATING ROOM

The components of a safe and effective sign-out can be summarized using the acronym *ANTICipate*:

Administrative data (e.g., patient's name, age, sex, medical record number, and location) must be accurate.
New clinical information must be updated (e.g., current status, critical laboratory values, recent changes).
Tasks to be performed by the covering provider must be clearly explained (e.g., vital sign frequency, intravenous fluid adjustment, wound observations).
Illness severity must be communicated (e.g., risks for complications must be specified).
Contingency plans for changes in clinical status must be outlined to assist cross-coverage in managing a patient (e.g., clarify role of surgeon, anesthesia provider in patient recovery, anticipate nurse staffing needs).

Adapted from Agency for Healthcare Research and Quality (AHRQ): *Patient safety primers: handoffs and signouts,* AHRQ October 2012, http://www.psnet.ahrq.gov/primer.aspx?primerID=9. Accessed November 19, 2013.

Complication Prevention

Patients are at high risk for a variety of complications following surgery. Prevention of respiratory and cardiac complications requires critical thinking and knowledge of the pulmonary and cardiovascular systems. Assessment begins in the preoperative area and continues through the postoperative period. Detection of breathing difficulties or airway issues requires you to have excellent assessment skills, anticipate and identify problems, and know a patient's risk. Quick intervention prevents significant problems.

Gylcemic Control and Infection Prevention

Evidence has shown that there is a relationship between wound and tissue infection and blood glucose levels. Poor control of blood glucose levels (specifically hyperglycemia) during surgery and afterward increases the risk for wound infection and patient mortality in certain types of surgery (Frisch et al., 2010; Rutan and Sommers, 2012). Perioperative nurses work with their medical colleagues to maintain normal glucose levels in the postoperative period to reduce the risk for wound and tissue infection.

Pressure Ulcer Prevention

Surgical patients pose a unique challenge in preventing pressure ulcers. Patients are at risk for pressure ulcer formation intraoperatively as a result of sustained pressure from positioning on OR tables. Pressure compresses skin and muscle between bones and the OR bed, resulting in tissue ischemia. Anesthetic agents lower blood pressure, altering tissue perfusion. Factors such as shear force, negativity from multiple layers of drapes, and moisture on the OR bed add to the risk for ulcer formation (Bulfone et al., 2012). OR nurses prevent pressure ulcers intraoperatively by careful positioning and use of pressure-relieving surfaces. After surgery nurses perform careful skin assessment and intervene by using low-air-loss or pressure-reduction beds and mattresses and frequent repositioning for those unable to move themselves.

CRITICAL THINKING

Synthesis

You will apply elements of critical thinking whenever you perform the nursing process with patients. Consider the scientific knowledge you have learned, your experience, critical thinking attitudes, and standards to ensure an individualized approach to patient care.

Knowledge. It is essential to have a strong knowledge base in anatomy and physiology, principles of aseptic technique (see Chapter 14), pharmacology (see Chapter 17), and teaching-learning principles (see Chapter 12). In addition, understanding the effect that surgical procedures and medications have on different body systems is essential. It is also important to understand the normal stress response to anticipate potential complications during the perioperative experience (see Chapter 25). Effective preoperative teaching requires a knowledge base of teaching and communication principles and the planned surgical procedure.

Experience. Any personal experience with surgery helps you understand the anxiety of patients and their families and explain some of the physical sensations that patients experience. Past experiences with surgical patients enable you to anticipate questions that a patient and family will ask and focus preoperative teaching. In addition, experience helps you recognize physiological changes in patients more quickly so you are able to initiate preventive and corrective measures early.

Attitudes. A key attitude for a perioperative nurse is responsibility. As a perioperative nurse, you are responsible for following perioperative care standards and being a patient advocate. When a patient consents to surgery and receives an anesthetic agent that alters the level of consciousness, health care providers have the responsibility to protect a patient. You are responsible for maintaining the rights of a patient when a patient cannot speak on his or her own behalf.

Perioperative nurses who are creative apply evidence in the plan of care to deal with individual patient differences. For example, to promote venous return, a nurse positions a pregnant patient on the operating table with a positioning wedge under the right hip to displace the uterus to the left. Assess each patient and use the most appropriate padding and positioning techniques possible to prevent injury.

Your attitude about the discipline of nursing is also important when caring for surgical patients. A patient experiences numerous routines for preparation for surgery and an efficient and optimal recovery. Systematically follow the current standards of practice to ensure high-quality care for each patient.

Standards. The application of critical thinking intellectual standards is important for a patient having surgery, particularly if a patient has preexisting physical or psychological factors that will influence surgical outcomes. Be very precise, accurate, and complete in gathering assessment data; and use a logical, relevant, and well–thought out approach in making clinical decisions because a patient's condition can change quickly.

The Association of periOperative Registered Nurses (AORN) established standards and recommended practice for nurses in perioperative clinical practice. The standards and position statements cover practices to ensure patient safety, appropriate monitoring and evaluation, infection control practices, and timely and effective nursing interventions. These standards are incorporated in the content of this chapter. As a perioperative nurse you are responsible for following these standards (AORN, 2012). The Joint Commission's 2014 Hospital National Patient Safety Goals include two sets of recommendations for perioperative care: prevent infection and prevent mistakes in surgery (TJC, 2014). Specifically, perioperative nurses use evidence-based guidelines to prevent infection after surgery, which includes cleansing the operative site before an incision and wound care after surgery. Surgical nurses prevent mistakes in surgery by making sure that a patient undergoes the correct surgery, marking the place on a patient's body where surgery is to be done, and pausing before surgery to make sure that a mistake is not made.

PREOPERATIVE SURGICAL PHASE

Patients having surgery enter a health care setting in different stages of health. Some patients enter the facility feeling relatively healthy while awaiting elective surgery. Other patients enter in great distress when facing emergency surgery. Many tests and procedures are often necessary to ensure that surgery is indicated and that a patient is in an optimum condition. During these tests and procedures a patient meets many health care personnel who play a role in his or her care and recovery. Family members or friends also play an important role by providing support and education reinforcement, but they also face many of the same stressors as patients.

Some patients have preoperative preparation several days before the day of surgery. Preadmission testing is often done in the hospital, surgeon's office, or outpatient laboratory. With this testing completed, patients usually enter a hospital the day that surgery is performed. Many hospitals have special outpatient or "ambulatory" surgery centers for elective surgery, where patients come to the center, have surgery, and return home on the same day. Outpatient surgery is also performed in freestanding clinics. At times a patient enters the hospital the day before surgery. Be able to properly prepare a patient for surgery, regardless of where he or she enters the health care setting.

NURSING PROCESS

ASSESSMENT

Your preoperative assessment of a patient establishes a normal baseline for a patient before surgery and alerts you to special needs and potential intraoperative and postoperative complications. Use effective communication skills to gather information and screen patients for potential risk factors for surgery (Kiernan, 2012).

Nursing History. The preoperative history includes key elements that are relevant to a patient's risks and needs (Box 39-2). In the ambulatory surgical setting the history is often less detailed than when a patient is hospitalized the evening before surgery; however, the basic information outlined in the following paragraphs is necessary for competent care in each setting. Interview family members or significant others if a patient is unable to relate all needed information. As with any admission to a health care facility, include information concerning advance directives. Ask if a patient has a durable power of attorney for health care and a living will (see Chapter 5) and include a copy in the chart. The law requires advance directive identification for patients of all ages and for all surgical procedures. Often directives are modified during the perioperative period but are reestablished after postoperative stabilization.

Medical History. A review of a patient's medical history includes past illnesses and the primary reason for seeking medical care. A history screens candidates for surgery for major medical conditions that increase the risk for complications (Table 39-2). If a patient is at increased risk, surgery as an outpatient may not be advisable. For example, ask women of childbearing age about the date of their last menstrual period (LMP), if their last period was "typical" for them, and if they have had unprotected sex in the last month. Because many women do not know they are pregnant early in the first trimester, many institutions require a pregnancy test when a patient of childbearing age is scheduled for surgery and has not had surgical sterilization. Inquire about family history for anesthetic complications because an adverse reaction called **malignant hyperthermia** is an inherited disorder. Malignant hyperthermia is a life-threatening complication resulting in high carbon dioxide levels, tachypnea, tachycardia, heart rhythm irregularities, and muscular rigidity with elevated temperature in the late stages (Johns et al., 2012).

Previous Surgeries. Review of a patient's past experience with surgery reveals physical and psychological responses that may occur during the current planned procedure. Complications such as anaphylaxis or malignant hyperthermia during previous surgery alert you to the need for preventive measures and availability of emergency equipment. A history of postoperative complications such as persistent vomiting or uncontrolled pain alerts you to the possible need for different medications. Reports of severe anxiety before a previous surgery identify the need for additional emotional support, medications, and preoperative teaching. Inform the surgeon of your findings when you believe that medications are indicated.

Medication History. Review whether a patient is taking any medications that predispose him or her to surgical complications (Table 39-3). Many medications interact unpredictably with anesthetic agents during surgery (Lehne, 2013). If a patient regularly uses prescription or over-the-counter (OTC) medications or herbal supplements, some surgeons temporarily discontinue them before surgery or adjust the dosages. Instruct patients to ask their surgeons whether they should take their usual medications the morning of surgery. If a patient is having inpatient surgery, all prescription drugs taken before surgery are automatically discontinued after surgery unless reordered. Be vigilant in reviewing a surgeon's preoperative orders so you do not forget any medication that a patient needs to take before the operation. It is important that, as a patient moves through different areas (e.g., holding area to OR), a complete list of his or her medications is accurately communicated from nurse to nurse (TJC, 2013).

Allergies. Allergies to medications, topical agents used to prepare the skin for surgery, and latex create significant risks for surgical patients. An allergic response to any agent is potentially fatal, depending on its severity. Latex allergies are on the rise (see Chapter 14). A latex allergy manifests as contact dermatitis with redness, inflammation, and blisters; as contact urticaria with pruritus, redness, and swelling; or as hay fever–like symptoms and anaphylaxis.

All health care workers need to know about their patient's allergies. In most agencies patients who have allergies receive an allergy identification band at the time of admission that

BOX 39-2 SYNTHESIS IN PRACTICE

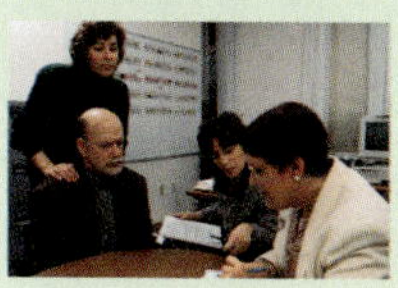

As Sue prepares to conduct Mr. Korloff's preadmission assessment, she recalls what she has learned regarding risk factors for patients undergoing surgery. Mr. Korloff has a history of heart disease. Five years ago he was treated for a cardiac rhythm irregularity but has had no further problems. Sue applies the critical thinking attitude by questioning Mr. Korloff thoroughly about any potential cardiac symptoms. She plans to have his daughters present during the discussion.

Sue's knowledge of laparoscopic surgery helps her anticipate the types of postoperative problems that Mr. Korloff is likely to develop such as food intolerance and abdominal or referred pain from the carbon dioxide gas used during laparoscopy. Sue's experience with her own father after surgery helps her to explain some of the sensations that Mr. Korloff will experience such as a sore throat from the breathing tube used for administering anesthesia. She also needs to draw on her experiences with patients for whom she cared after laparoscopic surgeries during her previous rotation on a general surgery floor. She informs Mr. Korloff and his daughters that he will have intravenous (IV) fluids infusing until he tolerates oral fluids and that he will likely experience mild discomfort. Mr. Korloff will be able to get out of bed the evening of surgery; and, if all goes well, he will likely be discharged the next day.

TABLE 39-2 MEDICAL CONDITIONS THAT INCREASE THE RISKS OF SURGERY

TYPE OF CONDITION	REASON FOR RISK
Bleeding disorders (thrombocytopenia, hemophilia)	Disorders increase risk for hemorrhaging during and after surgery.
Diabetes mellitus	Diabetes increases susceptibility to infection and impairs wound healing from altered glucose metabolism and associated circulatory impairment. Fluctuating blood glucose levels cause central nervous system alterations during anesthesia. Stress of surgery causes increases in blood glucose levels.
Heart disease (recent myocardial infarction, dysrhythmias, congestive heart failure) and peripheral vascular disease	Stress of surgery causes increased demands on myocardium to maintain cardiac output. General anesthetic agents depress cardiac function.
Hypertension	Hypertension increases risk for cardiovascular complications during anesthesia (e.g., stroke, inadequate tissue oxygenation).
Upper respiratory infection	Infection increases risk for respiratory complications during anesthesia (e.g., pneumonia, spasm of laryngeal muscles).
Renal disease	Renal disease alters excretion of anesthetic drugs and their metabolites and acid-base balance, increasing risk for surgical complications.
Liver disease	Liver disease alters metabolism and elimination of drugs administered during surgery and impairs wound healing and clotting time because of alterations in protein metabolism.
Fever	Fever predisposes patient to fluid and electrolyte imbalances and often indicates underlying infection.
Chronic respiratory disease (emphysema, bronchitis, asthma)	Respiratory disease reduces patient's ability to compensate for acid-base alterations. Anesthetic agents reduce respiratory function, increasing risk for severe hypoventilation.
Immunological disorders (leukemia, acquired immunodeficiency syndrome [AIDS], bone marrow depression, organ transplantation, and use of chemotherapeutic drugs)	Immunological disorders increase risk for infection and delay wound healing after surgery.
Abuse of alcohol and street drugs	Patients who abuse drugs sometimes have underlying disease (human immunodeficiency virus [HIV], hepatitis) and altered wellness, which affect healing. Alcohol addiction causes unpredictable reactions to anesthesia. People go into withdrawal during and after surgery.
Chronic pain	Regular use of pain medications often results in higher tolerance. Increased doses of opioids frequently are necessary to achieve postoperative pain control.

remains on until discharge. Allergies are also listed on the front of patients' charts, on medical order sheets, and on patients' medication administration records. Verify your patient's allergies before, during, and after surgery.

Smoking Habits. A patient who smokes is at a greater risk for postoperative pulmonary complications than a patient who does not smoke. Smoking decreases ciliary movement of mucus from the lower airways upward, increases mucus production, and causes bronchial constriction, thus increasing airway obstruction. After surgery patients have greater difficulty clearing the airways of mucus secretions and are at increased risk for **bronchospasm** and **laryngospasm.** Use this information to plan aggressive postoperative **pulmonary hygiene,** including more frequent turning, deep breathing, coughing, use of incentive spirometry, and chest physical therapy (PT) if ordered. Smoking causes hypercoagulability of the blood and increased risk for clot formation (Black and Hawks, 2009). Provide measures to decrease the risk for clot formation such as pneumatic compression stockings, deep breathing, leg exercises, and early ambulation.

Alcohol and Controlled Substance Use and Abuse. The surgical team needs to be aware of the use of alcohol and controlled substances by patients to prepare for adverse reactions such as withdrawal that may occur during surgery. Increased tolerance to opioids occurs with chronic opioid use, resulting in an increased need for anesthesia and postoperative analgesics (Black and Hawks, 2009).

Family Support. Determine if and to what extent a patient will have support from family members or friends. Surgery often results in temporary disability that requires direct care

TABLE 39-3 MEDICATIONS WITH SPECIAL IMPLICATIONS FOR THE SURGICAL PATIENT

DRUG CLASS	EFFECTS DURING SURGERY
Antibiotics	Potentiate action of anesthetic agents. If taken within 2 weeks before surgery, aminoglycosides (gentamicin, tobramycin, neomycin) cause mild respiratory depression from depressed neuromuscular transmission.
Antidysrhythmics	Reduce cardiac contractility and heart rate and impair cardiac conduction during anesthesia.
Anticoagulants	Alter normal clotting factors, increasing risk for hemorrhage during and after surgery. Discontinue them at least 48 hours before surgery. Aspirin is a common medication that alters clotting mechanisms.
Anticonvulsants	Long-term use of certain anticonvulsants (e.g., phenytoin [Dilantin], phenobarbital) alters metabolism of anesthetic agents.
Antihypertensives	Interact with anesthetic agents and cause bradycardia, hypotension, and impaired circulation. They inhibit synthesis and storage of norepinephrine in sympathetic nerve endings.
Corticosteroids	Prolonged use of corticosteroids causes adrenal atrophy, which reduces the ability of the body to withstand stress and results in hypotension during surgery. Dosages are sometimes temporarily increased before and during surgery.
Insulin	Patients with diabetes often need different insulin doses after surgery. Their nutritional intake is decreased immediately after surgery; however, stress response and intravenous administration of glucose solutions increase blood sugar. Thus regulating blood sugars with insulin after surgery is challenging.
Diuretics	Potentiate electrolyte imbalances (particularly potassium), increasing the risk for dysrhythmias during and after surgery.
Nonsteroidal antiinflammatory drugs (NSAIDs)	Inhibit platelet aggregation and prolong bleeding time, increasing susceptibility to bleeding during and after surgery.

and assistance from significant others during recovery. A patient does not always immediately assume the same level of physical activity and often returns home with dressings to change or exercises to perform. Ask questions to determine the condition of a patient's home environment, the availability of resources (family or friends as caregivers), and how a patient's expected limitations will affect his or her ability to perform activities of daily living. For example, a patient receives discharge instructions that state the need to use an incentive spirometer every 2 hours. When talking with the patient, you discover that he or she has difficulty using the device. In this case you make sure that the patient's family understands how to help him or her use the incentive spirometer until the patient demonstrates using the device without assistance.

Occupation. Surgery often results in physical alterations that prevent a person from returning to work. Assess a patient's occupational history to anticipate the effect that surgery will have on convalescence and eventual work performance. Explain any restrictions that a patient will have when returning to work.

Feelings. Surgery causes anxiety and a feeling of loss of control for most patients. Many families are concerned about the ability of a patient to return to a productive life and the impact that recovery will have on the family. Assess a patient's feelings about having surgery from both verbal and nonverbal cues. A patient who is fearful may ask many questions or be very quiet, may seem uneasy when strangers enter the room, or may actively seek the company of friends and relatives.

It is difficult to assess patients' feelings thoroughly before ambulatory surgery is scheduled. You have limited time to spend with a patient. As a nurse in an outpatient surgical program, telephone the patient at home before surgery or interview him or her during a preadmission testing visit. For patients in the hospital, choose a time for discussion after preliminary admitting or diagnostic tests are complete. A patient's ability to share feelings depends in part on your willingness to ask questions, listen, be supportive, and clarify misconceptions.

Cultural and Spiritual Factors. Cultural beliefs, attitudes, and traditions affect how patients respond to any health care problem; surgery is no exception. Differences in the use of both verbal and nonverbal communication require you to validate interpretation of cues with a patient and family (Box 39-3). This is especially important after you conduct the initial preoperative assessment and then look for changes in a patient's status after surgery. For example, patients from Asian cultures often remain silent out of respect, not fear. However, you cannot assume that every Asian patient will be the same. Learn how to form relationships that enable you to understand a person's culture and preferences. Ask questions such as, "Tell me about what this surgery means to you and your family?" "Having surgery may make you feel afraid; tell me your concerns." In some cultures women follow the directives of the significant male member of the family; therefore it is very

BOX 39-3 PATIENT-CENTERED CARE

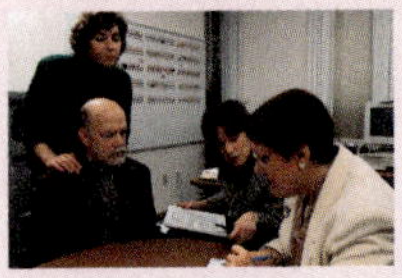

In preparing a preoperative plan of care, Sue needs to explore Mr. Korloff's experiences, beliefs, and preferences about surgery (Starkweather, 2010). Studies have shown that some Russian Americans expect the nurse to be friendly, using open, inviting, nonverbal postures and a friendly smile. Sue learns that this is the case for Mr. Korloff by the way that he reacts to her communication. Sue must also learn if Mr. Korloff is willing to share his health problems with her. Russian Americans are sometimes willing to follow teaching provided by nurses when they believe that they are sincere, competent, and trustworthy. They value receiving immediate information and answers from health care workers and follow health care instructions when they fully understand them. It is clear to Sue that Mr. Korloff has strong family ties and values. The Russian American father usually plays a primary role in the function of the family. Using this knowledge, Sue develops a patient-centered plan of care.

IMPLICATIONS FOR PRACTICE

- Assess Mr. Korloff's opinions about surgery first and then include his family.
- Assess the level of involvement of the family in his surgical preparation and care.
- Provide preoperative teaching in a warm, caring, open manner using frequent smiles and hand gestures.
- Speak slowly and clearly in a low, calm voice using simple words.
- Provide an explanation of the importance of postoperative exercises so Mr. Korloff understands why the exercises are important and will be more willing to do them after surgery.
- Determine if family members are close to Mr. Korloff and include them in the teaching session.

important to explain everything to your female patient's husband, father, or brother for her to participate in the plan of care (Giger, 2013). When doing this, make sure to have permission from a patient to share personal health information. Many cultural and religious taboos exist concerning the body, who cares for the physical needs of others, and treatments appropriate for healing; thus it is important to explore these issues with a patient and/or family. Although it is important to recognize and plan for differences based on culture, remember that not all members of one family hold the same beliefs or practices. Asking relevant questions of each patient concerning his or her spiritual beliefs and expectations about surgery further individualizes your nursing care (see Chapters 20 and 21). Patients' spiritual beliefs help in coping with fears and anxieties related to the upcoming surgery. Help a patient obtain the spiritual help requested before surgery. For example, contact the hospital chaplain per patient request before going to surgery.

Coping Resources. Assessment of patients' feelings and self-concept reveals whether they have the ability to cope with the stress of surgery. It is also valuable to ask patients about stress management. If a patient has had previous surgery, discuss the behaviors that helped to resolve past tension or nervousness. You sometimes instruct a patient in relaxation exercises (see Chapter 25) to help control anxiety.

Body Image. Surgical removal of a diseased tissue or organ often leaves permanent disfigurement or alteration in body function. Concern over mutilation, change in sexuality, or loss of a body part adds to a patient's fears. Individuals react differently, depending on age, culture, occupation, self-image, and self-esteem. Encourage patients to express these concerns so you can offer support (see Chapter 23).

Patient Expectations. It is important to identify a patient's and family's perceptions and expectations regarding surgery, recovery, and health care providers. This information allows you to plan interventions for teaching and emotional preparation and provides the basis for evaluation of care. For example, some patients have expectations regarding pain control and the use of pain medications that are unrealistic. Patients who are prepared to experience pain and know the proper use of pharmacological and nonpharmacological pain-relief measures tend to require less medication (Rothrock, 2011).

Patients and family members often have misconceptions about surgery. *For example, it is important to discuss with Mr. Korloff's daughters their understanding of his ability to perform activities at home that require lifting or moving heavy objects in the immediate postoperative period. Sue learns that Mr. Korloff has a 40-lb older dog at home. He will not be able to lift the dog as he usually does when taking the dog in the car with him.* When a patient is well prepared and knows what to expect in day-to-day activities, his or her knowledge is reinforced.

You face an ethical dilemma when a patient is unaware of the actual reason for surgery. In such a case, speak with the surgeon before revealing specific information related to the medical diagnosis to prevent confusion and identify the need for clarification.

Physical Examination. You conduct a partial or complete physical examination (see Chapter 16), depending on the setting and nature of the surgery. The assessment focuses on findings found in a patient's medical history and on body systems that surgery or anesthesia will affect (Table 39-4).

General Survey. Gestures and body movements often reflect decreased energy or weakness caused by illness. Height and body weight are important indicators of nutritional status and are used to calculate medication dosages. Preoperative vital signs provide a baseline for intraoperative and postoperative comparison because anesthetic agents and medications can alter vital signs. Preoperative assessment of vital signs is also important to detect fluid and electrolyte abnormalities (see Chapter 18).

An elevated temperature is cause for concern. If a patient has an underlying infection, elective surgery is often postponed until the infection is treated or resolved. An elevated body temperature also alters drug metabolism and increases the risk for fluid and electrolyte imbalances.

Head and Neck. Assessment of oral mucous membranes reveals the level of hydration. Dehydration increases the risk for the development of serious fluid and electrolyte imbalances during surgery. During the oral examination

TABLE 39-4 FOCUSED PATIENT ASSESSMENT

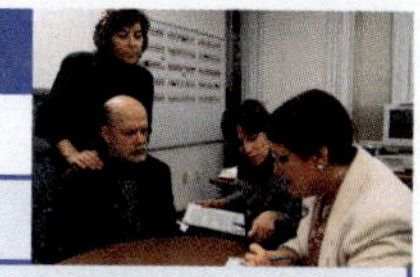

Preoperative Assessment

FACTORS TO ASSESS	QUESTIONS	PHYSICAL ASSESSMENT
Significant medical history and previous surgeries	Do you have any bleeding disorders; diabetes; heart, lung, renal, or liver disease; or any immune disorder?	Monitor vital signs and note any abnormalities. Inspect neck for jugular vein distention (cardiac disease, fluid overload).
	Have you had a recent fever or upper respiratory infection?	Inspect skin for turgor, dryness, rashes, skin breakdown. Auscultate heart and lungs for abnormal sounds (murmurs, congestion, bruits).
	Do you experience chronic pain?	Perform pain assessment with pain tool, including severity, location, description, measures used to relieve. Assess extremities for decreased sensation, hair loss, clubbed fingers, deformed nails, sluggish capillary reflex, color.
Medication history and allergies	Which prescription, over-the-counter, and herbal medications are you currently taking? What instructions were you given from your surgeon about taking or omitting medications before surgery?	Inspect any medication containers brought in by patient or family.
	Do you have any personal and/or family history of allergic responses to medications (including anesthetics) or environmental factors (e.g., latex, foods)?	Monitor laboratory values for any evidence of side effects of medications or drug levels, if ordered.

identify loose or capped teeth because they often become dislodged during endotracheal intubation. Note any dentures or partial plates that your patient uses, remove them when necessary, and give to a family member to prevent loss or damage.

Inspection of the soft palate and nasal sinuses sometimes reveals sinus drainage indicative of respiratory or sinus infection. To rule out the possibility of local or systemic infection, palpate for cervical lymph node enlargement. Also inspect the jugular veins for distention. Excess fluid within the circulatory system or failure of the heart to contract efficiently frequently leads to jugular vein distention. A patient with heart disease or fluid overload is at risk for cardiovascular complications during surgery.

Skin. Thoroughly inspect a patient's skin overlying all body parts, especially bony prominences. During surgery a patient lies in a fixed position, often for several hours. Avoid positioning him or her over an area where the skin shows signs of pressure over bony prominences. A patient is susceptible to skin breakdown if the skin is thin or dry or has poor turgor (see Chapter 37).

Thorax and Lungs. A decline in ventilatory function, assessed through breathing pattern and chest excursion, indicates a patient's risk for respiratory complications. Serious pulmonary congestion often causes postponement of surgery. For example, narrowing of the airways, as occurs with chronic lung disease (CLD, formerly known as chronic obstructive pulmonary disease [COPD]), increases the risk for airway obstruction because of bronchospasm related to endotracheal intubation and anesthesia.

Heart and Vascular System. If a patient has heart disease, assess the apical pulse. After surgery compare the pulse rate and rhythm with preoperative baseline values. Assessment of peripheral pulses, color, and temperature of extremities is particularly important for a patient undergoing vascular or orthopedic surgery and when applying constricting bandages or casts to an extremity after surgery. Postoperative changes in skin color and sensation or development of a weak or absent pulse in a patient who had adequate circulation before surgery indicates impaired circulation.

Abdomen. Alterations in gastrointestinal function after surgery often result in decreased or absent bowel sounds and abdominal distention. Assess a patient's usual abdominal anatomy to assess for distention. Assessment of preoperative bowel sounds and normal elimination pattern is useful as a baseline. If surgery requires manipulation of portions of the gastrointestinal tract or if a general anesthetic is used, normal peristalsis sometimes does not return, and bowel sounds are absent or diminished for hours to several days.

Neurological Status. A patient's level of consciousness changes as a result of general anesthesia. However, after the effects of anesthesia disappear, expect a patient to return to his or her preoperative level of responsiveness. Spinal or epidural anesthesia causes temporary paralysis of the lower extremities. Be aware of preexisting weakness or impaired mobility of the lower extremities to avoid becoming alarmed when full motor function does not return immediately after a procedure.

Risk Factors. Knowledge of preoperative risk factors discussed earlier enables you to take necessary precautions in planning care.

TABLE 39-5 COMMON LABORATORY BLOOD TESTS

TEST	NORMAL VALUES*	SIGNIFICANCE: LOW	SIGNIFICANCE: HIGH
Complete Blood Count (CBC)			
Hemoglobin (Hgb)	Female: 12-16 g/dL; male: 14-18 g/dL	Anemia	Polycythemia (elevated red blood cell count)
Hematocrit (Hct)	Female: 37%-47%; male: 42%-52%	Fluid overload	Dehydration
Platelet count	150,000-400,000/mm^3	Decreased clotting	Increased risk of blood clot
White blood cell count	5,000-10,000/mm^3	Decreased ability to fight infection	Infection
Blood Chemistry			
Sodium (Na)	136-145 mEq/L	Fluid overload	Dehydration
Potassium (K)	3.5-5.0 mEq/L	Cardiac rhythm irregularities	Cardiac rhythm irregularities
Chloride (Cl)	98-106 mEq/L	Follows shifts in sodium blood levels	Follows shifts in sodium blood levels
Carbon dioxide (CO_2)	23-30 mEq/L	Affects acid base balance in blood	Affects acid base balance in blood
Blood urea nitrogen (BUN)	10-20 mg/dL	Liver disease/fluid overload	Renal disease/dehydration
Glucose	70-110 mg/dL fasting	Insulin reaction, inadequate glucose intake	Diabetes mellitus and stress of surgery
Creatinine	Female: 0.5-1.1 mg/dL; male: 0.6-1.2 mg/dL	Malnutrition	Renal disease
Coagulation Studies			
International Normalized Ratio (INR)	0.76-1.27	Risk of clot	Risk of bleeding
Prothrombin time (PT)	11-12.5 sec; 85%-100%	Risk of clot	Risk of bleeding
Partial thromboplastin time (PTT)	60-70 sec	Risk of clot	Risk of bleeding
Activated PTT (APTT)	30-40 sec	Risk of clot	Excess heparin; risk of spontaneous bleeding

From Pagana KD, Pagana TJ: *Mosby's diagnostic and laboratory test reference,* ed 11, St Louis, 2013, Mosby.
*Normal ranges vary slightly among laboratories.

Diagnostic Screening. Patients undergo diagnostic test screening for preexisting abnormalities before surgery. Patients scheduled for elective surgery have testing as an outpatient on or before the morning of surgery. If tests reveal severe problems, the surgeon or anesthesiologist cancels surgery until the condition stabilizes. As the preoperative nurse coordinate the completion of tests and verify that a patient is prepared properly. Review diagnostic results when available, alert the surgeon and/or anesthesiologist to findings, and intervene as appropriate.

Screening tests depend on a patient's condition and the nature of the surgery. Table 39-5 summarizes routine screening tests. In addition, a patient needs a blood type and screen if transfusions are anticipated. Additional preoperative tests include a urinalysis screen for urinary tract infections (UTIs), renal disease, or diabetes mellitus and a 12-lead electrocardiogram to analyze heart rate and rhythm.

Older Adult Considerations. Older patients are at greater surgical risk as a result of physiologic changes related to aging (see Chapter 22). A chest x-ray film to assess the size and shape of the heart, presence of lung lesions and chest wall abnormalities, and position of the diaphragm and aorta is a common preoperative test for older adults and those with cardiovascular or pulmonary abnormalities. An older patient's physical capacity to adapt to the stress of surgery lessens because of deterioration of certain body functions (Table 39-6).

NURSING DIAGNOSIS

After you obtain assessment data, cluster defining characteristics to identify appropriate nursing diagnoses and related factors. The nature and type of surgery and a patient's age and health status suggest defining characteristics for many

TABLE 39-6 PHYSIOLOGICAL FACTORS THAT PLACE OLDER ADULTS AT RISK DURING SURGERY

ALTERATIONS	RISKS	NURSING IMPLICATIONS
Cardiovascular System		
Degeneration of myocardium and valves	Reduces cardiac reserve	Assess baseline vital signs and patient's fluid volume status.
Rigid arteries and reduction in sympathetic and parasympathetic innervation to heart	Predisposes patient to postoperative hemorrhage and hypertension	Instruct patient in techniques for performing leg exercises and proper turning.
Increase in calcium and cholesterol deposits within small arteries; thickened arterial walls	Increases risk for clot formation in lower extremities	Apply antiembolism stockings, sequential compression devices.
Integumentary System		
Decreased subcutaneous tissue and increased fragility of skin	Patient prone to pressure ulcers and skin tears	Assess skin every 2 hours or more often; pad all bony prominences during surgery. Turn or reposition every 2 hours if possible.
Pulmonary System		
Rib cage stiffened and reduced in size	Reduces vital capacity	Instruct patient in proper technique for coughing, deep breathing, splinting incision, and use of incentive spirometer.
Reduced range of movement in diaphragm	Greater residual capacity or volume of air left in lung after normal breath, reducing amount of new air brought into lungs with each inspiration	When possible have patient ambulate and sit in chair frequently.
Stiffened lung tissue and enlarged air spaces	Reduces blood oxygenation levels	Provide supplemental oxygen when ordered.
Decreased ability to cough and clear upper airway	Increases risk for postoperative pulmonary infection	Have patient cough, deep breathe, and use incentive spirometer every 2 hours.
Renal System		
Reduced blood flow to kidneys	Increases risk for damage to renal tissues	For patients hospitalized before surgery, determine baseline urinary output for 24 hours.
Reduced glomerular filtration rate and excretory times	Limits ability to eliminate drugs or toxic substances	Maintain adequate hydration.
Reduced bladder capacity	Voiding frequency increases, and larger amount of urine stays in bladder after voiding	Instruct patient to notify nurse immediately when sensation of bladder fullness develops.
	Sensation of need to void sometimes does not occur until bladder is full	Keep call light and bedpan within easy reach.
Neurological System		
Sensory losses, including reduced tactile sense and increased pain tolerance	Patient less able to respond to early warning signs of surgical complications	Orient patient to surrounding environment. Observe for nonverbal signs of pain.
Decreased reaction time	Patient becomes easily confused after anesthesia	Reorient frequently. Keep side rails up and room free from clutter.
Metabolic System		
Reduced number of red blood cells and hemoglobin levels	Reduces ability to carry adequate oxygen to tissues	Administer necessary blood products. Monitor blood test results.
Change in total amounts of body potassium and water volume	Increases risk for fluid or electrolyte imbalance	Monitor fluid and electrolyte levels.

Normal ranges vary slightly among laboratories.

nursing diagnoses. The diagnoses establish direction for care during one or all of the surgical phases. For example, a patient's restlessness, poor eye contact, and expressed concern about the results of surgery point to the diagnosis of *Anxiety.* However, you need to validate the assessment to avoid misdiagnosis. In the foregoing assessment restlessness may also indicate pain. Therefore you need to ensure that you identify the nursing diagnosis that best fits your patient's problem. Possible nursing diagnoses for the preoperative patient include the following:

- *Anxiety*
- *Compromised Family Coping*
- *Ineffective Coping*
- *Fear*
- *Risk for Imbalanced Fluid Volume*
- *Deficient Knowledge*
- *Risk for Imbalanced Nutrition: More Than Body Requirements*
- *Powerlessness*
- *Ineffective Role Performance*
- *Risk for Spiritual Distress*

A diagnosis and its related factors offer direction to the most effective nursing interventions for a patient. Ensure that related factors are accurate to avoid inappropriate interventions. For example, *Anxiety related to deficient knowledge of perioperative routines* requires you to offer thorough instruction before surgery and immediately after surgery. However, *Anxiety related to threat of ineffective role performance* requires counseling and coaching during postoperative recovery.

PLANNING

Always include a patient and family in any discussions before surgery. Patient-centered care integrates patient and family preferences and values in how you teach and inform. Involving them early minimizes surgical risks and postoperative complications because they can inform you of factors to monitor and consider. Structured preoperative teaching reduces the amount of anesthesia and postoperative pain medication needed, decreases the occurrence of postoperative urinary retention, promotes an earlier return to normal oral intake, and decreases length of hospital stay (Rothrock, 2011). Patients who understand what to expect about their surgical experience are less likely to be fearful and are better prepared for expected outcomes.

Goals and Outcomes. The plan of care begins in the preoperative phase, and you modify it as needed during the intraoperative and postoperative phases (see Care Plan). The goals of care for the surgical patient include the following:

- Understanding the physiological and psychological responses to surgery
- Understanding intraoperative and postoperative events
- Achieving emotional and physiological comfort and rest
- Achieving return of normal physiological function after surgery (e.g., return of normal vital signs, fluid and electrolyte balance, muscle function)
- Remaining free of surgical wound infection
- Remaining safe from harm during the perioperative period

Outcomes established for each goal of care provide measurable ways to determine a patient's progress toward meeting stated goals. For example, in the case of "understanding intraoperative and postoperative events," outcomes include "Patient describes postoperative exercises," or "Patient explains positioning during surgery."

Setting Priorities. Establish individualized care by prioritizing nursing diagnoses and interventions based on the assessed needs of each patient. Setting priorities requires clinical judgment. For example, your patient has two nursing diagnoses, *Anxiety* and *Deficient Knowledge.* You determine the priority is Deficient Knowledge for this patient because, in this case, patient instruction will likely relieve the anxiety. Be thorough in your plan and be sure that it reflects your understanding of the implications of a patient's age, physical and psychological health, educational level, previous experience with surgery, cultural and religious practices, and stated and/or written wishes concerning advance directives.

Collaborative Care. Perioperative care requires collaboration with other health care disciplines. Consider which members of the health care team (e.g., dietitians, occupational therapists) you need to involve while planning patient care. For example, patients who require aggressive pulmonary rehabilitation such as those having thoracic surgery need a referral to a respiratory therapist. Many patients and their families benefit from referral to pastoral care, especially if the procedure is an emergency or is life threatening. You anticipate patient and family needs on discharge based on information learned in the initial assessment.

The preoperative planning phase for ambulatory surgical patients usually occurs in an outpatient setting before or on the morning of surgery. Ideally it begins in the surgeon's office and continues in the home. This gives a patient and family time to reflect on the surgical experience, make necessary physical preparations, and ask questions about postoperative procedures. Well-planned preoperative care ensures that a patient and family are well informed and actively participate during recovery.

IMPLEMENTATION

Preoperative nursing interventions focus on patient education and physical preparation of a patient for surgery.

Informed Consent. A surgeon cannot legally perform surgery nor can an anesthesia care provider administer an anesthetic until a patient understands the need for the procedure and the steps, risks, expected results, and alternative treatments involved. Chapter 5 summarizes issues and guidelines for informed consent. Patients need to sign all consent forms before you administer any preoperative medications that alter their consciousness. The primary responsibility for informing a patient rests with the surgeon and anesthesia provider. However, if a patient is confused or uncertain about a procedure, you are ethically obligated to contact the

CARE PLAN

Surgery

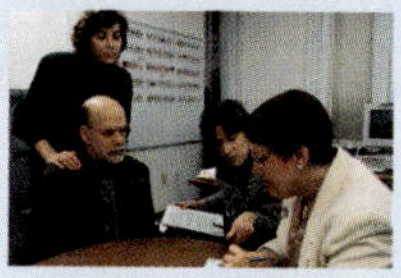

ASSESSMENT

As Mr. Korloff enters the preadmission center for testing, Sue greets him and his daughters. She explains the need to gather a history and asks Mr. Korloff if he wishes to have his daughters join him. He smiles and says, "Yes, my daughters will be my nurses for a few days." The nursing staff report that Mr. Korloff's daughters have been calling on the phone and asking many questions about intraoperative and postoperative events. Mr. Korloff is alert and attentive and answers appropriately. His vision and hearing are normal. This will be his first experience having surgery.

ASSESSMENT ACTIVITIES	FINDINGS/DEFINING CHARACTERISTICS*
Ask Mr. Korloff what he has been told regarding surgery by his surgeon.	He states that **he knows very little about the surgery.**
Ask Mr. Korloff what he understands about preoperative preparation and what to expect after surgery.	He says **he knows few specifics and asks if he will have an intravenous (IV) line.**
Ask Mr. Korloff what concerns him about having surgery.	He repeatedly says, "Oh, I'm not worried," but then **asks many questions, often repeatedly.**

*__Defining characteristics__ are shown in **bold type.**

NURSING DIAGNOSIS: Deficient Knowledge regarding implications of surgery (cholecystectomy) related to first surgical experience and inadequate preparation

PLANNING

GOAL

- Mr. Korloff will understand preoperative, intraoperative, and postoperative events before the day of surgery.

EXPECTED OUTCOMES (NOC)†

Knowledge: Treatment Procedure

- Patient and his daughters describe events that commonly occur in the holding area and operating room on the day before surgery.
- Patient and his daughters describe routine postoperative nursing procedures on the day of admission.
- Patient and his daughters describe ways to participate in postoperative care on the day of admission.

†Outcomes classification labels from Moorhead S, et al, editors: *Nursing outcomes classification (NOC)*, ed 5, St Louis, 2013, Mosby.

INTERVENTIONS (NIC)‡ ***Teaching: Procedure/Treatment***	RATIONALE
• Give Mr. Korloff a copy of the teaching booklet *Your Surgical Experience.*	Patients who are prepared for surgery experience less anxiety and report a greater sense of psychological well-being and satisfaction (Haufler and Harrington, 2011; Makki et al., 2011).
• Provide planned teaching session for Mr. Korloff and his daughters after preadmission testing. Explain events that will occur in holding area (e.g., insertion of IV catheter, vital sign check) and in operating room (e.g., positioning, anesthesia). Use visual aids to help Mr. Korloff understand the laparoscopic procedure.	Teaching focused on information that patient will need to know on morning of admission decreases anxiety and allows patient and family to better participate in care (Haufler and Harrington, 2011; Makki et al., 2011).
• Allow Mr. Korloff to express his feelings and fears related to surgery.	Expressing feelings and fears decreases anxiety related to the surgical experience for patient teaching to be more effective.
• Provide planned teaching session on day of admission with Mr. Korloff and his daughters to answer questions, explain common events that occur after surgery, and demonstrate postoperative exercises.	Preoperative teaching improves patient's ability to ambulate, participate in care activities, and resume activities of daily living after surgery. Demonstration is an effective method in teaching psychomotor skills.
• Have Mr. Korloff perform return demonstration of postoperative exercises.	Return demonstration verifies that learning has occurred and patient is able to correctly perform exercises to reduce postoperative complications.

‡Interventions classification label from Bulechek GM, et al, editors: *Nursing interventions classification (NIC)*, ed 6, St Louis, 2013, Mosby.

Continued

CARE PLAN—cont'd

Surgery

EVALUATION

NURSING ACTIONS	PATIENT RESPONSE/FINDING	ACHIEVEMENT OF OUTCOME
Ask Mr. Korloff and his daughters to identify the basic purpose of the surgery and changes to expect afterward.	Mr. Korloff describes the surgical procedure and explains why he needs the surgery.	Mr. Korloff demonstrates a good understanding of the surgery.
Ask Mr. Korloff and his daughters to identify routine types of postoperative monitoring and treatment.	He describes postoperative exercises to perform after surgery but is not able to discuss monitoring activities.	Mr. Korloff describes postoperative exercises, requires further instruction on monitoring activities.
Observe Mr. Korloff perform postoperative exercises.	Mr. Korloff demonstrates coughing, deep breathing, and use of leg exercises. Has difficulty using incentive spirometer. Mr. Korloff's daughters remind him to hold his breath for 2 to 3 seconds with use of incentive spirometer.	Mr. Korloff demonstrates coughing, deep breathing, and leg exercises appropriately. Requires further demonstration and assistance from his daughters in use of incentive spirometer.

surgeon and/or anesthesia provider so further discussion and clarification are offered. A patient always has the right to refuse surgery or treatment even after giving written consent.

Health Promotion. Health promotion activities during the preoperative phase focus on prevention of complications, health maintenance, and support of possible rehabilitation needs after surgery.

Preoperative Teaching. Patient education relieves anxiety, increases patient satisfaction, speeds up the recovery process, decreases the amount of perceived pain, and facilitates a more rapid return to work or normal functioning (Lewis et al., 2011). Systematic, structured, and interactive **preoperative teaching** has a positive influence on patients' recoveries. Structured teaching often influences the following postoperative factors:

1. *Ventilatory function:* Teaching improves the ability and willingness to deep breathe and cough effectively.
2. *Physical functional capacity:* Teaching increases understanding and willingness to ambulate and resume activities of daily living.
3. *Sense of well-being:* Patients who are prepared for surgery experience less anxiety and report a greater sense of psychological well-being (Haufler and Harrington, 2011).
4. *Length of hospital stay:* Teaching frequently reduces a patient's length of hospital stay by preventing or minimizing postoperative complications.
5. *Anxiety about pain and amount of pain medication needed for comfort:* Patients who learn about pain and ways to relieve it before surgery are less anxious about the pain, ask for what they need, and actually require less pain medication after surgery (Grawe et al., 2010).

The most effective type of teaching program for surgical patients covers the entire surgical experience. Box 39-4 outlines the parameters for perioperative preparation. Because many patients are not admitted to the hospital before surgery, preoperative teaching often occurs in the home, surgeon's office, or preadmission unit. Offer printed literature, DVDs, or videotapes to patients. Call patients before surgery to provide education and clarify questions (Black and Hawks, 2009).

Always include family members and significant others in preoperative preparation. They are frequently the coaches for postoperative exercises when a patient returns from surgery. If family members and significant others do not understand routine postoperative events, their anxiety heightens a patient's fears or concerns. Reduce misunderstanding and anxiety with thoughtful preparation. However, if a patient does not wish to include them, respect the request for privacy.

Timing. Preoperative teaching is most useful when started the week before admission and reinforced immediately before surgery. Teaching performed when a patient is less anxious results in more effective learning. Anxiety and fear are barriers to learning. Assess the surgical patient's readiness and ability to learn (see Chapter 12). Always present information in a logical sequence beginning with preoperative events and advancing to intraoperative and postoperative routines. Preoperative teaching checklists offer helpful guidelines for presenting patients with a comprehensives set of instructions.

Content. Preoperative teaching includes information to help a patient, family, and significant others prepare for the surgical experience and participate in the plan of care (Kearney et al., 2011).

Surgical Procedure. After the surgeon explains the basic purpose of the surgical procedure and its steps, a patient may ask you additional questions. While answering questions, avoid using technical medical terms because this adds to a patient's confusion. Avoid saying anything that contradicts the surgeon's explanation. One way to avoid contradictions is to first ask what the surgeon told a patient. If a patient has little or no understanding about the surgery, refer him or her back to the surgeon for additional information.

BOX 39-4 PATIENT TEACHING

Perioperative Patient Preparation

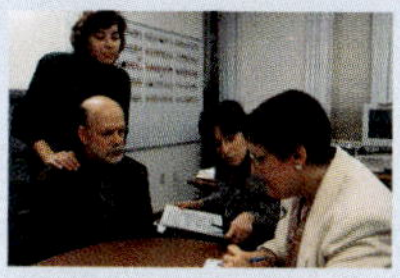

Sue plans time after completing Mr. Korloff's assessment to discuss the planned surgery with him and his daughters. She begins by asking Mr. Korloff to describe what he thinks the procedure will involve, share any concerns, and identify the type of information he wants to understand. This shows Sue's cultural sensitivity, which makes teaching more appropriate.

OUTCOME

At the end of the teaching session Mr. Korloff will be able to:

- Describe preoperative, intraoperative, and postoperative procedures to anticipate for a laparoscopic procedure
- Demonstrate postoperative exercises

TEACHING STRATEGIES

Preoperative Procedures

- State time to arrive at facility and time of surgery (approximate time or if his case is "to follow" a previous surgery).
- Explain extent and purpose of food and fluid restrictions.
- Explain or review informed consent.
- Teach about physical preparation required (e.g., bowel or skin preparation).
- Explain about procedures performed in preanesthesia just before transport to operating room (IV line insertion, urinary catheterization or voiding, preoperative medications).

Intraoperative Procedures

- Describe preanesthesia care environment and activities.
- Describe operating room environment.
- Explain about the roles of circulating nurse, scrub nurse, and anesthesia care provider.

Postoperative Procedures

- Describe postanesthesia care environment and activities.
- Teach about pain control and other comfort measures.
- Explain purpose of any anticipated tubes, drains, or IV lines.
- Emphasize importance of postoperative exercises (see Skill 39-1).
- Demonstrate exercises and have patient perform return demonstration.
- Encourage Mr. Korloff and family to verbalize any concerns.
- Assess Mr. Korloff and his family's understanding of perioperative preparation and respond appropriately.

EVALUATION STRATEGIES

- Have Mr. Korloff describe his understanding of preoperative, intraoperative, and postoperative procedures.
- Have Mr. Korloff demonstrate coughing, deep-breathing, and turning exercises.

IV, Intravenous.

Preoperative Routines. Explain the preoperative routines that a patient will undergo. For example, if your patient needs an enema, explain why it is necessary. Knowing which tests and procedures are planned and why increase a patient's sense of control.

The anesthesiologist visits with a patient to complete a preanesthesia assessment either during the preoperative admission process or in the presurgical care unit. A patient and family need to know about this visit so they can ask any questions and be prepared to provide necessary information such as previous experience with anesthesia.

Explain to a patient and family the importance of the patient following oral intake instructions for food and liquids as provided by the surgeon and anesthesiologist. The American Society of Anesthesiologists (ASA) provides recommendations on fluid and food intake before procedures requiring general anesthesia, regional anesthesia, or sedation/analgesia. These recommendations include fasting from intake of clear liquids for 2 or more hours, breast milk for 4 hours, formula and nonhuman milk for 6 hours, and a light meal of toast and clear liquids for 6 hours. A patient also cannot have any meat or fried foods 8 hours before surgery, unless explicitly specified by the anesthesiologist or surgeon (ASA Committee on Standards and Practice Parameters, 2011). *Despite these regulations, many facilities still have patients maintain nothing by mouth after midnight.* Ensure that you follow the health care provider's orders. During the use of general anesthesia, the muscles relax, and gastric contents can reflux into the esophagus. The anesthetic eliminates a patient's ability to gag. Therefore a patient is at risk for aspiration of food or fluids from the stomach into the lungs. The surgeon's orders provide additional guidance for routines to explain to a patient (e.g., intravenous [IV] therapy, preoperative medications, or insertion of a urinary catheter or a nasogastric [NG] tube).

Intraoperative Routines. The scheduled operative time is only an anticipated time. Unanticipated delays occur for many reasons that have nothing to do with your patient. Emphasize that the scheduled time is a rough estimate and the actual time can be sooner or later than the scheduled time. Tell family members where to wait and inform them that the surgeon will speak to them when the surgery is completed. Communicate excessive delays to the family if they occur.

Postoperative Routines. A patient and family want to know about postoperative events. If they understand routine postoperative vital sign monitoring, they are less likely to worry when nurses perform these assessments. Also explain if a patient is to have IV lines, dressings, or drainage tubes. Do not overprepare or underprepare a patient and family. You cannot predict all of a patient's requirements, and a patient may be misinformed about a therapy that may not be initiated. Contradictions between your explanations and reality cause anxiety.

Sensory Preparation. Provide a patient with information about sensations typically experienced before, during, and after surgery. Preparatory information helps them anticipate the steps of a procedure and form a realistic image of the surgical experience. When sensations occur as predicted, a patient is better at coping with the experiences. For example, warn that the OR room is very bright and cool. Explain that you will apply a cuff for a noninvasive blood pressure monitor to the patient's arm. This monitor makes a hum and a beep, and the cuff tightens around the arm. Informing a patient about these and other sensations in the OR reduces anxiety before the patient is anesthetized, which helps to decrease the amount of anesthetic needed for induction. Other postoperative sensations to describe include blurred vision from ophthalmic ointment, dryness of the mouth or the sensation of a sore throat resulting from an endotracheal tube, pain at the incision site, tightness of the dressings, and feeling cold.

Pain Relief. One of the surgical patient's greatest fears is pain. The family is also concerned about a patient's comfort. Preoperative preparation regarding pain and pain-control measures helps patients cope with pain. Patient-controlled analgesia (PCA) is common and provides patients with control over pain. Explain to a patient how to operate a pump and the importance of administering medication as soon as pain becomes persistent (see Chapter 32). In one study, Wu et al. (2005) found epidural analgesia overall provided superior postoperative analgesia compared with IV PCA. Patients who receive epidural analgesia need a thorough understanding of how this affects movement and sensation (see Chapter 32).

Oral and parenteral analgesics do not provide adequate pain relief if a patient waits until the pain becomes excruciating before using or requesting an analgesic. Even though around-the-clock (ATC) analgesia is more effective, most patients still have analgesics ordered prn (as needed). Pain control is essential for a surgical patient to recover quickly. Encourage a patient to use analgesics as needed and not be fearful of any dependence on them following surgery. Explain the schedule for administration of all analgesics. If analgesics are not ordered continuous or ATC, encourage a patient to inform nurses as soon as pain becomes a persistent discomfort. A patient also needs to know that it takes time for a drug to act and that the drug rarely eliminates all the discomfort. In addition, inform a patient and family of other therapies available for pain relief such as focused breathing and relaxation, distraction, and the use of heat or cold compresses.

Postoperative Exercises. Every preoperative teaching program includes explanation and demonstration of postoperative exercises, including diaphragmatic breathing, incentive spirometry, controlled coughing, turning, and leg exercises (see Skill 39-1). Diaphragmatic breathing improves lung expansion and oxygen delivery without using excess energy. A patient learns to use the diaphragm during deep breathing to take slow, deep, and relaxed breaths. Eventually a patient's lung volume improves. Deep breathing also helps to clear any anesthetic gases from the airways. To facilitate deep breathing a health care provider often orders an incentive spirometer for a patient (see Chapter 30). Incentive spirometry encourages forced inspiration. The therapy is effective in preventing atelectasis after surgery.

Coughing helps to remove retained mucus in the airways. A deep, productive cough is more beneficial than merely clearing the throat. A patient needs to anticipate postoperative discomfort and understand the importance of coughing, even when it is difficult. Teach a patient to splint an abdominal or thoracic incision to minimize pain during coughing. Pain control is essential for effective deep breathing and coughing; educate a patient to ask for pain medications as needed.

Leg exercises and turning improve blood flow to the extremities and thus reduce venous stasis, reducing the risk for clot formation and subsequent pulmonary emboli. Contractions of lower leg muscles promote venous return, making it difficult for clots to form. Turning also helps to mobilize pulmonary secretions and increases ventilation and perfusion of the lungs. After explaining each exercise, demonstrate it. Then, while acting as a coach, ask a patient to demonstrate each exercise. Show family members how they can become coaches as well. Also explain that a patient is likely to have compression hose stockings after surgery to reduce risk of deep vein thrombosis.

Activity Resumption. The type of surgery affects how quickly a patient is able to resume normal physical activity and regular eating habits. Explain that it is normal for a patient to progress gradually in activity and eating. If a patient tolerates activity and diet well, activity levels progress more quickly. For example, if a patient is not nauseated following cholecystectomy, encourage ambulation the night of surgery.

Promotion of Nutrition. A surgical patient is vulnerable to fluid and electrolyte imbalances as a result of inadequate preoperative intake, excessive fluid loss during surgery, and the stress response. A patient usually takes nothing by mouth for several hours before surgery to reduce risks for vomiting and aspirating emesis during surgery. Instruct a patient to eat and drink sufficient amounts before fasting to ensure adequate fluid and nutrient intake. Make sure that his or her diet includes foods high in protein with sufficient amounts of carbohydrates, fat, and vitamins. Instruct a patient and family members regarding preoperative fasting requirements and oral medication use. Notify the surgeon and anesthesiologist as soon as possible if a patient eats or drinks during the fasting period.

For patients who are hospitalized, remove all fluids and solid foods from the bedside and post a sign over the bed to alert hospital personnel and family members about fasting restrictions. Instruct patients to rinse their mouths with water or mouthwash and brush their teeth but not to swallow anything, even clear liquids. Patients may take oral medications with sips of water if ordered by the health care provider. Notify the dietary department to cancel meals. A patient who is at home the evening before surgery needs to understand the importance of not taking food or fluids, when to start fasting, and be willing to follow restrictions.

Promotion of Rest. Rest is essential for normal healing. Anxiety about surgery interferes with the ability to relax or sleep. The underlying conditions requiring surgery are often painful, further impairing rest. Frequent visits by staff members, diagnostic testing, and physical preparation for surgery take a long time; and a patient has few opportunities to reflect on events. Make sure that a patient's individual needs are met. The patient and family need time to express feelings about surgery, either together or separately. A patient's level of anxiety influences the frequency of discussions, and you need to encourage expression of these concerns.

Attempt to make a patient's environment quiet and comfortable. The surgeon occasionally orders a sedative-hypnotic or antianxiety agent for the night before surgery. Sedative-hypnotics affect and promote sleep. Antianxiety agents act on the cerebral cortex and limbic system to relieve anxiety. An advantage to ambulatory surgery or same-day surgical admissions is that a patient is able to sleep at home the night before surgery.

Acute Care. The degree of preoperative physical preparation depends on a patient's health status, the surgery, and the surgeon's preferences. Seriously ill patients receive more supportive care than patients facing less serious elective procedures.

Minimize Risk for Surgical Wound Infection. The risk for developing a surgical wound infection depends on the amount and type of microorganisms contaminating a wound, the susceptibility of the host, and the condition of the wound at the end of the operation (Box 39-5). All three factors interact, determining the risk for infection (see Chapter 14). The skin is a favorite site for microorganisms to grow and multiply. Without proper skin preparation, the risk for postoperative wound infection is high. Many surgeons have patients bathe or shower with an antimicrobial soap such as chlorhexidene the evening before surgery. Often patients have to bathe or shower more than once, whereas others give special attention to cleansing the proposed operative site with special cleansing pads. If the surgical procedure involves the head, neck, or upper chest area, a patient also is required to shampoo the hair. Surgeons generally order hair removal only if the hair has the potential to interfere with exposure, closure, or dressing of the surgical site. Remove hair as close to the time of surgery as possible (AORN, 2012). Instruct patients not to shave the surgical area because shaving leaves nicks in the skin that can harbor infectious microorganisms.

Prevention of Bowel Incontinence and Contamination. A patient often receives a bowel preparation (e.g., a cathartic or an enema) if surgery involves the lower gastrointestinal system. Manipulation of portions of the gastrointestinal tract during surgery results in absence of peristalsis for 24 hours and sometimes longer. Enemas (see Chapter 35) and cathartics cleanse the gastrointestinal tract to prevent problems with incontinence or constipation. An empty bowel reduces risk for injury to the intestines and minimizes contamination of the operative wound in case a portion of the bowel is incised or opened.

Interventions on Day of Surgery. On the morning of surgery complete the routine procedures discussed in the following sections before releasing a patient for surgery.

Documentation. Before a patient goes to the OR, check the medical record to be sure that all relevant laboratory and test results are present. Check all consent forms for completeness and accuracy of information. A preoperative checklist provides guidelines for ensuring completion of all nursing interventions. Check the nurses' notes to be sure that documentation is current, especially if a patient experienced unpredicted problems the night before surgery.

Assessment of Vital Signs. Make a final assessment of vital signs and document them on the preoperative flowsheet or checklist and in the nurses' notes. If the vital signs are abnormal, notify the surgeon.

Hygiene. Basic hygiene measures remove skin contamination and increase a patient's comfort. If a patient is unwilling or unable to take a complete bath, a partial bath is refreshing and removes irritating secretions or drainage from the skin. Because a patient cannot wear personal nightwear to the OR, provide a clean hospital gown and instruct him or her to remove all other articles of clothing, including undergarments. After having nothing by mouth throughout the night, a patient usually has a very dry mouth. Offer mouthwash and toothpaste and caution a patient not to swallow anything.

BOX 39-5 EVIDENCE-BASED PRACTICE

PICO Question: Does the type and timing of aseptic technique practices used in the perioperative setting compared with standard hospital practice decrease the risk of infection in the postoperative patient?

SUMMARY OF EVIDENCE

Postoperative surgical wound infections result in the disruption of the anticipated recovery time and contribute to increased morbidity and mortality rates. The increased length of time and medications required to treat postoperative wound infections is also a concern (Lipke et al., 2010). Implementation of strategies to control the environment during the perioperative experience decreases the risk for infection. Handwashing is the most important tool in the prevention of infection. Everyone is responsible for safe patient-centered care, regardless of his or her role (Roesler et al., 2010; Starkweather, 2010). Interventions to prevent surgical wound infection include the clipping of hair (versus shaving), disinfection of the skin with an antiseptic agent such as chlorhexidene immediately before the incisional cut, administration of a prophylactic antibiotic, delay of dressing change until 48 hours following surgery, and adherence to principles of asepsis. Evidence demonstrates a direct relationship between the use of these preventive measures and decreased postoperative wound infection (Gregson, 2011; Kiernan, 2012). Nurses working in perioperative areas play a significant role in preventing and detecting postoperative wound infection as they ensure that key interventions are implemented for all patients in all situations.

APPLICATION TO NURSING PRACTICE

- Develop a safe, patient-centered plan of care that is known to all staff involved in the care of the surgical patient (Roesler et al., 2010).
- Check a patient for clinical signs of infection (Kiernan, 2012).
- Implement multiple strategies to reduce the risk for surgical site infections (Lipke et al., 2010).

Preparation of Hair and Removal of Cosmetics. During major surgery the anesthesiologist positions a patient's head to put an endotracheal tube into the airway (see Chapter 30). This involves manipulation of the hair and scalp. To avoid injury, ask a patient to remove hairpins or clips. In addition, have patients remove hairpieces or wigs. Patients can braid long hair and wear disposable hats to contain hair before entering the OR.

During and after surgery the anesthesia provider and nurses assess skin and mucous membranes to determine a patient's level of oxygenation, circulation, and fluid balance. A pulse oximeter is often applied to a finger to monitor oxygen saturation of the blood (see Chapter 15). Anesthesia providers are also using end-tidal carbon dioxide, by way of capnography, to assess patients' physiological stability. When using a pulse oximeter, have patients remove all makeup (lipstick, powder, blush, nail polish) and at least one artificial fingernail to expose normal skin and nail coloring. Anything in or around the eye irritates or injures the eye during surgery. Have patients remove contact lenses, false eyelashes, and eye makeup. Eyeglasses usually remain in the room or you can give them to the family immediately before a patient enters the OR.

Removal of Prostheses. It is easy for any type of prosthetic device to become lost or damaged during surgery. Have patients remove all removable prosthetics for safekeeping. If a patient has a brace or splint, check with his or her surgeon to determine whether it should remain with a patient to be reapplied after surgery. Although patients need to remove hearing aids, eyeglasses, and contact lenses, do not have them do this until just before the surgery. Allowing patients to wear these aids facilitates communication and increases a patient's sense of control. Refer to institution policies for clarification.

For many patients removing dentures is embarrassing. If a patient removes dentures before surgery, provide him or her privacy. Place dentures in special containers and label with a patient's name for safekeeping to prevent breakage. Assess a patient for loose teeth. A broken tooth can become dislodged during insertion of an endotracheal tube and obstruct the airway.

Inventory and secure all prosthetic devices. Give prosthetics to family members or significant others or keep the devices at a patient's bedside. Follow agency policy and document the devices' location.

Preparation of Bowel and Bladder. Some patients receive an enema or cathartic the morning of surgery (see Chapter 35). If so, give it at least 1 hour before a patient leaves for surgery, allowing time for a patient to defecate without rushing.

Instruct a patient to void just before leaving for the OR. If a patient is unable to void, enter a notation on the preoperative checklist. An empty bladder minimizes incontinence and injury to the bladder during surgery. An empty bladder also makes abdominal organs more accessible. The surgeon orders an indwelling catheter if the surgery is long or the incision is in the lower abdomen (see Chapter 34).

Application of Antiembolism Devices. Many surgeons order **antiembolic stockings** or sequential compression stockings for patients to wear during surgery. When correctly sized and properly applied, these devices reduce the risk for deep vein thrombosis (see Chapter 36). Antiembolic stockings maintain compression of small veins and capillaries of the lower extremities. The constant compression forces blood into larger vessels, thus promoting venous return and preventing venous stasis. **Sequential compression stockings** are attached to an air pump that inflates and deflates the stockings, applying intermittent pressure sequentially from the ankle to the knee and alternating calves, mimicking the venous return process of walking.

Promotion of Patient's Dignity. During preoperative preparations care becomes depersonalized unless you maintain a patient's privacy and reduce sources of anxiety. Ambulatory and same-day surgical-admission patients often sit in a waiting room before surgery. To protect patients' modesty, allow them to wear underclothes when possible and provide cover robes. Ensure hospitalized patients their privacy by closing room curtains or doors during preoperative preparation. Allow family to stay until a patient goes to the OR.

Performing Special Procedures. Sometimes a patient's condition requires special interventions before surgery. On the surgeon's order start IV infusions (see Chapter 18), insert a Foley catheter (see Chapter 34), insert a **nasogastric (NG) tube** for gastric decompression (see Chapter 35), or administer medications (see Chapter 17).

Safeguarding Valuables. If a patient has valuables, give them to family members or secure them for safekeeping in a designated location. Many facilities require patients to sign a release to free the institution of responsibility for lost valuables. Prepare a list with a description of items, place a copy with a patient's chart, and give a copy to a designated family member. Patients are often reluctant to remove wedding rings or religious medals. Tape a wedding band in place; however, do not create a tourniquet with the tape. If there is a risk that a patient will experience swelling of the hand or fingers, remove the band. Many hospitals allow patients to pin religious medals to their gowns, although the risk for loss increases (Phillips, 2013).

Administering Preoperative Medications. Typically the surgeon or anesthesia provider orders preoperative drugs for you to give before a patient leaves for the OR. Complete all nursing care measures before giving the preoperative medications. Preoperative drugs such as benzodiazepines, opioids, antiemetics, and anticholinergics usually do not induce sleep; but they can cause dry mouth, drowsiness, and dizziness. If the drug causes drowsiness or dizziness, keep the side rails in the up position, the bed in the low position, and the call bell within easy reach for a patient. Instruct a patient to remain in bed until the surgical nursing assistant or transporter arrives to take a patient to the OR and to call for assistance if there is a need to get out of bed. A patient can easily fall, thinking that nothing is wrong, only to realize that the medications have seriously hampered the ability to walk steadily.

Never allow a patient to sign an informed consent document while under the influence of an opioid or sedative.

EVALUATION

Evaluation of the preoperative goals and outcomes of the plan of care begins before surgery and extends into the postoperative period, providing direction for future interventions. For some patients surgery is an emergency. Others require procedures up until surgery. This leaves little time for evaluation. For some measures such as those to prevent infection, evaluate after surgery when you are able to determine the outcome.

Patient Care. Determine if a patient and family have adequate preoperative preparation by asking the patient to describe the surgical procedure, its purpose, and the postoperative care (Box 39-6). For example, by having a patient and family describe the reasons for postoperative exercises and incentive spirometry, you evaluate the patient's understanding of the physiological and psychological responses to surgery. Evaluate adequacy of preoperative teaching by asking a patient to demonstrate exercises. Evaluate anxiety by monitoring pulse and blood pressure, facial expressions, and verbal interactions. In addition, ask a patient if he or she remains anxious or fearful of any aspect of the surgery.

Patient Expectations. Determine if a patient's and family's expectations have been met up to this point. Spend time talking with them to learn if they are satisfied with their preparation. Knowing this information allows you to help a patient redefine realistic expectations. In emergency situations this becomes more difficult to evaluate. The family often becomes the focus of the evaluation if a patient is unable to respond or is in a condition that prevents a meaningful discussion.

BOX 39-6 EVALUATION

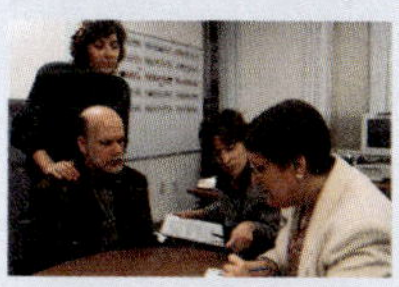

It is the morning of Mr. Korloff's surgery, and Sue admits him to the hospital with the help of one of his daughters. She checks that the informed consent has been signed and witnessed. She completes his physical assessment, which focuses on assessing breath sounds, condition of his skin, and vital signs. Sue also completes the preoperative checklist. She asks Mr. Korloff if he has any questions about the nature or purpose of the surgery. At times he still seems a bit anxious about what to expect. Sue also reviews with Mr. Korloff and his daughter the events that will occur in the holding area and the postanesthesia care unit. She asks if they are frightened about any aspect of the procedure or routine, and she addresses their concerns. Sue then reviews with Mr. Korloff the exercises that were in the booklet he received in the preadmission testing center. She has Mr. Korloff demonstrate coughing and deep breathing while reinforcing its importance once surgery is over. She then gives Mr. Korloff a hospital gown and cover-up and shows him to the changing area. After he has removed his clothes and put on the hospital gown, Sue accompanies Mr. Korloff and his daughter to the holding area.

DOCUMENTATION NOTE

"Admitted for scheduled laparoscopic cholecystectomy. Blood pressure, 142/84 mm Hg; pulse, 88 beats/min; respirations, 18 breaths/min; temperature, 98.9° F. Lungs clear to auscultation bilaterally with normal excursion. Skin warm and dry; no evidence of lesions. Remained NPO during the night. Reviewed instructions on postoperative exercises and is able to demonstrate coughing and deep breathing. Has some difficulty holding incentive spirometer in mouth. Daughters will be in waiting area during procedure."

Transport to the Operating Room

Personnel in the **operating room (OR)** notify the nursing unit or preoperative surgery holding area when it is time for surgery. In many hospitals a nursing assistant or a transporter brings a wheelchair or stretcher for transporting patients. The transporter checks a patient's identification bracelet against a patient's medical record to be sure that the correct person is going to surgery. When using a stretcher to transport a patient, the nurses and transporter help the patient safely transfer from bed to stretcher. The ambulatory surgery patient, if able and not medicated, often walks to the OR, providing more control over the event.

Give the family the opportunity to visit before a patient goes to the OR. Then direct the family to the appropriate waiting area. If a patient has been hospitalized before surgery and will be returning to the same nursing unit, prepare the bed and room for his or her return. You are better prepared for postoperative care if the room is ready before a patient's return. Include the following in a postoperative bedside unit:

1. Sphygmomanometer, stethoscope, and thermometer
2. Emesis basin
3. Clean gown
4. Washcloth, towel, and facial tissues
5. IV pole and pump
6. Suction equipment (if needed)
7. Oxygen equipment (if ordered)
8. Extra pillows for positioning a patient comfortably
9. Bed pads to protect bed linen from drainage
10. PCA (see Chapter 32) pump and tubing (if ordered)
11. Bed raised to stretcher height, bed linen turned back, and furniture moved to accommodate the stretcher

Preanesthesia Care Unit. In most hospitals a patient enters a **preanesthesia care unit** or **presurgical care unit (PSCU)** (sometimes called a *holding area*) outside the OR, where preoperative preparations are completed. Nurses in the PSCU are usually part of the OR room staff and wear surgical scrub suits. If an IV catheter is not already present, a nurse, nurse anesthetist, or anesthesiologist inserts a catheter into a patient's vein to establish a route for fluid replacement, IV drugs, or blood or blood products. He or she also administers preoperative medications and/or conscious sedation at this time.

If a patient needs to have hair removed around the surgical site, perform this procedure in a private area near the OR immediately before surgery. AORN-recommended practices include the use of electric or battery-operated clippers for preoperative hair removal. Clippers minimize the risk for irritation and small cuts, which predispose a patient to infection. Follow manufacturer guidelines if you use a depilatory to remove hair (AORN, 2012).

INTRAOPERATIVE SURGICAL PHASE

Care of a patient during surgery requires careful preparation and knowledge of the events that will occur during a surgical procedure.

NURSE'S ROLE DURING SURGERY

A nurse usually assumes one of two roles in the OR: **circulating nurse** or **scrub nurse** (Figure 39-1). The circulating nurse, who is a licensed registered nurse (RN), cares for a patient in the OR by completing a preoperative assessment, establishing and implementing the intraoperative plan of care, evaluating the care, and providing for the continuity of care after surgery. The circulating nurse assists the anesthesia provider with endotracheal intubation, calculating blood loss and urinary output, and administering blood. This nurse monitors sterile technique of surgical team members and a safe OR environment. A nurse also assists the surgeon and scrub nurse by operating nonsterile equipment, providing additional instruments and supplies; maintaining accurate and complete documentation; and tracking sponge, needle, and instrument counts.

The scrub person is an RN, a licensed practical nurse (LPN), or a surgical technician. Like the surgeon, the scrub person performs a hand scrub and applies sterile gown and gloves for a procedure. The scrub person maintains the sterile field during a surgical procedure and adheres to strict surgical asepsis. This person assists with applying surgical drapes and hands the surgeon instruments, sponges, sutures, and other supplies.

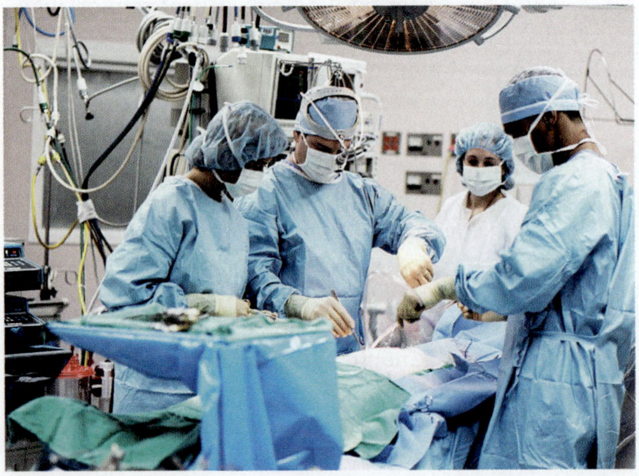

FIGURE 39-1 Nurses in operating room. (© 2011 Jupiterimages Corporation.)

NURSING PROCESS

ASSESSMENT

As a circulating nurse in the PSCU and OR, conduct a special preoperative assessment to verify that a patient is ready for surgery and to plan intraoperative care. Ask a patient his or her name and date of birth and compare the response with the identification band and medical record. Review consent forms, allergies, medical history, physical assessment findings, and test results. Verify with a patient the type of surgery and the surgical site (Table 39-7). Pay special attention to a patient's psychological comfort. Also perform a brief assessment of key body systems.

NURSING DIAGNOSIS

Review preoperative nursing diagnoses and modify them to individualize the care plan in the OR. Add diagnoses and related factors based on a patient's condition, specific surgical intervention, and method and type of anesthesia. Nursing diagnoses for the intraoperative patient often include the following:

- *Risk for Latex Allergy Response*
- *Risk for Aspiration*
- *Decreased Cardiac Output*
- *Risk for Deficient Fluid Volume*
- *Impaired Gas Exchange*
- *Risk for Infection*
- *Risk for Perioperative-Positioning Injury*
- *Impaired Skin Integrity*
- *Ineffective Thermoregulation*
- *Ineffective Peripheral Tissue Perfusion*

Nursing care in the OR routinely includes monitoring for *Latex Allergy Response* and prevention of *Risk for Perioperative-Positioning Injury.* These diagnoses provide direction for the intraoperative and postoperative care of patients who have them.

PLANNING

Goals and Outcomes. Some patient-centered outcomes of preoperative care extend into the intraoperative phase. These include remaining free of infection and achieving psychological and physical comfort. Additional goals include maintaining skin integrity, therapeutic body temperature, and fluid and electrolyte balance. Measure goal achievement through outcome criteria such as the presence of intact skin, without redness or irritation; body temperature within a patient's normal range; stable vital signs; and adequate urinary output.

Priority setting and continuity of care come from the plan of care and any additional information from oral and written reports of the preadmission area and/or the presurgical care unit.

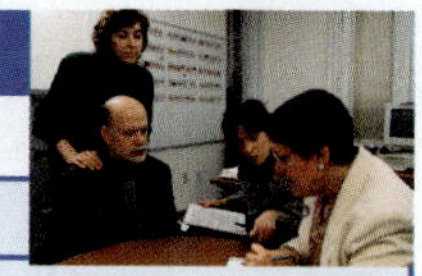

TABLE 39-7 FOCUSED PATIENT ASSESSMENT

Intraoperative Assessment

FACTORS TO ASSESS	QUESTIONS	PHYSICAL ASSESSMENT
Right patient	What is your full name?	Ask patient to state name. Inspect patient identification band for patient name and date of birth and compare with medical record.
Right surgical procedure on right body part	For which surgery are you here? Compare answer with operative permit.	Inspect and palpate body part to add any physical evidence of need for surgery (redness, edema, pain). Sometimes there is none, depending on the nature of the surgery. Observe for surgical site marking if laterality of body part involved (i.e., right ankle marked with "yes"). Marking is often performed in presurgical care unit by surgeon.
Right set of data in chart	Verify and clarify with patient any medical, surgical, medication, and allergy history found in preoperative assessment. Review findings from laboratory reports, diagnostic tests, x-ray films, and electrocardiogram.	Inspect skin for stated surgical scars. Observe for the presence and patency of ordered tubes and lines (NG, Foley, IV).
Right frame of mind of patient	What do you expect as an outcome of surgery? How do you feel about surgery? If patient changes mind about surgery, notify surgeon. Surgery will be canceled or postponed.	Observe for signs of fear and anxiety. Monitor vital signs for indications of excessive anxiety. Compare vital signs to baseline.

IV, Intravenous; *NG,* nasogastric.

IMPLEMENTATION

A major focus of intraoperative care is to prevent injury and complications related to anesthesia, surgery, positioning, and use of equipment. As the perioperative nurse advocate for patients during surgery. Protect patients' dignity and rights at all times.

Acute Care

Admission to the Operating Room. After assessing a patient, the circulating nurse transfers a patient into the OR. A patient is usually still awake and notices health care providers wearing surgical masks, protective eyewear, and gowns. Carefully transfer a patient to the operating bed, being sure that the stretcher and bed are locked in place. After being transferred to the bed, the OR team secures a patient with safety straps. Just before starting the surgical procedure, the surgical team takes a "time out" for a final verification of the right patient, right procedure, and right site. This final "time out" is part of TJC's Universal Protocol for Eliminating Wrong Site, Wrong Procedure, and Wrong Person Surgery (TJC, 2014).

Physical Preparation. After securing a patient safely, first apply small plastic electrodes on the chest and extremities for continuous electrocardiographic (ECG) monitoring during surgery. A monitor displays the electrical activity of the heart. Next apply a blood pressure cuff around a patient's arm for the anesthesiologist to measure the blood pressure. Attach a pulse oximeter sensor to a patient's finger or earlobe for measurement of the oxygen saturation of the blood and an evaluation of ventilation.

Intraoperative Warming. Intraoperative warming is designed to prevent hypothermia during surgery and thus prevent postoperative complications such as shivering, cardiac arrest, need for blood transfusion, and pressure ulcers. The nurse in the OR applies warm blankets, forced-air warmers, or circulating water mattresses over a patient. Evidence in the literature indicates that circulating water-garment systems are most effective in maintaining patient body temperature (Poveda, Martinez, and Galvão, 2012). The use of warming devices reduces postoperative pain levels, offers thermal comfort, and reduces treatment costs.

Psychological Support. Entering the OR is stressful for most patients. Reassure them and remain at a patient's side until after anesthesia is induced. Offering a hand to hold is often helpful. If a patient is awake during surgery, give support throughout the surgical procedure.

Positioning. Positioning typically occurs after relaxation from anesthesia has been achieved. For example, when using general anesthesia, the nursing personnel and surgeon usually do not position a patient until the anesthesia provider notifies them that he or she is intubated and has entered the stage of complete relaxation. Proper positioning of a patient provides good access to and exposure of the operative site and promotes adequate circulatory and respiratory function. Ensure that positioning does not impair neuromuscular structures

TABLE 39-8 INTRAOPERATIVE NURSING CARE

OUTCOMES	INTERVENTIONS
Patient is free of infection.	Maintain Standard Precautions. Monitor surgical asepsis during surgical case. Perform surgical skin scrub.
Patient is free of pressure ulcer.	Use appropriate pressure-relieving strategies in operating room, especially for high-risk patients (e.g., very obese, nutritionally depleted, long surgical procedure). Strategies such as type of mattress, headrest, protectors, supports, and pillows reduce postoperative pressure ulcer incidence (Bulfone et al., 2012).
Patient is free of injury.	Apply sterile surgical drapes. Perform accurate sponge, needle, and instrument counts. Provide grounding for electrosurgical cautery. Provide eye protection when using a laser.
Patient maintains body temperature.	Monitor body temperature. Warm irrigating solutions. Apply warming blanket or garment intraoperatively if possible or immediately after surgery.
Patient maintains fluid and electrolyte balance.	Monitor blood loss, NG drainage, and urinary output. Provide blood products as ordered. Monitor type and flow rate of IV fluids.

IV, Intravenous; *NG*, nasogastric.

or skin integrity. Most ORs now use a variety of pressure-relieving surfaces to reduce the incidence of pressure ulcers intraoperatively (see Chapter 37).

Consider a patient's comfort and safety. It is sometimes difficult for a patient to understand why he or she feels a wide range of discomfort after surgery. If a joint is extended too far in an alert person, pain stimuli warn the individual that muscle and joint strain is too great and the individual changes position. In an anesthetized patient normal defense mechanisms do not guard against joint damage and muscle stretch and strain. A patient's muscles are so relaxed that it is relatively easy to place him or her in a position that he or she normally does not assume while awake. A patient often remains in the same position for several hours. Once he or she awakens, musculoskeletal pain is significant. Intraoperative nursing care includes interventions to prevent infection and injury to a patient, maintain fluid and electrolyte balance, and control a patient's temperature (Table 39-8).

Introduction of Anesthesia. The nature and extent of a patient's surgery and current physical status influence the type of anesthesia administered in surgery. It is especially important after surgery that you know the complications to anticipate after a patient receives anesthesia (Table 39-9).

TABLE 39-9 EXAMPLES OF COMPLICATIONS OF ANESTHESIA

TYPE	COMPLICATIONS
General anesthesia	Aspiration of vomitus, cardiac irregularities, decreased cardiac output, hypotension, hypothermia, hypoxemia, laryngospasm, malignant hyperthermia, nephrotoxicity, respiratory depression
Regional anesthesia	Hypotension
Epidural	Hypothermia
Spinal	Injury to spinal cord, injury to numb legs, respiratory paralysis, spinal headache
Local anesthesia	Anaphylactic shock, hives, rash
Conscious sedation	Aspiration, decreased level of consciousness, hypoxemia, respiratory depression

General Anesthesia. Under **general anesthesia** a patient loses all sensations, consciousness, and reflexes, including gag and blink reflexes. A patient's muscles relax, and he or she experiences amnesia. General anesthesia is administered during major procedures requiring extensive tissue manipulation or any time that analgesia, muscle relaxation, immobility, and control of the autonomic nervous system are required. This includes minor procedures, especially with children.

Regional Anesthesia. **Regional anesthesia** results in loss of sensation in an area of the body by anesthetizing sensory pathways. This type of anesthesia is accomplished by injecting a local anesthetic along the pathway of a nerve from the spinal cord (Rothrock, 2011). Administration techniques include peripheral nerve blocks and spinal, epidural, and caudal blocks. A patient requires careful monitoring during and immediately after regional anesthesia for return of sensation and movement distal to the regional anesthesia. The nurse must ensure that the limb is protected from harm until full sensation has returned.

Local Anesthesia. Local anesthesia involves loss of sensation at the desired surgical site by inhibiting peripheral nerve conduction. It is used during minor procedures performed in ambulatory surgery. Local anesthetics are also used in addition to general or regional anesthesia. Long-acting local anesthetics are sometimes injected into the incision at the end of a patient's surgery for postoperative pain relief (see Chapter 32).

Moderate Sedation (Conscious Sedation). IV **moderate sedation/analgesia** or **conscious sedation** is routinely used for diagnostic or therapeutic procedures (e.g., colonoscopy or certain laparoscopies) that do not require complete anesthesia but simply a decreased level of consciousness. A patient needs to maintain respirations and respond appropriately to physical and verbal stimuli. Advantages to IV conscious sedation include adequate sedation, diminished anxiety, amnesia, pain relief, mood alteration, enhanced patient cooperation, stable vital signs, and rapid recovery with minimal risk (Fullwood and Sargent, 2010).

The administration of conscious sedation generally requires facility certification to care for these patients. The ability to assess, diagnose, and intervene if a complication arises is essential, including skills in airway management, oxygen delivery, and use of resuscitation equipment (AORN, 2012). Document vital signs, oxygen saturation, assessment of breath sounds and heart rhythm, and level of consciousness every 15 minutes during the procedure and the immediate recovery period (AORN, 2012) (see agency policy).

Support any patient who remains awake by explaining procedures, encouraging questions, and warning a patient when unpleasant sensations will be experienced. Some settings provide music to mask unpleasant sounds and promote relaxation and pain relief.

Documentation of Intraoperative Care. During the intraoperative phase continue the established plan of care and modify it as needed. Throughout the surgical procedure keep an accurate record of patient care activities and procedures performed by OR personnel. This record provides useful data for the nurse who cares for a patient after surgery.

EVALUATION

Evaluation of many interventions implemented during the intraoperative phase occurs in the postoperative phase because complications (e.g., infection) often arise days after surgery.

Patient Care. After surgery perform a postoperative evaluation of a patient before he or she leaves the OR (Box 39-7). Inspect the skin under the grounding pad and areas of the skin where equipment or positioning has exerted pressure. Monitor body temperature immediately after surgery to assess thermoregulation. Obtain vital signs and auscultate lung sounds to assess pulmonary and fluid and electrolyte status.

Patient Expectations. Frequently ask patients who did not receive general anesthesia during a procedure about pain, numbness, and perceived room temperature. This determines if the analgesia is adequate and if a patient is comfortable in regard to position and temperature.

When a patient is having major surgery, it is very important to keep the family informed. Typically family members want to know if surgery is progressing without problems. Most hospitals provide phones within waiting areas that allow nursing staff to reach families and explain the progress of the surgery. If you are on the surgical nursing unit, give the families updates and support in the waiting areas.

BOX 39-7 EVALUATION

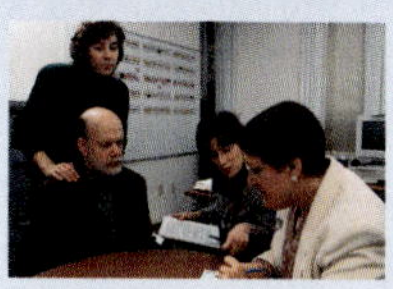

Mr. Korloff's surgery is complete, and he is transferred to the PACU. Sue accompanies him into the PACU. She reviews the operative record. Mr. Korloff received general anesthesia, and the procedure was uneventful. Mr. Korloff did not receive any blood or blood products. He received Ringer's lactate solution intravenously via a catheter in the left lower forearm. Sue examines the IV site, and it is without signs of phlebitis or infiltration. Small gauze dressings were applied to the four small abdominal puncture wounds, with no drainage at this time. Sue positions Mr. Korloff to maintain a patent airway and notes that his respirations are 12 breaths/min and unlabored. Airway is clear of secretions. There are no signs of pressure over bony prominences.

IV, Intravenous; *PACU*, postanesthesia care unit.

POSTOPERATIVE SURGICAL PHASE

Following surgery a patient's postoperative course involves two phases: the immediate recovery period and convalescence. For a patient following ambulatory surgery, the immediate recovery period normally lasts only 1 to 2 hours, and convalescence occurs at home. For a hospitalized patient the immediate postoperative period often lasts a few hours, with convalescence taking 1 or more days, depending on the extent of surgery and a patient's response.

RECOVERY

During recovery it is important to be very conscientious in monitoring a patient and making the clinical judgments necessary to determine if the patient is progressing as expected. This is a time when a patient's condition can change very quickly. Immediately after surgery a patient goes to the postanesthesia care unit (PACU) for close monitoring. Before a patient arrives, the PACU nurse receives a report from the surgical team in the OR to relay a patient's most current status, nursing care priorities, and the need for special equipment. The report includes information about anesthetic agents given during surgery; IV fluids and blood products administered; status of the wound, including the presence of drainage devices; and whether a patient had any surgical complications such as excessive blood loss. While a patient is in the PACU, conduct ongoing assessments every 15 minutes or per protocol.

POSTANESTHESIA CARE IN AMBULATORY SURGERY

The postanesthesia care of patients having ambulatory surgery occurs in two phases. Phase 1 is essentially the same as described for hospitalized patients in the PACU. However, phase 2 prepares patients for discharge and self-care. A patient receiving only local anesthesia is usually admitted directly to the phase 2 area. In phase 2 encourage a patient to gradually sit up on the stretcher or recliner and begin to take ice chips or sips of water or other clear liquids after regaining full alertness.

BOX 39-8 INFORMATION GIVEN TO AMBULATORY SURGICAL PATIENTS

- Health care provider's office telephone number (24-hour answer)
- Telephone number for surgery center
- Follow-up appointment date and time
- Review of prescribed medications and discussion of when to take and side effects for which to observe.
- Guidelines related to specific surgery and surgeon's preference: dressing and wound care, activity restrictions
- Guidelines related to anesthesia: diet and fluid resumption, activity restrictions
- Warning signs of complications

Phase 2 postanesthesia care occurs in a room equipped with medical recliner chairs, side tables, and footrests. Kitchen facilities for preparing light snacks and beverages are in the area, along with bathrooms. The phase 2 environment promotes a patient's and family's comfort and well-being until discharge. Continue to monitor a patient but not at the same intensity as in phase 1. In phase 2 initiate postoperative teaching with patients and family members (Box 39-8). When a patient's condition remains stable in the sitting position and there is no nausea or dizziness, he or she is discharged.

RECOVERY PHASE

Once a patient is stable, usually within 2 to 3 hours, the anesthesia provider or surgeon transfers the hospitalized patient to a postoperative nursing unit, whereas the ambulatory surgical patient returns home. Unstable patients remain in the PACU or go to an intensive care unit for more intense monitoring and care. During recovery or convalescence consider the goals of care established during the preoperative and intraoperative phases to help a patient return to normal physiological function. In addition, direct your nursing care toward facilitating a patient's smooth transition home. Encourage family participation in a patient's plan of care. The family provides coaching during postoperative exercises and important psychosocial support to a patient.

NURSING PROCESS

ASSESSMENT

The parameters you assess for a patient following surgery are basically the same during recovery and convalescence. When patients enter the PACU, perform a rapid assessment of the respiratory and circulatory status and attach electronic monitors. Conduct assessments while considering patients' surgical risks and the type of surgery performed. For example, if a patient has a history of smoking and had abdominal surgery involving a high abdominal incision, focus on his or her respiratory status. A patient's pain could potentially reduce ventilation, leading to the development of atelectasis.

Once a patient reaches a postoperative nursing unit, perform vital sign measurements and assessments less often, usually every 15 to 30 minutes initially, then hourly, and then less often per surgeon's or health care provider's orders. Check the institution policy on vital signs following surgery. Table 39-10 summarizes a focused postoperative assessment.

Respiration. Assess the quality of a patient's respirations and the patency of the airway. A patient receiving a general anesthetic often has an artificial airway still in place when arriving in the PACU. Certain anesthetic agents and opioids often continue to affect ventilation. Thus be especially alert for slow, shallow breathing. Assess respiratory rate, rhythm, depth, and quality of ventilatory movement. Auscultate the lungs for adventitious sounds such as crackles, which do not clear with coughing, and for wheezing, which results from air squeezed through passageways narrowed almost to closure from secretions (Jarvis, 2012). If breathing is unusually shallow, place your hand over a patient's face or mouth to feel exhaled air. Pulse oximetry reflecting 92% to 100% saturation is within normal limits unless the surgeon or anesthesia care provider orders other limits (see Chapter 15).

Once a patient is on a surgical nursing unit, respirations have usually stabilized. Frequent auscultation of lung sounds is still important because a patient is still at risk for developing pneumonia unless he or she follows postoperative exercises routinely. Remember that pain control is important during convalescence so a patient is able to cough and deep breathe with relative ease.

Circulation. A patient is at risk for cardiovascular complications from actual or potential blood loss at the surgical site, side effects of anesthesia, electrolyte imbalances, and depression of normal circulatory regulating mechanisms. Continuous ECG monitoring is routine in the PACU to detect rhythm and rate disturbances. Assessment of heart rate and rhythm and blood pressure monitors a patient's cardiovascular status. Compare preoperative vital signs with postoperative values to assess a patient's status.

Assess circulatory perfusion, especially for patients who have had procedures that impair circulation such as vascular surgery, use of a tourniquet, or application of casts or tight dressings. Always be alert to the amount of bleeding that occurs after surgery and the possibility of hemorrhage. The risk for hemorrhage continues for several days after surgery. Blood loss occurs externally through a drain or incision or internally within the surgical site. Either type of hemorrhage is indicated by a fall in blood pressure; elevated heart and respiratory rates; a thready pulse; cool, clammy, pale skin; and restlessness.

Temperature Control. The OR environment is cool, and a patient's depressed level of body function results in a lowering of metabolism and fall in body temperature. When patients begin to awaken in the PACU, they often complain of feeling cold and uncomfortable. Shivering is not always a sign of hypothermia but rather a side effect of certain anesthetic agents. Measure body temperature to plan for interventions. On a surgical unit monitoring body temperature is important for detecting early occurrence of infection (e.g.,

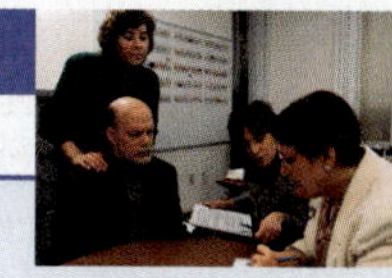

TABLE 39-10 FOCUSED PATIENT ASSESSMENT

Postoperative Assessment

FACTORS TO ASSESS	QUESTIONS/RECORD REVIEW	PHYSICAL ASSESSMENT
Respirations	Ask if patient feels short of breath or has discomfort during breathing.	Monitor respiratory rate, rhythm, and depth every 15 min × 4 or until stable, then every 30 min × 2, and then every hour × 4. Compare with baseline findings.
	Review medical history for conditions involving respiratory system, medications taken, and any allergies.	Observe for symmetry of chest wall movements, color of skin and mucous membranes.
	Review report of type of anesthesia and agents used during surgery.	Auscultate breath sounds for rales, wheezing, decreased or absent sounds.
	Review report of any medications given during surgery or in PACU that affect respiratory function (analgesics, antianxiety agents).	Apply pulse oximeter to detect oxygen saturation.
Circulation	Review baseline heart rate for current comparison.	Monitor pulse rate and rhythm and blood pressure at same frequency as respiratory rate or more often as patient's condition warrants. Maintain continuous ECG monitoring if ordered.
	Review report of amount of blood loss and any replacement blood or blood products in the OR and PACU.	Assess level of consciousness and symptoms of restlessness or altered mental status.
	Review current IV orders as to type of fluid and infusion rate.	Observe skin, nail beds, and mucous membranes for color and hydration.
	Ask if patient is having any dizziness or visual disturbances when changing positions.	Palpate peripheral pulses distal to surgical site, tight dressing, or cast if present.
		Inspect for amount of bleeding on dressing, in drainage systems (NG suction, Hemovac, Jackson-Pratt drain, Foley catheter), and underneath patient.
Infection control	Review patient's risk factors for infection and poor wound healing (contaminated surgical site, history of diabetes mellitus, HIV, or use of immunosuppressing drugs [prednisone]).	Monitor patient temperature and white blood cell count as indicated.
	Ask if patient is having any burning or pain with urination.	Inspect any urine output, note color, consistency, and odor.
	Ask if patient is having extreme tenderness at wound site.	Observe surgical wound for redness, edema, warmth, drainage, and dehiscence. Note the character of the drainage (e.g., color, odor, consistency).
Gastrointestinal function	Review report for history of problems with gastrointestinal function.	Inspect for abdominal distention.
	Are you having any nausea, abdominal cramping? How's your appetite?	Auscultate for bowel sounds in all four quadrants at least every shift until discharge.
	Have you passed any gas or had a bowel movement today? How was the stool compared to your normal stool?	Palpate abdomen for firmness.
		Monitor NG tube for patency and NG tube output for color and amount of drainage (if present).
		Observe patient's ability and willingness to tolerate fluids and food.
Comfort	Review symptoms of pain before surgery, type of anesthesia, location of surgery, and expected level of pain associated with this type of surgery.	Observe for signs and symptoms of discomfort (restlessness, elevated pulse, respirations and blood pressure, grimaces, guarding).
	Review any history of alcohol or illicit drug use.	Assess for any side effects of pain medication (altered mental status, depressed respirations, bradycardia, orthostatic hypotension, nausea or vomiting, urinary retention, constipation).
	Ask patient to rate pain on a 0-10 scale. Inquire about pain level before and after each administration of pain medication.	Observe patient's expressions, body position, ability to rest or sleep.

ECG, Electrocardiogram; *HIV,* human immunodeficiency virus; *IV,* intravenous; *NG,* nasogastric; *OR,* operating room; *PACU,* postanesthesia care unit.

wound or lung). If a patient develops a fever, report it to the surgeon immediately.

Neurological Function. A patient is usually drowsy in the PACU but reacts to verbal commands. However, drugs, electrolyte and metabolic changes, pain, reduced oxygen saturation, and emotional factors influence level of consciousness. Normally as anesthetic agents are metabolized, a patient's reflexes return, he or she regains muscle strength, and a normal level of orientation returns. Check for pupillary and gag reflexes, hand grasp, and movements of the extremities (see Chapter 16). If a patient had surgery involving a portion of the neurological system, conduct a more thorough neurological assessment.

Once a patient returns to a surgical nursing unit, a sudden change in consciousness is not normal. However, routine detailed neurological assessment is unnecessary unless a patient is slow to awaken fully or has had surgery involving the neurological system.

Fluid and Electrolyte Balance. Because of a surgical patient's risk for fluid and electrolyte abnormalities, assess hydration status and monitor cardiac and neurological function for signs of electrolyte alterations (see Chapter 18). Routinely inspect the IV catheter and insertion site to verify patency, absence of signs of phlebitis and infiltration, and proper infusion of IV fluids. It is important that a good venous access is available in case a patient requires fluid and/or blood replacement. IV fluids continue on the surgical nursing unit, sometimes for several days. Duration of IV catheter use depends on the type of surgery, the medications received, and how well a patient tolerates resumption of oral fluids and food.

Monitor and accurately record intake and output to assess fluid balance and renal and cardiac function. Measure all sources of input (e.g., IV fluids and oral intake) and output (e.g., NG tubes, drains, diarrhea, and urine) and consult with the surgeon if appropriate.

Skin Integrity and Condition of the Wound. Thoroughly assess the condition of a patient's skin. A rash often indicates a drug sensitivity or allergy. Abrasions or petechiae result from inadequate padding during positioning or securing on the operating bed. If a patient has burns or serious injury to the skin, communicate this information by completing an incident or occurrence report (see Chapter 5).

The surgical wound sometimes has no dressing, or it is covered with gauze or transparent dressing that protects the wound site. For open wounds or during the changing of a dressing, observe the appearance of the suture line and note the color, odor, and consistency of any drainage (see Chapter 37). Estimate the amount of drainage by noting the extent and area of the dressing covered (e.g., lower half of dressing saturated with sanguineous drainage). If a patient has a wound drainage system, monitor the output and character of drainage routinely. Keep the drainage tubes patent by removing any kinks. A sudden increase in drainage indicates possible hemorrhage.

A critical time for wound healing is 24 to 72 hours after surgery (see Chapter 37). A patient exerts physical stress on a wound from coughing, vomiting, or movement in bed. Inadequate nutrition, impaired circulation, and metabolic alterations further impair healing. Observe the incision for signs of dehiscence and evisceration (Table 39-11). Notify the surgeon of any area of dehiscence. Evisceration is a medical emergency. In the event of evisceration, cover any exposed abdominal contents with gauze soaked with sterile normal saline. Prepare an IV infusion set for rapid infusion of IV fluids.

If a wound becomes infected, it usually occurs 3 to 6 days after surgery, when a patient is at home. Ongoing observation of a wound includes inspection for redness, increased warmth, edema, and purulent drainage. Instruct a patient or family caregiver on how to assess the wound at home and to immediately report any signs and symptoms of wound infection to the surgeon.

Genitourinary Function. Spinal anesthesia often prevents a patient from feeling bladder fullness or distention and may cause urinary retention for up to 6 to 8 hours. Palpate the lower abdomen just above the symphysis pubis for bladder distention. Use a bladder scanner to determine if urine has accumulated in the bladder (see Chapter 34). A full bladder is painful and often the cause of a patient's restlessness, agitation, or high blood pressure. If a patient has an indwelling urinary catheter (see Chapter 34), monitor urine output and expect at least 30 mL/hr in adults or 1 to 2 mL/kg/hr in infants and children. Observe the color and odor of urine. Surgery involving portions of the urinary tract normally causes bloody urine for at least 12 to 24 hours.

Gastrointestinal Function. Anesthetics slow gastrointestinal motility and cause nausea. In addition, manipulation of the intestines during abdominal surgery further impairs peristalsis. Faint or absent bowel sounds are typical during the immediate recovery phase. Normal bowel sounds usually return in about 24 hours, unless major abdominal surgery was performed. Paralytic ileus (i.e., loss of function of the intestine), which causes abdominal distention, is always a possibility after abdominal surgery. On the surgical nursing unit ask whether a patient is passing flatus, an important sign indicating return of normal bowel function that may be more indicative of postoperative gastrointestinal function return in patients undergoing abdominal surgery than presence of bowel sounds (Massey, 2012). Inspect the abdomen for distention caused by gas. Distention also develops if internal bleeding occurs in patients who have had abdominal surgery. If an NG tube is in place for decompression, assess the patency of the tube (see Chapter 35) and the color and amount of drainage.

Comfort. As a patient awakens from general anesthesia, the sensation of discomfort often becomes prominent. Some patients perceive pain before regaining full consciousness. Acute incisional pain causes patients to become restless and frequently causes changes in vital signs. Pain management is one of the most important priorities in postoperative care. Appropriate pain management enables patients to deep breathe and cough more effectively and initiate ambulation. If a patient has PCA or PCEA, have him or her begin using

TABLE 39-11 COMMON POSTOPERATIVE COMPLICATIONS

COMPLICATION	CAUSE
Respiratory System	
Atelectasis: Collapse of alveoli with retained mucus secretions. Signs and symptoms: elevated respiratory rate, dyspnea, fever, crackles over involved lobes of lungs, productive cough.	Caused by inadequate lung expansion. Greater risk in patients with upper abdominal surgery who have pain during inspiration and repress deep breathing.
Pneumonia: Inflammation of alveoli caused by infectious process. Usually develops in lower dependent lobes of lung if patient is immobilized. Signs and symptoms: fever, chills, productive cough, chest pain, purulent mucus, dyspnea.	Caused by poor lung expansion with retained secretions. *Streptococcus pneumoniae,* a resident bacterium in the respiratory tract, causes most cases of pneumonia.
Hypoxemia: Inadequate concentration of oxygen in arterial blood. Signs and symptoms: restlessness, dyspnea, hypertension, tachycardia, diaphoresis, cyanosis.	Respirations depressed by anesthetics or analgesics. Increased retention of mucus with impaired ventilation occurs from pain, poor positioning, or poor coughing and deep breathing.
Pulmonary embolism: Clot blocks pulmonary artery and disrupts blood flow to one or more lobes of lung. Signs and symptoms: dyspnea, sudden chest pain, cyanosis, tachycardia, hypotension.	Patients who are immobilized and have preexisting circulatory or coagulation disorders are at high risk. Patients with pelvic and abdominal cancer surgeries are at higher risk.
Circulatory System	
Hemorrhage: Loss of large amount of blood externally or internally in short period of time. Signs and symptoms: same as for hypovolemic shock.	Slipping of suture or dislodged clot at incisional site. Patients with coagulation disorders are at greater risk.
Hypovolemic shock: Reduced perfusion of tissues and cells from loss of circulatory fluid volume. Signs and symptoms: hypotension, weak and rapid pulse, cool and clammy skin, rapid breathing, restlessness, reduced urine output.	Hemorrhage usually causes hypovolemic shock following surgery.
Thrombophlebitis: Inflammation of vein (usually in leg), often accompanied by clot formation. Signs and symptoms: swelling and inflammation of involved site, aching or cramping pain. Vein feels hard, cordlike, and sensitive to touch.	Venous stasis is aggravated by prolonged sitting or immobilization, trauma to vessel wall, and hypercoagulability of blood.
Thrombus: Formation of clot attached to interior wall of vein or artery, which occludes vessel lumen. Symptoms include localized tenderness along vein, swollen calf or thigh in affected leg. Decreased pulse below thrombus (if arterial).	Venous stasis and vessel trauma. Venous injury is usually common after surgery of legs, abdomen, pelvis, and major vessels. Patients with major surgery or trauma to these areas are at risk for thrombus formation.
Embolus: Piece of thrombus that has dislodged and circulates in bloodstream until it lodges in another vessel, commonly lungs, heart, or brain.	Thrombi also form from increased coagulability of blood.
Gastrointestinal System	
Paralytic ileus: Nonmechanical obstruction of the bowel caused by physiological, neurogenic, or chemical imbalance; it may be associated with decreased peristalsis. Common in initial hours following surgery.	Handling of intestines during surgery can lead to loss of peristalsis for a few hours to several days.
Abdominal distention: Retention of air within intestines. Signs and symptoms: increased abdominal girth, complaint of fullness and "gas pains."	Caused by slowed peristalsis from anesthesia, bowel manipulation, or immobilization.
Nausea and vomiting: Symptoms of improper gastric emptying or chemical stimulation of vomiting center. Patient complains of gagging or feeling full or sick to stomach.	Caused by severe pain, abdominal distention, fear, medications, eating or drinking before peristalsis returns, and initiation of gag reflex.

Continued

TABLE 39-11 COMMON POSTOPERATIVE COMPLICATIONS—cont'd

COMPLICATION	CAUSE
Genitourinary System	
Urinary retention: Involuntary accumulation of urine in bladder as result of loss of muscle tone. Signs and symptoms: inability to void, restlessness, and bladder distention occurring 6-8 hours after surgery.	Caused by effects of anesthesia, opioid analgesics; local manipulation of tissues surrounding bladder; and poor positioning of patient, which impairs voiding reflex.
Urinary tract infection caused by bacteria or yeast entering through urethra. Possible symptoms: pain, itching, burning, urgency, and frequency.	A health care–acquired urinary tract infection can occur after bladder catheterization, with poor adherence to catheter care, and if catheter remains in place too long.
Integumentary System	
Wound infection: An invasion of deep or superficial wound tissues by pathogenic microorganisms. Signs and symptoms: warm, red, and tender skin around incision, fever and chills, purulent drainage. It usually appears 3-6 days after surgery.	Caused by poor aseptic technique intraoperatively or during postoperative dressing changes, contaminated wound before surgical exploration. Patients who are chronically ill, obese, or immunosuppressed are at high risk.
Wound dehiscence: Separation of wound edges at suture line. Signs and symptoms: increased drainage and appearance of underlying tissues occurring 6-8 days after surgery.	Caused by malnutrition, obesity, preoperative radiation to surgical site, old age, poor circulation to tissues, and unusual strain on suture line from coughing.
Wound evisceration: Protrusion of internal organs and tissues through incision. It usually occurs 6-8 days after surgery.	Develops following dehiscence (see Wound dehiscence).
Nervous System	
Intractable pain: Pain that is not amenable to analgesia or pain-relief measures.	Related to wound healing, type of dressing, anxiety, or patient positioning.

the device as soon as possible. The American Society of Anesthesiologists (2012) recommends that a postoperative patient should receive systemic, as opposed to intramuscular, analgesics ATC and not prn.

A patient who has regional or local anesthesia usually does not experience pain initially because the incisional area is still anesthetized. You need to be skilled at assessing levels of pain and alert to a patient's need for pain medication. Pain scales are an effective method of assessing pain, evaluating the response to analgesics, and objectively documenting the severity of a patient's pain (see Chapter 32).

NURSING DIAGNOSIS

Based on your assessment and information gathered from the reports of members of the surgical team, identify nursing diagnoses that apply to your patient. Nursing diagnoses that give direction to the continuing care of a patient in the PACU and on the surgical nursing unit after surgery include the following:

- *Ineffective Airway Clearance*
- *Anxiety*
- *Disturbed Body Image*
- *Ineffective Breathing Pattern*
- *Risk for Deficient Fluid Volume*
- *Risk for Infection*
- *Impaired Physical Mobility*
- *Nausea*
- *Acute Pain*
- *Delayed Surgical Recovery*

Analyze and validate assessment data and cluster defining characteristics to identify correct nursing diagnoses. For example, a finding of *Anxiety* manifested by restlessness, glancing about or facial tension could be related to *Acute Pain, Urinary Retention,* or *Ineffective Peripheral Tissue Perfusion.* Further assessment and clustering of findings leads to the correct diagnosis and then the appropriate interventions.

PLANNING

Because of the critical nature of the immediate postoperative period, the plan of care in the PACU involves close monitoring of a patient and frequent assessments to ensure stable physiological function. On the surgical nursing unit focus care on facilitating a patient's recovery (Box 39-9). Base your nursing care on your nursing assessment and the surgeon's postoperative orders. Typical postoperative orders include the following:

1. Frequency of vital signs monitoring and special assessments
2. Types of IV fluids and rate of infusion
3. Postoperative medications (including those for pain, nausea, and antibiotic prophylaxis)
4. Oxygen therapy or incentive spirometry
5. Fluids and food allowed by mouth
6. Level of activity that a patient is allowed to resume

BOX 39-9 SYNTHESIS IN PRACTICE

Postoperative Assessment and Planning

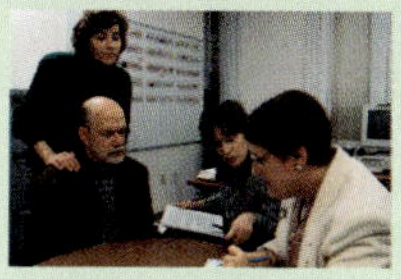

Mr. Korloff's stay in the PACU is uneventful except for pain in the right shoulder. Sue explains to Mr. Korloff that air is put into the abdominal cavity during a laparoscopy. The air causes referred pain. In the PACU Mr. Korloff's pain was a 7 on a scale of 0 to 10.

It is the evening of the day of Mr. Korloff's surgery. Mr. Korloff is in the nursing division for an overnight stay because of his previous cardiac history. He performs deep-breathing and coughing exercises and, after a few demonstrations by Sue, uses the incentive spirometer as ordered. Because he is ambulating frequently in the hall with the assistance of his daughters, he is not performing postoperative leg exercises. The IV fluids were discontinued just before he left the PACU. Mr. Korloff was able to tolerate a clear liquid diet and is passing flatus. He rates his pain as 5 on a scale of 0 to 10, continuing to note some discomfort in the shoulder area. His pain has been controlled with an oral pain medication, acetaminophen with codeine, which he receives every 3 to 4 hours around the clock. His vital signs are within normal limits compared with preoperative values, and his lungs are clear on auscultation. The four small abdominal puncture wounds are without drainage or redness.

IV, Intravenous; *PACU,* postanesthesia care unit.

7. Position that patient is to maintain while in bed
8. Intake and output measures
9. Laboratory tests and x-ray film studies

Goals and Outcomes. During recovery in the PACU goals of care include returning a patient to normal physiological functioning without complications and maintaining physical and psychological comfort. Examples of outcomes include stable vital signs within a patient's normal range, patent airway, palpable peripheral pulses, oxygen saturation over 95%, an intact incision with minimal wound drainage, and balanced intake and output. Another outcome is for a patient to be awake and oriented to the PACU environment with the ability to move all extremities and verbalize pain relief and decreased anxiety.

Once a patient is on the surgical nursing unit, goals are more long term. Maintenance of pain control with improvement in physiological function is still a priority. Adequate wound healing without the presence of infection, restoration of nutrition, a patient's return to a functional state of health, and maintenance of self-concept and body image are additional goals. Examples of measurable outcomes include the following: patient states that level of pain relief is acceptable and appetite has improved; nutritional intake returns to previous or improved caloric intake; and patient states willingness to participate in discharge instruction.

Setting Priorities. While in the PACU a patient's priorities usually center on physiological needs. As you review preoperative and intraoperative data and your ongoing assessments in the PACU, you determine how a patient is progressing and set priorities on developing needs. For example, if a patient begins to awaken without complications but urinary output is less than normal, consult with the surgeon or anesthesia provider to determine if IV fluids need to be increased to prevent dehydration. Data indicating any immediate postoperative complications such as hemorrhage require alteration in the plan of care and implementation of necessary emergency measures.

A patient's physical status often changes on the surgical nursing unit; thus it remains important to be alert for developing complications. Focus priorities on returning a patient to preoperative functioning or better. Patients generally have many nursing diagnoses (Figure 39-2). However, management of acute pain is often the priority of postoperative nursing care. If a surgical patient's pain is properly managed, ambulation begins earlier, deep breathing and coughing are less difficult, and a patient has a better sense of well-being. In addition, begin to prepare a patient for discharge by providing a patient and family necessary instruction and ensuring that adequate resources are available in the home. Research has shown that it is highly important to inform patients and families about what to do about pain and side effects after discharge (Kastanias et al., 2009) because patients place high importance on information about the pain experience, the pain-management plan after discharge, and side-effect management. Monitoring a patient for any psychosocial problems such as body image disturbance or altered coping is also important during convalescence.

Continuity of Care. Continuity of nursing care between the OR, the PACU, and the surgical nursing unit depends on good hand-off communication among all members of the nursing and surgical team. Nursing staff within each area must convey clear and accurate information about a patient's status, treatments, and medications to the next nurse who assumes care for a patient. For example, you need to thoroughly describe the condition of a wound so each nurse knows what to anticipate during wound assessment and care. In that way all staff are able to detect any signs of poor wound healing early.

The ambulatory surgical patient will likely be discharged home with family members or friends. It is essential that a patient and family understand a patient's continuing care needs. Usually the ambulatory surgery nursing staff has discharge instruction sheets available. When caring for patients on surgical nursing units, consider their continuing care needs in the home. For example, referral to home care services or a clinical nurse specialist in wound care or ostomy care provides valuable assistance.

IMPLEMENTATION

Critical thinking is important in the postoperative care of patients. Consider the interrelationship of all body systems and the effect of therapies. A patient remains at risk for a variety of postoperative complications (see Table 39-11) unless aggressive care is provided and a patient becomes actively involved in recovery and convalescence. Review a

CONCEPT MAP

Nursing Diagnosis: Deficient Knowledge
- First experience with surgery
- Primary language of Russian affects ability to understand medical terms
- Has questions about procedure

Interventions
- Provide planned teaching sessions (including daughters) in preadmission
- Use visual teaching aids showing laparoscopy method and positioning in surgery
- Provide reinstruction morning of surgery, focusing on areas about which the patient and daughters remain uncertain

Nursing Diagnosis: Anxiety
- Expresses concerns about surgery
- States, "I am just worried about how this will affect me over the next few weeks."
- Requires repeat explanations on aspects of preoperative instruction

Interventions
- After preadmission tests, sit down with the patient and daughters and discuss their specific concerns
- Teach relaxation exercise to the patient and have him return demonstrate
- Suggest to daughters the use of distraction by having conversations with the patient and bringing business magazines for the patient to read after surgery

Primary Health Problem: Elective laparoscopic surgery—cholecystectomy
Priority Assessments: Readiness to learn, level of knowledge, coping strategies, ability to understand questions

Nursing Diagnosis: Impaired Verbal Communication
- Sometimes looks away from nurse during discussion and turns to daughters instead
- Ability to speak in English reduced when discussing medical terms
- Hesitates to find words when asking questions

Interventions
- Have a professional interpreter present when explaining medical procedures
- Ask the patient if there is anything about his culture that will influence his acceptance of postoperative care
- Incorporate the patient's values into how postoperative care is delivered: when to involve daughters, how to manage pain

—— Link between medical diagnosis and nursing diagnosis - - - - Link between nursing diagnoses

FIGURE 39-2 Concept map.

patient's perioperative teaching and reinforce as needed (Box 39-10). If a patient is an older adult, use gerontological nursing practice guidelines (Box 39-11).

Respiration. Following general anesthesia a patient in the PACU often has an oral or nasal airway present from the OR to maintain a patent airway until regular breathing at a normal rate resumes. This airway is not taped in place. As respiratory function returns, a patient spits out the airway. A patient's ability to do so signifies a return of a normal gag reflex.

BOX 39-10 PATIENT TEACHING

Postoperative Teaching

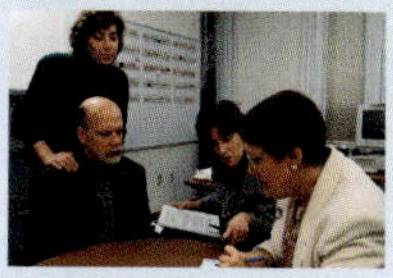

Mr. Korloff tells Sue that the plan is for discharge tomorrow. In their conversation he tells Sue that he hopes he will remember everything that she taught him before surgery. Sue develops the following teaching plan for Mr. Korloff.

OUTCOME

At the end of the teaching session, Mr. Korloff will be able to:

- Verbalize understanding of pain-relief approaches and wound-care practices.

TEACHING STRATEGIES

- Explain the rationale for postoperative exercises so Mr. Korloff knows how the exercises benefit him.
- Encourage Mr. Korloff to practice postoperative exercises every 1 to 2 hours.
- Reinforce the need to take pain medication before pain becomes severe.
- Encourage him to avoid smoking because nicotine accelerates the metabolism of pain medication, resulting in shorter duration of effect.
- Teach nonpharmacological means of pain control such as slow deep breathing, progressive relaxation with music, and use of tactile stimulation such as back rubs (see Chapter 31).
- Teach the names, purpose, and timing of medications and possible side effects so Mr. Korloff can continue medications safely at home.
- Teach signs and symptoms of hemorrhage and wound infection.
- Instruct in proper hand hygiene.
- Demonstrate wound care techniques that are necessary after discharge (see Chapter 37).
- Review high-protein foods needed for wound healing.

EVALUATION STRATEGIES

- Have Mr. Korloff provide return demonstration of the coughing, deep-breathing, and leg exercises; hand hygiene; and wound care techniques.
- Ask Mr. Korloff to identify foods to include in his diet.
- Have Mr. Korloff verbalize wound care and signs and symptoms of abnormal wound healing to report to the health care provider.

BOX 39-11 CARE OF THE OLDER ADULT

Principles of Postoperative Care

- Discuss cognitive and sensory functioning such as decision-making processes, vision, and hearing in the preoperative phase of education; design appropriate strategies after surgery.
- Older adults are at greatest risk for complications related to transitions of care, especially in the ambulatory care setting. The likelihood of the older adult having multiple care providers and co-morbidities can compromise safety (Nelson and Carrington, 2011).
- If a patient will be on bed rest for more than 24 hours, an order for subcutaneous heparin or enoxaparin is necessary to prevent deep vein thrombosis.
- Intake and output is maintained longer after surgery because perfusion of kidneys is compromised and the older adult frequently decreases oral intake of fluids to minimize voiding frequency.
- Any fluid, electrolyte, or acid-base imbalance quickly alters mental status. Older adults often need to be closer to the nurses' station and monitored more frequently for confusion, disorientation, or decreased level of consciousness. Fall precautions are necessary.
- Patients with increased pain tolerance need to be medicated appropriately when they indicate that they have pain. Ask patients often to rate their pain and give them treatment options. Offer pain medications before painful procedures (e.g., dressing changes, walking in the hallway, getting up in a chair).
- Pain medication is more likely to cause altered mental status in older adults, increasing the need to monitor for confusion and disorientation.
- Metabolism of drugs is slowed in older patients; thus the effects of medication persist for a longer period of time.
- Nutritional deficits are common; and diets high in protein, calcium, and vitamins B and C are necessary for wound healing and positive nitrogen balance. Carbohydrate intake is essential for energy and to spare protein use for wound healing. Increase iron intake if a patient is anemic.
- Older adults have more difficulty with constipation because of decreased peristalsis, decreased activity, weakening of abdominal muscles, and the risk for dehydration. Orders for a stool softener and/or extra fiber are accompanied by increased fluid intake despite the resulting increased need to void.

One of the greatest concerns following surgery is airway obstruction resulting from weakness of pharyngeal or laryngeal muscle tone (from the effects of anesthetics); aspiration of emesis; accumulation of secretions in the pharynx, trachea, or bronchial tree; or laryngeal or subglottic edema. Often the tongue causes airway obstruction. The following measures maintain airway patency:

1. *Position a patient on one side with the face downward and the neck slightly extended* (Figure 39-3). A small, folded towel supports the head. Neck extension prevents pharyngeal occlusion of the airway. When the face

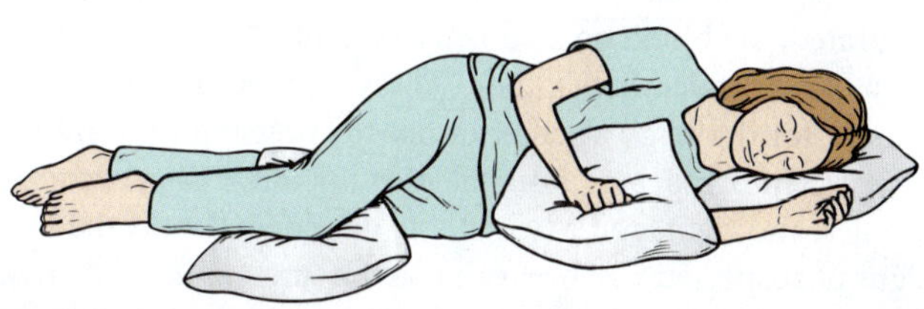

FIGURE 39-3 Position of patient during recovery from general anesthesia. (From Lewis SL, et al: *Medical-surgical nursing: assessment and management of clinical problems,* ed 8, St Louis, 2011, Mosby.)

is angled downward, the tongue moves forward, and mucus secretions flow out of the mouth instead of accumulating in the pharynx. If the nature of the surgery prevents turning a patient on one side, elevate the head of the bed and slightly extend a patient's neck with the head turned to the side. Never position patients with arms over or across their chest because this reduces maximum chest expansion.

2. *Suction the artificial airway and oral cavity for mucus secretions as necessary* (see Chapter 30). Avoid continually eliciting the gag reflex, which causes vomiting. Before removing an airway, suction the back of the airway to remove any mucous plugs or mucus secretions.
3. *Begin deep breathing and coughing exercises* as soon as a patient responds to instructions.
4. *Administer oxygen as ordered* and monitor oxygen saturation with a pulse oximeter.

Once a patient reaches a surgical nursing unit, begin aggressive pulmonary hygiene. A patient participates actively if preoperative instruction was effective. Remember, have the family help coach patients in completing their exercises. Encourage diaphragmatic breathing exercises every hour while a patient is awake. Follow diaphragmatic breathing by having a patient use the incentive spirometer. Encourage a patient to reach the inspiratory volume achieved before surgery on the spirometer. Proper use of the spirometer ensures a maximum inspiration. Encourage regular turning and early ambulation. Walking stimulates an increased respiratory rate and improves circulation. Assist patients who are restricted to bed to turn side-to-side every 1 to 2 hours while awake and to sit when possible. If a patient develops pulmonary secretions, encourage coughing exercises followed by deep breathing at least once an hour. Maintain pain control so a patient achieves a full, productive cough. Provide frequent oral hygiene to help a patient expectorate mucus easily. If a patient is not allowed to have anything by mouth (NPO) or is on a limited fluid intake, the mouth easily becomes dry. Initiate postural drainage and suctioning if a patient is too weak or unable to cough secretions (see Chapter 30).

Circulation. In the PACU it is important to monitor for changes in blood pressure or heart rate. The surgeon usually writes an order indicating which changes to report. However, use critical thinking and notify the surgeon when there is a significant change or a continuous negative trend in vital signs. If hemorrhage is external, observe for increased bloody drainage on dressings or through drains. If a dressing becomes saturated, the blood oozes down a patient's sides and collects in a pool under bedclothes. Always check underneath a patient for drainage whether or not the dressing is saturated. When hemorrhage is internal, the operative site becomes swollen and tight, and a hematoma develops. Report the first signs of suspected hemorrhaging to the surgeon immediately. Maintain the IV infusion, monitor vital signs continuously, continue oxygen, and raise a patient's legs in a modified Trendelenburg's position to promote venous return until a patient's condition stabilizes.

Early measures directed at preventing venous stasis are aimed at preventing deep vein thrombosis (DVT) during convalescence. On the surgical nursing unit begin these interventions as soon as possible:

1. *Encourage patients to perform leg exercises* at least every hour while awake unless contraindicated by surgery.
2. *Apply antiembolism stockings or sequential compression stockings as ordered by the surgeon* (see Chapter 36). Often you apply these devices on a patient in the OR. Remove the stockings every 8 hours and leave off for 1 hour. Thoroughly assess the skin of the legs at this time.
3. *Encourage early ambulation.* Most patients are ordered to ambulate the evening of surgery, depending on the severity of surgery and their condition. The degree of activity allowed progresses as a patient's condition improves. Before ambulation assess vital signs. Abnormalities often contraindicate ambulation. If vital signs are normal, first help a patient sit on the side of the bed. Dizziness is a sign of postural hypotension (see Chapter 15). Check a patient's blood pressure again and ensure that he or she is not dizzy to determine if ambulation is safe. Help with ambulation by standing at a patient's side and helping to either hold or move equipment. During the first few times out of bed, a patient often walks only a few feet. Tolerance improves each time. Evaluate a patient's tolerance to activity by periodically assessing pulse rate.
4. *Avoid positioning a patient in a manner that interrupts blood flow to the extremities.* While a patient is in bed, do not place pillows or rolled blankets directly under the knees. Compression of the popliteal vessels causes a thrombus to form. When sitting in a chair, have a patient elevate the legs on a footstool, avoiding hyperextension of the knee. Never allow a patient to sit with one leg crossed over the other.
5. *Administer anticoagulant drugs if ordered.* Small doses of anticoagulants such as low-molecular-weight heparin given subcutaneously reduce risk for thrombus formation.
6. *Promote adequate fluid intake orally or intravenously.* Adequate hydration prevents the concentration of platelets and red blood cells and thus prevents formation of small clots within blood vessels. Adequate hydration also promotes tissue healing and liquefies respiratory secretions.

Temperature Control. As a result of the cool temperature in the OR and evaporative heat loss, a patient is usually cool when arriving in the PACU. An exception is when intraoperative warming is provided. If no device is in place, provide warmed blankets or other warming devices (e.g., heated air blankets). Increasing body warmth raises a patient's metabolism, and circulatory and respiratory functions improve. Patients often still feel cold when reaching a surgical nursing unit. Offer extra blankets or apply a loose-fitting pair of socks to the feet.

Neurological Function. Deep breathing and coughing help to expel retained anesthetic gases and increase a patient's level of consciousness. Try to arouse a patient by calling his or her name in a moderate tone of voice, noting whether he or she responds appropriately. If the patient remains asleep or is unresponsive, waken him or her through touch or by gently moving a body part. If you need a painful stimulus to wake a patient, notify the anesthesia provider. Orientation to the environment is important in maintaining alertness. Explain that surgery is complete and describe all procedures and nursing measures performed.

Fluid and Electrolyte Balance. A patient's only source of fluid intake immediately after surgery is IV; therefore it is important to maintain a patent IV catheter (see Chapter 18). You typically remove the IV catheter once a patient awakens after ambulatory surgery and is able to tolerate water without gastrointestinal upset. A more seriously ill patient requires an IV catheter to receive fluids until hydration and electrolyte balance are achieved. Some patients require blood products, depending on the amount of blood lost during surgery. A surgeon orders a prescribed solution and rate for each IV infusion. Infuse IV solutions through an infusion pump to ensure correct volume delivery.

Genitourinary Function. A full bladder is painful and causes a patient awakening from surgery to become restless or agitated. Patients who have abdominal surgery or surgery of the urinary system frequently have indwelling catheters inserted until voluntary control of urination returns. If a catheter is in place and urinary output is less than 30 mL/hr in an adult patient and 1 to 2 mL/kg/hr in infants and children, check for catheter occlusion or kinking. Notify the surgeon if measured output does not improve. The following measures promote normal urinary elimination after surgery (see Chapter 34):

- Help the patient assume normal positions for voiding.
- Check the patient frequently for the need to void when a catheter is not in place. The feeling of bladder fullness and urgency to void is often sudden, and you need to respond promptly when a patient calls for assistance.
- Assess for bladder distention. A patient's surgeon usually orders a straight urinary catheter to be inserted if a patient does not void within 8 hours of surgery or sooner if the bladder is distended. Even if a patient has been NPO for hours, IV fluids give the renal system sufficient fluid to excrete urine. Continued difficulty in voiding requires an indwelling catheter, which increases the patient's risk for catheter-associated urinary tract infections (CAUTI) (see Chapter 34).
- Monitor intake and output. If a patient's urine is dark and concentrated, notify the surgeon. A patient easily becomes dehydrated. Remember, the minimum urine output is 30 mL/hr in adults or 1 to 2 mL/kg/hr in infants and children. Notify the surgeon if output is less than these ranges.

Gastrointestinal Function. Minimize a patient's nausea during recovery in the PACU by avoiding sudden movement. If a patient has an NG tube, maintain tube patency per protocol or as ordered (see Chapter 35). Occlusion of an NG tube causes the accumulation of gastric contents in the stomach. Because stomach emptying slows under anesthesia, the accumulated contents cannot escape, and nausea and vomiting develop. Normally a patient does not receive fluids to drink in the PACU because of the risk for vomiting and altered mental status from general anesthesia. Use a moist swab to relieve dryness of a patient's lips and mouth. If a patient is nauseated, give prescribed medication to prevent vomiting and aspiration.

Interventions for preventing gastrointestinal complications promote the return of normal elimination and faster resumption of normal nutritional intake. It takes several days for a patient who has surgery on gastrointestinal structures to resume a normal dietary intake. Normal peristalsis does not usually return for 24 to 48 hours. In contrast, a patient whose gastrointestinal tract is unaffected directly by surgery simply recovers from the effects of anesthesia before resuming dietary intake. Follow these guidelines:

1. *Maintain a gradual progression in dietary intake.* Patients having ambulatory surgery can generally resume their diet immediately after surgery. Patients requiring an intraoperative IV line receive only IV fluids initially. Once a surgeon orders resumption of oral intake, first provide clear liquids such as water, apple juice, or decaffeinated tea or coffee after nausea subsides. Overloading with large amounts of fluids leads to distention and vomiting. If a patient tolerates liquids without nausea, advance the diet to full liquids, followed by a light diet of solid foods and finally a regular diet, stressing the importance of foods that are high in protein and vitamin C. Patients who have had abdominal surgery are usually NPO the first 24 hours or until the passage of flatus.
2. *Promote ambulation and exercise.* Physical activity stimulates a return of peristalsis. A patient who suffers abdominal distention and "gas pain" often obtains relief while walking.
3. *Maintain an adequate fluid intake.* Fluids keep fecal material soft for easy passage.
4. *Administer fiber supplements, stool softeners, enemas, and rectal suppositories as ordered.* Constipation or distention often develops after surgery related to side effects of anesthetic agents and pain medication and dehydration.
5. *Stimulate a patient's appetite* by removing sources of noxious odors and providing small servings of nonspicy foods.
6. *Help a patient sit* (if possible) during mealtime to minimize pressure on the abdomen.
7. *Provide frequent oral hygiene.*
8. *Provide meals when a patient is rested and free from pain.* A patient often loses interest in eating if he or she is exhausted by activities such as ambulation before mealtime.

Comfort. The anesthesiologist or nurse anesthetist orders medications for pain management in the PACU. Intravenous (IV) opioid analgesics such as morphine sulfate are the drugs of choice for the immediate postoperative period. Titrate IV morphine as ordered until pain relief is achieved. Morphine can depress level of consciousness and vital signs, but at appropriate doses this is rare. Assess a patient for the proper dose of analgesic and monitor for possible side effects. Once a patient is awake, a PCA or PCEA pump may be initiated. If a patient has an epidural catheter, use caution in giving additional analgesics (see Chapter 32).

A patient's pain increases as the effects of anesthesia wear off; this often occurs once a patient reaches the surgical nursing unit. A patient becomes more aware of surroundings and more perceptive of discomfort. The incisional area is only one source of pain. Irritation from drainage tubes, tight dressings, or casts and the muscular strains caused from positioning on the operating bed also cause discomfort. Air insufflation during laparoscopic surgery can cause significant discomfort, especially in the shoulder area.

Pain significantly slows recovery. Assess a patient's pain thoroughly. Do not assume that it is incisional in origin. When a patient requests pain medication, determine the nature and character of the pain. Patients have the most surgical pain during the first 24 to 48 hours after surgery. Provide analgesics as often as allowed. IV or epidural PCA systems allow patients to administer analgesics from specially prepared pumps (see Chapter 32). A PCA device is attached to the IV line, or the analgesic is given via an epidural catheter, as with fentanyl or morphine. A patient controls the amount of analgesia received within set doses and times ordered by the surgeon or anesthesia provider. Program the doses and frequencies of pain medication into the pump. PCA medication is delivered at a preprogrammed basal rate, a bolus dose at specified intervals as needed, or both. Continuous epidural analgesia is frequently used after surgery for thoracic and abdominal surgical procedures. Several research studies have shown continuous epidural analgesia to provide superior pain relief in terms of less analgesic use, better postoperative pain relief, and faster gastrointestinal function (McCarthy et al., 2010; Zingg et al., 2009).

Notation of respirations and level of consciousness is important for a patient receiving pain medications through a PCA pump or an epidural catheter. Documentation of frequent objective pain assessment using a pain scale, appropriate nursing interventions, and evaluation of a patient's response must be in every patient's medical record; this standard was set in January 2001 by TJC 2000 standards, and they continue today (TJC, 2013).

Promoting Wound Healing. Surgical dressings remain in place the first 24 hours after surgery to reduce the risk for infection. During this time add an extra layer of gauze on top of the original dressing if drainage develops. Mark or draw around the drainage on the dressing and date and time the marking. This provides a means to monitor increasing amounts of drainage. Notify the surgeon if bleeding is excessive. In certain types of surgery the surgeon chooses to use no dressing at all (see Chapter 37).

Closely observe the surgical wound. If a wound becomes infected, it usually occurs 3 to 6 days after surgery. Always use aseptic technique during dressing changes and wound care. Surgical drains need to remain patent so accumulated secretions are removed from the incision site. Observation of the wound identifies early signs and symptoms of infection.

To ensure continuity of care be sure that all staff are aware of the proper materials to use in a dressing change. It is common for patients to feel discomfort during an extensive dressing change; therefore offer pain medication 5 to 30 minutes before a procedure. Time the procedure to begin when the pain medication begins to work. For example, oral pain medications take about 30 minutes to begin working; therefore give oral pain medication 30 minutes before a procedure. IV pain medications given IV push usually only take 5 to 10 minutes to work. Give IV pain medication 5 to 10 minutes before a dressing change.

If you anticipate that a patient will need to continue dressing changes in the home, plan instruction when a patient is alert and comfortable and family caregivers are present. Before discharge ensure that a patient knows how to obtain the materials needed for the dressing change.

Maintaining Self-Concept. During a patient's recovery, the appearance of wounds, bulky dressings, and extruding drains and tubes threaten the self-concept. The nature of the surgery often also creates a permanent change in body image. If surgery leads to impairment in body function, a patient's role within the family and community often changes significantly. Observe a patient for alterations in self-concept (see Chapter 23). Some patients show revulsion toward their appearance by refusing to look at an incision or carefully covering dressings with bedclothes. The fear of not being able to return to a functional role in the family or to a previously held job even causes a patient to avoid participating in the care plan.

The family or significant other frequently plays an important role in efforts to improve a patient's self-concept. Help the family to accept a patient's needs and still encourage independence. The following measures maintain a patient's self-concept:

1. *Provide privacy* during dressing changes or wound inspection by closing room curtains and draping a patient so only the dressing and incisional area are exposed.
2. *Maintain a patient's hygiene.* A complete bath the first day after surgery usually makes a patient feel renewed. Offer a clean gown and washcloth if the gown becomes soiled. Keep a patient's hair neatly combed and offer frequent oral hygiene, every 2 hours while awake, especially for a patient who is NPO.
3. *Prevent drains from overflowing.* Measure drainage every 8 hours for output recording. Empty and measure them more often if drainage is excessive.

4. *Maintain a pleasant environment.* Store or remove all unused supplies and keep the bedside orderly and clean.
5. *Offer opportunities for a patient to discuss feelings about appearance.* Patients worry about permanent scarring. When a patient chooses to look at an incision for the first time, make sure that the area is clean. Eventually a patient will care for the incision site by applying simple dressings or bathing.
6. *Give the family opportunities to discuss ways to promote a patient's self-concept.* Encouraging independence is difficult for a family member who has a strong desire to help a patient in any way. By knowing about the appearance of a wound or incision, family members can be supportive during dressing changes.

Restorative and Continuing Care. Other postoperative care activities promote a patient's return to a functional state of health. Promote a patient's independence and active participation in care. When a patient is in pain or suffers from postoperative complications, motivation for self-care is sometimes low. The goals set for a patient's involvement need to be realistic. It is unrealistic to involve a patient if movement is highly restricted or if participation increases his or her discomfort.

Keep a patient and family informed of progress made toward recovery. Many patients become depressed if they think recovery is slow. Explain the length of time expected to reach a level of maximal recovery. For some patients surgery also causes permanent physical limitations that require time to accept.

Plan care daily, keeping in mind the ultimate goals for recovery. From the moment a patient enters the hospital, anticipate and plan for his or her return home. Be sure to involve any family caregivers in that plan of care. Involvement of family members in the care plan facilitates early discharge and adequate care at home. Instruct family members in care activities such as dressing changes, how to assist with ambulation, and medication management. If family members are unable to help a patient, work with the surgeon, social worker, and/or discharge planner for referrals to home care agencies to provide services at home.

EVALUATION

Patient Care. In the PACU continuously evaluate the effectiveness of interventions and a patient's response. A patient's condition can change quickly. Evaluation of a patient's status involves ongoing measurement of vital signs, pulse oximetry, wound drainage, intake and output, and other physical assessments. The modified Aldretti score evaluates a patient's level of consciousness and return of motor function. Determine frequency of assessments based on a patient's response to anesthesia. If evaluation reveals that a patient is recovering from anesthesia, the surgeon or anesthesia provider discharges a patient from the PACU.

On the surgical nursing unit evaluate the effectiveness of care on the basis of expected outcomes resulting from nursing interventions. Evaluation occurs over several days. It is important to evaluate a patient's clinical progress and readiness for discharge by observing his or her participation in postoperative exercises, self-care activities, and ambulation (Box 39-12). Evaluate the ambulatory surgical patient's outcomes by making a postoperative telephone call to the patient's home. The call, usually placed 24 hours after surgery, reassures a patient and allows for evaluation of recovery progress and the opportunity to answer any questions from a patient or family.

Patient Expectations. In the PACU some patients are not able to voice expectations. However, evaluation of pain is critical. Because pain is subjective, validate it by frequently asking a patient how he or she feels. If possible, use a pain-assessment scale. Note a patient's movement and positioning because nonverbal behaviors indicate if a patient is comfortable. If pain is not adequately relieved, change the dosage or type of medication. In addition, evaluate a patient's level of anxiety by assessing presence of any concerns or fears. Further explanation of postoperative progress and procedures reduces anxiety.

As a patient recovers, physical and psychological comfort continues to be a typical expectation of patients and families. Also evaluate if a patient feels prepared for discharge from the acute care facility. Is a patient able to explain the required care that is to be continued following discharge? Have a patient demonstrate any procedures such as wound care or medication administration. Give a patient and family numerous opportunities to ask questions about what to anticipate once a patient returns home.

BOX 39-12 EVALUATION

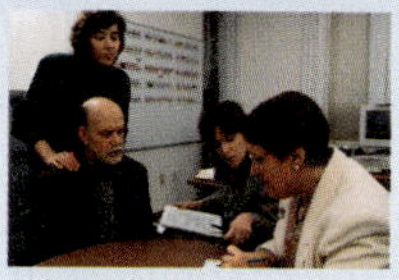

Mr. Korloff progressed well and is ready for discharge the day after surgery. He expresses relief that everything went well and that he will be able to return to work, hopefully by next week. Sue continues to care for him on the surgical patient care unit. She explains how to remove the gauze on the puncture sites and tells him to bathe and shower tomorrow. Symptoms for which Mr. Korloff and his daughters need to watch include redness, swelling, bile-colored drainage or pus from the abdominal wounds, severe abdominal pain, nausea, vomiting, and fever with a temperature greater than 37.7° C (100° F) or chills. Any of these symptoms needs to be reported to Mr. Korloff's surgeon immediately. His daughters observed the puncture sites and are able to identify symptoms of complications. Mr. Korloff is ready for discharge and plans to stay with one of his daughters over the weekend. Sue makes a follow-up surgical appointment for Mr. Korloff and gives him the surgeon's phone number in case he has any questions or concerns once he returns home.

DOCUMENTATION NOTE

"Abdominal puncture sites dry and intact, without redness. Discharge teaching provided to patient and daughters. Repeated signs and symptoms of complications; wound care instructions; activity restrictions; and follow-up appointment time, date, and place. Patient and daughters verbalize understanding of all discharge instructions."

SAFETY GUIDELINES FOR NURSING SKILLS

Ensuring patient safety is an essential role of the professional nurse. To ensure patient safety, communicate clearly with members of the health care team, assess and incorporate the patient's priorities of care and preferences, and use the best evidence when making decisions about your patient's care. When performing the skill in this chapter, follow these safety guidelines:

- Know if a patient will have any activity restrictions after surgery that prevent performance of postoperative exercises or require adaptation of skill.
- Be sure that patient uses proper body mechanics when performing exercises for turning.

SKILL 39-1 TEACHING POSTOPERATIVE EXERCISES

View Video!

DELEGATION CONSIDERATIONS

The skill of postoperative exercise teaching cannot be delegated to nursing assistive personnel (NAP). The nurse guides NAP to:

- Help patients perform postoperative exercises, reinforcing information.

EQUIPMENT

- Pillow (*optional;* used to splint surgical incision when coughing)
- Incentive spirometer (IS)
- Positive expiratory pressure device

STEP	EVOLVE
ASSESSMENT	
1. Identify patient using two identifiers (e.g., name and birthday or name and account number) according to agency policy. Compare identifiers with information on patient's medication administration record (MAR) or medical record.	Ensures correct patient. Complies with The Joint Commission requirements for patient safety (TJC, 2014).
2. Assess patient's risk for postoperative respiratory complications: Review medical history to identify presence of chronic pulmonary condition (e.g., emphysema, asthma), any condition that affects chest wall movement, history of smoking, and presence of reduced hemoglobin (low red blood cell [RBC] count).	General anesthesia contributes to respiratory problems because lungs do not fully inflate during surgery, cough reflex is suppressed, and mucus collects within airway passages. After surgery patient has reduced lung volume and requires greater effort to deep breathe and cough; inadequate lung expansion leads to atelectasis and pneumonia. Patient is at greater risk for developing respiratory complications if chronic lung conditions are present (Sifain and Papadakos, 2011). Smoking damages ciliary clearance and increases mucus secretion. A reduced hemoglobin level leads to inadequate oxygenation.
3. Auscultate lungs.	Establishes baseline for postoperative comparison.
4. Assess patient's ability to cough and deep breathe by having him or her take a deep breath and observing movement of shoulders, chest wall, and abdomen. Palpate chest excursion during a deep breath. Ask patient to cough after taking a deep breath.	Reveals maximum potential for chest expansion and ability to cough forcefully; serves as baseline to measure patient's ability to perform exercises after surgery.
5. Assess patient's risk for postoperative thrombus formation (e.g., older patients, those with active cancer, patients who are immobilized, those with personal or family history of clots, women over 35 years who smoke and are taking oral contraceptives). Observe the calves for redness, warmth, and tenderness; swollen calf or thigh; calf swelling more than 3 cm compared with asymptomatic leg; pitting edema in symptomatic leg; and collateral superficial veins. Compare legs for bilateral equality.	Determines baseline circulation status. Thrombus forms when venous stasis, hypercoagulability, and vein trauma exist simultaneously (Lewis et al., 2011). Following general anesthesia circulation slows, resulting in a greater tendency for clot formation. Immobilization results in decreased muscular contraction in lower extremities, which promotes venous stasis. The physical stress of surgery creates a hypercoagulable state in most individuals. Manipulation and positioning during surgery sometimes cause trauma to leg veins.

Clinical Decision Point: **If you suspect a thrombus, notify surgeon and refrain from manipulating extremity any further. Surgery is usually postponed. Graduated compression stockings or intermittent pneumatic compression stockings may be ordered for patients at risk for thrombus formation.**

STEP	EVOLVE
6. Assess patient's ability to move independently while in bed. Have patient turn and move all extremities.	Patients confined to bed rest, even for limited periods, need to turn regularly. Determines existence of any mobility restrictions.
7. Assess patient's willingness and capability to learn exercises; note attention span, anxiety, level of consciousness, and language level.	Ability to learn depends on readiness, ability, and learning environment.
8. Assess family members' or significant other's willingness to learn and support patient after surgery.	Encourage family member or significant other to coach patient on exercise performance.
9. Assess patient's medical orders before and after surgery.	Some patients require adaptations in method of performing exercises.
PLANNING	
1. Prepare equipment as needed.	
2. Plan teaching sessions to occur when patient is not in pain.	Decreased levels of pain enhance patient learning.
3. Plan to explain postoperative exercises to patient and any family caregiver, including importance to recovery and physiological benefits.	Information allows patient to understand significance of exercises and motivates learning. Promotes patient cooperation and decreases anxiety.
4. Prepare room for teaching.	Environment needs to be conducive to learning (see Chapter 12).
IMPLEMENTATION	
1. Demonstrate Exercises	
A. **Diaphragmatic Breathing**	
(1) Help patient to comfortable semi-Fowler's position in bed or sitting position on side of bed or in chair.	Upright position facilitates diaphragmatic excursion.
(2) Stand or sit facing patient.	Allows patient to observe breathing exercise.
(3) Instruct patient to place palms of hands across from one another, down, and along lower borders of anterior rib cage; place fingers lightly together on upper abdomen (see illustration). Demonstrate for patient.	Position of hands allows patient to feel movement of chest and abdomen as diaphragm descends and lungs expand.
(4) Instruct patient to take slow, deep breaths, inhaling through nose and pushing abdomen against hands. Tell patient to feel middle fingers separate during inhalation. Explain that patient will feel normal downward movement of diaphragm while inhaling and that abdominal organs descend and chest wall expands. Demonstrate for patient.	Slow, deep breaths prevent panting or hyperventilation. Inhaling through nose warms, humidifies, and filters air. Diaphragmatic breathing allows air to pass by, partially obstructing mucous plug, thus increasing the force to expel the mucus. Explanation and demonstration focus on normal ventilatory movement of chest wall. Patient learns how diaphragmatic breathing feels.
(5) Instruct patient to avoid using chest and shoulders while inhaling.	Using auxiliary chest and shoulder muscles during breathing wastes energy and does not promote full lung expansion.

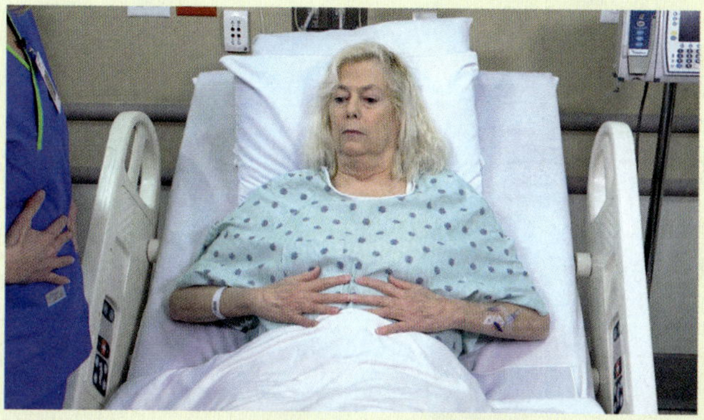

STEP 1A(3) Deep-breathing exercise: placement of hands during inhalation.

SKILL 39-1 TEACHING POSTOPERATIVE EXERCISES—cont'd

STEP	EVOLVE
(6) Instruct patient to take a slow, deep breath, hold for count of three, and slowly exhale through mouth as if blowing out a candle (through pursed lips). Demonstrate for patient. Tell patient that middle fingertips will touch as chest wall contracts during exhalation.	Pursed-lip exhalation allows for gradual expulsion of air.
(7) Repeat complete breathing exercise 3 to 5 times.	Allows patient to observe slow, rhythmical breathing pattern. Repetition reinforces learning.
(8) Have patient practice exercise. Instruct patient to take 10 slow, deep breaths every hour while awake during postoperative period.	Regular deep breathing prevents postoperative complications.
B. Incentive Spirometry (IS)	
(1) Perform hand hygiene.	Reduces transmission of microorganisms.
(2) Instruct patient to assume semi-Fowler's or high-Fowler's position.	Promotes optimal lung expansion.
(3) For patient who is obese, consider the reverse Trendelenburg's position.	Patients who are obese are often able to move their diaphragm better in this position.
(4) Indicate to patient on the IS the volume level to obtain with each inhalation. Use manufacturer guidelines to set volume for patient.	Establishes goal of volume level necessary for adequate lung expansion.
(5) Demonstrate and then have patient place mouthpiece of IS so lips completely cover mouthpiece (see illustration).	Demonstration is reliable technique for teaching psychomotor skill and enables patient to ask questions.
(6) Instruct patient to inhale slowly while maintaining constant flow through unit until he or she reaches goal volume. Once maximal inspiration is reached, have patient hold his or her breath for 2 to 3 seconds (see illustration) and exhale slowly (Davis, 2012). Make sure that the number of breaths does not exceed 10 to 12 per minute.	Maintains maximal inspiration and reduces risk for progressive collapse of individual alveoli. Slow breathing (less than 12 breaths/min) prevents or minimizes pain from sudden pressure changes in chest.
(7) Instruct patient to breathe normally for short period between each of the 10 breaths on the spirometer.	Prevents hyperventilation and fatigue.
(8) Have patient repeat maneuver until goals are achieved.	Ensures correct use of spirometer.
(9) Perform hand hygiene.	Reduces transmission of microorganisms.
C. Positive Expiratory Pressure Therapy and "Huff" Coughing	
(1) Perform hand hygiene.	Reduces transmission of microorganisms.
(2) Set positive expiratory pressure (PEP) device for setting ordered.	Higher settings require more ventilatory effort.

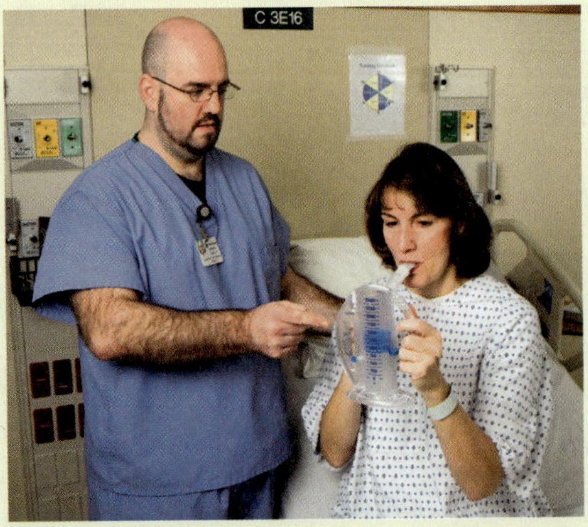

STEP 1B(5) Patient demonstrating incentive spirometry.

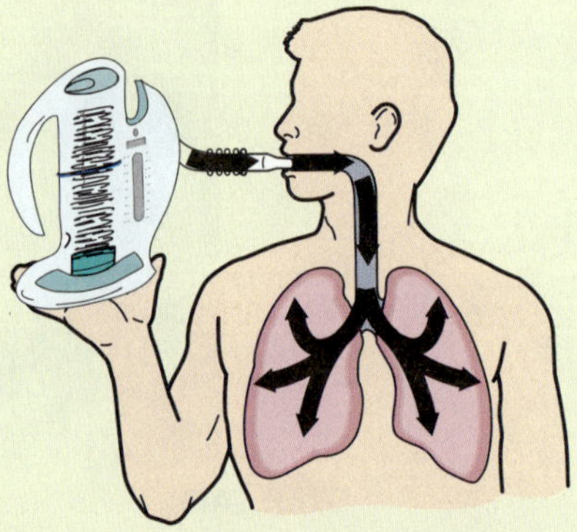

STEP 1B(6) Diagram of use of incentive spirometer.

STEP	EVOLVE
(3) Instruct patient to assume semi-Fowler's or high-Fowler's position and place nose clip on his or her nose (see illustration).	Promotes optimum lung expansion, enabling patient to expectorate mucus.
(4) Have patient place lips around mouthpiece or demonstrate placement. Instruct patient to take a full breath and exhale through device 2 or 3 times longer than inhalation. Repeat pattern for 10 to 20 breaths.	Ensures that patient does all breathing through mouth and uses device properly.
(5) Remove device from mouth and have patient take a slow, deep breath; hold for 3 seconds; cough in quick, short, forced "huffs."	Promotes lung expansion before coughing. Forced expiratory technique, promotes bronchial hygiene by increasing expectoration of secretions.
D. Controlled Coughing	
(1) Explain importance of maintaining an upright position.	Facilitates diaphragm excursion and enhances thorax expansion.
(2) If surgical incision will be either abdominal or thoracic, teach patient to place pillow or bath blanket over incisional area and place hands over pillow to splint incision. During breathing and coughing exercises, have patient press gently against incisional area for splinting or support (see illustrations).	Surgical incision cuts through muscles, tissues, and nerve endings. Deep-breathing and coughing exercises place additional stress on suture line and cause discomfort. Splinting incision with hands or pillow provides firm support and reduces incisional pulling.
(3) Demonstrate coughing. Instruct patient to take two slow, deep breaths, inhaling through nose and exhaling through mouth.	Deep breaths expand lungs fully so air moves behind mucus and facilitates effects of coughing.
(4) Instruct patient to inhale deeply a third time, hold breath to count of three, and cough fully for two or three consecutive coughs without inhaling between coughs. (Tell patient to push all air out of lungs.)	Consecutive coughs help remove mucus more effectively and completely than one forceful cough.

Clinical Decision Point: **Coughing is often contraindicated after brain, spinal, head, neck, or eye surgery because of a potential increase in intracranial or intraocular pressure.**

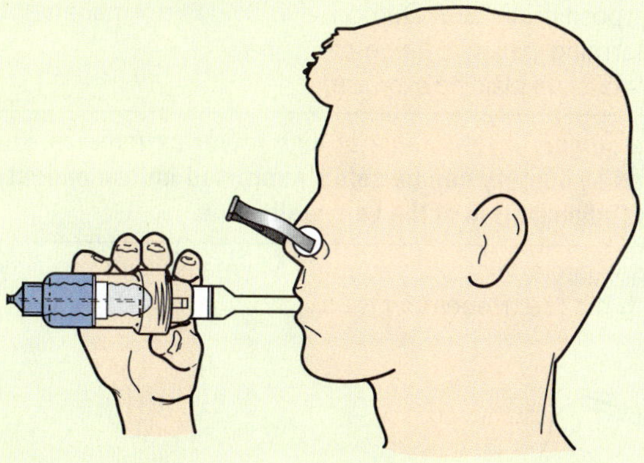

STEP 1C(3) Diagram of use of positive expiratory pressure device.

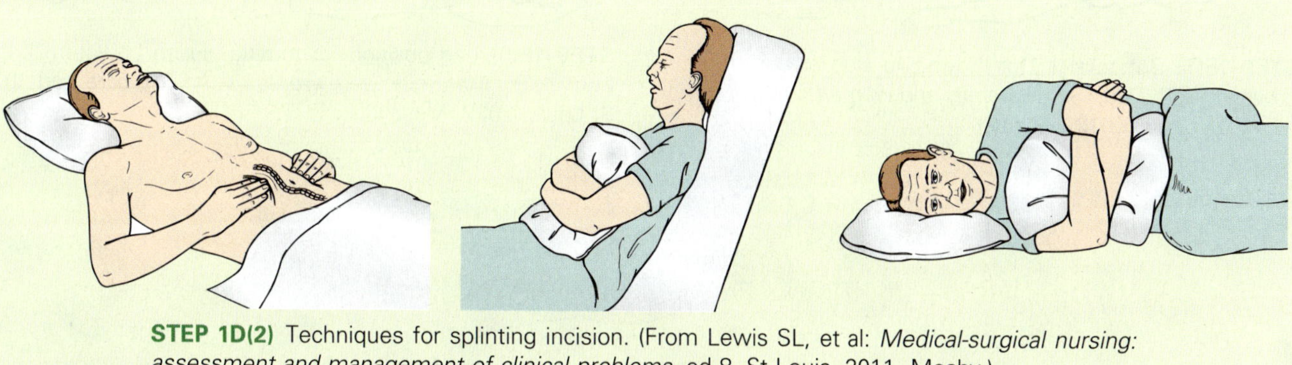

STEP 1D(2) Techniques for splinting incision. (From Lewis SL, et al: *Medical-surgical nursing: assessment and management of clinical problems*, ed 8, St Louis, 2011, Mosby.)

SKILL 39-1 TEACHING POSTOPERATIVE EXERCISES—cont'd

STEP	EVOLVE
(5) Caution patient against just clearing throat instead of coughing. Explain that coughing does not cause injury to incision.	Clearing throat does not remove mucus from deeper airways. Postoperative incisional pain makes it harder to cough effectively.
(6) Have patient continue to practice coughing exercises, splinting imaginary incision. Instruct patient to cough 2 to 3 times every 2 hours while awake.	Stresses value of deep coughing with splinting to effectively expectorate mucus with minimal discomfort.
(7) Instruct patient and family caregiver to examine sputum for consistency, odor, amount, and color changes.	Sputum characteristics indicate the presence of a pulmonary complication such as pneumonia.
E. Turning	
(1) Instruct patient to assume supine position and move to side of bed (left side in this example) by bending knees and pressing heels against mattress to raise and move buttocks (see illustration).	Positioning begins on one side of bed so turning to other side does not cause patient to roll toward edge of bed. Buttocks lift prevents shearing force from body movement against sheets.

Clinical Decision Point: **If patient has decreased strength or mobility on one side, have him or her assume position on the other side of the bed. Also use safe patient handling to turn patient.**

STEP	EVOLVE
(2) Instruct patient to place right hand over incisional area to splint it *(optional)*.	Splinting incision supports and minimizes pulling on suture line during turning.
(3) Instruct patient to keep right leg straight and flex left knee up (see illustration).	Straight leg stabilizes patient's position. Flexed left leg shifts weight for easier turning.

Clinical Decision Point: **Patients who have had back surgery, brain surgery, or vascular repair are often restricted from flexing their legs. They need to logroll or require assistance for positioning.**

STEP	EVOLVE
(4) Have patient grab right side rail with left hand, pull toward right, and roll onto right side.	Pulling toward side rail reduces effort needed for turning.
(5) Instruct patient to turn every 2 hours while awake.	Reduces risk for vascular and pulmonary complications.
F. Leg Exercises	
(1) Have patient assume supine position in bed. Demonstrate leg exercises by performing passive range-of-motion exercises and simultaneously explaining exercise.	Provides normal anatomical position of lower extremities.

Clinical Decision Point: **If patient's surgery involves one or both lower extremities, surgeon must order leg exercises in postoperative period. Leg unaffected by surgery can be safely exercised unless patient has preexisting thrombosis (blood clot formation) or thrombophlebitis (inflammation of the vein wall).**

STEP	EVOLVE
(2) Rotate each ankle in complete circle. Instruct patient to draw imaginary circles with big toe. Repeat 5 times (see illustration).	Maintains joint mobility and promotes venous return.

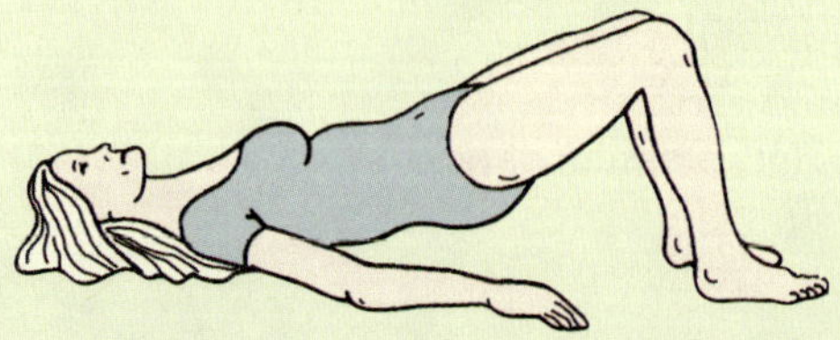

STEP 1E(1) Buttocks lift for moving to side of bed. (From Lowdermilk D, Perry SE: *Maternity and women's health care,* ed 10, St Louis, 2012, Mosby.)

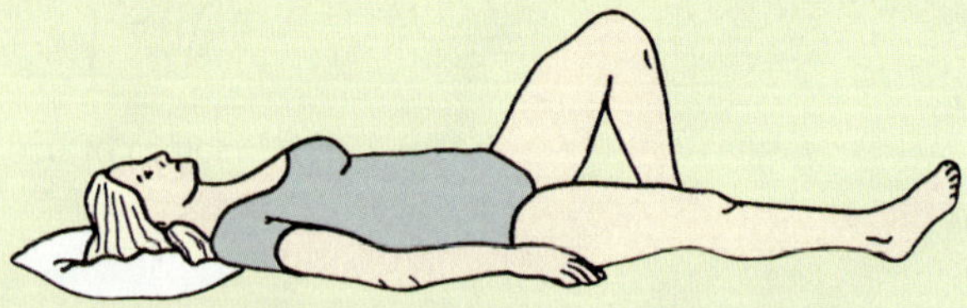

STEP 1E(3) Leg position for turning. (From Lowdermilk D, Perry SE: *Maternity and women's health care,* ed 10, St Louis, 2012, Mosby.)

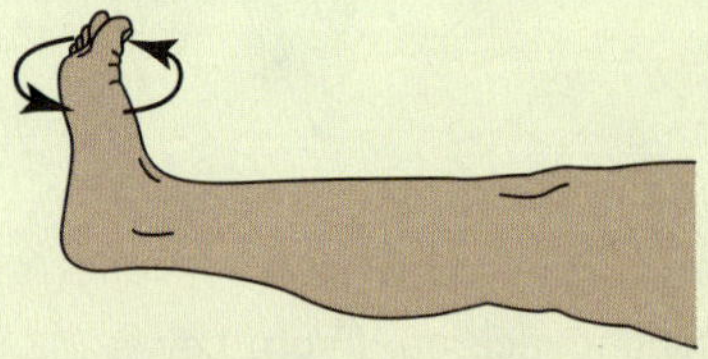

STEP 1F(2) Foot circles. (From Ignatavicius DD, Workman ML: *Medical-surgical nursing: patient-centered collaborative care,* ed 7, St Louis, 2013, Saunders.)

STEP	EVOLVE
(3) Alternate dorsiflexion and plantar flexion of both feet. Direct patient to feel calf muscles contract and relax alternately (see illustration). Repeat 5 times.	Stretches and contracts gastrocnemius muscles, improving venous return.
(4) Perform quadriceps setting by tightening thigh and bringing knee down toward mattress, then relaxing. Repeat 5 times.	Contracts muscles of upper legs, maintains knee mobility, and enhances venous return.
(5) Have patient alternately raise each leg up from bed surface, keeping legs straight, and have patient bend leg at hip and knee (see illustration). Repeat 5 times.	Contracts and relaxes quadriceps muscles and prevents venous pooling. Bending leg reduces strain on back.
2. Have patient continue to practice exercises at least every 2 hours while awake. Instruct patient to coordinate turning and leg exercises with diaphragmatic breathing, incentive spirometry, and coughing exercises.	Repetition of exercise sequence reinforces learning. Establishes routine for exercises that develops habit for performance. Sequence of exercises is leg exercises, turning, breathing, and coughing.
EVALUATION	
1. Observe patient performing all four exercises independently.	Provides opportunity for practice and return demonstration of exercises. Ensures that patient has learned correct technique.
2. Observe family members or significant others' ability to coach patient.	Family members or significant others can assist positively or interfere with correct technique.
3. Observe patient's chest excursion.	Determines extent of lung expansion.
4. Auscultate patient's lungs.	Reveals presence of abnormal lung sounds.
5. Palpate calves gently for redness, warmth, and tenderness. Assess pedal pulses.	Absent signs and normal pulses usually indicate that no venous thrombosis is present.
6. Use Teach Back—State to patient, "I want to be sure that you understand why I want you to sit upright and deep breathe and cough every hour and move your extremities." Revise your instruction now or develop plan for revised patient teaching to be implemented at an appropriate time if patient is not able to teach back correctly.	Evaluates what the patient is able to explain or demonstrate.

RECORDING AND REPORTING

- Record which exercises you have demonstrated to patient and if patient performs exercises independently or needs continued assistance.
- Evaluate learning. Report any problems patient has in practicing exercises to nurse assigned to patient on next shift for follow-up.
- Document your evaluation of patient learning.

UNEXPECTED OUTCOMES AND RELATED INTERVENTIONS

- Patient is unable to perform exercises correctly before surgery.
  - Assess for the presence of anxiety, pain, and fatigue.
  - Teach patient stress-reduction techniques and/or pain-management strategies.
  - Repeat teaching using more demonstration or redemonstration at time when family member is present.
- Patient is unwilling to perform exercises after surgery because of incisional pain of thorax or abdomen (deep breathing, coughing, and turning) or because of surgery in

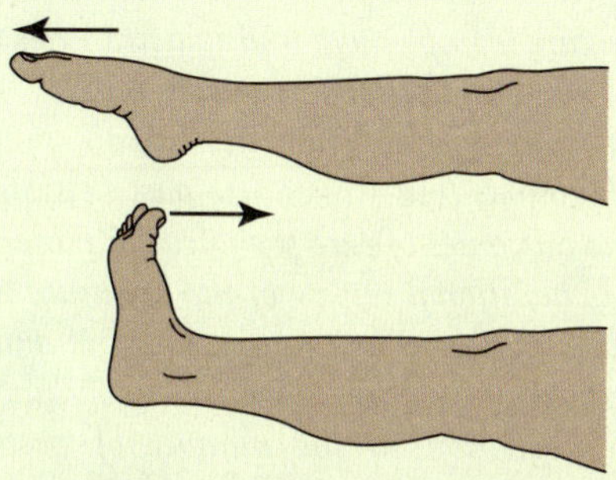

STEP 1F(3) Alternate dorsiflexion and plantar flexion. (From Ignatavicius DD, Workman ML: *Medical-surgical nursing: patient-centered collaborative care,* ed 7, St Louis, 2013, Saunders.)

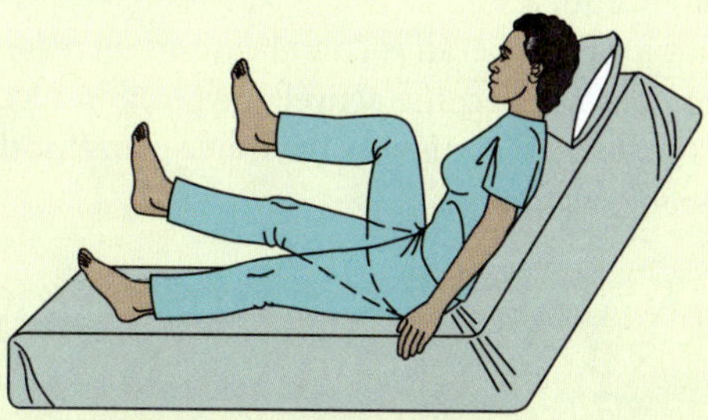

STEP 1F(5) Hip and knee movements. (From Ignatavicius DD, Workman ML: *Medical-surgical nursing: patient-centered collaborative care,* ed 7, St Louis, 2013, Saunders.)

SKILL 39-1 TEACHING POSTOPERATIVE EXERCISES—cont'd

lower abdomen, groin, buttocks, or legs (leg exercises, turning) (Valkenet et al., 2011).
  - Instruct patient to ask for pain medication 30 minutes before performing postoperative exercises or to use patient-controlled analgesia (PCA) a few minutes before exercising.
  - Report to surgeon inadequate pain relief and need to change analgesic or increase dose.
- Patient develops pulmonary complications after surgery.
  - Assess breath sounds in all lobes and compare bilaterally.
  - Place patient in upright position.
  - Notify surgeon of findings.
  - Be prepared to start oxygen or intravenous (IV) antibiotics as ordered.
- Patient develops circulatory complications such as venous stasis or thrombophlebitis after surgery.
  - Notify health care provider of findings.
  - Place patient on bed rest with affected leg elevated.
  - Continue to have patient do exercises with unaffected leg.

KEY POINTS

- Previous illnesses and past surgeries affect a patient's ability to tolerate surgery.
- Older-adult patients are at greater surgical risk because of the physiological changes associated with aging.
- All medications taken before surgery are automatically discontinued after surgery unless a health care provider reorders the drugs.
- Family members and significant others are important in assisting patients with physical limitations and providing emotional support after surgery.
- Preoperative assessment of vital signs and physical findings provides a baseline with which to compare postoperative assessment data.
- Primary responsibility for informed consent rests with the surgeon.
- Structured preoperative teaching positively influences postoperative recovery.
- In ambulatory surgery nurses use the limited time available to assess, prepare, and educate patients for surgery.
- Nurses within the OR focus on protecting a patient from potential harm.
- Postoperative assessment centers on the body systems most likely to be affected by surgery.
- Because a surgical patient's condition may change rapidly during recovery, monitor a patient's status at least every 15 minutes until stable.
- Postoperative nursing interventions focus on prevention of complications.
- The risk for postoperative complications increases when a patient does not become actively involved in recovery.
- From the time of admission, the nurse plans for the surgical patient's discharge.

CLINICAL DECISION-MAKING EXERCISES

A perioperative nurse will care for Mr. Korloff throughout the three surgical phases. Recall that he is having laparoscopic gallbladder surgery (cholecystectomy). This procedure will create four small puncture wounds in his right upper quadrant for the gallbladder to be removed.

1. Preoperative assessment includes consideration of cultural and spiritual factors that influence patients' health care outcomes. Which implications for practice should you consider for Mr. Korloff?
2. On arrival to the postanesthesia care unit (PACU), Mr. Korloff has an oral airway in place. You suction the mucus accumulating in his mouth and airway. His respirations are even at a rate of 12 per minute. Which interventions do you perform, given your knowledge of the immediate needs of a postoperative patient?
3. Six hours after he has returned from surgery, you notice that one of Mr. Korloff's dressings has a 3-cm area of serosanguineous drainage on it. Which nursing interventions should you perform at this time?

evolve
Answers to Clinical Decision-Making Exercises can be found on the Evolve website.

QSEN ACTIVITY: QUALITY IMPROVEMENT

Sue is working on a surgical unit that is implementing a quality improvement (QI) project focused on prevention of postsurgical site infections. Sue's review of the literature reinforces the importance for all health care team members involved in a patient's postoperative care to implement multiple strategies to reduce the risk for surgical site infections (Lipke et al., 2010). She recognizes that she, along with other health care professionals of varying backgrounds and values, are part of system processes that affect the outcomes of care provided for patients and their families. Sue's additional review of the literature regarding QI projects reveals that consistent communication and implementation of the plan of care are imperative to obtain the expected outcome of prevention in the number of postsurgical site infections.

What is the best method(s) for Sue to communicate her findings and strategies for prevention of postsurgical site infections to all health care providers and family participating in Mr. Korloff's care? How does Sue identify gaps between local and best practice?

Which measures could Sue use to evaluate if change has taken place?

evolve

Answers to QSEN Activities can be found on the Evolve website.

REVIEW QUESTIONS

1. When preparing a 6-month-old patient for surgery, which surgical risks should the nurse consider?
    1. Congestive heart failure
    2. Prolonged wound healing
    3. High risk for hypothermia or hyperthermia
    4. Gastrointestinal interferences
2. When developing a list of home care instructions for a patient who had abdominal surgery, which of the following would be the least important for a nurse to include in his discharge plan of care?
    1. Deep-breathing exercises
    2. Wound care
    3. Activity restrictions
    4. Follow-up care
3. The nurse should be aware of the following surgical risk associated with a patient who has diabetes mellitus:
    1. Respiratory depression
    2. Altered metabolism and drug excretion
    3. Fluid and electrolyte imbalance
    4. Slow wound healing
4. Which of the following preoperative medications is prescribed to decrease pulmonary and oral secretions?
    1. Anticholinergic
    2. Narcotic analgesic
    3. Histamine receptor antihistaminic
    4. Neuroleptic analgesic
5. The following patient preparation is recommended immediately before surgery:
    1. Administer enemas until clear.
    2. Ensure that a patient is well nourished and hydrated.
    3. Shave the incisional area with a straight razor.
    4. Allow no food or drink for 8 to 12 hours before surgery.
6. What is the most common postanesthesia emergency in the postanesthesia care unit (PACU)?
    1. Cardiac distress
    2. Dehydration
    3. Wound infection
    4. Airway obstruction
7. Which action should be taken after surgery to prevent the formation of vascular thrombus?
    1. A patient should not be turned until pain subsides.
    2. A patient should be instructed to cough regularly every hour.
    3. A patient should be instructed to perform leg exercises.
    4. A patient should eat a liquid diet.
8. Which of the following should a nurse include in the preoperative teaching of a patient in the use of an incentive spirometer?
    1. A patient should be in a semi- or high-Fowler's position.
    2. A patient should hold his or her breath for 15 seconds after maximum inspiration.
    3. A patient should keep a loose seal between the lips and mouthpiece.
    4. A patient should inhale as rapidly as possible.
9. Which of the following are significant abnormal findings associated with presurgical screening tests? (Select all that apply.)
    1. Increased hemoglobin, indicating infection
    2. Elevated blood urea nitrogen or creatinine, indicating risk for cardiac problems
    3. Decreased hematocrit and hemoglobin levels, indicating bleeding or anemia
    4. Elevated white blood count, indicating an infection
    5. Abnormal urinalysis, indicating infection or fluid imbalances
10. Arrange the following instructions for teaching a patient effective coughing exercises in the order in which they should be performed.
    1. Instruct a patient to cough fully for three short breaths.
    2. Instruct a patient to repeat the exercise every 2 hours while awake.
    3. Help a patient to a semi-Fowler's position with a pillow or bath blanket to splint the incision.
    4. Instruct a patient to cough deeply once or twice and take another deep breath.
    5. Instruct a patient to take a quick breath with mouth open.
    6. Instruct a patient to inhale and exhale deeply and slowly 3 times through the nose.
    7. Instruct a patient to take a deep breath and hold it for 3 seconds.

evolve

Rationales for Review Questions can be found on the Evolve website.

1. 3; **2.** 1; **3.** 4; **4.** 1; **5.** 2; **6.** 4; **7.** 3; **8.** 1; **9.** 3, 4, 5; **10.** 3, 6, 7, 1, 5, 4, 2

REFERENCES

American Society of Anesthesiologists (ASA) Committee on Standards and Practice Parameters: Practice guidelines for preoperative fasting and the use of pharmacologic agents to reduce the risk of pulmonary aspiration: application to healthy patients undergoing elective procedures, *Anesthesiology* 114(3):495, 2011.

American Society of Anesthesiologists (ASA) Committee on Standards and Practice Parameters: Practice guidelines for acute pain management in the perioperative setting: an updated report by the American Society of Anesthesiologists Task Force on Acute Pain Management, *Anesthesiology* 116(2):248, 2012.

Association of periOperative Registered Nurses (AORN): *Perioperative standards and recommended practices*, Denver, 2012, The Association.

Black JM, Hawks JH: *Medical-surgical nursing: clinical management for positive outcomes*, ed 8, St Louis, 2009, Saunders.

Bulfone G, et al: A longitudinal study of the incidence of pressure sores and the associated risks and strategies adopted in Italian operating theatres, *J Perioperative Pract* 22(2):50, 2012.

Cvetic E: Communication in the perioperative setting, *AORN J* 94(3):261, 2011.

Davis S: Incentive spirometry after abdominal surgery, *Nurs Times* 108(26):22, 2012.

Frisch A, et al: Prevalence and clinical outcome of hyperglycemia in the perioperative period in noncardiac surgery, *Diabetes Care* 33(8):1783, 2010.

Fullwood D, Sargent S: An overview of sedation for adult patients in hospital, *Nurs Stand* 24(39):48, 2010.

Giger JN: *Transcultural nursing: assessment and intervention*, ed 6, St Louis, 2013, Mosby.

Grawe JS, et al: Impact of preoperative patient education on postoperative pain in consideration of the individual coping style, *Der Schmerz* 24(6):575, 2010.

Gregson H: Reducing surgical site infection following caesarean section, *Art Sci* 24(50):35, 2011.

Haufler K, Harrington M: Using nurse-to-patient telephone calls to reduce day-of-surgery cancellations, *AORN J* 94(1):19, 2011.

Jarvis C: *Physical examination and health assessment*, ed 6, St Louis, 2012, Saunders.

Johns CD, et al: Malignant hyperthermia: a crisis response plan, *OR Manager* 28(6):18, 2012.

Kastanias P, et al: What do adult surgical patients really want to know about pain and pain management? *Pain Manage Nurs* 10(1):22, 2009.

Kearney M, et al: Effects of preoperative education on patient outcomes after joint replacement surgery, *Orthop Nurs* 30(6):391, 2011.

Kiernan M: Reducing the risk of surgical site infection, *Nurs Times* 108(27):12, 2012.

Lehne RA: *Pharmacology for nursing care*, ed 8, St Louis, 2013, Saunders.

Lewis S, et al: *Medical-surgical nursing: assessment and management of clinical problems*, ed 8, St Louis, 2011, Mosby.

Lipke VL, et al: Reducing surgical site infections by bundling multiple risk reduction strategies and active surveillance, *AORN J* 92(3):288, 2010.

Makki D, et al: The efficacy of patient information sheets in wrist arthroscopy: a randomized controlled trial, *J Orthop Surg* 19(1):85, 2011.

Massey RL: Return of bowel sounds indicating an end of postoperative ileus: is it time to cease this long-standing nursing tradition? *Medsurg Nurs* 21(3):146, 2012.

McCarthy GC, et al: Impact of intravenous lidocaine infusion on postoperative analgesia and recovery from surgery, *Drugs* 70(9):1149, 2010.

Nelson JM, Carrington JM: Transitioning the older adult in the ambulatory care setting, *AORN J* 94(4):348, 2011.

Nugent KM, Phy M, Raj R: Obstructive sleep apnea and post-operative complications: single center data, review of literature and guidelines for practicing internists and surgeons, *Surg Sci* 3(2):65, 2012.

Phillips B: Postoperative complications in patients with obstructive sleep apnea, *Hosp Med Alert* 7(3):17, 2012.

Phillips N: *Berry and Kohn's operating room technique*, ed 12, St Louis, 2013, Mosby.

Poveda VB, Martinez EZ, Galvão CM, Active cutaneous warming systems to prevent intraoperative hypothermia: a systematic review, *Rev Lat Am Enfermagem* 20(1):183, 2012.

Roesler R, et al: Chasing zero: Our journey to preventing surgical site infections, *AORN J* 91(2):224, 2010.

Rothrock J: *Alexander's care of a patient in surgery*, ed 14, St Louis, 2011, Mosby.

Rutan L, Sommers K: Hyperglycemia as a risk factor in the perioperative patient, *AORN J* 95(3):352, 2012.

Sifain A, Papadakos PJ: Pump lung: the conundrum of cardiopulmonary bypass, *Can J Respir Ther* 47(3):29, 2011.

Starkweather A: Improving patient-centered medical-surgical nursing practice with quality-of-life assessment, *Medsurg Nurs* 19(4):224, 2010.

The Joint Commission (TJC): *2013 Hospital accreditation standards*, Oakbrook Terrace, IL, 2013, The Joint Commission.

The Joint Commission (TJC): *National Patient Safety Goals*, Oakbrook Terrace, IL, 2014, The Commission. Available at http://www.jointcommission.org/standards_information/npsgs.aspx.

Valkenet K, et al: The effects of preoperative exercise therapy on postoperative outcome: a systematic review, *Clin Rehabil* 25:99, 2011.

Wu C, et al: Efficacy of postoperative patient-controlled and continuous infusion epidural analgesia versus intravenous patient-controlled analgesia with opioids: a meta-analysis, *Anesthesiology* 103(5):1079, 2005.

Zingg U, et al: Influence of thoracic epidural analgesia on postoperative pain relief and ileus after laparoscopic colorectal resection, *Surg Endosc* 23:276, 2009.

A

abduction Movement of a limb away from the body.

abrasion Scraping or rubbing away of epidermis; may result in localized bleeding and later weeping of serous fluid.

absorption Passage of drug molecules into the blood. Factors influencing drug absorption include route of administration, ability of the drug to dissolve, and conditions at the site of absorption.

acceptance Fifth stage of Kübler-Ross's stages of grief and dying. An individual comes to terms with a loss rather than submitting to resignation and hopelessness.

accessory muscles Muscles in the thoracic cage that assist with respiration.

accommodation Process of responding to the environment through new activity and thinking and changing the existing schema or developing a new schema to deal with the new information. For example, a toddler whose parent consistently corrected him when he called a horse a "doggie" accommodates and forms a new schema for horses.

accountability State of being answerable for one's actions—a nurse answers to himself or herself, the patient, the profession, the employing institution such as a hospital, and society for the effectiveness of nursing care performed.

accreditation Process whereby a professional association or nongovernmental agency grants recognition to a school or institution for demonstrated ability to meet predetermined criteria.

acculturation The process of adapting to and adopting a new culture.

acne Inflammatory, papulopustular skin eruption, usually occurring on the face, neck, shoulders, and upper back.

acromegaly Chronic metabolic condition caused by overproduction of growth hormone and characterized by gradual, marked enlargement and elongation of bones of the face, jaw, and extremities.

active error Errors that occur at the point of contact between a human and some aspect of a larger system (e.g., a human-machine interface).

active listening Listening attentively with the whole person—mind, body, and spirit. It includes listening for main and supportive ideas, acknowledging and responding, giving appropriate feedback, and paying attention to the other person's total communication, including the content, the intent, and the feelings expressed.

active range-of-motion (ROM) exercise Completion of exercise to the joint by the patient while doing activities of daily living or during joint assessment.

active strategies of health promotion Activities that depend on the patient's being motivated to adopt a specific health program.

active transport Movement of materials across the cell membrane by means of chemical activity that allows the cell to admit larger molecules than would otherwise be possible.

activities of daily living (ADLs) Activities usually performed in the course of a normal day in the patient's life, such as eating, dressing, bathing, brushing the teeth, or grooming.

activity tolerance Kind or amount of exercise or work a person is able to perform.

actual loss Loss of an object, person, body part or function, or emotion that is overt and easily identifiable.

actual nursing diagnosis A judgment that is clinically validated by the presence of major defining characteristics.

acuity recording Mechanism by which entries describing patient care activities are made over a 24-hour period. The activities are then translated into a rating score, or acuity score, that allows for a comparison of patients who vary by severity of illness.

acute care Pattern of health care in which a patient is treated for an acute episode of illness, for the sequelae of an accident or other trauma, or during recovery from surgery.

acute illness Illness characterized by symptoms that are of relatively short duration, are usually severe, and affect the functioning of the patient in all dimensions.

adduction Movement of a limb toward the body.

adolescence The period in development between the onset of puberty and adulthood. It usually begins between 11 and 13 years of age.

adult day care centers Facility for the supervised care of older adults, providing activities such as meals and socialization during specified day hours.

advanced sleep phase syndrome Common in older adults, a disturbance in sleep manifested as early waking in the morning with an inability to get back to sleep. It is thought that this syndrome is caused by advancing of the body's circadian rhythm.

adventitious sounds Abnormal lung sounds heard with auscultation.

adverse effect Harmful or unintended effect of a medication, diagnostic test, or therapeutic intervention.

adverse reaction Any harmful, unintended effect of a medication, diagnostic test, or therapeutic intervention.

advocacy Process whereby a nurse objectively provides patients with the information they need to make decisions and supports the patients in whatever decisions they make.

afebrile Without fever.

affective learning Acquisition of behaviors involved in expressing feelings in attitudes, appreciation, and values.

afterload Resistance to left ventricular ejection; the work the heart must overcome to fully eject blood from the left ventricle.

age-related macular degeneration Progressive disorder in which the macula (the specialized portion of the retina responsible for central vision) degenerates as a result of aging and loses its ability to function efficiently. First signs include blurring of reading matter, distortion or loss of central vision, sensitivity to glare, and distortion of objects.

agnostic Individual who believes that any ultimate reality is unknown or unknowable.

Airborne Precautions Safeguards designed to reduce the risk of transmission of infectious agents through the air a person breathes.

alarm reaction Mobilization of the defense mechanisms of the body and mind to cope with a stressor. The initial stage of the general adaptation syndrome.

aldosterone Mineralocorticoid steroid hormone produced by the adrenal cortex with action in the renal tubule to regulate sodium and potassium balance in the blood.

allergic reactions Unfavorable physiological response to an allergen to which a person has previously been exposed and to which the person has developed antibodies.

alopecia Partial or complete loss of hair; baldness.

Alzheimer's disease Disease of the brain parenchyma that causes a gradual and progressive decline in cognitive functioning.

AMBULARM Device used for the patient who climbs out of bed unassisted and is in danger of falling. This device is worn on the leg and signals when the leg is in a dependent position such as over the side rail or on the floor.

amino acid Organic compound of one or more basic groups and one or more carboxyl groups. Amino acids are the building blocks that construct proteins and the end products of protein digestion.

anabolism Constructive metabolism characterized by conversion of simple substances into more complex compounds of living matter.

analgesic Relieving pain; drug that relieves pain.

analogies Resemblances made between things otherwise unlike.

anaphylactic reactions Hypersensitive condition induced by contact with certain antigens.

aneurysm Localized dilations of the wall of a blood vessel, usually caused by atherosclerosis, hypertension, or a congenital weakness in a vessel wall.

anger Second stage of Kübler-Ross's stages of grief and dying. During this stage an individual resists loss by expressing extreme displeasure, indignation, or hostility.

angiotensin Polypeptide occurring in the blood, causing vasoconstriction, increased blood pressure, and the release of aldosterone from the adrenal cortex.

anion gap Difference between the concentrations of serum cations and anions, determined by measuring the concentrations of sodium cations and chloride and bicarbonate anions.

anions Negatively charged electrolytes.

anthropometric measurements Body measures of height, weight, and skinfolds to evaluate muscle atrophy.

anthropometry Measurement of various body parts to determine nutritional and caloric status, muscular development, brain growth, and other parameters.

antibodies Immunoglobulins, essential to the immune system, that are produced by lymphoid tissue in response to bacteria, viruses, or other antigens.

anticipatory grief Grief response in which the person begins the grieving process before an actual loss.

antidiuretic hormone (ADH) Hormone that decreases the production of urine by increasing the reabsorption of water by the renal tubules. ADH is secreted by cells of the hypothalamus and stored in the posterior lobe of the pituitary gland.

antiembolic stockings Elasticized stockings that prevent formation of emboli and thrombi, especially after surgery or during bed rest.

antigen Substance, usually a protein, that causes the formation of an antibody and reacts specifically with that antibody.

antipyretic Substance or procedure that reduces fever.

anxiolytics Drugs used primarily to treat episodes of anxiety.

aphasia Abnormal neurological condition in which language function is defective or absent; related to injury to speech center in cerebral cortex, causing receptive or expressive aphasia.

apical pulse Heartbeat as listened to with the bell or diaphragm of a stethoscope placed on the apex of the heart.

apnea Cessation of airflow through the nose and mouth.

apothecary system System of measurement. The basic unit of weight is a grain. Weights derived from the grain are the gram, ounce, and pound. The basic measure for fluid is the minim. The fluidram, fluid ounce, pint, quart, and gallon are measures derived from the minim.

approximate To come close together, as in the edges of a wound.

arcus senilis Opaque ring, gray to white in color, that surrounds the periphery of the cornea. The condition is caused by deposits of fat granules in the cornea. Occurs primarily in older adults.

asepsis Absence of germs or microorganisms.

aseptic technique Any health care procedure in which added precautions are used to prevent contamination of a person, object, or area by microorganisms.

assault Unlawful threat to bring about harmful or offensive contact with another.

assertive communication Type of communication based on a philosophy of protecting individual rights and responsibilities. It includes the ability to be self-directive in acting to accomplish goals and advocate for others.

assessment First step of the nursing process; activities required in the first step are data collection, data validation, data sorting, and data documentation. The purpose is to gather information for health problem identification.

assimilation To become absorbed into another culture and to adopt its characteristics.

assisted living Residential living facilities in which each resident has his or her own room and shares dining and social activity areas.

associative play Form of play in which a group of children participates in similar or identical activities without formal organization, direction, interaction, or goals.

atelectasis Collapse of alveoli, preventing the normal respiratory exchange of oxygen and carbon dioxide.

atheist Individual who does not believe in the existence of God.

atherosclerosis Common arterial disorder characterized by yellowish plaques of cholesterol, lipids, and cellular debris in the inner layers of the walls of the large- and medium-size arteries.

atrioventricular (AV) node A portion of the cardiac conduction system located on the floor of the right atrium; it receives electrical impulses from the atrium and transmits them to the bundle of His.

atrophied Wasted or reduced size or physiological activity of a part of the body caused by disease or other influences.

attachment Initial psychosocial relationship that develops between parents and the neonate.

attentional set Internal state of the learner that allows focusing and comprehension.

auditory Related to, or experienced through, hearing.

auscultation Method of physical examination; listening to the sounds produced by the body, usually with a stethoscope.

auscultatory gap Disappearance of sound when obtaining a blood pressure; typically occurs between the first and second Korotkoff sounds.

authority The right to act in areas in which an individual has been given and accepts responsibility.

autologous transfusion Procedure in which blood is removed from a donor and stored for a variable period before it is returned to the donor's own circulation.

autonomy Ability or tendency to function independently.

B

back-channeling Active listening technique that prompts a respondent to continue telling a story or describing a situation. Involves use of phrases such as "Go on," "Uh huh," and "Tell me more."

bacteriuria Presence of bacteria in the urine.

balance Position when the person's center of gravity is correctly positioned so that falling does not occur.

bandages Available in rolls of various widths and materials including gauze, elasticized knit, elastic webbing, flannel, and muslin. Gauze bandages are lightweight and inexpensive, mold easily around contours of the body, and permit air circulation to underlying skin to prevent maceration. Elastic bandages conform well to body parts but can also be used to exert pressure over a body part.

bargaining Third stage of Kübler-Ross's stages of grief and dying. A person postpones the reality of a loss by attempting to make deals in a subtle or overt manner with others or with a higher being.

baridi A condition among the Bena people of Tanzania, this illness is attributed to disrespectful behavior within the family or transgression of cultural taboos. The person experiences physical and psychological symptoms and is usually treated by a traditional healer, who has the person make a public admission or an apology or who treats the person with herbal remedies.

basal cell carcinoma Malignant epithelial cell tumor that begins as a papule and enlarges peripherally, developing a central crater that erodes, crusts, and bleeds. Metastasis is rare.

basal metabolic rate (BMR) Amount of energy used in a unit of time by a fasting, resting subject to maintain vital functions.

battery Legal term for touching of another's body without consent.

bed boards Boards placed under the mattress of a bed that provide extra support to the mattress surface.

bed rest Placement of the patient in bed for therapeutic reasons for a prescribed period.

benchmarking Identifying best practices and comparing them to the organization's current practices for the purpose of improving performance. This process helps to support the institution's claims of quality care delivery.

beneficence Doing good or active promotion of doing good. One of the four principles of the ethical theory of deontology.

benign breast disease (fibrocystic) A benign condition characterized by lumpy, painful breasts and sometimes nipple discharge. Symptoms are more apparent before the menstrual period. Known to be a risk factor for breast cancer.

bereavement Response to loss through death; a subjective experience that a person suffers after losing a person with whom there has been a significant relationship.

biases and prejudices Beliefs and attitudes associating negative permanent characteristics to people who are perceived as different from oneself.

bilineally Kinship that extends to both the mother's and father's sides of the family.

binders Bandages made of large pieces of material to fit specific body parts.

bioethics Branch of ethics within the field of health care.

biological clock Cyclical nature of body functions; functions controlled from within the body are synchronized with environmental factors; same meaning as biorhythm.

biotransformation The chemical changes that a substance undergoes in the body, such as by the action of enzymes.

blanchable hyperemia Redness of the skin due to dilation of the superficial capillaries. When pressure is applied to the skin, the area blanches, or turns a lighter color.

body image Persons' subjective concept of their physical appearance.

body mechanics Coordinated efforts of the musculoskeletal and nervous systems to maintain proper balance, posture, and body alignment.

bone resorption Destruction of bone cells and release of calcium into the blood.

borborygmi Audible abdominal sounds produced by hyperactive intestinal peristalsis.

botanica Place that sells religious and herbal remedies.

bradycardia Slower-than-normal heart rate; heart contracts fewer than 60 times per minute.

bradypnea Abnormally slow rate of breathing.

bronchospasm An excessive and prolonged contraction of the smooth muscle of the bronchi and bronchioles resulting in an acute narrowing and obstruction of the respiratory airway.

bruit Abnormal sound or murmur heard while auscultating an organ, gland, or artery.

buccal Of or pertaining to the inside of the cheek or the gum next to the cheek.

buccal cavity Consists of the lips surrounding the opening of the mouth, the cheeks running along the side walls of the cavity, the tongue and its muscles, and the hard and soft palate.

buffer Substance or group of substances that can absorb or release hydrogen ions to correct an acid-base imbalance.

bundle of His A portion of the cardiac conduction system that arises from the distal portion of the atrioventricular (AV) node and extends across the AV groove to the top of the intraventricular septum, where it divides into right and left bundle branches.

C

cachexia Malnutrition marked by weakness and emaciation, usually associated with severe illness.

capitation Payment mechanism in which a provider (e.g., health care network) receives a fixed amount of payment per enrollee.

carbohydrates Dietary classification of foods comprising sugars, starches, cellulose, and gum.

carbon monoxide Colorless, odorless, poisonous gas produced by the combustion of carbon or organic fuels.

cardiac index The adequacy of the cardiac output for an individual. It takes into account the body surface area (BSA) of the patient.

cardiac output (CO) Volume of blood expelled by the ventricles of the heart, equal to the amount of blood ejected at each beat, multiplied by the number of beats in the period of time used for computation (usually 1 minute).

cardiopulmonary rehabilitation Actively assisting the patient with achieving and maintaining an optimal level of health through controlled physical exercise, nutrition counseling, relaxation and stress management techniques, prescribed medications and oxygen, and compliance.

cardiopulmonary resuscitation (CPR) Basic emergency procedures for life support consisting of artificial respiration and manual external cardiac massage.

care To feel concern or interest in one who has sorrow or difficulties.

caring Universal phenomenon that influences the way we think, feel, and behave in relation to one another.

carriers Persons or animals who harbor and spread an organism that causes disease in others but do not become ill.

case management Organized system for delivering health care to an individual patient or group of patients across an episode of illness and/or a continuum of care; includes assessment and development of a plan of care, coordination of all services, referral, and follow-up; usually assigned to one professional.

case management plan A multidisciplinary model for documenting patient care that usually includes plans for problems, key interventions, and expected outcomes for patients with a specific disease or condition.

catabolism Breakdown of body tissue into simpler substances.

cataplexy Condition characterized by sudden muscular weakness and loss of muscle tone.

cataracts An abnormal progressive condition of the lens of the eye characterized by loss of transparency.

cathartics Drugs that act to promote bowel evacuation.

catheterization Introduction of a catheter into a body cavity or organ to inject or remove fluid.

cations Positively charged electrolytes.

center of gravity Midpoint or center of the weight of a body or object.

centigrade Denotes temperature scale in which 0° is the freezing point of water and 100° is the boiling point of water at sea level; also called Celsius.

cerumen Yellowish or brownish waxy secretion produced by sweat glands in the external ear.

chancres Skin lesions or venereal sores (usually primary syphilis) that begin at the site of infection as papules and develop into red, bloodless, painless ulcers with a scooped-out appearance.

change-of-shift report Report that occurs between two scheduled nursing work shifts. Nurses communicate information about their assigned patients to nurses working on the next shift of duty.

channel Method used in the teaching-learning process to present content: visual, auditory, taste, smell. In the communication process, a method used to transmit a message: visual, auditory, touch.

charting by exception (CBE) Charting methodology in which data are entered only when there is an exception from what is normal or expected. Reduces time spent documenting in charting. It is a shorthand method for documenting normal findings and routine care.

chemical restraints Medications, such as anxiolytics and sedatives, that are used to manage a patient's behavior and are not a standard treatment for a patient's condition.

chest percussion Striking of the chest wall with a cupped hand to promote mobilization and drainage of pulmonary secretions.

chest physiotherapy (CPT) Group of therapies used to mobilize pulmonary secretions for expectoration.

chest tube A catheter inserted through the thorax into the chest cavity for removing air or fluid, used after chest or heart surgery or pneumothorax.

chronic illness Illness that persists over a long time and affects physical, emotional, intellectual, social, and spiritual functioning.

circadian rhythm Repetition of certain physiological phenomena within a 24-hour cycle.

circulating nurse Assistant to the scrub nurse and surgeon whose role is to provide necessary supplies, dispose of soiled instruments and supplies, and keep an accurate count of instruments, needles, and sponges used.

civil law Statutes concerned with protecting a person's rights.

climacteric Physiological, developmental change that occurs in the male reproductive system between the ages of 45 and 60.

clinical criteria Objective or subjective signs and symptoms, clusters of signs and symptoms, or risk factors.

clinical decision making A problem-solving approach that nurses use to define patient problems and select appropriate treatment.

clinical decision support system (CDSS) Computerized programs used within a health care setting to guide interventions.

closed-ended question A form of question that limits a respondent's answer to one or two words.

clubbing Bulging of the tissues at the nail base that is caused by insufficient oxygenation at the periphery, resulting from conditions such as chronic emphysema and congenital heart disease.

code of ethics Formal statement that delineates a profession's guidelines for ethical behavior; a code of ethics sets standards or expectations for the professional to achieve.

cognitive learning Acquisition of intellectual skills that encompass behaviors such as thinking, understanding, and evaluating.

collaborative interventions Therapies that require the knowledge, skill, and expertise of multiple health care professionals.

collaborative problem Physiological complication that require the nurse to use nursing-prescribed and physician-prescribed interventions to maximize patient outcomes.

colloid osmotic pressure Abnormal condition of the kidney caused by the pressure of concentrations of large particles, such as protein molecules, that will pass through a membrane.

colon Portion of the large intestine from the cecum to the rectum.

colonization The presence and multiplication of microorganisms without tissue invasion or damage.

comforting Acts toward another individual that display both an emotional and physical calm. The use of touch, establishing presence, the therapeutic use of silence, and the skillful and gentle performance of a procedure are examples of comforting nursing measures.

common law One source for law that is created by judicial decisions as opposed to those created by legislative bodies (statutory law).

communicable disease Any disease that can be transmitted from one person or animal to another by direct or indirect contact or by vectors.

communication Ongoing, dynamic series of events that involves the transmission of meaning from sender to receiver.

community health nursing A nursing approach that combines knowledge from the public health sciences with professional nursing theories to safeguard and improve the health of populations in the community.

community-based nursing The acute and chronic care of individuals and families to strengthen their capacity for self-care and promote independence in decision making.

compassion fatigue A condition that is a combination of secondary traumatic stress and burnout. A health care provider experiences the trauma of caring for those who are suffering and perceives the demands of caregiving exceeding the resources available.

competence Specific range of skills necessary to perform a task.

complete bed bath Bath in which the entire body of a patient is washed in bed.

compress Soft pad of gauze or cloth used to apply heat, cold, or medications to the surface of a body part.

computer-based patient record Comprehensive computerized system used by all health care practitioners to permanently store information pertaining to a patient's health status, clinical problems, and functional abilities.

concentration Relative content of a component within a substance or solution.

concentration gradient Gradient that exists across a membrane separating a high concentration of a particular ion from a low concentration of the same ion.

concept map A care-planning tool that assists in critical thinking and forming associations between a patient's nursing diagnoses and interventions.

confianza Trust.

confidentiality The act of keeping information private or secret; in health care, the nurse only shares information about a patient with other nurses or health care providers who need to know private information about a patient in order to provide care for the patient; information can only be shared with the patient's consent.

conjunctivitis Highly contagious eye infection. The crusty drainage that collects on eyelid margins can easily spread from one eye to the other.

connectedness Having close spiritual relationships with oneself, others, and God or another spiritual being.

connotative meaning The shade or interpretation of a word's meaning influenced by the thoughts, feelings, or ideas people have about the word.

conscious sedation Administration of central nervous system depressant drugs and/or analgesics to provide analgesia, relieve anxiety, and/or provide amnesia during surgical, diagnostic, or interventional procedures.

constipation Condition characterized by difficulty in passing stool or an infrequent passage of hard stool.

consultation Process in which the help of a specialist is sought to identify ways to handle problems in patient management or in the planning and implementing of programs.

Contact Precautions Safeguards designed to reduce the risk of transmission of epidemiologically important microorganisms by direct or indirect contact.

continent urinary diversion Surgical diversion of the drainage of urine from a diseased or dysfunctional bladder. Patient uses a catheter to drain the pouch.

convalescence Period of recovery after an illness, injury, or surgery.

coping Making an effort to manage psychological stress.

core temperature Temperature of deep structures of the body.

cough Sudden, audible expulsion of air from the lungs. The person breathes in, the glottis is partially closed, and the accessory muscles of expiration contract to expel the air forcibly.

counseling A problem-solving method used to help patients recognize and manage stress and to enhance interpersonal relationships; it helps patients examine alternatives and decide which choices are most helpful and appropriate.

crackles Fine bubbling sounds heard on auscultation of the lung; produced by air entering distal airways and alveoli, which contain serous secretions.

crime Act that violates a law and that may include criminal intent.

criminal law Concerned with acts that threaten society but may involve only an individual.

crisis Transition for better or worse in the course of a disease, usually indicated by a marked change in the intensity of signs and symptoms.

crisis intervention Use of therapeutic techniques directed toward helping a patient resolve a particular and immediate problem.

critical pathways Tools used in managed care that incorporate the treatment interventions of caregivers from all disciplines who normally care for a patient. Designed for a specific care type, a pathway is used to manage the care of a patient throughout a projected length of stay.

critical period of development A specific phase or period when the presence of a function or reasoning has its greatest effect on a specific aspect of development.

critical thinking The active, purposeful, organized, cognitive process used to carefully examine one's thinking and the thinking of other individuals.

crutch gait A gait achieved by a person using crutches.

cue Information that a nurse acquires through hearing, visual observations, touch, and smell.

cultural and linguistic competence A set of congruent behaviors, attitudes, and policies that come together in a system, agency, or among professionals that enables effective work in cross-cultural situations.

cultural assessment A systematic and comprehensive examination of the cultural care values, beliefs, and practices of individuals, families, and communities.

cultural awareness Gaining in-depth awareness of one's own background, stereotypes, biases, prejudices, and assumptions about other people.

cultural care accommodation or negotiation Adapting or negotiating with the patient/families to achieve beneficial or satisfying health outcomes.

cultural care preservation or maintenance Retaining and/or preserving relevant care values so that patients are able to maintain their well-being, recover from illness, or face handicaps and/or death.

cultural care repatterning or restructuring Reordering, changing, or greatly modifying a patient's/family's customs for new, different, and beneficial health care pattern.

cultural competence Process in which the health care professional continually strives to achieve the ability and availability to work effectively with individuals, families, and communities.

cultural encounters Engaging in cross-cultural interactions; refining intercultural communication skills; gaining in-depth understanding of others and avoiding stereotypes; and cultural conflict management.

cultural imposition Using one's own values and customs as an absolute guide in interpreting behaviors.

cultural knowledge Obtaining knowledge of other cultures; gaining sensitivity to, respect for, and appreciation of differences.

cultural pain The feeling a patient has after a health care worker disregards the patient's valued way of life.

cultural skills Communication, cultural assessment, and culturally competent care.

culturally congruent care Care that fits the people's valued life patterns and sets of meanings generated from the people themselves. Sometimes this differs from the professionals' perspective on care.

culturally ignorant or blind Uneducated about other cultures.

culture Integrated patterns of human behavior that include the language, thoughts, communications, actions, customs, beliefs, values, and institutions of racial, ethnic, religious, or social groups.

culture-bound syndromes Illnesses restricted to a particular culture or group because of its psychosocial characteristics.

culture care theory Leininger's theory that emphasizes culturally congruent care.

culturological nursing assessment A systematic and comprehensive examination of the cultural care values, beliefs, and practices of individuals, families, and communities.

cutaneous stimulation Stimulation of a person's skin to prevent or reduce pain perception. A massage, warm bath, hot and cold therapies, and transcutaneous electrical nerve stimulation are some ways to reduce pain perception.

cyanosis Bluish discoloration of the skin and mucous membranes caused by an excess of deoxygenated hemoglobin in the blood or a structural defect in the hemoglobin molecule.

D

DAR (data, action, patient response) The format used in focus charting for recording patient information.

data analysis Logical examination of and professional judgment about patient assessment data; used in the diagnostic process to derive a nursing diagnosis.

data cluster A set of signs or symptoms that are grouped together in logical order.

database Store or bank of information, especially in a form that can be processed by computer.

debridement Removal of dead tissue from a wound.

decentralized management An organizational philosophy that brings decisions down to the level of the staff. Individuals best informed about a problem or issue participate in the decision-making process.

decision making Process involving critical appraisal of information that results from recognition of a problem and ends with the generation, testing, and evaluation of a conclusion. Comes at the end of critical thinking.

defecation Passage of feces from the digestive tract through the rectum.

defendant Individual or organization against whom legal charges are brought in a court of law.

defining characteristics Related signs and symptoms or clusters of data that support the nursing diagnosis.

dehiscence Separation of a wound's edges, revealing underlying tissues.

dehydration Excessive loss of water from the body tissues, accompanied by a disturbance of body electrolytes.

delegation Process of assigning another member of the health care team to be responsible for aspects of patient care; for example, assigning nurse assistants to bathe a patient.

delirium An acute confusional state, which is potentially reversible and is often due to a physical cause.

dementia A generalized impairment of intellectual functioning that interferes with social and occupational functioning.

denial Unconscious refusal to admit an unacceptable idea.

denotative meaning Meaning of a word shared by individuals who use a common language. The word "baseball" has the same meaning for all individuals who speak English, but the word "code" denotes cardiac arrest primarily to health care providers.

dental caries Abnormal destructive condition in a tooth caused by a complex interaction of food, especially starches and sugars, with bacteria that form dental plaque.

denture stomatitis Inflammation of oral mucosa in contact with a denture surface.

deontology Traditional theory of ethics that proposes to define actions as right or wrong based on the characteristics of fidelity to promises, truthfulness, and justice. The conventional use of ethical terms such as *justice, autonomy, beneficence,* and *nonmaleficence* constitutes the practice of deontology.

depression (1) A reduction in happiness and well-being that contributes to physical and social limitations and complicates the treatment of concomitant medical conditions. It is usually reversible with treatment. (2) Fourth stage of Kübler-Ross's stages of grief and dying. In this stage the person realizes the full impact and significance of the loss.

dermis Sensitive vascular layer of the skin directly below the epidermis composed of collagenous and elastic fibrous connective tissues that give the dermis strength and elasticity.

determinants of health The many variables that influence the health status of individuals or communities.

detoxify To remove the toxic quality of a substance; the liver acts to detoxify chemicals in drug compounds.

development Qualitative or observable aspects of the progressive changes one makes in adapting to the environment.

developmental crises Crises associated with normal and expected phases of growth and development, for example, the response to menopause; same as maturational crises.

diabetic retinopathy A disorder of retinal blood vessels. Pathological changes secondary to increased pressure in the blood vessels of the retina result in decreased vision or vision loss due to hemorrhage and macular edema.

diagnosis-related group (DRG) Group of patients classified to establish a mechanism for health care reimbursement based on length of stay; classification is based on the following variables: primary and secondary diagnosis, comorbidities, primary and secondary procedures, and age.

diagnostic process Mental steps (data clustering and analysis, problem identification) that follow assessment and lead directly to the formulation of a diagnosis.

diagnostic reasoning Process that enables an observer to assign meaning and to classify phenomena in clinical situations by integrating observations and critical thinking.

diaphoresis Secretion of sweat, especially profuse secretion associated with an elevated body temperature, physical exertion, or emotional stress.

diaphragmatic breathing Respiration in which the abdomen moves out while the diaphragm descends on inspiration.

diarrhea Increase in the number of stools and the passage of liquid, unformed feces.

diastolic Pertaining to diastole, or the blood pressure at the instant of maximum cardiac relaxation.

dietary reference intake (DRI) Information on each vitamin or mineral to reflect a range of minimum to maximum amounts that avert deficiency or toxicity.

diffusion Movement of molecules from an area of high concentration to an area of lower concentration.

digestion Breakdown of nutrients by chewing, churning, mixing with fluid, and chemical reactions.

direct care interventions Treatments performed through interaction with the patient. For example, a patient may require medication administration, insertion of an intravenous infusion, or counseling during a time of grief.

discharge planning Activities directed toward identifying future proposed therapy and the need for additional resources before and after returning home.

discrimination Prejudicial outlook, action, or treatment.

disease Malfunctioning or maladaptation of biological or psychological processes.

disinfection Process of destroying all pathogenic organisms, except spores.

disorganization and despair One of Bowlby's four phases of mourning in which an individual endlessly examines how and why the loss occurred.

distress Damaging stress; one of the two types of stress identified by Selye.

disuse osteoporosis Reductions in skeletal mass routinely accompanying immobility or paralysis.

diuresis Increased rate of formation and excretion of urine.

documentation Written entry into the patient's medical record of all pertinent information about the patient. These entries validate the patient's problems and care and exist as a legal record.

dominant culture The customs, values, beliefs, traditions, and social and religious views held by a group of people that prevail over another secondary culture.

dorsiflexion Flexion toward the back.

drainage evacuators Convenient portable units that connect to tubular drains lying within a wound bed and exert a safe, constant, low-pressure vacuum to remove and collect drainage.

Droplet Precautions Safeguards designed to reduce the risk of droplet transmission of infectious agents.

dysmenorrhea Painful menstruation.

dysphagia Difficulty in swallowing, commonly associated with obstructive or motor disorders of the esophagus.

dyspnea Sensation of shortness of breath.

dysrhythmia Deviation from the normal pattern of the heartbeat.

dysuria Painful urination resulting from bacterial infection of the bladder and obstructive conditions of the urethra.

E

ecchymosis Discoloration of the skin or bruise caused by leakage of blood into subcutaneous tissues as a result of trauma to underlying tissues.

ectropion Eversion of the eyelid, exposing the conjunctival membrane and part of the eyeball.

edema Abnormal accumulation of fluid in interstitial spaces of tissues.

edentulous Without teeth.

egocentric Developmental characteristic wherein a toddler is only able to assume the view of his or her own activities and needs.

electrocardiogram (ECG) Graphic record of the electrical activity of the myocardium.

electrolyte Element or compound that, when melted or dissolved in water or other solvent, dissociates into ions and can carry an electrical current.

electronic infusion device A piece of medical equipment that delivers intravenous fluids at a prescribed rate through an intravenous catheter.

embolism Abnormal condition in which a blood clot (embolus) travels through the bloodstream and becomes lodged in a blood vessel.

emic worldview An insider or native perspective.

empathy Understanding and acceptance of a person's feelings and the ability to sense the person's private world.

endogenous infections Infections produced within a cell or organism.

endorphins Hormones that act on the mind like morphine and opiates, producing a sense of well-being and reducing pain.

enema Procedure involving introduction of a solution into the rectum for cleansing or therapeutic purposes.

enteral nutrition (EN) Provision of nutrients through the gastrointestinal tract when the patient cannot ingest, chew, or swallow food but can digest and absorb nutrients.

entropion Condition in which the eyelid turns inward toward the eye.

environment All of the many factors, such as physical and psychological, that influence or affect the life and survival of a person.

epidermis Outer layer of the skin that has several thin layers of skin in different stages of maturation; shields and protects the underlying tissues from water loss, mechanical or chemical injury, and penetration by disease-causing microorganisms.

epidural infusion Type of nerve block anesthesia in which an anesthetic is intermittently or continuously injected into the lumbosacral region of the spinal cord.

erythema Redness or inflammation of the skin or mucous membranes that is a result of dilation and congestion of superficial capillaries; sunburn is an example.

eschar A thick layer of dead, dry tissue that covers a pressure ulcer or thermal burn; it may be allowed to be sloughed off naturally or it may need to be surgically removed.

ethical dilemma Dilemma existing when the right thing to do is not clear. Resolution requires the negotiation of differing values among those involved in the dilemma.

ethical principles Set of guidelines for a profession's expectations and standards of behavior for its members.

ethics Principles or standards that govern proper conduct.

ethics of care Delivery of health care based on ethical principles and standards of care.

ethnicity A shared identity related to social and cultural heritage such as values, language, geographical space, and racial characteristics.

ethnocentrism A tendency to hold one's own way of life as superior to others.

ethnohistory Significant historical experiences of a particular group.

etic worldview An outsider's perspective.

etiology Study of all factors that may be involved in the development of a disease.

eupnea Normal respirations that are quiet, effortless, and rhythmical.

eustress Stress that protects health; one of the two types of stress identified by Selye.

evaluation Determination of the extent to which established patient goals have been achieved.

evidence-based knowledge Knowledge that is derived from the integration of best research, clinical expertise, and patient values.

evidence-based practice The use of current best evidence from nursing research, clinical expertise, practice trends, and patient preferences to guide nursing decisions about care provided to patients.

evisceration Protrusion of visceral organs through a surgical wound.

exacerbations Increases in the seriousness of a disease or disorder as marked by greater intensity in signs or symptoms.

excessive daytime sleepiness Extreme fatigue felt during the day. Signs of this include falling asleep at inappropriate times, such as while eating, talking, or driving. May indicate a sleep disorder.

excoriation Injury to the skin's surface caused by abrasion.

exhaustion stage Phase that occurs when the body can no longer resist the stress; when the energy necessary to maintain adaptation is depleted.

exogenous infection Infection originating outside an organ or part.

exostosis An abnormal benign growth on the surface of a bone.

expected outcomes Expected conditions of a patient at the end of therapy or of a disease process, including the degree of wellness and the need for continuing care, medications, support, counseling, or education.

extended care facility An institution devoted to providing medical, nursing, or custodial care for an individual over a prolonged period, such as during the course of a chronic disease or during the rehabilitation phase after an acute illness.

extension Movement by certain joints that increases the angle between two adjoining bones.

extracellular fluid (ECF) Portion of body fluids composed of the interstitial fluid and blood plasma.

exudate Fluid, cells, or other substances that have been slowly discharged from cells or blood vessels through small pores or breaks in cell membranes.

F

face-saving A way of speaking or acting that preserves dignity.

Fahrenheit Denotes temperature scale in which 32° is the freezing point of water and 212° is the boiling point of water at sea level.

faith Set of beliefs and a way of relating to self, others, and a supreme being.

fajita Cotton binder used on a newborn's abdomen among Hispanics and Filipinos to prevent gas and umbilical hernia.

family Group of interacting individuals composing a basic unit of society.

family as context Nursing perspective in which the family is viewed as a unit of interacting members having attributes, functions, and goals separate from those of the individual family members.

family diversity The unique needs and characteristics of each member in a family.

family durability A system of support for a family that includes immediate and extended family members.

family forms Patterns of people considered by family members to be included in the family.

family functioning Processes families use to achieve their goals.

family hardiness Internal strengths and durability of the family unit; characterized by a sense of control over the outcome of life events and hardships, a view of change as beneficial and growth-producing, and an active rather than passive orientation in responding to stressful life events.

family health Determined by the effectiveness of the family's structure, the processes that the family uses to meet its goals, and internal and external forces.

family as patient A nursing approach that takes into consideration the effect of one intervention on all members of a family.
family resiliency A family's ability to cope with expected and unexpected stressors.
family structure Based on organization (i.e., ongoing membership) of the family and the pattern of relationships.
farmacia Place to obtain prescribed medications.
febrile Pertaining to or characterized by an elevated body temperature.
fecal impaction Accumulation of hardened fecal material in the rectum or sigmoid colon.
fecal incontinence Inability to control passage of feces and gas from the anus.
fecal occult blood test (FOBT) Measures microscopic amounts of blood in the feces.
feces Waste or excrement from the gastrointestinal tract.
feedback Process in which the output of a given system is returned to the system.
felony Crime of a serious nature that carries a penalty of imprisonment or death.
feminist ethics Ethical approach that focuses on relationships of those involved in an ethical dilemma rather than traditional abstract principles of deontology.
fever Elevation in the hypothalamic set point, so that body temperature is regulated at a higher level.
fictive Nonblood kin; considered family in some collective cultures.
fidelity The agreement to keep a promise.
fight-or-flight response The total physiological response to stress that occurs during the alarm reaction stage of the general adaptation syndrome. Massive changes in all body systems prepare a human being to choose to flee or to remain and fight the stressor.
filtration The straining of fluid through a membrane.
fistula Abnormal passage from an internal organ to the body surface or between two internal organs.
flashback A recollection so strong that the individual thinks he or she is actually experiencing the trauma again or seeing it unfold before his or her eyes.
flatus Intestinal gas.
flora Microorganisms that live on or within a body to compete with disease-producing microorganisms and provide a natural immunity against certain infections.
flow sheets Documents on which frequent observations or specific measurements are recorded.
fluid volume deficit (FVD) A fluid and electrolyte disorder caused by failure of the body's homeostatic mechanisms to regulate the retention and excretion of body fluids. The condition is characterized by decreased output of urine, high specific gravity of urine, output of urine that is greater than the intake of fluid in the body, hemoconcentration, and increased serum levels of sodium.
fluid volume excess (FVE) A fluid and electrolyte disorder characterized by an increase in fluid retention and edema, resulting from failure of the body's homeostatic mechanisms to regulate the retention and excretion of body fluids.
focus charting A charting methodology for structuring progress notes according to the focus of the note, for example, symptoms and nursing diagnosis. Each note includes data, actions, and patient response.
focused cultural assessment Method of evaluating a patient's ethnohistory, biocultural history, social organization, and religious and spiritual beliefs to find issues that are most relevant to the problem at hand.
food poisoning Toxic processes resulting from the ingestion of a food contaminated by toxic substances or by bacteria-containing toxins.
foot boots Soft, foot-shaped devices designed to reduce the risk of footdrop by maintaining the foot in dorsiflexion.
footdrop An abnormal neuromuscular condition of the lower leg and foot, characterized by an inability to dorsiflex, or evert, the foot.
friction Effects of rubbing or the resistance that a moving body meets from the surface on which it moves; a force that occurs in a direction to oppose movement.
functional health illiteracy The inability of an individual to obtain, interpret, and understand basic information about health.
functional health patterns Method for organizing assessment data based on the level of patient function in specific areas, for example, mobility.
functional nursing Method of patient care delivery in which each staff member is assigned a task that is completed for all patients on the unit.
future orientation Time dimension emphasized by dominant American culture. It is characterized by direct communication and is focused on task achievement, whereas past orientation communication is circular and indirect and is focused on group harmony.

G

gait Manner or style of walking, including rhythm, cadence, and speed.
gastrostomy feeding tube The insertion of a feeding tube, through a stoma, into the stomach for the purpose of providing enteral nutrition.
general adaptation syndrome (GAS) Generalized defense response of the body to stress, consisting of three stages: alarm, resistance, and exhaustion.
general anesthesia Intravenous or inhaled medications that cause the patient to lose all sensation and consciousness.
geriatrics Branch of health care dealing with the physiology and psychology of aging and with the diagnosis and treatment of diseases affecting older adults.
gerontology The study of all aspects of the aging process and its consequences.
gingivae Gums of the mouth; a mucous membrane with supporting fibrous tissue that overlies the crowns of unerupted teeth and encircles the necks of those teeth that have erupted.
glaucoma An abnormal condition of elevated pressure within an eye caused by obstruction of the outflow of aqueous humor. Often results in peripheral visual loss, decreased visual acuity with difficulty adapting to darkness, and a halo effect around lights, if untreated.
globalization Worldwide scope or application.
glomerulus Cluster or collection of capillary vessels within the kidney involved in the initial formation of urine.
gluconeogenesis Formation of glucose or glycogen from substances that are not carbohydrates, such as protein or lipid.
glucose The primary fuel for the body, needed to carry out major physiological functions.
glycogen Polysaccharide that is the major carbohydrate stored in animal cells.
glycogenesis The process for storage of glucose in the form of glycogen in the liver.
goals Desired results of nursing actions, set realistically by the nurse and patient as part of the planning stage of the nursing process.
Good Samaritan laws Legislation enacted in some states to protect health care professionals from liability in rendering emergency aid, unless there is proven willful wrong or gross negligence.
graduated measuring container Receptacle for volume measurement.
granny midwives Amateur health practitioners that assist in labor and delivery.
granulation tissue Soft, pink, fleshy projections of tissue that form during the healing process in a wound not healing by primary intention.
graphic record Charting mechanism that allows for the recording of vital signs and weight in such a manner that caregivers can quickly note changes in the patient's status.
grief Form of sorrow involving the person's thoughts, feelings, and behaviors, occurring as a response to an actual or perceived loss.
grieving process Sequence of affective, cognitive, and physiological states through which the person responds to and finally accepts an irretrievable loss.
grounded Connection between the electric circuit and the ground, which becomes part of the circuit.
growth Measurable or quantitative aspect of an individual's increase in physical dimensions as a result of an increase in number of cells. Indicators of growth include changes in height, weight, and sexual characteristics.
guided imagery Method of pain control in which the patient creates a mental image, concentrates on that image, and gradually becomes less aware of pain.
gustatory Pertaining to the sense of taste.

H

halal Foods permissible for Muslims to eat.
hand rolls Rolls of cloth that keep the thumb slightly adducted and in opposition to the fingers.

hand-wrist splints Splints individually molded for the patient to maintain proper alignment of the thumb, slight adduction of the wrist, and slight dorsiflexion.

haram Foods prohibited by Muslim religious standards.

health Dynamic state in which individuals adapt to their internal and external environments so that there is a state of physical, emotional, intellectual, social, and spiritual well-being.

health belief model Conceptual framework that describes a person's health behavior as an expression of the person's health beliefs.

health beliefs Patient's personal beliefs about levels of wellness, which can motivate or impede participation in changing risk factors, participating in care, and selecting care options.

health care–acquired infection An infection that was not present or incubating at the time of admission to a health care setting.

health care problems Any conditions or dysfunctions that the patient experiences as a result of illness or treatment of an illness.

health promotion Activities such as routine exercise and good nutrition that help patients maintain or enhance their present levels of health and reduce their risk of developing certain diseases.

health promotion model Defines health as a positive, dynamic state, not merely the absence of disease. The health promotion model emphasizes well-being, personal fulfillment, and self-actualization rather than reacting to the threat of illness.

health status Description of health of an individual or community.

heat exhaustion Abnormal condition caused by depletion of body fluid and electrolytes resulting from exposure to intense heat or the inability to acclimatize to heat.

heat stroke Continued exposure to extreme heat raising the core body temperature to 40.5° C (105° F) or higher.

hematemesis Vomiting of blood, indicating upper gastrointestinal bleeding.

hematoma Collection of blood trapped in the tissues of the skin or an organ.

hematuria Abnormal presence of blood in the urine.

hemolysis Breakdown of red blood cells and release of hemoglobin that may occur after administration of hypotonic intravenous solutions, causing swelling and rupture of erythrocytes.

hemoptysis Coughing up blood from the respiratory tract.

hemorrhoids Permanent dilation and engorgement of veins within the lining of the rectum.

hemostasis Termination of bleeding by mechanical or chemical means or by the coagulation process of the body.

hemothorax Accumulation of blood and fluid in the pleural cavity between the parietal and visceral pleurae.

hernia Protrusion of an organ through an abnormal opening in the muscle wall of the cavity that surrounds it.

hilots Amateur health practitioners that assist in labor and delivery among Filipinos.

holistic Of or pertaining to the whole; considering all factors.

holistic health Comprehensive view of the person as a biopsychosocial and spiritual being.

home care Health service provided in the patient's place of residence for the purpose of promoting, maintaining, or restoring health or minimizing the effects of illness and disability.

homeostasis State of relative constancy in the internal environment of the body, maintained naturally by physiological adaptive mechanisms.

hope Confident, yet uncertain, expectation of achieving a future goal.

hospice System of family-centered care designed to help terminally ill persons be comfortable and maintain a satisfactory lifestyle throughout the terminal phase of their illness.

Hoyer lift A mechanical device that uses a canvas sling to easily lift dependent patients for transfer.

humidification Process of adding water to gas.

humor Coping strategy based on an individual's cognitive appraisal of a stimulus that results in behavior such as smiling, laughing, or feelings of amusement that lessen emotional distress.

hydrocephalus Abnormal accumulation of cerebrospinal fluid in the ventricles of the brain.

hydrostatic pressure Pressure caused by a liquid.

hypercalcemia Greater-than-normal amount of calcium in the blood.

hypercapnia Greater-than-normal amounts of carbon dioxide in the blood; also called hypercarbia.

hyperextension Position of maximal extension of a joint.

hyperglycemia Elevated serum glucose levels.

hypertension Disorder characterized by an elevated blood pressure persistently exceeding 120/80 mm Hg.

hyperthermia Situation in which body temperature exceeds the set point.

hypertonic Situation in which one solution has a greater concentration of solute than another solution; therefore the first solution exerts greater osmotic pressure.

hypertonicity Excessive tension of the arterial walls or muscles.

hyperventilation Respiratory rate in excess of that required to maintain normal carbon dioxide levels in the body tissues.

hypnotics Class of drug that causes insensibility to pain and induces sleep.

hypostatic pneumonia Pneumonia that results from fluid accumulation as a result of inactivity.

hypotension Abnormal lowering of blood pressure that is inadequate for normal perfusion and oxygenation of tissues.

hypothermia Abnormal lowering of body temperature below 35° C, or 95° F, usually caused by prolonged exposure to cold.

hypotonic Situation in which one solution has a smaller concentration of solute than another solution; therefore the first solution exerts less osmotic pressure.

hypotonicity Reduced tension of the arterial walls or muscles.

hypoventilation Respiratory rate insufficient to prevent carbon dioxide retention.

hypovolemia Abnormally low circulating blood volume.

hypoxemia Arterial blood oxygen level less than 60 mm Hg; low oxygen level in the blood.

hypoxia Inadequate cellular oxygenation that may result from a deficiency in the delivery or use of oxygen at the cellular level.

I

identity Component of self-concept characterized by one's persisting consciousness of being oneself, separate and distinct from others.

idiosyncratic reaction Individual sensitivity to effects of a drug caused by inherited or other bodily constitution factors.

illness (1) Abnormal process in which any aspect of a person's functioning is diminished or impaired compared with that person's previous condition. (2) The personal, interpersonal, and cultural reaction to disease.

illness behavior Ways in which people monitor their bodies, define and interpret their symptoms, take remedial actions, and use the health care system.

illness prevention Health education programs or activities directed toward protecting patients from threats or potential threats to health and toward minimizing risk factors.

imam Muslim priest.

immobility Inability to move about freely, caused by any condition in which movement is impaired or therapeutically restricted.

immunity The quality of being insusceptible to or unaffected by a particular disease or condition.

immunization A process by which resistance to an infectious disease is induced or augmented.

implementation Initiation and completion of the nursing actions necessary to help the patient achieve health care goals.

impression management The ability to interpret the others' behavior within their own context of meanings and behave in a culturally congruent way to achieve desired outcomes of communication.

incentive spirometry Method of encouraging voluntary deep breathing by providing visual feedback to patients of the inspiratory volume they have achieved.

incident rates The rate of new cases of a disease in a specified population over a defined period of time.

incident report Confidential document that describes any patient accident while the person is on the premises of a health care agency. (See occurrence report.)

independent practice association (IPA) Managed care organization that contracts with physicians or health care providers who usually are members of groups and whose practices include fee-for-service and capitated patients.

indirect care interventions Treatments performed away from the patient but on behalf of the patient or group of patients.

induration Hardening of a tissue, particularly the skin, because of edema or inflammation.

infection The invasion of the body by pathogenic microorganisms that reproduce and multiply.

inference (1) A judgment or interpretation of informational cues. (2) Taking one proposition as a given and guessing that another proposition follows.

infiltration Dislodging an intravenous catheter or needle from a vein into the subcutaneous space.

inflammation Protective response of body tissues to irritation or injury.

informed consent Process of obtaining permission from a patient to perform a specific test or procedure, after describing all risks, side effects, and benefits.

infusion pump Device that delivers a measured amount of fluid over a period of time.

infusions Introduction of fluid into the vein, giving intravenous fluid over time.

inhalation Method of medication delivery through the patient's respiratory tract. The respiratory tract provides a large surface area for drug absorption. Inhalation can be through the nasal or oral route.

injections Parenteral administration of medication; four major sites of injection: subcutaneous, intramuscular, intravenous, and intradermal.

insensible water loss Water loss that is continuous and is not perceived by the person.

insomnia Condition characterized by chronic inability to sleep or remain asleep through the night.

inspection Method of physical examination by which the patient is visually systematically examined for appearance, structure, function, and behavior.

instillation To cause to enter drop by drop, or very slowly.

institutional ethics committee An interdisciplinary committee that discusses and processes ethical dilemmas that arise within a health care institution.

instrumental activities of daily living (IADLs) Activities that are necessary to be independent in society beyond eating, grooming, transferring, and toileting and include such skills as shopping, preparing meals, banking, and taking medications.

integrated delivery network (IDN) Set of providers and services organized to deliver a coordinated continuum of care to the population of patients served at a capitated cost.

interpersonal communication Exchange of information between two persons or among persons in a small group.

interstitial fluid Fluid that fills the spaces between most of the cells of the body and provides a substantial portion of the liquid environment of the body.

interview Organized, systematic conversation with the patient designed to obtain pertinent health-related subjective information.

intracellular fluid Liquid within the cell membrane.

intradermal (ID) Injection given between layers of the skin, into the dermis. Injections are given at a 5- to 15-degree angle.

intramuscular (IM) Injections given into muscle tissue. The intramuscular route provides a fast rate of absorption that is related to the muscle's greater vascularity. Injections are given at a 90-degree angle.

intraocular Method of medication delivery that involves inserting a medication disk, similar to a contact lens, into the patient's eye.

intrapersonal communication Communication that occurs within an individual; that is, persons "talk with themselves" silently or form an idea in their own mind.

intravascular fluid Fluid circulating within blood vessels of the body.

intravenous Injection directly into the bloodstream. Action of the drug begins immediately when given intravenously.

intubation Insertion of a breathing tube through the mouth or nose into the trachea to ensure a patent airway.

intuition The inner sensing that something is so.

irrigation Process of washing out a body cavity or wounded area with a stream of fluid.

ischemia Decreased blood supply to a body part, such as skin tissue, or to an organ, such as the heart.

isolation Separation of a seriously ill patient from others to prevent the spread of an infection or to protect the patient from irritating environmental factors.

isometric exercises Activities that involve muscle tension without muscle shortening, do not have any beneficial effect on preventing orthostatic hypotension, but may improve activity tolerance.

isotonic Situation in which two solutions have the same concentration of solute; therefore both solutions exert the same osmotic pressure.

J

jaundice Yellow discoloration of the skin, mucous membranes, and sclera caused by greater-than-normal amounts of bilirubin in the blood.

jejunostomy tube Hollow tube inserted into the jejunum through the abdominal wall for administration of liquefied foods to patients who have a high risk of aspiration.

joint contracture Abnormality that may result in permanent condition of a joint, is characterized by flexion and fixation, and is caused by disuse, atrophy, and shortening of muscle fibers and surrounding joint tissues.

joints Connections between bones; classified according to structure and degree of mobility.

judgment Ability to form an opinion or draw sound conclusions.

justice The ethical standard of fairness.

K

Kardex Trade name for card-filing system that allows quick reference to the particular need of the patient for certain aspects of nursing care.

karma Asian Indian belief that attributes mental illness to past deeds in one's previous life.

Korotkoff sound Sound heard during the taking of blood pressure using a sphygmomanometer and stethoscope.

kyphosis Exaggeration of the posterior curvature of the thoracic spine.

L

la cuarantena Period of rest and restricted physical activity after childbirth that usually lasts 40 days.

la dieta Diet.

laceration Torn, jagged wound.

language Code that conveys specific meaning as words are combined.

laryngospasm Sudden uncontrolled contraction of the laryngeal muscles, which in turn decreases airway size.

latent error Less apparent failures of organization or design that contribute to the occurrence of adverse events/medical errors or allow them to cause harm to patients.

law Rule, standard, or principle that states a fact or a relationship between factors.

laxatives Drugs that act to promote bowel evacuation.

learning Acquisition of new knowledge and skills as a result of reinforcement, practice, and experience.

learning objective Written statement that describes the behavior a teacher expects from an individual after a learning activity.

left-sided heart failure Abnormal condition characterized by impaired functioning of the left ventricle due to elevated pressures and pulmonary congestion.

leukoplakia Thick, white patches observed on oral mucous membranes.

licensed practical nurse (LPN) Also known as the licensed vocational nurse (LVN), or in Canada, registered nurse's assistant (RNA); trained in basic nursing skills and the provision of direct patient care.

licensed vocational nurse (LVN) The LVN is the same as a licensed practical nurse (LPN), an individual trained in the United States in basic nursing techniques and direct patient care who practices under the supervision of a registered nurse. The LVN is licensed by a board after completing what is usually a 12-month educational program and passing a licensure examination. In Canada an LVN is called a certified nursing assistant.

lipids Compounds that are insoluble in water but soluble in organic solvents.

lipogenesis Process during which fatty acids are synthesized.

living wills Instruments by which a dying person makes wishes known.

local anesthesia Loss of sensation at the desired site of action.

logroll Maneuver used to turn a reclining patient from one side to the other or completely over without moving the spinal column out of alignment.

lordosis Increased lumbar curvature.

M

maceration Softening and breaking down of skin from prolonged exposure to moisture.

mal de ojo Evil eye.

malignant hyperthermia Autosomal dominant trait characterized by often fatal hyperthermia in affected people exposed to certain anesthetic agents.

malpractice Injurious or unprofessional actions that harm another.

malpractice insurance Type of insurance to protect the health care professional. In case of a malpractice claim, the insurance pays the award to the plaintiff.

managed care Health care system in which there is administrative control over primary health care services. Redundant facilities and services are eliminated, and costs are reduced. Preventive care and health education are emphasized.

Maslow's hierarchy of needs A model, developed by Abram Maslow, used to explain human motivation.

matrilineal Kinship that is limited to only the mother's side.

maturation The genetically determined biological plan for growth and development. Physical growth and motor development are a function of maturation.

maturational loss Loss, usually of an aspect of self, resulting from the normal changes of growth and development.

Medicaid State medical assistance to people with low incomes, based on Title XIX of the Social Security Act. States receive matching federal funds to provide medical care and services to people meeting categorical and income requirements.

medical asepsis Procedures used to reduce the number of microorganisms and prevent their spread.

medical diagnosis Formal statement of the disease entity or illness made by the physician or health care provider.

medical record Patient's chart; a legal document.

Medicare Federally funded national health insurance program in the United States for people over 65 years of age. The program is administered in two parts. Part A provides basic protection against costs of medical, surgical, and psychiatric hospital care. Part B is a voluntary medical insurance program financed in part from federal funds and in part from premiums contributed by people enrolled in the program.

medication abuse Maladaptive pattern of recurrent medication use.

medication allergy Adverse reaction to a medication such as rash, chills, or gastrointestinal disturbances. Once a drug allergy occurs, the patient can no longer receive that particular medication.

medication dependence Maladaptive pattern of medication use in the following patterns: using excessive amounts of the medication, increased activities directed toward obtaining the medication, withdrawal from professional or recreational activities, and so on.

medication error Any event that could cause or lead to a patient's receiving inappropriate drug therapy or failing to receive appropriate drug therapy.

medication interaction The response when one drug modifies the action of another drug. The interaction can potentiate or diminish the actions of another drug, or it may alter the way a drug is metabolized, absorbed, or excreted.

melanoma Group of malignant neoplasms, primarily of the skin, that are composed of melanocytes. Common in fair-skinned people having light-colored eyes and in persons who have had a sunburn.

melena Abnormal black, sticky stool containing digested blood, indicative of gastrointestinal bleeding.

menarche Onset of a girl's first menstruation.

Meniere's disease A chronic disease of the inner ear characterized by recurrent episodes of vertigo, progressive sensorineural hearing loss, which may be bilateral, and tinnitus.

menopause Physiological cessation of ovulation and menstruation that typically occurs during middle adulthood in women.

message Information sent or expressed by sender in the communication process.

metabolic acidosis Abnormal condition of high hydrogen ion concentration in the extracellular fluid caused by either a primary increase in hydrogen ions or a decrease in bicarbonate.

metabolic alkalosis Abnormal condition characterized by the significant loss of acid from the body or by increased levels of bicarbonate.

metabolism Aggregate of all chemical processes that take place in living organisms, resulting in growth, generation of energy, elimination of wastes, and other functions concerned with the distribution of nutrients in the blood after digestion.

metacommunication Dependent not only on what is said but also on the relationship to the other person involved in the interaction. It is a message that conveys the sender's attitude toward the self and the message and the attitudes, feelings, and intentions toward the listener.

metastasize Spread of tumor cells to distant parts of the body from a primary site, for example, lung, breast, or bowel.

metered-dose inhaler (MDI) Device designed to deliver a measured dose of an inhalation drug.

metric system Logically organized decimal system of measurement; metric units can easily be converted and computed through simple multiplication and division. Each basic unit of measurement is organized into units of 10.

microorganisms Microscopic entities, such as bacteria, viruses, and fungi, capable of carrying on living processes.

micturition Urination; act of passing or expelling urine voluntarily through the urethra.

milliequivalent per liter (mEq/L) Number of grams of a specific electrolyte dissolved in 1 L of plasma.

mind mapping A graphic approach to represent the connections between concepts and ideas (e.g., nursing diagnoses) that are related to a central subject (e.g., the patient's health problems).

minerals Inorganic elements essential to the body because of their role as catalysts in biochemical reactions.

minimum data set (MDS) Required by the Omnibus Budget Reconciliation Act of 1987, the MDS is a uniform data set established by the Department of Health and Human Services. The MDS serves as the framework for any state-specified assessment instruments used to develop a written and comprehensive plan of care for newly admitted residents of nursing facilities.

misdemeanor Lesser crime than a felony; the penalty is usually a fine or imprisonment for less than 1 year.

mobility Person's ability to move about freely.

moderate sedation/analgesia/conscious sedation Administration of central nervous system depressant drugs and/or analgesics to provide analgesia, relieve anxiety, and/or provide amnesia during surgical, diagnostic, or interventional procedures. Routinely used for diagnostic or therapeutic procedures that do not require complete anesthesia but simply a decreased level of consciousness.

monounsaturated fatty acid A fatty acid in which some of the carbon atoms in the hydrocarbon chain are joined by double or triple bonds. Monounsaturated fatty acids have only one double or triple bond per molecule and are found as components of fats in such foods as fowls, almonds, pecans, cashew nuts, peanuts, and olive oil.

morals Personal conviction that something is absolutely right or wrong in all situations.

motivation Internal impulse that causes a person to take action.

mourning The process of grieving.

mucositis Painful inflammation of oral mucous membranes.

murmurs Blowing or whooshing sounds created by changes in blood flow through the heart or by abnormalities in valve closure.

muscle tone Normal state of balanced muscle tension.

myocardial contractility Measure of stretch of the cardiac muscle fiber. It can also affect stroke volume and cardiac output. Poor contraction decreases the amount of blood ejected by the ventricles during each contraction.

myocardial infarction Necrosis of a portion of cardiac muscle caused by obstruction in a coronary artery.

myocardial ischemia Condition that results when the supply of blood to the myocardium from the coronary arteries is insufficient to meet the oxygen demands of the organ.

N

NANDA International North American Nursing Diagnosis Association, organized in 1973, which formally identifies, develops, and classifies nursing diagnoses.

narcolepsy Syndrome involving sudden sleep attacks that a person cannot inhibit; uncontrollable desire to sleep may occur several times during a day.

nasogastric (NG) tube Tube passed into the stomach through the nose for the purpose of emptying the stomach of its contents or for delivering medication and/or nourishment.

nebulization Process of adding moisture to inspired air by the addition of water droplets.

necessary losses Losses that every person experiences.

necrotic Of or pertaining to the death of tissue in response to disease or injury.

negative health behaviors Practices actually or potentially harmful to health, such as smoking, drug or alcohol abuse, poor diet, and refusal to take necessary medications.

negative nitrogen balance Condition occurring when the body excretes more nitrogen than it takes in.

negligence Careless act of omission or commission that results in injury to another.

neonate Stage of life from birth to 1 month of age.

nephrons Structural and functional units of the kidney containing renal glomeruli and tubules.

neurotransmitter Chemical that transfers the electrical impulse from the nerve fiber to the muscle fiber.

never events Particularly shocking medical errors (such as wrong-site surgery) that should never occur. The list of Never Events has expanded to signify adverse events that are unambiguous (clearly identifiable and measurable), serious (resulting in death or significant disability), and usually preventable.

nociceptors Somatic and visceral free nerve endings of thinly myelinated and unmyelinated fibers. They usually react to tissue injury but may also be excited by endogenous chemical substances.

nocturia Urination at night; can be a symptom of renal disease or may occur in persons who drink excessive amounts of fluids before bedtime.

nonblanchable hyperemia Redness of the skin due to dilation of the superficial capillaries. The redness persists when pressure is applied to the area, indicating tissue damage.

nonmaleficence The fundamental ethical agreement to do no harm. Closely related to the ethical standard of beneficence.

nonrapid eye movement (NREM) sleep Sleep that occurs during the first four stages of normal sleep.

nonshivering thermogenesis Occurs primarily in neonates. Because neonates cannot shiver, a limited amount of vascular brown adipose tissue present at birth can be metabolized for heat production.

nonverbal communication Communication using expressions, gestures, body posture, and positioning rather than words.

normal sinus rhythm (NSR) The wave pattern on an electrocardiogram that indicates normal conduction of an electrical impulse through the myocardium.

numbing One of Bowlby's four phases of mourning. It is characterized by the lack of feeling or feeling stunned by the loss. May last a few days or many weeks.

Nurse Practice Acts Statutes enacted by the legislature of any of the states or by the appropriate officers of the districts or possessions that describe and define the scope of nursing practice.

nurse-initiated interventions The response of the nurse to the patient's health care needs and nursing diagnoses. This type of intervention is an autonomous action based on scientific rationale that is executed to benefit the patient in a predicted way related to the nursing diagnosis and patient-centered goals.

nursing diagnosis Formal statement of an actual or potential health problem that nurses can legally and independently treat. The second step of the nursing process, during which the patient's actual and potential unhealthy responses to an illness or condition are identified.

nursing health history Data collected about a patient's present level of wellness, changes in life patterns, sociocultural role, and mental and emotional reactions to illness.

nursing intervention Any treatment, based upon clinical judgment and knowledge, that a nurse performs to enhance patient outcomes.

nursing process Systematic problem-solving method by which nurses individualize care for each patient. The five steps of the nursing process are assessment, diagnosis, planning, implementation, and evaluation.

nursing-sensitive outcomes Outcomes that are within the scope of nursing practice; consequences or effects of nursing interventions that result in changes in the patient's symptoms, functional status, safety, psychological distress, or costs.

nurturant Behavior that involves caring for or fostering the well-being of another individual.

nutrients Foods that contain elements necessary for body function, including water, carbohydrates, proteins, fats, vitamins, and minerals.

O

obesity Abnormal increase in the proportion of fat cells, mainly in the viscera and subcutaneous tissues of the body.

objective data Information that can be observed by others; free of feelings, perceptions, prejudices.

occurrence report Confidential document that describes any patient accident while the person is on the premises of a health care agency. (See incident report.)

olfactory Pertaining to the sense of smell.

oncotic pressure The total influence of the protein on the osmotic activity of plasma fluid.

open-ended question A form of question that prompts a respondent to answer in more than one or two words.

operating bed Table for surgery.

operating room (1) Room in a health care facility in which surgical procedures requiring anesthesia are performed. (2) Informal: a suite of rooms or an area in a health care facility in which patients are prepared for surgery, undergo surgical procedures, and recover from the anesthetic procedures required for the surgery.

ophthalmic Drugs given into the eye, in the form of either eye drops or ointments.

ophthalmoscope Instrument used to illuminate the structures of the eye in order to examine the fundus, which includes the retina, choroid, optic nerve disc, macula, fovea centralis, and retinal vessels.

opioid Drug substance, derived from opium or produced synthetically, that alters perception of pain and that with repeated use may result in physical and psychological dependence (narcotic).

oral hygiene Condition or practice of maintaining the tissues and structures of the mouth.

orthopnea Abnormal condition in which a person must sit or stand up to breathe comfortably.

orthostatic hypotension Abnormally low blood pressure occurring when a person stands up.

osmolality Concentration or osmotic pressure of a solution expressed in osmoles or milliosmoles per kilogram of water.

osmolarity Osmotic pressure of a solution expressed in osmoles or milliosmoles per kilogram of the solution.

osmoreceptors Neurons in the hypothalamus that are sensitive to the fluid concentration in the blood plasma and regulate the secretion of antidiuretic hormone.

osmosis Movement of a pure solvent through a semipermeable membrane from a solution with a lower solute concentration to one with a higher solute concentration.

osmotic pressure Drawing power for water, which depends on the number of molecules in the solution.

osteoporosis Disorder characterized by abnormal rarefaction of bone, occurring most frequently in postmenopausal women, in sedentary or immobilized individuals, and in patients on long-term steroid therapy.

ostomy Surgical procedure in which an opening is made into the abdominal wall to allow the passage of intestinal contents from the bowel (colostomy) or urine from the bladder (urostomy).

otoscope Instrument, with a special ear speculum, used to examine the deeper structures of the external and middle ear.

ototoxic Having a harmful effect on the eighth cranial (auditory) nerve or the organs of hearing and balance.

outcome Condition of a patient at the end of treatment, including the degree of wellness and the need for continuing care, medication, support, counseling, or education.

outliers Patients with extended lengths of stay beyond allowable inpatient days or costs.

outpatient Patient who has not been admitted to a hospital but receives treatments in a clinic or facility associated with the hospital.

oxygen saturation The amount of hemoglobin fully saturated with oxygen, given as a percent value.

oxygen therapy Procedure in which oxygen is administered to a patient to relieve or prevent hypoxia.

P

pain Subjective, unpleasant sensation caused by noxious stimulation of sensory nerve endings.

palliative care A level of care that is designed to relieve or reduce intensity of uncomfortable symptoms but not to produce a cure. Palliative care relies on comfort measures and use of alternative therapies to help individuals become more at peace during end of life.

pallor Unnatural paleness or absence of color in the skin.

palpation Method of physical examination whereby the fingers or hands of the examiner are applied to the patient's body for the purpose of feeling body parts underlying the skin.

palpitations Bounding or racing of the heart associated with normal emotions or a heart disorder.

Papanicolaou (Pap) smear Painless screening test for cervical cancer. Specimens are taken of squamous and columnar cells of the cervix.

parallel play Form of play among a group of children, primarily toddlers, in which each one engages in an independent activity that is similar but not influenced by or shared with the others.

paralytic ileus Usually temporary paralysis of intestinal wall that may occur after abdominal surgery or peritoneal injury and that causes cessation of peristalsis. Leads to abdominal distention and symptoms of obstruction.

parenteral administration Giving medication by a route other than the gastrointestinal tract.

parenteral nutrition (PN) The administration of a nutritional solution into the vascular system.

parteras Lay midwives.

partial bed bath Bath in which body parts that might cause the patient discomfort if left unbathed (i.e., face, hands, axillary areas, back, and perineum) are washed in bed.

passive range-of-motion (PROM) exercises Range of movement through which a joint is moved with assistance.

passive strategies of health promotion Activities that involve the patient as the recipient of actions by health care professionals.

pathogenicity Ability of a pathogenic agent to produce a disease.

pathogens Microorganisms capable of producing disease.

pathological fractures Fractures resulting from weakened bone tissue; frequently caused by osteoporosis or neoplasms.

patient-centered care Concept to improve work efficiency by changing the way patient care is delivered.

patient-controlled analgesia (PCA) Drug delivery system that allows patients to self-administer analgesic medications when they want.

patrilineal, patrilineally Kinship that is limited to only the father's side.

peak The time it takes for a medication to reach its highest effective concentration.

perceived loss Loss that is less obvious to the individual experiencing it. Although easily overlooked or misunderstood, a perceived loss results in the same grief process as an actual loss.

perception Persons' mental image or concept of elements in their environment, including information gained through the senses.

percussion Method of physical examination whereby the location, size, and density of a body part is determined by the tone obtained from the striking of short, sharp taps of the fingers.

perfusion (1) Passage of a fluid through a specific organ or an area of the body. (2) Therapeutic measure whereby a drug intended for an isolated part of the body is introduced via the bloodstream.

perineal care Procedure prescribed for cleaning the genital and anal areas as part of the daily bath or after various obstetrical and gynecological procedures.

perioperative nursing Refers to the role of the operating room nurse during the preoperative, intraoperative, and postoperative phases of surgery.

peripherally inserted central catheter (PICC) Alternative intravenous access when the patient requires intermediate-length venous access greater than 7 days to 3 months. Intravenous access is achieved by inserting a catheter into a central vein by way of a peripheral vein.

peristalsis Rhythmical contractions of the intestine that propel gastric contents through the length of the gastrointestinal tract.

peritonitis Inflammation of the peritoneum produced by bacteria or irritating substances introduced into the abdominal cavity by a penetrating wound or perforation of an organ in the gastrointestinal tract or the reproductive tract.

PERRLA Acronym for "pupils equal, round, reactive to light, accommodation"; the acronym is recorded in the physical examination if eye and pupil assessments are normal.

petechiae Tiny purple or red spots that appear on skin as minute hemorrhages within dermal layers.

pharmacokinetics Study of how drugs enter the body, reach their site of action, are metabolized, and exit from the body.

phlebitis Inflammation of a vein.

physician-initiated interventions Based on the physician's response to a medical diagnosis, the nurse responds to the physician's written orders.

PIE note Problem-oriented medical record; the four interdisciplinary sections are the database, problem list, care plan, and progress notes.

placebos Dosage form that contains no pharmacologically active ingredients but may relieve pain through psychological effects.

plaintiff Individual who files formal charges against an individual or organization for a legal offense.

planning Process of designing interventions to achieve the goals and outcomes of health care delivery.

plantar flexion Toe-down motion of the foot at the ankle.

pleural friction rub Adventitious lung sound caused by inflamed parietal and visceral pleura rubbing together on inspiration.

pneumothorax Collection of air or gas in the pleural space.

point of maximal impulse (PMI) Point where the heartbeat can most easily be palpated through the chest wall. This is usually the fourth intercostal space at the midclavicular line.

point of view A way of looking at issues that reflects an individual's culture and societal influences.

poison Any substance that impairs health or destroys life when ingested, inhaled, or absorbed by the body in relatively small amounts.

poison control center One of a network of facilities that provides information regarding all aspects of poisoning or intoxication, maintains records of their occurrence, and refers patients to treatment centers.

polypharmacy Use of a number of different drugs by a patient who may have one or several health problems.

polyunsaturated fatty acid Fatty acid that has two or more carbon double bonds.

population A collection of individuals who have in common one or more personal or environmental characteristics.

positive health behaviors Activities related to maintaining, attaining, or regaining good health and preventing illness. Common positive health behaviors include immunizations, proper sleep patterns, adequate exercise, and nutrition.

postanesthesia care unit (PACU) Area adjoining the operating room to which surgical patients are taken while still under anesthesia.

postmortem care Care of a patient's body after death.

postural drainage Use of positioning along with percussion and vibration to drain secretions from specific segments of the lungs and bronchi into the trachea.

postural hypotension Abnormally low blood pressure occurring when an individual assumes the standing posture; also called orthostatic hypotension.

posture Position of the body in relation to the surrounding space.

power of attorney for health care A person designated by the patient to make health care decisions for the patient if the patient becomes unable to make his or her own decisions.

preadolescence Transitional developmental stage that occurs between childhood and adolescence.

preanesthesia care unit Area outside the operating room where preoperative preparations are completed.

preload Volume of blood in the ventricles at the end of diastole, immediately before ventricular contraction.

preoperative teaching Instruction regarding a patient's anticipated surgery and recovery given before surgery. Instruction includes, but is not limited to, dietary and activity restrictions, anticipated assessment activities, postoperative procedures and pain relief measures.

presbycusis Hearing loss associated with aging. It usually involves both a loss of hearing sensitivity and a reduction in the clarity of speech.

presbyopia Gradual decline in ability of the lens to accommodate or to focus on close objects. Reduces ability to see near objects clearly. This condition commonly develops with advancing age.

prescriptions Written directions for a therapeutic agent (e.g., medication, drugs).

presence The deep physical, psychological, and spiritual connection or engagement between a nurse and patient.

present time orientation Time dimension that focuses on what is happening here and now. Communication patterns are circular, and this time orientation is in conflict with the dominant organizational norm in health care that emphasizes punctuality and adherence to appointments.

pressure ulcer Inflammation, sore, or ulcer in the skin over a bony prominence.

presurgical care unit (PSCU) Area outside the operating room where preoperative preparations are completed.

preventive nursing actions Nursing actions directed toward preventing illness and promoting health to avoid the need for primary, secondary, or tertiary health care.

primary appraisal Evaluating an event for its personal meaning related to stress.

primary care First contact in a given episode of illness that leads to a decision regarding a course of action to resolve the health problem.

primary intention Primary union of the edges of a wound, progressing to complete scar formation without granulation.

primary nursing Method of nursing practice in which the patient's care is managed, for the duration, by one nurse, who directs and coordinates other nurses and health care personnel. When on duty, the primary nurse cares for the patient directly.

primary prevention First contact in a given episode of illness that leads to a decision regarding a course of action to prevent worsening of the health problem.

problem identification One of the steps of the diagnostic process in which the patient's health care problem is recognized as a result of data analysis based on professional knowledge and experience.

problem solving Methodical, systematic approach to explore conditions and develop solutions, including analysis of data, determination of causative factors, and selection of appropriate actions to reverse or eliminate the problem.

problem-oriented medical record (POMR) Method of recording data about the health status of a patient that fosters a collaborative problem-solving approach by all members of the health care team.

productive cough Sudden expulsion of air from the lungs that effectively removes sputum from the respiratory tract and helps clear the airways.

professional standards review organization (PSRO) Focuses on evaluation of nursing care provided in a health care setting. The quality, effectiveness, and appropriateness of nursing care for the patient is the focus of evaluation.

prone Position of the patient lying face down.

proprioception The body's ability to sense its position and movement in space.

prospective payment system (PPS) Payment mechanism for reimbursing hospitals for inpatient health care services in which predetermined rate is set for treatment of specific illnesses.

prostaglandins Potent hormonelike substances that act in exceedingly low doses on target organs. They can be used to treat asthma and gastric hyperacidity.

proteins Any of a large group of naturally occurring, complex, organic nitrogenous compounds. Each is composed of large combinations of amino acids containing the elements carbon, hydrogen, nitrogen, oxygen, usually sulfur, and occasionally phosphorus, iron, iodine, or other essential constituents of living cells. Protein is the major source of building material for muscles, blood, skin, hair, nails, and the internal organs.

proteinuria Presence in the urine of abnormally large quantities of protein, usually albumin. Persistent proteinuria is usually a sign of renal disease or renal complications of another disease, or hypertension or heart failure.

protocol Written and approved plan specifying the procedures to be followed during an assessment or in providing treatment.

pruritus Symptom of itching; an uncomfortable sensation leading to the urge to scratch.

psychomotor learning Acquisition of ability to perform motor skills.

ptosis Abnormal condition of one or both upper eyelids in which the eyelid droops, caused by weakness of the levator muscle or paralysis of the third cranial nerve.

puberty Developmental period of emotional and physical changes, including the development of secondary sex characteristics and the onset of menstruation and ejaculation.

public health nursing A nursing specialty that requires the nurse to care for the needs of populations or groups.

public communication Interaction of one individual with large groups of people.

pulmonary hygiene More frequent turning, deep breathing, coughing, use of incentive spirometry, and chest physical therapy (PT) if ordered.

pulse deficit Condition that exists when the radial pulse is less than the ventricular rate as auscultated at the apex or seen on an electrocardiogram. The condition indicates a lack of peripheral perfusion for some of the heart contractions.

pulse pressure Difference between the systolic and diastolic pressures, normally 30 to 40 mm Hg.

Purkinje network Complex network of muscle fibers that spread through the right and left ventricles of the heart and carry the impulses that contract those chambers almost simultaneously.

pursed-lip breathing Deep inspiration followed by prolonged expiration through pursed lips.

pyrexia Abnormal elevation of the temperature of the body above 37° C (98.6° F) because of disease; same as fever.

pyrogens Substances that cause a rise in body temperature, as in the case of bacterial toxins.

Q

quality improvement Monitoring and evaluation of processes and outcomes in health care or any other business to identify opportunities for improvement.

quality indicator Quantitative measure of an important aspect of care that determines whether quality of service conforms to requirements or standards of care.

R

race The common biological characteristics shared by a group of people.

Ramadan A religious observance held during the ninth month of the Islamic calendar year. It involves fasting from sunrise to sunset.

range of motion (ROM) Range of movement of a joint, from maximum extension to maximum flexion, as measured in degrees of a circle.

rapid eye movement (REM) sleep Stage of sleep in which dreaming and rapid eye movements are prominent; important for mental restoration.

reaction Component of the pain experience that may include both physiological responses, such as in the general adaptation syndrome, and behavioral responses.

reality orientation Therapeutic modality for restoring an individual's sense of the present.

receiver Person to whom message is sent during the communication process.

reception Neurophysiological components of the pain experience, in which nervous system receptors receive painful stimuli and transmit them through peripheral nerves to the spinal cord and brain.

record Written form of communication that permanently documents information relevant to health care management.

recovery A period of time immediately postoperative when the patient is closely observed for effects of anesthesia, changes in vital signs, and bleeding. The area is usually in the postanesthesia care unit.

referent Factor that motivates a person to communicate with another individual.

reflection Process of thinking back or recalling an event to discover the meaning and purpose of that event. Useful in critical thinking.

refractive error Defect in the ability of the lens of the eye to focus light, such as occurs in nearsightedness and farsightedness.

regional anesthesia Loss of sensation in an area of the body supplied by sensory nerve pathways.

registered nurse (RN) In the United States a nurse who has completed a course of study at a state approved, accredited school of nursing and has passed the National Council Licensure Examination (NCLEX-RN).

regression Return to an earlier developmental stage or behavior.

regulatory agencies Local, state, provincial, or national agencies that inspect and certify health care agencies as meeting specified standards. These agencies can also determine the amount of reimbursement for health care delivered.

rehabilitation Restoration of an individual to normal or near-normal function after a physical or mental illness, injury, or chemical addiction.

reinforcement Provision of a contingent response to a learner's behavior that increases the probability of the behavior's recurring.

related factor Any condition or event that accompanies or is linked with the patient's health care problem.

relaxation Act of being relaxed or less tense.

reminiscence Recalling the past for the purpose of assigning new meaning to past experiences.

remissions Partial or complete disappearances of the clinical and subjective characteristics of chronic or malignant disease; remission may be spontaneous or the result of therapy.

renal calculi Calcium stones in the renal pelvis.

renin Proteolytic enzyme, produced by and stored in the juxtaglomerular apparatus that surrounds each arteriole as it enters a glomerulus. The enzyme affects the blood pressure by catalyzing the change of angiotensinogen to angiotensin, a strong repressor.

reorganization The last phase Bowlby's phases of mourning. During this phase, which sometimes requires a year or more, the person begins to accept unaccustomed roles, acquire new skills, and build new relationships.

reports Transfer of information from the nurses on one shift to the nurses on the following shift. Report may also be given by one of the members of the nursing team to another health care provider, for example, a physician or therapist.

reservoir A place where microorganisms survive, multiply, and await transfer to a susceptible host.

residual urine Volume of urine remaining in the bladder after a normal voiding; the bladder normally is almost completely empty after micturition.

resistance stage Third stage of the stress response, when the person attempts to adapt to the stressor. The body stabilizes, hormone levels stabilize, and heart rate, blood pressure, and cardiac output return to normal.

resource utilization group (RUG) Method of classification for health care reimbursement for long-term care facilities.

respeto Respectful.

respiratory acidosis Abnormal condition characterized by increased arterial carbon dioxide concentration, excess carbonic acid, and increased hydrogen ion concentration.

respiratory alkalosis Abnormal condition characterized by decreased arterial carbon dioxide concentration and decreased hydrogen ion concentration.

respite care Short-term health services to dependent older adults either in their home or in an institutional setting.

responsibility Carrying out duties associated with a particular role.

restorative care Health care settings and services where patients who are recovering from illness or disability receive rehabilitation and supportive care.

restraint Device to aid in the immobilization of a patient or patient's extremity.

return demonstration Demonstration after the patient has first observed the teacher and then practiced the skill in mock or real situations.

rhonchi Abnormal lung sound auscultated when the patient's airways are obstructed with thick secretions.

right-sided heart failure Abnormal condition that results from impaired functioning of the right ventricle characterized by venous congestion in the systemic circulation.

risk factor Any internal or external variable that makes a person or group more vulnerable to illness or an unhealthy event.

risk management A function of administration of a hospital or other health facility directed toward identification, evaluation, and correction of potential risks that could lead to injury of patients, staff members, or visitors and result in property loss or damage.

risk nursing diagnosis Describes human responses to health conditions/life processes that may develop in a vulnerable individual, family, or community.

role performance The way in which a person views his or her ability to carry out significant roles.

root cause analysis A process of data collection and analysis that aids in finding the real cause of the problem and working on dealing with it rather than just dealing with the effects of the problem.

S

Sabbath From sundown on Friday to sundown on Saturday, this religious observance is a day of rest and worship for Jews and some Christian sects.

sandbags Sand-filled plastic tubes that can be shaped to body contours. They can immobilize an extremity or maintain body alignment.

saturated fatty acid Fatty acid in which each carbon in the chain has an attached hydrogen atom.

scientific method Codified sequence of steps used in the formulation, testing, evaluation, and reporting of scientific ideas.

scientific rationale Reason, based on supporting literature, why a specific nursing action was chosen.

scoliosis Lateral spinal curvature.

scrub nurse Registered nurse or operating room technician who assists surgeons during operations.

secondary appraisal Evaluating one's possible coping strategies when confronted with a stressor.

secondary intention Wound closure in which the edges are separated, granulation tissue develops to fill the gap, and, finally, epithelium grows in over the granulation, producing a larger scar than results with primary intention.

secondary prevention Level of preventive medicine that focuses on early diagnosis, use of referral services, and rapid initiation of treatment to stop the progress of disease processes.

sedatives Medications that produce a calming effect by decreasing functional activity, diminishing irritability, and allaying excitement.

segmentation Alternating contraction and relaxation of gastrointestinal mucosa.

self-concept Complex, dynamic integration of conscious and unconscious feelings, attitudes, and perceptions about one's identity, physical being, worth, and roles; how a person perceives and defines self.

self-esteem Feeling of self-worth characterized by feelings of achievement, adequacy, self-confidence, and usefulness.

self-transcendence Sense of authentically connecting to one's inner self.

sender Person who initiates interpersonal communication by conveying a message.

sensible water loss Loss of fluid from the body through the secretory activity of the sweat glands and the exhalation of humidified air from the lungs.

sensory deficits Defects in the function of one or more of the senses, resulting in visual, auditory, or olfactory impairments.

sensory deprivation State in which stimulation to one or more of the senses is lacking, resulting in impaired sensory perception.

sensory overload State in which stimulation to one or more of the senses is so excessive that the brain disregards or does not meaningfully respond to stimuli.

sequential compression stockings Plastic stockings attached to an air pump that inflates and deflates the stockings, applying intermittent pressure sequentially from the ankle to the knee.

serious reportable events Adverse events (including never events), that occur in hospitals, and that are serious, largely preventable, and of concern to both the public and health care providers.

serum half-life Time needed for excretion processes to lower the serum drug concentration by half.

sexual dysfunction Inability or difficulty in sexual functioning caused by physiological or psychological factors or both.

sexual orientation Clear, persistent erotic preference for a person of one sex or the other.

sexuality "A function of the total personality . . . concerned with the biological, psychological, sociological, spiritual and culture variables of life . . ." (Sex Information and Education Council of the United States, 1980).

sexually transmitted infection Infectious process spread through sexual contact, including oral, genital, or anal sexual activity.

shear Force exerted against the skin while the skin remains stationary and the bony structures move.

side effect Any reaction or consequence that results from medication or therapy.

side rails Bars positioned along the sides of the length of the bed or stretcher to reduce the patient's risk of falling.

simpatia Friendly.

sinoatrial (SA) node Called the "pacemaker of the heart" because the origin of the normal heartbeat begins at the SA node. The SA node is in the right atrium next to the entrance of the superior vena cava.

situational crisis Unexpected crisis that arises suddenly in response to an external event or a conflict concerning a specific circumstance.

situational loss Loss of a person, thing, or quality resulting from a change in a life situation, including changes related to illness, body image, environment, and death.

sitz bath Bath in which only the hips or buttocks are immersed in fluid.

skilled nursing facility Institution or part of an institution that meets criteria for accreditation established by the sections of the Social Security Act that determine the basis for Medicaid and Medicare reimbursement for skilled nursing care, including rehabilitation and various medical and nursing procedures.

skin tears Traumatic wounds in which the epidermis separates from the dermis.

sleep State marked by reduced consciousness, diminished activity of the skeletal muscles, and depressed metabolism.

sleep apnea Cessation of breathing for a time during sleep.

sleep deprivation Condition resulting from a decrease in the amount, quality, and consistency of sleep.

SOAP note Progress note that focuses on a single patient problem and includes subjective and objective data, analysis, and planning; most often used in the POMR.

socializing Interacting with friends or other people; communicating with others to form relationships and help people feel relaxed.

solute Substance dissolved in a solution.

solution Mixture of one or more substances dissolved in another substance. The molecules of each of the substances disperse homogeneously and do not change chemically. A solution may be a liquid, gas, or solid.

solvent Any liquid in which another substance can be dissolved.

source record Organization of a patient's chart so that each discipline (e.g., nursing, medicine, social work, or respiratory therapy) has a separate section in which to record data. Unlike POMR, the information is not organized by patient problems. The advantage of a source record is that caregivers can easily locate the proper section of the record in which to make entries.

sphygmomanometer Device for measuring the arterial blood pressure that consists of an arm or leg cuff with an air bladder connected to a tube and a bulb for pumping air into the bladder and a gauge for indicating the amount of air pressure being exerted against the artery.

spiritual distress State of being out of harmony with a system of beliefs, a supreme being, or God.

spiritual well-being Individual's spirituality that enables a person to love, have faith and hope, seek meaning in life, and nurture relationships with others.

spirituality Spiritual dimension of a person, including the relationship with humanity, nature, and a supreme being.

standard of care Minimum level of care accepted to ensure high-quality care to patients. Standards of care define the types of therapies typically administered to patients with defined problems or needs.

Standard Precautions Guidelines recommended by the Centers for Disease Control and Prevention (CDC) to reduce risk of transmission of blood-borne and other pathogens in hospitals.

standardized care plans Written care plans that are based on an institution's standards of practice and established guidelines and are used to care for patients with similar health problems. These care plans assist in accurate and efficient documentation.

standing order Written and approved documents containing rules, policies, procedures, regulations, and orders for the conduct of patient care in various stipulated clinical settings.

statutory law Of or related to laws enacted by a legislative branch of the government.

stenosis Abnormal condition characterized by the constriction or narrowing of an opening or passageway in a body structure.

stereotypes Generalizations that are made about individuals without further assessment.

sterilization (1) Rendering a person unable to produce children; accomplished by surgical, chemical, or other means. (2) A technique for destroying microorganisms using heat, water, chemicals, or gases.

stoma Artificially created opening between a body cavity and the body's surface; for example, a colostomy, formed from a portion of the colon pulled through the abdominal wall.

stress Physiological or psychological tension that threatens homeostasis or a person's psychological equilibrium.

stressor Any event, situation, or other stimulus encountered in a person's external or internal environment that necessitates change or adaptation by the person.

striae Streaks or linear scars that result from rapid development of tension in the skin.

stroke volume (SV) Amount of blood ejected by the ventricles with each contraction. It can be affected by the amount of blood in the left ventricle at the end of diastole (preload), the resistance to left ventricular ejection (afterload), and myocardial contractility.

subacute care Level of medical specialty care provided to patients who need a greater intensity of care than that provided in a skilled nursing facility but who do not require acute care.

subcultures Various ethnic, religious, and other groups with distinct characteristics from the dominant culture.

subcutaneous (Sub-Q) Injection given into the connective tissue, under the dermis. The subcutaneous tissue absorbs drugs more slowly than those injected into muscle. Injections are usually given at an angle of 45 degrees.

subjective data Information gathered from patient statements; the patient's feelings and perceptions. Not verifiable by another except by inference.

sublingual Route of medication administration in which the medication is placed underneath the patient's tongue.

Sunrise Model A model developed by Leininger that aids the health care practitioner in designing care decisions and actions in a culturally congruent fashion.

supine Position of the patient in which the patient is resting on his or her back.

suprainfection Secondary infection usually caused by an opportunistic pathogen.

suprapubic catheter Catheter surgically inserted through abdomen into bladder.

surfactant Chemical produced in the lung by alveolar type 2 cells that maintains the surface tension of the alveoli and keeps them from collapsing.

surgical asepsis Procedures used to eliminate any microorganisms from an area. Also called sterile technique.

sympathy Concern, sorrow, or pity felt by the nurse for the patient in which the nurse personally identifies with the patient's needs. Sympathy is a subjective look at another person's world that prevents a clear perspective of all sides of the issues confronting that person.

synapse Region surrounding the point of contact between two neurons or between a neuron and an effector organ.

syncope A brief lapse in consciousness caused by transient cerebral hypoxia.

synergistic effect Effect resulting from two drugs acting synergistically; the effect of the two drugs combined is greater than the effect that would be expected if the individual effects of the two drugs acting alone were added together.

systolic Pertaining to or resulting from ventricular contraction.

T

tachycardia Rapid regular heart rate ranging between 100 and 150 beats per minute.

tachypnea Abnormally rapid rate of breathing.

tactile Relating to the sense of touch.

tactile fremitus Tremulous vibration of the chest wall during breathing that is palpable on physical examination.

teaching Implementation method used to pre-sent correct principles, procedures, and techniques of health care; to inform patients about their health status; and to refer patients and family to appropriate health or social resources in the community.

team nursing Decentralized system in which the care of a patient is distributed among the members of a team. The charge nurse delegates authority to a team leader, who must be a professional nurse.

teratogens Chemical or physiological agents that may produce adverse effects in the embryo or fetus.

tertiary prevention Activities directed toward rehabilitation rather than diagnosis and treatment.

therapeutic communication Process in which the nurse consciously influences a patient or helps the patient to a better understanding through verbal and/or nonverbal communication.

therapeutic effect Desired benefit of a medication, treatment, or procedure.

thermoregulation Internal control of body temperature.

threshold Point at which a person first perceives a painful stimulus as being painful.

thrill Continuous palpable sensation like the purring of a cat.

thrombus Accumulation of platelets, fibrin, clotting factors, and the cellular elements of the blood attached to the interior wall of a vein or artery, sometimes occluding the lumen of the vessel.

tinnitus Ringing heard in one or both ears.

tissue ischemia Point at which tissues receive insufficient oxygen and perfusion.

tolerance Point at which a person is not willing to accept pain of greater severity or duration.

tort Act that causes injury for which the injured party can bring civil action.

total patient care A nursing delivery of care model originally developed during Florence Nightingale's time. In the model a registered nurse (RN) is responsible for all aspects of care for one or more patients. The nurse works directly with the patient, family, physician or health care provider, and health care team members. The model typically has a shift-based focus.

touch To come in contact with another person, often conveying caring, emotional support, encouragement, or tenderness.

toxic effect Effect of a medication that results in an adverse response.

transcendence The belief that there is a positive force outside of and greater than oneself that exists beyond the material world.

transcultural Concept of care extending across cultures that distinguishes nursing from other health disciplines.

transcultural nursing A distinct discipline developed by Leininger that focuses on the comparative study of cultures to understand similarities and differences among groups of people.

transcutaneous electrical nerve stimulation (TENS) Technique in which a battery-powered device blocks pain impulses from reaching the spinal cord by delivering weak electrical impulses directly to the skin's surface.

transdermal disk Medication delivery device in which the medication is saturated on a waferlike disk, which is affixed to the patient's skin. This method ensures that the patient receives a continuous level of medication.

transfer report Verbal exchange of information between caregivers when a patient is moved from one nursing unit or health care setting to another. The report includes information necessary to maintain a consistent level of care from one setting to another.

transfusion reaction Systemic response by the body to the administration of blood incompatible with that of the recipient.

trapeze bar Metal triangular-shaped bar that can be suspended over a patient's bed from an overhanging frame; permits patients to move up and down in bed while in traction or some other encumbrance.

trimester Referring to one of the three phases of pregnancy.

trochanter roll Rolled towel support placed against the hips and upper leg to prevent external rotation of the legs.

trough The lowest serum concentration of a medication before the next medication dose is administered.

turgor Normal resiliency of the skin caused by the outward pressure of the cells and interstitial fluid.

U

unsaturated fatty acid Fatty acid in which an unequal number of hydrogen atoms are attached and the carbon atoms attach to each other with a double bond.

ureterostomy Diversion of urine away from a diseased or defective bladder through an artificial opening in the skin.

urinal Receptacle for collecting urine.

urinary diversion Surgical diversion of the drainage of urine, such as a ureterostomy.

urinary incontinence Inability to control urination.

urinary reflux Abnormal, backward flow of urine.

urinary retention Retention of urine in the bladder; condition frequently caused by a temporary loss of muscle function.

urine hat Receptacle for collecting urine that fits toilet.

urometer Device for measuring frequent and small amounts of urine from an indwelling urinary catheter system.

urosepsis Organisms in the bloodstream.

utilitarianism Ethic that proposes that the value of something is determined by its usefulness. The greatest good for the greatest number of people constitutes the guiding principle for action in a utilitarian model of ethics.

utilization review (UR) committees Physician-supervised committees to review admissions, diagnostic testing, and treatments provided by physicians or health care providers to patients.

V

validation Act of confirming, verifying, or corroborating the accuracy of assessment data or the appropriateness of the care plan.

Valsalva maneuver Any forced expiratory effort against a closed airway, such as when an individual holds the breath and tightens the muscles in a concerted, strenuous effort to move a heavy object or to change positions in bed.

value Personal belief about the worth of a given idea or behavior.

valvular heart disease Acquired or congenital disorder of a cardiac valve characterized by stenosis and obstructed blood flow or valvular degeneration and regurgitation of blood.

variances The unexpected event that occurs during patient care and that is different from what is predicted on a CareMap. Variances or exceptions are interventions or outcomes that are not achieved as anticipated. Variance may be positive or negative.

variant Differing from a set standard.

vascular access devices Catheters, cannulas, or infusion ports designed for long-term, repeated access to the vascular system.

vasoconstriction Narrowing of the lumen of any blood vessel, especially the arterioles and the veins in the blood reservoirs of the skin and abdominal viscera.

vasodilation Increase in the diameter of a blood vessel caused by inhibition of its vasoconstrictor nerves or stimulation of dilator nerves.

venipuncture Technique in which a vein is punctured transcutaneously by a sharp rigid stylet (e.g., a butterfly needle), a cannula (e.g., an angiocatheter that contains a flexible plastic catheter), or a needle attached to a syringe.

ventilation Respiratory process by which gases are moved into and out of the lungs.

verbal communication The sending of messages from one individual to another or to a group of individuals through the spoken word.

vertigo Sensation of dizziness or spinning.

vibration Fine, shaking pressure applied by hands to the chest wall only during exhalation.

virulence The ability of an organism to rapidly produce disease.

visual Related to, or experienced through, vision.

vital signs Temperature, pulse, respirations, and blood pressure.

vitamins Organic compounds essential in small quantities for normal physiological and metabolic functioning of the body. With few exceptions, vitamins cannot be synthesized by the body and must be obtained from the diet or dietary supplements.

voiding The process of urinating.

vulnerable populations A collection of individuals who are more likely to develop health problems as a result of excess risks, limits in access to health care services, or being dependent on others for care.

W

wellness Dynamic state of health in which an individual progresses toward a higher level of functioning, achieving an optimum balance between internal and external environments.

wellness education Activities that teach people how to care for themselves in a healthy manner.

wellness nursing diagnosis Clinical judgment about an individual, group, or community in transition from a specific level of wellness to a higher level of wellness.

wheezes, wheezing Adventitious lung sound caused by a severely narrowed bronchus.

workaround Patterns and actions that health care staff adopt to bypass either safety steps in procedures or safety features of medical equipment. Although workarounds may temporarily "fix a problem," the system remains unaltered and thus continues to present potential safety hazards for future patients.

work redesign Formal process used to analyze the work of a certain work group and to change the actual structure of the jobs performed.

worldview A cognitive stance or perspective about phenomena characteristic of a particular cultural group.

wound culture Specimen collected from a wound to determine the specific organism that is causing an infectious process.

X

xerosis Abnormal dryness of the skin.

Y

yearning and searching The second phase of Bowlby's phases of mourning. It is characterized by emotional outbursts of tearful sobbing and acute distress.

Z

Z-track injection Technique for injecting irritating preparations into muscle without tracking residual medication through sensitive tissues.

INDEX

b indicates boxes, f indicates illustrations, and t indicates tables.

F

I

N

S

T

U

V

W

X

Y

PATIENT TEACHING

CARE OF THE OLDER ADULT

CARE PLAN